Laboratory Test Handbook

4th Edition

with
Key Word Index

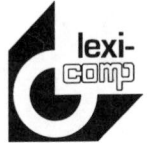

IN MEMORY OF – PAUL R. FINLEY, MD

The University of Arizona was in need of a pathologist to head up clinical chemistry when Dr Paul Finley dropped in one day. He was interested in relocating to the southwest because his wife, Cici, an accomplished potter, wanted to be near the well-springs of southwestern pottery. With his roots in private practice, Paul was deeply suspicious of academic medicine. We emphasized that our department was indeed clinically oriented, but I still remember, after a recruitment outing, a colleague whispering "I'm pretty sure she's bought the farm, but I still don't know about him." Paul did join us in 1972 and remained on the job until his death in 1994.

A native of St Paul, Minnesota, Paul graduated in medicine from the University of Minnesota, interned in Seattle, and did his pathology residency at the University of Minnesota. After advanced work in clinical chemistry in London, England, Paul returned to Minnesota as Director of Clinical Laboratories for the Fairview Hospital system. Twelve years later, he came to us, already well known on the national scene in clinical chemistry, as well as in the brand new applications of computers to clinical pathology. He was a great and ingenious methodologist. Once persuaded that he should let the world know about his innovations, he produced over a hundred scientific papers. The Chemistry chapter of the 3rd edition of the *Laboratory Test Handbook*, 1994, is among his many accomplishments. Paul was particularly active in therapeutic drug monitoring, polymerase chain reaction technology, and DNA fingerprinting. In the last 10 years, he took up music again (he had led a dance band in college) and played clarinet in various jazz, swing, and symphonic groups in Tucson.

Always the best of colleagues and friends, Paul was a keen observer of humanity, with a puckish sense of humor and an irreverent attitude that enlivened many faculty meetings. He was always ready to help with someone else's project, no matter how busy he was. God knows, we miss him.

Douglas W. Huestis, MD

Laboratory Test Handbook

4th Edition

with
Key Word Index

David S. Jacobs, MD, FACP, FCAP
Editor-in-Chief
President, Pathologists Chartered
Consultant in Pathology and Laboratory Medicine
Overland Park, Kansas

Wayne R. DeMott, MD, FCAP
Consultant in Pathology and Laboratory Medicine
Shawnee Mission, Kansas

Harold J. Grady, PhD
Editor
Professor of Pathology
University of Missouri Kansas City School of Medicine
Kansas City, Missouri

Rebecca T. Horvat, PhD
Assistant Professor of Pathology and Laboratory Medicine
University of Kansas Medical Center
Kansas City, Kansas

Douglas W. Huestis, MD
Emeritus Professor of Pathology
University of Arizona College of Medicine
Tucson, Arizona

Bernard L. Kasten, Jr, MD, FCAP
Vice President–Medical Director
Corning Clinical Laboratories
Teterboro, New Jersey

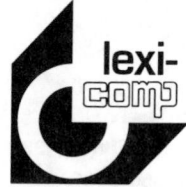

LEXI-COMP INC
Hudson (Cleveland)
1996

CREDITS

Medical Editor: Diane M. Harbart, MT(ASCP)

Production Manager: Barbara F. Kerscher

Production Assistants: Jacqueline L. Mizer, Jil R. Neuman, and Jeanne E. Wilson

Graphic Designer: Tracey J. Reinecke

Systems Analysts: David C. Marcus, Dennis P. Smithers, Kenneth Hughes

NOTICE

This handbook is intended to serve as a useful reference and not as a complete laboratory testing resource. The explosion of information in many directions, in multiple scientific disciplines, with advances in laboratory techniques, and continuing evolution of knowledge requires constant scholarship. The publication covers common, as well as many esoteric testing procedures. The authors, editors, reviewers, contributors, and publishers cannot be responsible for the continued currency of the information or for any errors or omissions in this book or for any consequences arising therefrom. Because of the dynamic nature of laboratory medicine as a discipline, readers are advised that decisions regarding diagnosis and treatment must be based on the independent judgment of the clinician. The editors are not responsible for any inaccuracy of quotation or for any false or misleading implication that may arise due to the text.

Previous editions copyrighted 1984, 1988, 1990, and 1994

This manual was produced using the Pathfinder™ Program – a complete publishing service of Lexi-Comp Inc.

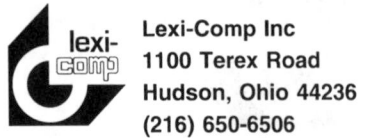

Lexi-Comp Inc
1100 Terex Road
Hudson, Ohio 44236
(216) 650-6506

ISBN 0-916589-35-8 (soft bound)
ISBN 0-916589-36-6 (case bound)

CPT codes and descriptions only are Copyright © 1995 American Medical Association.
All rights reserved.

TABLE OF CONTENTS

FOREWORD

The first version of this publication, released in 1984, was an effort by four community-based pathologists to include in a single volume all the routine and many of the more specialized analyses available in a modern clinical laboratory. The next edition represented the efforts of additional authors. The number of contributors to this edition has been considerably expanded. All are respected authorities in their fields of expertise. It is hoped that this enlarged edition is at once current and more comprehensive.

As in the previous edition, information about each laboratory procedure is presented in a standardized format, including **test name** and **synonyms**, **patient care** recommendations, **specimen requirements**, **reference ranges**, **interpretive** information, **footnotes**, and **references**. Each entry is complete in itself, but the whole work is extensively cross-referenced and indexed. The handbook is intended as a convenient reference resource for clinicians, pathologists, residents, medical and nursing students, medical technologists, ancillary medical personnel, and medical records staff.

We have devoted a great deal of effort to **clinical relevance**. We have been fortunate to have available to us the Lexi-Comp Pathfinder™ system, the Medline® system, and the computer publishing expertise of Lexi-Comp Inc. These assets have made possible extensive internal cross-referencing of entries, the inclusion, even late in the publishing process, of the most current references, and the Key Word Index.

The new edition has greatly expanded coverage of laboratory assays directly and indirectly related to molecular pathology; other additions include expanded treatments of clinical virology and therapeutic drug monitoring, and many new entries in the realm of clinical immunology and other subspecialties of clinical laboratory medicine. A new addition, Cytogenetic test listings, reflects exciting contemporary advances in laboratory medicine.

To survive in today's atmosphere of change in healthcare, clinicians must order the **needed** test, obtain reliable and accurate results, and have access to current clinical laboratory information. This book, we hope, will assist with ordering and such access. To attain accurate and reliable test results will depend in large measure upon quality attributes of the laboratory performing the analyses.

It is the authors' desire that this newest edition serve as a guide for the clinician and laboratorian, assist in obtaining the appropriate specimen for analysis, and provide avenues toward interpretation and relevance in the interest of optimal patient care.

ACKNOWLEDGMENTS

The *Laboratory Test Handbook with Key Word Index* exists in its present form as the result of the concerted efforts of many individuals. The publisher and president of Lexi-Comp Inc, Mr Robert D. Kerscher, deserves much credit for bringing the concept of such a book to fruition. His dedication to the project and his support and development of the many unique and innovative features included in the book (eg, format, internal cross-references, comprehensive indexing and Key Word Index) contribute substantially to the content and usefulness of the book.

Diane M. Harbart, MT (ASCP), medical editor, provided invaluable contributions, and her patience with the author's enumerable drafts, revisions, deletions, additions, and enhancements deserves special commendation.

Other members of the Lexi-Comp staff whose contributions were invaluable and whose efforts are especially appreciated include Barbara F. Kerscher, production manager; Lynn D. Coppinger, managing editor; Alexandra J. Hart, composition specialist; Leonard L. Lance, pharmacist; John Janosik, PharmD; Jacqueline L. Mizer, Jil R. Neuman, Jeanne E. Wilson, Tracey Reinecke, Leslie Ruggles, Beth Daulbaugh, and Julie Weekes, production assistants; Jeff J. Zaccagnini, Jerry M. Reeves, and Brian B. Vossler, sales managers; Edmund A. Harbart, vice-president, custom publishing division; Jack L. Stones, vice-president, reference publishing division; and Jay L. Katzen, product manager. The complex computer programming required for the production of this book was provided by Dennis P. Smithers, David C. Marcus, Kenneth Hughes, and Sean Conrad, system analysts, under the direction of Thury L. O'Connor, vice-president.

Lowell L. Tilzer, MD, PhD deserves special commendation and expression of appreciation. Dr Tilzer provided insight in a number of his areas of expertise, orchestrated many portions of the *Laboratory Test Handbook*, and provided valuable author recommendations. Unanticipated professional obligations prevented him from providing all the contributions he had intended.

The editors express appreciation to Charles W. Gorodetzky, MD, PhD for his review and contributions to the Therapeutic Drug Monitoring entries.

ABOUT THE AUTHORS

Julia A. Bridge, MD

Dr Bridge received her MD degree from the University of Nebraska Medical Center (UNMC) in Omaha, Nebraska. She completed her training in pathology at the University of Kansas Medical Center followed by a fellowship in clinical cytogenetics at the University of Nebraska Medical Center (UNMC) and a fellowship in molecular genetics at the Southwest Biomedical Research Institute under the directorship of Avery A. Sandberg, MD in Scottsdale, Arizona. She is certified in Anatomic Pathology and Clinical Cytogenetics and is currently an Associate Professor in the Department of Pathology/Microbiology, Pediatrics, and Orthopaedic Surgery at the University of Nebraska Medical Center, a position she has held since completion of her fellowship in 1990.

Dr Bridge is Associate Director of the Clinical Cytogenetics Laboratory and Director of the Molecular Diagnostic Laboratory and the Solid Tumor Bank at UNMC. She also regularly performs cytopathology and surgical pathology duties. She is on the Editorial Board of *Cancer Genetics and Cytogenetics* and has authored or coauthored over 60 papers, book chapters, and books.

Christopher F. Bryan, PhD

Dr Bryan received both his masters and doctoral degrees in Immunogenetics at Texas A & M in College Station, Texas, and did a postdoctoral fellowship at Sloan Kettering in New York in Clinical Immunobiology. Dr Bryan is currently Laboratory Director of Midwest Organ Bank, Kansas City.

Melanie J. Castelli, MD

Dr Castelli received her MD degree from the Loyola Stritch School of Medicine, Chicago, Illinois. She completed an internship in Internal Medicine at Hines Veterans Administration Hospital, Hines, Illinois prior to her combined Anatomic/Clinical Pathology residency training at Loyola Hospital. A 1-year fellowship in Surgical Pathology at Loyola followed.

In 1984 Dr Castelli became Director of Cytopathology at Loyola University Hospital. Development of an active fine needle aspiration service and cytopathology fellowship ensued and remain her primary interests.

Dr Castelli is presently Associate Professor of Pathology at Loyola University Hospital and Medical School. She is board certified in Anatomic and Clinical Pathology with subspecialty certification in Cytopathology. She is a fellow of the College of American Pathologists and the American Society of Clinical Pathologists as well as medical member of the American Society of Cytology and Illinois Society of Cytology.

Wayne R. DeMott, MD

Dr DeMott is a graduate of the University of Oregon Medical School (1959). He completed his internship at Madigan General Hospital outside Tacoma, Washington. After service in the U.S. Air Force as a General Medical Officer, he completed the pathology residency program at the University of California San Francisco Medical Center (1967). He was certified in Anatomic and Clinical Pathology by the American Board of Pathology in 1968.

As a practicing pathologist at Providence Medical Center from 1968-1994, Dr DeMott gave special attention to the areas of Hematology and Coagulation. He had participated in research activities involving separation of white cells from peripheral blood, measurement of zinc levels in peripheral blood leukocytes utilizing atomic absorption spectrophotometry, and separation of neutrophil enzymes by isoelectric focusing. He was a very active contributor to the Providence Medical Center (formerly Providence-St Margaret Health Center) School of Medical Technology, is a past president of the Medical Staff of Providence Medical Center, and was chairman or a member of several of the hospital professional committees, including the Cancer Committee.

Dr DeMott is a member of the American Society of Clinical Pathologists, College of American Pathologists, American Association for Clinical Chemistry, American Medical Association, Kansas Society of Pathologists, and Kansas City Society of Pathologists.

Susan B. Yokota Dubey, CT (ASCP), CMIAC

Ms Dubey is Clinical Instructor for the School of Cytotechnology at Truman Medical Center. Ms Dubey has published a number of cytologic articles as well as given lectures and workshops at state and national cytology conferences. During her 25-year career, she has been active in several state and national cytology organizations. She has served as president of the American Society for Cytotechnology and was a member of both the Executive Committee and the Cytotechnology Advisory Committee of the American Society of Cytopathology. She is currently serving as bylaws chairman for the American Society for Cytotechnology.

Sandra B. Earle, PharmD, BCPS

Dr Earle is a Clinical Pharmacist Specialist in Ambulatory Care at the Portland Veterans Administration Medical Center and an Adjunct Assistant Professor of Clinical Pharmacy at Oregon State University. She received her Doctor of Pharmacy at Ohio State University and completed a post-doctoral fellowship in Clinical Pharmacokinetics at Ohio State University with Dr Janis MacKichan. She was Board Certified as a Pharmacotherapy Specialist in 1992. Before coming to Portland in 1995, Dr Earle was an Associate Professor of Clinical Pharmacy at Ohio Northern University and Clinical Coordinator at Mt. Sinai Medical Center in Cleveland.

Her research interests include pharmacokinetic drug interactions involving protein binding alterations, as well as stereoselective interactions. She is a member of the American College of Clinical Pharmacy, American Association of Colleges of Pharmacy, American Society of Health Care Systems Pharmacists, and Oregon Society of Hospital Pharmacists.

Russell M. Fiorella, MD

Dr Fiorella received his undergraduate degree from Tulane University and his MD degree from the University of Missouri School of Medicine at Kansas City. He completed his anatomic/clinical pathology residency at Kansas University Medical Center, as well as a surgical pathology/cytopathology fellowship at the same institution. Dr Fiorella is certified in anatomic and clinical pathology, as well as having subspecialty certification in cytopathology. Currently, he is an associate professor of pathology at the University of Missouri Kansas City School of Medicine as well as the Director of Anatomic Pathology and Diagnostic Services for Truman Medical Center.

Paolo Gattuso, MD

Dr Gattuso received his MD degree from the University of Messina, Sicily. He completed a combined residency in Anatomic and Clinical Pathology at Loyola University Medical Center, Maywood, Illinois, followed by a fellowship in cytopathology at Loyola. Dr Gattuso is board certified in Anatomic and Clinical Pathology and also has subspecialty board certification in Cytopathology.

Presently, he is Assistant Professor of Pathology at Loyola University Medical Center and Associate Director of the Pathology Residency Training Program. His main areas of interest are fine needle aspiration biopsy and flow cytometry of solid tumors. Dr Gattuso has published extensively.

Charles W. Gorodetzky, MD, PhD

After completing his undergraduate work at MIT (BS, 1958), Dr Gorodetzky earned his MD degree at Boston University School of Medicine (1962), followed by an Internal Medicine internship at Boston City Hospital, and a PhD in Pharmacology at the University of Kentucky (1975).

Dr Gorodetzky spent 21 years in intramural NIH research in substance abuse at the National Institute on Drug Abuse, Addiction Research Center in Lexington, Kentucky (1963-1984). His major research interests were the human pharmacology and metabolism of drugs of abuse. He served as the director of the Lexington Center from 1979 to 1984. In 1984, Dr Gorodetzky joined the pharmaceutical industry and is currently Vice President of Global Therapeutic Area, CNS in the Drug Development Department at Hoechst Marion Roussel Inc in Kansas City, Missouri.

Dr Gorodetzky has authored or co-authored over 100 papers, book chapters, and books and has served on numerous government committees, including an FDA advisory committee and grant review committees. He holds or has held adjunct full professorships at the medical schools of the University of Kentucky, University of Louisville, and University of North Carolina. He served as an advisor and consultant to the Special Action Office on Drug Abuse Prevention, CDC and NIDA in the development and implementation of the Proficiency Testing Program for Drugs of Abuse.

Harold J. Grady, PhD

Dr Grady received his PhD from St Louis University. He joined the staff of the University of Kansas Medical Center in 1950 as Assistant Professor and Director of Clinical Chemistry. He became Full Professor of Pathology in 1965. During this period he was a consultant in Clinical Chemistry to several area hospitals.

He left the Medical Center in 1970 to become Director of Clinical Chemistry for Baptist Medical Center. He retired from this position in 1988.

He is currently Full Professor of Pathology at the University of Missouri Kansas City School of Medicine and Co-Director of Clinical Chemistry at Truman Medical Center.

Dr Grady is a member of the American Association for Clinical Chemistry and has been on the Board of Directors of that organization. He is a member of the American Chemical Society. He is on the Board of Directors of the American Board of Clinical Chemistry and is certified by that body in Clinical Chemistry and Toxicological Chemistry.

Larry D. Gray, PhD

Dr Gray received his bachelor's degree from the University of North Carolina at Chapel Hill and his master's and doctorate degrees from Wake Forest University (Bowman Gray School of Medicine). He received his postdoctoral training in Clinical Microbiology and Infectious Diseases at the Mayo Clinic.

Dr Gray has been the Director of Microbiology at Bethesda Hospitals in Cincinnati, Ohio for the last 5 years. He is a Volunteer Associate Professor of Pathology and Laboratory Medicine at the University of Cincinnati College of Medicine, is a Diplomate of the American Board of Medical Microbiology, and is on the editorial board of the *Journal of Clinical Microbiology*. In addition, he is an active member of the American Society for Microbiology, the American Board of Medical Microbiology, and the South Central Association for Clinical Microbiology.

Dr Gray's background includes 12 years of research in the pathogenesis of infectious diseases (ocular and pulmonary bacterial infections, electron microscopy) and the publication of many research, review, chapter, and book publications.

Steven H. Hinrichs, MD

Dr Hinrichs received his MD degree at the University of North Dakota and completed his residency at the University of California, Davis Medical Center. Following certification in Anatomic and Clinical Pathology, he was awarded a two-year fellowship in molecular pathology at the National Institutes of Health.

Dr Hinrichs is an Associate Professor in the Department of Pathology and Microbiology at the University of Nebraska Medical Center (UNMC) in Omaha, Nebraska. He also holds joint appointments in the Department of Orthopedics and the Eppley Cancer Research Institute for Cancer and Allied Diseases. Dr Hinrichs is Director of Clinical Microbiology and Virology at UNMC and is also Director of the Molecular Diagnostics Group which coordinates development of molecular diagnostic assays and establishes validation criteria. His clinical research involves the role of viruses in the immune-compromised host with particular emphasis on bone marrow transplant and solid organ recipients.

Dr Hinrichs' research interests focus on the role of viruses in oncogenesis, specifically how viruses disrupt cellular control of transcription. Current funded studies investigate the structural interaction between transcription factors and their DNA-binding motifs.

Rebecca T. Horvat, PhD

Dr Horvat received her doctorate from the University of Kansas Medical Center, Department of Microbiology. After completing her doctorate, Dr Horvat was awarded a postdoctoral fellowship from the American Cancer Society. Subsequent to her postdoctoral fellowship she worked as a Technical Director in the Clinical Laboratories at the University of Kansas Medical Center. In this capacity, she worked with Virology, Microbiology, and Hematology in developing new diagnostic tests based on nucleic acid analysis. Currently, Dr Horvat is an Assistant Professor in the Department of Pathology and Laboratory Medicine at the University of Kansas Medical Center in Kansas City, Kansas.

Dr Horvat's research interest involves the investigation of human herpes viruses in the development of leukemias and lymphomas. She is also interested in the diagnostic potential of nucleic acid detection, especially in immunocompromised patients. In her current position, she assists in the administration of the Microbiology and Virology sections of the clinical laboratories. This involves the education and teaching of residents and medical students, developing and instituting new diagnostic technology, and coordinating quality assurance in the Microbiology and Virology sections. In addition, Dr Horvat is the Clinical Microbiology consultant at the Dwight D. Eisenhower Veterans Administration Medical Center in Leavenworth, Kansas.

Dr Horvat is a member of the American Association of Immunologists (AAI) and the American Society for Microbiology (ASM).

Douglas W. Huestis, MD

Dr Huestis received his MD degree from McGill University, Montreal, Canada, in 1948 and did postgraduate training in pathology and related fields in Canada, Sweden, England, and the U.S.A. After a few years of general hospital pathology, he began concentrating on the field of blood transfusion and immunohematology in Chicago in 1960 then moved to Tucson to the then new medical school at the University of Arizona in 1969.

His major work while in Chicago was on erythrocyte antigens and antibodies and their relationship to difficulties and complications of blood transfusion. He also did some early work on the development of frozen blood systems, including the use of a unique vaporphase liquid nitrogen storage freezer and a simplified thawing-deglycerolizing system utilizing invert sugar. In Arizona, he developed a procedure for the collection of granulocytes by intermittent flow centrifugation and applied this to the special transfusion support of patients with cancer and leukemia. He has had much to do with the development of technical procedures with blood cell separators for the collection of white blood cells and platelets for transfusion, and for the treatment of leukemic patients with a dangerous excess of white blood cells or platelets. Most recently, he has been increasingly involved in transplantation immunology and in the rapidly developing field of plasma exchange. These various activities have resulted in over 90 scientific articles.

Dr Huestis has served as a director and vice-president of the American Association of Blood Banks and on many of its committees and was editor of two editions of its *Technical Manual*. He received the John Elliott award of that association for such activities. He has been an associate editor of the journal *Transfusion* since 1968. He has served on several advisory committees for the National Institutes of Health, has been a consultant to the U.S. Army and Air Force, and took part in two scientific exchange visits to the Soviet Union under the Soviet-American Health Exchange.

He considers one of his most important achievements to be the textbook *Practical Blood Transfusion*, coauthored with Joseph R. Bove and John Case and published by Little, Brown & Co. The 4th edition of this book appeared in 1988.

Daniel H. Jacobs, MD

Dr Daniel H. Jacobs is Assistant Professor of Neurology at Tufts University in Boston, Massachusetts. Dr Jacobs is specialized in behavioral neurology and higher cortical function and has published original research in the fields of aphasia, attention and neglect, and higher cortical function problems of patients with epilepsy.

Dr Jacobs received an AB in history from Stanford University and an MD from the University of Kansas. Dr Jacobs has residency training in psychiatry at the University of Iowa (1 year), in medicine at Francis Scott Key Hospital and Johns Hopkins Hospital, and in neurology at the University of Kansas. He has fellowship training in behavioral neurology and neuropsychology from Dr Kenneth Heilman at the University of Florida.

Dr Jacobs is a member of the Behavioral Neurology Society, the International Neuropsychological Association, the American Epilepsy Society, and the American Board of Psychiatry and Neurology.

David S. Jacobs, MD, FACP

Dr Jacobs was Director of Laboratories at Providence Medical Center for 29 years, leaving that position in 1994. He served as a member of the institutional Credentials Committee for 20 years. During Dr Jacobs' tenure as Director, then Medical Director of the School of Medical Technology, 173 medical technologists graduated from 1965 to 1990.

He remains Clinical Professor at the University of Kansas and the University of Missouri-Kansas City Schools of Medicine. He is a Fellow of the American College of Physicians and of the College of American Pathologists. He is a member of the International Academy of Pathology, the AMA, and the Kansas Medical Society. He is a member of the Editorial Board of *Kansas Medicine* and is Book Review Editor of that journal. Dr Jacobs is past President of the Kansas Society of Pathologists, the Kansas City Society of Pathologists, and of the Medical Staff of the Providence Medical Center (formerly Providence-St Margaret Health Center). He held a position on the Board of Directors of the Wyandotte County Medical Society for several years, and for many years served as an inspector for both the College of American Pathologists and for the American Association of Blood Banks.

Dr Jacobs' special interests include general pathology, particularly surgical pathology, interpretation of clinical laboratory tests, and transfusion medicine. His publications address topics in surgical pathology and the clinical relevance of laboratory testing.

He received his premedical education at the University of Michigan. Entering the UM Medical School in the "Letters and Medicine" program, Dr Jacobs remained at Michigan as a general rotating intern, then did his residency in Anatomic and Clinical Pathology at the same institution. Following service in the U.S. Army Medical Corps as a pathologist with 13 months residency, he returned to Ann Arbor and completed the pathology program under Drs A. J. French and M. R. Abell. He then spent an additional year in Chicago in clinical pathology with Drs Israel Davidsohn and Douglas Huestis. Dr Jacobs is certified in both Anatomic and Clinical Pathology by the American Board of Pathology.

Dr Jacobs presently is active as a consultant in pathology and laboratory medicine.

Bernard L. Kasten, Jr, MD

Dr Kasten is a graduate of Miami University, Oxford, Ohio and the Ohio State University College of Medicine. He interned at the University of Miami, Florida and served his residency in Clinical Pathology at the National Institute of Health Clinical Center followed by a fellowship at the National Cancer Institute Laboratory of Pathology. His staff appointments have included service in the Division of Laboratory Medicine at the Cleveland Clinic and as Associate Director of Pathology and Laboratory Services at Bethesda Hospitals in Cincinnati. He is now Vice President–Medical Director at Corning Clinical Laboratories, Teterboro, New Jersey. Dr Kasten is active as a fellow in the College of American Pathologists, in which he participates in the Inspection and Accreditation Program, Strategic Planning Committee, Management Resource Committee, and is past Chairman of the Publications Committee and past Chairman of the Editorial Board of *CAP Today*. In 1993, he received the Frank W. Hartman Award in recognition of his service to the College of American Pathologists.

Dr Kasten was a principal author of the first edition of the *Laboratory Test Handbook* and the author of the *Physicians DRG Handbook* and a principal author of the *Infectious Diseases Handbook*. His writings include articles on the use of bar codes in the clinical laboratory, optical storage of laboratory data and the computerized medical record. He has presented numerous lectures and seminars on the subjects of improving workflow in the laboratory, and total quality management. He is a member of the editorial board for Lexi-Comp Inc's medical publishing.

Phillip A. Munoz, MD

Dr Munoz received his MD degree from the University of Kansas Medical Center. He completed his first year of pathology training at Northwestern University and continued his training as a Research Associate in Immunology at the National Institutes of Health. He completed his training in Pathology at the University of Kansas Medical Center, then joined the medical faculty for the next 6 years. During that time, he developed a focus on hybridoma technology and cell marker studies applied to hematopathology and general surgical pathology. He is currently an Associate Pathologist and Director of Hematology and the Cell Marker Laboratories at Research Medical Center, Kansas City, Missouri.

In his current position, Dr Munoz oversees various laboratory aspects of an active hematology/oncology patient population in a large private hospital that serves as the center of a multihospital Kansas City based healthcare network. In addition to general surgical pathology and hematology services, he maintains an integrated immunocytochemistry and flow cytometry laboratory that serves as a reference laboratory for the healthcare system and other hospitals in the Kansas City area.

Dr Munoz is a member of the Kansas City Society of Pathologists, College of American Pathologists, American Society of Clinical Pathologists, American Pathology Foundation, and American Medical Association.

Patricia D. Murphy, PhD

Dr Murphy received her BA in physics from Colby College, Maine and her PhD in human genetics from Yale University in 1984. Dr Murphy remained at Yale as Assistant Clinical Professor and, subsequently held positions with the New York State Department of Health, State University of New York at Albany, and Genica Pharmaceuticals Corporation in Worcester, Massachusetts. Since 1994, she has been Vice-President and Director of Laboratory Operations at OncorMed, Inc, Gaithersburg, Maryland, and Adjunct Assistant Professor at the University of Maryland. She is a Diplomat, American Board of Medical Genetics in Clinical Cytogenetics (1987) and Molecular Genetics (1993).

Eugene S. Olsowka, MD, PhD

Dr Olsowka is a pathologist at the Institute of Pathology, Saginaw, Michigan. He is a fellow of the College of American Pathologists and the American Society of Clinical Pathologists.

Dr Olsowka studied mathematics as an undergraduate at the University of Chicago. He entered medical school at the University of Illinois in 1977 and was accepted into the MD, PhD program in 1978. He received his MD degree in 1984 and a PhD in Nutritional Sciences from the University of Illinois in 1989. Dr Olsowka was a pathology resident at The McGaw School of Medicine at Northwestern University in Chicago, from 1986 to 1990. He was a fellow in Surgical Pathology at Rush-Presbyterian-St Luke's Medical Center in Chicago from 1990 to 1991, then served as pathologist at the Providence Medical Center, Kansas City, Kansas. He is board certified in Anatomic and Clinical Pathology and is a fellow of the College of American Pathologists.

Dr Olsowka's interests are general pathology including surgical pathology, chemistry, and cytology.

Mark D. Ost, MD

Dr Ost received his MD degree from the University of Kansas in 1958 and completed his residency in pathology at Kansas City General Hospital (now Truman Medical Center, Kansas City, Missouri). Dr Ost is a Board Diplomate of the American Board of Pathology in Anatomic and Clinical Pathology and in Dermatopathology and is Clinical Professor at the University of Missouri at Kansas City School of Medicine.

Christopher J. Papasian, PhD

Dr Papasian received his doctorate in Microbiology from the State University of New York at Buffalo, School of Medicine and completed his postdoctoral training in Medical and Public Health Microbiology at Erie County Medical Center in Buffalo, New York. He is a Board-Certified Diplomate of the American Academy of Microbiology.

Dr Papasian is an Associate Professor of Pathology at the University of Missouri, (Kansas City) School of Medicine and is Director of Diagnostic Microbiology and Immunology Laboratories at Truman Medical Center in Kansas City, Missouri. He emphasizes cost-effective, clinically relevant microbiology in practice and in education, and has authored or coauthored over 40 original articles, book chapters, and abstracts.

Diane L. Persons, MD

Dr Persons received her Masters in Microbiology and Doctor of Medicine at the University of Kansas. She became board certified in Anatomic Pathology following a residency at the University of Kansas Medical Center. Following a three year combined research and clinical fellowship in Cytogenetics at the Mayo Clinic, she returned to the University of Kansas and is currently the Director of the Cytogenetics Laboratory and Assistant Professor of Pathology.

Dr Persons' research interests involve the study of cancer genetics including molecular cytogenetic characterization of tumors, gene amplification in solid tumors, and the interaction of oncogenes and cytokines in chemotherapeutic resistance in solid tumors.

Dr Persons is a member of the College of American Pathologists, American Society of Human Genetics, American Association for Cancer Research, and the American Association for the Advancement of Science.

Fred V. Plapp, MD, PhD

Dr Plapp received his MD and PhD degrees in a combined medical scientist program at the University of Kansas Medical Center. He completed an internship at the University of Chicago and pathology residency at the University of Kansas Medical Center. He practiced as an Associate Professor of Pathology at the University of Kansas Medical Center and then as Assistant Medical Director of the Community Blood Center of Greater Kansas City. Subsequently, he became a clinical pathologist at Saint Luke's Hospital of Kansas City, Kansas City, Missouri.

Lowell Tilzer, MD, PhD

Dr Tilzer received his medical degree and PhD in a combined medical science program from the Kansas University Medical Center in Kansas City, Kansas and did his residency in Anatomic and Clinical Pathology there. Certified in both Anatomic and Clinical Pathology, Dr Tilzer served at Kansas University Medical Center as associate Medical Director for 14 years and became full Professor, in charge of Hematology, Blood Bank, Clinical Chemistry, and Lab Computer. His research interests included laboratory computing (especially use of bar codes in specimen management, which he pioneered in the United States) and diagnostic Molecular Biology. He has extensive teaching experience with medical technology students, medical students, graduate students, and pathology residents. He holds several patents in the molecular biology field.

In 1992, Dr Tilzer moved to the Community Blood Center of Greater Kansas City in Kansas City, Missouri. He is Associate Medical Director. He is working on stem cell collection and bone marrow processing.

Dr Tilzer is a member of the American Association of Blood Banks, College of American Pathologists, American Association of Clinical Chemists, American Association for the Advancement of Science, and the Metropolitan Medical Society of Kansas City.

Patricia G. Tweeddale, Ed D, CT(ASCP)

Dr Tweeddale is the general supervisor of cytology at Hays Pathology Laboratories, Hays, Kansas. She received her cytology training at Muhlenberg Hospital, Plainfield, New Jersey in 1973, and her doctorate in Educational Administration from East Texas State University in 1991. She has served as President of the New Jersey State Society of Cytotechnology, established the first Cytology Department in Saudia Arabia, and was a founding member of the American Society for Cytotechnology.

Glen R. Willie, MD

Dr Willie earned his Masters in Biochemistry and Doctor of Medicine at the University of Minnesota in 1976 with research studying the receptor on the bacterial ribosome binding the antibiotic fusidic acid. He then completed his residency in Internal Medicine at Sinai Hospital of Detroit and a Nephrology Fellowship at Henry Ford Hospital in Detroit.

Since then, he has held teaching positions at Texas A&M University School of Medicine in Nephrology and Nutrition, currently as Assistant Professor of Medicine. Special areas of interest include nutrition, trace metals, metabolic bone disease, and applications of computers to the practice of medicine.

Dr Willie is a member of the American College of Physicians, Texas Medical Association, Renal Physicians Association, and the International Society of Nephrology.

HOW TO USE THIS HANDBOOK

The *Laboratory Test Handbook with Key Word Index* is arranged alphabetically by major clinical laboratory disciplines: Anatomic Pathology, Chemistry, Coagulation, Cytogenetics, Cytopathology, Hematology, Immunology and Serology, Microbiology, Molecular Pathology, Therapeutic Drug Monitoring/Toxicology/Drugs of Abuse, Trace Elements, Transfusion Service (Blood Bank), Urinalysis and Clinical Microscopy, and Virology. A general section, Specimen Collection, precedes the individual laboratory monographs. A section providing overviews of selected topics, including statistics, is entitled "Statistics, the Normal Range and the Ulysses Syndrome". The laboratory tests are listed alphabetically within each section and cross-referenced with synonyms referring the user to the actual test name. A brief introduction before each section provides general information about each major discipline.

Each individual test listing is arranged in a consistent format providing specific types of information. The fields of information include the following. The **test name**; the **current procedural terminology (CPT) code** is listed for most tests **related information** which lists other tests that may be of interest and the page number where these tests can be found; **synonyms** or other common names for a test are noted; topics or procedures which are not exact synonyms but have similar instructions or require similar consideration are referred to under the **applies to** heading; tests **replaced by** a current procedure are noted; a definition of procedures included within the named test is given under **test includes**; an **abstract** or overview of the test is often provided; patient **preparation** includes patient care considerations prior to the collection of specimen or performance of a test; **aftercare** includes patient care considerations following the collection of a specimen or performance of a procedure; the specific **specimen** required, the **container, sampling time**, specific **collection** instructions, specimen **storage instructions, causes for rejection** of the specimen by the laboratory, **turnaround time** when relevant, and **special instructions** indicating additional pertinent considerations relating to the specimen are all listed; a discussion of basic information relevant to the clinical application of the test, including **reference** (or normal) **range, critical values,** and **possible panic ranges,** specific **use** of the test, **limitations** of the test method, specific test **methodology** where appropriate, **contraindications** to the test, and **additional information** which may contribute to the interpretation or utilization of a test are given.

Footnotes and References

The bibliographic information provided with test listings may include footnotes referring to specific literature quotations, specific points of information, or opinions. Selected general references are provided as sources of information concerning the individual test listings. Footnotes and references are intended, as well, to expedite access to useful literature. Many are current, but the alert reader will find an important reference from 1785.

Acronyms and Abbreviations Glossary

This glossary provides a useful listing of many acronyms and abbreviations commonly associated with laboratory medicine. We offer this glossary not as an exhaustive authoritative list, but more as a guide to assist in interpreting frequently used terminology.

Key Word Index

The Key Word Index is not intended in any way to suggest patterns of physicians' orders, nor is it complete. Rather, it is the intent of the authors and editors to make information easier to find and utilize in order to support better patient care.

The Key Word Index provides a reference to test names based on a diagnostic property, disease entity, organ system, or syndrome for which the test may be useful. It provides lists of specific tests. Some may support possible clinical diagnoses or help to rule out other diagnostic possibilities.

Each laboratory test which may be relevant to the indexed diagnosis is listed and weighted. Two symbols (••) indicate that the test strongly supports a diagnosis or entity, that is, it significantly contributes to documentation of the diagnosis if the expected result is found. A single symbol (•) indicates a test frequently used in the diagnosis or management of the particular disease. The other listed tests may be useful on a selective basis with consideration of clinical factors and specific aspects of the case. A negative laboratory test result can be, and frequently is, highly relevant in the practice of medicine.

Clinical diagnosis is determined following history, physical examination, and usual laboratory investigation with selected additional tests. Complete blood count (CBC) with differential, urinalysis, and a basic chemistry profile are not only good medicine, they are in fact cost effective. Thus, these basic tests are excluded from much of the Key Word Index.

Diagnoses with *International Classification of Disease—Ninth Revision—Clinical Modification* (ICD-9-CM) codes are indicated within the [ ] symbol.

CPT Index

CPT codes are provided with each test for reference, as a basis for documentation of diagnostic procedures performed and to facilitate financial and patient record keeping. The codes are current. Applications of codes may vary by region of the country and in some instances the application of a specific code to a given procedure is a matter of individual interpretation.

Any five-digit numeric Physicians' **Current Procedural Terminology**, (CPT) codes service descriptions, instructions and/or guidelines are Copyright 1995 American Medical Association. All rights reserved.

CPT is a listing of descriptive terms and five-digit numeric identifying codes and modifiers for reporting medical services performed by physicians. This presentation includes only CPT descriptive terms, numeric identifying codes and modifiers for reporting medical services, and procedures that were selected by Lexi-Comp Inc for inclusion in this publication.

The most current CPT is available from the American Medical Association.

No fee schedules, basic unit values, relative value guides, conversion factors or scales or components thereof are included in CPT.

Lexi-Comp has selected certain CPT codes and service/procedure descriptions and assigned them to various specialty groups. The listing of a CPT service or procedure description and its code number in this publication does not restrict its use to a particular specialty group. Any procedure or service in this publication may be used to designate the services rendered by any qualified physician.

The AMA assumes no responsibility for the consequences attributable to or related to any use or interpretation of any information or views contained in or not contained in this publication.

Alphabetical Index

The most expedient method for locating a given test is the Alphabetical Index in the last section of this handbook. Test names and synonyms are listed and the page number on which the test description may be found is indicated.

STATISTICS, THE NORMAL RANGE, AND THE ULYSSES SYNDROME

or

A TEST IN SEARCH OF A DISEASE

David S. Jacobs, MD

Eugene S. Olsowka, MD, PhD

During and after the Trojan War, Ulysses was away from home 20 years. While traveling, he was involved in a series of frequently dangerous and sometimes needless adventures. The syndrome[1] was named for Ulysses because patients with it, although healthy at the beginning, journey through clinical investigations and undergo a number of experiences new to them before they once again reach the safe harbor of being considered healthy.

The bottom line of complex clinical, technical, and statistical data leads to a decision – whether or not a given laboratory report is normal for a particular patient.

The College of American Pathologists, in setting standards for their Inspection and Accreditation Program for Clinical Laboratories, advocates that reference values (normal values) for each test should be provided when possible. Two modern laboratory realities must be recognized:

1. A reference range is required for the interpretation of most laboratory tests, and
2. It may not be possible to provide an appropriate reference range in all cases.

It is important to recognize that laboratory methods and types of equipment greatly influence the outcome of any given test. The most relevant reference ranges are those generated by the laboratory performing the assay. Ability of a laboratory to provide meaningful reference ranges is limited by many factors.

Purely statistical approaches are unsatisfactory. For instance, since coronary arterial disease is rampant in present day America, we cannot base "normal" ranges for serum lipids on a Gaussian distribution.

Most tests do not have sharp cutoff points between normal and abnormal. "Normal" curves can be bell shaped, but they are often skewed.

Nominally, "normal" findings may have diagnostic significance in an appropriate setting.[2] Thus, efforts to increase our knowledge of the significance of normal range, and thus narrow the normal range for a given patient, can add value to "normal" results.

The effects of drugs on clinical laboratory tests have been exhaustively reviewed[3] and are therefore not emphasized in this book.

With computers, laboratories can stratify normal ranges by age and sex. We would no more expect a college varsity athlete and a great-grandmother to have the same normal ranges for clinical laboratory examinations, than we would expect them to have the same hat or shoe size. Such stratification remains at the fringe of clinical documentation, and relatively few published studies are available which are pertinent to normal ranges for all of the tests done by most laboratories. Clinical input is continually needed to improve available normal ranges.

Special situations in which computer generated normal ranges may be inappropriate, misleading, or nonexistent include the following.

1. **Glucose:** A computer may only be provided with normal ranges for fasting plasma glucose. Blood sugar levels have not been done in laboratories in years; serum and plasma are used.

2. **Pregnancy:** The well known increases in alkaline phosphatase, plasma volume, glomerular filtration rate, and hepatic protein synthesis, decreases in urea nitrogen, sodium, osmolality, albumin, and other changes accompanying pregnancy are not always taken into consideration when normal ranges are reported in pregnant individuals. (The laboratory is commonly not aware if an individual is pregnant, and if so, the length of gestation. Many laboratories do not have normal ranges for pregnancy available.) Cortisol, alpha$_1$-fetoprotein, alpha$_1$-antitrypsin, amylase, cholesterol, and triglycerides may increase.

3. **Athletes and Exercise:** Athletes are apt to have slight elevations of urea nitrogen and LD, as well as depressions of pulse rate.[4] After physical exercise, significant elevations of total CK are commonplace and creatinine, potassium, uric acid, bilirubin, leukocyte count, haptoglobin, transferrin, and BUN may increase. Exercise increases HDLC, lactate, and may increase aldolase.

4. **The First Month of Life:** Tremendous shifts in normal ranges occur during the first month of life. Some tests ideally should be stratified depending on whether the patient is premature or term, and others (hemoglobin, bilirubin) change significantly during the first month. Many computers cannot stratify in so many intervals. For such tests, a number of normal ranges exist depending upon the age in days in the first month of life, prematurity or term, and other factors.

5. **Posture:** Posture is reported to change the normal range for a number of tests – total protein, albumin, calcium, hemoglobin and hematocrit, plasma renin activity, urinary catecholamines, and perhaps alkaline phosphatase, cholesterol,[5] ALT (SGPT), and iron. Levels of such substances have been described as being higher in an upright position than in a reclining position. Consider that in the reclining individual, interstitial fluid enters the vascular compartment, diluting constituents which the clinical laboratory measures. On standing, the venous pressure in the lower part of the body increases, capillary pressure increases, and some plasma is ultrafiltered into the interstitial space. Cells and constituents such as protein, which do not readily pass the capillary

endothelium, increase. So do substances wholly or partly bound to protein (eg, calcium). Urea nitrogen, on the other hand, is so diffusible that patient posture makes no difference.

6. **Body Weight:** Some laboratory computer software makes no allowance for body weight. Creatinine clearance and blood volumes require this data. Positive weight dependencies are described for uric acid, glucose, and cholesterol; many subjects with high concentrations of such analytes are prone to be found in the high-weight group. Males, but not females, have such body weight associations for creatinine, protein, hemoglobin, and AST (SGOT). Inverse relationships are reported for phosphate and, in females, for calcium.[6]

7. **Topics Requiring Medical Judgment:** The significance of a few red cells in urine depends upon the clinical setting (voided versus catheterized urine, sex, menstruation or not); therefore, some tests cannot be classified as "normal" or "abnormal" by computer, but only by the physician caring for that particular patient.

Tests having no normals – because **positivity** in any quantity is itself abnormal – include:

> Serum acetone
> Porphobilinogen
> Alcohol and certain other toxins
> Urine glucose, ketones, blood, bile, nitrite
> ART, VDRL, and other serologic tests for syphilis
> Nucleated RBC/100 WBC, blasts, promyelocytes, myelocytes in diff
> LE slide test
> Test for sickling
> Malaria smear

Laboratory data must always be considered in light of the physician's clinical impression. If the clinician considers acute infarct of myocardium likely, and the early laboratory data do not support his initial impression, the patient should be treated as if he indeed had an infarct. (Laboratory data may be normal or inconclusive early in myocardial infarct; this is a particularly good example of the importance of the physician's clinical diagnosis.) When laboratory results are abnormal but not supported by clinical findings, the physician should thoroughly consider the laboratory reports before dismissing them as inconsequential.

Laboratory data suggest clues to unsuspected disease in about 12% of patients studied in a university hospital series.[7]

8. **Food and Nutrition:** Tests requiring the **fasting state** include fasting blood sugar, lipid profile, iron, iron binding capacity, B_{12}/folate levels, carotene, d-xylose, lactose, and glucose tolerance tests, Schilling test, most insulins, serum bile acids, and gastrin. Serum bile acids are sometimes measured before and after a meal. **Prolonged fasting** may increase serum bilirubin (up to 240% after a 48-hour fast) and cause decreases of plasma glucose and proteins (albumin, transferrin, and complement C3). Samples for PKU (chemical test), FTA-ABS, and antibodies for virus, fungal, and *Mycoplasma* agents should be clear serum, fasting if necessary.

Blood drawn immediately after a meal is apt to have elevated potassium and depressed phosphorus and later elevated triglycerides. Alkaline phosphatase may be elevated 2-4 hours after a fatty meal, especially in people who are Lewis-positive secretors of blood type O or B. Increased turbidity in postprandial blood can interfere with certain other tests, including bilirubin, LD (LDH), and total protein. Increased turbidity might depress uric acid and BUN, depending on methodology.

High protein diet can elevate BUN, ammonia, and urate. Purines increase uric acid. High intake of **bananas, pineapples, tomatoes,** and **avocados** may elevate 5-HIAA. **Caffeine** elevates catecholamines, as does **theophylline**.

9. **Drugs: Ethanol** causes immediate increases of uric acid, lactate, and acetone. Intermediate effects include increases of GGT (GGTP) and to a lesser degree ALT (SGPT). Actually, a short-chain carbohydrate, ethanol may induce increases in triglycerides. More chronic alcoholism may be manifested by increases of bilirubin, AST (SGOT), alkaline phosphatase, as well as GGT, and a decrease of folate. Although considerable information is available, a great deal more is needed.

Oral contraceptives increase T_4 (RIA) and decrease T_3 uptake. They are reported to increase alpha$_1$-antitrypsin (half of alpha$_1$ in serum protein electrophoresis), iron, triglycerides, ALT (SGPT), and GGT; to decrease albumin; and to affect as many as 100 laboratory tests.

10. **Hemolysis** from hemolytic anemia or venipuncture causes increases in LD, bilirubin, AST (SGOT), CK, potassium, ALT (SGPT), magnesium, and acid phosphatase. Hemolysis from traumatic venipuncture may be associated with release of thromboplastins and may invalidate the results of coagulation tests in some cases. Hemolysis has a less marked effect on total protein, alkaline phosphatase, iron, and phosphorus. Hemolysis will mask hemolyzing antibodies in the antibody screen and crossmatch.

11. **Circadian Rhythms:** Circadian (approximately 24-hour) rhythms have implications for physiology, measurement of many laboratory tests, drug excretion (eg, salicylates, sulfonamides), and responses to therapy. Levels fluctuating very significantly during the 24-hour cycle include cortisol (which has different normals for 8 AM and 8 PM), growth hormone, serum acid phosphatase, aldosterone (high 6 AM to 3 PM), transferrin (maximum 4 PM to 8 PM), ACTH, serum iron, serum creatinine (7 PM values 130% of 7 AM concentration), eosinophils (low in afternoon), lymphocytes (maximum early AM), WBC (maximum in early AM), leukocyte function and urine urobilinogen (maximum excretion in afternoon). Urinary excretion of potassium, LH, FSH, TSH, testosterone, and some less commonly ordered hormones have some diurnal variation. Parathyroid hormone is best drawn at 8 AM.

Triglyceride is higher in the afternoon, as is phosphate, BUN, and the hematocrit. Bilirubin falls in the PM, but overnight fasting itself causes bilirubin to increase.[8]

The waves which characterize circadian rhythms may be square shaped or may occur as a series of pulses. The latter pattern is seen with plasma cortisol concentration, which begins to increase during sleep. A large difference exists between this level and that found in the evening. Still another pattern is a single daily pulse such as occurs with growth hormone secretion.[9]

The magnitude of the effect of circadian rhythms is greater than is generally recognized. Although only 10% variation exists for plasma potassium concentration, urinary potassium excretion can vary fivefold during the day.[10]

Some hormone secretion cycles are longer (infradian) – eg, the menstrual cycle.

12. **Clots** in specimens which should lead to specimen rejection. Tiny clots may go unnoticed and generate misleading results (eg, CBC).

13. **Prolonged contact with the clot**, in the physician's office or in the laboratory, causes glucose to decrease and alkaline phosphatase to change somewhat. Iron, potassium, and LD increase, and AST (SGOT) increases slightly, but ALT (SGPT) and total CK remain constant. The greatest changes are in glucose, potassium, and LD.[11] We have seen some tubes left on a radiator a day or two with characteristic chemistry profile patterns: phosphorus very high, LD high, and no glucose.

14. **Other specimen mishandling** potentially causing misleading results includes blood tube exposure to **sunlight** which can cause misleading increases in white blood cell count, platelet count, and abnormalities in sedimentation rate.[12] Sunlight causes bilirubin to decrease in the test tube as it does in the neonate.

15. **Sampling Problems: It is best not to draw from an extremity in which there is an I.V. infusion site.** Rarely, there is no other place to draw, and such samples are apt to have dilutional changes resulting in invalid test results, especially for electrolytes and glucose, and factitious changes in coagulation parameters. A recommendation to wait 3 minutes after the I.V. has been shut off may lead to misleading results for glucose.[13] Drawing from indwelling venous catheters may present dilutional and many other artifacts.

A **tourniquet**, with patient clenching and unclenching his hand, will lead to build-up of high potassium and lactic acid from the hand muscles, and pH will decrease. It is best to avoid a tourniquet for pH, pCO_2, electrolytes, and lactic acid. Hand clenching is best avoided for such tests.

Capillary punctures can be done for CBC, differential, platelet count, reticulocyte count, electrolytes, gases, and many chemistry tests but may introduce tissue juices which result in possibly misleading conclusions.

Arterial specimens, compared to venous, have different normal ranges for lactic acid, pO_2 and oxygen saturation, and only slightly different ranges in the vast majority of well and sick patients for pH and pCO_2.

Unusual sites of venous sampling (other than anticubital veins) may lead to misleading results. Sampling from foot veins, for instance, may lead to results which differ from established levels based on conventional vein draws. With rare exceptions such as drug addicts and obese individuals, foot veins are not accessed. They are saved as a last resort. Such attempts are often unsuccessful.

Inappropriate specimen collection tubes (eg, for trace metals or coagulation tests), incorrect sample collection procedures, and incorrect choice of anticoagulant (eg, as in fibrinopeptide A and beta-thromboglobulin procedures) are potential mistakes inexperienced laboratorians may make.

16. **Lipemic specimens** may present a number of problems.

17. **Instruments:** Some are electronic marvels. Nevertheless, anyone who has ever purchased an automobile, refrigerator, or light bulb is aware that instruments can fail. This phenomenon is best expressed by Murphy's Law, third corollary: "If there is a possibility of several things going wrong, the one that will cause the most damage will be the one to go wrong."[14] Systems are relevant as well.[15]

18. **Genetic variations** exist in how individuals metabolize drugs and major variations occur.

19. **Aging** is accompanied by differences in normal ranges from those established for younger individuals.[16,17]

20. **Other variables** include sex, stress, menstrual cycle, menopause, and altitude.[18]

21. **Normal Range – A Guideline:** The reference or normal ranges in this book are merely guidelines. A great deal of variation exists between methods, instruments, reaction temperatures, and other parameters among laboratories, thus, reported reference ranges vary widely. The most relevant normal ranges for most assays are those developed and reported by the laboratory performing the assay. In situations where the normal range is extremely method dependent, it seemed prudent not to provide a normal range that would differ markedly from that encountered by many readers and thus might be potentially misleading.

Physicians confront dilemmas as they order and interpret tests. Third parties may not support clinical decisions, expanding technology provides increasingly complex investigations, and the literature is inconsistent in description of test properties.[19,20]

Although we read a great deal about cost-effective testing and care, with further reasons to continue to diminish laboratory evaluation, few call to our attention the costs of not testing. Gambino is among those who recognizes such follies, pointing out that a patient is unlikely to be treated for a disease which has gone untested and undiagnosed. Laboratory investigation can recognize the presence or absence of hypothyroidism or hyperthyroidism, for instance, prior to clinical recognition. Gambino provides further examples of the damage of not testing, discussing HIV, HbA_{1c}, and investigation of hepatitis B and C.

Evaluation of results of a given test over time may be more meaningful than a single result.

Cost-effective policies are less risky in theory than at the bedside.[21]

Statistical Review

Statistics is a branch of mathematics often much maligned by many current day savants. One often hears the incorrect expression, "You can say anything you like by using statistics." Substitution of the word "using" for the more accurate "misusing" corrects an incorrect expression. It is by the misuse of statistics (intentional or otherwise) that facts may be misconstrued. More colloquially, "statistics don't lie, people do." As our common everyday statistics and hypothesis testing are ultimately derived from probabilistic equations, discussion of statistics must necessarily include a discussion of probability. Following are some of the more common definitions and equations that are used daily in laboratory medicine, often hidden from conscious thought.

Sample Space: A collection of objects or outcomes of interest. As an example, in an unbiased single coin toss the sample space consists of the outcome heads or tails.

Relative Frequency: The ratio of the number of times an event occurs to the total number of observations. Relative frequencies are unstable for a small number of observations. For example, the relative frequency of obtaining a heads or a tails in an unbiased coin toss is 50% for a large number of tosses. It may be different for a limited number of tosses – say four.

Probability: The stable (over a large number of observations) relative frequency associated with an event. The probability of event A is usually denoted by the symbol P(A).

Random Variable: Given a sample space S with elements s and a function X, X is called a random variable if it assigns to each element s in the sample space S one and only one real number. Put mathematically, the random function X acting on sample space S is defined by the set of real numbers [x: x=X(s), s is an element of S]. One of the major problems for applied statisticians is to define such functions. As an example: To determine the effect of a diet on development of an animal, we may choose to look at total body weight gain, bone or organ growth, or times to maturation or senescence.

Statistic: A function of the elements of a random sample that does not depend upon any unknown parameters of the sample. Mean, median, mode, range, and variance of a given sample are all statistics.

Median: The middle most number in a data set (assuming set is arranged in ascending or descending order).

Mode: Most frequently occurring result or measurement in a data set.

Population Mean: Usually denoted by the symbol μ.

Population Variance: Usually denoted by the symbol σ^2. Typically μ and σ^2 are unknown and are estimated from $\overline{X}$ and S^2 – the sample mean and variance.

Mean of a Sample: Denoted by:

$$\overline{X} = 1/n \left(\sum_{i=1}^{n} X_i \right)$$

Variance of a Sample: Denoted by:

$$S^2 = (1/n) \sum_{i=1}^{n} (X_i - \overline{X})^2$$

or

$$S^2 = \left((1/n) \sum_{i=1}^{n} X_i^2 \right) - \overline{X}^2$$

Note: Using 1/n yields the variance of the empirical (sample) distribution. Use of 1/n-1 yields the unbiased estimator of σ^2. 1/n+1 yields the minimum mean square error estimator of σ^2. Standard deviation σ is the square root of the variance σ^2

Biased Statistic: A statistic is said to be biased if it is not equal to the parameter it is intended to measure, eg, if the mean $\overline{x}$ of a sampling distribution is not equal to the population mean μ, then the mean $\overline{x}$ is said to be biased. Conversely, if the mean $\overline{x}$ equals the parameter μ, then $\overline{x}$ is said to be unbiased.

Binomial Probability Function: Let p be a probability of success for a certain event. Then the probability of failure of the event is q = 1 – p. If n = total number of trials and x = the number of successes, the probability (p) of the number of successes in n trials is:

$$P(x) = \left(n! / x!(n-x)! \right) p^x q^{n-x}$$

Example: If each assay in a particular laboratory has a 1 in 100 chance of being erroneous, find the probability of finding 3 erroneous results in a batch of 10. Here n = 10, x = 3, p = 0.01, and q = 1 - 0.01 = 0.99. Probability of 3 erroneous results in a batch of 10 in this laboratory is given by:

$P(3) = (10!/3! \, (7)!) \, 0.01^3 \, 0.99^7$
$P(3) = (3628800/6 \, (5040)) \, 10^{-6} 0.9321$
$P(3) = 120 \, (9.321 \times 10^{-7})$
$P(3) = 0.000112$

Example: Under the above error rate assumptions, find the probability of an error with 5 replicated tests being made. Here the 10 tests consist of 5 tests with replication. With 10 tests, there is a total of 45 pairs of tests that could be in error; (10!/2! 8!) however, we are constrained to 5 combinations of replicate tests. The probability is given by:

$P(error) = 5 \, (0.01^2) \, 0.99^8 = 5 \, (10^{-4}) \, 0.9227$
$P(error) = 5 \, (9.23 \times 10^{-5}) = 0.0046$

Poisson Distribution: A special adaptation of the binomial distribution, given by the formula:

where λ is equal to both the mean and the variance of the poisson distribution (the probability of a given event occurring in a short time h must be λh). This distribution may be used to calculate the probabilities of the number of

$$P(X=x) = \lambda^x e^{-\lambda}/x!$$

or

$$P(X \leq x) = \sum_{k=0}^{x} (\lambda^k e^{-\lambda}/k!)$$

times particular events occur in a given time or on a given object. For example this distribution may be used to calculate the probability of obtaining defective cuvettes over a period of time in a manufacturing process. If a manufacturer of cuvettes expects 2 bad cuvettes every 5 minutes, what is the probability of 5 or more bad cuvettes in 15 minutes? Here, the average number of bad cuvettes in 15 minutes is 6, ie, $\lambda = 6$. If we assume a Poisson process then

$$P(X \geq 5) = 1 - P(X=4) = \sum_{i=0}^{4} 6^i e^{-6}$$

$$= 1 - 0.285 = 0.715 \text{ or } 71\%$$

Normal (Bell-Shaped) Distribution: Let μ = mean of the normal random variable, x, σ = standard deviation, π = 3.1416, and e = 2.71828, then the probability density function of a normal distribution is given by the equation:

$$f(x) = (1/\sigma\sqrt{2\pi})\, e^{-((x-\mu)^2/2\sigma^2)}$$

The z score gives the distance between a measurement and the mean in units equal to the standard deviation, ie, $z = (x - \mu)/\sigma$. The distribution of z scores also known as a standard normal distribution always has a mean of 0 and a standard deviation of 1.

Student's t Distribution: Let Z be a random variable that is normally distributed with mean 0 and variance 1, and let U be a random variable that is chi-square distributed with r degrees of freedom. If Z and U are independent, then

$$T = Z/\sqrt{U/r}$$

has a t distribution with r degrees of freedom. The probability density function is a rather complicated gamma function and the interested reader is encouraged to seek it in more specialized statistical textbooks. Figure 1 compares a normal distribution with mean 0 and variance 1 with a t distribution with 4 degrees of freedom. Note that the t distribution has more extreme probability than the normal distribution.

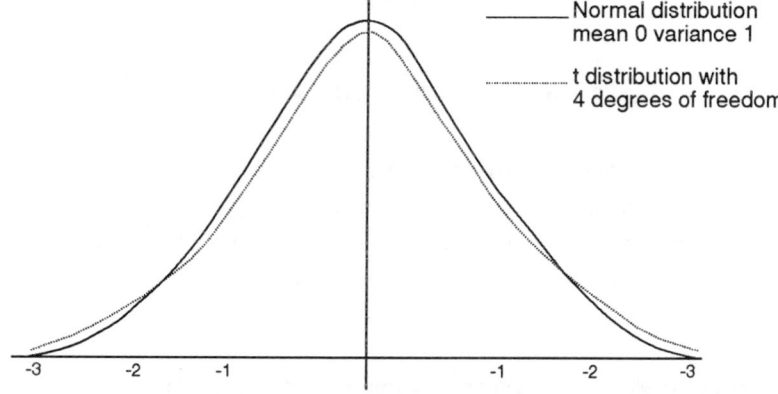

Figure 1. t distribution with 4 degrees of freedom compared with a normal distribution of mean 0 and variance 1

The Gamma Distribution: The random variable X is said to have a gamma distribution if its probability density function is defined by the equation

$$F(x) = \begin{cases} \dfrac{1}{\Upsilon(\alpha)\theta^\alpha}\, X\alpha^{-1}e^{-x/\theta} & 0 \leq x < \infty \\ 0 & x < 0 \end{cases}$$

where the gamma function is defined as:

$$\Upsilon(t) = \int_0^\infty y^{t-1}e^{-y}dy \qquad t > 0$$

The Chi-Square Distribution: Let X have a gamma distribution with $\theta = 2$ and $\alpha = r/2$ where r is a positive integer called the "degrees of freedom". X is chi-square distributed if its probability density function is given by:

The mean and variance of a chi-square distribution are

$$u = \alpha\theta = r \quad \text{and} \quad \sigma^2 = \alpha\theta^2 = 2r$$

$$f(x) = \begin{cases} \dfrac{1}{\Upsilon(r/2)2^{r/2}} x^{r/2-1} e^{-x/2} & 0 \le x < \infty \\ 0 & x < 0 \end{cases}$$

ie, the mean is equal to the number of degrees of freedom and the variance is equal to twice the number of the degrees of freedom.

The F Distribution: Let U and V be independent chi-square variables with r1 and r2 degrees of freedom. Then F is said to have an F distribution with r1 and r2 degrees of freedom when defined as:

$$F = \frac{U/r1}{V/r2}$$

The probability density function is complicated and the reader is encouraged to seek out advanced statistical textbooks. Graphs of some typical F distributions are seen in figure 2. Note that this distribution is assymetric and skewed. F distributions have many uses. They may be used to test equality of variances and linearity in regression analysis, among other uses.

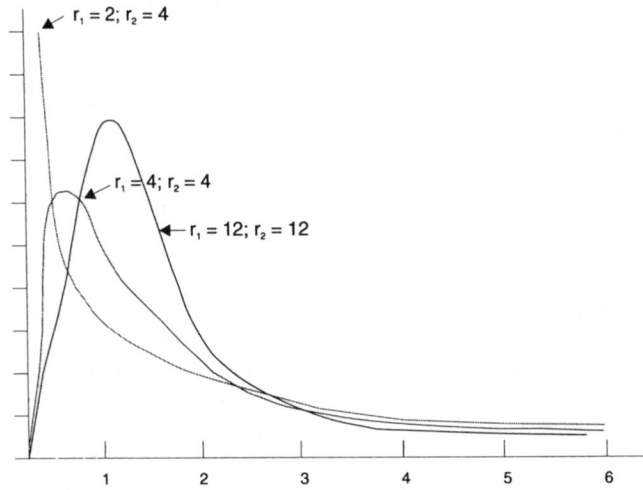

Figure 2. F distribution with r_1 and r_2 degrees of freedom

Brief Review of Simple Tests of Comparison

t Test: Given two means u_1 with sample size n_1 and u_2 with sample size n_2 and equal variances ($\sigma_1^2 = \sigma_2^2$).

To test null hypothesis that means u_1 and u_2 are equal against the hypothesis that $u_1 - u_2 \ne 0$, use the formula

$$t = \overline{x_1} - \overline{x_2} / \sqrt{sp^2(1/n_1 + 1/n_2)}$$

This statistic has a t distribution with $n_1 + n_2 - 2$ degrees of freedom. The pooled variance sp^2 may be estimated from the following formula:

$$sp^2 = \left[\sum_{i=1}^{n1} (X_{1i} - \overline{X_1})^2 + \sum_{j=1}^{n2} (X_{2j} - \overline{X_2})^2 \right] / (n_1 + n_2 - 2)$$

The t test may be used to answer such questions as to whether mean effects of two treatments are equal. The test may be one tailed or two tailed depending upon the question one is asking.

The F Test: May be used to test the (null) hypothesis that population means do not differ. Let MST be the mean square for a group of k treatments (sum of squares/k-1). Let MSE be the mean square for error given by sum of squares for error/n-k, where n = number of measurements. Then to compare the two sources of variability – source of variability among treatment means with that due to differences within samples, one may use the statistic:

F = MST/MSE

with k-1 and n-k degrees of freedom. This test assumes that all k populations are normally distributed, the k population variances are equal, and samples are randomly and independently selected. In the case of determining linearity in a single variable regression, the error may be partitioned into that of the regression and residual. An F test defined as:

F = MS(regression)/MS(residual)

may be used to determine whether there is a true linear effect. Note that as assays become more precise mean square residual error decreases which tends to increase the ratio. Thus as assays become more precise, the F test may appear to magnify subtle departures from linearity. This helps to explain the observation that with very precise assays that a clinically acceptable linear assay may not pass a statistical test of linearity. As the F test typically involves a comparison of two sources of variance, procedures utilizing F tests may be referred to as "analysis of variance."

The F test may be used to test for equal variances. Assay variance is also termed "imprecision" or "precision". The larger the variance (hence, standard deviation and coefficient of variability), the less precise the assay is said to be. One may then use the F test to determine if one assay is as imprecise as another.

Example: Assay 1 was compared with assay 2 for 21 days. The variance (S^2) of a series of measurements was 1432 for assay 1 and 3500 for assay 2. Is the imprecision of each assay comparable?

Answer: The test statistic here is denoted by:

$$F = \frac{\text{Larger sample variance}}{\text{smaller sample variance}} = \frac{3500}{1432} = 2.44$$

From published tables, the critical value of $F_{0.5}$ with 20 degrees of freedom in the numerator and denominator is 2.12 and $F_{0.01}$ is 2.94. Thus at the $\alpha=0.05$ significance level, we conclude that asay 1 is more precise (less imprecise) than assay 2. If we were held to more stringent significance levels, say $\alpha=0.01$, we could not conclude that the variances of the two assays were different (null hypothesis: $S_1^2 - S_2^2 = 0$).

Completely random design:

Let:

N = total number of observations
b = number of blocks
K = number of treatments
T_i = treatment total for a given block
B_i = block totals

Assume:

1. Distribution are normal
2. Variances are equal

An example is taken from McClove and Dietrich[22] with figures representing serum creatinine and blocks representing laboratories rather than supermarkets. The different treatments represent different assay methods. Here there are four treatments and ten blocks.

Serum Creatinine (mg/dL)

Lab	A	B	C	D	Total
1	2.43	2.47	2.47	2.41	9.78
2	2.48	2.52	2.53	2.48	10.01
3	2.38	2.44	2.42	2.35	9.59
4	2.40	2.47	2.46	2.39	9.72
5	2.35	2.42	2.44	2.32	9.53
6	2.43	2.49	2.47	2.42	9.81
7	2.55	2.62	2.64	2.56	10.37
8	2.41	2.49	2.47	2.39	9.76
9	2.53	2.60	2.59	2.49	10.21
10	2.35	2.43	2.44	2.36	9.58
Total	24.31	24.95	24.93	24.17	98.36

Is there a difference in the assay values from a standard serum creatinine among the assay methods A to D?

SS(Total) = 0.22936
SST = 0.05000
SSB = 0.17451
SSE = SS(Total)-SST-SSB = 0.00485

$$MST = \frac{SST}{K-1} = \frac{0.05}{3} = 0.01667$$

$$MSB = \frac{SSB}{b-1} = \frac{0.17451}{9} = 0.01939$$

$$MSE = \frac{SSE}{(b-1)(K-1)} = \frac{0.00485}{(9)(3)} = \frac{0.00485}{27} = 0.00017963$$

$$\text{Then } F = \frac{MST}{MSE} = \frac{0.01667}{0.00017963} = 92.8$$

Here the critical F for an $\alpha=0.05$ is 2.96

Thus, F = 92.8 > 2.96, and we conclude that at least two of the assay means are different.

Detection of Laboratory Error

If result of a particular assay is viewed as (blindly) selecting a value from a distribution with a particular mean and variation, then it is expected that one may get a value that is statistically different from that mean. In other words, given the myriads of results a laboratory reports per day, it is expected that a small fraction of these results may be erroneous. As some errors are truly random, there is no way to detect them. Can true errors be minimized? Three maneuvers may help to minimize such errors.

1. **Repeat Testing (Replicate):** Such repeat testing is another sampling with the same probability for error. As the probability for two errors is less than for a single error, replicate testing may help to minimize errors.

Then:

$$SS(Total) = \text{Total sum of squares}$$

$$= \Sigma x^2 - \frac{(\Sigma x)^2}{N}$$

SST $= $ Sum of squares for treatments

$$= \frac{\Sigma (\text{treatment totals})^2}{b} = \frac{T_i^2 + \ldots + T_k^2}{b} = SS(Total)$$

SSB $= $ Sum of squares for blocks

$$= \frac{\Sigma (Bi)^2}{K} - SS(Total)$$

SSE $= $ Sum of squares for error

$$= SS(Total) - SST - SSB$$

$$\text{Mean square for treatments} = MST = \frac{SST}{K-1}$$

$$\text{Mean square for blocks} = MSE = \frac{SSE}{(b-1)(K-1)}$$

Then: $F = \dfrac{MST}{MSE}$

2. **Analysis of Outliers:** Such maneuvers allow one to discard a result if it is more than a predefined number of standard deviations from a population mean. It is recognized by many that diseases such as metabolic blocks may produce values that are well beyond the population mean (sometimes 10 deviations). A highly unusual result may attract attention but be a true result. Repeat testing of an outlier may be a good way of minimizing error, but a dilemma exists if the repeat value is markedly different from the first – which is the true result?

3. **Comparison of a Current Value With the Last Value**—the so called delta check. Anyone who has followed serum enzymes for myocardial infarct knows that such a procedure may be misleading. However, one of the authors has had an experience in urinalysis in which a 1 g/dL urine glucose was properly questioned because the five previous urinalyses had glucose concentrations of 0. Used properly, delta checks may be very helpful. They are not particularly helpful with potentially labile analytes such as serum enzymes, blood gases, or electrolytes.

The above discussion applies to random laboratory error. Errors that are systemic (ie, resulting from faulty technique or equipment) are likely to be picked up by a reasonably good laboratory quality assurance program.

Thus, a wide variety of causes of erroneous or inaccurate laboratory results can cause a patient to begin a journey that may have more than a passing resemblance to Ulysses'.[23]

Laboratory Lament[24]

To the Editor:

Oh, what a tangled web is weavable
When clinical chemistry's not believable.

Digoxin dosage is not titratable.
Coronary risk becomes debatable.

The bottom line will be inscrutable
If based on tests that are disputable!

Footnotes

1. Rang M, "The Ulysses Syndrome," *Can Med Assoc J*, 1972, 106:122-3.
2. Gorry GA, Pauker SG, and Schwartz WB, "The Diagnostic Importance of the Normal Finding," *N Engl J Med*, 1978, 298:486-9.
3. Young DS, *Effects of Drugs on Clinical Laboratory Tests*, 4th ed, Washington, DC: AACC Press, 1995.
4. Solomon JG, "Abnormal Laboratory Results in Runners," *JAMA*, 1979, 241:2262, (letter).
5. Dixon M and Paterson CR, "Posture and the Composition of Plasma," *Clin Chem*, 1978, 24:824:6.
6. Munan L, Kelly A, PetitClerc C, et al, "Associations With Body Weight of Selected Chemical Constituents in Blood: Epidemiologic Data," *Clin Chem*, 1978, 24:722-7.
7. Young DS, "Why There Is a Laboratory," *Clin Chem*, Young, Hicks, Nipper, et al, eds, AACC, 1979, 3-22.
8. Pocock SJ, Ashby D, Shaper AG, et al, "Diurnal Variation in Serum Biochemical and Haematological Measurements," *J Clin Pathol*, 1989, 42(2):172-9.
9. Moore-Ede MC, Czeisler CA, and Richardson GS, "Circadian Timekeeping in Health and Disease, Part 1. Basic Properties of Circadian Pacemakers," *N Engl J Med*, 1983, 309:469-76.
10. Moore-Ede MC, Czeisler CA, and Richardson GS, "Circadian Timekeeping in Health and Disease, Part 2. Clinical Implications of Circadian Rhythmicity," *N Engl J Med*, 1983, 309:530-6.
11. Laessig RH, Indriksons AA, Hassemer DJ, et al, "Changes in Serum Chemical Values as a Result of Prolonged Contact With the Clot," *Am J Clin Pathol*, 1976, 66:598-604.

12. O'Bannon RH, "The Effects of Improper Specimen Handling on Lab Tests," *Med Lab Observer*, Nov 1988, 42-7.

13. Read DC, Viera H, and Arkin C, "Effect of Drawing Blood Specimens Proximal to an In-Place but Discontinued Intravenous Solution," *Am J Clin Pathol*, 1988, 90(6):702-6.

14. Block A, *Murphy's Law and Other Reasons Why Things Go Wrong!* Los Angeles, CA: Price/Stern/Sloan Publishers, Inc, 1977.

15. Gambino R, "Most Laboratory Errors Are System Dependent – Not People Dependent," *Lab Med*, 1989, 123.

16. Dietz AA, ed, *Aging – Its Chemistry*, Washington, DC: The American Association for Clinical Chemistry, 1980.

17. Rochman H, *Clinical Pathology in the Elderly*, Basel, Switzerland: Karger, 1988.

18. Siest G, Henny J, Schiele F, et al, eds, *Interpretation of Clinical Laboratory Tests*, Foster City, CA: Biomedical Publications, 1985.

19. Jaeschke R, Guyatt G, and Sackett DL, "Users' Guides to the Medical Literature. III. How to Use an Article About A Diagnostic Test. A. Are the Results of the Study Valid?" *JAMA*, 1994, 271(5):389-91.

20. Mills JL, "Data Torturing," *N Engl J Med*, 1993, 329(16):1196-9.

21. Gambino R, "The Value of Laboratory Tests to the Patient," *Lab Report*, 1995, 17(Suppl):S1-6.

22. McClove JT and Dietrich FH 2nd, "Analysis of Variance: Comparing More Than Two Means," *Statistics*, Chapter 9, San Francisco, CA: Dellen Publishing Co, 1985, 421-3.

23. Kasten BL, "Ulysses Comes Home – at Last," *CAP Today*, May 1987.

24. Goldman P, "Laboratory Lament," *New Engl J Med*, 1985, 312:865.

References

Adrogué HJ, Rashad MN, Gorin AB, et al, "Assessing Acid-Base Status in Circulatory Failure: Differences Between Arterial and Central Venous Blood," *N Engl J Med*, 1989, 320(20):1312-6.

Creer MH and Ladenson J, "Analytical Errors Due to Lipemia," *Lab Med*, 1983, 14:351-5.

Diamond I, "The Clinical Purposes of Laboratory Testing," *Arch Pathol Lab Med*, 1988, 112(4):377-8.

Fraser CG, Wilkinson SP, Neville RG, et al, "Biologic Variation of Common Hematologic Laboratory Quantities in the Elderly," *Am J Clin Pathol*, 1989, 92(4):465-70.

Friedman RB and Young DS, *Effects of Disease on Clinical Laboratory Tests*, 2nd ed, Washington, DC: AACC Press, 1989.

Gambino R, "Posture and Lab Tests," *Lab Report for Physicians*, 1981, 3:81-2.

Herr RD and Swanson T, "Pseudometabolic Acidosis Caused by Underfill of Vacutainer® Tubes," *Ann Emerg Med*, 1992, 21(2):177-80.

Hogg RV and Tanis EA, *Probability and Statistical Inference*, New York, NY: Macmillan Publishing Co Inc, 1977.

McClave JT and Dietrich FH, II, *Statistics*, 3rd ed, San Francisco, CA: Dellen Publishing Company, 1985.

Priest JB, Oei TO, and Moorehead WR, "Exercise-Induced Changes in Common Laboratory Tests," *Am J Clin Pathol*, 1982, 77:285-9.

Rosner B, *Fundamentals of Biostatistics*, Boston, MA: Dexbury Press, 1986.

Speicher CE, "All Laboratory Tests Are Not Created Equal," *Arch Pathol Lab Med*, 1985, 109(8):709-10.

Speicher CE and Smith JW, *Choosing Effective Laboratory Tests*, Philadelphia, PA: WB Saunders Co, 1983.

Valenstein PN, "Evaluating Diagnostic Tests With Imperfect Standards," *Am J Clin Pathol*, 1990, 93(2):252-8.

Watts NB, "Medical Relevance of Laboratory Tests," *Arch Pathol Lab Med*, 1988, 112(4):379-82.

Welch MJ and Hertz HS, "The How and Why of an Accuracy Base for Proficiency Testing Programs," *Arch Pathol Lab Med*, 1988, 112(4):343-5.

Yücel D and Dalva K, "Effect of *In Vitro* Hemolysis on 25 Common Biochemical Tests," *Clin Chem*, 1992, 38(4):575-7.

Zweig MH, "Evaluation of the Clinical Accuracy of Laboratory Tests," *Arch Pathol Lab Med*, 1988, 112(4):383-6.

SPECIMEN COLLECTION

Eugene S. Olsowka, MD, PhD

Harold J. Grady, PhD

Contributor: David S. Jacobs, MD

Proper specimen collection is pivotal for provision of meaningful clinical laboratory information.

Although rigorous laboratory quality assurance procedures are required to assure technically accurate results, such techniques cannot safeguard against incorrectly labeled tubes or improperly drawn specimens. If the specimen is not representative or has been compromised by improper collection or inappropriate handling, results may be misleading or potentially dangerous. As an example, a study reported that preanalytical sources of variation from behavioral, clinical, and sampling sources constituted about 60% of the total variation in a reported lipid measurement of an individual.[1] **The laboratory must have an optimum, properly labeled specimen.**

This section includes general information pertaining to the collection of laboratory specimens. Listings for common methods of blood and urine collection are outlined as general considerations. Specimen collection information specific for each individual test is provided with the detailed discussion of the test within the sections of the text. A discussion of the special requirements for collection of specimens for detection of **drugs of abuse and therapeutic drug levels** is presented in the introduction to the Therapeutic Drug Monitoring/Toxicology/Drugs of Abuse chapter *on page 527*, and a typical **chain-of-custody** form is illustrated in the Therapeutic Drug Monitoring/Toxicology/Drugs of Abuse appendix *on page 581*. The unique considerations required for the collection of specimens for **trace element** testing are discussed in the introduction of the Trace Elements chapter *on page 585*. Specifically, specimens submitted for trace elements must be submitted in heavy metal-free containers or metal-free Vacutainers®. The contaminating role of air in the procurement of blood samples for trace metals analysis has been discussed.[2] **Transfusion service** needs are addressed in the introduction of that chapter *on page 597*. Special requirements exist for **coagulation** testing, as described in that chapter.

Overview and Regulatory Considerations

Every healthcare employee, from nurse to housekeeper, has some (albeit small) risk of exposure to HIV and other viral agents such as hepatitis B and Jakob-Creutzfeldt agent. The incidence of HIV-1 transmission associated with a percutaneous exposure to blood from an HIV-1 infected patient is approximately 0.3% per exposure.[3] In 1989, it was estimated that 12,000 United States healthcare workers acquired hepatitis B annually.[4] An understanding of the appropriate procedures, responsibilities, and risks inherent in the collection and handling of patient specimens is necessary and is required by Occupational Safety and Health Administration (OSHA) regulations.

The Occupational Safety and Health Administration published its "Final Rule on Occupational Exposure to Bloodborne Pathogens" in the Federal Register on December 6, 1991. OSHA has chosen to follow the Centers for Disease Control (CDC) definition of universal precautions. The Final Rule provides full legal force to universal precautions and requires employers and employees to treat blood and certain body fluids as if they were infectious. The Final Rule mandates that healthcare workers must avoid parenteral contact and must avoid splattering blood or other potentially infectious material on their skin, hair, eyes, mouth, mucous membranes, or on their personal clothing. Hazard abatement strategies must be used to protect workers. Such plans typically include, but are not limited to, the following:

- safe handling of sharp items ("sharps") and disposal of such into puncture resistant containers
- gloves required for employees handling items soiled with blood or equipment contaminated by blood or other body fluids
- provisions of protective clothing when more extensive contact with blood or body fluids may be anticipated (eg, surgery, autopsy, or deliveries)
- resuscitation equipment to reduce necessity for mouth to mouth resuscitation
- restriction of HIV-1 or hepatitis B-exposed employees to noninvasive procedures

OSHA has specifically defined the following terms: **Occupational exposure** means reasonably anticipated skin, eye mucous membrane, or parenteral contact with blood or other potentially infectious materials that may result from the performance of an employee's duties. **Other potentially infectious materials** are human body fluids including semen, vaginal secretions, cerebrospinal fluid, synovial fluid, pleural fluid, pericardial fluid, peritoneal fluid, amniotic fluid, saliva in dental procedures, and body fluids that are visibly contaminated with blood, and all body fluids in situations where it is difficult or impossible to differentiate between body fluids; any unfixed tissue or organ (other than intact skin) from a human (living or dead); and HIV-containing cell or tissue cultures, organ cultures, and HIV- or HBV-containing culture medium or other solutions, and blood, organs, or other tissues from experimental animals infected with HIV or HBV. An **exposure incident** involves specific eye, mouth, other mucous membrane, nonintact skin, or parenteral contact with blood or other potentially infectious materials that results from the performance of an employee's duties.[5] It is important to understand that some exposures may go unrecognized despite the strictest precautions. Two simple techniques that decrease the risk of infection while obtaining blood for hematocrit and bilirubin measurements in neonates have been proposed.[6]

A written Exposure Control Plan is required. Employers must provide copies of the plan to employees and to OSHA upon request. Compliance with OSHA rules may be accomplished by the following methods.

- **Universal precautions (UPs)** means that all human blood and certain body fluids are treated as if known to be infectious for HIV, HBV, and other bloodborne pathogens. UPs do not apply to feces, nasal secretions, sputum, sweat, tears, urine, or vomitus unless they contain visible blood.
- **Engineering controls (ECs)** are physical devices which reduce or remove hazards from the workplace by eliminating or minimizing hazards or by isolating the worker from exposure. Engineering control devices include sharps disposal containers, self-resheathing syringes, etc.

- **Work practice controls (WPCs)** are practices and procedures that reduce the likelihood of exposure to hazards by altering the way in which a task is performed. Specific examples are the prohibition of two-handed recapping of needles, prohibition of storing food alongside potentially contaminated material, discouragement of pipetting fluids by mouth, encouraging handwashing after removal of gloves, safe handling of contaminated sharps, and appropriate use of sharps containers.
- **Personal protective equipment (PPE)** is specialized clothing or equipment worn to provide protection from occupational exposure. PPE includes gloves, gowns, laboratory coats (the type and characteristics will depend upon the task and degree of exposure anticipated), face shields or masks, and eye protection. Surgical caps or hoods and/or shoe covers or boots are required in instances in which gross contamination can reasonably be anticipated (eg, autopsies, orthopedic surgery). If PPE is penetrated by blood or any contaminated material, the item must be removed immediately or as soon as feasible. **The employer must provide and launder or dispose of all PPE at no cost to the employee.** Gloves must be worn when there is a reasonable anticipation of hand contact with potentially infectious material, including a patient's mucous membranes or nonintact skin. Disposable gloves must be changed as soon as possible after they become torn or punctured. Hands must be washed after gloves are removed.

Housekeeping protocols: OSHA requires that all bins, cans, and similar receptacles, intended for reuse which have a reasonable likelihood for becoming contaminated, be inspected and decontaminated immediately or as soon as feasible upon visible contamination and on a regularly scheduled basis. Broken glass that may be contaminated must not be picked up directly with the hands. Mechanical means (eg, brush, dust pan, tongs, or forceps) must be used. Broken glass must be placed in a proper sharps container.

Employers are responsible for teaching appropriate clean-up procedures for the work area and personal protective equipment. A 1:10 dilution of household bleach is a popular and effective disinfectant. It is necessary for employers to maintain signatures or initials of employees who have been properly educated. If one does not have written proof of education of universal precautions teaching, then by OSHA standards, such education never happened.

Pre-exposure and postexposure protocols: OSHA's Final Rule includes the provision that employees, who are exposed to contamination, be offered the hepatitis B vaccine at no cost to the employee. Employees may decline; however, a declination form must be signed. The employee must be offered free vaccine if he/she changes his/her mind. Vaccination to prevent the transmission of hepatitis B in the healthcare setting is widely regarded as sound practice.[7] In the event of exposure, a confidential medical evaluation and follow-up must be offered at no cost to the employee. Follow-up must include collection and testing of blood from the source individual for HBV and HIV if permitted by state law if a blood sample is available. If a postexposure specimen must be specially drawn, the individual's consent is usually required. Some states may not require consent for testing of patient blood after accidental exposure. One must refer to state and/or local regulations for proper guidance.

The employee follow-up must also include appropriate postexposure prophylaxis, counseling, and evaluation of reported illnesses. The employee has the right to decline baseline blood collection and/or testing. If the employee gives consent for the collection but not the testing, the sample must be preserved for 90 days in the event that the employee changes his/her mind within that time. Confidentiality related to blood testing must be ensured. **The employer does not have the right to know the results** of the testing of either the source individual or the exposed employee.[5]

Communication of Hazards

Communication regarding the dangers of bloodborne infections through the use of labels, signs, information, and education is required. Storage locations (eg, refrigerators and freezers, waste containers) that are used to store, dispose of, transport, or ship blood or other potentially infectious materials require labels. The label background must be red or bright orange with the biohazard design and the word biohazard in a contrasting color. The label must be part of the container or affixed to the container by permanent means.

Education provided by a qualified and knowledgeable instructor is mandated. The sessions for employees must include:[5]

- accessible copies of the regulation
- general epidemiology of bloodborne diseases
- modes of bloodborne pathogen transmission
- an explanation of the exposure control plan and a means to obtain copies of the written plan
- an explanation of the tasks and activities that may involve exposure
- the use of exposure prevention methods and their limitations (eg, engineering controls, work practices, personal protective equipment)
- information on the types, proper use, location, removal, handling, decontamination, and disposal of personal protective equipment)
- an explanation of the basis for selection of personal protective equipment
- information on the HBV vaccine, including information on its efficacy, safety, and method of administration and the benefits of being vaccinated (ie, the employee must understand that the vaccine and vaccination will be offered free of charge)
- information on the appropriate actions to take and persons to contact in an emergency involving exposure to blood or other potentially infectious materials
- an explanation of the procedure to follow if an exposure incident occurs, including the method of reporting the incident
- information on the postexposure evaluation and follow-up that the employer is required to provide for the employee following an exposure incident
- an explanation of the signs, labels, and color coding
- an interactive question-and-answer period

Record Keeping

The OSHA Final Rule requires that the employer maintain both education and medical records. Medical records must be kept confidential and be maintained for the duration of employment plus 30 years. They must contain a copy of the employee's HBV vaccination status and postexposure incident information. Education records must be maintained for 3 years from the date the program was given.

OSHA has the authority to conduct inspections without notice. Penalties for cited violation may be assessed as follows.[5]

Serious violations. In this situation, there is a substantial probability of death or serious physical harm, and the employer knew, or should have known, of the hazard. A violation of this type carries a mandatory penalty of up to $7000 for each violation.

Other-than-serious violations. The violation is unlikely to result in death or serious physical harm. This type of violation carries a discretionary penalty of up to $7000 for each violation.

Willful violations. These are violations committed knowingly or intentionally by the employer and have penalties of up to $70,000 per violation with a minimum of $5000 per violation. If an employee dies as a result of a willful violation, the responsible party, if convicted, may receive a personal fine of up to $250,000 and/or a 6-month jail term. A corporation may be fined $500,000.

Large fines frequently follow visits to laboratories, physicians' offices, and healthcare facilities by OSHA Compliance Safety and Health Offices (CSHOs). Regulations are vigorously enforced. A working knowledge of the final rule and implementation of appropriate policies and practices is imperative for all those involved in the collection and analysis of medical specimens.

Effectiveness of universal precautions in averting exposure to potentially infectious materials has been documented.[8] Compliance with appropriate rules, procedures, and policies, including reporting exposure incidents, is a matter of personal professionalism and prudent self-preservation.

Footnotes

1. Cooper GR, Myers GL, Smith SJ, et al, "Blood Lipid Measurements. Variations and Practical Utility," *JAMA*, 1992, 268:985-6.
2. Chappuis P, Pineau A, Guillard O, et al, "Practical Advice Concerning Biological Fluids for Analysis of Trace-Elements," *Ann Biol Clin*, 1994, 52(2):103-9.
3. Henderson DK, Fahey BJ, Willy M, et al, "Risk for Occupational Transmission of Human Immunodeficiency Virus Type 1 (HIV-1) Associated With Clinical Exposures. A Prospective Evaluation," *Ann Intern Med*, 1990, 113(10):740-6.
4. Niu MT and Margolis HS, "Moving Into a New Era of Government Regulation: Provisions for Hepatitis B Vaccine in the Workplace, *Clin Lab Manage Rev*, 1989, 3:336-40.
5. Bruning LM, "The Bloodborne Pathogens Final Rule – Understanding the Regulation," *AORN Journal*, 1993, 57(2):439-40.
6. Leistikow EA, Mack WN, de Sierra TM, et al, "Reducing Risk of Infection When Obtaining Hematocrit and Bilirubin Determinations: Beyond Universal Precautions," *J Perinatol*, 1995, 15(1):7-9.
7. Schaffner W, Gardner P, and Gross PA, "Hepatitis B Immunization Strategies: Expanding the Target," *Ann Intern Med*, 1993, 118(4):308-9.
8. Wong ES, Stotka JL, Chinchilli VM, et al, "Are Universal Precautions Effective in Reducing the Number of Occupational Exposures Among Healthcare Workers?" *JAMA*, 1991, 265:1123-8.

References

Buehler JW and Ward JW, "A New Definition for AIDS Surveillance," *Ann Intern Med*, 1993, 118(5):390-2.

Brown JW and Blackwell H, "Complying With the New OSHA Regs, Part 1: Teaching Your Staff About Biosafety," *MLO*, 1992, 24(4):24-8. Part 2: "Safety Protocols No Lab Can Ignore," 1992, 24(5):27-9. Part 3: "Compiling Employee Safety Records That Will Satisfy OSHA," 1992, 24(6):45-8.

Department of Labor, Occupational Safety and Health Administration, "Occupational Exposure to Bloodborne Pathogens; Final Rule (29 CFR Part 1910.1030),"*Federal Register*, December 6, 1991, 64004-182.

Gold JW, "HIV-1 Infection: Diagnosis and Management," *Med Clin North Am*, 1992, 76(1):1-18.

"Hepatitis B Virus: A Comprehensive Strategy for Eliminating Transmission in the United States Through Universal Childhood Vaccination," *MMWR Morb Mortal Wkly Rep*, 1991, 40(RR-13):1-25.

"Mortality Attributable to HIV Infection/AIDS – United States," *MMWR Morb Mortal Wkly Rep*, 1991, 40(3):41-4.

National Committee for Clinical Laboratory Standards, "Protection of Laboratory Workers From Infectious Disease Transmitted by Blood, Body Fluids, and Tissue," NCCLS Document M29-T, Villanova, PA: NCCLS, 1989, 9(1).

"Nosocomial Transmission of Hepatitis B Virus Associated With a Spring-Loaded Fingerstick Device – California", *MMWR Morb Mortal Wkly Rep*, 1990, 39(35):610-3.

Polish LB, Shapiro CN, Bauer F, et al, "Nosocomial Transmission of Hepatitis B Virus Associated With the Use of a Spring-Loaded Fingerstick Device," *N Engl J Med*, 1992, 326(11):721-5.

"Recommendations for Preventing Transmission of Human Immunodeficiency Virus and Hepatitis B Virus to Patients During Exposure-Prone Invasive Procedures," *MMWR Morb Mortal Wkly Rep*, 1991, 40(RR-8):1-9.

"Update: Acquired Immunodeficiency Syndrome – United States," *MMWR Morb Mortal Wkly Rep*, 1992, 41(26):463-8.

"Update: Transmission of HIV Infection During an Invasive Dental Procedure – Florida, " *MMWR Morb Mortal Wkly Rep*, 1991, 40(2):21-7, 33.

"Update: Universal Precautions for Prevention of Transmission of Human Immunodeficiency Virus, Hepatitis B Virus, and Other Bloodborne Pathogens in Healthcare Settings," *MMWR Morb Mortal Wkly Rep*, 1988, 37(24):377-82, 387-8.

Acquired Immunodeficiency Syndrome Precautions, Specimen Collection *see* Blood and Fluid Precautions, Specimen Collection *on this page*

AIDS Precautions, Specimen Collection *see* Blood and Fluid Precautions, Specimen Collection *on this page*

Allen Test *see* Arterial Blood Collection *on this page*

Alternate Site Testing (AST) *see* Point-of-Care Testing *on page 27*

Ancillary Testing *see* Point-of-Care Testing *on page 27*

Arterial Blood Collection

CPT 36600

Related Information
Blood and Fluid Precautions, Specimen Collection *on this page*
Specimen Identification Requirements *on page 29*

Synonyms Arterial Puncture

Applies to Allen Test

Test Commonly Includes Brachial, radial, or femoral artery puncture by trained personnel to obtain arterial blood most frequently for blood gas analysis

Patient Preparation The patient should be resting for 20-30 minutes before collection of the specimen.

Aftercare Direct pressure must be applied to the arterial puncture site and should be maintained for a minimum of 10 minutes. Patients with bleeding tendency due to anticoagulation, platelet deficiency, factor deficiency, or liver disease may bleed excessively and form a hematoma. Such patients should be monitored carefully after the procedure to be sure bleeding has been controlled. Arterial spasm preventing aspiration of the specimen and thrombosis of the punctured artery can occur.

Specimen Arterial blood

Container Heparinized syringe with 21- or 23-gauge needle. Alternatively, a 21- or 23-gauge Butterfly® infusion set may be used.

Collection The experienced arterial puncturist should carefully select an appropriate artery. If the radial artery is used, **Allen's test** to assure collateral circulation to the hand from the ulnar artery is performed: the hand is closed tightly by the patient or by an assistant to form a fist. Pressure is then applied at the wrist, compressing and obstructing both the radial and ulnar arteries. The hand is then opened (but not fully extended), revealing a blanched palm and fingers. The obstructing pressure is next removed from only the ulnar artery while the palm and fingers, including thumb, are observed; they should become flushed within 15 seconds as the blood from the ulnar artery refills the empty capillary bed. If the ulnar artery does not adequately supply the entire hand (a negative Allen test), the radial artery should not be used as a puncture site; an alternate artery should be selected.[1] Recent studies have confirmed the efficacy and usefulness of this test.[2,3]

Careful preparation of the puncture site is performed with 70% alcohol (isopropanol) using a circular motion working out from the site. Dry with gauze or let air dry. The artery is stabilized by holding with a finger. Take care not to contaminate the puncture site. The artery is punctured at a 30° angle for the radial artery, 45° angle for the brachial, 45° or 90° angle for the femoral. The bevel of the needle or Butterfly® should be pointed toward the direction of blood flow. The syringe should fill spontaneously. Small bore needles or plastic syringes may require gentle slow suction. Be sure no air bubbles are aspirated into the syringe. After adequate sample volume is obtained quickly remove the needle and apply pressure. See Aftercare. Place specimen on ice after sealing the needle into a piece of hard rubber or plastic. Deliver to the laboratory within 15 minutes of collection.

Storage Instructions Keep the specimen air tight and water tight in a container of ice. This slows the metabolic rate of white cells in the specimen and reduces oxygen consumption. The specimen must be analyzed rapidly. Results are often needed urgently.

Causes for Rejection Clots in the specimen

Use Obtain arterial blood for analysis. **See listing Blood Gases, Arterial on page 87.**

Limitations Arterial puncture should be performed by persons familiar with the procedure and the potential complications. For example, forearm compartment syndrome occurs after percutaneous arterial blood sampling and is usually associated with anticoagulation therapy. This syndrome has occurred once in a young woman with Goodpasture's syndrome.[4] Liquid sodium heparin should be used sparingly only to fill the needle and dead space. Excess heparin in the sample will lower the pH and pCO_2. pO_2 may be variably affected, and acid base calculations will be erroneous. Air bubbles in the syringe can greatly alter pO_2.

Additional Information The evaluation of alveolar pO_2 is routinely done by assuming that the respiratory gas exchange ratio is equal to 0.8. A study of the respiratory gas exchange ratio in patients undergoing arterial puncture revealed that in approximately 25% of cases, there is a transient change in alveolar ventilation associated with arterial puncture that may cause a change in the gas exchange ratio and lead to at least a 10 mm Hg error in estimating alveolar pO_2.[5] Evidently, some patients respond to arterial puncture by transient breath holding or by taking rapid shallow breaths. Arterialized capillary blood is addressed in the listing Skin Puncture Blood Collection *on page 28*.

Footnotes
1. National Committee for Clinical Laboratory Standards, "Percutaneous Collection of Arterial Blood for Laboratory Analysis," Approved Standard, ANSI/NCCLS H11-A-2985, Villanova, PA: National Committee for Clinical Laboratory Standards, 1985.
2. Fuhrman TM, Reilley TE, and Pippin WD, "Comparison of Digital Blood Pressure, Plethysmography, and the Modified Allen's Test as Means of Evaluating the Collateral Circulation to the Hand," *Anaesthesia*, 1992, 47(11):959-61.
3. Choudhury RP and Cleator SJ, "An Examination of Needlestick Injury Rates, Hepatitis B Vaccination Uptake and Instruction on "Sharps" Technique Among Medical Students," *J Hosp Infect*, 1992, 22(2):143-8.
4. Safran MR, Bernstein A, and Lesavoy MA, "Forearm Compartment Syndrome Following Brachial Arterial Puncture in Uremia," *Ann Plast Surg*, 1994, 32(5):535-8.
5. Cinel D, Markwell K, Lee R, et al, "Variability of the Respiratory Gas Exchange Ratio During Arterial Puncture," *Am Rev Respir Dis*, 1991, 143(2):217-8.

Arterialized Capillary Blood *see* Skin Puncture Blood Collection *on page 28*

Arterial Puncture *see* Arterial Blood Collection *on this page*

Bacteriology Specimen Identification *see* Specimen Identification Requirements *on page 29*

Bedside Testing *see* Point-of-Care Testing *on page 27*

Blood and Fluid Precautions, Specimen Collection

Related Information
Arterial Blood Collection *on this page*
Hepatitis B Surface Antigen *on page 399*
Phlebotomist Procedures *on page 27*
Skin Puncture Blood Collection *on page 28*
Venous Blood Collection *on page 30*

Synonyms Acquired Immunodeficiency Syndrome Precautions, Specimen Collection; AIDS Precautions, Specimen Collection; HIV Precautions, Specimen Collection; Isolation Patients, Precautions for Specimen Collection

Patient Preparation The **Occupational Safety and Health Administration (OSHA)** Final Rule requires that the risk to healthcare workers of accidental exposure to infection be minimized. By careful planning and thoughtful attention to detail an appropriate and representative specimen can be safely collected. See Overview and Regulatory Considerations, discussed in the Specimen Collection Introduction *on page 21*.

Before entering the isolation room or drawing area:

Put on gloves.

Read the isolation sign on the door or patient's chart. It will explain the type of isolation and what you must wear and do. **Follow these directions carefully.**

Check your orders and assemble the equipment needed for this patient. Remember that anything taken into the room must be left there, discarded, or carefully cleansed if taken out of the room.

Find out if it is necessary to take a tourniquet and/or a plastic holder into the room. Many times these items will be there already.

Take in the minimum equipment needed: tourniquet; plastic holder; evacuated tube needle; alcohol sponges; evacuated blood collection tubes or blood culture media; glass slides (if a blood smear is to be made).

In the room:
- Put on gloves.
- Place paper towels on table and place your equipment on these towels.
- Obtain blood samples in the usual manner, avoiding any unnecessary contact with the patient and the bed.
- After obtaining blood samples, leave tourniquet and plastic holder in room and discard needle in proper container.
- Wash hands.
- Place several clean paper towels on the table, one on top of the other. If the outside of the tubes is contaminated, follow established laboratory decontamination procedures.
- If blood smears were made, place smears on two clean paper towels. When ready to leave, wrap smears and tubes in the top paper towel and discard the bottom paper towel.
- Label specimens for proper identification (see listing Specimen Identification Requirements *on page 29*) as directed by institutional policy. Label specimens for infectious hazards in a distinctive manner as required by institutional policy. Since the implementation of

universal blood and body fluid precautions for **all** patients, special labeling for specific patients may be eliminated, depending upon institutional policies and local regulations. In any case, **universal precautions must be observed.**

• Bring specimens to the laboratory.[1]

Special Instructions

Precautions for laboratories: Blood and other body fluids from **all** patients should be considered infective. To supplement the universal blood and body fluid precautions, the following precautions are recommended for healthcare workers in clinical laboratories.

All specimens of blood and body fluids should be put in a well-constructed container with a secure lid to prevent leaking during transport. Care should be taken when collecting each specimen to avoid contamination of the outside of the container and of the laboratory form accompanying the specimen.

All persons collecting and processing blood and body fluid specimens should wear gloves. Masks, protective eyewear, and laboratory coats or gowns should be worn if contact with blood or body fluids is anticipated. Gloves should be changed and hands washed after completion of specimen processing.

For routine procedures, such as histologic and pathologic studies or microbiologic culturing, a biological safety cabinet is not necessary. However, biological safety cabinets (class I or II) should be used whenever procedures are conducted that have a high potential for generating droplets. These include activities such as blending, sonicating, and vigorous mixing. Mechanical pipetting devices must be used for manipulating all liquids in the laboratory. **Mouth pipetting must not be done.**

Use of needles and syringes should be limited to situations in which there is no alternative, and the recommendations for preventing injuries with needles outlined under universal precautions must be followed.

Laboratory work surfaces should be decontaminated with an appropriate chemical germicide after a spill of blood or other body fluids and when work activities are completed.

Contaminated materials used in laboratory tests should be decontaminated before reprocessing or be placed in bags and disposed of in accordance with institutional policies for disposal of infective waste.

Scientific equipment that has been contaminated with blood or other body fluids should be decontaminated and cleaned before being repaired in the laboratory or transported to the manufacturer.

All persons must wash their hands after completing laboratory activities and should remove personal protective equipment before leaving the laboratory.

Implementation of universal blood and body fluid precautions for **all** patients eliminates the need for warning labels on specimens since blood and other body fluids from all patients should be considered infective. OSHA rules require "Biohazard" labeling or color coding of containers of regulated waste, refrigerators and freezers containing blood or other potentially infectious material, and containers used to store, transport, or ship such materials.

Additional Information Human immunodeficiency virus (HIV), the virus that causes acquired immunodeficiency syndrome (AIDS), is transmitted through sexual contact, exposure to infected blood or blood components, and perinatally from mother to neonate. HIV has been isolated from blood, semen, vaginal secretions, saliva, tears, breast milk, cerebrospinal fluid, amniotic fluid, and urine and is likely to be isolated from other body fluids, secretions, and excretions. However, epidemiologic evidence has implicated only blood, semen, vaginal secretions, and possibly breast milk in transmission.

The increasing prevalence of HIV infection increases the risk that healthcare workers will be exposed to blood from patients infected with HIV, especially when blood and body fluid precautions are not followed for all patients. Thus, the Centers for Disease Control (CDC) in its recommendations for prevention of HIV transmission in healthcare settings[2] emphasizes the need for healthcare workers to consider **all** patients as potentially infected with HIV and/or other blood-borne pathogens and to adhere rigorously to infection control precautions for minimizing the risk of exposure to blood and body fluids of all patients.

The CDC universal precaution recommendations and the OSHA Final Rule regulations[2,3] have been developed for use in healthcare settings and emphasize the need to treat blood and other body fluids from **all** patients as potentially infective. These same prudent precautions also should be taken in other settings in which persons may be exposed to blood or other body fluids.

Precautions to Prevent Transmission of HIV - Universal Precautions: Since medical history and examination cannot reliably identify all patients infected with HIV or other blood-borne pathogens, blood and body fluid precautions should be consistently used for **all** patients. This approach, recommended by CDC and referred to as "universal blood

and body fluid precautions" or "universal precautions," must be used in the care of **all** patients as a result of OSHA's Final Rule.[3]

All healthcare workers must routinely use appropriate barrier precautions to prevent skin and mucous membrane exposure when contact with blood or other body fluids of any patient is anticipated. Gloves should be worn for touching blood and body fluids, mucous membranes, or nonintact skin of all patients, for handling items on surfaces soiled with blood or body fluids, and for performing venipuncture and other vascular access procedures. Gloves should be changed after contact with each patient. Masks and protective eyewear or face shields should be worn during procedures that are likely to generate droplets of blood or other body fluids to prevent exposure of mucous membranes of the mouth, nose, and eyes. Laboratory coats, gowns, or aprons should be worn during procedures that are likely to generate splashes of blood or other body fluids.

Hands and other skin surfaces should be washed immediately and thoroughly if contaminated with blood or other body fluids. Hands should be washed immediately after gloves are removed.

All healthcare workers must take precautions to prevent injuries caused by needles, scalpels, and other sharp instruments or devices during procedures; when cleaning used instruments; during disposal of used needles; and when handling sharp instruments after procedures. To prevent needlestick injuries, needles must not be recapped, purposely bent or broken by hand, removed from disposable syringes, or otherwise manipulated by hand. After they are used, disposable syringes and needles, scalpel blades, and other sharp items must be placed in puncture-resistant containers for disposal; the puncture-resistant containers should be located as close as possible to the area of use. Large-bore reusable needles should be placed in a puncture-resistant container for transport to the reprocessing area.

Two simple procedures are described to decrease the risk of exposure while obtaining specimens for hematocrit and bilirubin measurement.[4]

Although saliva has not been implicated in HIV transmission, to minimize the need for emergency mouth-to-mouth resuscitation, mouthpieces, resuscitation bags, or other ventilation devices should be available for use in areas in which the need for resuscitation is predictable.

Healthcare workers who have exudative lesions or weeping dermatitis should refrain from all direct patient care and from handling patient care equipment until the condition resolves.

Pregnant healthcare workers are not known to be at greater risk of contracting HIV infection than healthcare workers who are not pregnant; however, if a healthcare worker develops HIV infection during pregnancy, the infant is at risk of infection resulting from perinatal transmission. Because of this risk, **pregnant healthcare workers should be especially familiar with and strictly adhere to precautions to minimize the risk of HIV transmission.**

Implementation of universal blood and body fluid precautions for **all** patients eliminates the need for use of the isolation category of "Blood and Body Fluid Precautions" previously recommended by CDC for patients known or suspected to be infected with blood-borne pathogens. Isolation precautions (eg, enteric, AFB) should be used as necessary if associated conditions, such as infectious diarrhea or tuberculosis, are diagnosed or suspected.

Environmental Considerations for HIV Transmission: No environmentally mediated mode of HIV transmission has been documented. Nevertheless, the precautions described should be taken routinely in the care of **all** patients.

Sterilization and Disinfection: Standard sterilization and disinfection procedures for patient care equipment currently recommended for use in a variety of healthcare settings, including hospitals, medical and dental clinics and offices, hemodialysis centers, emergency care facilities, and long-term nursing care facilities, are adequate to sterilize or disinfect instruments, devices, or other items contaminated with blood or other body fluids from persons infected with blood-borne pathogens including HIV.

Cleaning and Decontaminating Spills of Blood or Other Body Fluids: Chemical germicides that are approved for use as "hospital disinfectants" and are tuberculocidal when used at recommended dilutions can be used to decontaminate spills of blood and other body fluids. Strategies for decontaminating spills of blood and other body fluids in a patient care setting are different than for spills of cultures or other materials in clinical, public health, or research laboratories. In patient care areas, visible material should first be removed and then the area should be decontaminated. With large spills of cultured or concentrated infectious agents in the laboratory, the contaminated area should be flooded with a liquid germicide before cleaning, then decontaminated with fresh germicidal chemical. In both settings, gloves should be worn during the cleaning and decontaminating procedures.

Studies have shown that HIV is inactivated rapidly after being exposed to commonly used chemical germicides at concentrations that are much
(Continued)

Blood and Fluid Precautions, Specimen Collection (Continued)

lower than used in practice. Embalming fluids (formalin preparations) are similar to the types of chemical germicides that have been tested and found to completely inactivate HIV. Formalin may not rapidly inactivate hepatitis B virus nor quickly kill bacteria. It is a slow-acting antiseptic agent requiring 18 hours or more to kill microorganisms. In addition to commercially available chemical germicides, a solution of sodium hypochlorite (household bleach) prepared daily is an inexpensive and effective germicide. Concentrations ranging from approximately 500 ppm (1:100 dilution of household bleach) sodium hypochlorite to 5000 ppm (1:10 dilution of household bleach) are effective depending on the amount of organic material (eg, blood, mucus) present on the surface to be cleaned and disinfected. Disinfecting surfaces in cases of known Jakob-Creutzfeld agent may require full strength bleach. Commercially available chemical germicides may be more compatible with certain medical devices that might be corroded by repeated exposure to sodium hypochlorite.

Housekeeping: Environmental surfaces such as walls, floors, and other surfaces are not associated with transmission of infections to patients or healthcare workers. Therefore, extraordinary attempts to disinfect or sterilize these environmental surfaces are not necessary. However, cleaning and removal of soil should be done routinely.

Cleaning schedules and methods vary according to the area of the hospital or institution, type of surface to be cleaned, and the amount and type of soil present. Horizontal surfaces (eg, bedside tables and hard-surfaced flooring) in patient care areas are usually cleaned on a regular basis, when soiling or spills occur, and when a patient is discharged. Cleaning of walls, blinds, and curtains is recommended only if visibly soiled. Disinfectant fogging is an unsatisfactory method of decontaminating air and surfaces and is not recommended.

Disinfectant detergent formulations registered by EPA may be used for cleaning environmental surfaces, but the actual physical removal of microorganisms by scrubbing is probably as important as any antimicrobial effect of the cleaning agent. Therefore, cost, safety, and acceptability by housekeepers can be the main criteria for selecting any such registered agent. The manufacturers' instructions for appropriate use should be followed.

Laundry: Although soiled linen has been identified as a source of large numbers of certain pathogenic microorganisms, the risk of actual disease transmission is negligible. Rather than rigid procedures and specifications, hygienic and common sense storage and processing of clean and soiled linen are recommended. Soiled linen should be handled as little as possible with minimum agitation to prevent gross microbial contamination of the air and persons handling the linen. All soiled linen should be bagged at the location where it was used; it should not be sorted or rinsed in patient care areas. Linen soiled with blood or body fluids must be placed and transported in bags that prevent leakage.

Infective Waste: There is no epidemiologic evidence to suggest that most hospital waste is any more infective than residential waste. Moreover, there is no epidemiologic evidence that hospital waste has caused disease in the community as a result of improper disposal. Therefore, identifying wastes for which special precautions are indicated is largely a matter of judgment about the relative risk of disease transmission. The most practical approach to the management of infective waste is to identify those wastes with the potential for causing infection during handling and disposal and for which some special precautions appear prudent. Hospital wastes for which special precautions are required include microbiology laboratory waste, pathology waste, blood specimens or blood products, and other potentially infectious material. Any item that has had contact with blood, exudates, or secretions may be potentially infective. Infective waste, in general, should either be incinerated or should be autoclaved before disposal in a sanitary landfill. Bulk blood, suctioned fluids, excretions, and secretions may be carefully poured down a drain connected to a sanitary sewer. Sanitary sewers may also be used to dispose of other infectious wastes capable of being ground and flushed into the sewer.

Survival of HIV in the Environment: The most extensive study on the survival of HIV after drying involved greatly concentrated HIV samples (ie, 10 million tissue culture infectious doses/mL). This concentration is at least 100,000 times greater than that typically found in the blood or serum of patients with HIV infection. HIV was detectable by tissue culture techniques 1-3 days after drying, but the rate of inactivation was rapid. Studies performed at CDC have also shown that drying HIV causes a rapid (within several hours) 1-2 log (90% to 99%) reduction in HIV concentration. In tissue culture fluid, cell-free HIV could be detected up to 15 days at room temperature, up to 11 days at 37°C (98.6°F), and up to 1 day if the HIV was cell-associated.

When considered in the context of environmental conditions in healthcare facilities, these results do not require any changes in currently recommended sterilization, disinfection, or housekeeping strategies. When medical devices are contaminated with blood or other body fluids, existing recommendations include the cleaning of these instruments followed by disinfection or sterilization, depending on the type of medical device. These protocols assume "worst case" conditions of extreme virologic and microbiologic contamination and whether or not viruses have been inactivated after drying plays no role in formulating these strategies. Consequently, no changes in the published procedures for cleaning, disinfecting, or sterilizing need to be made.

Risk to Healthcare Workers of Acquiring HIV in Healthcare Settings: Healthcare workers with documented percutaneous or mucous membrane exposures to blood or body fluids of HIV-infected patients have been prospectively evaluated to determine the risk of infection after such exposures. The risk of HIV-1 transmission associated with a percutaneous exposure to blood from an HIV-1 infected patient is approximately 0.3% per exposure (95 CI, 0.13% to 0.70%). The risks associated with occupational mucous membrane and cutaneous exposures are likely to be substantially smaller. Universal precautions are widely considered effective in reducing the risk of occupational exposures among healthcare workers,[5] and in a prospective study, physicians on a medical service.[6]

Footnotes

1. Bennett BD, Cox RS, Davis CM, et al, eds, *So You're Going to Collect a Blood Specimen: An Introduction to Phlebotomy*, 5th ed, Northfield, IL: College of American Pathologists, 1992.
2. "Leads From the *MMWR*. Update: Universal Precautions for Prevention of Transmission of Human Immunodeficiency Virus, Hepatitis B Virus, and Other Bloodborne Pathogens in Healthcare Settings," *JAMA*, 1988, 260(4):462-5.
3. Department of Labor, Occupational Safety and Health Administration, "Occupational Exposure to Bloodborne Pathogens; Final Rule (29 CFR Part 1910.1030)," *Federal Register*, 1991, 64004-182.
4. Leistikow EA, Mach WN, de Sierra, et al, "Reducing Risk of Infection When Obtaining Hematocrit and Bilirubin Determinations: Beyond Universal Precautions," *J Perinatol*, 1995, 15(1):7-9.
5. Henderson DK, Fahey BJ, Willy M, et al, "Risk for Occupational Transmission of Human Immunodeficiency Virus Type 1 (HIV-1) Associated With Clinical Exposures - A Prospective Evaluation," *Ann Intern Med*, 1990, 113(10):740-6.
6. Wong ES, Stotka JL, Chinchilli VM, et al, "Are Universal Precautions Effective in Reducing the Number of Occupational Exposures Among Healthcare Workers? A Prospective Study of Physicians on a Medical Service," *JAMA*, 1991, 265(9):1123-8.

References

"Agent Summary Statement for Human Immunodeficiency Viruses (HIVs) Including HTLV-III, LAV, HIV-1, and HIV-2," *MMWR Morb Mortal Wkly Rep*, 1988, 37(Suppl 4):1-17.

Blood Collection Tube Information

Related Information

Chain-of-Custody Protocol *on page 542*
Phlebotomist Procedures *on next page*
Venous Blood Collection *on page 30*

Synonyms Blood Container Description; Vacutainer® Tube Description

Special Instructions See individual listings throughout this book for particular test requirements.

Tube Codes

Color	Optimum Volume/ Minimum Volume	Additive
Blue	4.5 mL/4.5 mL	Sodium citrate
Blue/navy	7 mL	No additive (for trace metals) Heparin (for trace metals)
Culture (yellow)	8.3 mL/8.3 mL	SPS
FSP (blue)	2 mL/2 mL	Thrombin, trypsin inhibitor
Gray	5 mL/5 mL 7 mL/7 mL	Potassium oxalate, sodium fluoride
Green	10 mL/3.5 mL	Heparin
Lavender	7 mL/2 mL	EDTA
Orange	10 mL/NA	Thrombin
Red	10 mL/NA	None
Red/gray (gel)	10 mL/NA	Inert barrier material; clot activator
Yellow	5 mL/NA	ACD
Yellow/black	7 mL	Thrombin
Pediatric Tubes		
Blue	2.7 mL/2.7 mL	Sodium citrate
Culture (yellow)	3.3 mL/3.3 mL	SPS
Green	2 mL/2 mL	Heparin
Lavender	2 mL/0.6 mL 3 mL/0.9 mL 4 mL/1 mL	EDTA
Red	2 mL/NA 3 mL/NA 4 mL/NA	None

Additional Information The table describes standard color codes, optimum and minimum volumes required, and additives contained in common vacuum draw tubes. **It is important to be certain that a tube is filled with the prescribed minimum volume in order to avoid spurious results due to an inappropriate anticoagulant to specimen ratio.**

Special needs exist for specimens for coagulation testing. See the Coagulation Introduction *on page 225*.

See Transfusion Service Introduction *on page 597* for specimen requirements.

The Trace Metals Introduction *on page 585* provides information for specimens drawn for those substances.

See the Therapeutic Drug Monitoring/Toxicology/Drugs of Abuse Introduction *on page 527* for appropriate specimen requirements. It addresses anticonvulsants (antiepileptic drugs), antibiotic and cardiac drug levels, peaks and troughs, as well as collections for drugs of abuse. Chain-of-Custody Protocol information *on page 542* is provided as a listing and is in the Therapeutic Drug Monitoring/Toxicology/Drugs of Abuse Appendix *on page 581*.

Blood Collection, Venous *see* Venous Blood Collection *on page 30*

Blood Container Description *see* Blood Collection Tube Information *on previous page*

Blood Specimen Identification *see* Specimen Identification Requirements *on page 29*

Body Fluid Identification *see* Specimen Identification Requirements *on page 29*

Capillary Blood Collection *see* Skin Puncture Blood Collection *on page 28*

Cytology Smear Identification *see* Specimen Identification Requirements *on page 29*

Decentralized Testing *see* Point-of-Care Testing *on this page*

Fingerstick Blood Collection *see* Skin Puncture Blood Collection *on next page*

Heelstick Blood Collection *see* Skin Puncture Blood Collection *on next page*

HIV Precautions, Specimen Collection *see* Blood and Fluid Precautions, Specimen Collection *on page 24*

Identification Requirements, Specimen *see* Specimen Identification Requirements *on page 29*

Isolation Patients, Precautions for Specimen Collection *see* Blood and Fluid Precautions, Specimen Collection *on page 24*

Near Patient Testing (NPT) *see* Point-of-Care Testing *on this page*

Pathology Specimen Identification *see* Specimen Identification Requirements *on page 29*

Peripheral Blood Smear Preparation *see* Skin Puncture Blood Collection *on next page*

Phlebotomist Procedures

Related Information
Blood and Fluid Precautions, Specimen Collection *on page 24*
Blood Collection Tube Information *on previous page*
Skin Puncture Blood Collection *on next page*
Specimen Identification Requirements *on page 29*
Venous Blood Collection *on page 30*

Synonyms Specimen Collection Policy, Phlebotomist

Collection Phlebotomists are generally required to adhere to the following procedures. Phlebotomists are only allowed to obtain samples from patients who have been positively identified. See listing Specimen Identification Requirements *on page 29*. Phlebotomists are limited to attempting venipunctures in upper extremities unless so ordered by the physician. **Phlebotomists may not perform a venipuncture above an I.V. site or in an arm with a heparin lock or shunt.** Only by a physician's order may a trained phlebotomist collect a sample from a fistula or shunt. Phlebotomists should not collect a sample from an arm which is on the same side as a recent mastectomy. Phlebotomists are generally limited to two attempts to obtain a blood sample. After two unsuccessful tries, the phlebotomist must call another phlebotomist or supervisor. If the second phlebotomist is unsuccessful, the physician or responsible nurse will be notified. Phlebotomists are not allowed to force a patient to have blood drawn. If a patient refuses, the phlebotomist will notify the responsible nurse or physician. The phlebotomist will perform skin punctures when ordered by the physician (with some exceptions) or if venipuncture is unsuccessful or prohibited (due to I.V., etc), provided the procedure requested can be performed on a skin puncture specimen. (Dependent on the policy and equipment available in laboratory receiving the specimen.) See Skin Puncture Blood Collection *on page 28*.

Special Instructions The perception of pain associated with venipuncture in children increases with anxiety and is inversely correlated with the patient's age.[1] Strategies to reduce the child's and parents' distress during venipuncture are important considerations.[2,3] Use of topical anesthetics has also been suggested.[4,5] More than 33% of adult patients report needle discomfort greater than expected.[6] Every effort should be made to improve patient satisfaction by reducing discomfort from phlebotomy procedures.

Additional Information See Sampling Problems in Statistics, the Normal Range, and the Ulysses Syndrome *on page 11*.

Footnotes

1. Lander J, Fowler-Kerry S, and Oberle S, "Children's Venipuncture Pain: Influence of Technical Factors," *J Pain Symptom Manage*, 1992, 7(6):343-9.
2. Manne SL, Redd WH, Jacobsen PB, et al, "Behavioral Intervention to Reduce Child and Parent Distress During Venipuncture," *J Consult Clin Psychol*, 1990, 58(5):565-72.
3. Harrison A, "Preparing Children for Venous Blood Sampling," *Pain*, 1991, 45(3):299-306.
4. Woolfson AD, McCafferty DF, and Boston V, "Clinical Experiences With a Novel Percutaneous Amethocaine Preparation: Prevention of Pain Due to Venipuncture in Children," *Br J Clin Pharmacol*, 1990, 30(2):273-9.
5. Joyce TH 3d, "Topical Anesthesia and Pain Management Before Venipuncture," *J Pediatr*, 1993, 122(5 Pt 2):S24-9.
6. Howanitz PJ, Cembrowski GS, and Bachner P, "Laboratory Phlebotomy - College of American Pathologists Q-Probe Study of Patient Satisfaction and Complications in 23,783 Patients," *Arch Pathol Lab Med*, 1991, 115(9):867-72.

References

Bennett BD, Cox RS, Davis CM, et al, eds, *So You're Going to Collect a Blood Specimen: An Introduction to Phlebotomy*, 5th ed, Northfield, IL: College of American Pathologists, 1992.

Phlebotomy, Venous *see* Venous Blood Collection *on page 30*

POCT *see* Point-of-Care Testing *on this page*

Point-of-Care Testing

Related Information
Glucose, Fasting *on page 137*
Glucose, Random *on page 138*
Glycated Hemoglobin *on page 140*

Synonyms Alternate Site Testing (AST); Ancillary Testing; Bedside Testing; Decentralized Testing; Near Patient Testing (NPT); POCT

Test Commonly Includes Depending on physician needs, point-of-care assays may include one or more of the following analytes: hematocrit, hemoglobin, glucose, β-hCG, CK-MB, blood gases (pH, pCO_2, pO_2), electrolytes (Na^+, K^+, Cl^-), ionized calcium, ionized magnesium, lactate, blood urea nitrogen, creatinine, drugs of abuse, and activated clotting time.

Abstract Development of diagnosis-related groups (DRG's), manufacturer's incentives to provide instrumentation to less regulated sites (eg, physicians' office laboratories prior to CLIA '88),[1] advancing technology[1] including development of biosensors with improved electronics[2] and evolving requirements for abbreviated turnaround times have driven interest in near patient testing. Point-of-care testing (POCT) ultimately will find its niche in terms of clinical utility. It has been proven practicable and some aspects are desirable,[3] but it is not always cost-effective.

Specimen Whole blood, urine

Turnaround Time Minutes

Reference Range See reference range for each particular analyte.

Critical Values See each analyte listing for critical values and panic ranges.

Use Bedside glucose monitoring to guide insulin administration; intensive care and surgical theaters and other settings in which need for rapid turnaround times is great or desirable.

Limitations Point-of-care testing generally is more expensive than analysis of specimens in a centralized laboratory. Expense is related in part to volume of testing and the number of personnel involved in such testing; handheld bedside-type devices tend to be less precise than larger instruments in centralized laboratories; *vide infra*. Information handling, storage, and billing may become problematical. Such challenges may be overcome by incorporation of radiofrequency and infrared links to the central laboratory as part of the point-of-care testing devices. Some scientists observe that such devices are used by personnel who may not be fully trained to use them, nor have they backgrounds which support a quality improvement mind-set. Others argue that these objections may be balanced by strict oversight of personnel using point-of-care devices.
(Continued)

Point-of-Care Testing (Continued)

Inspection and accreditation requirements, quality assurance and proficiency testing, supervision and management for POCT continue to evolve. Difficulties include as well needs to monitor such programs and requirements to maintain standards[4] with training and competency requirements.[5]

Methodology Methodology ranges from reflectance measurements of glucose oxidase strips for some of the simplest bedside glucometers to microelectrode technology for some of the most sophisticated devices measuring electrolytes and blood gases.

Additional Information Point-of-care testing (POCT) or alternate site testing (AST) is an emerging area in which laboratory tests are performed outside of the central laboratory. Tests are often performed by personnel with little or no formal training in laboratory technology, nor exposure to the concepts of quality control or continuous quality improvement. Laboratory testing has until recently been delivered by increasingly large centralized entities, predominantly sophisticated laboratories including those in hospitals. Assay equipment for most of the recent past was composed of ever increasingly complex large automated instruments with interfaced information systems. This complex of large machines with an associated cadre of highly-trained professional personnel has created laboratories with ability to generate large amounts of test data at a relatively low cost per test. Bachner[6] reviews the history of such laboratory testing. He relates that the growth of large central laboratories has been a direct result of the linkage of technological development and the increase in the number and size of American hospitals. Recently the advent of microminiature electronics and very powerful microprocessors has led to a new generation of compact portable instruments that are relatively easy to use and provide reasonable precision even in the hands of relatively inexperienced users. Such devices are not inexpensive, nor are they foolproof. In many ways technological trends have driven instrumentation to a central location and then recently, have begun to move them away to more peripheral (hopefully essential) sites.

The concept of POCT remains controversial. Proponents argue that the need for decreased turnaround times in areas such as anticoagulation during balloon angioplasty, bedside coagulation monitoring and bedside glucose testing to guide insulin therapy has driven the site of testing from the central laboratory to the bedside, at which turnaround times may be as little as 3 minutes.[7] While decentralized testing tends to be more expensive than centralized analysis, some have argued that the cost structure for POCT is different from that of the centralized laboratory.[8] Others have pointed out that cost analyses to date have not included the "costs of failure" which such items as the loss of ability to make timely clinical decisions, unnecessary stat orders induced by slow specimen transport to the laboratory, and poor communication between laboratory and clinical care providers.[9] Laposata et al[10] have studied costs for bedside glucose monitoring and report that increased POCT costs relate to the volume of alternate site testing performed and the number of healthcare workers performing such tests. Reagent and instrument costs also are relevant. Limiting POCT to units in which glucose testing is performed five times or more per day and limiting the number of personnel doing such testing minimizes the expense of bedside glucose monitoring. However, such limits preclude POCT application in many community hospital settings. Limitations of POCT to more active services supports enhancement of competence by those performing bedside testing.

Other issues that likely will remain controversial include selection of performance standards for POCT, definition of acceptable reproducibility (precision), information handling, reporting and billing issues, responsibility for POCT programs in hospitals and definition of realistic turnaround times. A recent report on timeliness of clinical laboratory tests[11] makes it clear that the perception of reasonable turnaround time is much different for clinical care providers than for laboratory staff.

An important paper provides recommendations for bedside glucose monitoring programs, essentially outlining organizational structure and requirements for successful programs. First among these is specific designation of responsible individual(s) and whenever possible, involvement of laboratory personnel in administration and quality assurance. Written procedures, organized training programs, defined maintenance, regular quality control testing with two levels of control material, and standards for acceptable performance are needed. Orchestrated, regular comparisons of POC results with corresponding specimens analyzed in the clinical laboratory and with performance standards are recommended. Participation in external proficiency testing programs, recognition of glucose concentration limits of POC instruments, specified out-of-limits requirements for central laboratory glucose assays and acknowledgment of effects of the hematocrit, appropriate clinical restrictions, and determination of instrument bias are needed.[12]

Footnotes

1. Handorf CR, "Background-Setting the Stage for Alternate-Site Laboratory Testing," *Clin Lab Med*, 1994, 14(3):451-8.
2. Woo J and Henry JB, "The Advance of Technology as a Preclude to the Laboratory of the Twenty-First Century," *Clin Lab Med*, 1994, 14(3):459-71.
3. Handorf CR, "Quality Control and Quality Management of Alternate-Site Testing," *Clin Lab Med*, 1994, 14(3):539-57.
4. Travers EM, Wolke JC, and Sitak MM, "Consolidating Ancillary Testing in Multihospital Systems," *Clin Lab Med*, 1994, 14(3):493-524.
5. Allred TJ and Steiner L, "Alternate-Site Testing. Consider the Analyst," *Clin Lab Med*, 1994, 14(3):569-604.
6. Bachner P, "Alternate Site Testing. The Old and New Paradigm or the Past Is Prologue," *Arch Pathol Lab Med*, 1995, 119(10):881-5.
7. Becker RC, "Exploring the Medical Need for Alternate Site Testing. A Clinician's Perspective," *Arch Pathol Lab Med*, 1995, 119(10):894-7.
8. De Cresce RP, Phillips DL, and Howanitz PJ, "Financial Justification of Alternate Site Testing," *Arch Pathol Lab Med*, 1995, 119(10):898-901.
9. Fuhrman SA, Travers EM, and Handorf CR, "The Mobile Laboratory in Alternative Site Testing," *Arch Pathol Lab Med*, 1995, 119(10):939-42.
10. Laposata M and Lewandrowski KB, "Near Patient Blood Glucose Monitoring," *Arch Pathol Lab Med*, 1995, 119(10):926-8.
11. Steindel SJ, "Timeliness of Clinical Laboratory Tests. A Discussion Based on Five College of American Pathologists Q-Probe Studies," *Arch Pathol Lab Med*, 1995, 119(10):918-23.
12. Jones BA, Bachner P, and Howanitz PJ, "Bedside Glucose Monitoring: A College of American Pathologists Q-Probes Study of the Program Characteristics and Performance in 605 Institutions," *Arch Pathol Lab Med*, 1993, 117(11):1080-7.

References

Auerbach DM, "Alternate Site Testing - Information Handling and Reporting Issues," *Arch Pathol Lab Med*, 1995, 119(10):924-5.
Belanger AC, "Alternate Site Testing - The Regulatory Perspective," *Arch Pathol Lab Med*, 1995, 119(10):902-6.
Felder RA, Savory J, Margrey KS, et al, "Development of a Robotic Near Patient Testing Laboratory," *Arch Pathol Lab Med*, 1995, 119(10):948-51.
Fraser CG and Petersen PH, "Desirable Performance Standards for Imprecision and Bias in Alternate Sites - The Views of Laboratory Professionals," *Arch Pathol Lab Med*, 1995, 119(10):909-13.
Green M, "Successful Alternatives to Alternate Site Testing - Use of a Pneumatic Tube System to the Central Laboratory," *Arch Pathol Lab Med*, 1995, 119(10):943-7.
Hamlin WB, "Regulatory and Accreditation Implications of Alternate-Site Laboratory Testing," *Clin Lab Med*, 1994, 14(3):605-22.
Jones BA, "Testing at the Patient's Bedside," *Clin Lab Med*, 1994, 14(3):473-91.
Lamb LS Jr, "Responsibilities in Point-of-Care Testing - An Institutional Perspective," *Arch Pathol Lab Med*, 1995, 119(10):886-9.
Santrach PJ and Burritt MF, "Point-of-Care Testing," *Mayo Clin Proc*, 1995, 70(5):493-4.
Watts NB, "Reproducibility (Precision) in Alternate Site Testing, a Clinician's Perspective," *Arch Pathol Lab Med*, 1995, 119(10)914-7.
Weiss SL, Cembrowski GS, and Mazze RS, "Patient and Physician Analytic Goals for Self-Monitoring Blood Glucose Instruments," *Am J Clin Pathol*, 1994, 102(5):611-5.

Rejection Criteria, Specimen *see* Specimen Rejection Criteria *on next page*

Requisition Information *see* Specimen Identification Requirements *on next page*

Skin Puncture Blood Collection

CPT 36415

Related Information

Blood and Fluid Precautions, Specimen Collection *on page 24*
Phlebotomist Procedures *on previous page*
Specimen Identification Requirements *on next page*

Synonyms Capillary Blood Collection; Fingerstick Blood Collection; Heel-stick Blood Collection

Applies to Arterialized Capillary Blood; Peripheral Blood Smear Preparation

Test Commonly Includes Obtaining capillary blood from finger tip of an adult or heel in infants

Patient Preparation

Heel puncture: Select a site on the medial or lateral portion of the plantar surface of the foot. Do not puncture greater than 2.4 mm. Do not puncture the posterior curvature of the heel.[1] Do not repuncture previous puncture sites because of the possibility of infection.

Finger puncture: Select a site on the palmar aspect on the center of distal phalanx. Do not puncture the side or tip of the phalanx because the skin is much thinner.

Skin preparation: The skin site selected should be cleaned with 70% alcohol (isopropanol) and dried with sterile gauze. Infection is a frequent complication of fingersticks. Prepare the skin site carefully. Do not use iodine, which interferes with many assays.

Arterialized blood: Warming the site with a moist towel at temperatures not to exceed 42°C produces an increase in blood flow and **arterializes the capillary blood.** pH and blood gas determinations are usually performed on arterialized capillary blood in infants and children.

Aftercare Elevate the site above the body and apply direct pressure to the puncture site with sterile gauze until bleeding stops. Bandaids or bandages are generally not applied because of the risk of skin sensitization to tape and the risk of aspiration, should the bandage come loose.

Specimen Capillary blood or arterialized capillary blood

Container Capillary tube or microtube

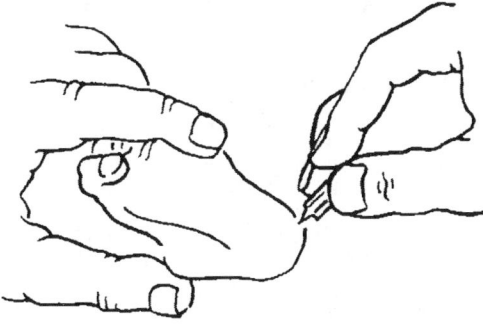

Gloves should be worn when collecting capillary blood specimens. From JD Bauer, *Clinical Laboratory Methods*, 9th ed, St. Louis, MO: Mosby-Year Book Inc, 1982, with permission.

Collection Patient identification: Confirm that the patient being drawn is the correct one by comparing the requisition with the identification wristband. After preparation of the selected site, the skin should be punctured at a slight angle. A disposable skin puncture lancet should be used rather than a surgical blade because a surgical blade may make too deep an incision and damage underlying tissues. The first drop should be wiped away as it may contain tissue fluid. Blood flow will be increased by holding the site downward. Slight pressure may be applied to the surrounding tissue. **Squeezing or milking should not be done.** Tubes should be sealed quickly to avoid exposure to atmospheric oxygen. Specimen identification: The specimen should be labeled with the patient's name, hospital number, room number, date and time of collection, and initials or identification of the person collecting the specimen.

Special Instructions Avoid injury to the calcaneus (heel bone). Be aware of the volume of specimens being collected from newborns. The limited blood volumes of neonates makes extensive testing hazardous. Such caution includes specimens for blood gas analysis.

Use Obtain capillary or arterialized capillary blood for analysis. Collection of blood from infants and children, patients who have had repeated venipunctures or whose veins are damaged or inadequate. Procedure of choice for preparing peripheral blood smears for morphologic examinations.

Limitations Technically, a specimen obtained by skin puncture consists of a mixture of arterial, capillary and venous blood, and tissue fluid. Specimen volume is limited. Repeat determinations often require repeat blood collection. Finger tips are sensitive; the procedure may be painful. Infection, particularly in debilitated hosts, may occur. Cell counts (ie, RBC, WBC, and platelets) are not accurate on capillary specimens.

Contraindications Use of surgical blades may create a wound deeper and larger than necessary and are contraindicated. **Finger punctures should not be performed on infants because the distance from the skin to the bone is less than 1.5 mm.**

Footnotes

1. Blumenfeld TA, Turi GK, and Blanc WA, "Recommended Sites and Depth of Newborn Heel Skin Punctures Based on Anatomic Measurements and Histopathology," *Lancet*, 1979, 1:230-3.

References

National Committee for Clinical Laboratory Standards, *Procedures for the Collection of Diagnostic Blood Specimens by Skin Puncture*, 2nd ed, Approved Standard, NCCLS Publication H14-A2, Villanova, PA: National Committee for Clinical Laboratory Standards, 1990.

Specimen Collection Policy, Phlebotomist *see* Phlebotomist Procedures *on page 27*

Specimen Identification Requirements

Related Information

Arterial Blood Collection *on page 24*
Chain-of-Custody Protocol *on page 542*
Phlebotomist Procedures *on page 27*
Skin Puncture Blood Collection *on previous page*
Urine Collection, 24-Hour *on next page*
Venous Blood Collection *on next page*

Synonyms Identification Requirements, Specimen

Applies to Bacteriology Specimen Identification; Blood Specimen Identification; Body Fluid Identification; Cytology Smear Identification; Pathology Specimen Identification; Requisition Information; Spinal Fluid Identification; Urine Specimen Identification

Causes for Rejection Laboratories must reserve the right to refuse improperly labeled specimens. Accurate specimen identification is critical to the provision of accurate results. Specimens must be provided in appropriate containers with correct preservatives; see individual test listings.

Special Instructions Patient identification: Inpatient: Compare the information on the request form with the patient's identification band and room and bed number. Confirm identification by asking the patient to state his/her full name. If the patient cannot state his/her name, ask a nurse or patient's relative to confirm the patient's identity. Confirm that the specimen label information is identical to the wristband and request form information. Label specimens as indicated below. Outpatient: Confirm identification by asking the patient to state his/her full name. If the patient cannot state his/her name, ask a nurse or patient's relative to confirm the patient's identity. Confirm the specimen label information is identical to the wristband and request form information. The requirements for labeling specimens and requisitions are as follows.

Blood specimens: All blood specimens received by the laboratory must have a permanently attached label with the following information written in black indelible ink: patient's name, hospital number, date and time of collection, initials of person drawing the specimen. Person obtaining blood sample must perform the proper identification check. Draw the sample of blood. Label all the tubes at the patient's bedside. Certain blood tests require special or immediate handling after collection. Consult the individual test listings for specific information and also the Transfusion Service (Blood Bank) Introduction *on page 597* for specifics on Blood Bank patient identification.

Urine specimens: All urine specimens received by the laboratory must have the following information fixed to the container (not cover): patient's name, hospital number, date and time of collection. Urine specimens delivered to the laboratory usually must be placed in the specimen refrigerator. Certain urine tests require special or immediate handling after collection; eg, crystalluria is best evaluated on a fresh, warm specimen. Consult the individual test listings for specific information.

Cerebrospinal fluids: Each tube submitted must be labeled with the patient's name, hospital number, source of specimen, date and time of collection, tube identification number (#1, #2, #3 according to the order of collection). Spinal fluid tests are usually considered to be stat procedures because spinal fluid constituents are unstable and cells degrade quickly, and because some may be samples from patients with meningitis. Consequently, spinal fluid must be taken to the laboratory immediately after collection and handed to a technologist or receptionist. Consult the individual test listings for specific information; most such listings in this book bear designations beginning "Cerebrospinal Fluid...".

Body fluids: All body fluids must be labeled with the patient's name, hospital number, date and time of collection, source of fluid. Body fluid constituents are unstable, and thus, expeditious handling is required. Some may derive from patients with medical emergencies or catastrophies. Consult individual test listings for specific information; many in this book bear designations beginning "Body Fluid...".

Cytology smears: All slides for cytologic examination should be appropriately and immediately fixed, labeled with the patient's name, and placed in a cardboard folder with the cytology requisition slip containing patient's name, patient information, and physician's name wrapped around it. Further information is provided in the Cytopathology Introduction *on page 285*.

Bacteriology specimens: All specimens for bacteriology testing must be labeled with the patient's name, hospital number, date and time of collection, source of material. Bacteriology specimens should be delivered to the laboratory as soon after collection as possible to preserve the viability of bacteria or viruses and to provide optimal patient care.

Pathology (surgical) specimens: All specimens for pathology must be labeled with the patient's name, hospital number, name of physician, name of surgeon, and source of specimen. Further information is available in the Anatomic Pathology Introduction *on page 33*. For many but not all specimens, the listing Histopathology provides detailed information. Consult individual test listings for specific information pertinent to specimens requiring special handling.

Chain-of-custody specimens: Specimens for drugs of abuse screening and specimens which may be used as legal evidence (eg, bullets removed surgically) must be collected according to a chain-of-custody protocol. For further information, see the listing Chain-of-Custody Protocol *on page 542*, as well as the Therapeutic Drug Monitoring/Toxicology/Drugs of Abuse Appendix *on page 581*.

Specimen Rejection Criteria

Synonyms Rejection Criteria, Specimen; Unsatisfactory Specimens Criteria

Causes for Rejection Criteria for specimen rejection are dependent on individual tests. Generally, specimens received by a laboratory are not discarded until the physician ordering the test or responsible nursing unit is notified. Events which may lead to the rejection of a specimen include specimen improperly labeled or unlabeled, specimen improperly collected and/or preserved, specimen sample volume not sufficient for (Continued)

Specimen Rejection Criteria (Continued)

requirement of test protocol, outside of container contaminated by specimen (ie, infectious hazard), or patient not properly prepared for test requirements. Examples of the last include nonfasting state for assays in which fasting is needed, and recent radioisotope scan in a patient in whom a test is ordered which is done by radioimmunoassay.

Some information is provided under Causes for Rejection in individual test listings, but most requirements are provided under appropriate fields such as Preparation.

It is ultimately the responsibility of the ordering physician to make certain that the laboratory is provided with a properly collected and identified specimen for analysis. Communications regarding less than optimal specimens generally should be oriented toward concern for patient welfare rather than nonavailability or unwillingness to provide laboratory service.

Spinal Fluid Identification *see* Specimen Identification Requirements *on previous page*

Timed Urine Collection *see* Urine Collection, 24-Hour *on this page*

Twenty-Four Hour Urine Collection *see* Urine Collection, 24-Hour *on this page*

Unsatisfactory Specimens Criteria *see* Specimen Rejection Criteria *on previous page*

Urine Collection, 12-Hour, 2-Hour, and Timed *see* Urine Collection, 24-Hour *on this page*

Urine Collection, 24-Hour

Related Information
Specimen Identification Requirements *on previous page*

Synonyms Twenty-Four Hour Urine Collection

Applies to Timed Urine Collection; Urine Collection, 12-Hour, 2-Hour, and Timed

Collection Twenty-four hour urine collections are often a problem for both patient and laboratory. A good collection regimen is as follows: Discard first morning specimen on day one. Collect all specimens during the remainder of the day and evening. Collect the first morning specimen on day two. Stop collection. Label specimen with patient's name, hospital number, room number, and date and time of collection. This presumes that time of arising is the same on day one and day two. Alternate regimen: Patient is to empty his/her bladder completely at a designated time (for example, 8 AM). This specimen is discarded. All urine is saved throughout the day and evening. Patient is to empty his/her bladder at the same time on day two as in step 1 above (for example, 8 AM). This specimen is combined with the rest of the collection for the previous 24 hours. Stop collection. Label specimen with patient's name, hospital number, room number, date and time of collection. Urines must be kept chilled at 5°C if bacteriologic activity will adversely affect results (eg, Schilling's test).

Normal fluid intake is allowed during 24-hour urine collections. Dietary restrictions are required for some procedures and are specified in the individual test listing. Since results are based on total volume, it is critical that the volume be measured accurately and the information included with the paper or electronic test requisition. Clearance tests require an estimate of body surface area; patient's height and weight must be available to the laboratory or provided to the laboratory when a clearance is requested.

Special Instructions See instructions in the particular listings listed above under Related Information for urine collections for trace metals. See specific instructions elsewhere in this book under specific listings for collection procedures for other substances. For information on urine collection procedures for drugs of abuse testing, see the Therapeutic Drug Monitoring/Toxicology/Drugs of Abuse Introduction *on page 527.*

Limitations Some tests require a critical minimal volume for accuracy. For example, some Schilling test protocols require a minimum of 500 mL/24 hours, and are unreliable for reduced urine volumes. Consult individual test listings for information on critical urine volumes.

Additional Information The procedure may be followed for other timed collections (ie, 12-hour, etc) as follows: Discard the initial specimen. Record time. Collect all specimens voided within the requested time frame. Label the specimen with patient's name, hospital number, room number, and date and time of collection.

Urine Specimen Identification *see* Specimen Identification Requirements *on previous page*

Vacutainer® Tube Description *see* Blood Collection Tube Information *on page 26*

Venipuncture, Venous *see* Venous Blood Collection *on this page*

Venous Blood Collection

CPT 36415

Related Information
Blood and Fluid Precautions, Specimen Collection *on page 24*
Blood Collection Tube Information *on page 26*
Phlebotomist Procedures *on page 27*
Specimen Identification Requirements *on previous page*

Synonyms Blood Collection, Venous; Phlebotomy, Venous; Venipuncture, Venous

Test Commonly Includes Routine method for obtaining blood when anticoagulants or larger volumes than can be obtained by capillary blood collection are required

Patient Preparation Select a suitable site for venipuncture. Prepare the site by scrubbing with 70% alcohol (isopropanol) using a circular motion working out from the site. Dry with gauze or let air dry. Do not touch site after cleansing until blood drawing is complete. Special requirements exist for alcohol levels; see Alcohol, Blood or Urine *on page 531.* Avoid hand pumping.

Aftercare Apply pressure to the venipuncture site and elevate the arm until bleeding stops. If bleeding persists, apply a pressure dressing to the site.

Specimen Venous blood

Container Syringe with a 20- or 21-gauge needle for volumes up to 10 mL, 18-gauge for larger volumes to assure adequate blood flow. Use a Vacutainer® or similar system for multiple specimens or anticoagulants. A 20- or 21-gauge Butterfly® infusion set may be used for difficult draws or blood cultures with multiple tubes.

Sampling Time Some samples for analytes that exhibit diurnal variation should be drawn at specific times of the day. See individual test listings.

Collection If one must be used at all, apply tourniquet 4-6 inches above drawing site. Do not leave tourniquet applied for more than 1 minute. Cleanly puncture the vein, loosen the tourniquet, and apply gentle suction or insert Vacutainer® tube into holder to fill tubes. Remove the needle and fill the tubes without delay.

If blood is being drawn for venous pH, pCO_2, lactic acid, or electrolytes, it is best to draw blood without a tourniquet. If one is needed, leave it in place while the sample is drawn. Alternatively, if a tourniquet must be used, sample blood 1-2 minutes after the hand is relaxed and the tourniquet removed. **Avoid hand clenching for these tests, especially for potassium and lactic acid determinations.** The first aliquot is best for pH.

Gently invert tubes 10 times to assure mixing of anticoagulants.

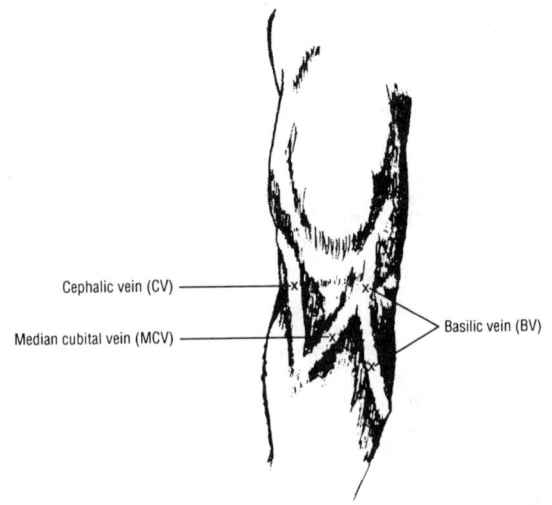

Cephalic vein (CV)

Median cubital vein (MCV)

Basilic vein (BV)

From JD Bauer, *Clinical Laboratory Methods,* 9th ed, St. Louis, MO: Mosby-Year Book Inc, 1982, with permission.

Causes for Rejection Samples collected for coagulation studies which have <90% of the expected fill may be rejected. Samples collected for coagulation studies may require additional anticoagulant if the hematocrit is low. Grossly hemolyzed specimens may be rejected depending on tests requested. Specimens that are not properly identified cannot be accepted.

Use Obtain venous blood for analysis

Limitations Venipuncture is technically difficult in obese patients, infants, children, patients with collapsed veins such as those in shock, and occasionally, other subjects as well. Hemolysis may occur as a result of excessive suction during collection, violent mixing of the specimen, or vigorous transfer of the specimen from syringe to tube.

Contraindications Fist clenching will alter potassium, pH and pCO_2 studies. If a tourniquet is applied but released before blood is aspirated, K^+ and lactic acid are washed out and results will be even more misleading.[1]

Additional Information Draw EDTA tube last. Hematology tubes contain K-EDTA. Any contamination can raise potassium and decrease pH.

See individual test listings for specific specimen collection requirements. To avoid contamination with tissue thromboplastins released by the venipuncture, a two-syringe or two-tube collection technique, in which the first tube is discarded, is required for coagulation specimens (eg, prothrombin time, activated partial thromboplastin time, etc). Blood collection for cytokine measurements needs particular attention to prevent possible contamination by endotoxins which can trigger cytokine production after sampling.[2]

Footnotes

1. Gambino R, "The Correct Way to Draw Venous Blood - Does Stasis Matter?" *Lab Rep*, 1996, 18(1):1-3.

2. Bienvenu J, Doche C, and Gutowski MC, "Methods for Studying Cytokines in Biologic Media," *Allerg Immunol* 1995, 27(4):116, 119-22.

References

Bennett BD, Cox RS, Davis CM, et al, eds, *So You're Going to Collect a Blood Specimen: An Introduction to Phlebotomy*, 5th ed, Northfield, IL: College of American Pathologists, 1992.

National Committee for Clinical Laboratory Standards, *Collection, Transport, and Preparation of Blood Specimens for Coagulation Testing and Performance of Coagulation Assays*, Approved Guideline, NCCLS Document H21-A, Villanova, PA: National Committee for Clinical Laboratory Standards, 1986.

National Committee for Clinical Laboratory Standards, *Procedures for the Collection of Diagnostic Blood Specimens by Venipuncture*, 2nd ed, Approved Standard, NCCLS Publication H3-A2, Villanova, PA: NCCLS, 1984.

National Committee for Clinical Laboratory Standards, *Procedures for the Handling and Processing of Blood Specimens, Approved Guideline*, NCCLS Publication H18-A, Villanova, PA: National Committee for Clinical Laboratory Standards, 1990.

National Committee for Clinical Laboratory Standards, *Procedures for the Collection of Diagnostic Blood Specimens by Venipuncture*, 3rd ed, Approved Standard, H3-A3, Villanova, PA: NCCLS, 1991.

ANATOMIC PATHOLOGY

Phillip A. Munoz, MD

David S. Jacobs, MD

Contributors:
    Steven H. Hinrichs, MD
    Mark D. Ost, MD

The specialty of anatomic pathology is the morphologic study, both gross and microscopic, of the effects of disease on tissue. It forms the basis of much of our current knowledge on the form and cause of disease. The discipline has been greatly enhanced by increases in sophistication of instruments and technology, including the quality and capabilities of our reagents.

The autopsy is the ultimate quality control procedure in the care of patients. It remains the validator or the invalidator of the results of many of the more recent diagnostic modalities.

As anatomic pathology has become more complex, it has become increasingly difficult for any single pathologist to remain easily familiar with all current information about all of its branches. Contributors to previous editions have included Jaime A. Diaz, MD, Raoul Fresco, MD, John G. Gruhn, MD, Michael S. Handler, MD, and David F. Keren, MD. We hope this book provides useful information, perhaps not quickly found elsewhere.

Acute Leukemia *see* MIC2 *on page 52*

Alpha Fetoprotein *see* Immunoperoxidase Procedures *on page 43*

Aneuploidy *see* Tumor Aneuploidy by Flow Cytometry *on page 57*

Automated Cytophotometry *see* Image Analysis *on page 43*

Autopsy

CPT 88000 (necropsy (autopsy), gross examination only without CNS); 88005 (with brain); 88007 (with brain and spinal cord); 88012 (infant with brain); 88014 (stillborn or newborn with brain); 88016 (macerated stillborn); 88020 (necropsy (autopsy), gross and microscopic without CNS); 88025 (with brain); 88027 (with brain and spinal cord); 88028 (infant with brain); 88029 (stillborn or newborn with brain); 88036 (necropsy (autopsy) limited, gross and/or microscopic, regional); 88037 (single organ); 88040 (necropsy (autopsy) forensic examination); 88045 (coroner's call); 88099 (unlisted necropsy (autopsy) procedure)

Synonyms Necropsy; Postmortem Examination

Applies to Cause of Death; Coroner's Case; Death Certificate; Disease Reporting; Medical Examiner's Case; Quality Assurance in the Practice of Medicine; Vital Statistics

Abstract The expression **"autopsy"** means to see for oneself, or to see with one's own eyes.

Special Instructions Consent: A hospital autopsy is not usually performed until the pathologist has, in hand, a properly signed autopsy permit. A valid permit must contain the signature of the highest ranking survivor in the next-of-kin lineage. A commonly used decreasing order of responsibility: spouse, adult children, parents, adult brothers and sisters, relatives, and then anyone who will accept responsibility for the body for purposes of burial. (State laws are not uniform.) Witnesses are often required to sign necropsy permits. **It is desirable as well as courteous for the attending physician to discuss the clinical particulars with the pathologist before the dissection is begun.** In regard to physician attendance at autopsy, some of the most important clinicopathologic correlations and in-depth investigations occur in autopsies at which clinicians attend. There are frequently matters discussed which are not in the chart and morphologic findings may provide immediate feedback to a clinician in a way unavailable to him/her from even a lengthy autopsy report. Clinician attendance at autopsy is always rewarding to everyone involved. Particularly in autopsies on individuals who are not hospital inpatients, critical clinical facts are likely to be unavailable, fragmentary, or completely unknown. The presence of the attending physician at such autopsies compensates to some degree for the lack of a well worked up chart. It is usually the responsibility of the attending physician to obtain permission for the autopsy from the next-of-kin. Except in coroner's cases, it is usually the responsibility of the attending physician to complete the death certificate.

Use Validated for over a century, the autopsy is a great deal more than an educational tool. It determines the cause and manner of death, determines severity of disease, represents an effort to preserve the quality of medical practice and to support excellence in medicine (quality assurance). It enhances medical knowledge, provides insight to understand pathogenesis and recognition of hereditary/familial diseases relevant to genetic counseling and possibly pertinent to surviving relatives, and permits diagnosis of contagious diseases and exposure to toxic entities. The autopsy provides valid comparisons between premortem and postmortem diagnoses. It produces valid statistics not otherwise available. Autopsies provide information on certain environmental or occupational exposures, provide data relevant to the public health and vital statistics, yield information on the success or failure of therapy, and provide data for evaluation of new procedures and new drugs not obtained by other means. A teaching instrument of great value, the autopsy remains a component of good medical care. It has been described as a vital clinical quality control measure,[1] a definitive monitor of quality of care given to the patient or by the medical system;[2] *vide infra*. The autopsy may support or provide recognition of emerging medical entities, such as acquired immunodeficiency syndrome (AIDS), toxic shock syndrome, microbiology of Legionnaires' disease, and sudden infant death syndrome (SIDS). It may provide recognition of changes taking place in old ones.

Contraindications Improperly completed written permission

Methodology Gross organ and microscopic tissue examination with subsequent special procedures as indicated

Additional Information

CORONER'S CASES

In possible medical legal cases, the Coroner's Office or Medical Examiner should be contacted before any suggestion regarding autopsy permission is made to the family of the deceased. Cases falling under the jurisdiction of the coroner usually include all unnatural deaths including sudden unexpected or unexplained death, death due to accident and violence (death following injury immediately or delayed for an indefinite time), cases of suspected homicide or suicide, unusual or suspicious circumstances, and cases falling in the public interest (ie, meningitis or other contagious diseases). The Coroner's Office should be notified in the event of all deaths in which a physician was not recently attending the patient (usually defined as the 48 hours prior to death) or in which the personal physician is unwilling to sign the death certificate. The Coroner's or Medical Examiner's office should be notified of unexpected deaths of children younger than 1 year of age and of all drug deaths, save for anesthetic deaths in most jurisdictions or complications of legitimate therapy. Deaths in custody (jail, psychiatric facilities, and other custodial situations) should elicit notification. Deaths due to abortion, whether self-induced or otherwise, require notification. Deaths related to employment may require notification. Such deaths need not be immediate. Persons who have knowledge of such deaths are usually required to notify the medical examiner or coroner. Failure to do so may be a misdemeanor.

The autopsy may resolve insurance questions, including addressing diagnoses of suicide or homicide.

THE AUTOPSY MAY SUPPORT RISK MANAGEMENT

It may eliminate suspicion and provide reassurance to families; it may provide facts instead of conjecture, and support malpractice defense and reduce medicolegal claims as well as improve the quality of care.[3]

QUALITY ASSURANCE AND THE AUTOPSY

The declining rate of autopsies is a cause for concern by the Council on Scientific Affairs of the American Medical Association, which has emphasized the lack of change in class I error in spite of better clinical techniques.[4] (Class I error is one in which a different diagnosis before death may have prolonged life.) This *JAMA* paper reported that the House of Delegates of the American Medical Association reaffirmed that autopsies are of fundamental importance in any quality assurance program.[4]

In 1987, the Council on Long Range Planning and Development of the American Medical Association published a paper in which this sentence appears: "Both organized medicine and society at large are in a position to demand autopsy services **in an effort to preserve the quality of medical practice.**"[5]

About 10% of autopsies in referral hospitals reveal a major diagnosis which bears upon therapy and survival. Overreliance on new procedures such as scans, ultrasound, and computerized tomography occasionally leads to missed diagnoses. The value of the autopsy has not been diminished.

A study of 2145 autopsies reported an overall rate of major discrepancies of 29%. The most often misdiagnosed or missed entities in this series included infections and malignancies. The most frequently overlooked immediate causes of death included pulmonary embolism and gastrointestinal hemorrhage.[6] Missed diagnoses of infections include fungal infections.[7]

Discrepancies between antemortem and postmortem diagnoses are found in 25% of cases, leading to skepticism about critical health statistics not based on autopsy findings. Cabot had questioned the accuracy of death certificates in 1912; such questions have persisted in the United Kingdom, in the United States, and in a number of other Western countries for good reasons.

Deficiencies in statistics, because of the "astonishing inaccuracy" of death certificates, can lead to "wrong priorities and wrong policies."[8]

It is not currently possible to predict which autopsy cases will have high yields.[9,10] Overwhelming data document the need for the autopsy in quality assurance.[11] The autopsy service provides information relevant to quality of care in an institution, the most optimal quality assurance mechanism. It is fallacious to preselect deaths for a postmortem evaluation. Ideally cases to be autopsied should be randomly selected to exclude bias.

Guidelines for request for postmortem examination may include:
- unanticipated death
- cause of death obscure
- death occurring while the patient is being treated with a new therapy, drug or regime
- intraoperative or intraprocedural death
- death occurring within 48 hours after surgery or an invasive diagnostic procedure
- death related to pregnancy or within 7 days of delivery
- death during a psychiatric admission
- death in admitted infants and children with congenital malformations

HAZARDS OF THE AUTOPSY

Hazards of necropsies include tuberculosis, hepatitis B, acquired immune deficiency syndrome (AIDS), and Jakob-Creutzfeldt disease.[12]

Formalin does not kill the etiologic agent of Jakob-Creutzfeldt disease, and it may not kill mycobacteria promptly.

Footnotes

1. Scottolini AG and Weinstein SR, "The Autopsy in Clinical Quality Control," *JAMA*, 1983, 250:1192-4.
2. Lundberg GD, "Medical Students, Truth, and Autopsies," *JAMA*, 1983, 250:1199-1200.
3. Valaske MJ, "Loss Control/Risk Management. A Survey of the Contribution of Autopsy Examination," *Arch Pathol Lab Med*, 1984, 108(6):462-8.
4. "Autopsy. A Comprehensive Review of Current Issues. Council on Scientific Affairs," *JAMA*, 1987, 258(3):364-9.
5. "The Future of Pathology. Council on Long Range Planning and Development," *JAMA*, 1987, 258(3):370-7.
6. Stevanovic G, Tucakovic G, Dotlic R, et al, "Correlation of Clinical Diagnosis With Autopsy Findings: A Retrospective Study of 2145 Consecutive Autopsies," *Hum Pathol*, 1986, 17(12):1225-30.
7. Goldman L, "Diagnostic Advances *vs* the Value of the Autopsy," *Arch Pathol Lab Med*, 1984, 108(6):501-5.
8. Hill RB and Anderson RE, "Is a Valid Quality Assurance Program Possible Without the Autopsy?" *Hum Pathol*, 1988, 19(10):1125-6.
9. Friederici HH and Sebastian M, "Autopsies in a Modern Teaching Hospital. A Review of 2,537 Cases," *Arch Pathol Lab Med*, 1984, 108(6):518-21.
10. Lundberg GD, "Now Is the Time to Emphasize the Autopsy in Quality Assurance," *JAMA*, 1988, 260(23):3488.
11. Landefeld CS, Chren MM, Myers A, et al, "Diagnostic Yield of the Autopsy in a University Hospital and a Community Hospital," *N Engl J Med*, 1988, 318(19):1249-54.
12. Orenstein JM, "Guidelines for High Risk or Potentially High Risk Autopsy Cases," *Pathologist*, 1984, 33-4.

References

Burke MC, Aghababian RV, and Blackbourne B, "Use of Autopsy Results in the Emergency Department Quality Assurance Plan," *Ann Emerg Med*, 1990, 19(4):363-6.
Friederici HH, "Reflections on the Postmortem Audit," *JAMA*, 1988, 260(23):3461-5.
Geller SA, "Religious Attitudes and the Autopsy," *Arch Pathol Lab Med*, 1984, 108(6):494-6.
Hill RB and Anderson RE, *The Autopsy - Medical Practice and Public Policy*, Boston, MA: Butterworth's Publishers, 1988.
Hirsch CS, "Talking to the Family After an Autopsy," *Arch Pathol Lab Med*, 1984, 108(6):513-4.
Lundberg GD, "Medicine Without the Autopsy," *Arch Pathol Lab Med*, 1984, 108(6):449-54.
Michigan Association of Medical Examiners, "The Duties and Organization of Michigan County Medical Examiners," 1993.
Sanner M, "A Comparison of Public Attitudes Toward Autopsy, Organ Donation, and Anatomic Dissection. A Swedish Survey," *JAMA*, 1994, 271(4):284-8.
Sarode VR, Datta BN, Banerjee AK, et al, "Autopsy Findings and Clinical Diagnoses: A Review of 1000 Cases," *Hum Pathol*, 1993, 24(2):194-8.
Stehbens WE, "An Appraisal of the Epidemic Rise of Coronary Heart Disease and Its Decline," *Lancet*, 1987, 1(8533):606-11.
Stothert JC Jr, Gbaanador GB, and Herndon DN, "The Role of Autopsy in Death Resulting From Trauma," *J Trauma*, 1990, 30(8):1021-5.
Wagner BM, "Mortality Statistics Without Autopsies: Wonderland Revisited," *Hum Pathol*, 1987, 18(9):875-6.

Basement Membrane Zone Antibodies *see* Skin Biopsy, Immunofluorescence *on page 56*

Biopsy *see* Histopathology *on page 42*

Biopsy, Breast *see* Breast Biopsy *on this page*

B-Lymphocyte Analysis by Flow Cytometry *see* Immunophenotypic Analysis of Tissues by Flow Cytometry *on page 45*

Brain Biopsy *see* Electron Microscopy *on page 37*

BRCA1 *see* Breast Biopsy *on this page*

BRCA2 *see* Breast Biopsy *on this page*

Breast Biopsy

CPT 88305; 88307 (breast, mastectomy - partial/simple); 88309 (breast, mastectomy - with regional lymph nodes)

Related Information

Ataxia-Telangiectasia, Chromosome Breakage Study *on page 274*
Breast Cancer, Hereditary (BRCA1) *on page 504*
CA 15-3 *on page 93*
Carcinoembryonic Antigen *on page 100*
Cyst Fluid Cytology *on page 292*
Estrogen and Progesterone Receptor Assay *on page 38*
Fine Needle Aspiration, Superficial Palpable Masses *on page 294*
Frozen Section *on page 41*
Histopathology *on page 42*
Immunoperoxidase Procedures *on page 43*
Immunophenotypic Analysis of Tissues by Flow Cytometry *on page 45*
Nipple Discharge Cytology *on page 297*
p53, Functional Assay/Sequencing *on page 522*
Tumor Aneuploidy by Flow Cytometry *on page 57*

Synonyms Biopsy, Breast

Applies to BRCA1; BRCA2; Cathepsin D; c-erb-B2; DNA; DNA Ploidy; Epidermal Growth Factor Receptor; Flow Cytometry; Gross Cystic Disease Fluid Protein-15 (GCDFP-15); HER-2/neu; Oncogene Expression; Ploidy; S Phase

Abstract Breast biopsies are among the most common and complex specimens received in the surgical pathology laboratory. In recent years, increasing emphasis on early detection and conservative treatment has generated a new approach to the management of breast biopsies with particular emphasis on indicators of prognosis. Favorable prognostic factors in breast carcinoma include tumor size of <1 cm, low histologic grade, negative axillary lymph nodes, and positive estrogen receptors (ER) and progesterone receptors (PR). Surgical margins, presence or absence of vascular invasion, tumor type, staging, grading, ploidy S phase fraction, cathepsin D, epidermal growth factor receptor, *p53*, and c-erb-B2 (HER-2/neu or HER-2) oncogene are relevant to survival. The first priority is histopathologic diagnosis. Other studies are secondary. The differential diagnosis of carcinoma of breast includes radial scar, microglandular adenosis, sclerosing adenosis and other entities which can present difficulty in distorted, extremely small, previously frozen, or crushed specimens.

Patient Preparation Appropriate history and clinical information should be provided with the specimen. A strong family or personal history is relevant. History of prior biopsy or trauma may explain fibroplasia that might be mistaken for tumor desmoplasia. History of current or recent pregnancy may be extremely helpful. Whether or not nipple discharge was present and whether the lesion was detected by palpation, mammography, or both should be recorded. Tumor location may be especially important for lesions in proximity to the nipple, where nipple duct adenoma (florid papillomatosis) may occur. For needle localization studies, the original mammograms with x-rays of the needle localization are desirable.

Specimen Breast biopsies are commonly sent fresh for immediate evaluation. Open biopsy specimens should be sent intact so that orientation can be established and dye applied to margins. Frozen section and/or imprints of grossly evident tumor may confirm the presence of carcinoma and establish the basis to allocate tissues for hormone receptor assays and DNA studies. **Frozen sections of very small tumors should be discouraged,** as diagnosis and classification are more important than accessory studies. If needed, hormone receptor and DNA studies can be performed on paraffin-embedded tissues. Experienced surgeons often recognize benign specimens such as fibroadenomas and fix them in formalin. Image-guided needle biopsies are being used with increased frequency and may allow for better preoperative, cost-effective treatment planning.[1]

Container Fresh specimens of breast tissue should be sent in a clean, dry, labeled container on ice (to preserve receptors)[2] and placed in the hands of a pathologist or histotechnician.

Causes for Rejection Contraindications for frozen section on a breast specimen: insufficient tissue to sacrifice for frozen section examination; a biopsy done for calcification without a mass should not be frozen; lack of a gross lesion suspicious for carcinoma

Use Establish the presence of breast disease and classify the process. The first priority of breast biopsy examination is histopathologic diagnosis. Confirm the presence of calcifications noted in preoperative mammograms and characterize them. Specimen radiography is commonly performed to confirm that the biopsied tissue contains the calcific structures, but their etiology can only be evaluated histologically. Since many women presently request breast-conserving surgical procedures, evaluation of resection margins has assumed major importance in the early evaluation of the breast biopsy and efficacy of extent of the surgical procedure. For malignant diseases, lumpectomy (tylectomy) is presently followed by radiation therapy in many cases.[3]

Limitations Shortcomings of needle biopsies include potential for false-negative results related to problems of sampling. Other problems include crush artifact and lack of opportunity to visualize the lesion and its relationship to its environs. Needle localization is most often used as a guide to open biopsy.[2] Local recurrence may complicate lumpectomy. **Multiple foci of carcinoma** are considered contraindications to breast-conserving therapy.

Methodology *Vide infra*

Additional Information The pathologist determines the extent of the tumor and its relationship to its corresponding resection margins. Specimen orientation by the surgeon may be desirable for direction of potential further surgery. When the surgeon requires a report reflecting the relationship of the tumor to resection margins, it is necessary to clearly identify margins (superior, inferior, lateral, medial, deep, superficial) in a combination appropriate for the setting of a given neoplasm. The pathologist often identifies surgical margins of lumpectomy and of re-excision specimens with India ink and colored dyes.[4] So as not to interfere with receptor assays, tissues submitted for receptor analysis should be free of ink or dye.[5] Sections can then be taken to provide margin evaluation on microscopy. The complex geometry of lumpectomy margins has been addressed in a variety of ways.[2,4,6,7] Connolly and others conclude that **frozen section evaluation of margins which are grossly free of** (Continued)

Breast Biopsy (Continued)

tumor has no significant role in intraoperative management. It may compromise evaluation of margins in permanent sections. In up to 33% of breast biopsies done for microcalcifications in which carcinoma is found, the calcifications are in adjacent benign breast tissue and not in the tumor. Therefore, tissue **adjacent** to focal microcalcifications is often included in the biopsy and should be sampled for microscopy. Studies addressing outcomes in receptor-negative and receptor-positive conservatively treated tumors have been reported by the National Surgical Adjuvant Breast and Bowel Project (NSABP).[8,9]

Risks of local recurrence in patients treated with conservative surgery are influenced by several important factors.[10] These factors include patient age (which is inversely related to the rate of local recurrence). The adequacy of resection is borne out by studies noting a higher local recurrence rate in specimens with narrow margins (tumorectomies) than in specimens with very wide margins (quadrantectomies). The presence of extensive intraductal carcinoma, especially comedocarcinoma, or of infiltrating lobular carcinoma represents major risk factors for local recurrence, probably owing to the multicentric nature of these diseases. Factors which limit adjuvant radiation therapy also predispose to an increased recurrence rate.

The risk of regional or distant recurrence is also dependent on a number of factors, the most important of which is stage of disease. Favorable histopathologic tumor types include pure mucinous (colloid), pure tubular, invasive cribriform carcinoma, and the rare adenoid cystic carcinoma of breast. Inflammatory carcinoma and carcinosarcoma are aggressive but uncommon. Histopathologic features associated with an aggressive clinical course include poorly differentiated tumors (high histologic grade), tumor necrosis, frequent mitoses, and vascular invasion. Principles of histologic grading proposed by Bloom and Richardson have repeatedly shown predictive value.[11,12,13] The role of tumor angiogenesis and the associated risk of dissemination is becoming increasingly appreciated.[14]

In the absence of axillary lymph node metastases, the 10-year surgical failure rate is about 20%. Immunochemical methods are useful in selected cases for detection of occult lymph node metastases though the finding of micrometastatic disease is not clearly associated with worse overall survival.[15] Micrometastases are more likely when the primary breast carcinomas are larger than 2 cm. Vascular invasion is significantly related to recurrence and metastasis, but is subject to interobserver variation.[12] Immunostains for factor VIII-related antigen have sometimes been used to highlight the presence of neoplastic cells within vascular spaces.

In addition to providing accurate pathological staging information, the pathologist is also becoming increasingly pivotal for provision of studies of therapeutic and prognostic significance. **Estrogen receptor (ER) expression** in breast cancer has the unique characteristic of having both prognostic and therapeutic implications. **Progesterone receptor (PR) expression** has indirect therapeutic implications but may have a more direct bearing on prognosis. The frequency of ER expression tends to increase with age as does the level of ER expression.[16] (See listing Estrogen and Progesterone Receptor Assay on page 38.) PR expression is induced by estrogen and in part reflects functional integrity of the estrogen regulatory pathway.[17] Accordingly, ER-, PR+ phenotype is very uncommon. Although some conflicting data have been reported, there is consensus that presence of ER is correlated with longer disease-free survival and overall survival. Such differences tend to be most significant at follow-up of 5 years or less. Survival curves tend to merge with longer term follow-up. Stage-matched patients with higher expression of ER tend to follow a more favorable clinical course than do patients with low levels of expression. Generally, both ER and PR expression tend to reflect tumor growth rate rather than metastatic potential.

ER expression is highly associated with response to endocrine therapy. Tumor-static responses are associated with ER, with the greatest likelihood of response in those with high levels of ER expression and those with coexpression of PR. Some studies have suggested a more favorable course in patients with PR expression while other studies show no added benefit over that associated with ER expression. Patterns of metastasis in ER-positive and ER-negative patients may differ. Patients with ER-negative tumors have a higher rate of visceral involvement while patients with ER-positive tumors have a predilection for bony metastasis.[18]

Estrogen and progesterone receptor assay information is provided as a separate listing. Expression of both hormone receptors may be measured in several ways. The time honored dextran-coated charcoal (DCC) method is based on the binding of radioactive hormone to a cytosol extract of the tumor and does not detect the true intranuclear form of the receptor. More recently, an enzyme immunoassay (EIA) for both hormones has gained favor. Enzyme immunoassays employ monoclonal antibodies to the respective hormone receptors measuring only the cytosol receptor fraction. Receptors are quantitated by a colorimetric

enzyme amplified signal. Enzyme immunoassays require less tissue than DCC and are not subject to interference by endogenous or exogenous hormones. When dealing with very small tumors or tissue biopsies, an immunocytochemical stain (ICC) may be employed to qualitatively measure hormone receptor expression. These stains allow direct morphologic correlation of hormone receptor activity with cell type and detect the true intranuclear form of receptor expression. Immunocytochemical studies have demonstrated a surprising degree of heterogeneity in hormone receptor expression, the significance of which is being actively investigated.

Flow cytometric determination of DNA ploidy and S-phase fraction (SPF) have gained wide acceptance in evaluation of breast carcinoma. Such studies may be obtained on tissues submitted for hormone receptor assays or from paraffin blocks. Up to 66% of breast cancers are aneuploid and 30% to 40% are regarded as high SPF tumors. Several studies have demonstrated shorter time to relapse and worse overall survival in stage 1 patients with aneuploid tumors or those with high SPF. Patients with stage 1, low SPF tumors enjoyed a significantly reduced chance for relapse and longer survival.[19,20] When considered separately, tetraploid tumors tend to behave more like diploid tumors than other aneuploid tumors.[21] Aneuploidy and high SPF tumors tend to demonstrate high nuclear grade and are more frequently hormone receptor negative.

Other prognostic markers being actively investigated include **cathepsin D, epidermal growth factor receptor, and c-erb-B2 (HER-2/neu)** oncogene expression. **Cathepsin D** is a ubiquitous lysosomal protease capable of digesting basement membranes and other stromal elements of breast tissue. In normal breast, expression of cathepsin D is estrogen regulated. The possibility that such proteases may serve to promote tumor dissemination has led to studies investigating its prognostic utility. Using tissue extracts assayed by the Western blot procedure in a group of node-negative breast cancer patients, Tandon et al showed a strong correlation between high levels of cathepsin D and shorter disease-free intervals and overall survival.[22] In this study, cathepsin D was correlated with aneuploidy but showed no other significant associations with other clinical and prognostic variables. Another study utilizing immunocytochemical detection of cathepsin D produced conflicting results.[23] Henry et al found an overall increase in mean time to relapse and increased overall survival. In node-negative patients, they found no significant prognostic advantage while node-positive patients showed longer disease-free interval and improved overall survival. Armas et al found no significant correlation between survival and immunohistochemical detection in patients with limited stage disease.[24] Thus, the prognostic significance of cathepsin D remains ambiguous.

Epidermal growth factor receptor (EGFR) is a 170 kD transmembrane glycoprotein with tyrosine kinase activity and is intimately related to proliferation and differentiation of a wide variety of epithelia.[25] Based on an intensive literature review summarizing the results of 40 laboratories, Klijn et al found that about 48% of 5232 breast tumors were regarded as EGFR-positive. Expression of EGFR was correlated with estrogen and progesterone receptor negativity, high grade nuclear morphology, aneuploidy, increased S-phase fraction, and lymph node metastases. Expression in premenopausal patients may be increased. Generally, overall survival and relapse-free survival are thought to be worse for patients with increased EGFR expression. Further, EGFR status may identify prognostic subcategories in ER-negative patients.[26] Estrogen receptor-negative, EGFR-positive patients have a relatively poorer prognosis while ER-negative, EGFR-negative patients follow a clinical course more like that of ER-positive patients. Strategies to interrupt this stimulatory pathway are being investigated.[27]

It has also been suggested that the **c-erb-B2 (HER-2/neu) oncogene** has prognostic and therapeutic significance in patients with breast carcinoma. This gene encodes for a transmembrane receptor with tyrosine kinase activity. The exact function of this receptor is unknown but it shares structural similarities with EGFR. A variety of studies have indicated worse overall prognosis in patients with overexpression of c-erb-B2[28,29,30] while others have failed to confirm its value as an independent prognostic factor.[31,32] Expression of this marker may also have therapeutic value. In a large study, overexpression of c-erb-B2 was associated with poor response to conventional chemotherapy.[33] Overexpression may represent a marker for selection of patients more likely to benefit from high doses of adjuvant chemotherapy.[34,35] Clinical trials addressing the efficacy of monoclonal antibodies against this protein are underway.[27]

The *p53* tumor-suppressor gene functions to regulate control of the cell cycle. Mutations in the *p53* gene result in loss of its down regulatory functions and accumulation of the gene product which can be detected by immunohistochemistry. This protein can be detected in approximately 20% to 40% of breast carcinomas and is associated with other histologic and cell marker findings of overall worse prognosis.[36] Barnes et al suggest that prognostic value of *p53* may be second only to lymph node status.[37]

In the setting of metastatic carcinoma, immunoreactivity for gross cystic disease fluid protein (GCDFP-15) and ER are useful to confirm a breast primary.[38]

Isolation of susceptibility genes for breast cancer BRCA1 and BRCA2 represent exciting new information breakthroughs.[39]

See listing Breast Cancer, Hereditary (BRCA1) *on page 504.*

Footnotes

1. Parker SH, "Percutaneous Large Core Breast Biopsy," *Cancer*, 1994, 74(1 Suppl):256-62.
2. Carter D, "Interpretation of Breast Biopsies," *Biopsy Interpretation Series*, 2nd ed, New York, NY: Raven Press, 1990, 14.
3. Fisher B, Redmond C, Poisson R, et al, "Eight-Year Results of a Randomized Clinical Trial Comparing Total Mastectomy and Lumpectomy With or Without Irradiation in the Treatment of Breast Cancer," *N Engl J Med*, 1989, 320(13):822-8.
4. Carter D, "Margins of "Lumpectomy" for Breast Cancer," *Hum Pathol*, 1986, 17(4):330-2.
5. Muensch H and Maslow WC, "Interference of O.C.T. Embedding Compound With Hormone Receptor Assays," *Am J Clin Pathol*, 1984, 82(1):89-92.
6. Connolly JL and Schnitt SJ, "Evaluation of Breast Biopsy Specimens in Patients Considered for Treatment by Conservative Surgery and Radiation Therapy for Early Breast Cancer," *Pathol Annu*, 1988, 23(Pt 1):1-23.
7. Frazier TG, Wong RW, and Rose D, "Implications of Accurate Pathologic Margins in the Treatment of Primary Breast Cancer," *Arch Surg*, 1989, 124(1):37-8.
8. Fisher B, Redmond C, Dimitrov NV, et al, "A Randomized Clinical Trial Evaluating Sequential Methotrexate and Fluorouracil in the Treatment of Patients With Node-Negative Breast Cancer Who Have Estrogen-Receptor-Negative Tumors," *N Engl J Med*, 1989, 320(8):473-8.
9. Fisher B, Costantino J, Redmond C, et al, "A Randomized Clinical Trial Evaluating Tamoxifen in the Treatment of Patients With Node-Negative Breast Cancer Who Have Estrogen-Receptor-Positive Tumors," *N Engl J Med*, 1989, 320(8):479-84.
10. Osteen RT, "Selection of Patients for Breast Conserving Procedures," *Cancer*, 1994, 74(1 Suppl):366-71.
11. Elston CW, "Grading of Invasive Carcinoma of the Breast," *Diagnostic Histopathology of the Breast*, Page DL and Anderson TJ, eds, New York, NY: Churchill Livingstone, 1987, 300-11.
12. Tavassoli FA, *Pathology of the Breast*, New York, NY: Elsevier/North Holland Biomedical Press, 1992, 36-43.
13. Simpson JF and Page DL, "Status of Breast Cancer Prognostication Based on Histopathologic Data," *Am J Clin Pathol*, 1994, 102(4 Suppl 1):S3-8.
14. Hayes DF, "Angiogenesis and Breast Cancer," *Hematol Oncol Clin North Am*, 1994, 8(1):51-71.
15. Nasser IA, Lee AK, Bosari S, et al, "Occult Axillary Lymph Node Metastases in "Node-Negative" Breast Carcinoma," *Hum Pathol*, 1993, 24(9):950-7.
16. Clark GM, Osborne CK, and McGuire WL, "Correlations Between Estrogen Receptor, Progesterone Receptor, and Patient Characteristics in Human Breast Cancer," *J Clin Oncol*, 1984, 2(10):1102-9.
17. Osborne CK, "Receptors," *Breast Diseases*, Harris JR, Hellman S, Henderson IC, et al, eds, Philadelphia, PA: JB Lippincott Co, 1991, 210-32.
18. Clark GM, Sledge GW, Osborne CK, et al, "Survival From First Recurrence: Relative Importance of Prognostic Factors in 1015 Breast Cancer Patients," *J Clin Oncol*, 1988, 37:221-6.
19. Dressler LG, Seamer LC, Owens MA, et al, "DNA Flow Cytometry and Prognostic Factors in 1331 Frozen Breast Cancer Specimens," *Cancer*, 1988, 61(3):420-7.
20. Clark GM, Dressler LM, Owens MA, et al, "Prediction of Relapse or Survival in Patients With Node Negative Breast Cancer by DNA Flow Cytometry," *N Engl J Med*, 1989, 320(10):627-33.
21. Witzig TE, Gonchoroff NJ, Therneau T, et al, "DNA Content Flow Cytometry as a Prognostic Factor for Node Positive Breast Cancer. The Role of Multiparameter Ploidy Analysis and Specimen Sonication," *Cancer*, 1991, 68(8):1781-8.
22. Tandon AK, Clark GM, Chamness GC, et al, "Cathepsin D and Prognosis in Breast Cancer," *N Engl J Med*, 1990, 322(5):297-302.
23. Henry JA, McCarthy AL, Angus B, et al, "Prognostic Significance of the Estrogen-Regulated Protein, Cathepsin D, in Breast Cancer," *Cancer*, 1990, 65(2):265-71.
24. Armas OA, Gerald WL, Lesser ML, et al, "Immunohistochemical Detection of Cathepsin D in T2NOMO Breast Carcinomas," *Am J Surg Pathol*, 1994, 18(2):158-66.
25. Klijn JG, Berns PM, Schmitz PI, et al, "The Clinical Significance of Epidermal Growth Factor Receptor (EGF-R) in Human Breast Cancer: A Review of 5232 Patients," *Endocr Rev*, 1992, 13(1):3-17.
26. Sainsbury JR, Needham GK, Farndon JR, et al, "Epidermal-Growth-Factor Receptor Status as Predictor of Early Recurrence of and Death From Breast Cancer," *Lancet*, 1987, 1(8547):1398-402.
27. Tripathy D and Benz C, "Growth Factors and Their Receptors," *Hematol Oncol Clin North Am*, 1994, 8(1):29-50.
28. Van de Vijver MJ, Peterse JL, Mooi WJ, et al, "neu-Protein Overexpression in Breast Cancer," *N Engl J Med*, 1988, 319(19):1239-45.
29. Tandon AK, Clark GM, Chamness GC, et al, "HER-2/neu Oncogene Protein and Prognosis in Breast Cancer," *J Clin Oncol*, 1989, 7(8):1120-8.
30. Battifora H, Gaffey M, Esteban J, et al, "Immunohistochemical Assay of neu/c-erbB-2 Oncogene Product in Paraffin-Embedded Tissues in Early Breast Cancer: Retrospective Follow-Up Study of 245 Stage I and II Cases," *Mod Pathol*, 1991, 4(4):466-74.
31. Wong WW, Vijayakumar S, and Weichselbaum RR, "Prognostic Indicators in Node Negative Early Stage Breast Cancer," *Am J Med*, 1992, 92(5):539-48.
32. Elledge RM, McGuire WL, and Osborne CK, "Prognostic Factors in Breast Cancer," *Semin Oncol*, 1992, 19(3):244-53.
33. Gusterson BA, Gelber RD, Goldhirsch A, "Prognostic Importance of c-erbB-2 Expression in Breast Cancer," *J Clin Oncol*, 1992, 10(7):1049-56.
34. Muss HB, Thor AD, Berry DA, et al, "c-erbB-2 Expression and Response to Adjuvant Therapy in Women With Node-Positive Early Breast Cancer," *N Engl J Med*, 1994, 330(18):1260-6.
35. Goldhirsch A and Gelber RD, "Understanding Adjuvant Chemotherapy for Breast Cancer," *N Engl J Med*, 1994, 330(18):1308-9.
36. Porter-Jordan K and Lippman ME, "Overview of the Biologic Markers of Breast Cancer," *Hematol Oncol Clin North Am*, 1994, 8(1):73-100.
37. Barnes DM, Dublin EA, Fisher CJ, et al, "Immunohistochemical Detection of p53 Protein in Mammary Carcinoma: An Important New Independent Indicator of Prognosis?" *Hum Pathol*, 1993, 24(5):469-76.
38. Roche PC, "Immunohistochemical Stains for Breast Cancer," *Mayo Clin Proc*, 1994, 69(1):57-8.
39. Weber BL, "Susceptibility Genes for Breast Cancer," *N Engl J Med*, 1994, 331(22):1523-4.

References

Allred DC, Clark GM, Molina R, et al, "Overexpression of HER-2/neu and Its Relationship With Other Prognostic Change During the Progression of *In Situ* to Invasive Breast Cancer," *Hum Pathol*, 1992, 23(9):974-9.

Azzopardi JG, "Problems in Breast Pathology," *Major Problems in Pathology*, Vol 11, Philadelphia, PA: WB Saunders Co, 1979.

Banks PM, "Pathology Is More Than Just Microscopy," *Am J Clin Pathol*, 1995, 103(1):3.

Bellamy CO, McDonald C, Salter DM, et al, "Noninvasive Ductal Carcinoma of the Breast: The Relevance of Histologic Categorization," *Hum Pathol*, 1993, 24(1):16-23.

Bland KI and Copeland EM 3d, *The Breast. Comprehensive Management of Benign and Malignant Disease*, Philadelphia, PA: WB Saunders Co, 1991.

Fechner RE, "Frozen Section Examination of Breast Biopsies - Practice Parameter," *Am J Clin Pathol*, 1995, 103(1):6-7.

Frierson HF Jr, "Grade and Flow Cytometric Analysis of Ploidy for Infiltrating Ductal Carcinomas," *Hum Pathol*, 1993, 24(1):24-9.

Lay SF, Crump JM, Frykberg ER, et al, "Breast Biopsy. Changing Patterns During a Five-Year Period," *Am J Surg*, 1990, 56(2):79-85.

Livolsi VA, "A Surgical Pathologist Views Practice Parameters," *Am J Clin Pathol*, 1995, 103(1):1-2.

Ngai JH, Zelles GW, Rumore GJ, et al, "Breast Biopsy Techniques and Adequacy of Margins," *Arch Surg*, 1991, 126(11):1343-7.

Page DL and Anderson TJ, *Diagnostic Histopathology of the Breast*, New York, NY: Churchill Livingstone, 1987.

Bronchial Biopsy *see* Histopathology *on page 42*

Cardiac Biopsy *see* Electron Microscopy *on this page*

Cathepsin D *see* Breast Biopsy *on page 35*

Cause of Death *see* Autopsy *on page 34*

Cell Cycle Analysis of Tumors *see* Tumor Aneuploidy by Flow Cytometry *on page 57*

Cell Sorting Fluorescence Activation *see* Lymph Node Biopsy *on page 50*

Centrocytic Lymphoma *see* Mantle Cell Lymphoma *on page 51*

c-erb-B2 *see* Breast Biopsy *on page 35*

Chromogranin *see* Immunoperoxidase Procedures *on page 43*

Computerized Interactive Morphometry *see* Image Analysis *on page 43*

Copper, Hepatic *see* Liver Biopsy *on page 48*

Coroner's Case *see* Autopsy *on page 34*

Cytokeratins *see* Immunoperoxidase Procedures *on page 43*

Death Certificate *see* Autopsy *on page 34*

Dermatitis Herpetiformis Antibodies *see* Skin Biopsy, Immunofluorescence *on page 56*

Desmin *see* Immunoperoxidase Procedures *on page 43*

Disease Reporting *see* Autopsy *on page 34*

DNA *see* Breast Biopsy *on page 35*

DNA Content *see* Tumor Aneuploidy by Flow Cytometry *on page 57*

DNA in Tumor Nuclei *see* Image Analysis *on page 43*

DNA Ploidy *see* Breast Biopsy *on page 35*

DNA Ploidy Studies *see* Immunophenotypic Analysis of Tissues by Flow Cytometry *on page 45*

DNA Synthesis Phase *see* Tumor Aneuploidy by Flow Cytometry *on page 57*

Electron Microscopy

CPT 88348 (diagnostic); 88349 (scanning)

Related Information

Electron Microscopic Examination for Viruses, Stool *on page 665*
Fine Needle Aspiration, Deep Seated Lesions *on page 294*
Fine Needle Aspiration, Superficial Palpable Masses *on page 294*
Kidney Biopsy *on page 47*
MIC2 *on page 52*
Microsporidia Diagnostic Procedures *on page 487*
Muscle Biopsy *on page 53*
Skin Biopsy *on page 54*

Synonyms EM; Transmission Electron Microscopy; Ultrastructural Study

Applies to Brain Biopsy; Cardiac Biopsy; Viral Diseases by EM

Abstract A major application of electron microscopy is to delineate histogenesis of poorly differentiated neoplasms when light microscopy is equivocal and when proper therapy and prognosis depend on precise diagnosis. Although applications have diminished with development of immunoperoxidase methods, EM remains useful and provides information which otherwise cannot be obtained.

Specimen Fresh unfixed tissue, blood, bone marrow aspirate
(Continued)

Electron Microscopy *(Continued)*

Container Vial containing glutaraldehyde or other appropriate fixative, depending upon institution or reference laboratory. Blood and bone marrow aspirate may be collected in heparinized or EDTA tubes and submitted immediately.

Collection Specimen obtained by surgical biopsy should be cut within minutes of excision, minced into cubes 1 mm or less, and placed in glutaraldehyde, paraformaldehyde, or other special fixative. (See listing Kidney Biopsy *on page 47.*) Two percent to 4% phosphate or cacodylate-buffered glutaraldehyde is recommended. Formaldehyde-fixed tissue may be used if glutaraldehyde is not available. All EM fixatives, particularly glutaraldehyde, should be refrigerated until used to retard oxidative damage to fixative. Discard if a precipitate forms.

Causes for Rejection Specimen placed in formalin or not quickly placed in appropriate EM fixative. Lack of appropriate fixative is a relative cause for rejection, depending on the information required.

Use In adults, the distinction between poorly differentiated carcinoma, amelanotic melanoma, and lymphoma can be established by ultrastructural findings. Demonstration of desmosomes or tight junctions often characterize epithelial neoplasms while the presence of premelanosomes characterize amelanotic melanoma. Lack of such findings support a diagnosis of lymphoma. The presence of rare neurosecretory granules may distinguish small cell carcinoma (oat cell carcinoma) from various poorly differentiated nonsmall cell carcinomas. Other neuroendocrine neoplasms (eg, anterior pituitary tumors, insulinoma, and other APUDomas) are characterized by their numerous neurosecretory granules. Mesotheliomas characteristically display elongated villous cell borders. Diagnosis of poorly differentiated leukemias, some lymphomas, and of Langerhans cell (eosinophilic) granulomatosis (histiocytosis-X) is sometimes enhanced by electron microscopy with demonstration of Birbeck granules as well as characteristic nuclear convolution.[1] EM demonstration of platelet peroxidase in the nuclear envelope of the blast cells aids in the diagnosis of megakaryoblastic leukemias (M7).[2] When limited material is available, such as fine needle aspiration biopsies, electron microscopy may allow a more precise classification in selected cases.[3,4]

Electron microscopy is useful in certain viral and other infectious diseases. In AIDS encephalopathy, EM of brain biopsies helps to determine the responsible agent (ie, HIV, CMV, herpes, Jakob Creutzfeldt, progressive multifocal leukoencephalopathy, etc). EM may be invaluable in the evaluation of muscle biopsies (eg, mitochondrial myopathies) and peripheral nerve biopsies. Storage/metabolic diseases sometimes are well evaluated with EM. Ceroid lipofuscinoses and Pompe's type II glycogenosis bear characteristic inclusions in peripheral blood lymphocytes by EM. Many other lysosomal storage diseases can be identified by EM of skin, conjunctival, or gum biopsies.[5] The immotile cilia syndrome is diagnosed by the absence of one or both dynein arms in cross sections of ciliary microtubules in nasal or bronchial biopsies.[6] Some liver biopsies have lesions in which EM may be useful (eg, Dubin-Johnson syndrome, Rotor's disease). With heart biopsy, EM can reveal Adriamycin® cardiotoxicity.

Limitations EM is labor intensive and limited by cost and sampling errors. This method is usually not useful to distinguish benign from malignant neoplasms. Utility is diminished by poor fixation, crush or drying artifact. The role of EM has recently been eroded by rapid advances in immunocytochemistry for the differential diagnosis of tumors and infectious agents. For instance immunodiagnostic methods are definitive and rapid for herpes encephalitis, but EM supports diagnosis.

Methodology Properly fixed tissues are embedded in a high density plastic polymer from which thick sections (1 micron) are cut and stained to select the best areas for ultrastructural studies. Thin sections are subsequently prepared and stained with electron dense materials such as uranyl acetate. The specimens are then ready to examine in a transmission electron microscope.

Additional Information Concomitant light microscopic evaluation is usually required for ultrastructural correlation. Often light microscopic findings lead to a decision of whether or not EM is indicated (eg, tumors). EM is not a substitute for light microscopy. When renal biopsies are obtained, immunofluorescence studies are recommended, as well as light microscopy. Immunofluorescence and EM are mutually complementary.

Footnotes
1. Lieberman PH, Jones CR, Steinman RM, et al, "Langerhans Cell (Eosinophilic) Granulomatosis - A Clinicopathologic Study Encompassing 50 Years," *Am J Surg Pathol*, 1996, 20(5):519-552.
2. Koike T, "Megakaryoblastic Leukemia: The Characterization and Identification of Megakaryoblasts," *Blood*, 1984, 64(3):683-92.
3. Strausbauch P, Neill J, Dabbs DJ, et al, "The Impact of Fine Needle Aspiration Biopsy on a Diagnostic Electron Microscopy Laboratory," *Arch Pathol Lab Med*, 1989, 113(12):1354-6.

4. Yazdi HM and Dardick I, "Techniques for Specimen Processing," *Guides to Clinical Aspiration Biopsy, Diagnostic Immunocytochemistry, and Electron Microscopy*, New York, NY: Igaku-Shoin, 1991, 11-25.
5. Dolman CL, "Diagnosis of Neurometabolic Disorders by Examination of Skin Biopsies and Lymphocytes," *Semin Diag Pathol*, 1984, 1(2):82-97.
6. Afzelius BA, "The Immotile-Cilia Syndrome and Other Ciliary Diseases," *Int Rev Exp Pathol*, 1979, 19:1-43.

References
Azar HA, *Pathology of Human Neoplasms: An Atlas of Diagnostic Electron Microscopy and Immunohistochemistry*, New York, NY: Raven Press, 1988.

Dickersin GR, *Diagnostic Electron Microscopy: A Text/Atlas*, New York, NY: Igaku-Shoin, 1988.

Dvorak AM, *Diagnostic Ultrastructural Pathology*, Vol I, Boca Raton, FL: CRC Press, Inc, 1992.

Erlandson RA, *Diagnostic Transmission Electron Microscopy of Human Tumors With Clinicopathological, Immunohistochemical, and Cytogenetic Correlations*, New York, NY: Raven Press, 1994.

Ghadially FN, *Ultrastructural Pathology of the Cell and Matrix*, London, UK: Butterworths, 1988.

EM *see* Electron Microscopy *on previous page*

Endoscopic Biopsy *see* Histopathology *on page 42*

Epidermal Growth Factor Receptor *see* Breast Biopsy *on page 35*

Epithelial Membrane Antigen (EMA) *see* Immunoperoxidase Procedures *on page 43*

ER *see* Estrogen and Progesterone Receptor Assay *on this page*

ER-ICA *see* Estrogen and Progesterone Receptor Assay *on this page*

ER/PR *see* Estrogen and Progesterone Receptor Assay *on this page*

Estradiol Receptor *see* Estrogen and Progesterone Receptor Assay *on this page*

Estradiol Receptor (Immunocytochemical) *see* Estrogen and Progesterone Receptor Assay *on this page*

Estrogen and Progesterone Receptor Assay

CPT 84233 (estrogen receptor cytosol assay); 84234 (progesterone receptor cytosol assay); 88342 (estrogen or progesterone receptor immunocytochemical stain)

Related Information
Breast Biopsy *on page 35*
Histopathology *on page 42*
Image Analysis *on page 43*
Immunophenotypic Analysis of Tissues by Flow Cytometry *on page 45*
Tumor Aneuploidy by Flow Cytometry *on page 57*

Synonyms ER; ER-ICA; ER/PR; Estradiol Receptor; Estradiol Receptor (Immunocytochemical); Estrogen Binding Protein ERICA; Estrogen Binding Protein (Immunocytochemical); PgR; PgRICA or PgR(ICA); PR; PRICA or PR(ICA); Progesterone Binding Protein (Immunocytochemical); Progestogen Receptor (Immunocytochemical)

Applies to Tamoxifen

Test Commonly Includes Receptors are a part of pathologic evaluation to accurately stage breast carcinoma. DNA ploidy and S phase analysis are highly desirable, done on the same tissue specimen separately employing flow cytometry or image analysis. Many laboratories also provide panels of other prognostic markers (see listing Breast Biopsy *on page 35*). Hormone receptor analysis may provide similar information for other neoplasms, particularly ovarian and endometrial carcinoma and meningioma.

Abstract Estrogen receptor (ER) and progesterone receptor (PR) studies provide invaluable information primarily used to select patients most likely to benefit from endocrine therapy while also providing prognostic information. The method of analysis is dependent on the nature of sampled tissue.

Patient Preparation Antiestrogen preparations within 3 weeks may cause false-negative ER results. Exogenous hormones taken for contraceptive purposes, or menopausal estrogens, are related to lower receptor levels in competitive binding assays (*vide infra*). Therefore, hormone use including tamoxifen should be discontinued for about 3 weeks before breast biopsy.[1]

Specimen Receptor assays should be done on all primary breast carcinomas and may also be done on metastases. Send fresh tumor to the laboratory immediately on ice for frozen and permanent sections. Indicate that ER/PR studies are to be performed following confirmation by frozen section of diagnosis of breast cancer.

Container Liquid tight specimen container preferably sent in ice bath; **no formalin or other fixative.** Container must be labeled at least with patient's name, age, site of specimen (eg, right or left breast), and date.

The receptor assay request forms must be completed with patient information.

Collection It is imperative that the fresh specimen be kept on ice and sent to the laboratory **immediately** as a fresh specimen; receptor proteins are heat labile and should be frozen immediately by the pathologist. Ideally, tissues should be snap frozen in liquid nitrogen. If a dry ice acetone mixture is used for rapid freezing, do not permit tissue to touch this mixture. Instead, put the tissue in a labeled plastic screw-cap container. Acetone in direct contact with the tissue will denature receptor proteins. Quick freezing can also be done in the cryostat. Avoid contact with frozen section embedding media such as O.C.T.®[2] Anecdotal reports exist of pigments such as India ink causing interference with ER assay. If margins are marked with pigments, it may be prudent to trim away such edges of tissue submitted for receptor assay.

Storage Instructions -70°C freezer or colder. Avoid cyclic temperature fluctuations and prolonged storage. Dry ice is recommended for transportation.

Causes for Rejection Benign neoplasms; cytosol-based assays should not be performed on small primary neoplasms, those with extensive necrosis, or specimens contaminated by fixatives or heavily cauterized. Immunocytochemical examination can be performed on malignant specimens including those not suitable for cytosol assays.

Turnaround Time Cytosol assays may be sent frozen to reference laboratories, most of which can provide turnaround time of less than a week. Immunocytochemical analysis can usually be completed in a similar time frame.

Special Instructions Even short delays without proper cold packing can alter the results. A frozen section must be performed to document presence of viable carcinoma in the tissue to be analyzed. If tumor is sampled away from the frozen section site, then a permanent section of the area adjacent to the sampling site should be processed for permanent sections and designated as such. If the specimen is excised at a satellite facility, it should be quickly frozen, packed in sufficient ice to prevent thawing, and transported to reference laboratory frozen.

Reference Range For cytosol-based assays, <3 fmol/mg cytosol protein usually indicates no estrogen receptor activity; >10 fmol/mg usually indicates positivity; >100 fmol/mg cytosol protein is strongly positive. Reference ranges for progesterone cytosol assays are similar with <5 fmol/mg protein considered negative, >10 fmol/mg protein considered positive, and >100 fmol/mg considered strongly positive. Immunocytochemical stains are visually appraised and semiquantitated in a fashion similar to that previously reported.[3] Alternatively, a more precise evaluation may be performed by image analysis.[4,5,6,7] (See listing Image Analysis *on page 43*.)

Use The frequency of hormone receptor positivity is influenced by menopausal status, as depicted in the table.[8]

Receptor Status

	Premenopausal	Postmenopausal
ER+,PR+	45%	63%
ER+,PR-	12%	15%
ER-,PR-	28%	17%
ER-,PR+	15%	5%

ER and PR provide independent prognostic data.[9,10] In a multivariate analysis of women with recurrent or metastatic breast cancer, only the ER concentration was significant in predicting the response to tamoxifen.[11] Hormone receptor positivity is more common in postmenopausal women and is correlated with better histopathologic differentiation, longer disease-free interval, and with longer overall survival.[12,13,14] Progesterone receptor is reported by McGuire and Clark to be the second most critical factor after the number of positive nodes and to be a more significant prognostic factor than the presence or absence of ER.

More importantly, hormone receptor status has significant therapeutic implications. Patients with positive hormone receptor status are candidates for antiestrogen therapy. In patients treated with tamoxifen, the response rate is approximately 50% in ER-positive tumors and 60% to 70% in patients with both ER- and PR-positive tumors. Responses are observed in only approximately 8% of patients with ER-negative tumors.[15] In a multicenter study of 2644 node-negative patients, tamoxifen-treated patients enjoyed a longer disease-free survival, a lower incidence of second primary neoplasms in the contralateral breast, a lower incidence of recurrent local disease following lumpectomy, and an overall reduced incidence of treatment failure when combined with chemotherapy.[16] Although most breast carcinomas responding to endocrine therapy contain receptors, the presence of estrogen receptors does not assure response to endocrine management. Owing to its apparent protective role, tamoxifen therapy is often recommended even if other prognostic factors indicate a low chance for recurrence.

Patients whose breast carcinomas lack estrogen receptors are often candidates for chemotherapy. This decision is often based on multiple factors, the most important of which is stage of disease.

The detection of hormone receptors in metastatic tumors of unknown origin provide useful clues to predict primary tumor of breast.[17,18]

Neoplasms other than breast carcinoma may also express hormone receptors. Such tissue includes meningiomas,[19] soft tissue tumors,[20,21] endometrial hyperplasias, carcinomas, and other gynecologic tumors.[22,23] Adenocarcinomas of lung, melanomas and hepatocellular carcinomas are among other tumors in which ER may be detected.[24,25,26,27] Neoplastic proliferation of cervical squamous cells induced by HPV may be associated with reduced ER and increased PR expression.[28]

Limitations Technical and biological factors limit the utility of hormone receptor assays. Estrogen receptors are thermolabile with a highly variable half-life ranging from 30 minutes to 6 hours.[8] Progesterone receptors are somewhat more stable than estrogen receptors but are significantly subject to decay over short periods to time.[29] Thus, false-negative assays may occur when tissues are not rapidly frozen. Even brief contamination by fixative renders cytosol assays unreliable. Tissues submitted for cytosol assays should be meticulously selected to avoid contamination with benign breast tissue. Tissue adequacy is optimized when samples are selected by a pathologist with frozen section control. Desmoplastic tumors contain proportionally more stroma than cancer cells and may negatively bias cytosol assays. Extensively necrotic neoplasms produce a similar effect. The volume of tissue required for cytosol assays is such that extremely small carcinomas should not be submitted for cytosol assays and should be entirely allocated for tissue diagnosis. Estrogen and progesterone receptor immunocytochemical assays provide reasonable alternatives with some advantages compared to conventional cytosolic measurements of estrogen and progesterone receptors (*vide infra*).

Although stromal elements do not appear to significantly contribute to the ER content of breast carcinoma, they may contribute to the PR content. Phase of the menstrual cycle also influences the hormone receptor content of tissues with progressively decreasing ER content during the mid and late phases of the cycle. Mean ER is highest in proliferative phase. Elevated estrogen and progesterone levels in younger patients appear to decrease measured receptor levels by several mechanisms. Exogenous hormone therapy may alter the measured receptor content of a given tissue. Tamoxifen also results in diminished estrogen receptor expression. Thus, imperfect correlation exists between receptor positivity and response to endocrine therapy. Hormone replacement therapy or tamoxifen should have been discontinued for about 3 weeks prior to biopsy for optimal analysis.[8]

Contraindications Benign neoplasms, stromal or lymphoid tumors

Methodology Cytosol preparations generally recommend approximately 1 g (a mass slightly less than 1 x 1 x 1 cm) of fresh neoplastic tissue free of fat, necrotic tissue, and normal breast tissue, especially if ploidy studies are to be performed concurrently. The minimal amount of tissue required for assay is laboratory dependent but is about 150 mg. Biochemical measurements employ a cytosol extract of the tissue homogenate and are based on competitive binding of radiolabeled ligands. The choice of ligands and assay conditions allow accurate quantitation and assessment of receptor-ligand affinity. However, such methods are most subject to interference by endogenous and exogenous hormones. More recently, **enzyme immunoassays (EIA)** have been developed which utilize monoclonal antibodies specific for epitopes of receptor proteins apart from the hormone binding site. They are not subject to interference by exogenous hormones, do not employ radioisotopes, and are becoming the favored technology.

Immunocytochemical (ICC) procedures utilize monoclonal antibodies to estrogen and progesterone receptors (see listing Immunoperoxidase Procedures *on page 43*). Tissue examined may be paraffin sections, frozen (cryostat) sections, or touch imprints. One of the greatest advantages of ICC over conventional cytosolic assays is the ability to detect hormone receptors in small breast carcinomas not subject to receptor quantitation by cytosolic methods. Tumors composed predominantly of stroma and few tumor cells are also better assayed by this method. ICC assays are not adversely affected by endogenous or exogenous hormone competing for binding sites though down regulation of receptor expression remains a pitfall. True estrogen receptor positivity is conferred by nuclear but not cytoplasmic staining for the antiestrogen antibody H222 (Abbott Laboratories).[30] Using this antibody, studies comparing ERICA on frozen sections with cytosolic methods have generally shown good agreement[6,31,32,33,34,35,36,37] ranging from 79% to 95% concordance. Comparisons of paraffin-embedded sections with frozen sections show slightly less agreement, usually between 80% and 85%. Discrepancies may be attributable to presence of normal epithelium adjacent to ERICA-negative tumor cells, scant tumor cells in sample, and competitive inhibition by circulating hormones.[34] Recently (Continued)

Estrogen and Progesterone Receptor Assay
(Continued)

developed monoclonal antibodies have included several with more reliable staining characteristics in routinely fixed tissues[35] and are gaining wider application.

Relative Merits of Hormone Receptor Assay Techniques

Attribute	DCC/EIA	ICC
Quantitative result	yes	no
Clinically significant cutoff	yes	no
Sample size	larger	smaller
Morphologic correlation	no	yes
Determine heterogeneity	no	yes
Receptor assayed	cytosol	nuclear

Additional Information The ER exists as a 65 kilodalton monomeric protein concentrated within the cellular nucleus. ER is composed of several functional domains, one of which is responsible for binding estrogen passively transferred through the cytoplasm. Following estrogen binding, the estrogen receptor is phosphorylated to form a homodimer which apparently interacts with other yet unidentified proteins to develop high affinity interactions with specific sequences of DNA using a domain distinct from that occupied by estrogen. The family of heat shock proteins is thought to play a critical role in promoting the binding of ligand-receptor complex to its DNA receptor. The net result of this interaction is the transcription of DNA and the activation of other genes regulating cell growth and differentiation. These pathways include synthesis of the insulin-like growth factor-1, transforming growth factor alpha, progesterone receptor, epidermal growth factor receptor, and c-erb-B2. Such pathways function in concert to maintain an orderly state of cellular proliferation and differentiation. Perturbations of these pathways may lead to autocrine and paracrine "short-circuits" and ultimately to the neoplastic state.

Antiestrogens, such as tamoxifen, are used to down regulate estrogen dependent cell growth but do not confer cytotoxic activity. Tamoxifen does so by displacing estrogen but inhibiting the conformational changes required for DNA binding. However, tamoxifen resistance occurs, usually owing to primary lack of ER expression. Tumors which initially express ER may lose this ability, perhaps by mutation of the ER gene. Nomura et al report diminution and loss of ER and PR as the malignant state progresses and with endocrine therapy.[38] Other possible mechanisms include altered metabolism of antiestrogenic compounds, changes in estrogen pathway cofactors that influence ER-mediated transcription and activation of other pathways that bypass ER-mediated cell regulation.[39] A more complete understanding of these pathways and development of new drugs influencing these interactions may lead to significant advances in the control of breast cancer.

Footnotes

1. Lesser ML, Rosen PP, Senie RT, et al, "Estrogen and Progesterone Receptors in Breast Carcinoma: Correlations With Epidemiology and Pathology," *Cancer*, 1981, 48:299-309.
2. Muensch H and Maslow WC, "Interference of O.C.T. Embedding Compound With Hormone Receptor Assays," *Am J Clin Pathol*, 1984, 82(1):89-92.
3. Wilbur DC, Willis J, Mooney RA, et al, "Estrogen and Progesterone Receptor Detection in Archival Formalin-Fixed, Paraffin-Embedded Tissue From Breast Carcinoma: A Comparison of Immunohistochemistry With the Dextran-Coated Charcoal Assay," *Mod Pathol*, 1992, 5(1):79-84.
4. Aziz DC, "Quantitation of Estrogen and Progesterone Receptors by Immunocytochemical and Image Analyses," *Am J Clin Pathol*, 1992, 98(1):105-11.
5. El-Badawy N, Cohen C, Derose PB, et al, "Immunohistochemical Progesterone Receptor Assay - Measurement by Image Analysis," *Am J Clin Pathol*, 1991, 96(6):704-10.
6. Esteban JM, Kandalaft PL, Mehta P, et al, "Improvement of the Quantification of Estrogen and Progesterone Receptors in Paraffin-Embedded Tumors by Image Analysis," *Am J Clin Pathol*, 1993, 99(1):32-8.
7. Bacus S, Flowers JL, Press MF, et al, "The Evaluation of Estrogen Receptor in Primary Breast Carcinoma by Computer-Assisted Image Analysis," *Am J Clin Pathol*, 1988, 90(3):233-9.
8. Whittliff JL, Pasic R, and Bland KI, "Steroid and Peptide Receptor Identification in Breast Tissue," *The Breast. Comprehensive Management of Benign and Malignant Disease*, Bland KI and Copeland EM, eds, Philadelphia, PA: WB Saunders Co, 1991.
9. Chevallier B, Heintzmann F, Mosseri V, et al, "Prognostic Value of Estrogen and Progesterone Receptors in Operable Breast Cancer," *Cancer*, 1988, 62(12):2517-24.
10. McGuire WL and Clark GM, "Role of Progesterone Receptors in Breast Cancer," *J Clin Oncol*, 1984, 2:414-9.
11. Bezwoda WR, Esser JD, Dansey R, et al, "The Value of Estrogen and Progesterone Receptor Determinations in Advanced Breast Cancer - Estrogen Receptor Level but Not Progesterone Receptor Level Correlates With Response to Tamoxifen," *Cancer*, 1991, 68(4):867-72.
12. Rochman H, Conniff ES, and Kuk-Nagle KT, "Age and Incidence of Estrogen Receptor Positive Breast Tumors," *Ann Clin Lab Sci*, 1985, 15(2):106-8.
13. Mohammed RH, Lakatua DJ, Haus E, et al, "Estrogen and Progesterone Receptors in Human Breast Cancer - Correlation With Histologic Subtype and Degree of Differentiation," *Cancer*, 1986, 58(5):1076-81.
14. Clark GM, McGuire WL, Hubay CA, et al, "Progesterone Receptors as a Prognostic Factor in Stage II Breast Cancer," *N Engl J Med*, 1983, 309:1343-7.
15. Valavaara R, Tuominen J, and Johansson R, "Predictive Value of Tumor Estrogen and Progesterone Receptor Levels in Postmenopausal Women With Advanced Breast Cancer Treated With Toremifene," *Cancer*, 1990, 66(11):2264-9.
16. Fisher B, Constantino J, Redmond C, et al, "A Randomized Clinical Trial Evaluating Tamoxifen in the Treatment of Patients With Node Negative Breast Cancer Who Have Estrogen Positive Tumors," *N Engl J Med*, 1989, 320(8):479-84.
17. Bhatia SK, Saclarides TJ, Witt TR, et al, "Hormone Receptor Studies in Axillary Metastases From Occult Breast Cancers," *Cancer*, 1987, 59(6):1170-2.
18. Deamant FD, Pombo MT, and Battifora H, "Estrogen Receptor Immunohistochemistry as a Predictor of Site of Origin in Metastatic Breast Cancer," *Appl Immunohistochem*, 1993, 1(3):188-92.
19. Grunberg SM, Weiss MH, Spitz IM, et al, "Treatment of Unresectable Meningiomas With the Antiprogesterone Agent Mifepristone," *J Neurosurg*, 1991, 74(6):861-6.
20. Weiss SW, Langloss JM, Shmookler BM, et al, "Estrogen Receptor Protein in Bone and Soft Tissue Tumors," *Lab Invest*, 1986, 54(6):689-94.
21. Lim CL, Walker MJ, Mehta RR, et al, "Estrogen and Antiestrogen Binding Sites in Dermoid Tumor," *Eur J Cancer Clin Oncol*, 1986, 22(5):583-7.
22. Farley AL, O'Brien T, Moyer D, et al, "The Detection of Estrogen Receptors in Gynecologic Tumors Using Immunoperoxidase and the Dextran-Coated Charcoal Assay," *Cancer*, 1982, 49:2153-60.
23. Sabini G, Chumas JC, and Mann WJ, "Steroid Hormone Receptors in Endometrial Stromal Sarcomas - A Biochemical and Immunohistochemical Study," *Am J Clin Pathol*, 1992, 97(3):381-6.
24. Beattie CW, Hansen NW, and Thomas PA, "Steroid Receptors in Human Lung Cancer," *Cancer Res*, 1985, 45(9):4206-14.
25. Walker MJ, Ronan SG, Han MC, et al, "Interrelationship Between Histopathologic Characteristics of Melanoma and Estrogen Receptor Status," *Cancer*, 1991, 68(1):184-8.
26. Nagasue N, Ito A, Yukaya H, et al, "Estrogen Receptors in Hepatocellular Carcinoma," *Cancer*, 1986, 57(1):87-91.
27. Nagasue N, Kohno H, Chang Y-C, et al, "Androgen and Estrogen Receptors in Hepatocellular Carcinoma and the Surrounding Liver in Women," *Cancer*, 1989, 63(1):112-6.
28. Konishi I, Fujii S, Nonogaki H, et al, "Immunohistochemical Analysis of Estrogen Receptors, Progesterone Receptors, Ki-67 Antigen, and Human Papillomavirus DNA in Normal and Neoplastic Epithelium of the Uterine Cervix," *Cancer*, 1991, 68(6):1340-50.
29. Ellis LM, Wittliff JL, Bryant MS, et al, "Lability of Steroid Hormone Receptors Following Devascularization of Breast Tumors," *Arch Surg*, 1989, 124(1):39-42.
30. O'Keane JC, Okon E, Moroz K, et al, "Antiestradiol Immunoperoxidase Labeling of Nuclei, Not Cytoplasm, in Paraffin Sections, Determines Estrogen Receptor Status of Breast Cancer," *Am J Surg Pathol*, 1990, 14(2):121-7.
31. Cudahy TJ, Boeryd BR, Franlund BK, et al, "A Comparison of Three Different Methods for the Determination of Estrogen Receptors in Human Breast Cancer," *Am J Clin Pathol*, 1988, 90(5):583-90.
32. Tesch M, Shawwa A, and Henderson R, "Immunohistochemical Determination of Estrogen and Progesterone Receptor Status in Breast Cancer," *Am J Clin Pathol*, 1993, 99(1):8-12.
33. Ozzello L, DeRosa C, Habif DV, et al, "An Immunohistochemical Evaluation of Progesterone Receptor in Frozen Sections, Paraffin Sections, and Cytologic Imprints of Breast Carcinomas," *Cancer*, 1991, 67(2):455-62.
34. Parl FF and Posey YF, "Discrepancies of the Biochemical and Immunohistochemical Estrogen Receptor Assays in Breast Cancer," *Hum Pathol*, 1988, 19(8):960-6.
35. Kell DL, Kamel OW, and Rouse RV, "Immunohistochemical Analysis of Breast Carcinoma Estrogen and Progesterone Receptors on Paraffin-Embedded Tissue. Correlation of Clones ER1D5 and 1A6 With a Cytosol-Based Hormone Receptor Assay," *Appl Immunohistochem*, 1993, 1(4):275-81.
36. Shimada A, Kimura S, Abe K, et al, "Immunocytochemical Staining of Estrogen Receptor in Paraffin Sections of Human Breast Cancer by Use of Monoclonal Antibody: Comparison With That in Frozen Sections," *Proc Natl Acad Sci U S A*, 1985, 82(14):4803-7.
37. Hanna W and Mobbs BG, "Comparative Evaluation of ER-ICA and Enzyme Immunoassay for the Quantitation of Estrogen Receptors in Breast Cancers," *Am J Clin Pathol*, 1989, 91(2):182-6.
38. Nomura Y, Tashiro H, and Shinozuka K, "Changes of Steroid Hormone Receptor Content by Chemotherapy and/or Endocrine Therapy in Advanced Breast Cancer," *Cancer*, 1985, 55(3):546-51.
39. Brown M, "Estrogen Receptor Molecular Biology," *Hematol Oncol Clin North Am*, 1994, 8(1):101-12.

References

Allred DC, "Should Immunohistochemical Examination Replace Biochemical Hormone Receptor Assays in Breast Cancer?" *Am J Clin Pathol*, 1993, 99(1):1-3.

Battifora H, Mehta P, Ahn C, et al, "Estrogen Receptor Immunohistochemistry Assay in Paraffin-Embedded Tissue: A Better Gold Standard?" *Appl Immunohistochem*, 1993, 1(1):39-45.

Brown M, "Estrogen Receptor Molecular Biology," *Hematol Oncol Clin North Am*, 1994, 8(1):101-12.

Cohen C, Unger ER, Sgoutas D, et al, "Automated Immunohistochemical Estrogen Receptor in Fixed Embedded Breast Carcinomas - Comparison With Manual Immunohistochemistry on Frozen Tissues," *Am J Clin Pathol*, 1989, 92(5):669-72.

Harding M, Cowan S, Hole D, et al, "Estrogen and Progesterone Receptors in Ovarian Cancer," *Cancer*, 1990, 65(3):486-91.

Horwitz KB, "Hormone-Resistant Breast Cancer or "Feeding the Hand That Bites You"," *Prog Clin Biol Res*, 1994, 387:29-45.

Kiang DT, "The Presence of Steroid Receptors in "Nontarget" Tissues and Its Significance," *Am J Clin Pathol*, 1993, 99(2):120-2.

Masood S, "Prognostic and Diagnostic Implications of Estrogen and Progesterone Receptor Assays in Cytology," *Diagn Cytopathol*, 1994, 10(3):263-7.

Masood S, "Use of Monoclonal Antibody for Assessment of Estrogen Receptor Content in Fine-Needle Aspiration Biopsy Specimen From Patients With Breast Cancer," *Arch Pathol Lab Med*, 1989, 113(1):26-30.

Menendez-Botet CJ and Schwartz MK, "Estrogen and Progesterone Receptor Proteins in Patients With Breast Cancer," *Adv Clin Chem*, 1993, 30:185-225.

Pierce VE Jr, Rives DA, Sisley JF, et al, "Estradiol and Progesterone Receptors in a Case of Fibromatosis of the Breast," *Arch Pathol Lab Med*, 1987, 111(9):870-2.

Tavassoli FA, *Pathology of the Breast*, Norwalk, CT: Appleton & Lange, 1992.

Tesch M, Shawwa A, and Henderson R, "Immunohistochemical Determination of Estrogen and Progesterone Receptor Status in Breast Cancer," *Am J Clin Pathol*, 1993, 99(1):8-12.

Thornton JG and Wells M, "Oestrogen Receptor in Glands and Stroma of Normal and Neoplastic Human Endometrium: A Combined Biochemical, Immunohistochemical, and Morphometric Study," *J Clin Pathol*, 1987, 40(12):1437-42.

Winek RR, Jiang N-S, and Wold LE, "Estrogen and Progesterone Receptors in Benign Breast Tissue," *Am J Clin Pathol*, 1987, 88:526-7.

Wolf RM, Schneider SL, Pontes JE, et al, "Estrogen and Progestin Receptors in Human Prostatic Carcinoma," *Cancer*, 1985, 55(10):2477-81.

Estrogen Binding Protein ERICA *see* Estrogen and Progesterone Receptor Assay *on page 38*

Estrogen Binding Protein (Immunocytochemical) *see* Estrogen and Progesterone Receptor Assay *on page 38*

Ewing's Sarcoma *see* MIC2 *on page 52*

Factor VIII Related Antigen *see* Immunoperoxidase Procedures *on page 43*

Flow Cytometry *see* Immunophenotypic Analysis of Tissues by Flow Cytometry *on page 45*

Flow Cytometry *see* Breast Biopsy *on page 35*

Flow Cytometry of Tumor Aneuploidy *see* Tumor Aneuploidy by Flow Cytometry *on page 57*

Fluorescein-Tagged Antibodies *see* Kidney Biopsy *on page 47*

Fluorescence Activated Cell Sorting *see* Immunophenotypic Analysis of Tissues by Flow Cytometry *on page 45*

Frozen Section

CPT 88331 (single); 88332 (each additional)

Related Information

Breast Biopsy *on page 35*
Histopathology *on next page*
Lymph Node Biopsy *on page 50*
Virus, Direct Detection by Fluorescent Antibody *on page 682*

Synonyms FS; Intraoperative Consultation, Pathology; Pathology Operating Room Consultation; Surgical Pathology Consultation

Test Commonly Includes Gross examination, specimen evaluation, and possible frozen section with interpretation, followed by histopathology report. Imprints and smears may be made from fresh tissue. Further studies may be initiated depending on clinical input, gross observations, and frozen section and/or cytologic findings.

Abstract Provision of immediate intraoperative diagnosis when consultation is needed to enhance patient care. Intraoperative consultation may not require a frozen section at all. It is the pathologist's responsibility to do that which is in the best interest of the patient. Tissue freezing may actually be contraindicated. **When patient care is not enhanced, a frozen section is not indicated.** More sampling limitations and technical problems exist than are experienced with fixed, permanent sections.[1]

Patient Preparation Pertinent clinical history should be provided to the pathologist.

Specimen Fresh tissue with **no** added fixative or fluid, rapidly submitted in a sterile container

Container Sterile towel, Petri dish, or jar with appropriate attention to biohazard containment

Collection Container must be labeled with patient's name, date, operating room, and name of the surgeon requesting frozen section.

Causes for Rejection Specimen in fixative, bone. See Limitations and Contraindications.

Use Establish rapid histopathologic diagnosis of a pathologic process;[2] provision of rapid intraoperative diagnosis to support immediate intraoperative decisions.[3] The frozen section diagnosis should respond to a clear, unambiguous surgical question.[1] FS may be used to ascertain if cultures are indicated and, if so, to provide indication of the type of cultures needed; procure tissue for fat stains; procure tissue for direct immunofluorescent examination (eg, products of immune activation, viral antigens); rapid evaluation for direction of fresh tissues for possible subsequent special studies such as lymphocyte markers, flow cytometry, receptor assays, and/or electron microscopy. Determination of extent of disease may be accomplished with frozen sections in selected settings; for instance, evaluation of margins of surgical resection. An example may be given of pelvic lymph node examination prior to radical prostatectomy, one of the applications of frozen sections in which false-negatives from sampling errors occur. Surgeons sometimes request frozen sections to evaluate unanticipated findings (eg, a nodule in the liver).

Limitations Limitations are imposed by the type and size of tissue, intrinsic difficulties associated with certain types of diseases, and extent of examination required within a limited time frame. Bone or heavily

calcified tissue cannot be cut. Tissues dominated by fat are technically difficult and may not be amenable to frozen section. Fixed tissues are technically difficult to manage for frozen section. Small biopsies pose technical difficulties and may significantly compromise evaluation of corresponding permanent sections.

Some lesions require permanent sections for definitive diagnosis, such as many lymphoid lesions and occasional problematic breast lesions (eg, papillary lesions, instances of lobular and intraductal hyperplasias). Frozen sections are more useful to provide diagnosis of a visible lesion than to rule out a possibility of an entity of microscopic proportions such as lobular carcinoma *in situ* (LCIS). LCIS, in fact, usually should not be diagnosed on frozen section but only on good quality paraffin sections. The problems of frozen section for thyroid surgery include the differential diagnosis between instances of follicular adenoma versus carcinoma,[4] as well as identification of the occasional relatively small papillary carcinoma. Differential diagnosis between reactive gliosis and low grade glioma has been a problem for many experienced surgical pathologists and may continue to pose difficulties in high quality paraffin sections. In these setting, false-negative responses are more frequent than false-positive ones.

Sampling errors are important pitfalls in application of frozen sections.[3,5,6,7] Patients usually should not be kept anesthetized while multiple frozen section blocks are processed, cut, stained, and examined when paraffin sections would serve as well, or better.

Margins of specimens in resections for cancer may be a problem for which surgeons may request frozen section support. Negative margins in tumor resections may be of very limited value, especially when such margins are of substantial size, by virtue of sampling problems. Special problems in the breast are touched upon in the listing Breast Biopsy *on page 35*. The presence of fat, the geometry of multiple irregular surfaces in specimens, multiplicity of specimens in some cases, and time limitation while the patient remains under anesthesia all limit the significance of a negative frozen section report of margins. Absence of positive margins does not guarantee local control of the tumor, nor is it in any way a reliable guide to tumor behavior. Luna's head and neck series showed a relationship between **positive** margins and patient survival. If frozen section margins were positive, only 1 of 20 patients lived 2 years.[8]

False-negative frozen section diagnoses relate to the limited sampling possible within the abbreviated time available. Pathologists recognize the potential gravity of false-positive frozen section diagnosis of cancer. In some series, a zero incidence of false-positives is reported.[6] The poorest accuracy reported from George Washington University was associated with thyroid and parathyroid glands, related in the former to the ease with which microscopic foci of papillary carcinoma or the presence of capsular or vascular invasion can be missed.[5] Intraoperative consultation on diseases of the parathyroid glands may be challenging.[9] Silverberg wisely observes that those who publish results of frozen section examinations (false-positives, false-negatives, deferrals) are invariably those who have a great deal of experience with the technique.[10]

In addition to sampling errors, Luna recognizes three other types of errors: interpretive, communicative, and technical.[8] Misinterpretation as a cause of diagnostic error at the Mayo Clinic involved mostly false-negative errors, but false-positive errors occurred as well.[3] Lack of proper clinical information (eg, history of prior irradiation) can lead to interpretive error.

Reasons to defer diagnosis at frozen section include need for more extensive sampling, lack of adequate epithelium lining cysts, twisted and infarcted lesions,[6] and need for special stains, immunohistochemistry, and optimal sections. In some cases, diagnosis must be delayed for permanent sections. Silverberg acknowledges the need for deferral in some cases and recognizes that the frequency of false-positive diagnoses relates inversely to that of deferral of diagnosis.[5,10]

Contraindications Tissue is consumed in the process of frozen section. Tiny critical specimens (for example, possible breast carcinomas less than 5 mm in diameter) are best not risked. Breast specimens not grossly suspicious should not be frozen.[1] The freezing process may distort lymphoid as well as other tissues. Therefore, for suspected lymphoma, it is advisable to await proper fixation of the lymph node and paraffin sections for definitive diagnosis, but frozen sections are commonly utilized for immunohistochemical evaluation of lymphoid lesions. See listing Lymph Node Biopsy *on page 50* for further details. Frozen section artifact in paraffin sections subsequently processed may preclude definitive diagnosis. If frozen section diagnosis is unnecessary for immediate patient management, Silverberg[10] and many others[7] recognize that it should not be performed. Silverberg comments on the role of the frozen section in provision of instant gratification to the surgeon, observing that charges are made and that information should be of value in patient management. Frozen sections are considered contraindicated when the patient is known to be HIV positive, to avoid contamination of the cryostat.[5] In such instances, imprints and smears (Continued)

Frozen Section *(Continued)*

can sometimes replace frozen sections.[11] Luna and others include small melanocytic lesions among contraindications to frozen section.[8,11]

Methodology Freezing tissues in liquid nitrogen is better and faster than carbon dioxide. A vacuum bottle containing liquid nitrogen may be kept in the frozen section room. A slice of the specimen on an object holder, placed onto O.C.T.® compound, is lowered into the vacuum bottle with a metal clamp. Cryobaths with a refrigerant such as 2-methyl butane chilled to -70°C also give satisfactory results. Rapid H & E stains are commonly used. Some cases are adequately evaluated with a single rapid supravital dye such as toluidine blue.

Additional Information Direct communication between pathologist and surgeon must occur at the time of frozen section diagnosis, according to requirements both of regulatory agencies and of good patient care. **Imprints** may be stained with H & E, Wright's stain, or by other methods. They sometimes are extremely helpful in interpretation of frozen sections. Occasionally, imprints are more diagnostic than the frozen section. They are especially helpful with lymphoid specimens, occasional breast specimens, and in diagnosis of meningioma.

Footnotes

1. Page DL and Gray GF Jr, "Intraoperative Consultations by Pathologists at the Mayo Clinic: A Unique Experience," *Mayo Clin Proc*, 1995, 70(12):1222-3.
2. Sawady J, Berner JJ, and Siegler EE, "Accuracy of and Reasons for Frozen Sections: A Correlative, Retrospective Study," *Hum Pathol*, 1988, 19(9):1019-23.
3. Ferreiro JA, Myers JL, and Bostwick DG, "Accuracy of Frozen Section Diagnosis in Surgical Pathology: Review of a 1-Year Experience With 24,880 Cases at Mayo Clinic Rochester," *Mayo Clin Proc*, 1995, 70(12):1137-41.
4. Shaha A, Gleich L, DiMaio T, et al, "Accuracy and Pitfalls of Frozen Section During Thyroid Surgery," *J Surg Oncol*, 1990, 44(2):84-92.
5. Oneson RH, Minke JA, and Silverberg SG, "Intraoperative Pathologic Consultation. An Audit of 1000 Recent Consecutive Cases," *Am J Surg Pathol*, 1989, 13(3):237-43.
6. Obiakor I, Maiman M, Mittal K, et al, "The Accuracy of Frozen Section in the Diagnosis of Ovarian Neoplasms," *Gynecol Oncol*, 1991, 43(1):61-3.
7. Prey MU, Vitale T, and Martin SA, "Guidelines for Practical Utilization of Intraoperative Frozen Sections," *Arch Surg*, 1989, 124(3):331-5.
8. Luna MA, "Uses, Abuses, and Pitfalls of Frozen Section Diagnoses of Diseases of the Head and Neck," *Surgical Pathology of the Head and Neck*, Vol 1, Barnes L, ed, New York, NY: Marcel Dekker Inc, 1985, 7-22.
9. LiVolsi VA and Hamilton R, "Intraoperative Assessment of Parathyroid Gland Pathology. A Common View From the Surgeon and the Pathologist," *Am J Clin Pathol*, 1994, 102(3):365-73.
10. Silverberg SG, *Principles and Practice of Surgical Pathology*, 2nd ed, Vol 1, Chapter 1, New York, NY: Churchill Livingstone, 1990, 1-12.
11. Reyes MG, Homsi MF, McDonald LW, et al, "Imprints, Smears, and Frozen Sections of Brain Tumors," *Neurosurgery*, 1991, 29(4):575-9.

References

Fechner RE, "Frozen Section (Intraoperative Consultation)," *Hum Pathol*, 1988, 19(9):999-1000.

Gephardt GN and Rice TW, "Utility of Frozen-Section Evaluation of Lymph Nodes in the Staging of Bronchogenic Carcinoma at Mediastinoscopy and Thoracotomy," *J Thorac Cardiovasc Surg*, 1990, 100(6):853-9.

Silva EG and Kraemer BB, *Intraoperative Pathologic Diagnosis: Frozen Sections and Other Techniques*, Baltimore, MD: Williams & Wilkins, 1987.

Zarbo RJ, Hoffman GG, and Howanitz PJ, "Interinstitutional Comparison of Frozen-Section Consultation. A College of American Pathologists Q-Probe Study of 79,647 Consultations in 297 North American Institutions," *Arch Pathol Lab Med*, 1991, 115(12):1187-94.

FS *see* Frozen Section *on previous page*

G₁ Phase *see* Tumor Aneuploidy by Flow Cytometry *on page 57*

G₂M *see* Tumor Aneuploidy by Flow Cytometry *on page 57*

GCDFP-15 *see* Immunoperoxidase Procedures *on next page*

Glial Fibrillary Acidic Protein *see* Immunoperoxidase Procedures *on next page*

G₀ Phase *see* Tumor Aneuploidy by Flow Cytometry *on page 57*

Grocott's-Methanamine Silver Stain *see* Skin Biopsy *on page 54*

Gross and Microscopic Pathology *see* Histopathology *on this page*

Gross Cystic Disease Fluid Protein-15 *see* Immunoperoxidase Procedures *on next page*

Gross Cystic Disease Fluid Protein-15 (GCDFP-15) *see* Breast Biopsy *on page 35*

hCG *see* Immunoperoxidase Procedures *on next page*

β-hCG *see* Immunoperoxidase Procedures *on next page*

HER-2/neu *see* Breast Biopsy *on page 35*

Histopathology

CPT 88300 (level I - surgical pathology, gross examination only); 88302 (level II - surgical pathology, gross and microscopic examination of presumptively normal tissue(s) for identification and record purposes); 88304 (level III - surgical pathology, gross and microscopic examination of presumptively abnormal tissue(s) uncomplicated specimen); 88305 (level IV - single complicated or multiple uncomplicated specimens without complex dissection); 88307 (level V - single complicated specimen requiring complex dissection or multiple complicated specimens); 88309 (level VI - complex diagnostic problems with or without extensive dissection)

Related Information

Aluminum, Bone *on page 586*

Bacterial Culture, Biopsy or Body Fluid *on page 456*

Breast Biopsy *on page 35*

Chromosome Analysis, Lymph Node and Solid Tumor *on page 279*

Chromosome *In Situ* Hybridization *on page 281*

Electron Microscopic Examination for Viruses, Stool *on page 665*

Estrogen and Progesterone Receptor Assay *on page 38*

Fine Needle Aspiration, Superficial Palpable Masses *on page 294*

Frozen Section *on previous page*

Fungal Culture, Biopsy or Body Fluid *on page 476*

Gene Rearrangement for Leukemia and Lymphoma *on page 512*

Human Papillomavirus DNA Probe Test *on page 516*

Immunophenotypic Analysis of Tissues by Flow Cytometry *on page 45*

Liver Biopsy *on page 48*

Lymph Node Biopsy *on page 50*

Mantle Cell Lymphoma *on page 51*

MIC2 *on page 52*

Muscle Biopsy *on page 53*

Mycobacterial Culture, Biopsy or Body Fluid *on page 487*

N-*myc* Amplification *on page 522*

p53, Functional Assay/Sequencing *on page 522*

Retinoblastoma Gene DNA Detection *on page 524*

Skin Biopsy *on page 54*

Tumor Aneuploidy by Flow Cytometry *on page 57*

Viral Culture *on page 675*

Viral Culture, Tissue *on page 680*

Virus, Direct Detection by Fluorescent Antibody *on page 682*

Synonyms Biopsy; Gross and Microscopic Pathology; Pathologic Examination; Surgical Pathology; Tissue Examination

Applies to Bronchial Biopsy; Endoscopic Biopsy; Lung Biopsy; Medical Legal Specimens

Test Commonly Includes Gross and microscopic examination and diagnosis. Imprints may be made if the tissue is fresh and unfixed and if indications for imprints exist.

Abstract Surgical pathology has been defined as the discipline which deals with the anatomic pathology of tissues removed from living patients.[1] Smears, aspirates, special stains, immunocytochemistry, flow cytometry, and molecular pathology may be included.

Patient Preparation It is essential that each specimen be accompanied by an adequate description of what it is thought to represent, as well as an appropriate clinical history.[1]

Specimen Fresh tissue, tissue fixed in phosphate-buffered formalin or other appropriate fixative. Each specimen container must be labeled to include source as well as patient's name. Each specimen from a different anatomic site must be placed in a separate, correctly labeled container, designated "left," "right," "proximal," "distal," "ventral," "dorsal," and so forth.

Container Jars of assorted sizes, containing formalin or another appropriate fixative; the neck of the container should not be smaller than its diameter. Fresh specimens should be submitted on a sterile gauze pad moistened with sterile saline and should not be left on countertops; they must be placed in the hands of a responsible person.

Collection Small biopsy specimens are to be placed immediately in fixative, unless special needs such as frozen section exist. Use approximately 5 to 20 times as much fixative solution as the bulk of the tissue. Small tissues such as those from bronchoscopic biopsy, bladder biopsy, and endometrium can be ruined in a very short time by drying out.

Storage Instructions Fixation in formalin solution or other appropriate fixative

Causes for Rejection Mislabeled specimen container, unlabeled specimen

Turnaround Time Biopsy reports commonly require a day or more. Delays are caused by need for clinical information, deeper sections, decalcification, or special stains.

Special Instructions See specific handling instructions in test listings such as Muscle Biopsy *on page 53*, Estrogen and Progesterone Receptor Assay *on page 38*, Frozen Section *on page 41*, Kidney Biopsy *on page 47*, and Liver Biopsy *on page 48*. Consult the Pathology Department prior to beginning the procedure for specific instructions. Requisition should state operative diagnosis and source of specimen, as well as patient's name, age, sex, room or location, name of surgeon, and names of other physicians who will need a copy of the pathology report.

Use Histopathologic diagnosis; evaluate extent of lesions and provision of classification and, when appropriate, grading in the case of tumors

Limitations Tissue fixed in formalin **cannot** be used for microbial culture, chemical estrogen or progesterone receptor assay, certain types of histochemistry, frozen sections, gene rearrangement, or optimal electron microscopy.

Additional Information A major advantage of conventional over frozen sections is that extensive sampling of the entire specimen can take place.

Cultures of tissue are best taken in the O.R., where a sterile field exists. A piece of tissue (eg, a curetting of a fistulous tract) should be placed in an appropriate sterile tube with requests for smear, culture, anaerobic culture, AFB, and fungus culture if appropriate. It should be immediately taken to the Microbiology Laboratory. See Microbiology listings.

Routine tissues are brought in fixative. Fixatives should be picked up prior to the biopsy. Commonly used fixatives include modified Zenker's fluid (for tiny specimens, eg, endometrial curettage, liver, and other needle biopsies, **not** skin), and formalin (for specimens thicker than 3 mm).

Bullets, shotgun pellets, and other metallic objects require special handling, but no fixative is needed. Of major importance in handling bullets and other specimens of possible forensic significance, including vaginal swabs obtained in rape cases, is the scrupulous maintenance of a chain-of-custody. Specimens must be accurately labeled, and transfer and receipt must be documented. Specimens must be kept under safeguards in the laboratory until turned over to law enforcement officials. See listing Chain-of-Custody Protocol *on page 542.*

Bone biopsy for metabolic bone disease requires special handling.

Materials sometimes not sent for histopathologic examination, depending on the institution, include bullets, shotgun pellets, neonatal foreskins, grossly unremarkable placentas from uneventful deliveries, and orthopedic appliances. If a specimen is not sent to the Pathology Department, the surgeon should carefully describe the specimen in the operative report.

Footnotes
1. Silverberg SG, *Principles and Practice of Surgical Pathology,* 2nd ed, Vol 1, Chapter 1, New York, NY: Churchill Livingstone, 1990, 1-12.

References
Coulson WF, *Surgical Pathology,* 2nd ed, Vols 1 and 2, Philadelphia, PA: JB Lippincott Co, 1988.
Sternberg SS, Antonioli DA, Carter D, et al, *Diagnostic Surgical Pathology,* Vol 1 and 2, New York, NY: Raven Press, 1989.

HMB-45 *see* Immunoperoxidase Procedures *on this page*

Image Analysis
CPT 88399
Related Information
Estrogen and Progesterone Receptor Assay *on page 38*
Fine Needle Aspiration, Superficial Palpable Masses *on page 294*
Tumor Aneuploidy by Flow Cytometry *on page 57*

Synonyms Automated Cytophotometry; Computerized Interactive Morphometry; Image Morphometry; Static Image Analysis

Applies to DNA in Tumor Nuclei; Immunocytochemistry; Ploidy; S Phase

Test Commonly Includes Use of computerized imaging system to contribute information which may be useful in determination of prognostic and therapeutic factors of tumors. Such factors may include quantitation, tumor ploidy, DNA content, oncogene protein content, hormone receptor expression and cellular proliferative proteins.

Abstract This is a means of quantifying microscopic images by digital conversion and computer analysis.[1] Affordable memory devices with microprocessors and quality cameras make image processing and statistical image analysis practical. The system can selectively measure a neoplastic cell population.[2] Such information from optical physics and engineering appears in pathology journals.[3,4,5,6,7]

Specimen Fresh tissue is the best specimen; 1 cm^2 or less fresh tumor tissue or 1 mL body fluid for concentration by cytospin. Freshly excised tumor made into "touch preps" (tissue touched or spotted lightly on glass slides that allow for release of cells from the connective tissue framework to the slide) allow best separation of cells. Frozen section slides and paraffin sections may also be used. Exfoliative cytology specimens and body fluids, concentrated or unconcentrated, may be used.

Turnaround Time 2-5 days are needed to prepare the specimen, stain it appropriately, evaluate the cells, interpret the results, and produce a report. Turnaround time may vary with individual laboratories, depending on technical assistance available. Only large hospitals and medical centers may have the equipment and expertise at the time of this writing.

Reference Range For DNA index, normal is 0.8-1.2 or the diploid state. Normal proliferation index (Ki-67 positivity of tumor cells) is <10%; S phase should be <7%.

Use Image analysis is an emerging method which is used to evaluate tumor aggressiveness and patient prognosis. The concept of image analysis holds that the further dedifferentiated a tumor becomes, the further it deviates from the normal diploid state. This may be expressed as a tetraploid or aneuploid state according to the amount of DNA in the Feulgen-stained nuclei. In terms of ploidy, this is expressed as a DNA index between 1.0 and 2.0. The amount of cells in the S phase of the cell cycle is also a parameter that can be measured by image analysis. In general, the more cells in S phase (DNA synthesis phase), the more aggressive the tumor.

Image analysis, in combination with immunohistochemistry, may be used to study antigens expressed by tumor cells that are important in cancer prognosis. Estrogen and progesterone receptors[5] may be semi-quantitated with immunochemical staining of breast cancer cells with subsequent study by image analysis. Other proteins such as HER-2/neu, Ki-67, and proliferative antigen have been developed for better prognostication of tumors from many sources. Recently, for instance, even gene suppressor products have been found to be helpful in evaluation of tumors of the thyroid.[6]

Limitations While flow cytometry assays 10,000-20,000 or more nuclei, in image analysis only a few hundred nuclei are counted.[7] Image analysis is labor intensive. Equipment is not inexpensive.

Methodology Essentially, a computer is used to analyze digitized microscopic images. Reproducibility can be achieved with presently available equipment. Commercial systems are available and personally compiled systems are described.[3]

Additional Information Analysis can be restricted to counting only cells of interest (eg, keratin-positive cells in instances of epithelial tumors).[7]

Footnotes
1. Sebo TJ, "Digital Image Analysis," *Mayo Clin Proc,* 1995, 70(1):81-2.
2. Geradts J and McLendon WW, "Pathology and Laboratory Medicine," *JAMA,* 1994, 271(21):1700-1.
3. Wells WA, Rainer RO, and Memoli VA, "Basic Principles of Image Processing," *Am J Clin Pathol,* 1992, 98(5):493-501.
4. Wells WA, Rainer RO, and Memoli VA, "Equipment, Standardization, and Applications of Image Processing," *Am J Clin Pathol,* 1993, 99(1):48-56.
5. El-Badawy N, Cohen C, Derose PB, et al, "Immunohistochemical Progesterone Receptor Assay, Measurement by Image Analysis," *Am J Clin Pathol,* 1991, 96(6):704-10.
6. Figge J, Bakst G, Weisheit D, et al, "Image Analysis Quantitation of Immunoreactive Retinoblastoma Protein in Human Thyroid Neoplasms With a Streptavidin-Biotin-Peroxidase Staining Technique," *Am J Pathol,* 1991, 139(6):1213-9.
7. Robinson RA, "Defining the Limits of DNA Cytometry," *Am J Clin Pathol,* 1992, 98(3):275-7.

References
Bosari S, Wiley BD, Hamilton WM, et al, "DNA Measurement by Image Analysis of Paraffin-Embedded Breast Carcinoma Tissue - A Comparative Investigation," *Am J Clin Pathol,* 1991, 96(6):698-703.
Elsheikh TM, Silverman JF, McCool JW, et al, "Comparative DNA Analysis of Solid Tumors by Flow Cytometric and Image Analyses of Touch Imprints and Flow Cell Suspensions," *Am J Clin Pathol,* 1992, 98(3):296-304.
Marchevsky AM and Bartels PH, *Image Analysis. A Primer for Pathologists,* New York, NY: Raven Press, 1994.
Martin-Reay DG, Kamentsky LA, Weinberg DS, et al, "Evaluation of a New Slide-Based Laser Scanning Cytometer for DNA Analysis of Tumors. Comparison With Flow Cytometry and Image Analysis," *Am J Clin Pathol,* 1994, 102(4):432-8.
Salmon I and Kiss R, "Relationship Between Proliferative Activity and Ploidy Level in a Series of 530 Human Brain Tumors, Including Astrocytomas, Meningiomas, Schwannomas, and Metastases," *Hum Pathol,* 1993, 24(3):329-35.

Image Morphometry *see* Image Analysis *on this page*

Immunocytochemistry *see* Immunoperoxidase Procedures *on this page*

Immunocytochemistry *see* Image Analysis *on this page*

Immunofluorescence *see* Immunoperoxidase Procedures *on this page*

Immunofluorescence Skin Biopsy *see* Skin Biopsy, Immunofluorescence *on page 56*

Immunohistochemistry *see* Immunoperoxidase Procedures *on this page*

Immunomicroscopy *see* Immunoperoxidase Procedures *on this page*

Immunoperoxidase Procedures
CPT 88342
Related Information
Body Fluid Cytology *on page 286*
Breast Biopsy *on page 35*
CA 19-9 *on page 93*
CA 125 *on page 94*
Calcitonin *on page 96*
(Continued)

Immunoperoxidase Procedures (*Continued*)

Synonyms Immunocytochemistry; Immunohistochemistry; Immunomicroscopy; Immunostains; Peroxidase-Antiperoxidase (PAP)

Applies to Alpha Fetoprotein; Chromogranin; Cytokeratins; Desmin; Epithelial Membrane Antigen (EMA); Factor VIII Related Antigen; GCDFP-15; Glial Fibrillary Acidic Protein; Gross Cystic Disease Fluid Protein-15; hCG; β-hCG; HMB-45; Immunofluorescence; *In Situ* Hybridization; Intermediate Filaments; Kappa Light Chains; Ki-67; Lambda Light Chains; Lectins; Leukocyte Common Antigen; Leu M1; Light Chains; Lysozyme; Monoclonal Immunoglobulins; Myoglobin; Myosin; PCNA; Peptide Hormones; Prostate Specific Acid Phosphatase; S100; Synaptophysin; Thyroglobulin; Tissue Antigens; T Lymphocytes; Vimentin

Test Commonly Includes Antigen localization in tissue sections

Abstract Immunocytochemistry is a major diagnostic tool employed in surgical pathology, cytopathology, immunopathology, and hematopathology. Evaluation of tumor with unknown primary site is often expedited by immunocytochemical investigation.

Specimen Blood, bone marrow, or cytology smears; paraffin, plastic or frozen sections; fresh tissue remains important for work-up of possible lymphoma

Container Petri dish ideally containing fresh tissue, immediately delivered to optimize choice of fixatives and to permit the laboratory to snap freeze tissue if indicated.

Storage Instructions Deliver fresh specimens, not in fixative.

Causes for Rejection Extensive drying of specimen, very extensive necrosis, tissue left unfixed or unrefrigerated for prolonged periods

Special Instructions Place fresh specimen in the hands of a histotechnician or pathologist.

Use Immunoperoxidase techniques are used to identify and localize antigens in tissue sections. The results allow pathologists to determine the major lineage of poorly differentiated neoplasms, sometimes distinguish benign from malignant lymphoid proliferations, subclassify lymphoreticular and hematopoietic neoplasms, document elaboration of tumor-associated markers of potential use in monitoring the course of disease, and identify or confirm the presence of infectious agents. Information on oncogene expression has shed insights on molecular mechanisms of tumor biology and offers tools of potential prognostic significance.[1]

Perhaps the most common application is the investigation of the cellular lineage of poorly differentiated neoplasms based on the phenotypic profile of the tumor. This is most reliably done by the use of a panel of immunostains performed simultaneously to provide complementary positive and negative results. In some situations, the use of overly restricted panels may lead to false interpretation of results (ie, S100 positive carcinomas, as in breast). Examples of common applications are shown in Table 1.

Cancer-specific antibodies are not yet commercially available, but the potential is highlighted by the antibody HMB-45 for melanoma.[2] Antibodies to oncofetal antigens such as carcinoembryonic antigen (CEA) or the B72.3 antigen are selectively expressed by carcinomas but are not tissue specific.[3] The detection of tissue-specific antigens may establish the site of origin of a metastatic neoplasm, such as prostate specific antigen (PSA) and prostate specific acid phosphatase (PSAP) for prostatic adenocarcinoma or thyroglobulin for thyroid carcinoma. Gross cystic disease fluid protein (GCDFP-15) has proven useful in confirming carcinoma of breast origin.[4,5] In selected settings, the cytokeratin profile may narrow the differential diagnosis to choices which can be more readily established on a clinical basis.[6,7] Antigens which may be detected in tissues and monitored by serological studies to reflect tumor burden include CEA in carcinoma, monoclonal immunoglobulins in plasma cell dyscrasias, and some lymphomas, α-fetoprotein and β-hCG for certain types of germ cell tumors, and peptide hormones in neuroendocrine malignancies. The utility of immunostains in the evaluation of lymphoreticular and hematopoietic neoplasms is discussed in the test

listing Lymph Node Biopsy *on page 50*. Type and subtype specific antibodies allow detection and classification of viruses and other infectious agents such as cytomegalovirus and herpes virus. Markers such as progesterone receptor, c-erb-B2 (HER-2/neu), and epithelial growth factor receptor may prove useful prognostic markers in breast cancer while estrogen receptor expression has both prognostic and therapeutic implications.[1] Proliferation markers such as Ki-67 and proliferation-associated nuclear antigen (PCNA) are useful prognostic markers for a variety of tumors.[8]

Limitations Deficient basic histology. Unknown or undesirable cross reactivities of different antibodies. The need for utilization of different fixatives to optimally preserve the broadest range of antigens of interest for a particular case. The intrinsic variability of antigen expression owing to the neoplastic state. Variable specificity and sensitivity of different staining procedures owing to differences in commercial sources of primary antibodies, detection systems, incubation conditions, and modifications adapted to suit the needs of individual laboratories. Relative lack of quality assurance programs. Limited number of technical personnel are adept in a broad range of immunohistochemistry procedures. Expense is substantial relative to conventional special stains. Several semiautomated and automated instruments may help circumvent many of these intrinsic limitations but cost remains significant.

Methodology There are many modifications based on the following theme (see figure):

- Intrinsic tissue enzyme activity is blocked.
- The primary antibody, which conveys the specificity of the stain, is applied to tissue sections, incubated, and unbound antibody is washed free.
- An enzyme-linked detection system specific for the primary antibody is applied to the tissues, incubated, and unbound reagents washed free.
- A substrate for the enzyme detection system is incubated, producing an insoluble product which can be visualized by light microscopy.

Primary antibodies of diagnostic importance are available from a variety of commercial sources, as monoclonal antibodies derived from mouse or rat, and polyclonal antibodies usually derived from rabbits or goats. Most commercial systems employ a second antibody with specificity for the primary antibody to serve as a link to the enzyme. The two most common detection methods are the peroxidase-antiperoxidase (PAP) technique or the biotin-avidin technique, to specifically introduce the enzyme into the complex. See figure.

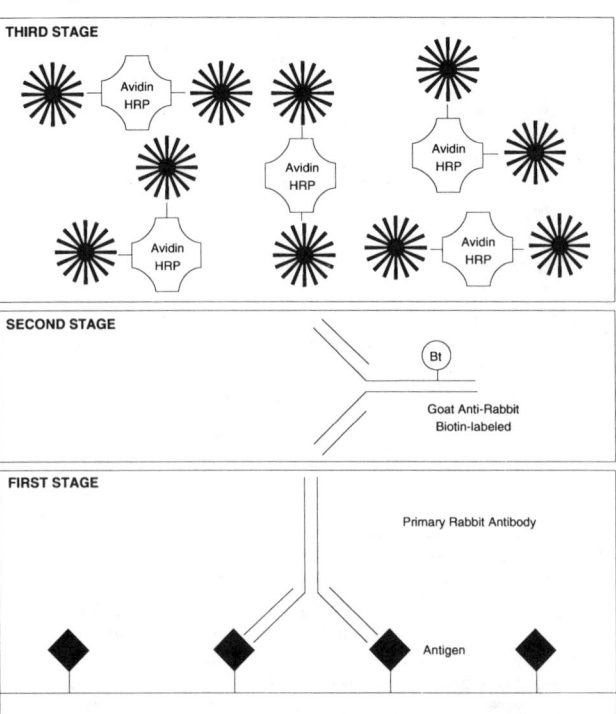

General scheme for performing immunoperoxidase stains: Tissue sections are deparaffinized and blocked to suppress endogenous peroxidase activity and nonspecific protein binding. For some stains (eg, cytokeratin), antigenic determinants are unmasked by protease digestion or microwave techniques. The first stage, incubation with the primary antibody, confers the specificity of the stain. The second stage antibody is covalently labeled with biotin for which avidin has an extraordinarily high affinity. Horse radish peroxidase (HRP) may be covalently coupled to avidin and after incubation with an appropriate substrate, antigens are localized.

Table 1. Characteristic Phenotypic Profile of Neoplasms Based on Histogenesis*

| | Intermediate Filaments | | | | | Chromgrn | NSE | EMA | S100 | LCA | Muscle Actin | A₁ ACT |
	Cytokeratin	Vimentin	Desmin	NF	GFAP							
Carcinoma, NOS†	+	-/+	-	-	-	-	-/+	+	-/+	-	-	-/+
neuroendocrine§	+/-	-/+	-	-/+	-	+	+	+/-	-	-	-	-
Lymphoma#	-	-/+	-	-	-	-	-/+	-	-	+	-	-
Melanoma•	-	+	-	-	-	-	+/-	-	+	-	-	-/+
Soft tissue tumors												
fibrous histiocytoma	-	+	-	-	-	-	-	-	-	-	-/+	+
nerve sheath	-	+	-	-	-	-	-	-	-	-	-	-
muscle	-	+	+	-	-	-	-	-	-	-	+	-
vascular**	-	+	-	-	-	-	-	-	-	-	-	-
Glioma	-	+	-	-	+	-	-	-	+	-	-	-

Abbreviations: NF: neurofilament; GFAP: glial fibrillary acidic protein; Chromgrn: chromogranin A; NSE: neuron-specific enolase; EMA: epithelial membrane antigen; LCA: leukocyte common antigen; A₁ ACT: alpha₁-antichymotrypsin. Designated reactions: +: characteristically positive; +/-: characteristically positive but may be negative; -/+: characteristically negative but may be positive; -: characteristically negative.

Footnotes:

*There are many exceptions to the indicated reactions. The phenotypic profile must always be put into perspective with the light microscopy and other special studies.

†Cytokeratin profile, coexpression of S100 or other tissue specific markers may help identify origin of metastatic carcinoma.

§Expression of various peptide hormones may further aid in the clinicopathologic classification of the neoplasm.

#For additional information, see listing on Lymph Node Biopsy and Immunophenotypic Analysis of Tissues by Flow Cytometry.

•Melanoma associated antigen HMB-45 may help differentiate it from some nerve sheath tumors.

**Many vascular tumors are also positive for factor VIII-related antigen, for the lectin UEA-1, CD31, and CD34.

Specificity and sensitivity of the primary antibody and the detection system should always be verified by testing on a limited library of tissues, which include known positives and negatives. When validated for diagnostic testing, careful attention must be continuously rendered to appropriately fixed control tissues and to internal controls which may be present in the test tissues. A valid positive immunostain will have a clean background and discrete reaction. A negative reaction is equally valid if properly controlled and if it complements a positive reaction for another mutually exclusive antigen. The use of antigen retrieval systems has greatly improved the reliability of immunostains in routinely processed tissues. These methods often employ the use of microwave radiation in citrate buffers.[9]

Additional Information Immunofluorescent procedures address similar issues but require a relatively expensive fluorescence microscope, are less sensitive, lack the resolution afforded by light microscopy, and do not produce an archivable slide. However, immunofluorescence is the method of choice for the localization of immunoglobulins, complement, and fibrin in the evaluation of renal biopsies and inflammatory dermatoses. Lectins, plant proteins with specificity for given carbohydrate moieties, are useful for antigen localization and can be used much like a primary antibody. More recently, *in situ* **hybridization** has been employed to identify nucleic acid sequences in cells. Using techniques generally similar to immunoperoxidase stains, biotin-labeled, genetically-engineered sequences of nucleic acids are used to localize viruses or oncogenes of potential pathologic significance.

Footnotes

1. Elledge RM, McGuire WL, and Osborne CK, "Prognostic Factors in Breast Cancer," *Semin Oncol*, 1992, 19(3):244-53.
2. Gown AM, Vogel AM, Hoak D, et al, "Monoclonal Antibodies Specific for Melanocytic Tumors Distinguish Subpopulations of Melanocytes," *Am J Pathol*, 1986, 123(2):195-203.
3. Esteban JM, Paxton R, Mehta P, et al, "Sensitivity and Specificity of Gold Types 1 to 5 Anticarcinoembryonic Antigen Monoclonal Antibodies: Immunohistologic Characterization in Colorectal Cancer and Normal Tissues," *Hum Pathol*, 1993, 24(3):322-8.
4. Mazoujian G, Parish TH, and Haagensen DE Jr, "Immunoperoxidase Localization of GCDFP-15 With Mouse Monoclonal Antibodies Versus Rabbit Antiserum," *J Histochem Cytochem*, 1988, 36(4):377-82.
5. Wick MR, Lilemoe TJ, Copland GT, et al, "Gross Cystic Disease Fluid Protein-15 as a Marker for Breast Cancer: Immunohistochemical Analysis of 690 Human Neoplasms and Comparison with Alpha-Lactalbumin," *Hum Pathol*, 1989, 20(3):281-7.
6. Cooper D, Schermer A, and Sun TT, "Classification of Human Epithelia and Their Neoplasms Using Monoclonal Antibodies to Keratins: Strategies, Applications, and Limitations," *Lab Invest*, 1985, 52(3):243-56.
7. Kahn HJ, Thorner PS, Yeger H, et al, "Distinct Keratin Patterns Demonstrated by Immunoperoxidase Staining of Adenocarcinomas, Carcinoids, and Mesotheliomas Using Polyclonal and Monoclonal Antikeratin Antibodies," *Am J Clin Pathol*, 1986, 86(5):566-74.
8. Riley RS, "Cellular Proliferation Markers in the Evaluation of Human Cancer," *Clin Lab Med*, 1992, 12(2):163-99.
9. Gown AM, deWever N, and Battifora H, "Microwave-Based Antigenic Unmasking. A Revolutionary New Technique for Routine Immunohistochemistry," *Appl Immunohistochem*, 1993, 1(4):256-66.

References

Battifora H, "Clinical Applications of Immunohistochemistry of Filamentous Proteins," *Am J Surg Pathol*, 1988, 12(Suppl 1):24-42.

Colvin RB, Bhan AK, and McCluskey RT, *Diagnostic Immunopathology*, 2nd ed, New York, NY: Raven Press, 1995.

De Lellis RA and Kwan P, "Technical Considerations in the Immunohistochemical Demonstration of Intermediate Filaments," *Am J Surg Pathol*, 1988, 12(Suppl 1):17-23.

Grogan TM, Casey TT, Miller PC, et al, "Automation of Immunohistochemistry," *Advances in Pathology and Laboratory Medicine*, Vol 6, St Louis, MO: CV Mosby Co, 1993, 253-83.

Nagle RB, "Intermediate Filaments: A Review of the Basic Biology," *Am J Surg Pathol*, 1988, 12(Suppl 1):4-16.

Swanson PE, "Foundations of Immunohistochemistry," *Am J Clin Pathol*, 1988, 90(3):333-9.

Wolfe HJ, "DNA Probes in Diagnostic Pathology," *Am J Clin Pathol*, 1988, 90(3):340-4.

Immunophenotypic Analysis of Tissues by Flow Cytometry

CPT 88180 (each cell surface marker); 88182 (cell cycle or DNA analysis)

Related Information

Body Fluid Cytology on page 286
Breast Biopsy on page 35
Cerebrospinal Fluid Cytology on page 290
Chromosome Analysis, Lymph Node and Solid Tumor on page 279
Estrogen and Progesterone Receptor Assay on page 38
Fine Needle Aspiration, Deep Seated Lesions on page 294
Fine Needle Aspiration, Superficial Palpable Masses on page 294
Gene Rearrangement for Leukemia and Lymphoma on page 512
Histopathology on page 42
Immunoperoxidase Procedures on page 43
Leukocyte Immunophenotyping on page 414
Lymph Node Biopsy on page 50
Mantle Cell Lymphoma on page 51
MIC2 on page 52
Terminal Deoxynucleotidyl Transferase on page 349
Tumor Aneuploidy by Flow Cytometry on page 57

Synonyms Flow Cytometry; Fluorescence Activated Cell Sorting; Lymphocyte Immunophenotyping

Applies to B-Lymphocyte Analysis by Flow Cytometry; DNA Ploidy Studies; Kappa Light Chain Analysis by Flow Cytometry; Lambda Light Chain Analysis by Flow Cytometry; Leukemia Analysis by Flow Cytometry; Light Chain Analysis by Flow Cytometry; Lymphocyte Analysis by Flow Cytometry; Lymphocyte Markers; Lymphoma Analysis by Flow Cytometry; Solid Tumors Analysis by Flow Cytometry; T-Lymphocyte Analysis by Flow Cytometry

Abstract Flow cytometry provides important immunophenotypic and DNA cycle information of both diagnostic and prognostic interest in hematopathology, cytopathology, and general surgical pathology.

Specimen Fresh tissues, fresh frozen tissues, body fluids; formalin-fixed paraffin-embedded tissue may be used for DNA studies

Container Fresh tissues are best submitted in a Petri dish, test tube, or jar containing saline or tissue culture media. Frozen tissue submitted for DNA ploidy studies should not be embedded in O.C.T.®

Storage Instructions Fresh tissues submitted for immunophenotypic studies are sufficiently stable to be transported by overnight courier on ice pack to a reference laboratory. Frozen tissue submitted for DNA ploidy studies should be maintained frozen during transport to a reference laboratory.

Reference Range Flow cytometry provides immunophenotypic data and/or DNA cell cycle data, depending on the desired information and (Continued)

Immunophenotypic Analysis of Tissues by Flow Cytometry *(Continued)*

processing methodologies. More information on DNA cell cycle studies is available in the listing Tumor Aneuploidy by Flow Cytometry *on page 57*. Immunophenotypic studies are most useful in evaluation of hematologic or lymphoid tissues. Individual cell populations may be selected based on size or antigen expression to minimize preparatory steps. For example, information relating to cell size (forward light scatter) and internal complexity (90° light scatter) can be used to evaluate a population of interest. In a lymph node containing small and large lymphoid cells, independent analysis may show a reactive population of small T cells and a monoclonal population of large B cells. Flow cytometry is not well suited for evaluation of nonhematopoietic neoplasms, but lack of CD45 (leukocyte common antigen) expression on a cellular population should be regarded as suspicious for involvement by another process.

Approximately 80% of non-Hodgkin's lymphomas are derived from monoclonal B cells. Characteristically, B-cell lymphomas will express pan B-cell antigens and express either kappa or lambda immunoglobulin light chains, proving clonality.[1] B-cell lymphomas never express both kappa and lambda light chains, but approximately 5% to 10% of lymphomas are surface immunoglobulin negative.[2] The presence of a significant population of surface immunoglobulin negative B cells is also substantial proof of clonality. Loss of normal pan B-cell antigen expression or acquisition of T-cell antigen expression represents phenotypic aberrancy and satisfies minor criteria for malignancy. B-cell lymphomas which coexpress the T-cell antigen CD5 characterize lymphomas of small lymphocytic and mantle cell (intermediately differentiated) lymphocytic varieties. Expression of CD10 is commonly documented in follicular lymphomas. B-cell lymphomas lacking HLA-Dr expression are thought to represent a poor prognostic group.

Approximately 20% of non-Hodgkin's lymphomas are derived from T cells. For these neoplasms, proof of clonality is more challenging. Clonality may be inferred by documenting abnormal pan T-cell antigen expression, abnormal T-cell subset antigen expression, or expression of thymocyte antigens.[3] For atypical T-cell lymphoproliferative disorders in which flow cytometry cannot prove clonality, use of gene rearrangement

Frequently Used Lymphocyte Differentiation Antigens for Flow Cytometry

Lineage Association	Antigenic Specificity/ Predominate Antigen Distribution
B-cell associated markers	
CD19	Pan B cell
CD20	Pan B cell
CD21	C3d and EBV receptor, resting B cell
CD10	CALLA, follicular center cells
Kappa, lambda	Mature B cells
Ig heavy chains	Mature B cells
T-cell associated antigens	
CD2	Sheep erythrocyte receptor, pan T cell
CD3	T-cell antigen receptor complex, pan T cell
CD5	Pan T cell, B-CLL, B-cell small lymphocytic lymphoma, B-cell mantle cell lymphoma
CD7	Pan T cell
CD4	Helper/inducer subset
CD8	Cytotoxic, suppressor subset
CD1	Cortical thymocyte
Myeloid/monocytic antigens	
CD13	Predominately myeloid
CD15	Predominately myeloid, Reed-Sternberg cells
CD14	Predominately monocytic
CD33	Predominately monocytic
Miscellaneous antigens	
CD11c	Predominately granulocytic/monocytic; hairy cell leukemia, some CLL
CD25	IL-2 receptor, activated T cells, hairy cell leukemia
HLA-Dr	Immune response associated antigen, most B cells, activated T cells, early granulocytic and most monocytic cells
Glycophorin A	Erythroid precursors
CDw41	GPIIb/IIIa complex, megakaryocytes

See also a tabular presentation of lymphocyte markers used in paraffin sections in the listing Lymph Node Biopsy. CD indicates cluster designations.

studies may be invaluable; see listing Gene Rearrangement for Leukemia and Lymphoma *on page 512*.

Flow cytometric studies of cases of Hodgkin's disease are generally nondiagnostic. Typically, the majority of cells are reactive mature T cells with variable numbers of polyclonal B cells. This pattern cannot be distinguished from a totally benign reactive hyperplasia. Immunophenotypic verification of Hodgkin's disease is best accomplished in paraffin section using an appropriate panel of antibodies correlated with morphological features of the neoplastic cells.

When considering the possibility of a neoplasm of granulocytic/monocytic precursors, expression of CD13, CD14, or CD33 is usually documented. Additionally, expression of CD45 is characteristically weaker than that typically seen in lymphoid neoplasms. Lack of reactivity for other markers of T- or B-cell lineage is also expected. A panel of commonly utilized lymphocyte markers for the evaluation of lymphoma and leukemia is listed in the table.

Limitations Flow cytometry is of limited use when nonlymphoid or nonhematopoietic neoplasms are evaluated. The nature of the tissue may also confer severe limitations. Generally, endoscopic biopsies are too small to extract sufficient cells for a meaningful evaluation. However, blood, bone marrow, and body fluids are readily suitable for flow cytometric studies. Tissues which are fibrotic or sclerotic, such as skin, are frequently too difficult to dissociate and extract enough viable cells for evaluation. Additionally, necrotic tissues frequently produce poor results. Finally, important diagnostic morphologic and architectural features are lost when single cell suspensions are made. Therefore, the suitability of each biopsy needs to be individually considered before tissues are allocated for special studies beyond that of conventional histopathology. Interpretation of the phenotypic profile must always be correlated with pathological features of individual cases.[4] In those cases in which flow cytometry fails to demonstrate clonality, the use of gene rearrangement studies may be helpful.

Methodology A single cell suspension is required for flow cytometric evaluation. When using tissues, cells are isolated from stromal elements by gentle mechanical dissociation.[5] Most lymphoid tissues release lymphocytes with relative ease while other tissues, such as skin, pose significant difficulties in extracting viable lymphocytes. Isolated lymphocytes are washed and viability may be enriched by density gradient centrifugation. In some specimens, overnight culture is useful to decrease nonspecific staining caused by cytophilic antibody binding mediated by immunoglobulin Fc receptors expressed by lymphoid and other inflammatory cells. However, necrotic tissues and those with high grade neoplasm often lose viable tumor cells and become enriched by reactive T cells. Therefore, discretion is necessary to optimize the preparatory aspects of tissue processing. Ultimately, the single cell suspension is stained with fluorochrome conjugated antibodies, washed, and analyzed on the flow cytometer. Panels of antibodies are utilized to quantitate the numbers of B cells, T cells, and myelomonocytic cells. B-cell clonality is assessed with immunoglobulin light chains while T-cell clonality is inferred by abnormal expression of T-cell antigens.

Footnotes

1. Huh YO and Andreeff M, "Flow Cytometry. Clinical and Research Applications in Hematologic Malignancies," *Hematol Oncol Clin North Am*, 1994, 8(4):703-23.
2. Little JV, Foucar K, Horvath A, et al, "Flow Cytometric Analysis of Lymphoma and Lymphoma-Like Conditions," *Semin Diagn Pathol*, 1989, 6(1):37-54.
3. Picker LJ, Weiss LM, Medeiros LJ, et al, "Immunophenotypic Criteria for the Diagnosis of Non-Hodgkin's Lymphoma," *Am J Pathol*, 1987, 128(1):181-201.
4. Foucar K, Chen IM, and Crago S, "Organization and Operation of a Flow Cytometric Immunophenotyping Laboratory," *Semin Diagn Pathol*, 1989, 6(1):13-36.
5. Visscher DW and Crissman JD, "Dissociation of Intact Cells From Tumors and Normal Tissues," *Methods Cell Biol*, 1994, 41:1-13.

References

Coon JS and Weinstein RS, *Diagnostic Flow Cytometry*, Baltimore, MD: Williams & Wilkins, 1991.

Johnson RL, "Flow Cytometry. From Research to Clinical Laboratory Applications," *Clin Lab Med*, 1993, 13(4):831-52.

Keren DF, *Flow Cytometry in Clinical Diagnosis*, Chicago, IL: American Society of Clinical Pathologists, 1989.

Kipps TJ, Meisenholder G, and Robbins BA, "New Developments in Flow Cytometric Analysis of Lymphocyte Markers," *Clin Lab Med*, 1992, 12(2):237-75.

Knowles DM, *Neoplastic Hematopathology*, Baltimore, MD: Williams & Wilkins, 1992.

Immunostains *see* Immunoperoxidase Procedures *on page 43*

***In Situ* Hybridization** *see* Immunoperoxidase Procedures *on page 43*

Intercellular Substance Antibodies *see* Skin Biopsy, Immunofluorescence *on page 56*

Intermediate Filaments *see* Immunoperoxidase Procedures *on page 43*

Intermediate Lymphocytic Lymphoma *see* Mantle Cell Lymphoma *on page 51*

Intraoperative Consultation, Pathology *see* Frozen Section *on page 41*

Jones Stain *see* Kidney Biopsy *on this page*

Kappa Light Chain Analysis by Flow Cytometry *see* Immunophenotypic Analysis of Tissues by Flow Cytometry *on page 45*

Kappa Light Chains *see* Immunoperoxidase Procedures *on page 43*

Ki-67 *see* Immunoperoxidase Procedures *on page 43*

Kidney Biopsy

CPT 88305 (surgical pathology); 88307 (kidney, partial/total nephrectomy); 88312 (special stains, each); 88346 (immunofluorescence, each antibody); 88348 (electron microscopy)

Related Information
Adult Polycystic Kidney Disease DNA Detection *on page 502*
Antihyaluronidase Titer *on page 365*
Antineutrophil Cytoplasmic Antibody *on page 367*
Antinuclear Antibody *on page 368*
Creatinine Clearance *on page 117*
Electron Microscopy *on page 37*
Factor B *on page 393*
Fat, Urine *on page 635*
Glomerular Basement Membrane Antibody *on page 395*
Hemoglobin, Qualitative, Urine *on page 637*
Kidney Profile *on page 153*
Protein, Quantitative, Urine *on page 649*
Protein, Semiquantitative, Urine *on page 650*
Scleroderma Antibody *on page 430*
Urea Nitrogen, Blood *on page 213*
Urinalysis *on page 658*

Synonyms Renal Biopsy

Applies to Fluorescein-Tagged Antibodies; Jones Stain; Michael's Solution; Zeus Fixative

Test Commonly Includes Light microscopy: H & E, PAS, methenamine silver, trichrome, congo red, and other stains; immunofluorescent studies; electron microscopy

Patient Preparation CBC, prothrombin time, activated thromboplastin time, and urine Gram's stain are prerequisite, with appropriate imaging and sometimes with a template bleeding time.[1]

Specimen Fresh kidney tissue obtained by percutaneous needle biopsy or open surgery.

Specimen handling: The core of renal tissue or a wedge obtained by open biopsy is immediately placed in a Petri dish containing physiologic saline solution or sterile culture media to prevent drying. An alternative is wrapping the specimen in saline-moistened gauze. The specimen should be sent to the laboratory within 5-10 minutes. If the specimen cannot be sent to the laboratory within this time frame, it should be divided into three parts and prepared in the appropriate fixative for light microscopy, electron microscopy, and immunofluorescence. Avoid compression of the specimen.

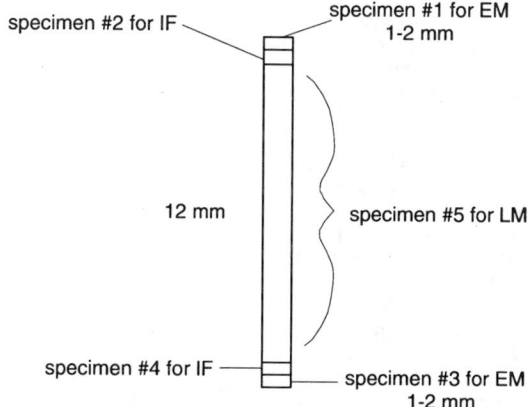

specimen #2 for IF — specimen #1 for EM 1-2 mm
12 mm — specimen #5 for LM
specimen #4 for IF — specimen #3 for EM 1-2 mm

Specimen separation: When dividing the specimen, each part must contain glomeruli. A suggested method is:

A. If an open biopsy or three or more tissue cores are obtained, one core or fragment of the wedge biopsy is submitted for immunofluorescence, one for electron microscopy, and the remainder for light microscopy.

B. If two tissue cores are obtained, one is submitted for light microscopy, and the second core is divided as follows:
- Cut four 1-2 mm fragments with a sharp razor blade. Two from each end of the core to avoid lack of cortex for ultrastructural examination.

Submit two fragments for electron microscopy and the other two for immunofluorescence. The central portion of the core is submitted for light microscopy (see illustration).

C. If only one tissue core is obtained and it is small (<8 mm), submit it for light microscopy. If it is larger than 8 mm, divide it and submit as B. When dividing a small biopsy, priority usually is given to: 1) light microscopy, 2) immunofluorescence, and 3) electron microscopy in this order, or at the discretion of the clinician depending on the clinical situation. A hand lens or a dissecting scope can be useful in recognizing the difference between renal cortex and medulla (glomeruli in the cortex appears as red dots, cortex is darker than medulla and is proximal within the needle used for biopsy).

Specimen preparation: Several means of collection may be used. For immunofluorescence studies, one core or portion of a wedge (open biopsy) is placed in a foil or plastic bag, frozen in liquid nitrogen or in a cryostat, shipped on dry ice to the laboratory, and stored at -76°C until processed. The frozen state must be maintained. An alternative method is to immerse the biopsy in a half-saturated ammonium sulfate buffer at room temperature. Michael's solution is used to transport the specimen to another institution. Zeus fixative is sometimes used. The tissue should not be held in this fixative for more than 5 days, preferably less. For **light microscopy**, the second core or fragment is commonly fixed in 4% formaldehyde that is 10 times the volume of the tissue, but a variety of fixatives are in use. For **electron microscopy**, the third core or fragment is fixed in 2.5% glutaraldehyde fixative.

Possible problems:
- Drying of the specimen. In order to avoid drying, place the specimen, immediately after the biopsy is obtained, in normal saline. Keep it in saline until it is frozen or placed in fixative.
- Absence of cortex. If glomeruli are not identified in the tissue, a repeat biopsy is necessary. If glomeruli are only present in the specimen submitted for immunofluorescence or electron microscopy, the remaining tissue may be cut and slides made for light microscopy.
- Too few glomeruli present in the biopsy. A minimum of 8-10 glomeruli is considered to be adequate for proper evaluation of a renal biopsy. This is particularly important in focal glomerular disease. The probability of finding abnormal glomeruli is closely related to the total number of glomeruli present. For evaluation of severity of disease, an adequate number of glomeruli is necessary.[2]

Causes for Rejection Drying of specimen due to lack of fixative

Special Instructions Adequate clinical history, differential diagnosis, and laboratory findings are essential for proper interpretation of renal biopsies and should be received with the specimen.

Use There are no absolute indications for renal biopsy. Clinical judgment is required to determine necessity of biopsy. A single disease can lead to different patterns of abnormality, and several disease entities can cause similar clinical presentations. In general, renal biopsy is useful to establish diagnosis in subjects with renal dysfunction, ascertain prognosis, evaluate disease severity and extent,[1] and guide therapy[3] in conditions which include the following:
- acute renal failure in cases in which clinical diagnosis cannot be established and/or which are unresponsive
- asymptomatic non-nephrotic progressive proteinuria
- nephrotic syndrome in adults, especially including SLE; selected diabetic patients
- nephrotic syndrome in children with minimal change disease, who do not respond to therapy as anticipated
- acute nephritic syndrome; characteristics of acute nephritic syndrome include acute onset of hematuria with red cell casts, hypertension, and proteinuria often with deteriorating renal function. Causes include postinfectious glomerulonephritis, antiglomerular basement membrane disease, membranoproliferative glomerulonephritis, IgA nephropathy, Henoch-Schönlein purpura, SLE, and vasculitis.[1]
- hematuria of uncertain etiology, selected cases
- systemic diseases with renal involvement
- drug toxicity
- candidacy for renal transplantation in patients in chronic renal failure
- evaluation of dysfunction in recipients of renal allografts; transplantation reactions, rejection, or failure

Contraindications
- Bleeding diathesis
- Neoplasm
- Cystic disease, large cysts
- Obstructive uropathy
- Acute pyelonephritis
- Abscess
- Uncontrolled hypertension
- Solitary kidney present (although biopsies of solitary renal allografts are often obtained without serious complications[1])
- Anatomic abnormalities
- Pregnancy
- Uncooperative patient

(Continued)

47

Kidney Biopsy *(Continued)*

- Chronic renal disease with very small kidneys
- Renal arterial aneurysm

This list of contraindications is more relative than absolute. In several of these situations, the patient may be considered for biopsy after receiving appropriate therapy. In some cases, an open biopsy may be performed.

Methodology Light microscopy: Specimen is embedded in paraffin, sections are cut at 2-4 microns and stained with H & E, Gomori trichrome, PAS, and silver methenamine (Jones stain). Additional stains such as amyloid, fibrin, and so forth are occasionally needed. In the H & E and PAS stain, the basic pattern of the disease process is determined, and the extent and distribution of morphologic change is noted. Glomeruli, tubules, interstitium, and blood vessels are examined separately and any abnormality noted. The degrees of glomerular sclerosis, interstitial fibrosis, tubular atrophy, and vascular changes are quantitatively estimated. Such parameters are important in determination of the degree of chronicity, severity of the renal disease, and overall prognosis. The **PAS stain** is helpful in studying glomerular and tubular basement membranes and the mesangium. PAS stain highlights hyaline and fibrinoid changes, and the presence of glomerular and arterial sclerosis (all stain red). It supports diagnoses of mesangial proliferative glomerulonephritis, focal segmental glomerulosclerosis, and diabetic nephropathy, and usually reacts with light chains.[1] The **trichrome stain** is used to determine the presence of interstitial fibrosis and glomerular and vascular sclerosis. It may show immune deposits and fibrin (the collagen stains blue; muscle, immune deposits, and fibrin stain red). The **silver stain (Jones stain)** is used especially to study glomerular and tubular basement membranes. It also brings out the mesangium and demonstrates the presence of glomerular sclerosis (all appear black). **Congo red** for amyloid is often used.

Immunofluorescence: The specimen is snap frozen and sectioned. A battery of fluorescein-tagged antibodies against different immunoglobulins and complement is used. The most commonly used are IgG, IgM, IgA, C3, C4, C1q, properdin, fibrinogen, albumin, and kappa and lambda light chains. Sections are then examined under fluorescence microscopy. Intensity, pattern, and distribution of immunoglobulins are noted. Normal renal biopsy usually shows no immunoglobulin depositions. Immunofluorescence allows for classification of renal disease, demonstrating immune complex deposition in glomerular diseases. One may ascertain the degree of immunologic activity in immune diseases, suggest systemic entities (eg, SLE) and establish certain diagnoses (eg, IgA nephropathy).

Electron microscopy (EM): The specimen is embedded in plastic. Ultrathin sections are treated with osmium. Electron microscopy is useful for localization and quantitation of immune deposits. Abnormalities of the basement membrane and the presence of cellular inclusions may be detected. Survey sections 1 μm thick are stained with 1% toluidine blue. EM is necessary to establish some diagnoses (eg, Alport's syndrome, thin basement membrane nephritis, and the fibrillary glomerulonephritis).

Light microscopy, immunofluorescence, and electron microscopy are complementary and necessary in most cases. EM is essential in about 25% of cases and helpful in half.[1]

Additional Information Complications of renal biopsy:

- Hematuria: Microscopic hematuria is a common complication seen in most patients. It resolves spontaneously. Gross hematuria is seen in 5% to 9% of the cases and is more common in patients with uncontrolled hypertension or uremia. It usually resolves spontaneously in 2-3 days. In 0.5% of the patients, hematuria will persist for 2-3 weeks, occasionally occurring a few days after the biopsy. Blood transfusions are only necessary in about 1% to 3% of the cases, and nephrectomy for massive or persistent bleeding is necessary in only 1 of 2000-5000 cases.
- Perinephric hematoma is not uncommon, however, only 1% to 2% of patients develop a local mass, hypotension, or diminution in hematocrit. The hematoma usually resolves within a few months.
- Arteriovenous fistula is considered frequent in arteriographic studies. Most cases are clinically silent and resolve spontaneously within 2 years.
- Other complications: Postbiopsy aneurysm appears in <1% of patients. Other rare complications that have been described include infection; ileus; lacerations of the liver, spleen, pancreas, gallbladder, intestine, visceral and subcostal arteries; pancreatitis; pneumothorax; and dissemination of carcinoma. Death has occurred in 0.12% of patients.[1]

In summary, renal biopsy is relatively safe and useful in diagnosis and management of significant renal disease.

Footnotes

1. Radford MG Jr, Donadio JV Jr, Holley KE, et al, "Renal Biopsy in Clinical Practice," *Mayo Clin Proc*, 1994, 69(10):983-4.
2. Madaio MP, "Renal Biopsy," *Kidney Int*, 1990, 38(3):529-43.

3. Vidt DG, "Recognition and Management of Reversible Renal Failure," *South Med J*, 1994, 87(10):1018-27.

References

Alon U, "Hemorrhagic Complications of Kidney Biopsy," *Clin Pediatr (Phila)*, 1991, 30(6):391.

Espinel CH, "Diagnosis of Acute and Chronic Renal Failure," *Clin Lab Med*, 1993, 13(1):89-102.

Glassock RJ, Hirschman GH, and Striker GE, "Workshop on the Use of Renal Biopsy in Research on Diabetic Nephropathy: A Summary Report," *Am J Kidney Dis*, 1991, 18(5):589-92.

Levison SP, "Renal Disease in the Elderly: The Role of the Renal Biopsy," *Am J Kidney Dis*, 1990, 16(4):300-6.

Mauer SM, Chavers BM, and Steffes MW, "Should There Be an Expanded Role for Kidney Biopsy in the Management of Patients With Type I Diabetes?" *Am J Kidney Dis*, 1990, 16(2):96-100.

McLaughlin J, Gladman DD, Urowitz MB, et al, "Kidney Biopsy in Systemic Lupus Erythematosus. II. Survival Analyses According to Biopsy Results," *Arthritis Rheum*, 1991, 34(10):1268-73.

Menon SK and Kirchner KA, "The Role of Percutaneous Renal Biopsy in Clinical Nephrology," *Curr Opin Nephrol Hypertens*, 1993, 2(6):968-73.

Modesto-Segonds A, Ah-Soune MF, Durand D, et al, "Renal Biopsy in the Elderly," *Am J Nephrol*, 1993, 13(1):27-34.

Rance CP, "When Should Renal Biopsy Be Done?" *Clin Pediatr (Phila)*, 1990, 29(11):653-66.

Solez K, Racusen LC, and Olsen S, "New Approaches to Renal Biopsy Assessment in Acute Renal Failure: Extrapolation From Renal Transplantation," *Kidney Int Suppl*, 1994, 44:S65-9.

Striker LJ, "Modern Renal Biopsy Interpretation: Can We Predict Glomerulosclerosis?" *Semin Nephrol*, 1993, 13(5):508-15.

Lambda Light Chain Analysis by Flow Cytometry *see* Immunophenotypic Analysis of Tissues by Flow Cytometry *on page 45*

Lambda Light Chains *see* Immunoperoxidase Procedures *on page 43*

LE Antibodies *see* Skin Biopsy, Immunofluorescence *on page 56*

Lectins *see* Immunoperoxidase Procedures *on page 43*

Leukemia Analysis by Flow Cytometry *see* Immunophenotypic Analysis of Tissues by Flow Cytometry *on page 45*

Leukocyte Common Antigen *see* Immunoperoxidase Procedures *on page 43*

Leu M1 *see* Immunoperoxidase Procedures *on page 43*

Light Chain Analysis by Flow Cytometry *see* Immunophenotypic Analysis of Tissues by Flow Cytometry *on page 45*

Light Chains *see* Immunoperoxidase Procedures *on page 43*

Liver Biopsy

CPT 88307

Related Information

Acetaminophen, Serum *on page 530*
Alanine Aminotransferase *on page 65*
Alcohol, Blood or Urine *on page 531*
Alkaline Phosphatase, Serum *on page 69*
Alpha$_1$-Antitrypsin Phenotyping *on page 362*
Amiodarone, Serum *on page 532*
Antimitochondrial Antibody *on page 366*
Antinuclear Antibody *on page 368*
Aspartate Aminotransferase *on page 84*
Bilirubin, Total *on page 86*
Ceruloplasmin *on page 107*
Copper, Serum *on page 589*
Copper, Urine *on page 590*
Ferritin, Serum *on page 127*
Hepatitis B$_e$ Antigen *on page 397*
Hepatitis B Surface Antibody *on page 398*
Hepatitis B Surface Antigen *on page 399*
Hepatitis C RNA Detection *on page 513*
Hepatitis C Serology *on page 399*
Histopathology *on page 42*
Iron and Total Iron Binding Capacity/Transferrin *on page 150*
Liver/Kidney Microsomal Type 1 Antibodies *on page 415*
Liver Profile *on page 161*
Phlebotomy, Therapeutic *on page 614*
Q Fever Titer *on page 426*
Smooth Muscle Antibody *on page 431*

Synonyms Needle Biopsy of Liver

Applies to Copper, Hepatic; Transjugular Needle Biopsy of the Liver

Test Commonly Includes The liver may be biopsied as a percutaneous or transjugular needle biopsy. One to a few 2 cm cores of liver tissue are excised. Investigation includes light microscopy, commonly with a number of special stains. Immunohistochemistry is often helpful. Electron microscopy is occasionally needed. *In situ* hybridization techniques may be helpful. Microbiologic culture may be required. Liver biopsy is a valuable and time-honored means for diagnosis of diffuse liver parenchymal disease as well as disseminated focal disease.

Patient Preparation Procedures and risks of the procedure are explained and consent is required. Procedure entails overnight hospitalization in most cases. All aspirin products and nonsteroidal agents must be discontinued at least 7 days beforehand. If taking oral anticoagulants (Coumadin®), hospitalization is required to convert to heparin therapy before biopsy. Screening laboratory studies ordered 24-48 hours in advance commonly include CBC, PT/PTT, BUN, bleeding time, type and screen or type and crossmatch for possible transfusion, additional to careful history and physical examination. Electrolytes are usually optional. If pneumonia or pleural effusion is suspected on examination, PA and lateral chest x-ray is obtained.

Aftercare In general, patient is monitored in a recovery area with frequent vital signs postbiopsy. If hypotension, tachycardia, fever, rigidity of abdomen, or uncontrolled pain occurs, physician should be notified immediately and an intravenous line placed. Some physicians recheck hematocrit 24 hours after procedure before approving hospital discharge.

Specimen At least two to three liver cores, each >2 cm in length are desirable.

Collection Tissue fixation for light microscopy: specimen is usually fixed in 10% buffered formalin within 1 minute, Zenker's fluid or a Zenker modification. A specimen from subjects with cystinosis should be separately alcohol-fixed and so labeled. For transmission electron microscopy, 1 mm cubes of specimen are fixed immediately in glutaraldehyde, but EM is not often needed. For Wilson's disease, handling has recently been outlined.[1]

Use This procedure, by nature, is invasive. In most cases, noninvasive imaging studies such as CT scan or ultrasound are obtained first. **Indications for liver biopsy include:**
- chronic hepatitis, with or without cirrhosis, to identify cases of autoimmune hepatitis, and the entities included in its differential diagnosis; evaluation of disease severity (eg, hepatitis C)
- suspected cases of liver cirrhosis, to confirm the diagnosis and, if possible, establish etiology (eg, alcohol, alpha₁-antitrypsin deficiency, primary biliary cirrhosis, hemochromatosis, etc); assess and stage level of activity; assess complications
- portal hypertension
- persistently elevated liver-related enzyme tests
- cholestasis of unknown etiology, in which other studies of biliary obstruction are negative
- disorders of bilirubin metabolism (eg, Dubin-Johnson syndrome)
- selected cases of fever of unknown origin (eg, tuberculosis, brucellosis); a portion of biopsy can be cultured for appropriate organisms[2]
- suspected liver disease in the known alcoholic patient, to confirm alcoholic liver disease, exclude alternative causes of liver disease, stage and assess disease activity
- diagnosis of benign and malignant tumors (eg, hepatoma, metastatic neoplasms)

Types of Toxic Reactions Occurring in the Liver

Type of Reaction	Examples of Agents
Direct reaction	Acetaminophen, carbon tetrachloride, mushrooms, phosphorus
Idiosyncratic reaction	Isoniazid, disulfiram, propylthiouracil*
Toxic-allergic reaction	Halothane, isoflurane, ticrynafen
Allergic hepatitis	Phenytoin, amoxicillin-clavulanic acid, sulfonamides
Cholestatic reaction	Chlorpromazine, erythromycin estolate, estradiol, captopril, sulfonamides
Granulomatous reaction	Diltiazem, quinidine, phenytoin, procainamide
Chronic hepatitis	Nitrofurantoin, methyldopa, isoniazid, trazodone
Alcoholic hepatitis-like reaction	Amiodarone, perhexiline maleate, valproic acid
Microvesicular steatosis	Tetracyclines, aspirin, zidovudine, didanosine, fialuridine
Fibrosis or cirrhosis alone	Methotrexate, vitamin A, methyldopa
Veno-occlusive disease	Cyclophosphamide, other chemotherapeutic agents, herbal teas
Ischemic damage	Cocaine, sustained-release nicotinic acid, methylenedioxyamphetamine

*There are hundreds of other agents that can cause idiosyncratic reactions.
From Lee WM, "Drug-Induced Hepatotoxicity," *N Engl J Med*, 1995, 333(17):1121, with permission.

- recognition and staging of lymphoma
- suspected multisystem disease with liver involvement in which other diagnostic techniques have not been fruitful (eg, sarcoidosis, amyloidosis, tuberculosis, glycogen storage disease)
- unexplained hepatomegaly
- selected cases of hepatitis of unknown etiology, in order to try to differentiate viral from drug-induced etiologies (not always possible) or to assess complications, such as cholestasis; differential diagnosis of drug-induced hepatic disease;[3] see table.
- acute hepatitis without explained etiology; in protracted cases
- infectious disease (eg, Q fever); extrapulmonary *P. carinii* infection is reported in liver and spleen in immunocompromised individuals[4]
- evaluation of response to treatment (eg, patients on methotrexate)
- following bone marrow or liver transplantation
- investigate inborn error of metabolism (eg, Wilson's disease, α₁-antitrypsin deficiency, glycogen storage disease, Gaucher's disease, other storage diseases)
- instances of vascular abnormalities (eg, veno-occlusive disease)

Liver biopsy is less useful in:
- acute hepatitis A or B infection, unless the diagnosis is in question
- extrahepatic biliary obstruction in which percutaneous transhepatic cholangiography and ERCP are considered first-line procedures
- fluid-filled liver cysts detected on ultrasound or CT scan, probably more amenable to guided thin needle aspiration first

Limitations Mahal et al (1979) noted that failure to heed accepted contraindications led directly to 22 bleeding episodes in 3800 percutaneous liver biopsies.

Contraindications include:
- impaired hemostasis, accepted as prothrombin time more than 3 seconds over control, PTT more than 20 seconds over control, thrombocytopenia, or markedly prolonged bleeding time
- severe anemia (Hgb <9.5 g/dL)
- local infection near needle entry site, such as right sided pleural effusion or empyema, right lower lobe pneumonia, local cellulitis, infected ascites or peritonitis
- tense ascites (low yield technically, risk of leakage)
- high-grade extrahepatic biliary obstruction with jaundice (increased risk of bile peritonitis)
- septic cholangitis
- possible hemangioma, other vascular tumors
- possible echinococcal (hydatid) cyst
- lack of adequate facilities for blood transfusion
- uncooperative patient
- liver biopsy is more hazardous when performed on outpatients who have cirrhosis or neoplasms, since these are the categories associated with mortality (from hemoperitoneum)

Complications:

Significant morbidity has been estimated at 1%. Fatality rate of up to 0.1% is recognized with thick needle biopsy.[5] More commonly seen complications include:
- pain
- hemorrhage - minor episodes are common. Significant hemorrhage is infrequent but is the most common cause of death from liver biopsy. Several series have estimated an incidence of approximately 0.2%, but Sherlock (1984) reported 40 patients out of 6379 who required transfusion for intraperitoneal bleeding. Specific sites include the abdominal cavity (hemoperitoneum), liver capsule (capsular hematoma), liver parenchyma (intrahepatic hematoma), biliary tree (hemobilia), or into the pleural space. Postulated risk factors include cirrhosis, coagulopathy, amyloid liver, hepatocellular injury, hemangioma and vascularized tumor. However, bleeding may be massive even when no risk factors are present.
- bile leakage with peritonitis - associated with severe obstruction of the larger bile ducts.
- laceration of internal organs and viscera - right kidney, gallbladder, colon, pancreas, and others
- others: right-sided pneumothorax, bacteremia, sepsis, arteriovenous fistula, drug toxicity

Contraindications Frozen section is usually contraindicated for needle biopsy material except for recognition of tumor in the course of open surgical procedures.

Methodology Several biopsy needles are available: Menghini needle, "Trucut" needle, Vim-Silverman needle.
- Tissue stains including: **H & E** for general histopathology; **reticulin** preparation; **Masson's trichrome** - fibrosis, cirrhosis in concert with a reticulin preparation; **pentachrome** may be helpful; **iron stain** - useful for hemosiderosis, hemochromatosis, and to distinguish these from hemofuchsin and bile pigments; **PAS stain** with and without diastase - useful for alpha₁-antitrypsin globules, bile ducts; **orcein** - for hepatitis B surface antigen; stains for amyloid and various stains for organisms; other stains occasionally needed as well. Immunohistochemistry is sometimes needed (eg, CEA).

(Continued)

Liver Biopsy (Continued)

- Cytologic preparation - fluid from aspirating syringe may be smeared on clean microscope slide, fixed, and sent to Cytology Laboratory
- Microbiological culture - send specimen without fixative in sterile container. Special stains (AFB, KOH, etc) and cultures (tuberculosis, viral, *Brucella*, parasites, fungi) as needed. See listings Bacterial Culture, Abscess *on page 454*;[2] *Entamoeba histolytica* Serological Test *on page 391*;[1] Bacterial Culture, Biopsy or Body Fluid *on page 456*; Fungal Culture, Biopsy or Body Fluid *on page 476*; Mycobacterial Culture, Biopsy or Body Fluid *on page 487*. Liver biopsies are most likely to contain acid-fast organisms in HIV-positive subjects when the patient is febrile, AIDS is longstanding and serum alkaline phosphatase is very high.[6]

Additional Information Although **fine needle aspiration** is useful for the diagnosis of carcinoma, it is not usually adequate for evaluation of other hepatic disease entities. Fine needle aspiration is used to confirm malignant tumors with less morbidity and mortality than is encountered with thick needle biopsies. Guided (by imaging techniques) biopsies bear increased diagnostic yield both for thick and thin needle aspirations.

In Wilson's disease, tissue copper values are >250 µg/g (4 µmol/g) dry weight, while in other entities characterized by increased copper (chronic cholestatic liver diseases including primary biliary cirrhosis and primary sclerosing cholangitis) liver copper concentration is <80 µg/g (1.26 µmol/g) dry weight. The only other entity with very high copper levels, Indian childhood cirrhosis, is extremely rare in the U.S. If copper levels are needed, specific paraffins are required to embed the needle biopsy.[1] See listings Copper, Serum *on page 589*; Copper, Urine *on page 590*; and Ceruloplasmin *on page 107*.

Footnotes

1. Ludwig J, Moyer TP, and Rakela J, "The Liver Biopsy Diagnosis of Wilson's Disease. Methods in Pathology," *Am J Clin Pathol*, 1994, 102(4):443-6.
2. Pitt HA, "Surgical Management of Hepatic Abscesses," *World J Surg*, 1990, 14(4):498-504.
3. Lee WM, "Drug-Induced Hepatotoxicity," *N Engl J Med*, 1995, 333(17):1118-27.
4. "Case Records of the Massachusetts General Hospital. Weekly Clinicopathological Exercises. Case 3-1995. A 29-Year-Old Man With AIDS and Multiple Splenic Abscesses," *N Engl J Med*, 1995, 332(4):249-57.
5. Saul SH, "Masses of the Liver," *Diagnostic Surgical Pathology*, 2nd ed, Chapter 37, Sternberg SS, ed, New York, NY: Raven Press, 1994, 1517-80.
6. Christie JD and Callihan DR, "The Laboratory Diagnosis of Mycobacterial Diseases. Challenges and Common Sense," *Clin Lab Med*, 1995, 15(2):279-306.

References

Bird GL, "Investigation of Alcoholic Liver Disease," *Baillieres Clin Gastroenterol*, 1993, 7(3):663-82.

Burgart LJ, Batts KP, Ludwig J, et al, "Recent-Onset Autoimmune Hepatitis. Biopsy Findings and Clinical Correlations," *Am J Surg Pathol*, 1995, 19(6):699-708.

Froehlich F, Lamy O, Fried M, et al, "Practice and Complications of Liver Biopsy. Results of a Nationwide Survey in Switzerland," *Dig Dis Sci*, 1993, 38(8):1480-4.

Herrera JL, "Abnormal Liver Enzyme Levels. Clinical Evaluation in Asymptomatic Patients," *Postgrad Med*, 1993, 93(2):119-20, 125, 129-32.

John TG and Garden OJ, "Needle Track Seeding of Primary and Secondary Liver Carcinoma After Percutaneous Liver Biopsy," *HPB Surg*, 1993, 6(3):199-204.

Lefkowitch JH, "Pathologic Diagnosis of Liver Disease," *Hepatology: A Textbook of Liver Disease*, 2nd ed, Chapter 29, Zakim D and Boyer TD, eds, Philadelphia, PA: WB Saunders Co, 1990, 711-32.

Maddrey WE, "Percutaneous Needle Biopsy of the Liver," *Shackelford's Surgery of the Alimentary Tract*, 3rd ed, Chapter 25, Zuidema GD, ed, Philadelphia, PA: WB Saunders Co, 1991, 292-5.

Mahal AS, Knauer CM, and Gregory PB, "Bleeding After Liver Biopsy," *West J Med*, 1981, 134(1):11-4.

McGill DB, Rakela J, Zinsmeister AR, et al, "A 21-Year Experience With Major Hemorrhage After Percutaneous Liver Biopsy," *Gastroenterology*, 1990, 99(5):1396-400.

Perrault J, McGill DB, Ott BJ, et al, "Liver Biopsy: Complications in 1000 Inpatients and Outpatients," *Gastroenterology*, 1978, 78(1):103-6.

Piccinino F, Sagnelli E, Pasquale G, et al, "Complications Following Percutaneous Liver Biopsy," *J Hepatol*, 1986, 2(2):165-73.

Rubin RA, Falestiny M, and Malet PF, "Chronic Hepatitis C. Advances in Diagnostic Testing and Therapy," *Arch Intern Med*, 1994, 154(4):387-92.

Scheuer PJ and Lefkowitch JH, *Liver Biopsy Interpretation*, 5th ed, Philadelphia, PA: WB Saunders Co, 1994.

Schiff L and Schiff ER, *Diseases of the Liver*, 7th ed, Vol 1, Philadelphia, PA: JB Lippincott Co, 1993.

Sherlock S, "Needle Biopsy of the Liver," *Diseases of the Liver and Biliary System*, 7th ed, Chapter 3, Oxford, England: Blackwell Scientific Publications, 1985, 28-37.

Sherlock S, Dick R, and van Leeuwen DJ, "Liver Biopsy Today. The Royal Free Hospital Experience," *J Hepatol*, 1984, 1(1):75-85.

Thung SN and Gerber MA, "Liver," *Histology for Pathologists*, Chapter 32, Sternberg SS, ed, New York, NY: Raven Press, 1992, 625-38.

Van Ness MM and Diehl AM, "Is Liver Biopsy Useful in the Evaluation of Patients With Chronically Elevated Liver Enzymes?" *Ann Intern Med*, 1989, 111(6):473-8.

Van Thiel DH, Gavaler JS, Wright H, et al, "Liver Biopsy. Its Safety and Complications as Seen at a Liver Transplant Center," *Transplantation*, 1993, 55(5):1087-90.

Zamcheck N and Klausenstock O, "Liver Biopsy. II. The Risk of Needle Biopsy," *N Engl J Med*, 1953, 249(26):1062-3.

Lung Biopsy *see* Histopathology *on page 42*

Lupus Band Test *see* Skin Biopsy, Immunofluorescence *on page 56*

Lymph Node Biopsy

CPT 88180 (flow cytometry each cell surface marker); 88305 (surgical pathology); 88307 (lymph nodes, regional resection); 88312 (special stains each); 88342 (immunoperoxidase stains each antibody); 88346 (immunofluorescence each antibody); 88348 (electron microscopy)

Related Information

Bacterial Culture, Biopsy or Body Fluid *on page 456*
bcl-2 Gene Rearrangement *on page 503*
Bloom's Syndrome, Chromosome Breakage Study *on page 274*
Bone Marrow *on page 307*
Buffy Coat Smear Study of Peripheral Blood *on page 309*
Cat Scratch Disease Serology *on page 375*
Chromosome Analysis, Blood *on page 276*
Chromosome Analysis, Bone Marrow *on page 277*
Chromosome Analysis, Lymph Node and Solid Tumor *on page 279*
Chromosome *In Situ* Hybridization *on page 281*
Complete Blood Count *on page 312*
Epstein-Barr Virus Culture *on page 666*
Frozen Section *on page 41*
Gene Rearrangement for Leukemia and Lymphoma *on page 512*
Histopathology *on page 42*
Immunofixation Electrophoresis *on page 408*
Immunoperoxidase Procedures *on page 43*
Immunophenotypic Analysis of Tissues by Flow Cytometry *on page 45*
Infectious Mononucleosis Screening Test *on page 410*
Leishmaniasis Serological Test *on page 413*
Leukocyte Immunophenotyping *on page 414*
Mantle Cell Lymphoma *on next page*
Muramidase, Blood and Urine *on page 333*
Peripheral Blood: Differential Leukocyte Count *on page 336*
Skin Biopsy *on page 54*
Tartrate Resistant Leukocyte Acid Phosphatase *on page 349*
Terminal Deoxynucleotidyl Transferase *on page 349*
Tularemia Agglutinins *on page 436*
White Blood Count *on page 353*

Applies to Cell Sorting Fluorescence Activation; Lymphocyte Markers

Test Commonly Includes Microscopic examination of frozen sections, paraffin and/or plastic sections, and touch preparations. Immunoperoxidase studies for immunoglobulin heavy and light chains are best done on snap-frozen cryostat sections rather than paraffin sections.

Abstract Lymph nodes may harbor malignant lymphomas, metastatic carcinomas and sarcomas, hyperplasias, and a variety of proliferative, inflammatory, reactive, infiltrative, immunodeficiency and degenerative entities.

Specimen Lymph node or other tissues suspected of harboring lymphoma or other abnormality, ideally submitted fresh within minutes of the biopsy

Container Sterile saline moistened sponge or Petri dish

Collection Optimal selection of site of biopsy and the lymph nodes to be biopsied enhance ultimate correct diagnosis. Supraclavicular and cervical biopsies will most likely provide diagnostic specimens. The most accessible lymph nodes are not always the best choice.[1] The whole, intact lymph node with its capsule and adjacent fat or other tissue provides an optimal specimen.[1]

Proper initial triage of the tissue is of utmost importance in establishing the correct diagnosis. Ideally, sufficient tissue must be available for permanent sections and immunophenotypic analysis in frozen sections or by flow cytometry. Tissues allocated for immunotypic studies are also suitable for genotypic studies if necessary. Routine histopathology remains the gold standard in diagnostic hematopathology, and optimal histology begins with proper fixation. Fine nuclear detail is best achieved using B5, zinc formalin, or a Zenker's-like fixative. These fixatives are also best for cell marker analysis in paraffin section. An ever expanding selection of antibodies is useful for establishing lineage of hematopoietic cells in paraffin section (see table).[2,3] However, phenotypic indicators of clonal proliferation are most reliably established in frozen section or by flow cytometry. As morphologic detail in frozen sections is intrinsically limited, every precaution to minimize artifacts must be taken. Snap freezing small, thin slices of tissue using liquid nitrogen-cooled isopentane yields tissues free of freezing artifacts. Special attention to fine details of cryostat sectioning is necessary to yield interpretable results. If a frozen section evaluation is necessary to initiate a "lymphoma protocol," the tissues used for this rapid diagnosis are often unsuitable for immunophenotypic analysis. If the size of biopsy is limiting, a routine frozen section evaluation should be discouraged as freezing distorts lymphoid tissue and may result in errors in final interpretation.

If tissues are to be sent to a reference laboratory for immunotyping, three basic options are available. First, the tissues may be snap frozen and

Lymphocyte Markers Useful in Paraffin Section*

	LCA (CD45)	EMA	LN-2 (CD71w)	L26 (CD20)	UCHL-1 (CD45RO)	CD3	Leu-M1 (CD15)	Mono Ig's	Lysozyme	KP1 (CD68)	CAE
Non-Hodgkin's lymphoma											
B-cell lymphoma†	+	-	+	+	-	-	-	+	-	-	-
T-cell lymphomas§	+	-/+	-	-	+	+	-/+	-	-	-	-
Hodgkin's disease (NS, MC, LD)	-	-	+	-	-	-	+	-	-	-	-
Hodgkin's disease, LP	+	+/-	+	+	-	-	-	-	-	-	-
Myeloma/plasmacytoma	-/+	-/+	-	-	-	-	-	+	-	-	-
Granulocytic sarcoma#	+/-	-	-/+	-	-	-	+/-	-	+	+	+
True histiocytic lymphoma#	+/-	-/+	-/+	-	-	-	-	-	+	+	-

Abbreviations: LCA: leukocyte common antigen; EMA: epithelial membrane antigen; Mono Ig's: monoclonal immunoglobulins; CAE: chloroacetate esterase (an enzyme cytochemical stain rather than an immunostain); Hodgkin's disease (NS, MC, LD): nodular sclerosing, mixed cellularity, and lymphocyte depleted subtypes, respectively; Hodgkin's disease, LP: lymphocyte predominate subtype. Designated reactions: +: characteristically positive; +/-: characteristically positive but may be negative; -/+: characteristically negative but may be positive; -: characteristically negative.

Footnotes:

*Most lymphomas characteristically contain neoplastic and non-neoplastic lymphoid elements in variable proportions. Caution must be exercised in determining the phenotype of the neoplastic cells.

†Monoclonal immunoglobulins are best detected in frozen section. Large cell lymphomas and those with plasmacytic differentiation are more likely to display a convincing staining in paraffin section than other subtypes.

§T-cell clonal proliferation cannot be determined in paraffin section alone. The best phenotypic expression of clonal proliferation is aberrant expression of pan T-cell antigens which can be detected only by frozen section immunohistology, by flow cytometry using cell suspensions, or by gene rearrangement.

#Enzyme cytochemical profile using touch preparations is extremely useful in establishing these diagnoses.

stored at -70°C or colder until immunotyping is considered necessary. If facilities for proper snap freezing and storage are not available, this option should be discouraged. Second, the tissues may be delivered in carrier media or saline-soaked gauze on ice immediately by courier to the reference laboratory, where experienced personnel will process the tissue. Third, tissues may be placed in a carrier media which may circumvent the need for immediate action for up to 24 hours without significantly compromising the immunologic studies. However, delayed fixation will compromise histologic and cytologic detail. Primary and reference laboratories should establish a standing agreement upon such options.

Storage Instructions Snap frozen tissues should be maintained at -70°C or colder until immunophenotypic analysis can be performed. If frozen tissues are to be transported to a reference laboratory, they should be shipped on dry ice, using an overnight courier if necessary. Tissues placed in carrier media should be maintained on wet ice or at room temperature and packaged in insulated containers to avoid large fluctuations in temperature if sent to a reference laboratory.

Causes for Rejection Desiccated specimen, excessive freezing artifact, formalin exposure or excessive necrosis may compromise evaluation of light chain restriction.

Special Instructions Relevant information including history, clinical differential diagnosis, and significant laboratory findings are critical for optimal handling of the fresh lymph node. The specimen should not be placed in fixative if it can be delivered immediately to the laboratory. Intrinsic diagnostic difficulties are compounded by poor fixation and improper handling. Lymph node biopsies should be immediately delivered to the Histology Laboratory uncut in a small sterile jar or Petri dish. Requests for all examinations including bacteriology should accompany the specimen. All such specimens should be brought to the immediate attention of a pathologist. Bone marrow, blood studies sometimes including serologic test for infectious mononucleosis, and clinical information are commonly needed for appropriate work-up.

Use Diagnose various lymphadenopathies, including reactive and inflammatory entities, malignant lymphoma and metastatic neoplasia.

Limitations Formalin-fixed tissue cannot be used for culture or imprints and is suboptimal for evaluation of light chain restriction and electron microscopy. Childhood lymphoma is likelier to occur in extranodal sites, including mediastinum, abdomen, head, and neck.[4]

Methodology Quality conventional histology is of paramount importance in the evaluation of the lymph node biopsy. Interpretive errors are often due to deficient basic histopathology.[2] Touch preparations should always be obtained and are often invaluable for final diagnosis. Representative tissues should be allocated for immunotyping, taking the necessary precautions to minimize morphologic artifacts while maintaining maximal antigenicity. Immunoperoxidase stains on paraffin or frozen sections are accomplished according to the general procedures outlined in the test listing Immunoperoxidase Procedures *on page 43*. Immunologic markers on touch preparations and bone marrow smears are often best demonstrated by using an alkaline phosphatase enzyme detection system to minimize background staining. Cultures for infectious agents are sometimes indispensable.

Additional Information Correlation with peripheral blood, bone marrow, and other clinical laboratory studies is often desirable and sometimes mandatory. Flow cytometry on dissociated tissues or body fluids is often utilized instead of immunohistology for cell marker analysis. See listings Immunophenotypic Analysis of Tissues by Flow Cytometry *on page 45* and Leukocyte Immunophenotyping *on page 414*. This methodology offers a more quantitative approach to cell markers but only at the critical expense of destruction of immunoarchitecture. In general, immunohistology provides the best approach for typing tissues while flow cytometry is best suited for blood, bone marrow, and other body fluids. Properly acquired and frozen tissue is suitable for gene probe analysis (gene rearrangement studies), which may be necessary to document B- or T-cell clonal proliferation in rare cases.

See also a tabular presentation of frequently used **lymphocyte differentiation antigens** in the listing Immunophenotypic Analysis of Tissues by Flow Cytometry *on page 45*.

Footnotes
1. Ioachim HL, *Lymph Node Biopsy*, Philadelphia, PA: JB Lippincott Co, 1982, 17-8.
2. Warnke RA and Rouse RV, "Limitations Encountered in the Application of Tissue Section Immunodiagnosis to the Study of Lymphomas and Related Disorders," *Hum Pathol*, 1985, 16(4):326-31.
3. Chittal SM, Caveriviere P, Schwarting R, et al, "Monoclonal Antibodies in the Diagnosis of Hodgkin's Disease - The Search for a Rational Panel," *Am J Surg Pathol*, 1988, 12(1):9-21.
4. Sandlund JT, Downing JR, and Crist WM, "Non-Hodgkin's Lymphoma in Childhood," *N Engl J Med*, 1996, 334(19):1238-48.

References
Chan JK, Banks PM, Cleary ML, et al, "A Revised European-American Classification of Lymphoid Neoplasms Proposed by the International Lymphoma Study Group: A Summary Version," *Am J Clin Pathol*, 1995, 103(5):543-60.
Dehner LP, "Here We Go Again: A New Classification of Malignant Lymphomas: A Viewpoint From the Trenches," *Am J Clin Pathol*, 1995, 103(5):539-40.
Jaffe ES, "Surgical Pathology of the Lymph Nodes and Related Organs," *Major Problems in Pathology*, Vol 16, Philadelphia, PA: WB Saunders Co, 1995.
Knowles DM, *Neoplastic Hematopathology*, Baltimore, MD: Williams & Wilkins, 1992.
Warnke RA, Weiss LM, Chan JKC, et al, "Tumors of the Lymph Nodes and Spleen," *Atlas of Tumor Pathology*, 3rd Series, Fascicle 14, Washington, DC: Armed Forces Institute of Pathology, 1995.

Lymphocyte Analysis by Flow Cytometry *see* Immunophenotypic Analysis of Tissues by Flow Cytometry *on page 45*

Lymphocyte Immunophenotyping *see* Immunophenotypic Analysis of Tissues by Flow Cytometry *on page 45*

Lymphocyte Markers *see* Immunophenotypic Analysis of Tissues by Flow Cytometry *on page 45*

Lymphocyte Markers *see* Lymph Node Biopsy *on previous page*

Lymphoma *see* MIC2 *on next page*

Lymphoma Analysis by Flow Cytometry *see* Immunophenotypic Analysis of Tissues by Flow Cytometry *on page 45*

Lymphoma of Intermediate Differentiation *see* Mantle Cell Lymphoma *on this page*

Lysozyme *see* Immunoperoxidase Procedures *on page 43*

Mantle Cell Lymphoma
CPT 88306
Related Information
Histopathology *on page 42*
(Continued)

Mantle Cell Lymphoma *(Continued)*

Immunoperoxidase Procedures *on page 43*
Immunophenotypic Analysis of Tissues by Flow Cytometry *on page 45*
Leukocyte Immunophenotyping *on page 414*
Lymph Node Biopsy *on page 50*

Synonyms Centrocytic Lymphoma; Intermediate Lymphocytic Lymphoma; Lymphoma of Intermediate Differentiation

Test Commonly Includes Histologic characterization of abnormal lymphoid tissue based on key morphologic and cytologic features. Immunohistochemistry and immunophenotyping are used to support the histologic diagnosis. Chromosome analysis is typically ordered separately.

Abstract Lymphomas are classified on the basis of morphologic features as well as immunophenotypes. Prognosis and therapy are based on the classification of the lymphoma. Mantle cell lymphoma (MCL) is a distinctive subtype of lymphoma which is believed to arise from lymphocytes in the primary lymphoid follicles and mantle zones of secondary follicles.[1] A number of well-studied series with detailed descriptions of the morphologic and clinical features of MCL have been published.[2] The neoplastic cells of MCL have an immature monoclonal B cell phenotype and commonly have a characteristic cytogenetic abnormality, t(11;14)(q13;q32).[3]

Specimen A biopsy of a lymph node is typically performed to obtain fresh tissue. The diagnosis may also be made from splenic tissue involved with lymphoma.

Turnaround Time Processing and histologic review typically require 1-2 days, however, immunohistochemistry and molecular assays may delay final interpretation.

Reference Range A pathologist typically provides an interpretative report that describes the key features present in the lesion that provide for classification. In addition the pathologist will summarize and integrate data from the other essential assays performed, such as immunohistochemistry, flow analysis, and chromosome or molecular studies.

Use Histopathologic characterization and molecular assay provide information related to prognosis and treatment of the specific entity, mantle cell lymphoma

Methodology Histologic classification is based on the presence of key morphological features and characteristic results by immunophenotyping.

Additional Information The classification of non-Hodgkin's lymphomas involves multiple parameters, however is based principally on morphologic and cytologic key features. Immunophenotyping of cells is also an important adjunct. Recently, molecular assays have been utilized to aid in the diagnosis of specific tumor types. When a specific chromosomal translocation is associated with the pathologic entity. Mantle cell lymphoma is an illustrative example of the complexity of modern day classification of non-Hodgkin's lymphoma. The non-Hodgkin's of mantle cell type consist of atypical small lymphoid cells with either a nodular or diffuse pattern of growth. The lesion was first described in the 1980s by two separate groups as a type of follicular lymphoma characterized by the proliferation of atypical small lymphoid cells in wide mantles around benign germinal centers. Current belief is that mantle cell lymphomas represent a closely related spectrum of lymphomas arising from lymphocytes of primary lymphoid follicles or mantle zones of secondary follicles. The nodularity which may be present in approximately 30% of cases of MCL may lead to confusion with a follicular center cell lymphoma of the small-cleaved cell type. Cytologically, MCL shows atypical intermediate cell type of morphology of atypical small to medium sized lymphoid cells with irregular and indented nuclei, moderately coarse chromatin, inconspicuous nucleoli, and scant cytoplasm. Neoplastic cells may not only infiltrate lymph node but also bone marrow and commonly spleen. A diagnosis of MCL should not be based solely on peripheral blood or bone marrow findings. Involvement of other organs by MCL is common since patients usually have advanced stage disease at the time of diagnosis.

MCL has a characteristic cytogenetic abnormality of t(11,14) q(14,q8) which has recently been shown to involve an error in VDJ joining during IgG heavy gene rearrangement.[3] The translocation results in movement of a punitive cellular oncogene adjacent to bcl-1 into proximity of the enhancer region of Ig heavy chain gene (14q32)[4]. The gene involved in the MCL breakpoint is named PRAD1 and more recently CCND1.[5] The gene encodes for cyclin D1 and is overexpressed in nearly all cases of MCL. Overexpression of cyclin D1 results in a shortened D1 phase. Thus, this specific type of lymphoma demonstrates how different types of B-cell neoplasia result from the interference with normal differentiation at stages in the cell cycle.

Immunologic features identified by flow cytometry may be very useful in the identification of the typical immature monoclonal B cell phenotype. These cells almost always bear surface IgM with surface IgD and IgG

less common. Sixty percent of the cases express monoclonal lambda light chain. In addition to the typical pan B-cell markers of CD19, 22, and 24, the tumors also carry the pan T-cell antigen CD5 and are negative for CD10. The lack of CD23 may be useful for distinction from small lymphocytic lymphoma and chronic lymphocytic leukemia. Molecular assays for detection of the characteristic fusion sequence have been developed.[6]

MCL comprises 2% to 4% of non-Hodgkin's lymphoma in the U.S. and 7% to 9% of lymphomas in Europe. The median age at first diagnosis is approximately 60 years and males predominant 4 to 1 over females.[7] Generalized lymphadenopathy is a typical presentation (stage III/IV) including both bone marrow and liver involvement. The median survival of patients with MCL range is between 3 and 4 years. Current proposals are for MCL to be considered a low-grade lymphoma (KIEL classification) when it is predominantly nodular and composed of small lymphoid cells, but when MCL is diffuse, it is to be considered an intermediate grade lymphoma.

Footnotes

1. Weisenburger DD, Nathwani BN, Diamond LW, et al, "Malignant Lymphoma, Intermediate Lymphocytic Type. A Clinicopathologic Study of 42 Cases," *Cancer*, 1981, 48:1415.
2. Pittaluga S, Wlodarska I, Stul MS, et al, "Mantle Cell Lymphoma: A Clinicopathologic Study of 55 Cases," *Histopathology*, 1995, 26(1):17-24.
3. Williams ME, Swerdlow SH, and Meeker TC, "Chromosome t(11;14)(q13;q32) Breakpoints in Centrocytic Lymphoma are Highly Localized at the bcl-1 Major Translocation Cluster," *Leukemia*, 1993, 7(9):1437-40.
4. Segal GH, Masih AS, Fox AC, et al, "CD5-Expressing B-Cell Non-Hodgkin's Lymphomas With bcl-1 Gene Rearrangement Have a Relatively Homogeneous Immunophenotype and Are Associated With an Overall Poor Prognosis," *Blood*, 1995, 85(6):1570.
5. Bosch F, Jares P, Campo E, et al, "PRAD1/Cyclin D1 Gene Overexpression in Chronic Lymphoproliferative Disorders: A Highly Specific Marker of Mantle Cell Lymphoma," *Blood*, 1994, 84(8):2726-32.
6. Rimokh R, Berger F, Delsol G, et al, "Detection of the Chromosomal Translocation in t(11;14) by Polymerase Chain Reaction in Mantle Cell Lymphomas," *Blood*, 1994, 83(7):1871.
7. Zucca E, Roggero E, Pinotti G, et al, "Patterns of Survival in Mantle Cell Lymphoma," *Ann Oncol*, 1995, 6(3):257-62.

References

Norton AJ, Mathews J, Pappa V, et al, "Mantle Cell Lymphoma: Natural History Defined in a Serially Biopsied Population Over a 20-Year Period," *Ann Oncol*, 1995, 6(3):249-56.
Pittaluga S, Verhoef G, Criel A, et al, "Small B-Cell Non-Hodgkin's Lymphomas With Splenomegaly at Presentation Are Either Mantle Cell Lymphoma or Marginal Zone Cell Lymphoma - A Study Based on Histology, Cytology, Immunohistochemistry, and Cytogenetic Analysis," *Am J Surg Pathol*, 1996, 20(2):211-223.
Swerdlow SH, Zukerberg LR, Yang WI, et al, "The Morphologic Spectrum of Non-Hodgkin's Lymphomas With BCL1/Cyclin D1 Gene Rearrangements," *Am J Surg Pathol*, 1996, 20(5):627-40.

Medical Examiner's Case see Autopsy *on page 34*

Medical Legal Specimens see Histopathology *on page 42*

MIC2

CPT 88342

Related Information

Chromosome Analysis, Lymph Node and Solid Tumor *on page 279*
Electron Microscopy *on page 37*
Histopathology *on page 42*
Immunoperoxidase Procedures *on page 43*
Immunophenotypic Analysis of Tissues by Flow Cytometry *on page 45*

Applies to Acute Leukemia; Ewing's Sarcoma; Lymphoma; Peripheral Epithelioma; Primitive Neuroectodermal Tumor; Small Blue Cell Tumors

Test Commonly Includes Histopathology and may include electron microscopic examination and cytogenetic studies. MIC2 immunoperoxidase stains should always be evaluated in context of other cell marker studies.

Abstract MIC2 is a surface glycoprotein expressed by the Ewing's/primitive neuroectodermal tumors (PNET) group of sarcomas. It is reliably detected by immunoperoxidase methods in routinely processed tissues. Identification of this protein is highly useful in the classification of small round blue cell tumors of childhood and related tumors in the adult.

Specimen Routinely processed formalin-fixed, paraffin-embedded tissue; MIC2 antigen survives decalcification

Causes for Rejection Inadequate tumor sampling, extensive necrosis

Use Differential diagnosis of Ewing's sarcoma and other small round cell tumors

Limitations Occasional negative reactions occur despite optimal immunohistology. Other neoplasms in the differential diagnosis of Ewing's sarcoma are immunoreactive (*vide infra*).

Methodology MIC2 is detected by ordinary immunoperoxidase procedures. See test listing Immunoperoxidase Procedures *on page 43*. The antigen is optimally stained in B5 fixed tissues but produces acceptable results in formalin-fixed tissues. MIC2 also survives decalcification, making it suitable for evaluation of bone tumors and bone marrow biopsies.

Additional Information MIC2 is a 30/32 kilodalton surface glycoprotein thought to play a role in cell adhesion. MIC2 is normally expressed at low density by a variety of cells and can be detected by immunohistology in normal thymic cortex and pancreatic islets. However, in other tissues, MIC2 expression is sufficiently weak such that it is undetectable by immunohistology. Overexpression of this protein was first discovered in precursor T-cell malignancies[1] and Ewing's sarcoma.[2]

A unique chromosomal abnormality, t(11,22)(q24;q12), has been consistently demonstrated in Ewing's sarcoma. Subsequently, extraskeletal Ewing's sarcomas, primitive (peripheral) neuroectodermal tumors (PNET), Askin's tumors, and neuroepitheliomas were also shown to demonstrate the identical karyotypic marker. These tumors share overlapping characteristics including ultrastructural differentiation, cell culture behavior, and patterns of antigen and proto-oncogene expression, supporting the view that these tumors are derived from the mesenchymal "stem cell," differing only in the extent of differentiation along a common pathway. The relationship between this unique translocation and overexpression of MIC2 is unclear. MIC2 expression has been noted in cases lacking molecular evidence of the abnormal fusion gene product.[3]

By immunohistochemistry, MIC2 is detected in >90% of skeletal and extraskeletal Ewing's sarcoma. It is also expressed to an equal frequency in PNET, Askin's tumors, and neuroepitheliomas.[4,5,6,7,8] Characteristically, neoplastic cells show strong membrane staining which is generally diffuse but sometimes focal in distribution. However, antigen expression is not restricted to this family of tumors. MIC2 is occasionally found in other soft tissue tumors including alveolar rhabdomyosarcoma and mesenchymal chondrosarcoma. In these cases, MIC2 expression is usually weak and patchy. To date, neuroblastoma, small cell osteosarcoma, abdominal desmoplastic round cell tumor and so called "primitive sarcoma of bone" have been consistently negative. In adults, MIC2 is only rarely positive in small cell carcinoma[9] but may be more commonly positive in Merkel cell carcinoma.[10]

Special note should be made of MIC2 expression in lymphoid neoplasms, especially as lymphoma commonly enters the differential diagnosis of pediatric small round cell tumors. MIC2 is normally expressed early during lymphocyte ontogeny.[11] Cortical thymocytes and circulating precursor T cells normally express MIC2 at high density while CD34 positive precursor B cells are also strongly positive. Granulocytic and monocytic precursors as well as natural killer cells also express MIC2. Consequently, lymphomas and lymphoblastic leukemias, particularly of precursor T-cell origin, are immunoreactive for MIC2. Thus, MIC2 should be used in conjunction with a panel of other markers to exclude lymphoma and acute leukemia.

The MIC2 antigen is detected by three different monoclonal antibodies designated 12E7, HBA-71, and O13. At this time 12E7 and HBA-71 are commercially available. A direct comparison of these antibodies has not been published.

MIC2 has proven to be a highly useful and discriminating marker for the Ewing's/PNET group of tumors but should be used in conjunction with other immunologic markers to optimize its diagnostic utility.

Footnotes
1. Levy R, Dilley J, Fox RI, et al, "A Human Thymus Leukemia Antigen Defined by Hybridoma Monoclonal Antibodies," *Proc Natl Acad Sci USA*, 1979, 76:6552-6.
2. Hamilton G, Fellinger EJ, Schratter I, et al, "Characterization of a Human Endocrine Tissue and Tumor Associated Ewing's Sarcoma Antigen," *Cancer Res*, 1988, 48(21):6127-34.
3. Ladanyi M, Lewis R, Garin-Chesa P, et al, "EWS Rearrangement in Ewing's Sarcoma and Peripheral Neuroectodermal Tumor. Molecular Detection and Correlation With Cytogenetic Analysis and MIC2 Expression," *Diagn Mol Pathol*, 1993, 2(3):141-6.
4. Fellinger EJ, Garin-Chesa P, Triche TJ, et al, "Immunohistochemical Analysis of Ewing's Sarcoma Cell Surface Antigen p30/32 MIC2," *Am J Pathol*, 1991, 139(2):317-25.
5. Fellinger EJ, Garin-Chesa P, Glasser DB, et al, "Comparison of Cell Surface Antigen HBA-71 (p30/32 MIC2), Neuron Specific Enolase and Vimentin in Immunohistochemical Analysis of Ewing's Sarcoma of Bone," *Am J Surg Pathol*, 1992, 16(8):746-55.
6. Perlman EJ, Dickman PS, Askin FB, et al, "Ewing's Sarcoma - Routine Diagnostic Utilization of MIC2 Analysis: A Pediatric Oncology Group/Children's Cancer Group Intergroup Study," *Hum Pathol*, 1994, 25(3):304-7.
7. Ramani P, Rampling D, and Link M, "Immunocytochemical Study of 12E7 in Small Round-Cell Tumours of Childhood: An Assessment of Its Sensitivity and Specificity," *Histopathology*, 1993, 23(6):557-61.
8. Devaney K, Abbondanzo SL, Shekitka KM, et al, "MIC2 Detection in Tumors of Bone and Adjacent Soft Tissues," *Clin Orthop*, 1995, 310:176-87.
9. Lumadue JA, Askin FB, and Perlman EJ, "MIC2 Analysis of Small Cell Carcinoma," *Am J Clin Pathol*, 1994, 102(5):692-4.
10. Perlman EJ, Lumadue JA, Hawkins AL, et al, "Primary Cutaneous Neuroendocrine Tumors. Diagnostic Use of Cytogenetic and MIC2 Analysis," *Cancer Genet Cytogenet*, 1995, 82(1):30-4.
11. Dworzak MN, Fritsch G, Buchinger P, et al, "Flow Cytometric Assessment of Human MIC2 Expression in Bone Marrow, Thymus, and Peripheral Blood," *Blood*, 1994, 83(2):415-25.

References
Enzinger FM and Weiss SW, *Soft Tissue Tumors*, St Louis, MO: CV Mosby Co, 1995.

Michael's Solution *see* Kidney Biopsy *on page 47*

Monoclonal Immunoglobulins *see* Immunoperoxidase Procedures *on page 43*

Muscle Biopsy

CPT 88305 (surgical pathology); 88312 (special stains each); 88313 (trichrome stain); 88346 (immunofluorescence each antibody); 88348 (electron microscopy)

Related Information

Aldolase, Serum *on page 66*
Chromosome Analysis, Lymph Node and Solid Tumor *on page 279*
Creatine Kinase *on page 115*
Duchenne/Becker Muscular Dystrophy DNA Detection *on page 509*
Electron Microscopy *on page 37*
Histopathology *on page 42*
Inherited Diseases of Metabolism and Cell Structure Tests *on page 327*
Jo-1 Antibody *on page 411*
Myoglobin, Blood *on page 167*
Myoglobin, Qualitative, Urine *on page 644*
Myositis-Specific Autoantibody *on page 420*
Striational Antibodies *on page 432*
Trichinosis Serology *on page 436*

Synonyms Skeletal Muscle Biopsy

Test Commonly Includes For optimal evaluation of muscle biopsies, enzyme histochemistry often must be included.

Abstract Diagnosis and classification of muscle disease includes medical history, examination, laboratory assessment, electromyogram with nerve conduction studies, and muscle biopsy.[1]

Patient Preparation Clinical data is required and should include the patient's age and sex; the pattern, severity, duration, and tempo of the muscle involvement; relevant laboratory results (ie, CPK, ESR); nerve conduction and electromyographic (EMG) findings; and the presence of significant related conditions (ie, dermatitis, neoplasm, steroid or AZT therapy, AIDS); and the muscle biopsied. Family history may prove invaluable.

Sampling Time The biopsy should be performed early in the day as the specimen will immediately require special handling and should arrive when histotechnical personnel are available. The requisition should provide a brief clinical history, pertinent laboratory findings, and the location of the biopsy site.

Collection Selection of muscle biopsy site: The site for muscle biopsy should be one that bears well characterized features (ie, quadriceps femoris or biceps brachii (preferred)[1] or deltoid or gastrocnemius).[2] Unusual muscle groups such as oculomotor or pharyngeal muscles should be avoided, as they have several unique and potentially confusing features. Biopsy should be from an accessible muscle that is involved by the disease but has not reached "end-stage" atrophy. If more distal muscles are involved, a more distal biopsy site may be required. EMG or injection sites and sites near the myotendinous junction should be avoided as these biopsies commonly exhibit artifactual changes. It is the muscle belly that should be sampled, not the tendon insertion.

Surgical technique: Except for children or exceptional adult cases, the procedure is done with local anesthesia. A biopsy volume of at least 0.5 cm^3 usually is optimal. Additional muscle tissue may be needed for studies such as mitochondrial enzyme and DNA analysis.[1] Ideally, the biopsied muscle should not be allowed to contract because this creates microscopic artifacts. To achieve an isometric specimen, it is best to use a surgical muscle clamp that prevents contraction; some authors find the Price clamp satisfactory.[1] If no clamp is available, the specimen may be tied or pinned to a tongue blade to prevent contraction. A portion of the muscle, in continuity with that held in the clamp, should extend from the clamp so it may be cut off for freezing and histochemistry. A small piece should be placed in 1% glutaraldehyde for electron microscopy. Deliver on a saline-moistened gauze pad immediately to the Pathology Department. Moistened gauze is used to prevent drying. The specimen must not become saturated as this will cause severe ice crystal artifact during snap freezing. **The tissue should not be frozen or placed in fixative.** It should ideally reach the Pathology Laboratory within 30 minutes to retain enzyme activity.

Storage Instructions At least a small portion of the fresh material should be snap frozen for possible later use in biochemical assays (eg, quantitation of glycogen, enzymes, or dystrophin levels).

Use Evaluate muscle disease in terms of hereditary and acquired neurogenic atrophy, hereditary muscular dystrophies, myositis (infectious and "idiopathic," or autoimmune), hereditary and acquired metabolic and endocrine myopathies, ischemic, traumatic, and drug-induced problems, acquired diseases of the neuromuscular junction, and congenital/hereditary myopathies and enzyme deficiencies. A muscle biopsy may shed light on a systemic condition such as systemic vasculitis in the absence (Continued)

Muscle Biopsy (Continued)

of overt clinical muscle disease, but a low yield of abnormalities is found in such specimens.

Limitations Normal morphometric features vary with age, sex, and the muscle biopsied.[2] End stage atrophy is likely to provide only nonspecific findings. Placement of an unclamped muscle biopsy specimen directly into fixative creates artifact.[1] Muscle pathology has become a complex subspecialty.

Methodology A portion of the clamped muscle is oriented, frozen in isopentane/liquid nitrogen, and transverse sections are obtained for H & E, trichrome, and various histochemical preparations, some of which are listed below.

- Adenosine triphosphate (ATPase): At differing pHs, used to differentiate type I, IIa, and IIb myofibers and reveal abnormal fiber type distributions and diseases that selectively involve certain myofiber types.
- Succinate dehydrogenase (SDH): Stains mitochondria and shows abnormal aggregates or loss. Nicotinamide adenine dinucleotide-tetrazolium reductase (NADH-TR) may be used, but it is less sensitive.
- Oil red O: Stains lipids to detect abnormal accumulations.
- Periodic acid-Schiff (PAS): Used to detect glycogen in glycogenoses (ie, McArdle's disease, Pompe's disease, etc).

Extra frozen sections should be obtained and held in case additional more specific, enzyme preparations are needed (ie, cytochrome C oxidase, phosphofructokinase, phosphorylase). The remaining muscle tissue is formalin-fixed, paraffin-embedded, and stained with H & E and trichrome. Such preparations are used to detect small foci of myositis or vasculitis which may be missed on cryostat-cut sections, which are, of necessity, much smaller.

Footnotes

1. DeGirolami U, Smith TW, Chad D, et al, "Skeletal Muscle," *Principles and Practice of Surgical Pathology*, Silverberg SG, ed, New York, NY: Churchill Livingstone, 1990, 545-92.
2. Pearl GS and Ghatak NR, "Muscle Biopsy," *Arch Pathol Lab Med*, 1995, 119(4):303-6.

References

Brooke MH, "Disorders of Skeletal Muscle," *Neurology in Clinical Practice*, Bradley WG, Daroff RB, Fenichel GM, et al, eds, Boston, MA: Butterworth-Heinemann, 1991, 1843-86.

Carpenter S, "Light-Microscopic Pathology of Skeletal Muscle," *Disorders of Voluntary Muscle*, 6th ed, Walton J, Karpati G, Hilton-Jones D, eds, Edinburgh, England: Churchill Livingstone, 1994, 233-59.

Cullen MF, Hudgson P, and Mastaglia FL, "Ultrastructural Studies of Diseased Muscle," *Disorders of Voluntary Muscle*, 6th ed, Walton J, Karpati G, Hilton-Jones D, eds, Edinburgh, England: Churchill Livingstone, 1994, 319-80.

Dalakas MC, Illa I, Dambrosia JM, et al, "A Controlled Trial of High-Dose Intravenous Immune Globulin Infusions as Treatment for Dermatomyositis," *N Engl J Med*, 1993, 329(27):1993-2000.

Heffner RR Jr, "Skeletal Muscle," *Histology for Pathologists*, Sternberg SS, ed, New York, NY: Raven Press, 1992, 81-108.

Hoffman EP, Fischbeck KH, Brown RH, et al, "Characterization of Dystrophin in Muscle-Biopsy Specimens From Patients With Duchenne's or Becker's Muscular Dystrophy," *N Engl J Med*, 1988, 318(21):1363-8.

Plotz PH, "Not Myositis: A Series of Chance Encounters," *JAMA*, 1992, 268(15):2074-7.

Sewry CA and Dubowitz V, "Histochemical and Immunocytochemical Studies in Neuromuscular Diseases," *Disorders of Voluntary Muscle*, 6th ed, Walton J, Karpati G, Hilton-Jones D, eds, Edinburgh, England: Churchill Livingstone, 1994, 261-318.

Varga J, Uitto J, and Jimenez SA, "The Cause and Pathogenesis of the Eosinophilia-Myalgia Syndrome," *Ann Intern Med*, 1992, 116(2):140-7.

Myoglobin *see* Immunoperoxidase Procedures *on page 43*

Myosin *see* Immunoperoxidase Procedures *on page 43*

Necropsy *see* Autopsy *on page 34*

Needle Biopsy of Liver *see* Liver Biopsy *on page 48*

Oncogene Expression *see* Breast Biopsy *on page 35*

p53 *see* Breast Biopsy *on page 35*

PAS Stain *see* Skin Biopsy *on this page*

Pathologic Examination *see* Histopathology *on page 42*

Pathology Operating Room Consultation *see* Frozen Section *on page 41*

PCNA *see* Immunoperoxidase Procedures *on page 43*

Peptide Hormones *see* Immunoperoxidase Procedures *on page 43*

Peripheral Epithelioma *see* MIC2 *on page 52*

Peroxidase-Antiperoxidase (PAP) *see* Immunoperoxidase Procedures *on page 43*

PgR *see* Estrogen and Progesterone Receptor Assay *on page 38*

PgRICA or PgR(ICA) *see* Estrogen and Progesterone Receptor Assay *on page 38*

Ploidy *see* Breast Biopsy *on page 35*

Ploidy *see* Image Analysis *on page 43*

Ploidy *see* Tumor Aneuploidy by Flow Cytometry *on page 57*

Ploidy Analysis of Tumors *see* Tumor Aneuploidy by Flow Cytometry *on page 57*

Postmortem Examination *see* Autopsy *on page 34*

PR *see* Estrogen and Progesterone Receptor Assay *on page 38*

PRICA or PR(ICA) *see* Estrogen and Progesterone Receptor Assay *on page 38*

Primitive Neuroectodermal Tumor *see* MIC2 *on page 52*

Progesterone Binding Protein (Immunocytochemical) *see* Estrogen and Progesterone Receptor Assay *on page 38*

Progestogen Receptor (Immunocytochemical) *see* Estrogen and Progesterone Receptor Assay *on page 38*

Proliferative Indices *see* Tumor Aneuploidy by Flow Cytometry *on page 57*

Prostate Specific Acid Phosphatase *see* Immunoperoxidase Procedures *on page 43*

Quality Assurance in the Practice of Medicine *see* Autopsy *on page 34*

Renal Biopsy *see* Kidney Biopsy *on page 47*

S100 *see* Immunoperoxidase Procedures *on page 43*

Skeletal Muscle Biopsy *see* Muscle Biopsy *on previous page*

Skin Biopsy

CPT 88302 (plastic repair); 88304 (cyst/tag/debridement); 88305 (other than cyst/tag/debridement)

Related Information

Antinuclear Antibody *on page 368*
Bloom's Syndrome, Chromosome Breakage Study *on page 274*
Cat Scratch Disease Serology *on page 375*
Electron Microscopic Examination for Viruses, Stool *on page 665*
Electron Microscopy *on page 37*
Fungal Culture, Skin *on page 478*
Fungus Smear, Stain *on page 481*
Gene Rearrangement for Leukemia and Lymphoma *on page 512*
Gram's Stain *on page 481*
Herpes Cytology *on page 296*
Herpes Simplex Virus Antigen Detection *on page 667*
Histopathology *on page 42*
Immunoperoxidase Procedures *on page 43*
KOH Preparation *on page 485*
Leishmaniasis Serological Test *on page 413*
Lymph Node Biopsy *on page 50*
Mycobacterial Culture, Cutaneous and Subcutaneous Tissue *on page 489*
Oral Cavity Cytology *on page 298*
Pemphigus-Like Antibodies *on page 422*
Scleroderma Antibody *on page 430*
Skin Biopsy, Immunofluorescence *on page 56*
Varicella-Zoster Virus Culture *on page 675*
Varicella-Zoster Virus Serology *on page 437*
Viral Culture *on page 675*
Viral Culture, Dermatological Symptoms *on page 679*
Xeroderma Pigmentosum, Chromosome Breakage Study *on page 283*

Applies to Grocott's-Methanamine Silver Stain; PAS Stain

Abstract This section deals with sampling and procurement techniques and with a selected group of diagnostic skin problems.

Container 10% neutral formalin is satisfactory for submission of most specimens, but there are special requirements for immunofluorescence and electron microscopy. See also Histopathology *on page 42*, Electron Microscopy *on page 37*, and Immunoperoxidase Procedures *on page 43*.

Collection Techniques for procuring skin specimens:

Shave biopsy: A technique for obtaining superficial samples of predominantly epidermal or projecting lesions by cutting them flush with adjacent skin is illustrated in Figure 1. This technique is usually used for nonmalignant lesions but may be useful for the patch phase of mycosis fungoides. **Since shave biopsy provides the most limited specimen, a serious potential for histopathologic misdiagnosis exists, especially in regard to melanocytic lesions.**

Punch biopsy: Very popular with dermatologists because it can be done easily, quickly, and repetitively at low cost in office practice. Biopsy punches, illustrated in Figure 2, range from 3-6 mm in size. The punch is pressed into the skin and rotated. It yields a plug or core of tissue which

Figure 1. Shave Biopsy

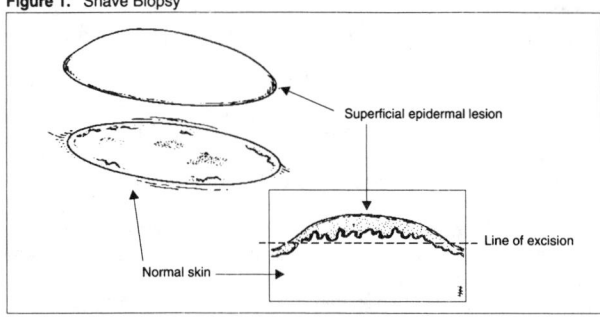

is cut from its base by scissors as the punch is withdrawn. It may be difficult to adequately sample subcutanea by punch. Pathologists prefer the largest possible sample.

Figure 2. Punch Biopsy

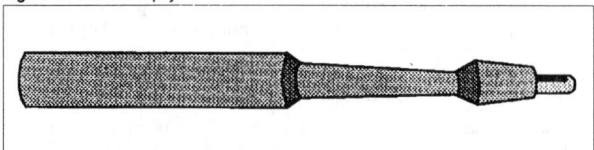

Excisional biopsy: This usually implies total removal of a skin lesion, most commonly a tumor, with a scalpel as illustrated in Figure 3. It is a preferred technique for removal of pigmented lesions and tumors.

Figure 3. Excisional Biopsy by Scalpel

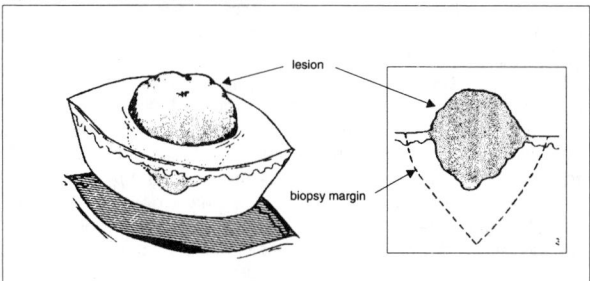

Incisional biopsy: Removal of a portion of a lesion by scalpel is illustrated in Figure 4. It is performed when a non-neoplastic lesion (eg, necrobiosis lipoidica) is too large to be totally excised but definitive diagnosis mandates a large sample to evaluate overall architectural detail. It may be used selectively in the case of tumors for which complete excision would require extensive surgery and/or would produce cosmetic deformity that would not be warranted, until accurate histopathologic diagnosis is established.

Figure 4. Incisional Biopsy by Scalpel

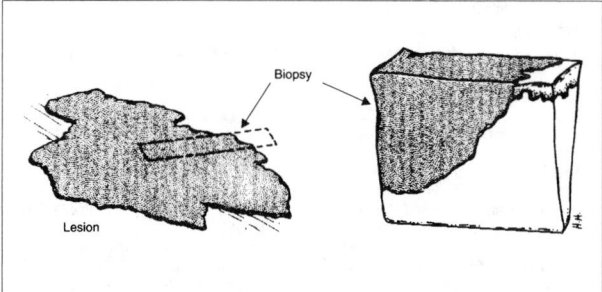

Smears and/or aspirates: Wright or Giemsa type stains may suffice to demonstrate polymorphonuclear leukocytes or eosinophils (as in toxic erythema or pustular melanosis of newborns). Gram's, acid-fast, PAS, and Grocott's methenamine-silver (GMS) stains, and cultures are used to study bacterial or fungal organisms. Finding appropriate multinucleated giant cells in smears in a proper clinical context suggests herpes or related viral infection. Smears of *Molluscum contagiosum* may be diagnostic. Aspirates may be adequate for cultures for bacteria, fungi, and viruses. Scrapings are often utilized to evaluate dermatophytoses. Negative KOH examination does not exclude the diagnosis of fungal infection.

Cytologic techniques (Tzanck smears) are rarely used in practice to evaluate acantholytic processes or tumors.

Curettings: Most frequently used when nodular basal cell carcinoma is suspected, and used as well for actinic and seborrheic keratoses. **Contraindicated for suspicious melanotic lesions.**

Storage Instructions See listing Histopathology *on page 42.*

Use Diagnosis of dermatologic disease

Additional Information Selected Problems in Dermatopathology:

A. Specimens of Pigmented Lesions and Tumors
1. In general, pigmented lesions and tumors should not be needled, aspirated, curetted, shaved, or punched, but should be excised, *in toto*, including margins, whenever possible, to permit comprehensive evaluation and measurements appropriate if melanoma.

B. Specimens of Vesiculobullous Lesions
1. If the diagnostic impression is pemphigus or pemphigoid, fresh lesions are preferred. Figure 5 illustrates appropriate biopsy technique.

Figure 5. Punch Biopsy Pemphigus or Pemphigoid

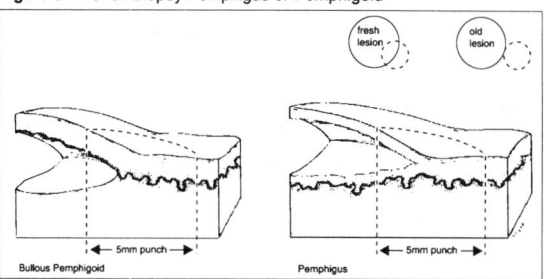

2. If the diagnostic impression is dermatitis herpetiformis, take the biopsy at the edge of the lesion (to study the change in dermal papillae) as shown in Figure 6, rather than the lesion itself.

Figure 6. Punch Biopsy: Dermatitis Herpetiformis

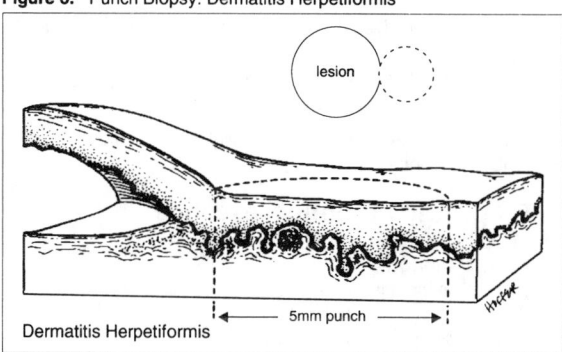

3. If the diagnostic impression is epidermolysis bullosa, the clinician should be aware of availability of four special regional reference centers in the USA for special studies of mechanobullous lesions. The Epidermolysis Registry Center is located in Chapel Hill, North Carolina. Contact phone number is (919) 966-2007.
4. Immunofluorescent studies of vesiculobullous lesions: Vesiculobullous lesions which require biopsy should be considered for immunofluorescent studies (IF). In many laboratories, skin samples for immunofluorescent studies are separately submitted in vials of isopentane prior to snap freezing in liquid nitrogen by the laboratory. Some reference laboratories provide special solutions such as Michael's solution or Zeus fixative to store specimens for their analysis. See listing Skin Biopsy, Immunofluorescence *on page 56.*

C. Specimens for Lupus Erythematosus (LE)
1. Direct immunofluorescence was first utilized on cutaneous biopsies in LE. The procedure (lupus band test) was widely utilized to study systemic lupus erythematosus (SLE), discoid lupus erythematosus (DLE), and mixed connective tissue disorder (MCTD). Recent data suggests the band test is much less specific and sensitive than previously thought. It is not clinically useful in discrimination of SLE

Biopsy Site	SLE	DLE
Lesional Tissue	+	+
Uninvolved, Sun-exposed	+	-

(Continued)

Skin Biopsy *(Continued)*

from other connective tissue (CT) disorders or in predicting which patients with undifferentiated CT disease would develop SLE. Serologic evaluation is more sensitive, efficient, and cost-effective in discriminating DLE and SLE.[1]

D. Specimens of Epidermolysis Bullosa Acquisita (EBA)
  1. Recent studies suggest that from 5% to 10% of patients regarded as bullous pemphigoid by routine direct immunofluorescence can be shown to be EBA based on indirect immunofluorescence on salt-split skin.[2]

E. Special Studies for Hematopoietic Disorders
  1. Special studies for T and B cells and lymphocyte markers are considered elsewhere. See Lymph Node Biopsy *on page 50* and Immunoperoxidase Procedures *on page 43*.

Pitfalls and artifacts to avoid: The biopsy technique should provide adequate and representative lesional tissue. Specimens should be handled gently without crushing by forceps. Cautery of lesions may burn or coagulate tissue making pathologic diagnosis impossible. If specimens are mailed to a reference laboratory in freezing weather, they may freeze after fixation. Formation of ice crystals may render interpretation hazardous if not impossible. Send in Lillie's "winter fixative" (acetic acid alcohol and formaldehyde).[3]

Footnotes
1. Harrist T, *Selected Topics in Cutaneous Immunofluorescence*, Boston, MA: International Academy of Pathology, 1990.
2. Logan RA, Bhogal B, Das AK, et al, "Localization of Bullous Pemphigoid Antibody - An Indirect Immunofluorescence Study of 228 Cases Using a Split-Skin Technique," *Br J Dermatol*, 1987, 117(4):471-8.
3. Lillie RD, *Histopathologic Technique and Practical Histochemistry*, Blakiston Co, 1954.

References
Elder DE and Murphy GF, "Melanocytic Tumors of the Skin," *Atlas of Tumor Pathology*, Washington, DC: Armed Forces Institute of Pathology, 1990.
Lever WF and Schaumburg-Lever G, *Histopathology of the Skin*, 7th ed, Philadelphia, PA: JB Lippincott Co, 1990.
Murphy GF and Elder DE, "Nonmelanocytic Tumors of the Skin," *Atlas of Tumor Pathology*, Washington, DC: Armed Forces Institute of Pathology, 1991.
Pariser DM, Caserio RJ, and Eaglstein WH, *Techniques for Diagnosis of Skin and Hair Disease*, 2nd ed, New York, NY: Thieme Inc, 1986.

Skin Biopsy Antibodies *see* Skin Biopsy, Immunofluorescence *on this page*

Skin Biopsy For Bullous or Collagen Disease *see* Skin Biopsy, Immunofluorescence *on this page*

Skin Biopsy For Pemphigus/Pemphigoid *see* Skin Biopsy, Immunofluorescence *on this page*

Skin Biopsy, Immunofluorescence

CPT 88346 (each antibody)

Related Information
Endomysial Antibodies *on page 391*
Oral Cavity Cytology *on page 298*
Pemphigus-Like Antibodies *on page 422*
Skin Biopsy *on page 54*
Viral Culture *on page 675*
Viral Culture, Dermatological Symptoms *on page 679*

Synonyms Immunofluorescence Skin Biopsy

Applies to Basement Membrane Zone Antibodies; Dermatitis Herpetiformis Antibodies; Intercellular Substance Antibodies; LE Antibodies; Lupus Band Test; Skin Biopsy Antibodies; Skin Biopsy For Bullous or Collagen Disease; Skin Biopsy For Pemphigus/Pemphigoid

Test Commonly Includes Anti-IgG, anti-IgA, anti-IgM, anti-C3, antifibrin immunofluorescence

Abstract There are two methods of immunofluorescence in dermatopathology. Antibodies against specific antigens in skin help distinguish between several bullous dermatoses. **Indirect testing** using serum and **direct testing** on appropriately sampled, labeled, and handled skin biopsies can provide invaluable information for the differential diagnosis of bullous and vasculitic diseases.

Patient Preparation Steroid therapy can convert findings to negative in previously positive patients.

Specimen 3 mm³ skin punch biopsy and serum

Container Covered Petri dish, or screw-cap glass vial; red top tube for blood

Collection Take biopsies from the following sites: If **pemphigus** or **bullous pemphigoid** is suspected, take a perilesional biopsy. If **dermatitis herpetiformis** is suspected, take biopsy of uninvolved area, 0.5-1.0 cm from lesion. Repeated biopsies are sometimes necessary to confirm dermatitis herpetiformis. If **systemic lupus erythematosus** or **discoid LE** is suspected, take biopsy of involved skin for diagnosis. Uninvolved skin, preferably of the wrist, is indicated to distinguish between discoid

and systemic LE. Biopsies from lesions may be positive in both SLE and discoid LE while normal appearing sun-exposed skin yields positive findings in SLE only. Lesions older than 6 weeks should be biopsied in suspected SLE. Nonexposed skin may be biopsied to **rule out** SLE. In **vasculitis**, biopsy of lesion less than 24 hours old is recommended.

Biopsy must be kept moist on saline soaked gauze or filter paper. Do not put specimen in formalin, Zenker's solution, or other usual fixatives. Deliver to the laboratory on ice immediately upon completion of biopsy. Label each specimen as exposed or nonexposed skin, involved or not involved, and so forth.

Storage Instructions Either snap freezing or placement in transport medium is usually satisfactory. Fixation in N-ethylmaleimide requires subsequent removal of fixative and frozen section. Consult the laboratory prior to obtaining specimen. Background immunofluorescence due to IgG staining is often a problem. It is largely due to deposition of the interstitial IgG and can be considerably reduced by an overnight incubation in phosphate-buffered saline.

Causes for Rejection Specimen in fixative, drying out of specimen

Use Useful in differential diagnosis of bullous skin diseases including epidermolysis bullosa acquisita, SLE, DLE, pemphigus, bullous pemphigoid, herpes gestationis and dermatitis herpetiformis, other skin entities, and for small vessel vasculitis

Limitations Many skin lesions which may clinically resemble SLE and DLE also have deposits of immunoglobulins at the basement membrane. These include psoriasis, polymorphous light eruption, and drug eruptions. Low titer anti-intercellular substance antibodies must be interpreted cautiously in the diagnosis of pemphigus. This is a complex subject which is difficult even to summarize. For instance, electron microscopy may be needed for diagnosis of **epidermolysis bullosa**. In the blistering disease **porphyria cutanea tarda**, uroporphyrinogen, uroporphyrin, and coproporphyrin urinary excretion is increased.

Contraindications Specimen should not be taken from heavily keratinized body areas if possible. Failure to demonstrate IgG in some biopsies may be due to a secondary change in the tissue due to infection and inflammatory reaction.

Methodology Direct fluorescent antibody (DFA) is done on skin and mucosal biopsies, examined for IgG, IgM, and IgA, C3, and fibrin. Indirect fluorescent antibody (IFA) is done using patient serum to detect antibodies on test tissues, such as monkey esophagus.

Additional Information Distinctive patterns of IgG, IgA, IgM, fibrin, and complement components in epidermis, basement membrane, and dermal vessels may contribute to the differential diagnosis of bullous skin diseases, discoid and systemic lupus erythematosus, and other entities.

Serum antibodies to skin components can be demonstrated, using a tissue substrate (usually monkey or guinea pig esophagus). Such observations must be correlated with clinical and histopathologic facets as well as findings on direct immunofluorescence.[1] In bullous disease antibody levels often reflect disease activity and rising titers may foretell clinical relapse, but such correlation is imperfect.

See listing Endomysial Antibodies *on page 391*, relevant to dermatitis herpetiformis and coeliae disease. See listing Antinuclear Antibody *on page 368* relevant to systemic lupus erythematosus and mixed connective tissue disease.

Immunoglobulins or complement depositions in vessels may be found in skin biopsies in instances of vasculitis.

Footnotes
1. Leavelle DE, *Mayo Medical Laboratories Interpretive Handbook*, Rochester, MN: Mayo Medical Laboratories, 1994, 157-8, 473-5.

References
Alcocer J, Moreno J, Garcia-Torres R, et al, "Immunofluorescent Skin Band Test in the Differential Diagnosis of Systemic Lupus Erythematosus," *J Rheumatol*, 1979, 6:196-203.
Brown C, Lieu TS, and Sontheimer RD, "Correlation Between Dermal Interstitial Immunoglobulin G and Hypergammaglobulinemia," *J Invest Dermatol*, 1991, 97(2):373-7.
Farmer ER and Provost TT, "Immunologic Studies of Skin Biopsy Specimens in Connective Tissue Diseases," *Hum Pathol*, 1983, 14:316-25.
Gammon WR, Kowalewski C, Chorzelski TP, et al, "Direct Immunofluorescence Studies of Sodium Chloride-Separated Skin in the Differential Diagnosis of Bullous Pemphigoid and Epidermolysis Bullosa Acquisita," *J Am Acad Dermatol*, 1990, 22(4):664-70.
Harrist TJ and Mihm MC, "Cutaneous Immunopathology. The Diagnostic Use of Direct and Indirect Immunofluorescence Techniques in Dermatologic Disease," *Hum Pathol*, 1979, 10:625-53.
Izuno GT, "Cutaneous Immunofluorescence," *Clin Lab Med*, 1986, 6(1):85-102.
Wick MR, Ritter JH, Humphrey PA, et al, "Immunopathology of Nonneoplastic Skin Disease. A Brief Review," *Am J Clin Pathol*, 1996, 105(4):417-29.

Small Blue Cell Tumors *see* MIC2 *on page 52*

Solid Tumors Analysis by Flow Cytometry *see* Immunophenotypic Analysis of Tissues by Flow Cytometry *on page 45*

S Phase *see* Breast Biopsy *on page 35*

S Phase *see* Image Analysis *on page 43*

S Phase see Tumor Aneuploidy by Flow Cytometry on this page

Static Image Analysis see Image Analysis on page 43

Surgical Pathology see Histopathology on page 42

Surgical Pathology Consultation see Frozen Section on page 41

Synaptophysin see Immunoperoxidase Procedures on page 43

Tamoxifen see Estrogen and Progesterone Receptor Assay on page 38

Thymidine Labeling Index see Tumor Aneuploidy by Flow Cytometry on this page

Thyroglobulin see Immunoperoxidase Procedures on page 43

Tissue Antigens see Immunoperoxidase Procedures on page 43

Tissue Examination see Histopathology on page 42

T-Lymphocyte Analysis by Flow Cytometry see Immunophenotypic Analysis of Tissues by Flow Cytometry on page 45

T Lymphocytes see Immunoperoxidase Procedures on page 43

Transjugular Needle Biopsy of the Liver see Liver Biopsy on page 48

Transmission Electron Microscopy see Electron Microscopy on page 37

Tumor Aneuploidy by Flow Cytometry

CPT 88358

Related Information
Body Fluid Cytology on page 286
Breast Biopsy on page 35
Cerebrospinal Fluid Cytology on page 290
Chromosome Analysis, Lymph Node and Solid Tumor on page 279
Estrogen and Progesterone Receptor Assay on page 38
Fine Needle Aspiration, Superficial Palpable Masses on page 294
Histopathology on page 42
Homovanillic Acid, Urine on page 145
Image Analysis on page 43
Immunophenotypic Analysis of Tissues by Flow Cytometry on page 45
Lymphocyte Transformation Test on page 416
Urine Cytology on page 301

Synonyms Cell Cycle Analysis of Tumors; Flow Cytometry of Tumor Aneuploidy; Ploidy Analysis of Tumors

Applies to Aneuploidy; DNA Content; DNA Synthesis Phase; G_1 Phase; G_2M; G_0 Phase; Ploidy; Proliferative Indices; S Phase; Thymidine Labeling Index

Test Commonly Includes Assessment of nuclear DNA for aneuploid clones; estimation of percentage of cells in S phase ("replicating fraction," "S phase fraction")

Abstract Assessment of ploidy may be helpful to estimate prognosis and to plan therapy for patients from whom tumors have been sampled or excised.

Specimen Portion of tissue, fresh or paraffin-embedded, needle aspiration of neoplasm. Fresh tissue is better than formalin-fixed, paraffin-embedded specimen.[1]

Reference Range Almost all specimens of benign, non-neoplastic tissue show a dominant population of diploid nuclei with an amount of stainable DNA designated "2C." There are approximately 10% cells actively synthesizing DNA, "S phase fraction," and only a small number of premitotic cells with double the normal diploid DNA content, "4C." See diagram.

Use Quantitate nuclear DNA content and replicative activity of neoplastic cells. The presence of aneuploid peaks, representing nuclei with abnormal amounts of DNA and/or an increased percentage of cells actively synthesizing DNA, may be prognostically significant and may be independent of tumor grade and stage, depending on the primary neoplasm.

Limitations This assay is not in itself diagnostic of malignancy. Results must be interpreted with caution and experience. Results are most meaningful when applied to a sample in which the diagnosis of malignancy has already been established by histopathology. Neoplasms with diploid cell lines, even if malignant, may be indistinguishable by this technique from benign or normal tissue. Some neoplasms may harbor multiple stem lines, some aneuploid, some not. Some neoplasms have "near-diploid" stem lines which may be difficult or impossible to identify as abnormal. **Some benign adenomas may contain aneuploid cells,**

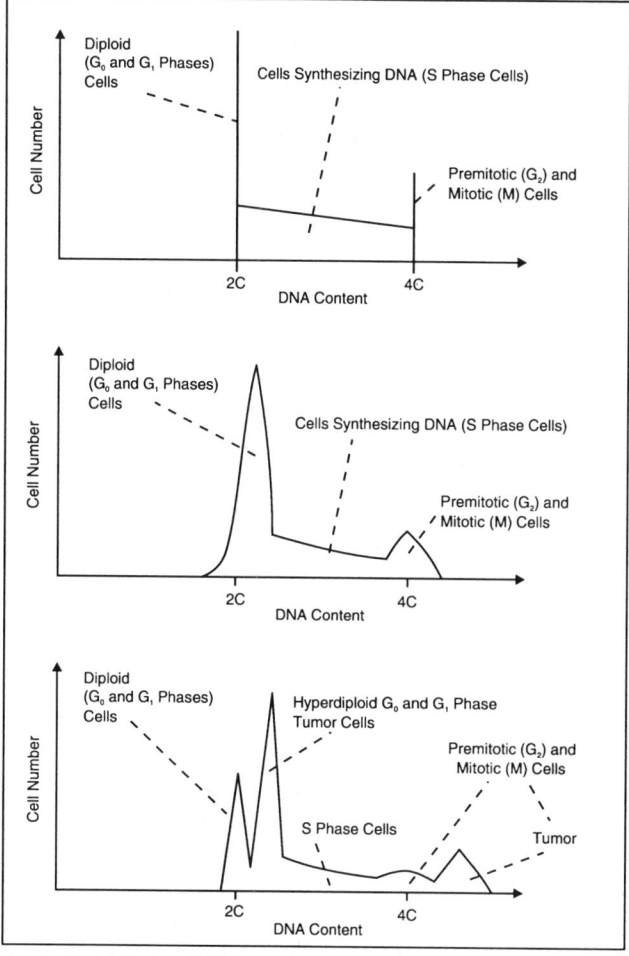

Top: An ideal distribution of DNA content in a cell population. Center: A distribution more typical of those actually obtained by flow cytometry. Bottom: A distribution such as is obtained from a tumor exhibiting DNA aneuploidy.
From Shapiro, "DNA Content," *Arch Pathol Lab Med*, 1989, 113:592, with permission.

and the DNA content of some carcinomas of the same tissue may be diploid (eg, adrenal cortical adenomas and adenocarcinomas).[2]

Use of poorly fixed blocks or improperly stored blocks may lead to artifacts which may be interpreted as aneuploid peaks. Avoid use of blocks processed with precipitating fixatives such as B5 or Zenker's fluid, as such fixatives tend to produce poor coefficients of variation and possibly uninterpretable total nuclear protein and light scatter data.[3,4] If possible, a separate block of tumor should be fixed in nonbuffered formalin.

Flow cytometry from formalin-fixed, paraffin-embedded tissue may not always detect aneuploid cell populations, when compared to analysis of fresh tissue.[5] DNA analysis by flow cytometry, compared to image analysis, has shown high concordance. Discordant results do occur.[6,7]

Methodology Flow cytometry (FC) of tumor cell suspension stained with an intercalating dye which binds quantitatively to DNA (usually ethidium bromide or propidium iodide). The nuclear stain fluoresces when excited by the cytometer's laser in direct linear proportion to the amount of nuclear DNA and is quantitated by the instrument's photomultiplier tubes. When sufficient nuclei have been analyzed (usually 5000-10,000), a histogram is generated (see diagrams) plotting the numbers of nuclei with given amounts of DNA. Much the same information can be developed on a quantitative image analysis system consisting of a light microscope interfaced with a computer for data analysis. Image analysis systems typically gather information on hundreds of cells, rather than thousands.

Additional Information That many cancers have abnormal amounts of nuclear DNA comes as no surprise to anyone who has looked at malignant tissue microscopically. Indeed, this is largely the basis for the prognostic significance of histologic grading systems, in which tumors which "look bad" connote a worse prognosis. If flow cytometry offered no more than quantified confirmation of this phenomenon, it would be only an expensive, elegant redundancy.
(Continued)

Tumor Aneuploidy by Flow Cytometry *(Continued)*

CELL CYCLE

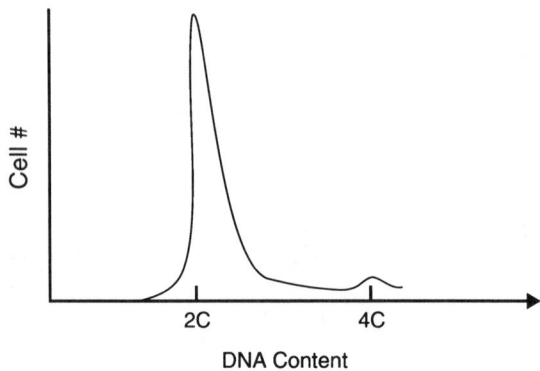

Diploid cells, slowly replicating

Aneuploid cells, rapid replication

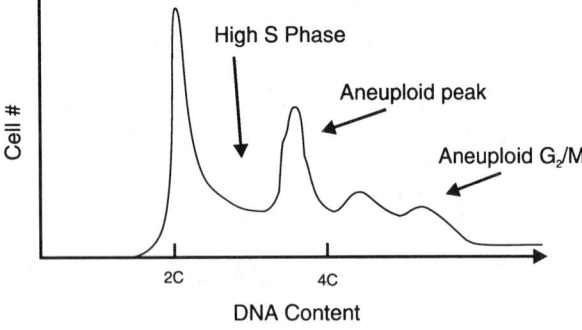

Flow cytometry is used to divide tumors into euploid **(diploid)** or **aneuploid** types. A tumor is classified as diploid if the DNA distribution has a major proliferation node at the normal diploid DNA value. Such a normal diploid value is typically derived from a cell culture fibroblast line or normal cells processed in the same block as the tumor. DNA measurement by flow cytometry is relatively insensitive, and it is well known that the gain or loss of several chromosomes or minor deletions might go undetected.

The powers of flow cytometric analysis of ploidy are that aneuploid cell lines or increased proliferative capacity can be detected even in histologically low grade neoplasms.[8] Stage for stage and grade for grade, neoplasms with aneuploid nuclei are generally prognostically worse than those which are diploid.[9] The prognostic value of DNA flow cytometry is largely dependent upon tumor type. Predictive value by flow cytometry is most solidly established for cancers of the breast,[10,11,12,13,14] prostate,[15,16] and colon.[17] It is less clearly true for cancers of the ovary, lung, and kidney.

For a few neoplasms (acute lymphoblastic lymphoma, neuroblastoma), the presence of aneuploid cell lines is prognostically favorable.

Flow cytometry may also be of prognostic value in patients with transitional cell carcinoma of bladder.[18,19,20,21] Some have advocated the use of bladder washings to follow up patients with transitional cell carcinomas. This presupposes an adequately cellular specimen, and the assurance that the neoplasm being followed had an aneuploid line or other detectable abnormality to begin with. Such circumstances may not consistently be so for well differentiated papillary carcinomas.

Measurement of S phase fraction (DNA synthesis phase) is advocated for breast carcinoma. SPF correlates with thymidine labeling index, which is a measure of cellular proliferation.

In most clinical laboratories, SPF is determined by statistical modeling rather than direct measurement. For many specimens a reliable estimate cannot be determined because of cellular/nuclear debris ("dirty specimen") or overlapping of peaks. Selection of the appropriate mathematical model and variability introduced by the sample or sample preparation lead to significant interlaboratory disparity in reported SPF.[22] Alternative methods to directly measure SPF are being investigated but have yet to significantly penetrate the clinical laboratory setting.[23]

Hedley developed a method of retrieving tissue from paraffin blocks, making possible analysis of archival material.[24] Thus, if a specimen is small, it can be totally processed for microscopy with the assurance that DNA analysis can be done later from the block, if necessary. The Hedley technique also lets one be confident that the material being analyzed indeed represents the cancer. Various modifications of the Hedley technique have been proposed.[25,26,27]

Footnotes

1. Robinson RA, "Defining the Limits of DNA Cytometry," *Am J Clin Pathol*, 1992, 98(3):275-7 (editorial).
2. Medeiros LJ and Weiss LM, "New Developments in the Pathologic Diagnosis of Adrenal Cortical Neoplasms," *Am J Clin Pathol*, 1992, 97(1):73-83.
3. Herbert DJ, Nishiyama RH, Bagwell CB, et al, "Effects of Several Commonly Used Fixatives on DNA and Total Nuclear Protein Analysis by Flow Cytometry," *Am J Clin Pathol*, 1989, 91(5):535-41.
4. Esteban JM, Sheibani K, Owens M, et al, "Effects of Various Fixatives and Fixation Conditions on DNA Ploidy Analysis. A Need for Strict Internal DNA Standards," *Am J Clin Pathol*, 1991, 95(4):460-6.
5. Frierson HF Jr, "Flow Cytometric Analysis of Ploidy in Solid Neoplasms: Comparison of Fresh Tissues With Formalin-Fixed Paraffin-Embedded Specimens," *Hum Pathol*, 1988, 19(3):290-4.
6. Elsheikh TM, Silverman JF, McCool JW, et al, "Comparative DNA Analysis of Solid Tumors by Flow Cytometric and Image Analyses of Touch Imprints and Flow Cell Suspensions," *Am J Clin Pathol*, 1992, 98(3):296-304.
7. Ghali VS, Liau S, Teplitz C, et al, "A Comparative Study of DNA Ploidy in 115 Fresh-Frozen Breast Carcinomas by Image Analysis Versus Flow Cytometry," *Cancer*, 1992, 70(11):2668-72.
8. Frierson HF Jr, "Grade and Flow Cytometric Analysis of Ploidy for Infiltrating Ductal Carcinomas," *Hum Pathol*, 1993, 24(1):24-9.
9. Merkel DE, Dressler LG, and McGuire WL, "Flow Cytometry, Cellular DNA Content, and Prognosis in Human Malignancy," *J Clin Oncol*, 1987, 5(10):1690-703.
10. Dressler LG, Seamer LC, Owens MA, et al, "DNA Flow Cytometry and Prognostic Factors in 1331 Frozen Breast Cancer Specimens," *Cancer*, 1988, 61(3):420-7.
11. Clark GM, Dressler LG, Owens MA, et al, "Prediction of Relapse or Survival in Patients With Node-Negative Breast Cancer by DNA Flow Cytometry," *N Engl J Med*, 1989, 320(10):627-33.
12. Lewis WE, "Prognostic Significance of Flow Cytometric DNA Analysis in Node-Negative Breast Cancer Patients," *Cancer*, 1990, 65(10):2315-20.
13. Bosari S, Lee AK, Tahan SR, et al, "DNA Flow Cytometric Analysis and Prognosis of Axillary Lymph Node-Negative Breast Carcinoma," *Cancer*, 1992, 70(7):1943-50.
14. Hedley DW, Clark GM, Cornelisse CJ, et al, "Consensus Review of the Clinical Utility of DNA Cytometry in Carcinoma of the Breast. Report of the DNA Cytometry Consensus Conference," *Cytometry*, 1993, 14(5):482-5.
15. Jones EC, McNeal J, Bruchovsky N, et al, "DNA Content in Prostatic Adenocarcinoma. A Flow Cytometry Study of the Predictive Value of Aneuploidy for Tumor Volume, Percentage Gleason Grade 4 and 5, and Lymph Node Metastases," *Cancer*, 1990, 66(4):752-7.
16. Shankey TV, Kallioniemi OP, Koslowski JM, et al, "Consensus Review of the Clinical Utility of DNA Content Cytometry in Prostate Cancer," *Cytometry*, 1993, 14(5):497-500.
17. Bauer KD, Bagwell CB, Giaretti W, et al, "Consensus Review of the Clinical Utility of DNA Flow Cytometry in Colorectal Cancer," *Cytometry*, 1993, 14(5):486-91.
18. Farsund T, Hoestmark JG, and Laezum OD, "Relation Between Flow Cytometric DNA Distribution and Pathology in Human Bladder Cancer. A Report on 69 Cases," *Cancer*, 1984, 54(9):1771-7.
19. Murphy WM, "DNA Flow Cytometry in Diagnostic Pathology of the Urinary Tract," *Hum Pathol*, 1987, 18(4):317-9.
20. Blomjous EC, Schipper NW, Baak JP, et al, "The Value of Morphometry and DNA Flow Cytometry in Addition to Classic Prognosticators in Superficial Urinary Bladder Carcinoma," *Am J Clin Pathol*, 1989, 91(3):243-8.
21. Wheeless LL, Badalament RA, de Vere White RW, et al, "Consensus Review of the Clinical Utility of DNA Cytometry in Bladder Cancer. Report of the DNA Cytometry Consensus Conference," *Cytometry*, 1993, 14(5):478-81.
22. Coon JS, Paxton H, Lucy L, et al, "Interlaboratory Variation in DNA Flow Cytometry. Results of the College of American Pathologists' Survey," *Arch Pathol Lab Med*, 1994, 118(7):681-5.
23. Meyer JS, Koehm SL, Hughes JM, et al, "Bromodeoxyuridine Labeling for S-Phase Measurement in Breast Carcinoma," *Cancer*, 1993, 71(11):3531-40.
24. Hedley DW, Friedlander ML, Taylor IW, et al, "Method for Analysis of Cellular DNA Content of Paraffin-Embedded Pathological Material Using Flow Cytometry," *J Histochem Cytochem*, 1983, 31:1333-5.
25. Weaver DL, Bagwell CB, Hitchcox SA, et al, "Improved Flow Cytometric Determination of Proliferative Activity (S Phase Fraction) From Paraffin-Embedded Tissue," *Am J Clin Pathol*, 1990, 94(5):576-84.
26. Babiak J and Poppema S, "Automated Procedure for Dewaxing and Rehydration of Paraffin-Embedded Tissue Sections for DNA Flow Cytometric Analysis of Breast Tumors," *Am J Clin Pathol*, 1991, 96(1):64-9.
27. Schultz DS and Zarbo RJ, "Comparison of Eight Modifications of Hedley's Method for Flow Cytometric DNA Ploidy Analysis of Paraffin-Embedded Tissue," *Am J Clin Pathol*, 1992, 98(3):291-5.

References

Arber DA, Cook PD, Moser LK, et al, "Variation in Reference Cells for DNA Analysis of Paraffin-Embedded Tissue," *Am J Clin Pathol*, 1992, 97(3):387-92.

Danova M, Riccardi A, Mazzini G, et al, "Flow Cytometric Analysis of Paraffin-Embedded Material in Human Gastric Cancer," *Anal Quant Cytol Histol*, 1988, 10(3):200-6.

Duque RE, Andreeff M, Braylan RC, et al, "Consensus Review of the Clinical Utility of DNA Flow Cytometry in Neoplastic Hematopathology," *Cytometry*, 1993, 14(5):492-6.

Herman CJ, Hedley D, Wheeless LL, et al, "DNA Cytometry in Cancer Prognosis," *PPO Updates*, 1993, 7(3).

Homburger HA and Wold LE, "College of American Pathologists Conference XV on Analytical Cytology and Immunohistochemistry," *Arch Pathol Lab Med*, 1989, 113:577-683.

Joensuu H, Klemi PJ, and Eerola E, "Diagnostic Value of Flow Cytometric DNA Determination Combined With Fine Needle Aspiration Biopsy in Thyroid Tumors," *Anal Quant Cytol Histol*, 1987, 9(4):328-34.

Khoo SK, Hurst T, Kearsley J, et al, "Prognostic Significance of Tumor Ploidy in Patients With Advanced Ovarian Carcinoma," *Gynecol Oncol*, 1990, 39(3):284-8.

Landay AL, Ault KA, Bauer KD, et al, eds, *Clinical Flow Cytometry*, Vol 677, New York, NY: The New York Academy of Sciences, 1993.

Listinsky CM, Bonfiglio TA, and Leary J, "Variable Ploidy of Ovarian Clear Cell Carcinomas," *Anal Quant Cytol Histol*, 1988, 10(1):21-7.

Look AT, Douglass EC, and Meyer WH, "Clinical Importance of Near-Diploid Tumor Stem Lines in Patients With Osteosarcoma of an Extremity," *N Engl J Med*, 1988, 318(24):1567-72.

McCarthy RC and Fetterhoff TJ, "Issues for Quality Assurance in Clinical Flow Cytometry," *Arch Pathol Lab Med*, 1989, 113(6):658-66.

Radio SJ, Woodridge TN, and Linder J, "Flow Cytometric DNA Analysis of Malignant Fibrous Histiocytoma and Related Fibrohistiocytic Tumors," *Hum Pathol*, 1988, 19(1):74-7.

Stonesifer KJ, Xiang JH, Wilkinson EJ, et al, "Flow Cytometric Analysis and Cytopathology of Body Cavity Fluids," *Acta Cytol* 1987, 31(2):125-30.

Tsushima K, Stanhope CR, Gaffey TA, et al, "Uterine Leiomyosarcomas and Benign Smooth Muscle Tumors: Usefulness of Nuclear DNA Patterns Studied by Flow Cytometry," *Mayo Clin Proc*, 1988, 63(3):248-55.

van den Ingh HF, Griffioen G, and Cornelisse CJ, "Flow Cytometric Detection of Aneuploidy in Colorectal Adenomas," *Cancer Res*, 1985, 45(7):3392-7.

Ultrastructural Study *see* Electron Microscopy *on page 37*

Vimentin *see* Immunoperoxidase Procedures *on page 43*

Viral Diseases by EM *see* Electron Microscopy *on page 37*

Vital Statistics *see* Autopsy *on page 34*

Zeus Fixative *see* Kidney Biopsy *on page 47*

CHEMISTRY

Harold J. Grady, PhD

David S. Jacobs, MD

Eugene S. Olsowka, MD, PhD

Contributors:
    Wayne R. DeMott, MD
    Lowell L. Tilzer, MD, PhD

Major advances in analytical methods, reagents, and instrumentation have markedly improved the scope and efficiency of clinical chemistry laboratories. Most of the analytical techniques in these laboratories are now performed by automated or semi-automated analyzers. Many of these have menus of 30-50 tests which can be performed in random order and have stat-interrupt capability. A panel of 20 or more tests can typically be completed in a matter of minutes so that throughput is in the range of 500-800 tests per hour. Dwell time is usually a matter of 1-2 minutes so that stat-test analyzer time is frequently less than 5 minutes. This type of analyzer processes 90% to 95% of the clinical chemistry workload using exclusively spectrophotometric techniques, while the remaining tests are performed by more specialized automated systems employing principles of immunoassay, chromatography, isotopic assay, mass spectroscopy, ion counting, potentiometry, and coulometry. Some also involve spectrophotometry. As these systems have become more sophisticated, their accuracy and precision have also improved. Coefficients of variation (imprecision) for most tests are under 5% and for nearly all tests, under 10%. Bias (inaccuracy) is usually under 5%.

The above systems are typically coupled to laboratory information systems (LIS) which use computers and computer techniques to track and record the patient sample from order entry to the final printout of the analytical result at the site of data use. Computers also furnish automatic alerts for out-of-range sample results, as well as warnings of unacceptable control values. Many of the above chemical techniques are used for other specialized tests found in this book in the chapters entitled Molecular Pathology, Immunology and Serology, and Therapeutic Drug Monitoring/Toxicology/Drugs of Abuse. Use of point-of-care testing (POCT) or alternate site testing (AST) is increasing in an attempt to shorten turnaround time and decrease sample handling. Automated systems similar to the above have been designed for this purpose and are capable of whole blood analysis which minimizes the patient's loss of blood for laboratory samples. This is especially important for pediatric testing. The subject is discussed further in the chapter Specimen Collection under Point-of-Care Testing *on page 27*.

The Clinical Laboratory Improvement Act of 1988 (CLIA '88) is essentially fully implemented and defines regulations for all healthcare laboratories concerning laboratory and personnel accreditation, external proficiency testing, internal quality control, quality assurance, and method validation. Although a few simple tests are exempt from these regulations, all other testing is covered and all healthcare laboratories must meet the same strict standards. These regulations apply to clinical chemistry as well as to all other divisions of the clinical laboratory.

Turnaround time is essentially not discussed under the test entries in this chapter because it can be quite variable. It depends upon the instrumentation and laboratory organization. In general, in many modern laboratories, results from usual orders are available within 2 hours and from stats within 30-40 minutes. Most of this time is devoted to specimen procurement, transport, and preparation. Results from send outs (to reference laboratories) will often be available the next day (for tests done every day) or in 2-3 days (for tests done only several times per week).

Some terminology has been changed to meet current standards of acceptance. The somewhat ambiguous term "normal range" has been replaced with the more readily definable term "reference range" which can be used for any population provided a description of that population is furnished. CLIA regulations require that all laboratories acquire the data that justifies the applicability of their reference ranges to the population they serve. The information listed in the specimen field of each test reflects the sample type actually analyzed rather than the sample collected (eg, serum or plasma vs blood). However, when the name of the test entry contains a reference to a sample type, it will not always be the sample that is analyzed. Generally, SI units are given after the conventional units unless SI units are widely used, then only the SI units are used.

An extensive review of many of the factors involved in the decision as to whether or not a result is within the "normal" or "reference" range for a given patient is found in the chapter entitled Statistics, the Normal Range, and the Ulysses Syndrome *on page 11*.

Clinical problems are nearly always too complex to allow satisfactory interpretation of laboratory results without correlation with clinical data. Thus, a review of the patient's clinical and laboratory findings by an interested and knowledgable consultant (eg, internist, endocrinologist, nephrologist, clinical pathologist) will frequently increase the usefulness of laboratory determinations and enhance the contribution of laboratory data to patient care.

The revisions and new entries in this chapter, as well as in all other chapters, reflect the rapid increase in knowledge and expertise of laboratory practitioners and their dedication to the implementation of contemporary advances.

Dr Paul Finley was first author of the Chemistry test listings in the 3rd edition of the *Laboratory Test Handbook*.

βA4 Peptide *see* Apolipoprotein E *on page 82*

ABGs *see* Blood Gases, Arterial *on page 87*

ACE *see* Angiotensin Converting Enzyme *on page 80*

Acetaminophen *see* Liver Profile *on page 161*

Acetaminophen Hepatotoxicity *see* Aspartate Aminotransferase *on page 84*

Acetoacetate *see* Ketone Bodies, Blood *on page 152*

Acetone *see* Ketone Bodies, Blood *on page 152*

Acetylcholinesterase *see* Pseudocholinesterase, Serum *on page 196*

Acetylcholinesterase, Red Cell

CPT 82482

Related Information

Alpha$_1$-Fetoprotein, Amniotic Fluid *on page 71*
Alpha$_1$-Fetoprotein, Serum *on page 72*
Dibucaine Number *on page 122*
Pseudocholinesterase, Serum *on page 196*

Synonyms Cholinesterase, Erythrocytic; Cholinesterase I; Erythrocyte Cholinesterase; True Cholinesterase

Abstract The red cell enzyme (true cholinesterase) is specific for the substrate acetylcholine. The serum enzyme (pseudocholinesterase) hydrolyzes other choline esters.

Specimen Red blood cells

Container Green top (heparin) tube or heparinized capillary tubes

Storage Instructions Stable at 4°C to 25°C for 1 week only.

Reference Range Not well established, varies with method, age, sex, and use of oral contraceptives. Typical value: 30-40 units/g Hgb. Normally absent in amniotic fluid.

Use Erythrocyte cholinesterase is measured to diagnose organophosphate and carbamate toxicity and to detect atypical forms of the enzyme, although most frequently the serum enzyme (pseudocholinesterase) is used for this purpose. Cholinesterase is irreversibly inhibited by organophosphate insecticides and reversibly inhibited by carbamate insecticides. Serum or plasma pseudocholinesterase is commonly used to measure acute toxicity, while erythrocyte levels are better for chronic exposure. (Serum level returns to normal prior to normalizing of red cell level.) Persons with an atypical form of the enzyme (with low enzyme activity) exhibit prolonged apnea following the use of certain suxamethonium-type muscle relaxants in anesthesia (succinylcholine sensitivity - AA phenotype). These atypical forms may be detected by the use of fluoride or dibucaine inhibition. Again, the serum enzyme (pseudocholinesterase) is the one usually used for this purpose. Its presence in amniotic fluid in conjunction with increased alpha-fetoprotein is evidence for neural tube defects in the fetus.

Limitations Values decrease as erythrocytes become senescent. Activity in red blood cells may not always provide a good index of intoxication with acetylcholine inhibitors.[1]

High resolution ultrasonography may prove to be more cost effective and accurate than alpha-fetoprotein and acetylcholinesterase at second trimester amniocentesis in detection of congenital anomalies.[2]

Contraindications Pseudocholinesterase in serum is the indicated test for succinylcholine sensitivity.

Methodology Methods are based on determination of result (rate) of hydrolysis of an ester catalyzed by the enzyme acetylcholinesterase and include colorimetry, fluorometry, spectrophotometry based systems. Polyacrylamide gel electrophoresis is used for the qualitative demonstration of acetylcholinesterase in amniotic fluid. Screening methods are available.

Additional Information The cholinesterase activity in human red cells is highly, but not exclusively specific, for acetylcholine. It is referred to as true or specific cholinesterase. Cholinesterase activity present in the serum/plasma hydrolyses both choline and aliphatic esters, has a broader range of esterolytic activity and is referred to as "pseudo-" or "nonspecific" cholinesterase. It hydrolyses acetylcholine only slowly. The systematic name for acetylcholinesterase is acetylcholine acetylhydrolase. Systematic name for cholinesterase (serum/plasma) is acylcholine acylhydrolase. The different nature of the cholinesterases was first described in 1940. The plasma enzyme is synthesized by the liver, the red cell enzyme during erythropoiesis.

Cholinesterase activity is low at birth and higher in adult males than females. The enzyme is a large complex protein. There is evidence that it has a multiple subunit structure, four peptide chains that form two dimers. Because of the many constituent amino acids, many molecular variants are possible. The RBC level is **increased** in hemolytic states such as the thalassemias, spherocytosis, hemoglobin SS, and acquired hemolytic anemias. It is **decreased** in paroxysmal nocturnal hemoglobinuria and in relapse of megaloblastic anemia and it returns to normal with therapy. It is not widely regarded as useful as a test for paroxysmal nocturnal hemoglobinuria.

Potent inhibitors of cholinesterase may present important clinical toxicological problems. Systemic insecticides (eg, organophosphates or carbamates) are examples. Both RBC acetylcholinesterase and plasma cholinesterase are usually inhibited. The effect on the plasma enzyme is more marked, however, and serum levels are usually utilized in diagnosis and assessment of recovery. Recovery is best determined by looking for a plateau in erythrocyte cholinesterase activity. Toxic potency may vary, plasma versus red cell cholinesterase, such that in some cases erythrocyte levels may be needed for diagnosis and/or monitoring. If there is suspicion that a decrease in cholinesterase activity may not relate to the inhibitor effect of an organophosphate then red cell level of acetylcholinesterase should be obtained. If both serum and RBC levels are significantly decreased, findings are those of exogenous toxic effect.

True cholinesterase (acetylcholinesterase-RBC cholinesterase) is not normally present in amniotic fluid. Presence of acetylcholinesterase activity and increased levels of alpha-fetoprotein in amniotic fluid are presumptive evidence of an open neural tube defect (eg, anencephaly, open spina bifida, or omphalocele) in the fetus.

Footnotes

1. Igisu H, Matsumura H, and Matsuoka M, "Acetylcholinesterase in the Erythrocyte Membrane," *Sangyo Ika Daigaku Zasshi*, 1994, 16(3):253-62.
2. Sepulveda W, Donaldson A, Johnson RD, et al, "Are Routine Alpha-Fetoprotein and Acetylcholinesterase Determinations Still Necessary at Second-Trimester Amniocentesis? Impact of High-Resolution Ultrasonography," *Obstet Gynecol*, 1995, 85(1):107-12.

References

Burtis CA and Ashwood ER, *Tietz Textbook of Clinical Chemistry*, 2nd ed, Philadelphia, PA: WB Saunders Co, 1994, 877-82.
Datta C, Gupta J, and Sengupta D, "Interaction of Organophosphorus Insecticides Phosphamidon and Malathion on Lipid Profile and Acetylcholinesterase Activity in Human Erythrocyte Membrane," *Indian J Med Res*, 1994, 100:87-9.

Acid-Base Regulation *see* Delta Base, Blood *on page 121*

Acid-Base Status *see* pCO$_2$, Blood *on page 179*

Acid-Base Status Evaluation *see* Carbon Dioxide, Blood *on page 100*

Acid Phosphatase

CPT 84060

Related Information

Prostate Specific Antigen, Serum *on page 193*

Synonyms o-Phosphoric-Monoester Phosphohydrolase; PAP; Phosphatase, Acid; Prostatic Acid Phosphatase

Abstract Several acid phosphatases are present in serum from various sources. Acid phosphatase from the prostate is of most interest.

Patient Preparation Do not order immediately after rectal examination of the prostate, after TUR, or after prostatic massage. Fasting specimen is preferred, as lipemia may interfere.

Specimen Serum or plasma

Container Lavender top (EDTA) tube is preferred; red top tube is acceptable

Collection Morning collection is recommended, since diurnal variation exists (circadian rhythms). The sample should be drawn in EDTA anticoagulant to provide proper pH for stabilizing acid phosphatase. Due to the unstable nature of the enzyme, the test should be performed as soon as possible. Serum (red top tube) may also be used although it is possible to lose acid phosphatase activity within 1 hour.

Storage Instructions Separate sample and store on ice. Acidify and freeze sample if it cannot be run immediately. For acidification 50 μL of acetic acid (5M) per mL of serum is added. Crystalline disodium citrate monohydrate at a level of 10 mg/mL of serum can be used as an alternative. Stable frozen at -20°C for 6 months, or at -70°C indefinitely.

Reference Range Method dependent; males: 2-12 units/L (enzymatic, total); 0.2-3.5 units/L (enzymatic, prostatic); 2.5-3.7 ng/mL (RIA, prostatic). Enzymatic values are with use of 4-nitrophenyl phosphate as the substrate.

Use Staging of carcinoma of prostate, with other parameters; minimal role in establishing the diagnosis of primary carcinoma of prostate, helpful role in diagnosis of metastatic adenocarcinoma of prostate and/or extension beyond prostatic capsule; monitor therapy and follow patient's response to treatment. **Not a screening test** for prostatic adenocarcinoma. Used on vaginal material in work-up of alleged rape.[1] Used in immunocytochemistry.

Limitations Specimens stored for any length of time, even at 4°C, will lose activity especially if exposed to air. Acidification to pH 6 will stabilize the enzyme for 1 week at 4°C. When adenocarcinoma is confined within the prostate, acid phosphatase is usually normal. Occasionally in patients with extensive carcinoma of prostate, acid phosphatase levels may be within normal limits. Even immunoassay methods do not detect early carcinomas consistently and, like enzyme methods, there may be false-positives. Acid phosphatase may be **increased** in diseases other than adenocarcinoma of prostate (eg, in infarct). Increased serum PAP with normal serum PSA may provide indication of significant extraprostatic (nonprostatic) disease.[2] Moderate elevations of total acid phosphatase have been observed also with malignant invasion of bone from nonprostatic primaries, as well as with myelocytic leukemia, Gaucher's disease, and Niemann-Pick disease. However, the thymolphthalein monophosphate method is said to be more specific for prostatic acid phosphatase than are some other chemical substrates. Specimens drawn after recent rectal digital examination, TUR, bladder catheterization, and/or other manipulation of the prostate may have elevated values. The enzyme may be increased with prostatitis and may be increased with urinary retention. Acid phosphatase is increased by radioimmunoassay in up to 27% of patients with benign hypertrophy.[3] When using nonspecific substrates (eg, 4-nitrophenyl phosphate), the tartrate inhibition is measured. The inhibited fraction is considered to be of prostatic origin. In males, approximately half of the normal total acid phosphatase is of prostatic origin. Tartrate inhibition is not entirely specific. Acid phosphatase by RIA is not a screening test for carcinoma of prostate.[3] Acid phosphatase exhibits diurnal variation.[4] It has been suggested that routine screening for prostatic carcinoma using acid phosphatase is no longer justified.[5]

Methodology Immunoassays: Radioimmunoassay (RIA), enzyme immunoassay (EIA), counterimmunoelectrophoresis (CIE); chemical methods: hydrolysis of thymolphthalein monophosphate, alpha naphthylphosphate, other enzymatic methods; tartrate inhibition

Additional Information Exacerbations and remissions of adenocarcinoma of prostate are not always correlated with acid phosphatase levels. Other parameters are also needed to follow such patients (eg, serum alkaline phosphatase, PSA). The RIA method has little advantage over the enzymatic approach using alpha-naphthyl phosphate substrate. Normal results do not consistently distinguish between localized and more extensive neoplasm. RIA method may not be cost-effective,[6] but it does provide increased sensitivity over enzymatic approaches in following stage D patients.[3,6]

Done chemically, using alpha-naphthyl acid phosphate as substrate, Tavassoli et al reported acid phosphatase increases with bone metastases from nonprostatic primaries. They advocated acid phosphatase as a means of detection of skeletal metastasis.[7]

CK-BB, an isoenzyme of CK, may be detected in the serum of some patients with carcinoma of prostate. It is not a specific test.

Prostate-specific antigen is more sensitive than prostatic acid phosphatase, but neither test is specific for adenocarcinoma of prostate.[8] Neither is 100% sensitive. The organ specificity, sensitivity and diagnostic value of PSA is an advance which can be used with acid phosphatase in staging and follow-up of prostatic carcinoma.[9] Serum PSA is superior to PAP in predicting disease recurrence in stages C and D prostate cancer treated by combination endocrine therapy. **The assay of serum PAP does not add significantly to measurement of serum PSA alone.**[10] Rectal carcinoid tumors may show histochemically positive PAP.[11] Benign prostatic hyperplasia causes definite increase in PAP, whereas in intracapsular prostate cancer normal levels are found.[12]

Footnotes

1. Gomez RR, Wunsch CD, Davis JH, et al, "Qualitative and Quantitative Determinations of Acid Phosphatase Activity in Vaginal Washings," *Am J Clin Pathol*, 1975, 64:423-32.
2. Gambino R, "An Elevated Prostatic Acid Phosphatase (PAP) Level, in the Presence of a Normal Prostate-Specific Antigen (PSA) Level, Usually Indicates Serious Nonprostatic Disease," *Lab Rep*, 1994, 16(9):70-1.
3. Gittes RF, "Serum Acid Phosphatase and Screening for Carcinoma of the Prostate," *N Engl J Med*, 1983, 309:852-3.
4. Brenckman WD, Lastinger LB, and Sedor F, "Unpredictable Fluctuations in Serum Acid Phosphatase Activity in Prostatic Cancer," *JAMA*, 1981, 245:2501-4.
5. Nicoll CD, Jeffrey J, and Dreyer J, "Routine Acid Phosphatase Testing for Screening and Monitoring Prostate Cancer No Longer Justified," *Clin Chem*, 1993, 39(12):2540-1.
6. Mensink HJ, Marrink J, Hindriks FR, et al, "Prostatic Acid Phosphatase: Comparison of Radioimmunoassay and Enzyme Activity Assay," *J Urol*, 1983, 129:1136-40.
7. Tavassoli M, Rizo M, and Yam LT, "Elevation of Serum Acid Phosphatase in Cancers With Bone Metastasis," *Cancer*, 1980, 45:2400-3.
8. Stamey TA, Yang N, Hay AR, et al, "Prostate-Specific Antigen as a Serum Marker for Adenocarcinoma of the Prostate," *N Engl J Med*, 1987, 317(15):909-16.
9. Gittes RF, "Prostate-Specific Antigen," *N Engl J Med*, 1987, 317(15):954-5.
10. Dupont A, Cusan L, Gomez JL, et al, "Prostate Specific Antigen and Prostatic Acid Phosphatase for Monitoring Therapy of Carcinoma of the Prostate," *J Urol*, 1991, 146(4):1064-7.
11. Azumi N, Traweek ST, and Battifora H, "Prostatic Acid Phosphatase in Carcinoid Tumors. Immunohistochemical and Immunoblot Studies," *Am J Surg Pathol*, 1991, 15(8):785-90.
12. Salo JO, Rannikko S, and Haapiainen R, "Serum Acid Phosphatase in Patients With Localised Prostatic Cancer, Benign Prostatic Hyperplasia or Normal Prostates," *Br J Urol*, 1990, 66(2):188-92.

References

Kaplan LA, Chen IW, Sperling M, et al, "Clinical Utility of Serum Prostatic Acid Phosphatase Measurements for Detection (Screening), Diagnosis, and Therapeutic Monitoring of Prostatic Carcinoma; Assessment of Monoclonal and Polyclonal Enzymes and Radioimmunoassays," *Am J Clin Pathol*, 1985, 84(3):334-9.

Kroll MH and Nipper H, "Rapid Rise of Serum Acid Phosphatase After Irradiation of Metastatic Carcinoma of Prostate," *Urology*, 1987, 29:650-2.

Maatman TJ, Gupta MK, and Montie JE, "The Role of Serum Prostatic Acid Phosphatase as a Tumor Marker in Men With Advanced Adenocarcinoma of the Prostate," *J Urol*, 1984, 132(1):58-63.

Romas NA and Kwan DJ, "Prostatic Acid Phosphatase. Biomolecular Features and Assays for Serum Determination," *Urol Clin North Am*, 1993, 20(4):581-8.

Seiber PR and Rohner TJ, "Importance of Acid Phosphatase in Response Criteria for Prostate Cancer," *Urology*, 1987, 30:316-7.

ACTH *see* Adrenocorticotropic Hormone *on this page*

ACTH Infusion Test *replaced by* Cosyntropin Test *on page 114*

Actual Base Excess *see* Delta Base, Blood *on page 121*

ADA, Red Cells *see* Adenosine Deaminase, Serum, Red Cells *on this page*

ADA, Serum *see* Adenosine Deaminase, Serum, Red Cells *on this page*

Adenosine Deaminase, Serum, Red Cells

Synonyms ADA, Red Cells; ADA, Serum

Abstract This serum enzyme level is elevated in chronic liver disease and in tuberculosis and sarcoidosis. Red cell enzyme in severe combined immunodeficiency disease (SCID) in infants is deficient.

Specimen Serum or whole blood

Container Red top tube for serum, lavender top (EDTA) tube for red cells

Storage Instructions Stable at 4°C for 1 week.

Special Instructions Usually sent to reference specialty laboratory.

Reference Range Serum: 12-25 units/L; red cells: 0.8-1.3 units/g Hgb

Use Red cell enzyme levels decreased in red cells in severe combined immunodeficiency disease (SCID); likely to present with repeated infections and failure to thrive. About 50% of SCID patients have ADA deficiency.

Increases in red cell enzyme produces mild chronic hemolytic anemia. Changes of ADA levels occur in acute myelogenous leukemia.

Serum levels increased in exacerbation of chronic sarcoidosis and increased in tuberculosis in children.

Methodology Spectrophotometric, kinetic assay; fluorometric

Additional Information Elevations seen in patients with Parkinson's disease. ADA and its isoenzyme ADA-2 is thought to be important in regulation of immune function. Deficiency of ADA is the most frequent known cause of SCID. The enzyme is nearly always low in biliary tract disease but elevated in chronic liver disease.

References

Oosthuizen HM, Ungerer JP, and Bissbort SH, "Kinetic Determination of Serum Adenosine Deaminase," *Clin Chem*, 1993, 39(10):2182-5.

Patmasiriwat P, Anukarahanonta T, and Chinprasertsuk S, "Purine Degradative Enzymes and Terminal Transferase in Acute Myelogenous Leukemia: Clinical Relevance," *Ann Clin Lab Sci*, 1993, 23(4):281-9.

Adrenocorticotropic Hormone

CPT 82024

Related Information

Calcitonin *on page 96*
Carcinoembryonic Antigen *on page 100*
Cortisol, Blood *on page 112*
Cortisol, Urine *on page 113*
Follicle Stimulating Hormone *on page 129*
Growth Hormone *on page 141*
Luteinizing Hormone, Blood or Urine *on page 163*
Metyrapone Stimulation Test *on page 167*
Testosterone, Free and Total *on page 202*
Thyroid Stimulating Hormone *on page 204*
Thyroxine *on page 206*

Synonyms ACTH; Corticotropin

Applies to Corticotropin Release Hormone Stimulation Test; Corticotropin Stimulation Test; Dexamethasone Suppression

Abstract The most important regulator of corticotropin is corticotropin-releasing hormone (CRH) from the hypothalamus.[1] Corticotropin (ACTH) stimulates the adrenal cortices, which produce cortisol. In Cushing's syndrome, inappropriately increased ACTH stimulates the adrenal cortices to secrete excessive quantities of cortisol (**corticotropin-dependent Cushing's syndrome**), in which Cushing's disease (pituitary ACTH-dependent adrenal cortical hyperplasia) or the ectopic ACTH syndrome is present. In **corticotropin-independent Cushing's syndrome**, abnormal adrenal cortical tissue (adenoma, carcinoma, hyperplasia) suppresses secretion of both CRH and ACTH.[1] A battery of (Continued)

Adrenocorticotropic Hormone *(Continued)*

adrenal function tests and imaging procedures is recommended to establish the diagnosis of Cushing's syndrome.

Patient Preparation Avoid radioisotope scans or recently administered radioisotopes prior to collection of specimen.

Specimen Plasma

Container Use chilled syringe. Use two lavender top (EDTA) tubes or two green top (heparin) tubes, previously cooled in ice. (Check with laboratory for appropriate container.)

Sampling Time ACTH is normally characterized by diurnal variation. Most secretion occurs in the morning. Normal secretion, as well as that in Cushing's disease, is pulsatile and so may require multiple samples. For sequential follow-up, ACTH should always be drawn at the same time each day. For diagnosis of Cushing's syndrome and to distinguish between corticotropin-independent Cushing's syndrome, sampling corticotropin and cortisol midnight to 2 AM is ideal; these hormones are then at their lowest levels. Afternoon, 4 PM or later, usually is acceptable.

Collection Samples for demonstration of the normal circadian rhythm should be drawn between 6 AM and 10 AM and between 9 PM and 12 PM. Commonly collected simultaneously with cortisol level. Transport specimen **immediately** to the laboratory following collection.

Storage Instructions Separate plasma in refrigerated centrifuge and freeze immediately. Store frozen at -70°C in plastic tubes. Aprotinin (Trasylol®) 500 kU/mL should be added for long-term storage.

Reference Range Values at 5 AM to 7 AM by RIA (patient supine): 8-30 pg/mL (SI: 8-30 ng/L); by IRMA, same conditions: 9-50 pg/mL (SI: 9-50 ng/L). These would represent the highest values in the diurnal variation. Samples drawn between 9 AM and 12 noon have been recommended.[2] Evening samples normally are about one-half to two-thirds of the morning specimens. The normal daily circadian rhythm (periodicity) has diagnostic significance (ie, lack of change is abnormal).

Use Evaluate the etiology of Cushing's syndrome; differentiate pituitary from extrapituitary causes of corticosteroid excess and deficiency syndromes (ie, distinguish corticotropin-dependent from corticotropin-independent Cushing's syndrome); evaluate ectopic ACTH production by neoplasm; examine results of transsphenoidal surgery; follow up patients after bilateral adrenalectomy for diagnosis of Nelson syndrome. (Nelson syndrome is the development of a tumor of the anterior pituitary gland and skin pigmentation following bilateral adrenalectomy.) Signs and symptoms of hypopituitarism can be secondary to disease either of the pituitary or the hypothalamus. (Secondary endocrine deficiencies are target gland failures secondary to lack of stimulation by a pituitary hormone, eg, ACTH.[3]) The differential diagnosis of the obese, hirsute, hypertensive patient includes not only Cushing's syndrome but cushingoid obesity.

Limitations A single determination may be within normal limits in patients with either excessive production (Cushing's disease) or partial deficiency. Normal corticotropin assay in a subject with low serum cortisol is evidence of ACTH deficiency. The ACTH level is affected by stress, which may obscure the normal diurnal change. ACTH level must be correlated with cortisol levels. Tests in use include low-dose dexamethasone suppression test, high-dose dexamethasone suppression tests, metyrapone stimulation test, petrosal venous sinus catheterization, as well as imaging procedures.[1] Spurious elevation of immunoreactive ACTH is reported and an extraction is recommended.[4] A differential diagnosis includes entities of pseudo-Cushing's syndrome.[1]

Methodology Radioimmunoassay (RIA) after separatory step and immunoradiometric assay (IRMA); IRMA is most sensitive and specific

Additional Information Cortisol excess of any source is **"Cushing's syndrome."** Increased ACTH from a pituitary tumor, leading to bilateral adrenocortical hyperplasia and producing excessive cortisol, was described by Cushing and called **"Cushing's disease."** ACTH secretion is stimulated by insulin, metyrapone, and vasopressin and suppressed by dexamethasone. Cushing's disease usually demonstrates suppression of ACTH and cortisol by high-dose dexamethasone; whereas in adrenal adenomas, adrenal carcinomas, and ectopic ACTH-producing tumors, ACTH and cortisol are not suppressed by high-dose dexamethasone. ACTH levels in Cushing's disease may be elevated or in the high normal range (but inappropriately elevated for the patient's plasma cortisol level), with loss of the normal diurnal changes. ACTH levels in **ectopic ACTH syndrome** are usually very high; whereas in Cushing's syndrome due to adrenal adenoma or carcinoma, ACTH levels are very low to undetectable. Most cases of ectopic ACTH secretion are caused by small cell carcinoma of lung. ACTH was increased in 30% of patients with oat cell carcinoma and 26% with large cell carcinoma of lung in a series of 110 patients with lung cancer.[5] Ectopic ACTH production may derive from bronchial and other carcinoids as well, and from medullary carcinoma of thyroid or other neuroendocrine neoplasms.[1]

Measurement of plasma lipotropin provides an alternative index for diagnosis of Cushing's syndromes and follow-up of treated Cushing's diseases.[6] Elevated plasma ACTH in adrenal hyperplasia with no tumor is reported.[7]

In **primary adrenal insufficiency (Addison's disease)** due to destruction of the adrenal glands by tumor, infection or immune mechanisms, ACTH plasma concentrations are elevated and cortisol levels are depressed. ACTH increases are found with congenital adrenal hyperplasia (adrenogenital syndrome). In secondary adrenal insufficiency (secondary to pituitary insufficiency), ACTH and cortisol both are low.

Causes of **hypopituitarism** include pituitary adenomas, craniopharyngioma, meningioma, other primary and metastatic tumors, postirradiation states, hemorrhage, infiltrative diseases (eg, eosinophilic granuloma), inflammation (eg, lymphocytic and granulomatous hypophysitis), and other disease entities. Concentrations of ACTH, TSH, FSH, LH, growth hormone, and of target organ hormones (eg, thyroxine, cortisol, testosterone) are decreased. Partial deficiencies require dynamic tests, such as the **corticotropin stimulation test.**[3]

Urinary free **cortisol** is the test of choice for the separation of Cushing's syndrome from entities, including obesity, which mimic it.[8,9] The increased ACTH of **pseudo-Cushing's syndrome** does not exhibit normal circadian rhythms and fails to suppress with dexamethasone. Pseudo-Cushing's syndrome is a reversible entity sometimes related to alcohol abuse.[1,8]

Continuous (7-hour) dexamethasone infusion in patients with Cushing's syndrome is reported to identify 100% of patients with ACTH-secreting pituitary adenomas, with a specificity of 90% and diagnostic accuracy of 98%,[10] but investigation goes on.[11,12] The corticotropin release hormone (CRH) stimulation test has a 91% sensitivity and a 95% specificity for the pituitary Cushing's syndrome.[13] Its present role is addressed.[1]

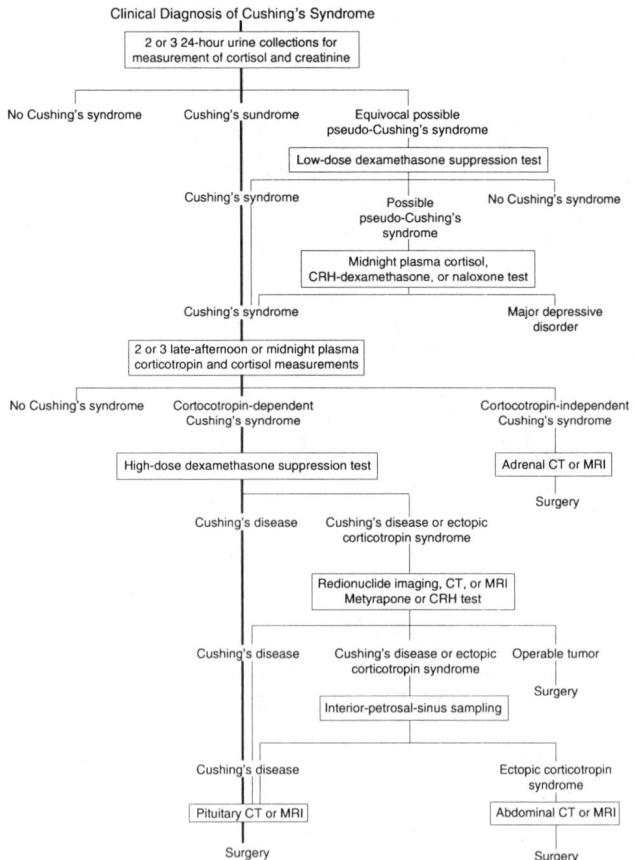

An approach to the diagnosis of Cushing's syndrome and its cause. The heavy line indicates the diagnostic path for the majority of patients who have Cushing's disease. CT denotes computed tomography and MRI magnetic resonance imaging.

From Orth DN, "Cushing's Syndrome," N Engl J Med, 1995, 332(12):795, with permission.

Footnotes

1. Orth DN, "Cushing's Syndrome," *N Engl J Med*, 1995, 332(12):791-803.

2. Leavelle DE, "Adrenocorticotropic Hormone (ACTH), Plasma," *Mayo Medical Laboratories Interpretive Handbook*, Rochester, MN: Mayo Medical Laboratories, 1994, 18.

3. Vance ML, "Hypopituitarism," *N Engl J Med*, 1994, 330(23):1651-62.

4. Wickus GG, Pagliara AS, and Caplan RH, "Spurious Elevation of Plasma Immunore-active Adrenocorticotropic Hormone in Cyclic Cushing's Syndrome," *Arch Pathol Lab Med*, 1989, 113(7):797-9.

5. Gropp C, Havemann K, and Scheuer A, "Ectopic Hormones in Lung Cancer Patients at Diagnosis and During Therapy," *Cancer*, 1980, 46:347-54.

6. Kuhn JM, Proeschel MF, Seurin DJ, et al, "Comparative Assessment of ACTH and Lipoprotein Plasma Levels in the Diagnosis and Follow-up of Patients With Cushing's Syndrome: A Study of 210 Cases," *Am J Med*, 1989, 86(6 Pt 1):678-84.

7. Ismail AA, Burn WA, Taylor NF, et al, "Elevated Plasma ACTH With Adrenal Hyperplasia: A New Factor in ACTH?" *J Clin Endocrinol Metab*, 1991, 73(4):752-7.

8. Grizzle WE and Dunlap N, "Cushing's Syndrome - Diagnosis of the Atypical Patient," *Arch Pathol Lab Med*, 1989, 113(7):727-8.

9. Flack MR, Oldfield EH, Cutler GB Jr, et al, "Urine Free Cortisol in the High-Dose Dexamethasone Suppression Test for the Differential Diagnosis of the Cushing Syndrome," *Ann Intern Med*, 1992, 116(3):211-7.

10. Biemond P, deJong FH, and Lamberts SW, "Continuous Dexamethasone Infusion for Seven Hours in Patients With the Cushing Syndrome. A Superior Differential Diagnostic Test," *Ann Intern Med*, 1990, 112(10):738-42.

11. Avgerinos PC, Yanovski JA, Oldfield EH, et al, "The Metyrapone and Dexamethasone Suppression Tests for the Differential Diagnosis of the Adrenocorticotropin-Dependent Cushing Syndrome: A Comparison," *Ann Intern Med*, 1994, 121(5):318-27.

12. Orth DN, "The Cushing Syndrome: Quest for the Holy Grail," *Ann Intern Med*, 1994, 121(5):377-8.

13. Kaye TB and Crapo L, "The Cushing Syndrome: An Update on Diagnostic Tests," *Ann Intern Med*, 1990, 112(6):434-4.

References

Becker M and Aron DC, " Ectopic ACTH Syndrome and CRH-Mediated Cushing's Syndrome," *Endocrinol Metab Clin North Am*, 1994, 23(3):585-606.

Blunt SB, Sandler LM, Burrin JM, et al, "An Evaluation of the Distinction of Ectopic and Pituitary ACTH Dependent Cushing's Syndrome by Clinical Features, Biochemical Tests and Radiological Findings," *Q J Med*, 1990, 77(283):1113-33.

"Case Records of the Massachusetts General Hospital. Weekly Clinicopathological Exercises. Case 25-1995. A 44-Year-Old Woman With Headache, Blurred Vision, and an Intrasellar Mass," *N Engl J Med*, 1995, 333(7):441-7.

Findling JW, "Eutopic or Ectopic Adrenocorticotropic Hormone-Dependent Cushing's Syndrome? A Diagnostic Dilemma," *Mayo Clin Proc*, 1990, 65(10):1377-80.

Findling JW and Doppman JL, "Biochemical and Radiologic Diagnosis of Cushing's Syndrome," *Endocrinol Metab Clin North Am*, 1994, 23(3):511-37.

Grinspoon SK and Biller BM, "Clinical Review 62: Laboratory Assessment of Adrenal Insufficiency," *J Clin Endocrinol Metab*, 1994, 79(4):923-31.

Jones KL, "The Cushing Syndromes," *Pediatr Clin North Am*, 1990, 37(6):1313-32.

Kreisberg R, "Clinical Problem-Solving. Half a Loaf," *N Engl J Med*, 1994, 330(18):1295-9.

Magiakou MA, Mastorakos G, Oldfield EH, et al, "Cushing's Syndrome in Children and Adolescents: Presentation, Diagnosis, and Therapy," *N Engl J Med*, 1994, 331(10):629-36.

Midgette AS and Aron DC, "High-Dose Dexamethasone Suppression Testing Versus Inferior Petrosal Sinus Sampling in the Differential Diagnosis of Adrenocorticotropin-Dependent Cushing's Syndrome: A Decision Analysis," *Am J Med Sci*, 1995, 309(3):162-70.

Siegel SF, Finegold DN, Lanes R, et al, "ACTH Stimulation Tests and Plasma Dehydroepiandrosterone Sulfate Levels in Women With Hirsutism," *N Engl J Med*, 1990, 323(13):849-54.

Snow K, Jiang NS, and Kao PC, "Biochemical Evaluation of Adrenal Dysfunction: The Laboratory Perspective," *Mayo Clin Proc*, 1992, 67(11):1055-65.

AFP *see* Alpha₁-Fetoprotein, Serum *on page 72*

AFP, Amniotic Fluid *see* Alpha₁-Fetoprotein, Amniotic Fluid *on page 71*

A/G Ratio *see* Albumin/Globulin Ratio *on next page*

ALA *see* Delta Aminolevulinic Acid, Urine *on page 121*

ALA Dehydratase *see* Delta Aminolevulinic Acid, Urine *on page 121*

Alanine Aminotransferase

CPT 84460

Related Information

Acetaminophen, Serum *on page 530*
Aspartate Aminotransferase *on page 84*
Bilirubin, Total *on page 86*
Hepatitis B Surface Antigen *on page 399*
Lactate Dehydrogenase *on page 153*
Liver Biopsy *on page 48*
Liver Profile *on page 161*
Risks of Transfusion *on page 623*

Synonyms ALT; Glutamic Pyruvate Transaminase; GPT; 2-Oxoglutarate Aminotransferase; SGPT; Transaminase

Applies to Aminotransferases

Replaces Cephalin Flocculation; Isocitric Dehydrogenase; Thymol Turbidity

Abstract Of the aminotransferases, AST and ALT are important, widely used enzymes. Increases over tenfold occur in some cases of hepatitis and shock.

Specimen Serum

Container Red top tube

Storage Instructions Stable 1 day at 25°C and 3 days at 4°C; refrigeration is preferable to freezing.

Causes for Rejection Excessive hemolysis

Reference Range Slightly increased ranges in infancy compared to adult normal range. Typical reference range: 10-35 units/L. Males have slightly higher alanine aminotransferase activity.

Use A liver function test, ALT is more sensitive for the detection of hepatocyte injury than for biliary obstruction. ALT is more specific for liver injury than AST (SGOT). Useful for hepatic cirrhosis, and other liver disease. Increased in Reye's syndrome, with AST.[1] Screening test for hepatitis. Acute hepatitis A, B, and C can be confirmed serologically. Negative serological findings in the presence of hepatitis-like chemistry abnormalities may suggest acute drug-induced hepatitis, an impression supported by resolution after removal of the offending agent.[2] The combination of increased AST and ALT with negative hepatitis markers occurs in a number of other entities including infectious mononucleosis. Sensitive to heart failure.

ALT has been used in combination with anti-HB$_c$ as an indirect screen for non-A, non-B hepatitis in blood donors,[3,4,5] but is no longer required. (Tests for antibody to hepatitis C provide identification of most donors with non-A, non-B hepatitis virus.[6]) As liver function tests, the transaminases play a role in evaluation of inborn errors of metabolism.

Limitations Grossly hemolyzed samples can generate somewhat spurious results. The activity in red cells is six times that of serum. Elevations are reported in trauma to striated muscle, rhabdomyolysis, polymyositis, and dermatomyositis, but the CK (CK-MM fraction) is increased in such patients and it is preferable to consider diseases of skeletal muscle. ALT is less sensitive than is AST to alcoholic liver disease. Increased ALT is found with obesity.

Methodology Spectrophotometry by rate assay

Additional Information Among entities in which AST and ALT increases occur are therapeutic applications of bovine or porcine heparin. LD (LDH) abnormality with elevation of hepatic fractions has also been reported.[7]

In children with acute lymphoblastic leukemia, high ALT activity at diagnosis is associated with rapidly progressive ALL.[8]

A number of drugs, including diphenylhydantoin, heparin therapy, and many others cause ALT increases. Acetaminophen hepatotoxicity may be potentiated in alcoholics, the alcohol-acetaminophen syndrome, in which coagulopathy and extremely abnormal ALT and AST are found.[9] The ALT and AST, about 9000 units/L in a study, distinguish the alcohol-acetaminophen syndrome from alcoholic or viral hepatitis. Such levels are found with overdose as well.[10] Drug effects are published.[11]

AST/ALT ratios are highest in alcoholic liver disease but are often above unity in nonalcoholic cirrhosis. AST/ALT ratios are commonly 0.5-0.8 with acute and chronic viral hepatitis.[12] Such ratios may be expected to vary between laboratories by virtue of differences in enzyme methods.

The hepatitis C virion has been detected by polymerase chain reaction and reverse transcriptase of HCV-RNA sequences in patients with elevated ALT and positive anti-HCV.[13]

Footnotes

1. "Diagnosis and Treatment of Reye's Syndrome," (Consensus Conference) *JAMA*, 1981, 246:2441-4.

2. Frank BB and Members of the Patient Care Committee of the American Gastroenterological Association, "Clinical Evaluation of Jaundice - A Guideline of the Patient Care Committee of the American Gastroenterological Association," *JAMA*, 1989, 262(21):3031-4.

3. Biswas R, "Post-transfusion Non-A, Non-B Hepatitis: Significance of Raised ALT and Anti-HB$_c$ in Blood Donors," *Vox Sang*, 1989, 56(1):63.

4. Friedman LS, Dienstag JL, Watkins E, et al, "Evaluation of Blood Donors With Elevated Serum Alanine Aminotransferase Levels," *Ann Intern Med*, 1987, 107:137-44 (published erratum appears in *Ann Intern Med*, 1987, 107(5):791).

5. Spurling CL and Saxena S, "Controversies in Transfusion Medicine. Alanine Aminotransferase Screening of Blood Donors," *Transfusion*, 1990, 30(4):368-73.

6. Desforges JF, "Infectious Disease Testing for Blood Transfusions," *NIH Consensus Statement*, 1995, 13(1):1-27.

7. Dukes GE Jr, Sanders SW, Russo J, et al, "Transaminase Elevations in Patients Receiving Bovine or Porcine Heparin," *Ann Intern Med*, 1984, 100(5):646-50.

8. Rautonen J and Siimes MA, "Elevated Serum Transaminase Activity at Diagnosis Is Associated With Rapidly Progressing Disease in Children With Acute Lymphoblastic Leukemia," *Cancer*, 1988, 61(4):754-7.

9. Seeff LB, Cuccherini BA, Zimmerman HJ, et al, "Acetaminophen Hepatotoxicity in Alcoholics, a Therapeutic Misadventure" *Ann Intern Med*, 1986, 104(3):399-404.

10. Lee WM, "Drug-Induced Hepatotoxicity," *N Engl J Med*, 1995, 333(17):1118-27.

11. Vincent-Viry M and Delwaide P, "Aspartate Aminotransferase and Alanine Aminotransferase," *Drug Effects on Laboratory Test Results Analytical Interferences and Pharmacological Effects*, Siest G and Galteau MM, eds, Littleton, MA: PSG Publishing Co Inc, 1988, 91-130.

12. Williams AL and Hoofnagle JH, "Ratio of Serum Aspartate to Alanine Aminotransferase in Chronic Hepatitis. Relationship to Cirrhosis," *Gastroenterology*, 1988, 95(3):734-9.

13. Ulrich PP, Romeo JM, Lane PK, et al, "Detection, Semiquantitation, and Genetic Variation in Hepatitis C Virus Sequences Amplified From the Plasma of Blood Donors With Elevated Alanine Aminotransferase," *J Clin Invest*, 1990, 86(5):1609-14.

References

Giesen P, Peltenburg HG, and de Zwaan C, "Greater Than Expected Alanine Aminotransferase Activities in Plasma and in Hearts of Patients With Acute Myocardial Infarction," *Clin Chem*, 1989, 35(2):279-83.

(Continued)

Alanine Aminotransferase *(Continued)*

Halevy A, Gold-Deutch R, Negri M, et al, "Are Elevated Liver Enzymes and Bilirubin Levels Significant After Laparoscopic Cholecystectomy in the Absence of Bile Duct Injury?" *Ann Surg*, 1994, 219(4):362-4.

Herlong HF, "Approach to the Patient With Abnormal Liver Enzymes," *Hosp Pract*, 1994, 29(11):32-8.

Kubo SH, Walter BA, John DH, et al, "Liver Function Abnormalities in Chronic Heart Failure. Influence of Systemic Hemodynamics," *Arch Intern Med*, 1987, 147(7):1227-30.

Patwardhan RV, Smith OJ, and Farmelant MH, "Serum Transaminase Levels and Cholescintigraphic Abnormalities in Acute Biliary Tract Obstruction," *Arch Intern Med*, 1987, 147(7):1249-53.

Saxena S, Korula J, Tse-Ling F, et al, "Are Gender-Specific ALT Cutoff Values Necessary?" *Lab Med*, 1995, 26(10):682-6.

Sherman KE, "Alanine Aminotransferase in Clinical Practice. A Review," *Arch Intern Med*, 1991, 151(2):260-5.

Van Ness MV and Diehl AM, "Is Liver Biopsy Useful in the Evaluation of Patients With Chronically Elevated Liver Enzymes?" *Ann Intern Med*, 1989, 111(6):473-8.

Albs-a *see* Body Fluid *on page 89*

Albumin, Ascites Fluid *see* Body Fluid *on page 89*

Albumin/Globulin Ratio

CPT 82040 (albumin); 84155 (protein, total)

Related Information

Albumin, Serum *on this page*

Synonyms A/G Ratio

Abstract A calculation derived from chemistry profiles.

Specimen Serum

Container Red top tube

Reference Range ≥1; high ratio is usually clinically insignificant.

Use Low A/G ratio is found in cirrhosis and other liver diseases, chronic glomerulonephritis and nephrotic syndromes, myeloma, macroglobulinemia of Waldenström, sarcoidosis and other granulomatous diseases, collagen diseases, severe infections and inflammatory states, cachexia, burns, ulcerative colitis and other chronic inflammatory states.

Limitations More chemically precise A/G ratio is derived from serum protein electrophoresis than from chemical methods, and electrophoresis provides considerably more information. The multilayer-film bromcresol green method for albumin measurement is significantly inaccurate when albumin/globulin ratio is <0.8.[1]

Methodology Electrophoretic or chemically determined albumin divided by [total protein minus albumin]

Additional Information Total protein minus albumin equals globulins. Albumin divided by globulins equals the ratio.

Footnotes

1. Leerink CB and Winckers EK, "Multilayer-Film Bromcresol Green Method for Albumin Measurement Significantly Inaccurate When Albumin/Globulin Ratio Is Less Than 0.8," *Clin Chem*, 1991, 37(5):766-8.

References

Ibrahim K, Zuberi SJ, and Husnain SN, "Serum Total Protein, Albumin, Globulin, and Their Ratio in Apparently Healthy Population of Various Ages and Sex in Karachi," *J Pak Med Assoc*, 1989, 39(1):12-6.

Nandedkar AK, Royal GC Jr, and Nandedkar MA, "Evaluation of Albumin-Globulin Ratio to Confirm the Clinical Stages of Sarcoidosis," *J Natl Med Assoc*, 1986, 78(10):969-71.

Albumin, Serum

CPT 82040

Related Information

Albumin/Globulin Ratio *on this page*
Liver Profile *on page 161*
Protein Electrophoresis, Serum *on page 424*
Protein, Total, Serum *on page 194*
Zinc, Serum *on page 595*

Applies to Globulin; Nutritional Status

Abstract Serum albumin is lower in liver disease, malnutrition and malabsorption (decreased synthesis), and in renal disease (increased loss in urine).

Specimen Serum

Container Red top tube or capillary tube

Reference Range 0-1 year: 2.9-5.5 g/dL (SI: 29-55 g/L); 1-31 years: 3.5-4.8 g/dL (SI: 35-50 g/L) with A/G ratio >1. After age 40, the normal range gradually decreases.

Possible Panic Range <1.5 g/dL (SI: <15 g/L)

Use Evaluate nutritional status, blood oncotic pressure, liver disease, renal disease with proteinuria, and other chronic illnesses. Serum albumin is reported as an independent risk factor in older subjects for mortality; hypoalbuminemia relates to increased risk.[1] Admission serum albumin in geriatric patients is a predictor of outcome.[2]

High albumin indicates dehydration. Look for increase in hemoglobin, hematocrit in such patients.

Low albumin is found with use of I.V. fluids, rapid hydration, overhydration; cirrhosis, other liver disease, including chronic alcoholism; in pregnancy and with oral contraceptive use; many chronic diseases, including the nephrotic syndromes, neoplasia, protein-losing enteropathies (including Crohn's disease and ulcerative colitis), peptic ulcer, thyroid disease, burns, severe skin disease, prolonged immobilization, heart failure, chronic inflammatory diseases such as autoimmune diseases and other chronic catabolic states.

Starvation, malabsorption, or malnutrition: In the absence of I.V. fluid therapy and in patients without liver or renal disease, low albumin may be regarded as an indication of inadequate body protein reserves. It is described as the most common nutrition-related abnormality in patients with infection.[3] Serum albumin has a half-life of about 18-20 days. Its half-life is decreased in patients with catabolic states: infection and with protein loss through the kidneys (eg, nephrosis), gastrointestinal tract, and skin (eg, burns). Its prognostic application is most useful in patients with weight loss, anorexia, surgical therapy, hemorrhage, and infection. Total iron binding capacity <240 µg/dL (SI: <43 µmol/L)[3] and/or low transferrin levels would support an impression of inadequate protein reserves. Absolute lymphocyte counts <1500/mm[3] may also be seen with protein malnutrition.[4] **In severe malnutrition**, albumin has been reported as <2.5 g/dL (SI: <25 g/L), total lymphocytes as <800/mm[3] and TIBC as <150 µg/dL.[4]

Albumin levels ≤2.0-2.5 g/dL (SI: ≤20-25 g/L) may be the cause of edema (eg, nephrotic syndrome, protein-losing enteropathies).

Albumin, prealbumin, and transferrin are regarded as "negative" acute phase reactants (ie, these proteins decrease with acute inflammatory/infectious processes).

Low albumin values are associated with longer hospital stay.[3]

Limitations Bromcresol green somewhat overestimates serum albumin and lacks specificity. Albumin level can decrease (up to 0.5 g/dL) (SI: 5.0 g/L) for patients in supine position. Decreased in highly icteric specimens by HABA method but not by bromcresol green.[5] Ampicillin added *in vitro* interferes with both methods.[5] Salicylates do not interfere with bromcresol green method.[5] Monochromatic measurement of albumin by bromcresol green overestimates albumin in heparinized plasma owing to fibrinogen. The artifact is avoided by using bichromatic wavelengths.[6] Increased albumin-bilirubin complexes (ie, icteric sera) causes an underestimation of albumin in the bromcresol purple method but not in the bromcresol green method.[7]

Methodology Bromcresol green (BCG) is widely used. It measures some alpha-globulins and therefore provides slightly higher figures than does serum protein electrophoresis.

Additional Information Twenty-four hour urine collection to measure protein loss is helpful in work-up of some patients with hypoalbuminemia.

Other tests useful in assessment of nutritional status include serum prealbumin, TIBC, transferrin, iron, absolute lymphocyte count, and vitamin B_{12}/folate levels.

Globulin may be provided as a calculation, total protein minus albumin = globulin. Total protein and albumin are commonly measured on chemistry profiling instruments. Globulins are measured by serum protein electrophoresis, immunoelectrophoresis, or immunofixation. Quantitative IgA, IgM, and IgG are more precise.

Footnotes

1. Corti MC, Guralnik JM, Salive ME, et al, "Serum Albumin Level and Physical Disability as Predictors of Mortality in Older Persons," *JAMA*, 1994, 272(13):1036-42.
2. McEllistrum MC, Collins JC, and Powers JS, "Admission Serum Albumin Level as a Predictor of Outcome Among Geriatric Patients," *South Med J*, 1993, 86(12):1360-1.
3. Anderson CF and Wochos DN, "The Utility of Serum Albumin Values in the Nutritional Assessment of Hospitalized Patients," *Mayo Clin Proc*, 1982, 57:181-4.
4. Shapiro M, Rhodes JB, and Beyer PL, "Malnutrition. Recognition and Correction by Enteral Nutrition," *Kans Med*, 1983, 341-5, 356.
5. Beng CG and Lim KL, "An Improved Automated Method for Determination of Serum Albumin Using Bromcresol Green," *Am J Clin Pathol*, 1973, 59:14-21.
6. Hallbach J, Hoffmann GE, and Guder WG, "Overestimation of Albumin in Heparinized Plasma," *Clin Chem*, 1991, 37(4):566-8.
7. Ihara H, Nakamura H, Aoki Y, et al, "Effects of Serum-Isolated vs Synthetic Bilirubin-Albumin Complexes on Dye-Binding Methods for Estimating Serum Albumin," *Clin Chem*, 1991, 37(7):1269-72.

References

Chu SY and MacLeod J, "Effect of Three-Day Clot Contact on Results of Common Biochemical Tests With Serum," *Clin Chem*, 1986, 32(11):2100.

Herbeth B, Diemert MC, and Galli A, "Albumin," *Drug Effects on Laboratory Test Results Analytical Interferences and Pharmacological Effects*, Siest G and Galteau MM, eds, Littleton, MA: PSG Publishing Co Inc, 1988, 52-66.

ALD *see* Aldolase, Serum *on this page*

Aldolase, Serum

CPT 82085

Related Information

Duchenne/Becker Muscular Dystrophy DNA Detection *on page 509*
Muscle Biopsy *on page 53*

Synonyms ALD; Fructose Biphosphate Aldolase

Abstract Very high elevations of this enzyme occur in certain diseases of skeletal muscle such as muscular dystrophy and dermatomyositis but not in diseases of neurogenic origin (eg, polio, multiple sclerosis).

Patient Preparation Patient should be fasting.

Specimen Serum

Container Red top tube

Storage Instructions Separate serum and freeze immediately. May be stored at -20°C until analysis. The addition of boric acid will stabilize aldolase.

Causes for Rejection Hemolysis (red cells contain aldolase)

Reference Range Newborns: up to four times adult levels; pediatrics: 10-24 months: 3.4-11.8 units/L, 25 months to 16 years: 1.2-8.8 units/L (method of Pinto et al[1]); adults: 1.7-4.9 units/L for assay at 30°C with patient at bedrest.

Use Evaluate muscle wasting processes. High levels are found in progressive Duchenne's muscular dystrophy (MD). Elevations occur in carriers of MD, in limb-girdle dystrophy and other dystrophies, in dermatomyositis, polymyositis, and trichinosis, but not in neurogenic atrophies (eg, myasthenia gravis).

Limitations As muscle mass diminishes, aldolase decreases. Serum aldolase elevation is not specific for muscle disease (see following discussion). In recent years the assay of creatine kinase (CK) has been preferred for evaluation of muscle disease. It is more specific for skeletal muscle degeneration. AST and LD are also more commonly ordered and also reflect damage to muscle, but lack specificity.

Elevated aldolase levels may be found with hepatitis, other liver diseases, myocardial infarction, hemorrhagic pancreatitis, gangrene, delirium tremens, and in some cases of neoplasia. In cases of acute viral hepatitis, increase in serum aldolase tends to parallel ALT (SGPT) levels. A small fraction of cases of measles in young adults have been reported to have significant elevations of serum CK and aldolase.[2,3] Aldolase is an ubiquitous enzyme and is thus not particularly useful in diagnostic work-ups.

Contraindications Aldolase levels are not frequently needed or ordered. Many laboratories do not offer this test.

Methodology Ultraviolet, kinetic, coupled enzymatic[4]

Additional Information In the progressive dystrophies, aldolase levels may be 10 to 15 times normal when muscle mass is relatively intact as in early stages of the disease. When advanced muscle wasting is present, values decline. In the inflammatory myopathies (eg, dermatomyositis) serum aldolase (as well as CK) levels may be applied to monitoring the response to steroid therapy. They are of particular value in guiding tapering of steroid administration.[1]

Aldolase is formed of two subunits. There are three different possible subunits designated A, B, and C, but just four isoenzymes. The molecular form AAAA is the predominant aldolase in skeletal muscle, BBBB predominates in liver, and CCCC in brain and other tissue. A hybrid isoenzyme, AAAC is present in tissues but at a lower concentration. The UV coupled enzymatic methods determine total enzyme activity and thus are not specific for muscle aldolase.

Radioimmunoassays for aldolase A, B, and C have been developed but are not widely available. Their clinical utility has not been established.

The level of serum aldolase B (RIA method) may be decreased (<20 ng/mL) in some patients with epithelial malignancy (cases studied included esophageal, hepatic, pancreatic, lung, and breast cancers).[5] After successful surgical resection, serum aldolase B levels recovered to normal range (20-60 ng/mL).

Serum aldolase and CK may be elevated in the serum of patients who have taken L-tryptophan and develop eosinophilia-myalgia syndrome.[6]

Footnotes

1. Visnapuu LA, Karlson LK, Dubinsky EH, et al, "Pediatric Reference Ranges for Serum Aldolase," *Am J Clin Pathol*, 1989, 91(4):476-7.
2. Harjanne A, "The Kinetic Measurement of Serum Aldolase," *Clin Chim Acta*, 1979, 92:311-3.
3. Leibovici L, Sharir T, Kalter-Leibovici O, et al, "An Outbreak of Measles Among Young Adults: Clinical and Laboratory Features in 461 Patients," *J Adolesc Health Care*, 1988, 9(3):203-7.
4. Gavish D, Kleinman Y, Morag A, et al, "Hepatitis and Jaundice Associated With Measles in Young Adults," *Arch Intern Med*, 1983, 143:674-7.
5. Asaka M, Kimura T, Nishikawa S, et al, "Decreased Serum Aldolase B Levels in Patients With Malignant Tumors," *Cancer*, 1988, 62(12):2554-7.
6. Kilbourne EM, Swygert LA, Philen RM, et al, "Interim Guidance on the Eosinophilia-Myalgia Syndrome," *Ann Intern Med*, 1990, 112(2):85-7.

References

Burtis CA and Ashwood ER, *Tietz Textbook of Clinical Chemistry*, 2nd ed, Philadelphia, PA: WB Saunders Co, 1994, 809-11.

Aldosterone, Blood

CPT 82088

Related Information

Aldosterone, Urine *on next page*

Potassium, Serum or Plasma *on page 188*
Potassium, Urine *on page 189*
Renin, Plasma *on page 197*

Abstract Aldosterone is a mineralocorticoid hormone produced in the adrenal zona glomerulosa under complex control by the renin-angiotensin system. Its action is on the renal distal tubule where it increases resorption of sodium and water at the expense of increased potassium excretion. Primary aldosteronism is characterized by hypersecretion of aldosterone, hypertension, renal potassium wasting with suppressed plasma renin activity. It is found in 1% of subjects with hypertension.

Patient Preparation No recent radioactive scans or other radioactivity. Diuretics, antihypertensive drugs, cyclic progestogens, estrogens, and licorice should be terminated 2-4 weeks before testing. Patient should be on a normal sodium diet for 2-4 weeks (135 mmol or 3 g sodium/day). Supine sample should be drawn early, before the inpatient arises. If an upright sample is indicated, patient should have been sitting up for 2 hours or more. Replacement of potassium deficit is recommended before samples for aldosterone are taken. **A random measurement of aldosterone is of no diagnostic utility unless plasma renin activity is determined simultaneously.** The diagnosis of hyperaldosteronism requires the demonstration of persistent hyperaldosteronemia in the presence of saline loading or steroid administration.

Specimen Serum or plasma, peripheral blood and if indicated, percutaneous catheterization for sampling adrenal vein aldosterone and cortisol

Container Red top tube, green top (heparin) tube, or lavender top (EDTA) tube

Collection Specify exact source of specimen. Specify patient's posture. Renin levels are often indicated in the same clinical settings requiring measurement of aldosterone; consider obtaining sufficient blood for both assays. Plasma renin and aldosterone are sampled before and during upright posture.

Storage Instructions Transport at once to the laboratory on ice. Freeze serum or plasma in a plastic vial as soon as possible after sampling.

Reference Range Varies with sodium intake, with time of day, source of specimen (eg, peripheral vein, adrenal vein), and with posture (upright posture is accompanied by higher aldosterone values). Reference ranges differ with laboratory, but vary from 7-30 ng/dL (SI: 190-832 pmol/L) in upright individuals, on unrestricted salt intake, peripheral venous blood. Prolonged heparin therapy decreases serum levels. Aldosterone may be low in diabetics. Aldosterone decreases with higher altitudes and with pre-eclampsia.[1] In supine position reference range is 3-16 ng/dL (SI: 80-440 pmol/L).

Critical Values Ratio of plasma aldosterone to renin activity >50 is significant.[2]

Use The principal use for aldosterone measurements is in the diagnosis of primary hyperaldosteronism, which is most commonly caused by a specific type of adrenal adenoma. Primary aldosteronism caused by adrenal tumor is Conn's syndrome. Another type of primary aldosteronism is idiopathic hyperaldosteronism (bilateral hyperplasia of zona glomerulosa). A few patients have unilateral nodular adrenal hyperplasia. Secondary aldosteronism is more common. Work-up is especially indicated in the patient with hypertension and hypokalemia not induced by diuretic agents. Criteria of serum potassium ≤3.6 mmol/L, 24-hour urine potassium ≥40 mmol/L is used to begin work-up of a hypertensive patient for aldosteronism.[2] Suppressed plasma renin activity suggests primary aldosteronism and provides indication for aldosterone measurement in a hypertensive subject with renal potassium wasting. The diagnosis of primary aldosteronism is supported by suppressed plasma renin activity, increased 24-hour urinary aldosterone, increased ratio of plasma aldosterone to renin activity, adrenal vein sampling for aldosterone and cortisol and other studies. The clinical and biochemical features are characterized by diversity.[2] Secondary aldosteronism may occur in congestive heart failure, cirrhosis with ascites, nephrosis, potassium loading, sodium-depleted diet, toxemia of pregnancy and other states of contraction of plasma volume and Bartter's syndrome. Renin is high in secondary aldosteronism, low in primary aldosteronism.

Limitations Decreased perfusion of the kidneys leads to increased aldosterone and renin. Aldosterone may be falsely elevated in chronic renal failure when assayed by direct RIA.[3]

Contraindications Hypokalemia caused by thiazide diuretics can resemble primary aldosteronism.

Methodology Radioimmunoassay (RIA), chemiluminescence assay (CIA)[4]

Additional Information Syndromes of primary aldosterone excess are characterized by hypokalemia. Conversely, increased serum potassium levels act to increase aldosterone output. Renin also acts to increase aldosterone secretion through a feedback loop including angiotensins I and II. Aldosterone accounts for about 50% of the mineralocorticoid activity in the serum. Most subjects with primary aldosteronism are 30-50 (Continued)

Aldosterone, Blood *(Continued)*

years of age and ≤90% have hypokalemia. Potassium is often only moderately decreased, 3.0-3.5 µmol/L. An increased ratio of aldosterone to plasma renin activity supports the diagnosis of primary aldosteronism in the absence of chronic renal insufficiency. The role of aldosterone in salt-wasting and hypertensive forms of congenital adrenal hyperplasia, aldosterone synthase deficiency, adrenoleukodystrophy, congenital adrenal hypoplasia, adrenal insufficiency, acquired immunodeficiency syndrome, pseudohypoaldosteronism, glucocorticoid-suppressible hyperaldosteronism, and apparent mineralocorticoid excess have been reviewed recently.[5]

Footnotes
1. Blumenfeld JD, Sealey JE, Schlussel Y, et al, "Diagnosis and Treatment of Primary Hyperaldosteronism," *Ann Intern Med*, 1994, 121(11):877-85.
2. August P, Lenz T, Ales KL, et al, "Longitudinal Study of the Renin-Angiotensin-Aldosterone System in Hypertensive Pregnant Women: Deviations Related to the Development of Superimposed Pre-eclampsia," *Am J Obstet Gynecol*, 1990, 163(5 Pt 1):1612-21.
3. Koshida H, Miyamori I, Miyazaki R, et al, "Falsely Elevated Plasma Aldosterone Concentration by Direct Radioimmunoassay in Chronic Renal Failure," *J Lab Clin Med*, 1989, 114(3):294-300.
4. Stabler TV and Siegel AL, "Chemiluminescence Immunoassay of Aldosterone in Serum," *Clin Chem*, 1991, 37(11):1987-9.
5. White PC, "Disorders of Aldosterone Biosynthesis and Action," *N Engl J Med*, 1994, 331(4):250-8.

References
Bortolotto LA, Silva HB, Lopes HF, et al, "Primary Hyperaldosteronism and Adrenal Tumors. Clinico-Surgical Experience With 9 Patients," *Arq Bras Cardiol*, 1994, 62(3):165-9.
Bravo EL, "Primary Aldosteronism," *Urol Clin North Am*, 1989, 16(3):481-6.
Canzanello VJ and Textor SC, "Noninvasive Diagnosis of Renovascular Disease," *Mayo Clin Proc*, 1994, 69(12):1172-81.
Gregoire JR, "Adjustment of the Osmostat in Primary Aldosteronism," *Mayo Clin Proc*, 1994, 69(11):1108-10.
McKenna TJ, Sequeira SJ, Heffernan A, et al, "Diagnosis Under Random Conditions of All Disorders of the Renin-Angiotensin-Aldosterone Axis, Including Primary Hyperaldosteronism," *J Clin Endocrinol Metab*, 1991, 73(5):952-7.
McLeod MK, Thompson NW, Gross MD, et al, "Idiopathic Aldosteronism Masquerading as Discrete Aldosterone-Secreting Adrenal Cortical Neoplasms Among Patients With Primary Aldosteronism," *Surgery*, 1989, 106(6):1161-7.
Miyamoto S, Shimokawa H, Sumioki H, et al, "Circadian Rhythm of Plasma Atrial Natriuretic Peptide, Aldosterone, and Blood Pressure During the Third Trimester in Normal and Pre-eclamptic Pregnancies," *Am J Obstet Gynecol*, 1988, 158(2):393-9.
Radin DR, Manoogian C, and Nadler JL, "Diagnosis of Primary Hyperaldosteronism: Importance of Correlating CT Findings With Endocrinologic Studies," *Am J Roentgenol*, 1992, 158(3):553-7.
Stabler TV and Siegel AL, "Chemiluminescence Immunoassays of Aldosterone in Serum," *Clin Chem*, 1991, 37(11):1987-9.
Torres VE, Young WF Jr, Offord KP, et al, "Association of Hypokalemia, Aldosterone, and Renal Cysts," *N Engl J Med*, 1990, 322(6):345-51.
Weinberger MH and Fineberg NS, "The Diagnosis of Primary Aldosteronism and Separation of Two Major Subtypes," *Arch Intern Med*, 1993, 153(18):2125-9.
Young WF Jr, Hogan MJ, Klee GG, et al, "Primary Aldosteronism: Diagnosis and Treatment," *Mayo Clin Proc*, 1990, 65(1):96-110.

Aldosterone, Urine

CPT 82088

Related Information
Aldosterone, Blood *on previous page*
Electrolytes, Urine *on page 124*
Potassium, Serum or Plasma *on page 188*
Renin, Plasma *on page 197*
Urine Collection, 24-Hour *on page 30*

Abstract Investigation for hypertension begins with history and physical examination, urinalysis, BUN and creatinine, serum or plasma potassium, and ECG. When hyperaldosteronism is suspected, 24-hour urine for potassium provides a useful screening test following repletion of potassium and adequate salt intake.[1]

Patient Preparation Diuretics, antihypertensive drugs, cyclic progestogens, estrogens, and licorice should be terminated for at least 2 weeks and preferably 4 weeks prior to testing. Patient should be on a diet containing 135 mmol (3 g) sodium/day for at least 2 weeks and preferably 30 days prior to testing. No recent radioactive scans. Potassium deficiencies should be corrected before specimen is collected.[1]

Specimen 24-hour urine

Collection Boric acid preservative is used by some laboratories. Other laboratories require 20 mL of 33% acetic acid added to the container prior to starting the collection. Urine pH should be between 2 and 4. Do not use strong mineral acid. Check with laboratory. Instruct the patient to void at 8 AM and discard the specimen. Then collect all urine including the final specimen voided at the end of the 24-hour collection period (ie, 8 AM the next morning). Refrigerate during collection. Label.

Storage Instructions Freeze

Special Instructions A 24-hour urine collection or an aliquot from same, indicating total volume is required.

Reference Range Reference ranges vary at different laboratories; approximately 3-19 µg/24 hours (SI: 8-53 nmol/day) in a normal adult on normal salt intake. 1.5-20 µg/g creatinine is sometimes used. Salt

loading in a normal individual will decrease aldosterone secretion. Black children secrete less aldosterone.[3]

Use A portion of the investigation for hyperaldosteronism. The major causes of primary aldosteronism are aldosterone-producing adenoma (Conn's syndrome); idiopathic hyperaldosteronism (bilateral hyperplasia of zona glomerulosa); unilateral nodular adrenal hyperplasia; adrenocorticol carcinoma, glucocorticoid-remediable hyperaldosteronism, and indeterminate disorders.[1,2] Plasma and urine aldosterone are high, plasma renin and potassium low with primary aldosteronism. Aldosterone and renin are high, plasma potassium low with secondary aldosteronism.

Limitations Urinary aldosterone measurements alone are of very limited value in the diagnosis of hyperaldosteronism. Cushing's syndrome must be excluded with investigation for hyperaldosteronism.[1]

Methodology Radioimmunoassay (RIA) following extraction

Footnotes
1. "Case Records of the Massachusetts General Hospital. Weekly Clinicopathological Exercises. Case 24-1992. A 52-Year-Old Man With Hypertension, Hypokalemia, and an Adrenal Mass," *N Engl J Med*, 1992, 326(24):1617-23.
2. White PC, "Disorders of Aldosterone Biosynthesis and Action," *N Engl J Med*, 1994, 331(4):250-8.
3. Pratt JH, Jones JJ, Miller JZ, et al, "Racial Differences in Aldosterone Excretion and Plasma Aldosterone Concentrations in Children," *N Engl J Med*, 1989, 321(17):1152-7.

References
Blumenfeld JD, Sealey JE, Schlussel Y, et al, "Diagnosis and Treatment of Primary Hyperaldosteronism," *Ann Intern Med*, 1994, 121:877-85.
Mattingly D, Martin H, and Tyler CM, "Estimation of Urinary Aldosterone Using Thin Layer Chromatography and Fluorimetry," *J Clin Pathol*, 1993, 46(12):1109-12.

Alkaline Phosphatase, Heat Stable

CPT 84078

Related Information
Alkaline Phosphatase Isoenzymes *on next page*
Alkaline Phosphatase, Serum *on next page*
Gamma Glutamyl Transferase *on page 133*

Synonyms Fractionated Alkaline Phosphatase; Heat Stable Alkaline Phosphatase

Test Commonly Includes Total alkaline phosphatase and heat stable alkaline phosphatase as a percent of total.

Abstract The placental isoenzyme is very heat stable as is the Regan isoenzyme (a placental-like fetal form occurring in some carriers). Liver isoenzyme is more stable than the bone form. GGT is often helpful and more definitive than this fractionation of alkaline phosphatase. GGT is increased with hepatobiliary disease.

Patient Preparation Patient should be fasting.

Specimen Serum

Container Red top tube

Storage Instructions Refrigerate serum.

Reference Range In nonpregnant subjects, heating at 55°C for 15 minutes resulting in percent residual activity >25% favors hepatic origin; <10% favors bone origin. The addage "bone burns, liver lives" makes the differentiation easier to remember. If >90% of stability, probably a placental form is present.

Use Differentiate liver and bone diseases in patients with increased alkaline phosphatase. Preferred method for this purpose is separation of isoenzyme by electrophoresis. See Alkaline Phosphatase Isoenzymes.

Limitations Sometimes misleading. Prolonged storage at room temperature can increase alkaline phosphatase activity. Hemolysis causes false elevation of alkaline phosphatase. If intestinal ALP or other more heat stable isozymes (eg, placental) of ALP are present, percentage of liver fraction may be falsely increased. Serum GGT, leucine aminopeptidase, and 5′ nucleotidase may be more helpful in differentiating between osseous and hepatobiliary etiologies of elevated alkaline phosphatase.

Contraindications Total alkaline phosphatase not elevated

Methodology Heat inhibition at 56°C. Liver fraction is more resistant to heat and urea inactivation than is the bone isoenzyme. The bone fraction is very heat labile, while placental and cancer (Regan, Nagao) isoenzymes are extremely stable to heat (90% stable).[1] Heating serum at 65°C for 5 minutes results in loss of activity of all ALP fractions with the exception of placental ALP. Heating at 55°C for 15 minutes results in 50% loss of intestinal fraction activity, 60% loss of hepatic fraction, and 90% loss of bone ALP activity. Heat inactivation, when used alone, is an inferior technique, since sharp demarcations of the heat stability of the ALP isoenzymes do not occur. The presence of very heat-stable forms (Regan) may give unusually high half-life values. Extremely close temperature control is required. The preferred method is electrophoresis in polyacrylamide gel or high resolution agarose.[2]

Additional Information Heat stable alkaline phosphatase provides an alternative to alkaline phosphatase electrophoresis. Postmenopausal females generally have slightly elevated total alkaline phosphatase and a low percentage of heat stable fraction, indicating osseous origin.

Footnotes

1. Wolf PL, "Clinical Significance of an Increased or Decreased Serum Alkaline Phosphatase Level," *Arch Pathol Lab Med*, 1978, 102:497-501.
2. Day AP, Saward S, Royle CM, et al, "Evaluation of Two New Methods for Routine Measurement of Alkaline Phosphatase Isoenzymes," *J Clin Pathol*, 1992, 45(1):68-71.

References

Farley JR, Hall SL, Herring S, et al, "Reference Standards for Quantification of Skeletal Alkaline Phosphatase Activity in Serum by Heat Inactivation and Lectin Precipitation," *Clin Chem*, 1993, 39(9):1878-84.

Alkaline Phosphatase Isoenzymes

CPT 84080

Related Information

Alkaline Phosphatase, Heat Stable *on previous page*
Alkaline Phosphatase, Serum *on this page*
Osteocalcin, Serum *on page 174*

Synonyms ALP Isoenzymes; Isoenzymes of Alkaline Phosphatase

Test Commonly Includes Total ALP level with or without neuraminidase and with or without pretreatment by monoclonal antibody to intestinal fraction ALP. May include combinations of heat and/or L-phenylalanine inactivation with or without electrophoretic differentiation.

Abstract Electrophoresis plus use of selective inhibitors allows identification of the principle isoenzymes of alkaline phosphatase, which include those from bone, liver, intestine, and placenta.

Patient Preparation Patient should be fasting.

Specimen Serum

Container Red top tube

Turnaround Time Method dependent, ordinarily at least 2-3 days

Use Evaluate contribution of liver, bone, placental, and Regan isoenzymes to total alkaline phosphatase. Bone fraction is increased in Paget's disease of bone. In the usual chemistry panel, marked isolated increase of alkaline phosphatase in a nonpregnant, older patient who has no healing fracture, with other tests within normal range, is likeliest to indicate Paget's disease of bone. Osteoblastic tumor can also cause increased alkaline phosphatase. If gamma glutamyl transferase is elevated, the source of the elevated ALP is most likely the liver.

Limitations For evaluation of biliary tract, the alternatives of GGT, LAP (leucine aminopeptidase), and 5' nucleotidase as well as radiologic imaging techniques are generally preferred, rather than alkaline phosphatase isoenzymes. Availability of test is limited.

Contraindications Normal total alkaline phosphatase level

Methodology Differential susceptibility of alkaline phosphatase to inhibition by L-phenylalanine and inactivation by heat. Intestinal and placental ALP are inhibited by L-phenylalanine. Skeletal and intestinal ALP are sensitive to inactivation by heat. Polyacrylamide gel electrophoresis with or without pretreatment of sample with neuraminidase and/or monoclonal antibody to the intestinal fraction of ALP (I-ALP). Intestinal fraction can be measured using a method involving sequestration of I-ALP by a monoclonal antibody.[1] Partial digestion with neuraminidase enhances subsequent electrophoretic separation of bone and liver fractions. Pretreatment of samples with monoclonal antibody to I-ALP will retard movement of the latter, allowing for separation of the bone fraction.[2] Isoelectric focusing over a pI range of 3.01-4.86 has separated ALP isoenzymes into 12 bands reflecting at least 12 cellular components. It is claimed that the availability and application of this methodology to clinical problems will render the above manipulations unnecessary.[3,4]

Additional Information In the majority of cases, elevation in serum total alkaline phosphatase (T-ALP) is reasonably well defined on the basis of other already established clinical-pathologic findings. The usually more readily available LD (LDH) isoenzyme fractionation or serum gamma glutamyl transferase activity frequently serves to define the clinical problem sufficiently that recourse to ALP separation is not necessary. In a minority of patients, elevation of T-ALP resists explanation. Here, application of ALP isoenzyme studies may indicate whether T-ALP is increased on the basis of contributions from liver, bone, intestinal, placental, endothelial cell, or pathologic (tumor markers Regan and Nagao) fractions.

Total liver and bone ALP are increased in hyperthyroid patients. B-ALP is most commonly and significantly increased. I-ALP is not elevated in the hyperthyroid state.[5] Thyroid hormone has a direct stimulatory action on osteoblasts.[6]

T-ALP may be elevated in rheumatic diseases (30% to 50% of cases) (eg, rheumatoid arthritis and ankylosing spondylitis).[7] Osteoarthritis and inactive RA are nearly always associated with normal T-ALP. A few cases of RA have increase in liver AP. Increase in T-ALP and in bone fraction has been shown to correlate with disease activity and the number of involved joints.[7]

Cobalamin (vitamin B_{12}) deficient patients have reduced bone ALP. The degree of megaloblastic anemia has been found to correlate with the decrease in enzyme level.[8] T-ALP level, however, is usually within normal range in B_{12} deficient patients.

A number of ALP isoenzymes have been described (rarely) in association with carcinoma. They are most commonly seen with hepatocellular cancer or carcinoma metastatic to liver. They include Regan, Magoo, Regan variant, Kashahara, fetal intestinal, and Timperley types. The Regan isoenzyme, which is similar to placental ALP, is seen in 1% to 3% of carcinomas (varying in primary site of origin) metastatic to liver.

Footnotes

1. Brock DJ, Barron L, Bedgood D, et al, "Prenatal Diagnosis of Cystic Fibrosis Using a Monoclonal Antibody Specific for Intestinal Alkaline Phosphatase," *Prenat Diagn*, 1984, 4(6):421-6.
2. Tibi L, Collier A, Patrick AW, et al, "Plasma Alkaline Phosphatase Isoenzymes in Diabetes Mellitus," *Clin Chim Acta*, 1988, 177(2):147-55.
3. Griffiths J and Black J, "Separation and Identification of Alkaline Phosphatase Isoenzymes and Isoforms in the Serum of Healthy Persons by Isoelectric Focusing," *Clin Chem*, 1987, 33(12):2171-7.
4. Griffiths J, "Alkaline Phosphatases: Newer Concepts in Isoenzymes and Clinical Applications," *Clin Lab Med*, 1989, 9(4):717-30.
5. Tibi L, Patrick AW, Leslie P, et al, "Alkaline Phosphatase Isoenzymes in Plasma in Hyperthyroidism," *Clin Chem*, 1989, 35(7):1427-30.
6. Sato K, Han DC, Fujii Y, et al, "Thyroid Hormone Stimulates Alkaline Phosphatase Activity in Cultured Rat Osteoblastic Cells (ROS 17/2.8) Through 3,5,3'-Triiodo-L-Thyronine Nuclear Receptors," *Endocrinology*, 1987, 120(5):1873-81.
7. Siede WH, Seiffert UB, Merle S, et al, "Alkaline Phosphatase Isoenzymes in Rheumatic Diseases," *Clin Biochem*, 1989, 22(2):121-4.
8. Carmel R, Lau, KH, Baylink DJ, et al, "Cobalamin and Osteoblast-Specific Proteins," *N Engl J Med*, 1988, 319(2):70-5.

References

Chamberlain BR, Buttery JE, Pannall PR, "A Simple Electrophoretic Method for Separating Elevated Liver and Bone Alkaline Phosphatase Isoenzymes in Plasma After Neuraminidase Treatment," *Clin Chim Acta*, 1992, 208(3):219-24.
Domar U, Danielsson A, Hirano K, et al, "Alkaline Phosphatase Isozymes in Non-Malignant Intestinal and Hepatic Diseases," *Scand J Gastroenterol*, 1988, 23(7):793-800.
Fisken J, Leonard RC, Shaw G, et al, "Serum Placental-Like Alkaline Phosphatase (PLAP): A Novel Combined Enzyme Linked Immunoassay for Monitoring Ovarian Cancer," *J Clin Pathol*, 1989, 42(1):40-5.
Panteghini M and Pagani F, "Reference Intervals for Two Bone-Derived Enzyme Activities in Serum: Bone Isoenzyme of Alkaline Phosphatase (ALP) and Tartrate-Resistant Acid Phosphatase (TR-ACP)," *Clin Chem*, 1989, 35(1):180-1.
Schreiber WE and Sadro LC, "Agarose Gel Patterns of ALkaline Phosphatase Isoenzymes Before and After Treatment With Neuraminidase," *Am J Clin Pathol*, 1988, 90(2):181-6.
Seabrook RN, Bailyes EM, Price CP, et al, "The Distinction of Bone and Liver Isoenzymes of Alkaline Phosphatase in Serum Using a Monoclonal Antibody," *Clin Chim Acta*, 1988, 172(2-3):261-6.

Alkaline Phosphatase, Serum

CPT 84075

Related Information

Alkaline Phosphatase, Heat Stable *on previous page*
Alkaline Phosphatase Isoenzymes *on this page*
Aspartate Aminotransferase *on page 84*
Bilirubin, Total *on page 86*
Gamma Glutamyl Transferase *on page 133*
Hydroxyproline, Total, Urine *on page 148*
Kidney Stone Analysis *on page 640*
Leucine Aminopeptidase *on page 158*
Liver Biopsy *on page 48*
5' Nucleotidase *on page 171*
Osteocalcin, Serum *on page 174*

Synonyms ALP; Phosphatase, Alkaline

Replaces BSP

Abstract Serum alkaline phosphatase (ALP) activity normally originates from liver and bone. Other sources include intestine and placenta. ALP is excreted in bile. Serum total ALP level provides a useful but nonspecific indication of liver or bone disease. With biliary tract obstruction, the rise in ALP parallels increase in serum bilirubin. Heating serum at 56°C causes significant inactivation of ALP of bone origin, but electrophoresis (see Alkaline Phosphatase Isoenzymes) or determination of serum gamma glutamyl transferase are probably better tests for determination of the source of the elevated ALP. GGT is more readily available.

Patient Preparation Patient should be fasting.

Specimen Serum

Container Red top tube or capillary tube

Storage Instructions Refrigerate. Serum alkaline phosphatase increases slowly with storage. Increases of 5% to 10% can be expected after less than 4 hours storage at 4°C. For this reason, it is best to analyze on the day of collection.

Reference Range Normal values are higher for pediatric patients and in pregnancy. Levels are two to three or more times adult range in children and are increased in puberty compared to adult range. During episodes of very rapid growth, levels as high as 1000 units/L may be normal. The high level of ALP in childhood results from increase in bone fraction. Postpuberty, serum ALP is mostly of liver origin. Adult normal range is approximately 50-120 units/L (IFCC reference method at 37°C). Values (Continued)

Alkaline Phosphatase, Serum *(Continued)*

in adult males are slightly higher than in adult females. With menopause and after, values in women increase, are similar to or higher than those in men, and are higher than in younger subjects.

Use Causes of **high alkaline phosphatase** include nonfasting specimen, bone growth, healing fracture, acromegaly, osteogenic sarcoma, liver or bone metastases, leukemia, myelofibrosis, and rarely myeloma. Alkaline phosphatase is used as a tumor marker.[1,2] Elevations occur especially 2-4 hours after a fatty meal, especially in people who are Lewis positive secretors of blood type O or B. (See Additional Information.) Standing of blood specimen before analysis; up to 30% increase with storage of serum.

In rickets and osteomalacia, serum calcium and phosphorus are low to normal; and alkaline phosphatase may be normal or increased.

Hypervitaminosis D may cause elevations in alkaline phosphatase, as may vitamin D malabsorption (eg, celiac sprue).

In Paget's disease of bone, there is often isolated elevation of ALP, some among the highest levels seen.

Hyperthyroidism, by its effects upon bone, may elevate alkaline phosphatase. There is evidence that thyroid hormone (T_3) acts to stimulate bone alkaline phosphatase activity through an osteoblast nuclear receptor-mediated process.[3]

Hyperparathyroidism, in some patients; pseudohyperparathyroidism.

Chronic alcohol ingestion (in chronic alcoholism, alkaline phosphatase may be normal or increased, but often with high AST (SGOT) and/or high bilirubin and especially with high GGT; MCV may be high).

Biliary obstruction (eg, tenfold increase may be seen with carcinoma of head of pancreas, choledocholithiasis); cholestasis; GGT also high. Cholecystitis with cholangitis. In most patients with cholecystitis and cholangitis who do not have a common duct stone, alkaline phosphatase is within normal limits or only slightly increased. Sclerosing cholangitis (eg, with ulcerative colitis), although 3% of cases of symptomatic sclerosing cholangitis may have normal serum ALP.[4] Endoscopic retrograde cholangiography might be considered then in patients with diseases known to be associated with primary sclerosing cholangitis and with appropriate symptomatology even though ALP level is normal.

Autoimmune cholangiopathy includes features of primary biliary cirrhosis or primary sclerosing cholangitis, pruritus with high ALP without antimitochondrial antibodies.[5]

With primary or metastatic tumor in the liver, there may be a marked increase in alkaline phosphatase and GGT. Only three laboratory markers were consistently abnormal, in screening for metastatic carcinoma of breast, prior to clinical detectability of metastases: these were alkaline phosphatase, GGT, and CEA.[2]

Cirrhosis, especially in primary biliary cirrhosis, in which fivefold or more increases are seen.

Gilbert's syndrome;[6] postoperative cholestasis, pancreatitis, carcinoma of pancreas, cystic fibrosis.

Hepatitis: Moderate increases in alkaline phosphatase occur in viral hepatitis, but greater elevations of the transaminases (AST (SGOT), ALT (SGPT)) are usually found.

Fatty metamorphosis of liver (moderate increase occurs in acute fatty liver).

Diabetes mellitus, diabetic hepatic lipidosis.

Infiltrative liver diseases (eg, sarcoid, TB, amyloidosis, metastatic cancer, abscess).

Sepsis and certain viral diseases including infectious mononucleosis and cytomegalovirus infections.

Pulmonary infarct (1-3 weeks after embolism. Healing infarcts in other organs, including kidney, may also cause increased ALP); other situations in which angiofibroplasia occurs, such as healing in a large decubitus ulcer.

Tumors, especially hypernephroma; neoplastic ectopic production (Regan, Nagao isoenzymes).

Fanconi syndrome, familial hyperphosphatasemia, idiopathic.

Peptic ulcer, erosion; intestinal strangulation or obstruction, or ulcerative lesion; steatorrhea, malabsorption (from bone, secondary to vitamin D deficiency); ulcerative colitis with pericholangitis, other erosive lesions of colon.

Congestive heart failure, parenteral hyperalimentation of glucose, intravenous albumin administration.

Drugs - estrogens (large doses), birth control agents, methyltestosterone, phenothiazines, oral hypoglycemic agents, erythromycin, or any drug producing hypersensitivity or toxic cholestasis. Many commonly and uncommonly used drugs elevate alkaline phosphatase, and tenfold increases may be seen with drug cholestasis.

Causes of **low alkaline phosphatase** are said to include: Hypothyroidism - but most hypothyroid patients have normal alkaline phosphatase.

Pernicious anemia - in very few patients.

Hypophosphatasia: Very low ALP values are found in the presence of normocalcemia or hypocalcemia. This diagnosis may be confirmed by quantitation of urinary phosphoethanolamine.

Malnutrition has been reported to relate to low values, but in practice, diseases causing malnutrition relate often to high ALP (eg, disseminated neoplasia).

Some drugs (clofibrate, azathioprine, estrogens and estrogens in combination with androgens) lower serum ALP activity.

Limitations Normal ranges dependent upon methodology, age, and sex. Used alone, alkaline phosphatase may be misleading.

Methodology Some original spectrophotometric methods and their modifications (eg, King-Armstrong, described in 1934 and using the substrate phenylphosphate[7]) have been largely supplanted by more recent end point, kinetic spectrophotometric or fluorescent procedures. Most current assays use *p*-nitrophenyl phosphate (pNPP) as substrate (eg, Bessey-Lowry-Brock). More recent techniques utilize chromogenic substrates (eg, methylumbelliferyl phosphate) and improved buffer systems with resultant increased sensitivity. A reference method using pNPP as substrate has been proposed by the American Association of Clinical Chemistry.[8]

Additional Information Serum ALP is a member of a family of zinc metalloprotein enzymes that function to split off a terminal phosphate group from an organic phosphate ester. This enzyme functions in an alkaline environment (optimum pH of 10). Active center of ALP enzymes includes a serine residue. Magnesium and zinc ions are required for minimal activity. Enzyme activity is localized in the brush border of the proximal convoluted tubule of the kidney, intestinal mucosal epithelial cells, hepatic sinusoidal membranes, vascular endothelial cells, and osteoblasts of bone. There are distinctive forms of ALP in the placenta and small intestine; hepatic, renal, and osteoblast (bone) ALP are similar molecules.

Serum ALP activity of intestinal origin occurs only in individuals of ABO blood type O or A. They are secretors of ABH RBC antigens and also carry the Lewis red cell antigen. Serum intestinal ALP level increases in these individuals about 2 hours following consumption of a fatty meal.

Increased in cholestasis and inflammatory liver disease as well as in infiltrative liver disease, ALP is sensitive to obstructive biliary processes, even small secondary bile duct obstruction, and thus may be increased in those patients when bilirubin is normal due to compensatory bilirubin excretion by the rest of the liver. ALP may be helpful in localized obstructive problems such as hepatic metastases. An electrophoretically slow moving isoenzyme with high relative mass may occur in some patients with bile duct obstruction and hepatic metastases and may result in false elevation of CK-MB.[9]

To confirm biliary abnormality, an additional useful test is GGT. GGT is elevated in hepatobiliary disease, not in uncomplicated bone disease.

Serum ALP is increased during pregnancy. Marked decline of high ALP of pregnancy is seen with placental insufficiency and imminent fetal demise.

A characteristic of acute liver failure in Wilson's disease is the combination of a very high bilirubin, >30 mg/dL (>513 μmol/L) with decreased serum alkaline phosphatase activity. The ratio of ALP to bilirubin <2.0 is relatively distinctive.[10]

Footnotes

1. Narayanan S, "Alkaline Phosphatase as Tumor Marker," *Ann Clin Lab Sci*, 1983, 13:133-6.
2. Coombes RC, Powles TJ, Gazet JC, et al, "Screening for Metastases in Breast Cancer: An Assessment of Biochemical and Physical Methods," *Cancer*, 1981, 48:310-5.
3. Sato K, Han DC, Fujii Y, et al, "Thyroid Hormone Stimulates Alkaline Phosphatase Activity in Cultured Rat Osteoblastic Cells (ROS 17/2.8) Through 3,5,3'-Triiodo-L-Thyronine Nuclear Receptors," *Endocrinology*, 1987, 120(5):1873-81.
4. Cooper JF and Brand EJ, "Symptomatic Sclerosing Cholangitis in Patients With a Normal Alkaline Phosphatase: Two Case Reports and a Review of the Literature," *Am J Gastroenterol*, 1988, 83(3):308-11.
5. Krawitt EL, "Autoimmune Hepatitis," *N Engl J Med*, 1996, 334(14):897-903.
6. Lieverse AG, van Essen GG, Beukeveld GJ, et al, "Familial Increased Serum Intestinal Alkaline Phosphatase: A New Variant Associated With Gilbert's Syndrome," *J Clin Pathol*, 1990, 43(2):125-8.
7. King EJ and Armstrong AR, "A Convenient Method for Determining Serum and Bile Phosphatase Activity," *Can Med Assoc J*, 1934, 31:376-81.
8. Tietz NW, Burtis CA, Duncan P, et al, "A Reference Method for Measurement of Alkaline Phosphatase Activity in Human Serum," *Clin Chem*, 1983, 29:751-61.

9. Butch AW, Goodnow TT, Brown WS, et al, "Stratus Automated Creatine Kinase - MB Assay Evaluated: Identification and Elimination of Falsely Increased Results Associated With High-Molecular-Mass Form of Alkaline Phosphatase," *Clin Chem*, 1989, 35(10):2048-53.

10. Lee WM, "Acute Liver Failure," *N Engl J Med*, 1993, 329(25):1862-72.

References

Epstein S, "Serum and Urinary Markers for Bone Remodeling: Assessment of Bone Turnover," *Endocr Rev*, 1988, 9(4):437-49.

Gordon T, "Factors Associated With Serum Alkaline Phosphatase Level," *Arch Pathol Lab Med*, 1993, 117(2):187-90.

Kihn L, Dinwoodie A, and Stinson RA, "High-Molecular-Weight Alkaline Phosphatase in Serum Has Properties Similar to the Enzyme in Plasma Membranes of the Liver," *Am J Clin Pathol*, 1991, 96(4):470-8.

Reichling JJ and Kaplan MM, "Clinical Use of Serum Enzymes in Liver Disease," *Dig Dis Sci*, 1988, 33(12):1601-14.

Van Hoof VO, Hoylaerts MF, Geryl H, et al, "Age and Sex Distribution of Alkaline Phosphatase Isoenzymes by Agarose Electrophoresis," *Clin Chem*, 1990, 36(6):875-8.

Vincent-Viry M and Galteau MM, "Alkaline Phosphatases," *Drug Effects on Laboratory Test Results Analytical Interferences and Pharmacological Effects*, Siest G and Galteau MM, eds, Littleton, MA: PSG Publishing Co Inc, 1988, 67-90.

Wilson JW, "Inherited Elevation of Alkaline Phosphatase Activity in the Absence of Disease," *N Engl J Med*, 1979, 301:983-4.

Allergen Profile see Allergen Specific IgE Antibody *on this page*

Allergen Specific IgE Antibody

CPT 86003 (quantitative or semiquantitative); 86005 (qualitative)

Synonyms Allergen Profile; Allergy Screen; IgE Allergen Specific; Radioallergosorbent Test (RAST®)

Test Commonly Includes *Alternaria tenuis*, bermuda grass, cat epithelium, common ragweed, *Dermatophagoides farinae*, dog epithelium, egg white, English plantain, house dust, maple, oak, timothy, or specific mini panels of grasses, foods, animal danders, etc

Abstract Radiolabeled anti-IgE is used to detect binding of patient's IgE to specific allergens present on a paper disk.

Patient Preparation No radioisotopes administered 24 hours prior to collection of specimen.

Specimen Serum

Container Red top tube

Storage Instructions Separate serum and refrigerate.

Turnaround Time 1 week (test is commonly performed by a reference laboratory)

Reference Range Each allergen scored from 0-4, 0 meaning no IgE detected, 1 meaning a borderline result, and 2-4 increasing IgE against allergen

Use Detect possible allergic responses to various substances in the environment such as animals, antibiotics, foods, grasses, house dust, mites, insects, insulin, molds, smuts, trees, and weeds. Evaluate hay fever, extrinsic asthma, atopic eczema, respiratory allergy.

Radioallergosorbent test (RAST®) is indicated when:
- specific allergic sensitivity is needed to allow immunotherapy ("desensitization shots") to be initiated
- testing for food or chemical sensitivity, where skin testing is unreliable
- there is a history of severe allergic reaction to skin testing
- testing infants
- evaluating patients who refuse skin tests or who are unable to have them because of dermatopathic conditions
- immunotherapy or other therapeutic measures based on skin testing results have not led to a satisfactory remission of symptoms

Limitations RAST® results should be interpreted in the context of all available clinical and laboratory findings. False-negative results are possible and may reflect the timing of the blood sample relative to the previous adverse reaction. High levels of total IgE (>3000 IU/mL as may be seen due to parasitic infestation) may result in nonspecific binding and thus, false-positive RAST® results. Total quantitative IgE level must usually be ordered separately. Not all IgE allergens can be tested at this time. Levels less than the geometric mean of IgE probably will not have significant RAST® results.

Contraindications Recently administered radioisotopes will interfere with this test, causing spurious results.

RAST® is contraindicated when:
- all skin tests are negative
- the patient has only mild symptoms or can be successfully treated with medication and avoidance
- IgE levels are <10 IU/mL unless there is strong clinical suggestion of allergic disease
- patients have successfully responded to immunotherapy
- evaluating non-IgE mediated disease, such as certain drug and food reactions

Methodology Radioallergosorbent test (a radioimmunoassay); in this procedure specific allergen is adsorbed on a paper disk; immunospecific IgE, if present in the test (patient's) serum will bind to the disk; detection

is effected by radiolabeled anti-IgE. Different scoring systems comparing test results with the absolute binding of a negative control are in use. Commonly, the Fadal/Nalebuff modified RAST® procedure is followed with overnight incubation and resultant greater sensitivity.[1] Monoclonal anti-IgE techniques are useful in the detection of specific IgE in serum.[2] Also, multiallergen dipstick screening test has been introduced recently.[3]

Additional Information IgE is elevated 4 to 30 times normal in various diseases, among which atopic disorders and parasitic infections are most prominent. The principal limitation of this test is the wide and overlapping range of IgE values between atopic and nonatopic disease states. A positive value is usually meaningful; a negative value is equivocal. RAST® test is valuable on patients who do not respond to environmental control or conservative medical management and where skin tests are contraindicated.

Over 20 years have passed since RAST® testing has been available. Identification of allergen or allergens in patients with atopic disease may be approached clinically by history, avoidance of the offender, by skin testing and/or by RAST® studies. Numerous reports comparing skin testing and RAST® have accumulated in the literature, generally to assess which method has the better sensitivity/specificity. The results appear to vary with the allergen, that is, the relative performance of the two different methods is allergen-dependent.[4] This finding has provided the stimulus for expanded allergen specific comparison studies in the decade of the eighties. A brief summary of a subset of such studies follows.
- With dog and cat as allergens, sensitivity/specificity are similar but negative predictive value of either skin test or RAST® is much greater than positive predictive value.[5]
- Sensitivity of skin test vs RAST® in studies of shrimp allergens is somewhat comparable. There are apparent species-specific shrimp allergens possibly explaining intermittent nature of symptoms in some patients. Test sensitivity may be increased by use of extracts from more than one species of shrimp.[6]
- A comparison of fresh food skin prick tests and RAST® for a variety of vegetables, fruits, and nuts in patients with oral allergy syndrome showed generally variable specificity but better sensitivity with skin testing. RAST® showed better sensitivity only with hazelnut.[7]
- A comparison of RAST® with skin prick testing results in wasp venom allergy found systemic reaction to correlate with a positive paper RAST®. There was relatively good specificity with paper RAST® and skin prick testing, nearly all patients with a systemic reaction had positive paper RAST®.[8]

New assays for the detection of specific IgE are of recent development and include RIA, EIA, and immunofluorometric based systems.[9]

Footnotes

1. King WP, "Efficacy of a Screening Radioallergosorbent Test," *Arch Otolaryngol Head Neck Surg*, 1982, 108:781-6.

2. Duc J, Peitrequin R, and Pecoud AR, "Clinical Evaluation of a New Enzymo-Assay for Allergen Specific IgE," *Ann Allergy*, 1989, 62(6):503-6.

3. Twiggs JT, Gray RL, Pichler K, et al, "Evaluation of Multiallergen Dipstick Screening Test," *Ann Allergy*, 1989, 63(3):225-8.

4. Wittig HJ and Blaiss MS, "How Helpful Is the Radioallergosorbent Test in the Diagnosis of Allergic Disease?" *South Med J*, 1982, 75:820-3.

5. Ferguson AC and Murray AB, "Predictive Value of Skin Prick Tests and Radioallergosorbent Tests for Clinical Allergy to Dogs and Cats," *Can Med Assoc J*, 1986, 134(12):1365-8.

6. Morgan JE, O'Neil CE, Daul CB, et al, "Species-Specific Shrimp Allergens: RAST® and RAST®-Inhibition Studies," *J Allergy Clin Immunol*, 1989, 83(6):1112-7.

7. Ortolani C, Ispano M, Pastorello EA, et al, "Comparison of Results of Skin Prick Tests (With Fresh Foods and Commercial Food Extracts) and RAST® in 100 Patients With Oral Allergy Syndrome," *J Allergy Clin Immunol*, 1989, 83(3):683-900.

8. Heinig JH, Mosbech H, Engel T, et al, "A Comparison of Two RAST® Methods and Skin Prick Testing in the Diagnosis of Wasp Venom Allergy," *Allergy*, 1989, 44(4):260-3.

9. Gueant JL, Moneret-Vautrin DA, Dejardin G, et al, "Comparative Evaluation of RAST® and FAST for 11 Allergens in 288 Patients," *Allergy*, 1989, 44(3):204-8.

References

Canadian Paediatric Society, Allergy Section, "Blood Tests for Allergy in Children," *Can Med Assoc J*, 1990, 142(11):1207-8.

Kelso JM, Sodhi N, Gosselin VA, et al, "Diagnostic Performance Characteristics of the Standard Phadebas RAST®, Modified RAST®, and Pharmacia CAP System Versus Skin Testing," *Ann Allergy*, 1991, 67(5):511-4.

Ownby DR, "Allergy Testing: *In Vivo* Versus *In Vitro*," *Pediatr Clin North Am*, 1988, 35(5):995-1009.

Shearer WT, "Specific Diagnostic Modalities: IgE, Skin Tests, and RAST®," *J Allergy Clin Immunol*, 1989, 84(6 Pt 2):1112-6.

Van Arsdel PP Jr and Larson EB, "Diagnostic Tests for Patients With Suspected Allergic Disease," *Ann Intern Med*, 1989, 110(4):304-12.

Yunginger JW, "Allergens: Recent Advances," *Pediatr Clin North Am*, 1988, 35(5):981-93.

Allergy Screen see Allergen Specific IgE Antibody *on this page*

ALP see Alkaline Phosphatase, Serum *on page 69*

Alpha₁-Fetoprotein, Amniotic Fluid

CPT 82106

Related Information

Acetylcholinesterase, Red Cell *on page 62*
(Continued)

Alpha₁-Fetoprotein, Amniotic Fluid (Continued)

Alpha₁-Fetoprotein, Serum *on this page*

Amniotic Fluid, Chromosome and Genetic Abnormality Analysis *on page 273*

Chromosome *In Situ* Hybridization *on page 281*

Cystic Fibrosis DNA Detection *on page 507*

Duchenne/Becker Muscular Dystrophy DNA Detection *on page 509*

Synonyms AFP, Amniotic Fluid

Applies to Amniotic Fluid Acetylcholinesterase

Abstract Alpha-fetoprotein (AFP) is a glycoprotein produced by the fetal liver, gastrointestinal tract, and the yolk sac. Amniotic fluid AFP testing is done following positive maternal screening, but it is also done when the maternal or family history is positive for neural tube defect.

Patient Preparation Since interpretation depends on gestational age, diagnostic ultrasound is more desirable than calculated gestational age.[1] (Ultrasound may also delineate other important information, eg, twins.)

Specimen Amniotic fluid

Container Sterile syringe

Collection The optimal time to collect amniotic fluid for AFP is between the 16th and 18th week of gestation. Include the gestational age on the requisition. If the amniotic fluid is traumatic (bloody), a maternal blood specimen should also be submitted. One or two drops of blood in amniotic fluid can give false-positive results.

Causes for Rejection Sample determined not to be amniotic fluid; contamination of amniotic fluid with maternal or fetal blood; recently administered radioisotopes if RIA is used for assay; urine urea nitrogen (UUN) of maternal urine >100 g/day, that of normal amniotic fluid is much less.

Reference Range Interlaboratory differences exist. Ranges are stratified by weeks of gestation, decreasing with increasing maturity. It is essential that the reference ranges supplied by the laboratory performing the assay be used to interpret results, which are expressed as "multiples of the median" (MOM) and are generally >0.5 MOM and <2.5 MOM. Most authorities, however, regard MOM >2.0 as abnormal until proven otherwise. MOM is **not** corrected for maternal race, maternal weight, and maternal insulin-dependent diabetes mellitus. Amniotic fluid AFP peak differs from that of maternal serum.

Use Analyze second trimester amniotic fluid for detection of neural tube defects: anencephaly, spina bifida (with ultrasound), myelocele, hydrocephaly

Limitations Amniotic fluid alpha-fetoprotein may also be increased in non-neural tube anomalies (such as congenital nephrosis, esophageal atresia, duodenal atresia) and fetal bleeding into the amniotic space. The Kleihauer-Betke stain can detect fetal blood contamination of the tap but requires that fetal intact red cells be present. Fetal serum contains mg/mL levels of AFP. Closed neural tube defects are generally not detected by alpha-fetoprotein testing. When an amniotic fluid alpha-fetoprotein level is elevated, confirmatory testing, such as **high resolution ultrasonography** and measurement of **amniotic fluid acetylcholinesterase**, should be undertaken to confirm the neural tube defect. Acetylcholinesterase is independent of gestational age and is not affected by fetal blood contamination.

Measurement of AFP and acetylcholinesterase in second trimester amniotic fluid specimens appears to be low yield and may not be as effective as high resolution ultrasonography.[2]

Methodology Immunoassay, solid-phase and enzyme-labeled monoclonal antibody directed to different epitopes

Additional Information Levels of amniotic fluid AFP >2.5 MOM are generally regarded as abnormally high.

When evaluating amniotic fluid AFP and acetylcholinesterase levels in twin gestations in which only one fetus is affected, placental anatomy appears to be important.[1] With diamniotic-dichorionic twin placentas, amniotic fluid AFP and acetylcholinesterase are within normal range for the unaffected fetus, and elevated in the affected fetus. With diamniotic-monochorionic twin placentas, the unaffected twin may demonstrate elevated amniotic fluid AFP and acetylcholinesterase levels, presumably due to diffusion across the amnion bilayer membrane from the affected site.

Fetal status can be assessed by ultrasound (high-resolution) and chorionic villus sampling by the end of the first trimester. The finding that determination of AFP (coupled with "cautious" interpretation of acetylcholinesterase) has application to detection of neural tube defects during this period has important value.[3] The expected level of α-fetoprotein in amniotic fluid between 11 and 15 weeks should not be determined by extrapolation backward from medians of later gestational age.[4,5] The laboratory must establish its own database for MOMs. The calculation is based on a smoothed weighted log-linear regression. The amniotic fluid MOM is uncorrected, whereas the serum MOM must be corrected for weight, race, and insulin-dependent diabetes.

AFP in amniotic fluid is of two sources, one from the fetal liver, the other originating from the fetal yolk sac. These two forms show varying affinity for concanavalin-A. As gestation advances, the yolk sac contribution to amniotic fluid decreases. The decrease in AFP in amniotic fluid surrounding fetuses with trisomy 21 involves proportionately equal reduction in the yolk sac subfraction and total AFP. No advantage in diagnostic efficiency has been found, therefore, in differential determination of the yolk sac subfractions.[6]

AFP levels in Down syndrome overlap normal values.[7] An excellent review is available.[8] A large percentage of open tube neural defects can be detected by maternal serum AFP measurement.[9] Prenatal assessment of serum alpha-fetoprotein with unconjugated estriol and β-hCG to screen for Down syndrome can be considered.[10]

Footnotes

1. Stiller RJ, Lockwood CJ, Belanger K, et al, "Amniotic Fluid Alpha-Fetoprotein Concentrations in Twin Gestations: Dependence on Placental Membrane Anatomy," *Am J Obstet Gynecol*, 1988, 158(5):1088-92.
2. Sepulveda W, Donaldson A, Johnson RD, et al, "Are Routine Alpha-Fetoprotein and Acetylcholinesterase Determinations Still Necessary at Second-Trimester Amniocentesis? Impact of High-Resolution Ultrasonography," *Obstet Gynecol*, 1995, 85(1):107-12.
3. Drugan A, Syner FN, Greb A, et al, "Amniotic Fluid Alpha-Fetoprotein and Acetylcholinesterase in Early Genetic Amniocentesis," *Obstet Gynecol*, 1988, 72(1):35-8.
4. Crandall BF, Hanson FW, Tennant F, et al, "Alpha-Fetoprotein Levels in Amniotic Fluid Between 11 and 15 Weeks," *Am J Obstet Gynecol*, 1989, 160(5 Pt 1):1204-6.
5. Brumfield CG, Cloud GA, Davis RO, et al, "The Relationship Between Maternal Serum and Amniotic Fluid Alpha-Fetoprotein in Women Undergoing Early Amniocentesis," *Am J Obstet Gynecol*, 1990, 163(3):903-6.
6. Jones SR, Evans SE, and Gillan L, "Amniotic Fluid Alpha-Fetoprotein Subfractions in Fetal Trisomy 21 Affected Pregnancies," *Br J Obstet Gynaecol*, 1988, 95(4):327-9.
7. Wenk RE and Rosenbaum JM, "Analyses of Amniotic Fluid," *Todd-Sanford-Davidsohn Clinical Diagnosis and Management by Laboratory Methods*, 18th ed, Henry JB, ed, Philadelphia, PA: WB Saunders Co, 1991, 482-96.
8. Bock JL, "Current Issues in Maternal Serum Alpha-Fetoprotein Screening," *Am J Clin Pathol*, 1992, 97(4):541-54.
9. Burtis CA and Ashwood ER, *Tietz Textbook of Clinical Chemistry*, 2nd ed, Philadelphia, PA: WB Saunders Co, 1994, 2121-2.
10. Haddow JE, Palomaki GE, Knight GJ, et al, "Reducing the Need for Amniocentesis in Women 35 Years of Age or Older With Serum Markers for Screening," *N Engl J Med*, 1994, 330(16):1114-8.

References

Brumfield CG, Cloud GA, Finley SC, et al, "Amniotic Fluid Alpha-Fetoprotein Levels and Pregnancy Outcome," *Am J Obstet Gynecol*, 1987, 157(4 Pt 1):822-5.

Cuckle HS, "Screening for Neural Tube Defects," *Ciba Found Symp*, 1994, 181:253-69.

Drugan A, Syner FN, Belsky R, et al, "Amniotic Fluid Acetylcholinesterase: Implications of an Inconclusive Result," *Am J Obstet Gynecol*, 1988, 159(2):469-74.

Hogge WA, Thiagarajah S, Ferguson JE 2d, et al, "The Role of Ultrasonography and Amniocentesis in the Evaluation of Pregnancies at Risk for Neural Tube Defects," *Am J Obstet Gynecol*, 1990, 163(3):520-3.

Knight GJ, "Maternal Serum Alpha-Fetoprotein Screening," *Techniques in Diagnostic Human Biochemical Genetics*, Hommes FA, ed, New York, NY: Wiley-Liss, 1991, 491-518.

"Maternal Serum Alpha-Fetoprotein Screening Programs and Quality Control for Laboratories Performing Maternal Serum and Amniotic Fluid Alpha-Fetoprotein Assays: Policy Statement. American Society of Human Genetics," *Can Med Assoc J*, 1987, 136(12):1253-6.

Richards DS, Seeds JW, Katz VL, et al, "Elevated Maternal Serum Alpha-Fetoprotein With Oligohydramnios: Ultrasound Evaluation and Outcome," *Obstet Gynecol*, 1988, 72(3 Pt 1):337-41.

Stephens JD, "Amniotic Fluid Alpha-Fetoprotein and Acetylcholinesterase in Early Genetic Amniocentesis," *Obstet Gynecol*, 1989, 73(1):141-2.

Alpha₁-Fetoprotein, Serum

CPT 82105

Related Information

Acetylcholinesterase, Red Cell *on page 62*

Alpha₁-Fetoprotein, Amniotic Fluid *on previous page*

Body Fluid *on page 89*

CA 19-9 *on page 93*

Carcinoembryonic Antigen *on page 100*

Cyst Fluid Cytology *on page 292*

Human Chorionic Gonadotropin, Serum *on page 145*

Synonyms AFP

Applies to Inhibin A

Abstract A major protein of normal fetal plasma, very low levels of AFP are found in the serum of nonpregnant adults. It is increased in hepatic disorders attended by hepatocyte regenerative activity, in hepatoma, and in various germ cell derived tumors. With some neural tube congenital (developmental) defects (eg, spina bifida), AFP is elevated in amniotic fluid and therefore in the serum of the gravid woman, but not in all instances. With some fetal chromosomal abnormalities (Down syndrome, trisomy 21, trisomy 18), it is relatively low in the maternal serum. The risk of Down syndrome increases with advancing maternal age.

Patient Preparation Avoid radioisotope scan prior to collection of specimen if assay is performed.

Specimen Serum

Container Red top tube

Sampling Time The optimal time to draw **maternal serum** for AFP, for prenatal screening, is between the 16th week and 18th week of gestation.[1] Repeat 1 week or more later if a high result is found. Maternal serum can be collected between the 15th and 22nd weeks.

Storage Instructions Refrigerate

Causes for Rejection Recently administered radioisotopes if RIA is used for assay

Special Instructions Include maternal age, gestational age, maternal weight, race, and diabetic status with request.

Reference Range Normal adults: <10 ng/mL (SI: <10 µg/L) serum. Interlaboratory differences exist. The level in maternal serum increases to a maximum of 550 ng/mL (SI: 550 µg/L) during the third trimester of pregnancy. Normal values for maternal serum may vary from laboratory to laboratory. Normal is considered 0.5-2.5 multiples of the median (MOM), although some authorities recommend 0.5-2.0 MOM recently.[1] The MOM is always corrected for maternal weight, maternal race, and maternal insulin-dependent diabetes mellitus.

Use Diagnose **hepatocellular carcinoma:** With sensitive RIA procedures, elevation of AFP will occur in 90% of patients with hepatocellular carcinoma. Values in excess of 1000 ng/mL (SI: >1000 µg/L) are almost always secondary to hepatocellular carcinoma. However, overlap with AFP elevations caused by nonmalignant chronic liver diseases is widely recognized.

Gonadal and extragonadal germinal tumor types include endodermal sinus tumor (yolk sac tumor), embryonal carcinoma, teratocarcinoma, and choriocarcinoma. AFP increases occur as well from extragonadal locations, retroperitoneum, and mediastinum.

Monitor therapy with antineoplastic drugs, in patients being treated for hepatoma or germinal neoplasm.

Differential diagnosis of **neonatal hepatitis** versus biliary atresia in newborns.

Useful in **intrauterine** screening with other tests, including chorionic gonadotropins, unconjugated estriol and ultrasound. Elevated values are found in anencephaly, spina bifida (with ultrasound), myelomeningocele, and other open neural tube defects; fetal death; esophageal atresia; congenital nephrosis; diagnose multiple pregnancy; oligohydramnios; abruptio placentae; and pre-eclampsia.[2] Increased values of AFP in maternal serum can result from underestimated gestational age or from contamination with fetal plasma. Low values are associated with chromosomal abnormalities including trisomy 21 and trisomy 18.

Limitations High in some cases of nonmalignant liver disease (eg, massive hepatic necrosis, acute hepatitis, alcoholic cirrhosis, and chronic active hepatitis). American instances of hepatocellular carcinoma are not as consistently AFP rich, as are many cases from overseas.

Pure **seminomas, dysgerminomas, and teratomas** do not produce AFP, and increased AFP in a subject with seminoma by histology suggests nonseminomatous elements such as embryonal carcinoma, or hepatic metastasis.[3]

Elevations have been described in tyrosinemia, ataxia telangiectasia, and congenital nephrotic syndrome. A low incidence of elevations occurs in a variety of tumors, especially carcinoma of stomach, pancreas, and biliary tract.

Some maternal serum samples from women carrying fetuses with closed **neural tube defects** have normal levels of AFP. Maternal serum AFP detects about 75% of instances of spina bifida at 18-20 weeks.[4] False-positives for prenatal diagnosis of neural tube defects have been reported. Increased AFP in maternal serum can occur with twins, incorrect gestational age, any blockage of fetal gastrointestinal tract, fetal death, and other conditions.[5]

Elevations are reported with alcoholism.[6]

Contraindications Recently administered radioisotopes may interfere with RIA testing.

Methodology Radioimmunoassay (RIA), enzyme immunoassay (EIA), monoclonal immunofluorescent assay

Additional Information AFP is a major glycoprotein of fetal plasma, structurally similar to albumin with molecular weight of about 65,000. In the embryo it is synthesized by the yolk sac and later by the fetal liver. During the sixth week of gestation, AFP appears in fetal serum. It achieves peak concentration in fetal serum and amniotic fluid at 14-weeks gestation. In the maternal circulation, AFP is about 10 ng/mL (SI: 10 µg/L) at the 8th week, 60 ng/mL (SI: 60 µg/L) at 20 weeks and undergoes further rise to term.

Maternal screening for presence of open neural tube defects (eg, spina bifida) is based on the finding of elevated AFP in a maternal serum specimen ideally taken at the 16th to 18th week of gestation. The findings must be confirmed by amniotic fluid acetylcholinesterase study and ultrasound study of the fetal spine to detect the possibility of false-positive resulting from inaccurate dating, twins, threatened abortion, congenital nephrosis, and other causes.

Unexplained increase in maternal serum AFP with second trimester oligohydramnios is associated with an especially poor prognosis. There is evidence that serial ultrasound evaluations of amniotic fluid volume can assist in predicting pregnancy outcome.[7] With severe decrease in amniotic fluid (eg, severe oligohydramnios or no amniotic fluid), the majority (essentially all) of cases will have pulmonary hypoplasia, Potter deformities, renal developmental abnormalities (such as polycystic kidney), or neonatal death. Genetic testing may be indicated in cases of low values for correct gestational age.

AFP levels may be increased in cases of hepatic parenchymal regeneration (eg, following traumatic injury, associated with the viral hepatitides, and following recovery from exposure to hepatotoxins).

Extremely high AFP levels are found with endodermal sinus tumors (yolk sac tumors).[3] Such neoplasms occur in testis, ovary, and in extragonadal sites. Typically they occur in young subjects. Forty percent of patients with nonseminomatous germ cell tumor present with increased levels of hCG. Approximately 7% to 18% of patients with pure seminoma present or develop an elevated hCG in the course of their disease. Assay of hCG is useful in post-treatment prediction of survival. Pretreatment levels are also useful in prognosis and response to treatment.[3]

While some hepatocarcinomas are associated with very high AFP levels (>10,000 µg/L), there is evidence that tumors with such high levels are decreasing in prevalence while tumors with lower levels are becoming more common.[8] For size-matched cases of hepatocellular carcinoma, prognosis has been found to relate importantly to serum AFP levels. Patients with low levels of AFP (≤20 µg/L) had two- to threefold increase in survival as compared with patients having the highest (>10,000 µg/L) levels.[8]

Low serum levels of β-hCG and AFP are found in first and second trimesters in mothers with Down syndrome (trisomy 21) pregnancies. However, the test to screen for this condition has poor predictive value. Maternal serum AFP levels are decreased in other examples of fetal chromosomal abnormalities (trisomy 18).[9] Recently, the combination of maternal serum AFP with maternal serum human chorionic gonadotropin (hCG) and unconjugated estriol (UE$_3$) have been advocated to improve the predictive value of screening for Down syndrome.[10] This "triple test" can detect 60% to 75% of Down syndrome cases with a false-positive rate of about 6%. Some sources suggest that the UE$_3$ is not essential for the screen. Others have advocated the use of a free beta-hCG assay to improve predictive value. In the second trimester, the best detection rates have included AFP, β-hCG, inhibin A, and age. (Inhibin A is increased with Down syndrome). However, use of inhibin A failed to contribute to the detection of trisomy 18.[11] National surveys by the CAP found that larger laboratories tend to make the clinically important adjustments for maternal weight, race, and diabetic status more often than smaller laboratories.

AFP testing is useful in the detection of pregnancy complications such as intrauterine growth retardation, fetal distress, fetal demise, or in the presence of severe maternal pregnancy-induced hypertension. In all these instances, the serum AFP was increased >2.0 MOM. The use of this test was found to be more valuable in detecting these complications than in detecting neural tube defects.[1]

Footnotes

1. Lenke RR, Guerrieri J, Nemes JM, et al, "Elevated Maternal Serum Alpha-Fetoprotein Values: How Low Is High?" *J Reprod Med*, 1989, 34(8):511-6.
2. Milunsky A, Jick SS, Bruell CL, et al, "Predictive Values, Relative Risks, and Overall Benefits of High and Low Maternal Serum α-Fetoprotein Screening in Singleton Pregnancies: New Epidemiological Data," *Am J Obstet Gynecol*, 1989, 161(2):291-7.
3. Bajorin DF and Bosl GJ, "The Use of Serum Tumor Markers in the Prognosis and Treatment of Germ Cell Tumors," *Principles and Practice of Oncology*, 1992, 1-11.
4. Cuckle HS, "Screening for Neural Tube Defects," *Ciba Found Symp*, 1994, 181:253-69.
5. Cunningham FG and Gilstrap LC, "Maternal Serum Alpha-Fetoprotein Screening," *N Engl J Med*, 1991, 325(1):55-7.
6. Christiansen M, Andersen JR, Tørning J, et al, "Serum Alpha-Fetoprotein and Alcohol Consumption," *Scand J Clin Lab Invest*, 1994, 54(3):215-20.
7. Richards DS, Seeds JW, Katz VL, et al, "Elevated Maternal Serum Alpha-Fetoprotein With Oligohydramnios: Ultrasound Evaluation and Outcome," *Obstet Gynecol*, 1988, 72(3 Pt 1):337-41.
8. Nomura F, Ohnishi K, and Tanabe Y, "Clinical Features and Prognosis of Hepatocellular Carcinoma With Reference to Serum Alpha-Fetoprotein Levels," *Cancer*, 1989, 64(8):1700-7.
9. "Trisomy 18 Detected by MSAFP Screening," *Lab Med*, 1991, 22:605-7.
10. MacDonald ML, Wagner RM, and Slotnick RN, "Sensitivity and Specificity of Screening for Down Syndrome With Alpha-Fetoprotein, hCG, Unconjugated Estriol, and Maternal Age," *Obstet Gynecol*, 1991, 77(1):63-8.
11. Aitken DA, Wallace EM, Crossley JA, et al, "Dimeric Inhibin A as a Marker for Down's Syndrome in Early Pregnancy," *N Engl J Med*, 1996, 334(19):1231-6.

References

Bock JL, "Current Issues in Maternal Serum Alpha-Fetoprotein Screening," *Am J Clin Pathol*, 1992, 97(4):541-54.
Bosl GJ, Lange PH, Nochomovitz LE, et al, "Tumor Markers in Advanced Nonseminomatous Testicular Cancer," *Cancer*, 1981, 47:572-6.
Chen DS and Sung JL, "Serum Alpha-Fetoprotein in Hepatocellular Carcinoma," *Cancer*, 1977, 40:779-83.

(Continued)

Alpha₁-Fetoprotein, Serum (Continued)

Curtin JP, Rubin SC, Hoskins WJ, et al, "Second-Look Laparotomy in Endodermal Sinus Tumor: A Report of Two Patients With Normal Levels of Alpha-Fetoprotein and Residual Tumor at Reexploration," *Obstet Gynecol*, 1989, 73(4):893-5.

Eckfeldt JH and Long TA, "Influence of Laboratory Test Volume and Geographic Location on Maternal Alpha-Fetoprotein Results," *Arch Pathol Lab Med*, 1991, 115(7):647-53.

Haddow JE, Palomaki GE, Knight GJ, et al, "Reducing the Need for Amniocentesis in Women 35 Years of Age or Older With Serum Markers for Screening," *N Engl J Med*, 1994, 330(16):1114-8.

Macri JN, "Critical Issues in Prenatal Maternal Serum Alpha-Fetoprotein Screening for Genetic Abnormalities," *Am J Obstet Gynecol*, 1986, 155(2):240-6.

Sato Y, Nakata K, Kato Y, et al, "Early Recognition of Hepatocellular Carcinoma Based on Altered Profiles of Alpha-Fetoprotein," *N Engl J Med*, 1993, 328(25):1802-6.

Upton K, "Fetal Monitoring," *Clinical Laboratory Science: Strategies for Practice*, Chapter 41, Davis BG, Bishop ML, and Mass D, eds, Philadelphia, PA: JB Lippincott Co, 1989, 493-508.

Wu JT, "Serum Alpha-Fetoprotein and Its Lectin Reactivity in Liver Diseases: A Review," *Ann Clin Lab Sci*, 1990, 20(2):98-105.

Alpha₁ Lipoprotein Cholesterol *see* High Density Lipoprotein Cholesterol *on page 143*

Alpha-Hydroxybutyric Dehydrogenase (HBDH) *replaced by* Cardiac Enzymes/Isoenzymes *on page 102*

Alpha-Hydroxybutyric Dehydrogenase, Serum *replaced by* Lactate Dehydrogenase Isoenzymes *on page 154*

Alpha Tocopherol *see* Vitamin E, Serum *on page 219*

ALP Isoenzymes *see* Alkaline Phosphatase Isoenzymes *on page 69*

ALT *see* Alanine Aminotransferase *on page 65*

Amino Acid Screen *see* Amino Acid Screen, Qualitative, Urine *on next page*

Amino Acid Screen, Plasma

CPT 82128

Related Information

Amino Acid Screen, Qualitative, Urine *on next page*
Ammonia, Blood *on next page*
Ketone Bodies, Blood *on page 152*
Ketones, Urine *on page 639*
Phenylalanine, Blood *on page 181*

Synonyms Inborn Errors of Metabolism Screen; Metabolic Screen for Amino Acids

Applies to Biotinidase; Carnitine; Organic Acids, Urine

Test Commonly Includes Screening for the presence of all amino acids

Abstract Various metabolic disorders and genetic diseases produce alterations in the concentration of serum and urine amino acids.

Patient Preparation Infants: 4-hour fast; children and adults: 12-hour fast. Protein intake does not affect diurnal variation, but it influences absolute concentrations of amino acids in blood or urine. One day of fasting will decrease the excretion by 50%. Amphetamines, antihistamines, and phenothiazines are known to interfere with this assay. Patient should not take these drugs for at least 72 hours prior to specimen collection.

Specimen Plasma

Container Green top (heparin) tube

Sampling Time A marked circadian rhythm is exhibited with values highest in afternoon and lowest in early morning.

Collection Routine venipuncture

Storage Instructions Centrifuge. Transfer plasma to plastic vial and freeze within 1 hour of collection. Stable frozen for 2-4 weeks, analysis within 1 week is preferable.

Reference Range Established by each laboratory. The reference range must be correlated with the time of day used for collection.

Use Screen for inborn errors of metabolism of amino acids (eg, investigation of metabolic acidosis, ketosis, hyperammonemia, developmental impairment)

Limitations For some of these entities, investigation should include urine organic acids, amino acids, blood ammonia, biotinidase, and carnitine.

Methodology Plasma screen by single dimension thin-layer chromatography (TLC), amino acid analyzer (ion-exchange chromatography), gas chromatography (GC), and high performance liquid chromatography (HPLC) may have clinical application[1,2,3,4]

Additional Information Amino acid concentrations show a significant circadian rhythm with plasma level variation of 30%. Values are highest in midafternoon and lowest in the early morning. A variety of inherited metabolic disorders result in aminoacidemia/aminoaciduria. **Cystinuria** has an autosomal recessive mode of inheritance, is a disorder of amino acid transport involving renal tubules/GI tract and should be suspect in cases of urinary stone disease. It is characterized by the formation of radiopaque stones and by the presence of characteristic hexagonal crystals in the urine. **Lysinuric protein intolerance** is another disorder of membrane transport. As in some cases of cystinuria, cationic amino acids (lysine, arginine and ornithine) are involved. Lysine is present in large amounts in the urine but is normal or decreased in plasma. Patients have poor appetite, fail to thrive, develop hepatosplenomegaly, hypotonia, sparse hair, osteoporosis, mental retardation, and a variety of other problems. In **Hartnup disease**, there is impaired neutral amino acid transport involving the kidneys and small intestine. It is characterized clinically by pellagra-like features, mental retardation and/or psychotic behavior, intermittent ataxia and is inherited as an autosomal recessive. A comprehensive review of these and other amino acidurias is provided in the text edited by Scriver et al.

The usual approach is to screen urine for amino acids. However, urinary levels are variable: plasma is more definitive. Quantitative tests for plasma amino acids are available. In all cases in which an amino acid is elevated in blood, it will also be elevated in urine. CSF amino acids are

Congenital Disorders of Amino Acid Metabolism

Name	Enzyme or Metabolic Pathways	Clinical Findings	Laboratory Findings
Classic phenylketonuria	Phenylalanine hydroxylase	Mental retardation, psychiatric dysfunction	Plasma phenylalanine >15 mg/dL
Benign phenylalaninemia	Phenylalanine hydroxylase	Asymptomatic	Plasma phenylalanine <15 mg/dL
Malignant phenylalaninemia	Dihydropteridine reductase	Mental retardation, psychiatric dysfunction	Increased plasma phenylalanine
Malignant phenylalaninemia	GTP cyclohydrolase	Mental retardation, psychiatric dysfunction	Increased plasma phenylalanine
Hereditary tyrosinemia	p-hydroxy phenyl acetic acid hydroxylase	Hepatic cirrhosis, renal tubular dysfunction	Increased plasma tyrosine
Alkaptonuria	Homogentisic acid oxidase	Ochronosis, arthritis	Increased urinary homogentisic acid
Histidinemia	Histidine-ammonia lyase	Hearing and speech defect	Increased plasma and urine histidine
Branched-chain aminoacidemia	Branched-chain amino acid oxidase	Seizures, ketosis, mental retardation	Increased urine and branched-chain amino acids
Homocystinuria	Cystathionine synthase	Mental retardation, thromboembolism	Increased plasma and urine homocystine and methionine
Cystathioninuria	Cystathionase	Asymptomatic	Increased urine cystine and dibasic amino acids
Cystinuria	Renal transport system for cystine and dibasic amino acids	Cystine stones	Increased urine cystine and dibasic amino acids
Hyperglycinemias			
Ketotic form	Propionyl-CoA carboxylase	Ketosis, neutropenia, mental retardation	Increased urine and plasma glycine and propionic acid
Nonketotic form	Glycine decarboxylase	Developmental retardation	Increased urine and plasma glycine
Urea cycle abnormalities	Carbamoylphosphate synthase, ornithine-carbamoyltransferase, citrulline aspartate lyase, argininosuccinate arginine-lyase	Developmental retardation, vomiting, lethargy, seizures, hepatomegaly	Increased urine and plasma ammonia, glutamine, citrulline, and arginosuccinate
Glycinuria	Renal transport system for glycine and amino acids	Asymptomatic	Increased urine glycine, proline, and hydroxyproline
Hartnup disease	Renal transport system for neutral amino acids	Ataxia, retardation	Increased urine neutral amino acids
Fanconi syndrome	General renal transport deficiency	Acidosis and rickets	General aminoaciduria, glycinemia, phosphaturia

useful in the diagnosis of nonketotic hyperglycinemia. When urea cycle defects are suspected, plasma quantitative amino acids, urine orotic acids, and organic acids should be assessed.[5] See table.

Footnotes

1. Gamerith G, "Analysis of Amino Acids as Their N-TFA n-Propyl Esters," *Amino Acid Analysis by Gas Chromatography*, Vol II, Chapter 5, Zumwalt RW, Kuo KCT, and Gehrke CW, eds, Boca Raton, FL: CRC Press Inc, 1987, 117-39.
2. Desgrès J and Padieu P, "Gas-Liquid Chromatographic Analysis of Amino Acids as Isobutyl Esters, N(O)-Heptafluorobutyrate Derivatives: Applications to Clinical Biology," *Amino Acid Analysis by Gas Chromatography*, Vol I, Chapter 5, Gehrke CW, Kuo KCT, and Zumwalt RW, eds, Boca Raton, FL: CRC Press Inc, 1987, 119-42.
3. Hancock WS and Harding DR, "Review of Separation Conditions," *CRC Handbook of HPLC for the Separation of Amino Acids, Peptides, and Proteins*, Vol I, Hancock WS, ed, Boca Raton, FL: CRC Press Inc, 1984, 235-62.
4. Ishimitsu S, Fujimoto S, and Ohara K, "m- and O-Tyrosine," *CRC Handbook of HPLC for the Separation of Amino Acids, Peptides, and Proteins*, Vol I, Hancock WS, ed, Boca Raton, FL: CRC Press Inc, 1984, 263-73.
5. Lindor NM and Karnes PS, "Laboratory Medicine and Pathology: Initial Assessment of Infants and Children With Suspected Inborn Errors of Metabolism," *Mayo Clin Proc*, 1995, 70(10):987-8.

References

Cleary MA and Wraith JE, "Antenatal Diagnosis of Inborn Errors of Metabolism," *Arch Dis Child*, 1991, 66(7 Spec No):816-22.
Forman DT, "Role of the Laboratory in Diagnosis of Organic Acidurias," *Ann Clin Lab Sci*, 1991, 21(2):85-93.
National Academy of Clinical Biochemistry 14th Annual Symposium, "Diagnosis and Treatment of Inborn Errors of Metabolism," *Clin Biochem*, 1991, 24(4):289-381.
Rutledge JC and Rudy J, "HPLC Qualitative Amino Acid Analysis in the Clinical Laboratories," *Am J Clin Pathol*, 1987, 87(5):614-8.
Scriver CR, "Amino Acids," Part 4 and "Membrane Transport Systems," Part 15, *The Metabolic Basis of Inherited Disease*, 6th ed, Scriver CR, Beaudet AL, Sly WS, et al, eds, New York, NY: McGraw-Hill Inc, 1989, 495-771, 2479-580.
Shih VE, "Detection of Hereditary Metabolic Disorders Involving Amino Acids and Organic Acids," *Clin Biochem*, 1991, 24(4):301-9.
Slocum RH and Cummings JG, "Amino Acid Analysis of Physiological Samples," *Techniques in Diagnostic Human Biochemical Genetics*, Hommes FA, ed, New York, NY: Wiley-Liss, 1991, 87-126.
Verjee ZH, "Amino Acid Screen," *Methods in Clinical Chemistry*, Chapter 22, Pesce AJ and Kaplan LA, eds, St Louis, MO: Mosby-Year Book Inc, 1987, 146-53.

Amino Acid Screen, Qualitative, Urine

CPT 82128

Related Information
Amino Acid Screen, Plasma *on this page*
Phenylalanine, Blood *on page 181*

Synonyms Amino Acid Screen; Inborn Errors of Metabolism Screen; Metabolic Screen for Amino Acids

Test Commonly Includes Differences exist between laboratories. Examination may include beta-amino isobutyrate, cystathionine, cystine, glycine, homocystine, hydroxyproline, isoleucine, leucine, methionine, ornithine, phenylalanine, proline, tryptophan, tyrosine, and valine.

Abstract Urinary amino acid excretion is altered in certain metabolic diseases. Although amino acids filtered through the renal glomerulus are normally almost entirely reabsorbed, in Fanconi syndrome they are not, in spite of the presence of normal plasma concentrations.

Patient Preparation Amphetamines, norepinephrine, levodopa, and all antibiotics have been reported to interfere chemically with this test. Amino acid concentrations in urine are physiologically increased by aspirin, bismuth, hydrocortisone, insulin, lead poisoning, and triamcinolone.

Specimen Urine

Collection Random specimen acceptable, no preservative. Morning urine preferred.

Storage Instructions Freeze

Causes for Rejection Specific gravity of the urine must be ≥1.010

Reference Range Subjective interpretation based on comparison of patient, normal, and control urines of comparable age. Interpretation is age dependent. Urinary amino acids separated by thin-layer chromatography (TLC) are not usually quantitated. If any amino acids appear to be in high concentration compared to normals or controls, quantitation can be carried out by separate methodology.

Use Investigation of failure to thrive, acidosis, hypokalemia, hypophosphatemia, and abnormalities of vitamin D metabolism.[1] Screen for "inborn errors of metabolism" of amino acids, Fanconi syndrome, Wilson's disease, and Lowe's syndrome.

Limitations Dilute urines cannot be run. Must have concentrated urine.

Methodology Thin-layer chromatography (TLC)

Additional Information Excretion of certain amino acids is increased in several specific **aminoacidurias**, such as phenylketonuria and maple syrup urine disease. **Aminoacidopathies**, with ninhydrin-positive urinary amino acids, include phenylketonuria, nonketotic hyperglycinemia and homocystinuria. Their investigation includes urine organic acids and amino acids, plasma amino acids, blood NH_3^+, biotinidase, and carnitine.[1] Aminoaciduria may also be seen in a variety of other disorders, including viral hepatitis, multiple myeloma, rickets, hyperparathyroidism, and chronic renal failure. A positive test should be followed

up with quantitation on a 24-hour collection. See table under Amino Acid Screen, Plasma *on page 75*.

The Fanconi syndrome (FS), characterized by dysfunction of the proximal renal tubule, is caused by a variety of hereditary and acquired diseases. The former include primary idiopathic FS, cystinosis, Lowe's syndrome, tyrosinemia type 1, galactosemia, hereditary fructose intolerance, glycogen storage disease, Wilson's disease, and other entities. Acquired FS may be caused by aminoglycosides, outdated tetracyclines, cephalothins, valproic acid, streptozotocin, 6-mercaptopurine, azathioprine, and cisplatinum; toxins including heavy metals, toluene sniffing and paraquet. It may be found with nephrotic syndrome, myeloma, amyloidosis, antitubular basement membrane antibody, renal vein thrombosis, cancer, and following renal transplantation.[2]

Footnotes

1. Lindor NM and Karnes PS, "Initial Assessment of Infants and Children With Suspected Inborn Errors of Metabolism," *Mayo Clin Proc*, 1995, 70(10):987-8.
2. Brewer ED and Powell DR, "Pan-Proximal Tubular Dysfunction (Fanconi's Syndrome)," *Principles and Practice of Pediatrics*, 2nd ed, Oski FA, DeAngelis CD, Feigin RD, et al, eds, Philadelphia, PA: JB Lippincott Co, 1994, 1818-23.

References

Coe FL and Kathpalia S, "Hereditary Tubular Disorders," *Harrison's Principles of Internal Medicine*, 13th ed, Chapter 241, Isselbacher KJ, Braunwald E, Wilson JD, et al, eds, New York, NY: McGraw-Hill Inc, 1994, 1323-8.
Rosenberg LE, "Inherited Disorders of Amino Acid Metabolism and Storage," *Harrison's Principles of Internal Medicine*, 13th ed, Chapter 352, Isselbacher KJ, Braunwald E, Wilson JD, et al, eds, New York, NY: McGraw-Hill Inc, 1994, 2117-25.
Slocum RH and Cummings JG, "Amino Acid Analysis of Physiological Samples," *Techniques in Diagnostic Human Biochemical Genetics*, Hommes FA, ed, New York, NY: Wiley-Liss, 1991, 87-126.

Aminolevulinic Acid *see* Delta Aminolevulinic Acid, Urine *on page 121*

Aminoterminal Propeptide of Type III Procollagen *see* CA 125 *on page 94*

Aminotransferases *see* Alanine Aminotransferase *on page 65*

Aminotransferases *see* Aspartate Aminotransferase *on page 84*

Ammonia, Blood

CPT 82140

Related Information
Amino Acid Screen, Plasma *on previous page*
Cerebrospinal Fluid Glutamine *on page 105*
Complete Blood Count *on page 312*
Ketone Bodies, Blood *on page 152*
Ketones, Urine *on page 639*
Lactic Acid, Blood *on page 156*
Reducing Substances, Urine *on page 652*
Uric Acid, Serum *on page 213*
Valproic Acid *on page 577*

Synonyms NH_3, Blood

Applies to Ammonia, Cerebrospinal Fluid

Abstract May be useful for diagnosis of Reye's syndrome, urea cycle deficiencies, and to explain hepatic coma in liver disease

Patient Preparation Patient should avoid smoking prior to sampling.

Specimen Plasma

Container Green top (sodium or lithium heparin) tube or lavender top (EDTA) tube. One author, however, suggests that heparin will produce false low results.[1]

Collection Tube must be filled completely and kept tightly stoppered at all times. Avoid hemolysis, which increases plasma ammonia. Specimen must be placed on ice immediately and rotated, then centrifuged at 4°C. Plasma should be very promptly separated from the cells. Test must be performed within 20 minutes of the venipuncture, or the plasma frozen immediately. Concentration rapidly increases on standing. Never freeze whole blood.

Storage Instructions Ammonia is stable for several days at -70°C.

Reference Range Variations of reference ranges between laboratories exist for ammonia. See table for approximate ranges. Ammonia level in cerebrospinal fluid is about 33% to 50% of that in arterial blood.[2]

Ammonia N, Blood

Age	µg N/dL	SI: µmol/L
Neonates	90-150	64-107
<2 wk	79-129	56-92
Children	29-70	21-50
Adults	15-45	11-32

Note: Values are somewhat higher in capillary blood.

Use Ammonia is elevated in liver disease, urinary tract infection with distention and stasis, Reye's syndrome, inborn errors of metabolism *(Continued)*

Ammonia, Blood (Continued)

including deficiency of enzymes in the urea cycle, HHH syndrome (hyperornithinemia, hyperammonemia-homocitrullinuria), organic acidemias, some normal neonates (usually returning to normal in 48 hours), total parenteral nutrition, ureterosigmoidostomy, and sodium valproate therapy. Ammonia determination is indicated in neonates with neurological deterioration, subjects with lethargy and/or emesis not explained, and in patients with possible encephalopathy.

The diagnostic utility of ammonia measurements is limited. Ammonia is of use in the diagnosis of **urea cycle deficiencies** (to be considered in any neonate with unexplained nausea, vomiting, or neurological deterioration appearing after the first feeding). Investigation includes plasma amino acids, urine orotic and organic acids.[3]

In **Reye's syndrome**, threefold increases in AST, ALT, and serum ammonia are required for diagnosis with/or the diagnostic liver biopsy findings. Ammonia levels increase characteristically early; serum ammonia ≥100 µg/dL (SI: ≥59 µmol/L) reflects severe hepatic changes. Prothrombin time is increased in essentially all patients, prototypically three seconds longer than the control. Bilirubin is usually normal. Glucose should be monitored; hypoglycemia may develop. Hyperosmolality and acid-base imbalance may develop, lactate may increase, CK may increase and CK-MB may be elevated. Uric acid may increase.[4] Increased ammonia and prolonged prothrombin time provide indicators of disease progression.

Limitations The correlation between blood ammonia levels and **hepatic coma** is poor. Ammonia determinations are not reliable predictors of impending hepatic coma. Ammonia levels are not always high in all patients with urea cycle disorders. High protein diet may cause increased levels. Ammonia levels may also be elevated with **gastrointestinal hemorrhage**. If portal hypertension develops with cirrhosis, hepatic blood flow is altered, leading to elevated blood ammonia levels.

Methodology Laboratory contamination by NH_4OH, tobacco smoke, urine, formaldehyde must be avoided. Ion-selective electrode (ISE) methods are preferred; Ektachem® dry film method is also recommended. A number of methods for ammonia are found in standard texts. Many are in use. Some are obsolete. A recommendation to soak glassware in hypochlorite, 52.5 g/L and to then rinse it thoroughly with deionized water was provided to Paramax™ users.

Additional Information Ammonia and alpha-ketoglutarate with NADH yield glutamate; glutamate and ammonia yield glutamine. **Cerebrospinal fluid glutamine levels** are useful in hepatic encephalopathy and with Reye's syndrome. In the HHH syndrome hyperammonemia is intermittent; it presents in infancy often, but symptoms can be delayed.

Metabolic acidosis with ketosis are found in the **organic acidemias**, in which hyperammonemia is found. Plasma amino acids, urine organic acids, and amino acids are indicated with NH_3, biotinidase, and carnitine.[3]

Recommendations for laboratory investigation for an infant or child suspected of having an **inborn error of metabolism** include blood gases, glucose, urinary ketones, plasma ammonia, electrolytes, nonglucose urinary reducing substances, CBC, uric acid and liver-related enzymes, blood lactate, blood carnitine, free fatty acids, and β-hydroxybutyrate and acetoacetate.[3]

Footnotes
1. Dorwart WV and Saner M, "Heparinized Plasma Is an Unacceptable Specimen for Ammonia Determination," Clin Chem, 1992, 38(1):161.
2. Burtis CA and Ashwood ER, Tietz Textbook of Clinical Chemistry, 2nd ed, Philadelphia, PA: WB Saunders Co, 1994, 1485-8.
3. Lindor NM and Karnes PS, "Initial Assessment of Infants and Children With Suspected Inborn Errors of Metabolism," Mayo Clin Proc, 1995, 70(10):987-8.
4. Meythaler JM and Varma RR, "Reye's Syndrome in Adults: Diagnostic Considerations," Arch Intern Med, 1987, 147(1):61-4.

References
Cascino GD, Jensen JM, Nelson LA, et al, "Periodic Hyperammonemic Encephalopathy Associated With a Ureterosigmoidostomy," Mayo Clin Proc, 1989, 64(6):653-6.

Diamond DA, Blight A, Samuell CT, et al, "Ammonia Levels in Paediatric Ureterosigmoidostomy Patients: A Screen for Hyperammonaemia?" Br J Urol, 1991, 67(5):541-4.

Fine P, Adler K, and Gerstenfeld D, "Idiopathic Hyperammonemia After High-Dose Chemotherapy," Am J Med, 1989, 86(5):629.

Fishman RA, Cerebrospinal Fluid in Diseases of the Nervous System, 2nd ed, Philadelphia, PA: WB Saunders Co, 1992, 238-9.

Giacoia GP and Padilla-Lugo A, "Severe Transient Neonatal Hyperammonemia," Am J Perinatol, 1986, 3(3):249-54.

Green A, "When and How Should We Measure Plasma Ammonia?" Ann Clin Biochem, 1988, 25(Pt 3):199-204.

Hurwitz ES, "Reye's Syndrome," Epidemiol Rev, 1989, 11:249-53.

Miga DE and Roth KS, "Hyperammonemia: The Silent Killer," South Med J, 1993, 86(7):742-7.

Ammonia, Cerebrospinal Fluid see Ammonia, Blood on previous page

Amniotic Fluid Acetylcholinesterase see Alpha₁-Fetoprotein, Amniotic Fluid on page 71

Amniotic Fluid Analysis for Erythroblastosis Fetalis (OD 450)

CPT 82143

Related Information

Amniotic Fluid, Chromosome and Genetic Abnormality Analysis on page 273

Bilirubin, Neonatal on page 86

Cord Blood Screen on page 605

Hemolytic Disease of the Newborn, Antibody Identification on page 610

Prenatal Screen, Immunohematology on page 618

Synonyms Amniotic Fluid Analysis for Hemolytic Disease of the Newborn; Amniotic Fluid Spectral Analysis; Liley Test; OD 450 Method; Spectral Analysis, Amniotic Fluid

Replaces Amniotic Fluid Bilirubin

Test Commonly Includes Delta OD 450 spectral analysis, creatinine and total bilirubin

Abstract Amniocentesis is performed in selected instances, in the presence of a maternal antibody which may cause severe hemolytic disease of the newborn. Measurement of the 450 nm peak by scanning densitometry estimates the bilirubin level in amniotic fluid and hence the severity of the disease.

Aftercare If the amniotic tap of an Rh negative pregnant woman is bloody, draw a maternal blood specimen an hour later for a Kleihauer test, to ascertain need for RhIG.

Specimen Amniotic fluid, 5-10 mL

Container Brown sterile plastic or glass container which is put in a larger, opaque container. Alternatively, a glass container can be wrapped with opaque tape or aluminum foil.

Collection Amniocentesis performed by physician, usually after 30 weeks. Protect from light throughout. If possible collect on ice in order to allow an L/S determination, if ordered, on the same specimen.

Storage Instructions Centrifuge promptly and filter supernatant in the dark. Protect supernatant from light at 4°C.

Special Instructions Protect collected specimen from the light. Requisition should state date and length of pregnancy to date.

Reference Range Dependent on gestational age. The useful range is only clearly defined for Rh incompatibility and is only of use in the first sensitized pregnancy. OD at 450 nm (Delta A450) at the 40th week of 0.0-0.02 corresponds to Freda classification of 1+, normal or only slightly affected. At 28 weeks, Delta A450 is normal at <0.048.

Possible Panic Range Delta A450 of 0.25-0.35, Freda 3+, indicates severe fetal distress and danger; >0.40, Freda 4+, indicates impending fetal death.[1]

Use Evaluate fetal jeopardy in fetal-maternal irregular antibody incompatibility (in hemolytic disease of the newborn or erythroblastosis fetalis)

Limitations False-negatives and false-positives occur. Amniotic fluid contaminated with meconium can have significant elevations due to bilirubin content. Trends from sequential determinations are used (single results may be misleading). Amniotic fluid contaminated with maternal blood can give incorrect results. Maternal urine can be aspirated instead of amniotic fluid, but urinary urea nitrogen (UUN) and creatinine of maternal urine would be many times that of amniotic fluid. Diamniotic twin pregnancies contain two sacs; each should be sampled. Hazards exist for the fetus, but in experienced hands they are limited.

Methodology Spectral analysis of centrifuged amniotic fluid using a scanning spectrophotometer. The peak at 450 nm relates to bilirubin.

Additional Information The spectral analysis is based on the quantity of free bilirubin in amniotic fluid, which bears a relationship to the degree of hemolysis present in the fetus.[2] Useful figures are published by Huestis, Bove, and Case.[3] Amniotic fluid creatinine is useful for estimation of fetal age. The delta optical density measurement at 450 nm may be unreliable in patients with sickle cell disease.[4,5]

In the past, most cases of erythroblastosis fetalis caused by maternal antibody reacting with fetal erythrocytes were due to anti-D. With the widespread utilization of Rh immune globulin, the incidence of anti-D caused erythroblastosis fetalis has decreased. This has lead to a **relative** increase in the incidence of other antibodies, particularly other Rh antibodies and anti-Kell, as causes of hemolytic disease of the newborn. Liley curves are not as reliable in those instances.

Footnotes
1. Bauer JD, "Examination of Biologic Fluids, Sputum, and Pus," Clinical Laboratory Methods, 9th ed, St Louis, MO: Mosby-Year Book Inc, 1982, 750-79.
2. Dito WR, "Amniotic Fluid and Maternal Serum Assessment in Pregnancies at Risk," Gradwohl's Clinical Laboratory Methods and Diagnosis, 8th ed, Sonnenwirth AC and Jarett L, eds, St Louis, MO: Mosby-Year Book Inc, 1980, 469-77.
3. Huestis DW, Bove JR, and Case J, Practical Blood Transfusion, 4th ed, Boston, MA: Little, Brown and Co, 1988.
4. Hadi HA, Fadel HE, Nelson GH, et al, "The Unreliability of Amniotic Fluid Bilirubin Measurements in Isoimmunized Pregnancies in Sickle Cell Disease Patients," Obstet Gynecol, 1985, 65(5):758-60.

5. Lindsay MK and Lupo VR, "Nonpredictive Value of Measurements of Delta Optical Density at 450 nm in SS Disease," *Am J Obstet Gynecol*, 1985, 153(1):75-6.

References

Ananth U and Queenan JT, "Does Midtrimester ΔOD_{450} of Amniotic Fluid Reflect Severity of Rh Disease?" *Am J Obstet Gynecol*, 1989, 161(1):47-9.

Ananth U, Warsof SL, Coulehan JM, et al, "Midtrimester Amniotic Fluid Delta Optical Density at 450 nm in Normal Pregnancies," *Am J Obstet Gynecol*, 1986, 155(3):664-6.

Horger EO 3d and Moody LO, "Use of Indigo Carmine for Twin Amniocentesis and Its Effect on Bilirubin Analysis," *Am J Obstet Gynecol*, 1984, 150(7):858-60.

Kiltz RJ, Burke MS, and Porreco RP, "Amniotic Fluid Glucose Concentration as a Marker for Intra-amniotic Infection," *Obstet Gynecol*, 1991, 78(4):619-22.

Liley AW, "Liquor Amnio Analysis in the Management of the Pregnancy Complicated by Rhesus Sensitization," *Am J Obstet Gynecol*, 1961, 82:1359-70.

Wenk RE and Rosenbaum JM, "Analyses of Amniotic Fluid," *Todd-Sanford-Davidsohn Clinical Diagnosis and Management by Laboratory Methods*, 18th ed, Henry JB, ed, Philadelphia, PA: WB Saunders Co, 1991, 482-96.

Amniotic Fluid Analysis for Hemolytic Disease of the Newborn *see* Amniotic Fluid Analysis for Erythroblastosis Fetalis (OD 450) *on previous page*

Amniotic Fluid Bilirubin *replaced by* Amniotic Fluid Analysis for Erythroblastosis Fetalis (OD 450) *on previous page*

Amniotic Fluid Creatinine

CPT 82570

Related Information

Amniotic Fluid, Chromosome and Genetic Abnormality Analysis *on page 273*

Amniotic Fluid Lecithin/Sphingomyelin Ratio and Phosphatidylglycerol *on this page*

Body Fluid *on page 89*

Synonyms Creatinine, Amniotic Fluid

Applies to Amniotic Fluid Glucose; Amniotic Fluid Protein; Amniotic Fluid Urea Nitrogen

Abstract Amniotic fluid creatinine is a measure of fetal kidney maturity, which indirectly assesses lung maturity but it is not as useful as amniotic fluid L/S ratio.

Container Brown sterile plastic or glass bottle

Storage Instructions Keep on ice, protect from light. Freeze if analysis is delayed more than 24 hours.

Special Instructions Correlation of maternal serum and amniotic fluid creatinine levels is recommended.

Reference Range >2 mg/dL (SI: >177 µmol/L) at 37th to 38th week; results >2 mg/dL indicate maturity if maternal serum creatinine is normal. Concentrations of 1.6-1.8 mg/dL (SI: 141-159 µmol/L) are found at 36th week.

Possible Panic Range Creatinine in amniotic fluid <1.6 mg/dL (SI: <141 µmol/L) bears an implication that the fetus is immature or premature,[1] <2500 g.

Use Estimate fetal age in concert with other parameters. Creatinine of 2 mg/dL (SI: 177 µmol/L) is an indication of maturity. This test is rarely performed.

Limitations Oligohydramnios, related to fetal urinary tract obstruction or to renal agenesis, or polyhydramnios, may alter the usual amniotic fluid criteria set forth above.[1] Elevation of maternal creatinine may cause increases in the amniotic fluid creatinine level. Complications of amniocentesis may occur.

Contraindications Fetal age must be estimated from more than a single facet.

Methodology Colorimetry, Jaffé reaction

Additional Information Fetal lung and kidney development are related, and normal lung development is dependent on the normal development of the kidneys. Estimation of fetal kidney maturity by measuring amniotic fluid creatinine, therefore, provides an indirect assessment of fetal lung maturity. In addition to creatinine, **amniotic fluid urea nitrogen** has been suggested as a marker for fetal renal maturity and as a predictor of respiratory distress syndrome.[2] **Amniotic fluid glucose** when low, is a marker for intrauterine infection in women with preterm labor. Its specificity is 94% to 100%, but it has poor sensitivity.[3]

Amniotic fluid protein decreases with advancing maturity: a level ≤180 mg/dL (SI: ≤1.8 g/L) supports fetal age of 36 weeks or more. Uric acid in amniotic fluid can be used to project maturity and predict the Lesch-Nyhan syndrome.[1] **Amniotic fluid C-peptide** has been proposed as a parameter of intrauterine growth. Most laboratories utilize amniotic fluid phosphatidylglycerol and lecithin/sphingomyelin ratio as the primary tests for assessing fetal lung maturity and do not use the creatinine measurement.

Footnotes

1. Dito WR, "Amniotic Fluid and Maternal Serum Assessment in Pregnancies at Risk," *Gradwohl's Clinical Laboratory Methods and Diagnosis*, 8th ed, Sonnenwirth AC and Jarett L, eds, St Louis, MO: Mosby-Year Book Inc, 1980, 469-77.
2. Almeida OD and Kitay DZ, "Amniotic Fluid Urea Nitrogen in the Prediction of Respiratory Distress Syndrome," *Am J Obstet Gynecol*, 1988, 159(2):465-8.

3. Greig PC, Ernest JM, and Teot L, "Low Amniotic Fluid Glucose Levels Are a Specific But Not a Sensitive Marker for Subclinical Intrauterine Infections in Patients in Preterm Labor With Intact Membranes," *Am J Obstet Gynecol*, 1994, 171(2):365-71.

References

Darling RE and Zlatnik FJ, "Comparison of Amniotic Fluid Optical Density, L/S Ratio and Creatinine Concentration in Predicting Fetal Pulmonary Maturity," *J Reprod Med*, 1985, 30(6):460-4.

Raghav M, Vijay G, Chowdhary DR, et al, "Amniotic Fluid Amino Acids, Urea, Creatinine in Normal and Toxemic Pregnancies," *Indian J Med Sci*, 1985, 39(12):291-3.

Troccoli R, Stella C, Pachi A, et al, "Hydroxyproline and Creatinine Levels in Normal Amniotic Fluid," *Ric Clin Lab*, 1986, 16(1):37-41.

Tyden O, Eriksson U, Agren H, et al, "Estimation of Fetal Maturity by Amniotic Fluid Cytology, Creatinine, Lecithin/Sphingomyelin Ratio and Phosphatidylglycerol," *Gynecol Obstet Invest*, 1983, 16:317-26.

Amniotic Fluid Foam Test *see* Amniotic Fluid Pulmonary Surfactant *on next page*

Amniotic Fluid Glucose *see* Amniotic Fluid Creatinine *on this page*

Amniotic Fluid Lecithin/Sphingomyelin Ratio and Phosphatidylglycerol

CPT 83661 (L/S ratio); 84081 (phosphatidylglycerol)

Related Information

Amniotic Fluid, Chromosome and Genetic Abnormality Analysis *on page 273*

Amniotic Fluid Creatinine *on this page*

Amniotic Fluid Cytology *on page 286*

Amniotic Fluid Pulmonary Surfactant *on next page*

Nile Blue Fat Stain *on page 297*

Synonyms Lecithin/Sphingomyelin Ratio; L/S Ratio; Phospholipid Profile, Amniotic Fluid

Applies to Disaturated Phosphatidylcholine (DSPC); Fetal Lung Maturity Surfactant/Albumin Ratio Assay (FLM S/A); Phosphatidylglycerol; Phosphatidylinositol; Saturated Phosphatidylcholine (SPC)

Test Commonly Includes L/S ratio; may include qualitative determination of phosphatidylglycerol (PG).

Abstract Test for assessment of fetal lung maturity to attempt to ascertain the probability of development of respiratory distress syndrome (RDS), for which infants of diabetic mothers are at increased risk. The major component of pulmonary surfactant is disaturated phosphatidylcholine. The performance of FLM surfactant/albumin ratio assay (FLM S/A) is comparable to the L/S ratio; it uses fluorescence polarization.

Aftercare Kleihauer-Betke should be done on maternal blood after amniocentesis on Rh negative patients. If result is increased, Rh immune globulin (human) (RhIG) is recommended. Others bypass the Kleihauer-Betke after amniocentesis on Rh negative patients and directly give RhIG.

Specimen Amniotic fluid, 10 mL

Container Sterile brown plastic or glass tube protected from light; aluminum foil is useful

Storage Instructions Specimen may be light sensitive, a point for which documentation is obscure. Record color and, if present, any mucus or heavy precipitate. Centrifuge specimen only at low speed for 10 minutes and transfer supernatant to a clean glass tube. It can be stored at 4°C for up to 10 days, and it can be stored frozen indefinitely.

Special Instructions Send sample to the laboratory **immediately** after collection.

Reference Range The incidence of respiratory distress syndrome (RDS) is very low when the L/S ratio is >3:1, in the presence of PG. L/S ratio >3.5 for fetuses of diabetic mothers; L/S ratio <3:1 or lack of PG provides indication of increased risk.[1] Borderline: L/S ratio 1.5-1.9 with risk of respiratory distress syndrome (RDS). The L/S ratio is 1.0 at 32 weeks and reaches 2.0 by 35 weeks. While sphingomyelin tends to decrease from the 32nd week, lecithin increases. Caution is necessary in interpretation of results from the diabetic patient, in whom misleading evidence for pulmonary maturity has been reported.[2] Presence of phosphatidylglycerol (PG) is evidence that the fetus is within 2-6 weeks of full-term. Levels of saturated phosphatidylcholine (SPC) >500 µg/dL suggest maturity. FLM S/A ≥70 mg/g at or near term indicates absence of RDS. Levels of disaturated phosphatidylcholine (DSPC) >1000 µg/dL indicate fetal lung maturity in infants of mothers with insulin-dependent diabetes mellitus.

Possible Panic Range Immature lung: L/S ratio <1.5. This level predicts RDS on delivery and bears an implication of 34 weeks or less gestation.

Use Attempt to prevent respiratory distress syndrome (RDS) from low surfactant in early delivery, by evaluation of fetal pulmonary maturation. Amniotic fluid test for fetal maturity; indicator to determine optimal time for obstetrical intervention in cases of possible fetal distress: maternal diabetes, toxemia, hemolytic disease of the newborn (erythroblastosis fetalis), postmaturity.

(Continued)

Amniotic Fluid Lecithin/Sphingomyelin Ratio and Phosphatidylglycerol (Continued)

Limitations Conventional testing is not automated and is technically difficult. The L/S ratio is labor intensive. Results are less objective than are many other laboratory tests and require experience in performance and interpretation. False-negative results (L/S <2.0 but no lung disease) occur in 5% of cases; false-positive results occur in 0.6% of cases. False predictions of maturity using the L/S ratio are recognized in diabetic gestations. Measurement of PG improves diagnostic accuracy. Maternal blood contamination of the specimen decreases the ratio and reliability of the result. Fetal plasma contains a large amount of lecithin, and fetal blood falsely elevates the L/S ratio. Heavy contamination by meconium distorts the ratio. However, fluid contaminated by blood or meconium can still be analyzed for PG.

Methodology Thin-layer chromatography (TLC). PG may also be measured by immunologic and enzymatic assays.[3] FLM S/A can be measured by fluorescence polarization using the Abbott TDx. SPC can be measured by a spectrophotometric method using amniotic fluid.

Additional Information Repeat sampling weekly or in 2 weeks, as clinically indicated, when the L/S ratio indicates transitional phase of maturation (ratio 1.5-1.9). Lecithin increases sharply in amniotic fluid during the last weeks of gestation. PG appears at about 35 weeks. The following factors may increase surfactant production: maternal diabetes, toxemia, hypertension, malnutrition, placenta previa, drug addiction, premature rupture of membranes, intrauterine growth retardation, female fetus, and hemoglobinopathy. The following factors may decrease surfactant production: anemia, polyhydramnios, hypothyroidism, male fetus, twins, isoimmune disease, liver disease, renal disease, advanced maternal age, syphilis, and toxoplasmosis. A **fluorescence polarization assay** (TDx analyzer, Abbott Laboratories) is a means of assessing fetal lung maturity comparable to the L/S ratio.[4,5,6] Fluorescence polarization in amniotic fluid reflects the ratio of phospholipid to albumin and saturation of phospholipids, but is not directly dependent on saturated phospholipid. Specificity problems and false-positives are described. A fetal lung maturity surfactant/albumin ratio assay based upon fluorescence polarization and gestational age may enhance decision making.[7] Addition of DSPC to FLM S/A was not helpful in a recent study.[8] A relationship between strong control of maternal glucose and fetal lung profiles is recognized.[8] SPC determination is said to be more reliable than L/S ratio when the results show immaturity.[9]

Footnotes

1. Leavelle DE, *Mayo Medical Laboratories Interpretive Handbook*, Rochester, MN: Mayo Medical Laboratories, 1994.
2. Ojomo EO and Coustan DR, "Absence of Evidence of Pulmonary Maturity at Amniocentesis in Term Infants of Diabetic Mothers," *Am J Obstet Gynecol*, 1990, 163(3):954-7.
3. Eisenbrey AB, Epstein E, Zak B, et al, "Phosphatidylglycerol in Amniotic Fluid. Comparison of an "Ultrasensitive" Immunologic Assay With TLC and Enzymatic Assay," *Am J Clin Pathol*, 1989, 91(3):293-7.
4. Ashwood ER, Tait JF, Foerder CA, et al, "Improved Fluorescence Polarization Assay for Use in Evaluating Fetal Lung Maturity. III. Retrospective Clinical Evaluation and Comparison With the Lecithin/Sphingomyelin Ratio," *Clin Chem*, 1986, 32(2):260-4.
5. Talt JF, Foerder CA, Ashwood ER, et al, "Prospective Clinical Evaluation of an Improved Fluorescence Polarization Assay for Predicting Fetal Lung Maturity," *Clin Chem*, 1987, 33(4):554-8.
6. Dubin SB, "The Laboratory Assessment of Fetal Lung Maturity," *Am J Clin Pathol*, 1992, 97(6):836-49.
7. Tanasijevic MJ, Wybenga DR, Richardson D, et al, "A Predictive Model for Fetal Lung Maturity Employing Gestational Age and Test Results," *Am J Clin Pathol*, 1994, 102(6):788-93.
8. Tanasijevic MJ, Winkelman JW, Wybenga DR, et al, "Prediction of Fetal Lung Maturity in Infants of Diabetic Mothers Using the FLM S/A and Disaturated Phosphatidylcholine Tests," *Am J Clin Pathol*, 1996, 105(1):17-22.
9. Burtis CA and Ashwood ER, *Tietz Textbook of Clinical Chemistry*, Philadelphia, PA: WB Saunders Co, 1994, 2132.

References

Apple FS, Bilodeau L, Presse LM, et al, "Clinical Implementation of a Rapid, Automated Assay for Assessing Fetal Lung Maturity," *J Reprod Med*, 1994, 39(11):883-7.

Darling RE and Zlatnik FJ, "Comparison of Amniotic Fluid Optical Density, L/S Ratio and Creatinine Concentration in Predicting Fetal Pulmonary Maturity," *J Reprod Med*, 1985, 30(6):460-4.

Garite TJ, Freeman RK, and Nageotte MP, "Fetal Maturity Cascade: A Rapid and Cost-Effective Method for Fetal Lung Maturity Testing," *Obstet Gynecol*, 1986, 67(5):619-22.

Hallman M, Arjomaa P, Mizumoto M, et al, "Surfactant Proteins in the Diagnosis of Fetal Lung Maturity. I. Predictive Accuracy of the 35 kD Protein, the Lecithin/Sphingomyelin Ratio, and Phosphatidylglycerol," *Am J Obstet Gynecol*, 1988, 158(3 Pt 1):531-5.

Jobe A, "Amniotic Fluid Tests of Fetal Lung Maturity," *Maternal-Fetal Medicine: Principles and Practice*, 2nd ed, Creasy RK and Resnik R, eds, Philadelphia, PA: WB Saunders Co, 1989, 426-33.

Nugent CE, Ayers JW, and Menon KM, "Comparison of Amniotic Fluid Desaturated Phosphatidylcholine and the Lecithin-Sphingomyelin Ratio in the Prediction of Fetal Lung Maturity," *Obstet Gynecol*, 1986, 68(4):541-5.

Parker CR Jr, Leveno KJ, Milewich L, et al, "Lecithin-Sphingomyelin Ratios in Amniotic Fluid of Pregnancies With an Anencephalic Fetus," *Obstet Gynecol*, 1986, 68(4):546-9.

Saad SA, Fadel HE, Fahmy K, et al, "The Reliability and Clinical Use of a Rapid Phosphatidylglycerol Assay in Normal and Diabetic Pregnancies," *Am J Obstet Gynecol*, 1987, 157(6):1516-20.

Shaver DC, Spinnato JA, Whybrew D, et al, "Comparison of Phospholipids in Vaginal and Amniocentesis Specimens of Patients With Premature Rupture of Membranes," *Am J Obstet Gynecol*, 1987, 156(2):454-7.

Teng SH, Andrews AG, and Horacek I, "Rapid Enzyme Analysis of Amniotic Fluid Phospholipids Containing Choline: A Comparison With the Lecithin to Sphingomyelin Ratio in Prenatal Assessment of Fetal Lung Maturity," *J Clin Pathol*, 1985, 38(11):1304-8.

Towers CV and Garite TJ, "Evaluation of the New Amniostat-FLM Test for the Detection of Phosphatidylglycerol in Contaminated Fluids," *Am J Obstet Gynecol*, 1989, 160(2):298-303.

Amniotic Fluid Protein *see* Amniotic Fluid Creatinine *on previous page*

Amniotic Fluid Pulmonary Surfactant

CPT 84999

Related Information

Amniotic Fluid, Chromosome and Genetic Abnormality Analysis *on page 273*

Amniotic Fluid Lecithin/Sphingomyelin Ratio and Phosphatidylglycerol *on previous page*

Cystic Fibrosis DNA Detection *on page 507*

Synonyms Pulmonary Surfactant; Shake Test

Applies to Amniotic Fluid Foam Test

Test Commonly Includes Semiquantitative estimate of pulmonary surfactant and fetal maturity

Abstract The assessment of fetal lung maturity is to determine the probability of development of respiratory distress syndrome, if the fetus was presently delivered. A low prevalence exists for this clinical entity.

Specimen Amniotic fluid

Container Clean glass or plastic tube

Use Evaluate fetal lung maturity, newborn risk for respiratory distress syndrome (hyaline membrane disease of newborn); manage high risk pregnancies, such as intrauterine growth retardation, maternal diabetes. Other tests are more useful; this test is not widely used.[1]

Limitations Contamination of specimen with blood or meconium can falsely increase results. Falsely decreased results can occur; negative tests occur with normal lungs.[2] Although the test generally correlates with the L/S ratio, **the shake test has serious limitations**. Interpretation is subjective; blood, meconium, and vaginal fluid may interfere, and the ratio of false-negatives is high (50%).

Methodology Dilutions of amniotic fluid are mixed with ethanol and then shaken.[2]

Additional Information The surfactant complex lowers surface tension in alveoli. It moves into amniotic fluid, a sample of which can provide projections of fetal lung maturity. An article discussed the theoretical effects of amniotic fluid volume changes on surfactant measurements.[3] Chronic oligohydramnios/polyhydramnios had minimal effect on the surfactant concentration measurement in the amniotic fluid. Acute oligohydramnios/polyhydramnios may significantly affect the amniotic fluid surfactant measurement if the acute change in volume is due to decreased/increased volume of inflow. Acute oligohydramnios/polyhydramnios due to increased/decreased volume of outflow had much less effect on the amniotic fluid surfactant measurement.

Footnotes

1. Dubin SB, "The Laboratory Assessment of Fetal Lung Maturity," *Am J Clin Pathol*, 1992, 97(6):836-49.
2. Jobe A, "Amniotic Fluid Tests of Fetal Lung Maturity," *Maternal-Fetal Medicine: Principles and Practice*, 2nd ed, Creasy RK and Resnik R, eds, Philadelphia, PA: WB Saunders Co, 1989, 426-33.
3. Nelson GH and Nelson SJ, "Theoretical Effects of Amniotic Fluid Volume Changes on Surfactant Concentration Measurements," *Am J Obstet Gynecol*, 1985, 152(7 Pt 1):870-8.

References

Nakamura Y, Yamamoto I, Funatsu Y, et al, "Decreased Surfactant Level in the Lung With Oligohydramnios: A Morphometric and Biochemical Study," *J Pediatr*, 1988, 112(3):471-4.

Sher G, Statland B, and Freer DE, "Clinical Evaluation of the Quantitative Foam Stability Index Test," *Obstet Gynecol*, 1980, 55:617-20.

Statland BE and Sher G, "Reliability of Amniotic Fluid Surfactant Measurements," *Am J Clin Pathol*, 1985, 83(3):382-4.

Amniotic Fluid Spectral Analysis *see* Amniotic Fluid Analysis for Erythroblastosis Fetalis (OD 450) *on page 76*

Amniotic Fluid Urea Nitrogen *see* Amniotic Fluid Creatinine *on previous page*

AMP, Cyclic, Plasma *see* Cyclic AMP, Plasma *on page 119*

AMP, Cyclic, Urine *see* Cyclic AMP, Urine *on page 119*

Amylase, Body Fluid *see* Body Fluid Amylase *on page 91*

Amylase/Creatinine Ratio *see* Amylase, Urine *on next page*

Amylase, Peritoneal Fluid *see* Body Fluid Amylase *on page 91*

Amylase, Pleural Fluid *see* Body Fluid Amylase *on page 91*

Amylase, Serum

CPT 82150

Related Information

Amylase, Urine *on this page*
Bilirubin, Total *on page 86*
Body Fluid Amylase *on page 91*
Lipase, Serum *on page 158*

Synonyms 1,4-α-D Glucanohydrolase, Serum

Abstract Amylase is a group of enzymes (hydrolases) from the exocrine pancreas. Serum amylase is usually a sensitive and useful diagnostic method in those patients with acute pancreatitis who present within hours of the onset of pain. Lipase assay provides somewhat better sensitivity and specificity and is best used with amylase determination. Pancreatitis is a disease which varies from mild to the most formidible of catastrophies.[1]

Specimen Serum

Container Red top tube

Collection Anticoagulants other than heparin diminish amylase activity

Storage Instructions Amylase is stable for 1 week at 25°C and 2 months at 4°C.

Special Instructions Dilution of lipemic sera may cause amylase values to increase.

Reference Range 23-85 units/L (SI: 0.39-1.45 μkat/L) (Du Pont ACA values). Method dependent. Newborns' serum shows little amylase activity. Much of this activity is apparently of salivary origin. Children up to 2 years of age have virtually no pancreatic isoamylase. Markedly low values may not rise to adult values until the end of the second year of life.

Possible Panic Range Over three times the upper limit of normal for a given method probably indicates a significant increase.

Use Useful in diagnosis of acute pancreatitis. Serum amylase is used to work up abdominal pain, epigastric tenderness, nausea, and vomiting, findings which characterize acute pancreatitis as well as acute surgical emergencies such as gastrointestinal perforation (eg, peptic ulcer with perforation) or bowel infarct. Pancreatitis in an individual may or may not be related to alcoholism. Amylase levels tend to be higher in instances not related to alcohol. Hypercalcemia related to pancreatitis is recognized with hyperparathyroidism and other entities. About 80% of subjects with acute pancreatitis have increased serum amylase within 24 hours.

Limitations Poor specificity. Oxalate or citrate depress results. Lipemic sera (hypertriglyceridemia) may contain inhibitors which falsely depress results. About 20% of patients with acute pancreatitis have abnormal lipids. Normal serum amylase may occur in pancreatitis, especially relapsing and chronic pancreatitis. (Subjects in whom pseudocysts complicate chronic pancreatitis often do have elevations of the pancreatic enzymes.) The entire pancreas can be destroyed in pancreatitis; in such cases serum amylase will derive from other structures (eg, the salivary glands). Urinary amylase increases often persist longer than do those of serum. High levels in alcoholics, in pregnancy, and in diabetic ketoacidosis are of salivary rather than pancreatic origin. Salivary type amylase makes up about 60% of the serum enzyme, while it is the pancreatic fraction that is of clinical interest.[2] The expression "salivary amylase" includes other nonpancreatic sources of the enzyme. Serum amylase is cleared by renal excretion. Serum amylase may increase one to two times upper limit of normal in renal failure without diagnostic significance. In such cases, urine amylase is normal or low.

Methodology Amyloclastic, saccharogenic, chromolytic; up to 200 methods exist

Additional Information Causes of **high serum amylase** include acute pancreatitis, pancreatic pseudocyst, pancreatic ascites, pancreatic abscess, neoplasm in or adjacent to pancreas, trauma to pancreas, and common duct stones.

Nonpancreatic causes of hyperamylasemia can confuse interpretation in some cases. They include inflammatory salivary lesions (eg, mumps), perforated peptic ulcer involving pancreas or not, intestinal obstruction and infarction, afferent loop syndrome, biliary tract disease usually including stones, but uncommonly occurring in gallbladder disease even without pancreatitis; aortic aneurysm, peritonitis, acute appendicitis, cerebral trauma, burns and traumatic shock, the postoperative state (with and without pancreatitis), diabetic ketoacidosis, and extrapancreatic carcinomas (especially of esophagus, lung, ovary). Amylase levels more than 25-fold the upper limit of normal may be found when metastatic tumors produce ectopic amylase. Such levels are higher than those usually found in cases of pancreatitis.[3] In renal insufficiency amylase is usually not more than three times the upper limit of normal. Moderate increases may be reported in normal pregnancy. Increases may be found with tubo-ovarian abscess, ruptured ectopic pregnancy, macroamylasemia, and with a substantial number of drugs, including morphine. Relationships between pancreatitis and hyperlipidemias types

I, IV, and V are described. Amylasemia may be associated with hyperparathyroidism.

Macroamylase is a high molecular weight material, normal amylase complexed to high molecular weight protein such as immunoglobulin. It is characterized by high serum amylase and low to normal urine amylase. Macroamylase occurs in normal as well as abnormal subjects.[4]

Other tests: In **pancreatitis**, varying percentages of patients have the following other abnormalities in varying combinations: elevation of triglyceride, alkaline phosphatase, AST (SGOT), total bilirubin, white blood cell count, left shift. Alanine aminotransferase (ALT) (SGPT), increased to three times baseline or more, provides indication for gall-induced etiology of pancreatitis. Calcium levels should be followed in fulminant pancreatitis, since extremely low serum calcium levels can evolve. **Serum lipase** assay provides somewhat greater sensitivity and sensitivity in acute pancreatitis. Both may be valuable. Although determination of serum methemalbumin has been advocated as a test for acute hemorrhagic pancreatitis, it is cumbersome and is not done in many American laboratories.

Laboratory and other factors useful to project severity are published.[1]

Isoenzymes of amylase exist: pancreatic and salivary type, as noted under Limitations. They can be separated by polyacrylamide gel or agarose film electrophoresis, isoelectric focusing, ion exchange chromatography, and plant isoamylase inhibitors. A monoclonal antibody approach is described.[3,5] Amylase isoenzymes are separated in few laboratories. Where available the procedure is an expensive one. It is useful in assessing the decrease of pancreatic function in cystic fibrosis, in children older than 5 years of age, who may be candidates for enzyme replacement.

Footnotes

1. Steinberg W and Tenner S, "Acute Pancreatitis," *N Engl J Med*, 1994, 330(17):1198-210.
2. Ellis C, Koehler DF, Eckfeldt JH, et al, "Evaluation of an Inhibitor Assay to Determine Serum Isoamylase Distribution," *Dig Dis Sci*, 1982, 27:897-901.
3. Eckfeldt JH and Levitt MD, "Diagnostic Enzymes for Pancreatic Disease," *Clin Lab Med*, 1989, 9(4):731-43.
4. Van Gossum A, "Macroamylasemia: A Biochemical or Clinical Problem?" *Dig Dis*, 1989, 7(1):19-27.
5. Warshaw AL and Hawboldt MM, "Puzzling Persistent Hyperamylasemia, Probably Neither Pancreatic Nor Pathologic," *Am J Surg*, 1988, 155(3):453-6.

References

Agarwal N, Pitchumoni CS, and Sivaprasad AV, "Evaluating Tests for Acute Pancreatitis," *Am J Gastroenterol*, 1990, 85(4):356-66.
Borgström A and Bohe M, "Severe Acute Pancreatitis and Normal Serum Amylase Activity Due to Pancreatic Isoamylase Deficiency," *Dig Dis Sci*, 1989, 34(4):644-6.
Clavien PA, Burgan S, and Moossa AR, "Serum Enzymes and Other Laboratory Tests in Acute Pancreatitis," *Br J Surg*, 1989, 76(12):1234-43.
Corsetti JP, Cox C, Schulz TJ, et al, "Combined Serum Amylase and Lipase Determinations for Diagnosis of Suspected Acute Pancreatitis," *Clin Chem*, 1993, 39(12):2495-9.
Dougherty SH, Saltzstein EC, Peacock JB, et al, "Rapid Resolution of High Level Hyperamylasemia as a Guide to Clinical Diagnosis and Timing of Surgical Treatment in Patients With Gallstones," *Surg Gynecol Obstet*, 1988, 166(6):491-6.
Dubick MA, Conteas CN, Billy HT, et al, "Raised Serum Concentrations of Pancreatic Enzymes in Cigarette Smokers," *Gut*, 1987, 28(3):330-5.
Eckfeldt JH and Kershaw MJ, "Hyperamylasemia Following Methyl Alcohol Intoxication: Source and Significance," *Arch Intern Med*, 1986, 146(1):193-4.
Gumaste VV, Dave PB, Weissman D, et al, "Lipase/Amylase Ratio. A New Index That Distinguishes Acute Episodes of Alcoholic From Nonalcoholic Acute Pancreatitis," *Gastroenterology*, 1991, 101(5):1361-6.
Humphries LL, Adams LJ, Eckfeldt JH, et al, "Hyperamylasemia in Patients With Eating Disorders," *Ann Intern Med*, 1987, 106(1):50-2.
Kleinman DS and O'Brien JF, "Macroamylase," *Mayo Clin Proc*, 1986, 61(8):669-70.
Justice AD, DiBenedetto RJ, and Stanford E, "Significance of Elevated Pancreatic Enzymes in Intracranial Bleeding," *South Med J*, 1994, 87(9):889-93.
King LG, Seelig CB, and Ramney JE, "The Lipase to Amylase Ratio in Acute Pancreatitis," *Am J Gastroenterol*, 1995, 90(1):67-9.
Kurzweil SM, Shapiro MJ, Andrus CH, et al, "Hyperbilirubinemia Without Common Bile Duct Abnormalities and Hyperamylasemia Without Pancreatitis in Patients With Gallbladder Disease," *Arch Surg*, 1994, 129(8):829-33.
Lott JA and Lu CJ, "Lipase Isoforms and Amylase Isoenzymes: Assays and Application in the Diagnosis of Acute Pancreatitis," *Clin Chem*, 1991, 37(3):361-8.
Orebaugh SL, "Normal Amylase Levels in the Presentation of Acute Pancreatitis," *Am J Emerg Med*, 1994, 12(1):21-4.
Ruzena S, "Normal Serum Amylase in Acute Pancreatitis," *Dig Dis Sci*, 1989, 34(6):960-1.
Simon HK, Muehlberg A, and Linakis JG, "Serum Amylase Determinations in Pediatric Patients Presenting to the ED With Acute Abdominal Pain or Trauma," *Am J Emerg Med*, 1994, 12(3):292-5.
Wilson C and Imrie CW, "Amylase and Gut Infarction," *Br J Surg*, 1986, 73(3):219-21.

Amylase, Urine

CPT 82150

Related Information

Amylase, Serum *on this page*
Body Fluid Amylase *on page 91*
Lipase, Serum *on page 158*

Synonyms 1,4-α-D Glucanohydrolase, Urine

Applies to Amylase/Creatinine Ratio; Trypsin, Immunoreactive

Abstract Urine amylase is elevated early and reaches high levels in acute pancreatitis. However, diagnostic utility of serum amylase is said to be superior.[1]

(Continued)

Amylase, Urine *(Continued)*

Specimen 2-hour urine specimen is preferred, no preservative

Collection Collect timed specimen. Instruct the patient to void at the beginning of the collection period and discard the specimen. Collect all urine including the final specimen voided at the end of the collection period. Centrifugation to provide optically clear specimen is desirable.

Storage Instructions Keep refrigerated.

Special Instructions Requisition should include date and time collection started, date and time collection finished.

Reference Range 4-37 units/2 hours (Du Pont ACA units). Method dependent. Normals for random urine specimens have not been established.

Use Work up abdominal pain, epigastric tenderness, nausea, and vomiting. An enzyme with molecular weight of 45,000-55,000 daltons, the role of increased urinary amylase in the differential diagnosis of acute pancreatitis has become controversial, save for diagnosis of macroamylasemia.[2] It is also elevated in about 25% of patients with carcinoma of pancreas. It is very useful in diagnosis of pseudocyst of the pancreas, in which the urine amylase may remain elevated for weeks after the serum amylase has returned to normal, after a bout of acute pancreatitis.

Methodology Maltopentose, other methods also available

Additional Information Macroamylasemia is characterized by high serum amylase but normal urine amylase. The **amylase/creatinine ratio** remains useful for the diagnosis of macroamylasemia, but its nonspecificity has otherwise left it with few other applications. In macroamylasemia the clearance is very low.[3] Unlike serum amylase, urine amylase levels are normal with renal failure. While serum amylase usually returns to normal within 3-5 days, without complications urine amylase is increased longer than serum amylase in acute pancreatitis. Two-hour collections are more practical and provide results sooner than longer collections. The major test for pancreatitis additional to serum and urine amylase is serum lipase. It has good specificity and its laboratory analysis is greatly improved from the 1960s. Also, some patients with pancreatitis have very high triglyceride levels. **Immunoreactive trypsin** is not available stat and is not widely available at all.

Footnotes
1. Burtis CA and Ashwood ER, *Tietz Textbook of Clinical Chemistry*, 2nd ed, Philadelphia, PA: WB Saunders Co, 1994, 854.
2. Steinberg W and Tenner S, "Acute Pancreatitis," *N Engl J Med*, 1994, 330(17):1198-210.
3. Eckfeldt JH and Levitt MD, "Diagnostic Enzymes for Pancreatic Disease," *Clin Lab Med*, 1989, 9(4):731-43.

References
Bertholf RL, Winn-Deen ES, and Bruns DE, "Amylase in Urine as Measured by a Single-Step Chromolytic Procedure," *Clin Chem*, 1988, 34(4):754-7.

Androstenedione, Serum

CPT 82157

Related Information

Dehydroepiandrosterone Sulfate *on page 120*

17-Hydroxyprogesterone, Blood or Amniotic Fluid *on page 148*

Testosterone, Free and Total *on page 202*

Abstract An androgen precursor for peripheral conversion to testosterone and dihydrotestosterone, produced by the adrenals and gonads

Patient Preparation Fasting morning specimen is preferred. Collect 1 week before or after menstrual period.

Specimen Serum or EDTA plasma

Container Red top tube

Storage Instructions Freeze serum.

Causes for Rejection Recently administered radioisotopes

Reference Range Variation exists between laboratories. **Male:** 1-3 months: 20-45 ng/dL (SI: 0.7-1.6 nmol/L), 3-5 months: 10-40 ng/dL (SI: 0.3-1.4 nmol/L), adults: 75-205 ng/dL (SI: 2.6-7.2 nmol/L); **female:** 1-3 months: 15-25 ng/dL (SI: 0.5-0.9 nmol/L), 3-5 months: 10-15 ng/dL (SI: 0.3-0.5 nmol/L), adults: 85-275 ng/dL (SI: 3.0-9.6 nmol/L).[1] Values are higher in pregnancy, highest at delivery. These represent peak values (early morning samples). A marked diurnal variation exists, with a peak around 7 AM and a nadir around 4 PM. Levels rise sharply after puberty to peak at about 20 years of age. An abrupt decline occurs after menopause.

Possible Panic Range >1000 ng/dL (SI: >34.9 nmol/L) suggests a virilizing tumor

Use Evaluate androgen production in hirsute females; less useful in evaluation of other aspects of virilization. Greatly elevated in the most common type of congenital adrenal hyperplasia due to C_{21}-hydroxylase deficiency, in which in infancy elevated 17-hydroxyprogesterone, progesterone, urinary 17-ketosteroids, renin, and ACTH with low serum cortisol are anticipated.

Limitations Poor correlation of plasma levels with clinical severity

Methodology Radioimmunoassay (RIA)

Additional Information Androstenedione is a major precursor in the biosynthesis of androgens and estrogens. It serves as prohormone for testosterone and estrone, particularly in menopausal females. Androstenedione is a weak androgen produced in equal amounts by adrenal glands and ovaries in normal women. The predominant androgens in the female are androstenedione and dehydroepiandrosterone. Androstenedione is increased in cases of hirsutism, including Stein-Leventhal syndrome, ovarian stromal hyperplasia, congenital adrenal hyperplasia, Cushing's syndrome and ectopic ACTH-producing tumor. Luteinized stromal cells produce hormones in ovarian tumors with functioning stroma. About 60% of cases of female hirsutism show elevations of androstenedione. Peripheral conversion of androstenedione to estrogen takes place in adipose tissue of obese women, who may develop endometrial hyperplasia.

Concentrations of androstenedione as well as testosterone and dihydrotestosterone were increased in a case report of the entity, massive ovarian edema with virilization.[2]

Prenatal diagnosis of congenital adrenal hyperplasia due to 21-hydroxylase deficiency is possible. Laboratory investigation includes measurement of 17-hydroxyprogesterone, androstenedione, testosterone, 21-deoxycortisol and HLA typing.[3] Early diagnosis can now be made with molecular genetic studies from chorionic villus sampling.[4]

Footnotes
1. Burtis CA and Ashwood ER, *Tietz Textbook of Clinical Chemistry*, 2nd ed, Philadelphia, PA: WB Saunders Co, 1994, 2178.
2. van den Brule F, Bourque J, Gaspard UJ, et al, "Massive Ovarian Edema With Androgen Secretion. A Pathological and Endocrine Study With Review of the Literature," *Horm Res*, 1994, 41(5-6):209-14.
3. Levine LS and Pang S, "Prenatal Diagnosis and Treatment of Congenital Adrenal Hyperplasia," *J Pediatr Endocrinol*, 1994, 7(3):193-200.
4. Forest MG, David M, and Morel Y, "Prenatal Diagnosis and Treatment of 21-Hydroxylase Deficiency," *J Steroid Biochem Mol Biol*, 1993, 45(1-3):75-82.

References
Adashi EY, "The Climacteric Ovary as a Functional Gonadotropin-Driven Androgen-Producing Gland," *Fertil Steril*, 1994, 62(1):20-7.
Gompel A, Wright F, Kuttenn F, et al, "Contribution of Plasma Androstenedione to 5 Alpha-Androstanediol Glucuronide in Women With Idiopathic Hirsutism," *J Clin Endocrinol Metab*, 1986, 62(2):441-4.
Mahlck CG, Backstrom T, Kjellgren O, et al, "Plasma Progesterone and Androstenedione in Relation to Changes in Tumor Volume and Recurrence in Women With Ovarian Carcinoma," *Gynecol Obstet Invest*, 1986, 22(3):157-64.
Ylikorkala O, Stenman UH, and Halmesmaki E, "Testosterone, Androstenedione, Dehydroepiandrosterone Sulfate, and Sex-Hormone-Binding Globulin in Pregnant Alcohol Abusers," *Obstet Gynecol*, 1988, 71(5):731-5.

Androsterone *see* 17-Ketosteroids Fractionation, Urine *on page 152*

Angiotensin *see* Renin, Plasma *on page 197*

Angiotensin Converting Enzyme

CPT 82164

Synonyms ACE; Angiotensin-I-Converting Enzyme

Applies to Angiotensin Converting Enzyme, CSF; Cerebrospinal Fluid Angiotensin Converting Enzyme

Abstract ACE is a dipeptidyl carboxypeptidase. It functions to split dipeptides from the free carboxy end of a variety of polypeptides including angiotensin I and bradykinin. It is especially known for its generation of the octapeptide angiotensin II by releasing the dipeptide histidyl-leucine from angiotensin I. The major site of ACE production is the pulmonary bed of endothelial cells.

Patient Preparation Patient need not be fasting.

Specimen Serum or plasma

Container Red top tube or green top (heparin) tube

Storage Instructions Separate serum (or plasma) immediately. Stable 1 week at 4°C, 6 months at -20°C.

Reference Range 8-53 units/L (SI: 0.14-0.88 μkat/L)

Use High in sarcoidosis, more often when the disease is active. Of value in assessing the response of sarcoidosis to corticosteroid therapy. Changes in serum ACE correlate with clinical status and results of gallium scans (which reflect presence and activity of inflammatory granulomatous lesions). Falling ACE level is a favorable prognostic sign. Rising levels may reflect activity uncontrolled by therapy. It also is used in investigation for Gaucher's disease.

Limitations Test lacks specificity and sensitivity for diagnosis of sarcoidosis. Elevations have been reported in about 35% to 80% of cases of sarcoidosis (see reference by Jordan et al for entry to the somewhat older literature on this subject). ACE levels are less likely to be increased with chronic sarcoidosis. Different admixtures of acute and chronic cases may explain some of the apparent variation in reported incidence of elevation in sarcoidosis. Elevations have been found in patients with diabetes mellitus, Gaucher's disease and leprosy. Twenty-five percent of 86 patients with acute histoplasmosis had elevated levels.[1] Increased in some patients with primary biliary cirrhosis, amyloidosis, myeloma, Melkersson-Rosenthal syndrome, some alpha$_1$-antitrypsin variants, and hyperthyroidism. It has been found increased in some cases of hyperparathyroidism and in some instances of oncogenic hypercalcemia. Thus, it is not a specific marker for the diagnosis of sarcoidosis.[2] Positives are also reported in patients with extrinsic allergic alveolitis, coccidioidomycosis, beryllium disease, asbestosis, silicosis, and alcoholic liver disease.[3] ACE activity is decreased during starvation, independent of the level of thyroid activity (as monitored by T$_3$ levels).[4] ACE is physiologically decreased by administration of captopril, enalapril, and lisinopril. Hemolysis and lipemia interfere with these methods.

Methodology Spectrofluorometric or radioimmunoassay (RIA), spectrophotometric utilizing synthetic substrates

Additional Information Other abnormalities found in some sarcoidosis patients include elevations of serum alkaline phosphatase, calcium, gamma globulin with polyclonal gammapathy, and hypercalciuria. Serum angiotensin converting enzyme is elevated in half of the cases of sarcoidosis but usually not in cases of active tuberculosis or Hodgkin's disease. Increases are less frequent when sarcoidosis is inactive.[2] Some 80% to 90% of patients with demonstrably active sarcoidosis have elevated serum ACE. Angiotensin converting enzyme activity is also increased in sarcoid lymph node homogenate. The diagnosis of sarcoidosis is a histopathologic/clinical complex. Noncaseating granulomas must be proven not to be caused by tuberculosis, histoplasmosis, or other microbiologic entities. Berylliosis is a very rare cause of such granulomas.

Thyroid hormone may modulate ACE activity. Both patients with low T$_3$ levels (and clinical hypothyroidism) and patients with anorexia nervosa with associated findings of hypothyroidism may have low serum ACE activity.[5,6] Monitoring of ACE levels may have application in assessing risk of pulmonary damage due to use of some antineoplastic agents, in particular bleomycin.[7] Serum ACE is decreased in some patients with bronchogenic carcinoma. With response to chemotherapy/radiation therapy the ACE level has been noted to normalize.[8] Cerebrospinal fluid ACE is useful in patients with neurosarcoidosis.

Elevated serum ACE levels in a case of the uncommon entity, Melkersson-Rosenthal syndrome, probably relate to the sarcoid-like noncaseating granulomas that are found in this condition. ACE levels normalized after successful (clinical management) therapy with methotrexate.[9]

Serum ACE abnormality has been reported in 20% to 30% of alpha$_1$-antitrypsin variants (MZ, ZZ, and MS Pi types) but in only about 1% of individuals with normal MM Pi type.[10] There is evidence that paraquat poisoning (because of its effect on pulmonary capillary endothelium) is associated with elevated serum ACE.[11]

Footnotes
1. Ryder KW, Jay SJ, Kiblawi SO, et al, "Serum Angiotensin Converting Enzyme Activity in Patients With Histoplasmosis," *JAMA*, 1983, 249:1888-9.
2. Lufkin EG, DeRemee RA, and Rohrbach MS, "The Predictive Value of Serum Angiotensin Converting Enzyme Activity in the Differential Diagnosis of Hypercalcemia," *Mayo Clin Proc*, 1983, 58:447-51.
3. Studdy PR, Lapworth R, and Bird R, "Angiotensin Converting Enzyme and Its Clinical Significance - A Review," *J Clin Pathol*, 1983, 36:938-47.
4. Butkus NE, Burman KD, and Smallridge RC, "Angiotensin-Converting Enzyme Activity Decreases During Fasting," *Horm Metab Res*, 1987, 19(2):76-9.
5. Matsubayashi S, Tamai H, Kobayashi N, et al, "Angiotensin Converting Enzyme and Anorexia Nervosa," *Horm Metab Res*, 1988, 20(12):761-4.
6. Smallridge RC, Rogers J, and Verma PS, "Serum Angiotensin Converting Enzyme: Alterations in Hyperthyroidism, Hypothyroidism, and Subacute Thyroiditis," *JAMA*, 1983, 250:2489-93.
7. Nussinovitch N, Peleg E, Yaron A, et al, "Angiotensin Converting Enzyme in Bleomycin-Treated Patients," *Int J Clin Pharmacol Ther Toxicol*, 1988, 26(6):310-3.
8. Schweisfurth H, Schmidt M, Brugger E, et al, "Alterations of Serum Carboxypeptidases N and Angiotensin-I-Converting Enzyme in Malignant Diseases," *Clin Biochem*, 1985, 18(4):242-6.
9. Leicht S, Youngberg G, and Modica L, "Melkersson-Rosenthal Syndrome: Elevations in Serum Angiotensin Converting Enzyme and Results of Treatment With Methotrexate," *South Med J*, 1989, 82(1):74-6.
10. Lieberman J and Sastre A, "Serum Angiotensin Converting Enzyme Levels in Patients With Alpha$_1$-Antitrypsin Variants," *Am J Med*, 1986, 81(5):821-4.
11. Hollinger MA, Potwell SW, Zuckerman JE, et al, "Effect of Paraquat on Serum Angiotensin Converting Enzyme," *Am Rev Respir Dis*, 1980, 121:795-8.

References
Alhenc-Gelas F, Richard J, Courbon D, et al, "Distribution of Plasma Angiotensin Converting Enzyme in Healthy Men: Relationship to Environmental and Hormonal Parameters," *J Lab Clin Med*, 1991, 117(1):33-9.
Beneteau-Burnat B, Baudin B, Morgant G, et al, "Serum Angiotensin-Converting Enzyme in Healthy and Sarcoidotic Children: Comparison With the Reference Interval for Adults," *Clin Chem*, 1990, 36(2):344-6.
Jordan DR, Anderson RL, Nerad JA, et al, "The Diagnosis of Sarcoidosis," *Can J Ophthalmol*, 1988, 23(5):203-7.
Lieberman J, "Enzymes in Sarcoidosis: Angiotensin Converting Enzyme (ACE)," *Clin Lab Med*, 1989, 9(4):745-55.
Sharma OP, "Sarcoidosis," *Dis Mon*, 1990, 36(9):469-535.
Seidman MD, Lewandowski CA, Sarpa JR, et al, "Angioedema Related to Angiotensin-Converting Enzyme Inhibitors," *Otolaryngol Head Neck Surg*, 1990, 102(6):727-31.
Thomas PD and Hunninghake GW, "Current Concepts of the Pathogenesis of Sarcoidosis," *Am Rev Respir Dis*, 1987, 135(3):747-60.

Thompson AB, Cale WF, and Lapp NL, "Serum Angiotensin-Converting Enzyme Is Elevated in Association With Underground Coal Mining," *Chest*, 1991, 100(4):1042-5.

Angiotensin Converting Enzyme, CSF *see* Angiotensin Converting Enzyme *on previous page*

Angiotensin-I-Converting Enzyme *see* Angiotensin Converting Enzyme *on previous page*

Anion Gap

Related Information

Synonyms Electrolyte Gap; Gap; Ion Gap

Applies to Anion Gap, Urine

Test Commonly Includes A calculation from electrolytes, sodium, potassium, HCO$_3^-$, and chloride to ascertain quantities of unmeasured cations and anions

Abstract The anion gap is useful in evaluation of patients with acid-base abnormalities. The sum of anions and cations must be equal in the blood. This calculation (anion gap) is a measure of undetermined anions.

Specimen Serum

Container Red top tube

Reference Range 8-16 mmol/L (SI: 8-16 mmol/L); slight differences may be established in different laboratories. This value is applicable for calculation of anion gap as follows: $[Na^+] - [HCO_3^- + Cl^-]$. If K is included with the cations the reference range is 10-20 mmol/L (SI: 10-20 mmol/L). Electrolytes for the above were done mostly by flame photometry. As ion-selective electrodes have come into wider use, reference ranges for anion gap tend to be slightly lower (eg, 3-14 mmol/L) (SI: 3-14 mmol/L).

Use Extensively used for quality control in the laboratory, the widest clinical application of the anion gap is in the diagnosis of types of metabolic acidosis. Unmeasured cations include Ca^{2+} and Mg^{2+}. Unmeasured anions include protein, PO_4^{3-}, SO_4^{2-}, and organic acids.[2] Organic acidosis includes lactic acidosis and ketoacidosis.

A marked elevation of anion gap, >30 mmol/L suggests **metabolic acidosis**.[3] Increased anion gaps are found in states such as renal failure and toxic ingestions. Above 30 mmol/L gap increase is commonly secondary to **lactic acidosis** or ketoacidosis but can be caused also by rhabdomyolysis or nonketotic hyperglycemic coma.

In **diabetic ketoacidosis** plasma glucose is high, often much >300 mg/dL (SI: >16.7 mmol/L), pH is <7.3, and ketones are found in blood and urine. Increased serum osmolality and increased calculated osmolality (osmolar gap) are found, and serum sodium is often decreased.

In **alcoholic ketoacidosis** glucose may be increased, normal or low, but a high alcohol level may be found, and amylase and uric acid may be increased.

Limitations Differences in formula are used by different laboratories. A spurious increase may follow excessive exposure of the sample to room air as well as underfilling the Vacutainer® tube.[4] Some gaps remain unexplained. All metabolic abnormalities are not detected by abnormal gaps (eg, isopropanol ingestion is accompanied by normal gap, but ketone bodies are positive). There are a number of causes of normal anion gap acidosis associated with hyperchloremia. Anion gap is unsuitable as a quick screen for lactic acidosis. Still useful, the anion gap should not replace assay for lactate, creatinine, ketone bodies, or osmolality. In one study, only 66% of patients with an anion gap of 20-29 mmol/L could be proven to have an organic acidosis.[1]

Methodology

Calculation: $(Na^+ + K^+) - (Cl^- + HCO_3^-)$ or $Na^+ - (Cl^- + HCO_3^-)$ = anion gap; actually determined by the difference between concentrations of anions and cations. The calculation using Na^+ as the only cation is used most often.

Additional Information Anion gap represents approximately the sum of the unmeasured anions minus the unmeasured cations. (Measured anions are chloride and bicarbonate. Measured cations are sodium.)

Anion gap high: Caused by high unmeasured anions. With **pH high**: extracellular volume contraction; massive transfusion (with renal failure
(Continued)

Anion Gap *(Continued)*

and/or volume contraction); carbenicillin, penicillin (large doses), salts of organic acids such as citrate. With **pH low:** uremia: most common cause; abnormal anion gap in uremia is usually seen only when creatinine is >4.0 mg/dL (SI: >354 μmol/L). Uremic acidosis is rare without hyperphosphatemia. Nonketotic hyperglycemic coma and rhabdomyolysis may cause high anion gap metabolic acidosis. Lactic acidosis and diabetic or alcoholic ketoacidosis characteristically fall into this group. With **normal osmolal gap:** salicylate and paraldehyde toxicity; with **increased osmolal gap:** methanol and ethylene glycol toxicity.

High anion gap metabolic acidosis without elevated lactic acid or acetone; consider: ketoacidosis with negative or slightly positive "acetone" if patient is hypoxic and/or has alcoholic ketoacidosis, such ketoacidosis may be life-threatening;[3] salicylate toxicity; methanol toxicity (paint thinners); ethylene glycol toxicity (antifreeze) - urinary sediment contains abundant calcium oxalate and/or hippurate crystals; paraldehyde intoxication (may have positive ketone reactions); toluene toxicity[5] (transmission fluid, paint thinner inhalation or sniffing). See listing Osmolality, Calculated *on page 172*.

Anion gap low: Caused by retained unmeasured anions. Most common cause is hypoalbuminemia (eg, in nephrosis, cirrhosis), dilution, hypernatremia, very marked hypercalcemia, very severe hypermagnesemia, IgG myeloma and polyclonal gamma globulin increases[6] - hyperviscosity with certain lab instruments, lithium toxicity, bromism (low anion gap may not be present). Decreased anion gap with spurious hyperchloremia and with hyponatremia is reported in hyperlipidemia.[7] Dilution of extracellular fluid may cause a decreased gap.[8] The finding of a **low anion gap** is perceived as an unreliable diagnostic parameter but should be strongly considered as an **indication of laboratory error.**

Normal anion gap may occur with **metabolic acidosis,** causes have been published.[3] They include diarrhea, renal tubular acidosis, hyperalimentation, ureteroileostomy, ureterosigmoidostomy, external drainage of pancreaticobiliary fluids, NH₄Cl and other drugs.

The urinary anion gap is used in the diagnosis of hyperchloremic metabolic acidosis[9] and evaluation of renal potassium wasting.[10]

Footnotes

1. Badrick T and Hickman PE, "The Anion Gap: A Reappraisal," *Am J Clin Pathol*, 1992, 98(2):249-52.
2. Oh MS and Carroll HJ, "The Anion Gap," *N Engl J Med*, 1977, 297:814-7.
3. Emmett M and Narins RG, "Clinical Use of the Anion Gap," *Medicine*, 1977, 56:38-54.
4. Herr RD and Swanson T, "Pseudometabolic Acidosis Caused by Underfill of Vacutainer® Tubes," *Ann Emerg Med*, 1992, 21(2):177-80.
5. Fischman CM and Oster JR, "Toxic Effects of Toluene: A New Cause of High Anion Gap Metabolic Acidosis," *JAMA*, 1979, 241:1713-5.
6. Keshgegian AA, "Anion Gap and Immunoglobulin Concentration," *Am J Clin Pathol*, 1980, 74:282-4.
7. Graber ML, Quigg RJ, et al, "Spurious Hyperchloremia and Decreased Anion Gap in Hyperlipidemia," *Ann Intern Med*, 1983, 98:607-9.
8. Preuss HG, "Fundamentals of Clinical Acid-Base Evaluation," *Clin Lab Med*, 1993, 13(1):103-16.
9. Battle DC, Hizon M, Cohen E, et al, "The Use of the Urinary Anion Gap in the Diagnosis of Hyperchloremic Metabolic Acidosis," *N Engl J Med*, 1988, 318(10):594-9.
10. Oster JR, Perez GO, and Materson BJ, "Use of the Anion Gap in Clinical Medicine," *South Med J*, 1988, 81(2):229-37.

References

Adams SL, "Alcoholic Ketoacidosis," *Emerg Med Clin North Am*, 1990, 8(4):749-60.
Baker RJ, "Biochemical Gaps: Osmolal and Anion," *Curr Surg*, 1987, 44(5):378-81.
Cembrowski GS, Westgard JO, and Kurtycz DF, "Use of the Anion Gap for the Quality Control of Electrolyte Analyzers," *Am J Clin Pathol*, 1983, 79:688-96.
Hertford JA, McKenna JP, and Chamovitz BN, "Metabolic Acidosis With an Elevated Anion Gap," *Am Fam Physician*, 1989, 39(4):159-68.
Rothenberg DM, Berns AS, Barkin R, et al, "Bromide Intoxication Secondary to Pyridostigmine Bromide Therapy," *JAMA*, 1990, 263(8):1121-2.
"Urinary Anion Gap in Hyperchloremic Metabolic Acidosis," *N Engl J Med*, 1988, 319(9):585-7.
Wrenn K, "The Delta (Delta) Gap: An Approach to Mixed Acid-Base Disorders," *Ann Emerg Med*, 1990, 19(11):1310-3.
Wrenn KD, Slovis CM, Minion GE, et al, "The Syndrome of Alcoholic Ketoacidosis," *Am J Med*, 1991, 91(2):119-28.

Anion Gap, Urine *see Anion Gap on previous page*

Apo A-I *see Apolipoprotein A and B on this page*

Apo A-II *see Apolipoprotein A and B on this page*

Apo B *see Apolipoprotein A and B on this page*

APOE *see Apolipoprotein E on this page*

apo E *see Apolipoprotein E on this page*

Apolipoprotein A and B

CPT 82172

Related Information

Apolipoprotein E *on this page*
Cholesterol, Serum *on page 110*
High Density Lipoprotein Cholesterol *on page 143*
Lipid Profile *on page 159*
Lipoprotein (a) *on page 160*
Lipoprotein Electrophoresis *on page 161*
Low Density Lipoprotein Cholesterol *on page 162*
Triglycerides *on page 209*

Synonyms Apo A-I; Apo A-II; Apo B; Apolipoprotein A-I

Abstract Apolipoprotein A is the principle protein (90%) associated with the HDL particle. Apo B is an important constituent of all lipoprotein particles other than HDL (chylomicrons, VLDC, and LDL).

Patient Preparation Patient must be fasting 12-14 hours.

Specimen Serum

Container Red top tube

Storage Instructions Separate serum and refrigerate. **Do not freeze.** Stable 1 week at 4°C.

Causes for Rejection Specimen from nonfasting patient, frozen specimen

Reference Range Apolipoprotein A: male: 80-151 mg/dL, female: 80-170 mg/dL; apolipoprotein B: male: 49-123 mg/dL, female: 26-119 mg/dL

Use Evaluate the risk of coronary artery disease

Limitations Significant differences in Apo A-II were not found in diabetic subjects between those with and without coronary arterial disease.[1]

Methodology Immunonephelometry (preferred), enzyme-linked immunosorbent assay (ELISA), radioimmunoassay (RIA). Apo A and Apo B have recently been standardized, and all commercial assays should conform to the new calibrator standards.[2] The precision of the nephelometric assays is superior (2% to 3% CV). Both ELISA and RIA have high sensitivity. Immunomagnetic separation is described.[3]

Additional Information Apolipoproteins are the protein components of the lipoprotein complexes. Apolipoprotein A is the main protein component of HDL. Measurement of apolipoprotein A is more useful than the measurement of HDL in predicting patients with high risk of coronary artery disease. Levels of apolipoprotein A are inversely correlated with the risk of premature coronary artery disease. Apolipoprotein B is the major component of low density lipoproteins (VLDL and LDL). The relative proportion of apolipoprotein B to apolipoprotein A is more effective in differentiating those with or without ischemic heart disease than the measurement of lipid or lipoprotein cholesterol. An adverse Apo B/Apo A profile at a young age is potentially a marker for coronary heart disease.

Footnotes

1. Wentworth MA, O'Brien T, Rastogi A, et al, "Apolipoprotein A-II Levels and Coronary Artery Disease in Subjects With and Without Diabetes: A Study With Use of a Specific Radioimmunoassay for Apolipoprotein A-II," *Mayo Clin Proc*, 1993, 68(6):556-60.
2. Albers JJ and Marcovina SM, "Standardization of Apolipoprotein B and A-I Measurements," *Clin Chem*, 1989, 35(7):1357-61.
3. Rastogi A, Bren ND, Hallaway BJ, et al, "Immunomagnetic Separation of Subpopulations of Apolipoprotein A-I," *Mayo Clin Proc*, 1994, 69(2):137-43.

References

Boerwinkle E, Brown SA, Rohrbach K, et al, "Role of Apolipoprotein E and B Gene Variation in Determining Response of Lipid, Lipoprotein, and Apolipoprotein Levels to Increased Dietary Cholesterol," *Am J Hum Genet*, 1991, 49(6):1145-54.
Genest JJ Jr, Bard JM, Fruchart JC, et al, "Plasma Apolipoprotein A-I, A-II, B, E, and C-III Containing Particles in Men With Premature Coronary Artery Disease," *Atherosclerosis*, 1991, 90(2-3):149-57.
Paulweber B, Friedl W, Krempler F, et al, "Association of DNA Polymorphism at the Apolipoprotein B Gene Locus With Coronary Heart Disease and Serum Very Low Density Lipoprotein Levels," *Arteriosclerosis*, 1990, 10(1):17-24.
Shephard MD, Hester J, Walmsley RN, et al, "Variation in Plasma Apolipoprotein A-1 and B Concentrations Following Myocardial Infarction," *Ann Clin Biochem*, 1990, 27(Pt 1):9-14.
Walmsley TA, Grant S, and George PM, "Effect of Plasma Triglyceride Concentrations on the Accuracy of Immunoturbidimetric Assays of Apolipoprotein B," *Clin Chem*, 1991, 37(5):748-53.
Williams KJ, Petrie KA, Brocia RW, et al, "Lipoprotein Lipase Modulates Net Secretory Output of Apolipoprotein B *In Vitro*. A Possible Pathophysiologic Explanation for Familial Combined Hyperlipidemia," *J Clin Invest*, 1991, 88(4):1300-6.
Young SG, "Recent Progress in Understanding Apolipoprotein B," *Circulation*, 1990, 82(5):1574-94.

Apolipoprotein A-I *see Apolipoprotein A and B on this page*

Apolipoprotein A-I *see High Density Lipoprotein Cholesterol on page 143*

Apolipoprotein E

CPT 82172

Related Information

Apolipoprotein A and B *on this page*
Cerebrospinal Fluid Amyloid Precursor Protein and Amyloid β-Protein *on page 376*
Cerebrospinal Fluid Oligoclonal Bands *on page 379*
Cerebrospinal Fluid Tau Protein *on page 382*
Cholesterol, Serum *on page 110*
Lipid Profile *on page 159*
Lipoprotein (a) *on page 160*
Lipoprotein Electrophoresis *on page 161*

Synonyms APOE; apo E; Apoprotein E

Applies to βA4 Peptide; Neurofibrillary Tangles

Test Commonly Includes ε2, ε3, and ε4

Abstract Apolipoprotein E (apoE) acts as a ligand for (binds) the low density lipoprotein (LDL) and other receptors and thus, modulates LDL metabolism. There are multiple molecular forms of apoE. This polymorphism is expressed with the common alleles, ε2, ε3, and ε4.[1] Apoε4 predisposes to coronary artery disease (CAD) and to Alzheimer's dementia. Mechanisms of action involve effects on cholesterol metabolism and concentration (CAD) and differential interaction with β-amyloid (Alzheimer's disease).

Specimen Plasma

Container Lavender top (EDTA) tube

Storage Instructions Store at 2°C to 8°C. Do not freeze.

Causes for Rejection Hemolysis, heparinized blood collected, specimen frozen

Special Instructions Test will usually be performed by a reference laboratory. Correlate/schedule patient sample requirements, handling, and timing with local and/or referral laboratories.

Reference Range Variation in and lack of standardization of methodology has resulted in wide variation of reported **mean** values in healthy individuals (30-120 mg/L), see reference by Seist et al.

Use Evaluate abnormal lipid metabolism associated with coronary artery disease; study predisposing factors to the development of Alzheimer's disease (AD); aid in the differential diagnosis of AD

Methodology Quantitative methods for total apoE include radioimmunoassay (RIA), immunonephelometry, radial immunodiffusion (RID), and electroimmunoassay. ApoE identification (phenotyping) can be performed using polyacrylamide gel isoelectric focusing (PAGE-IEF) or PAGE-IEF of plasma followed by immunoblotting[2] or immunofixation.[3] Because of technical problems, presence of rare variants and of post-translational modifications, isoelectric focusing is less desirable than apoE genotyping for determination of apoE polymorphism. ApoE genotyping is generally performed by restriction enzyme isoform genotyping (restriction isotyping) which utilizes polymerase chain reaction amplification of the genomic sequence containing the apoE polymorphic sites followed by restriction endonuclease (HhaI) digestion and PAGE electrophoresis of the resultant fragments.[4] "MADGE" (microplate array diagonal gel electrophoresis) should allow lower cost, large scale apoE genotyping.[5]

Additional Information Apolipoprotein E (apoE) is produced largely in the liver and circulates in the blood as a 299 amino acid single chain protein. Isoelectric focusing (phenotypic analysis) confirmed by direct sequencing of cDNA (genotyping) has shown that apoE is present as three major isoforms, ε2, ε3, and ε4, with rarely encountered variants. The three isoforms result in six different phenotypes, ε2/2, ε3/3, ε4/4 (homozygotes) and ε2/3, ε2/4, and ε3/4 (heterozygotes). ApoE polymorphism has its structural basis in variation at amino acids 112 and 158, the alleles ε2, ε3, and ε4 encoding Cys-Cys, Cys-Arg, and Arg-Arg, respectively.

Apolipoprotein E plays a variety of roles in lipid metabolism with increasing evidence of significance in both vascular and central nervous system (Alzheimer) degenerative disease.

ApoE and Vascular Disease

ApoE mediates removal of chylomicron and very low density lipoprotein (VLDL) remnants from plasma by binding of these particles to low density lipoprotein (LDL). ApoE binds to (is a ligand for) the LDL receptor, a function dependent upon basic amino acids present between apoE residues 136 and 150. In this role, apoE modulates cholesterol transport and is a component of cholesterol-rich lipoproteins (low density lipoprotein, LDL) functioning in the removal of such circulating particles through a specific hepatocyte plasma membrane receptor. Fully functioning apoE (eg, apoε3) is associated with decreased plasma cholesterol levels as compared to apoE forms with impaired LDL ligand function (eg, apoε4) which are associated with increased plasma cholesterol levels and development of premature atherosclerosis.[6] ApoE isoforms affect plasma concentration of cholesterol and LDL (apoε4 being associated with elevated levels). Isoform type is perhaps the most important lipid risk factor for coronary artery disease.[7] While apoE mediates metabolism of LDL plasma cholesterol levels, other lipoproteins are involved in the absorption and assimilation of dietary cholesterol (eg, apolipoprotein A-IV).[8] Rare mutant apoE isoforms have been associated with aberrant lipid metabolism (eg, apoε3' with double pre-β very low density lipoprotein[9] and apoε7 with xanthomas of the Achilles tendon and coronary artery disease[10]).

The apoε2/ε2 phenotype (apoε3 deficient) is associated with type III hyperlipidemia (in which there is chylomicronemia, increased plasma triglyceride, cholesterol, and β-VLDL, and risk of peripheral and coronary arterial disease). The ε2/ε2 genotype is uncommon (about 1% of individuals) and, as additional risk factors are involved, only 2% to 5% of ε2/ε2 individuals develop type III hyperlipidemia. Presence of the amino acid cysteine at sites 112 and 158 (see above) are considered to impair binding to the LDL receptor resulting in impaired clearance of plasma

intermediate density lipoprotein. The ε4 allele is present in 10% to 15% of individuals in the population but compared to the ε3 allele, it is over-represented in association with coronary heart disease.[11] While the average effect of the ε2 allele is to decrease cholesterol and apolipoprotein B levels, both apoε2 and ε4 alleles may be associated with increased cholesterol and/or triglyceride levels. The lowest cholesterol levels are associated with ε3/ε3 phenotype. There is compelling evidence that apoE polymorphism is a major determinant of risk for development of atherosclerotic vascular disease and its complications.[6] Demand for apoE genotype and/or phenotype determination is likely to increase, in particular, if therapeutic modulation of the effect of apoε4 is developed.

ApoE and Alzheimer's Disease

Since 1993, there have been some 90 reports worldwide confirming an association between Alzheimer's disease (AD) and apoε4. The allele frequency of apoε4 is increased in patients with late-onset AD and in cases of sporadic AD.[12] In a study of elderly patients with mild cognitive impairment, many (24% by 18 months, 44% by 36 months, and 55% by 54 months) progressed to dementia with apoε4 a strong predictor of progression.[13] Until a reliable phenotypic marker of AD is available (eg, see listing Cerebrospinal Fluid Tau Protein *on page 382*), however, it has been emphasized that while apoE genotyping is a major contribution to the differential evaluation of an older individual with dementia, apoE genotype cannot be used for predicting the development of AD.[12] Reduced rate of glucose metabolism in certain areas of the brain (eg, posterior cingulate gyrus) utilizing positron-emission tomography has been associated with preclinical evidence of AD in homozygotes for the ε4 allele.[14]

A functional role of apoE in the pathogenesis of late-onset AD is suggested by the finding that apoE is localized (immunochemically) in senile plaques, vascular amyloid and neurofibrillary tangles (neuropathologic morphologic hallmarks of AD).[15] In addition, cerebrospinal fluid has been shown to bind synthetic βA4 peptide *in vitro*. βA4 peptide is the primary constituent of senile plaques.[15]

In a series of randomly selected (85 year old or older) individuals with neuropathologic autopsy support for the the diagnosis of AD, 28 of 33 carriers of the apoε4 allele had dementia and confirmation of AD. The other 5 carriers had no cognitive impairment indicating that presence of apoε4, while an important risk factor for AD, does not mean that dementia is inevitable.[16] The ε4 allele frequency was 30% in subjects with AD but only 8% in those without dementia.

Functional aspects of apoE in relation to tau protein may underlie the increased risk for AD shown by individuals who bear the apoε4 allele. Normally, apoε3 binds to tau protein and is believed to slow the initial rate of phosphorylation of tau protein and self assembly to form paired helical filaments (PHFs) of neurofibrillary tangles (NFTs). NFTs are pathologic intracellular formations composed of PHFs made of hyperphosphorylated tau protein. Apoε4 does not bind to tau protein, may allow hyperphosphorylation of tau which is then unable to bind and stabilize microtubules.[17] See listing Cerebrospinal Fluid Tau Protein *on page 382*.

Other contenders for a role in the pathophysiology of AD include clusterin (apoJ), a multifunctional apolipoprotein which is associated with amyloid β-peptide (Aβ) in senile plaques of AD. It has been considered that slowly sedimenting Aβ complexes (formed in the presence of clusterin) may contribute to the neurotoxicity of Aβ deposits.[18]

In search of a phenotypic marker of AD that could be paired with the results of apoE genotyping, it is of interest that cerebrospinal fluid (CSF) Aβ42 levels have been reported to be significantly lower in AD patients as compared to controls.[19] Aβ42 has been shown to preferentially deposit in the brains of AD patients. The study of Aβ42 CSF levels, however, found no association of CSF Aβ42 or tau protein with apoE genotype.[19]

Footnotes

1. Hill JS and Pritchard PH, "Improved Phenotyping of Apolipoprotein E: Application to Population Frequency Distribution," *Clin Chem*, 1990, 36(11):1871-4.
2. Kataoka S, Paidi M, and Howard BV, "Simplified Isoelectric Focusing/Immunoblotting Determination of Apoprotein E Phenotype," *Clin Chem*, 1994, 40(1):11-3.
3. Hackler R, Schafer JR, Motzny S, et al, "Rapid Determination of Apolipoprotein E Phenotypes From Whole Plasma by Automated Isoelectric Focusing Using Phast-System™ and Immunofixation," *J Lipid Res*, 1994, 35(1):153-8.
4. Hixson JE and Vermier DT, "Restriction Isotyping of Human Apolipoprotein E by Gene Amplification and Cleavage With HhaI," *J Lipid Res*, 1990, 31(3):545-8.
5. Bolla MK, Haddad L, Humphries SE, et al, "High-Throughput Methods for Determination of Apolipoprotein E Genotypes With Use of Restriction Digestion Analysis by Microplate Array Diagonal Gel Electrophoresis," *Clin Chem*, 1995, 41(11):1599-604.
6. Davignon J, Gregg RE, and Sing CF, "Apolipoprotein E Polymorphism and Atherosclerosis," *Arteriosclerosis*, 1988, 8(1):1-21.
7. Wilson PW, Myers RH, Larson MG, et al, "Apolipoprotein E Alleles, Dyslipidemia, and Coronary Heart Disease: The Framingham Offspring Study," *JAMA*, 1994, 272(21):1666-71.
8. McCombs RJ, Marcadis DE, Ellis J, et al, "Attenuated Hypercholesterolemic Response to a High-Cholesterol Diet in Subjects Heterozygous for the Apolipoprotein A-IV-2 Allele," *N Engl J Med*, 1994, 331(11):706-10.
9. Minnich A, Weisgraber KH, Newhouse Y, et al, "Identification and Characterization of a Novel Apolipoprotein E Variant, Apolipoprotein ε3' (Arg → His): Association With

(Continued)

Apolipoprotein E (Continued)

Mild Dyslipidemia and Double Pre-β Very Low Density Lipoproteins," *J Lipid Res*, 1995, 36(1):57-66.

10. Ueyama Y, Nozaki S, Yanagi K, et al, "Familial Hypercholesterolaemia-Like Syndrome With Apolipoprotein E-7 Associated With Marked Achilles Tendon Xanthomas and Coronary Artery Disease: A Report of Two Cases," *J Intern Med*, 1994, 235(2):169-74.

11. Luc G, Bard JM, Arveiler D, et al, "Impact of Apolipoprotein E Polymorphism on Lipoproteins and Risk of Myocardial Infarction. The ECTIM Study," *Arterioscler Thromb*, 1994, 14(9):1412-9.

12. Roses AD, "Apolipoprotein E Genotyping in the Differential Diagnosis, Not Prediction, of Alzheimer's Disease," *Ann Neurol*, 1995, 38(1):6-14.

13. Petersen RC, Smith GE, Ivnik RJ, et al, "Apolipoprotein E Status as a Predictor of the Development of Alzheimer's Disease in Memory-Impaired Individuals," *JAMA*, 1995, 273(16):1274-8.

14. Reiman EM, Caselli RJ, Yun LS, et al, "Preclinical Evidence of Alzheimer's Disease in Persons Homozygous for the ε4 Allele for Apolipoprotein E," *N Engl J Med*, 1996, 334(12):752-8.

15. Strittmatter WJ, Saunders AM, Schmechel D, et al, "Apolipoprotein E: High-Avidity Binding to β-Amyloid and Increased Frequency of Type 4 Allele in Late-Onset Familial Alzheimer Disease," *Proc Natl Acad Sci USA*, 1993, 90(5):1977-81.

16. Hyman BT and Tanzi R, "Molecular Epidemiology of Alzheimer's Disease," *N Engl J Med*, 1995, 333(19):1283-4 (editorial).

17. Strittmatter WJ, Weisgraber KH, Goedert M, et al, "Hypothesis: Microtubule Instability and Paired Helical Filament Formation in the Alzheimer Disease Brain Are Related to Apolipoprotein E Genotype," *Exp Neurol*, 1994, 125(2):163-71.

18. Oda T, Wals P, Osterburg HH, et al, "Clusterin (apoJ) Alters the Aggregation of Amyloid β-Peptide (Aβ₁-₄₂) and Forms Slowly Sedimenting Aβ Complexes That Cause Oxidative Stress," *Exp Neurol*, 1995, 136(1):22-31.

19. Motter R, Vigo-Pelfrey C, Kholodenko D, et al, "Reduction of β-Amyloid Peptide₄₂ in the Cerebrospinal Fluid of Patients With Alzheimer's Disease," *Ann Neurol*, 1995, 38(4):643-8.

References

Bird TD, "Apolipoprotein E Genotyping in the Diagnosis of Alzheimer's Disease: A Cautionary View," *Ann Neurol*, 1995, 38(1):2-4.

Davignon J, Gregg RE, and Sing CF, "Apolipoprotein E Polymorphism and Atherosclerosis," *Arteriosclerosis*, 1988, 8(1):1-21.

Deng J, Rudick V, and Dory L, "Lysosomal Degradation and Sorting of Apolipoprotein E in Macrophages," *J Lipid Res*, 1995, 36(10):2129-40.

Dyer CA, Cistola DP, Parry GC, et al, "Structural Features of Synthetic Peptides of Apolipoprotein E That Bind the LDL Receptor," *J Lipid Res*, 1995, 36(1):80-8.

O'Brien KD, Deeb SS, Ferguson M, et al, "Apolipoprotein E Localization in Human Coronary Atherosclerotic Plaques by *In Situ* Hybridization and Immunohistochemistry and Comparison With Lipoprotein Lipase," *Am J Pathol*, 1994, 144(3):538-48.

Polvikoski T, Sulkava R, Haltia M, et al, "Apolipoprotein E, Dementia, and Cortical Deposition of β-Amyloid Protein," *N Engl J Med*, 1995, 333(19):1242-7.

Reddick RL, Zhang SH, and Maeda N, "Atherosclerosis in Mice Lacking Apo E. Evaluation of Lesional Development and Progression," *Arterioscler Thromb*, 1994, 14(1):141-7.

Siest G, Pillot T, Regis-Bailly A, et al, "Apolipoprotein E: An Important Gene and Protein to Follow in Laboratory Medicine," *Clin Chem*, 1995, 41(8 Pt 1):1068-86.

Apoprotein E see Apolipoprotein E on page 82

Apoproteins see Lipid Profile on page 159

Arterial-Ascitic Fluid pH Gradient see Body Fluid pH on page 92

Arterial Blood Gases see Blood Gases, Arterial on page 87

Arylamidase see Leucine Aminopeptidase on page 158

Arylamidase Naphthylamidase see Leucine Aminopeptidase on page 158

Ascitic Fluid Analysis see Body Fluid on page 89

Ascorbic Acid, Blood

CPT 82180

Related Information

Oxalate, Urine *on page 174*
Urinalysis *on page 658*

Synonyms Vitamin C

Abstract The functions of vitamin C include roles in collagen synthesis, stimulation of neutrophil chemotaxis, lipid and protein metabolism, as an antioxidant and in wound healing.[1] The principle disease associated with vitamin C deficiency is scurvy. Decreased serum levels indicate nutritional deficiency. An individual on a diet totally deficient in vitamin C will develop scurvy in 60-90 days.

Patient Preparation Patient should be fasting.

Specimen Plasma, serum, or leukocytes, or urine following a loading test; Lee et al write that a fundamental question is what ought to be measured.[2]

Container Green top (heparin) tube preferred; red top tube, lavender top (EDTA) tube, or gray top (sodium fluoride) tube also acceptable; check with the laboratory.

Collection Draw blood in chilled tube. Keep specimen on ice.

Storage Instructions Freeze separated plasma (serum). Stable 30 minutes at 25°C. Stable 4 days at -20°C.

Causes for Rejection Specimen not frozen

Reference Range Plasma or serum: 0.6-2.0 mg/dL (SI: 34-114 μmol/L); leukocytes: 20-50 μg/10⁸ WBC

Critical Values <0.3 mg/dL (SI: <17 μmol/L) in plasma provides evidence for least the risk of deficiency and <0.2 mg/dL (SI: <11 μmol/L) indicates deficiency. Clinical scurvy appears when total body stores diminish to <300 mg.[1]

Use Evaluate vitamin C deficiency. Principal clinical findings in scurvy include bleeding gums, petechiae, follicular hyperkeratosis, perifollicular hemorrhages beginning on the lower thighs, muscle aches, easy fatiguability, effusions, and emotional changes. The metabolite product of hypervitaminosis C, oxalate, may lead to renal oxalate calculi.

Contraindications Ascorbic acid therapy

Methodology High-performance liquid chromatography (HPLC),[3] acidic 2,4-dinitrophenylhydrazine with photometry

Additional Information Plasma or serum levels of vitamin C are an adequate measurement of clinical status, although leukocyte levels are superior but more difficult to obtain. Vitamin C is a cofactor for protocollagen hydroxylase; it promotes the conversion of tropocollagen to collagen. Low values occur in scurvy, malabsorption, alcoholism, pregnancy, hyperthyroidism, and renal failure. Smokers have lower levels than nonsmokers. The disease scurvy and its treatment, from Tierra del Fuego in 1519 to the present, represents a tapestry of naval and world history. The defeat of the French and Spanish at Trafalgar and the successful blockade of the French at Brest may have been supported by the interest in prevention and treatment of scurvy by the British Admiralty, limited as that interest may have been.[1]

Footnotes

1. Cuppage FE, *James Cook and the Conquest of Scurvy*, Westport, CT: Greenwood Press, 1994.

2. Lee W, Davis KA, Rettmer RL, et al, "Ascorbic Acid Status: Biochemical and Clinical Considerations," *Am J Clin Nutr*, 1988, 48(2):286-90.

3. Leavelle DE, *Mayo Medical Laboratories Interpretive Handbook*, Rochester, MN: Mayo Medical Laboratories, 1994.

References

Basu J, Vermund SH, Mikhail M, et al, "Plasma Reduced and Total Ascorbic Acid in Healthy Women: Effects of Smoking and Oral Contraception," *Contraception*, 1989, 39(1):85-93.

Dhariwal KR, Hartzell WO, and Levine M, "Ascorbic Acid and Dehydroascorbic Acid Measurements in Human Plasma and Serum," *Am J Clin Nutr*, 1991, 54(4):712-6.

Garry PJ, Vander Jagt DJ, and Hunt WC, "Ascorbic Acid Intakes and Plasma Levels in Healthy Elderly," *Ann N Y Acad Sci*, 1987, 498:90-9.

Henson DE, Block G, and Levine M, "Ascorbic Acid: Biologic Functions and Relation to Cancer," *J Natl Cancer Inst*, 1991, 83(8):547-50.

Jacob RA, Otradovec CL, Russell RM, et al, "Vitamin C Status and Nutrient Interactions in a Healthy Elderly Population," *Am J Clin Nutr*, 1988, 48(6):1436-42.

Levine M, Dhariwal KR, Washko PW, et al, "Ascorbic Acid and In Situ Kinetics: A New Approach to Vitamin Requirements," *Am J Clin Nutr*, 1991, 54(6 Suppl):1157S-1162S.

Schorah CJ, Bishop N, Wales JK, et al, "Blood Vitamin C Concentrations in Patients With Diabetes Mellitus," *Int J Vitam Nutr Res*, 1988, 58(3):312-8.

Vander Jagt DJ, Garry PJ, and Bhagavan HN, "Ascorbic Acid Intake and Plasma Levels in Healthy Elderly People," *Am J Clin Nutr*, 1987, 46(2):290-4.

Zilva JF and Pannall PR, *Clinical Chemistry in Diagnosis and Treatment*, 4th ed, Chicago, IL: Year Book Medical Publishers Inc, 1985, 451-3.

Aspartate Aminotransferase

CPT 84450

Related Information

Acetaminophen, Serum *on page 530*
Alanine Aminotransferase *on page 65*
Alkaline Phosphatase, Serum *on page 69*
Bilirubin, Total *on page 86*
Gamma Glutamyl Transferase *on page 133*
Hepatitis B Surface Antigen *on page 399*
Lactate Dehydrogenase *on page 153*
Liver Biopsy *on page 48*
Liver Profile *on page 161*

Synonyms AST; Glutamic Oxaloacetic Transaminase, Serum; GOT; L-Aspartate: 2-Oxoglutarate Aminotransferase; SGOT; Transaminase

Applies to Acetaminophen Hepatotoxicity; Aminotransferases

Replaces Cephalin Flocculation; Thymol Turbidity

Abstract AST and ALT are widely used enzymes. They are increased in diseases of the liver and in many other diseases.

Specimen Serum

Container Red top tube

Storage Instructions Stable 3 days at 25°C and 1 week at 4°C; fairly stable refrigerated or frozen.

Causes for Rejection Hemolysis

Reference Range Levels in infancy are two to three times those found in adults. Ranges decrease during childhood years. Typical adult reference range: 20-48 units/L (SI: 0.32-0.82 μkat/L). AST reference values are higher in males.

Use A wide range of disease entities alters AST (SGOT), with origin from many organs. When an increased AST is from the liver, it is likely to relate to disease of the hepatocyte. Other enzymes, including alkaline phosphatase and GGT, are more sensitive indicators of biliary obstruction.

Causes of low AST: uremia, vitamin B_6 deficiency (this can be corrected), metronidazole, trifluoperazine.

Causes of high AST: chronic alcohol ingestion, not limited to overt chronic alcoholism; cirrhosis. In alcoholic hepatitis, AST values usually are <300 units/L, but transaminases are extremely high in the alcohol-acetaminophen syndrome; *vide infra*. In viral hepatitis, look for high AST/LD (LDH) ratio, >3, and very high AST peaking at 500-3000 units/L in acute viral hepatitis (ie, in clinical acute viral hepatitis the transaminases may be increased ten times or more above their upper limits of normal). AST increases are found in other types of liver disease, including earlier stages of hemochromatosis and chemical injury (eg, necrosis related to toxins such as carbon tetrachloride). Some instances of cholecystitis cause increased AST. A mean 1.8-fold increase in AST was found 24 hours following laparoscopic cholecystectomy in 73% of patients, in 82% a 2.2-fold increment in ALT.[1]

AST and ALT (SGPT) are increased in Reye's syndrome.[2,3] In infectious mononucleosis, LD (LDH) is commonly considerably higher than AST. Trauma (including head trauma and including surgery) and other striated muscle diseases, including dystrophy, dermatomyositis, trichinosis, polymyositis, and gangrene cause AST increases. Both AST and ALT elevations are found with Duchenne's muscular dystrophy. Look for high CK in myositis, high LD_5 (or isomorphic pattern in some instances of polymyositis) on LD isoenzymes. See listing Myositis-Specific Autoantibody *on page 420.*

In myocardial infarction AST peaks about 24 hours after infarct and returns to normal 3-7 days later. In acute MI without shock or heart failure, ALT is not apt to increase significantly. AST increases in congestive failure with centrilobular liver congestion, in which high LD_5 on LD isoenzymes is found, and in pericarditis, myocarditis, pancreatitis, and other inflammatory states including Legionnaires' disease. In renal infarction LD is usually high, out of proportion to AST.[4] Lung infarction and other disease entities leading to necrosis including large, necrotic tumors cause increased AST; LD is commonly also increased in such instances. Shock (LD also usually increased); hypothyroidism (LD and/or CK not infrequently increased in myxedema); hemolytic anemias (LD high with increased LD_1) and certain CNS diseases may increase AST.

Drugs: A large number of commonly used drugs have been reported to elevate AST: isoniazid, phenothiazines, erythromycin, progesterone, anabolic-androgenic steroids, halothane, methyldopa, opiates, indomethacin, salicylates in children, and other drugs. Hepatotoxicity from drugs may cause high aminotransferase activity with elevation of AST/ALT ratio.[5]

Acetaminophen hepatotoxicity deserves special mention. In alcoholics, apparently moderate doses of the analgesic have caused severe hepatotoxicity.[6] Doses of 2.6-16.5 g/24 hours are reported with total bilirubin 1.3-23.9 mg/dL (SI: 22-409 µmol/L), AST 1,960-29,700 units/L, and ALT 12,000-12,550 units/L. The characteristic pattern included mild to severe coagulopathy and AST greater than ALT by a considerable margin.[7] The pH <7.3, prothrombin time >100 seconds, and creatinine >34 mg/dL in patients with grade III-IV encephalopathy are criteria for need for liver transplantation or prediction of death.[8]

Macroenzyme causing unexplained increase of AST is described with normal levels of CK and ALT.[9]

Limitations Gross hemolysis causes falsely high values.

Methodology Spectrophotometry, kinetic assay, malate dehydrogenase; like ALT, AST can be measured at 25°C, 30°C, 32°C, and 37°C.[5] The best assays used pyridoxal-5'-phosphate (a coenzyme) supplementation of the reaction mixture. Assays in the United States are almost always done at 37°C.

Additional Information AST has origin from heart, liver, skeletal muscle, kidney, pancreas, spleen, and lung. Very high values, >500 units/L, usually suggest hepatitis or other types of hepatocellular necrosis but can also be found with large necrotic tumors, other types of necrosis or extensive hypoxia, congestive failure, and shock. Unexplained AST elevations should first be investigated with ALT and GGT. Mitochondrial AST (m-AST) may be useful in the diagnosis of alcoholic liver disease; it is reviewed by Rej.[5]

Laboratory findings supportive of the diagnosis of **acute liver failure** include high aminotransferase and low glucose concentrations and evidence of respiratory alkalosis.[8]

Footnotes
1. Halevy A, Gold-Deutch R, Negri M, et al, "Are Elevated Liver Enzymes and Bilirubin Levels Significant After Laparoscopic Cholecystectomy in the Absence of Bile Duct Injury?" *Ann Surg*, 1994, 219(4):362-4.
2. Lichtenstein PK, Heubi JE, Daugherty CC, et al, "Grade I Reye's Syndrome. A Frequent Cause of Vomiting and Liver Dysfunction After Varicella and Upper Respiratory Tract Infection," *N Engl J Med*, 1983, 309:133-9.
3. DeVivo DC, "How Common Is Reye's Syndrome?" *N Engl J Med*, 1983, 309:179-81.
4. Winzelberg GG, Hull JD, Agar JW, et al, "Elevation of Serum Lactate Dehydrogenase Levels in Renal Infarction," *JAMA*, 1979, 242:268-9.
5. Rej R, "Aminotransferase in Disease," *Clin Lab Med*, 1989, 9(4):667-87.
6. Lee WM, "Drug-Induced Hepatotoxicity," *N Engl J Med*, 1995, 333(17):1118-27.
7. Seeff LB, Cuccherini BA, Zimmerman HJ, et al, "Acetaminophen Hepatotoxicity in Alcoholics. A Therapeutic Misadventure," *Ann Intern Med*, 1986, 104(3):399-404.
8. Lee WM, "Acute Liver Failure," *N Engl J Med*, 1993, 329(25):1862-72.
9. Litin SC, O'Brien JF, Pruett S, et al, "Macroenzyme as a Cause of Unexplained Elevation of Aspartate Aminotransferase," *Mayo Clin Proc*, 1987, 62(8):681-7.

References
Rosenthal P and Haight M, "Aminotransferase as a Prognostic Index in Infants With Liver Disease," *Clin Chem*, 1990, 36(2):346-8.
Rotenberg Z, Weinberger I, Davidson E, et al, "Does Determination of Serum Aspartate Aminotransferase Contribute to the Diagnosis of Acute Myocardial Infarction?" *Am J Clin Pathol*, 1989, 91(1):91-4.
Schölmerich J, Gross V, Johannesson T, et al, "Detection of Biliary Origin of Acute Pancreatitis. Comparison of Laboratory Tests, Ultrasound, Computed Tomography, and ERCP," *Dig Dis Sci*, 1989, 34(6):830-3.
Vincent-Viry M and Delwaide P, "Aspartate Aminotransferase and Alanine Aminotransferase," *Drug Effects on Laboratory Test Results Analytical Interferences and Pharmacological Effects*, Siest G and Galteau MM, eds, Littleton, MA: PSG Publishing Co Inc, 1988, 91-130.
Williams AL and Hoofnagle JH, "Ratio of Serum Aspartate to Alanine Aminotransferase in Chronic Hepatitis. Relationship to Cirrhosis," *Gastroenterology*, 1988, 95(3):734-9.

AST *see* Aspartate Aminotransferase *on previous page*

AST/ALT Ratio *see* Cardiac Enzymes/Isoenzymes *on page 102*

Baby Bilirubin *see* Bilirubin, Neonatal *on next page*

Base Excess *see* Delta Base, Blood *on page 121*

Beta-Carotene *see* Carotene, Serum *on page 103*

Beta-Hexosaminidase, Serum

Synonyms Beta-N-Acetylglucosaminidase; Beta-N-Acetylhexosaminidase; β-Hexosaminidase, Serum; NAG

Test Commonly Includes May include isolation of isoenzyme hexosaminidase A, B, and S. Patients with Tay-Sachs disease lack hexosaminidase A, while B may be normal or elevated.

Abstract Tay-Sachs disease is a fatal autosomal recessive lysosomal sphingolipid storage disorder characterized by hypotonia, blindness, seizures, and dementia. The enzyme includes the isoenzymes, hexosaminidase A, hexosaminidase B, and hexosaminidase S. In Tay-Sachs disease, isoenzyme A is missing and B and S may be increased. In Sandhoff disease, A and B are absent. This entity is clinically similar to Tay-Sachs disease.

Specimen Serum, plasma, white blood cells, cultured fibroblasts

Container Red top tube

Storage Instructions Store at -20°C.

Special Instructions Usually sent to reference laboratory.

Reference Range Hexosaminidase A isoenzyme: noncarriers, 450-600 µmol/hour/mL; Tay-Sachs homozygotes: none present; heterozygotes: 200-300 µmol/hour/mL. If isoenzyme A is <50% of total activity, carrier status is indicated.

Use Isoenzyme A is absent in serum of Tay-Sachs homozygotes. Isoenzyme A and B are absent in Sandhoff disease.

Limitations Total hexosaminidase levels are not useful for evaluation of Tay-Sachs disease. A mutant allele may prevent reliable measurement of enzyme activity when artificial substrates are employed.

Methodology DEAE chromatography followed by photometric or fluorometric assay of appropriate isoenzyme

Additional Information Hexosaminidase A can be measured in plasma, cultured fibroblasts or leukocytes as well as serum. Prenatal diagnosis of Tay-Sachs disease is done with amniocentesis or chorionic villus sampling.

References
Kaback M, Lim-Steele J, Dabholkar D, et al, "Tay-Sachs Disease - Carrier Screening, Prenatal Diagnosis, and the Molecular Era. An International Perspective, 1970 to 1993," *JAMA*, 1993, 270(19):2307-15.
Peleg L and Goldman B, "Detection of Tay-Sachs Disease Carriers Among Individuals With Thermolabile Hexosaminidase B," *Eur J Clin Chem Clin Biochem*, 1994, 32(2):65-9.
Wappner RS and Brandt IK, "Inborn Errors of Metabolism," *Principles and Practice of Pediatrics*, Oski F, DeAngelis CD, Feigin RD, et al, eds, Philadelphia, PA: JB Lippincott Co, 1994, 115-30.

Beta-Hydroxybutyrate *see* Ketone Bodies, Blood *on page 152*

Beta Lipoproteins *see* Low Density Lipoprotein Cholesterol *on page 162*

Beta-N-Acetylglucosaminidase *see* Beta-Hexosaminidase, Serum *on this page*

Beta-N-Acetylhexosaminidase *see* Beta-Hexosaminidase, Serum *on this page*

Beta Subunit, hCG *see* Human Chorionic Gonadotropin, Serum *on page 145*

Beta-Subunit Human Chorionic Gonadotropin Urine or Serum *see* Pregnancy Test *on page 190*

Beutler Test *see* Galactose Screening Tests for Galactosemia *on page 132*

BGP *see* Osteocalcin, Serum *on page 174*

Bicarbonate *see* HCO₃, Blood *on page 142*

Bicarbonate *see* Carbon Dioxide, Blood *on page 100*

Bilirubin, Conjugated *see* Bilirubin, Direct *on this page*

Bilirubin, Direct

CPT 82250

Related Information

Bile, Urine *on page 631*

Urobilinogen, 2-Hour Urine *on page 660*

Synonyms Bilirubin, Conjugated; Direct Bilirubin

Abstract The mono- and diconjugated bilirubin and delta bilirubin (tightly bound to albumin) account for the "direct" value. Elevated direct bilirubin is evidence of hepatobiliary disease.

Specimen Serum

Container Red top tube, red top Microtainer™ for babies

Collection Pediatrics: Blood drawn from a heelstick

Storage Instructions Store in refrigerator. **Protect from light.**

Causes for Rejection Specimen not protected from light, gross hemolysis

Special Instructions Transport promptly.

Reference Range Newborns: varies with age in days, prematurity vs maturity; adults: ≤0.4 mg/dL (SI: ≤7 µmol/L)

Use Evaluate liver and biliary disease. Increased direct bilirubin occurs with biliary diseases, including both intrahepatic and extrahepatic lesions. Hepatocellular causes of elevation include hepatitis, cirrhosis, and advanced neoplastic states. Increased with cholestatic drug reactions, Dubin-Johnson syndrome, and Rotor syndrome. In the latter two syndromes, the level is usually <5 mg/dL.

Limitations Cord blood samples may yield elevated values. Visibly hemolyzed samples may yield spurious results by some methods.

Contraindications Measurement of direct bilirubin is usually not necessary when the total bilirubin is <1.2 mg/dL (SI: <21 µmol/L).

Methodology Diazo reaction with spectrophotometry, high performance liquid chromatography (HPLC)

Additional Information Theoretically, direct bilirubin should not be increased in hemolytic anemias, in which bilirubin increase should be in the indirect bilirubin fraction in the absence of complications. In practice, some increase in the direct fraction may be encountered in patients with hemolytic anemia in whom complications have not been proven. Some methods have shown the direct bilirubin to be spuriously high. This may be due to different concentrations of sodium nitrite, which may convert some of the unconjugated bilirubin to conjugated bilirubin.[1,2] Direct bilirubin is the water soluble (conjugated) fraction. When conjugated bilirubin is increased in serum, bilirubin should become positive in the urine. Physiologic jaundice, occurring 2-4 days after birth, is due to lack of liver glucuronyl transferase.

Footnotes

1. Chan KM, Scott MG, Wu TW, et al, "Inaccurate Values for Direct Bilirubin With Some Commonly Used Direct Bilirubin Procedures," *Clin Chem*, 1985, 31(9):1560-3.
2. Mair B and Klempner LB, "Abnormally High Values for Direct Bilirubin in the Serum of Newborns as Measured With the Du Pont aca®," *Am J Clin Pathol*, 1987, 87(5):642-4.

References

Franquemont DW, Sutphen JL, Herold DA, et al, "Characterization of Sulfasalazine's Interference in the Measurement of Conjugated Bilirubin by the Ektachem® Slide Method," *Clin Chem*, 1989, 35(8):1760-2.

Newman TB, Hope S, and Stevenson DK, "Direct Bilirubin Measurements in Jaundiced Term Newborns. A Re-Evaluation," *Am J Dis Child*, 1991, 145(11):1305-9.

Rosenthal P, Keefe MT, Henton D, et al, "Total and Direct-Reacting Bilirubin Values by Automated Methods Compared With Liquid Chromatography and With Manual Methods for Determining Delta Bilirubin," *Clin Chem*, 1990, 36(5):788-91.

Bilirubin, Neonatal

CPT 82251

Related Information

Amniotic Fluid Analysis for Erythroblastosis Fetalis (OD 450) *on page 76*

Cord Blood Screen *on page 605*

Hemolytic Disease of the Newborn, Antibody Identification *on page 610*

Synonyms Baby Bilirubin; Microbilirubin; Total Bilirubin, Neonatal

Abstract Used to monitor diseases causing jaundice in the newborn, chiefly erythroblastosis fetalis

Specimen Serum

Container Microbilirubin tube

Collection Draw blood from heel using capillary pipette.

Storage Instructions Protect sample from light; bilirubin is photosensitive.

Reference Range Normal range depends on whether baby is premature or term, and age in days. See table.

Bilirubin, Neonatal Upper Reference Limit (mg/dL)

Age	Premature	Full-Term
Cord	2.9	2.5
<24 h	8.0	6.0
<48 h	12.0	10.0
3-5 d	15.0	12.0
7 d	15.0	10.0

Note: At 7 days, occasional premature infants may develop kernicterus at 10.0-12.0 mg/dL of bilirubin.

Possible Panic Range >15.0 mg/dL (SI: >257 µmol/L) in term infants, 10.0-15.0 mg/dL (SI: 171-257 µmol/L) in premature babies

Use Monitor erythroblastosis fetalis (hemolytic disease of the newborn), which usually causes jaundice in the first 2 days of life.[1] Other causes of neonatal jaundice include physiologic jaundice, hematoma/hemorrhage, hypothyroidism, Crigler-Najjar syndrome, and obstructive jaundice. Time sequences and differential diagnosis have been outlined.[1]

Limitations Only total bilirubin is measured with "neonatal bilirubin." Procedure is not utilized for patients older than 10 days of age due to formation of endogenous carotenoids. Ten percent fat emulsion has been reported to interfere with neonatal bilirubin measurement.[2]

Contraindications Request regular total bilirubin for infants older than 10 days of age.

Methodology Spectrophotometric, direct (bichromatic)

Additional Information Erythroblastosis fetalis occurs from Rh₀(D), other Rh antibodies, ABO incompatibility, and antibodies involving additional blood groups including Kidd, Kell and Duffy.

Causes of neonatal jaundice also include galactosemia, sepsis, syphilis, toxoplasmosis, cytomegalovirus, and rubella. Red cell enzyme problems include G-6-PD and pyruvate kinase deficiencies. Spherocytosis can lead to neonatal icterus.[3]

Drugs may displace bilirubin from albumin. It is the so-called "free" form of bilirubin, thus displaced, which crosses the blood-brain barrier.[4]

Jaundice may also be seen in babies who are breast feeding. Mothers sometimes want to stop breast feeding because of such jaundice. They should not be encouraged to cease breast feeding prematurely.[5]

Phototherapy reduces the need for exchange transfusions in premature babies who are Coombs' negative. In infants who weigh more than 2500 g and who are Coombs' positive, phototherapy was not significantly beneficial over control babies, and did not reduce the need for exchange transfusions.[6]

Footnotes

1. Thaler MM, "Jaundice in the Newborn," *Using the Clinical Laboratory in Medical Decision-Making*, Lundberg GD, ed, Chicago, IL: American Society of Clinical Pathologists, 1983, 33-9.
2. Moore JJ, Sax SM, and DeFranc S, "Liposyn® Interference With Neonatal Bilirubin Measurements," *Clin Chem*, 1982, 28:2334-5.
3. Polesky HF, "Diagnosis, Prevention, and Therapy in Hemolytic Disease of the Newborn," *Clin Lab Med*, 1982, 2:107-22.
4. Walker PC, "Neonatal Bilirubin Toxicity: A Review of Kernicterus and the Implication of Drug-Induced Bilirubin Displacement," *Clin Pharmacokinet*, 1987, 13(1):26-50.
5. Kemper K, Forsyth B, and McCarthy P, "Jaundice, Terminating Breast Feeding, and the Vulnerable Child," *Pediatrics*, 1989, 84(5):773-8.
6. Maurer HM, Kirkpatrick BV, McWilliams NB, et al, "Phototherapy for Hyperbilirubinemia of Hemolytic Disease of the Newborn," *Pediatrics*, 1985, 75(2 Pt 2):407-12.

References

Benaron DA and Bowen FW, "Variation of Initial Serum Bilirubin Rise in Newborn Infants With Type of Illness," *Lancet*, 1991, 338(8759):78-81.

Cashore WJ, "Neonatal Hyperbilirubinemia," *N Y State J Med*, 1991, 91(11):476-7.

Graziani LJ, Mitchell DG, Kornhauser M, et al, "Neurodevelopment of Preterm Infants: Neonatal Neurosonographic and Serum Bilirubin Studies," *Pediatrics*, 1992, 89(2):229-34.

Newman TB and Maisels MJ, "Bilirubin and Brain Damage: What Do We Do Now?" *Pediatrics*, 1989, 83(6):1062-5.

Scheidt PC, Graubard BI, Nelson KB, et al, "Intelligence at Six Years in Relation to Neonatal Bilirubin Levels: Follow-Up of the National Institute of Child Health and Human Development Clinical Trial of Phototherapy," *Pediatrics*, 1991, 87(6):797-805.

Seidman DS and Stevenson DK, "Neonatal Bilirubin," *Lancet*, 1992, 339(8784):65-6.

Bilirubin, Total

CPT 82250

Related Information

Alanine Aminotransferase *on page 65*

Alkaline Phosphatase, Serum *on page 69*

Amylase, Serum *on page 79*

Aspartate Aminotransferase *on page 84*

Bile, Urine *on page 631*

Gamma Glutamyl Transferase *on page 133*

Lipase, Serum *on page 158*

Liver Biopsy *on page 48*

Liver Profile *on page 161*
Urobilinogen, 2-Hour Urine *on page 660*

Synonyms Total Bilirubin

Applies to Fasting Bilirubin Test

Abstract Used to monitor diseases of the liver. Bilirubin may also be elevated in hemolytic diseases.

Specimen Serum

Container Red top tube; capillary tube for babies

Collection Blood drawn from a heelstick for babies.

Storage Instructions Protect sample from light.

Causes for Rejection Grossly hemolyzed specimen, specimen not protected from light

Reference Range Newborns: see table under Bilirubin, Neonatal *on page 86*; adults: 0.3-1.0 mg/dL (SI: 5-17 μmol/L)

Use Causes of **high bilirubin:** Liver disease: hepatitis, cholangitis, cholecystitis, even without common duct calculi; cirrhosis, other types of liver disease (including primary or secondary neoplasia); alcoholism (usually with high AST (SGOT), GGT, MCV, or some combination of these findings); biliary obstruction (intrahepatic or extrahepatic); infectious mononucleosis (look also for increased LD (LDH), lymphocytosis); Dubin-Johnson syndrome; Gilbert's disease[1] (familial hyperbilirubinemia) is encountered as a moderate elevation with otherwise unremarkable chemistries.

Anorexia or prolonged fasting: 36 hours or more may cause moderate rise.

Pernicious anemia, hemolytic anemias, erythroblastosis fetalis, other neonatal jaundice, hematoma and following a blood transfusion, especially if several units are given in a short time or with delayed hemolytic transfusion reaction.

Pulmonary embolism and/or infarct, congestive heart failure.

Drugs: A large number of drugs can cause jaundice by *in vivo* action or by chemistry methodology. Drugs causing cholestasis and/or hepatocellular damage include diphenylhydantoin, azathioprine, phenothiazines, erythromycin, penicillin, sulfonamides, oral contraceptives, anabolic-androgenic steroids, halothane, aminosalicylic acid, isoniazid, methyldopa, indomethacin, pyrazinamide, and others.

Limitations Differential diagnosis of liver diseases requires total and direct bilirubin values, as well as other tests. Visibly hemolyzed sera and lipemia can produce erroneous results.

Methodology Diazo reaction for adults; differential spectrophotometry for neonates (not useful for infants >10 days old)

Additional Information Total bilirubin is commonly available in chemistry multitest profiling instruments, in which it is a useful parameter. Interpretation of increased bilirubin is greatly enhanced by other chemistry results. In acute viral hepatitis with jaundice, for instance, the transaminases ALT (SGPT) and AST (SGOT) are consistently increased, while an isolated elevation of bilirubin is seen in Gilbert's disease.[1] **Obstruction** causes increases in bilirubin and alkaline phosphatase greater than and out of proportion to the transaminases.[2] Amylase and lipase are useful in differential diagnosis of obstructive jaundice. In **intrahepatic cholestasis,** the transaminases are not as increased, relative to bilirubin, as they are in hepatitis.[3] Work-up of jaundice has been outlined.[4,5]

Nicotinic acid increases the formation of bilirubin in the spleen, leading to a rise in unconjugated bilirubin. This can be used as a test for **Gilbert's disease**[1] in which there is a decreased hepatic clearance of unconjugated bilirubin with the criterion of basal total bilirubin >1.2 mg/dL. Although the indirect bilirubin level is increased in normal controls when nicotinic acid is given, the increase is greater in patients with Gilbert's disease. The **fasting bilirubin test** can be used to support the diagnosis of constitutional hyperbilirubinemia. It involves fasting for 24 hours following a light breakfast, with only 100 g of sucrose and water allowed. Unconjugated bilirubin increases 1 mg/dL in subjects with Gilbert's disease, or 1.5 mg/dL increase of total bilirubin.[6]

Acute liver failure caused by **Wilson's disease** is characterized by very high bilirubin, often >30 μg/dL (513 μmol/L) with decreased alkaline phosphatase. A ratio of alkaline phosphatase to bilirubin <2.0 is fairly distinctive.[7] In the **Crigler-Najjar** syndrome type I, the unconjugated bilirubin is >20 μg/dL. In type II, the level is <20 μg/dL.

Footnotes

1. Ohkubo H and Okuda K, "The Nicotinic Acid Test in Constitutional Conjugated Hyperbilirubinemia and Effects of Corticosteroids," *Hepatology*, 1984, 4(6):1206-8.
2. Scharschmidt BF, Goldberg HI, and Schmid R, "Current Concepts in Diagnosis. Approach to the Patient With Cholestatic Jaundice," *N Engl J Med*, 1983, 308:1515-9.
3. Goldberg DM, Spooner RJ, Ellis G, et al, "Biochemical Features of Intrahepatic Cholestasis," *Am J Clin Pathol*, 1979, 71:557-63.
4. Ostrow JD, "Jaundice in Older Children and Adults," *Using the Clinical Laboratory in Medical Decision Making*, Lundberg GD, ed, Chicago, IL: American Society of Clinical Pathologists, 1983, 41-8.

5. Fischer MG, Gelb AM, and Weingarten LA, "Cholestatic Jaundice in Adults," *Using the Clinical Laboratory in Medical Decision Making*, Lundberg GD, ed, Chicago, IL: American Society of Clinical Pathologists, 1983, 49-54.
6. Baldassare V and Ricci GL, "Specific Pattern of Unconjugated Bilirubin During Fasting Can Identify Constitutional Hyperbilirubinemia," *Ital J Gastroenterol*, 1993, 25(7):375-9.
7. Lee WM, "Acute Liver Failure," *N Engl J Med*, 1993, 329(25):1862-72.

References

Adachi Y, Katoh H, Fuchi I, et al, "Serum Bilirubin Fractions in Healthy Subjects and Patients With Unconjugated Hyperbilirubinemia," *Clin Biochem*, 1990, 23(3):247-51.

Donnachie EM, Seccombe DW, Urquhart NI, et al, "Indocyanine Green Interference in the Kodak Ektachem® Determination of Total Bilirubin," *Clin Chem*, 1989, 35(5):899-900.

Frank BB, "Clinical Evaluation of Jaundice - A Guideline of the Patient Care Committee of the American Gastroenterological Association," *JAMA*, 1989, 262(21):3031-4.

Helzberg JH and Spiro HM, "LFTs Test More Than the Liver," *JAMA*, 1986, 256(21):3006-7.

Kurzweil SM, Shapiro MJ, Andrus CH, et al, "Hyperbilirubinemia Without Common Bile Duct Abnormalities and Hyperamylasemia Without Pancreatitis in Patients With Gallbladder Disease," *Arch Surg*, 1994, 129(8):829-33.

Lepage L and Trivin F, "Total Bilirubin," *Drug Effects on Laboratory Test Results Analytical Interferences and Pharmacological Effects*, Siest G and Galteau MM, eds, Littleton, MA: PSG Publishing Co Inc, 1988, 131-47.

Westwood A, "The Analysis of Bilirubin in Serum," *Ann Clin Biochem*, 1991, 28(Pt 2):119-30.

Biotin *see* Lactic Acid, Blood *on page 156*

Biotinidase *see* Amino Acid Screen, Plasma *on page 74*

Blood Gases, Arterial

CPT 82803

Related Information

Arterial Blood Collection *on page 24*
Carbon Dioxide, Blood *on page 100*
Carboxyhemoglobin *on page 541*
HCO_3, Blood *on page 142*
Lactic Acid, Blood *on page 156*
Methemoglobin *on page 166*
Oxygen Saturation, Blood *on page 175*
pCO_2, Blood *on page 179*
pH, Blood *on page 180*
Phlebotomy, Therapeutic *on page 614*

Synonyms ABGs; Arterial Blood Gases; Gases, Arterial

Applies to Oxygen Content; Oxygen Saturation; pCO_2; pH; pO_2

Test Commonly Includes Measured results include pH, pCO_2 ($PaCO_2$), pO_2 (PaO_2), hematocrit, and may also include electrolytes, and ionized calcium. Calculated values include total carbon dioxide (TCO_2), bicarbonate (HCO_3^-), oxygen saturation, base excess, alveolar-arterial (A-a) gradient, and P_{50} (pO_2 at half saturation of hemoglobin) offered by some laboratories. Standard bicarbonate concentration (SBc), base excess of extracellular fluid, carboxyhemoglobin, methemoglobin, normalized calcium, hemoglobin content, and anion gap and osmolality (if electrolytes measured) may also be provided as calculations.

Abstract These measurements are used to evaluate oxygen and carbon dioxide exchange, respiratory function, and some aspects of acid-base balance.

Patient Preparation Patient should be supine, relaxed. The patient's temperature should be recorded.

Aftercare Watch for bleeding, hematoma. Ideally, extremity punctured should be kept up for 10 minutes with pressure applied to the puncture site if the patient is not on anticoagulants. If patient is receiving heparin, pressure must be applied to puncture site for a minimum of 15 minutes. Arterial puncture may be especially hazardous in the anticoagulated patient. However, there is frequently simultaneous need for arterial blood gases and for anticoagulation. See listing Arterial Blood Collection *on page 24.*

Specimen Whole blood

Container Heparinized syringe or through an indwelling arterial line

Collection Very small diameter needles are used. Specimen is drawn into air-free heparinized syringe, then stoppered. The radial artery is commonly used, utilizing the Allen test. The Allen test is used to assess the presence of normal collateral circulation. The brachial artery is the second choice. **All specimens should be on ice and brought to the laboratory immediately.** Mode of oxygen delivery or room air must be indicated. Rapid changes may occur if collected immediately after exercise.[1] Avoid excessive heparin. Strict anaerobiosis must be maintained. **Blood drawn from a vein or capillary can provide helpful information including pH, pCO_2, and, occasionally, pO_2.**

Storage Instructions Place on ice. The following *in vitro* changes occur in blood gas parameters:[2] pH, 0.001/10 minutes at 4°C, pCO_2, 0.1 mm Hg/10 minutes at 4°C, pO_2, 3 mm Hg/10 minutes at 4°C. No difference exists between glass and plastic syringes.

(Continued)

Blood Gases, Arterial (Continued)

Causes for Rejection Specimen **not** received on ice, air bubbles or clots in syringe

Special Instructions Sample obtained just after a change in inspired oxygen concentration (FiO_2) (eg, room air or quantity of therapeutic oxygen delivered) is apt to generate confusing results.

Reference Range Arterial pH: 7.35-7.45; TCO_2: 23-29 mmol/L; pCO_2: 35-45 mm Hg; pO_2: adult: 80-95 mm Hg, newborn: 60-70 mm Hg; O_2: 95% to 99% saturation. Such ranges must be interpreted in light of the FiO_2 and other parameters.

Possible Panic Range pH <7.2, >7.55; pCO_2 <20 mm Hg, >60 mm Hg; pO_2 <40 mm Hg

Use Evaluate oxygen and carbon dioxide gas exchange, respiratory function including hypoxia, and acid-base status. Assess asthma, chronic obstructive pulmonary disease (COPD), and other types of lung disease,[3] embolism including fat embolism, and coronary arterial bypass surgical cases.

ARTERIAL BLOOD GAS QUALITY ASSURANCE AND APPROPRIATENESS REVIEW:

In the following lists, clinical judgment is required. Many of the clinical entities listed do not necessarily require blood gas analysis.

Criteria:

Severe cardiorespiratory disturbances:
- shock
- cardiac arrest
- coma
- acute respiratory failure
- acute infarct, myocardium with complications
- severe congestive heart failure
- pulmonary edema
- serious disturbances of cardiac rhythm
- unexplained right heart failure
- suspected R-L shunt evaluation
- evaluate V/Q abnormality

Investigate cardiorespiratory, metabolic, central nervous system disturbances:
- shortness of breath by history, if indicated
- unexplained tachypnea, if indicated
- unexplained dyspnea, if indicated
- lung disease, if indicated
- decompensated established lung disease
- deep vein thrombus
- suspected pulmonary embolism, including fat embolism
- pneumonia
- unexplained polycythemia, erythrocytosis
- unexplained mental status abnormalities
- cyanosis
- smoke inhalation, possibly with CO intoxication
- toxin ingestion (CN, ASA, methanol, ethylene glycol)
- rule out carboxyhemoglobinemia or methemoglobinemia
- monitor oxygen therapy as medically needed
- home oxygen management, selected instances
- exercise, oxygen therapy
- occasional fracture
- metabolic acidosis and alkalosis, selected instances
- electrolyte disturbances (abnormal bicarbonate level, anion gap), selected cases
- change in patient's clinical status
- rest and exercise pulmonary function testing
- sleep disorder work-up

Miscellaneous medical/surgical conditions:
- change in ventilatory settings, if indicated
- contemplated prolonged anesthesia
- contemplated major abdominal surgery, if indicated
- contemplated pulmonary resection
- chest pain, pleurisy, if indicated
- abnormal chest x-ray with clinical indications
- follow-up abnormal ABG, if indicated
- follow O_2 prescription if needed
- during or following surgery, if indicated
- abnormal oxygen saturation, if indicated
- during dialysis, if needed
- after prescription of $NaHCO_3$ or Na citrate, if indicated
- Kussmaul respiration
- uncontrolled diabetes with suspected acidosis, as medically indicated
- previous pH <7.35 or 7.30, if indicated
- renal failure (creatinine >4 mg/dL (SI: >353 μmol/L) or creatinine clearance <25 mL/min), if indicated
- profuse diarrhea, if indicated
- history of renal tubular acidosis (RTA), if indicated
- ureterosigmoidostomy, if indicated
- pancreatic, small bowel or biliary drainage, if indicated
- nausea/vomiting, nasogastric drainage, if indicated
- hypokalemia, diuretic use, if indicated

In ill adults who are stable, blood gas analysis is considered when a change in clinical management is considered or when an alteration in the patient's clinical status develops.

Limitations Arterial puncture may be extremely difficult in some individuals. O_2 saturation is calculated on assumption of 100% A hemoglobin. Reported value may be misleading when hemoglobins with different dissociation curves are present. Calculations commonly assume body temperature of 37°C.

When hemoglobin is reported with blood gases, it usually is a screening hemoglobin, which is less reliable than a conventional hemoglobin ordered as such.

Variability of results occurs;[3,4] changes in pO_2 in isolated reports must be interpreted cautiously and in light of data trends, oxygen delivery, and the patient's clinical appearance. Such variation occurs without change in FiO_2 or the patient's clinical status.

Correlation of arterial gases with pulmonary function testing and with severity in asthma was reported as poor.[5]

ABGs are of little value in treatment decisions for carbon monoxide poisoning.[6]

Complications of arterial puncture potentially include hematoma, bleeding, arterial occlusion, infection, and, very rarely, gangrene.

Although normal pO_2 diminishes the likelihood of pulmonary embolism, the former does not rule out the latter. (Alveolar-arterial gradient usually is widened in pulmonary embolism.)

Methodology Selective electrodes measuring pH, pCO_2, and pO_2

Additional Information The pH, pCO_2 and pO_2 are measured directly while the hemoglobin, carboxyhemoglobin, and methemoglobin are measured and calculated using spectrophotometric analysis at specific wavelengths and electronic representation of mathematical relationships. It is assumed that largely normal A hemoglobin is present (most importantly that there are no significant levels of fetal hemoglobin.)
Methemoglobin levels <10% are subject to about a 1% error; but with methemoglobin levels >10%, the error is at about the 10% level. (See listing Methemoglobin on page 166.) High serum bilirubin levels do not contribute to error. Methylene blue (used in treatment of some forms of methemoglobinemia) may interfere and result in nonrepresentative methemoglobin and other hemoglobin measurements. Sulfhemoglobin is a cause of spectral interference.

"Hypoxemia" can be defined as pO_2 <80 mm Hg, but other, more sophisticated definitions are available.[7]

Raffin points out that few studies are available to indicate how many arterial samples are actually indicated. He observes that a complete list of clinical settings involving ill patients in whom blood gas studies might be indicated would include much of the tables of contents of general medicine texts.[7]

The combination of pH values <7.25 without elevation of pCO_2, may indicate need for a lactic acid determination.

Nonsurvivors in a group of COPD patients had lower arterial oxygen tension and higher carbon dioxide tension.[8,9]

The **acute respiratory distress syndrome (ARDS)** is usually initially characterized by respiratory alkalosis and hypoxemia. This complex response to pulmonary injury requires insight to enhance survival.[10]

Exercise testing with ABG has been advocated for patients in congestive heart failure. Hypoxemia is rare on exercise in subjects in stable congestive failure. Hypoxemia on exercise may indicate an alternative diagnosis.[11] Assessment of acid-base status of tissues in patients in circulatory failure may be misleading if only arterial blood gas data is available. Adrogué presents data supporting the need for information on **mixed venous** as well as arterial gases in care of critically ill patients.[12]

Footnotes

1. Ries AL, Fedullo PF, and Clausen JL, "Rapid Changes in Arterial Blood Gas Levels After Exercise in Pulmonary Patients," *Chest*, 1983, 83:454-6.
2. Bruegger BB and Sherwin JE, "Blood Gas Analysis and Oxygen Saturation," *Methods in Clinical Chemistry*, Chapter 8, Pesce AJ and Kaplan LA, eds, St Louis, MO: Mosby-Year Book Inc, 1987, 54-66.
3. Thorson SH, Marini JJ, Pierson PJ, et al, "Variability of Arterial Blood Gas Values in Stable Patients in the ICU," *Chest*, 1983, 84:14-8.
4. Sasse SA, Chen PA, and Mahutte CK, "Variability of Arterial Blood Gas Values Over Time in Stable Medical ICU Patients," *Chest*, 1994, 106(1):187-93.
5. Nowak RM, Tomlanovich MC, Sarkar DD, et al, "Arterial Blood Gases and Pulmonary Function Testing in Acute Bronchial Asthma. Predicting Patient Outcomes," *JAMA*, 1983, 249:2043-6.
6. Myers RA and Britten JS, "Are Arterial Blood Gases of Value in Treatment Decisions for Carbon Monoxide Poisoning?" *Crit Care Med*, 1989, 17(2):139-42.
7. Raffin TA, "Indications for Arterial Blood Gas Analysis," *Ann Intern Med*, 1986, 105(3):390-8.

8. Kawakami Y, Kishi F, Yamamoto H, et al, "Relation of Oxygen Delivery, Mixed Venous Oxygenation, and Pulmonary Hemodynamics to Prognosis in Chronic Obstructive Pulmonary Disease," *N Engl J Med*, 1983, 308:1045-9.
9. Bergofsky EH, "Tissue Oxygen Delivery and Cor Pulmonale in Chronic Obstructive Pulmonary Disease," *N Engl J Med*, 1983, 308:1092-4.
10. Kollef MH and Schuster DP, "The Acute Respiratory Distress Syndrome," *N Engl J Med*, 1995, 332(1):27-37.
11. Clark AL and Coats AJ, "Usefulness of Arterial Blood Gas Estimations During Exercise in Patients With Chronic Heart Failure," *Br Heart J*, 1994, 71(6):528-30.
12. Adrogué HJ, Rashad MN, Gorin AB, et al, "Assessing Acid-Base Status in Circulatory Failure: Differences Between Arterial and Central Venous Blood," *N Engl J Med*, 1989, 320(20):1312-6.

References
Anderson S, "ABGs. Six Easy Steps to Interpreting Blood Gases," *Am J Nurs*, 1990, 90(8):42-5.
Charan NB, Marks M, and Carvalho P, "Use of Plasma for Arterial Blood Gas Analysis in Leukemia," *Chest*, 1994, 105(3):954-5.
Courtney SE, Weber KR, Breakie LA, et al, "Capillary Blood Gases in the Neonate. A Reassessment and Review of the Literature," *Am J Dis Child*, 1990, 144(2):168-72.
Delclaux B, Orcel B, Housset B, et al, "Arterial Blood Gases in Elderly Persons With Chronic Obstructive Pulmonary Disease (COPD)," *Eur Respir J*, 1994, 7(5):856-61.
Eichhorn JH, "Performance Characteristics for Devices Measuring pO_2 and pCO_2 in Blood Samples," *National Committee for Clinical Laboratory Standards*, 1989.
Hansen JE, "Arterial Blood Gases," *Clin Chest Med*, 1989, 10(2):227-37.
Hibbard JU, Hibbard MC, and Whalen MP, "Umbilical Cord Blood Gases and Mortality and Morbidity in the Very Low Birth Weight Infant," *Obstet Gynecol*, 1991, 78(5 Pt 1):768-73.
Meyer BA, Dickinson JE, Chambers C, et al, "The Effect of Fetal Sepsis on Umbilical Cord Blood Gases," *Am J Obstet Gynecol*, 1992, 166(2):612-7.
Pierson DJ, "Pulse Oximetry Versus Arterial Blood Gas Specimens in Long-Term Oxygen Therapy," *Lung*, 1990, 168(Suppl):782-8.
Ribbert LS, Snijders RJ, Nicolaides KH, et al, "Relation of Fetal Blood Gases and Data From Computer-Assisted Analysis of Fetal Heart Rate Patterns in Small for Gestation Fetuses," *Br J Obstet Gynaecol*, 1991, 98(8):820-3.

Blood Gases, Capillary

CPT 82803

Related Information

Carbon Dioxide, Blood *on page 100*

pCO_2, Blood *on page 179*

pH, Blood *on page 180*

Synonyms Capillary Blood Gases

Test Commonly Includes Measured results include pH, pCO_2 ($PaCO_2$), pO_2 (PaO_2), hematocrit, and may also include electrolytes, and ionized calcium. Calculated values include total carbon dioxide (TCO_2), bicarbonate (HCO_3^-), oxygen saturation, oxygen content, base excess, alveolar-arterial (A-a) gradient, and P_{50} offered by some laboratories. Standard bicarbonate concentration (SBc), base excess of extracellular fluid, carboxyhemoglobin, methemoglobin, normalized calcium, hemoglobin content, and anion gap and osmolality (if electrolytes measured) may also be provided as calculations.

Abstract Capillary pH and pCO_2 are entirely adequate for many purposes. Usually used for monitoring blood gases in neonates or other patients in whom arterial puncture is not practical

Patient Preparation Nursing staffs have traditionally, in many hospitals, prewarmed the heel. However, *vide infra*. The puncture should be deep enough to allow a free flow of blood. Blood is then collected in heparinized capillary tubes, which should be filled as much as possible, capped and mixed well.

Aftercare Apply pressure on site for 5-10 minutes, apply bandaid.

Specimen Whole blood

Container Two heparinized 250 µL capillary tubes capped tightly with internal mixing flea

Collection Fill both tubes completely excluding any air bubbles, mix immediately with heparin to avoid clotting. A 2.5 mm x 1.5 mm microlancet may be used for skin punctures. See listing Skin Puncture Blood Collection *on page 28*.

Storage Instructions Immediately put in iced water.

Causes for Rejection No heparin, sample clotted, specimen not received on ice

Reference Range pH: 7.35-7.45, pO_2: >90 mm Hg, pCO_2: 26.4-41.2 mm Hg, O_2 saturation: 95% to 99%

Use Acid base balance. Although capillary blood is satisfactory for most purposes for pH and pCO_2, the role of capillary pO_2 is limited to exclusion of hypoxia.[1] Capillary blood sampling is less likely to cause complications than is arterial puncture.

Methodology Specific electrodes

Additional Information Warming the heel, a traditional practice, made no difference in a study from Leeds.[1]

Footnotes

1. McLain BI, Evans J, Dear PR, et al, "Comparison of Capillary and Arterial Blood Gas Measurements in Neonates," *Arch Dis Child*, 1988, 63(7 Spec No):743-7.

References
Couriel JM, "Interpretation of Blood Gas Analysis," *Indian J Pediatr*, 1988, 55(5):656-60.
Dong SH, Liu HM, Song GW, et al, "Arterialized Capillary Blood Gases and Acid-Base Studies in Normal Individuals From 29 Days to 24 Years of Age," *Am J Dis Child*, 1985, 139(10):1019-22.

Blood Gases, Venous

CPT 82803

Related Information

Carbon Dioxide, Blood *on page 100*

pH, Blood *on page 180*

Synonyms Venous Blood Gases

Applies to Central Venous Blood

Test Commonly Includes Measured results include pH, pCO_2 ($PaCO_2$), pO_2 (PaO_2), hematocrit, and may also include electrolytes, and ionized calcium. Calculated values include total carbon dioxide (TCO_2), bicarbonate (HCO_3^-), oxygen saturation, oxygen content, base excess, alveolar-arterial (A-a) gradient, and P_{50} offered by some laboratories. Standard bicarbonate concentration (SBc), base excess of extracellular fluid, carboxyhemoglobin, methemoglobin, normalized calcium, hemoglobin content, and anion gap and osmolality (if electrolytes measured) may also be provided as calculations.

Abstract Determination of pH and pCO_2 can be done reliably from venous blood in most clinical situations, but measurements involving oxygen are not usually useful when done on venous blood.

Patient Preparation The patient should be supine, relaxed.

Specimen Whole blood

Container Heparinized syringe, green top (heparin) tube

Collection Draw specimen into air-free heparinized syringe or green top vacuum blood collection tube. If a vacuum blood collection tube is used, it must be removed from needle before needle is removed from patient's arm. Keep sample on ice. Indicate specimen source (ie, venous) and mode of oxygen delivery or room air if applicable on requisition.

Storage Instructions Keep specimen on ice.

Causes for Rejection Specimen **not** received on ice, specimen clotted

Reference Range Venous pH: 7.32-7.43, TCO_2: 23-30 mmol/L, pCO_2: 38-50 mm Hg, pO_2 should be about 40 mm Hg, O_2 saturation should be about 75%.

Use Evaluate cellular hypoxia, acid-base balance. A major use is to obtain pH in infants, children, and adults in whom oxygen parameters are not needed, without arterial puncture. In many metabolic situations a venous pH is adequate for pH, and arterial puncture is unnecessary. Both arterial and central venous blood samples play a role in assessment of acid-base status in subjects in critical hemodynamic compromise. With severe hypoperfusion central venous blood better detects hypercapnia and acidemia.[1] The pO_2, pCO_2, and pH from pulmonary arterial samples correlate with central venous specimens.[2]

Limitations In hypotensive subjects with severe circulatory failure, Adrogué et al describe substantial differences between mean arterial and central venous pH and pCO_2.[1]

Methodology Specific electrodes

Additional Information The arteriovenous pH difference is usually extremely small (0.01-0.03), except in patients in congestive heart failure and in shock. The differences in pH and pCO_2 widen only slightly with moderate cardiac failure.[1] Total CO_2 values are slightly higher in venous blood than in arterial blood. Arterial blood, however, must be used to accurately measure pO_2 and oxygen saturation.

Footnotes

1. Adrogué HJ, Rashad MN, Gorin AB, et al, "Assessing Acid-Base Status in Circulatory Failure: Differences Between Arterial and Central Venous Blood," *N Engl J Med*, 1989, 320(20):1312-6.
2. Eichhorn JH, "Accuracy and Comparisons in Blood Gas Measurements," *Chest*, 1988, 94(1):1-2.

Blood Gas P-50 *see* P-50 Blood Gas *on page 176*

Blood Lactate *see* Lactic Acid, Blood *on page 156*

Blood pH *see* pH, Blood *on page 180*

Blood Spot Screen for Galactose/Galactose-1-Phosphate *see* Galactose Screening Tests for Galactosemia *on page 132*

Blood Sugar, Fasting *see* Glucose, Fasting *on page 137*

Blood Urea Nitrogen *see* Urea Nitrogen, Blood *on page 213*

Body Fluid

CPT 89051 (cell count with differential)

Related Information

Alpha$_1$-Fetoprotein, Serum *on page 72*

Amniotic Fluid Creatinine *on page 77*

Bacterial Culture, Biopsy or Body Fluid *on page 456*

Body Fluid Amylase *on page 91*

Body Fluid Analysis, Cell Count *on page 306*

Body Fluid Cytology *on page 286*

Body Fluid Glucose *on page 91*

Body Fluid Lactate Dehydrogenase *on page 92*

Body Fluid pH *on page 92*

(Continued)

Body Fluid (Continued)

Synonyms Ascitic Fluid Analysis; Fluid, Peritoneal; Fluid, Pleural; Paracentesis Fluid Analysis; Pericardial Fluid Analysis; Peritoneal Fluid Analysis; Pleural Fluid Analysis; Thoracentesis Fluid Analysis

Applies to Albs-a; Albumin, Ascites Fluid; CEA, Body Fluid; Cyst Fluid Chemistry; Lactic Acid, Body Fluid; LD, Body Fluid; Protein, Body Fluids; Rheumatoid Factor, Body Fluid; Serum-Ascites Albumin Gradient

Test Commonly Includes Tests commonly helpful in work-up of a fluid include **cell count** and differential, hemoglobin/hematocrit, **glucose, LDH, albumin**, specific gravity, **amylase** and pH. **Protein** quantitation, as in the table, is somewhat useful for pleural fluid but is less reliable for peritoneal fluid. **Cultures** are commonly indicated, require a sterile specimen, and generally are ordered for routine, anaerobic, TB and sometimes fungi. **Gram's and acid-fast smears** are often desirable. **Cytology** and **tumor markers** may be indicated.

Abstract The differential diagnosis of fluid collections from pericardial, pleural, and peritoneal spaces includes entities which include malignancy, bacterial, and viral infection, other inflammatory disorders (eg, pancreatitis), hepatic cirrhosis, prior irradiation, and (in the case of the pericardial sac) uremia.

Patient Preparation Usual aseptic aspiration procedure

Specimen Body fluid (ie, ascitic fluid, pleural fluid, etc)

Container Red top tube, lavender top (EDTA) tube, and green top (heparin) tube; sterile containers for microbiologic cultures

Collection Body fluids are usually worked up in several laboratory sections. A common error is not to provide sufficient quantity of fluid for adequate examinations. A simultaneous blood specimen drawn for serum chemistry is often needed (eg, for albumin to calculate the serum ascites albumin gradient).

Special Instructions Laboratory must be made aware of the source of the specimen.

Reference Range Pathologic fluids: When such fluids as pleural or peritoneal transudates or exudates are examined, no normal ranges exist because such fluids by their very nature are not normal.

Use Evaluate effusions; diagnose transudate versus exudate. Transudates are colorless to yellow, clear, and do not clot. Exudates may be opaque to purulent, contain fibrinogen, and may clot (thus, green top tubes are needed for cytology). Causes of **transudates** include hepatic cirrhosis, congestive heart failure, and the nephrotic syndromes. **Exudates** are caused by various types of infection including TB, esophageal or other hollow viscus rupture, abscess such as subphrenic or liver abscess, neoplasia, the rheumatoid arthritis state, pancreatitis, embolization or lung infarct, trauma, and systemic LE.[1]

Limitations Postural changes are significant for measurement of pH, LDH, red blood cells, and protein in exudates but not in transudates in pleural effusions.[2]

Additional Information Cytology is often critically important. Lung and breast carcinoma are the two most common tumors causing pleural effusion. **CEA, CA 15-3, and CA 19-9** may be useful, additional to exfoliative cytology, in work-up for cancer.[3] Additionally, **CA 125** can be helpful in selected cases.

Other tests sometimes helpful include **pH**, especially in chest fluids. **Urea nitrogen (BUN)** is helpful if a question of bladder content versus ascitic fluid exists.

Test green fluids for **bilirubin**; if positive, consider perforated intestine, peptic ulcer, or gallbladder.

Bloody fluids, if not caused by traumatic tap, are exudates. TB as well as infarct or cancer must be considered. **Hematocrit** of the fluid is useful for diagnosis of hemothorax or hemoperitoneum (eg, trauma).

Chylous fluids appear milky. Chylous effusion contains chylomicrons and has very high **triglycerides**. Such effusions relate to trauma and lymphoma; carcinoma and tuberculosis also are reported to cause chylous effusion.[1]

High levels of **rheumatoid factor** in a pleural fluid support a diagnosis of rheumatoid effusion, while in SLE, rheumatoid factor titers are apt to be only about 1:40.[4]

Peritoneal and pleural fluid **lactic acid** is increased with infection. In uninfected ascites, ascitic fluid lactate was 15±5 mg/dL (SI: 1.7±0.6

mmol/L), while in bacterial peritonitis, 14 patients ranged 45±37 mg/dL (SI: 5.0±4.1 mmol/L). A cutoff >25 mg/dL (SI: >2.8 mmol/L) is suggested.[5] Lactic acid may also be increased in malignant disease in body fluids.

The differential diagnosis of ascites includes cancer and hepatic cirrhosis. The **ratio of LD (LDH)** in serum to that of ascitic fluid is helpful. Ratios of less than unity occur with malignant disease, while ratios >1 are reported mostly with cirrhosis, when these two groups are compared.[6] However, a few instances of cancer have ratios greater than unity.[6] The LD of the ascitic fluid of cirrhosis is usually <60% that of serum.[7]

Albumin in body fluids is the main determinant of oncotic pressure. Calculate the **serum-ascites albumin gradient** by subtraction of albumin value of the fluid from that of serum. The gradient between serum and ascites may be expressed as **"Albs-a"**, referring to albumin concentration. It correlates with portal pressure, the pressure gradient between the portal capillaries and the peritoneal cavity.[8,9] Gradients ≥1.1 g/dL (SI: 11 g/L) correlate with portal hypertension. Serum/ascites albumin gradient is greater in transudates (1.6±0.5 g/dL) than exudates (0.6±0.4 g/dL).[1] According to serum-ascites albumin gradient, disease states related to high gradients (albs-a ≥1.1 g/dL) include cirrhosis, alcoholic hepatitis, cardiac failure, massive liver metastases, fulminant hepatic failure, Budd-Chiari syndrome, portal vein thrombosis, veno-occlusive disease, fatty liver of pregnancy, and myxedema.[10] Constrictive pericarditis is usually associated with high gradient. **Low gradients** are found with peritoneal carcinomatosis and tuberculosis, pancreatic and biliary ascites, nephrotic syndrome, serositis, and bowel obstruction or infarct.[10] Other diseases reported with low gradients include myxedema, SLE, certain ovarian diseases, and severe hypoalbuminemia.[7,8]

"High protein ascites," >2.5 g total protein/dL (SI: >25 g/L), is found in 15% to 20% of subjects who have hepatic disease, while a similar fraction of patients with malignant disease have **"low protein ascites."**[8]

Since **secondary peritonitis** often requires surgery, its distinction from spontaneous peritonitis is critical. Secondary peritonitis is characterized by total protein ≥1.0 g/dL, fluid LDH greater than upper limit of normal for serum, glucose <50 mg/dL, and polymicrobial infection.[10] See, as well, the listing Body Fluid Amylase *on page 91*.

Cholesterol levels have been studied in pleural[11] and ascitic[12] fluids and may prove useful in differential diagnosis of body fluids. Discrimination between ascites of hepatocellular carcinoma and other malignant entities is supported by assays of ascitic fluid cholesterol and LDH.[13] The usefulness of fluid cholesterol has recently been questioned.[10] See table.

Body Fluid

	Transudate	Exudate
WBC/mm³	<100/mm³	>1000/mm³
Specific gravity	<1.016	>1.016
Total protein	<2.5-3.0 g/dL	>3.0 g/dL
LD (LDH)	Similar to serum LD or lower	Fluid LD to serum LD ratio >0.6 or LD >200 units/L
Glucose		Low – especially in rheumatoid effusion
Cholesterol pleural	<60 mg/dL (SI: <1.55 mmol/L)	>60 mg/dL (SI: >1.55 mmol/L)
Cholesterol ascitic	<46 mg/dL (SI: <1.19 mmol/L)	>46 mg/dL (SI: >1.19 mmol/L)

The separation between transudate and exudate is blurring; Albs-a (serum-ascites albumin difference) provides useful information – see text.

Malignant tumors give rise to fluids commonly more similar to **exudates** than to **transudates**. Although cytology is more useful than chemistry for tumor diagnosis, false-negatives are not uncommon; sensitivity is only 40% to 60%.

Tumor markers are also useful in body fluids, including CEA[14] and CA 125.[14,15] CEA increases occur with many carcinomas primary in the gastrointestinal tract, breast, and lung. CEA level is normal with lymphoma and mesothelioma. CA 125 increased without high CEA is consistent with primary carcinoma of ovary, fallopian tube or endometrium, but may occur with stage III or IV endometriosis.[15] CEA is commonly negative in müllerian carcinomas but positive with mucinous cystadenocarcinoma of ovary.[11] (Adenocarcinoma primary in the endocervix is often CEA positive.) Normal CEA and CA 125 in malignant fluids suggest possible mesothelioma, melanoma, or lymphoma.[14]

Hepatocellular carcinoma gives rise to ascites, but implants of malignant cells are only rarely found in the peritoneum. Chemical analysis is useful.[13]

Pericardial fluid specimens are usually exudates. (Such fluids are selected by having been tapped. Pericarditis related to the uremic state is not usually sampled, for instance.) Significant palliation may be achieved with diagnosis and therapy of some malignant effusions (eg, of pericardium, in which primaries include lung, breast, esophagus, and lymphoma).[16]

In descending order, **causes of ascites** in the U.S. are listed as cirrhosis (predominantly alcohol related), cancer, heart failure, tuberculosis, dialysis, and pancreatic disease.[10]

Footnotes

1. Kjeldsberg CR and Knight JA, *Body Fluids - Laboratory Examination of Amniotic, Cerebrospinal, Seminal, Serous, and Synovial Fluids*, 3rd ed, Chicago, IL: American Society of Clinical Pathologists, 1993, 159-253, 186-7.
2. Brandstetter RD, Velazquez V, Viejo C, et al, "Postural Changes in Pleural Fluid Constituents," *Chest*, 1994, 105(5):1458-61.
3. Couch WD, "Combined Effusion Fluid Tumor Marker Assay, Carcinoembryonic Antigen (CEA) and Human Chorionic Gonadotropin (hCG), in the Detection of Malignant Tumors," *Cancer*, 1981, 48:2475-9.
4. Dines DE, "Studies on Pleural Fluid," *Mayo Clin Proc*, 1981, 56:460.
5. Garcia-Tsao G, Conn HO, and Lerner E, "The Diagnosis of Bacterial Peritonitis: Comparison of pH, Lactate Concentration and Leukocyte Count," *Hepatology*, 1985, 5(1):91-6.
6. Greene LS, Levine R, Gross MJ, et al, "Distinguishing Between Malignant and Cirrhotic Ascites by Computerized Step-Wise Discriminant Functional Analysis of Its Biochemistry," *Am J Gastroenterol*, 1978, 70:448-54.
7. Rector WG Jr, "An Improved Diagnostic Approach to Ascites," *Arch Intern Med*, 1987, 147(2):215.
8. Marshall JB and Vogele KA, "Serum-Ascites Albumin Differences in Tuberculous Peritonitis," *Am J Gastroenterol*, 1988, 83(11):1259-61.
9. Rector WG Jr and Reynolds TB, "Superiority of the Serum-Ascites Albumin Difference Over the Ascites Total Protein Concentration in Separation of "Transudative" and "Exudative" Ascites," *Am J Med*, 1984, 77(1):83-5.
10. Runyon BA, "Care of Patients With Ascites," *N Engl J Med*, 1994, 330(5):337-42.
11. Hamm H, Brohan U, Bohmer R, et al, "Cholesterol in Pleural Effusions. A Diagnostic Aid," *Chest*, 1987, 92(2):296-302.
12. Prieto M, Gómez-Lechón MJ, Hoyos M, et al, "Diagnosis of Malignant Ascites: Comparison of Ascitic Fibronectin, Cholesterol, and Serum-Ascites Albumin Difference," *Dig Dis Sci*, 1988, 33(7):833-8.
13. Castaldo G, Oriani G, Cimino L, et al, "Total Discrimination of Peritoneal Malignant Ascites From Cirrhosis- and Hepatocarcinoma-Associated Ascites by Assays of Ascitic Cholesterol and Lactate Dehydrogenase," *Clin Chem*, 1994, 40(3):478-83.
14. Pinto MM, Bernstein LH, Brogan DA, et al, "Immunoradiometric Assay of CA 125 in Effusions: Comparison With Carcinoembryonic Antigen," *Cancer*, 1987, 59(2):218-22.
15. Dawood MY, Khan-Dawood FS, and Ramos J, "Plasma and Peritoneal Fluid Levels of CA 125 in Women With Endometriosis," *Am J Obstet Gynecol*, 1988, 159(6):1526-31.
16. Wilkes JD, Fidias P, Vaickus L, et al, "Malignancy-Related Pericardial Effusion. 127 Cases From the Roswell Park Cancer Institute," *Cancer*, 1995, 76(8):1377-87.

References

Bac DJ, Siersema PD, and Wilson JH, "Paracentesis. The Importance of Optimal Ascitic Fluid Analysis," *Neth J Med*, 1993, 43(3-4):147-55.
Horowitz ML, Schiff M, Samuels J, et al, "*Pneumocystis carinii* Pleural Effusion. Pathogenesis and Pleural Fluid Analysis," *Am Rev Respir Dis*, 1993, 148(1):232-4.
Kiltz RJ, Burke MS, and Porreco RP, "Amniotic Fluid Glucose Concentration as a Marker for Intra-amniotic Infection," *Obstet Gynecol*, 1991, 78(4):619-22.
Paavonen T, Liippo K, Aronen H, et al, "Lactate Dehydrogenase, Creatine Kinase, and Their Isoenzymes in Pleural Effusions," *Clin Chem*, 1991, 37(11):1909-12.
Rocco VK and Ware AJ, "Cirrhotic Ascites," *Ann Intern Med*, 1986, 105(4):573-85.
Rodriguez-Panadero F and Lopez-Mejias J, "Low Glucose and pH Levels in Malignant Pleural Effusions. Diagnostic Significance and Prognostic Value in Respect to Pleurodesis," *Am Rev Respir Dis*, 1989, 139(3):663-7.

Body Fluid Amylase

CPT 82150

Related Information

Amylase, Serum *on page 79*
Amylase, Urine *on page 79*
Body Fluid *on page 89*
Body Fluid Analysis, Cell Count *on page 306*
Body Fluid Cytology *on page 286*
Lipase, Serum *on page 158*

Synonyms Amylase, Body Fluid; Amylase, Peritoneal Fluid; Amylase, Pleural Fluid

Abstract High pleural fluid amylase is found with pancreatitis and its complications, rupture of the esophagus and with tumors, especially adenocarcinoma of lung and ovary. Peritoneal fluid work-up may resolve diagnostic issues.

Specimen Body fluid (ie, ascitic fluid, pleural fluid, etc); simultaneously drawn serum for amylase. Often, fluid for cytopathology is indicated.

Container Clean container, no preservative

Collection Peritoneal fluid may be obtained by peritoneal lavage.[1] Centrifugation is desirable.

Storage Instructions Amylase is fairly stable at normal levels.

Reference Range Elevation of fluid amylase bears an implication of an increase in the serum level. Body fluid (peritoneal or pleural) levels may reach many times the upper limit for serum amylase in pancreatitis. Reference values are not applicable since the presence of the body fluids in any quantity is itself abnormal.

Use Pancreatitis with or without pseudocyst formation or pancreatic pleural fistula is the most common cause of amylase elevation in pleural fluid. Rupture of the esophagus is the second most common group and malignant effusion is the third.[3] Other causes include pancreatic ascites and pancreatic duct trauma. Defect in the wall of the gastrointestinal tract (eg, perforated peptic ulcer) will allow pancreatic secretion to enter the

peritoneal cavity. Similarly, peritoneal fluid amylase elevations may be found in the presence of necrotic bowel. Peritoneal fluid, containing such amylase, can find its way into a pleural space.

Limitations In collection of ascitic fluid, the localization of the catheter is likely to affect the chemistry result.[1] Oxalate or citrate depress results. Lipemic sample may contain inhibitors which falsely depress results. Benign ovarian cyst fluids may have significant amylase activity. In about 10% of instances of pancreatic disease, ascitic fluid, as well as serum amylase, may be within normal limits.[2]

Methodology Photometric using hydrolysis of small oligosaccharides or "defined" substrates

Additional Information Most patients with pancreatic ascites have high peritoneal fluid amylase as well as amylase and lipase elevations in serum. Pancreatitis may present with pleural effusion. Of 34 patients who had high amylase in pleural fluid associated with neoplasms, 18 had carcinoma of lung. Other tumors were gynecologic, gastrointestinal, lymphoma, breast, and malignancy of unknown origin.[3]

Dark, prune juice-like peritoneal fluid is described as characteristic of severe, necrotizing pancreatitis.[4]

The presence of bacteria in a foul smelling peritoneal fluid indicates perforated viscus in the differential diagnosis of pancreatitis[4] and peritonitis.

Footnotes

1. Robert JH, Meyer P, and Rohner A, "Can Serum and Peritoneal Amylase and Lipase Determinations Help in the Early Prognosis of Acute Pancreatitis?" *Ann Surg*, 1986, 203(2):163-8.
2. Kjeldsberg CR and Knight JA, *Body Fluids - Laboratory Examination of Amniotic, Cerebrospinal, Seminal, Serous, and Synovial Fluids*, 3rd ed, Chicago, IL: American Society of Clinical Pathologists, 1993, 159-222.
3. Kramer MR, Saldana MJ, Cepero RJ, et al, "High Amylase Levels in Neoplasm-Related Pleural Effusion," *Ann Intern Med*, 1989, 110(7):567-9.
4. Steinberg W and Tenner S, "Acute Pancreatitis," *N Engl J Med*, 1994, 330(17):1198-210.

Body Fluid GGT see Gamma Glutamyl Transferase *on page 133*

Body Fluid Glucose

CPT 82947

Related Information

Body Fluid *on page 89*
Body Fluid Analysis, Cell Count *on page 306*
Body Fluid Cytology *on page 286*
Body Fluid pH *on next page*
Carcinoembryonic Antigen *on page 100*
Cerebrospinal Fluid Glucose *on page 105*
Glucose, Fasting *on page 137*
Rheumatoid Factor *on page 427*
Synovial Fluid Analysis *on page 656*

Synonyms Glucose, Body Fluid

Abstract Decreased pleural fluid glucose may be found in bacterial infection, tuberculosis, rheumatoid effusion and with malignant disease.

Specimen Body fluid; simultaneously drawn plasma glucose

Container Sterile container

Reference Range Fluid glucose concentration is usually similar to plasma glucose concentration. Levels <60 mg/dL or 40 mg/dL less than the plasma level drawn simultaneously, are considered decreased.[1]

Use Decreased fluid glucose concentration is usually associated with septic or inflammatory processes; in pleural effusion, very low glucose is a facet of rheumatoid effusion: pleural fluid glucose <50 mg/dL (SI: <2.8 mmol/L) characterizes rheumatoid effusion. It is often much less. In contrast, fluid glucose in SLE is usually >60 mg/dL. Pleural fluid glucose levels <60 mg/dL indicate grossly purulent parapneumonic effusion or rheumatoid effusion. Pericardial effusions with decreased glucose are reported with malignant disease and with bacterial endocarditis.[1] Ascitic fluid glucose is often decreased in tuberculous peritonitis and with malignant disease but is usually normal with cirrhosis or congestive failure.

Limitations Garcia-Tsao et al found glucose the least reliable of the tests they evaluated for the diagnosis of bacterial peritonitis; ascitic fluid glucose in their series ranged from 0-418 mg/dL (SI: 0-23 mmol/L). They also found poor correlation with blood glucose levels. This group recognized the more consistent glucose decrease found in smaller, sequestered fluid collections such as those of meningitis (cerebrospinal fluid) and empyema (pleural fluid).[2]

Methodology Enzymatic with photometry

Additional Information Potts et al describe loculated effusions or empyemas with low glucose and low pH. Low glucose is found with empyema, tuberculosis, neoplasia, as well as rheumatoid effusion.[3] In cases of malignant pleural effusions, when there is low pleural fluid glucose, <60 mg/dL (SI: <3.3 mmol/L), and pH <7.30, a probability of 90% that the cytologic yield will be positive was reported.[4]

(Continued)

Body Fluid Glucose *(Continued)*

Footnotes
1. Kjeldsberg CR and Knight JA, *Body Fluids - Laboratory Examination of Amniotic, Cerebrospinal, Seminal, Serous, and Synovial Fluids*, 3rd ed, Chicago, IL: American Society of Clinical Pathologists, 1993, 159-222.
2. Garcia-Tsao G, Conn HO, and Lerner E, "The Diagnosis of Bacterial Peritonitis: Comparison of pH, Lactate Concentration and Leukocyte Count," *Hepatology*, 1985, 5(1):91-6.
3. Potts DE, Taryle DA, and Sahn SA, "The Glucose-pH Relationship in Parapneumonic Effusions," *Arch Intern Med*, 1978, 138:1378-80.
4. Rodriguez-Panadero F and Lopez-Mejias JL, "Low Glucose and pH Levels in Malignant Pleural Effusions. Diagnostic Significance and Prognostic Value in Respect to Pleurodesis," *Am Rev Respir Dis*, 1989, 139(3):663-7.

Body Fluid Lactate Dehydrogenase

CPT 83615

Related Information
Body Fluid *on page 89*
Body Fluid Analysis, Cell Count *on page 306*
Body Fluid Cytology *on page 286*
Body Fluid pH *on this page*
Cerebrospinal Fluid LD *on page 106*
Lactate Dehydrogenase *on page 153*
Synovial Fluid Analysis *on page 656*

Synonyms Lactate Dehydrogenase, Variable; LD, Fluid; LD Variable

Applies to Protein, Body Fluids

Abstract Elevated body fluid LD levels are higher than serum levels in malignant effusions, unlike cases of benign effusions. Elevations are found in inflammatory states.[1]

Specimen Body fluid; simultaneously drawn serum

Container Sterile container

Special Instructions Source of fluid must be made known to the laboratory.

Reference Range Fluid LD activity is normally much less than the plasma LD activity.

Use Differential diagnosis of effusions, includes work-up for rheumatoid effusion and classification as transudate or exudate; aid in differential diagnosis of traumatic tap vs central nervous system (CNS) hemorrhage in newborns

Limitations This test has limited usefulness due to its nonspecificity. Like use of total protein, LDH fails to classify fluids accurately as transudate or exudate.[2]

Methodology Lactate to pyruvate monitored at 340 nm

Additional Information Lactate dehydrogenase (LD) is a normal component of CSF. LD_1 and LD_2 are decreased in lavage fluid in pulmonary alveolar proteinosis.[3] With ascitic fluid cholesterol, ascitic fluid LDH is helpful in the differential diagnosis of hepatocellular carcinoma versus ascites from other malignant neoplasms.[4] See listing Body Fluid *on page 89* for more information.

Footnotes
1. Kjeldsberg CR and Knight JA, *Body Fluids - Laboratory Examination of Amniotic, Cerebrospinal, Seminal, Serous, and Synovial Fluids*, 3rd ed, Chicago, IL: American Society of Clinical Pathologists, 1993, 159-222.
2. Runyon BA, "Care of Patients With Ascites," *N Engl J Med*, 1994, 330(5):337-42.
3. Hoffman RM and Rogers RM, "Serum and Lavage Lactate Dehydrogenase Isoenzymes in Pulmonary Alveolar Proteinosis," *Am Rev Respir Dis*, 1991, 143(1):42-6.
4. Castaldo G, Oriani G, Cimino L, et al, "Total Discrimination of Peritoneal Malignant Ascites From Cirrhosis- and Hepatocarcinoma-Associated Ascites by Assays of Ascitic Cholesterol and Lactate Dehydrogenase," *Clin Chem*, 1994, 40(3):478-83.

References
Brandstetter RD, Velazquez V, Viejo C, et al, "Postural Changes in Pleural Fluid Constituents," *Chest*, 1994, 105(5):1458-61.

Body Fluid Lipase *see* Lipase, Serum *on page 158*

Body Fluid pH

CPT 83986

Related Information
Bacterial Culture, Biopsy or Body Fluid *on page 456*
Body Fluid *on page 89*
Body Fluid Analysis, Cell Count *on page 306*
Body Fluid Cytology *on page 286*
Body Fluid Glucose *on previous page*
Body Fluid Lactate Dehydrogenase *on this page*
Fungal Culture, Biopsy or Body Fluid *on page 476*
Mycobacterial Culture, Biopsy or Body Fluid *on page 487*

Applies to Arterial-Ascitic Fluid pH Gradient; Peritoneal Fluid pH; Body Fluid; Pleural Fluid pH; Thoracentesis Fluid pH

Abstract A role exists for determination of pH among tests done on pleural and peritoneal fluids.

Specimen Pleural fluid

Container Sample should be collected anaerobically. A green top (lithium heparin) tube to prevent clotting should be used, especially if the syringe has not been rinsed with heparin. Keep on ice and promptly analyze for pH. A syringe rinsed with 0.2 mL of heparin, 1:1000 may be used; collect anaerobically.

Collection If the specimen is collected in a syringe, all air should be expelled and needle sealed and capped. The pH should be measured anaerobically without delay.

Storage Instructions Keep the specimen refrigerated.

Reference Range Serous fluid pH about 7.4-7.64; since body fluid accumulations are themselves abnormal, provision of a digital "range" would be misleading.

Use Determine pH of body fluid to work up diagnosis (eg, pleuritis, empyema, bacterial peritonitis, rheumatoid effusion, carcinoma, esophageal rupture)

Methodology pH meter

Additional Information pH of pleural fluid <6.0 is highly suggestive of rupture of esophagus.[1] Pleural fluid amylase is very helpful for this diagnosis as well. pH <7.3 relates to exudates: in empyema and in loculated effusions pleural fluid pH is <7.2-7.3.[1,2]

The pH is often <7.2 and consistently <7.3[1] in rheumatoid pleural effusion, which is characterized by low glucose, high LD (LDH), and high rheumatoid factor titer. pH >7.3 is in general a feature of transudates. Low pH and low glucose together are found with loculated effusion or with empyema.[3] Effusions related to lupus erythematosus generally have a pH >7.35.[1]

Effusions of tuberculosis usually have pH <7.3,[1] usually with increased lymphocytes. In the single patient with proven tuberculous peritonitis in the series of Garcia-Tsao et al, ascitic fluid pH was 7.33.[4]

In bacterial peritonitis pH is decreased: cutoff <7.35 is useful, especially with PMNs >500/mm^3. The mean pH of infected ascitic fluid is reported as 7.24. The **arterial-ascitic fluid pH gradient** >0.10 with >500 PMNs is described as virtually diagnostic of bacterial peritonitis.[4]

Reduction of pH and in some, but not all, series increments of PMN counts may be found also with peritoneal metastases.[4,5] Low pleural fluid pH with negative cytologic examination may indicate lack of recognizable malignant cells in a sample of malignant effusion but may point to tuberculosis or rheumatoid effusion. Differences in survival exist between patients with low pH and normal pH in malignant pleural effusions, a significant inverse relationship.[5]

A transudative low pH (<7.30) pleural fluid in which the pleural fluid/serum creatinine ratio is >1 points toward urinothorax, a possibility which may be considered in patients with obstructive uropathy.[6]

Footnotes
1. Kjeldsberg CR and Knight JA, *Body Fluids - Laboratory Examination of Amniotic, Cerebrospinal, Seminal, Serous, and Synovial Fluids*, 3rd ed, Chicago, IL: American Society of Clinical Pathologists, 1993, 186-7.
2. Dines DE, "Studies on Pleural Fluid," *Mayo Clin Proc*, 1981, 56:460.
3. Potts DE, Taryle DA, and Sahn SA, "The Glucose-pH Relationship in Parapneumonic Effusions," *Arch Intern Med*, 1978, 138:1378-80.
4. Garcia-Tsao G, Conn HO, and Lerner E, "The Diagnosis of Bacterial Peritonitis: Comparison of pH, Lactate Concentration, and Leukocyte Count," *Hepatology*, 1985, 5(1):91-6.
5. Sahn SA and Good JT, "Pleural Fluid pH in Malignant Effusions: Diagnostic, Prognostic, and Therapeutic Implications," *Ann Intern Med*, 1988, 108(3):345.
6. Miller KS, Wooten S, and Sahn SA, "Urinothorax: A Cause of Low pH Transudative Pleural Effusions," *Am J Med*, 1988, 85(3):448-9.

References
el-Touny M, Osman L, Abd-el-Hamid T, et al, "Re-Evaluation of the Value of Ascitic Fluid pH Lactate Dehydrogenase and Total Proteins in the Diagnosis of Spontaneous Bacterial Peritonitis (SBP)," *J Trop Med Hyg*, 1989, 92(1):6-9.
Halla JT, Schrohenloher RE, and Volanakis JE, "Immune Complexes and Other Laboratory Features of Pleural Effusions: A Comparison of Rheumatoid Arthritis, Systemic Lupus Erythematosus, and Other Diseases," *Ann Intern Med*, 1980, 92:748-52.

Bone GLA Protein *see* Osteocalcin, Serum *on page 174*

Bovine ACTH *replaced by* Cosyntropin Test *on page 114*

Breath Hydrogen *see* Lactose Tolerance Test *on page 157*

Bromism *see* Chloride, Serum *on page 108*

BSP *replaced by* Alkaline Phosphatase, Serum *on page 69*

BSP *replaced by* Gamma Glutamyl Transferase *on page 133*

BSP *replaced by* 5' Nucleotidase *on page 171*

BUN *see* Urea Nitrogen, Blood *on page 213*

BUN/Creatinine Ratio

CPT 82565 (creatinine); 84520 (BUN)

Related Information
Creatinine, Serum *on page 118*
Urea Nitrogen, Blood *on page 213*

Synonyms Urea Nitrogen/Creatinine Ratio

Test Commonly Includes Serum creatinine and urea nitrogen

Abstract Most automated analyzers calculate this ratio from the serum concentrations of each constituent. Used with other investigation to distinguish between prerenal failure, intrinsic failure, and obstruction.

Specimen Serum

Reference Range 10-20; about 14 for a person on a normal diet. The ratio is usually normal with intrinsic renal failure.

Critical Values Ratio is generally >20:1 in prerenal failure (decreased renal blood flow, decreased perfusion) or in urinary tract obstruction

Use High BUN/creatinine ratio is found in overproduction or lowered excretion of urea nitrogen.[1] High ratios occur with prerenal azotemia[2] (eg, congestive heart failure), decreased renal perfusion, shock, volume depletion, hypotension, and dehydration. Often the BUN/creatinine ratio is greatly elevated in gastrointestinal bleeding and with swallowed blood from the upper airway. A BUN/creatinine ratio >36 suggests upper gastrointestinal bleeding, whereas a ratio <36 is not helpful in locating the source of the bleeding.[3] It may be increased with high protein diet, with ileal conduit, with catabolic states, and with urinary tract obstruction.[4] It may also be increased with tetracyclines or steroids. These conditions frequently occur with normal serum creatinine levels. In postrenal obstruction and in prerenal azotemia superimposed on renal disease a high BUN/creatinine ratio is present with elevated serum creatinine.

Low BUN/creatinine ratio may be found in low protein diet, malnutrition, pregnancy, liver disease, rhabdomyolysis, prolonged I.V. fluid therapy, ketosis (acetoacetic acid interferes with and falsely elevates creatinine), repeated hemodialysis, inappropriate secretion of antidiuretic hormone, with drugs which increase creatinine but not urea nitrogen (eg, cimetidine, trimethoprim), and with tetracycline use (antianabolic effect).

Limitations Patients' variability in protein intake and mass of voluntary muscle can cause this ratio to be misleading.[2]

Footnotes

1. Maher JF, "Disparity in BUN and Plasma Creatinine Test Results in Patient," *JAMA*, 1977, 237:2535.
2. Beck LH, "Hypouricemia in the Syndrome of Inappropriate Secretion of Antidiuretic Hormone," *N Engl J Med*, 1979, 301:528-30.
3. Richards RJ, Donica MB, and Grayer D, "Can the Blood Urea Nitrogen/Creatinine Ratio Distinguish Upper From Lower Gastrointestinal Bleeding?" *J Clin Gastroenterol*, 1990, 12(5):500-4.
4. Dossetor JB, "Creatininemia Versus Uremia: The Relative Significance of Blood Urea Nitrogen and Serum Creatinine Concentrations in Azotemia," *Ann Intern Med*, 1966, 65:1287-99.

References

Lindeman RD, "Assessment of Renal Function in the Old: Special Considerations," *Clin Lab Med*, 1993, 13(1):269-77.

Olsen LH and Andreassen KH, "Stools Containing Altered Blood-Plasma Urea: Creatinine Ratio as a Simple Test for the Source of Bleeding," *Br J Surg*, 1991, 78(1):71-3.

CA 15-3

CPT 86316

Related Information

Body Fluid *on page 89*
Breast Biopsy *on page 35*
Breast Cancer, Hereditary (BRCA1) *on page 504*
CA 19-9 *on this page*
CA 125 *on next page*
Carcinoembryonic Antigen *on page 100*

Synonyms Carbohydrate Antigen 15-3

Applies to CA 549, CA M26, CA M29, Mucin-Like Carcinoma-Associated Antigen (MCA)

Test Commonly Includes CA 19-9, CEA, TAG 72

Abstract The measurement of CA 15-3, a carbohydrate epitope, has greatest utility in monitoring recurrent carcinoma of breast.

Specimen Serum

Container Red top tube

Storage Instructions Refrigerate serum. Stable at 4°C for 2 weeks.

Reference Range <30 kU/mL (SI: <30 kU/L)

Use CA 15-3 is used to monitor patients for systemic recurrence of breast carcinoma[1] after diagnosis and initial therapy.[2] With CEA, CA 15-3 is helpful to monitor therapeutic response but CA 15-3 is more sensitive than CEA for detection of recurrent breast carcinoma.[2] It is **not** suitable as a screening test. Ninety-six percent of patients with combined local and systemic disease had increased CA 15-3 levels.[1]

Limitations Like CEA, CA 15-3 fails as a reliable marker for early breast cancer. It has limited sensitivity.[3]

Methodology Immunoradiometric (IRMA)

Additional Information The use of CA 15-3 in the evaluation of pelvic masses in women is less effective than the measurement of CA 125. The employment of multiple markers facilitates the separation of benign from malignant masses.[4] There is good correlation of CA 15-3 levels with tumor stage of breast cancer, and CA 15-3 is better than CEA in detection of metastases from carcinoma of breast.[5]

Markers for breast carcinoma include **CA 15-3, CA 549, CA M26, CA M29, and mucin-like carcinoma-associated antigen (MCA)**. Sensitivity of each is limited. They reflect tumor burden and prognosis. Panels of markers and sequential testing may enhance their limited clinical utility.[3] Of this group, the best single marker is CA 15-3. Possible combinations of markers may include CEA, CA 15-3, and ESR.[2] CA 15-3 is superior to MCA for metastatic breast carcinoma.[6]

Footnotes

1. Geraghty JG, Coveney EC, Sherry F, et al, "CA 15-3 in Patients With Locoregional and Metastatic Breast Carcinoma," *Cancer*, 1992, 70(12):2831-4.
2. Lamerz R, Stieber P, and Fateh-Moghadam A, "Serum Marker Combinations in Human Breast Cancer," *In Vivo*, 1993, 7(6B):607-13.
3. Werner M, Faser C, and Silverberg M, "Clinical Utility and Validation of Emerging Biochemical Markers for Mammary Adenocarcinoma," *Clin Chem*, 1993, 39(11 Pt 2):2386-96.
4. Soper JT, Hunter VJ, Daly L, et al, "Preoperative Serum Tumor-Associated Antigen Levels in Women With Pelvic Masses," *Obstet Gynecol*, 1990, 75(2):249-54.
5. Safi F, Kohler I, Rottinger E, et al, "The Value of the Tumor Marker CA 15-3 in Diagnosing and Monitoring Breast Cancer. A Comparative Study With Carcinoembryonic Antigen," *Cancer*, 1991, 68(3):574-82.
6. O'Brien DP, Gough DB, Skehill R, et al, "Simple Method for Comparing Reliability of Two Serum Tumour Markers in Breast Carcinoma," *J Clin Pathol*, 1994, 47(2):134-7.

References

Dnistrian AM, Schwartz MK, Greenberg EJ, et al, "CA 15-3 and Carcinoembryonic Antigen in the Clinical Evaluation of Breast Cancer," *Clin Chim Acta*, 1991, 200(2-3):81-93.

Ferroni P, Szpak C, Greiner JW, et al, "CA 72-4 Radioimmunoassay in the Diagnosis of Malignant Effusions. Comparison of Various Tumor Markers," *Int J Cancer*, 1990, 46(3):445-51.

Gion M, Plebani M, Mione R, et al, "Serum CA549 in Primary Breast Cancer: Comparison With CA15.3 and MCA," *Br J Cancer*, 1994, 69(4):721-5.

Hayes DF, "Tumor Markers for Breast Cancer," *Ann Oncol*, 1993, 4(10):807-19.

Jacobs IJ, Oram DH, and Bast RC Jr, "Strategies for Improving the Specificity of Screening for Ovarian Cancer With Tumor-Associated Antigens CA 125, CA 15-3, and TAG 72.3," *Obstet Gynecol*, 1992, 80(3 Pt 1):396-9.

Kiang DT, Greenberg LJ, and Kennedy BJ, "Tumor Marker Kinetics in the Monitoring of Breast Cancer," *Cancer*, 1990, 65(2):193-9.

Robertson JF, Pearson D, Price MR, et al, "Objective Measurement of Therapeutic Response in Breast Cancer Using Tumour Markers," *Br J Cancer*, 1991, 64(4):757-63.

Shinozaki T, Chigira M, and Kato K, "Multivariate Analysis of Serum Tumor Markers for Diagnosis of Skeletal Metastases," *Cancer*, 1992, 69(1):108-12.

CA 19-9

CPT 86316

Related Information

Alpha$_1$-Fetoprotein, Serum *on page 72*
Body Fluid *on page 89*
CA 15-3 *on this page*
CA 125 *on next page*
Carcinoembryonic Antigen *on page 100*
Immunoperoxidase Procedures *on page 43*

Synonyms Carbohydrate Antigen 19-9

Applies to CA 50; CA 242; TAG-72; Tissue Polypeptide Antigen; TPA

Abstract A tumor marker, CA 19-9 is a carbohydrate antigen, a monosialoganglioside. Its widest use has been work-up for and monitoring of carcinoma of pancreas. Some small carcinomas of the pancreas may be detected with CA 19-9, SPan-1, and imaging.[1]

Specimen Serum

Container Red top tube

Storage Instructions Freeze to ship.

Reference Range <37 kU/mL (Centocor assay). This value is arbitrary and statistically derived.

Use Although the diagnostic accuracy of CA 19-9 for pancreatic cancers was superior to that of other markers, experience with patients who have early carcinoma of pancreas has been limited; its diagnostic value in early cases has been low.[2] It is used to monitor gastrointestinal cancers, head and neck tumors, and gynecologic tumors; predict the recurrence of stomach, pancreatic, and colorectal malignancies, liver, gallbladder, cholangiocarcinoma, and urothelial tumors.

Limitations CA 19-9 has so far been evaluated in highly selected populations. It is described as inferior to **CEA** as a marker for colorectal carcinoma.[3] **Tissue polypeptide antigen (TPA)** has been found to provide a closer relationship to clinical status than CEA or CA 19-9 in subjects with bronchogenic carcinoma.[4] False-positive CA 19-9 and alpha-fetoprotein (AFP) assays are described with hepatic cirrhosis. CA 19-9 is described as inferior to AFP in detection of carcinoma arising in cirrhosis.[5] Its sensitivity and specificity in other settings needs to be established. It is **not** a screening test.

Methodology Immunoradiometric assay (IRMA). Like CEA, it is used immunocytochemically as well.

Additional Information CA 19-9, a carbohydrate antigen, is related to Lewis blood group antigen. Individuals who are Lewis (a-b-) phenotype (6% of the population) cannot synthesize CA 19-9, CA 50, and CA 195; and this may account for the lesser diagnostic value of these markers compared to CEA, in the diagnosis of colorectal cancer.[6] CA 19-9 is helpful in post-therapeutic monitoring to determine success of therapy or (Continued)

CA 19-9 (Continued)

development of recurrence when used serially. CA 19-9 has been reported as positive in 70% to 80% of pancreatic carcinomas, 50% to 60% of gastric cancers, 60% of hepatobiliary cancers, 30% of colorectal cancers, and few lung, breast, renal cell, or prostate cancers. Serum levels may differentiate pancreatic cancer from pancreatitis, but a study of 54 patients with pancreatic adenocarcinoma and 27 patients with chronic pancreatitis showed that serum levels of CA 19-9 were less accurate than CT-guided pancreatic fine-needle aspiration biopsy and ultrasound in distinguishing the two entities.[7]

The test may also be positive in patients with non-neoplastic disease, particularly inflammatory bowel disease, cirrhosis, and autoimmune conditions including rheumatoid arthritis (33%), systemic lupus erythematosus (32%), and scleroderma (33%). The prognostic value of serum CA 19-9 levels in histologically proven pancreatic adenocarcinoma was studied.[8] Levels correlate with pancreatic cancer staging. Levels were significantly lower in patients with tumors <5 cm in diameter than in those with tumors >5 cm. Average survival time was longer in those patients whose levels returned to normal after resection than in those whose level decreased but did not return to normal. In those who underwent resection, recurrent elevation of CA 19-9 preceded changes detected by computed tomography or clinical examination by 2-9 months. In those patients who died of pancreatic carcinoma, 65% had a definite rise in CA 19-9 levels before death.

CA 19-9 and **CA 50** are useful in distinguishing hepatocellular carcinoma from cholangiocarcinoma. CA 19-9 and CA 50 antigens are normal constituents of bile ducts. In a small series of cases, 9 out of 10 cholangiocarcinomas stained (immunoperoxidase) for CA 50 and 8 out of 10 for CA 19-9. Eleven cases of hepatocellular carcinomas were negative for both markers by immunoperoxidase technique.[9] This combination of antigen assays has been recommended with ultrasound for diagnosis of pancreatic cancer.[10]

In a large study of carcinoma of gallbladder in a high-risk population in Mexico and Bolivia, it was found that serum levels of CA 19-9 had superior sensitivity (79.4%) than serum CEA levels (50.0%). Use of the tests in parallel did not improve results.[11]

Another marker, **CA 242**, shows promise as a marker for colorectal, pancreatic, and hepatobiliary carcinoma. Its sensitivity and specificity exceeds that of CEA, CA 19-9, and CA 50.[12,13] Tumor-associated glycoprotein (TAG-72) (CA 72-4) has been used with CA 15-3, CEA, enzymes, and cytopathology in aspirates from pancreatic cysts. TAG-72 levels were markedly increased in fluid from mucinous cystadenocarcinomas.[14]

Footnotes

1. Satake K, Chung YS, Umeyama K, et al, "The Possibility of Diagnosing Small Pancreatic Cancer (Less Than 4.0 cm) by Measuring Various Serum Tumor Markers," Cancer, 1991, 68(1):149-52.
2. Gullo L, "CA 19-9: The Italian Experience," Pancreas, 1994, 9(6):717-9.
3. Quentmeier A, Möller P, Schwarz V, et al, "Carcinoembryonic Antigen, CA 19-9, and CA 125 in Normal and Carcinomatous Human Colorectal Tissue," Cancer, 1987, 60(9):2261-6.
4. Buccheri GF, Ferrigno D, Sartoris AM, et al, "Tumor Markers in Bronchogenic Carcinoma. Superiority of Tissue Polypeptide Antigen to Carcinoembryonic Antigen and Carbohydrate Antigenic Determinant 19-9," Cancer, 1987, 60(1):42-50.
5. Fabris C, Basso DA, Leandro G, et al, "Serum CA 19-9 and Alpha-Fetoprotein Levels in Primary Hepatocellular Carcinoma and Liver Cirrhosis," Cancer, 1991, 68(8):1795-8.
6. van der Schouw YT, Verbeek AL, Wobbes T, et al, "Comparison of Four Serum Tumour Markers in the Diagnosis of Colorectal Carcinoma," Br J Cancer, 1992, 66(1):148-54.
7. DelMaschio A, Vanzulli A, Sironi S, et al, "Pancreatic Cancer Versus Chronic Pancreatitis: Diagnosis With CA 19-9 Assessment, US, CT, and CT-Guided Fine-Needle Biopsy," Radiology, 1991, 178(1):95-9.
8. Tian F, Appert HE, Myles J, et al, "Prognostic Value of Serum CA 19-9 Levels in Pancreatic Adenocarcinoma," Ann Surg, 1992, 215(4):350-5.
9. Haglund U, Lindgren J, Roberts PJ, et al, "Difference in Tissue Expression of Tumour Markers CA 19-9 and CA 50 in Hepatocellular Carcinoma and Cholangiocarcinoma," Br J Cancer, 1991, 63(3):386-9.
10. Bovo P, Rigo L, Togni M, et al, "Rapid Diagnosis of Pancreatic Cancer by Combination of Ultrasonography and Serum Tumour Markers CA 19-9 and CA 50," Ital J Gastroenterol, 1993, 25(9):477-81.
11. Strom BL, Maislin G, West SL, et al, "Serum CEA and CA 19-9: Potential Future Diagnostic or Screening Tests for Gallbladder Cancer?" Int J Cancer, 1990, 45(5):821-4.
12. Nilsson O, Johansson C, Glimelius B, et al, "Sensitivity and Specificity of CA 242 in Gastrointestinal Cancer. A Comparison With CEA, CA 50, and CA 19-9," Br J Cancer, 1992, 65(2):215-21.
13. Kuusela P, Haglund C, and Roberts PJ, "Comparison of A New Tumour Marker CA 242 With CA 19-9, CA 50, and Carcinoembryonic Antigen (CEA) in Digestive Tract Diseases," Br J Cancer, 1991, 63(4):636-40.
14. Alles AJ, Warshaw AL, Southern JF, et al, "Expression of CA-72-4 (TAG-72) in the Fluid Contents of Pancreatic Cysts. A New Marker to Distinguish Malignant Pancreatic Cystic Tumors From Benign Neoplasms and Pseudocysts," Ann Surg, 1994, 219(2):131-4.

References

Barillari P, Sammartino P, Cardi M, et al, "Gastrointestinal Cancer Follow-Up: The Effectiveness of Sequential CEA, TPA, and CA 19-9 Evaluation in the Early Diagnosis of Recurrences," Aust N Z J Surg, 1991, 61(9):675-80.

Beretta E, Malesci A, Zerbi A, et al, "Serum CA 19-9 in the Postsurgical Follow-Up of Patients With Pancreatic Cancer," Cancer, 1987, 60(10):2428-31.

Casetta G, Piana P, Cavallini A, et al, "Urinary Levels of Tumour Associated Antigens (CA 19-9, TPA and CEA) in Patients With Neoplastic and Non-neoplastic Urothelial Abnormalities," Br J Urol, 1993, 72(1):60-4.

Collazos J, "Serum CA 19-9 and Alpha-Fetoprotein Levels in Primary Hepatocellular Carcinoma and Liver Cirrhosis," Cancer, 1992, 70(5):1202-3.

Foutch PG, "A Diagnostic Approach to Pancreatic Cancer," Dig Dis, 1994, 12(3):129-38.

Ho JJ and Kim YS, "Serological Pancreatic Tumor Markers and the MUC1 Apomucin," Pancreas, 1994, 9(6):674-91.

Konishi I, Fujii S, Nanbu Y, et al, "Mucin Leakage Into the Cervical Stroma May Increase Lymph Node Metastasis in Mucin-Producing Cervical Adenocarcinomas," Cancer, 1990, 65(2):229-37.

Kouri M, Pyrhönen S, and Kuusela P, "Elevated CA 19-9 as the Most Significant Prognostic Factor in Advanced Colorectal Cancer," J Surg Oncol, 1992, 49(2):78-85.

Loy TS, Sharp SC, Andershock CJ, et al, "Distribution of CA 19-9 in Adenocarcinomas and Transitional Cell Carcinomas. An Immunohistochemical Study of 527 Cases," Am J Clin Pathol, 1993, 99(6):726-8.

Lucarotti ME, Habib NA, Kelly SB, et al, "Clinical Evaluation of Combined Use of CEA, CA 19-9, and CA 50 in the Serum of Patients With Pancreatic Carcinoma," Eur J Surg Oncol, 1991, 17(1):51-3.

Pleskow DK, Berger HJ, Gyves J, et al, "Evaluation of a Serologic Marker, CA 19-9, in the Diagnosis of Pancreatic Cancer," Ann Intern Med, 1989, 110(9):704-9.

Richter JM, Christensen MR, Rustgi AK, et al, "The Clinical Utility of the CA 19-9 Radioimmunoassay for the Diagnosis of Pancreatic Cancer Presenting as Pain or Weight Loss - A Cost-Effective Analysis," Arch Intern Med, 1989, 149(10):2292-7.

Satake K, Kanazawa G, Kho I, et al, "Evaluation of Serum Pancreatic Enzymes, Carbohydrate Antigen 19-9, and Carcinoembryonic Antigen in Various Pancreatic Diseases," Am J Gastroenterol, 1985, 80(8):630-6.

Sell S, "Detection of Cancer by Tumor Markers in the Blood: A View to the Future," Crit Rev Oncog, 1993, 4(4):419-33.

Shimomura C, Eguchi K, Kawakami A, et al, "Elevation of a Tumor-Associated Antigen CA 19-9 Levels in Patients With Rheumatic Diseases," J Rheumatol, 1989, 16(11):1410-5.

Steinberg W, "The Clinical Utility of the CA-19-9 Tumor-Associated Antigen," Am J Gastroenterol, 1990, 85(4):350-5.

Warshaw AL and Fernández-del Castillo C, "Pancreatic Carcinoma," N Engl J Med, 1992, 326(7):455-64.

Wobbes T, Thomas CM, Segers MF, et al, "Evaluation of Seven Tumor Markers (CA 50, CA 19-9, CA 19-9 TruQuant, CA 72-4, CA 195, Carcinoembryonic Antigen, and Tissue Polypeptide Antigen) in the Pretreatment Sera of Patients With Gastric Carcinoma," Cancer, 1992, 69(8):2036-41.

CA 50 see CA 19-9 on previous page

CA 125

CPT 86316

Related Information

Body Fluid on page 89
Body Fluid Analysis, Cell Count on page 306
Body Fluid Cytology on page 286
CA 15-3 on previous page
CA 19-9 on previous page
Carcinoembryonic Antigen on page 100
Cyst Fluid Cytology on page 292
Immunoperoxidase Procedures on page 43

Synonyms Cancer Antigen 125

Applies to Aminoterminal Propeptide of Type III Procollagen; OVX1; PIIINP; Placental Alkaline Phosphatase; TAG 72

Abstract The antigen CA 125 is recognized by a monoclonal antibody, OC-125. The CA 125 antigen is expressed in derivatives of fetal coelom such as müllerian epithelia (epithelium of fallopian tubes, endometrium and endocervix), pleura and peritoneum. Peritoneal irritation (eg, ruptured ectopic pregnancy) may contribute to CA 125 concentration. Its clinical application is marred by production of CA 125 from benign tissue (eg, benign ovarian cysts, irritated peritoneum) as well as by carcinoma.[1] It is found with certain gynecologic tumors and is advocated postoperatively and preoperatively for prognostic information. Used serially, it may be useful in detection of relapse and as a monitor of patient response to chemotherapeutic agents. Doubling or halving of its serum level correlates with tumor regression, progression, tumor status following therapy, and detection of recurrence. CA 125 must be used with additional markers to play a role as a diagnostic adjunct to differentiate carcinoma from benign ovarian tumors and from subjects with carcinoma of colon.[2] Its sensitivity is enhanced with serial application and when combined with imaging.

Specimen Serum

Container Red top tube

Storage Instructions Refrigerate within 2 hours of collection. Freeze at -20°C for long-term storage.

Reference Range <35 kU/mL (SI: <35 kU/L); levels >35 kU/mL (SI:>35 kU/L) are highly correlated with malignancy

Critical Values Levels >65 units/mL are associated with malignancy in >90% of cases with pelvic masses.

Use Useful tumor marker for serially monitoring of certain gynecologic tumors, including nonmucinous (serous) neoplasms of ovary, adenocarcinoma, and adenosquamous carcinoma of cervix, and adenocarcinoma of endometrium. Not a screening test for ovarian cancer, it is insensitive early. It is among the markers for evaluation of women with metastatic carcinoma of unknown primary site. Persistently increasing levels indicate progressive neoplasia.

Limitations CA 125 is not specific for tumors of the ovary and cannot distinguish benign from malignant tumors. It is **not** a screening test. False-positive CA 125 values have been reported in patients who developed antibodies against mouse immunoglobulins when monoclonal-based double determinant immunoradiometric assays were used. Such interference can be removed by affinity chromatography on columns designed to remove human IgG.

Lack of elevation of CA 125 does not provide reliable information that a patient is tumor-free, but rising levels do indicate poor prognosis. Hysterectomy and menopausal status effect levels.[3] Fifty percent of the patients with stage I ovarian cancer have normal levels of CA 125, although most subjects with advanced stage tumor have elevations. Elevations bear correlation with tumor stage but normal levels have been reported with large volume tumors.[4] High levels are described with hepatic cirrhosis[5] and tuberculous peritonitis.[6]

False elevations are reported following irradiation therapy for adenocarcinoma of endometrium.[7]

Methodology Enzyme immunoassay (EIA), radioimmunoassay (RIA), immunoradiometric assay (IRMA); immunohistochemical methods are in use

Additional Information CA 125 is a 220 kD glycoprotein expressed by more than 80% of nonmucinous ovarian epithelial neoplasms. It is also expressed by other coelomic epithelial derivatives and other gynecologic neoplasms such as endometrial and fallopian tube carcinoma, and some tumors of the pancreas, liver, colon, breast, and lung (in smaller percentages). It can also be detected in pregnancy, abruptio placentae, tubo-ovarian abscess, advanced endometriosis, and benign teratomas (dermoids).

CA 125 is most useful in monitoring progression or recurrence in cases of known ovarian carcinoma. For this purpose, levels >35 IU/mL may be significant; although a lower level does not replace a second-look operation. Although elevations have been recognized 3 months before clinical recurrence, about 25% of patients have CA 125 levels <35 IU/mL before second-look laparotomy despite the presence of residual tumor. However, some women with a negative second-look procedure reverted to a positive CA 125 within 1 month. Therefore, CA 125 remains a useful tool to follow these patients.

A long-term (3-7 years) follow-up study of 33 patients with advanced nonmucinous epithelial ovarian carcinoma after primary treatment, using monthly determination of CA 125, showed a sensitivity of 95% in detecting early recurrence.[8] A similar study showed that serial monitoring was useful, and the elevations in progressive disease preceded clinical diagnosis by a median time of 6 months.[9]

Because of the high frequency of false-positive results associated with common benign conditions, CA 125 is not useful as a screening test for ovarian carcinoma. Such benign conditions include menstruation, pregnancy, benign pelvic tumors, pelvic inflammatory disease, ovarian hyperstimulation syndrome, and peritonitis.[10]

Studying tissue sections, 68% of adenocarcinomas of endometrium express CA 125 and another 8% contain focal reactivity.[11] Fifty-eight percent of patients with recurrent carcinoma of endometrium had increased concentration of CA 125. Use of CA 125 has led to detection of endometrial carcinoma. If elevated at diagnosis, CA 125 is a marker for projection of recurrence, including papillary serous carcinoma of endometrium.[7]

The use of CA 125 in management of endometriosis is published.[12,13,14]

Use of additional markers, such as CA 15-3, TAG 72, and placental alkaline phosphatase, with CA 125 has been advocated to enhance specificity.[15] OVX1 has recently been advocated as the most useful additional marker. It is detected by an immunoradiometric assay.[16]

In effusion fluids, elevation of CA 125 without increases of CEA are in keeping with a primary in ovary, fallopian tube, or endometrium. Increased CEA without elevation of CA 125 may be found with mucinous adenocarcinoma of lung, breast, gastrointestinal tract, as well as ovary.[17]

Footnotes

1. Bischof P, "What Do We Know About the Origin of CA 125?" *Eur J Obstet Gynecol Reprod Biol*, 1993, 49(1-2): 93-8.
2. Kenemans P, Yedema CA, Bon GG, et al, "CA 125 in Gynecological Pathway - A Review," *Eur J Obstet Gynecol Reprod Biol*, 1993, 49(1-2):115-24
3. Grover S, Quinn MA, Weideman P, et al, "Factors Influencing Serum CA 125 Levels in Normal Women," *Obstet Gynecol*, 1992, 79(4):511-4.
4. Patsner B, Orr JW Jr, Mann WJ Jr, et al, "Does Serum CA 125 Level Prior to Second-Look Laparotomy for Invasive Ovarian Adenocarcinoma Predict Size of Residual Disease?" *Gynecol Oncol*, 1990, 38(3):373-6.
5. Ruibal A and Siuriana R, "Evidence of A Relationship Between High Serum CA 125 and Liver Failure Pattern in Cirrhotic Patients Without Ascites and Jaundice," *Int J Biol Markers*, 1989, 1(1):55-6.
6. O'Riordan DK, Deery A, Dorman A, et al, "Increased CA 125 in a Patient With Tuberculosus Peritonitis: Case Report and Review of Published Works," *Gut*, 1995, 36(2):303-5.
7. Rose PG, Sommers RM, Reale FR, et al, "Serial Serum CA 125 Measurements for Evaluation of Recurrence in Patients With Endometrial Carcinoma," *Obstet Gynecol*, 1994, 84(1):12-6.
8. Hogberg T and Kagedal B, "Long-Term Follow-Up of Ovarian Cancer With Monthly Determinations of Serum CA 125," *Gynecol Oncol*, 1992, 46(2):191-8.
9. Sevelda P, Rosen A, Denison U, et al, "Is CA 125 Monitoring Useful in Patients With Epithelial Ovarian Carcinoma and Preoperative Negative CA 125 Serum Levels?" *Gynecol Oncol*, 1991, 43(2):154-8.
10. Daoud E and Bodor G, "CA 125 Concentrations in Malignant and Nonmalignant Disease," *Clin Chem*, 1991, 37(11):1968-74.
11. Podczaski E, Kaminski PF, and Zaino R, "CA 125 and CA 19-9 Immunolocalization in Normal, Hyperplastic, and Carcinomatous Endometrium," *Cancer*, 1993, 71(8):2551-6.
12. Pittaway DE, "The Use of Serial CA 125 Concentrations to Monitor Endometriosis in Infertile Women," *Am J Obstet Gynecol*, 1990, 163(3):1032-7.
13. Koninckx PR, Muyldermans M, Meuleman C, et al, "CA 125 in the Management of Endometriosis," *Eur J Obstet Gynecol Reprod Biol*, 1993, 49(1-2):109-13.
14. Fedele L, Vercellini P, Arcaini L, et al, "CA 125 in Serum, Peritoneal Fluid, Active Lesions and Endometrium of Patients With Endometriosis," *Am J Obstet Gynecol*, 1988, 158(1):166-70.
15. Bast RC Jr, Knauf S, Epenetos A, et al, "Coordinate Elevation of Serum Markers in Ovarian Cancer but Not in Benign Disease," *Cancer*, 1991, 68(8):1758-63.
16. Berek JS and Bast RC Jr, "Ovarian Cancer Screening. The Use of Serial Complementary Tumor Markers to Improve Sensitivity and Specificity for Early Detection," *Cancer*, 1995, 76:2092-6.
17. Rudolph RA, Pinto MM, and Bernstein LH, "Measuring Decision Values for CEA and CA 125 in Effusions," *Lab Med*, 1990, 21(9):574-8.

References

Bersinger NA and Rageth JC, "A Comparison Between Pregnancy-Associated α_2-Glycoprotein (α_2-PAG), Carcin-Embryonic Antigen (CEA), CA 125, and CA 15-3 as Tumor Markers in Breast Cancer," *Eur J Gynaecol Oncol*, 1990, 11(2):135-9.

Brand E and Lidor Y, "The Decline of CA 125 Level After Surgery Reflects the Size of Residual Ovarian Cancer," *Obstet Gynecol*, 1993, 81(1):29-32.

Buller RE, Berman ML, Bloss JD, et al, "CA 125 Regression: A Model for Epithelial Ovarian Cancer Response," *Am J Obstet Gynecol*, 1991, 165(2):360-7.

Cruickshank DJ, Paul J, Lewis CR, et al, "An Independent Evaluation of the Potential Clinical Usefulness of Proposed CA 125 Indices Previously Shown to Be of Prognostic Significance in Epithelial Ovarian Cancer," *Br J Cancer*, 1992, 65(4):597-600.

Diez M, Cerdàn FJ, Ortega MD, et al, "Evaluation of Serum CA 125 as a Tumor Marker in Non-Small Cell Lung Cancer," *Cancer*, 1991, 67(1):150-4.

Duk JM, De Bruijn HW, Groenier KH, et al, "Adenocarcinoma of the Uterine Cervix - Prognostic Significance of Pretreatment Serum CA 125, Squamous Cell Carcinoma Antigen, and Carcinoembryonic Antigen Levels in Relation to Clinical and Histopathologic Tumor Characteristics," *Cancer*, 1990, 65(8):1830-7.

Finkler NJ, Benacerraf B, Lavin PT, et al, "Comparison of Serum CA 125, Clinical Impression, and Ultrasound in the Preoperative Evaluation of Ovarian Masses," *Obstet Gynecol*, 1988, 72(4):659-64.

Gadducci A, Ferdighini M, Ceccarini T, et al, "A Comparative Evaluation of the Ability of Serum CA 125, CA 19-9, CA 15-3, CA 50, CA 72-4, and TATI Assays in Reflecting the Course of Disease in Patients With Ovarian Carcinoma," *Eur J Gynaecol Oncol*, 1990, 11(2):127-33.

Ghazizadeh M, Sasaki Y, Oguro T, et al, "Combined Immunohistochemical Study of Tissue Polypeptide Antigen and Cancer Antigen 125 in Human Ovarian Tumours," *Histopathology*, 1990, 17(2):123-8.

Granai CO, "Ovarian Cancer - Unrealistic Expectations," *N Engl J Med*, 1993, 327(3):197-200.

Helzisouer KJ, Bush TL, Alberg AJ, et al, "Prospective Study of Serum CA 125 Levels as Markers of Ovarian Cancer," *JAMA*, 1993, 269(9):1123-6.

Hising C, Anjegard IM, and Einhorn N, "Clinical Relevance of the CA 125 Assay in Monitoring of Ovarian Cancer Patients," *Am J Clin Oncol*, 1991, 14(2):111-4.

Hosono MN, Endo K, Sakahara H, et al, "Different Antigenic Nature in Apparently Healthy Women With High Serum CA 125 Levels Compared With Typical Patients With Ovarian Cancer," *Cancer*, 1992, 70(12):2851-6.

Hunter VJ, Daly L, Helms M, et al, "The Prognostic Significance of CA 125 Half-Life in Patients With Ovarian Cancer Who Have Received Primary Chemotherapy After Surgical Cytoreduction," *Am J Obstet Gynecol*, 1990, 163(4 Pt 1):1164-7.

Ismail MA, Rotmensch J, Mercer LJ, et al, "CA-125 in Peritoneal Fluid From Patients With Nonmalignant Gynecologic Disorders," *J Reprod Med*, 1994, 39(7):510-2.

Jacobs IJ, Oram DH, and Bast RC Jr, "Strategies for Improving the Specificity of Screening for Ovarian Cancer With Tumor-Associated Antigens CA 125, CA 15-3, and TAG 72.3," *Obstet Gynecol*, 1992, 80(3 Pt 1):396-9.

Kamiya N, Mizuno K, Kawai M, et al, "Simultaneous Measurement of CA 125, CA 19-9, Tissue Polypeptide Antigen, and Immunosuppressive Acidic Protein to Predict Recurrence of Ovarian Cancer," *Obstet Gynecol*, 1990, 76 (3 Pt 1):417-21.

Koomen GC, Betjes MG, Zemel D, et al, "Cancer Antigen 125 Is Locally Produced in the Peritoneal Cavity During Continuous Ambulatory Peritoneal Dialysis," *Perit Dial Int*, 1994, 14(2):132-6.

Maggino T, Gadducci A, D'Addario V, et al, "Prospective Multicenter Study on CA 125 in Postmenopausal Pelvic Masses," *Gynecol Oncol*, 1994, 54(2):117-23.

Motoyama T, Watanabe H, Takeuchi S, et al, "Cancer Antigen 125, Carcinoembryonic Antigen, and Carbohydrate Determinant 19-9 in Ovarian Tumors," *Cancer*, 1990, 66(12):2628-35.

O'Shaughnessy A, Check JH, Nowroozi K, et al, "CA 125 Levels Measured in Different Phases of the Menstrual Cycle in Screening for Endometriosis," *Obstet Gynecol*, 1993, 81(1):99-103.

Podczaski E, Whitney C, Manetta A, et al, "Use of CA 125 to Monitor Patients With Ovarian Epithelial Carcinomas," *Gynecol Oncol*, 1989, 33(2):193-7.

Richardson GS, "Ovarian Cancer," *JAMA*, 1993, 269(9):1163.

Sichel F, Salaun V, Bar E, et al, "Biological Markers and Ovarian Carcinomas," *Clin Chim Acta*, 1994, 227(1-2):87-96.

Tseng PC, Sprance HE, Carcangiu ML, et al, "CA 125, NB/70K, and Lipid-Associated Sialic Acid in Monitoring Uterine Papillary Serous Carcinoma," *Obstet Gynecol*, 1989, 74(3 Pt 1):384-7.

Turpeinen U, Lehtovirta P, Alfthan H, et al, "Interference by Human Antimouse Antibodies in CA 125 Assay After Immunoscintigraphy: Anti-idiotypic Antibodies Not Neutralized by Mouse IgG but Removed by Chromatography," *Clin Chem*, 1990, 36(7):1333-8.

van Nagell JR Jr, "Ovarian Cancer Screening," *Cancer*, 1991, 68(4):679-80.

Witt BR, Miles R, Wolf GC, et al, "CA 125 Levels in Abruptio Placentae," *Am J Obstet Gynecol*, 1991, 164(5 Pt 1):1225-8.

Zurawski VR Jr, Sjovall K, Schoenfeld DA , et al, "Prospective Evaluation of Serum CA 125 Levels in a Normal Population, Phase I: The Specificities of Single and Serial Determinations in Testing for Ovarian Cancer," *Gynecol Oncol* , 1990, 36(3):299-305.

CA 242 *see CA 19-9 on page 93*

CA 549, CA M26, CA M29, Mucin-Like Carcinoma-Associated Antigen (MCA) *see CA 15-3 on page 93*

Ca, Blood *see Calcium, Serum on next page*

Calcitonin

CPT 82308

Related Information

Adrenocorticotropic Hormone *on page 63*
Catecholamines, Fractionation, Plasma *on page 103*
Catecholamines, Fractionation, Urine *on page 104*
Immunoperoxidase Procedures *on page 43*
Multiple Endocrine Neoplasia/Familial Medullary Thyroid Carcinoma *on page 519*
Phosphorus, Urine *on page 183*

Synonyms Thyrocalcitonin

Applies to Calcium Stimulation Test; Pentagastrin Stimulation Test

Abstract A hypocalcemic polypeptide made by the normal C cells (parafollicular cells) of the thyroid gland, by tumors of the C cells (medullary carcinoma of thyroid), and by certain other neoplasms (lung, breast, pancreas).

Patient Preparation Patient should fast overnight. Avoid recent isotope scan or other exposure to radioactivity.

Specimen Serum or plasma

Container Red top tube or green top (heparin) tube

Collection Avoid hemolysis.

Storage Instructions Collect into chilled tube. Process within 10 minutes of collection. Separate in a refrigerated centrifuge. Separate serum (plasma) into plastic tube and freeze.

Reference Range <19 pg/mL (SI: <19 ng/L) basal for a sensitive RIA assay or column chromatography. Normal ranges for calcium/pentagastrin stimulation tests are available. For stimulation tests, values <350 pg/mL in men and <100 pg/mL in women are expected.

Possible Panic Range Elevated levels are not diagnostic of medullary carcinoma of thyroid (MCT). However, some patients with MCT have values >500 pg/mL.

Use Calcitonin concentrations are increased in both the sporadic and the familial types of MCT and in its precursors, C-cell hyperplasia and microscopic medullary carcinoma. Among the most significant of tumor markers, calcitonin levels roughly correlate with tumor weight or extent of disease, and are used in postoperative patients to monitor for residual, recurrent, and/or metastatic carcinoma. Postoperative levels have prognostic application. The doubling time of serum levels correlates with recurrence.[1]

Multiple endocrine neoplasia (MEN) type 2A includes medullary carcinoma of thyroid, pheochromocytoma, and sometimes, parathyroid adenoma. This is Sipple's syndrome. MEN type 2B includes medullary carcinoma of thyroid, pheochromocytoma, mucosal neuromas, marfanoid habitus, and intestinal ganglioneuromatosis. Medullary carcinoma is found without such other tumors in familial medullary carcinoma.

An important use of calcitonin assay additional to follow-up of patients with medullary carcinoma is investigation of their families to detect early, subclinical cases which may exist as C-cell hyperplasia, microscopic or larger MCT. Indications for calcitonin assay include family history of unspecified type of thyroid cancer, calcified thyroid mass, thyroid tumor associated with hypercalcemia and/or pheochromocytoma, amyloid-containing metastatic carcinoma with unknown primary site and the presence of mucosal neuromas.

Limitations In numbers of patients with MCT (especially those with familial medullary carcinoma of thyroid) the baseline calcitonin may be normal; however, an abnormally large calcitonin response may follow secretagogues, provocative infusion of calcium and/or pentagastrin.[2] A combined calcium pentagastrin test is described. These tests are much more useful than random plasma levels of calcitonin for the diagnosis of MCT. Most subjects with microscopic medullary carcinoma and all with C-cell hyperplasia have normal basal calcitonin levels; provocative testing is needed. Serum calcitonin levels usually cannot differentiate between C-cell hyperplasia alone, and that complicated by emerging microscopic MCT.

Occasional spurious high results are encountered. Hemolysis can cause spurious high levels. Misleading results are recognized. The purity of standards may vary and antibodies in various assays may lack uniform specificities. Calcitonin in patients' sera lacks immunoreactive uniformity. Side effects take place.

DNA analysis identifies carriers of MEN 2A without ambiguity;[3] see listing Multiple Endocrine Neoplasia/Familial Medullary Thyroid Carcinoma *on page 519.*

Methodology Radioimmunoassay (RIA), immunoradiometric assay (IRMA)[4]

Additional Information High concentrations of calcitonin occur not only in patients with malignant parafollicular or C-cell tumors (medullary thyroid carcinoma) but may also be found in patients with small cell carcinomas of the lung; carcinoids; in some individuals with carcinoma of breast, islet cell tumors, APUDomas, in patients with pancreatitis, thyroiditis, and in renal failure. Hypergastrinemia may account for calcitonin elevations in the Zollinger-Ellison syndrome and in pernicious anemia. Medullary carcinoma arises from thyroid C cells (parafollicular cells). C-cell hyperplasia is a preneoplastic state in patients with MEN. Early diagnosis of MCT is needed; total thyroidectomy is curative if the tumor is treated early.

Calcitonin was increased in 48% of patients with small cell (oat cell) carcinoma in a study of 110 patients with lung cancer.

Calcitonin gene-related peptide (CGRP) has been suggested as a useful test together with calcitonin, as tumor markers in MEN type 2.[5]

CEA is next most useful, after calcitonin, as a marker for medullary carcinoma. CEA generates less fluctuation than calcitonin in calculation of doubling time.[1] Histaminase is elevated in most patients with medullary carcinoma. Medullary carcinomas may produce other substances, including ACTH and serotonin. Such ectopic ACTH secretion may cause Cushing's syndrome.

If there are preoperative findings to suggest MCT (eg, family history of unspecified type of thyroid cancer) in a patient with a thyroid mass, then calcitonin level, metanephrines, catecholamines, and CAT scan of the adrenals for pheochromocytoma should be considered. Medullary carcinomas of the thyroid gland have a variable histologic picture. Correlation between serum calcitonin levels and immunoperoxidase staining of the neoplastic thyroid tissue for calcitonin may assist in confirming the diagnosis in difficult cases.

The direct manifestation of high calcitonin levels is secretory diarrhea in 30% of patients with medullary thyroid carcinoma.

Increased calcitonin has been found in systemic mast cell disease.[6]

Footnotes

1. Miyauchi A, Matsuzuka F, Kuma K, et al, "Evaluation of Surgical Results and Prediction of Prognosis in Patients With Medullary Thyroid Carcinoma by Analysis of Serum Calcitonin Levels," *World J Surg*, 1988, 12(5):610-5.
2. Guilloteau D, Perdrisot R, Calmettes C, et al, "Diagnosis of Medullary Carcinoma of the Thyroid (MCT) by Calcitonin Assay Using Monoclonal Antibodies: Criteria for the Pentagastrin Stimulation Test in Hereditary MCT," *J Clin Endocrinol Metab*, 1990, 71(4):1064-7.
3. Lips CJ, Landsvater RM, Höppener JW, et al, "Clinical Screening as Compared With DNA Analysis in Families With Multiple Endocrine Neoplasma Type 2A," *N Engl J Med*, 1994, 331(13):828-35.
4. Perdrisot R, Bigorgne JC, Guilloteau D, et al, "Monoclonal Immunoradiometric Assay of Calcitonin Improves Investigation of Familial Medullary Thyroid Carcinoma," *Clin Chem*, 1990, 36(2):381-3.
5. Schifter S, "Calcitonin Gene-Related Peptide and Calcitonin as Tumour Markers in MEN 2 Family Screening," *Clin Endocrinol (Oxf)*, 1989, 30(3):263-70.
6. Yocum MW, Butterfield JH, and Gharib H, "Increased Plasma Calcitonin Levels in Systemic Mast Cell Disease," *Mayo Clin Proc*, 1994, 69(10):987-90.

References

Boultwood J, Wynford-Thomas D, Richards GP, et al, "*In Situ* Analysis of Calcitonin and CGRP Expression in Medullary Thyroid Carcinoma," *Clin Endocrinol (Oxf)*, 1990, 33(3):381-90.
Carter WB, Taylor RL, Kao PC, et al, "Determination of Plasma Calcitonin Gene-Related Peptide Concentrations by a New Immunochemiluminometric Assay in Normal Persons and Patients With Medullary Thyroid Carcinoma and Other Neuroendocrine Tumors," *J Clin Endocrinol Metab*, 1991, 72(2):327-35.
Gautvik KM, "Medullary Carcinoma of the Thyroid. An Uptake of Diagnostic and Prognostic Factors," *Scand J Clin Lab Invest Suppl*, 1991, 206:85-92.
Ghillani PP, Motte P, Troalen F, et al, "Identification and Measurement of Calcitonin Precursors in Serum of Patients With Malignant Diseases," *Cancer Res*, 1989, 49(23):6845-51.
Rosai J, Carcangiu ML, and Delellis RA, "Tumors of the Thyroid Gland," *Atlas of Tumor Pathology*, Washington, DC: Armed Forces Institute of Pathology, 1992.
Rougier P, Calmettes C, LaPlanche A, et al, "The Values of Calcitonin and Carcinoembryonic Antigen in the Treatment and Management of Nonfamilial Medullary Thyroid Carcinoma," *Cancer*, 1983, 51:855-62.
Sanchez GJ, Venkataraman PS, Pryor RW, et al, "Hypercalcitoninemia and Hypocalcemia in Acutely Ill Children: Studies in Serum Calcium, Blood Ionized Calcium, and Calcium-Regulating Hormones," *J Pediatr*, 1989, 114(6):952-6.

Calcitriol *see Vitamin D₃, Serum on page 218*

Calcium/Creatinine Ratio *see Calcium, Urine on page 99*

Calcium, Ionized

CPT 82330

Related Information

Calcium, Serum *on next page*
Kidney Stone Analysis *on page 640*
Parathyroid Hormone *on page 178*

Synonyms Ionized Calcium

Abstract This is the physiologically active portion of serum calcium and represents about half of total calcium.

Patient Preparation Patient should be recumbent for 30 minutes prior to collection.

Specimen Whole blood (preferred), serum, or plasma

Container Green top (heparin) tube if whole blood or plasma is used or red top tube

Collection Collect anaerobically, leave stoppers in; do not use tourniquet. Heparin syringe is best; 1 unit of heparin/mL of blood lowers ionized calcium 0.01 mmol/L. The use of dry, electrolyte balanced heparin virtually eliminates the heparin interference.[1]

Storage Instructions Store anaerobically. Such specimens can be stored 48 hours at 4°C.

Special Instructions Controversy exists over the ideal specimen for ionized calcium determination. Concern exists that ionized calcium values may be altered by clotting (serum) or by heparin binding of calcium (plasma). However, serum and plasma have been found to give generally similar values, while whole blood is 1% to 2% higher.

Most large laboratories have instrumentation (selective ion electrode) for direct measurement of ionized calcium. Adjusting pH to 7.4 is not necessary if blood is collected anaerobically.

Reference Range See table.

Calcium, Ionized

Age	Reference Range (Whole Blood)	
	Conventional units (mg/dL)	SI units (mmol/L)
Cord blood	5.20-5.84	1.30-1.46
3-24 h	4.32-5.12	1.08-1.28
24-48 h	4.00-4.72	1.00-1.18
Adults	4.60-5.08	1.12-1.32

Critical Values Replacement may begin when the ionized calcium value is <0.8 mmol/L.[2]

Possible Panic Range <0.70 mmol/L[2]

Use Ionized calcium is usually ordered to avoid hypocalcemia. Ionized calcium measurements are used to evaluate nonbound calcium; it is a measure of physiologically active calcium fraction. Ionized calcium is increased with hyperparathyroidism, ectopic parathyroid hormone-producing neoplasms, and with excessive vitamin D.

Ionized calcium is measured in patients with renal failure and/or transplantation, in whom problems include secondary hyperparathyroidism. It is indicated for patients with sepsis, with magnesium deficiency, and in pancreatitis. Hypocalcemia occurs following administration of citrate (eg, liver transplantation) or infusion of other fluids during extracorporeal membrane oxygenation or surgery, and measurement of ionized calcium is needed to ascertain balance in dialysis patients.[2]

Ill premature infants with hypoproteinemia and acidosis. Occasionally useful when hypercalcemia coexists with abnormal protein state such as myeloma, in disturbances of acid base balance; in cirrhosis.

Low in hypoparathyroidism, vitamin D deficiency, pseudohypoparathyroidism.

A role for ionized calcium levels exists in cardiothoracic surgery and heart transplantation and in patients in cardiac arrest.[3]

Limitations Total calcium remains the first line test for evaluation of calcium abnormality.

Methodology Ion-selective electrode (ISE)

Additional Information Calcium in serum exists ionized, bound to organic anions such as phosphate and citrate, and bound to proteins (mainly albumin). Of these, ionized calcium is the physiologically important form.

Measurement of serum ionized calcium provides insight into the effect of total protein and albumin on serum calcium levels. A patient can have high total calcium, with normal ionized calcium and increased total protein and/or albumin, as in dehydration or in myeloma.

Women have greater circadian variation of ionized calcium and intact PTH than men.[4]

An inverse relationship between ionized calcium and phosphate concentration exists.[5]

Footnotes

1. Toffaletti J, Ernst P, Hunt P, et al, "Dry Electrolyte-Balanced Heparinized Syringes Evaluated for Determining Ionized Calcium and Other Electrolytes in Whole Blood," *Clin Chem*, 1991, 37:(10 Pt 1)1730-3.
2. Toffaletti J, "Physiology and Regulation. Ionized Calcium, Magnesium and Lactate Measurements in Critical Care Settings," *Am J Clin Pathol*, 1995, 104(4 Suppl 1):S88-94.
3. Urban P, Scheidegger D, Buchmann B, et al, "Cardiac Arrest and Blood Ionized Calcium Levels," *Ann Intern Med*, 1988,.109(2):110-3.
4. Calvo MS, Eastell R, Offord KP, et al, "Circadian Variation in Ionized Calcium and Intact Parathyroid Hormone: Evidence for Sex Differences in Calcium Homeostasis," *J Clin Endocrinol Metab*, 1991, 72(1):69-76.
5. Lehmann M and Mimouni F, "Serum Phosphate Concentration. Effect on Serum Ionized Calcium Concentration In Vitro," *Am J Dis Child*, 1989, 143(11):1340-1.

References

Cooper RS and Shamsi N, "Ionized Serum Calcium in Black Hypertensives: Absence of a Relationship With Blood Pressure," *J Clin Hypertens*, 1987(4), 3:514-9.
Forman DT and Lorenzo L, "Ionized Calcium: Its Significance and Clinical Usefulness," *Ann Clin Lab Sci*, 1991, 21(5):297-304.
Loughead JL, Mimouni F, and Tsang RC, "Serum Ionized Calcium Concentrations in Normal Neonates," *Am J Dis Child*, 1988, 142(5):516-8.
Rasmussen N, Frolich A, Hornnes PJ, et al, "Serum Ionized Calcium and Intact Parathyroid Hormone Levels During Pregnancy and Postpartum," *Br J Obstet Gynaecol*, 1990, 97(9):857-9.
Roelofsen JM, Berkel GM, Uttendorfsky OT, et al, "Urinary Excretion Rates of Calcium and Magnesium in Normal and Complicated Pregnancies," *Eur J Obstet Gynecol Reprod Biol*, 1988, 27(3):227-36.
Rosen IB and Pollard A, "Ionized Calcium in Monitoring Effective Parathyroidectomy: A Preliminary Report," *World J Surg*, 1988, 12(5):630-4.
Thode J, Holmegaard SN, Transbol I, et al, "Adjusted Ionized Calcium (at pH 7.4) and Actual Ionized Calcium (at Actual pH) in Capillary Blood Compared for Clinical Evaluation of Patients With Disorders of Calcium Metabolism," *Clin Chem*, 1990, 36(3):541-4.
Wu AH, Bracey A, Bryan-Brown CW, et al, "Ionized Calcium Monitoring During Liver Transplantation," *Arch Pathol Lab Med*, 1987, 111(10):935-8.

Calcium Oxalate, Urine see Oxalate, Urine on page 174

Calcium, Serum

CPT 82310

Related Information

Aluminum, Bone on page 586
Aluminum, Serum on page 586
Calcium, Ionized on previous page
Calcium, Urine on page 99
Concentration Test, Urine on page 633
Cyclic AMP, Urine on page 119
Kidney Stone Analysis on page 640
Magnesium, Serum on page 164
Magnesium, Urine on page 165
Multiple Endocrine Neoplasia/Familial Medullary Thyroid Carcinoma on page 519
Osteocalcin, Serum on page 174
Parathyroid Hormone on page 178
Phosphorus, Serum on page 182
Phosphorus, Urine on page 183
Potassium, Serum or Plasma on page 188
Vitamin D₃, Serum on page 218

Synonyms Ca, Blood; Total Calcium, Serum

Applies to Chloride/Phosphorus Ratio; Parathyroid Hormone-Related Protein

Abstract The two most common causes of hypercalcemia (beyond slight increases from dehydration) are primary hyperparathyroidism (HPT) and malignancy. Activation of osteoclasts by parathormone or parathyroid hormone-related protein leads to hypercalcemia through bone resorption.[1]

Disorders of calcium metabolism are initially evaluated with measurements of serum phosphorus, alkaline phosphatase, albumin, chloride, total protein and commonly, parathormone assays as well as serum and often 24-hour urine calcium levels.

Specimen Serum

Container Red top tube

Sampling Time Morning, fasting sample is desirable, since some diurnal variation exists (which may reflect postural changes).

Collection Pediatrics: Blood drawn from heelstick for capillary. Since about half of serum calcium is bound to proteins, there is variation with posture. Venous stasis in sampling causes misleading results.

Storage Instructions Refrigerate in stoppered vials, not in sample cups.

Causes for Rejection Gross hemolysis

Reference Range Infant to 1 month: 7.0-11.5 mg/dL (SI: 1.75-2.87 mmol/L); 1 month to 1 year: 8.6-11.2 mg/dL (SI: 2.15-2.79 mmol/L) normal range slowly descends. Up to 60 years: 8.2-10.2 mg/dL (SI: 2.05-2.54 mmol/L). It decreases slightly in older years. These ranges bear an assumption of normal serum albumin concentration. If albumin is increased, adjust calcium downward and if albumin is diminished, adjust serum calcium upwards. Calcium can be adjusted 0.8 mg/dL (0.20 mmol/L) for each 1.0 g/dL by which albumin is above or <4 g/dL.[1]

Critical Values <7.0 mg/dL (SI: <1.75 mmol/L) may lead to tetany. Calcium >12.0 mg/dL (SI: >2.99 mmol/L) may induce coma, although some patients tolerate higher levels.

Possible Panic Range Possibly life-threatening levels: ≤6.0 mg/dL (SI: ≤1.50 mmol/L); **severe hypercalcemia** is defined as ≥14.0 mg/dL (SI: ≥3.5 mmol/L). Hypercalcemia leads to polyuria, anorexia, and nausea. Extremely high levels may be found with primary parathyroid carcinomas, which are very uncommon.
(Continued)

Calcium, Serum *(Continued)*

Use Work-up for coma, investigation of pancreatitis and other gastrointestinal problems, nephrolithiasis, polydipsia, polyuria, azotemia, multiple endocrine adenomatosis.

Causes of high calcium:

- Primary hyperparathyroidism (HPT) - look also for high ionized calcium, measured or calculated. Hyperparathyroidism may coexist with other endocrine tumors (multiple endocrine adenomatosis syndromes).
- Carcinoma, with or without bone metastases. Humoral hypercalcemia of malignancy (HHM), tumor induced hypercalcemia is seen especially in primary squamous cell carcinoma of lung, head and neck, but other important tumors include primaries in the breast, kidney, liver, bladder, and ovary. It is usually caused by **parathyroid hormone-related protein**, for which assays exist. Hypercalcemia can also result from conversion of 25-hydroxy vitamin D to 1,25-dihydroxy vitamin D by neoplasm.[1] The most common solid tumors causing bone metastases are primaries in the breast and lung. Other neoplasms may also cause hypercalcemia, especially myeloma. Differences between HPT and humoral hypercalcemia of malignancy include low dihydroxy vitamin D, reduced calcium absorption, and the presence of a nonparathyroid tumor. Hypercalcemia with alkaline phosphatase more than twice its upper limit is more suggestive of **cancer** than of hyperparathyroidism. Especially if there is only a brief duration of symptoms, anemia, increased LDH and alkaline phosphatase, hypoalbuminemia, and other findings suggestive of malignant disease, chloride/phosphorus ratio <29 mmol/L, chloride <100 mmol/L, high serum LD (LDH) and/or phosphorus, think first of malignant neoplasm.[2] **The chloride/phosphorus ratio** is predominantly of value when it is <29 mmol/L, to provide evidence **against** a diagnosis of primary hyperparathyroidism.[2] **Parathyroid hormone-related protein** is a 141-amino acid peptide with limited homology to PTH itself. Both peptides activate the PTH receptor to produce hypercalcemia. PTH-related protein is now recognized as the cause of hypercalcemia in most solid tumors, particularly squamous and renal carcinomas.[3]
- Myeloma, leukemia, lymphoma; especially T-cell[4] lymphoma/leukemia and Burkitt's lymphoma.
- Dehydration is an extremely common cause of slight increases of calcium.
- Sarcoidosis (10% to 20% of patients have high serum calcium; usually without low serum phosphorus). About 50% have hypercalciuria.
- Chronic hypervitaminosis D; ectopic production of 1,25-dihydroxy vitamin D; vitamin A intoxication, isotretinoin (a vitamin A derivative).[5]
- Prolonged immobilization (uncommon), in patient with increased bone turnover (eg, Paget's disease of bone, malignancy, children).
- TB, histoplasmosis, coccidioidomycosis, berylliosis, leprosy, Wegener's granulomatosis (increased 1,25-dihydroxy vitamin D production)
- Milk-alkali syndrome: prolonged use of calcium-containing materials and alkali (eg, $CaCO_3$) or other absorbable alkali ulcer remedies with high milk intake (now rare).
- Idiopathic hypercalcemia of infancy (uncommon)
- Endocrine: hyperthyroidism; Addison's disease; acromegaly; pheochromocytoma (rare cause of hypercalcemia); vasoactive intestinal polypeptide hormone-producing tumor
- Advanced chronic liver disease
- Bacteremia
- Familial hypocalciuric hypercalcemia[6] (dominant inheritance); the best test for familial benign hypercalciuria (FBH) is a plot of fasting serum PTH against fasting urine calcium excretion[7]
- Aluminum-induced renal osteomalacia
- Parenteral nutrition
- Renal insufficiency
- Drugs: calcium salts, lithium, thiazide/chlorthalidone therapy, other diuretics; antiestrogens and estrogens (rapid increase in patients with breast carcinoma).

In any case of hypercalcemia, it is desirable to measure magnesium and potassium levels.

Causes of low calcium:

- Low albumin and low total protein relate to common, usually slight decreases of calcium. The usual method measures **total** calcium, about half of which is bound to plasma proteins. Since the metabolically active form of calcium is the ionized state, the patient's serum protein level should be considered when interpreting a calcium result. For example, a patient's ionized calcium may be normal when the total calcium is elevated in the presence of elevated proteins and, conversely, may also be normal when the total calcium is low and the proteins are low.
- High phosphorus: renal insufficiency, hypoparathyroidism, pseudohypoparathyroidism

- Vitamin D deficiency, rickets, osteomalacia (Alkaline phosphatase is a screening test for osteomalacia. Calcium, phosphorus, and alkaline phosphatase can all be normal in osteomalacia.)
- Milkman's syndrome
- Malabsorption or malnutrition with interference with vitamin D and/or calcium absorption
- Renal tubular acidosis
- Pancreatitis, acute
- Dilutional: I.V. fluids
- Bacteremia
- Hypomagnesemia
- Anticonvulsants and other common drugs, most by *in vivo* action, can depress calcium. Barbiturates in elderly may cause calcium decrease; other drugs including calcitonin, corticosteroids, gastrin, glucagon, glucose, insulin, magnesium salts, methicillin, and tetracycline in pregnancy.

The differential diagnosis is shown in a graph presented in the listing Parathyroid Hormone *on page 178*, in which PTH is plotted against calcium.

Limitations Sodium citrate, EDTA, and NaF potassium oxalate interfere. Gross hemolysis falsely elevates results.

Methodology Cresolphthalein complexone; complexone is required to minimize effect of hemolysis[8]; atomic absorption (AA) is not used extensively, but remains the reference method.

Additional Information In the differential diagnosis of hypercalcemia, serum calcium should be measured on at least three occasions. In **primary hyperparathyroidism**, parathyroid hormone, serum chloride, and urine calcium are increased. Rarely, in HPT the hypercalcemia is accompanied by a low-normal PTH.[9] In HPT, calcium rises, then phosphorus falls, then alkaline phosphatase rises. Alkaline phosphatase is usually not more than twice its upper limit in HPT. Measured ionized calcium and calculated ionized calcium may be helpful. Primary hyperparathyroidism and cancer with or without metastases cause 95% of instances of hypercalcemia.

Twenty-four hour urinary calcium is increased in HPT, low in **familial hypocalciuric hypercalcemia** (FHH) which is characterized by hypercalcemia and hypocalciuria. An autosomal dominant, it apparently has no complications. Ratio of renal calcium clearance to creatinine clearance <0.01 suggests this genetic disease. The calcium/creatinine clearance ratio is said to discriminate between FHH and hyperparathyroidism.[2] Family studies are highly desirable.

Hypocalcemia, rather then hypercalcemia, occur with rhabdomyolysis - induced acute renal failure.[10,11]

Footnotes

1. Bilezikian JP, "Management of Acute Hypercalcemia," *N Engl J Med*, 1992, 326(18):1196-1203.
2. Wong ET and Freier EF, "The Differential Diagnosis of Hypercalcemia. An Algorithm for More Effective Use of Laboratory Tests," *JAMA*, 1982, 247:75-80.
3. Strewler GJ and Nissenson RA, "Hypercalcemia in Malignancy," *West J Med*, 1990, 153(6):635-40.
4. Sirianni SR, Mora ME, Sands AM, et al, "Malignant Lymphoma Presenting With Severe Hypercalcemia," *N Y State J Med*, 1989, 89(9):533-5.
5. Valentic JP, Elias AN, and Weinstein GD, "Hypercalcemia Associated With Oral Isotretinoin in the Treatment of Severe Acne," *JAMA*, 1983, 250:1899-900.
6. Marx SJ, "Familial Hypocalciuric Hypercalcemia," *N Engl J Med*, 1980, 303:810-1.
7. Gunn IR and Wallace JR, "Urine Calcium and Serum Ionized Calcium, Total Calcium and Parathyroid Hormone Concentrations in the Diagnosis of Primary Hyperparathyroidism and Familial Benign Hypercalcaemia," *Ann Clin Biochem*, 1992, 29(Pt 1):52-8.
8. Corns CM, "Interference by Haemoglobin With the Cresolphthalein Complexone Method for Serum Calcium Measurement," *Ann Clin Biochem*, 1990, 27(Pt 2):152-5.
9. Hollenberg AN and Arnold A, "Hypercalcemia With Low-Normal Serum Intact PTH: A Novel Presentation of Primary Hyperparathyroidism," *Am J Med*, 1991, 91(5):547-8.
10. Llach F, Felsenfeld AJ, and Haussler MR, "The Pathophysiology of Altered Calcium Metabolism in Rhabdomyolysis-Induced Acute Renal Failure, Interactions of Parathyroid Hormone, 25-Hydroxycholecalciferol, and 1,25-Dihydroxycholecalciferol," *N Engl J Med*, 1981, 305:117-23.
11. Knochel JP, "Serum Calcium Derangements in Rhabdomyolysis," *N Engl J Med*, 1981, 305:161-3.

References

Aderka D, Schwartz D, Dan M, et al, "Bacteremic Hypocalcemia - A Comparison Between the Calcium Levels of Bacteremic and Nonbacteremic Patients With Infection," *Arch Intern Med*, 1987, 147(2):232-6.

Balland M and Trivin F, "Total Calcium," *Drug Effects on Laboratory Test Results Analytical Interferences and Pharmacological Effects*, Siest G and Galteau MM, eds, Littleton, MA: PSG Publishing Co Inc, 1988, 148-64.

Bourke E and Delaney V, "Assessment of Hypocalcemia and Hypercalcemia," *Clin Lab Med*, 1993, 13(1):157-81.

Broadus AE, Mangin M, Ikeda K, et al, "Humoral Hypercalcemia of Cancer. Identification of a Novel Parathyroid Hormone-Like Peptide," *N Engl J Med*, 1988, 319(9):556-63.

Budayr AA, Nissenson RA, Klein RF, et al, "Increased Serum Levels of a Parathyroid Hormone-like Protein in Malignancy-Associated Hypercalcemia," *Ann Intern Med*, 1989, 111(10):807-12.

Chasan SA, Pothel LR, and Huben RP, "Management and Prognostic Significance of Hypercalcemia in Renal Cell Carcinoma," *Urology*, 1989, 33(3):167-70.

Gerhardt A, Greenberg A, Reilly JJ Jr, et al, "Hypercalcemia - A Complication of Advanced Chronic Liver Disease," *Arch Intern Med*, 1987, 147(2):274-7.

Gibbs WN, Lofters WS, Campbell M, et al, "Non-Hodgkin Lymphoma in Jamaica and Its Relation to Adult T-Cell Leukemia-Lymphoma," *Ann Intern Med*, 1987, 106(6):361-8.

Hruska KA and Teitelbaum SL, "Renal Osteodystrophy," *N Engl J Med*, 1995, 333(3):166-74.

Jayabose S, Iqbal K, Newman L, et al, "Hypercalcemia in Childhood Renal Tumors," *Cancer*, 1988, 61(4):788-91.

Klee GG, Kao PC, and Heath H 3d, "Hypercalcemia," *Endocrinol Metab Clin North Am*, 1988, 17(3):573-600.

Law WM Jr and Heath H 3d, "Familial Benign Hypercalcemia (Hypocalciuric Hypercalcemia)," *Ann Intern Med*, 1985, 102(4):511-9.

Law WM Jr, Wahner HW, and Heath H ed, "Bone Mineral Density and Skeletal Fractures in Familial Benign Hypercalcemia (Hypocalciuric Hypercalcemia)," *Mayo Clin Proc*, 1984, 59(12):811-5.

Lobaugh B, Neelon FA, Oyama H, et al, "Circadian Rhythms for Calcium, Inorganic Phosphorus, and Parathyroid Hormone in Primary Hyperparathyroidism: Functional and Practical Considerations," *Surgery*, 1989, 106(6):1009-16.

Samaan NA, Ouais S, Ordonez NG, et al, "Multiple Endocrine Syndrome Type I: Clinical, Laboratory Findings, and Management in Five Families," *Cancer*, 1989, 64(3):741-52.

Sanchez GJ, Venkataraman PS, Pryor RW, et al, "Hypercalcitoninemia and Hypocalcemia in Acutely III Children: Studies in Serum Calcium, Blood Ionized Calcium, and Calcium-Regulating Hormones," *J Pediatr*, 1989, 114(6):952-6.

Zaloga GP, Chernow B, and Eil C, "Hypercalcemia and Disseminated Cytomegalovirus Infection in the Acquired Immunodeficiency Syndrome," *Ann Intern Med*, 1985, 102(3):331-3.

Calcium Stimulation Test *see* Calcitonin *on page 96*

Calcium, Urine

CPT 82340

Related Information

Calcium, Serum *on page 97*

Kidney Stone Analysis *on page 640*

Magnesium, Urine *on page 165*

Parathyroid Hormone *on page 178*

Phosphorus, Urine *on page 183*

Uric Acid, Urine *on page 215*

Urine Collection, 24-Hour *on page 30*

Vitamin D₃, Serum *on page 218*

Applies to Calcium/Creatinine Ratio

Abstract Used to investigate effects of vitamin D, parathyroid hormone, and parathyroid hormone-related protein. When bone resorption is accelerated, the kidney defends against hypercalcemia by enhanced calciuria. Symptoms of hypercalciuria include polyuria, polydipsia, and sometimes nephrocalcinosis and nephrolithiasis.[1]

Patient Preparation In stone evaluation, urinary calcium results are more meaningful if the patient initially is on his/her usual diet for 3 days prior to urine collection. Drugs affecting mineral metabolism include antacids, phosphates, glucocorticoids, carbonic anhydrase inhibitors, anticonvulsants, and diuretics including thiazides. Thiazides are used therapeutically to lower urine calcium excretion. If the patient is on a stone prevention regime and test is for follow-up, then medications should **not** be stopped for the test.

Specimen 24-hour urine

Container Plastic urine container or acid-washed glass bottle

Reference Range Varies with diet; based on average calcium intake of 600-800 mg/24 hours (SI: 15-20 mmol/day): excretion may be 100-250 mg/24 hours (SI: 2.5-6.2 mmol/day). On a diet of 400-800 mg/24 hours of calcium daily (SI: 10-20 mmol/day), others set the upper limit at 200 mg/24 hours of calcium (SI: 5 mmol/day) in a 24-hour urine collection. More than 4 mg/kg is associated with increased prevalence of stone formation. Low calcium diet: <150 mg/24 hours (SI: <3.7 mmol/day) excreted. High calcium diet: 250-300 mg/24 hours (SI: 6.2-7.5 mmol/day) excreted. Hypercalciuria has been defined as calcium excretion in excess of 250 mg/24 hours (SI: 6.2 mmol/day) for women, 300 mg/24 hours (SI: 7.5 mmol/day) for men.[2] Calcium excretion, like other laboratory results, must be related to the individual patient. The rate of calcium excretion can also be expressed as a calcium/creatinine ratio. In healthy individuals with constant muscle mass, urinary calcium (mg/dL)/creatinine (mg/dL) is <0.14 (SI: calcium (mmol/L)/creatinine (mmol/L) is <0.40). Values >0.20 (mg/dL) or >0.57 (mmol/L units) suggest hypercalciuria.

Use Reflects intake, rates of intestinal calcium absorption, bone resorption, and renal loss. Those processes relate to parathyroid hormone, parathyroid hormone-related protein, and vitamin D levels. Evaluate bone disease, calcium metabolism, renal stones (nephrolithiasis)[3] and idiopathic hypercalciuria.[4] Follow up patients on calcium therapy for osteopenia.

High in 30% to 80% of instances of primary hyperparathyroidism, but urinary calcium excretion does not consistently, reliably distinguish hyperparathyroidism from other entities. High in about 50% of patients with sarcoidosis. Increased with immobilization, with steroid therapy, with Paget's disease of bone, and in primary (idiopathic) hypercalciuria.[5] Increased with entities causing high ultrafiltrable calcium: humoral hypercalcemia of malignancy, some cases of renal tubular acidosis, Fanconi syndrome, increased calcium intake, vitamin D intoxication, hyperthyroidism, diabetes mellitus, acromegaly, glucocorticoid excess, some cases of Crohn's disease and ulcerative colitis, myeloma, some

instances of leukemia and lymphoma, and carcinoma metastatic to bone. Reported relationship to hematuria in children.[6]

Low in familial hypocalciuric hypercalcemia, for which urine calcium measurements are mandatory; low with thiazide diuretics, vitamin D deficiency, renal osteodystrophy, vitamin D resistant rickets, hypoparathyroidism, pseudohypoparathyroidism and pre-eclampsia.[7]

Limitations Decreased in patients on oral contraceptives. Lacks specificity for hyperparathyroidism when increased. Five percent of the population have hypercalciuria.[5]

Methodology Cresolphthalein complexone, atomic absorption (AA)

Additional Information Hypercalcemia leads to polyuria through interference with renal reabsorption of sodium and water.[1]

Twenty percent to 25% of patients who form calcium stones have hyperuricosuria. Urinary calcium reflects in part the relation between GFR and tubular reabsorption.

Footnotes

1. Bilezikian JP, "Management of Acute Hypercalcemia," *N Engl J Med*, 1992, 326(18):1196-1203.
2. Palmieri GM, "Calcium, Phosphate, and Magnesium Metabolism," *The Laboratory in Clinical Medicine. Interpretation and Application*, 2nd ed, Halsted JA and Halsted CH, eds, Philadelphia, PA: WB Saunders Co, 1981, 688-96.
3. Silverberg SJ, Shane E, Jacobs TP, et al, "Nephrolithiasis and Bone Involvement in Primary Hyperparathyroidism," *Am J Med*, 1990, 89(3):327-34.
4. Lemann J Jr and Gray RW, "Idiopathic Hypercalciuria," *J Urol*, 1989, 141(3 Pt 2):715-8.
5. Erickson SB, "Hypercalciuria," *Mayo Clin Proc*, 1981, 56:579.
6. Stark H, Tieder M, Eisenstein B, et al, "Hypercalciuria as a Cause of Persistent or Recurrent Haematuria," *Arch Dis Child*, 1988, 63(3):312-3.
7. Taufield PA, Ales KL, Resnick LM, et al, "Hypocalciuria in Preeclampsia," *N Engl J Med*, 1987, 316(12):715-8.

References

"Case Records of the Massachusetts General Hospital. Weekly Clinicopathological Exercises. Case 50-1981. A 76 Year Old Woman With Intermittent Hypercalcemia," *N Engl J Med*, 1981, 305:1457-64.

Friedman RB and Young DS, *Effects of Disease on Clinical Laboratory Tests*, Washington, DC: American Association of Clinical Chemistry Press, 1989.

Gunn IR and Wallace JR, "Urine Calcium and Serum Ionized Calcium, Total Calcium and Parathyroid Hormone Concentrations in the Diagnosis of Primary Hyperparathyroidism and Familial Benign Hypercalcaemia," *Ann Clin Biochem*, 1992, 29(Pt 1):52-8.

Lemann J Jr, Pleuss JA, Gray RW, et al, "Potassium Administration Reduces and Potassium Deprivation Increases Urinary Calcium Excretion in Healthy Adults," *Kidney Int*, 1991, 39(5):973-83.

Lemann J Jr, Worcester EM, and Gray RW, "Hypercalciuria and Stones," *Am J Kidney Dis*, 1991, 17(4):386-91.

Marx SJ, Stock JL, Attie MF, et al, "Familial Hypocalciuric Hypercalcemia: Recognition Among Patients Referred After Unsuccessful Parathyroid Exploration," *Ann Intern Med*, 1980, 92:351-6.

Sanchez-Ramos L, Jones DC, and Cullen MT, "Urinary Calcium as an Early Marker for Pre-eclampsia," *Obstet Gynecol*, 1991, 77(5):685-8.

cAMP, Plasma *see* Cyclic AMP, Plasma *on page 119*

cAMP, Urine *see* Cyclic AMP, Urine *on page 119*

Cancer Antigen 125 *see* CA 125 *on page 94*

Capillary Blood Gases *see* Blood Gases, Capillary *on page 89*

Captopril Test *see* Renin, Plasma *on page 197*

Carbohydrate Antigen 15-3 *see* CA 15-3 *on page 93*

Carbohydrate Antigen 19-9 *see* CA 19-9 *on page 93*

Carbohydrate Deficient Glycoprotein *see* Carbohydrate Deficient Transferrin *on this page*

Carbohydrate Deficient Glycoprotein Syndrome *see* Carbohydrate Deficient Transferrin *on this page*

Carbohydrate Deficient Transferrin

CPT 82644

Synonyms Carbohydrate Deficient Glycoprotein Syndrome

Applies to Carbohydrate Deficient Glycoprotein

Abstract Serum transferrin with fewer than the normal number of attached sialic acid groups is found in a genetic disorder of infancy and childhood.

Specimen Serum

Container Red top tube

Storage Instructions Freeze immediately; ship on dry ice.

Special Instructions Usually sent to reference laboratory.

Reference Range Normal values are reported as percentage of total transferrin: pentasialo: 13% to 23%; tetrasialo: 38% to 49%; trisialo: 17% to 31%; disialo: 2% to 15%; monosialo: 0% to 5%

Use Potential marker for excessive alcohol consumption. It may prove to be a useful marker for relapse. It is used to diagnose a newly recognized genetic disease, carbohydrate deficient glycoprotein syndrome, which involves a central nervous system developmental disorder characterized by muscular weakness and hypotonia.

Methodology Affinity chromatography and isoelectric focusing

(Continued)

Carbohydrate Deficient Transferrin (Continued)

Additional Information This test is not generally affected by liver disease.

References

Fagerberg B, Agewall S, Berglund A, et al, "Is Carbohydrate-Deficient Transferrin in Serum Useful for Detecting Excessive Alcohol Consumption in Hypertensive Patients?" Clin Chem, 1994, 40(11 Pt 1):2057-63.

Hagberg B, Blennow G, Kristiansson B, et al, "Carbohydrate-Deficient Glycoprotein Syndromes: Peculiar Group of New Disorders," Pediatr Neurol, 1993, 9(4):255-62.

Jaeken J and Carchon H, "The Carbohydrate-Deficient Glycoprotein Syndromes: An Overview," J Inherit Metab Dis, 1993, 16(5):813-20.

Leavelle DE, Mayo Medical Laboratories Interpretive Handbook, Rochester, MN: Mayo Medical Laboratories, 1994.

Rosman AS and Lieber CS, "Diagnostic Utility of Laboratory Tests in Alcoholic Liver Disease," Clin Chem, 1994, 40(8):1641-51.

Carbon Dioxide, Blood

CPT 82374

Related Information

Blood Gases, Arterial on page 87

Blood Gases, Capillary on page 89

Blood Gases, Venous on page 89

Chloride, Serum on page 108

Electrolytes, Serum or Plasma on page 123

HCO_3, Blood on page 142

Kidney Stone Analysis on page 640

pCO_2, Blood on page 179

pH, Blood on page 180

Synonyms CO_2 Content; CO_2T; tCO_2

Applies to Acid-Base Status Evaluation; Bicarbonate

Abstract Used principally for evaluation of acid-base balance, CO_2T includes bicarbonate, carbonic acid, and CO_2 in solution. It is used most often on venous serum to estimate bicarbonate.

Specimen Whole blood; plasma or serum

Container Green top (heparin) tube

Collection Specimen should be kept tightly closed, as CO_2 will diffuse out, causing erroneous values. This loss may amount to 6 mmol/hour.[1] Anaerobic conditions are best.

Reference Range Whole blood - infancy to 2 years: 18-28 mmol/L (SI: 18-28 mmol/L); 2 years and older: arterial: 23-29 mmol/L (SI: 23-29 mmol/L); venous: 22-26 mmol/L (SI: 22-26 mmol/L). Plasma or serum - venous: 23-29 mmol/L (SI: 23-29 mmol/L).

Possible Panic Range <15 mmol/L (SI: <15 mmol/L), >50 mmol/L (SI: >50 mmol/L).

Use Evaluate the total carbonate buffering system in the body, acid-base balance. High results may represent respiratory acidosis with CO_2 retention (eg, advanced pulmonary emphysema) or metabolic alkalosis (eg, prolonged vomiting). Low value may indicate respiratory alkalosis as in hyperventilation or metabolic acidosis (eg, diabetes with ketoacidosis).

Limitations Interpretation requires clinical information and evaluation of the other electrolytes.

Methodology Colorimetry, enzyme assay, or pCO_2 electrode. TCO_2 can be calculated from blood gas measurements. Organic acids interfere (positively) in the total carbon dioxide as measured on the Kodak Ektachem® 700.[1,2]

Additional Information "Total carbon dioxide" consists of CO_2 in solution or bound to proteins, HCO_3^-, CO_3^{2-}, and H_2CO_3. In practice, 80% to 90% is present as bicarbonate (HCO_3^-). "Hypercapnia" means excessive carbon dioxide in the blood. Impaired elimination of CO_2 reflects interaction of abnormalities in mechanisms controlling respiratory drive, the muscles of respiration, and the function of the lung. Elimination of carbon dioxide from the lung involves alveolar ventilation but not dead-space ventilation. Partitioning of these spaces is expressed as a ratio between dead space and total volume per breath: the tidal volume. The tidal volume normally is <0.30. These and other aspects of pulmonary gas exchange, ventilation and their consequences are addressed as the partial pressure of arterial carbon dioxide, $PaCO_2$, a part of arterial blood gases.[3]

Footnotes

1. Rifai N, Hyde J, Iosefsohn M, et al, "Organic Acids Interfere in the Measurement of Carbon Dioxide Concentration by the Kodak Ektachem® 700," Ann Clin Biochem, 1992, 29(Pt 1):105-8.
2. O'Leary TD and Langton SR, "Calculated Bicarbonate or Total Carbon Dioxide?" Clin Chem, 1989, 35(8):1697-700.
3. Weinberger SE, Schwartzstein RM, and Weiss JW, "Hypercapnia," N Engl J Med, 1989, 321(18):1223-31.

References

Henneman PL, Gruber JE, Marx JA, et al, "Development of Acidosis in Human Beings During Closed-Chest and Open-Chest CPR," Ann Emerg Med, 1988, 17(7):672-5.

McLain BI, Evans J, Dear PR, et al, "Comparison of Capillary and Arterial Blood Gas Measurements in Neonates," Arch Dis Child, 1988, 63(7 Spec No):743-7.

Zenger M, Brenner M, Hua P, et al, "Measuring Oxygen Uptake and Carbon Dioxide Production in Critically Ill Patients Using a Standard Blood Gas Analyzer," Crit Care Med, 1994, 22(5):783-8.

Carbonic Anhydrase III see Myoglobin, Blood on page 167

Carcinoembryonic Antigen

CPT 82378

Related Information

Adrenocorticotropic Hormone on page 63

Alpha$_1$-Fetoprotein, Serum on page 72

Body Fluid on page 89

Body Fluid Analysis, Cell Count on page 306

Body Fluid Cytology on page 286

Body Fluid Glucose on page 91

Breast Biopsy on page 35

CA 15-3 on page 93

CA 19-9 on page 93

CA 125 on page 94

Colon Cancer, Hereditary Nonpolyposis Type on page 506

Cyst Fluid Cytology on page 292

Homovanillic Acid, Urine on page 145

Immunoperoxidase Procedures on page 43

Occult Blood, Stool on page 645

Synonyms CEA

Abstract One of the first tumor markers, CEA is an oncofetal glycoprotein antigen. It is not organ specific. Abnormalities are found in a wide range of tumor types, but application is widest with adenocarcinomas of the gastrointestinal tract.

Patient Preparation Avoid radioisotope scan prior to collection of specimen (if radioisotope based procedure is used or if method by which CEA is to be determined is unknown).

Specimen Serum or plasma, effusion fluid, bronchoalveolar lavage[1]

Container Red top tube or lavender top (EDTA) tube, avoid heparin anticoagulant

Sampling Time Preoperative; approximately 4 weeks postoperative and subsequently

Storage Instructions Separate serum (or plasma) from cells and refrigerate if assayed within 24 hours. For longer storage, freeze at -20°C.

Reference Range Adult: nonsmoker: <2.5 ng/mL (SI: <2.5 µg/L), smoker: ≤5.0 ng/mL (SI: ≤5.0 µg/L)

Use CEA remains the best tumor marker available as an independent factor to project prognosis and is most useful as a chemical monitor of recurrence and of therapy in patients with gastrointestinal carcinomas, especially colorectal neoplasms. It is the best marker available to follow postoperative patients regardless of whether or not preoperative CEA was increased; and it is the most useful means of detection of hepatic metastases. The National Cancer Institute feels that CEA is the best noninvasive method to monitor colorectal cancer. Increase bears an implication of treatment failure or recurrence and is a signal for second-look procedures. Detection of locally recurrent carcinoma, lung or hepatic metastasis, especially from colorectal primaries, may lead to resection of recurrent or metastatic carcinoma for cure. The highest levels occur with metastases to liver or bone. Marker for monitoring effectiveness of therapy. CEA is also useful for other primary carcinomas of entodermal origin, including stomach and pancreas. Significant elevations may be found with primaries of breast and lung. High CEA occurs with medullary carcinoma of thyroid. Increases have been reported with giant cell carcinomas of thyroid, with neuroblastoma, and with some tumors of ovary. Work-up of effusion fluids for carcinoma.

Limitations CEA levels are elevated in smokers; patients with inflammation including infections, inflammatory bowel disease, and pancreatitis; some patients with hypothyroidism; cirrhosis; and in some patients with noncolorectal neoplasms especially gastric, pancreatic, breast, and some ovarian primaries. CA 15-3 is a better marker than CEA in breast cancer.[2] CEA is **not** a screening test for occult cancer. Many negatives occur in patients with early carcinoma. Doubtful cost-effectiveness for many patients. **CEA is negative in some patients with even metastatic colorectal and other neoplasms:** a minority of such patients do not have high CEA levels. CEA testing may be less sensitive with poorly differentiated tumors. Correlation between tumor burden and CEA level is imperfect, especially with lung primaries. Hepatotoxicity of antineoplastic drugs, as well as tumor cell necrosis or membrane damage may permit escape of CEA into the circulation and cause CEA increase; simultaneous evaluation of liver-related tests has been advocated for the former. Radiation therapy may also induce a transient rise in CEA. As patients are followed, CEA testing should be repeated by the same laboratory, by the same method, for all assays. Benign diseases usually do not cause CEA levels >5-10 ng/mL (SI: >5-10 µg/L). When longitudinal monitoring is carried out, use the same method for all samples.

Methodology Radioimmunoassay (RIA), enzyme immunoassay (EIA). Patients who received diagnostic presurgical radioimmunoscintigraphy with ^{111}In-labeled anti-CEA murine monoclonal antibody and who had no clinical evidence of disease after resection showed an increase in CEA concentrations. In these cases, CEA was measured with a double-antibody enzyme immunoassay. This increase, in many cases, is an artifact, and the artifact can be eliminated by adding polyclonal IgG or a mixture of IgG_1, IgG_{2a}, and IgG_{2b} monoclonal antibodies before assay. This correction is critical in the follow-up of patients who receive murine monoclonal antibodies for diagnosis or treatment. The role of antimurine antibody (HAMA) should be considered in all such cases.[3,4]

Additional Information CEA is present in embryonic tissues and certain epithelial malignancies as described above. Chemical heterogeneity in the carbohydrate portion of the CEA molecule is the basis for a family of molecules varying in immunologic specificity. CEA may vary in different tissues and individuals. Preoperative CEA levels project differences in 5-year survival in Dukes stages B and C colorectal adenocarcinoma, and may distinguish a subgroup who will benefit from adjuvant chemotherapy. Progressive elevations of CEA may herald tumor recurrence 3-36 months before clinical evidence of metastases. A small rise may signal local recurrence, a large rise hepatic metastasis. Postoperative CEA elevation following hepatic resection of metastatic colorectal carcinoma provides indication for further therapy. Important monitors for breast and colon cancer patients include GGT, alkaline phosphatase, and CEA. CEA is not specific for any one type of cancer; however, values >20 ng/mL (SI: >20 µg/L) are most significantly correlated with metastatic disease and/or with primary pancreatic and colorectal carcinoma.

CEA is more sensitive to recurrence of **colonic** than **rectal** primaries.[5] It is positive in about 63% of patients having a colorectal carcinoma; about 20% of patients with Dukes A, 58% with Dukes B, 68% with Dukes C.[6]

Hepatic scans have become positive months after a rise in CEA; lack of sensitivity of liver scans for early, resectable metastases is widely recognized, as is their expense. Similarly, serum alkaline phosphatase has been disappointing, but its value may be enhanced in concert with GGT and CEA. Monthly testing for these three is desirable for the first 1-2 years after resection, followed by progressively less frequent testing until 5 years have elapsed.

Shorter time delays between confirmed CEA increase and second look procedure relate to resectability rate for cure. Mean time delays for resectable cases were 1.4 months, and 4.5 months for unresectable patients, in a Memorial Sloan-Kettering series.[7]

Although 37 of 118 tumor-free patients had CEA false-positive at >5 ng/mL (SI: >5 µg/L) on at least one occasion, CEA remains the most sensitive means to detect recurrent colon cancer. CEA may be more sensitive to distant metastasis of colon cancer than to local recurrence.[8]

Of a relatively small group of patients with detectable recurrence who are resectable, 30% to 50% survive 5 years after resection.[9]

Preoperative level of serum CEA is a prognostic indicator (of survival) in patients with colorectal cancer.[10] Median survival rate and disease-free interval were better in those whose preoperative CEA elevations returned to normal following hepatic reaction for metastatic disease.[11] CEA has prognostic significance for **gastric carcinoma** as well.[12]

On the other hand, an immunocytochemistry study of 180 primary **breast carcinomas** utilizing antisera to CEA and CEA/NCA (nonspecific cross reacting antigen) showed no correlation between positivity of CEA immunocytochemistry and histologic grade, lymph node stage, disease-free interval or patient survival.[13] As concerns circulating levels of CA 15-3 and CEA, a study of 173 patients with advanced breast carcinoma found that elevated CEA levels correlated with extent of disease but not with survival.[14]

Earlier studies have shown that plasma CEA is elevated in 60% to 70% of patients with metastatic breast cancer and that CEA level tends to reflect tumor burden.[15] Disparate conclusions, however, have been reached concerning prognostic significance.[15,16,17] Measurement of CEA levels in nipple discharge from patients with nonpalpable breast cancer has been reported to have value in separating malignant from benign disease. Cases of breast cancer generally had nipple discharge levels >100 ng/mL (SI: >100 µg/L).[18]

CEA is one of a number of oncofetal antigens (adenocarcinoma-associated antigens) to which radiolabeled monoclonal antibodies have been prepared and utilized in the radioimmunodetection and therapy of colorectal cancer.[19,20,21,22]

As the measurement of CEA and other oncofetal antigens has not been useful in screening for presence of colon cancer, attention is currently focused on utilization of molecular biologic techniques and genotypic markers. The familial adenomatous polyposis syndrome (Gardner syndrome) as well as some sporadic colorectal carcinomas have 5q chromosome defects (Gardner's interstitial deletion of 5q13-q22).

See listing Colon Cancer, Hereditary Nonpolyposis Type *on page 506.*

Footnotes

1. deDiego A, Compte L, Sanchis J, et al, "Usefulness of Carcinoembryonic Antigen Determination in Bronchoalveolar Lavage Fluid. A Comparative Study Among Patients With Peripheral Lung Cancer, Pneumonia, and Healthy Individuals," *Chest*, 1991, 100(4):1060-3.
2. Safi F, Kohler I, Rottinger E, et al, "The Value of the Tumor Marker CA 15-3 in Diagnosing and Monitoring Breast Cancer. A Comparative Study With Carcinoembryonic Antigen," *Cancer*, 1991, 68(3):574-82.
3. Price T, Beatty BG, Beatty JD, et al, "Human Antimurine Antibody Interference in Measurement of Carcinoembryonic Antigen Assessed With a Double-Antibody Enzyme Immunoassay," *Clin Chem*, 1991, 37(1):51-7.
4. Hardman N, Gill LL, DeWinter RF, et al, "Generation of a Recombinant Mouse-Human Chimaeric Monoclonal Antibody Directed Against Human Carcinoembryonic Antigen," *Int J Cancer*, 1989, 44(3):424-33.
5. Welch CE and Malt RA, "Abdominal Surgery (Second of Three Parts)," *N Engl J Med*, 1983, 308:685-95.
6. Martin EW Jr, James KK, Hurtubise PE, et al, "The Use of CEA as an Early Indicator for Gastrointestinal Tumor Recurrence and Second-Look Procedures," *Cancer*, 1977, 39:440-6.
7. Attiyeh FF and Stearns MW Jr, "Second-Look Laparotomy Based on CEA Elevations in Colorectal Cancer," *Cancer*, 1981, 47:2119-25.
8. Beart RW Jr and O'Connell MJ, "Postoperative Follow-Up of Patients With Carcinoma of the Colon," *Mayo Clin Proc*, 1983, 58:361-3.
9. Sener SF, Imperato JP, Chmiel J, et al, "The Use of Cancer Registry Data to Study Preoperative Carcinoembryonic Antigen Level as an Indicator of Survival in Colorectal Cancer," *CA*, 1989, 39(1):50-7.
10. Slentz K, Senagore A, Hibbert J, et al, "Can Preoperative and Postoperative CEA Predict Survival After Colon Cancer Resection?" *Ann Surg*, 1994, 60(7):528-31.
11. Hohenberger P, Schlag PM, Gerneth T, et al, "Pre- and Postoperative Carcinoembryonic Antigen Determinations in Hepatic Resection for Colorectal Metastases: Predictive Value and Implications for Adjuvant Treatment Based on Multivariate Analysis," *Ann Surg*, 1994, 219(2):135-43.
12. Nakane Y, Okamura S, Akehira K, et al, "Correlation of Preoperative Carcinoembryonic Antigen Levels and Prognosis of Gastric Cancer Patients," *Cancer*, 1994, 73(11):2703-8.
13. Robertson JFR, Ellis IO, Bell J, et al, "Carcinoembryonic Antigen Immunocytochemistry in Primary Breast Cancer," *Cancer*, 1989, 64(8):1638-45.
14. Colomer R, Ruibal A, and Salvador L, "Circulating Tumor Marker Levels in Advanced Breast Carcinoma Correlate With the Extent of Metastatic Disease," *Cancer*, 1989, 64(8):1674-81.
15. Waalkes TP, Enterline JP, Shaper JH, et al, "Biological Markers for Breast Carcinoma," *Cancer*, 1984, 53(3 Suppl):644-51.
16. Mansour EG, Hastert M, Park CH, et al, "Tissue and Plasma Carcinoembryonic Antigen in Early Breast Cancer: A Prognostic Factor," *Cancer*, 1983, 51:1243-8.
17. Cohen C, Sharkey FE, Shulman G, et al, "Tumor-Associated Antigens in Breast Carcinomas. Prognostic Significance," *Cancer*, 1987, 60(6):1294-8.
18. Inaji H, Yayoi E, Maeura Y, et al, "Carcinoembryonic Antigen Estimation in Nipple Discharge as an Adjunctive Tool in the Diagnosis of Early Breast Cancer," *Cancer*, 1987, 60(12):3008-13.
19. Murray JL and Unger MW, "Radioimmunodetection of Cancer With Monoclonal Antibodies: Current Status, Problems, and Future Directions," *Crit Rev Oncol Hematol*, 1988, 8(3):227-53.
20. Schlom J, "Innovations in Monoclonal Antibody Tumor Targeting: Diagnostic and Therapeutic Implications," *JAMA*, 1989, 261(5):744-6.
21. Dillman RO, "Monoclonal Antibodies for Treating Cancer," *Ann Intern Med*, 1989, 111(7):592-603.
22. Kaplan EH, "New Perspectives in Large Bowel Cancer: The Diagnostic and Therapeutic Use of Monoclonal Antibodies in Colorectal Cancer," *Hematol Oncol Clin North Am*, 1989, 3:125-31.

References

Ballesta AM, Molina R, Filella X, et al, "Carcinoembryonic Antigen in Staging and Follow-up of Patients With Solid Tumors," *Tumour Biol*, 1995, 16(1):32-41.

Bhayana V and Diamandis EP, "A Double Monoclonal Time-Resolved Immunofluorometric Assay of Carcinoembryonic Antigen in Serum," *Clin Biochem*, 1989, 22(6):433-8.

Carl J, Brunsgaard N, Kjaer M, et al, "Estimated Treatment Responses in Metastatic Colorectal Carcinoma Based on Longitudinal Carcinoembryonic Antigen Series," *Scand J Clin Lab Invest*, 1993, 53(8):829-34.

Casetta G, Piana P, Cavallini A, et al, "Urinary Levels of Tumour Associated Antigens (CA 19-9, TPA and CEA) in Patients With Neoplastic and Non-Neoplastic Urothelial Abnormalities," *Br J Urol*, 1993, 72(1):60-4.

Cohen AM and Paty P, "CEA for Monitoring Colon Cancer," *JAMA*, 1994, 271(5):346.

Fritsche HA, "Serum Tumor Markers for Patient Monitoring: A Case Oriented Approach Illustrated With Carcinoembryonic Antigen," *Clin Chem*, 1993, 39(11 Pt 2):2431-4.

Greiner JW, Guadagni F, Goldstein D, et al, "Evidence for the Elevation of Serum Carcinoembryonic Antigen and Tumor-Associated Glycoprotein-72 Levels in Patients Administered Interferons," *Cancer Res*, 1991, 51(16):4155-63.

Ichiki H, Shishido M, Nishitani K, et al, "Evaluation of CEA, SLX, and CA125 in Active Pulmonary Tuberculosis," *Nippon Kyobu Shikkan Gakkai Zasshi*, 1993, 31(12):1522-7.

Ikemoto S, Iimori H, Nishimoto K, et al, "Two Cases of Urothelial Tumor With High Serum Level of Carcinoembryonic Antigen and TA-4," *Urol Int*, 1993, 51(2):105-7.

Kiang DT, Greenberg LJ, and Kennedy BJ, "Tumor Marker Kinetics in the Monitoring of Breast Cancer," *Cancer*, 1990, 65(2):193-9.

Kudo R, Sasano H, Koizumi M, et al, "Immunohistochemical Comparison of New Monoclonal Antiody 1C5 and Carcinoembryonic Antigen in the Differential Diagnosis of Adenocarcinoma of the Uterine Cervix," *Int J Gynecol Pathol*, 1990, 9(4):325-36.

Lamerz R, Stieber P, and Fateh-Moghadam A, "Serum Marker Combinations in Human Breast Cancer," *In Vivo*, 1993, 7(6B):607-13.

McCall JL, Black RB, Rich CA, et al, "The Value of Serum Carcinoembryonic Antigen in Predicting Recurrent Disease Following Curative Resection of Colorectal Cancer," *Dis Colon Rectum*, 1994, 37(9):875-81.

Norton JA, "Carcinoembryonic Antigen. New Applications for an Old Marker," *Ann Surg*, 1991, 213(2):95-7.

Pectasides D, Bourazanis J, Economides N, et al, "Squamous Cell Carcinoma Antigen (SCC), Carcinoembryonic Antigen (CEA), and Tumour-Associated Trypsin Inhibitor (TATI) for Monitoring Head and Neck Cancer," *Int J Biol Markers*, 1993, 8(2):81-7.

Primus FJ, Newell KD, Blue A, et al, "Immunological Heterogeneity of Carcinoembryonic Antigen: Antigenic Determinants on Carcinoembryonic Antigen Distinguished by Monoclonal Antibodies," *Cancer Res*, 1983, 43:686-92.

(Continued)

Carcinoembryonic Antigen *(Continued)*

Rocklin MS, Senagore AJ, and Talbott TM, "Role of Carcinoembryonic Antigen and Liver Function Tests in the Detection of Recurrent Colorectal Carcinoma," *Dis Colon Rectum*, 1991, 34(9):794-7.

Steele G Jr, Zamcheck N, Wilson R, et al, "Results of CEA-Initiated Second-Look Surgery for Recurrent Colorectal Cancer," *Am J Surg*, 1980, 139:544-8.

Tatsuta M, Iishi H, Ichii M, et al, "Diagnosis of Gastric Cancers With Fluorescein-Labeled Monoclonal Antibodies to Carcinoembryonic Antigen," *Lasers Surg Med*, 1989, 9(4):422-6.

Theriault RL, Hortobagyi GN, Fritsche HA, et al, "The Role of Serum CEA as a Prognostic Indicator in Stage II and III Breast Cancer Patients Treated With Adjuvant Chemotherapy," *Cancer*, 1989, 63(5):828-35.

Torosian MH, "The Clinical Usefulness and Limitations of Tumor Markers," *Surg Gynecol Obstet*, 1988, 166(6):567-79.

Wang JY, Tang R, and Chiang JM, "Value of Carcinoembryonic Antigen in the Management of Colorectal Cancer," *Dis Colon Rectum*, 1994, 37(3):272-7.

Cardiac Enzymes/Isoenzymes

CPT 82550 (CK); 83615 (LD); 84450 (AST); 84460 (ALT)

Related Information

Creatine Kinase *on page 115*

Creatine Kinase Isoenzymes/Isoforms *on page 115*

Lactate Dehydrogenase *on page 153*

Lactate Dehydrogenase Isoenzymes *on page 154*

Myoglobin, Blood *on page 167*

Troponin *on page 212*

Applies to AST/ALT Ratio; CK Isoenzymes; LD Isoenzymes; Myocardial Infarct Panel

Replaces Alpha-Hydroxybutyric Dehydrogenase (HBDH)

Test Commonly Includes CK with isoenzymes, LD (LDH) with the five LD isoenzymes; some recommend that AST (SGOT) remain included with cardiac enzymes, especially for diagnosis of patients who present subsequent to the CK-MB peak. In this setting AST supports evidence of abnormal LD isoenzymes. Presently, cardiac troponin I (cTnI) is coming into use. It is very likely to significantly replace other assays.

Abstract Measurement of these enzymes and isoenzymes can detect presence of acute myocardial infarction.

Specimen Serum

Container Red top tube

Sampling Time Samples are usually taken on admission, then in a sequence, depending on clinical history, initial results, and perceptions of the attending physician. Some suggest sampling on admission and at 6 and 12 hours which may permit earlier diagnosis. The *Clinical Practice Guideline* from the National Heart, Lung, and Blood Institute recommends that total CK and CK-MB should be measured every 6-8 hours for the first 24 hours after admission. Serial LDH isoenzymes are useful in subjects who present between 24 and 72 hours following onset of symptoms, if serial CK and CK isoenzymes are normal.[2] Further information on timing is provided in the listing Creatine Kinase Isoenzymes/Isoforms *on page 115*. A case is made for sampling on admission and at 16 hours after onset for CK-MB peak.[1] See listing Troponin *on page 212* for recommendations for sampling for this assay; cTnI remains elevated for up to 5-7 days.

Collection Avoid hemolysis, which causes false increase of LD and may cause false $LD_1:LD_2$ inversion.

Storage Instructions Separate serum; freeze serum for CK isoenzymes (but store LD isoenzymes at room temperature) if not done same day.

Causes for Rejection Hemolysis

Special Instructions Isoenzymes should be run, if acute MI is suspected, even if total enzyme(s), CK and/or LD, are within normal limits[3], unless they are so low (eg, <80% of upper limit of reference range) that a given laboratory does not feel that attempted separation is practical.

Reference Range Decision limits are extensively discussed in the literature. They are method dependent. Each laboratory should evaluate its own methods and experience in concert with cardiologists and with active chart review. Problems relevant to decision limits in cardiac enzymes and isoenzymes are shared with many other laboratory tests, as problems of sensitivity versus specificity. Arguments which claim that in some patients the diagnosis of AMI is missed include cases of fatal AMI.[1]

Use Diagnosis of acute infarct of myocardium (acute MI, or AMI)

Limitations At onset of acute infarction of myocardium, all enzymes and isoenzymes are normal. It is desirable to draw cardiac enzymes at onset for a baseline. $LD_1:LD_2$ flip (inversion) and CK-MB elevation have been reported during marathon training with increases of total LD and CK.[4] Elevations of total CK with increased CK-MB and CK-BB, was found with necrotic intestine in experimental animals.[5] Myositis, various myopathies, rhabdomyolysis, and Reye's syndrome are reported to cause elevations of CK-MB. In these situations CKMB is elevated and remains elevated for days, while the values peak in about 1 day after AMI and then begin to decline. Thus, the test is not entirely specific for AMI, and

confirmation by LD isoenzyme studies may be indicated.[6] High LD occurs in a variety of diseases. LD isoenzyme separations greatly improve the diagnostic specificity of an elevated LD value.

Methodology Isoenzymes have been done mostly by electrophoretic separation. Other techniques such as immunoassays and immunoinhibition have been introduced which are more rapid, sensitive, and specific than electrophoresis (regarding CK-MB).[7] Immunochemical CK-2 is very commonly used and reported in mass units. It has a distinct advantage over electrophoresis because of a short turnaround time (15-20 minutes).

Additional Information Acute MI: CK and CK-MB (CKMB2) have been widely considered to peak about 1 day following onset, as does AST in usual hospital practice. However, see Sampling Time in the listing Creatine Kinase Isoenzymes/Isoforms *on page 115*. LD_1 usually peaks at the second day, when $LD_1:LD_2$ inversion (flip) is most commonly found. CK and CK isoenzymes can be discontinued after MB returns to normal. LD isoenzymes should be stopped after $LD_1:LD_2$ flip with elevation of LD_1 is found.

CK-MB, LD_1, $LD_1:LD_2$ ratio, total CK and total LD classically increase with acute MI. CK-MB and LD_1 increase in percentage and absolutely (each isoenzyme percent times the respective total enzyme), peak, then decrease. More information is provided in the individual test listings.

New investigational tests which may allow for much earlier detection of acute myocardial injury include CK-MM and CK-MB isoforms,[8,9,10] quantitation of human ventricular myosin light chains in the blood, and an assay of troponin. These newer tests may have particular value in determining candidates for and monitoring response to thrombolytic therapy (tissue plasminogen activator, streptokinase).[11]

The literature continues to call attention to the poor sensitivity of the ECG for acute myocardial infarction.[1]

The use of AST (SGOT) in diagnosis of AMI includes its application with ALT (SGPT). However, transaminases are no longer frequently used in MI work-up. Myocardial injury can generate an AST/ALT ratio ≥3.1, or a twofold increase in this ratio. Only certain kinds of hepatocellular injury can also cause such AST/ALT ratio abnormality; they include acetaminophen or ethanol toxicity, hepatoma or metastatic carcinoma to liver, marked hepatocellular congestion, cirrhosis, and severe injury to striated muscle.[1] Further, AST and ALT are usually available on a stat basis.

AST (aspartate aminotransferase) with LD and LD isoenzymes is advocated when the patient reaches medical attention 48-72 hours after onset of a possible acute myocardial infarct.[12,13]

Footnotes

1. Pappas NJ Jr, "Enhanced Cardiac Enzyme Profile," *Clin Lab Med*, 1989, 9(4):689-716.
2. Braunwald E, Mark DB, Jones RH, et al, *Unstable Angina: Diagnosis and Management*, U.S. Department of Health and Human Services, 1994.
3. Scottolini AG, Zaim MT, and Bhagavan NV, "Acute Myocardial Infarction With Normal Total Cardiac Enzymes and Specific Isoenzyme Patterns," *Prac Cardiol*, 1983, 9:193-202.
4. Apple FS and McGue MK, "Serum Enzyme Changes During Marathon Training," *Am J Clin Pathol*, 1983, 79:716-9.
5. Graeber GM, O'Neill JF, Wolf RE, et al, "Elevated Levels of Peripheral Serum Creatine Phosphokinase With Strangulated Small Bowel Obstruction," *Arch Surg*, 1983, 118:837-40.
6. Wolf PL, "Common Causes of False-Positive CK-MB Test for Acute Myocardial Infarction," *Clin Lab Med*, 1986, 6(3):577-81.
7. Gibler WB, Lewis LM, Erb RE, et al, "Early Detection of Acute Myocardial Infarction in Patients Presenting With Chest Pain and Nondiagnostic ECGs: Serial CK-MB Sampling in the Emergency Department," *Ann Emerg Med*, 1990, 19(12):1359-66.
8. Puleo PR, Meyer D, Wathen C, et al, "Use of a Rapid Assay of Subforms of Creatine Kinase MB to Diagnose or Rule Out Acute Myocardial Infarction," *N Engl J Med*, 1994, 331(9):561-6.
9. Puleo PR, Guadagno P, Scheel M, et al, "Diagnostic Accuracy of a Rapid MB-CK Subform Assay in the Early Hours of Myocardial Infarction," *Clin Chem*, 1989, 35:1119.
10. Wu AH, Gornet TG, Wu VH, et al, "Early Diagnosis of Acute Myocardial Infarction by Rapid Analysis of Creatine Kinase Isoenzyme-3 (CK-MM) Sub-Types," *Clin Chem*, 1987, 33(3):358-62.
11. Apple FS, Sharkey SW, Werdick M, et al, "Analyses of Creatine Kinase Isoenzymes and Isoforms in Serum to Detect Reperfusion After Acute Myocardial Infarction," *Clin Chem*, 1987, 33(4):507-11.
12. Rotenberg Z, Weinberger I, Davidson E, et al, "Does Determination of Serum Aspartate Aminotransferase Contribute to the Diagnosis of Acute Myocardial Infarction?" *Am J Clin Pathol*, 1989, 91(1):91-4.
13. Faulkner WR, "Aspartate Aminotransferase and Acute Myocardial Infarction," *Lab Report for Physicians*, 1989, 11:92-3.

References

Adams JE 3d, Sicard GA, Allen BT, et al, "Diagnosis of Perioperative Myocardial Infarction With Measurement of Cardiac Troponin I," *N Engl J Med*, 1994, 330(10):670-4.

Galbraith LV, Leung FY, Jablonsky G, et al, "Time-Related Changes in the Diagnostic Utility of Total Lactate Dehydrogenase, Lactate Dehydrogenase Isoenzyme-1, and Two Lactate Dehydrogenase Isoenzyme-1 Ratios in Serum After Myocardial Infarction," *Clin Chem*, 1990, 36(7):1317-22.

Goldman L, "Assessment of Perioperative Cardiac Risk," *N Engl J Med*, 1994, 330(10):707-9.

Jensen AE, Reikvam A, Nordgard S, et al, "Diagnostic Accuracy of Kodak Creatine Kinase MB, Stratus Creatine Kinase MB, and Lactate Dehydrogenase Isoenzyme 1 in Serum After Acute Myocardial Infarction," *Clin Chem*, 1990, 36(10):1847-8.

Karagounis L, Moreno F, Menlove RL, et al, "Effects of Early Thrombolytic Therapy (Anistreplase Versus Streptokinase) on Enzymatic and Electrocardiographic Infarct Size in Acute Myocardial Infarction. Team-2 Investigators," *Am J Cardiol*, 1991, 68(9):848-56.

Lee TH, Juarez G, Cook EF, et al, "Ruling Out Acute Myocardial Infarction. A Prospective Multicenter Validation of A 12-Hour Strategy for Patients at Low Risk," *N Engl J Med*, 1991, 324(18):1239-46.

Manzo V, Sun T, and Lien YY, "Misdiagnosis of Acute Myocardial Infarction," *Ann Clin Lab Sci*, 1990, 20(5):324-8.

Cardiac Troponin see Troponin *on page 212*

Carnitine see Amino Acid Screen, Plasma *on page 74*

β-Carotene see Carotene, Serum *on this page*

Carotene, Serum
CPT 82380
Related Information
Fat, Semiquantitative, Stool *on page 634*
Vitamin A, Serum *on page 217*
Vitamin E, Serum *on page 219*

Synonyms Beta-Carotene; β-Carotene

Abstract The use of the test is controversial. Precursors of vitamin A, carotenes when measured do not often provide high levels of diagnostic information. Beta-carotene is a retinoid found in fresh fruits and vegetables, a fat-soluble provitamin. It is the best known of a group of carotenoids which have antioxidant activity. Further research is needed. Beta-carotene represents approximately a quarter of the total of serum carotenoids. Antioxidant properties are not uniform among the different carotenoids.[1]

Patient Preparation Patient must fast a minimum of 8 hours.

Specimen Serum

Container Red top tube

Storage Instructions Separate serum from clot. Freeze in plastic vial. Prevent exposure to light.

Causes for Rejection Hemolysis

Reference Range 10-85 µg/dL (SI: 0.2-1.6 µmol/L); varies with diet and between laboratories (*vide infra*). Levels vary in infancy and childhood.[2]

Use Confirm the diagnosis of carotenoderma; screen for fat malabsorption, depressed carotene levels may be found in cases of steatorrhea. A role for total carotenoid serum levels may be evolving in projection of coronary events, but further study is needed, *vide infra*.[1] Carotenemia may be confused with jaundice.

Limitations High levels are useful to rule out steatorrhea but lower values lack specificity.

The gold standard for confirmation of a diagnosis of malabsorption remains fat measurement of a 72-hour stool specimen. There is poor sensitivity. High in the serum of those ingesting large amounts of vegetables. Variability of reference ranges and poor technical precision at lower levels, which are the decision levels, have led to recommendations to discontinue use of this test, which is not a reliable indicator of vitamin A status.

Methodology High performance liquid chromatography (HPLC), colorimetry with extraction step to eliminate other carotenoids

Additional Information Vitamin A or carotene serum levels do not correlate well with liver stores. It is also reported high with some cases of diabetes mellitus, myxedema, chronic nephritis, nephrotic syndrome,[3,4] liver disease, hypothyroidism, type I, IIA, and IIB hyperlipoproteinemia, and in a group of amenorrheic hypogonadotropic women.[3] High carotene levels have been found in the serum of faddists ingesting large amounts of vegetables. Oral leukoplakia has been reported to have responded to beta-carotene therapy.[4]

Attention has recently been directed at the antioxidants, including beta carotene and vitamin E. Efficacy of these substances has not been proven at present to prevent colorectal tumors[5] or lung carcinoma in smokers.[6] A possible decreased risk of age-related macular degeneration by consumption of certain carotenoid-containing foods requires further study.[7] A decreased risk of coronary heart disease was reported for individuals with high serum total carotenoid concentrations. (Serum levels of total carotenoids were studied, not beta-carotene exclusively.)[1]

Further investigation is required.

See listing Vitamin A, Serum *on page 217*.

Footnotes
1. Morris DL, Kritchevsky SB, and Davis CE, "Serum Carotenoids and Coronary Heart Disease - The Lipid Research Clinics Coronary Primary Prevention Trial and Follow-Up Study," *JAMA*, 1994, 272(18):1439-44.
2. Leung AK, Siu TO, Chiu AS, et al, "Serum Carotene Concentrations in Normal Infants and Children," *Clin Pediatr (Phila)*, 1990, 29(10):575-8.
3. Kemmann E, Pasquale SA, and Skaf R, "Amenorrhea Associated With Carotenemia," *JAMA*, 1983, 249:926-9.
4. Garewal HS, Meyskens FL Jr, Killen D, et al, "Response of Oral Leukoplakia to Beta-Carotene," *J Clin Oncol*, 1990, 8(10):1715-20.

5. Greenberg ER, Baron JA, Tosteson TD, et al, "A Clinical Trial of Antioxidant Vitamins to Prevent Colorectal Adenoma," *N Engl J Med*, 1994, 331(3):141-7.
6. "The Effect of Vitamin E and Beta Carotene on the Incidence of Lung Cancer and Other Cancers in Male Smokers. The Alpha-Tocopherol, Beta Carotene Cancer Prevention Study Group," *N Engl J Med*, 1994, 330(15):1029-35.
7. Seddon JM, Ajani UA, Sperduto RD, et al, "Dietary Carotenoids, Vitamins A, C, and E, and Advanced Age-Related Macular Degeneration," *JAMA*, 1994, 272(18):1413-20.

References
Hallfrisch J, Muller DC, and Singh VN, "Vitamin A and E Intakes and Plasma Concentrations of Retinol, Beta Carotene, and Alpha Tocopherol in Men and Women of the Baltimore Longitudinal Study of Aging," *Am J Clin Nutr*, 1994, 60(2):176-82.
Hankinson S and Stampfer MJ, "All That Glitters Is Not Beta Carotene," *JAMA*, 1994, 272(18):1455-6.

Catecholamines see Metanephrines *on page 165*

Catecholamines, Fractionation, Plasma
CPT 82383 (total); 82384 (fractionated)
Related Information
Calcitonin *on page 96*
Homovanillic Acid, Urine *on page 145*
Metanephrines *on page 165*
Vanillylmandelic Acid, Urine *on page 216*

Synonyms Epinephrine, Norepinephrine, Dopamine; Pressor Amines

Applies to Chromogranin A, Plasma; Clonidine Suppression Test; Plasma Neuropeptide Y

Test Commonly Includes Plasma catecholamines, total and fractionated (epinephrine, norepinephrine, dopamine)

Abstract In medical context, the expression "catecholamines" is a collective term for epinephrine, norepinephrine, and dopamine. They are produced chiefly by the chromaffin cells of the adrenal medulla but also by the sympathetic nervous system.

Pheochromocytoma, the tumor of chromaffin cells, is a curable cause of hypertension. Undiagnosed, it is a potentially life-threatening neoplasm.

Patient Preparation Patient should be fasting for 4 or more hours without smoking. Walnuts, bananas, and alpha methyldopa (Aldomet®) should be avoided for a week prior to sampling. Other drug interference may occur, including epinephrine and epinephrine-like drugs (eg, nosedrops, sinus and cough preparations, bronchodilators, appetite suppressants). Test is unreliable in subjects on levodopa or methenamine mandelate. It is best to communicate with the laboratory which will do the test with regard to other sources of interference, including drug interference. Avoid exposure to radioactivity (eg, scans) if laboratory will use a radioenzymatic procedure. Avoid patient stress.[1] See Limitations.

Specimen Plasma

Container EDTA-sodium metabisulfite tube. Some laboratories request a green top (heparin) tube, which is reported to enhance stability.[2]

Collection An indwelling heparinized venous catheter is advocated, since venipuncture can cause an increase in the substances for which testing is being done. Patient should remain supine in quiet surroundings for at least 30 minutes. Some laboratories require a chilled, special container; invert to mix blood with preservatives and place in an ice bath.

Storage Instructions Spin blood in a refrigerated centrifuge. Chill carriers if a refrigerated centrifuge is not available. Separate plasma into a plastic vial and freeze immediately in an upright position at -70°C. Do not let specimen thaw during transit.[3] Others report considerable stability for catecholamines.[4]

Reference Range Reference ranges vary among laboratories, but typical supine values for HPLC methodology are: epinephrine <50 pg/mL, norepinephrine <410 pg/mL, dopamine <90 pg/mL. Values for specimens taken when the subject is standing are higher than the ranges for supine posture for norepinephrine and epinephrine but not for dopamine. Depending on cutoff levels of epinephrine and norepinephrine, the diagnostic efficacy in diagnosing pheochromocytoma ranges from 85% to 95% (sensitivity) and 95% to 98% (specificity).

Use Diagnose pheochromocytoma and those paragangliomas which may secrete epinephrine, norepinephrine or both. Such tumors may cause paroxysmal or persistent hypertension. Investigation of hypertensive patients, especially younger individuals, particularly when hypertension is paroxysmal, suggesting pheochromocytoma. Plasma catecholamines with urinary metanephrines and VMA have been a recommended test battery for pheochromocytoma.[5] Others recommend plasma catecholamines when urinary collections are not diagnostic. Plasma and urine catecholamines (and plasma chromogranin A) are recommended to screen for pheochromocytoma in family members among two disorders bearing autosomal dominant inheritance mode: von Hippel-Lindau disease and multiple endocrine adenomatosis (MEN), type II.[6] Used also in diagnosis of disorders related to the nervous system and in assessment of resuscitation.[2]

Limitations Plasma levels are useful if elevated, especially during or immediately following an episode of hypertension, but false-negatives
(Continued)

Catecholamines, Fractionation, Plasma
(Continued)

occur when the specimen is drawn during an uneventful period. Elevations are usually >1000 pg/mL. Normotensive pheochromocytoma has been reported. False-positive results are common. Epinephrine secretion increases in response to cold and hypoglycemia. Depending on methods, drugs which may affect plasma norepinephrine levels include alpha- and beta-adrenergic blockers, vasodilators, clonidine, bromocriptine, theophylline, phenothiazine, tricyclic antidepressants, labetalol, calcium channel blockers, converting enzyme inhibitors, bromocriptine, chlorpromazine, haloperidol, and cocaine. Plasma catecholamines are less sensitive than are urinary catecholamines.[3] In general, urinary fractionated catecholamines result in values more consistent than those from plasma. **Although normal plasma metanephrine concentrations are reported to rule out pheochromocytoma, normal plasma catecholamine concentrations and normal urine metanephrine assays do not.**[7]

Methodology High performance liquid chromatography (HPLC) with electrochemical detection is the method of choice.[8] Other methods include high performance liquid chromatography (HPLC) with fluorometric or spectrophotometric detection, radioimmunoassay (RIA), and radiochemical assays.[9]

Additional Information The adrenal medullary catecholamines (epinephrine, norepinephrine, and their precursor, dopamine) are rapidly metabolized materials with intense vasoactivity, among many other properties. They can be synthesized by extra-adrenal cells or neoplasms of the APUD system. They are pathogenic in the episodic hypertension of pheochromocytoma, and will be elevated during and immediately after such a paroxysm. However, levels may be normal during asymptomatic intervals. Urine catecholamines, metanephrines (normetanephrine and metanephrine), VMA and HVA provide additive information. Plasma metanephrine concentrations are reported to be more consistent than are plasma catecholamine assays.[8]

Extra-adrenal pheochromocytomas may represent 15% of adult and 30% of childhood pheochromocytomas; the most common location is the superior para-aortic region between the diaphragm and lower renal poles.[10]

A clonidine-suppression test has been described; failure to suppress plasma catecholamines with clonidine supports the diagnosis.[11]

Plasma neuropeptide Y, a 36 amino acid peptide, is a marker for nervous system tissue. Its value remains to be established. Plasma levels can be assayed by immunoradiometric methods. Increased levels have been found with pheochromocytomas, neuroblastomas, and in some subjects with other neuroendocrine tumors such as carcinoids, medullary carcinoma of thyroid, and small cell carcinoma of lung.[12]

Footnotes
1. Sheps SG, Jiang N-S, Klee GG, et al, "Recent Developments in the Diagnosis and Treatment of Pheochromocytoma," *Mayo Clin Proc*, 1990, 65(1):88-95.
2. D'Alesandro MM, Reed HL, Robertson R, et al, "Simplified Method of Collecting and Processing Whole Blood for Quantitation of Plasma Catecholamines," *Lab Med*, 1990, 26-9.
3. Rumley AG, "The *In Vitro* Stability of Catecholamines in Whole Blood," *Ann Clin Biochem*, 1988, 25(Pt 5):585-86.
4. Boomsma F, Alberts G, Van Eijk L, et al, "Optimal Collection and Storage Conditions for Catecholamine Measurements in Human Plasma and Urine," *Clin Chem*, 1993, 39(12):2503-8.
5. Knight JA and Wu JT, "Catecholamines and Their Metabolites: Clinical and Laboratory Aspects," *Lab Med*, 1987, 18:153-8.
6. Neumann HP, Berger DP, Sigmund G, et al, "Pheochromocytomas, Multiple Endocrine Neoplasia Type 2, and von Hippel-Lindau Disease," *N Engl J Med*, 1993, 329(21):1531-8.
7. Lenders JW, Keiser HR, Goldstein DS, et al, "Plasma Metanephrines in the Diagnosis of Pheochromocytoma," *Ann Intern Med*, 1995, 123(2):101-9.
8. Koller M, "Results for 74 Substances Tested for Interference With Determination of Plasma Catecholamines by "High Performance" Liquid Chromatography With Electrochemical Detection," *Clin Chem*, 1988, 34(5):947-9.
9. Moyer TP, Jaing NS, Tyce GM, et al, "Analysis for Urinary Catecholamines by Liquid Chromatography With Amperometric Detection: Methodology and Clinical Interpretation of Results," *Clin Chem*, 1979, 25:256-63.
10. Whalen RK, Althausen AF, and Daniels GH, "Extra-adrenal Pheochromocytoma," *J Urol*, 1992, 147(1):1-10.
11. Bravo EL and Gifford RW Jr, "Current Concepts. Pheochromocytoma: Diagnosis, Localization, and Management," *N Engl J Med*, 1984, 311(20):1298-303.
12. Grouzmann E, Comoy E, and Bohuon C, "Plasma Neuropeptide Y Concentrations in Patients With Neuroendocrine Tumors," *J Clin Endocrinol Metab*, 1989, 68(4):808-13.

References
Gerlo EA and Sevens C, "Urinary and Plasma Catecholamines and Urinary Catecholamine Metabolites in Pheochromocytoma: Diagnostic Value in 19 Cases," *Clin Chem*, 1994, 40(2):250-6.

Leavelle DE, *Mayo Medical Laboratories Interpretive Handbook*, Rochester, MN: Mayo Medical Laboratories, 1994.

Rogers PJ, Tyce GM, Weinshilboum RM, et al, "Catecholamine Metabolic Pathways and Exercise Training. Plasma and Urine Catecholamines, Metabolic Enzymes, and Chromogranin-A," *Circulation*, 1991, 84(6):2346-56.

Tyce GM, Ahlskog JE, Carmichael SW, et al, "Catecholamines in CSF, Plasma, and Tissue After Autologous Transplantation of Adrenal Medulla to the Brain in Patients With Parkinson's Disease," *J Lab Clin Med*, 1989, 114(2):185-92.

Yoshino K, Takahashi K, Shirai T, et al, "Changes in Plasma Catecholamines and Pulsatile Patterns of Gonadotropin Release in Subjects With a Normal Ovulatory Cycle and With Polycystic Ovary Syndrome," *Int J Fertil*, 1990, 35(1):34-9.

Catecholamines, Fractionation, Urine

CPT 82382 (total); 83835 (metanephrines); 84585 (VMA)

Related Information
Calcitonin *on page 96*
Homovanillic Acid, Urine *on page 145*
Metanephrines *on page 165*
Urine Collection, 24-Hour *on page 30*
Vanillylmandelic Acid, Urine *on page 216*

Synonyms Free Catecholamine Fractionation, Urine

Applies to Dopamine, Urine; Epinephrine, Urine; Norepinephrine, Urine

Replaces Total Urinary Catecholamines

Abstract This is a collection term for the biogenic amines epinephrine, norepinephrine, and dopamine.

Patient Preparation Avoid patient stress, exercise, smoking, and pain. Many drugs (reserpine and α-methyldopa, levodopa, monoamine oxidase inhibitors, and sympathomimetic amines) may interfere and should be discontinued 2 weeks prior to specimen collection. Nose drops, sinus and cough medicines, bronchodilators and appetite suppressants, α_2-agonists, calcium channel blockers, converting enzyme inhibitors, bromocriptine, phenothiazine, tricyclic antidepressants, alpha and beta blockers, labetolol may interfere.[1] Mandelamine® interferes, but thiazides do not. Drug effects may be difficult to anticipate. Caffeine products should be avoided before and during collection. The patient should not be subjected to hypoglycemia or exertion. Increased intracranial pressure and clonidine withdrawal can also cause false-positive results.[1]

Specimen 24-hour urine

Container Brown urine container. Adjust to pH 4 with acetic or hydrochloric acid.

Storage Instructions Refrigerate during and after collection.

Reference Range Adults: approximate range, urine: epinephrine: 0-20 µg/24 hours (SI: 0-118 nmol/day); norepinephrine: 15-80 µg/24 hours (SI: 89-473 nmol/day); dopamine: 65-400 µg/24 hours (SI: 420-2600 nmol/day). Ranges given here are not identical among all laboratories but are those associated with HPLC methodology.

Critical Values >50 µg/24 hours (SI: >297 nmol/day) of epinephrine secretion may be the only abnormality in subjects who have the multiple endocrine adenomatosis syndrome.

Use Work up neuroblastoma; diagnose pheochromocytoma; evaluate possible multiple endocrine adenomatosis type II. Pheochromocytomas and occasional paragangliomas may cause persistent or paroxysmal hypertension. Work up of palpitation, severe headache, diaphoresis. Urine collections are preferred to blood sampling when there is suspicion for tumor, when hypertension is not paroxysmal.

Limitations False-negatives and false-positives occur. Many interfering substances exist for fluorometric assays. Plasma and urine assays for metanephrines are among the best tests for pheochromocytoma.[2,3] Plasma metanephrines are more sensitive.[3] Sheps et al used urinary catecholamine fractionation as confirmation, following a metanephrine screen.[1] Neuroblastoma is better worked up with urinary collections for HVA and VMA. MHPG (3-methoxy-4-hydroxyphenylethylene glycol) is a major metabolite of norepinephrine in the central nervous system; it is a metabolite of some neuroblastomas.

Methodology High performance liquid chromatography (HPLC) with electrochemical detection, trihydroxyindole methods after boric acid elution or resin exchange column extraction. Alumina absorption methods displayed the poorest intralaboratory precision in a CAP urine chemistry survey.[4]

Additional Information The expression "free" in free catecholamine fractionation means unconjugated. This assay is of most value for pheochromocytoma when specimen is collected during a hypertensive episode. Since a 24-hour urine collection represents a longer sampling time than a random, or symptom-directed serum sample, and because catecholamine secretion by pheochromocytomas is intermittent, the urine test may detect some cases missed by a blood level.

See also Catecholamines, Fractionation, Plasma *on page 103*.

Footnotes
1. Sheps SG, Jiang N-S, Klee GG, et al, "Recent Developments in the Diagnosis and Treatment of Pheochromocytoma," *Mayo Clin Proc*, 1990, 65(1):88-95.
2. Knight JA and Wu JT, "Catecholamines and Their Metabolites: Clinical and Laboratory Aspects," *Lab Med*, 1987, 18:153-8.
3. Lenders JW, Keiser HR, Goldstein DS, et al, "Plasma Metanephrines in the Diagnosis of Pheochromocytoma," *Ann Intern Med*, 1995, 123(2):101-9.
4. Weaver DK and Glenn GC, "The Urine Chemistry Survey - Series 2: 5 Years Experience With and Interlaboratory Comparison Program," *Arch Pathol Lab Med*, 1989, 113(7):713-22.

References

"Case Records of the Massachusetts General Hospital. Weekly Clinicopathological Exercises. Case 45-1989. A 48 Year-Old Woman With Acute Respiratory Failure and a Left Suprarenal Mass," *N Engl J Med*, 1989, 321(19):1316-29.

Cleland JG and Dargie HJ, "Arrhythmias, Catecholamines and Electrolytes," *Am J Cardiol*, 1988, 62(2):55A-9A.

Gerlo EA and Sevens C, "Urinary and Plasma Catecholamines and Urinary Catecholamine Metabolites in Pheochromocytoma: Diagnostic Value in 19 Cases," *Clin Chem*, 1994, 40(2):250-6.

Rosano TG, Swift TA, and Hayes LW, "Advances in Catecholamine and Metabolite Measurements for Diagnosis of Pheochromocytoma," *Clin Chem*, 1991, 37(10 Pt 2):1854-67.

Weinkove C, "Measurement of Catecholamines and Their Metabolites in Urine," *J Clin Pathol*, 1991, 44(4):269-75.

Catecholamines, Plasma *replaced by* Metanephrines *on page 165*

CEA *see* Carcinoembryonic Antigen *on page 100*

CEA, Body Fluid *see* Body Fluid *on page 89*

Central Venous Blood *see* Blood Gases, Venous *on page 89*

Cephalin Flocculation *replaced by* Alanine Aminotransferase *on page 65*

Cephalin Flocculation *replaced by* Aspartate Aminotransferase *on page 84*

Cerebrospinal Fluid Angiotensin Converting Enzyme *see* Angiotensin Converting Enzyme *on page 80*

Cerebrospinal Fluid Glucose

CPT 82947

Related Information

Bacterial Antigens, Rapid Detection Methods *on page 454*
Bacterial Culture, Cerebrospinal Fluid *on page 460*
Body Fluid Glucose *on page 91*
Cerebrospinal Fluid Analysis *on page 309*
Cerebrospinal Fluid Lactic Acid *on next page*
Cerebrospinal Fluid LD *on next page*
Cerebrospinal Fluid Protein *on page 380*
Fungal Culture, Cerebrospinal Fluid *on page 477*
Glucose, Fasting *on page 137*
Gram's Stain *on page 481*
Mycobacterial Culture, Cerebrospinal Fluid *on page 489*
Viral Culture, Central Nervous System Symptoms *on page 677*

Synonyms CSF Glucose; Glucose, Cerebrospinal Fluid; Spinal Fluid Glucose

Abstract For diagnosis of meningitis, culture and then Gram's staining have priority over all other testing, when only a small quantity of cerebrospinal fluid (CSF) is available. Cell count with differential deserve the next priority, followed by glucose and protein.

Patient Preparation Blood (ie, plasma) glucose is needed also. Ideally, it should be drawn 2 hours before the lumbar puncture, the equilibration time.

Specimen Cerebrospinal fluid

Container Clean, sterile CSF tube

Collection Tubes should be labeled with patient's identification, date, time of collection, and with numbers indicating the sequence in which tubes were obtained.

Special Instructions A plasma glucose should be drawn.

Reference Range 50-80 mg/dL (SI: 2.8-4.4 mmol/L) in fasting patients, should be interpreted with plasma glucose. Values may be somewhat higher in children, 45-100 mg/dL (SI: 2.5-5.6 mmol/L).[1] CSF glucose should be 60% to 70% of plasma glucose. However, equilibration between plasma and CSF glucose levels may require several hours. In premature and newborn infants, CSF glucose may be 80% or more of plasma glucose, possibly due to greater permeability of the blood-brain barrier and/or increased rate of cerebral blood flow.

Critical Values Less than 40% of simultaneously analyzed serum glucose

Possible Panic Range <40 mg/dL (SI: <2.2 mmol/L), especially with increased cells and/or protein

Use Evaluate viral, bacterial, tuberculous, and other types of meningitis; neoplastic involvement of meninges; other neurological disorders. Diagnose neuroglycopenia, even in presence of normal plasma glucose. While the finding of glucose in clear nasal discharge has in past years been considered indicative of CSF rhinorrhea,[2] studies have shown that glucose may be present in non-CSF nasal fluids.[3,4]

Limitations Falsely decreased levels may result due to cellular and bacterial utilization of glucose if the test is not performed immediately. Visibly xanthochromic samples may give misleading results. The sensitivity of CSF glucose for bacterial meningitis was only 72% in a series from Rochester, Minnesota, inferior to the sensitivity of the nucleated

blood cell count.[5] Bloody taps cause falsely increased glucose, since there is more glucose in blood.

Methodology Same procedures as used for blood glucose (eg, glucose oxidase, hexokinase reactions); a reagent strip and a handheld analyzer method have been reported as reliable for use in the bedside determination of CSF glucose.[6]

Additional Information Elevation implies hyperglycemia 2-4 hours earlier. Significantly decreased cerebrospinal fluid glucose levels are <40 mg/dL (SI: <2.2 mmol/L) in fasting patient with normal plasma glucose. The frequency of low CSF glucose in bacterial meningitis varies somewhat between series. A major textbook of pediatrics points out that acute viral meningitis is often differentiated from acute bacterial meningitis, because the latter is characterized by a CSF glucose <30 mg/dL, a CSF glucose-to-blood glucose ratio <0.2-0.3 as well as a protein >200 mg/dL, a CSF PMN count >1000/mm^3, and an 80% to 90% likelihood of positive Gram's stain in an illness often occurring during the winter in a child younger than 2 years of age.[7] The magnitude of the seasonal curves for viral versus bacterial meningitis (the former more frequent in the summer) is greater than most clinicians appreciate.[8] In 134 Gram's stain positive cases, CSF glucose was 14.4/30.6/50.4 mg/dL, 25th/percentile median/75th percentile.[8] **The gold standard for the diagnosis of bacterial meningitis is the culture,**[5,9] which is fundamental to appropriate diagnosis and treatment.[10] Decreased CSF glucose is characteristically but not invariably found in tuberculous, fungal, and amebic meningitis (*Naegleria*) as well as in bacterial meningitis. Glucose is usually normal in viral meningitis, but in herpes or mumps meningoencephalitis, lymphocytic choriomeningitis, and with enterovirus infection, glucose may be low. Sarcoidosis and neurosyphilis are reported causes of low CSF glucose. Other very uncommon causes of low CSF glucose include meningeal cysticercosis, trichinosis, and with the chemical meningitis which accompanies intrathecal therapy. Low CSF glucose may also occur in subarachnoid hemorrhage and neoplasia (eg, medulloblastoma). Low CSF glucose may be found in CNS leukemia. Decrease has led to the diagnosis of insulinoma presenting with CNS symptoms. Rheumatoid meningitis and lupus myelopathy may cause low CSF glucose.[10] CSF glucose levels ≤20 mg/dL are highly correlated with bacterial meningitis.[11]

Lactic acid may be useful in the diagnosis of bacterial meningitis, but values overlap those found with viral meningitis (aseptic meningitis).[10]

Footnotes

1. Knight JA, Dudek SM, and Haymond RE, "Early (Chemical) Diagnosis of Bacterial Meningitis-Cerebrospinal Fluid Glucose, Lactate, and Lactate Dehydrogenase Compared," *Clin Chem*, 1981, 27:1431-4.
2. Beckhardt RN, Setzen M, and Carras R, "Primary Spontaneous Cerebrospinal Fluid Rhinorrhea," *Otolaryngol Head Neck Surg*, 1991, 104(4):425-32.
3. Hull HF and Morrow G, "Glucorrhea Revisited: Prolonged Promulgation of Another Plastic Pearl," *JAMA*, 1975, 234:1052-3.
4. Steedman DJ and Gordon M, "CSF Rhinorrhoea: Significance of the Glucose Oxidase Strip Test," *Injury*, 1987, 18(5):327-8.
5. Rodewald LE, Woodin KA, Szilagyi PG, et al, "Relevance of Common Tests of Cerebrospinal Fluid in Screening for Bacterial Meningitis," *J Pediatr*, 1991, 119(3):363-9.
6. Slovis CM, Negus RA, Amerson SM, et al, "Bedside Cerebrospinal Fluid Glucose Analysis," *Ann Emerg Med*, 1989, 18(9):931-3.
7. Behrman RE, Kliegman RM, Nelson WE, et al, *Nelson Textbook of Pediatrics*, 14th ed, Philadelphia, PA: WB Saunders Co, 1992, 683-91.
8. Spanos A, Harrell FE Jr, and Durack DT, "Differential Diagnosis of Acute Meningitis. An Analysis of the Predictive Value of Initial Observations," *JAMA*, 1989, 262(19):2700-7.
9. Smith AL, "Bacterial Meningitis," *Pediatr Rev*, 1993, 14(1):11-8.
10. Fishman RA, *Cerebrospinal Fluid in Diseases of the Nervous System*, 2nd ed, Philadelphia, PA: WB Saunders Co, 1992, 219-21.
11. Greenlee JE, "Approach to Diagnosis of Meningitis - Cerebrospinal Fluid Evaluation," *Infect Dis Clin North Am*, 1990, 4(4):583-98.

References

Avery GM, "Measurement of Glucose in Cerebrospinal Fluid With Reagent Strips and a Reflectance Photometer," *Clin Chem*, 1991, 37(4):590-1.

Bonadio WA and Smith D, "Cerebrospinal Fluid Changes After 48 Hours of Effective Therapy for *Haemophilus influenzae* Type B Meningitis," *Am J Clin Pathol*, 1990, 94(4):426-8.

Brumback RA, "Collecting Cerebrospinal Fluid: Chemistry," *The Cerebrospinal Fluid*, Chapter 4, Herndon RM and Brumback RA, eds, Boston, MA: Kluwer Academic Publishers, 1989, 222-6.

Gray LD and Fedorko DP, "Laboratory Diagnosis of Bacterial Meningitis," *Clin Microbiol Rev*, 1992, 5(2):130-45.

Cerebrospinal Fluid Glutamine

CPT 82975

Related Information

Ammonia, Blood *on page 75*

Synonyms CSF Glutamine; Glutamine, Spinal Fluid; Spinal Fluid Glutamine

Abstract Ammonia is toxic to the nervous system. It combines with alpha-ketoglutarate to yield glutamine. Such glutamine formation serves to protect the nervous system.[1]

Specimen Cerebrospinal fluid

Container Clean, sterile CSF tube

(Continued)

Cerebrospinal Fluid Glutamine (Continued)

Collection Tube should be labeled with the number indicating the sequence in which tubes were obtained.

Storage Instructions With immediate ethanol deproteinization CSF samples may be stored for 9 months at -80°C.[2]

Causes for Rejection Samples contaminated with red blood cells

Special Instructions Specimen must be transported **immediately** to the laboratory.

Reference Range Enzymatic: adults: 8-10 mg/dL (SI: 550-685 µmol/L), for adults, enzymatic; infants: 2-19 mg/L[3] (SI: 164-1321 µmol/L); isotachophoresis method: adults: 2-10 mg/dL (SI: 137-685 µmol/L)[4]

Use Evaluate hepatic encephalopathy and aid in assessment of its severity; evaluate coma; increased in many instances of Reye's syndrome (20 of 27 cases);[5] work up hyperammonemic encephalopathies. Levels from 25-95 mg/dL are seen with hepatic coma. Values >35 mg/dL are almost always related to encephalopathy.[1]

Limitations Higher levels are reported with parenteral nutrition, meningitis, and in cerebral hemorrhage.[2]

Methodology Enzymatic, amino acid analyzer, high performance liquid chromatography (HPLC), capillary-isotachophoresis.[4] Glutamine/glutamate levels vary widely with different methods and in particular with specimen handling and preparation prior to analysis. This may be due importantly to *in vitro* hydrolysis of glutamine to glutamate. Immediate deproteinization of CSF with ethanol may circumvent this problem.[2]

Additional Information Glutamine is the most prominent amino acid in CSF. CSF glutamine levels are used with blood ammonia, determinations in diagnosis of hepatic encephalopathy. In hepatic encephalopathy, plasma glutamine values correlate better with the clinical course than do values for blood ammonia but imperfect correlation exists with CSF ammonia levels.[1] There is evidence that CSF glutamine levels are within normal range in a variety of infectious, inflammatory, degenerative and metabolic neurologic disorders.[4] Levels are increased in some cases of meningitis and associated with CSF pleocytosis. Elevated CSF total protein (>40 mg/dL (SI: >0.4 g/L)), in which some examples of loss of integrity of the blood-brain-CSF would be expected, is not accompanied by increase in CSF glutamine unless cell count is also increased. With response of meningitis to therapy (and fall in CSF cell count), CSF glutamine also declines.[4] Increase in CSF glutamine relating to pleocytosis is of a much lesser magnitude than the high levels occurring in cases of hepatic coma.

Footnotes

1. Fishman RA, *Cerebrospinal Fluid in Diseases of the Nervous System*, 2nd ed, Philadelphia, PA: WB Saunders Co, 1992, 238-9.
2. Alfredsson G, Wiesel FA, and Lindberg M, "Glutamate and Glutamine in Cerebrospinal Fluid and Serum From Healthy Volunteers - Analytical Aspects," *J Chromatogr*, 1988, 424(2):378-84.
3. Boeckx RL, Iosefsohn M, and Hicks JM, "Reference Values for Cerebrospinal Fluid Glutamine Concentration in Infants," *Clin Chem*, 1980, 26:601-3.
4. Hiraoka A, Miura I, Tominaga I, et al, "Capillary-Isotachophoretic Determination of Glutamine in Cerebrospinal Fluid of Various Neurological Disorders," *Clin Biochem*, 1989, 22(4):293-6.
5. Romshe CA, "Laboratory Diagnosis of Reye's Syndrome," *Reye's Syndrome*, Pollack JD, ed, New York, NY: Grune and Stratton Inc, 1975, 15-26.

References

Fernstrom MH and Fernstrom JD, "Rapid Measurement of Free Amino Acids in Serum and CSF Using High Performance Liquid Chromatography," *Life Sci*, 1981, 29:2119-30.

Mizock BA, Sabelli HC, Dubin A, et al, "Septic Encephalopathy. Evidence for Altered Phenylalanine Metabolism and Comparison With Hepatic Encephalopathy," *Arch Intern Med*, 1990, 150(2):443-9.

Teerlink T, Hennekes MW, Van Leeuwen PA, et al, "Rapid Determination of Glutamine in Biological Samples by High Performance Liquid Chromatography," *Clin Chim Acta*, 1993, 218(2):159-68.

Cerebrospinal Fluid Lactic Acid

CPT 83605

Related Information

Bacterial Culture, Cerebrospinal Fluid *on page 460*
Cerebrospinal Fluid Analysis *on page 309*
Cerebrospinal Fluid Glucose *on previous page*
Cerebrospinal Fluid Protein *on page 380*
Gram's Stain *on page 481*
Viral Culture, Central Nervous System Symptoms *on page 677*

Synonyms CSF Lactic Acid; Lactic Acid, Cerebrospinal Fluid; Spinal Fluid Lactic Acid

Abstract Interest in CSF lactic acid is related to increases in bacterial meningitis and partially treated bacterial meningitis, in contrast to the usual finding of normal lactic acid with viral meningitis. However, overlapping concentrations in tuberculous, other bacterial and viral meningitis have limited its diagnostic value.[1,2]

Specimen Cerebrospinal fluid

Container Clean, sterile CSF tube

Storage Instructions Unstable at room temperature[3]

Reference Range Increased in first 2 weeks of life. A recent article suggests a reference range of 4.5-28.8 mg/dL (SI: 0.5-3.2 mmol/L).[4]

Possible Panic Range Lactic acid >30.1 mg/dL (SI: >3.34 mmol/L) is present in essentially all instances of bacterial meningitis, inversely related to CSF glucose. Lower results are reported in partially treated bacterial meningitis.

Use The role of CSF lactic acid determinations is controversial. CSF lactic acid has been used in differentiation of bacterial and nonbacterial meningitis. Rutledge et al reported that with equivocal clinical and spinal fluid findings, CSF lactic acid failed to distinguish between bacterial and nonbacterial infections.[5] CSF lactate must not be used in place of the traditional laboratory evaluation of meningitis. CSF lactate was elevated in all patients (group of 21) with culture proven tuberculous meningitis.[6] It was also elevated in cases of biopsy proven Creutzfeldt-Jakob disease (CJD) and has been suggested as a biochemical marker of that disease.[7] CSF lactic acid increase is a characteristic finding of acute infarct of cerebrum. Increased levels are found with cerebral hemorrhage, subarachnoid hemorrhage, primary CSF acidosis, malignant hypertension, hepatic encephalopathy, diabetes mellitus, hypoglycemia coma, and in the first 3 days following head injury.[1] An entity of developmental delay with infantile seizures and with depressed CSF glucose and lactate levels is noteworthy, because it responds to a special diet.[1]

Limitations Increases must be interpreted in light of the clinical setting and in concert with conventional parameters of meningitis work-up (glucose, protein, cell count, Gram's stain, and culture). Slight increases have been described with craniocerebral trauma, stroke, seizures (up to 81.1 mg/dL (9.0 mmol/L)), and brain tumor. Results from neurosurgical cases must be interpreted cautiously. It is reported as elevated in fungal infections,[1] but levels have been reported to be erratic in cryptococcal meningitis. *Staphylococcus epidermidis* meningitis after shunt installation and very early neonatal bacterial meningitis have been described without increased lactic acid levels. Overlapping results limit the value of lactate levels in differential diagnosis between viral meningitis, partially treated bacterial meningitis, and tuberculous meningitis. The assay for lactic acid has not been shown to contribute to accuracy of diagnosis in instances of possible meningitis.[1]

Methodology Enzymatic, gas-liquid chromatography (GLC), amperometric utilizing a lactate-sensitive electrode[3]

Additional Information A linear increase in CSF lactate in relation to lactate producing inflammatory cells with high levels at cell counts >350/mm[3] has been noted.[8] It is implied that increase in CSF lactate results from CSF pleocytosis. Antimicrobial therapy given prior to collection of spinal fluid may decrease reliability of the usual diagnostic tests (Gram's stain, cell count, culture, protein, and glucose levels). Equivocal results of tests in some instances of aseptic meningitis may lead to an erroneous diagnosis of bacterial etiology. The Gram's stain may be negative in as many as 25% of culture-proven bacterial meningitides. Lactate determination may provide an indicator of the presence or absence of bacterial meningitis. Lactic acid in viral meningitis will occasionally fall between 2.78-3.34 mmol/L. Relapse has been detected by lactic acid assay, which may be of value in calibration of therapeutic response. In early stage of tuberculous meningitis, elevated CSF lactate persists even with adequate antituberculous therapy.[8] Spinal fluid lactate levels are said to be independent of plasma levels.

Footnotes

1. Fishman RA, *Cerebrospinal Fluid in Diseases of the Nervous System*, 2nd ed, Philadelphia, PA: WB Saunders Co, 1992.
2. Feigin RD, "Bacterial Meningitis Beyond the Newborn Period," *Principles and Practice of Pediatrics*, Oski FA, DeAngelis CD, Feigin RD, et al, eds, Chapter 54, Philadelphia, PA: JB Lippincott Co, 1990, 1028-35.
3. Brook I, "Stability of Lactic Acid in Cerebrospinal Fluid Specimens," *Am J Clin Pathol*, 1982, 77:213-6.
4. Cameron PD, Boyce JM, and Ansori BM, "Cerebrospinal Fluid Lactate in Meningitis and Meningocarcemia," *J Infect*, 1993, 26(3):245-52.
5. Rutledge J, Benjamin D, Hood L, et al, "Is the CSF Lactate Measurement Useful in the Management of Children With Suspected Bacterial Meningitis?" *J Pediatr*, 1981, 98:20-4.
6. Tang LM, "Serial Lactate Determinations in Tuberculous Meningitis," *Scand J Infect Dis*, 1988, 20(1):81-3.
7. Awerbuch G, Peterson P, and Sandyk R, "Elevated Cerebrospinal Fluid Lactic Acid Levels in Creutzfeldt-Jakob Disease," *Int J Neurosci*, 1988, 42(1-2):1-5.
8. Kolmel HW and von Maravic M, "Correlation of Lactic Acid Level, Cell Count and Cytology in Cerebrospinal Fluid of Patients With Bacterial and Nonbacterial Meningitis," *Acta Neurol Scand*, 1988, 78(1):6-9.

References

Latcha S and Cunha BA, "*Listeria monocytogenes* Meningoencephalitis: The Diagnostic Importance of CSF Lactic Acid," *Heart Lung*, 1994, 23(2):177-9.

Cerebrospinal Fluid LD

CPT 83615

Related Information

Bacterial Culture, Cerebrospinal Fluid *on page 460*
Body Fluid Lactate Dehydrogenase *on page 92*
Cerebrospinal Fluid Analysis *on page 309*

Cerebrospinal Fluid Cytology *on page 290*
Cerebrospinal Fluid Glucose *on page 105*
Cerebrospinal Fluid Protein *on page 380*

Synonyms Cerebrospinal Fluid LDH; CSF LDH; Lactate Dehydrogenase, Cerebrospinal Fluid; Spinal Fluid LDH

Applies to Lactic Acid Dehydrogenase, Fluid

Abstract Lactate dehydrogenase (LD) is a normal component of cerebrospinal fluid (CSF). Overlapping values between cases of bacterial and viral meningitis limit the usefulness of CSF LD in differential diagnosis of meningitis.

Specimen Cerebrospinal fluid

Container Clean, sterile CSF tube

Reference Range CSF LD (LDH) activity is normally much less than the plasma LD activity. Normal spinal fluid LD levels are about 10% of serum values (<20 units/L). In children, the reference range is 0-23.5 units/L.[1]

Use A high fluid LD activity, nearly equal to the serum activity is usually associated with inflammatory processes. Increased amounts may occur in association with ischemic necrosis, meningitis, leukemia, metastatic cancer of the CNS, and lymphoma. High fluid LD level, greater than the serum level, is found with neoplasm and with inflammation. Spinal fluid LD has been used by some to identify bacterial meningitis,[1] but overlapping with results in cases of viral meningitis is recognized.[2] CSF lactate, LD (LDH), and LD isoenzymes do not provide definitive data for a diagnosis of bacterial meningitis in childhood.[3]

With CK and AST (SGOT), cerebrospinal fluid LD has been advocated to distinguish cortical from lacunar stroke. These three enzymes are increased in cases of cortical stroke. While CK and AST are not increased with lacunar stroke, LD is only slightly elevated. CSF LD is increased in patients with severe brain injury but is not useful (as is CK-BB) in assessing the degree of injury or in monitoring outcome.[4]

Another application of LD measurement is the differential diagnosis of intracranial hemorrhage in neonates versus traumatic tap. Lactate dehydrogenase is elevated in proportion to severity of CNS hemorrhage, but unchanged by traumatic tap. CSF LDH is higher in stroke than in transient ischemic attack.[5]

Limitations This test has very limited usefulness alone due to its nonspecificity.

Additional Information A tabulation of CSF enzymes in neurological diseases is available.[2]

Footnotes

1. Knight JA, Dudek SM, and Haymond RE, "Early (Chemical) Diagnosis of Bacterial Meningitis-Cerebrospinal Fluid Glucose, Lactate, and Lactate Dehydrogenase Compared," *Clin Chem*, 1981, 27:1431-4.
2. Fishman RA, *Cerebrospinal Fluid in Diseases of the Nervous System*, 2nd ed, Philadelphia, PA: WB Saunders Co, 1992, 215-6.
3. Castro-Gago M, Couce ML, Losada MC, et al, "C-Reactive Protein, Lactate, and LDH Isoenzymes in the Cerebrospinal Fluid in the Diagnosis in Childhood Meningitis," *An Esp Pediatr*, 1988, 28(1):31-3.
4. Paşaoğlu A and Paşaoğlu H, "Enzymatic Changes in the Cerebrospinal Fluid as Indices of Pathological Change," *Acta Neurochir*, 1989, 97(1-2):71-6.
5. Lampl Y, Paniri Y, Eshel Y, et al, "Cerebrospinal Fluid Lactate Dehydrogenase Levels in Early Stroke and Transient Ischemic Attacks," *Stroke*, 1990, 21(6):854-7.

References

Donnan GA, Zapf P, Doyle AE, et al, "CSF Enzymes in Lacunar and Cortical Stroke," *Stroke*, 1983, 14:266-9.
Lampl Y, Paniri Y, Eshel Y, et al, "LDH Isoenzymes in Cerebrospinal Fluid in Various Brain Tumours," *J Neurol Neurosurg Psychiatry*, 1990, 53(8):697-9.
Nolli ML, Picinni P, Polamarasetti T, et al, "Cerebrospinal Fluid Examination as a Possible Predictor of Neurological Outcome in Patients With Acute Liver Failure," *Transplant Proc*, 1993, 25(3):2218-9.

Cerebrospinal Fluid LDH *see* Cerebrospinal Fluid LD *on previous page*

Ceruloplasmin

CPT 82390

Related Information

Copper, Serum *on page 589*
Copper, Urine *on page 590*
Liver Biopsy *on page 48*

Abstract This is the copper-containing protein of plasma. It is decreased in Wilson's disease, Menkes' syndrome, and nutritional deficiency. It is an acute phase reactant and as such is increased in infections, malignancy, in pregnancy, with estrogens, and in trauma. Wilson's disease is an autosomal recessive abnormality of copper metabolism. Its diagnosis can sometimes be made on the basis of hypoceruloplasminemia, hypocupremia, and hypercupruria,[1] with abnormalities in liver-related tests. Liver biopsy may be necessary for diagnosis of Wilson's disease.

Specimen Serum

Container Red top tube

Collection Draw in chilled tube. Keep specimen on ice. Prolonged storage at room temperature leads to decreased levels. Although serum copper and serum ceruloplasmin are normally parallel one with the other, both are needed in Wilson's disease and with acute copper toxicity.

Storage Instructions Separate serum and freeze.

Reference Range Neonatal levels are lower than adults. Adult levels are reached 3-6 months after birth. Adults: 20-40 mg/dL (SI: 1.26-2.52 µmol/L). Ranges depend on methods, but <10 mg/dL (SI: <0.63 µmol/L) is strong evidence for Wilson's disease.

Use Decreased in most instances of Wilson's disease (hepatolenticular degeneration); hence, ceruloplasmin is used in differential diagnosis of autoimmune hepatitis, cirrhosis and other liver disease. In Wilson's disease, there is decreased ability to incorporate copper into apoceruloplasmin. As a result, free copper levels in plasma and in tissue, especially liver and brain, are greatly increased.

Should be considered in cases of central nervous system disease of obscure etiology. Neurological symptoms include problems of coordination.

Ceruloplasmin is **low** in Menkes' kinky hair syndrome (in Menkes' syndrome the defect is secondary to poor absorption and utilization of dietary copper), and with protein loss such as the nephrotic syndrome, malabsorption, and with some cases of advanced liver disease in which decreases of serum proteins have occurred.

Ceruloplasmin is **high** in a variety of neoplastic and inflammatory states, since it behaves as an acute phase reactant, although levels rise more slowly than more widely recognized "acute phase reactants". Increases are described with carcinomas, leukemias, Hodgkin's disease, primary biliary cirrhosis, and with SLE and rheumatoid arthritis. High levels occur in pregnancy, with estrogens, and with oral contraceptive use when the agent contains estrogen as well as progesterone. Increased with copper intoxication.

Limitations A normal ceruloplasmin does not rule out Wilson's disease, especially in childhood cases. Serum and often liver copper should be measured in addition. Discrepancies occur between immunologic and enzymatic assays in serum of patients with Wilson's disease.

Methodology Spectrophotometric, nephelometric, radial immunodiffusion. Multiplying ceruloplasmin level (mg/L) by three gives the binding protein's contribution to serum copper (µg/L). This may be as great as 90% to 95% of total serum copper. Performing this maneuver allows the clinician to exert a measure of quality control on the laboratory results.

Additional Information Ceruloplasmin is an α_2-globulin containing copper. About 70% or more of total serum copper is associated with ceruloplasmin, 7% with a high MW protein, transcuprein, 19% with albumin, and 2% with amino acids.[2]

Liver biopsy is sometimes needed. In addition to H & E microscopy, tissue copper concentrations, when necessary, can confirm the diagnosis of Wilson's disease.[1] Demonstration of failure to incorporate radiolabeled copper into ceruloplasmin is a definitive test for Wilson's disease. Liver and CNS manifestations of Wilson's disease need not both be present. Kayser-Fleischer rings are extremely helpful findings, but are often absent.

Excessive therapeutic zinc may lead to block of intestinal absorption of copper and a copper deficiency syndrome characterized by hypochromic microcytic anemia with leukopenia/neutropenia and zero level of ceruloplasmin. A prolonged period of time may be required to eliminate the excess zinc, overcome the block of intestinal copper absorption, and obtain increase in serum copper and ceruloplasmin levels.[3]

More information relevant to serum and urine copper, Wilson's disease, and other states is provided in the entries Copper, Serum *on page 589* and Copper, Urine *on page 590*.

Footnotes

1. Ludwig J, Moyer TP, and Rakela J, "The Liver Biopsy Diagnosis of Wilson's Disease," *Am J Clin Pathol*, 1994, 102(4):443-6.
2. Barrow L and Tanner MS, "Copper Distribution Among Serum Proteins in Pediatric Liver Disorders and Malignancies," *Eur J Clin Invest*, 1988, 18(6):555-60.
3. Hoffman HN II, Phyliky RL, and Fleming CR, "Zinc-Induced Copper Deficiency," *Gastroenterology*, 1988, 94(2):508-12.

References

Houwen RH, Van Hattum J, and Hoogenraad T, "Wilson's Disease," *Neth J Med*, 1993, 43(1-2):26-37.
Lockitch G, Halstead AC, Quigley G, et al, "Age and Sex Specific Pediatric Reference Intervals: Study Design and Methods Illustrated by Measurement of Serum Proteins With the Behring LN Nephelometer," *Clin Chem*, 1988, 34(8):1618-21.
Menkes JH, "Kinky Hair Disease: Twenty-Five Years Later," *Brain Dev*, 1988, 10(2):77-9.
Milne DB and Johnson PE, "Assessment of Copper Status: Effect of Age and Gender on Reference Ranges in Healthy Adults," *Clin Chem*, 1993, 39(5):883-7.

Chemistry Profile

CPT 80012 (12 tests)

Applies to Health Fairs; Wellness Programs

Test Commonly Includes The tests present in the Chemistry Profile vary widely among laboratories. Often included are total protein, albumin, calcium, phosphorus, glucose, urea nitrogen (BUN), uric acid, creatinine, total bilirubin, alkaline phosphatase, LD (LDH), AST (SGOT), (Continued)

Chemistry Profile *(Continued)*

electrolytes (often, but not always), and calculated ionized calcium (occasionally). A/G ratio may be provided as calculations. Other calculations which may be offered include urea N/creatinine ratio, globulins, anion gap, and osmolarity. Chemistry profiles may be done by a variety of instruments and include a variable number of tests. The previous list is one of a large number of possible configurations. **Such chemistry profiles should be significantly less expensive than when the same tests are individually carried out.**

Abstract This is a collection of commonly automated serum tests which can be as extensive as 20-25 tests. Frequently used as an admission panel. **The significance of the normal result is much greater than is generally recognized. The value of a baseline set of serum chemistry tests is understood by physicians who review records to care for their patients.** Obvious examples of need for baseline chemistry results include the differential diagnosis of acute infarct of myocardium, lung, or kidney.

Patient Preparation 8- to 12-hour fast is preferred.

Specimen Serum

Container Red top tube

Storage Instructions Separate serum promptly and refrigerate.

Causes for Rejection Gross hemolysis

Reference Range See individual profile tests.

Use Multiple organ system survey, admission profile; establishment of baseline values; evaluation of patients who present as possible diagnostic problems

Limitations More meaningful results are obtained if the specimen is collected after an 8- to 12-hour fast. Lipemia will interfere with some tests. This battery of tests may be or may have been intended for screening, but many laboratories operate their chemistry profiles as definitive tests. Current HCFA policy does not support reimbursement for tests in a large panel unless each can be medically justified.

Methodology Most tests are spectrophotometric except electrolytes which use ion-selective electrodes (ISE)

Additional Information Additional tests can be ordered if indicated. The tests listed are those which the authors feel are desirable, inclusive of creatinine. Provision of chemistry profile with rapid turnaround on hospital patients enhances good care and cost-containment. In many institutions, chemistry profiles are cost-effective; we agree that **fewer tests may increase overall hospital costs[1] by prolonging hospitalization prior to diagnosis.** In wellness programs and health fairs, cholesterol and glucose are often selected. A case for ferritin and thyroid testing can be made,[2] but those are not included in many profiles.

Footnotes

1. Horvath B, Pecci J, and Gay W, "Fewer Tests May Cost More," *N Engl J Med*, 1985, 312(25):1645-6.
2. Witte DL, Angstadt DS, and Schweitzer JK, "Chemistry Profiles in "Wellness Program": Test Selection and Participant Outcomes," *Clin Chem*, 1988, 34(7):1447-50.

References

Berwick DM, "Screening in Health Fairs - A Critical Review of Benefits, Risks, and Costs," *JAMA*, 1985, 254(11):1492-8.

Collen MF, Dales LG, Friedman GD, et al, "Multiphasic Check-Up Evaluation Study. 4. Preliminary Cost Benefit Analysis for Middle-Aged Men," *Prev Med*, 1973, 2:236-46.

Ring AM, "Multiphasic Screening: Panacea or Diagnostic Nightmare?" *JAMA*, 1985, 254(11):1499.

Speicher CE, "So Duplicate Chemistry Profiles Correlate With Multiple Physicians: Let's Not Blame the Doctors," *Arch Pathol Lab Med*, 1988, 112(3):235-6.

Young DS, "Why There Is a Laboratory," *Clinical Chemistry*, Young DS, Hicks J, Nipper H, et al, eds, Washington, DC: American Association of Clinical Chemistry, 1979.

Chloride/Phosphorus Ratio *see* Calcium, Serum *on page 97*

Chloride, Serum

CPT 82435

Related Information

Anion Gap *on page 81*
Bromide, Serum *on page 538*
Carbon Dioxide, Blood *on page 100*
Electrolytes, Serum or Plasma *on page 123*
Kidney Stone Analysis *on page 640*
Potassium, Serum or Plasma *on page 188*
Sodium, Blood *on page 199*

Synonyms Cl, Serum

Applies to Bromism

Abstract Used as part of serum electrolyte evaluation, chloride is needed for calculation of the anion gap.

Specimen Serum

Container Red top tube. Green top (heparin) tube is acceptable, but use of anticoagulants other than heparin may alter electrolyte composition.

Collection Pediatrics: Blood drawn from heelstick for capillary.

Storage Instructions Refrigerate

Reference Range Premature: 95-110 mmol/L (SI: 95-110 mmol/L); fullterm: 96-106 mmol/L (SI: 96-106 mmol/L); children and adults: 97-107 mmol/L (SI: 97-107 mmol/L)

Possible Panic Range <80 mmol/L (SI: <80 mmol/L), >115 mmol/L (SI: >115 mmol/L)

Use Electrolyte evaluation; investigation of acid-base balance, water balance, and ketosis. Chloride generally increases and decreases with plasma or serum sodium.

Chloride is **increased** in dehydration, with ammonium chloride administration, with renal tubular acidosis (hyperchloremic metabolic acidosis), and with excessive infusion of normal saline. Chloride is higher in hyperparathyroidism than in some of the other causes of hypercalcemia, but a great deal of overlap exists.

Chloride is **decreased** with overhydration, congestive failure, syndrome of inappropriate secretion of ADH, vomiting, gastric suction, chronic respiratory acidosis, Addison's disease, salt-losing nephritis, burns, metabolic alkalosis, and in some instances of diuretic therapy.

Differential diagnosis of acidemias and alkalemias; an important use of chloride is in application of the anion gap. Consult the listing Anion Gap *on page 81* for more information.

Limitations Interference from bromide occurs in hospital patients, in some of whom bromide concentrations are detectable.[1,2] Chloride is not used independently, but only with sodium and commonly with potassium and carbon dioxide.

Methodology Coulometry, colorimetry, mercuric thiocyanate, ion-selective electrode (ISE)

Additional Information Like other electrolytes, chloride cannot be interpreted without clinical knowledge of the patient. A diagnostic approach to the evaluation of hyperchloremic metabolic acidosis includes use of the urinary anion gap in conjunction with measurement of plasma potassium and urinary pH.[3] Direct (no dilution) ISE method is free of the volume displacement error that occurs with specimens with high lipid or protein content.

Footnotes

1. Wenk RE, Lustagarten JA, Pappas NJ, et al, "Serum Chloride Analysis, Bromide Detection, and the Diagnosis of Bromism," *Am J Clin Pathol*, 1976, 65:49-57.
2. Rehak NN and Andersen TE, "Evaluation of Gilford Chemistry Control Interference With the Chloride Method in the Beckman Synchron CX3 System Analyzer: Cumulative Effect of Bromide on Chloride Results," *Clin Chem*, 1989, 35(7):1538.
3. Battle DC, Hizon M, Cohen E, et al, "The Use of the Urinary Anion Gap in the Diagnosis of Hyperchloremic Metabolic Acidosis," *N Engl J Med*, 1988, 318(10):594-9.

References

Koch SM and Taylor RW, "Chloride Ion in Intensive Care Medicine," *Crit Care Med*, 1992, 20(2):227-40.

Lowe RA, Wood AB, Burney RE, et al, "Rational Ordering of Serum Electrolytes: Development of Clinical Criteria," *Ann Emerg Med*, 1987, 16(3):260-9.

McCleane GJ, "Urea and Electrolyte Measurement in Preoperative Surgical Patients," *Anaesthesia*, 1988, 43(5):413-5.

Rothenberg DM, Berns AS, Barkin R, et al, "Bromide Intoxication Secondary to Pyridostigmine Bromide Therapy," *JAMA*, 1990, 263(8):1121-2.

Wrenn KD, Slovis CM, Minion GE, et al, "The Syndrome of Alcoholic Ketoacidosis," *Am J Med*, 1991, 91(2):119-28.

Chloride, Sweat

CPT 82435 (analysis); 89360 (collection)

Related Information

Cystic Fibrosis DNA Detection *on page 507*
d-Xylose Absorption Test *on page 122*

Synonyms Cystic Fibrosis Sweat Test; Iontophoresis; Sweat, Chloride

Applies to Sodium, Sweat; Trypsin Activity, Stool; Trypsinogen, Immunoreactive

Test Commonly Includes Sodium level may also be measured.

Abstract The disease cystic fibrosis is characterized by broad clinical heterogenicity.[1] The usual application of this test is as an aid in the diagnosis of cystic fibrosis. Typically pilocarpine is iontophoresed into a small area of skin to induce localized sweating. Resulting sweat is collected onto filter paper or gauze, diluted, and analyzed for sodium and/or chloride concentration(s).

Specimen Sweat

Reference Range 5-40 mmol/L (SI: 5-40 mmol/L). Sweat chloride and sodium levels >70 mmol/L are essentially diagnostic of cystic fibrosis in children, but all values must be interpreted with the family history and clinical presentation to include the presence of chronic obstructive pulmonary disease or documentation of pancreatic exocrine insufficiency.[2] Intermediate range is 40-60 mmol/L.[2] Adult values up to 50 mmol/L may be normal. In adults, >70 mmol/L is diagnostic,[3] and >60 mmol/L is diagnostic when other criteria are present.[2]

Critical Values More than 60 mmol/L is considered diagnostic up to about 20 years of age. In older adults, >70 mmol/L is diagnostic.[3]

Use Establish the diagnosis of cystic fibrosis (mucoviscidosis); evaluate frequent and/or foul stools, diarrhea, malabsorption, pancreatic insufficiency, history of meconium ileus, neonatal intestinal obstruction, rectal prolapse, infant celiac disease, other chronic problems of gastrointestinal tract and/or lung disease in children; work up chronic pulmonary disease, asthma, chronic cough, mucoid *Pseudomonas*, and other bronchitis in children;[4] work up children for failure to thrive and of young adult males for aspermia;[4] evaluation for absence of vas deferens.

Limitations Duplicate tests should always be done. Skin covered by rashes or lesions will cause higher chloride levels. Elevations have been reported in adrenal insufficiency, pseudohypoaldosteronism, ectodermal dysplasia, hereditary nephrogenic diabetes insipidus, hypothyroidism, malnutrition, fucosidosis, glucose-6-phosphatase deficiency, mucopolysaccharidosis and other entities. Shwachman and Mahmoodian emphasize that in some of the diseases listed, sweat chloride and sodium elevations lack the constancy that is found in cystic fibrosis.[3] False low results have been described with edema, hypoproteinemia, and excessive sweating. Results are highly variable in adults, especially women in whom sweat chloride levels vary with the menstrual cycle. Sweat chloride levels in adults must be interpreted cautiously: false-positives and negatives may occur.

Borderline tests must be repeated.[5] Even negative tests should be repeated if the clinical picture suggests mucoviscidosis. Warwick and Hansen are among those who have advocated subsequent confirmation of positives.[6] Sweat chloride test does not identify carriers (heterozygotes). Reliability in the first weeks of life is questionable.[2]

Standards for sweat electrolytes are not widely available as standards are for other chemistry assays, but can be made locally. A small fraction of cystic fibrosis patients do not have diagnostic sweat chloride patterns.[1,2,4,7] The measurement of sodium and the determination of the Na/Cl ratio may be useful. An application of evolving pathology involves isolation of DNA with amplification utilizing the polymerase chain reaction: see listing Cystic Fibrosis DNA Detection *on page 507*. Molecular recombinant DNA diagnostic techniques may be the best way to diagnose the disease and the carrier states.

Different clinical facets of cystic fibrosis are recognized. Mutations which cause less severe pancreatic disease are known, and a mutation associated with mild lung disease is described.[10]

Contraindications Dermatitis. Do not collect sweat from the palm of the hand, or from any site following excessive sweating such as following high temperature or heavy exercise. Improper placement of pad or electrode can cause skin burn.[4]

Methodology Chloride in sweat from the forearm by pilocarpine-ionotophoresis.[2] It may be necessary in infants to use the upper back. Measurement by an ion-specific electrode (ISE). Schales and Schales method, Cotlove titration are acceptable. At least 50 mg of sweat must be collected for test validity.[2] Usual collections, using proper equipment producing exactly 1.5 ma, range from 100-400 mg of sweat. The Cystic Fibrosis Indicator System™ (Medtronic) may be promising.[8]

Additional Information Meconium ileus, very strongly associated with cystic fibrosis, is a separate entity from the meconium plug syndrome.

Other laboratory abnormalities in cystic fibrosis may include low total protein, prolongation of prothrombin time and abnormalities which may relate to evolving hepatic cirrhosis.

Normal sweat **sodium** level is 5-40 mmol/L. Sweat sodium >80 mmol/L also is evidence for cystic fibrosis. High sweat sodium may be found in Addison's disease, ectodermal dysplasia, hereditary nephrogenic diabetes insipidus, hypothyroidism, glucose-6-phosphatase deficiency, hypoparathyroidism, familial cholestasis,, pancreatitis, mucopolysaccharidoses, fucosidosis, and malnutrition.[2] Low sodium may be found with sodium depletion and in hyperaldosteronism.

Testing of stool samples for decreased trypsin activity (due to pancreatic exocrine dysfunction) has also been used as a screening test for cystic fibrosis in infants and young children. However, testing for stool trypsin activity is less reliable than the sweat chloride test and should not be used in its place. Assay of serum immunoreactive trypsinogen may be a useful test in cystic fibrosis screening programs.[9]

Different clinical facets of cystic fibrosis are recognized. Mutations which cause less severe pancreatic disease are known, and a mutation associated with mild lung disease is described.[10]

Footnotes

1. Highsmith WE, Burch LH, Zhou Z, et al, "A Novel Mutation in the Cystic Fibrosis Gene in Patients With Pulmonary Disease but Normal Sweat Chloride Concentrations," *N Engl J Med*, 1994, 331(15):974-80.
2. Behrman RE, Kliegman RM, and Nelson WE, *Nelson Textbook of Pediatrics*, 14th ed, Philadelphia, PA: WB Saunders Co, 1992, 1108-9.
3. Hall SK, Stableforth DE, and Green A, "Sweat Sodium and Chloride Concentrations - Essential Criteria for the Diagnosis of Cystic Fibrosis in Adults," *Ann Clin Biochem*, 1990, 27(Pt 4):318-20.
4. Schwachman H and Mahmoodian A, "The Sweat Test and Cystic Fibrosis," *Diagn Med*, 1982, 61-77.
5. Stern RC, Boat TF, Abramowsky CR, et al, "Intermediate-Range Sweat Chloride Concentration and *Pseudomonas* Bronchitis. A Cystic Fibrosis Variant With Preservation of Exocrine Pancreatic Function," *JAMA*, 1978, 239:2676-80.

6. Warwick WJ and Hansen L, "Measurement of Chloride in Sweat With the Chloride-Selective Electrode," *Clin Chem*, 1978, 24:2050-3.
7. Stewart B, Zabner J, Shuber AP, et al, "Normal Sweat Chloride Values Do Not Exclude the Diagnosis of Cystic Fibrosis," *Am J Respir Crit Care Med*, 1995, 151(3 Pt 1):899-903.
8. Warwick WJ, Hansen LG, and Werness ME, "Quantification of Chloride in Sweat With the Cystic Fibrosis Indicator System," *Clin Chem*, 1990, 36(1):96-8.
9. Hammond KB, Abman SH, Sokol RJ, et al, "Efficacy of Statewide Neonatal Screening for Cystic Fibrosis by Assay of Trypsinogen Concentrations," *N Engl J Med*, 1991, 325(11):769-74.
10. Gan KH, Veeze HJ, van den Ouweland AMW, et al, "A Cystic Fibrosis Mutation Associated With Mild Lung Disease," *N Engl J Med*, 1995, 333(2):95-9.

References

Abrons HL, "Cystic Fibrosis: Current Concepts," *W V Med J*, 1993, 89(6):236-40.

Durieu I, Bey-Omar F, Rollet J, et al, "Diagnostic Criteria for Cystic Fibrosis in Men With Congenital Absence of the Vas Deferens," *Medicine*, 1995, 74(1):42-7.

Hammond KB, Turcios NL, and Gibson LE, "Clinical Evaluation of the Macroduct Sweat Collection System and Conductivity Analyzer in the Diagnosis of Cystic Fibrosis," *J Pediatr*, 1994, 124(2):255-60.

Hanukoglu A, Bistritzer T, Rakover Y, et al, "Pseudohypoaldosteronism With Increased Sweat and Saliva Electrolyte Values and Frequent Lower Respiratory Tract Infections Mimicking Cystic Fibrosis," *J Pediatr*, 1994, 125(5 Pt 1):752-5.

Kirk JM, Keston M, McIntosh I, et al, "Variation of Sweat Sodium and Chloride With Age in Cystic Fibrosis and Normal Populations: Further Investigations in Equivocal Cases," *Ann Clin Biochem*, 1992, 29(Pt 2):145-52.

Larsen J, Campbell S, Faragher EB, et al, "Cystic Fibrosis Screening in Neonates - Measurement of Immunoreactive Trypsin and Direct Genotype Analysis for Delta F508 Mutation," *Eur J Pediatr*, 1994, 153(8):569-73.

LeGrys VA and Burnett RW, "Current Status of Sweat Testing in North America," *Arch Pathol Lab Med*, 1994, 118(9):865-7.

Meites S, *Pediatric Clinical Chemistry: Reference (Normal) Values*, 3rd ed, Washington, DC: American Association of Clinical Chemistry Press, 1989, 244-7.

Polack FP, Transue DJ, Belknap WM, et al, "Transient Evaluation of Sweat Chloride Concentration in a Malnourished Girl With the Mauriac Syndrome," *J Pediatr*, 1995, 126(2):261-3.

Ravnik-Glavac M, Glavac D, Chernick M, et al, "Screening for CF Mutations in Adult Cystic Fibrosis Patients With a Directed and Optimized SSCP Strategy," *Hum Mutat*, 1994, 3(3):231-8.

Rodrigues ME, Melo MC, Reis FJ, et al, "Concentration of Electrolytes in the Sweat of Malnourished Children," *Arch Dis Child*, 1994, 71(2):141-3.

Waters DL, Dorney SFA, Gaskin KJ, et al, "Pancreatic Function in Infants Identified as Having Cystic Fibrosis in a Neonatal Screening Program," *N Engl J Med*, 1990, 322(5):303-8.

Chloride, Urine

CPT 82436

Related Information

Electrolytes, Urine *on page 124*
Potassium, Serum or Plasma *on page 188*
Potassium, Urine *on page 189*
Sodium, Blood *on page 199*
Sodium, Urine *on page 199*
Urine Collection, 24-Hour *on page 30*

Synonyms Cl, Urine; Urine Cl

Abstract Used as an aid in evaluation of electrolyte balance, including metabolic alkalosis

Specimen Timed or random urine

Container No preservative

Reference Range 110-250 mmol/24 hours (SI: 110-250 mmol/day) in adults, lower values in infancy and childhood. Results depend on ingestion of chloride. In older adults, values may be somewhat lower.

Use Evaluate electrolyte composition of urine, acid-base balance studies. Distinguish whether or not a case of metabolic alkalosis is chloride-responsive (salt responsive). Sherman and Eisinger[1,2] discuss bicarbonate excretion, blood volume, potassium depletion, and the differential diagnosis of metabolic alkalosis with loss of gastric juice (emesis, intubation) and after diuretics. Chloride depleted patients excrete urine with low chloride, <10 mmol/L. Such patients are chloride-responsive (ie, they respond to chloride sufficient to return body stores to normal). Metabolic alkalosis with low urine chloride may also be found with villous tumors of the colon.

Endogenous or exogenous corticosteroids produce urine chloride values in excess of 20 mmol/L. Such patients are chloride resistant. The finding of chloride resistant metabolic alkalosis may provide a stimulus to identify an ACTH or aldosterone producing neoplasm (eg, Cushing's syndrome or Conn's syndrome). In Bartter's syndrome with metabolic alkalosis, there is usually increased urine chloride. The complex relationships of chronic pulmonary disease with metabolic alkalosis are mentioned by Sherman and Eisinger.

Limitations Halogens other than chloride (bromide), which are also present in urine, may erroneously elevate the chloride result. Isolated urine chloride, without urine sodium or potassium or without serum or plasma electrolytes, can provide misleading information. Discussion of electrolyte balance is beyond the scope of this manual (eg, effect of profound potassium depletion on impairment of chloride reabsorption). Fetal urinary electrolytes are an unreliable guide to evaluate fetal renal function.[3]

Methodology Coulometric titration, ion-selective electrode (ISE)
(Continued)

Chloride, Urine *(Continued)*

Additional Information Urine chloride is often ordered with sodium and potassium as a timed urine. The urinary anion gap $[Na^+ - (Cl^- + HCO_3^-)]$ or $[(Na^+ + K^+) - (Cl^-)]$ is useful in the initial evaluation of hyperchloremic metabolic acidosis.[4] In metabolic alkalosis, spot urine chloride in the presence of hypertension can provide important information.[5]

Footnotes

1. Sherman RA and Eisinger RP, "The Use (and Misuse) of Urinary Sodium and Chloride Measurements," *JAMA*, 1982, 247:3121-4.
2. Sherman RA and Eisinger RP, "Urinary Sodium and Chloride During Renal Salt Retention," *Am J Kidney Dis*, 1983, 3:121-3.
3. Elder JS, O'Grady JP, Ashmead G, et al, "Evaluation of Fetal Renal Function: Unreliability of Fetal Urinary Electrolytes," *J Urol*, 1990, 144(2 Pt 2):574-8.
4. Battle DC, Hizon M, Cohen E, et al, "The Use of the Urinary Anion Gap in the Diagnosis of Hyperchloremic Metabolic Acidosis," *N Engl J Med*, 1988, 318(10):594-9.
5. Preuss HG, "Fundamentals of Clinical Acid-Base Evaluation," *Clin Lab Med*, 1993, 13(1):103-16.

References

Harrington JT and Cohen JJ, "Measurement of Urinary Electrolytes - Indications and Limitations," *N Engl J Med*, 1975, 293:1241-3.

Jeffery RW, Mullenbach VA, Bjornson-Benson WM, et al, "Home Testing of Urine Chloride to Estimate Dietary Sodium Intake: Evaluation of Feasibility and Accuracy," *Addict Behav*, 1987, 12(1):17-21.

Kamel KS, Magner PO, Ethier JH, et al, "Urine Electrolytes in the Assessment of Extracellular Fluid Volume Contraction," *Am J Nephrol*, 1989, 9(4):344-7.

Pan WH, Chen JY, Chen YC, et al, "Diurnal Electrolyte Excretion Pattern Affects Estimates of Electrolyte Status Based on 24-Hour, Half-Day, and Overnight Urine," *Chin J Physiol*, 1994, 37(1):49-53.

Cholecalciferol *see* Vitamin D_3, Serum *on page 218*

Cholesterol/HDLC Ratio *see* Cholesterol, Serum *on this page*

Cholesterol/HDLC Ratio *see* High Density Lipoprotein Cholesterol *on page 143*

Cholesterol, Serum

CPT 82465

Related Information

Apolipoprotein A and B *on page 82*

Apolipoprotein E *on page 82*

High Density Lipoprotein Cholesterol *on page 143*

Lipid Profile *on page 159*

Lipoprotein Electrophoresis *on page 161*

Low Density Lipoprotein Cholesterol *on page 162*

Triglycerides *on page 209*

Applies to Cholesterol/HDLC Ratio

Abstract A causal relationship exists between hypercholesterolemia and risk for coronary artery disease, but other factors also are relevant.

Patient Preparation To support proper interpretation of lipid analysis:

- For optimum patient condition at the time of blood drawing: no change in diet for 3 weeks, stable body weight, and fasting (no food, except water and possibly black coffee without sugar in the morning) for 12 hours. (Fasting is not important before cholesterol analysis but is important when determining other lipids, eg, triglycerides.)
- Posture may be a significant factor: cholesterol values may be 10% to 15% lower after 20 minutes in a recumbent position. From standing to a sitting position values are about 6% lower after 20 minutes.
- Increases of 2% to 5% in cholesterol may be seen if tourniquet is applied for 2 minutes during sampling. Emotional and physical stress may also be factors influencing cholesterol levels.
- Abstinence from alcohol for 72 hours may be desirable, but only inconclusive information is available.

Specimen Serum

Container Red top tube

Reference Range Sharp inconsistencies are obvious when one studies published normal ranges of serum cholesterol in the United States through the 1970s and much of the 1980s. Cholesterol levels have decreased from 1980 to 1987 in a study by the Minnesota Heart Survey.[1]

Cord blood cholesterol: <100 mg/dL (SI: <2.59 mmol/L); >100 mg/dL (SI: >2.59 mmol/L) is indicative of type II hyperlipoproteinemia. 0-1 month: 45-100 mg/dL (SI: 1.16-2.59 mmol/L). Adults, 20 years and older: Although 100-200 mg/dL (SI: 2.59-5.43 mmol/L) would be regarded as a low normal range for American adults, an increase between ages 25 and 45 of about 25 mg/dL (SI: 0.65 mmol/L) is recognized.[2] Levels >180 mg/dL (SI: >4.65 mmol/L) are not desirable,[3] but are commonplace in the United States. Percentile values are provided in a LRC report.[4] The National Cholesterol Education Program (NCEP) suggested limit: <200 mg/dL (without age stratification) (SI: <5.1 mmol/L). See Classification Based on Total Cholesterol later in this discussion.

Cholesterol <115 mg/dL (SI: <2.97 mmol/L) in youthful subjects is in the 5th percentile for males, <119 mg/dL (SI: <3.08 mmol/L) for females 0-19 years. Cholesterol levels <50 mg/dL (SI: <1.29 mmol/L) are found in the Bassen-Kornzweig syndrome with triglycerides <30 mg/dL. Cholesterol levels <100 mg/dL are found in Tangier disease without low triglycerides. Each is an autosomal recessive disease.

Cholesterol >240 mg/dL (SI: >6.21 mmol/L) may indicate need for dietary or other intervention.[2,5] This level is excessive for young adults and even 220 mg/dL (SI: 5.69 mmol/L) is somewhat high for young adults, depending on LDL, HDL, family history, and other factors.

A national effort is underway to identify patients at risk for coronary heart disease due to elevated cholesterol levels. A key facet is standardization of cholesterol measurements traceable to the National Reference System for Cholesterol, rather than the customary instrument/method dependent "reference ranges." NBS (National Bureau of Standards) Standard Reference Material for Cholesterol in Human Serum was released to general laboratories in the first half of 1988 and has been valuable.[6] A collaborative study between the CAP and CDC to evaluate reference materials has been of great utility in the effort to determine specific instrument bias.[7]

Plasma cholesterol values are up to 10% lower than serum values. This difference should be considered when comparing patient values to published reference tables.

Critical Values Although cholesterol concentrations >300 mg/dL bear a strong relationship to coronary heart disease, only a fraction of individuals who have coronary occlusive disease have cholesterol that increased.[8]

Use Evaluate risk of coronary arterial occlusion, atherosclerosis, and myocardial infarction. **Increased** in primary hypercholesterolemia, secondary hyperlipoproteinemias including nephrotic syndrome, hypothyroidism, primary biliary cirrhosis, and some cases of diabetes mellitus. Increased cholesterol is found in 76% of adult cases of glycogen storage disease type 1a.[9] **Low levels** have been found in cases of malnutrition, malabsorption, hyperthyroidism, myeloma, macroglobulinemia of Waldenström, polycythemia vera, myeloid metaplasia, myelofibrosis, chronic myelocytic leukemia, analphalipoproteinemia (Tangier disease), abetalipoproteinemia (Bassen-Kornzweig syndrome) (acanthocytosis), and in some individuals who subsequently present with carcinoma. Levy has pointed out that the weak inverse relationship with cancer, mostly colon carcinoma, is limited to cholesterol levels <190 mg/dL (SI: <4.91 mmol/L) and is limited to men.[10] Hypocholesterolemia may occur with sideroblastic anemia or in the thalassemias. Severe liver disease may lower cholesterol dramatically.

Cholesterol and HDLC are major facets of coronary heart disease risk.[4] Since premature mortality from coronary arterial disease is rampant and since cholesterol levels are available as a test which can detect a modifiable risk factor, serum cholesterol remains a critical and genuinely newsworthy topic and an important screening test. Effective intervention is available when cholesterol studies identify subjects likely to benefit, asymptomatic persons as well as those with recognized coronary disease. A report of the Lipid Research Clinics (LRC) has provided reference ranges.[4]

Limitations Other risk factors for coronary arterial disease include hypertension, family history of premature coronary arterial disease, especially when it is premature; use of cigarettes, obesity (excess body weight >30%), physical inactivity, low HDLC, hypertension, diabetes mellitus, prior myocardial infarct, prior cerebrovascular or occlusive peripheral vascular disease, *vide infra*. Many heart attacks occur at levels of cholesterol considered "within normal limits." In fact, a majority of cases of heart disease are found in persons whose cholesterol levels are not worse than moderately elevated. The curves of those without and those with a coronary event heavily overlap when plotted against cholesterol levels. Random testing of TC, HDLC, and LDLC may fail to detect wide fluctuations in these levels (±20%). Variations of more than ±20% were seen in 75%, 65%, and 95% of a tested group.

Cholesterol values are altered by weight loss, pregnancy and (like HDL and apolipoproteins) acute illness, as well as by acute myocardial infarct. Inconsistencies exist between the serum cholesterol, the proportion of younger individuals who experience coronary occlusion, and the severity of atherogenesis. Nevertheless, cholesterol determinations done in good, well-standardized laboratories on samples from well subjects provide reliable information. The serum total cholesterol is insufficient as a screening tool for detection of elevated levels of low-density lipoprotein cholesterol in children and adolescents.[11] Elderly individuals, those in the late 70's and older, probably should not be screened.[12]

Methodology Enzymatic, ferric chloride-sulfuric acid, Leibermann-Burchardt reaction

Additional Information About 50% to 80% of plasma/serum cholesterol is carried as low density lipoprotein cholesterol (LDLC) (β-lipoprotein). Much of the remainder is found in HDL, with small quantities as VLDL and as chylomicrons. Cholesterol is a component of cell membranes and organelles. It is the precursor of steroid hormones.

Classification Based on Total Cholesterol

Desirable blood cholesterol: <200 mg/dL (SI: <5.17 mmol/L)
Borderline-high blood cholesterol: 200-239 mg/dL (SI: 5.17-6.18 mmol/L)
High blood cholesterol: ≥240 mg/dL (SI: ≥6.21 mmol/L)

- The total blood cholesterol level is the basis for initial patient classification.
- All blood cholesterol levels >200 mg/dL (SI: >5.17 mmol/L) should be confirmed by repeat measurements, with the average used to guide clinical decisions.
- Other CHD risk factors should be taken into account in selecting appropriate follow-up measures for patients with borderline-high cholesterol levels.
- All patients with a level ≥240 mg/dL (SI: ≥6.21 mmol/L), which is classified as high blood cholesterol, should receive a lipoprotein analysis. Patients with borderline-high blood cholesterol levels 200-239 mg/dL (SI: 5.17-6.18 mmol/L), who in addition have definite CHD or two other CHD risk factors, should also have a lipoprotein analysis performed.
- CHD risk factors as defined in the report include:
  - male sex
  - family history of premature CHD (definite myocardial infarction or sudden death before age 55 in a parent or sibling)
  - cigarette smoking (currently more than 10 cigarettes per day)
  - hypertension
  - low HDL cholesterol concentration, <35 mg/dL, (SI: <0.91 mmol/L) confirmed by repeat measurement
  - diabetes mellitus
  - history of definite cerebrovascular or occlusive peripheral vascular disease
  - severe obesity (≥30% overweight)
- In public screening programs, all patients with a level > 200 mg/dL (SI: >5.17 mmol/L) should be referred to their physician for remeasurement and evaluation.

"National Cholesterol Education Program, Adult Treatment Panel Report 1987," National Cholesterol Education Program, National Heart, Lung, and Blood Institute, National Institutes of Health, C-200, Bethesda, MD 20892, 1987.
Compare to the following table.
Note NCEP lack of age stratification. Some authorities suggest that stratification should be maintained.

Values for Selecting Adults at Moderate and High Risk Requiring Treatment

Age	Moderate Risk		High Risk	
	mg/dL	SI: mmol/L	mg/dL	SI: mmol/L
20-29 y	>200	>5.17	>220	>5.69
30-39 y	>220	>5.69	>240	>6.21
≥40 y	>240	>6.21	>260	>6.72

From "Lowering Blood Cholesterol to Prevent Heart Disease," *JAMA*, 1985, 253:2080-6, with permission.

Intervention Levels for Serum Cholesterol by Sex and Age*

Male				Female			
Age (y)	Percentile			Age (y)	Percentile		
	75th		90th		75th		90th
0-19	170	(4.40)	185	(4.80)	0-19	175	(4.50)	190	(4.90)
20-24	185	(4.80)	205	(5.30)	20-24	190	(4.90)	215	(5.55)
25-29	200	(5.15)	225	(5.80)	25-34	195	(5.05)	220	(5.70)
30-34	215	(5.55)	240	(6.20)	35-39	205	(5.30)	230	(5.95)
35-39	225	(5.80)	250	(6.45)	40-44	215	(5.55)	235	(6.05)
40-44	230	(5.95)	250	(6.45)	45-49	225	(5.80)	250	(6.45)
45-69	235	(6.05)	260	(6.70)	50-54	240	(6.20)	265	(6.85)
70+	230	(5.95)	250	(6.45)	55+	250	(6.45)	275	(7.10)

From the Lipid Research Clinics Data, with permission. *Arch Intern Med*, 1987, 147:357-60.

Values are given in mg/dL (mmol/L).

Cholesterol is included in lipid profiles. For optimal prediction of coronary atherosclerosis, cholesterol alone fails as an adequate evaluation of all adults' blood lipids. However, relationships between diet, serum cholesterol, and long-term risk of death from coronary arterial disease in middle-aged American men are widely recognized. Rifkind and Segal have pointed out that male subjects in the upper quintile of cholesterol levels had more than 50% of excessive coronary events related to high cholesterol.[4] Hyperlipoproteinemia type II (hypercholesterolemia) is recognizable at any age and can be recognized at birth from cord blood cholesterol. Cholesterol levels should not be drawn immediately after a myocardial infarct has occurred.

The National Cholesterol Education Program (NCEP) has defined a classification based on cholesterol. Unfortunately, this program did not provide age-adjusted normal ranges. He went on to discuss the disconcerting lack of data on older persons.[13] Palumbo discussed a lack of data on older persons.[12] Writing the Mayo editorial, he compared proposals of the NCEP with those of the Consensus Conference of 1985 for serum cholesterol levels. Dr. Palumbo recommended that "...the most prudent advice seems to be to adhere to the recommendations of the Consensus Conference of 1985"[14] and use the 75th and 90th percentile for serum cholesterol levels based on age as guidelines. See table.

"Hyperlipoproteinemia" indicates increased cholesterol and/or triglyceride. Intervention levels from the Lipid Research Clinics Data were presented by Kuske and Feldman.[15] See table.

An editorial in *JAMA* emphasized that for individuals older than 60 years intervention should be based on the judgment of the physician and patient preference.[16] Examining prevalence, about 60 million Americans' candidacy for medical advice and intervention has been projected.[17] The **cholesterol/HDLC ratio is significant**.[18,19] See listing High Density Lipoprotein Cholesterol *on page 143*.

The correlation between cases of hypercholesterolemia and instances of hypothyroidism is widely recognized.[20]

Footnotes

1. Burke GL, Sprafka JM, Folsom AR, et al, "Trends in Serum Cholesterol Levels From 1980 to 1987. The Minnesota Heart Survey," *N Engl J Med*, 1991, 324(14):941-6.
2. Hulley SB and Lo B, "Choice and Use of Blood Lipid Tests. An Epidemiologic Perspective," *Arch Intern Med*, 1983, 143:667-73.
3. Carleton RA, "Criterion for Cholesterol Norms - Healthy or Statistical?" *Am J Clin Pathol*, 1983, 79:402.
4. Rifkind BM and Segal P, "Lipid Research Clinics Program Reference Values for Hyperlipidemia and Hypolipidemia," *JAMA*, 1983, 250:1869-72.
5. "National Cholesterol Education Program, Adult Treatment Panel Report 1987," National Cholesterol Education Program, National Heart, Lung, and Blood Institute, National Institutes of Health, 1987, C-200, Bethesda, MD.
6. Bock JL, "Accuracy of Cholesterol Measurements," *Arch Intern Med*, 1991, 151(8):1677.
7. Myers GL, Schap D, Smith SJ, et al, "College of American Pathologists - Centers for Disease Control Collaborative Study for Evaluating Reference Materials for Total Serum Cholesterol Measurements," *Arch Pathol Lab Med*, 1990, 114(12):1199-205.
8. Talente GM, Coleman RA, Alter C, et al, "Glycogen Storage Disease in Adults," *Ann Intern Med*, 1994, 120(3):218-26.
9. O'Keefe JH Jr, Lavie CJ Jr, and McCallister BD, "Insights Into the Pathogenesis and Prevention of Coronary Artery Disease," *Mayo Clin Proc*, 1995, 70(1):69-79.
10. Levy RI, "Cholesterol and Disease - What Are the Facts?" *JAMA*, 1982, 248:2888-90.
11. Dennison BA, Kikuchi DA, Srinivasen SR, et al, "Serum Total Cholesterol Screening for the Detection of Elevated Low-Density Lipoprotein in Children and Adolescents: The Bogalusa Heart Study," *Pediatrics*, 1990, 85(4):472-9.
12. Hulley SB and Newman TB, "Cholesterol in the Elderly - Is It Important?" *JAMA*, 1994, 272(17):1372-4.
13. Palumbo PJ, "National Cholesterol Education Program: Does the Emperor Have Any Clothes?" *Mayo Clin Proc*, 1988, 63(1):88-90.
14. Consensus Conference, "Lowering Blood Cholesterol to Prevent Heart Disease," *JAMA*, 1985, 253(14):2080-6.
15. Kuske TT and Feldman EB, "Hyperlipoproteinemia, Atherosclerosis Risk, and Dietary Management," *Arch Intern Med*, 1987, 147(2):357-60.
16. Palumbo PJ, "Cholesterol Lowering for All: A Closer Look," *JAMA*, 1989, 262(1):91-2.
17. Sempos C, Fulwood R, Haines C, et al, "The Prevalence of High Blood Cholesterol Levels Among Adults in the United States," *JAMA*, 1989, 262(1):45-52.
18. Hostetter AL, "Screening for Dyslipidemia," *Am J Clin Pathol*, 1995, 103:380-5.
19. Grover SA, Palmer CS, and Coupal L, "Serum Lipid Screening to Identify High-Risk Individuals for Coronary Death," *Arch Intern Med*, 1994, 154(6):679-84.
20. Oettgen R, Ginsburg GS, Horowitz GL, et al, "Frequency of Hypothyroidism in Adults With Serum Total Cholesterol Levels 200 mg/dL," *Am J Cardiol*, 1994, 73(13):955-7.

References

American Academy of Pediatrics Committee on Nutrition, "Indications for Cholesterol Testing in Children," *Pediatrics*, 1989, 83(1):141-2.
Anderson KM, Castelli WP, and Levy D, "Cholesterol and Mortality - 30 Years of Follow-Up From the Framingham Study," *JAMA*, 1987, 257(16):2176-80.
Austin GE, Hollman J, Lynn MJ, et al, "Serum Lipoprotein Levels Fail to Predict Postangioplasty Recurrent Coronary Artery Stenosis," *Cleve Clin J Med*, 1989, 56(5):509-14.
Benfante R and Reed D, "Is Elevated Serum Cholesterol Level a Risk Factor for Coronary Heart Disease in the Elderly?" *JAMA*, 1990, 263(3):393-6.
Borhani NO, "Prevention of Coronary Heart Disease in Practice: Implications of the Results of Recent Clinical Trials," *JAMA*, 1985, 254(2):257-62.
Bradford RH and Rifkind BM, "Lowering Blood Cholesterol to Reduce Coronary Heart Disease Risk," *Clin Lab Med*, 1989, 9(1):1-6.
Christenson RH, Roeback JR Jr, Watson TE, et al, "Improving the Reliability of Total and High-Density Lipoprotein Cholesterol Measurements. Four Testing Strategies Compared in a High-Risk Population," *Arch Pathol Lab Med*, 1991, 115(12):1212-6.
Copeland BE, "Serum Cholesterol Methodology: 100 Years of Development," *Ann Clin Lab Sci*, 1990, 20(1):1-11.
Drown DJ and Engler MM, "New Guidelines for Blood Cholesterol by the National Cholesterol Education Program (NCEP). National Cholesterol Education Program (NCEP)," *Prog Cardiovasc News*, 1994, 9(1):43-4.
Garber AM, Sox HC Jr, and Littenberg B, "Screening Asymptomatic Adults for Cardiac Risk Factors: The Serum Cholesterol Level," *Ann Intern Med*, 1989, 110(8):622-39.
Goodman DS, "New Guidelines for Lowering Blood Cholesterol," *Clin Lab Med*, 1989, 9(1)17-27.
Goodman DS, Bradford RH, Brewer HB Jr, et al, "AHA Conference Report on Cholesterol. Diagnosis, Evaluation, and Treatment: Current Status and Issues," *Circulation*, 1989, 80(3):735-8.
Grundy SM, "Cholesterol and Coronary Heart Disease: A New Era," *JAMA*, 1986, 256(20):2849-58.

(Continued)

Cholesterol, Serum *(Continued)*

Hoeg JM, "Familial Hypercholesterolemia: What the Zebra Can Teach Us About the Horse," *JAMA*, 1994, 271(7):543-6.

Iso H, Jacobs DR Jr, Wentworth D, et al, "Serum Cholesterol Levels and Six-Year Mortality From Stroke in 350,977 Men Screened for the Multiple Risk Factor Intervention Trial," *N Engl J Med*, 1989, 320(14):904-10.

Kronmal RA, "Commentary on the Published Results of the Lipid Research Clinics Coronary Primary Prevention Trial," *JAMA*, 1985, 253(14):2091-3.

Laemmle P, Unger L, McCray C, et al, "Cholesterol Guidelines, Lipoprotein Cholesterol Levels, and Triglyceride Levels: Potential for Misclassification of Coronary Heart Disease Risk," *J Lab Clin Med*, 1989, 113(3):325-33.

Law MR, Walk NJ, and Thompson SG, "By How Much and How Quickly Does Reduction in Serum Cholesterol Concentration Lower Risk of Ischaemic Heart Disease?" *BMJ*, 1994, 308(6925):367-72.

Levine GN, Keaney JF Jr, and Vita JA, "Cholesterol Reduction in Cardiovascular Disease. Clinical Benefits and Possible Mechanisms," *N Engl J Med*, 1995, 332(8):512-21.

Naito HK, "The Need for Accurate Total Cholesterol Measurement: Recommended Analytical Goals, Current State of Reliability, and Guidelines for Better Determinations," *Clin Lab Med*, 1989, 9(1):37-60.

Steinmetz J, Jouanel P, and Delattre J, "Total Cholesterol," *Drug Effects on Laboratory Test Results Analytical Interferences and Pharmacological Effects*, Siest G and Galteau MM, eds, Littleton, MA: PSG Publishing Co Inc, 1988, 165-84.

Vanderlinde RE, Bowers GN Jr, Schaffer R, et al, "The National Reference System for Cholesterol," *Clin Lab Med* , 1989, 9(1):89-104.

Warnick GR, Leary ET, Ammirati EB, et al, "Cholesterol in Fingerstick Capillary Specimens Can Be Equivalent to Conventional Venous Measurements," *Arch Pathol Lab Med*, 1994, 118(11):1110-4.

Wilson PWF, Christiansen JC, Anderson KM, et al, "Impact on National Guidelines for Cholesterol Risk Factor Screening: The Framingham Offspring Study," *JAMA*, 1989, 262(1):41-4.

Cholinesterase, Erythrocytic *see* Acetylcholinesterase, Red Cell *on page 62*

Cholinesterase I *see* Acetylcholinesterase, Red Cell *on page 62*

Cholinesterase II *see* Pseudocholinesterase, Serum *on page 196*

Cholinesterase Inhibition by Dibucaine *see* Dibucaine Number *on page 122*

Cholinesterase, Serum *see* Pseudocholinesterase, Serum *on page 196*

Chorionic Gonadotropin, Beta Subunit *see* Human Chorionic Gonadotropin, Serum *on page 145*

Chorionic Somatomammotropin *see* Placental Lactogen, Human *on page 184*

Chromogranin A, Plasma *see* Catecholamines, Fractionation, Plasma *on page 103*

Chylomicrons *see* Triglycerides *on page 209*

CK *see* Creatine Kinase *on page 115*

CK-2 *see* Creatine Kinase Isoenzymes/Isoforms *on page 115*

CK Isoenzymes *see* Creatine Kinase Isoenzymes/Isoforms *on page 115*

CK Isoenzymes *see* Cardiac Enzymes/Isoenzymes *on page 102*

CK Isoforms *see* Creatine Kinase Isoenzymes/Isoforms *on page 115*

CK-MB and Total CK *see* Creatine Kinase Isoenzymes/Isoforms *on page 115*

Clomid® Test *see* Clomiphene Test *on this page*

Clomiphene Test

CPT 83001 (follicle stimulating hormone); 83002 (luteinizing hormone)

Related Information

Follicle Stimulating Hormone *on page 129*
Luteinizing Hormone, Blood or Urine *on page 163*

Synonyms Clomid® Test

Test Commonly Includes FSH analysis, post-clomiphene LH

Abstract Clomiphene is a very weak nonsteroidal antiestrogenic agent which competes with estradiol at the hypothalamus, thereby blocking the negative feedback of the endogenous gonadal steroids on the hypothalamus. In the presence of an intact hypothalamic-pituitary-gonadal axis, administration of clomiphene leads to increased secretion of LH and FSH, inducing ovulation in many anovulatory patients.

Patient Preparation Four weeks of basal body temperatures are recorded. Ascertain that the patient is not pregnant and that the ovaries are not enlarged. No isotopes administered 24 hours prior to venipuncture. Females initially take 50 mg clomiphene orally daily for 5 days beginning on the fifth day of the induced or spontaneous menstrual cycle.

Specimen Serum

Container Red top tube

Collection Females: draw 5-9 days after last oral dose.

Storage Instructions Refrigerate serum. LH and FSH stable at least 7 days in refrigerated serum.

Special Instructions Provide information if post-clomiphene sample(s).

Reference Range FSH and LH are expected to peak 5-9 days after completing Clomid®. FSH increase >40% above baseline; LH increase >120% above baseline. Ovulation assessed by basal body temperature or serum progesterone 2 weeks after last clomiphene dose.

Use Clomiphene may be used to evaluate the integrity of the hypothalamic-pituitary-gonadal axis and to enhance fertility in anovulatory patients with normal ovarian function.

Contraindications In females, observation of hyperstimulation of ovaries but unusual on doses <200 mg, and there is a small risk of multiple pregnancies, about 5%.

Methodology Radioimmunoassay (RIA)

References

Blankstein J and Quigley MM, "The Anovulatory Patient. An Orderly Approach to Evaluation and Treatment," *Postgrad Med*, 1988, 83(5):97-102.

Check JH, Chase JS, Nowroozi K, et al, "Empirical Therapy of the Male With Clomiphene in Couples With Unexplained Infertility," *Int J Fertil*, 1989, 34(2):120-2.

Cunha GR, Taguchi O, Namikawa R, et al, "Teratogenic Effects of Clomiphene, Tamoxifen, and Diethylstilbestrol on the Developing Human Female Genital Tract," *Hum Pathol*, 1987, 18(11):1132-43.

Dickey RP, Olar TT, Taylor SN, et al, "Relationship of Follicle Number and Other Factors to Fecundability and Multiple Pregnancy in Clomiphene Citrate-Induced Intrauterine Insemination Cycles," *Fertil Steril*, 1992, 57(3):613-9.

Fedele L, Brioschi D, Dorta M, et al, "Prediction and Self-Prediction of Ovulation in Clomiphene Citrate-Treated Patients," *Eur J Obstet Gynecol Reprod Biol*, 1988, 28(4):297-303.

Keenan JA, Herbert CM, Bush JR, "Diagnosis and Management of Out-of-Phase Endometrial Biopsies Among Patients Receiving Clomiphene Citrate for Ovulation Induction," *Fertil Steril*, 1989, 51(6):964-7.

Li TC and Warren MA, "Ovulation Induction for Luteal Phase Defects and Luteal Phase Defects After Ovulation Induction," *Baillieres Clin Obstet Gynaecol*, 1993, 7(2):389-419.

Scott RT, Leonardi MR, Hoffman GE, et al, "A Prospective Evaluation of Clomiphene Citrate Challenge Test. Screening of the General Infertility Population," *Obstet Gynecol*, 1993, 82(4 Pt 1):539-44.

Clonidine Suppression Test *see* Catecholamines, Fractionation, Plasma *on page 103*

Cl, Serum *see* Chloride, Serum *on page 108*

Cl, Urine *see* Chloride, Urine *on page 109*

CO₂ Content *see* Carbon Dioxide, Blood *on page 100*

CO₂T *see* Carbon Dioxide, Blood *on page 100*

Compound F *see* Cortisol, Blood *on this page*

Connecting Peptide Insulin *see* C-Peptide *on page 114*

Coproporphyrins *see* Porphyrins, Quantitative, Urine *on page 186*

Coronary Heart Disease Risk Index *see* Lipid Profile *on page 159*

Corticotropin *see* Adrenocorticotropic Hormone *on page 63*

Corticotropin Release Hormone Stimulation Test *see* Adrenocorticotropic Hormone *on page 63*

Corticotropin Stimulation Test *see* Adrenocorticotropic Hormone *on page 63*

Cortisol, Blood

CPT 82533

Related Information

Adrenocorticotropic Hormone *on page 63*
Cosyntropin Test *on page 114*
Estradiol, Serum *on page 125*
17-Hydroxycorticosteroids, Urine *on page 147*
17-Ketogenic Steroids, Urine *on page 151*
Metyrapone Stimulation Test *on page 167*
Testosterone, Free and Total *on page 202*
Thorn Test *on page 350*

Synonyms Compound F; Hydrocortisone, Serum

Applies to Dexamethasone Suppression Test; 17-Hydroxycorticosteroids

Abstract Cortisol, a glucocorticoid, stimulates catabolism of protein and fat, generating substrates for hepatic production of glucose.[1] Used to evaluate adrenocortical function, cortisol represents about 80% of the total 17-hydroxycorticosteroids in blood. Blood and urine cortisol with adrenocorticotropic hormone are the three most pivotal tests in investigation of Cushing's disease and syndrome.

Patient Preparation Prior radioisotopes may interfere if assay method is RIA.

Specimen Serum or plasma

Container Red top tube or green top (heparin) tube

Sampling Time AM and PM levels. The evening nadir is not found in subjects with Cushing's syndrome; midnight result <5 µg/dL (138 nmol/L) rules it out.

Collection Blood may be drawn at 8 AM and 4 PM to evaluate baseline diurnal variation. (Some prefer the evening draw at 11 PM.) Morning specimen, usually highest, is often ordered with ACTH level.

Storage Instructions Stable 7 days at 4°C to 25°C.

Special Instructions Dexamethasone suppression test requires administration of high-dose or low-dose dexamethasone and subsequent measurement of cortisol levels; *vide infra*.

Reference Range AM (8:00): 5-25 µg/dL (SI: 138-690 nmol/L), PM (4:00): 3-16 µg/dL (SI: 83-442 nmol/L) depending on the assay. At 8:00 PM, <50% of 8:00 AM specimen.

Use Low cortisol is found with adrenocortical insufficiency (Addison's disease), adrenogenital syndrome, and with hypopituitarism.

Investigation of weight gain, hypertension, glucose intolerance, oligomenorrhea, amenorrhea, decreased libido, hirsutism, leading to investigation for Cushing's syndrome, for which the initial step is demonstration of hypersecretion of cortisol. The 24-hour urinary excretion of cortisol is the most direct index.[1] **High cortisol** occurs in adrenocortical hypersecretion, adrenal cortical hyperplasia, adenoma, or carcinoma (Cushing's syndrome), and with excess pituitary ACTH (Cushing's disease) or ectopic ACTH syndrome (*vide infra*). **Not useful for following dosage of exogenous, synthetic corticosteroids.**

Limitations Random serum cortisol may be misleading because of circadian variation in secretion. Method may have a high cross reaction with corticosterone and with 11-deoxycortisol (compound S). Cortisol is physiologically increased in patients with hypoglycemia, stress, and in pregnancy. False-negatives occur. Normal values can be found with partial pituitary deficiency.

Contraindications Single samples taken under uncontrolled conditions for cortisol assays are worthless.

Methodology Immunoassay, radioimmunoassay (RIA)

Additional Information Cortisol is the major adrenal glucocorticoid steroid hormone and is normally under feedback control by pituitary ACTH and the hypothalamus.

Causes of **low cortisol** include pituitary destruction or failure, with resultant loss of ACTH to stimulate the adrenal, and metabolic errors or destruction of the adrenal gland itself (adrenogenital syndromes, primary adrenocortical insufficiency, Addison's disease, [idiopathic, tuberculosis, histoplasmosis]). The diagnosis of hypoadrenalism generally requires confirmation with ACTH stimulation, due to the circadian rhythms of cortisol and other factors. Causes of **increased cortisol**, which may present initially simply as loss of normal diurnal variation, include pituitary overproduction of ACTH; production of ACTH by a nonpituitary tumor (ectopic corticotropin syndrome, most caused by small cell carcinomas of lung); adrenal cortical adenomas, hyperplasias, and carcinomas (corticotropin-independent Cushing's syndrome). See listing Adrenocorticotropic Hormone *on page 63*.

Dexamethasone suppression test helps distinguish among causes of elevated cortisol.[1,2] Dexamethasone is a synthetic steroid which suppresses ACTH secretion. It is a potent analogue of cortisol which is not detectable in urine free cortisol or plasma cortisol testing.[3] Under normal circumstances decreased cortisol levels follow. Suppressibility of elevated cortisol shows that feedback regulation is intact, and usually rules out Cushing's syndrome. If there is no suppression **overnight** after 1 mg of dexamethasone, higher doses and longer times may suppress ACTH production by a pituitary adenoma, but will not suppress an adrenal adenoma. Measurement of ACTH may also be informative. (See also the listing Cortisol, Urine *on page 113*.)

The **dexamethasone suppression test (DST)** is abnormal in many psychiatric illnesses. The sensitivity of the DST in major depression is approximately 40% to 50%, but is higher (60% to 70%) in severe (especially psychotic) affective disorders.[4] False-positive results occur with alcoholism and with stress (eg, hospitalization). The high-dose dexamethasone suppression test is misleading in subjects who have bronchial carcinoids.[5] In critically ill subjects, transient decreases of corticotropin may occur. Cortisol <15 µg/dL provides indication of adrenal cortisol insufficiency.[6]

For the diagnosis of adrenocortical insufficiency, the **cosyntropin test** has been recommended. The **corticotropin-releasing hormone (CRH) stimulation test** (1 µg/kg ovine CRH by I.V. administration) works well as the standard high-dose dexamethasone suppression test in distinguishing pituitary Cushing's disease from ectopic ACTH secretion. The test is less time consuming and can be an outpatient test. Cortisol in ACTH response is measured at timed intervals. A positive response (four times baseline) occurs in pituitary Cushing's disease, and a negative response is seen in ectopic ACTH-secreting tumor. There is a 97% positive predictive value. Cushing's is excluded in only 70% if there is

nonresponse, however when both tests (dexamethasone suppression and CRH stimulation) show no response, there is a 100% predictive value for ectopic ACTH-secreting tumor. The stimulation test should not be used in hypoadrenalism. **For the diagnosis of Cushing's syndrome (hypercortisolism), the urinary free cortisol is the test of choice.**

Footnotes

1. Orth DN, "Cushing's Syndrome," *N Engl J Med*, 1995, 333(12):791-803.
2. Weiner MF, "Age and Cortisol Suppression by Dexamethasone in Normal Subjects," *J Psychiatr Res*, 1989, 23(2):163-8.
3. Snow K, Jiang N-S, and Kao PC, "Biochemical Evaluation of Adrenal Dysfunction: The Laboratory Perspective," *Mayo Clin Proc*, 1992, 67(11):1055-65.
4. "The Dexamethasone Suppression Test: An Overview of Its Current Status in Psychiatry," The APA Task Force on Laboratory Tests in Psychiatry, *Am J Psychiatry*, 1987, 144(10):1253-62.
5. Orth DN, "The Cushing Syndrome: Quest for the Holy Grail," *Ann Intern Med*, 1994, 121(5):377-8.
6. Kidess AI, Caplan RH, Reynertson RH, et al, "Transient Corticotropin Deficiency in Critical Illness," *Mayo Clin Proc*, 1993, 68(5):435-41.

References

Avgerinos PC, Yanovski JA, Oldfield EH, et al, "The Metyrapone and Dexamethasone Suppression Tests for the Differential Diagnosis of the Adrenocorticotropin-Dependent Cushing Syndrome: A Comparison," *Ann Intern Med*, 1994, 121(5):318-27.
Bergadá I, Verara M, Maglio S, et al, "Functional Adrenal Cortical Tumors in Pediatric Patients: A Clinicopathologic and Immunohistochemical Study of a Long-Term Follow-up Series," *Cancer*, 1996, 77:771-7.
Dam H, "Dexamethasone Suppression Test," *Acta Psychiatr Scand Suppl*, 1988, 345:38-44.
Faulkner WR, "Laboratory Diagnosis of Cushing's Syndrome," *Lab Rep*, 1996, 18(2):9-16.
Kirkman S and Nelson DH, "Alcohol-Induced Pseudo-Cushing's Disease: A Study of Prevalence With Review of the Literature," *Metabolism*, 1988, 37(4):390-4.
Macro M, Reznik Y, Leymarie P, et al, "The Effect of Intrathecal Dexamethasone Injection on Plasma Cortisol Level," *Br J Rheumatol*, 1991, 30(3):238.
Magiakou MA, Mastorakos G, Oldfield EH, et al, "Cushing's Syndrome in Children and Adolescents - Presentation, Diagnosis, and Therapy," *N Engl J Med*, 1994, 331(10):629-36.
Nierenberg AA and Feinstein AR, "How to Evaluate a Diagnostic Marker Test. Lessons From the Rise and Fall of Dexamethasone Suppression Test," *JAMA*, 1988, 259(11):1699-702.
Vance ML, "Hypopituitarism," *N Engl J Med*, 1994, 330(23):1651-62.

Cortisol Response to Cosyntropin see Cosyntropin Test *on next page*

Cortisol, Urine

CPT 82533

Related Information

Adrenocorticotropic Hormone *on page 63*
Creatinine Clearance *on page 117*
17-Ketogenic Steroids, Urine *on page 151*
Metyrapone Stimulation Test *on page 167*
Thorn Test *on page 350*
Urine Collection, 24-Hour *on page 30*

Synonyms Urinary Free Cortisol; Urine Cortisol

Test Commonly Includes Creatinine concentration and total volume, to support adequacy of collection

Abstract The diagnosis of Cushing's syndrome requires evidence of autonomous, inappropriate secretion of cortisol.

Patient Preparation Radioisotopes (eg, scans) may interfere if assay method is by RIA. Patient should avoid spironolactone or quinacrine. Avoid patient stress.

Specimen 24-hour urine

Container Plastic container, kept on ice. 20 mL of 33% acetic acid or 1 g boric acid added before start of the collection may be required. If preservative is used, it is not necessary to refrigerate during collection.

Sampling Time Two or three 24-hour collections may be needed to support the diagnosis of Cushing's syndrome.

Collection Instruct the patient to void at 8 AM and discard the specimen. Then collect all urine including the final specimen voided at the end of the 24-hour collection period (ie, 8 AM the next morning). Keep urine sample refrigerated during collection. A normal diurnal rhythm exists with highest levels in the morning, but this circadian rhythm is lost in Cushing's syndrome.[1] Creatinine excretion should be measured with each collection.

Storage Instructions Refrigerate during collection if preservative not used. Stable 7 days at 4°C if preservative used.

Reference Range Using radioimmunoassay (RIA) after extraction: 30-100 µg/24 hours (SI: 83-276 nmol/day) (normal adult); lower in infants and children as a function of decreased cortisol production. Urine cortisol is essentially all "free" or unbound. Another range is given as 12-40 µg cortisol/24 hours.[2]

Critical Values <10 µg/24 hours (SI: <28 nmol/day) in general excludes Cushing's syndrome[3]

Use The most reliable index of cortisol secretion is 24-hour urinary collection.[3] Evaluate pituitary and adrenal cortical function, especially hyperfunction. Evaluate hyperglycemia and hypokalemia. Evaluate obese or hypertensive subjects with glucose intolerance, plethora, round (Continued)

Cortisol, Urine (Continued)

face, hirsutism, striae, backache, irregular menses in various combinations, most of whom do not have Cushing's syndrome;[4] elevation of urinary free cortisol in a properly collected specimen in the unstressed patient is sufficient to diagnose Cushing's syndrome, and a normal result is strong evidence against that diagnosis. This is the screening test of choice for the diagnosis of Cushing's syndrome.[2] Urinary free cortisol is a more accurate reflection of cortisol secretion than a single serum specimen.[2,3] It is sensitive and specific.[1,3]

Limitations Low values do not necessarily mean adrenal hypofunction. Assays in Addison's disease may overlap with normal ranges. Vagaries of improper urine collection or renal disease may produce misleading results. Avoid stressing the patient during collection, which physiologically raises cortisol. Increased in pregnancy and with oral contraceptives. Increased excretion may be found with pseudo-Cushing's syndrome, trauma, or infection.[2]

Methodology Radioimmunoassay (RIA) after extraction, high performance liquid chromatography (HPLC)

Additional Information Urinary cortisol reflects the portion of serum free cortisol (ie, the approximately 6% of serum cortisol not bound to protein) filtered by the kidney. It correlates with cortisol secretion rate. Cushing's syndrome is caused by a tumor of pituitary or hyperplasia or tumor of adrenal cortex; ectopic production of ACTH includes that of small cell carcinomas of lung, carcinoids, and medullary thyroid carcinomas.[2] The **dexamethasone suppression test** is useful as well;[1,2,4] normal results rule out the diagnosis of Cushing's syndrome. Two-day and overnight tests are in use; dexamethasone substitutes for endogenous cortisol to suppress ACTH secretion.[2] Corticotropin-releasing hormone stimulation following low-dose dexamethasone administration was more accurate in distinguishing Cushing's syndrome from pseudo-Cushing's states.[5]

Footnotes
1. Dunlap NE, Grizzle WE, and Siegel AL, "Cushing's Syndrome: Screening Methods in Hospitalized Patients," *Arch Pathol Lab Med*, 1985, 109(3):222-9.
2. Orth DN, "Cushing's Syndrome," *N Engl J Med*, 1995, 332(12):791-803.
3. Watts NB and Keffer JH, "Adrenal Cortex," *Practical Endocrinology*, 4th ed, Philadelphia, PA: Lea & Febiger, 1989, 91-120.
4. Oxley DK, "Cushing's Syndrome," *Arch Pathol Lab Med*, 1985, 109(3):221.
5. Yanovski JA, Cutler GB, Chrousos GP, et al, "Corticotropin-Releasing Hormone Stimulation Following Low-Dose Dexamethasone Administration. A New Test to Distinguish Cushing's Syndrome From Pseudo-Cushing's States," *JAMA*, 1993, 269(17):2232--8.

References
Flack MR, Oldfield EH, Cutler GB Jr, "Urine Free Cortisol in the High-Dose Dexamethasone Suppression Test for the Differential Diagnosis of the Cushing Syndrome," *Ann Intern Med*, 1992, 116(3):211-7.
Gwirtsman HE, Kaye WH, George DT, et al, "Central and Peripheral ACTH and Cortisol Levels in Anorexia Nervosa and Bulimia," *Arch Gen Psychiatry*, 1989, 46(1):61-9.
Yeh J and Barbieri RL, "Twenty-Four Hour Urinary Free Cortisol in Premenopausal Cigarette Smokers and Nonsmokers," *Fertil Steril*, 1989, 52(6):1067-9.
Zis AP, Remick RA, Clark CM, et al, "Evening Urine Cortisol Excretion and DST Results in Depression and Anorexia Nervosa," *J Psychiatr Res*, 1989, 23(3-4):251-5.

Cortrosyn® Test *see* Cosyntropin Test *on this page*

Cosyntropin Test

CPT 80400

Related Information
Cortisol, Blood *on page 112*
Metyrapone Stimulation Test *on page 167*
Thorn Test *on page 350*

Synonyms Cortisol Response to Cosyntropin; Cortrosyn® Test; Rapid ACTH Test; Synthetic α 1-24-ACTH Stimulation Test

Replaces ACTH Infusion Test; Bovine ACTH

Abstract This is a synthetic polypeptide (α 1-24-ACTH with ACTH activity) used to assess adrenal cortical responsiveness in suspected adrenocortical insufficiency.

Patient Preparation Baseline serum cortisol is drawn. Procedural information is available.[1]

Aftercare Additional serum cortisol levels are collected after infusion or injection of cosyntropin. Failure of postinjection cortisol levels to increase is abnormal and must lead to further work-up.

Specimen Serum

Container Red top tube

Storage Instructions Separate serum and freeze.

Use A test for adrenal insufficiency to determine the response of the adrenals to ACTH.

Limitations Response may be abnormal after prolonged steroid therapy. In a 1992 review paper, this test was not pivotal in evaluation of adrenal dysfunction.[2]

Methodology Immunoassay

Additional Information Cosyntropin (Cortrosyn®) is a synthetic 1-24 amino acid ACTH and does not produce anaphylaxis as bovine ACTH

may. If the adrenal glands are physically intact, and normally responsive to ACTH, cortisol will rise significantly after administration of cosyntropin. Absence of such a rise is evidence for primary adrenal insufficiency. If the adrenals can respond to exogenous ACTH (cosyntropin), then a metyrapone stimulation test can evaluate the integrity of the pituitary-adrenal axis. Adrenocortical sensitivity to cosyntropin may be enhanced in patients with depression.[3,4,5] A new test involving pretreatment with low-dose dexamethasone followed by corticotropin-releasing hormone stimulation and measurement of plasma cortisol 15 minutes later, successfully separated all patients with mild Cushing's syndrome from those with pseudo-Cushing's states.[6]

Footnotes
1. Williams GH and Dluhy RG, "Diseases of the Adrenal Cortex," *Harrison's Principles of Internal Medicine*, 13th ed, Vol 2, Isselbacher KJ, Braunwald E, Wilson JD, et al, eds, New York, NY: McGraw-Hill Inc, 1994, 1953-76.
2. Snow K, Jiang N-S, and Kao PC, "Biochemical Evaluation of Adrenal Dysfunction: The Laboratory Perspective," *Mayo Clin Proc*, 1992, 67(11):1055-65.
3. Amsterdam JD, Maislin G, Berwish N, et al, "Enhanced Adrenocortical Sensitivity to Submaximal Doses of Cosyntropin (Alpha 1-24 Corticotropin) in Depressed Patients," *Arch Gen Psychiatry*, 1989, 46(6):550-4.
4. Jaeckle RS, Kathol RG, Lopez JF, et al, "Enhanced Adrenal Sensitivity to Exogenous Cosyntropin (ACTH Alpha 1-24) Stimulation in Major Depression. Relationship to Dexamethasone Suppression Test Results," *Arch Gen Psychiatry*, 1987, 44(3):233-40.
5. Clayton RN, "Diagnosis of Adrenal Insufficiency," *BMJ*, 1989, 298(6669):271-2.
6. Yanovski JA, Cutler GB, Chrousos GP, et al, "Corticotropin-Releasing Hormone Stimulation Following Low-Dose Dexamethasone Administration. A New Test to Distinguish Cushing's Syndrome From Pseudo-Cushing's States," *JAMA*, 1993, 269(17):2232-8.

C-Peptide

CPT 84681

Related Information
Glucose, Fasting *on page 137*
Glucose Tolerance Test *on page 139*
Insulin Antibody, Serum *on page 149*
Insulin, Blood *on page 149*

Synonyms Connecting Peptide Insulin; Insulin-Connecting Peptide; Insulin C-Peptide; Proinsulin C-Peptide

Applies to C-Peptide Suppression Test

Test Commonly Includes Glucose assay is usually needed at the time a C-peptide specimen is drawn.

Abstract Proinsulin is cleaved into insulin and a biologically inactive fraction. The latter is C-peptide. Its assay provides distinction between exogenous and endogenous circulating insulin.

Patient Preparation Patient should fast for a minimum of 10 hours for basal values. No recent scans or other radioactivity.

Specimen Serum

Container Red top tube

Collection Date and time must be absolutely correct. Draw in chilled tube. Keep specimen on ice. Trasylol® (2000 units/mL) may be added to prevent degradation.

Storage Instructions Spin in centrifuge at 4°C. Take off serum. Freeze immediately in a plastic tube.

Reference Range Fasting: 0.5-2.5 ng/mL (SI: 0.17-0.83 nmol/L). Varies between laboratories. After stimulation with glucose or glucagon, values rise to 5.6 ng/mL (SI: 1.87 nmol/L).

Use The principal use of C-peptide is in the evaluation of hypoglycemia. Patients with insulin-secreting neoplasms have high levels of both C-peptide and endogenous insulin; in contrast, patients with factitious hypoglycemia from exogenous insulin administration will have low C-peptide levels in the presence of elevated (exogenous) serum insulin. Ingestion of a sulfonylurea may mimic insulinoma, because these drugs stimulate insulin secretion, C-peptide, and proinsulin.[1] C-peptide may also be useful in evaluation of residual beta cell function in insulin-dependent diabetics, many of whom have antibodies that interfere with insulin assays. Glucagon-stimulated C-peptide concentration has been described as a discriminator between insulin-requiring and noninsulin-requiring diabetic patients.[2,3] The concentrations of C-peptide increase in the plasma with those of insulin with insulinoma, supporting the endogenous origin of insulin.[1] The diagnosis of islet cell tumor is supported by elevation of C-peptide when plasma glucose is ≤40 mg/dL (SI: ≤2.2 mmol/L). When an individual who is not diabetic develops symptoms of hypoglycemia, evaluation then should include plasma glucose, serum C-peptide, as well as samples for alcohol, other drugs and toxins, sulfonylurea, cortisol, and insulin.[4]

Limitations C-peptide levels are increased with renal failure. (C-peptide is normally excreted by the kidneys.) Instances of insulinoma have been described in which proinsulin was increased but insulin and C-peptide were not.

Methodology Radioimmunoassay (RIA)[5]

Additional Information Because of its longer half-life (about 35 minutes), the molar ratio of C-peptide to insulin is approximately 5:1.

The C-peptide suppression test depends on suppression of beta cell secretion during hypoglycemia to a lesser degree in patients with insulinoma than in normal individuals.[1]

Footnotes

1. Polonsky KS, "A Practical Approach to Fasting Hypoglycemia," *N Engl J Med*, 1992, 326(15):994-8 (editorial).
2. Koskinen PJ, Viikari JS, and Irjala KM, "Glucagon-Stimulated and Postprandial Plasma C-Peptide Values as Measures of Insulin Secretory Capacity," *Diabetes Care*, 1988, 11(4):318-22.
3. Laakso M, Sarlund H, Korhonen T, et al, "Stopping Insulin Treatment in Middle-Aged Diabetic Patients With High Postglucagon Plasma C-Peptide. Effect on Glycaemic Control, Serum Lipids and Lipoproteins," *Acta Med Scand*, 1988, 223(1):61-8.
4. Foster DW and Rubenstein AH, "Hypoglycemia," *Harrison's Principles of Internal Medicine*, 13th ed, Isselbacher KJ, Braunwald E, Wilson JD, et al, eds, New York, NY: McGraw-Hill Inc, 1994, 2000-6.
5. Myrick JE, Gunter EW, Maggio VL, et al, "An Improved Radioimmunoassay of C-Peptide and Its Application in a Multiyear Study," *Clin Chem*, 1989, 35(1):37-42.

References

Argoud GW, Schade DS, Eaton RP, et al, "C-Peptide Suppression Test and Recurrent Insulinoma," *Am J Med*, 1989, 86(3):335-7.

Beer SF, Parr JH, Temple RC, et al, "The Effect of Thyroid Disease on Proinsulin and C-Peptide Levels," *Clin Endocrinol (Oxf)*, 1989, 30(4):379-83.

Bonora E, Rizzi C, Lesi C, et al, "Insulin and C-Peptide Plasma Levels in Patients With Severe Chronic Pancreatitis and Fasting Normoglycemia," *Dig Dis Sci*, 1988, 33(6):732-6.

Karjalainen J, Salmela P, Ilonen J, et al, "A Comparison of Childhood and Adult Type I Diabetes Mellitus," *N Engl J Med*, 1989, 320(14):881-6.

Service FJ, "Hypoglycemic Disorders," *N Engl J Med*, 1995, 332(17):1144-52.

Van Cauter E, Mestrez F, Sturis J, et al, "Estimation of Insulin Secretion Rates From C-Peptide Levels. Comparison of Individual and Standard Kinetic Parameters for C-Peptide Clearance," *Diabetes*, 1992, 41(3):368-77.

C-Peptide Suppression Test *see* C-Peptide *on previous page*

CPK *see* Creatine Kinase *on this page*

CPK Isoenzymes *see* Creatine Kinase Isoenzymes/Isoforms *on this page*

Creatine Kinase

CPT 82550

Related Information

Cardiac Enzymes/Isoenzymes *on page 102*
Creatine Kinase Isoenzymes/Isoforms *on this page*
Duchenne/Becker Muscular Dystrophy DNA Detection *on page 509*
Lactate Dehydrogenase *on page 153*
Muscle Biopsy *on page 53*
Myoglobin, Blood *on page 167*
Myoglobin, Qualitative, Urine *on page 644*
Myositis-Specific Autoantibody *on page 420*
Troponin *on page 212*

Synonyms CK; CPK; Creatine Phosphokinase, Total, Serum

Abstract Creatine kinase occurs principally in striated muscle, brain, and heart tissue. Other tissues (eg, kidney) contain much lower levels of activity.

Patient Preparation Avoid exercise before venipuncture. Increases may be anticipated in the immediate postoperative period following surgical procedures involving incision through muscle.

Specimen Serum

Container Red top tube

Storage Instructions Separate serum from red cells. Store in refrigerator. Avoid hemolysis.[1]

Reference Range Method dependent, but for assays at 37°C (most current assays) usually 50-200 units/L for males. Females have levels 20% to 25% less than males. Infants to 1 year of age may have levels two times adult. On average, black females have higher levels than white males.

Use Test for acute myocardial infarct and for skeletal muscular disease or damage; elevated in some patients with myxedema (hypothyroidism). Although CK is elevated in some individuals who have malignant hyperthermia syndrome, interval screening is most effective to detect susceptible subjects. Elevated in muscular dystrophy: CK is a marker for Duchenne's muscular dystrophy, with elevations of 20 to 200 times normal.[2] CK is increased in female carriers of this X-linked disease, and in muscular stress, in polymyositis, dermatomyositis, and with muscle trauma. Elevated in myocarditis. Extremely high values are seen in some instances of myositis and in the postictal state, recent grand mal seizure. CK may be elevated in a number of entities, including the eosinophilia-myalgia syndrome.[3] Marked increases occur with rhabdomyolysis including that with cocaine intoxication.[4] CK is sometimes increased with cerebrovascular accident. Malignancy (advanced) may show increased CK.[5] Cardioversion with multiple shocks may release CK-MB and may result in a false-positive diagnosis of myocardial infarction.[6] Low CK may reflect decreased muscle mass. It has been reported with a number of entities, including metastatic neoplasia, patients with steroid therapy, with alcoholic liver disease[7] with connective tissue diseases,[8] in ectopic

---

pregnancy (without CK-MB increase), and with rheumatoid arthritis.[9] Overnight bedrest may lower CK 10% to 20%.

Limitations Intramuscular injections increase serum CK activity. Elevated following exercise. Increases in CK and CK-MB must be interpreted cautiously during the peripartum period.[10] **Normal at onset of acute MI** unless the subject has been exercising or doing physical work. Elevation of CK following acute MI may not be observed until 6 or more hours after onset. CK returns to normal in approximately 48-72 hours after acute MI. Total CK can be normal early in acute MI, when CK-MB is increased. Newer tests, especially cardiac troponin I (cTn I) may allow for better detection of myocardial injury/infarction than routine CK and CK-MB measurements. Troponin I has superior specificity. Creatine kinase isoforms are available and are elevated slightly earlier than CK-MB following an MI.[11,12] Low CK does not rule out myositis in patients with the connective tissue diseases.[7] Decreased with pregnancy.

Methodology Kinetic - UV spectrophotometric

Additional Information High CK is found after trauma, surgery, and exercise; these entities are not accompanied by elevation of CK-MB. To distinguish myoglobinuria from hemoglobinuria, serum CK and LD may be helpful. CK is normal with uncomplicated hemolysis but LD and LD_1 usually are increased. When myoglobin is released, 40-fold elevation of CK may be anticipated with only moderate increase in serum LD and increased LD_5.[13]

Footnotes

1. Greenson JK, Farber SJ, and Dubin SB, "The Effect of Hemolysis on Creatine Kinase Determination," *Arch Pathol Lab Med*, 1989, 113(2):184-5.
2. Rosalki SB, "Serum Enzymes in Disease of Skeletal Muscle," *Clin Lab Med*, 1989, 9(4):767-81.
3. Kilbourne EM, Swygert LA, Philen RM, et al, "Interim Guidance on the Eosinophilia-Myalgia Syndrome," *Ann Intern Med*, 1990, 112(2):85-7.
4. Roth D, Alarcón FJ, Fernandez JA, "Acute Rhabdomyolysis Associated With Cocaine Intoxication," *N Engl J Med*, 1988, 319(11):673-7.
5. Eng C, Skolnick AE, and Come SE, "Elevated Creatine Kinase and Malignancy," *Hosp Pract (Off Ed)*, 1990, 25(12):123, 126, 129-30.
6. O'Neill PG, Faitelson L, Taylor A, et al, "Time Course of Creatine Kinase Release After Termination of Sustained Ventricular Dysrhythmias," *Am Heart J*, 1991, 122(3 Pt 1):709-14.
7. Nanji AA and Blank D, "Low Serum Creatine Kinase Activity in Patients With Alcoholic Liver Disease," *Clin Chem* 1981, 27:1954.
8. Wei N, Pavlidis N, Tsokos G, et al, "Clinical Significance of Low Creatine Phosphokinase Values in Patients With Connective Tissue Diseases," *JAMA*, 1981, 246:1921-3.
9. Leiserowitz GS, Evans AT, Samuels SJ, et al, "Creatine Kinase and Its MB Isoenzyme in the Third Trimester and the Peripartum Period," *J Reprod Med*, 1992, 37(11):910-6.
10. Sanmarti R, Collado A, Gratacos J, et al, "Reduced Activity of Serum Creatine Kinase in Rheumatoid Arthritis: A Phenomenon Linked to the Inflammatory Response," *Br J Rheumatol*, 1994, 33(3):231-4.
11. Wu AH, Gornet TG, Wu VH, et al, "Early Diagnosis of Acute Myocardial Infarction by Rapid Analysis of Creatine Kinase Isoenzyme-3 (CK-MM) Sub-Types," *Clin Chem*, 1987, 33(3):358-62.
12. Apple FS, Sharkey SW, Werdick M, et al, "Analyses of Creatine Kinase Isoenzymes and Isoforms in Serum to Detect Reperfusion After Myocardial Infarction," *Clin Chem*, 1987, 33(4):507-11.
13. Faulkner WR, "Update on Myoglobinurias," *Lab Report for Physicians*, 1989, 11:91-2.

References

Beek AM, Verheugt FW, and Meyer A, "Usefulness of Electrocardiographic Findings and Creatine Kinase Levels on Admission in Predicting the Accuracy of the Interval Between Onset of Chest Pain of Acute Myocardial Infarction and Initiation of Thrombolytic Therapy," *Am J Cardiol*, 1991, 68(13):1287-90.

Crisp DE, Ziter FA, and Bray PF, "Diagnostic Delay in Duchenne's Muscular Dystrophy," *JAMA*, 1982, 247:478-80.

Gambino R, "Creatine Kinase in Tubal Pregnancy," *Lab Rep*, 1994, 16(11):89-90.

Leung FY, Griffith AP, Jablonsky G, et al, "Comparison of the Diagnostic Utility of Timed Serial (Slope) Creatine Kinase Measurements With Conventional Serum Tests in the Early Diagnosis of Myocardial Infarction," *Ann Clin Biochem*, 1991, 28(Pt 1):78-82.

Creatine Kinase Isoenzymes/Isoforms

CPT 82552

Related Information

Cardiac Enzymes/Isoenzymes *on page 102*
Creatine Kinase *on this page*
Lactate Dehydrogenase Isoenzymes *on page 154*
Myoglobin, Blood *on page 167*
Troponin *on page 212*

Synonyms CK-2; CK Isoenzymes; CK Isoforms; CK-MB and Total CK; CPK Isoenzymes; Creatine Phosphokinase-MB Isoenzyme and Total Creatine Phosphokinase, Serum

Test Commonly Includes Separation of enzyme CK into its isoenzymes

Abstract Significant EKG abnormalities are not always found in acute myocardial injury. Three isoenzymes may be seen on electrophoresis: CK-MM (CK-3), CK-MB (CK-2), and CK-BB (CK-1). CK-MB is the isoenzyme of most interest and is now commonly measured by immunoassay. Rarely, macro CK and mitochondrial CK may be present. A diagnostic rise in CK-MB isoenzyme in acute myocardial infarct is not usually found in the first six hours, but assay for subforms can support diagnosis earlier. CK and CK-MB presently are the major available standards available to assess injury to myocardium.[1]

(Continued)

Creatine Kinase Isoenzymes/Isoforms *(Continued)*

Specimen Serum

Container Red top tube

Sampling Time CK is **most commonly elevated in** acute myocardial infarction (AMI), in which it has its greatest usefulness. Collection of specimen at onset of symptoms to establish baseline values is needed. A patient at onset of acute myocardial infarction (AMI) will have normal results, but some patients reach medical attention at or beyond CK peak. The National Heart, Lung, and Blood Institute has recommended total CK and CK-MB every 6-8 hours for the first 24 hours after admission. LDH isoenzymes may be useful in subjects presenting between 24-72 hours after onset, if CK and CK-MB are normal.[2] The new mass concentration assays have improved sensitivity over the more cumbersome electrophoretic assays and are diagnostic earlier. Some have suggested sampling times at 0, 3, 6, and 12 hours, to detect the rise of CK-MB.[3] The same sampling times should be used to assess effective myocardial reperfusion after thrombolytic therapy. In this case the CK and CK-MB rise very early and very high compared to patients not reperfused.[4] CK-MB usually peaks between 15-20 hours after the onset of a myocardial infarction. The mass assay for CK-MB is diagnostic as early as 3 hours in half, and >90% are positive in 6 hours.[1]

When increased CK-MB values have returned to normal, CK isoenzyme determinations are usually no longer required.

Collection Avoid hemolysis.

Storage Instructions Separate serum from red cells and freeze.

Reference Range Method dependent. CK-MB normally is <6% of total CK. In many laboratories normal range of MB is zero. The most common cause of elevation of MB is acute infarct of myocardium. Most normal individuals have only MM. The best reference range is established with an individual patient's own baseline, followed by serial sampling[1]. Newer assays usually measure mass concentration of CK-MB rather than enzyme activity. Mass assay of CK-MB gives a reference range of 0-3 μg/mL with a relative index of 0-2.5. **Relative index** is the CK-MB value (in mass units) divided by the total CK (in enzyme units) times 100. An isoform ratio (CK-MB2/CK-MB1) >1.5 is indicative of MI. The reference ratio is near 1.0.

Use Diagnose acute myocardial infarction (AMI). Three fractions normally may be found, each an isoenzyme.

- MM is present in normal serum.
- MB is the myocardial fraction associated with MI. It occurs in certain other states. MB can be used in estimation of infarct size.

A study using the chemiluminescence mass concentration assay for CK-MB showed that a CK-MB ≥10 ng/mL and CK relative index >3.0 (ng/mL CK-MB per unit CK x 100) gave these results: sensitivity = 1.00; specificity = 0.97; positive predictive value = 1.00; diagnostic efficiency = 0.97.[5] Similar results are seen for isoforms and they show significant changes somewhat earlier.

MB increases have been reported with other entities which cause damage to the myocardium, such as myocarditis, some instances of cardiomyopathy, and with extensive rhabdomyolysis, Duchenne's muscular dystrophy, malignant hyperthermia, polymyositis, dermatomyositis, mixed connective tissue disease, myoglobinemia, Rocky Mountain spotted fever, Reye's syndrome, and rarely in rheumatoid arthritis with high titer RF.[6] CK-MB does not generally abruptly rise and fall in such nonacute MI settings, as it does in acute myocardial infarct (AMI).

- BB is rarely present. BB has been described as a marker for adenocarcinoma of prostate, breast, ovary, colon, adenocarcinomas of gastrointestinal tract, and for small cell anaplastic carcinoma of lung. BB has been reported with severe shock and/or hypothermia, infarction of bowel,[7] brain injury, stroke, as a genetic marker in some families with malignant pyrexia, and with MB in alcoholic myopathy.
- The tissue isoform (CK-MB2) is low in normal serum but increases rapidly after an MI. The CK-MB2/CK-MB1 (isoform) ratio is used as the most sensitive indicator.

Limitations Exercise, intramuscular injections, myxedema, grand mal seizures, prior trauma or surgery, and acute MI very early or late lead to the combination of increased total CK but usually normal CK-MB. False-positives occur, eg, increased CK-MB has been described in marathon runners without MI.[8]

CK isoenzyme analysis is not usually practical when the total CK is very low, although in elderly people with low muscle mass, the use of sensitive mass concentration assays may be useful, especially when used in conjunction with mass index calculation (see above). A single CK isoenzyme examination may be misleading, as may any other enzyme or isoenzyme for diagnosis of AMI. One should look for a pattern in serial CK isoenzyme analyses and seek confirmation with the isoenzymes of LD (LDH), ideally beginning with onset to establish the baseline. LD isoenzyme 1:2 flip is most consistently found about 2 days after onset of acute infarction of myocardium. **The diagnosis of myocardial injury should be supported by clinical findings, ECG, and often other laboratory parameters** (eg, confirmation by LD isoenzymes).[4] AST/ALT ratio is mentioned in the listing Cardiac Enzymes/Isoenzymes *on page 102.*

A disadvantage of electrophoretic separation is that most laboratories are able to do electrophoresis for CK isoenzymes only once daily. Mass assay for CK-MB is usually available stat, 24 hours a day.

Contraindications CK-MB is increased with cardiac surgery.

Methodology Electrophoresis with densitometry has been commonly used to separate isoenzymes of CK. The advent of monoclonal CK-MB antibody has allowed the use of sensitive immunoassays, including microparticulate fluorescence,[9] enhanced luminescence, fluorescence, and chemiluminescence. These all measure mass concentration rather than enzyme activity. A very rapid test is that of Hybritech®, which uses the immunocentration format (ICON™). Isoelectric focusing may be used to measure isoforms. Immunoinhibition assays are less specific and are less sensitive.

The technical difficulty and cost of isoform quantitation have brought its implementation as a 24-hour stat test into question[1].

Additional Information CK-MB is found in much higher concentrations in cardiac muscle than in ordinary skeletal muscle.

CK-MB is usually not elevated in exercise (total CK elevated); myxedema (total CK elevated in about half of cases); injections into muscle (total CK elevated); strokes, CVA, and other brain disorders in which total CK may be increased; pericarditis; pneumonias or other lung diseases; pulmonary embolus; seizures (CK may be very high but no great MB increase, if any). Although CK-MB is not usually increased in angina, some CK-MB elevations are recognized in angina patients, depending partly on laboratory methodology.

Atypical forms of CK occur. **Macro-CK** migrates between MM and MB and is composed of immunoglobulin complexes of normal isoenzymes. This is found mainly in elderly women and is of no clinical significance. **Mitochondrial-CK** migrates cathodal to MM and is found in seriously ill patients, especially those with metastatic carcinoma. Its presence is a poor prognostic sign.

CK-MM and CK-MB isoforms have been evaluated. They have potential value for early detection of acute myocardial infarction and for assessing myocardial reperfusion following AMI. (An isoform is a subtype of an individual isoenzyme.)[3,4,10,11,12,13] Sensitivity of CK-MB subforms has been reported to be superior to that of conventional CK-MB.[14] A disadvantage of this type of assay is that there is only one commercially available instrument for this measurement (Helena Laboratories).[15,16] Isoforms are not inexpensive and their assay is somewhat complex.[17] The specificity of cardiac troponin (cTnI) is superior to that of CK and CK-MB. It remains elevated for up to 5-7 days after onset of AMI.[18]

The leukocyte differential has been used as well to provide early diagnosis of AMI.[19]

A current outstanding review anticipates future roles for cTnI, CK-MB, and myoglobin.[1]

Footnotes

1. Keffer JH, "Myocardial Markers of Injury - Evolution and Insights," *Am J Clin Pathol*, 1996, 105:305-20.
2. Braunwald E, Mark DB, Jones RH, et al, *Unstable Angina: Diagnosis and Management*, U.S. Department of Health and Human Services, 1994.
3. Marin MM and Teichman SL, "Use of Rapid Serial Sampling of Creatine Kinase MB for Very Early Detection of Myocardial Infarction in Patients With Acute Chest Pain," *Am Heart J*, 1992, 123(2):354-61.
4. Lott JA and Stang JM, "Differential Diagnosis of Patients With Abnormal Serum Creatine Kinase Isoenzymes," *Clin Lab Med*, 1989, 9(4):627-42.
5. Pearson JR and Carrea F, "Evaluation of the Clinical Usefulness of a Chemiluminometric Method for Measuring Creatine Kinase MB," *Clin Chem*, 1990, 36(10):1809-11.
6. Wolf PL, "Common Causes of False-Positive CK-MB Test for Acute Myocardial Infarction," *Clin Lab Med*, 1986, 6(3):577-81.
7. Fried MW, Murthy UK, Hassig SR, et al, "Creatine Kinase Isoenzymes in the Diagnosis of Intestinal Infarction," *Dig Dis Sci*, 1991, 36(11):1589-93.
8. Seigel AJ, Silverman LM, and Evans WJ, "Elevated Skeletal Muscle Creatinine Kinase MB Isoenzyme Levels in Marathon Runners," *JAMA*, 1983, 250:2835-7.
9. Brandt DR, Gates RC, Eng KK, et al, "Quantifying the MB Isoenzyme of Creatine Kinase With the Abbott 'IMx' Immunoassay Analyzer," *Clin Chem*, 1990, 36(2):375-8.
10. Apple FS, Sharkey SW, Werdick M, et al, "Analyses of Creatine Kinase Isoenzymes and Isoforms in Serum to Detect Reperfusion After Myocardial Infarction," *Clin Chem*, 1987, 33(4):507-11.
11. Puleo PR, Guadagno P, Scheel M, et al, "Diagnostic Accuracy of a Rapid MB-CK Subform Assay in the Early Hours of Myocardial Infarction," *Clin Chem*, 1989, 35:1119.
12. Wu AH, Gornet TG, Wu VH, et al, "Early Diagnosis of Acute Myocardial Infarction by Rapid Analysis of Creatine Kinase Isoenzyme-3 (CK-MM) Sub-Types," *Clin Chem*, 1987, 33(3):358-62.
13. Apple FS, "Diagnostic Use of CK-MM and CK-MB Isoforms for Detecting Myocardial Infarction," *Clin Lab Med*, 1989, 9(4):643-54.
14. Puleo PR, Meyer D, Wathen C, et al, "Use of a Rapid Assay of Subforms of Creatine Kinase MB to Diagnose or Rule Out Acute Myocardial Infarction," *N Engl J Med*, 1994, 331(9):561-6.
15. Puleo PR, Guadagno PA, Roberts R, et al, "Early Diagnosis of Acute Myocardial Infarction Based on Assay for Subforms of Creatine Kinase-MB," *Circulation*, 1990, 82(3):759-64.

16. Abendschein DR, "Rapid Diagnosis of Myocardial Infarction and Reperfusion by Assay of Plasma Isoforms of Creatine Kinase Isoenzymes," *Clin Biochem*, 1990, 23(5):399-407.

17. Keffer JH, "The Revolution in Biochemical Assessment of Ischemic Myocardial Injury," 3rd Annual Progress in Clinical Pathology, University of Texas Southwestern Medical Center at Dallas, Sept 1995.

18. Adams JE 3rd, Sicard GA, Allen BT, et al, "Diagnosis of Perioperative Myocardial Infarction With Measurement of Cardiac Troponin I," *N Engl J Med*, 1994, 330(10):670-4.

19. Thomson SP, Gibbons RJ, Smars PA, et al, "Incremental Value of the Leukocyte Differential and the Rapid Creatine Kinase-MB Isoenzyme for the Early Diagnosis of Myocardial Infarction," *Ann Intern Med*, 1995, 122(5):335-41.

References

Adams J, Schechtman K, Landt J, et al, "Comparable Detection of Acute Myocardial Infarction by Creatine Kinase MB Isoenzyme and Cardiac Troponin I," *Clin Chem*, 1994, 40(7 Pt 1):1291-5.

Bakker AJ, Gorgels JP, Van Vlies B, et al, "Contribution of Creatine Kinase MB Mass Concentration at Admission to Early Diagnosis of Acute Myocardial Infarction," *Br Heart J*, 1994, 72(2):112-8.

Bhayana V, Cohoe S, Leung FY, et al, "Diagnostic Evaluation of Creatine Kinase-2 Mass and Creatine Kinase-3 and -2 Isoform Ratios in Early Diagnosis of Acute Myocardial Infarction," *Clin Chem*, 1993, 39(3):488-95.

Brush JE Jr, Brand DA, Acampora D, et al, "Relation of Peak Creatine Kinase Levels During Acute Myocardial Infarction to Presence or Absence of Previous Manifestations of Myocardial Ischemia (Angina Pectoris or Healed Myocardial Infarction)," *Am J Cardiol*, 1988, 62(9):534-7.

Davidson E, Weinberger I, Rotenberg Z, et al, "Elevated Serum Creatine Kinase Levels," *Arch Intern Med*, 1988, 148(10):2184-6.

Devries SR, Jaffe AS, Geltman EM, et al, "Enzymatic Estimation of the Extent of Irreversible Myocardial Injury Early After Reperfusion," *Am Heart J*, 1989, 117(1):31-6.

Gulbis B, Unger P, Lenaers A, et al, "Mass Concentration of Creatine Kinase MB Isoenzyme and Lactate Dehydrogenase Isoenzyme 1 in Diagnosis of Perioperative Myocardial Infarction After Coronary Bypass Surgery," *Clin Chem*, 1990, 36(10):1784-8.

Hamm CW, "New Serum Markers for Acute Myocardial Infarction," *N Engl J Med*, 1994, 331(9):607-8.

Hood D, Van Lente F, and Estes M, "Serum Enzyme Alterations in Chronic Muscle Disease. A Biopsy-Based Diagnostic Assessment," *Am J Clin Pathol*, 1991, 95(3):402-7.

Hossein-Nia M, Kallis P, Brown PA, et al, "Creatine Kinase MB Isoforms: Sensitive Markers of Ischemic Myocardial Damage," *Clin Chem*, 1994, 40(7 Pt 1):1265-71.

Kilpatrick WS, Wasornu D, McGuinness JB, et al, "Early Diagnosis of Acute Myocardial Infarction: CKMB and Myoglobin Compared," *Ann Clin Biochem*, 1993, 30(Pt 5):435-8.

King DT, Fu PC, and Wishon GM, "Persistent Creatine Kinase MB Isoenzyme Without Cardiac Disease," *Arch Pathol Lab Med*, 1978, 102:481-2.

Lee RT, Lee TH, Poole WK, et al, "Rate of Disappearance of Creatine Kinase-MB After Acute Myocardial Infarction: Clinical Determinants of Variability," *Am Heart J*, 1988, 116(6 Pt 1):1493-9.

Lewis BS, Ganz W, Laramee P, et al, "Usefulness of a Rapid Initial Increase in Plasma Creatine Kinase Activity as a Marker of Reperfusion During Thrombolytic Therapy for Acute Myocardial Infarction," *Am J Cardiol*, 1988, 62(1):20-4.

Nidorf SM, Thompson PL, Byrne A, et al, "The Creatine Kinase Ratio: A Useful Means of Detecting Early Peaking of the Creatine Kinase Curve After Acute Myocardial Infarction," *Am J Cardiol*, 1988, 62(13):961-3.

Nidorf SM, Thompson PL, de Klerk NH, et al, "Prognostic Significance of an Early Rise to Peak Creatine Kinase After Acute Myocardial Infarction," *Am J Cardiol*, 1988, 61(15):1178-80.

Pappas NJ Jr, "Enhanced Cardiac Enzyme Profile," *Clin Lab Med*, 1989, 9(4):689-716.

Piérard LA, Dubois C, Albert A, et al, "Prognostic Significance of a Low Peak Serum Creatine Kinase Level in Acute Myocardial Infarction," *Am J Cardiol*, 1989, 63(12):792-6.

Quale J, Kimmelstiel C, Lipschik G, et al, "Use of Sequential Cardiac Enzyme Analysis in Stratification of Risk for Myocardial Infarction in Patients With Unstable Angina," *Arch Intern Med*, 1988, 148(6):1277-9.

Sharkey SW, Apple FS, Elsperger KJ, et al, "Early Peak of Creatine Kinase-MB in Acute Myocardial Infarction With a Nondiagnostic Electrocardiogram," *Am Heart J*, 1988, 116(5 Pt 1):1207-11.

Smith RM and Neuman TS, "Elevation of Serum Creatine Kinase in Divers With Arterial Gas Embolization," *N Engl J Med*, 1994, 330(1):19-24.

Swaroop A, "CK Isoenzyme Variants in Electrophoresis," *Lab Med*, 1989, 20:305-10.

Thompson WG, Mahr RG, Yohannan WS, et al, "Use of Creatine Kinase MB Isoenzyme for Diagnosing Myocardial Infarction When Total Creatine Kinase Activity Is High," *Clin Chem*, 1988, 34(11):2208-10.

Vaidya HC, Maynard Y, Dietzler DN, et al, "Direct Measurement of Creatine Kinase-MB Activity in Serum After Extraction With a Monoclonal Antibody Specific to the MB Isoenzyme," *Clin Chem*, 1986, 32(4):657-63.

Voss EM, Sharkey SW, Gernert AE, et al, "Human and Canine Cardiac Troponin T and Creatine Kinase-MB Distribution in Normal and Diseased Myocardium, Infarct Sizing Using Serum Profiles," *Arch Pathol Lab Med*, 1995, 119(9):799-806.

Wu AH, Gornet TG, Harker CC, et al, "Role of Rapid Immunoassays for Urgent ("Stat") Determinations of Creatine Kinase Isoenzyme MB," *Clin Chem*, 1989, 35(8):1752-6.

Young GP and Green TR, "The Role of Single ECG, Creatine Kinase, and CKMB in Diagnosing Patients With Acute Chest Pain," *Am J Emerg Med*, 1993, 11(5):444-9.

Creatine Phosphokinase-MB Isoenzyme and Total Creatine Phosphokinase, Serum *see* Creatine Kinase Isoenzymes/Isoforms *on page 115*

Creatine Phosphokinase, Total, Serum *see* Creatine Kinase *on page 115*

Creatinine, 12- or 24-Hour Urine

CPT 82570

Related Information

Creatinine Clearance *on this page*
Uric Acid, Urine *on page 215*
Urine Collection, 24-Hour *on page 30*

Synonyms Urine Creatinine

Test Commonly Includes Urine creatinine in mg/dL and mg/24 hours or mg/12 hours

Abstract Timed urine collection is a portion of creatinine clearance.

Specimen 12- or 24-hour urine

Container Plastic urine container

Collection If the specimen is a 24-hour collection, instruct the patient to void at 8 AM and discard the specimen. Then collect all urine including the final specimen voided at the end of the 24-hour collection period (ie, 8 AM the next morning). Keep specimen on ice during collection. Container must be labeled with patient's name, date, and time collection started and date and time collection finished.

Storage Instructions Refrigerate

Causes for Rejection Incomplete collection

Reference Range Children: 2-3 years: 6-22 mg/kg/24 hours (SI: 52.8-193.6 µmol/kg/day), older than 3 years: 12-30 mg/kg/24 hours (SI: 105.0-264.0 µmol/kg/day); adults: male: 1-2 g/24 hours (SI: 8.8-17.7 mmol/day), female: 0.8-1.8 g/24 hours (SI: 7.1-15.9 mmol/day). Creatinine excretion decreases with advanced age as muscle mass diminishes. Normal age-adjusted values for anticipated creatinine excretion stratified for each sex by height are published. These tables assume ideal weight.[1]

Use Renal function test when used as part of creatinine clearance; crude marker for completeness of 24-hour urine collections when collected for other purposes. Useful as a renal function test only when done as part of a creatinine clearance.

Limitations Complete urine collections require vigilance on the part of nursing personnel. Ingestion of meat may increase creatinine values of urine collections as well as serum creatinine values. Application of urine creatinine excretion as a marker for complete collection is questioned.[2] **Drugs** interfering with tubular creatinine secretion include cimetidine, trimethoprim, and probenecid. Creatinine **reabsorption** occurs with very low urine flow rates. Entities in which reabsorption occurs include severe congestive heart failure, uncontrolled diabetes mellitus, and acute renal failure.[3]

Methodology Jaffé reaction (alkaline picrate); enzymatic, kinetic or endpoint

Additional Information Urine creatinine is not ordered alone. Creatinine clearance, which requires a serum creatinine, offers useful renal function data. Serum creatinine alone is not an adequate index of glomerular filtration rate.[3]

Footnotes

1. Walser M, "Creatinine Excretion as a Measure of Protein Nutrition in Adults of Varying Age," *J Parenter Enteral Nutr*, 1987, 11(5 Suppl):73S-8S.
2. Duarte CG, Elveback LR, and Liedeke RR, "Creatinine," *Renal Function Tests. Clinical Laboratory Procedures and Diagnosis*, Duarte CG, ed, Boston, MA: Little, Brown and Co, 1980, 1-28.
3. Levey AS, Perrone RD, and Madias NE, "Serum Creatinine and Renal Function," *Annu Rev Med*, 1988, 39:465-90.

References

Pesola G, Akhaven I, Carlton G, "Urinary Creatinine Excretion in the ICU: Low Excretion Does Not Mean Inadequate Collection," *Am J Crit Care*, 1993, 2(6):462-6.

Schwab SJ, Christensen RL, Dougherty K, et al, "Quantitation of Proteinuria by the Use of Protein-to-Creatinine Ratios in Single Urine Samples," *Arch Intern Med*, 1987, 147(5):943-4.

Creatinine, Amniotic Fluid *see* Amniotic Fluid Creatinine *on page 77*

Creatinine Clearance

CPT 82575

Related Information

Cortisol, Urine *on page 113*
Creatinine, 12- or 24-Hour Urine *on this page*
Creatinine, Serum *on next page*
Kidney Biopsy *on page 47*
Kidney Profile *on page 153*
Kidney Stone Analysis *on page 640*
Protein, Quantitative, Urine *on page 649*
Urea Nitrogen, Blood *on page 213*
Uric Acid, Serum *on page 213*
Urine Collection, 24-Hour *on page 30*

Applies to GFR

Replaces Urea Clearance; Urea Nitrogen Clearance

Test Commonly Includes Serum creatinine, urine creatinine

Abstract The most common test for evaluation of renal function is serum creatinine; the next is creatinine clearance.

Patient Preparation Avoid cephalosporins. If possible, drugs should be stopped beforehand. Have patient drink water before the clearance is begun and continue good hydration throughout the clearance. A meat-free diet is recommended.[1]

Specimen 24-hour urine and serum; test can be done for shorter periods

Container Urine container and red top tube

(Continued)

Creatinine Clearance (Continued)

Collection Instruct the patient to void at 8 AM and discard the specimen. Then collect all urine including the final specimen voided at the end of the 24-hour collection period (ie, 8 AM the next morning). Keep specimen on ice during collection. Bottle must be labeled with patient's name, date and time for a 24-hour collection. Especially for creatinine clearance, accuracy and precision of collection are important. Complete, carefully timed (usually 24-hour) collection is needed; 4- and 12-hour collections are acceptable. Urine flows >2 mL/minute are required for good clearance measurements.

Storage Instructions Refrigerate

Causes for Rejection No blood creatinine ordered, urine specimen not timed

Special Instructions Blood creatinine should be ordered at the same time. Patient's age, height, and weight are needed.

Reference Range A healthy 70 kg adult excretes about 1 g/day. Clearance for: children: 70-140 mL/minute/1.73 m^2 (SI: 1.17-2.33 mL/s/1.73 m^2); adults: male: 85-125 mL/minute/1.73 m^2 (SI: 1.42-2.08 mL/s/1.73 m^2), female: 75-115 mL/minute/1.73 m^2 (SI: 1.25-1.92 mL/s/1.73 m^2). For each age decades after 40, creatinine clearance decreases 6-7 mL/minute/1.73 m^2. When used in a series to evaluate completeness of collection for other substances (eg, urinary cortisol), up to about 10% variation is acceptable.

Critical Values Moderate renal impairment (adult): 30-40 mL/minute/1.73 m^2

Possible Panic Range Severe renal impairment (adult): <28 mL/minute/1.73 m^2

Use Renal function test to estimate glomerular filtration rate (GFR); evaluate renal function in small or wasted subjects; follow possible progression of renal disease; adjust dosages of medications in which renal excretion is pivotal (eg, aminoglycosides, methotrexate, cisplatin). Assay of creatinine is widely used to assess whether or not a 24-hour urine collection for another substance (eg, cortisol) is complete.

Limitations Exercise may cause increased creatinine clearance. The glomerular filtration rate is substantially increased in pregnancy. Ascorbic acid, ketone bodies (acetoacetate), hydantoin, numerous cephalosporins[2,3] and glucose may influence creatinine determinations. Trimethoprim, cimetidine, quinine, quinidine, procainamide reduce creatinine excretion. Icteric samples, lipemia and hemolysis may interfere with determination of creatinine. Since tubular secretion of creatinine is fractionally more important in progressing renal failure, the creatinine clearance overestimates GFR with high serum creatinine levels. While ingestion of cooked meats may cause some increase in creatinine level, in practice this seems to make a difference only occasionally. Intraindividual variation in creatinine clearance is about 15%. Males excrete more creatinine and have slightly higher clearance than females.

Serum creatinine and creatinine clearance are relatively insensitive indicators for glomerular filtration rate in diseases such as lupus nephritis; complement C50 and C3 depression have better correlation with progression in at least some patients with lupus nephritis. Urinalysis with urine sediment examination and protein excretion are important indicators for modification of therapy.[4]

Methodology Jaffé reaction (alkaline picrate) or enzymatic. The calculation for corrected creatinine clearance in mL/minute = [(urine volume per minute x urine creatinine)/serum creatinine] x (1.73/surface area of body in square meters). Body surface area is obtained from nomograms which require age, height, and weight.

Additional Information Glomerular filtration rate declines about 10% per decade after 50 years of age. Some patients with significant impairment of glomerular filtration rate have only slightly elevated serum creatinine.[5] Corrected creatinine clearance is calculated on the basis of the surface area of the patient. Corrected clearance = urine creat (mg/dL) x rate of urine flow (mL/minute) / plasma creat (mg/dL) x 1.73 / patient surface area in square meters. The estimated error of determining creatinine clearance utilizing serum and 24-hour urine collection has been found to be in the range of 10% to 15%. Any test requiring a 24-hour urine collection may also be run on this specimen (eg, protein, quantitative, 24-hour urine, cortisol).

Footnotes

1. Gambino R, "Crock-Pot Creatinine Revisited - Measure Creatinine Clearance While Patients Are on a Meat-Free Diet," *Lab Rep*, 1995, 17(2):15.
2. Swain RR and Briggs SL, "Positive Interference With the Jaffé Reaction by Cephalosporin Antibiotics," *Clin Chem*, 1977, 23:1340-2.
3. Levey AS, Perrone RD, and Madias NE, "Serum Creatinine and Renal Function," *Annu Rev Med*, 1988, 39:465-90.
4. Boumpas DT, Austin HA 3d, Fessler BJ, et al, "Systemic Lupus Erythematosus: Emerging Concepts. Part 1: Renal, Neuropsychiatric, Cardiovascular, Pulmonary, and Hematologic Disease," *Ann Intern Med*, 1995, 122(12):940-50.
5. Klahr S, "The Modifications of Diet in Renal Disease Study," *N Engl J Med*, 1989, 320(13):864-6.

References

Duarte CG and Preuss HG, "Assessment of Renal Function: Glomerular and Tubular," *Clin Lab Med*, 1993, 13(1):33-52.

Luke DR, Halstenson CE, Opsahl JA, et al, "Validity of Creatinine Clearance Estimates in the Assessment of Renal Function," *Clin Pharmacol Ther*, 1990, 48(5):503-8.

Payne RB, "Biological Variation of Serum and Urine Creatinine and Creatinine Clearance," *Ann Clin Biochem*, 1989, 26(Pt 6):565-6.

Sokoll LJ, Russell RM, Sodowski JA, et al, "Establishment of Creatinine Clearance Reference Values for Older Women," *Clin Chem*, 1994, 40(12):2276-81.

Van Lente F and Suit P, "Assessment of Renal Function by Serum Creatinine and Creatinine Clearance: Glomerular Filtration Rate Estimated by Four Procedures," *Clin Chem*, 1989, 35(12):2326-30.

Creatinine, Serum

CPT 82565

Related Information

Aminoglycosides *on page 531*
Amphotericin B *on page 535*
Anion Gap *on page 81*
BUN/Creatinine Ratio *on page 92*
Creatinine Clearance *on previous page*
Digoxin *on page 546*
Kidney Stone Analysis *on page 640*
Lactic Acid, Blood *on page 156*
Osmolality, Calculated *on page 172*
Urea Nitrogen, Blood *on page 213*
Uric Acid, Serum *on page 213*

Abstract A primary renal function test

Patient Preparation Fasting may be desirable. Certain cephalosporins, especially cefoxitin, cause misleading (high) results.[1]

Specimen Serum

Container Red top tube

Collection Pediatrics: Blood drawn from heelstick.

Causes for Rejection Hemolysis

Reference Range Children: 1-5 years: 0.3-0.5 mg/dL (SI: 27-44 µmol/L), 5-10 years: 0.5-0.8 mg/dL (SI: 44-71 µmol/L); adults: male: up to 1.2 mg/dL (SI: 106 µmol/L), female: up to 1.1 mg/dL (SI: 97 µmol/L).[2] Variation between sources for serum creatinine normal ranges is perhaps greater than for many other important tests. There are slight differences between the sexes with males higher, since the range relates to the amount of muscle mass present. The glomerular filtration rate increases in pregnancy; thus, serum creatinine should be slightly less during that period. In older patients, decrease of muscle mass must be considered in interpretation of results; the elderly have reduced creatinine generation. Similarly, other patients may have creatinine levels in which muscle abnormalities must be considered, including long-term corticosteroid therapy, hyperthyroidism, muscular dystrophy, paralysis, dermatomyositis, and polymyositis.

Use The most common clinical renal function test, providing a rough approximation of glomerular filtration.

Causes of high creatinine include renal diseases and insufficiency with decreased glomerular filtration (uremia or azotemia if severe); urinary tract obstruction; reduced renal blood flow including congestive heart failure, shock and dehydration; rhabdomyolysis causes high serum creatinine, which may be elevated out of proportion to BUN, or to the reduction in renal function.

Causes of low creatinine include small stature, debilitation, decreased muscle mass, some complex cases of severe hepatic disease. In advanced liver disease, low creatinine may result from decreased hepatic production of creatinine and inadequate dietary protein as well as reduced muscle mass.[1]

Index of fetal maturity in amniotic fluid analysis.

Limitations With reduced renal blood flow, creatinine rises less quickly than urea nitrogen. Concentration of creatinine only becomes abnormal when about half or more of the nephrons have stopped functioning in chronic progressive renal disease. Thus, it is not a sensitive indicator of early renal disease. Renal failure is underestimated by serum creatinine and creatinine clearance in patients with hepatic cirrhosis.[3]

Increased serum creatinine results may occur from noncreatinine substances, including meat ingestion, glucose, pyruvate, uric acid, fructose, guanidine, ketonemia (acetoacetate), hydantoin, ascorbic acid, and numerous cephalosporin antibiotics, especially cefoxitin. Cefoxitin levels fall in patients with normal kidney function, such that a sample can be drawn 2 hours after a dose but preferably, 4 hours or more afterwards.[4] With severe renal disease, creatinine is not reliable in the presence of cefoxitin therapy. There is less interference reported from the cephalosporins cephalothin, cephaloridine, cephadrile sodium, and cephaloglycin dihydrate.[5] Cefazolin and cefamandole may cause increased colorimetric values.[6] Cephapirin and moxalactam are described as not causing interference.[7] Differences in the interference of such cephalosporins between assay systems are published.[5,7] Methyldopa and trimethoprim may increase serum creatinine levels.[8] Lipemia, hemolysis, and bilirubin may interfere.[9,10] High creatinine in serum has been reported with methanol intoxication.[11] An antifungal drug, 5-flucytosine, and glucose interfere with the imidohydrolase method.[6] Tagamet® interferes with creatinine excretion in the renal tubule, causing a rise in creatinine without reduction in renal function. It may also cause an allergic nephritis with reduced renal function.

Moderate variation of results exists among chemistry analyzer systems.

Serum creatinine is only a crude guide to the progress of renal disease.[6] Moderate changes in the glomerular filtration rate (GFR) may not be detected by serum creatinine levels. Levey et al and others emphasize that the serum creatinine does **not** provide an adequate estimate of GFR.[6] A fraction of urine creatinine is from tubular secretion. Such tubular secretion increases with declining renal function.

Methodology Alkaline picrate (Jaffé reaction), enzymatic, *o*-nitrobenzaldehyde (Sakaguchi reaction), imidohydrolase (Ektachem®). Many interference problems are still unresolved in the Jaffé reaction.[12]

Additional Information Serum creatinine level is proportional to lean body muscle mass. It is unaffected by most diet or activity and is freely filtered by the glomerulus. Both BUN and creatinine are often ordered to follow renal problems. Creatinine overall is the more reliable index, but each has pitfalls. As creatinine increases in chronic renal failure, the hematocrit decreases, total carbon dioxide and bicarbonate fall, and serum phosphate and BUN increase.[13] Uric acid increases, usually subsequently. When serum creatinine increases postoperatively, a group of patients may be identified who are at risk for more severe renal failure. Creatinine clearances have a role in such investigations.[14] Serum creatinine has a role in determination of dosages of some drugs (eg, the aminoglycosides and digoxin), especially in elderly subjects.[15] Additional evaluation of renovascular disease may be needed.[16]

Footnotes
1. Takabatake T, Ohta H, Ishida Y, et al, "Low Serum Creatinine Levels in Severe Hepatic Disease," *Arch Intern Med*, 1988, 148(6):1313-5.
2. Savory DJ, "Reference Ranges for Serum Creatinine in Infants, Children, and Adolescents," *Ann Clin Biochem*, 1990, 27(Pt 2):99-101.
3. Caregaro L, Menon F, Angeli P, et al, "Limitations of Serum Creatinine Level and Creatinine Clearance as Filtration Markers in Cirrhosis," *Arch Intern Med*, 1994, 154(2):201-5.
4. Durham SR, Bignell AH, and Wise R, "Interference of Cefoxitin in the Creatinine Estimation and its Clinical Relevance," *J Clin Pathol*, 1979, 32:1148-51.
5. Saah AJ, Koch TR, and Drusano GL, "Cefoxitin Falsely Elevates Creatinine Levels," *JAMA*, 1982, 247:205-6.
6. Levey AS, Perrone RD, and Madias NE, "Serum Creatinine and Renal Function," *Annu Rev Med*, 1988, 39:465-90.
7. Kirby MG, Gal P, Baird HW, et al, "Cefoxitin Interference With Serum Creatinine Measurement Varies With the Assay System," *Clin Chem*, 1982, 28:1981.
8. Porter GA and Bennett WM, "Toxic Nephropathies," *The Kidney*, 2nd ed, Brenner BM and Rector FC Jr, eds, Philadelphia, PA: WB Saunders Co, 1981, 2045-108.
9. Bowers CD and Wong ET, "Kinetic Serum Creatinine Assays: A Critical Evaluation and Review," *Clin Chem*, 1980, 26:555-61.
10. Soldier SJ, Henderson L, and Hill JG, "The Effect of Bilirubin and Ketones on Reaction Rate Methods for the Measurement of Creatinine," *Clin Biochem*, 1978, 11:82-6.
11. Wu AH, Stout R, and McComb RB, "Falsely High Serum Creatinine Concentration Associated With Severe Methanol Intoxication," *Clin Chem*, 1983, 29:205-8.
12. Weber JA and van Zanten AP, "Interferences in Current Methods for Measurements of Creatinine," *Clin Chem*, 1991, 37(5):695-700.
13. Hakim RM and Lazarus JM, "Biochemical Parameters in Chronic Renal Failure," *Am J Kidney Dis*, 1988, 11(3):238-47.
14. Charlson ME, MacKenzie CR, Gold JP, et al, "Postoperative Changes in Serum Creatinine: When Do They Occur and How Much Is Important?" *Ann Surg*, 1989, 209(3):328-33.
15. Lindeman RD, "Assessment of Renal Function in the Old: Special Considerations," *Clin Lab Med*, 1993, 13(1):269-77.
16. Canzanello VJ and Textor SC, "Noninvasive Diagnosis of Renovascular Disease," *Mayo Clin Proc*, 1994, 69(12):1172-81.

References
Abuelo JG, "Benign Azotemia of Long-Term Hemodialysis: Increase in Blood Urea Nitrogen and Serum Creatinine Concentrations After the Initiation of Dialysis," *Am J Med*, 1989, 86(6 Pt 1):738-9.
Blijenberg BG, Brouwer HJ, Kuller TJ, et al, "Improvements in Creatinine Methodology: A Critical Assessment," *Eur J Chem Clin Biochem*, 1994, 32(7):529-37.
Duarte CG and Preuss HG, "Assessment of Renal Function: Glomerular and Tubular," *Clin Lab Med*, 1993, 13(1):33-52.
Fossati P, Ponti M, Passoni G, et al, "A Step Forward in Enzymatic Measurement of Creatinine," *Clin Chem*, 1994, 40(1):130-7.
Lemann J, Bidani AK, Bain RP, et al, "Use of the Serum Creatinine to Estimate Glomerular Filtration Rate in Health and Early Diabetic Nephropathy. Collaborative Study Group of Angiotensin Converting Enzyme Inhibition in Diabetic Nephropathy," *Am J Kidney Dis*, 1990, 16(3):236-43.
Lepage L and Galimany R, "Creatinine," *Drug Effects on Laboratory Test Results Analytical Interferences and Pharmacological Effects*, Siest G and Galteau MM, eds, Littleton, MA: PSG Publishing Co Inc, 1988, 198-210.
Narayanan S, "Creatinine: Review of Methods," *ASCP Check Sample®*, Gambino SR and Batsakis JG, eds, Chicago, IL: American Society of Clinical Pathologists, 1988, 4:1-10.

CSF Glucose *see* Cerebrospinal Fluid Glucose *on page 105*

CSF Glutamine *see* Cerebrospinal Fluid Glutamine *on page 105*

CSF Lactic Acid *see* Cerebrospinal Fluid Lactic Acid *on page 106*

CSF LDH *see* Cerebrospinal Fluid LD *on page 106*

cTnI (Troponin I) *see* Troponin *on page 212*

cTnT (Troponin T) *see* Troponin *on page 212*

3', 5'-Cyclic Adenosine Monophosphate, Plasma *see* Cyclic AMP, Plasma *on this page*

Cyclic Adenosine Monophosphate, Urine *see* Cyclic AMP, Urine *on this page*

3', 5'-Cyclic Adenosine Monophosphate, Urine *see* Cyclic AMP, Urine *on this page*

Cyclic AMP, Plasma
CPT 82030
Related Information
Parathyroid Hormone *on page 178*
Synonyms AMP, Cyclic, Plasma; cAMP, Plasma; 3', 5'-Cyclic Adenosine Monophosphate, Plasma
Applies to Nephrogenous Cyclic AMP
Abstract This test along with urinary cyclic AMP is sometimes used to evaluate hyperparathyroidism. Parathyroid hormone exerts its effect through cyclic AMP (cAMP) activity. It is a second messenger for a number of hormones, including parathormone, on target cells.[1]
Patient Preparation Avoid radioisotope scan prior to collection of specimen if RIA is used for assay.
Specimen Plasma
Container Lavender top (EDTA) tube; do not use heparin or citrate tube
Collection Stable 1 hour in plasma at 25°C, specimen should then be frozen[1] if longer storage is anticipated
Storage Instructions Separate plasma and freeze **immediately** upon receipt of the specimen.
Special Instructions Transport specimen to the laboratory **immediately** following collection.
Reference Range Male: 4.6-8.6 ng/mL (SI: 14-26 nmol/L); female: 4.3-7.6 ng/mL (SI: 13-23 nmol/L)
Use Differential diagnosis of hypercalcemia of hyperparathyroidism; calculate nephrogenous cAMP. Used to calculate the nephrogenous portion of total urinary cAMP.
Limitations Used with urine cAMP
Methodology Immunoassay or high performance liquid chromatography (HPLC)
Additional Information Serum and 2-hour urine collection for cAMP and creatinine in the recumbent, prepared patient are sometimes used in the differential diagnosis of hyperparathyroidism. In hyperparathyroidism and hypercalcemia of malignancy there are increased values for nephrogenous cyclic AMP. Utilization of cAMP in the diagnosis of hyperparathyroidism has been de-emphasized in recent years.[2] In patients with primary hyperparathyroidism, the loss of circadian rhythm of intact PTH and nephrogenous cyclic AMP occurs.[3]
Footnotes
1. Freissmuth M and Gilman AG, "G Proteins and the Regulation of Second Messenger Systems," *Harrison's Principles of Internal Medicine*, 13th ed, Isselbacher KJ, Braunwald E, Wilson JD, et al, eds, New York, NY: McGraw-Hill Inc, 1994, 426-31.
2. Watts NB and Keffer JH, *Practical Endocrine Diagnosis*, 4th ed, Philadelphia, PA: Lea & Febiger, 1989, 137-46.
3. Logue FC, Fraser WD, Gallacher SJ, et al, "The Loss of Circadian Rhythm for Intact Parathyroid Hormone and Nephrogenous Cyclic AMP in Patients With Primary Hyperparathyroidism," *Clin Endocrinol (Oxf)*, 1990, 32(4):475-83.
References
Levitzki A, "From Epinephrine to Cyclic AMP," *Science*, 1988, 241:800-6.

Cyclic AMP, Urine
CPT 82030
Related Information
Calcium, Serum *on page 97*
Parathyroid Hormone *on page 178*
Synonyms AMP, Cyclic, Urine; cAMP, Urine; Cyclic Adenosine Monophosphate, Urine; 3', 5'-Cyclic Adenosine Monophosphate, Urine
Applies to Nephrogenous Cyclic AMP
Abstract In conjunction with plasma cyclic AMP, this test is occasionally used to evaluate parathyroid function.
Patient Preparation Avoid radioisotope scan prior to collection of specimen. PTH or ADH may be administered as a provocative test.
Specimen Random urine
Storage Instructions Acidify to below pH 4 and freeze.
Reference Range 112-188 µg/L (SI: 340-570 nmol/L) or 0.3-3.6 mg/day (SI: 1.0-10.9 µmol/day). 6.6-15.5 µg/L (SI: 20-47 nmol/L) glomerular filtrate. Nephrogenous cAMP: <9.9 µg/L (SI: <30 nmol/L) glomerular filtrate. Also, 0.3-2.1 mg/g creatinine (SI: 106-723 µmol/mol creatinine).
Use Occasionally used in the differential diagnosis of hyperparathyroidism. In hyperparathyroidism there is increased cAMP in 24-hour urine specimens, also in humoral hypercalcemia of malignancy and
(Continued)

Cyclic AMP, Urine *(Continued)*

vitamin D deficiency. The plasma concentrations of immunoreactive parathyroid hormone-related protein correlate with levels of excreted cyclic AMP.[1] Must be used in conjunction with plasma cAMP.

Limitations There is some overlap between results of patients with hyperparathyroidism and those of normal subjects. Not all patients with hyperparathyroidism have abnormal urinary cAMP results. Urinary cAMP is reported increased in hypercalcemic cancer patients.

Methodology Radioimmunoassay (RIA)

Additional Information Please see Cyclic AMP, Plasma *on page 119* with citations. A role for cAMP excretion measurement in the evaluation of Zollinger-Ellison syndrome and differentiation of sporadic cases from those of multiple endocrine neoplasia type I may exist.[2] Assay of nephrogenous cyclic AMP has been applied to the monitoring of calcium intake in cases of osteoporosis.[3]

A target of parathyroid hormone (PTH) action is the renal tubule. The result is release of cAMP into the urine. Cyclic AMP output in the urine is thus an indirect measure of parathyroid action. PTH utilizes cyclic AMP to exert its effect on cells. Upon binding of PTH to its receptor, the latter undergoes a confirmational change which increases its affinity (through a second binding site) for a linking protein (Ns) which also binds guanosine triphosphate.

Type I pseudohypoparathyroidism (autosomal dominant inheritance), mimics hypoparathyroidism with hypocalcemia resistant to vitamin D and high serum phosphate and PTH levels. This condition appears to be due to a defect in linking protein (Ns) structure. Type I is characterized by defective renal tubular response to PTH and increased circulating and urinary cyclic AMP. Type II pseudohypoparathyroidism (autosomal dominant inheritance) has a normal cyclic AMP response.[4]

The level of urinary cAMP is the result of cAMP released by PTH, action of other hormones and plasma cAMP filtered by the renal glomerulus. "Nephrogenous cAMP" is the urinary excretion of cAMP minus that filtered by the glomerulus and correlates with the results of plasma PTH levels.[5]

Footnotes

1. Burtis WJ, Brady TG, Orloff JJ, et al, "Immunochemical Characterization of Circulating Parathyroid Hormone-Related Protein in Patients With Humoral Hypercalcemia of Cancer," *N Engl J Med*, 1990, 322(16):1106-12.
2. Mignon M and Bonfils S, "Diagnosis and Treatment of Zollinger-Ellison Syndrome," *Baillieres Clin Gastroenterol*, 1988, 2(3):677-98.
3. Licata A, Gall D, and Gupta M, "Monitoring Calcium Intake in Osteoporosis by Assay of Nephrogenous Cyclic AMP," *Am J Clin Nutr*, 1988, 47(6):1022-4.
4. Anderson DC and Braidman IP, "Hormone Receptor Disorders," *Subcellular Pathology of Systemic Disease*, Chapter 12, Peters TJ, ed, London, England: Chapman and Hall, 1987, 229-47.
5. Pollard A, Pritzker KPH, and Grynpas MD, "Disorders of Calcium, Magnesium, and Bone Metabolism," *Applied Biochemistry of Clinical Disorders*, 2nd ed, Chapter 17, Gornall AG, ed, Philadelphia, PA: JB Lippincott Co, 1986, 408-10.

Cysteine, Qualitative *see Cystine, Urine on this page*

Cyst Fluid Chemistry *see Body Fluid on page 89*

Cystic Fibrosis Sweat Test *see Chloride, Sweat on page 108*

Cystine, Urine

CPT 82615

Related Information

Kidney Stone Analysis *on page 640*
Urinalysis *on page 658*

Applies to Cysteine, Qualitative; Homocysteine, Qualitative; Nitroprusside Screening

Test Commonly Includes Homocystine, cysteine

Abstract Cystinuria is an inherited disease in which excessive cystine is excreted. Cystine is not soluble and causes stones. Patients with cystine stones face recurrent urolithiasis (33% recurrence rate) and repeated urinary tract infections.

Patient Preparation Penicillamine (a chelating agent) can cause false-negative results.

Specimen Random urine

Collection Random urine or 24-hour collection for quantitation

Storage Instructions Acidify to pH 2-3 or freeze specimen at -20°C, or 20 mL toluene can be added to the container prior to the start of a 24-hour collection.

Reference Range Normal: 40-60 mg cystine/g creatinine; heterozygotes: <300 mg/g; homozygotes: >250 mg/g[1]

Use Detect cystinuria, homocystinuria and other diseases related to the sulfur-containing amino acids. Work up nephrolithiasis.[2,3,4] Cystine stones account for 1% to 3% of renal calculi.[5] Early age at onset, positive family history, and recurrence of urolithiasis are features suggestive of cystine lithiasis.[6]

Limitations Cystinosis, a different entity from **cystinuria,** is not detected by this test. Patients with cystinosis are diagnosed with cystine

crystals in biopsies, corneal crystals on slit lamp examination or elevated leukocyte cystine levels.[7]

Methodology Microscopic examination of the sediment of a first morning urine sample can include the hexagonal crystals in samples from homozygotes.[1]

Nitroprusside screening test is positive with cystine or homocystine. The urine nitroprusside test reacts positively at levels of 75-125 mg cystine/g creatinine.[1] High performance liquid chromatography (HPLC), ion exchange chromatography are used.

Additional Information A positive screening test should be followed up by a quantitative procedure for cystine. In cystinosis, plasma cystine is usually normal, but increased cystine may be found in tissues. Therapy for cystinuria includes hydration, diet, urinary alkalinization (pH of urine maintained >7.5), chelation, surgery, and chemolysis. Cystine stones appear to be more resistant to lithotripsy than most stones.[5] Percutaneous ultrasonic lithotripsy is described for such patients.[6]

Footnotes

1. Coe FL and Favus MJ, "Nephrolithiasis," *Harrison's Principles of Internal Medicine*, 13th ed, Isselbacher KJ, Braunwald E, Wilson JD, et al, eds, New York, NY: McGraw-Hill Inc, 1994, 1329-33.
2. Wilson DM, "Clinical and Laboratory Approaches for Evaluation of Nephrolithiasis," *J Urol*, 1989, 141(3 Pt 2):770-4.
3. Pak CY, "Etiology and Treatment of Urolithiasis," *Am J Kidney Dis*, 1991, 18(6):624-37.
4. Sakhaee K, Poindexter JR, and Pak CY, "The Spectrum of Metabolic Abnormalities in Patients With Cystine Nephrolithiasis," *J Urol*, 1989, 141(4):819-21.
5. Singh A, Marshall FF, and Chang R, "Cystine Calculi: Clinical Management and *In Vitro* Observations," *Urology*, 1988, 31(3):207-10.
6. Knoll LD, Segura JW, Patterson DE, et al, "Long-Term Follow-up in Patients With Cystine Urinary Calculi Treated by Percutaneous Ultrasonic Lithotripsy," *J Urol*, 1988, 140(2):246-8.
7. Markello TC, Bernardini IM, and Gahl WA, "Improved Renal Function in Children With Cystinosis Treated With Cysteamine," *N Engl J Med*, 1993, 328(16):1157-62.

References

Singer A and Das S, "Cystinuria: A Review of the Pathophysiology and Management," *J Urol*, 1989, 142(3):669-73.

Cytochrome b5 Reductase (NADH-metHb Reductase) *see Methemoglobin on page 166*

Dehydroepiandrosterone *see 17-Ketosteroids Fractionation, Urine on page 152*

Dehydroepiandrosterone, Serum *see Dehydroepiandrosterone Sulfate on this page*

Dehydroepiandrosterone Sulfate

CPT 82627

Related Information

Androstenedione, Serum *on page 80*
17-Ketosteroids, Total, Urine *on page 153*
Prolactin *on page 192*
Testosterone, Free and Total *on page 202*

Synonyms DHEA-S; DHEAS

Applies to Dehydroepiandrosterone, Serum; DHEA

Abstract DHEA and its sulfate, DHEA-S, are the major precursors of 17-ketosteroids. Dehydroepiandrosterone is reported as a fraction in 17-ketosteroid fractionation of urine.[1] DHEA-S is perceived as a weak androgen but recently its effects have been reconsidered. In premenopausal women, it is either an estrogen antagonist or androgen. In men it is thought to act as an estrogen.[2] It is primarily synthesized in the adrenal, with a small amount from ovary. DHEA-S is the most abundant circulating C19 steroid and is a metabolite of dehydroepiandrosterone (DHEA).

Patient Preparation Avoid recently administered radioisotopes if assay method is RIA.

Specimen Serum or plasma

Container Red top tube or green top (heparin) tube

Storage Instructions Separate within 1 hour of collection. Serum or plasma stable 24 hours at 4°C. Freeze for longer storage.

Causes for Rejection Recently administered radioisotopes if RIA is used for assay

Special Instructions Ordered in work-up for hirsutism and/or infertility in women; related tests include 3-α-androstanediol glucuronide.

Reference Range Normal range varies between laboratories. Adult ranges may be approximate. See table. Infants and children have lower values.

Use Work up women with infertility, amenorrhea, or hirsutism, to identify the source of excessive androgen. Aid in evaluation of androgen excess (hirsutism and/or virilization), including congenital adrenal hyperplasia, adrenal tumor, and Stein-Leventhal syndrome. DHEA-S is not increased with hypopituitarism. It is low in Addison's disease.

Methodology Radioimmunoassay (RIA) or gas chromatography/mass spectrometry (GC/MS)

Dehydroepiandrosterone, Serum

DHEA (Unconjugated)	ng/mL	SI: nmol/L
Male	1.8-12.0	6.0-43.0
Female	1.3-10.0	4.0-34.0
DHEA-S	**μg/mL**	**SI: μmol/L**
Male	<4.0	<11.0
Female		
premenopausal	0.8-3.4	2.1-8.8
postmenopausal	0.3-2.6	0.8-7.0
term pregnancy	0.2-1.2	0.6-3.0

Additional Information DHEA is the major steroid of the fetal adrenal. DHEA is the principal adrenal androgen and is secreted together with cortisol under the control of ACTH and prolactin. DHEA-S is elevated with hyperprolactinemia.

Elevated levels may be found in the adrenogenital syndrome[3] as well as adrenocortical neoplasms. In females and children, DHEA excess causes masculinization.

Increased 3-α-androstanediol glucuronide indicates excessive androgen in peripheral tissues. Persistent anovulation, the polycystic ovary or Stein-Leventhal syndrome is characterized by increases of circulating levels of testosterone, androstenedione, dehydroepiandrosterone and DHEA-S. 17-hydroxyprogesterone and DHEA-S are only mildly increased compared to cases of adrenal hyperplasia. Patients with androgen-producing adrenal tumors also have moderate increases of 17-KS.

Testosterone is derived from ovaries, adrenals, and the peripheral tissues. Increased DHEA-S with normal testosterone provides evidence for an adrenal cause of excessive androgen. Low levels are found in amniotic fluid in Down syndrome.[4]

Footnotes
1. Leavelle DE, *Mayo Medical Laboratories Interpretive Handbook*, Rochester, MN: Mayo Medical Laboratories, 1994.
2. Ebeling P and Koivisto VA, "Physiological Importance of Dehydroepiandrosterone," *Lancet*, 1994, 343(8911):1479-81.
3. Pintor C, Genozanni AR, Carboni G, et al, "Adrenal Androgens and Pubertal Development in Physiological and Pathological Conditions," *Adrenal Androgens*, Genozanni AR, Thiossen JH, and Seiteri PK, eds, New York, NY: Raven Press, 1985, 816-90.
4. Cuckle HS, Wald NJ, Densem JW, et al, "Second Trimester Amniotic Fluid Oestriol, Dehydroepiandrosterone Sulphate, and Human Chorionic Gonadotropin Levels in Down Syndrome," *Br J Obstet Gynaecol*, 1991, 98(11):1160-2.

References
Meites S, *Pediatric Clinical Chemistry: Reference (Normal) Values*, 3rd ed, Washington, DC: American Association of Clinical Chemistry Press, 1989, 119-20.

Pang SY, Legido A, Levine LS, et al, "Adrenal Androgen Response to Metyrapone, Adrenocorticotropin, and Corticotropin-Releasing Hormone Stimulation in Children With Hypopituitarism," *J Clin Endocrinol Metab*, 1987, 65(2):282-9.

Snow K, Jiang N-S, Kao PC, et al, "Biochemical Evaluation of Adrenal Dysfunction: The Laboratory Perspective," *Mayo Clin Proc*, 1992, 67(11):1055-65.

Thomas G, Frenoy N, Legrain S, et al, "Serum Dehydroepiandrosterone Sulfate Levels as an Individual Marker," *J Clin Endocrinol Metab*, 1994, 79(5):1273-6.

Weykamp CW, Penders TJ, Schmidt NA, et al, "Steroid Profile for Urine: Reference Values," *Clin Chem*, 1989, 35(12):2281-4.

Delta-ALA *see* Delta Aminolevulinic Acid, Urine *on this page*

Delta Aminolevulinic Acid, Urine

CPT 82135

Related Information
Lead, Blood *on page 556*
Lead, Urine *on page 557*
Porphobilinogen, Qualitative, Urine *on page 185*
Porphyrins, Quantitative, Urine *on page 186*
Protoporphyrin, Free Erythrocyte *on page 195*
Protoporphyrin, Zinc, Blood *on page 196*
Urine Collection, 24-Hour *on page 30*

Synonyms ALA; Aminolevulinic Acid; Delta-ALA

Applies to ALA Dehydratase

Abstract ALA is a precursor of the porphyrins, uroporphyrin, coproporphyrin, and protoporphyrin. The acute neurological porphyrias are associated with ALA and PBG.

Specimen 24-hour urine

Container Dark urine container, kept on ice

Collection Acidify with acetic acid to pH 3-4.5; other laboratories use 2 g barbituric acid as a preservative. Sodium bicarbonate is appropriate as a preservative also for porphyrins and porphobilinogen.

Storage Instructions Protect from light and freeze.

Reference Range Normal: up to approximately 7 mg/24 hours urine (SI: 53 μmol/day), depending on method and laboratory

Possible Panic Range >20 mg/24 hours (SI: >153 μmol/day)

Use Diagnose porphyrias: delta-ALA may be increased in attacks of acute intermittent porphyria, hereditary coproporphyria, and porphyria variegata; evaluate certain neurological problems with abdominal pain; diagnose lead or mercury poisoning. Urinary delta-ALA is not a sensitive indicator of lead poisoning in children because it does not increase until blood lead concentration is 40 μg/dL, well above the recommended level of <15 μg/dL. ALA is increased also in tyrosinemia.[1] **Porphobilinogen, delta aminolevulinic acid, and uroporphyrinogen 1 synthase are the tests of choice for acute intermittent porphyria.** Molecular lesions have been identified in a severely affected homozygote with delta aminolevulinate dehydratase deficient porphyria.[2]

Limitations ALA may be normal during latent period of acute intermittent porphyria, hereditary coproporphyria, porphyria variegata. For the diagnosis of lead poisoning, measurement of blood and urine lead, free erythrocyte protoporphyrin and ALA dehydratase in red cells are other available options.

Methodology Ion-exchange resin columns, colorimetry

Additional Information Conversion of ALA to porphobilinogen is inhibited by lead and mercury; thus, **lead poisoning** causes increased urinary delta-ALA as well as increases of coproporphyrin, free erythrocyte protoporphyrin, and inhibition of ALA dehydratase. See listings Lead, Blood *on page 556* and Porphyrins, Quantitative, Urine *on page 186*.

Footnotes
1. "Hereditary Tyrosinaemia," *Lancet*, 1990, 335(8704):1500-1.
2. Plewinska M, Thunell S, Holmberg L, et al, "Delta-Aminolevulinate Dehydratase Deficient Porphyria: Identification of the Molecular Lesions in a Severely Affected Homozygote," *Am J Hum Genet*, 1991, 49(1):167-74.

References
Bird TD, Wallace DM, and Labbe RF, "The Porphyria, Plumbism, Pottery Puzzle," *JAMA*, 1982, 247:813-4.

Bloomer JR and Bonkovsky HL, "The Porphyrias," *Dis Mon*, 1989, 35(1):1-54.

Elder GH, Smith SG, and Smyth SJ, "Laboratory Investigation of the Porphyrias," *Ann Clin Biochem*, 1990, 27(Pt 5):395-412.

Takebayashi T, Omae K, Hosada K, et al, "Evaluation of Delta-Aminolevulinic Acid in Blood of Workers Exposed to Lead," *Br J Ind Med*, 1993, 50(1):49-54.

Delta Base, Blood

Related Information
pH, Blood *on page 180*

Synonyms Actual Base Excess; Base Excess

Applies to Acid-Base Regulation

Abstract An expression of metabolic acid-base imbalance.

Reference Range -3 to +3

Critical Values -5 or +5

Use A measure with which to assess abnormalities of metabolic or acute respiratory acidosis or alkalosis.

Limitations The validity of delta base is questioned by some.

Methodology Calculated from a Siggaard-Andersen curve nomogram or can be read directly from blood gas instruments which have computer calculation capabilities. Delta base represents deviation from normal buffer base.

Additional Information Delta base is the difference in concentration of strong base in whole blood and in the same blood titrated with strong acid or base to pH 7.40 at pCO_2 40 mm Hg and 37°C. This is an *in vitro* expression used mainly to describe situations with metabolic imbalance. Delta base below -3 indicates deficiency of fixed base or excess of acid (ie, metabolic acidosis). Delta base more than +3 indicates excess fixed base or deficit of nonvolatile acid (ie, metabolic alkalosis). Clinically, therapy is usually not given until -5 or +5 is reached. Umbilical cord blood gases do not predict morbidity in very low birth weight infants (500-1500 g).[1]

Footnotes
1. Hibbard JU, Hibbard MC, and Whalen MP, "Umbilical Cord Blood Gases and Mortality and Morbidity in the Very Low Birth Weight Infant," *Obstet Gynecol*, 1991, 78(5 Pt 1):768-73.

References
Burbea ZH, Gullans SR, and Ben-Yaakov S, "Delta Alkalinity: A Simple Method to Measure Cellular Net Acid-Base Fluxes," *Am J Physiol*, 1987, 253(4 Pt 1):C525-34.

Dickinson JE, Eriksen NL, Meyer BA, et al, "The Effect of Preterm Birth on Umbilical Cord Blood Gases," *Obstet Gynecol*, 1992, 79(4):575-8.

Dunham CM, Siegel JH, Weireter L, et al, "Oxygen Debt and Metabolic Acidemia as Quantitative Predictors of Mortality and the Severity of the Ischemic Insult in Hemorrhagic Shock," *Crit Care Med*, 1991, 19(2):231-43.

Economides DL, Johnson P, and MacKenzie IZ, "Does Amniotic Fluid Analysis Reflect Acid-Base Balance in Fetal Blood?" *Am J Obstet Gynecol*, 1992, 166(3):970-3.

11-Deoxycortisol *see* Metyrapone Stimulation Test *on page 167*

Dexamethasone Suppression *see* Adrenocorticotropic Hormone *on page 63*

Dexamethasone Suppression Test *see* Cortisol, Blood *on page 112*

Dexamethasone Suppression Test *see* Metyrapone Stimulation Test *on page 167*

Dexamethasone Suppression Test *see* Testosterone, Free and Total *on page 202*

1,4-α-D Glucanohydrolase, Serum *see* Amylase, Serum *on page 79*

1,4-α-D Glucanohydrolase, Urine *see* Amylase, Urine *on page 79*

DHEA *see* Dehydroepiandrosterone Sulfate *on page 120*

DHEA-S *see* Dehydroepiandrosterone Sulfate *on page 120*

DHEAS *see* Dehydroepiandrosterone Sulfate *on page 120*

Dialysis *see* Urea Nitrogen, Blood *on page 213*

Dibucaine Number

CPT 82638

Related Information

Acetylcholinesterase, Red Cell *on page 62*
Pseudocholinesterase, Serum *on page 196*

Synonyms Cholinesterase Inhibition by Dibucaine; Pseudocholinesterase Inhibition

Applies to Fluoride Inhibition of Cholinesterase

Abstract Dibucaine is a substance which inhibits the normal variant of the enzyme cholinesterase. Abnormal variants are less inhibited.

Specimen Serum or plasma

Container Red top tube or green top (heparin) tube

Collection Do not collect within 24 hours of administration of muscle relaxant.

Storage Instructions Serum cholinesterase (pseudocholinesterase) is stable and may be stored at 0°C to 4°C or at room temperature for 1 year or more and may be frozen/thawed a number of times without changing activity of the enzyme.[1]

Reference Range Normal individuals have normal (high) amounts of serum cholinesterase (pseudocholinesterase) activity which can be inhibited by dibucaine. Approximately 70% to 86% inhibition is normal; atypical enzyme shows resistance to inhibition, at about the level of only 20%. See normal range of laboratory doing the test.

Possible Panic Range Homozygotes for abnormal cholinesterase activity have low results (low percent inhibition) in assay for serum cholinesterase (pseudocholinesterase). Administration of succinylcholine by anesthesiologist may pose a risk to patients with abnormal pseudocholinesterase because there is abnormal persistence of the succinylcholine effect.

Use Assess presence of homozygous or heterozygous "atypical" cholinesterase variant in patients who have normal or low result (low inhibition) of serum cholinesterase assay and may be at risk of apnea when given succinylcholine muscle relaxant. Dibucaine inhibition provides identification of an abnormal allele. Sensitivity of pseudocholinesterase to dibucaine inhibition may distinguish congenital from acquired forms of abnormal pseudocholinesterase activity. About 4% of the population have abnormal inherited forms.[2]

Limitations No single simple test currently exists that can detect all enzyme variants. Traditional tests including dibucaine inhibition are not adequate to identify all variants. Instances of prolonged response to succinylcholine still go without explanation.

Methodology Hydrolysis of propionylthiocholine or butyrylthiocholine with and without dibucaine at 20°C to 40°C; fluoride inhibition at 25°C.[3,4,5,6]

Additional Information The degree of serum cholinesterase inhibition produced by dibucaine (and fluoride) is under genetic control. Sensitivity to succinylcholine is dependent upon at least four allelic genes. The most widely accepted system of classification (Motulsky) designates E_1 as the first locus for plasma cholinesterase (see table). The E_1^u gene codes for the most common form of the plasma enzyme. The E_1^a gene is responsible for the atypical enzyme which resists inhibition by dibucaine, E_1^f gene for the enzyme that is fluoride resistant, and the E_1^s (silent) gene results in an enzyme with little or no activity.[7] An international gene nomenclature conference has proposed a system designating the four alleles as "CHE1*U," "CHE1*A," "CHE1*F," and "CHE1*QO." Single quantitative cholinesterase determinations may not be reliable in detecting sensitivity to succinyl choline as variant enzymes exhibit qualitative and quantitative differences in substrate specificity. Another common phenotypic designation (of the 15 different phenotypes known) is those at risk, AF; FS and FF (moderate risk); and AA, AS, and SS (severe risk).

Dibucaine and fluoride numbers indicate the percent inhibition of enzyme activity by these agents when a serum sample is tested under standard conditions (inhibition expressed as a percent). This approach to

Dibucaine Number

Genotype	Phenotype	Previous Term
$E_1^u E_1^u$	U	Usual
$E_1^u E_1^a$	I	Intermediate
$E_1^a E_1^a$	A	Atypical
$E_1^u E_1^s$	U	Usual
$E_1^s E_1^s$	S	Silent
$E_1^u E_1^f$	UF	
$E_1^f E_1^f$	F	

screening for presence of serum cholinesterase variants does not entirely avoid the problem of variation in reactivity with some atypical enzymes. Individuals with the genotype E_1^u, E_1^f show resistance to fluoride inhibition (low fluoride number) but do not show resistance to dibucaine inhibition (the normal situation with high dibucaine number). This variant was published almost 30 years ago by Harris and Whittaker.[8] Prolonged apnea following hemodilutional cardiopulmonary bypass has been reported in a patient whose preoperative plasma cholinesterase level was slightly below the normal range.[9]

Footnotes

1. Huizenga JR, van der Belt K, Gips CH, et al, "The Effect of Storage at Different Temperatures on Cholinesterase Activity in Human Serum," *J Clin Chem Clin Biochem*, 1985, 23(5):283-5.
2. Holownia P, Newman DJ, Bruno C, et al, "Automated Dibucaine Number Measurement With DuPont Dimension® ES and AR Analyzers," *Clin Chem*, 1995, 41(5):664-7.
3. Abernethy MH, George PM, Herron JL, et al, "Plasma Cholinesterase Phenotyping With Use of Visible-Region Spectrophotometry," *Clin Chem*, 1986, 32(1 Pt 1):194-7.
4. Abernethy MH, George PM, and Melton VE, "A New Succinylcholine-Based Assay of Plasma Cholinesterase," *Clin Chem*, 1984, 30(2):192-5.
5. Evans RT and Wroe J, "Is Serum Cholinesterase Activity a Predictor of Succinyl Choline Sensitivity? An Assessment of Four Methods," *Clin Chem*, 1978, 24:1762-6.
6. Rostron P and Higgins T, "Serum Pseudocholinesterase and Dibucaine Numbers as Measured With the Technicon® RA-1000 Analyzer," *Clin Chem*, 1988, 34(9):1924-5.
7. Motulsky AG, "Pharmacogenetics," *Progressive Medical Genetics*, Vol 3, Chapter 2, Steinberg AG and Bearn AG, eds, New York, NY: Grune & Stratton, 1964, 49-52.
8. Harris H and Whittaker M, "Differential Inhibition of Human Serum Cholinesterase With Fluoride: Recognition of Two New Phenotypes," *Nature*, 1961, 496-8.
9. Jackson SH, Bailey GW, and Stevens G, "Reduced Plasma Cholinesterase Following Haemodilutional Cardiopulmonary Bypass," *Anaesthesia*, 1982, 37:319-20.

References

Kambam JR, Horton B, Parris WC, et al, "Pseudocholinesterase Activity in Human Cerebrospinal Fluid," *Anesth Analg*, 1989, 68(4):486-8.
Marrs TC, "Organophosphate Poisoning," *Pharmacol Ther*, 1993, 58(1):51-66.
Pantuck EJ, "Plasma Cholinesterase: Gene and Variations," *Anesth Analg*, 1993, 77(2):380-6.
Whittaker M, "Cholinesterase," *Monographs in Human Genetics*, Vol II, Beckman L, ed, Basel: Karger, 1986.

1,25-Dihydroxy Vitamin D₃ *see* Vitamin D₃, Serum *on page 218*

Direct Bilirubin *see* Bilirubin, Direct *on page 86*

Disaturated Phosphatidylcholine (DSPC) *see* Amniotic Fluid Lecithin/Sphingomyelin Ratio and Phosphatidylglycerol *on page 77*

Dopamine, Urine *see* Catecholamines, Fractionation, Urine *on page 104*

2,3-DPG *see* Oxygen Saturation, Blood *on page 175*

2,3-DPG *see* P-50 Blood Gas *on page 176*

d-Xylose Absorption Test

CPT 84620

Related Information

Chloride, Sweat *on page 108*
Cystic Fibrosis DNA Detection *on page 507*
Fat, Semiquantitative, Stool *on page 634*
Fecal Fat, Quantitative, 72-Hour Collection *on page 127*
Folic Acid, RBC *on page 317*
Lactose Tolerance Test *on page 157*
Meat Fibers, Stool *on page 642*
Methylene Blue Stain, Stool *on page 642*
Reducing Substances, Stool *on page 651*

Synonyms Xylose Absorption Test; Xylose Tolerance Test

Abstract d-Xylose is a five-carbon monosaccharide. It can be absorbed by the normal duodenum and jejunum, by a mechanism different from the absorption of other monosaccharides. It is used as a screening test for intestinal carbohydrate malabsorption by the mucosa of the proximal small intestine. Xylose absorption with measured serum and urine concentrations are among the indices of intestinal function, but the use of this test is somewhat controversial.

Patient Preparation Urea nitrogen, creatinine, and first morning urinalysis should be normal. Patient must fast a minimum of 8 hours prior to administration of d-xylose. Pediatric patients must be fasting for at least

4 hours. Patient must remain in supine position for duration of test. No food is permitted during the test. This substance, d-xylose, is a pentose. Patient should refrain from eating foods containing pentose. These include fruits, jams, jellies, and pastries. Many medications, including aspirin, indomethacin, other nonsteroidal anti-inflammatory drugs, neomycin, glipizide, or atropine interfere. These and preferably all medications should be discontinued for 24 hours prior to the test. No water restriction; in fact, patient should be encouraged to drink during the fasting period and during test. Start test at 8 AM. Instruct patient to void completely. Discard this urine. Draw fasting blood specimen.

Administer d-xylose: Adults, 25 g dose; for children under 12 years, a 5 g oral dose is recommended.[1] Others use weight-based dosage of d-xylose for children, oral administration: 0.5 g/kg body weight up to a maximum of 25 g, dissolved in water 10% (w/v) with a maximum of 250 mL. Have patient drink entire amount. Fill cup with 250 mL of water and have patient drink this also. Have patient drink another cup with 250 mL of water after 1 hour. Collect urine for 5 hours after administration of d-xylose.

Specimen Craig and Atkinson recommend a 25 g d-xylose absorption test with a 5-hour urine collection and a 1-hour serum specimen for adults, and the 1-hour serum test only for subjects with intermediate renal insufficiency.[1] Others, for 5-hour urine: blood specimens drawn at fasting, 30, 60, and 120 minutes in red top tubes. A 1-hour draw is also done, for infants and children in some institutions.

Container Brown, labeled urine container, red top tube

Special Instructions A 5-hour urine specimen is collected on patients 12 years of age or older as part of the test.

Reference Range Absorption and excretion of d-xylose increase with age; in geriatric patients the serum test is preferable. Renal excretion diminishes in patients older than 60 years of age.

Mean 5-hour urine excretion (% of load): pediatrics: Craig and Atkinson and others urge that urine tests be abandoned for children.[1,2] Some recommend 10% to 33% of dose ingested.

Older than 10 years: >16% (4 g) of a 25 g dose should be excreted; this criterion is widely used by Craig, Atkinson, and others.

Still others use ≥23% of a 5 g dose excreted over 5 hours as a criterion of normality. If <3 g is excreted, the diagnosis is most likely to be enterogenous malabsorption. In adults, the 5-hour urine collection was said to be more accurate in detecting intestinal malabsorption than the 1-hour blood test.[3]

Blood: For a 5 g dose, a level of blood d-xylose between 20-40 mg/dL (SI: 1.3-2.7 mmol/L) should be reached in 30-60 minutes and maintained for a further 60 minutes. Craig and Atkinson recognize a lower limit for adults of 25 mg/dL (SI: 1.7 mmol/L) for the 1-hour serum specimen and 20 mg for patients with intermediate renal insufficiency. For 1-hour sample, subjects up to 12 years of age: >20 mg/dL (SI: >1.3 mmol/L) following a 5 g oral d-xylose dose.

In malabsorption syndromes, the highest level in blood may be <20 mg/dL (SI: <1.3 mmol/L), following a 5 g oral d-xylose dose. Blood levels are especially important in older patients and in those with renal disease, liver disease with ascites and with delayed gastric emptying.

Use Use of the d-xylose test is mostly to work up gluten enteropathy, tropical sprue, and celiac disease. In general it is to evaluate possible enterogenous malabsorption syndromes; a test for functional integrity of the jejunum. Classically decreased in tropical and nontropical sprue (gluten-induced enteropathy, celiac disease). It may be abnormal in amyloidosis, lymphoma, small bowel ischemia, Whipple's disease, eosinophilic gastroenteritis, Zollinger-Ellison syndrome, radiation enteritis, scleroderma, following massive resection, bacterial overgrowth, and with certain parasitic infestations.

Limitations Poor renal function, vomiting, decreased or very rapid gastric emptying, hypomotility, intestinal stasis syndromes (eg, surgical blind loops), dehydration/hypovolemia, and certain drugs may cause low urine values **not** secondary to intestinal malabsorption. Normal results have been described with celiac disease. Renal function may present a problem in geriatric and other patients. The usefulness of the test has been somewhat controversial. Krawitt and Beeken studied urine excretion without blood levels and concluded in 1975 that no reason exists to do such d-xylose testing, when jejunal biopsies are available.[4]

Application of both blood and urine examination makes d-xylose considerably more reliable. Availability of small bowel mucosal biopsy by endoscopy must be considered, especially when results of blood and urine tests are inconsistent and before patient is committed to gluten-free diet.

It is not easy to reliably and accurately collect urine in children, leading Craig et al to prefer the 1-hour serum level after 5 g of d-xylose.[1]

Causes of low absorption: Small intestinal bacterial overgrowth, *Giardia lamblia* infestation, hookworm, schistosomiasis, viral gastroenteritis as well as recognized diseases causing malabsorption. Urinary

tests without blood levels have been shown to be misleading. The test may cause mild diarrhea.

Methodology Colorimetry; gas chromatography/mass spectrometry (GC/MS)[5]

Additional Information Normal renal function is necessary if urine values alone are determined. BUN and creatinine serum levels should be measured to exclude patients with renal impairment, resulting in poor xylose excretion and elevated blood xylose levels. Low blood and urine xylose levels indicate malabsorption. For this reason at least a 1- or 2-hour blood specimen is recommended. Elderly individuals with normal intestinal absorption may have elevated blood xylose levels and decreased urine xylose levels due to mild (subclinical) renal impairment. The [^{14}C] d-xylose breath test, if available, is useful for identifying malabsorption due to small intestinal bacterial overgrowth.[1] Pancreatic enzymes are not required for absorption of d-xylose. The d-xylose test is normal in the chronic nonspecific diarrhea syndrome of infancy.

Footnotes

1. Craig RM and Atkinson AJ Jr, "D-xylose Testing: A Review," *Gastroenterology*, 1988, 95(1):223-31.
2. Lifschitz CH and Polanco I, "The D-xylose Test in Pediatrics: Is It Useful?" *Gastroenterology*, 1989, 97(1):246-7.
3. Peled Y, Doron O, Laufer H, et al, "D-xylose Absorption Test. Urine or Blood?" *Dig Dis Sci*, 1991, 36(2):188-92.
4. Krawitt EL and Beeken WL, "Limitations of the Usefulness of the d-Xylose Absorption Test," *Am J Clin Pathol*, 1975, 63:261-3.
5. Deutsch JC, Kolli VR, Santhosh-Kumar CR, et al, "Serum Xylose Analysis by Gas Chromatography/Mass Spectrometry," *Am J Clin Pathol*, 1994, 102(5):595-9.

References

Casellas F, Chicharro L, and Malagelada JR, "Potential Usefulness of Hydrogen Breath Test With D-Xylose in Clinical Management of Intestinal Malabsorption," *Dig Dis Sci*, 1993, 38(2):321-7.
Casellas F and Malagelada JR, "Clinical Applicability of Shortened D-Xylose Breath Test for Diagnosis of Intestinal Malabsorption," *Dig Dis Sci*, 1994, 39(11):2320-6.
Ehrenpreis ED, Gulino SP, Patterson BK, et al, "Kinetics of D-xylose Absorption in Patients With Human Immunodeficiency Virus Enteropathy," *Clin Pharmacol Ther*, 1991, 49(6):632-40.
Hommes FA, ed, *Techniques in Diagnostic Human Biochemical Genetics*, New York, NY: Wiley-Liss, 1991.
Labib M, Gama R, and Marks V, "Predictive Value of D-xylose Absorption Test and Erythrocyte Folate in Adult Coeliac Disease: A Parallel Approach," *Ann Clin Biochem*, 1990, 27(Pt 1):75-7.

E$_2$, Unconjugated *see* Estradiol, Serum *on page 125*

Ecto-5′NT *see* 5′ Nucleotidase *on page 171*

Elastase, Serum *see* Lipase, Serum *on page 158*

Electrolyte Gap *see* Anion Gap *on page 81*

Electrolytes, Serum or Plasma

CPT 80004

Related Information

Anion Gap *on page 81*
Carbon Dioxide, Blood *on page 100*
Chloride, Serum *on page 108*
Drugs of Abuse Testing, Urine *on page 548*
HCO$_3$, Blood *on page 142*
Kidney Stone Analysis *on page 640*
Osmolality, Calculated *on page 172*
Osmolality, Serum *on page 172*
Potassium, Serum or Plasma *on page 188*
Sodium, Blood *on page 199*
Venous Blood Collection *on page 30*

Synonyms Plasma Electrolytes; Serum Electrolytes

Test Commonly Includes Sodium, potassium, chloride; often total CO_2, but in some laboratories pH and pCO_2 are measured and bicarbonate (HCO_3), and CO_2T calculated. Anion gap is reported with electrolytes by some laboratories.

Abstract Used to evaluate electrolyte and acid-base balance

Specimen Serum or plasma

Container Red top tube or green top (heparin) tube

Collection Best to collect without tourniquet if possible. Do **not** allow patient to clench-unclench his/her hand. See Venous Blood Collection *on page 30*.

Storage Instructions Do not freeze.

Reference Range Please see individual listings for test involved.

Use Monitor electrolyte status, screen water balance, diagnose respiratory and metabolic acid-base balance; evaluate hydrational status, diarrhea, dehydration, ketoacidosis in diabetes mellitus and other disorders; evaluate alcoholism and other toxicity states

Limitations Hemolysis and prolonged contact of serum with cells produces elevation of potassium. **The usual order for "electrolytes" does not include magnesium, osmolality, phosphorus, or lactic acid.**

(Continued)

Electrolytes, Serum or Plasma (Continued)

Methodology Ion-selective electrodes (ISE) or flame photometry are used for sodium and potassium. ISE measurement of chloride is common. Total CO_2 may be measured enzymatically and pCO_2 by potentiometric electrode. Sodium and potassium may also be measured by inductively-coupled plasma emission spectrometry.[1]

Additional Information May be performed on heparinized plasma but not on EDTA plasma. Knowledge of pertinent clinical criteria allows for more cost effective ordering of blood electrolytes in patients in whom the information will be clinically significant.[2] The **anion gap**, calculated Na^+ - $(Cl^- + HCO_3^-)$, provides useful information for interpreting acid-base disorders and may be useful for establishing a differential diagnosis in some conditions.[3]

Footnotes

1. Melton LA, Tracy ML, and Moller G, "Screening Trace Elements and Electrolytes in Serum by Inductively-Coupled Plasma Emission Spectrometry," *Clin Chem*, 1990, 36(2):247-50.
2. Lowe RA, Wood AB, Burney RE, et al, "Rational Ordering of Serum Electrolytes: Development of Clinical Criteria," *Ann Emerg Med*, 1987, 16(3):260-9.
3. Oster JR, Perez GO, and Materson BJ, "Use of the Anion Gap in Clinical Medicine," *South Med J*, 1988, 81(2):229-37.

References

Cleland JG and Dargie HJ, "Arrhythmias, Catecholamines and Electrolytes," *Am J Cardiol*, 1988, 62(2):55A-9A.

Ford HC, Lim WC, Chisnall WN, et al, "Renal Function and Electrolyte Levels in Hyperthyroidism: Urinary Protein Excretion and the Plasma Concentrations of Urea, Creatinine, Uric Acid, Hydrogen Ion, and Electrolytes," *Clin Endocrinol (Oxf)*, 1989, 30(3):293-301.

Graber M and Corish D, "The Electrolytes in Hyponatremia," *Am J Kidney Dis*, 1991, 18(5):527-45.

Kapsner CO and Tzamaloukas AH, "Understanding Serum Electrolytes. How to Avoid Mistakes," *Postgrad Med*, 1991, 90(8):151-4, 157-8, 161.

Lowe RA, Arst HF, and Ellis BK, "Rational Ordering of Electrolytes in the Emergency Department," *Ann Emerg Med*, 1991, 20(1):16-21.

McCleane GJ, "Urea and Electrolyte Measurement in Preoperative Surgical Patients," *Anaesthesia*, 1988, 43(5):413-5.

Olshaker JS and Mason JD, "The Usefulness of Serum Electrolytes in the Evaluation of Acute Adult Gastroenteritis," *Ann Emerg Med*, 1989, 18(3):258-60.

Shanbhogue LK, Sikdar T, Jackson M, et al, "Serum Electrolytes and Capillary Blood Gases in the Management of Hypertrophic Pyloric Stenosis," *Br J Surg*, 1992, 79(3):251-3.

Touitou Y, Touitou C, Bogdan A, et al, "Circadian and Seasonal Variations of Electrolytes," *Clin Chim Acta*, 1989, 180(3):245-54.

Electrolytes, Urine

CPT 80003

Related Information

Aldosterone, Urine *on page 68*
Chloride, Urine *on page 109*
Kidney Stone Analysis *on page 640*
Osmolality, Urine *on page 173*
Potassium, Urine *on page 189*
Renin, Plasma *on page 197*
Sodium, Urine *on page 199*
Urine Collection, 24-Hour *on page 30*

Synonyms Urine Electrolytes

Test Commonly Includes Sodium, potassium, and chloride on random or timed collections. Osmolality must be ordered as such.

Abstract Used to estimate fluid and electrolyte balance

Specimen Random, 12-, or 24-hour urine

Collection Specify whether random or timed collection.

Special Instructions Urine osmolality may be ordered with urine electrolytes, usually it must be specifically ordered.

Reference Range Please see individual listings for urine sodium, potassium, and chloride. There is a large diurnal variation in range for spot samples. Na^+/K^+ ratio: 0.90-3.88. Borderline Na^+/K^+ ratio: 0.3-6.0

Use Monitor kidney function, fluid and electrolyte balance, water balance, acid-base balance; evaluate electrolyte composition of urine, correlation with renin and aldosterone studies. Urine sodium levels are appropriate in patients with volume depletion, with acute oliguria, and with decreased plasma sodium. Urine potassium levels are needed in work-up of hypokalemia of unknown etiology (eg, primary aldosteronism, adrenal hyperplasia, Bartter's syndrome, renal tubular acidosis, Fanconi syndrome). Urine chloride is helpful to work up metabolic alkalosis in patients who are not on diuretics; assess dietary salt restriction. Urine electrolytes are used in work-up with aldosterone and renin assays.

Additional Information If a 24-hour timed specimen is collected, other tests which may be ordered simultaneously include Protein, Quantitative, 24-hour Urine and/or Creatinine Clearance (all of which can be collected together). Aldosterone and other adrenocortical steroids enhance reabsorption of sodium and promote excretion of potassium. In subjects with hyponatremia, normal blood volume, and urine Na^+ and Cl^- >40 mmol/L, the differential diagnosis includes hypothyroidism and the syndrome of inappropriate secretion of antidiuretic hormone. See listing Osmolality, Urine *on page 173*. Metabolic alkalosis, urinary chloride excretion, and relationships to Cushing's, Conn's, and Bartter's syndromes are discussed in the following references.

Fetal (amniotic fluid) electrolytes are not predictive of ultimate renal function.[1]

Footnotes

1. Elder JS, O'Grady JP, Ashmead G, et al, "Evaluation of Fetal Renal Function: Unreliability of Fetal Urinary Electrolytes," *J Urol*, 1990, 144(2 Pt 2):574-8.

References

Kamel KS, Ethier JH, Richardson RM, et al, "Urine Electrolytes and Osmolality: When and How to Use Them," *Am J Nephrol*, 1990, 10(2):89-102.

Kamel KS, Magner PO, Ethier JH, et al, "Urine Electrolytes in the Assessment of Extracellular Fluid Volume Contraction," *Am J Nephrol*, 1989, 9(4):344-7.

Knuiman JT, van Poppel G, Burema J, et al, "Multiple Overnight Urine Collections May Be Used for Estimating the Excretion of Electrolytes and Creatinine," *Clin Chem*, 1988, 34(1):135-8.

Sherman RA and Eisinger RP, "The Use (and Misuse) of Urinary Sodium and Chloride Measurements," *JAMA*, 1982, 247:3121-4.

Epinephrine see Metanephrines *on page 165*

Epinephrine, Norepinephrine, Dopamine see Catecholamines, Fractionation, Plasma *on page 103*

Epinephrine, Urine see Catecholamines, Fractionation, Urine *on page 104*

EPO see Erythropoietin, Serum *on this page*

Epoetin Beta see Erythropoietin, Serum *on this page*

Ergocalciferol (Vitamin D₂) see Vitamin D_3, Serum *on page 218*

Erythrocyte Cholinesterase see Acetylcholinesterase, Red Cell *on page 62*

Erythrocyte Porphobilinogen Deaminase see Porphobilinogen Deaminase, Erythrocyte *on page 185*

Erythrocyte Uroporphyrinogen I Synthase see Porphobilinogen Deaminase, Erythrocyte *on page 185*

Erythropoietin, Serum

CPT 82668

Related Information

Autologous Transfusion, Preoperative Deposit *on page 603*
Blood Volume *on page 306*
Ferritin, Serum *on page 127*
Hemoglobin *on page 323*
Iron and Total Iron Binding Capacity/Transferrin *on page 150*
Red Cell Count *on page 344*
Red Cell Mass *on page 345*
Viscosity, Blood *on page 350*
Vitamin B_{12} Unsaturated Binding Capacity *on page 352*

Synonyms EPO; S-Epo

Applies to Epoetin Beta

Test Commonly Includes Serum iron

Abstract A glycoprotein formed mainly in the kidney, erythropoietin (EP) has been purified and the gene cloned. The gene is found on chromosome 7. It stimulates erythropoiesis. Hypoxia increases erythropoietin production; bilateral nephrectomy drastically reduces erythropoietin synthesis and thereby inhibits erythropoiesis.

Cloning has led to the production of erythropoietin by recombinant technology (epoetin beta), now available therapeutically. Its benefits, risks, and optimal dosage are not as yet entirely defined.[1]

Patient Preparation Recent exposure to radioisotopes may interfere if assay method is by RIA.

Specimen Serum

Container Red top tube

Special Instructions Done only by a few laboratories

Reference Range Radioimmunoassay: 5-36 mU/mL[2] (SI: 5-36 IU/L); immunoassay: negative: <10 mU/mL (SI:<10 IU/L), equivocal: 11-48 mU/mL (SI: 11-48 IU/L), positive: >48 mU/mL (SI: >48 IU/L). EPO increases in pregnancy, in which significantly higher levels are found before the 24th week.[3] Reference values in children have been published.[4]

Use Investigate obscure anemias and the anemia of end-stage renal disease. The availability of assays for EP should provide means to identify cases in which epoetin beta therapy may become helpful.[5] Certain tumors may produce erythropoietin, giving rise to otherwise unexplained polycythemia (eg, hemangioblastoma of cerebellum, pheochromocytoma, hepatoma, nephroblastoma, and rarely leiomyomas, renal cysts, and renal adenocarcinoma). It may be used to differentiate secondary from primary polycythemia, but overlap exists between these groups.[6] S-Epo was below its reference range in 34 of 36 patients with polycythemia vera, elevated in cases of secondary polycythemia and normal in all but one of the cases of relative polycythemia.[7]

Limitations Hazards: Therapeutic administration of erythropoietin has been associated with vascular thrombosis with reports of neutropenia, thrombocytopenia, infection, and other possible complications in premature infants.[8] Serum erythropoietin levels may be increased by phlebotomy, androgens, TSH, ACTH, angiotensin, epinephrine, and growth hormone levels. Transfusions and estrogens may lower erythropoietin levels.

Methodology The development of recombinant erythropoietin[9] (epoetin beta) has made available assays from clinical specimens using radioimmunoassay (RIA),[10,11] enzyme-linked immunoassays (ELISA), immunoradiometric assays (IRMA),[6] and immunoprecipitin assays.[12]

Additional Information

Epoetin beta has diminished need for transfusions in very low birthweight infants, but further study is needed.[1,8]

Winearls et al[13] report 10 patients with end stage renal disease, all of whom responded with a good increase in their hemoglobin levels, but complications were recognized. Eschbach et al treated 25 patients with end-stage renal disease.[14] Eighteen had been previously treated with blood transfusions. Twelve of these 18 patients no longer needed blood transfusion. Iron therapy was also needed. Complications were seen.

In the anemia of renal disease the serum erythropoietin level is generally lower than expected. Plasma erythropoietin is inappropriately low in adult nephrotic syndrome mostly because of renal/urinary loss of the protein which contributes to the anemia.[15] In chronic iron deficiency the level of erythropoietin is increased, but the increase may not be as high as expected for the degree of anemia.

Erythropoietin has been used to improve the yield of autologous units of blood before orthopedic surgery. Erythropoietin was given twice a week for 21 days, 600 units/kg, intravenously.[16]

Erythropoietin response to anemia (excluding renal disease and pregnancy) in older subjects is similar to that of younger subjects.[17]

Footnotes
1. Strauss RG, "Erythropoietin and Neonatal Anemia," *N Engl J Med*, 1994, 330(17):1227-8.
2. Goldwasser E and Sherwood JB, "Radioimmune Assay of Erythropoietin," *Br J Haematol*, 1981, 48:359-63.
3. Riikonen S, Saijonmaa O, Jarvenpaa AL, et al, "Serum Concentrations of Erythropoietin in Healthy and Anemic Pregnant Women," *Scand J Clin Lab Invest*, 1994, 54(8):653-7.
4. Pressac M, Morgant G, Farnier MA, et al, "Enzyme Immunoassay of Serum Erythropoietin in Healthy Children: Reference Values," *Ann Clin Biochem*, 1991, 28(Pt 4):345-50.
5. Spivak JL, "The Clinical Physiology of Erythropoietin," *Semin Hematol*, 1993, 30(4 Suppl 6):2-11.
6. Casadevall N, "Determination of Serum Erythropoietin. Its Value in the Differential Diagnosis of Polycythemias," *Nouv Rev Fr Hematol*, 1994, 36(2):173-6.
7. Birgegard G and Wide L, "Serum Erythropoietin in the Diagnosis of Polycythaemia and After Phlebotomy Treatment," *Br J Haematol*, 1992, 81(4):603-6.
8. Maier RF, Obladen M, Scigalla P, et al, "The Effect of Epoetin Beta (Recombinant Human Erythropoietin) on the Need for Transfusion in Very-Low-Birth-Weight Infants. European Multicentre Erythropoietin Study Group," *N Engl J Med*, 1994, 330(17):1173-8.
9. Egrie JC, Cotes PM, Lane J, et al, "Development of Radioimmunoassays for Human Erythropoietin Using Recombinant Erythropoietin as Tracer and Immunogen," *J Immunol Methods*, 1987, 99(2):235-41.
10. Mason-Garcia M, Beckman BS, Brookins JW, et al, "Development of a New Radioimmunoassay for Erythropoietin Using Recombinant Erythropoietin," *Kidney Int*, 1990, 38(5):969-75.
11. Schlageter MH, Toubert ME, Podgorniak MP, et al, "Radioimmunoassay of Erythropoietin: Analytical Performance and Clinical Use in Hematology," *Clin Chem*, 1990, 36(10):1731-5.
12. Widness JA, Schmidt RL, Veng-Pedersen P, et al, "A Sensitive and Specific Erythropoietin Immunoprecipitation Assay: Application to Pharmacokinetic Studies," *J Lab Clin Med*, 1992, 119(3):285-94.
13. Winearls CG, Oliver DO, Pippard MJ, et al, "Effect of Human Erythropoietin Derived From Recombinant DNA on the Anaemia of Patients Maintained by Chronic Haemodialysis," *Lancet*, 1986, 2(8517):1175-8.
14. Eschbach JW, Egrie JC, Downing MR, et al, "Correction of the Anemia of End-Stage Renal Disease With Recombinant Human Erythropoietin. Results of a Combined Phase I and II Clinical Trial," *N Engl J Med*, 1987, 316(2):73-8.
15. Vaziri ND, Kaupke CJ, Barton CH, et al, "Plasma Concentration and Urinary Excretion of Erythropoietin in Adult Nephrotic Syndrome," *Am J Med*, 1992, 92(1):35-40.
16. Goodnough LT, Rudnick S, Price TH, et al, "Increased Preoperative Collection of Autologous Blood With Recombinant Human Erythropoietin Therapy," *N Engl J Med*, 1989, 321(17):1163-8.
17. Powers JS, Krantz SB, Collins JC, et al, "Erythropoietin Response to Anemia as a Function of Age," *J Am Geriatr Soc*, 1991, 39(1):30-2.

References

Beguin Y, Clemons GK, Pootrakul P, et al, "Quantitative Assessment of Erythropoiesis and Functional Classification of Anemia Based on Measurements of Serum Transferrin Receptor and Erythropoietin," *Blood*, 1993, 81(4):1067-76.
Greendyke RM, Sharma K, and Gifford FR, "Serum Levels of Erythropoietin and Selected Other Cytokines in Patients With Anemia of Chronic Disease," *Am J Clin Pathol*, 1994, 101(3):338-41.
Hubbard JD and Wheeler DJ, "Erythropoietin Measurement by EIA," *Lab Med*, 1989, 20:849-54.
Ifudu O, Feldman J, and Friedman EA, "The Intensity of Hemodialysis and the Response to Erythropoietin in Patients With End-Stage Renal Disease," *N Engl J Med*, 1995, 334:420-5.
Johnson GR, "Erythropoietin," *Br Med Bull*, 1989, 45(2):506-14.
Kario K, Matsuo T, and Nakao K, "Serum Erythropoietin Levels in the Elderly," *Gerontology*, 1991, 37(6):345-8.

Metcalf D, "Haemopoietic Growth Factors 1," *Lancet*, 1989, 1(8642):825-7.
Metcalf D, "Haemopoietic Growth Factors 2: Clinical Applications," *Lancet*, 1989, 1(8643):885-7.
Nissenson AR, "Erythropoietin Overview - 1993," *Blood Purif*, 1994, 12(1):6-13.
Ridley DM, Dawkins F, and Perlin E, "Erythropoietin: A Review," *J Natl Med Assoc*, 1994, 86(2):129-35.
Spivak JL, "Erythropoietin," *Blood Rev*, 1989, 3(2):130-5.
Tanebe M, Teshima S, Hanyu T, et al, "Rapid and Sensitive Method for Erythropoietin in Serum," *Clin Chem*, 1992, 38(9):1752-5.
Zanjani ED and Ascensao JL, "Erythropoietin," *Transfusion*, 1989, 29(1):46-57.

Estradiol, Serum

CPT 82670

Related Information

Cortisol, Blood *on page 112*
Estrogens, Nonpregnant, Urine *on next page*
Follicle Stimulating Hormone *on page 129*
Luteinizing Hormone, Blood or Urine *on page 163*
Prolactin *on page 192*

Synonyms E_2, Unconjugated

Abstract Estradiol is the most active endogenous estrogen. It is derived from ovaries, testes, and placentas[1] and is the principle estrogen of ovarian origin.

Patient Preparation Recent exposure to radioactivity (eg, scan) may interfere if assay method is RIA.

Specimen Serum

Container Red top tube

Sampling Time In females, the phase of the menstrual cycle may be needed for interpretation.

Collection Separate serum and freeze within 1 hour.[1]

Reference Range Children 6 months to 10 years: <15 pg/mL (SI: <55 pmol/L); adult males: 10-50 pg/mL (SI: 37-184 pmol/L); females: premenopausal: 30-400 pg/mL (SI: 110-1468 pmol/L) (depending on phase of menstrual cycle); postmenopausal: 0-30 pg/mL (SI: 0-110 pmol/L)

Use Estradiol provides indication of ovarian function. It may be useful to evaluate infertility, menstrual irregularities, and sexual precocity in females. Other conditions causing elevations include the polycystic ovary syndrome and feminizing tumors of the ovary or adrenals. Ovarian failure, hypogonadism, and Turner syndrome cause decreased levels. In males, estradiol may be useful to evaluate feminizing states. Oral contraceptives lower estradiol levels and clomiphene will increase them.

Limitations In menopausal females, order **estrogens** rather than estradiol. Estradiol increases with hepatic cirrhosis. Oral contraceptives increase serum levels. Estradiol level can be normal in women who have hypogonadism.[2]

Contraindications Should not be used in pregnant females or to evaluate fetal well-being because **it does not measure estriol.** Estriol comprises >90% of maternal estrogens. However, Guillaume et al report the use of estradiol in the effective diagnosis of ectopic pregnancy (low values are seen).[3]

Methodology Radioimmunoassay (RIA) following extraction; noncompetitive immunoassay[4]

Additional Information Estradiol measurements, in conjunction with gonadotropin levels, can be used to categorize amenorrhea syndromes, including anorexia nervosa. In premature ovarian failure, low serum or urine estrogens are accompanied by increased FSH and LH, in contrast to levels seen with hypothalamic or pituitary disease. Estradiol levels are very low in gonadal dysgenesis, and may be very high in hormonally active ovarian neoplasms.[5] Estradiol augments the amplitude of prolactin pulsatile secretion. Very high serum estradiol levels are not detrimental to clinical outcome of *in vitro* fertilization.[6]

Footnotes
1. Leavelle DE, "Estradiol, Serum," *Mayo Medical Laboratories Interpretive Handbook*, Rochester, MN: Mayo Medical Laboratories, 1994, 190.
2. Vance ML, "Hypopituitarism," *N Engl J Med*, 1994, 330(23):1651-62.
3. Guillaume J, Benjamin F, Sicuranza BJ, et al, "Serum Estradiol as an Aid in the Diagnosis of Ectopic Pregnancy," *Obstet Gynecol*, 1990, 76(6):1126-9.
4. Barnard G and Kohen F, "Idiometric Assay: Noncompetitive Immunoassay for Small Molecules Typified by the Measurement of Estradiol in Serum," *Clin Chem*, 1990, 36(11):1945-50.
5. Young RH and Scully RE, "Sex Cordstromal, Steroid Cell, and Other Ovarian Tumors With Endocrine, Parendocrine, and Paraneoplastic Manifestations," *Blaustein's Pathology of the Female Genital Tract*, 4th ed, Kurman RJ, ed, New York, NY: Springer-Verlag, 1994, 783-847.
6. Chenette PE, Sauer MV, and Paulson RJ, "Very High Serum Estradiol Levels Are Not Detrimental to Clinical Outcome of In Vitro Fertilization," *Fertil Steril*, 1990, 54(5):858-63.

References

Bouve J, De Boever J, Leyseele D, et al, "Direct Enzyme Immunoassay of Estradiol in Serum of Women Enrolled in an In Vitro Fertilization and Embryo Transfer Program," *Clin Chem*, 1992, 38(8 Pt 1):1409-13.
Darne J, McGarrigle HH, and Lachelin GC, "Saliva Oestriol, Oestradiol, Oestrone, and Progesterone Levels in Pregnancy: Spontaneous Labour at Term Is Preceded by a Rise in the Saliva Oestriol:Progesterone Ratio," *Br J Obstet Gynaecol*, 1987, 94(3):227-35.

(Continued)

Estradiol, Serum (Continued)

Kiel DP, Baron JA, Plymate SR, et al, "Sex Hormones and Lipoproteins in Men," *Am J Med*, 1989, 87(1):35-9.

Phillips GB, Yano K, and Stemmerman GN, "Decrease in Serum Estradiol Values With Storage," *N Engl J Med*, 1984, 311(25):1635.

Pont A, Goldman ES, Sugar AM, et al, "Ketoconazole-Induced Increase in Estradiol-Testosterone Ratio," *Arch Intern Med*, 1985, 145(8):1429-31.

Potischman N, Falk RT, Laiming VA, et al, "Reproducibility of Laboratory Assays for Steroid Hormones and Sex Hormone-Binding Globulin," *Cancer Res*, 1994, 54(20):5363-7.

Stewart MO, Whittaker PG, Persson B, et al, "A Longitudinal Study of Circulating Progesterone, Oestradiol, hCG and hPL During Pregnancy in Type 1 Diabetic Mothers," *Br J Obstet Gynaecol*, 1989, 96(4):415-23.

Studd J, Savvas M, Waston N, et al, "The Relationship Between Plasma Estradiol and the Increase in Bone Density in Postmenopausal Women After Treatment With Subcutaneous Hormone Implants," *Am J Obstet Gynecol*, 1990, 163(5 Pt 1):1474-9.

Veldhuis JD, Evans WS, and Stumpf PG, "Mechanisms That Subserve Estradiol's Induction of Increased Prolactin Concentrations: Evidence of Amplitude Modulation of Spontaneous Prolactin Secretory Bursts," *Am J Obstet Gynecol*, 1989, 161(5):1149-58.

Estriol, Free *see* Estriol, Unconjugated, Pregnancy, Blood or Urine on this page

Estriol, Unconjugated, Pregnancy, Blood or Urine

CPT 82677

Synonyms Estriol, Free; 16-Hydroxyestradiol; Unconjugated Estriol, Pregnancy

Abstract Estriol is the major estrogen of pregnancy, but it is no longer considered very useful for the detection of fetal distress.

Patient Preparation Avoid recently administered radioisotopes if assay method is RIA.

Specimen Serum or plasma, urine

Container Red top tube or green top (heparin) tube for blood; 24-hour urine container

Collection Since circadian rhythms exist, serum estriol should be drawn at the same time of day on each visit.

Causes for Rejection Recently administered radioisotopes if RIA is used for assay

Reference Range Urine concentrations of estriol increase with gestation, from 2 mg/24 hours (SI: 7 nmol/day) at 16 weeks gestation to 10-40 mg/24 hours (SI: 35-139 nmol/day) at term.[1,2] A wide normal range exists. **Serum** levels in the tables do not represent reference ranges for all laboratories. Different assays lead to wide differences of estriol in the same sample.

Normal Serum or Plasma Unconjugated Estriol Values[2,3,4] (Fetal Well-Being)

Weeks of Gestation	µg/L	SI: nmol/L
25	3.5-10.0	12-35
28	4.0-12.5	14-43
30	4.5-14.0	16-49
32	5.0-16.0	17-55
34	5.5-18.5	19-64
36	7.0-25.0	24-87
37	8.0-28.0	28-97
38	9.0-32.0	31-111
39	10.0-34.0	35-118
40	5.0-40.0	17-139

Note: This table is to be used to monitor fetal well-being.

Possible Panic Range Value of urinary estriol <4 mg/24 hours or 40% below mean of three prior values demands immediate evaluation of fetal well-being.

Use Serial estriol values, depending upon the integrity of the fetal-placental-maternal unit, have been thought to assess fetal well-being and placental function in later pregnancy, especially in high risk settings.[1,2] Estriol decreases in fetal adrenal aplasia or hypoplasia and anencephaly,[2] and increases with high fetal adrenocortical activity (eg, congenital adrenal hyperplasia).[3]

Limitations Single values are almost impossible to interpret; trends in a series of measurements are much more important. May be low in case of placental sulfatase deficiency in the presence of a healthy baby. Other causes of decreased estriol levels include subjects living at high altitudes, on penicillin or related drugs, corticosteroids, dexamethasone, betamethasone, diuretics, Mandelamine®, probenecid, estrogens, phenazopyridine, meprobamate, phenolphthalein, cascara, senna, and glutethimide.[2] It is decreased with anemia and severe liver disease.[2] Estriol may be increased with multiple pregnancy[2] and with oxytocin.[3] It

is not reliable in the presence of renal disease.[2,3] Use of the test has become controversial.[2] It is no longer done in a number of laboratories. **Few feel that a role for estriol remains with other more accurate and reliable means to monitor fetal well-being available.**

Serum Unconjugated Estriol Medians for Risk Prediction of Fetal Chromosomal Abnormalities

Weeks of Gestation	Median	
	µg/L	SI: nmol/L
15	0.82	2.83
16	1.16	4.01
17	1.45	5.02
18	1.73	5.98
19	2.06	7.13
20	2.36	8.16
21	2.70	9.34

Note: Data courtesy of Dr Linda Bradley, Director, Biochemical Genetics, Vivigen, Santa Fe, NM. (Every laboratory should establish their own reference data.)

Methodology Radioimmunoassay (RIA) or high performance liquid chromatography (HPLC)

Additional Information Estriol, E_3, is synthesized in the placenta from 16-α-hydroxydehydroepiandrosterone of fetal origin. Thus, normal production can serve as a measure of the integrity of the fetoplacental unit. Sequential monitoring of estriol in high risk pregnancy has made possible early intervention and fetal salvage. Chronically low estriol values are found in intrauterine growth retardation but also are sometimes seen in normal pregnancy. A decreasing trend is indicative of fetal distress. The sensitivity and specificity of this test for detecting fetal distress are very poor; **thus its use for this purpose has been largely abandoned.**

Since estriol comprises approximately 90% of the estrogen in the maternal urine in later pregnancy, many laboratories measure total urinary estrogen levels instead of estriol.

Combined evaluation of unconjugated serum estriol, maternal serum hCG, maternal serum AFP, and maternal age has value in predicting risk for fetal chromosomal abnormalities during pregnancy. The use of maternal serum AFP, hCG, and estriol predicts 65% of Down syndrome, as opposed to 28% if only serum AFP is used.[4,5,6] An opposing view of unconjugated estriol use is presented by Macri et al.[7]

Estriol/creatinine ratios have been advocated for evaluation of urinary estriol excretion. Total and unconjugated estriol levels by RIA are the most used plasma estriol assays.[8,9]

Footnotes

1. Knuppel RA and Goodlin RC, "Maternal-Placental-Fetal Unit; Fetal & Early Neonatal Physiology," *Current Obstetric & Gynecologic Diagnosis & Treatment 1987*, Pernoll ML and Benson RC, eds, Norwalk, CT: Appleton & Lange, 1987, 135-60.
2. Catanzarite VA, Perkins RP, and Pernoll ML, "Assessment of Fetal Well-Being," *Current Obstetric & Gynecologic Diagnosis & Treatment 1987*, Pernoll ML and Benson RC, eds, Norwalk, CT: Appleton & Lange, 1987, 279-302.
3. Speroff L, Glass RH, and Kase NG, *Clinical Gynecologic Endocrinology and Infertility*, 4th ed, Baltimore, MD: Williams & Wilkins, 1989.
4. White RS 3d, "Down Syndrome: Current Screening Technique," *South Med J*, 1989, 82(12):1483-6.
5. Heyl PS, Miller W, and Canick JA, "Maternal Serum Screening for Aneuploid Pregnancy by Alpha-Fetoprotein, hCG, and Unconjugated Estriol," *Obstet Gynecol*, 1990, 76(6):1025-31.
6. MacDonald ML, Wagner RM, and Slotnick RN, "Sensitivity and Specificity of Screening for Down Syndrome with Alpha-Fetoprotein, hCG, Unconjugated Estriol, and Maternal Age," *Obstet Gynecol*, 1991, 77(1):63-8.
7. Macri JN, Kasturi RV, Krantz DA, et al, "Maternal Serum Down Syndrome Screening: Unconjugated Estriol Is Not Useful," *Am J Obstet Gynecol*, 1990, 162(3):672-3.
8. Ray DA, "Biochemical Fetal Assessment," *Clin Obstet Gynecol*, 1987, 30(4):887-98.
9. Carroll JC, "Maternal Serum Screening," *Can Fam Physician*, 1994, 40:1756-64.

References

Macri JN, Kasturi RV, Krantz DA, et al, "Sensitivity and Specificity of Screening for Down Syndrome With Alpha-Fetoprotein, hCG, Unconjugated Estriol, and Maternal Age," *Obstet Gynecol*, 1991, 77(6):63-8.

Estrogens, Nonpregnant, Urine

CPT 82672

Related Information

Estradiol, Serum *on previous page*
Follicle Stimulating Hormone *on page 129*
Luteinizing Hormone, Blood or Urine *on page 163*
Progesterone *on page 191*
Urine Collection, 24-Hour *on page 30*

Synonyms Total Urinary Estrogens

Test Commonly Includes Urine volume, creatinine concentration and concentration of estradiol (E2), estrone (E1), estriol (E3), and estetrol (E4), unconjugated

Abstract In the normal cycle, estrogen increase begins in the middle of the proliferative phase.

Specimen 24-hour urine

Container No preservative

Collection Keep specimen on **ice** during collection.

Reference Range Children: <10 µg/24 hours (SI: <35 µmol/day); male: 15-40 µg/24 hours (SI: 52-139 µmol/day); female: menstruating: 15-80 µg/24 hours (SI: 52-277 µmol/day), postmenopausal: <20 µg/24 hours (SI: <69 µmol/day) (values at Mayo Medical Laboratories)

Use Predict ovulation; the increase of estrogen occurs before that of LH and progesterone;[1] evaluate hypoestrogenic and hyperestrogenic states, including hypopituitarism, hypogonadism, adrenal hyperplasia, neoplasms, anorexia nervosa, and stress

Contraindications This test is **not** used to assess fetal well-being.

Methodology Extraction and separation of estrogens, quantitation by spectroscopy or fluorometry. A method of estimation of urinary estrogen by competitive latex agglutination inhibition is described.[1]

Additional Information Urinary estrogens may be increased in adrenal hyperplasia and in functional ovarian neoplasms. Estrogens are excreted throughout pregnancy in increasing amounts. Estrogens are decreased in primary or secondary ovarian failure, with forms of gonadal dysgenesis, and with normal menopause. The use of this test is generally the same as that of serum or plasma estradiol. **With the advent of specific hormone immunoassays, total estrogen measurements have largely been replaced by more specific methods.**

Footnotes

1. Ishikawa M, Hoshiai H, Tozawa H, et al,"Monitoring Follicular Maturation Through Measurement of Urinary Estrogen Excretion by Latex Agglutination Inhibition Reaction," *Fertil Steril*, 1987, 48(4):688-90.

References

Avioli LV, "Hyperparathyroidism, Estrogens, and Osteoporosis," *Hosp Pract (Off Ed)*, 1991, 26(1):115-22, 127-8, 133-4.

Bartelsmeyer JA and Petrie RH, "Erythema Nodosum, Estrogens, and Pregnancy," *Clin Obstet Gynecol*, 1990, 33(4):777-81.

Goldin BR and Gorbach SL, "Effect of Diet on the Plasma Levels, Metabolism, and Excretion of Estrogens," *Am J Clin Nutr*, 1988, 48(3 Suppl):787-90.

Katsouyanni K, Boyle P, and Trichopoulos D, "Diet and Urine Estrogens Among Postmenopausal Women," *Oncology*, 1991, 48(6):490-4.

Longcope C, Goldfield SR, Brambilla DJ, et al, "Androgens, Estrogens, and Sex Hormone-Binding Globulin in Middle-Aged Men," *J Clin Endocrinol Metab*, 1990, 71(6):1442-6.

Longcope C, Herbert PN, McKinlay SM, et al, "The Relationship of Total and Free Estrogens and Sex Hormone-Binding Globulin With Lipoproteins in Women," *J Clin Endocrinol Metab*, 1990, 71(1):67-72.

Silberstein SD and Merriam GR, "Estrogens, Progestins, and Headache," *Neurology*, 1991, 41(6):786-93.

Stampfer MJ, "Smoking, Estrogen, and Prevention of Heart Disease in Women," *Mayo Clin Proc*, 1989, 64(12):1553-7.

Etiocholanolone *see* 17-Ketosteroids Fractionation, Urine *on page 152*

Fast Hemoglobins *see* Glycated Hemoglobin *on page 140*

Fasting Bilirubin Test *see* Bilirubin, Total *on page 86*

Fasting Blood Sugar *see* Glucose, Fasting *on page 137*

Fat, Quantitative, 72-Hour Stool Collection *see* Fecal Fat, Quantitative, 72-Hour Collection *on this page*

FBS *see* Glucose, Fasting *on page 137*

Fe and TIBC *see* Iron and Total Iron Binding Capacity/Transferrin *on page 150*

Fecal Fat, Quantitative, 72-Hour Collection

CPT 82710

Related Information

d-Xylose Absorption Test *on page 122*
Fat, Semiquantitative, Stool *on page 634*
Meat Fibers, Stool *on page 642*
Methylene Blue Stain, Stool *on page 642*
pH, Stool *on page 648*
Vitamin D₃, Serum *on page 218*

Synonyms Fat, Quantitative, 72-Hour Stool Collection; Quantitative Fecal Fat, 72-Hour Collection; Stool Fat, Quantitative

Abstract Nonspecific test for investigation of malabsorption and steatorrhea. If fat malabsorption occurs, the physician may consider the fat soluble vitamins A, D, E, and K. Of these, vitamin D lends itself to investigation not only with serum levels but with investigation of bone density as well.

Patient Preparation 100-150 g/day fat diet for 3 days before and during 72-hour collection period. Barium interferes.

Specimen 72-hour stool collection, usually in the fourth, fifth, and sixth days of the 100 g/day fat diet

Container Plastic stool container, preweighed

Sampling Time 72 hours; shorter collection periods are not usually acceptable

Collection Specimen should be refrigerated during its collection. A dietary fat intake of 50-150 g/day for **at least** 2 days before and during the collection period.

Storage Instructions Freeze on dry ice if analysis is not to be done promptly.

Causes for Rejection Improper container (ie, paper cartons, coffee cans, plastic bags, etc), foreign matter other than feces inside of container (ie, spoons, tongue depressors, plastic bags, toilet paper, etc), patient not on special diet, not 72-hour collection, inadequate labeling

Special Instructions Date and time collection started, date and time collection finished are needed.

Reference Range 2-7 g/24 hours (SI: 2-7 g/day); <20% of total solids

Use Diagnose the presence of steatorrhea, supporting a diagnosis of one of the malabsorption syndromes, including nontropical sprue, Crohn's disease, chronic pancreatitis, cystic fibrosis, Whipple's disease, or tuberculous enteropathy

Limitations Fecal fat collection does not provide a diagnostic explanation for the presence of steatorrhea. Stool fat collection is an unpleasant experience for the patient as well as others. It may be within normal limits in the presence of advanced loss of pancreatic parenchyma. Fecal fat measurement is regarded as unnecessary for investigation of pancreatic insufficiency.[1]

Contraindications Patient taking mineral oil

Methodology Extraction and titration of long chain fatty acids by sodium hydroxide. Fatty acids represent 60% to 80% of total fecal lipids.

Additional Information Identification of types of stool fat (eg, free fatty acids, triglycerides, neutral fats, phospholipids) is of little value. Fecal fat excretion >7 g/day is abnormal but nonspecific. Small intestinal, pancreatic or hepatobiliary diseases may cause such increased excretion. Increased fecal fat levels do not differentiate between pancreatic (maldigestion) and intestinal (malabsorption) steatorrhea.[2]

Mechanisms in the production of diarrhea include secretory and osmotic diarrhea and motility disorders. A summary of possible laboratory investigation of the first may include stool cultures, gastrin, 5-hydroxyindoleacetic acid, calcitonin, and vasoactive intestinal polypeptide. For the second, lactose tolerance test may be appropriate. The third category may include TSH and FT₄ for hyperthyroidism.

Footnotes

1. Holmes GK and Hill PG, "Do We Still Need to Measure Faecal Fat?" *Br Med J (Clin Res Ed)*, 1988, 296(6636):1552-3.
2. Bai JC, Andrush A, Matelo G, et al, "Fecal Fat Concentration in the Differential Diagnosis of Steatorrhea," *Am J Gastroenterol*, 1989, 84(1):27-30.

References

Beath S, Willis K, Hooley I, et al, "New Method for Determining Faecal Fat Excretion in Infancy," *Arch Dis Child*, 1993, 69(5):545-7.

Colombo C, Maiavacca R, Ronchi M, et al, "The Steatocrit: A Simple Method for Monitoring Fat Malabsorption in Patients With Cystic Fibrosis," *J Pediatr Gastroenterol Nutr*, 1987, 6(6):926-30.

"Dietary Fat Intake, 72-Hour Excretion, and Sudan Stain for Fecal Fat," *Gastroenterology*, 1989, 97(2):550-1.

Fine KD and Fordtran JS, "The Effect of Diarrhea on Fecal Fat Excretion," *Gastroenterology*, 1992, 102(6):1936-9.

Greenberger NJ and Isselbacher KJ, "Disorders of Absorption," *Harrison's Principles of Internal Medicine*, 13th ed, Isselbacher KJ, Braunwald E, Wilson JD, et al, eds, New York, NY: McGraw-Hill Inc, 1994, 1386-403.

Simko V and Michael S, "Absorptive Capacity for Dietary Fat in Elderly Patients With Debilitating Disorders," *Arch Intern Med*, 1989, 149(3):557-60.

Sokol RJ, Reardon MC, Accurso FJ, et al, "Fat-Soluble-Vitamin Status During the First Year of Life in Infants With Cystic Fibrosis Identified by Screening of Newborns," *Am J Clin Nutr*, 1989, 50(5):1064-71.

FEP *see* Protoporphyrin, Free Erythrocyte *on page 195*

Ferritin, Serum

CPT 82728

Related Information

Complete Blood Count *on page 312*
Erythropoietin, Serum *on page 124*
Hemoglobin *on page 323*
Iron and Total Iron Binding Capacity/Transferrin *on page 150*
Iron Stain, Bone Marrow *on page 328*
Lead, Urine *on page 557*
Liver Biopsy *on page 48*
Liver Profile *on page 161*
Protoporphyrin, Zinc, Blood *on page 196*
Red Cell Count *on page 344*
Transferrin *on page 209*

Applies to Hepatic Iron Index; HLA-A3; Liver Iron Concentration; Transferrin Receptor

Abstract Used as an aid in distinction of iron deficiency anemias from others, ferritin serum level generally reflects cellular iron stores. It is used (Continued)

Ferritin, Serum *(Continued)*

to support diagnosis and follow therapy of patients with hemochromatosis. Ferritin, an acute phase reactant, appears higher than is anticipated.

Patient Preparation No recent radioactive scans or other radioactivity if laboratory uses RIA for ferritin.

Specimen Serum

Container Red top tube

Storage Instructions Separate serum from clot and freeze immediately in plastic vial.

Reference Range 1 ng/mL of serum ferritin in normal subjects corresponds to approximately 8 mg of storage iron. Ferritin increases in adulthood in men to about the fifth decade and in women after the menopause. Typical reference range: male: 20-250 ng/mL (SI: 20-250 µg/L); female: younger than 40 years: 11-122 ng/mL (SI: 11-122 µg/L), older than 40 years: 12-263 ng/mL (SI: 12-263 µg/L).[1] Reference ranges of ferritin assays vary with age and sex. Values must be considered critically in the presence of inflammation.

Critical Values Iron deficiency: <10 ng/mL

Use Useful in the differential diagnosis of hypochromic, microcytic anemias. **Decreased** in iron deficiency anemia and increased in iron overload. Ferritin levels correlate with and are useful in evaluation of total body storage iron.

In hemochromatosis, both ferritin and iron saturation are increased. Ferritin levels in hemochromatosis may be >1000 ng/mL (SI: >1000 µg/L), but a normal serum ferritin cannot rule out homozygous hemochromatosis. Screening for hemochromatosis is better done with transferrin saturation. If saturation is >60% in men or >50% in women, serum ferritin should be assayed. If it is high for age and sex, liver biopsy may be considered.[2] Normal ferritin rules out iron deficiency anemia.[3]

Limitations Ferritin escapes from necrotic hepatocytes. It is more often increased in alcoholics who are actively abusing than in individuals with other liver diseases such as autoimmune hepatitis and hepatitis C. A quarter of patients with chronic hepatitis have increased ferritin.[4] In the presence of liver disease, with inflammation such as rheumatoid arthritis, with malignancy or with iron therapy, iron deficiency may not be reflected by low serum ferritin. Ferritin determinations are not reliable in infants on iron therapy. Bone marrow aspiration may be needed in some settings, such as low-normal ferritin and low serum iron in the presence of apparent anemia of chronic disease, low-normal ferritin in the presence of liver disease.[1]

Contraindications Ferritin is not of value to evaluate iron stores in alcoholics with liver disease. Ferritin is higher in abusing cirrhotics than in abstaining cirrhotics. The highest ferritin seen in a series was from a subject with acute hepatitis B.

Ferritin is elevated in hyperthyroidism.[6]

Methodology Radioimmunometric, radioimmunoassay (RIA), enzyme-linked immunosorbent assay (ELISA), fluoroenzymoimmunometric assay, colorimetric, immunoenzymometric[5]

Additional Information Other than a bone marrow examination, serum ferritin is the most reliable indicator of total body iron stores. When combined with serum iron and percent saturation of iron binding capacity/transferrin, it can usually differentiate the microcytic hypochromic anemias into iron deficiency anemia (ferritin low, iron low, saturation low, TIBC high, transferrin high), the anemia of chronic disease (ferritin normal or high, iron low, normal to low transferrin or TIBC), or thalassemia (ferritin normal or high). See Anemia Flow Chart in the Hematology Appendix *on page 355*. In iron deficiency, the **red cell distribution width** is increased, while it is normal with heterozygous alpha or beta thalassemia trait. The **MCV** is reduced in iron deficiency and alpha or beta thalassemia trait; each is normal with lead poisoning. Ferritin is low with combined iron deficiency and thalassemia. **In adults**, serum ferritin level ≤10 ng/mL indicates iron deficiency.

High serum ferritin may be associated with inflammation, liver disease, megaloblastic anemia, hemolytic anemia, sideroblastic anemia, thalassemia, iron overload (hemochromatosis, hemosiderosis), and malignant diseases. The latter include leukemia and malignant lymphoma. Very high levels usually indicate iron overload. Oral and injected iron increase ferritin levels. Increased serum ferritin is considered a risk factor in primary hepatocellular carcinoma.[2,7]

Primary hemochromatosis is inherited as an autosomal recessive trait, but clinically it is much more common in males. Only homozygotes bear full clinical expression of hemochromatosis. The frequency of homozygosity has been estimated at 3 to 10 per 1000 in some populations, but the frequency of hemochromatosis when liver biopsy is required for diagnosis is up to 3.7 per 1000. Hemochromatosis can be recognized before disease develops when only homozygosity for the mutant allele is required. The gold standard for diagnosis is liver biopsy with liver iron concentration and calculation of hepatic iron index (ratio of hepatic iron

to patient age).[8] Effective therapy (phlebotomies) is available.[2] **HLA-A3** alloantigen is found in about 70% of subjects who have hemochromatosis.[2] The genes are linked on the short arm of chromosome 6. Inappropriate increase in iron absorption and parenchymal tissue deposition may eventuate in hepatic cirrhosis, diabetes, testicular atrophy, and fine, soft, bronze to slate gray skin and very high serum ferritin levels (usually >1000 ng/mL).

Red cell ferritin in conjunction with plasma ferritin may be useful in distinguishing iron deficiency from iron overload in patients who have β-thalassemia.[9]

The decline in serum ferritin occurring during adolescence has been shown to be due to the onset of menarche rather than as a result of the accompanying growth spurt.[10]

Elevated serum ferritin levels in patients with cancer is associated with a poor prognosis which may be due in part to deleterious biological effects of tumor ferritins on lymphocyte and granulocyte function.[11] Data on the nature of isoferritins and their association with and possible utilization in the evaluation of malignant neoplasia is available.[12]

An immunoassay utilizing calibrated mixtures of anti-H and anti-L ferritin subunit monoclonal antibodies has been shown to recognize intermediate isoferritins but was not found to have significant application to tumor monitoring.[13]

Serum transferrin receptor measurements distinguish iron deficiency anemia from the anemia of chronic disease, used with assays of hemoglobin, hematocrit, and ferritin.[3,14,15,16]

Footnotes

1. Sheehan RG, Newton MJ, and Frenkel EP, "Evaluation of a Packaged Kit Assay of Serum Ferritin and Application to Clinical Diagnosis of Selected Anemias," *Am J Clin Pathol*, 1978, 70:79-84.
2. Edwards CQ and Kushner JP, "Screening for Hemochromatosis," *N Engl J Med*, 1993, 328(22):1616-20.
3. Cook JD, "Iron-Deficiency Anemia," *Baillieres Clin Haematol*, 1994, 7(4):787-804.
4. Bell H, Skinningsrud A, Raknerud N, et al, "Serum Ferritin and Transferrin Saturation in Patients With Chronic Alcoholic and Nonalcoholic Liver Diseases," *J Intern Med*, 1994, 236(3):315-22.
5. Ramm GA, Duplock LR, Powell LW, et al, "Sensitive and Rapid Colorimetric Immunoenzymometric Assay of Ferritin in Biological Samples," *Clin Chem*, 1990, 36(6):837-40.
6. Gambino R, "Serum Ferritin Levels Are Elevated in Hyperthyroidism," *Lab Rep*, 1994, 16(10):81
7. Hann HW, Kim CY, London WT, et al, "Increased Serum Ferritin in Chronic Liver Disease: A Risk Factor for Primary Hepatocellular Carcinoma," *Int J Cancer*, 1989, 43(3):376-9.
8. "Case Records of the Massachusetts General Hospital. Weekly Clinicopathological Exercises. Case 31-1994. A 25-Year Old Man With the Recent Onset of Diabetes Mellitus and Congestive Heart Failure," *N Engl J Med*, 1994, 331(7):460-6.
9. Van Der Weyden MB, Fong H, Hallam LJ, et al, "Red Cell Ferritin and Iron Overload in Heterozygous Beta-Thalassemia," *Am J Hematol*, 1989, 30(4):201-5.
10. Kagamimori S, Fujita T, Naruse Y, et al, "A Longitudinal Study of Serum Ferritin Concentration During the Female Adolescent Growth Spurt," *Ann Hum Biol*, 1988, 15(6):413-9.
11. Hann HW, Stahlhut MW, Lee S, et al, "Effects of Isoferritins on Human Granulocytes," *Cancer*, 1989, 63(12):2492-6.
12. Albertini A, Arosio P, Chiancone E, et al, "Ferritins and Isoferritins as Biochemical Markers," *Proceedings of Advanced Course on Ferritins and Isoferritins as Biochemical Markers*, Amsterdam, Holland: Elsevier/North Holland Biomedical Press, 1984.
13. Cozzi A, Levi S, Bazzigaluppi E, et al, "Development of an Immunoassay for All Human Isoferritins, and Its Application to Serum Ferritin Evaluation," *Clin Chim Acta*, 1989, 184(3):197-206.
14. Testa U, Pelosi E, and Peschle C, "The Transferrin Receptor," *Crit Rev Oncog*, 1993, 4(3):241-76.
15. Cook JD, Skikne BS, and Baynes RD, "Serum Transferrin Receptor," *Annu Rev Med*, 1993, 44:63-74.
16. Cook JD, Skikne BS, and Baynes RD, "Iron Deficiency: The Global Perspective," *Adv Exp Med Biol*, 1994, 356:219-28.

References

Brittenham GM, Cohen AR, McLaren CE, et al, "Hepatic Iron Stores and Plasma Ferritin Concentration in Patients With Sickle Cell Anemia and Thalassemia Major," *Am J Hematol*, 1993, 42(1):81-5.
Conrad ME and Umbreit JN, "A Concise Review: Iron Absorption - The Mucin-Mobilferrin-Integrin Pathway. A Competitive Pathway for Metal Absorption," *Am J Hematol*, 1993, 42(1):67-73.
Dawson DW, Fish DI, and Shackleton P, "The Accuracy and Clinical Interpretation of Serum Ferritin Assays," *Clin Lab Haematol*, 1992, 14(1):47-52.
Halliday CE, Halliday JW, and Powell LW, "The Clinical Manifestations of Chronic Iron Overload," *Baillieres Clin Haematol*, 1989, 2(2):403-21.
Hann HW, Lange B, Stahlhut MW, et al, "Prognostic Importance of Serum Transferrin and Ferritin in Childhood Hodgkin's Disease," *Cancer*, 1990, 66(2):313-6.
Holyoake TL, Stott DJ, McKay PJ, et al, "Use of Plasma Ferritin Concentration to Diagnose Iron Deficiency in Elderly Patients," *J Clin Pathol*, 1993, 46(9):857-60.
Oski FA, "Iron Deficiency in Infancy and Childhood," *N Engl J Med*, 1993, 329(3):190-3.
Stacy DL and Han P, "Serum Ferritin Measurement and the Degree of Agreement Using Four Techniques," *Am J Clin Pathol*, 1992, 98(5):511-5.
Vernet M, Revenant MC, Bied A, et al, "Rapid Determination of Ferritin in Serum by the "Stratus" Fluoroenzymoimmunometric Assay," *Clin Chem*, 1989, 35(4):672-3.
Witte D, "Ferritin Assays of the Past and Present," *CAP Today*, 1995, 1-2.

Fetal Lung Maturity Surfactant/Albumin Ratio Assay (FLM S/A) *see* Amniotic Fluid Lecithin/Sphingomyelin Ratio and Phosphatidylglycerol *on page 77*

Finasteride *see* Prostate Specific Antigen, Serum *on page 193*

Fluid, Peritoneal *see* Body Fluid *on page 89*

Fluid, Pleural *see* Body Fluid *on page 89*

Fluoride Inhibition of Cholinesterase *see* Dibucaine Number *on page 122*

Follicle Stimulating Hormone

CPT 83001

Related Information

Adrenocorticotropic Hormone *on page 63*
Ataxia-Telangiectasia, Chromosome Breakage Study *on page 274*
Clomiphene Test *on page 112*
Estradiol, Serum *on page 125*
Estrogens, Nonpregnant, Urine *on page 126*
Luteinizing Hormone, Blood or Urine *on page 163*
Prolactin *on page 192*
Testosterone, Free and Total *on page 202*

Synonyms Follitropin; FSH

Abstract LH and FSH are gonadotropic hormones, produced by the same pituitary cell type. They are glycoproteins. The alpha subunits of LH, FSH, TSH, and hCG are identical; specificity resides in the beta subunits.

Patient Preparation Avoid recently administered radioisotopes.

Specimen Serum or plasma, urine

Container Red top tube or green top (heparin) tube; plastic urine container with boric acid

Collection Refrigerate urine during collection.

Storage Instructions Separate and freeze serum or plasma; avoid hemolysis. FSH is stable 4 hours at 4°C to 25°C, 2 weeks at -20°C, 3 months at -70°C. In urine, stable 3 months at -20°C.[1,2]

Special Instructions For females, date of last menstrual period is necessary for evaluation.

Reference Range Normal ranges for FSH will vary among laboratories and are dependent upon which unit is used. Serum: prepubertal children: <10 IU/L (SI: <10 IU/L), adults: male: <22 IU/L (SI: <22 IU/L); adults: female: nonmidcycle: <20 IU/L (SI: <20 IU/L), midcycle surge: <40 IU/L (SI: <40 IU/L), (ovulatory midcycle peak about twice the basal level) postmenopause: 40-160 IU/L (SI: 40-160 IU/L).

Urine: male: 0-8 years of age: <5 IU/24 hours (SI: <5 IU/day), older than 9 years: <22 IU/24 hours (SI: <22 IU/day); female: 0-8 years: <5 IU/24 hours (SI: <5 IU/day), 9-15 years: <22 IU/24 hours (SI: <22 IU/day), older than 15 years: <30 IU/24 hours (SI: <30 IU/day), postmenopausal: two to three times cycling level.

Results must be interpreted in light of the clinical history. Even normal values are inappropriate, for instance, with amenorrhea or in men when the testosterone concentration is decreased.

Use Excessive FSH and LH are found in primary hypogonadism, anorchia, gonadal failure,[3] complete testicular feminization syndrome, Klinefelter syndrome, alcoholism, and castration. FSH and LH levels are high following menopause. FSH and LH are pituitary products, useful to distinguish primary gonadal failure from secondary (hypothalamic/pituitary) causes of gonadal failure. They are used in investigation of impotence, gynecomastia, menstrual disturbances including oligomenorrhea and amenorrhea. Useful in defining menstrual cycle phases in infertility evaluation of women and testicular dysfunction in men. FSH is commonly used with LH, which also is a gonadotropin. Both are **low in pituitary or hypothalamic (gonadotroph) failure.** Urinary collections for FSH escape the problems of pulsatile, episodic secretion. They are used mainly for children being worked up for precocious puberty and for cycles for *in vitro* fertilization.

Limitations Secretion of both LH and FSH are pulsatile, in response to the normal intermittent release of gonadotropin releasing hormone (GnRH). In addition, in females both FSH and LH vary over the course of the menstrual cycle, with peaks at time of ovulation. Thus, interpretation of a single determination may be difficult. It has been suggested that samples be obtained at 15- to 30-minute intervals and equal volumes of serum be pooled to decrease the effect of pulsatile excretion. Normal values do not exclude pituitary deficiency.

Methodology Radioimmunoassay (RIA)

Additional Information FSH and LH are under complex regulation by hypothalamic GnRH and by gonadal sex hormones, estrogen and progesterone in females, and testosterone. On the simplest level, FSH and LH are high in conditions in which sex hormones cannot be elaborated, and low in conditions of primary pituitary dysfunction. FSH acts on granulosa cells of the ovary and the Sertoli cells of testis. LH acts on Leydig (interstitial) cells of the gonads. Normally FSH increase occurs at an early stage of puberty and it is 2-4 years before LH reaches similar levels.

FSH **is high** in Klinefelter syndrome and in some subjects with precocious puberty. It is decreased with precocious puberty related to adrenal

tumors or congenital adrenal hyperplasia. Normal FSH in an adult nonovulating female, represents dysfunction at the central nervous system hypothalamic/pituitary level, and a "normal" value should in such a setting be considered pseudonormal.

High LH/FSH ratio (>1.5) is found in the polycystic ovary syndrome.[4]

Footnotes

1. Kubasik NP, Ricotta M, Hunter T, et al, "Effect of Duration and Temperature of Storage on Serum Analyte Stability - Examination of 14 Selected Radioimmunoassay Procedures," *Clin Chem*, 1982, 28:164-5.
2. Livesey JH, Hodgkinson SC, Roud MR, et al, "Effect of Time, Temperature, and Freezing on the Stability of Immunoreactive LH, FSH, TSH, Growth Hormone Prolactin and Insulin in Plasma," *Clin Biochem*, 1980, 13:151-5.
3. Layman LC, Wilson JT, Huey LO, et al, "Gonadotropin-Releasing Hormone, Follicle-Stimulating Hormone Beta, Luteinizing Hormone Beta Gene Structure in Idiopathic Hypogonadotropic Hypogonadism," *Fertil Steril*, 1992, 57(1):42-9.
4. Watts NB and Keffer JH, *Practical Endocrine Diagnosis*, 4th ed, Philadelphia, PA: Lea & Febiger, 1989.

References

Howanitz JH, "Review of the Influence of Polypeptide Hormone Forms on Immunoassay Results," *Arch Pathol Lab Med*, 1993, 1174(4):369-72.
Jaakkola T, Ding YQ, Kellokumpu-Lehtinen P, et al, "The Ratios of Serum Bioactive/Immunoreactive Luteinizing Hormone and Follicle-Stimulating Hormone in Various Clinical Conditions With Increased and Decreased Gonadotropin Secretion: Reevaluation by a Highly Sensitive Immunometric Assay," *J Clin Endocrinol Metab*, 1990, 70(6):1496-505.
Pandian MR, Odell WD, Carlton E, et al, "Development of Third-Generation Immunochemiluminometric Assays of Follitropin and Lutropin and Clinical Application in Determining Pediatric Reference Ranges," *Clin Chem*, 1993, 39(9):1815-9.
Taylor AE, Khoury RH, and Crowley WF Jr, "A Comparison of 13 Different Immunometric Assay Kits for Gonadotropins: Implications for Clinical Investigation," *J Clin Endocrinol Metab*, 1994, 79(1):240-7.
Vance ML, "Hypopituitarism," *N Engl J Med*, 1994, 330(23):1651-62.

Follitropin *see* Follicle Stimulating Hormone *on this page*

Follitropin *see* Luteinizing Hormone, Blood or Urine *on page 163*

Fractionated Alkaline Phosphatase *see* Alkaline Phosphatase, Heat Stable *on page 68*

Free Catecholamine Fractionation, Urine *see* Catecholamines, Fractionation, Urine *on page 104*

Free Erythrocyte Protoporphyrin *see* Protoporphyrin, Free Erythrocyte *on page 195*

Free T$_4$ *see* Thyroxine, Free *on page 208*

Free Testosterone *see* Testosterone, Free and Total *on page 202*

Free Thyroid Index *see* Free Thyroxine Index *on this page*

Free Thyroid Index *see* Thyroxine *on page 206*

Free Thyroxine *see* Thyroxine, Free *on page 208*

Free Thyroxine Index

CPT 84436 (T$_4$); 84479 (T$_3$ uptake)

Related Information

T$_3$ Uptake *on page 201*
Thyroid Antimicrosomal Antibody *on page 433*
Thyroid Stimulating Hormone *on page 204*
Thyrotropin Receptor Antibody *on page 434*
Thyroxine *on page 206*
Thyroxine Binding Globulin *on page 207*
Thyroxine, Free *on page 208*
Triiodothyronine *on page 211*

Synonyms Free Thyroid Index; FT$_4$I; FT$_4$ Index; FTI

Test Commonly Includes T$_3$ uptake and T$_4$

Abstract The free thyroxine index may be calculated as the product of T$_3$ resin uptake (RT$_3$U) and total T$_4$ level; it is usually proportional to actual FT$_4$. It is an imperfect measure but provides acceptable results with pregnant subjects and in a variety of other settings. A tendency exists for the free thyroxine index to provide low results in assays of subjects with nonthyroidal illness. In euthyroid elderly people, low FTIs may be found; and this may be due to a resetting of threshold of thyrotropin feedback suppression.[1] Presently the first line for diagnosis of thyroidal disorders is application of the sensitive TSH assays, often with T$_4$ or FT$_4$. In some clinical circumstances both sTSH and FTI are desirable.

Patient Preparation No recent administration of radioactive substances (eg, no recent scans) if RIA testing is in place. Schedule scans, if necessary, **after** thyroid profile is drawn. FT$_4$I may be increased with radiologic contrast agents, propranolol, amiodarone, and heparin.

Specimen Serum

Container Red top tube

Storage Instructions Separate within 48 hours; separated serum stable 1 week at 25°C

Reference Range 10 years to adult: normal: 5.0-13.0, low: ≤4.8, high: ≥14.0. Normal ranges will differ somewhat between laboratories. To (Continued)

Free Thyroxine Index (Continued)

prevent confusion with serum T_4 or T_3, these unitless values are sometimes labeled "index units".[2] The values are similar to total T_4 values.

Use In the basic thyroid work-up, the FT_4 index is a physiologic index of metabolic activity which generally correlates with free thyroxine. Costs of each should be compared. The FTI is presently used to monitor therapy for hyperthyroidism and to supplement the sTSH.

Limitations The "sick euthyroid syndrome" is an expression used to describe a euthyroid subject whose T_4 and FTI are decreased with severe illness.[3]

Free T_4 index based on T_3 binding to serum proteins (eg, T_3 uptake) is not entirely reliable when decreased serum thyroxine is caused by decreased thyroid hormone binding to thyroxine binding globulin (ie, the value of the free thyroxine index in the differential diagnosis of low total T_4 is minimal). The free thyroxine index and the T_4:TBG ratio are not a substitute for measurement of free T_4.[4]

Methodology Calculation from results of T_3 uptake and T_4. The FTI = (T_3U(%) of patient/T_3U(%) normal control mean) x T_4

Additional Information Calculation includes the T_4 and T_3 uptake values. T_3 uptake and T_4 are influenced by pregnancy, contraceptive pills, abnormalities of serum proteins and other factors, mostly in opposite directions. The free thyroxine index permits meaningful interpretation by balancing out most nonthyroidal factors.[5] For example, a pregnant euthyroid patient would have an increased T_4, but the FTI would be normal. An euthyroid patient with nephrotic syndrome may have a decreased T_4 (due to decreased levels by binding proteins), but the FTI would be normal. The FTI was described in 1983 as equal to the thyroid hormone/TBG ratio in hyperthyroidism and a better index in pregnancy, in thyroid binding globulin deficiency and in hypothyroidism.[6] The FT_4I is increased with levothyroxine.

Drugs that influence thyroid function are tabulated in the listing Thyroxine Binding Globulin *on page 207*. Thyroid binding globulin decreases with nicotinic acid.[4]

Footnotes

1. Lewis GF, Alessi CA, Imperial JG, et al, "Low Serum Free Thyroxine Index in Ambulating Elderly Is Due to a Resetting of the Threshold of Thyrotropin Feedback Suppression," *J Clin Endocrinol Metab*, 1991, 73(4):843-9.
2. Larsen PR, Alexander NM, Chopra IJ, et al, "Revised Nomenclature for Tests of Thyroid Hormones and Thyroid-Related Proteins in Serum," *Arch Pathol Lab Med*, 1987, 111(1):1141-5.
3. Feldkamp CS and Carey JL, "An Algorithmic Approach to Thyroid Function Testing in a Managed Care Setting - 3-Year Experience," *Am J Clin Pathol*, 1995, 105(1):11-6.
4. Nelson JC and Tomei RT, "Dependence of the Thyroxine/Thyroxine-Binding Globulin (TBG) Ratio and the Free Thyroxine Index on TBG Concentrations," *Clin Chem*, 1989, 35(4):541-4.
5. Nusynowitz ML, "Free Thyroxine Index," *JAMA*, 1975, 232:1050.
6. Wilke TJ, "Free Thyroid Hormone Index, Thyroid Hormone/Thyroxine-Binding Globulin Ratio, Triiodothyronine Uptake, and Thyroxine-Binding Globulin Compared for Diagnostic Value Regarding Thyroid Function," *Clin Chem*, 1983, 29:74-9.
7. Shakir KM, Kroll S, Aprill BS, et al, "Nicotinic Acid Decreases Serum Thyroid Hormone Levels While Maintaining a Euthyroid State," *Mayo Clin Proc*, 1995, 70(6):556-8.

References

Grund FM and Niewoehner CB, "Hyperthyroxinemia in Patients Receiving Thyroid Replacement Therapy," *Arch Intern Med*, 1989, 149(4):921-4.
Helfand M and Crapo LM, "Screening for the Thyroid Disease," *Ann Intern Med*, 1990, 112(11):840-9.
Mandel SJ, Larsen PR, Seely EW, et al, "Increased Need for Thyroxine During Pregnancy in Women With Primary Hypothyroidism," *N Engl J Med*, 1990, 323(2):91-6.

Free Thyroxine Index, Calculated *see* Thyroxine Binding Globulin *on page 207*

Fructosamine

CPT 82985

Related Information

Glucose, 2-Hour Postprandial *on page 136*
Glucose, Fasting *on page 137*
Glucose, Quantitative, Urine *on page 635*
Glycated Hemoglobin *on page 140*

Synonyms Glycated Albumin

Abstract A fructosamine is the result of glucose linking covalently with albumin or other proteins, producing a glycated product, a stable ketoamine.

Specimen Serum

Container Red top tube

Storage Instructions Refrigerate. Freeze sample if assay is not done within 2 hours.

Reference Range Normal ranges vary considerably according to method. Nondiabetics: 1.5-2.7 mmol/L; diabetics: ≥2.0-5.0 mmol/L depending on the degree of control.

Use Evaluate diabetic control, reflecting diabetic control over a shorter time period (2-3 weeks) than that represented by glycated hemoglobin

(hemoglobin A_{1c}) (4-8 weeks). Indicated as an index of longer term control than glucose levels, especially in diabetic subjects with abnormal hemoglobins, patients with gestational diabetes,[1] and in type I diabetes in children.[2] Fructosamine levels may be useful in screening geriatric populations.[3] Glycated albumin, because of its short half-life, lends itself as a test to monitor and control gestational diabetes.[1]

Limitations Fructosamine, like Hb A_{1c}, is probably not a useful test for screening for diabetes mellitus. Very low albumin concentrations (<3.0 g/dL) may result in falsely low fructosamine values. In practice, this test is not widely used.

Methodology Colorimetry or affinity chromatography. Methods suitable for automated analyzers have been described.[4]

Additional Information Fructosamine is found in the plasma of both normal and diabetic individuals. "Fructosamine" is the term used to describe proteins that have been glycated (ie, are derivatives of the nonenzymatic reaction product of glucose and albumin). It has been advocated as an alternative test to hemoglobin A_{1c} for the monitoring of long-term diabetic control. Fructosamine and hemoglobin A_{1c} do not measure exactly the same thing, since fructosamine has a shorter half-life and probably is somewhat more sensitive to short-term variations in glucose levels. However, this is not necessarily a disadvantage. Much of the development of fructosamine has occurred outside the United States. Although the tests are not identical, probably one or the other is sufficient in routine diabetic patients for the assessment of long-term control of hyperglycemia. It is not necessary to order both tests in all patients, although this may be a value in selective problem patients. Fructosamine is clearly superior in patients with abnormal hemoglobins because of the interference of abnormal hemoglobins in the anion-exchange chromatography methods for Hb A_{1c}. An ion-capture immunoassay (Abbott Laboratories) can measure Hb A_{1c} in the presence of abnormal hemoglobins.

Footnotes

1. Narayanan S, "Laboratory Monitoring of Gestational Diabetes," *Ann Clin Lab Sci*, 1991, 21(6):392-401.
2. Cefalu WT, Mejia E, Puente GR, et al, "Correlation of Serum Fructosamine Activity in Type I Diabetic Children," *Am J Med Sci*, 1989, 297(4):244-6.
3. Croxson SC, Absalom S, and Burden AC, "Fructosamine in Diabetes Screening of the Elderly," *Ann Clin Biochem*, 1991, 28(Pt 3):279-82.
4. Hill RP, Hindle EJ, Howey JE, et al, "Recommendations for Adopting Standard Conditions and Analytical Procedures in the Measurement of Serum Fructosamine Concentration," *Ann Clin Biochem*, 1990, 27(Pt 5):413-24.

References

Allgrove J and Cockrill BL, "Fructosamine or Glycated Haemoglobin as a Measure of Diabetic Control?" *Arch Dis Child*, 1988, 63(4):418-22.
Daubresse JC, Laurent E, Ligny C, et al, "The Usefulness of Fructosamine Determination in Diabetic Patients and Its Relation to Metabolic Control," *Diabete Metab* Paris, 1987, 13(3):217-21.
Desjarlais F, Comtois R, Beauregard H, et al, "Technical and Clinical Evaluation of Fructosamine Determination in Serum," *Clin Biochem*, 1989, 22(4):329-35.
Furnseth K, Bruusgaard D, Rutle O, et al, "Fructosamine Cannot Replace Hb A_{1c} in the Management of Type 2 Diabetes (NIDDM)," *Scand J Prim Health Care*, 1994, 12(3):219-24.
Gebhart SS, Wheaton RN, Mullins RE, et al, "A Comparison of Home Glucose Monitoring With Determinations of Hemoglobin A_{1c}, Total Glycated Hemoglobin, Fructosamine, and Random Serum Glucose in Diabetic Patients," *Arch Intern Med*, 1991, 151(6):1133-7.
Jerntorp P, Sundkvist G, Fex G, et al, "Clinical Utility of Serum Fructosamine in Diabetes Mellitus Compare With Hemoglobin A_{1c}," *Clin Chim Acta*, 1988, 175(2):135-42.
Kaufman HW, "Screening for Gestational Diabetes Mellitus," *Am Fam Physician*, 1989, 40(6):109-11.
Lapolla A, Poli T, Barison A, et al, "Fructosamine Assay: An Index of Medium-Term Metabolic Control Parameters in Diabetic Disease," *Diabetes Res Clin Pract*, 1988, 4(3):231-5.
Lloyd DR, Nott M, and Marples J, "Comparison of Serum Fructosamine With Glycosylated Serum Protein (Determined by Affinity Chromatography) for the Assessment of Diabetic Control," *Diabetic Med*, 1985, 2(6):474-8.
Miller JC, "Importance of Glycemic Index in Diabetes," *Am J Clin Nutr*, 1994, 59(3 Suppl):747S-52S.
Negoro H, Morley JE, and Rosenthal MJ, "Utility of Serum Fructosamine as a Measure of Glycemia in Young and Old Diabetic and Nondiabetic Subjects," *Am J Med*, 1988, 85(3):360-4.
Roberts AB, Baker JR, James AG, et al, "Fructosamine in the Management of Gestational Diabetes," *Am J Obstet Gynecol*, 1988, 159(1):66-71.
Yamanouchi T and Akanuma Y, "Serum 1,5-Anhydroglucitol (1,5 AG): New Clinical Marker for Glycemic Control," *Diabetes Res Clin Pract*, 1994, 24(Suppl):S261-8.

Fructose Biphosphate Aldolase *see* Aldolase, Serum *on page 66*

FSH *see* Follicle Stimulating Hormone *on previous page*

FT_4 *see* Thyroxine, Free *on page 208*

FT_4I *see* Free Thyroxine Index *on previous page*

FT_4 Index *see* Free Thyroxine Index *on previous page*

FTI *see* Free Thyroxine Index *on previous page*

Galactokinase, Blood

CPT 82759

Related Information

Galactose-1-Phosphate Uridyl Transferase, Erythrocyte *on this page*

Galactose Screening Tests for Galactosemia *on next page*

Synonyms RBC Galactokinase

Abstract The activity of this enzyme is decreased in galactokinase-deficient galactosemia.

Patient Preparation Avoid radioisotope scans or recently administered radioisotopes prior to collection of specimen.

Specimen Whole blood

Container Green top (heparin) tube

Collection Send blood immediately (on ice, not frozen) to the laboratory.

Storage Instructions Red blood cells must be washed repeatedly immediately after receipt in laboratory, therefore, transportation to the laboratory is critical.

Special Instructions Communicate with laboratory, as this test is not routinely available and may require referral.

Reference Range Children: 0-2 years: 11-150 mU/g Hgb (levels in infants are 3 to 4 times those of adults) 2-18 years: 11-54 mU/g Hgb; adults: 12-40 mU/g Hgb

Use Establish the diagnosis of galactokinase-deficiency galactosemia. Galactosemia may also be caused by a deficiency of galactose-1-phosphate uridyl transferase and uridine diphospho-glucose 4-epimerase.[1]

Methodology Radioisotopic: RBCs are hemolyzed and the hemolysate is incubated with radiolabeled galactose. The 1-^{14}C-galactose-1-phosphate is quantitated after binding to DEAE chromatography paper.

Additional Information This condition should enter into the differential consideration of any child with cataracts.[2] It is an autosomal recessive inherited enzyme deficiency, 0.2% of the population is heterozygous for the defect. Homozygotes have a form of galactosemia that is associated with cataracts but usually do not suffer mental retardation, liver disease, or problems in the newborn period resulting from galactose exposure (eg, failure to thrive, vomiting, or liver disease/jaundice). Heterozygotes are at risk for the development of cataracts in young adult life. In each of the different forms of galactosemia, an alternative route of galactose metabolism is utilized. Reduction (of galactose) to galactitol and oxidation to galactonate occurs. Galactitol accumulates in the lens, producing osmotic imbalance resulting in cataract formation. An incidence of 6.9% of galactokinase deficiency has been found in a group of idiopathic cataract patients 50 years of age or younger.[3] Heterozygotes have about 50% of the normal enzyme activity. Galactokinase deficiency is in the differential consideration of patients with pseudotumor cerebri.[4] Therapy, as for transferase deficiency, consists of galactose restriction.

Footnotes

1. Beutler E, "Galactosemia: Screening and Diagnosis," *Clin Biochem*, 1991, 24(4):293-300.
2. Stevens RE, Datiles MB, Srivastava SK, et al, "Idiopathic Presenile Cataract Formation and Galactosaemia," *Br J Ophthalmol*, 1989, 73(1):48-51.
3. Elman MJ, Miller MT, and Matalon R, "Galactokinase Activity in Patients With Idiopathic Cataracts," *Ophthalmology*, 1986, 93(2):210-5.
4. Litman N, Kanter A, and Finberg L, "Galactokinase Deficiency Presenting as Pseudotumor Cerebri," *J Pediatr*, 1975, 86:410-2.

References

Applegarth DA, Dimmick JE, and Toone JR, "Laboratory Detection of Metabolic Disease," *Pediatr Clin North Am*, 1989, 36(1):49-65.

Segal S and Berry GT, "Disorders of Galactose Metabolism: Galactokinase Deficiency Galactosemia," *The Metabolic and Molecular Bases of Inherited Disease*, 7th ed, Chapter 25, Scriver CR, Beaudet AL, Sly WS, et al, eds, New York, NY: McGraw-Hill Inc, 1995, 987-9.

Galactokinase Deficiency *see* Galactose-1-Phosphate Uridyl Transferase, Erythrocyte *on this page*

Galactose-1-Phosphate

CPT 84999

Related Information

Galactose-1-Phosphate Uridyl Transferase, Erythrocyte *on this page*

Galactose Screening Tests for Galactosemia *on next page*

Abstract Red cell concentration of galactose-1-phosphate is increased in patients with galactosemia. Used to monitor galactosemic patients.

Specimen Whole blood

Container Green top (heparin) tube

Storage Instructions Store at 4°C.

Causes for Rejection Specimen more than 3 hours old

Reference Range Usually <1 mg/dL galactose-1-phosphate/100 mL lysed packed red blood cells

Use Monitor galactosemic patients on a galactose-free diet

Limitations Analysis is offered by only a few specialized laboratories. Monitoring of galactose-free diet may be more simply achieved with less cost by using whole blood filter paper spot tests.

Methodology Enzymatic rate reaction (absorbance of NADH); normal red cells used as a source of galactose-1-phosphate uridyltransferase; galactose-1-phosphate of patient's red cells is limiting factor to which rate of reduction of NAD is proportional.[1] A method to detect galactose and galactose-1-phosphate from dried blood has been described.[2]

Additional Information Galactosemia, the result of an inherited cellular deficiency of galactokinase or uridine diphosphate galactose-4-epimerase, is characterized by galactosuria and increased red cell galactose-1-phosphate. The level of galactose in the blood relates to the dietary intake of lactose (as present in milk but also in foods containing lactose but not so labeled, ie, candy, breads, frankfurters, etc). Patients with congenital galactosemia maintained on a milk-free diet should have level of galactose-1-phosphate <2 mg/100 mL lysed packed red cells. If such patients are ingesting lactose (eg, drinking milk), levels of 9-20 mg/100 mL packed red cell lysate will be obtained.[1] A range of characteristic abnormalities result from galactose toxicity including failure to thrive, vomiting, abnormal liver function with resultant cirrhosis, and mental retardation.[3] Signs and symptoms (including even cataracts) will regress under the influence of a galactose-free diet. An increased frequency of hypergonadotropic hypogonadism in females (ovarian failure with decreased or absent ovarian tissue) has been reported[4] and occurs especially in subjects in whom diet therapy was delayed.

Footnotes

1. O'Brien D, Ibbott FA, and Rodgerson DO, *Laboratory Manual of Pediatric Micro-Biochemical Techniques*, 4th ed, New York, NY: Hoeber, 1968, 149-52.
2. Diepenbrock F, Heckler R, Schickling H, et al, "Colorimetric Determination of Galactose and Galactose-1-Phosphate From Dried Blood," *Clin Biochem*, 1992, 25(1):37-9.
3. Segal S and Berry GT, "Disorders of Galactose Metabolism," *The Metabolic and Molecular Bases of Inherited Disease*, 7th ed, Chapter 25, Scriver CR, Beaudet AL, Sly WS, et al, eds, New York, NY: McGraw-Hill Inc, 1995, 967-1000.
4. Kaufman FR, Kogut MD, Donnell GN, et al, "Hypergonadotropic Hypogonadism in Female Patients With Galactosemia," *N Engl J Med*, 1981, 304:994-8.

References

Applegarth DA, Dimmick JE, and Toone JR, "Laboratory Detection of Metabolic Disease," *Pediatr Clin North Am*, 1989, 36(1):49-65.

Beutler E, "Galactosemia: Screening and Diagnosis," *Clin Biochem*, 1991, 24(4):293-300.

Reichardt JK, Packman S, and Woo SL, "Molecular Characterization of Two Galactosemia Mutations: Correlation of Mutations With Highly Conserved Domains in Galactose-1-Phosphate Uridyl Transferase," *Am J Hum Genet*, 1991, 49(4):860-7.

Galactose-1-Phosphate Uridyl Transferase, Erythrocyte

CPT 82775

Related Information

Galactokinase, Blood *on this page*

Galactose-1-Phosphate *on this page*

Galactose Screening Tests for Galactosemia *on next page*

Applies to Galactokinase Deficiency; UDP Galactose-4-Epimerase Deficiency

Abstract Deficiency of this enzyme is the most common cause of galactosemia.

Patient Preparation Avoid radioisotope scans or recently administered radioisotopes prior to collection of specimen.

Specimen Erythrocytes

Container Green top (heparin) tube, lavender top (EDTA) tube

Storage Instructions Stable 14 days at room temperature, 4 weeks at 4°C; do not freeze.

Special Instructions A blood sample from a control individual is needed.

Reference Range 17-37 units (μmol/hour/g hemoglobin)

Use Diagnose galactosemia (galactose-1-phosphate uridyl transferase deficiency). Two other enzyme deficiencies cause galactosemia, galactokinase and UDP galactose-4-epimerase.

Methodology Radioactive with ^{14}C-galactose-1-phosphate as the substrate; colorimetric (dried blood)[1]

Additional Information Galactosemia is an autosomal recessive disorder of galactose metabolism most often caused by a deficiency of galactose-1-phosphate uridyl transferase, rarely by a deficiency of galactokinase or UDP galactose-4-epimerase. Molecular genetic studies have revealed molecular heterogeneity which is related to the variable clinical outcome observed in this disorder.[2] The resulting accumulation of galactitol and/or galactose-1-phosphate can result in juvenile cataracts, liver failure, failure to thrive, and mental retardation in galactose-1-phosphate uridyl transferase deficiency. Dietary restriction of galactose is a very effective treatment, and liver and lens changes are reversible. Quantitative assays, in addition to diagnosing transferase deficiency, can identify heterozygous transferase deficient carriers and homozygous transferase variants (Duarte variants). Blood for galactosemia screening should be (Continued)

Galactose-1-Phosphate Uridyl Transferase, Erythrocyte (Continued)

obtained as early in life as possible (less than 3-4 days) so that effective therapy can be instituted.

Footnotes

1. Diepenbrock F, Heckler R, Schickling H, et al, "Colorimetric Determination of Galactose and Galactose-1-Phosphate From Dried Blood," *Clin Biochem*, 1992, 25(1):37-9.
2. Reichardt JK, Packman S, and Woo SL, "Molecular Characterization of Two Galactosemia Mutations: Correlation of Mutations With Highly Conserved Domains in Galactose-1-Phosphate Uridyl Transferase," *Am J Hum Genet*, 1991, 49(4):860-7.

References

Kelley RI and Segal S, "Evaluation of Reduced Activity Galactose-1-Phosphate Uridyl Transferase by Combined Radioisotopic Assay and High-Resolution Isoelectric Focusing," *J Lab Clin Med*, 1989, 114(2):152-6.

Lagrou K and Declercq PE, "Simplified Assay of Galactose-1-Phosphate Uridyltransferase," *Clin Chem*, 1991, 37(12):2157-8.

Galactose Screening Tests for Galactosemia

CPT 82760

Related Information

Galactokinase, Blood *on previous page*

Galactose-1-Phosphate *on previous page*

Galactose-1-Phosphate Uridyl Transferase, Erythrocyte *on previous page*

Newborn Screen for T_4 *on page 170*

Synonyms Beutler Test; Blood Spot Screen for Galactose/Galactose-1-Phosphate; Paigen Test (*E. coli* Bacteriophage Resistance to Lysis Assay)

Test Commonly Includes Combinations of screening tests for red cell galactose/galactose-1-phosphate (increase) and red cell galactose-1-phosphate uridyltransferase (absence)

Abstract Effective screening test/tests for three inherited disorders causing galactosemia. The assumption that prompt treatment can provide long-term protection against central nervous system disorders, possibly including mental retardation, has recently come into question.

Specimen Whole blood, dried as a spot on filter paper; may use heparinized whole blood

Sampling Time Screening should be performed within the first 3 days of life but may be method/diet dependent.

Collection Drop of whole blood soaked into provided filter paper. See the listing Phenylalanine, Blood *on page 181* for collection details.

Storage Instructions Avoid exposure to high temperature during transit to the laboratory (eg, especially during heat of summer) (applies primarily to Beutler test).[1]

Causes for Rejection Insufficient or improper application of blood to filter paper spot, excessive exposure to heat, specimen paper without proper label/identification, blood collected in acid-citrate-dextrose or EDTA in some cases[2]

Reference Range Normal neonates: blood galactose <1 mg/dL (SI: <0.06 mmol/L) in 88%, 1-5 mg/dL (SI: 0.06-0.28 mmol/L) in 12% of cases. Galactosemic infants usually have blood galactose >20 mg/dL (SI: >1.11 mmol/L) (Paigen test);[3] presence of galactose transferase is the normal condition (Beutler-Baluda test).[2]

Use Detect galactosemia; monitor dietary therapy of galactosemia

Limitations Antibiotics present in the sample apparently do not cause a false-negative result in the Paigen test (*E. coli* bacteriophage resistance to lysis), see following information. The Beutler-Baluda test will detect transferase deficient cases of galactosemia only (galactose kinase and epimerase deficiencies although uncommon, would be missed). The Paigen screen for increased RBC galactose/galactose-1-phosphate, if positive, should be followed by a transferase screen (eg, Beutler test) which, if negative, would indicate a different cause for the galactosemia (eg, galactose kinase or epimerase deficiency, see following information). A galactose screening test that is not sensitive also to galactose-1-phosphate will require that the newborn have ingested milk prior to testing or a false-positive result may be obtained. **Transfusion may result in a false-negative Beutler-Baluda test for as long as 2-3 months.**

Methodology Urine can be screened for galactosuria by reagents usually commonly available in the Urinalysis and/or Chemistry sections of most clinical laboratories. Specimen is first tested for reducing substances by a cupric ion reduction method (eg, Benedict's Test, Clinitest® tablets). If positive, a glucose oxidase specific method is applied. If the specific test for glucose is negative, but a reducing substance is present, there is presumptive evidence for one of the three forms of galactosemia.

Screening programs for galactosemia have been established by most states in the United States and many countries of the world. Ease of specimen transport to high volume reference laboratories favors dried blood spot over urine testing. A variety of applicable tests utilizing whole blood samples spotted on filter paper have been described.[4]

The Beutler test has a fluorescent end point, tests for deficiency of galactose-1-phosphate uridyltransferase, and can be performed rapidly. Fluorescence may be delayed, however, in infants with partial enzyme deficiency (eg, heterozygotes for transferase deficiency or with the Duarte variant).[2]

The Paigen assay screens for increase in galactose and galactose-1-phosphate. It is the most effective **single** test available for all forms of galactosemia.[4] The procedure uses a strain of *E. coli* that resists C21 bacteriophage lysis in the presence of galactose. Thus, bacterial growth occurs around filter paper blood spots in cases of galactosemia. In the absence of galactose (normal nongalactosemic newborn), no growth occurs as the bacteria are killed by the phage. The diameter of the growth zone is proportional to the concentration of galactose.[3]

An enzymatic centrifugal analyzer chemical method has been developed. Galactose is determined by measuring the change in absorbance of reduced NADH at 340 nm after addition of galactose dehydrogenase.[5] A presumptive positive is defined as a blood galactose plus galactose-1-phosphate level >0.30 mmol/L. Each presumptive positive is also screened with a Beutler spot test to assess transferase activity. This method for galactosemia screening is rapid, sensitive and may be the method of choice for mass screening.[5] A microplate fluorometric method based on the GADH-NAD+/NADH system has similar advantages to the Manitoba system noted above, is rapid, reliable, and applicable to routine screening of newborns.[6]

Third generation cephalosporin antibiotics may cause false-positive results in *E. coli* W5 based tests (in which presence of galactose inhibits bacterial growth).[7] Presence of galactose, however, is not excluded, until another sample is appropriately tested by a different method.

Additional Information Galactosemia may occur with any of three metabolic abnormalities but is usually the result of an inherited deficiency of galactose-1-phosphate uridyltransferase activity. This condition, if undetected and untreated, is characterized clinically by failure to thrive, vomiting, cataracts, mental retardation, liver disease, and death. Incidence, generally is about 1:60,000 but estimates worldwide have ranged from 1:18,000 to 1:180,000. A number of starch gel electrophoretic variants have been defined of which the Duarte and Los Angeles variants are the most common.[8] The Duarte variant is characterized by intermediate levels of transferase (higher than those of the classical deficiency) and by an electrophoretically distinctive enzyme. Duarte form appears clinically benign. The Indiana variant is an unstable electrophoretically distinct enzyme. Individuals with Los Angeles variant do not have abnormal galactose metabolism.

Deficiency of cellular galactokinase results in a galactose toxicity that is usually milder and limited to development of cataracts.

The third cause of galactosemia, uridine diphosphate galactose-4-epimerase deficiency, occurs in two forms. One involves only red and white blood cells and is benign. The second form is unusual and requires care in dietary management. It manifests as does transferase deficiency and responds to dietary restriction of galactose. A low level of galactose must be maintained in the diet, however, since epimerase is involved in supplying UDP-galactose for complex carbohydrate, galactolipid and galactoprotein synthesis. While estimates of incidence of galactokinase and epimerase deficiencies have been in the 1:20,000 to 1:40,000 range, very few clinically deficient cases have been reported as compared to cases of transferase deficiency. The enzyme deficiencies responsible for galactosemia have an autosomal recessive mode of inheritance.

Galactose is present normally in blood and urine but in very low concentration, serum, 0.70 mg/dL (SI: 0.04 mmol/L); urine, 4 mg/dL (SI: 0.22 mmol/L). Urine from normal newborns may have levels of galactose as high as 60 mg/dL (SI: 3.33 mmol/L) urine (physiologic melituria); in premature infants this may occur over the first 2 weeks of life.[9] High level of milk intake may also produce galactosuria.[10] In cases of galactosemia, galactosuria may be intermittent (partly relating to the intake of milk) and may be missed if urine is very dilute. A screening program based on a copper reduction test, then, may result in false-negatives. Early identification and treatment of the infant with galactosemia is critical as cataracts, mental retardation, liver disease with hepatosplenomegaly, and death due to septicemia (in particular, *E. coli* septicemia) may occur in the untreated individual. Specific enzyme assays should be employed to define abnormalities detected by screening tests.

While dietary measures (galactose-restricted diets) control the acute life-threatening disorder, long-term outcome may be unfavorable. Developmental delay, learning disability, impaired motor function and balances, speech disorder, gonadal failure, and personality disorders occur in later years.[11]

Footnotes

1. "American Academy of Pediatrics, Committee on Genetics, Newborn Screening Fact Sheets," *Pediatrics*, 1989, 83(3):458-60.

2. Beutler E and Baluda MC, "A Simple Spot Screening Test for Galactosemia," *J Lab Clin Med*, 1966, 68:137-41.
3. Paigen K, Pacholec F, and Levy HL, "A New Method of Screening for Inherited Disorders of Galactose Metabolism," *J Lab Clin Med*, 1982, 88:895-907.
4. Levy HL and Hammersen G, "Newborn Screening for Galactosemia and Other Galactose Metabolic Defects," *J Pediatr*, 1978, 92:871-7.
5. Greenberg CR, Dilling LA, Thompson R, et al, "Newborn Screening for Galactosemia: A New Method Used in Manitoba," *Pediatrics*, 1989, 84(2):331-5.
6. Yamaguchi A, Fukushi M, Mizushima Y, et al, "Microassay for Screening Newborns for Galactosemia With Use of a Fluorometric Microplate Reader," *Clin Chem*, 1989, 35(9):1962-4.
7. Schunk JP, Bradley JS, Buist NR, et al, "Interference by Third Generation Cephalosporins With Neonatal Screening for Galactosemia," *J Pediatr*, 1988, 112(5):842.
8. Segal S and Berry GT, "Disorders of Galactose Metabolism," *The Metabolic and Molecular Bases of Inherited Disease*, 7th ed, Chapter 25, Scriver CR, Beaudet AL, Sly WS, et al, eds, New York, NY: McGraw-Hill Inc, 1995, 967-1000.
9. Dahlquist A and Svenningsen NW, "Galactose in the Urine of Newborn Infants," *J Pediatr*, 1969, 75:454.
10. Holl WK, Cravey CE, Chen PT, et al, "An Evaluation of Galactosuria," *J Pediatr*, 1970, 77:625.
11. Holton JB and Leonard JV, "Clouds Still Gathering Over Galactosaemia," *Lancet*, 1994, 344(8932):1242-3.

References

Applegarth DA, Dimmick JE, and Toone JR, "Laboratory Detection of Metabolic Disease," *Pediatr Clin North Am*, 1989, 36(1):49-65.
Berry HK and Croft CC, "Reagent That Restores Galactose-1-Phosphate Uridyltransferase Activity in Dry Blood Spots," *Clin Chem*, 1987, 33(8):1471-2.
Gitzelmann R and Steinmann B, "Galactosemia," *Eur J Pediatr*, 1995, 154(7 Suppl 2):S2-S105.
Kirby LT, Norman MG, Applegarth DA, et al, "Screening of Newborn Infants for Galactosemia in British Columbia," *Can Med Assoc J*, 1985, 132(9):1033-5.
Sokol RJ, McCabe ER, Kotzer AM, et al, "Pitfalls in Diagnosing Galactosemia: False-Negative Newborn Screening Following Red Blood Cell Transfusion," *J Pediatr Gastroenterol Nutr*, 1989, 8(2):266-8.

Gamma Glutamyl Transferase

CPT 82977

Related Information

Alkaline Phosphatase, Heat Stable *on page 68*
Alkaline Phosphatase, Serum *on page 69*
Aspartate Aminotransferase *on page 84*
Bilirubin, Total *on page 86*
Leucine Aminopeptidase *on page 158*
Liver Profile *on page 161*
5′ Nucleotidase *on page 171*

Synonyms Gamma Glutamyl Transpeptidase; GGT; GGTP; Glutamyl Transpeptidase; GT; GTP

Applies to Body Fluid GGT

Replaces BSP

Abstract This is a biliary excretory enzyme (a peptidase) useful in the diagnosis of certain liver diseases. It is especially responsive to obstructive disease and is sensitive to ethanol use.

Patient Preparation The patient ideally should fast for 8 hours prior to collection of the specimen. Since elevations may occur with phenytoin or phenobarbital therapy, one of the alternate tests, leucine aminopeptidase (LAP) or 5′ nucleotidase, is preferable in such patients.

Specimen Serum

Container Red top tube

Storage Instructions Hemolysis and prolonged contact with erythrocytes do not interfere. Stable 1 month at 4°C and 1 year at -20°C.

Reference Range Varies between laboratories. The following is appropriate only for some laboratories: higher in newborns, in first 3-6 months; male, 6 months and older: 2-30 units/L (SI: 0.03-0.51 µKat/L), female, 6 months and older: 1-24 units/L (SI: 0.02-0.41 µKat/L). Values in adult males are 25% higher than adult females.

Use A biliary enzyme that is especially useful in the diagnosis of obstructive jaundice, intrahepatic cholestasis, and pancreatitis.[1] A major application of GGT is in interpretation of increases of serum alkaline phosphatase.[2] GGT is more responsive to biliary obstruction than are aspartate aminotransferase (AST) (SGOT) and alanine aminotransferase (ALT) (SGPT). In obstructive disease values as high as 5 to 50 times upper limit of normal are seen. In infectious hepatitis, values seldom go above 5 times normal.

Increased in hepatoma and carcinoma of pancreas. Useful in diagnosis of metastatic carcinoma in the liver. Increasing levels in carcinoma patients relate to tumor progression and diminishing levels to response to treatment.[3] CEA, alkaline phosphatase, and GGT used together are useful markers for hepatic metastasis from breast and colon primaries. GGT is elevated in some instances of seminoma.

Useful in diagnosis of chronic alcoholic liver disease, but some heavy drinkers do not have GGT increases. Serial determinations of serum GGT, AST, and ALT levels can distinguish recovering alcoholics who resume drinking from those who remain abstinent.[4,5] Increase in body mass is positively correlated with increased GGT levels.[6] With MCV of red cells, GGT is useful as a screen for alcoholism.

GGT is the test for cholestasis during or immediately following pregnancy. Commonly elevated in cirrhosis and hepatitis. The transaminases, AST and ALT rise higher in acute viral hepatitis; these tests with GGT and other parameters are best used together in work-up of liver disease.

Increased in systemic lupus erythematosus.[3] Very high levels are common in primary biliary cirrhosis. High GGT is found in infants with biliary atresia. It is increased with hyperthyroidism and decreased in those with hypothyroidism. It was elevated in 93% of cases of adult glycogen storage disease.[7] GGT is comparable in many ways to two other biliary tests, LAP and 5′ nucleotidase. In some cases, five tests (including alkaline phosphatase and bilirubin) are necessary to evaluate the biliary tract. GGT usually is the most sensitive.

In **ascitic fluid**, very high GGT is increased in some, but not all cases of hepatoma, as opposed to cirrhosis or liver metastases. As in serum, it is high in the ascitic fluid of those with alcoholic cirrhosis.[8]

Limitations Acetaminophen toxicity has been reported to cause an *in vivo* increase. The combination of high alkaline phosphatase and normal GGT does not rule out liver disease completely. Activity is not significantly increased in sera of patients with lymphoma (unless there is hepatic involvement by the lymphoma). Used alone as a preoperative screening test for metastasis from colorectal carcinoma, GGT is unsatisfactory. As part of a screening battery for carcinoma patients, 19% of GGT results from patients with progressive disease were not abnormal, and 4% of values from patients without evidence of tumor were high.[3]

Methodology Kinetic by photometry

Additional Information GGT is a biliary excretory enzyme which is more specific for hepatic disease than is alkaline phosphatase. It is normal in most instances of renal failure.[9] GGT has no origin in bone or placenta, unlike alkaline phosphatase, and age beyond infancy does not influence GGT levels. Activity of GGT is highest in obstructive liver disease. It is commonly elevated in patients with infectious mononucleosis. When GGT and alkaline phosphatase are both high, but one is disproportionately elevated, suspect the possibility of drug-induced cholestasis (including alcoholism if it is GGT which is much higher). GGT, postprandial glucose, and triglyceride bear some correlation in certain groups of patients, including alcoholism and diabetes mellitus. Treatment of hypertriglyceridemia may also lead to decreased GGT. **GGT is normal** in normal children, adolescents, and in pregnant women. Unlike AST, it is not elevated in skeletal muscle disease. High levels of GGT are present in the prostate, which probably accounts for a higher reference range in males.

High levels have been reported in a family.[2]

Footnotes

1. Stein TA, Burns GP, and Wise L, "Diagnostic Value of Liver Function Tests in Bile Duct Obstruction," *J Surg Res*, 1989, 46(3):226-9.
2. Bibas M, Zampa G, Procopio A, et al, "High Serum Gamma-Glutamyltransferase Concentrations in a Family," *N Engl J Med*, 1994, 330(25):1832-3 (letter).
3. Sahm DF, Murray JL, Munson PL, et al, "Gamma Glutamyl Transpeptidase Levels as an Aid in the Management of Human Cancer," *Cancer*, 1983, 52:1673-8.
4. Irwin M, Baird S, Smith TL, et al, "Use of Laboratory Tests to Monitor Heavy Drinking by Alcoholic Men Discharged From a Treatment Program," *Am J Psychiatry*, 1988, 145(5):595-9.
5. Frimpong NA and Lapp JA, "Effects of Moderate Alcohol Intake in Fixed or Variable Amounts on Concentration of Serum Lipids and Liver Enzymes in Healthy Young Men," *Am J Clin Nutr*, 1989, 50(5):987-91.
6. Robinson D and Whitehead TP, "Effect of Body Mass and Other Factors on Serum Liver Enzyme Levels in Men Attending for Well Population Screening," *Ann Clin Biochem*, 1989, 26(Pt 5):393-400.
7. Talente GM, Coleman RA, Alter C, et al, "Glycogen Storage Disease in Adults," *Ann Intern Med*, 1994, 120(3):218-26.
8. Kjeldsberg CR and Knight JA, *Body Fluids - Laboratory Examination of Amniotic, Cerebrospinal, Seminal, Serous, and Synovial Fluids*, 3rd ed, Chicago, IL: American Society of Clinical Pathologists, 1993, 235.
9. Lum G and Gambino SR, "Serum Gamma Glutamyl Transpeptidase Activity as an Indicator of Disease of Liver, Pancreas, or Bone," *Clin Chem*, 1972, 18:358-62.

References

Burtis CA and Ashwood ER, *Tietz Textbook of Clinical Chemistry*, 2nd ed, Philadelphia, PA: WB Saunders Co, 1994, 847-50.
Gjerde H, Amundsen A, Skog OJ, et al, "Serum Gamma Glutamyltransferase: An Epidemiological Indicator of Alcohol Consumption?" *Br J Addict*, 1987, 82(9):1027-31.

Gamma Glutamyl Transpeptidase *see Gamma Glutamyl Transferase on this page*

Gap *see Anion Gap on page 81*

Gases, Arterial *see Blood Gases, Arterial on page 87*

Gastric Analysis

CPT 82926 (gastric acid, free and total single specimen); 89135 (gastric intubation aspiration and fractional collections, 1 hour); 89136 (2 hours); 89140 (2 hours with gastric stimulation, eg, pentagastrin); 89141 (3 hours with gastric stimulation)

Related Information

Gastrin, Serum *on page 135*
(Continued)

Gastric Analysis (Continued)

Helicobacter pylori Serology *on page 395*
Helicobacter pylori Urease Test and Culture *on page 484*
Intrinsic Factor Antibody *on page 411*
Parietal Cell Antibody *on page 421*

Synonyms Pentagastrin Stimulation Test; Peptavlon® Stimulation Test

Replaces Gastric Analysis, Nocturnal Acid Output; Histalog™ Stimulation Test; Tubeless Gastric Analysis

Test Commonly Includes Basal and four poststimulation specimens for pH, volume, and acid output

Abstract Acid (HCl) output of the stomach is relevant to peptic ulcer. Measurement of acid secretion in evaluation of selected ulcer patients is helpful in particular circumstances, but is not needed for diagnosis of peptic ulcer, and not indicated for most.

Patient Preparation Antacids and H_2-receptor antagonists should not be given to patient for 24-48 hours prior to testing. Drugs that affect gastric acid secretion, such as tricyclic antidepressants, anticholinergics, reserpine, and so forth should be discontinued overnight to 72 hours prior to testing. The patient must fast after the evening meal on the day prior to the test day, but may have water up to 1 hour before the test. After pentagastrin has been administered, medical supervision should be maintained since side reactions may occur.

Specimen Gastric secretions, four 15-minute basal and four 15-minute poststimulation collections. Entire volume collected. Longer periods are sometimes used (eg, 24-hour measurement) but are not well standardized and may be dangerous.

Container No preservative

Collection A cold lubricated gastric (Levine) tube is inserted orally or nasally while the patient is in a sitting or reclining position on his/her left side. The tube must have a radiopaque tip. Nasal intubation is used if the patient has a hyperactive gag reflex. It should be positioned in the stomach so that the tip is opposite the angularis or "re-entrant angle" in the most dependent portion of the stomach. In a patient who has had a subtotal gastrectomy, the tube should be placed well within the lumen of the stomach, below the fundus and above the anastomosis. Proper positioning of the tube is confirmed by fluoroscopy or x-ray. Wait 10-15 minutes for the patient to adjust to the tube. The patient should be in a sitting position. Gentle constant suction is needed, except for brief intervals when a small quantity of air can be injected to clear the tube. The first two or three specimens immediately following intubation (the first 15-30 minutes) should not be utilized as basal secretion as they do not accurately reflect the basal state. Give no liquids to the patient during the test and request that the patient expectorate saliva. The basal specimen is obtained by continuous aspiration of the gastric fluid with a Toomey syringe for 60 minutes as four 15-minute specimens. These are the **BAO (basal acid output)**. After the basal sample has been collected, pentagastrin is injected (see package insert). The collection of the poststimulation specimens must begin immediately. The gastric content is continuously aspirated for the next 60 minutes, during which time the gastric contents obtained from each of four 15-minute periods are collected into separate plastic containers labeled **poststimulation** number 1, 2, 3 and 4 respectively. Securely fasten the lids on the containers and send the eight specimens (four basal and four poststimulation) to the laboratory. The containers must identify the order in which the specimens were collected.

Storage Instructions Refrigerate if test delayed more than 4 hours.

Causes for Rejection Contamination of specimens with duodenal contents, indicated by the yellow color of bile

Reference Range Normal gastric juice may be clear or contain some bile. If red or black, test for blood.

A major disadvantage of gastric analysis is the breadth of values in normal individuals, overlapping results in those with duodenal and gastric ulcer. Normal BAO is up to 10.5 mmol/hour (men) and 5.6 mmol/hour (women). BAO represents gastric acid secretion in the absence of stimulation. It follows circadian rhythm and is highest from 2-11 PM. Brady et al define basal hypersecretion as basal acid output >11 mmol/hour (men) and 6 mmol/hour (women). They describe features of patients with *Helicobacter pylori* according to acid secretory status.[1] Lower ranges are provided by McGuigan.[2]

Normal MAO (maximal acid output) is up to 48 mmol/hour (men) and 30 mmol/hour (women). MAO is the sum of four 15-minute collections following pentagastrin.

Normal PAO (peak acid output) is 11-60 mmol/hour (men) and 8-40 mmol/hour (women).

Normal BAO to PAO is <0.29 (men) and <0.23 (women).

Critical Values More than 90% of patients with Z-E syndrome have BAO >15 mEq/hour if prior gastric surgery has not been done or >5 mEq/L if prior gastric resection or vagotomy had taken place.[3]

Use Evaluate gastric function. Support the diagnosis of pernicious anemia: provision of evidence of gastric mucosal atrophy; evaluation of recurrent peptic ulcer, Zollinger-Ellison (Z-E) syndrome, and Ménétrier's disease. **Gastrinoma/Zollinger-Ellison (ZE) syndrome** can lead to peptic ulcer with massive acid secretion. The Zollinger-Ellison syndrome includes the presence of nonbeta neuroendocrine tumors which secrete gastrin. The diagnosis of the Zollinger-Ellison syndrome is established by demonstration of gastric acid hypersecretion, basal acid secretion >15 mmol/hour in an unoperated subject with peptic ulcer, with fasting gastrin level >1000 pg/mL (SI: >1000 ng/L).[4] Fasting gastrin >1000 with pH <2.5 provides strong evidence for Z-E syndrome.[3]

Pernicious anemia: Anacidity has been an essential component for the diagnosis of PA. High gastrin levels are found, *vide infra*.

Gastritis: Severe gastritis with mucosal atrophy is associated with anacidity or is thought to produce progressive loss of secretory ability. Availability of superior endoscopy has diminished indications for gastric analysis for gastritis.

Ulcer recurrence: The explanation for ulcer recurrence following surgery may be sought with investigation of gastric acid secretion.

With hypergastrinemia: To separate entities causing gastric acid hypersecretion from achlorhydria.[2]

Gastric carcinoma: Few if any cases clinically, endoscopically and/or radiologically considered to be carcinoma, presently have gastric analysis. Gastric carcinoma and gastric polyps, classically, have often been associated with decreased-to-absent hydrochloric acid. Of course, carcinoma occurs without anacidity and anacidity occurs without carcinoma. The demonstration of complete anacidity to maximal stimulation (pentagastrin-fast achlorhydria) in the presence of a gastric ulcer supports (but does not prove) a diagnosis of malignancy. Patients with gastric ulcers generally show low to normal basal and maximum acid output.

Limitations Tube not in proper place for aspiration, incomplete volume collection. Losses of gastric juice into the duodenum occur, especially in patients who have had pyloroplasty or gastroenterostomy.

Gastric analysis itself is insufficient for the diagnosis of gastrinoma. Substantial overlap exists between patients with gastrinoma, with common duodenal ulcer and normal subjects in rates of gastric acid output.[4] Gastric analysis is time consuming, uncomfortable for the patient and it is expensive.

Contraindications Gastric intubation is contraindicated for patients with esophageal varices, diverticula, stenosis, malignant neoplasm of the esophagus, aortic aneurysm, severe gastric hemorrhage, and congestive heart failure. It is not necessary for the usual duodenal ulcer patient in whom the Zollinger-Ellison is not suspected.

Patient must not receive medication that influences gastric secretion; such contraindications include antacids, anticholinergic drugs, reserpine, alcohol, adrenergic blocking agents, and adrenocorticosteroids.

Histalog™ is contraindicated in patients with a history of asthma or paroxysmal hypertension, but asthmatics, severely hyperallergenic problems are thought not to be contraindications when pentagastrin (Pepavlon®) is used as the stimulant (see package insert). It contains the active carboxyterminal tetrapeptide amide part of gastrin. It is the preferred agent. Hypersensitivity or idiosyncrasy to pentagastrin is described. Histalog™ should not be given if the patient's systolic pressure is <110 mm Hg.

Methodology Volume measurement, pH measurement by pH meter. Do not use pH paper.[5] **Peak acid output (PAO)** is a calculation, in which the two highest 15-minute MAO specimens are combined and multiplied by 2.

Additional Information "Anacidity" is regarded as pH >6 following stimulation. If specimens become grossly bloody, physician should be contacted to ascertain if procedure should be continued. Confirm if indicated with a test for hemoglobin.

Basal gastric analysis: Specimens should be collected at 15-minute intervals for 1 hour, labeled basal 1, basal 2, etc, and sent to the laboratory.

Maximal stimulation gastric analysis: This measures the response to maximal stimulation by pentagastrin. This material is administered after collection of the basal specimens. Thirty minutes after administration of pentagastrin, four 15-minute specimens of gastric juice are aspirated as described, labeled "Max 1", "2", etc, and sent to the laboratory. The patient should be observed regularly, preferably by the physician. With proper precautions, side effects are rare.

Availability of assays for gastrin diminish the need for gastric analysis.

Contemporary work-up for pernicious anemia (PA) includes vitamin B_{12}/folate assays, Schilling test and sometimes, testing for antibodies to intrinsic factor and to parietal cells.

Of 36 subjects with *Helicobacter pylori* who underwent gastric analysis, 25 were normochlorhydric and 11 were hypochlorhydric. Nineteen normochlorhydric patients had ulcers (10 gastric and 9 duodenal). Two hypochlorhydric patients had gastric ulcers. These authors were unable to identify a consistent relationship between *Helicobacter pylori* and acid secretion.[1] Several studies showed that *H. pylori* is not a major contributing factor in duodenal ulcer associated with Z-E syndrome.[6,7]

Footnotes
1. Brady CE 3d, Hadfield TL, Hyatt JR, et al, "Acid Secretion and Serum Gastrin Levels in Individuals With *Campylobacter pylori*," *Gastroenterology*, 1988, 94(4):923-7.
2. McGuigan JE, "Peptic Ulcer and Gastritis," *Harrison's Principles of Internal Medicine*, 13th ed, Isselbacher KJ, Braunwald E, Wilson JD, et al, eds, New York, NY: McGraw-Hill Inc, 1994, 1363-82.
3. Jensen RT and Fraker DL, "Zollinger-Ellison Syndrome - Advances in Treatment of Gastric Hypersecretion and the Gastrinoma," *JAMA*, 1994, 271(18):1429-35.
4. Wolfe MM, "Diagnosis of Gastrinoma: Much Ado About Nothing?" *Ann Intern Med*, 1989, 111(9):697-9.
5. Caballero GA, Ausman RK, Quebbeman EJ, et al, "Gastric Secretion pH Measurement: What You See Is Not What You Get!" *Crit Care Med*, 1990, 18(4):396-9.
6. Saeed ZA, Evans DJ Jr, Evans DG, et al, "*Helicobacter pylori* and Zollinger-Ellison Syndrome," *Dig Dis Sci*, 1991, 36(1):15-8.
7. Fich A, Talley NJ, Shorter RG, et al, "Zollinger-Ellison Syndrome. Relation to *Helicobacter pylori*-Associated Chronic Gastritis and Gastric Acid Secretion," *Dig Dis Sci*, 1991, 36(1):10-4.

References
Berg CL and Wolfe MM, "Zollinger-Ellison Syndrome," *Med Clin North Am*, 1991, 75(4):903-21.
Malagelada JR, Davis CS, O'Fallon WM, et al, "Laboratory Diagnosis of Gastrinoma. 1. A Prospective Evaluation of Gastric Analysis and Fasting Serum Gastrin Levels," *Mayo Clin Proc*, 1982, 57:211-8.
Pisegna JR, Norton JA, Slimak GG, et al, "Effects of Curative Gastrinoma Resection on Gastric Secretory Function and Antisecretory Drug Requirement in the Zollinger-Ellison Syndrome," *Gastroenterology*, 1992, 102(3):767-78.
Segal HL, "Clinical Measurements of Gastric Secretion: Significance and Limitations," *Ann Intern Med*, 1960, 53:447.
Soybel DI and Modlin IM, "Sustained Suppression of Gastric Secretion and the Risk of Neoplasia in the Gastric Mucosa," *Am J Gastroenterol*, 1991, 86(12):1713-9.

Gastric Analysis, Nocturnal Acid Output *replaced by* Gastric Analysis *on page 133*

Gastrin, Serum
CPT 82941

Related Information
Gastric Analysis *on page 133*
Helicobacter pylori Urease Test and Culture *on page 484*
Schilling Test *on page 346*
Vitamin B$_{12}$ *on page 351*

Applies to Secretin Test

Abstract Gastrin is normally produced by cells in the gastric antral mucosa. The Zollinger-Ellison (Z-E) syndrome may be sporadic or familial. It is characterized by severe peptic ulcer disease, often with diarrhea. Esophageal complaints may be among early symptoms. In about 10% of cases, diarrhea is the only symptom. Basal gastrin levels are usually increased with the Z-E syndrome.[1] The original syndrome included extreme hypersecretion of gastric acid, refractory peptic ulcer disease, and nonbeta islet cell tumor.[2]

Patient Preparation The patient must be fasting overnight, preferably 12 hours or more. Protein meal can cause a marked increase in serum gastrin. No recent radioactive isotopes. Gastrin may be increased following gastroscopy.

Specimen Serum

Container Red top tube

Collection Transport specimen immediately to the laboratory following collection. Postprandial specimens should be so indicated.

Storage Instructions Separate in a refrigerated centrifuge and freeze immediately. Stable 4 hours at 4°C and 30 days at -20°C.

Causes for Rejection Avoid anticoagulated tubes for this assay.

Reference Range Fasting: up to 100 pg/mL (SI: 47.7 pmol/L) (up to 200 pg/mL (SI: 95.3 pmol/L) in some laboratories). Fasting values exhibit a circadian rhythm with lowest values between 0300 and 0700. Postprandial: 95-140 pg/mL (SI: 45.3-66.7 pmol/L) usually under 250 pg/mL (SI: 119.2 pmol/L). Normal basal concentrations usually rule out a diagnosis of gastrinoma.[1] Secretin stimulation is positive if the serum gastrin rises 200 pg/mL (SI: 95.3 pmol/L) or more anytime following secretin administration.[3]

Critical Values Basal serum gastrin is usually 3-100 times above normal in subjects with gastrinoma.[1] Fasting gastrin is increased but is <1000 in 60% of patients with Z-E syndrome.[2]

Use Diagnose Zollinger-Ellison (Z-E) syndrome; diagnose gastrinoma. Gastrin >1000 pg/mL (SI: >476.6 pmol/L) with gastric acid hypersecretion (basal acid secretion >15 mmol/hour in a patient with peptic ulcer who has not had surgery) establishes unequivocally the diagnosis of the Zollinger-Ellison syndrome.[4] Antral G-cell hyperplasia may relate to high gastrin levels and duodenal ulcer.

Limitations Gastric hyperacidity must be documented. Gastric ulcer, chronic renal failure, hyperparathyroidism, pyloric obstruction, carcinoma of stomach,[5] vagotomy without gastric resection, retained gastric antrum

and short bowel syndrome have been reported with moderate elevations of gastrin levels. Gastrin levels are increased with pernicious anemia. H$_2$-receptor blockers (cimetidine) may result in elevated levels. Overlap of serum gastrin values between gastrinoma and other states occurs. Up to 40% of Z-E patients have fasting gastrin values between 100-500 pg/mL (SI: 47.7-238.3 pmol/L), while a few patients with gastric or duodenal ulcer without gastrinoma, have results in this range. At least half of patients with the Z-E syndrome lack diagnostic serum gastrin levels, although in nearly all, fasting serum gastrin levels are increased.[4] Patients with Z-E syndrome with normal screening gastrin levels are described.[1,6]

Methodology Radioimmunoassay (RIA)

Additional Information Hypochlorhydria can induce hypergastrinemia. Gastrin is secreted by antral G cells and stimulates gastric acid production, antral motility, and secretion of pepsin and intrinsic factor. The principle forms of gastrin in blood are G-34 (big gastrin, half-life 5 minutes) and G-14 (minigastrin, half-life 5 minutes). Each of these polypeptides circulates in nonsulfated (I) or sulfated (II) forms. Instilling acid into the stomach normally inhibits gastrin secretion. Elevated gastrin levels should be interpreted in light of gastric acid secretion and other parameters. The neuroendocrine tumors associated with the Zollinger-Ellison syndrome are characterized by elevated rates of gastric HCl secretion and upper gastrointestinal ulcer disease. Gastrin levels >500-600 pg/mL (SI: >238-286 pmol/L) in a patient with basal acid hypersecretion often indicates gastrinoma, but antral G-cell hyperplasia cases can have gastrin levels >500 pg/mL and hyperchlorhydria. If gastrinoma is likely but fasting gastrin level is not diagnostic, the **secretin test** is the provocative test of choice. Absolute increase in serum gastrin level above the basal figure is preferred to percent change.[4] I.V. secretin normally diminishes gastrin, but serum gastrin increases in gastrinoma patients. Wolfe provides an explanation for this paradoxical effect.[4] Details of the secretin-injection test are available. It usually provides support for the diagnosis of gastrinoma, but false-positives are found with achlorhydria and hypergastrinemia.[1] Calcium infusion also stimulates gastrin release but does not distinguish other causes of ulcer as well as the secretin test. Protocols for stimulation tests are published.[7]

Up to 30% of Z-E patients have evidence of Werner's syndrome (multiple endocrine neoplasia type I (MEN-I)).[2] It may include hyperparathyroidism, pancreatic endocrine tumors including nonfunctional ones and others producing polypeptides, islet cell tumors of the pancreas, pituitary tumors, and Cushing's syndrome and 13% develop gastric carcinoid tumor.[2] Gastrinomas are malignant in 62% of cases, and 44% of patients have metastases.

Conditions associated with hypergastrinemia including chronic atrophic gastritis, Z-E syndrome with MEN-I and pernicious anemia all include significantly increased incidence of gastric carcinoids.[9]

No consistent relationship has been established between *Helicobacter pylori* and gastric acid secretion or serum gastrin levels.[3]

Features of gastrinoma additional to those of peptic ulcer may include steatorrhea.

Gastrinomas are often found in the pancreas but more than half are primary in the duodenum. A few cases in which a gastrinoma was primary in the stomach have been reported. The morphology is that of foregut carcinoids.[10]

Somatostatin inhibits the expression of gastrin mRNA.[11]

Footnotes
1. Zimmer T, Stölzel U, Bäder M, et al, "Brief Report: A Duodenal Gastrinoma in a Patient With Diarrhea and Normal Serum Gastrin Concentrations," *N Engl J Med*, 1995, 333(10):634-6.
2. Jensen RT and Fraker DL, "Zollinger-Ellison Syndrome - Advances in Treatment of Gastric Hypersecretion and the Gastrinoma," *JAMA*, 1994, 271(18):1429-35.
3. Brady CE 3d, Hadfield TL, Hyatt JR, et al, "Acid Secretion and Serum Gastrin Levels in Individuals With *Campylobacter pylori*," *Gastroenterology*, 1988, 94(4):923-7.
4. Wolfe MM, "Diagnosis of Gastrinoma: Much Ado About Nothing?" *Ann Intern Med*, 1989, 111(9):697-9.
5. Rakic S and Milicevic MN, "Serum Gastrin Levels in Patients With Intestinal and Diffuse Type of Gastric Cancer," *Br J Cancer*, 1991, 64(6):1189.
6. Yanda RJ, Ostroff JW, Ashbaugh CD, et al, "Zollinger-Ellison Syndrome in a Patient With Normal Screening Gastrin Level," *Dig Dis Sci*, 1989, 34(12):1929-32.
7. Malagelada JR, Glanzman SL, and GO VL, "Laboratory Diagnosis of Gastrinoma. II. A Prospective Study of Gastrin Challenge Tests," *Mayo Clin Proc*, 1982, 57:219-26.
8. Jensen RT, Gardner JD, Raufman JP, et al, "Zollinger-Ellison Syndrome: Current Concepts and Management," *Ann Intern Med*, 1983, 98:59-75.
9. Gilligan CJ, Lawton GP, Tang LH, et al, "Gastric Carcinoid Tumors: The Biology and Therapy of an Enigmatic and Controversial Lesion," *Am J Gastroenterol*, 1995, 90(3):338-52.
10. Wilander E, "Endocrine Cell Tumours," *Gastrointestinal and Oesophageal Pathology*, Whitehead R, ed, New York, NY: Churchill Livingstone, 1989, 629-41.
11. Karnik PS, Monahan SJ, and Wolfe MM, "Inhibition of Gastrin Gene Expression by Somatostatin," *J Clin Invest*, 1989, 83(2):367-72.

References
Bordi C, D'Adda T, Azzoni C, et al, "Hypergastrinemia and Gastric Enterochromaffin-Like Cells," *Am J Surg Pathol*, 1995, 19(Suppl 1):S8-19.
Fraker DL and Norton JA, "The Role of Surgery in the Management of Islet Cell Tumors," *Gastroenterol Clin North Am*, 1989, 18(4):805-30.

(Continued)

Gastrin, Serum (Continued)

Freston JW, Borch K, Brand SJ, et al, "Effects of Hypochlorhydria and Hypergastrinemia on Structure and Function of Gastrointestinal Cells. A Review and Analysis," *Dig Dis Sci*, 1995, 40(2 Suppl):50S-62S.

Green DW, Gomez G, and Greeley GH Jr, "Gastrointestinal Peptides," *Gastroenterol Clin North Am*, 1989, 18(4):695-733.

Lloyd KC, "Gut Hormones in Gastric Function," *Baillieres Clin Endocrinol Metab*, 1994, 8(1):111-36.

Malagelada JR, Davis CS, O'Fallon WM, et al, "Laboratory Diagnosis of Gastrinoma. I. A Prospective Evaluation of Gastric Analysis and Fasting Serum Gastrin Levels," *Mayo Clin Proc*, 1982, 57:211-8.

McQuaid KR, "Much Ado About Gastrin," *J Clin Gastroenterol*, 1991, 13(3):249-54.

Solcia E, Capella C, Fiocca R, et al, "The Gastroenteropancreatic Endocrine System and Related Tumors," *Gastroenterol Clin North Am*, 1989, 18(4):671-93.

Solcia E, Fiocca R, Villani L, et al, "Hyperplastic, Dysplastic, and Neoplastic Enterochromaffin-Like Cell Proliferations of the Gastric Mucosa Classification and Histogenesis," *Am J Surg Pathol*, 1995, 19(Suppl 1):S1-S7.

Solcia E, Rindi G, Silini E, et al, "Enterochromaffin-Like (ECL) Cells and Their Growths: Relationships to Gastrin, Reduced Acid Secretion and Gastritis," *Baillieres Clin Gastroenterol*, 1993, 7(1):149-65.

Warburton R and Close JR, "The *In Vitro* Stability of Gastrin in Serum and Whole Blood," *Ann Clin Biochem*, 1987, 24(Pt 3):320-1.

Wolfe MM, Jain DK, and Edgerton JR, "Zollinger-Ellison Syndrome Associated With Persistently Normal Fasting Serum Gastrin Concentrations," *Ann Intern Med*, 1985, 103(2):215-7.

Gestational Diabetes Screening Test see Glucose Tolerance Test on page 139

GFR see Creatinine Clearance on page 117

GGT see Gamma Glutamyl Transferase on page 133

GGTP see Gamma Glutamyl Transferase on page 133

GH see Growth Hormone on page 141

GHB see Glycated Hemoglobin on page 140

Globulin see Albumin, Serum on page 66

Globulin see Protein, Total, Serum on page 194

Glucagon see Vasoactive Intestinal Polypeptide on page 216

Glucagon, Plasma

CPT 82943

Related Information

Vasoactive Intestinal Polypeptide *on page 216*

Abstract A single chain polypeptide, glucagon provides primary defense against hypoglycemia.[1] Glucagonoma is an extremely rare endocrine tumor, some of which are found in multiple endocrine neoplasia type I (MEN-I).[2]

Patient Preparation Overnight fasting for basal levels. If diabetic, patient should be in good control before specimen is drawn. Avoid recent radioactive tracer (eg, for radioactive scan).

Specimen Plasma

Container Draw blood into a chilled lavender top (EDTA) tube. Deliver to the laboratory immediately.

Storage Instructions Freeze. Stable 2 months at -20°C.

Special Instructions Mix the blood immediately and centrifuge in a refrigerated centrifuge.

Reference Range ≤60 pg/mL (SI: ≤60 ng/L) at one laboratory, but other normal ranges are in use, eg, 20-100 pg/mL (RIA)

Critical Values Most patients with glucagonoma have levels >500 pg/mL (SI: >500 ng/L); >1000 pg/mL (SI: >1000 ng/L) is diagnostic.[1]

Use Diagnose glucagonoma. Glucagonoma may be present in three different syndromes. The first consists of a characteristic skin rash, necrolytic migratory erythema, diabetes mellitus or impaired glucose tolerance, weight loss, anemia, and venous thrombosis. This form usually is characterized by very high glucagon levels, >1000 pg/mL (SI: >1000 ng/L). The second form is associated with severe diabetes, and the third form is that with multiple endocrine neoplasia syndrome. This form may have relatively lower glucagon levels. It may be overproduced with neuroblastoma.

Contraindications Recent radioactive scan

Methodology Radioimmunoassay (RIA); ethanol extraction removes "big" glucagon, which is not considered biologically active.

Additional Information Glucagon is normally secreted by α_2-cells of pancreatic islets, and exerts a counterbalancing effect to insulin in regulation of glucose metabolism. Glucagon exists in "true" form (3500 daltons - biologically active form) and "big" form (160,000 daltons). This form may represent binding of the 3500-dalton glucagon to plasma protein, and rare families have increased amounts of "big" glucagon circulating. Very high levels of glucagon are seen with glucagonomas, and elevations are also seen in diabetic ketoacidosis, stress, uremia, hepatic cirrhosis, hyperosmolality, acute pancreatitis, burns, trauma, surgery, and hypoglycemia. Glucagonoma syndrome is reported with giant cell bronchogenic carcinoma.[3] Decreased values are found in cystic fibrosis, chronic pancreatitis, and in the postpancreatectomy state. Over 75% of glucagonomas have metastasized at time of diagnosis. After a glucose load, there is no suppression of glucagon in patients with glucagonoma (glucagon suppression test). In glucagon deficiency (cystic fibrosis, chronic pancreatitis) there is a failure of plasma glucagon to rise during arginine infusion.

Footnotes

1. Service FJ, "Hypoglycemic Disorders," *N Engl J Med*, 1995, 332(17):1144-52.
2. Kaplan LM, "Endocrine Tumors of the Gastrointestinal Tract and Pancreas," *Harrison's Principles of Internal Medicine*, 13th ed, Isselbacher KJ, Braunwald E, Wilson JD, et al, eds, New York, NY: McGraw-Hill Inc, 1994, 1535-42.
3. Hunstein W, Trümper LH, Dummer R, et al, "Glucagonoma Syndrome and Bronchial Carcinoma," *Ann Intern Med*, 1988, 109(11):920-1.

References

Boden G, "Glucagonomas and Insulinomas," *Gastroenterol Clin North Am*, 1990, 18(4):831-45.

Diem P, Redmon JB, Abid M, et al, "Glucagon, Catecholamine, and Pancreatic Polypeptide Secretion in Type I Diabetic Recipients of Pancreas Allografts," *J Clin Invest*, 1990, 86(6):2008-13.

Holst JJ, "Glucagonlike Peptide 1: A Newly Discovered Gastrointestinal Hormone," *Gastroenterology*, 1994, 107(6):1848-55.

Liu D, Moberg E, Kollind M, et al, "A High Concentration of Circulating Insulin Suppresses the Glucagon Response to Hypoglycemia in Normal Man," *J Clin Endocrinol Metab*, 1991, 73(5):1123-8.

Magnusson I, Rothman DL, Gerard DP, et al, "Contribution of Hepatic Glycogenolysis to Glucose Production in Humans in Response to a Physiological Increase in Plasma Glucagon Concentration," *Diabetes*, 1995, 44(2):185-9.

Rothe AJ, Young JW, Keramati B, et al, "The Value of Glucagon in Routine Barium Investigations of the Gastrointestinal Tract," *Invest Radiol*, 1987, 22(10):786-91.

Glucose, 2-Hour Postprandial

CPT 82950

Related Information

Fructosamine *on page 130*
Glucose, Quantitative, Urine *on page 635*
Glucose, Semiquantitative, Urine *on page 636*
Glycated Hemoglobin *on page 140*
Ketones, Urine *on page 639*
Microalbuminuria *on page 643*
Reducing Substances, Urine *on page 652*

Synonyms 2-Hour PP Glucose; Postprandial Glucose; PP, 2-Hour

Test Commonly Includes Glucose level 2 hours after meal or after measured glucose load

Abstract An important test used to establish the diagnosis of diabetes mellitus

Patient Preparation Adequate meal or glucose load 2 hours before "2-hour postprandial glucose," as specified by the patient's physician. Patient is allowed his/her usual meal (breakfast or lunch). Patient must complete meal within 15-20 minutes. Specimen is to be collected 2 hours from beginning of meal. It is preferable to administer 75 g glucose, for work-up for NIDDM, allowing 5 minutes for consumption. Gambino, among others, considers the 2-hour postload (75 g) glucose determination the best single sample for diabetes screening.[1]

Specimen Plasma or serum

Container Gray top (sodium fluoride) tube or red top tube

Collection Collect in morning after overnight fast and standard meal.

Reference Range <140 mg/dL (SI: <7.8 mmol/L). Some use 120 mg/dL 2 hours after a 75 g glucose load. In an unstressed nonpregnant patient not receiving any medication, a 2-hour postprandial glucose of 140-200 mg/dL (SI: 7.8-11.1 mmol/L) is classified as impaired. A 2-hour result >200 mg/dL, on at least two occasions, supports the diagnosis of diabetes mellitus. For the diagnosis of gestational diabetes mellitus, a plasma glucose >140 mg/dL (SI: >7.8 mmol/L) 1 hour after a 50 g glucose load is an indication for the glucose tolerance test recommended for gestational patients. A 2-hour postprandial glucose <105 mg/dL (SI: <5.8 mmol/L) is desirable.

Use Only a minority of patients with diabetes mellitus have the classic symptoms of polyuria, polyphagia, polydipsia, and weight loss. **The 2-hour postprandial glucose is extensively used to establish the diagnosis of diabetes mellitus**. It may be used along with FBS to follow patients with impaired glucose tolerance. Follow-up of women who had gestational diabetes, of whom most revert after delivery to normal glucose tolerance (up to half ultimately become diabetic). It is used as part of the work-up for impotence, hypertriglyceridemia, neuropathy, retinopathy, glycosuria and for certain types of renal diseases. Work-up of vulvovaginitis, blurred vision, fatigue, and some instances of urinary tract infections. **Causes of postprandial hypoglycemia** include alimentary type (commonly secondary to prior gastrointestinal surgery); reactive hypoglycemia without prior gastrointestinal surgery - alimentary or spontaneous, functional, idiopathic, indeterminate; some prediabetics; leucine-induced; fructose-induced; galactosemia; indeterminate group.

Additional Information Use of fasting and 2-hour postprandial glucose values are recommended to establish the diagnosis of diabetes mellitus.

Glycosylated hemoglobin is recommended for monitoring diabetes control. See chart.

Classification of Diabetes and Related Disorders

Diabetes mellitus (DM)			
Type I	IDDM	Insulin-dependent diabetes mellitus	Formerly called juvenile diabetes
Type II	NIDDM	Noninsulin-dependent diabetes mellitus	Formerly called adult-onset diabetes
Gestational diabetes			
Other types			
Diabetes with acromegaly			
Diabetes with Cushing's syndrome			
Diabetes with pancreatitis			
Diabetes with hemochromatosis			

Footnotes

1. Gambino R, "Criteria for Diagnosis of Diabetes," *Lab Report for Physicians*, 1987, 9:68-9.

References

Hanson RL, Nelson RG, McCance DR, et al, "Comparison of Screening Tests for Non-Insulin Dependent Diabetes Mellitus," *Arch Intern Med*, 1993, 153(18):2133-40.

Home P, "The OGTT: Gold That Does Not Shine," *Diabet Med*, 1988, 5(4):313-4.

Jarrett RJ, Keen H, and McCartney P, "The Whitehall Study: Ten Year Follow-Up Report on New With Impaired Glucose Tolerance With Reference to Worsening to Diabetics and Predictors of Death," *Diabet Med*, 1984, 1(4):279-83.

McCance DR, Hanson RL, Charles MA, et al, "Comparison of Tests for Glycated Haemoglobin and Fasting and Two-Hour Plasma Glucose Concentrations as Diagnostic Methods for Diabetes," *BMJ*, 1994, 308(6940):1323-8.

National Diabetes Data Group, "Classification and Diagnosis of Diabetes Mellitus and Other Categories of Glucose Intolerance," *Diabetes*, 1979, 28:1039-57.

Smart LM, Howie AF, Young RJ, et al, "Comparison of Fructosamine With Glycosylated Hemoglobin and Plasma Proteins as Measures of Glycemic Control," *Diabetes Care*, 1988, 11(5):433-6.

Glucose, Body Fluid see Body Fluid Glucose on page 91

Glucose, Cerebrospinal Fluid see Cerebrospinal Fluid Glucose on page 105

Glucose, Fasting

CPT 82947

Related Information

Alcohol, Blood or Urine *on page 531*
Body Fluid Glucose *on page 91*
Cerebrospinal Fluid Glucose *on page 105*
C-Peptide *on page 114*
Fructosamine *on page 130*
Glucose, Quantitative, Urine *on page 635*
Glucose, Semiquantitative, Urine *on page 636*
Glucose Tolerance Test *on page 139*
Glycated Hemoglobin *on page 140*
Insulin, Blood *on page 149*
Ketone Bodies, Blood *on page 152*
Microalbuminuria *on page 643*
Oxazepam, Serum *on page 566*
pH, Blood *on page 180*
Point-of-Care Testing *on page 27*
Reducing Substances, Urine *on page 652*

Synonyms Blood Sugar, Fasting; Fasting Blood Sugar; FBS; Sugar, Fasting

Applies to Glucose/Insulin Ratio; Tolbutamide Test

Abstract Used to evaluate disorders of carbohydrate metabolism. Fasting glucose is an insensitive method to screen for noninsulin dependent diabetes mellitus.

Patient Preparation Patient should be fasting for 8 hours.

Specimen Plasma or serum

Container Gray top (sodium fluoride) tube preferred; red top tube acceptable

Collection Neonatal: blood drawn from heelstick

Storage Instructions Glucose will drop 5-10 mg/dL per hour in unseparated, room temperature blood not collected with sodium fluoride (eg, red top tube).

Reference Range Premature infants: 40-65 mg/dL (SI: 2.2-3.6 mmol/L), 0-2 years: 60-110 mg/dL (SI: 3.3-6.1 mmol/L), 2 years to adult: 60-115 mg/dL (SI: 3.3-6.4 mmol/L). Normal range increases with age older than 50. Adult results between 115-140 mg/dL (SI: 6.4-7.8 mmol/L) bear re-examination, but if consistent, imply impairment of glucose tolerance. Some recommend oral glucose tolerance test (OGTT) for patients whose FBSs fall in this range, but most would first get additional FBS and 2-hour postprandial glucose. Fasting glucose (after an overnight fast) >140 mg/dL (SI: >7.8 mmol/L) on at least two occasions, indicates diabetes

mellitus in the unstressed, ambulatory nonpregnant adult, using conventional methods. **Hypoglycemia:** 47-60 mg/dL in adults, but young, lean, healthy women may have glucose levels as low as 40 mg/dL.[1]

Possible Panic Range Infants: <40 mg/dL (SI: <2.2 mmol/L); adults: male: <50 mg/dL (SI: <2.75 mmol/L), female: <40 mg/dL (SI: <2.2 mmol/L); adults: male and female: >400 mg/dL (SI: >22 mmol/L)

Use Establish the diagnosis of diabetes mellitus; evaluate disorders of carbohydrate metabolism, acidosis and ketoacidosis, dehydration, coma, hypoglycemia, and neuroglycopenia; plasma glucose is used to monitor therapy and support control[2] in diabetics; evaluate presence of insulinoma; work up patients with real or apparent alcoholism; investigate polyuria, polydipsia, polyphagia, weight loss, and dehydration

Limitations Mild glucose impairment can exist with fasting glucose within the normal range. Fasting glucose is not adequate to screen for noninsulin-dependent diabetes mellitus.[3] Measurement of plasma glucose without spinal fluid glucose can miss neuroglycopenia. To the extent that innovative new methods deviate from reference methods, such alternative techniques may be unreliable for certain patient care needs.[4] Fingerstick glucose determination in shock are lower than venous glucose and are dangerously misleading.[5]

Methodology Plasma (preferably) or serum glucose may be determined by enzyme-based assays, glucose oxidase or hexokinase. Glucose oxidase/oxygen consumption (Astra™ 8, Beckman Instruments), automated serum solid-phase glucose oxidase/peroxidase (Ektachem®, Eastman Kodak), serum solid-phase glucose oxidase/reflectance (Seralyzer®, Ames Co) and whole blood solid-phase glucose oxidase/reflectance (Dextrostix®, Ames Co) were compared with hexokinase (national reference method) by Gerson and Figoni. These authors expressed hope that considerations of cost may not be given priority over those of performance and patient care.[4] Portable glucose meters have been studied recently,[6] as well as four types of reagent strips, which performed well except Dextrostix®.[7] A favorable study on a reflectance meter has been published.[8] See listing Point-of-Care Testing *on page 27*.

Additional Information Like a fasting glucose level >140 mg/dL (SI: >7.8 mmol/L), a 2-hour postprandial glucose >200 mg/dL (SI: >11.1 mmol/L) is virtually diagnostic of diabetes mellitus and obviates the need for a glucose tolerance test. An oral glucose tolerance test (OGTT) is not necessary in the setting of sufficiently high fasting and 2-hour postprandial results.

Other causes of **high glucose** (serum or plasma) include nonfasting specimen; recent or current I.V. infusions of glucose; stress states such as myocardial infarct,[9] brain damage, CVA,[10] convulsive episodes, trauma, general anesthesia; Cushing's disease; acromegaly; pheochromocytoma; glucagonoma; severe liver disease; pancreatitis; drugs (thiazide and other diuretics, corticoids, many others are reported to affect glucose).

The danger of **hypoglycemia** (low glucose) is lack of a steady supply of glucose to the brain (neuroglycopenia). Causes of **low glucose:** Excess insulin, including rare insulin autoimmune hypoglycemia, surreptitious insulin injection, and sulfonylurea use; artifact secondary to leukemia; hemolysis; glycolysis in specimens overheated or old; serum permitted to stand on clot in red top tube for chemistry profile. Very prompt removal of plasma and analysis is needed in cases of marked leukocytosis. Hypoglycemia should be confirmed by specimens drawn in fluoride tubes (gray top tubes).

With hypoglycemia, symptoms must be correlated with plasma glucose.

Three major groups of hypoglycemia are defined: reactive, fasting, and surreptitious. The reactive group includes alimentary hyperinsulinism, prediabetic, endocrine deficiency, and idiopathic functional groups.[11] **Postprandial hypoglycemia** may occur after gastrointestinal surgery, and is described with hereditary fructose intolerance, galactosemia, and leucine sensitivity.

Fasting hypoglycemia is likelier to suggest serious organic disease. The overnight fasting glucose level rather than the glucose tolerance test is the optimal test, with glucose drawn during symptoms.

- Pancreatic islet cell tumors (insulinomas) - cause hypoglycemia in fasting individuals or after exercise. Measurement of simultaneous glucose, C-peptide, and insulin levels at the time of spontaneous hypoglycemia help to differentiate insulinoma from other conditions. The **glucose/insulin ratio** is useful in the diagnosis of insulinoma: insulin levels inappropriately increased for plasma glucose. An intravenous tolbutamide test with plasma glucose and serum insulin determinations may be used for evaluation of insulin-secreting islet cell tumors. The test is positive in approximately 75% of patients with these tumors.[11] Glucagon and leucine stimulation tests are less frequently utilized.
- Extrapancreatic tumors - rare bulky fibromas, sarcomas, mesotheliomas, and carcinomas, including hepatoma and adrenal tumors

(Continued)

Glucose, Fasting (Continued)

- Adrenal insufficiency (Addison's disease), including congenital adrenal hyperplasia
- Hypopituitarism, isolated growth hormone or ACTH deficiency
- Starvation, malabsorption - but starvation does not cause hypoglycemia in normal persons. The plasma glucose of normal fasting individuals may drop below 50 mg/dL.[1]
- Drugs including insulin (see above), oral hypoglycemic agents, and alcoholism, especially with starvation. Salicylates, quinine, haloperidol, and many other drugs, entities, and conditions[1] can depress glucose levels. Dispensing errors can occur. Anti-insulin antibodies, spontaneously produced, causing hypoglycemia are reported.[12]
- Liver damage, including fulminant hepatic necrosis (hepatitis, toxicity), and severe congestive failure
- Tumor-induced hypoglycemia appears to be caused by increased production of an insulin-like substance (insulin-like growth factor II) by the tumor. This substance induces increased utilization of glucose by the peripheral tissues and the tumor, and impairs the counterregulatory effect of growth hormone by suppressing growth hormone secretion.[13,14]

Infancy and childhood: Infants with tremor, convulsions and/or respiratory distress should have stat glucose, particularly in the presence of maternal diabetes, hemolytic disease of the newborn (erythroblastosis fetalis); babies too large or small for gestational age should also have glucose level measured in the first 24 hours of life. A large number of entities relate to neonatal and other hypoglycemia, including glycogen storage diseases,[15] galactosemia, hereditary fructose intolerance, ketotic hypoglycemia of infancy, fructose-1,6-diphosphatase deficiency, carnitine deficiency (a treatable disease presenting as Reye's syndrome), and nesidioblastosis. **Control of diabetes** is needed to avoid complications. Laboratory measures of importance include FBS, creatinine, BUN, glycated hemoglobin or fructosamine, and home measurements by capillary glucose.[2,16,17]

Footnotes

1. Service FJ, "Hypoglycemic Disorders," *N Engl J Med*, 1995, 332(17):1144-52.
2. Barbosa J, Steffes MW, Sutherland DER, et al, "Effect of Glycemic Control on Early Diabetic Renal Lesions - A 5-Year Randomized Controlled Clinical Trial of Insulin-Dependent Diabetic Kidney Transplant Recipients," *JAMA*, 1994, 272(8):600-6.
3. Modan M and Harris MI, "Fasting Plasma Glucose in Screening for NIDDM in the U.S. and Israel," *Diabetes Care*, 1994, 17(5):436-9.
4. Gerson B and Figoni MA, "Clinical Comparison of Glucose Quantitation Methods," *Arch Pathol Lab Med*, 1985, 109(8):711-5.
5. Atkin SH, Dasmahapatra A, Jaker MA, et al, "Fingerstick Glucose Determination in Shock," *Ann Intern Med*, 1991, 114:(12)1020-4.
6. Vallera DA, Bissell MG, and Barron W, "Accuracy of Portable Blood Glucose Monitoring. Effect of Glucose Level and Prandial State," *Am J Clin Pathol*, 1991, 95(2):247-52.
7. Cheeley RD and Joyce SM, "A Clinical Comparison of the Performance of Four Blood Glucose Reagent Strips," *Am J Emerg Med*, 1990, 8(1):11-5.
8. Yoo T and Chao J, "Screening for Gestational Diabetes Mellitus. Use and Accuracy of Capillary Blood Glucose Measured With a Reflectance Meter," *J Fam Pract*, 1989, 29(1):41-4.
9. Madsen JK, Haunsoe S, Helquist S, et al, "Prevalence of Hyperglycemia and Undiagnosed Diabetes Mellitus in Patients With Acute Myocardial Infarction," *Acta Med Scand*, 1986, 220(4):329-32.
10. Berger L and Hakim AM, "The Association of Hyperglycemia With Cerebral Edema in Stroke," *Stroke*, 1986, 17(5):865-71.
11. Field JB, "Hypoglycemia: A Systematic Approach to Specific Diagnosis," *Hosp Pract*, 1986, 21(9):187-94.
12. Polonsky KS, "A Practical Approach to Fasting Hypoglycemia," *N Engl J Med*, 1992, 326(15):994-8.
13. Daughaday WH, Emanuele MA, Brooks MH, et al, "Synthesis and Secretion of Insulin-Like Growth Factor II by a Leiomyosarcoma With Associated Hypoglycemia," *N Engl J Med*, 1988, 319(22):1434-40.
14. Axelrod L and Ron D, "Insulin-Like Growth Factor II and the Riddle of Tumor-Induced Hypoglycemia," *N Engl J Med*, 1988, 319(22):1477-9.
15. Talente GM, Coleman RA, Alter C, et al, "Glycogen Storage Disease in Adults," *Ann Intern Med*, 1994, 120(3):218-26.
16. Jones BA, Bachner P, and Howanitz PJ, "Bedside Glucose Monitoring. A College of American Pathologists Q-Probes Study of the Program Characteristics and Performance in 605 Institutions," *Arch Pathol Lab Med*, 1993, 117(11):1080-7.
17. Watts NB, "Bedside Monitoring of Blood Glucose in Hospitals. Speed vs Precision and Accuracy," *Arch Pathol Lab Med*, 1993, 117:1078-9.

References

Aono J, Ueda W, and Manabe M, "Alteration in Glucose Metabolism by Crying in Children," *N Engl J Med*, 1993, 329(15):1129.

Astles JR, Petros WP, Peters WP, et al, "Artifactual Hypoglycemia Associated With Hematopoietic Cytokines," *Arch Pathol Lab Med*, 1995, 119(8):713-6.

Atkinson MA and Maclaren NK, "The Pathogenesis of Insulin-Dependent Diabetes Mellitus," *N Engl J Med*, 1994, 331(21):1428-36.

Conrad PD, Sparks JW, Osberg I, et al, "Clinical Application of a New Glucose Analyzer in the Neonatal Intensive Care Unit: Comparison With Other Methods," *J Pediatr*, 1989, 114(2):281-7.

Li DF, Wong VC, O'Hoy KM, et al, "Evaluation of the WHO Criteria for 75 g Oral Glucose Tolerance Test in Pregnancy," *Br J Obstet Gynaecol*, 1987, 94(9):847-50.

Magni F, Paroni R, Bonini PA, et al, "Determination of Serum Glucose Concentration by a Candidate Definitive Method," *Clin Chem*, 1994, 40(10):1978-80.

Palardy J, Havrankova J, Lepage R, et al, "Blood Glucose Measurements During Symptomatic Episodes in Patients With Suspected Postprandial Hypoglycemia," *N Engl J Med*, 1989, 321(21):1421-5.

Singer DE, Coley CM, Samet JH, et al, "Tests of Glycemia in Diabetes Mellitus. Their Use in Establishing a Diagnosis and in Treatment," *Ann Intern Med*, 1989, 110(2):125-37.

Thomas S, Gough J, Benson N, et al, "Accuracy of Fingerstick Glucose Determination in Patients Receiving CPR," *South Med J*, 1994, 87(11):1072-5.

Vassault A and Cloarec A, "Glucose," *Drug Effects on Laboratory Test Results Analytical Interferences and Pharmacological Effects*, Siest G and Galteau MM, eds, Littleton, MA; PSG Publishing Co Inc, 1988, 241-68.

Glucose/Insulin Ratio see Glucose, Fasting on previous page

Glucose, Random

CPT 82947

Related Information

Drugs of Abuse Testing, Urine *on page 548*
Glucose, Quantitative, Urine *on page 635*
Glucose, Semiquantitative, Urine *on page 636*
Glycated Hemoglobin *on page 140*
Insulin, Blood *on page 149*
Ketone Bodies, Blood *on page 152*
Ketones, Urine *on page 639*
Point-of-Care Testing *on page 27*
Reducing Substances, Urine *on page 652*
Salicylate *on page 573*

Abstract Used to evaluate carbohydrate metabolism

Specimen Plasma or serum

Container Gray top (sodium fluoride) tube preferred; red top tube acceptable

Collection Pediatrics: Draw blood from heelstick.

Causes for Rejection Blood stored overnight on clot

Reference Range Dependent on time and content of last meal. Glucose >200 mg/dL (SI: >11.1 mmol/L) in a nonstressed, ambulatory subject supports the diagnosis of diabetes mellitus. Values in term neonates are published.[1]

Possible Panic Range Neonates: <40 mg/dL (SI: <2.2 mmol/L); adults: male: <50 mg/dL (SI: <2.8 mmol/L), >400 mg/dL (SI: >22.2 mmol/L); adults female: <40 mg/dL (SI: <2.2 mmol/L), >400 mg/dL (SI: >22.2 mmol/L)

Use Evaluate carbohydrate metabolism, acidosis and ketoacidosis, dehydration; work up alcoholism, or apparent alcoholism; work-up of coma, neuroglycopenia. **Hypoglycemia** if present should be investigated with C-peptide, insulin and proinsulin levels as well.[2] The diagnosis of **insulinoma** is established when random glucose <40 mg/dL is found with inappropriate plasma insulin levels following prolonged fasting.[3] For the diagnosis of **diabetes mellitus** in nonpregnant adult subjects, random glucose >200 mg/dL (SI: >11.1 mmol/L) is required, but random glucose is not adequate for this purpose. Other criteria exist. Determination of blood glucose on admission in patients who have had an out-of-hospital cardiac arrest can serve as a predictor of neurologic recovery. Higher levels are indicative of more severe brain ischemia and difficult resuscitation.[4] In pregnant women, a value >105 mg/dL usually prompts further investigation.

Limitations Glucose will decrease in samples left on the clot, and in tubes other than fluoride prior to analysis. Not satisfactory to screen for noninsulin-dependent diabetes mellitus.

Methodology Hexokinase, glucose oxidase, oxygen rate, ortho-toluidine

Additional Information Recall that **blood glucose** values are not equivalent to **plasma glucose**. Whole blood glucose is not normally measured in the hospital laboratory, but it is done by instruments designed for point-of-care monitoring. If glucose is >400 mg/dL (SI: >22.2 mmol/L), an acetone (ketone body) examination probably should be done. A fasting and a 2-hour postprandial specimen is preferable to a random specimen for evaluation of possible diabetes mellitus. The incidence of hypoglycemia in hospitalized patients appears to be significant, but may be better controlled if frequent monitoring of glucose levels is employed.[5] Wider utilization of bedside glucose testing may allow for closer patient monitoring, but the establishment of uniform quality control procedures is necessary to ensure valid results from this type of testing.[6,7,8] Evaluation of glycated hemoglobin and self-monitoring of blood glucose are means of assessing glycemia which have become widely available.[9]

Footnotes

1. Heck LJ and Erenberg A, "Serum Glucose Levels in Term Neonates During the First 48 Hours of Life," *J Pediatr*, 1987, 110(1):119-22.
2. Axelrod L, "Insulinoma: Cost-Effective Care in Patients With a Rare Disease," *Ann Intern Med*, 1995, 123(4):311-2.
3. Doppman JL, Chang R, Fraker DL, et al, "Localization of Insulinomas to Regions of the Pancreas by Intra-Arterial Stimulation With Calcium," *Ann Intern Med*, 1995, 123(4):269-73.
4. Longstreth WT Jr, Diehr P, Cobb LA, et al, "Neurologic Outcome and Blood Glucose Levels During Out-of-Hospital Cardiopulmonary Resuscitation," *Neurology*, 1986, 36(9):1186-91.
5. Fischer KF, Lees JA, and Newman JH, "Hypoglycemia in Hospitalized Patients. Causes and Outcomes," *N Engl J Med*, 1986, 315(20):1245-50.
6. Chu SY and Edney-Parker H, "Evaluation of the Reliability of Bedside Glucose Testing," *Lab Med*, 1989, 93-6.

7. Leroux ML and Desjardins PRE, "Establishment and Maintenance of a Hospital Glucose Meter Program," *Lab Med*, 1989, 97-9.

8. Bain OF, Brown KD, Sacher RA, et al, "A Hospital-Wide Blind Control Program for Bedside Glucose Meters," *Arch Pathol Lab Med*, 1989, 113(12):1370-5.

9. Singer DE, Coley CM, Samet JH, et al, "Tests of Glycemia in Diabetes Mellitus - Their Use in Establishing a Diagnosis and in Treatment," *Ann Intern Med*, 1989, 110(2):125-37.

References

Aono J, Ueda W, and Manabe M, "Alteration in Glucose Metabolism by Crying in Children," *N Engl J Med*, 1993, 329(15):1129.

Bolli GB and Fanelli CG, "Unawareness of Hypoglycemia," *N Engl J Med*, 1995, 333(26):1771-2.

Boyle PJ, Kempers SF, O'Connor AM, et al, "Brain Glucose Uptake and Unawareness of Hypoglycemia in Patients With Insulin-Dependent Diabetes Mellitus," *N Engl J Med*, 1995, 333(26):1726-31.

Brandt KR and Miles JM, "Relationship Between Severity of Hyperglycemia and Metabolic Acidosis in Diabetic Ketoacidosis," *Mayo Clin Proc*, 1988, 63(11):1071-4.

Gill GV, Hardy KJ, Patrick AW, et al, "Random Blood Glucose Estimation in Type 2 Diabetes: Does It Reflect Overall Glycaemic Control?" *Diabet Med*, 1994, 11(7):705-8.

Palardy J, Havrankova J, Lepage R, et al, "Blood Glucose Measurements During Symptomatic Episodes in Patients With Suspected Postprandial Hypoglycemia," *N Engl J Med*, 1989, 321(21):1421-5.

Weiner CP, Faustich M, Burns J, et al, "The Relationship Between Capillary and Venous Glucose Concentration During Pregnancy," *Am J Obstet Gynecol*, 1986, 155(1):61-4.

Glucose Tolerance Test

CPT 82951 (3 specimens); 82952 (each specimen beyond 3)

Related Information

Ataxia-Telangiectasia, Chromosome Breakage Study *on page 274*

Chromium, Serum *on page 587*

Chromium, Urine *on page 588*

C-Peptide *on page 114*

Glucose, Fasting *on page 137*

Glucose, Quantitative, Urine *on page 635*

Glucose, Semiquantitative, Urine *on page 636*

Insulin, Blood *on page 149*

Reducing Substances, Urine *on page 652*

Synonyms GTT; OGTT; Oral Glucose Tolerance Test

Applies to Gestational Diabetes Screening Test

Test Commonly Includes Fasting blood glucose, 30 minutes, first hour, second hour, and sometimes a third hour sample is drawn. Many delete the 30-minute specimen, and for noninsulin dependent diabetes mellitus only fasting, 1-hour, and 2-hour glucose are usually needed if GTT is done at all.

Abstract For detection of gestational diabetes, a 50 g glucose load followed in 1 hour by a plasma glucose assay has been recommended[1], but may be insensitive.[2] The 2-hour oral glucose tolerance test is a recommended method to screen for noninsulin-dependent diabetes mellitus.[3]

Patient Preparation Patient should not smoke due to glucose stimulation by nicotine. Patient should be active and have had adequate food intake with adequate carbohydrates (at least 150 g carbohydrate daily) for 3 days, and then fast 12 hours prior to test. Many drugs interfere. They include steroids, oral contraceptives, diuretics, and antihypertensive drugs including thiazides, furosemide, anticonvulsants, psychoactive drugs, antituberculous agents, and anti-inflammatory drugs including salicylates. Patient should not be stressed.

In pregnant subjects, indication for GTT is a positive **gestational diabetes screening test:** 50 g carbohydrate load, sample drawn in 1 hour. A positive usual gestational screening test is glucose >140 mg/dL (SI: >7.8 mmol/L).[4]

Specimen Plasma

Container Gray top (sodium fluoride) tube

Collection After fasting blood specimen and urine are obtained, administer oral glucose solution. Weigh patient for proper glucose loading dosage. Children receive 1.75 g/kg body weight up to 75 g. Usual adult dose is 75 g.

100 g may be used for possible gestational diabetes mellitus. Then draw blood at 30, 60, 90, and 120 minutes until specified hour. For gestational diabetes, the GTT is a 3-hour tolerance test, following positive screening test. The screening test for gestational diabetes is not necessarily done fasting.

Collect urine at 1, 2, and 3 hours if urine is to be collected; some delete urines for glucose. During the test, the patient should remain seated and consume nothing but water after the glucose solution is administered. Physical activity should be minimized and some recommend that the patient be kept supine throughout.[5] Vomiting or diarrhea may alter test results.

Causes for Rejection Time not marked on tubes, patient not appearing in the morning in the fasting state; stressed patient (following surgery, or with infection, or on corticosteroids) should not have GTT.

Reference Range Fasting: 60-115 mg/dL (SI: 3.3-6.4 mmol/L); 1 hour: ≤184 mg/dL (SI: ≤10.2 mmol/L); 2 hours: ≤138 mg/dL (SI: ≤7.7 mmol/L). Many different schemes have been offered to interpret the GTT. Some

were based on studies in atypical populations and tended to overdiagnose diabetes. The most often used classification currently is the one published by the National Diabetes Data Group, which states: fasting plasma glucose >140 mg/dL (SI: >7.8 mmol/L) or 2-hour postprandial plasma glucose >200 mg/dL (SI: >11.1 mmol/L) → GTT not necessary, patient has diabetes mellitus. GTT, 2-hour plasma glucose >200 mg/dL and at least one other value >200 mg/dL → patient has diabetes mellitus. 2-hour plasma glucose of 140-200 mg/dL and at least one other value >200 mg/dL → patient has **impaired glucose tolerance** but is not clearly diabetic.[6]

Use Indications vary somewhat between authorities. Some use the OGTT in individuals whose FBS varies between 115-139 mg/dL (SI: 6.4-7.7 mmol/L) on two or more occasions; others would use further fasting plasma glucose and 2-hour postprandial glucose determinations for such subjects. Some use the GTT infrequently or not at all.

The GTT only establishes the presence of glucose intolerance. It is used in patients with borderline fasting and postprandial glucose to support or rule out the diagnosis of diabetes mellitus. Some use it in unexplained hypertriglyceridemia, neuropathy, impotence, diabetes-like renal diseases, retinopathy, necrobiosis lipoidica diabeticorum, and re-evaluation of prior diagnosis made under substandard conditions. The OGTT is used to work up glycosuria without hyperglycemia (eg, to work up renal glycosuria). It is used to predict perinatal morbidity in pregnancy, to diagnose gestational diabetes. Risks of fetal abnormality and perinatal mortality are increased with abnormal carbohydrate metabolism in pregnancy.[7]

See listings Insulin, Blood *on page 149* and C-Peptide *on page 114* when patient has symptoms.

Glucose intolerance is due to obesity in some subjects. Abnormal curves may be caused by Cushing's syndrome, pheochromocytoma, or acromegaly.

Limitations Few indications still meet wide acceptance. Slight hyperglycemic effect is seen in patients on oral contraceptives. Failure to have patient on 3-day high carbohydrate diet may result in a false-positive GGT. Impaired glucose tolerance is **not** equivalent to diabetes mellitus. A normal result does not assure that diabetes will not subsequently develop. Criticisms of the OGTT include poor reproducability, patient inconvenience, and strong propensity for overdiagnosis of diabetes mellitus. The 5-hour oral glucose tolerance test is discredited.[8]

Proposals to abandon the OGTT have been published, to replace it with FBS and glycohemoglobin.[5] However, faults exist with each as a screen for diabetes. See listings Glucose, Fasting *on page 137* and Insulin, Blood *on page 149* for recommendations for work-up of hypoglycemia.

Contraindications FBS >140 mg/dL (SI: >7.8 mmol/L) on two occasions or postprandial blood glucose >200 mg/dL (SI: >11.1 mmol/L) on two occasions are indicative of diabetes mellitus, in the nonstressed subject, and obviate the need for an OGTT. OGTT is contraindicated in the presence of obvious diabetes mellitus.

Emesis is probably an indication to cancel the remainder of a GTT for that day; decision is up to the patient's physician.

Methodology Hexokinase, glucose oxidase, oxygen rate, ortho-toluidine

Additional Information Excessive growth hormone, adrenocortical and thyroid hormones and catecholamines cause decreased glucose tolerance. Diabetes is much more than glucose intolerance, but until now we have not been able to measure other factors pertinent to prediction of the complications of diabetes. The glucose tolerance test lacks specificity and sensitivity for the complications of diabetes mellitus. Some feel that it only determines glucose intolerance. **Impaired glucose tolerance** is a quasi-entity; 1% to 5% of such patients become overtly diabetic yearly. Such patients have increased risk for cardiovascular disease.

An increased prevalence of idiopathic hemochromatosis exists in the diabetic population compared to the general population.[9]

Criteria for interpretation for gestational diabetes mellitus: two or more of the following must be met. Fasting: ≥105 mg/dL (SI: ≥5.8 mmol/L); 1 hour: ≥190 mg/dL (SI: ≥10.5 mmol/L); 2 hour: ≥165 mg/dL (SI: ≥9.2 mmol/L); 3 hour: ≥145 mg/dL (SI: ≥8.0 mmol/L).[10,11] Pregnant women with an abnormal GTT are at risk for pre-eclampsia/eclampsia and delivery of a macrosomic infant.[12,13]

Nonketotic hyperglycemic syndrome is hyperglycemia, glucose >600 mg/dL with hyperosmolarity without significant ketonuria.[14]

Footnotes

1. McElduff A, Goldring J, Gordon P, et al, "A Direct Comparison of the Measurement of a Random Plasma Glucose and a Post-50-g Glucose Load Glucose in the Detection of Gestational Diabetes," *Aust N Z J Obstet Gynaecol*, 1994, 34(1):28-30.

2. van Turnhout HE, Lotgering FK, and Wallenburg HC, "Poor Sensitivity of the Fifty-Gram One-Hour Glucose Screening Test for Hyperglycemia," *Eur J Obstet Gynecol Reprod Biol*, 1994, 53(1):7-10.

3. Modan M and Harris MI, "Fasting Plasma Glucose in Screening for NIDDM in the U.S. and Israel," *Diabetes Care*, 1994, 17(5):436-9.

(Continued)

Glucose Tolerance Test (Continued)

4. Catalano PM, Vargo KM, Bernstein IM, et al, "Incidence and Risk Factors Associated With Abnormal Postpartum Glucose Tolerance in Women With Gestational Diabetes," *Am J Obstet Gynecol*, 1991, 165(4 Pt 1):914-9.
5. Gambino R, "Is It Time to Abandon the Oral Glucose Tolerance Test?" *Lab Rep*, 1995, 17(10):72.
6. National Diabetes Data Group, "Classification and Diagnosis of Diabetes Mellitus and Other Categories of Glucose Intolerance," *Diabetes*, 1979, 28:1039-57.
7. Forest JC, Garrido-Russo M, LeMay A, et al, "Reference Values for the Oral Glucose Tolerance Test at Each Trimester of Pregnancy," *Am J Clin Pathol*, 1983, 80:823-31.
8. Service FJ, "Hypoglycemic Disorders," *N Engl J Med*, 1995, 332(17):1144-52.
9. Phelps G, Chapman I, Hall P, et al, "Prevalence of Genetic Hemochromatosis Among Diabetic Patients," *Lancet*, 1989, 2(8657):233-4.
10. Singer DE, Coley CM, Samet JH, et al, "Tests of Glycemia in Diabetes Mellitus - Their Use in Establishing Diagnosis and in Treatment," *Ann Intern Med*, 1989, 110(2):125-37.
11. Hare JW, "Gestational Diabetes Mellitus. Levels of Glycemia as Management Goals," *Diabetes*, 1991, 40(Suppl 2):193-6.
12. Lindsay MK, Graves W, and Klein L, "The Relationship of One Abnormal Glucose Tolerance Test Value and Pregnancy Complications," *Obstet Gynecol*, 1989, 73(1):103-6.
13. Neiger R and Coustan DR, "The Role of Repeat Glucose Tolerance Tests in the Diagnosis of Gestational Diabetes," *Am J Obstet Gynecol*, 1991, 165(4 Pt 1):787-90.
14. Rother KI and Schwenk WF 2d, "An Unusual Case of the Nonketotic Hyperglycemic Syndrome During Childhood," *Mayo Clin Proc*, 1995, 70(1):62-5.

References

Astles JR, Petros WP, Peters WP, et al, "Artifactual Hypoglycemia Associated With Hematopoietic Cytokines," *Arch Pathol Lab Med*, 1995, 119(8):713-6.
Atkinson MA and Maclaren NK, "The Pathogenesis of Insulin-Dependent Diabetes Mellitus," *N Engl J Med*, 1994, 331(21):1428-36.
de Leacy EA and Cowley DM, "Evidence That the Oral Glucose Tolerance Test Does Not Provide a Uniform Stimulus to Pancreatic Islets in Pregnancy," *Clin Chem*, 1989, 35(7):1482-5.
Foster DW, "Diabetes Mellitus," *Harrison's Principles of Internal Medicine*, 13th ed, Isselbacher KJ, Braunwald E, Wilson JD, et al, eds, 1994, New York, NY: McGraw-Hill Inc, 1994, 1979-2000.
Gabbe SG, "Gestational Diabetes Mellitus," *N Engl J Med*, 1986, 315(16):1025-6.
Kritz-Silverstein D, Barrett-Connor E, and Wingard DL, "The Effect of Parity on the Later Development of Non-Insulin-Dependent Diabetes Mellitus or Impaired Glucose Tolerance," *N Engl J Med*, 1989, 321(18):1214-9.
Langer O, Brustman L, Anyaegbunam A, et al, "The Significance of One Abnormal Glucose Tolerance Test Value on Adverse Outcome in Pregnancy," *Am J Obstet Gynecol*, 1987, 157(3):758-63.
Neiger R and Coustan DR, "Are the Current ACOG Glucose Tolerance Test Criteria Sensitive Enough?" *Obstet Gynecol*, 1991, 78(6):1117-20.
Nelson RL, "Oral Glucose Tolerance Test: Indications and Limitations," *Mayo Clin Proc*, 1988, 63(3):263-9.
Nolan JJ, Ludvik B, Beersden P, et al, "Improvement in Glucose Tolerance and Insulin Resistance in Obese Subjects Treated With Troglitazone," *N Engl J Med*, 1994, 331(18):1188-93.
Sacks DA, Abu-Fadil S, Karten GJ, et al, "Screening for Gestational Diabetes With the One-Hour 50-g Glucose Test," *Obstet Gynecol*, 1987, 70(1):89-93.
Tallarigo L, Giampietro O, Penno G, et al, "Relation of Glucose Tolerance to Complications of Pregnancy in Nondiabetic Women," *N Engl J Med*, 1986, 315(16):989-92.

Glutamic Oxaloacetic Transaminase, Serum see Aspartate
Aminotransferase *on page 84*

Glutamic Pyruvate Transaminase see Alanine Aminotransferase
on page 65

Glutamine, Spinal Fluid see Cerebrospinal Fluid Glutamine *on page 105*

Glutamyl Transpeptidase see Gamma Glutamyl Transferase *on page 133*

Glycated Albumin see Fructosamine *on page 130*

Glycated Hemoglobin

CPT 83036

Related Information

Fructosamine *on page 130*
Glucose, 2-Hour Postprandial *on page 136*
Glucose, Fasting *on page 137*
Glucose, Quantitative, Urine *on page 635*
Glucose, Random *on page 138*
Glucose, Semiquantitative, Urine *on page 636*
Microalbuminuria *on page 643*
Point-of-Care Testing *on page 27*
Protein, Quantitative, Urine *on page 649*

Synonyms Fast Hemoglobins; GHB; HB$_{A1}$; Hemoglobin A$_{1a}$, A$_{1b}$, A$_{1c}$; Hemoglobin, Glycosylated

Abstract Glycated hemoglobin offers a weighted moving average that reflects prior plasma glucose levels.[1] **Glycemic control** ameliorates or prevents microangiopathic lesions of diabetes mellitus, including retinopathy and glomerulopathy. Such control includes regular assays of fasting glucose, Hb A$_1$, BUN/creatinine with ambulatory capillary glucose testing.[1,2]

Specimen Whole blood (washed erythrocytes or hemolysate)

Container Gray top (sodium fluoride) tube or lavender top (EDTA) tube, the latter for affinity column chromatography

Sampling Time Fasting specimens are not required. Testing at 3- to 4-month intervals is suggested for patients with type I diabetes. For patients with type II diabetes, glycated hemoglobins at diagnosis and at 6-month intervals are recommended.[1]

Storage Instructions Stable 7 days at 4°C.

Reference Range Dependent upon methodology. Diabetics in good control overlap the normal population. Reference range by affinity columns is reported as 4% to 7% of total hemoglobin for hemoglobin A$_1$.[3] For hemoglobin A$_{1c}$: 4% to 5.5% of total hemoglobin. There is no age dependence.

Critical Values The risk of microalbuminuria with insulin-dependent diabetes mellitus increases above hemoglobin A$_1$ of 10.1% (equivalent to A$_{1c}$ of 8.1%). This value corresponds with glucose levels <200 mg/dL (SI: <11.1 mmol/L).[4,5]

Use This is an irreversible glucose-protein bond which extends through the life of an erythrocyte. Glycated hemoglobin values are used to assess long-term glucose control in diabetes, especially in insulin-dependent diabetics whose glucose levels are labile, and in whom blood and urine glucose measurements exhibit significant daily variation. GHB measurements reflect the level of control present over the preceding 100-120 days; more recent levels have greater weight. GHB is especially helpful when renal thresholds are high or low. Glycosylated hemoglobin measurements are less frequently needed in stable diabetics. In such patients, whose fasting glucose concentrations are fairly consistent from day to day, there is a correlation between glycosylated hemoglobin and single fasting glucose levels. Continued high levels of blood glucose are reflected in high GHB concentrations. Singer et al suggested a diagnostic approach in which glycated hemoglobin may be substituted for the glucose tolerance test and advocated it as well as an adjunct in gestational diabetes.[1] Gambino too recently made this recommendation.[6] It is also useful in evaluation of fetal risk in known type II diabetics who become pregnant. Glycosylated hemoglobin predicts the progression of retinopathy.[7]

Limitations GHB measurements supplement but do not replace conventional urine and blood glucose levels. Chronic blood loss, hemolytic anemia, or other setting for decrease in RBC life span, results in a decrease in the glycated hemoglobin level. Pregnancy may lower glycated hemoglobin. Chronic renal failure with or without dialysis leads to decreased levels of glycated hemoglobin. Misleading high levels of glycated hemoglobin are found by ion exchange resin columns in patients who have elevated levels of fetal hemoglobin (Hb F);[8] high levels of Hb F are found in young children younger than 2 years of age and in some hemoglobinopathies. This is true also for hemoglobins H, I, J and N.[9] Low values derive from blood containing hemoglobin S, G, D, C, or E.[10] Such difficulties with abnormal hemoglobins do not apply to the affinity chromatography method.[3]

Contraindications Not useful more often than at 4- to 6-week intervals. Not widely accepted in diagnosis of diabetes.

Methodology Elution from resin columns, high performance liquid chromatography (HPLC), electrophoresis, isoelectric focusing, affinity chromatography, enzyme immunoassay (EIA).[11] Affinity columns avoid problems of temperature variations and abnormal hemoglobins F, S, C, D, G, and J do not generate misleading data.[12] Ion capture immunoassay shows no interference from abnormal hemoglobins.

Additional Information A useful test to reassure the patient who is well controlled, and to assess the status of insufficiently controlled patients. If a result does not seem consistent with the clinical findings, ask for a hemoglobin F level. Measurement of glycated hemoglobin by affinity chromatography permits better differentiation of the degree of blood glucose control among diabetics than does hemoglobin A$_{1c}$ or hemoglobin A$_1$ measurements.[13]

Footnotes

1. Singer DE, Coley CM, Samet JH, et al, "Tests of Glycemia in Diabetes Mellitus - Their Use in Establishing a Diagnosis and in Treatment," *Ann Intern Med*, 1989, 110(2):125-37.
2. Barbosa J, Steffes MW, Sutherland DE, et al, "Effect of Glycemic Control on Early Diabetic Renal Lesions. A 5-Year Randomized Controlled Clinical Trial of Insulin-Dependent Diabetic Kidney Transplant Recipients," *JAMA*, 1994, 272(8):600-6.
3. Fairbanks VF and Zimmerman BR, "Measurement of Glycosylated Hemoglobin by Affinity Chromatography," *Mayo Clin Proc*, 1983, 58:770-3.
4. Krolewski AS, Laffel LMB, Krolewski M, et al, "Glycosylated Hemoglobin and the Risk of Microalbuminuria in Patients With Insulin-Dependent Diabetes Mellitus," *N Engl J Med*, 1995, 332(19):1251-5.
5. Viberti G, "A Glycemic Threshold for Diabetic Complications?" *N Engl J Med*, 1995, 332(19):1293-4.
6. Gambino R, "Is It Time to Abandon the Oral Glucose Tolerance Test?" *Lab Rep*, 1995, 17(10):72.
7. Klein R, Klein BE, Moss SE, et al, "Glycosylated Hemoglobin Predicts the Incidence and Progression of Diabetic Retinopathy," *JAMA*, 1988, 260(19):2864-71.
8. Bergstrom RW, Kelley JR, and Ward WK, "Fetal Hemoglobin Alters Hemoglobin A$_{1c}$ Measurements," *Ann Intern Med*, 1991, 115(8):656.
9. Krauss JS and Khankhanian NK, "HPLC Determination of Hemoglobin A$_{1c}$ in the Presence of the Fast Hemoglobin F Philadelphia," *Clin Chem*, 1989, 35(3):494-5.
10. Holt GS, Wofford JL, and Velez R, "Hemoglobinopathies Affect Hemoglobin A$_{1c}$ Measurement," *Ann Intern Med*, 1991, 115(1):68-9.

11. Engbaek F, Christensen SE, and Jespersen B, "Enzyme Immunoassay of Hemoglobin A$_{1c}$: Analytical Characteristics and Clinical Performance for Patients With Diabetes Mellitus, With and Without Uremia," *Clin Chem*, 1989, 35(1):93-7.
12. Gascon F and Molina E, "Precision of Measurement of Glycated Hemoglobin by Affinity Chromatography on Regenerated Columns," *Clin Chem*, 1989, 35(1):191.
13. Teupe B, "Quantitative Determination of Glycated Hemoglobin Using Affinity Chromatography," *Symposium Proceedings: The Role of Glycated Hemoglobin in the Management of Diabetes*, Akron, OH: Isolab Inc, 1988, 9-16.

References
Allgrove J and Cockrill BL, "Fructosamine or Glycated Haemoglobin as a Measure of Diabetic Control," *Arch Dis Child*, 1988, 63(4):418-22.
Benjamin RJ and Sacks DB, "Glycated Protein Update: Implications of Recent Studies, Including the Diabetes Control and Complications Trial," *Clin Chem*, 1994, 40(5):683-7.
Bunn HF, Gabbay KH, and Gallop PM, "The Glycosylation of Hemoglobin: Relevance to Diabetes Mellitus," *Science*, 1978, 200:21-7.
Cox T, Hess PP, Thompson GD, et al, "Interference With Glycated Hemoglobin by Hemoglobin F May Be Greater Than Is Generally Assumed," *Am J Clin Pathol*, 1993, 99(2):137-41.
Goldstein DE, Little RR, Wiedmeyer HM, et al, "Is Glycohemoglobin Testing Useful in Diabetes Mellitus? Lessons From the Diabetes Control and Complications Trial," *Clin Chem*, 1994, 40(8):1637-40.
Jerntorp P, Sundkvist G, Fex G, et al, "Clinical Utility of Serum Fructosamine in Diabetes Mellitus Compare With Hemoglobin A$_{1c}$," *Clin Chim Acta*, 1988, 175(2):135-42.
Kilpatrick ES, Rumley AG, Dominiczak MH, et al, "Glycated Haemoglobin Values: Problems in Assessing Blood Glucose Control in Diabetes Mellitus," *BMJ*, 1994, 309(6960):983-6.
Kullberg CE and Arnqvist HJ, "Elevated Long-Term Glycated Haemoglobin Precedes Proliferative Retinopathy and Nephropathy in Type 1 (Insulin-Dependent) Diabetic Patients," *Diabetologia*, 1993, 36(10):961-5.
McCance DR, Hanson RL, Charles M, et al, "Comparison of Tests for Glycated Haemoglobin and Fasting and Two Hour Plasma Glucose Concentrations as Diagnostics Method for Diabetes," *BMJ*, 1994, 308(6940):1323-8.
Palumbo PJ, "Diabetes Control and Complications Trial: The Continuing Challenge Ahead," *Mayo Clin Proc*, 1993, 68(11):1126-7 (editorial).
Pickup JC, Crook MA, and Tutt P, "Blood Glucose and Glycated Haemoglobin Measurement in Hospital: Which Method?" *Diabet Med*, 1993, 10(5):402-11.

Glycolic Acid, Urine *see Oxalate, Urine on page 174*

Glyoxylic Acid, Urine *see Oxalate, Urine on page 174*

GnRH *see Human Chorionic Gonadotropin, Serum on page 145*

GOT *see Aspartate Aminotransferase on page 84*

GPT *see Alanine Aminotransferase on page 65*

Growth Hormone
CPT 83003
Related Information
Adrenocorticotropic Hormone *on page 63*
Phosphorus, Urine *on page 183*
Somatomedin-C *on page 201*

Synonyms GH; hGH; Somatotropin

Applies to Somatomedins

Abstract Growth hormone (GH), released by the anterior pituitary, promotes anabolism. Growth is stimulated through somatomedins. Causes of short stature related to GH include pituitary abnormality, hypothalamic dysfunction with secondary pituitary deficiency, insensitivity to growth hormone, and mutation in the GH gene.

Patient Preparation Avoid recent radioactive scan. Patient should be fasting and at complete rest for 30 minutes. Patient must not be stressed. Draw from rested patient.

Specimen Serum

Container Red top tube

Sampling Time GH increases with exercise; patient should be resting.

Storage Instructions Label tube with time and date of collection and identifying data. Separate serum and freeze in plastic container. Stable 4 hours at 25°C and 1 year at -20°C.[1]

Special Instructions Physiological state (feeding, fasting, sleep, activity) should be noted. Stimulation and suppression tests, and somatomedin C levels are often needed. Stimulation tests must be directed by a physician.

Reference Range Children: <20 ng/mL (SI: <880 pmol/L); adults: male: ≤5 ng/mL (SI: ≤220 pmol/L), female: <10 ng/mL (SI: <440 pmol/L); adults >60 years: male: <10 ng/mL, female: <14 ng/mL (SI: <616 pmol/L). Response to oral glucose administration is used in evaluation of acromegaly. Assays using a monoclonal antibody give lower results than those using polyclonal antibodies.

Use Pituitary function test useful in the diagnosis of hypothalamic disorders, hypopituitarism; deficiency leads to dwarfism in children, excess causes gigantism in children and acromegaly in adults.

Limitations A single fasting GH level is of limited value. Secretion of GH is episodic and pulsatile. GH has a half-life of 20-25 minutes. Testing for growth hormone deficiency in children is best done as part of a dynamic test that involves various stimuli. Patients with dysfunctional thyroids may have abnormal growth hormone release. Patients with GH-producing pituitary tumors often release GH in response to TRH or GnRH. Somatomedin C is used as a screening test for HGH deficiency,

but pitfalls exist.[2] Growth hormone levels may be increased in Laron dwarfism, but somatomedin-C is low.

Methodology Radioimmunoassay (RIA), immunoradiometric assay[3]

Additional Information Growth hormone secretion is influenced by deep sleep, arginine, glucagon, levodopa, low glucose and insulin, exercise and stress, vasopressin. Starvation increases HGH. In obesity, release of GH is reduced; and response of GH to insulin, sleep, or exercise may be impaired. Patients with acromegaly, even those with normal GH levels, will show no suppression of GH by oral glucose and may show a rise. In patients being evaluated for pituitary insufficiency, GH may be assayed after stimulation by administration of insulin, arginine, glucagon, vasopressin, or levodopa.[4] The defined normal response differs among laboratories. With the advent of recombinant growth hormone for treatment of short stature, assays for GH have increased. Somatomedins are produced in response to GH.[2] GH-binding proteins do not interfere significantly in assays commonly employed.[5] In children who are treated with GH and develop GH antibodies, the plasma GH measurement is factitiously elevated whereas the free GH is not.[6] Assays have been developed to measure GH in urine.[7,8]

Heterozygous missense mutation in the growth hormone gene is reported in a child with severe growth retardation.[9]

A current outstanding review of GH physiology and pathophysiology is available.[10]

Footnotes
1. Kabasik NP, Ricotta M, Hunter T, et al, "Effect of Duration and Temperature of Storage on Serum Analyte Stability: Examination of 14 Radioimmunoassay Procedures," *Clin Chem*, 1982, 28:164-5.
2. Watts NB and Keffer JH, "Anterior Pituitary and Hypothalamus," *Practical Endocrinology*, 4th ed, Chapter 2, Philadelphia, PA: Lea & Febiger, 1989, 11-36.
3. Pringle PJ, Jones J, Hindmarsh PC, et al, "Performance of Proficiency Survey Samples in Two Immunoradiometric Assays of Human Growth Hormone and Comparison With Patients' Sample," *Clin Chem*, 1992, 38(4):553-7.
4. Leavelle DE, *Mayo Medical Laboratories Interpretive Handbook*, Rochester, MN: Mayo Medical Laboratories, 1990.
5. Jan T, Shaw MA, and Baumann G, "Effects of Growth Hormone-Binding Proteins on Serum Growth Hormone Measurements," *J Clin Endocrinol Metab*, 1991, 72(2):387-91.
6. Pringle PJ, Hindmarsh PC, DiSilvio L, et al, "The Measurement and Effect of Growth Hormone in the Presence of Growth Hormone-Binding Antibodies," *J Endocrinol*, 1989, 121(1):193-9.
7. Evans AJ and Wood PJ, "Development of an Assay for Human Growth Hormone in Urine Using Commercially Available Reagents," *Ann Clin Biochem*, 1989, 26(Pt 4):353-7.
8. Hourd P and Edwards R, "Measurement of Human Growth Hormone in Urine: Development and Validation of a Sensitive and Specific Assay," *J Endocrinol*, 1989, 121(1):167-75.
9. Takahashi Y, Kaji H, Okimura Y, et al, "Brief Report: Short Stature Caused By a Mutant Growth Hormone," *N Engl J Med*, 1996, 334(7):432-6.
10. Laron Z, "Short Stature Due to Genetic Defects Affecting Growth Hormone Activity," *N Engl J Med*, 1996, 334(7), 463-5 (editorial).

References
Baumann G, Shaw MA, and Merimee TJ, "Low Levels of High-Affinity Growth Hormone-Binding Protein in African Pygmies," *N Engl J Med*, 1989, 320(26):1705-9.
Donaldson DL, Pan F, Hollowell JG, et al, "Reliability of Stimulated and Spontaneous Growth Hormone (GH) Levels for Identifying the Child With Low GH Secretion," *J Clin Endocrinol Metab*, 1991, 72(3):647-52.
Grumbach MM, "Growth Hormone Therapy and the Short End of the Stick," *N Engl J Med*, 1988, 319(4):238-41.
Ilondo MM, Vanderschueren-Lodeweyckx M, De Meyts P, et al, "Serum Growth Hormone Levels Measured by Radioimmunoassay and Radioreceptor Assay: A Useful Diagnostic Tool in Children With Growth Disorders?" *J Clin Endocrinol Metab*, 1990, 70(5):1445-51.
Kao PC, Abboud CF, and Zimmerman D, "Somatomedin C: An Index of Growth Hormone Activity," *Mayo Clin Proc*, 1986, 61(11):908-9.
Mercado M, Molitch ME, and Baumann G, "Low Plasma Growth Hormone Binding Protein in IDDM," *Diabetes*, 1992, 41(5):605-9.
Rose SR, Ross JL, Uriarte M, et al, "The Advantage of Measuring Stimulated as Compared With Spontaneous Growth Hormone Levels in the Diagnosis of Growth Hormone Deficiency," *N Engl J Med*, 1988, 319(4):201-7.

GT *see Gamma Glutamyl Transferase on page 133*

GTP *see Gamma Glutamyl Transferase on page 133*

GTT *see Glucose Tolerance Test on page 139*

Guthrie Test *see Phenylalanine, Blood on page 181*

HAP *see Haptoglobin, Serum on this page*

Haptoglobin, Serum
CPT 83010
Related Information
Hemoglobin, Plasma *on page 325*
Myoglobin, Blood *on page 167*

Synonyms HAP; HP; Hp

Abstract This is a hemoglobin-binding protein useful in work up of hemolytic states.

Specimen Serum

Container Red top tube

Causes for Rejection Hemolysis from traumatic venipuncture
(Continued)

Haptoglobin, Serum (Continued)

Reference Range 40-180 mg/dL (SI: 0.4-1.8 g/L) but method dependent. Newborns reach adult levels at approximately 4 months.

Possible Panic Range Low values, depending on the method, may be <40-50 mg/dL (SI: <0.4-0.5 g/L).

Use Decreased to absent levels occur more with intravascular than extravascular hemolysis: haptoglobin binds hemoglobin and carries it to the reticuloendothelial system. Thus, haptoglobin is useful in work-up for hemolytic states. It is low in the megaloblastic anemias, which have a hemolytic component. It is decreased in infectious mononucleosis. Decreases can occur with hematoma or tissue hemorrhage. Haptoglobin can be low with liver disease. Congenital absence occurs (small fraction of African-Americans and Orientals have ahaptoglobinemia, absence of detectable haptoglobin). Frequently **elevated** as an acute phase reactant, in inflammatory disorders (eg, collagen diseases, infections, tissue destruction), and with advanced malignant neoplasms.[1] Haptoglobin has been used as a genetic marker for forensic paternity exclusion.[2] A variety of α- and β-chain variants have been identified, 20 different α-chain haptoglobin phenotypes have been noted.

Limitations During inflammation or steroid therapy, normal concentrations do not rule out hemolysis; decreased with oral contraceptives; increased with androgens; haptoglobin normally higher in men; methods in use do not necessarily distinguish between haptoglobin phenotypes

Methodology Immunologic methods including radial immunodiffusion (RID), nephelometry, automated immunoprecipitation, hemoglobin binding capacity; in forensic (paternity exclusion) work, starch or acrylamide gel electrophoresis; one-dimensional isoelectric focusing/immunoblotting method has recently been assessed.[2] Differences in size of various haptoglobin phenotypes renders quantitation by RID inaccurate.

Additional Information Haptoglobin is a protein which binds free hemoglobin. Part of alpha$_2$ on serum protein electrophoresis, serum haptoglobin is a glycoprotein consisting of two pairs of nonidentical chains, α and β, made by the liver. The subunit structure is represented as $\alpha_2\beta_2$. The haptoglobin bound hemoglobin complex is removed rapidly by the reticuloendothelial system; its life is 10-30 minutes.[3] Too large to pass the renal glomeruli, the complex is metabolized to free amino acids and iron in just a few hours. This represents an efficient method for the conservation of iron. Low alpha$_2$ is commonly due to hemolysis and/or liver disease. Serum protein electrophoretic pattern showing low albumin, polyclonal increase in gamma globulin and decrease in alpha$_2$-globulin shown to be due to decreased haptoglobin has been correlated with poor prognosis in severe liver disease.[4] Haptoglobin is decreased for 2-3 days after only 25 mL of blood is lysed.[1] Thus, transfusions, which contain red blood cells which do not all survive in the recipient, can lower the level. The decrease in haptoglobin (after hemolysis) precedes any drop in hemopexin levels or the appearance of methemalbumin in serum or urine.

Myoglobin, unlike hemoglobin, is not bound by haptoglobin.

Immunohistochemical localization and haptoglobin in RNA in situ hybridization procedures have been developed.[5]

Fucosylated forms of the beta-chains of haptoglobins have been recently shown to be applicable to the monitoring of tumor burden in cancer patients and differentiating between active and inactive inflammatory (eg, rheumatoid) joint disease.[6] Elevated fucosylated haptoglobin levels, however, are not disease specific.[7]

Footnotes

1. Peters T Jr, "Proteins," *Chemical Diagnosis of Disease*, Brown SS, Mitchell FL, and Young DS, eds, Amsterdam, Holland: Elsevier/North Holland Biomedical Press, 1979, 311-62.
2. Teige B, Olaisen B, Pedersen L, et al, "Forensic Aspects of Haptoglobin: Electrophoretic Patterns of Haptoglobin Allotype Products and an Evaluation of Typing Procedure," *Electrophoresis*, 1988, 9(8):384-92.
3. Brittenham GM, "Disorders of Iron Metabolism: Iron Deficiency and Overload," *Hematology Basic Principles and Practice*, 2nd ed, Hoffman R, Benz EJ, Shattil SJ, et al, eds, New York, NY: Churchill Livingstone, 1995, 492-523.
4. Fitzmaurice M, Valenzuela R, and Winkelman EI, "Serum Protein Electrophoresis Pattern Associated With Decrease Serum Haptoglobin as a Poor Prognostic Indicator in Severe Liver Disease," *Am J Clin Pathol*, 1989, 91:365.
5. Bowman BH, Barnett DR, Lum JB, et al, "Haptoglobin," *Methods Enzymol*, 1988, 163:452-74.
6. Thompson S, Stappenbeck R, and Turner GA, "A Multiwell Lectin-Binding Assay Using *Lotus tetragonolobus* for Measuring Different Glycosylated Forms of Haptoglobin," *Clin Chim Acta*, 1989, 180(3):277-84.
7. Thompson S, Kelly CA, Griffiths ID, et al, "Abnormally-Fucosylated Serum Haptoglobins in Patients With Inflammatory Joint Disease," *Clin Chim Acta*, 1989, 184(3):251-8.

References

Patzelt D, Geserick G, and Schröder H, "The Genetic Haptoglobin Polymorphism: Relevance of Paternity Assessment," *Electrophoresis*, 1988, 9(8):393-7.

HB$_{A1}$ *see* Glycated Hemoglobin *on page 140*

hCG *see* Human Chorionic Gonadotropin, Serum *on page 145*

hCG, Slide Test, Stat *see* Pregnancy Test *on page 190*

hCG, Urine *see* Pregnancy Test *on page 190*

HCO$_3$, Blood

CPT 82374

Related Information

Anion Gap *on page 81*
Blood Gases, Arterial *on page 87*
Carbon Dioxide, Blood *on page 100*
Electrolytes, Serum or Plasma *on page 123*
Ketone Bodies, Blood *on page 152*
Osmolality, Calculated *on page 172*
pCO$_2$, Blood *on page 179*

Synonyms Bicarbonate

Test Commonly Includes Test is part of blood gases panel and electrolytes panel

Specimen Plasma or serum

Container Green top (heparin) tube, red top tube

Reference Range Newborns and infants: whole blood: 16-24 mmol/L (SI: 16-24 mmol/L); children and adults: serum or plasma: arterial: 21-28 mmol/L (SI: 21-28 mmol/L), venous: 22-29 mmol/L (SI: 22-29 mmol/L)

Possible Panic Range <10 mmol/L, >40 mmol/L

Use A measurement in acid-base and electrolyte status, bicarbonate is used in evaluation of fixed base. **Increased** with metabolic alkalosis (and with compensated respiratory acidosis). **Decreased** with metabolic acidosis and with compensated respiratory alkalosis (eg, low in ketoacidosis).

Limitations Calculated arterial bicarbonate was 10 mmol/L lower than directly measured venous bicarbonate, when the former was diluted with excessive heparin. In drawing arterial specimens, only sufficient heparin needed to fill the dead space of the syringe should be used to avoid dilution.[1] Inadequate filling of red top Vacutainer® tube will decrease apparent serum bicarbonate concentrations.[2]

Methodology Calculation is based on the Henderson-Hasselbalch equation when pH and pCO$_2$ are measured. Total carbon dioxide (TCO$_2$) (CO$_2$ content) equals carbonic acid plus bicarbonate. For venous blood electrolytes, methods to estimate HCO$_3$ are widely used. Calculated HCO$_3^-$ concentrations are accurate in pediatric and adult populations. In the vast majority of clinical settings, the calculated HCO$_3^-$ value is comparable to the measured TCO$_2$ for diagnostic and therapeutic considerations.[3] If only TCO$_2$ is measured (without pH) it is used interchangeably with bicarbonate. Any error using this estimate is ≤2 mmol/L.

Additional Information Most pediatric diabetic patients whose initial pH was ≥7.20 or whose bicarbonate concentration was ≥10 mmol/L had resolution of acidosis, mostly without hospitalization, while most patients whose pH was <7.20 and bicarbonate <10 mmol/L were hospitalized.[4] Rapid correction of metabolic acidosis in chronic renal failure patients may attenuate circulating PTH activity.[5]

Other laboratory tests needed in the work-up of diabetic ketoacidosis include the remaining electrolytes, plasma glucose, blood and urine ketone bodies, hematocrit, BUN, and sometimes osmolality.

Footnotes

1. Bloom SA, Canzanello VJ, Strom JA, et al, "Spurious Assessment of Acid-Base Status Due to Dilutional Effect of Heparin," *Am J Med*, 1985, 79(4):528-30.
2. Herr RD and Swanson T, "Serum Bicarbonate Declines With Sample Size in Vacutainer® Tubes," *Am J Clin Pathol*, 1992, 97(2):213-6.
3. Rivkees SA and Fine BP, "The Reliability of Calculated Bicarbonate in Clinical Practice," *Clin Pediatr (Phila)*, 1988, 27(5):240-2.
4. Bonadio WA, Gutzeit MF, Losek JD, et al, "Outpatient Management of Diabetic Ketoacidosis," *Am J Dis Child*, 1988, 142(4):448-50.
5. Lu KC, Shieh SD, Li BL, et al, "Rapid Correction of Metabolic Acidosis in Chronic Renal Failure; Effect on Parathyroid Hormone Activity," *Nephron*, 1994, 67(4):419-24.

References

O'Leary TD and Langton SR, "Calculated Bicarbonate or Total Carbon Dioxide?" *Clin Chem*, 1989, 35(8):1697-700.

Preuss HG, "Fundamentals of Clinical Acid-Base Evaluation," *Clin Lab Med*, 1993, 13(1):103-16.

hCS *see* Placental Lactogen, Human *on page 184*

HDL *see* High Density Lipoprotein Cholesterol *on next page*

HDLC *see* High Density Lipoprotein Cholesterol *on next page*

HDL Cholesterol *see* High Density Lipoprotein Cholesterol *on next page*

Health Fairs *see* Chemistry Profile *on page 107*

Heat Stable Alkaline Phosphatase *see* Alkaline Phosphatase, Heat Stable *on page 68*

Hemoglobin A$_{1a}$, A$_{1b}$, A$_{1c}$ *see* Glycated Hemoglobin *on page 140*

Hemoglobin, Glycosylated *see* Glycated Hemoglobin *on page 140*

Hemoglobin Saturation, Percent *see* Oxygen Saturation, Blood *on page 175*

Hepatic Iron Index *see* Ferritin, Serum *on page 127*

β-Hexosaminidase, Serum *see* Beta-Hexosaminidase, Serum *on page 85*

hGH *see* Growth Hormone *on page 141*

5-HIAA, Quantitative, Urine *see* 5-Hydroxyindoleacetic Acid, Quantitative, Urine *on page 147*

High Density Lipoprotein Cholesterol

CPT 83718

Related Information
Alcohol, Blood or Urine *on page 531*
Apolipoprotein A and B *on page 82*
Cholesterol, Serum *on page 110*
Lipid Profile *on page 159*
Lipoprotein Electrophoresis *on page 161*
Triglycerides *on page 209*

Synonyms Alpha$_1$ Lipoprotein Cholesterol; HDL; HDLC; HDL Cholesterol

Applies to Apolipoprotein A-I; Cholesterol/HDLC Ratio

Abstract A class of heterogeneous particles of varying sizes and densities, HDLC contains lipid and protein. It includes cholesterol esters and free cholesterol, triglycerides, phospholipids, and A, C, and E apoproteins. Two subclasses of HDL predominate: HDL$_2$ and smaller, denser HDL$_3$. HDL may function in so-called "reverse transport" of cholesterol to the liver. An independent, strong, inverse relationship of HDL cholesterol and coronary arterial disease (CAD) has been essentially confirmed in the industrial world.[1] Twenty percent to 30% of total cholesterol is HDLC.

Patient Preparation Patient ideally should be on a stable diet for 3 weeks and should fast for 9-10 hours prior to collection of specimen. Recent fat intake influences HDL. See Preparation in the listing Cholesterol, Serum *on page 110*. HDLC is usually done as part of lipid profile.

Specimen Serum

Container Red top tube

Storage Instructions Analysis promptly after sampling is best. The specimen can be refrigerated up to several days at 4°C or frozen for several weeks. For long-term storage use -70°C.[2]

Causes for Rejection Specimen collected in citrate or heparin anticoagulants

Reference Range Male: 15-34 years: 35-65 mg/dL (SI: 0.9-1.7 mmol/L); female: 35-80 mg/dL (SI: 0.9-2.0 mmol/L). HDLC levels in men <35 mg/dL (SI: <0.9 mmol/L) represent a coronary risk factor.[1,3] In women, HDLC <40 mg/dL is a risk factor. The 95th percentile increases to 70 mg/dL at age 45 years. HDL cholesterol values are about 20% to 30% of the total cholesterol and may be expressed as a percentage of total cholesterol. HDL after puberty is lower in males. African-Americans have higher HDL than do whites.

HDLC		Coronary Artery Disease Risk (times average)	
mg/dL	SI: mmol/L	Male	Female
25	0.65	2.0	
30	0.78	1.8	
35	0.91	1.5	
40	1.03	1.2	1.9
45	1.16	Average	1.6
50	1.29	0.8	1.3
55	1.42	0.7	Average
60	1.55	0.6	0.8
65	1.68	0.5	0.6
70	1.81		0.5
75	1.94	Longevity	

Note: Risk is inversely proportional to HDLC.

From Kannel WB, Castelli WP, and Gordon T, "Cholesterol in the Prediction of Atherosclerotic Disease," *Ann Intern Med*, 1979, 90:85, with permission.

Use A protective substance utilized for prediction of coronary arterial disease (CAD), especially useful in individuals with high serum cholesterol levels. Low HDLC is an important predictor of risk of coronary atherosclerosis and coronary heart disease. HDL may act as a protective scavenger molecule (reverse cholesterol transport). The liver is the major site of cholesterol **excretion**. When a slightly increased cholesterol is due to high HDL, therapy is not indicated.[3]

Limitations Increased levels are reported with estrogens and with birth control pills. Clofibrate, Atromid-S® therapy cause increases. There may

be interference from very high triglyceride concentrations. Standardization is not as good as that available for cholesterol in 1989 from CDC/NBS, and reliability everywhere may not equal that in published epidemiologic studies. Coefficients of variation are excessively high; the problems with lack of accuracy and precision of HDL are widely recognized. A new direct method for HDLC now available should improve precision. HCFA authorization for reimbursement is uncertain at this time. Only small mean differences are found between those with CAD and those who appear healthy. Bilirubin interferes; icteric specimens lead to underestimation of HDLC.

Methodology Ultracentrifugation; precipitation: heparin and 92 millimolar manganese followed by incubation, centrifugation in a refrigerated centrifuge; dextran sulfate and magnesium chloride; each followed by cholesterol analysis; phosphotungstate and magnesium ion also are used. A reflectance photometric technique with prior precipitation has been reported.[4] HDL$_2$ and HDL$_3$ cholesterol can be measured by precipitation and ultracentrifugation. Dextran sulfate produces lower results than other precipitating agents.

Additional Information Total cholesterol and triglycerides are required as well for determination of lipid risk factors for coronary artery disease. These tests with HDLC and LDLC are the usual lipid profile. HDLC is especially apt to be low in male subjects who are obese and sedentary, in those who smoke cigarettes, and in those who have diabetes mellitus. Uremia is also associated with lower HDLC. Exercise, appropriate diet, and moderate ethanol intake increase HDLC.

HDLC is useful with cholesterol in forecasting risk of coronary artery disease in the industrialized countries, possibly because of ingestion of high fat diets. LDLC, an excellent predictor, is usually a calculation. Those **at least risk** for development of CAD would have low cholesterol, low triglyceride, and high HDLC. Even in men with moderately low cholesterol, HDLC is protective against CAD.[5] Under a high fat diet, western women tend to have higher serum HDL than do western men. This may be explained by an increase of estradiol and estrone in high fat diets in women.[6]

Thiazides and nonselective beta-adrenergic blocking agents may decrease HDLC.[3]

Other coronary risk factors include glucose intolerance, increased systolic blood pressure, cigarette smoking, and left ventricular hypertrophy as well as cholesterol.[7]

Apolipoprotein A-I is the major protein of HDL. Apolipoprotein A-I determination may eventually be shown to be superior to HDLC; increased apoprotein A-I is associated with a diminished risk of atherogenesis. It is measured by RIA[8] and by nephelometry. Problems about apolipoproteins are discussed in the listing Lipid Profile *on page 159*. Essentially, current studies have not yet answered whether or not apoprotein A-I is a better discriminator than HDL.[9] HDL measurement has been considered preferable by Gordon and Rifkind.[1]

Factors contributing to decreased HDLC include:
- genetic factors: primary hypoalphalipoproteinemia[10]
- cigarette smoking[11]
- obesity[11]
- hypertriglyceridemia[11]
- lack of exercise
- steroids - androgens, progestogens, anabolic
- thiazides
- beta-adrenergic blockers
- probucol
- neomycin

Many other substances may affect risk of coronary artery disease, often by mechanisms not involving serum LDL cholesterol concentrations directly. Such substances include phytosterols, tocotrienols, arginine, and antioxidant vitamins.[12]

The rare entity, **Tangier disease**, is characterized by very low HDL, total cholesterol, and low lipoprotein cholesterol. Cholesterol esters accumulate in tissues. Severe coronary arterial sclerosis with extremely low HDL (1.4 mg/dL) was reported in a subject with Tangier disease.[13]

New information suggests that very active middle-aged men and women have higher plasma lipoprotein concentrations of HDL cholesterol and often moderately low levels of LDL cholesterol. Evidence suggests that fat loss by dieting alone or by exercising alone results in similar elevations of HDL cholesterol.[14]

Chylomicron remnants have been linked to CAD progression. This linkage is not explained by any relationship to the high density lipoprotein system and may indicate a direct atherogenic effect of chylomicron remnants themselves.[15] There is evidence, however, of beneficial effects of aggressive lipoprotein management.[16]

The **cholesterol to HDLC ratio** bears significant predictive value. An increase of one unit of this ratio bears association with increased risk of 53% following adjustment for nonlipid risk factors.[17]
(Continued)

High Density Lipoprotein Cholesterol *(Continued)*

The inverse relationship between moderate alcohol intake and risk of acute infarct of myocardium is thought to be mediated through HDL_2 and HDL_3.[18]

An association is perceived between low HDLC levels and propensity for restenosis following percutaneous transluminal coronary angioplasty.[19]

Footnotes

1. Gordon DJ and Rifkind BM, "High Density Lipoprotein - The Clinical Implications of Recent Studies," *N Engl J Med*, 1989, 321(19):1311-6.
2. Nanjee MN and Miller NE, "Evaluation of Long-Term Frozen Storage of Plasma for Measurement of High-Density Lipoprotein and Its Subfractions by Precipitation," *Clin Chem*, 1990, 36(5):783-8.
3. Betteridge DJ, "High Density Lipoprotein and Coronary Heart Disease," *BMJ*, 1989, 298(6679):974-5.
4. Ng RH, Sparks KM, and Statland BE, "Direct Measurement of High-Density Lipoprotein Cholesterol by the Reflotron Assay With No Manual Precipitation Step," *Clin Chem*, 1991, 37(3):435-7.
5. Kitamura A, Iso H, Naito Y, et al, "High-Density Lipoprotein Cholesterol and Premature Coronary Heart Disease in Urban Japanese Men," *Circulation*, 1994, 89(6):2533-9.
6. Kesteloot H and Sasaki S, "On the Relationship Between Nutrition, Sex Hormones and High-Density Lipoproteins in Women," *Acta Cardiol*, 1993, 48(4):355-63.
7. Kannel WB, Castelli WP, and Gordon T, "Cholesterol in the Prediction of Atherosclerotic Disease. New Perspectives Based on the Framingham Study," *Ann Intern Med*, 1979, 90:85-91.
8. Maciejko JJ, Holmes DR, Kottke BA, et al, "Apolipoprotein A-1 as a Marker of Angiographically Assessed Coronary Artery Disease," *N Engl J Med*, 1983, 309:385-9.
9. Miller NE, "Associations of High Density Lipoprotein Subclasses and Apolipoproteins With Ischemic Heart Disease and Coronary Atherosclerosis," *Am Heart J*, 1987, 113(2 Pt 2):589-97.
10. Grundy SM, Goodman DS, Rifkind BM, et al, "The Place of HDL in Cholesterol Management: A Perspective From the National Cholesterol Education Program," *Arch Intern Med*, 1989, 149(3):505-10.
11. Frohlich JJ and Pritchard PH, "The Clinical Significance of Serum High Density Lipoproteins," *Clin Biochem*, 1989, 22(6):417-23.
12. Fraser GE, "Diet and Coronary Heart Disease: Beyond Dietary Fats and Low Density Lipoprotein Cholesterol," *Am J Clin Nutr*, 1994, 59(5 Suppl):1117S-23S.
13. Mautner SL, Sanchez JA, Rader DJ, et al, "The Heart in Tangier Disease. Severe Coronary Atherosclerosis With Near Absence of High-Density Lipoprotein Cholesterol," *Am J Clin Pathol*, 1992, 98(2):191-8.
14. Wood PD, "Physical Activity, Diet, and Health: Independent and Interactive Effects," *Med Sci Sports Exerc*, 1994, 26(7):838-43.
15. Hamsten A, "Lipids as a Coronary Risk Factor: Analysis of Hyperlipidaemias," *Postgrad Med J*, 1993, 69(Suppl 1):S8-11.
16. Superko HR and Krauss RM, "Coronary Artery Disease Regression. Convincing Evidence for the Benefit of Aggressive Lipoprotein Management," *Circulation*, 1994, 90(2):1056-69.
17. Hostetter AL, "Screening for Dyslipidemia. Practice Parameter," *Am J Clin Pathol*, 1995, 103(4):380-5.
18. Gaziano JM, Buring JE, Breslow JL, et al, "Moderate Alcohol Intake, Increased Levels of High-Density Lipoprotein and its Subfractions, and Decreased Risk of Myocardial Infarction," *N Engl J Med*, 1993, 329(25):1829-34.
19. Roth A, Eshchar Y, Keren G, et al, "Serum Lipids and Restenosis After Successful Percutaneous Transluminal Coronary Angioplasty. Ichilov Magnesium Study Group," *Am J Cardiol*, 1994, 73(16):1154-8.

References

Asayama K, Miyao A, and Kato K, "High-Density Lipoprotein (HDL), HDL2, and HDL3 Cholesterol Concentrations Determined in Serum of Newborns, Infants, Children, Adolescents, and Adults by Use of a Micromethod for Combined Precipitation Ultracentrifugation," *Clin Chem*, 1990, 36(1):129-31.

Brunner D, Weisbort J, Meshulam N, et al, "Relation of Serum Total Cholesterol and High Density Lipoprotein Cholesterol Percentage to the Incidence of Definite Coronary Events: Twenty Year Follow-Up of the Donolo-Tel Aviv Prospective Coronary Artery Disease Study," *Am J Cardiol*, 1987, 59(15):1271-6.

Gordon DJ, Probstfield JL, Garrison RJ, et al, "High-Density Lipoprotein Cholesterol and Cardiovascular Disease: Four Prospective American Studies," *Circulation*, 1989, 79(1):8-15.

Kannel WB, "Low High Density Lipoprotein Cholesterol and What to Do About It," *Am J Cardiol*, 1992, 70(7):810-4.

Pocock SJ, Shaper AG, and Phillips AN, "Concentrations of High Density Lipoprotein Cholesterol, Triglycerides, and Total Cholesterol in Ischaemic Heart Disease," *Br Med J (Clin Res Ed)*, 1989, 298(6679):998-1002.

Rifkind BM, "High-Density Lipoprotein Cholesterol and Coronary Artery Disease: Survey of the Evidence," *Am J Cardiol*, 1990, 66(6):3A-6A.

Rosenson RS, "Low Levels of High Density Lipoprotein Cholesterol (Hypoalphalipoproteinemia). An Approach to Management," *Arch Intern Med*, 1993, 153(13):1528-38.

Schectmen G and Sasse E, "Variability of Lipid Measurements: Revelance for the Clinician," *Clin Chem*, 1993, 39(7):1495-503.

Steinmetz J and Delattre J, "High Density Lipoprotein Cholesterol," *Drug Effects on Laboratory Test Results Analytical Interferences and Pharmacological Effects*, Siest G and Galteau MM, eds, Littleton, MA: PSG Publishing Co Inc, 1988, 185-97.

Weitzman JB and Vladutiu AO, "Very High Values of Serum High Density Lipoprotein Cholesterol," *Arch Pathol Lab Med*, 1992, 116(8):831-6.

Hill Plots *see* P-50 Blood Gas *on page 176*

Histalog™ Stimulation Test *replaced by* Gastric Analysis *on page 133*

Histamine

CPT 83088

Applies to Methylimidazoleacetic Acid

Abstract A neurotransmitter molecule produced by mast cells and certain brain cells.

Patient Preparation Patient must be on a diet of microbially processed foods, such as cheeses or sauerkraut.

Specimen Urine

Collection Fifty percent acetic acid used as preservative at beginning of 24-hour urine collection to maintain pH 2.0-4.0.

Storage Instructions Store urine frozen.

Special Instructions Test is ordinarily available only from a few reference laboratories.

Reference Range Urine: 17-68 µg/24 hours (SI: 553-2210 nmol/L); <45 µg/g creatinine; considerably method variable

Use Evaluate possible systemic mastocytosis

Limitations Test is not very sensitive. There are false-positive results associated with urinary tract infections. Histamine level alone may not fully reflect the role of histamine in a disease process. Measurement of histamine and its metabolites may be necessary.[1]

Methodology Radioimmunoassay (RIA): gas chromatography (GC),[2] fluorometry,[3] radioisotope enzymatic,[4,5] high performance liquid chromatography (HPLC),[6,7] chemical ionization mass spectrometry

Additional Information Mast cells produce numerous biologically active materials, including histamine.[8] Histamine is often, but not consistently, elevated in cases of systemic mastocytosis,[9] and also in other myeloproliferative disorders such as chronic myelogenous leukemia and polycythemia vera. Some carcinoid tumors (particularly of gastric origin) produce excessive amounts of histamine. Measurement of urinary methylated and other histamine metabolites may be more sensitive and specific. In a study of 25 patients with urticaria pigmentosa, all cases of systemic mastocytosis were identified with investigation of methylimidazoleacetic acid, the major histamine metabolite (>4.1 mg/24 hours) while histamine was elevated in only 50% of cases.[10] In another study of systemic mast cell disease, urinary histamine was elevated in only 1 of 26 cases.[11] Histamine release from basophils and mast cells in response to allergen and reagin complex is generally recognized. There is also evidence that histamine is synthesized by T cells/macrophages *de novo* through the action of histidine decarboxylase.[12,13] There is evidence suggesting that basophils have an interleukin 1 receptor that can modulate the response to IgE-related signals.[14]

Serum histamine levels are decreased with HIV infection, a finding of possible prognostic significance. Splenectomy results in a rise in histamine levels in AIDS patients with thrombocytopenic purpura. Histamine levels have been reported decreased in some 60% of patients with malignant disease.[15]

Histamine is recognized as a true neurotransmitter. A neuronal system within the brain is well organized and is localized to a small area of the posterior hypothalamus. Histamine may be related to circadian rhythms.[16]

Uremic pruritus has been improved with erythropoietin therapy with lowering of plasma histamine concentrations.[17]

Footnotes

1. Green JP, Prell GD, Khandelwal JK, et al, "Aspects of Histamine Metabolism," *Agents Actions*, 1987, 22(1-2):1-15.
2. Khandelwal JK, Hough LB, Mornshow AM, et al, "Measurement of Tele-Methylhistamine and Histamine in Human Cerebrospinal Fluid, Urine, and Plasma," *Agents Actions*, 1982, 12:583-90.
3. Assem ES and Chong EK, "Simultaneous Fluorometric Assay of Histamine and Histidine in Biological Fluid Using an Automated Analyzer," *Agents Actions*, 1982, 12:26-9.
4. Horakova Z, Keiser HR, and Beaven MA, "Blood and Urine Histamine Levels in Normal and Pathological States as Measured by a Radiochemical Assay," *Clin Chim Acta*, 1977, 79:447-56.
5. Dyer J, Warren K, Merlin S, et al, "Measurement of Plasma Histamine: Description of an Improved Method and Normal Values," *J Allergy Clin Immunol*, 1982, 70:82-7.
6. Granerus G and Wass U, "Urinary Excretion of Histamine, Methylhistamine (1-MeHi), and Methylimidazoleacetic Acid (MeImAA) in Mastocytosis: Comparison of New HPLC Methods With Other Present Methods," *Agents Actions*, 1984, 14(3):341-5.
7. Liotet S, Meyohas MC, Batellier L, et al, "Blood Histamine Levels in Patients Infected With the Human Immunodeficiency Virus," *Presse Med*, 1988, 17(42):2240-2.
8. McBride P, Jacobs R, Bradley D, et al, "Use of Plasma Histamine Levels to Monitor Cutaneous Mast Cell Degranulation," *J Allergy Clin Immunol*, 1989, 83(2 Pt 1):374-80.
9. Friedman BS, Steinberg SC, Meggs WJ, et al, "Analysis of Plasma Histamine Levels in Patients With Mast Cell Disorders," *Am J Med*, 1989, 87(6):649-54.
10. Granerus G and Roupe G, "Increased Urinary Methylimidazoleacetic Acid (MeImAA) as an Indicator of Systemic Mastocytosis," *Agents Actions*, 1982, 12:29-31.
11. Webb TA, Li CY, and Yam LT, "Systemic Mast Cell Disease: A Clinical and Hematopathologic Study of 26 Cases," *Cancer*, 1982, 49:927-38.
12. Aoi R, Nakashima I, Kitamura Y, et al, "Histamine Synthesis by Mouse T Lymphocytes Through Induced Histidine Decarboxylase," *Immunology*, 1989, 66(2):219-23.
13. Oh C, Suzuki S, Nakashima I, et al, "Histamine Synthesis by Non-Mast Cells Through Mitogen-Dependent Induction of Histidine Decarboxylase," *Immunology*, 1988, 65(1):143-8.
14. Massey WA, Randall TC, Kagey-Sobotka A, et al, "Recombinant Human IL-1α and -1β Potentiate IgE-Mediated Histamine Release From Human Basophils," *J Immunol*, 1989, 143(6):1875-80.
15. Motoki T, Obara T, Ezoe H, et al, "Low Serum Histamine in Malignant Disease," *N Engl J Med*, 1984, 310(6):391-2.
16. Nowak JZ, "Histamine in the Central Nervous System: Its Role in Circadian Rhythmicity," *Acta Neurobiol Exp*, 1994, 54(Suppl):65-82.
17. De Marchi S, Cecchin E, Villalta D, et al, "Relief of Pruritus and Decreases in Plasma Histamine Concentrations During Erythropoietin Therapy in Patients With Uremia," *N Engl J Med*, 1992, 326(15):969-74.

References

Du Buske LM, "Introduction: Basophil Histamine Release and the Diagnosis of Food Allergy," *Allergy Proc*, 1993, 14(4):243-9.

Jacobs R, Kaliner M, Shelhamer JH, et al, "Blood Histamine Concentrations Are Not Elevated in Humans With Septic Shock," *Crit Care Med*, 1989, 17(1):30-5.

Keyzer JJ, de Monchy JG, van Doormaal JJ, et al, "Improved Diagnosis of Mastocytosis by Measurement of Urinary Histamine Metabolites," *N Engl J Med*, 1983, 309:1603-5.

HLA-A3 *see* Ferritin, Serum *on page 127*

Hoesch Test *see* Porphobilinogen, Qualitative, Urine *on page 185*

Holmes Formula *see* Osmolality, Calculated *on page 172*

Homocysteine, Qualitative *see* Cystine, Urine *on page 120*

Homovanillic Acid, Urine

CPT 83150

Related Information

Carcinoembryonic Antigen *on page 100*
Catecholamines, Fractionation, Plasma *on page 103*
Catecholamines, Fractionation, Urine *on page 104*
Metanephrines *on page 165*
N-*myc* Amplification *on page 522*
Tumor Aneuploidy by Flow Cytometry *on page 57*
Urine Collection, 24-Hour *on page 30*
Vanillylmandelic Acid, Urine *on page 216*

Synonyms HVA

Test Commonly Includes Measurement of creatinine excretion as well as HVA

Abstract HVA is a major terminal metabolite of dopamine. More than three fourths of patients with neuroblastoma excrete increased HVA and/or VMA.

Patient Preparation Patients should avoid aspirin, disulfiram, reserpine, and pyridoxine, if possible, at least 48 hours prior to collection of the specimen. Levodopa should be avoided for 2 weeks before collection.

Specimen 24-hour urine. Smaller collections are in use as well for pediatric patients.

Container Plastic urine container

Collection Urine specimen should not contact metal. Depending on laboratory, boric, acetic, or hydrochloric acid must initially be added to the container as a preservative. Check with your laboratory for volume and concentration.

Storage Instructions Measure 24-hour urine volume, adjust to pH 2-4 and aliquot 100 mL sample and refrigerate. Stable 7 days at 4°C.

Special Instructions For work-up for neuroblastoma, excretion of VMA should also be measured. Patient's age is needed.

Reference Range Adult normal range is usually <8.0 mg/24 hours (SI: <44.0 μmol/day). Pediatric values are up to 35.0 μg HVA/mg creatinine (SI: 22.0 mmol HVA/mol creatinine) in infancy. See table.

Homovanillic Acid, Urine

Age	μg HVA/mg creatinine	SI: mmol HVA/ mol creatinine
0-1 y	1.2-35.0	0.7-21.7
1-2 y	4.0-23.0	2.5-14.3
2-5 y	0.5-20.0	0.3-12.4
5-10 y	0.5-15.0	0.3-9.3
10-15 y	0.25-12.0	0.2-7.4
Adults	0.25-7.0	0.2-4.4

Adults: <8 mg/24 h.

Use Diagnose neuroblastoma, ganglioneuroblastoma, and pheochromocytoma; follow course of tumor treatment

Limitations Almost all patients with neuroblastoma have elevations of HVA, while only about 80% have elevations of urinary catecholamines. Increased HVA levels, however, are not specific for neuroblastoma.

Normal plasma levels of **metanephrines** are reported to rule out pheochromocytoma.[1] However, even that test is not without problems.[2]

Methodology High performance liquid chromatography (HPLC), solvent extraction, and colorimetry[3,4]

Additional Information HVA is the major terminal metabolite of the dopamine pathway. VMA is the major terminal metabolite of the norepinephrine pathway. HVA is often excreted in excess amounts by neuroblastomas, ganglioneuroblastomas, pheochromocytomas, and in Riley-Day syndrome. Excretion may be intermittent. Plasma HVA is increased in schizotypal personality disorders.[5] Approximately 20% of subjects with neuroblastoma do not have increased VMA.[3]

Carcinoembryonic antigen is an additional marker found in many patients with neuroblastoma. Relevant to neuroblastoma, see also listings N-*myc* Amplification *on page 522* and Tumor Aneuploidy by Flow Cytometry *on page 57*.

Depressed patients who have attempted suicide have been reported to have decreased urinary HVA compared to patients who have not attempted suicide.[6]

Footnotes

1. Lenders JW, Keiser HR, Goldstein DS, et al, "Plasma Metanephrines in the Diagnosis of Pheochromoctyoma," *Ann Intern Med*, 1995, 123(2):101-9.
2. Krakoff LR, "Searching for Pheochromocytoma: A New and Better Test?" *Ann Intern Med*, 1995, 123(2):150-1, editorial.
3. Rothstein A, "Determination of Urinary Homovanillic Acid Using the Nitrosonaphthol Reaction," *Am J Clin Pathol*, 1987, 87(5):644-8.
4. Davidson DF, "Simultaneous Assay for Urinary 4-Hydroxy-3-Methoxy-Mandelic Acid, 5-Hydroxyindoleacetic Acid and Homovanillic Acid by Isocractic HPLC With Electrochemical Detection," *Ann Clin Biochem*, 1989, 26(Pt 4):137-43.
5. Siever LJ, Amin F, Coccaro EF, et al, "Plasma Homovanillic Acid in Schizotypal Personality Disorder," *Am J Psychiatry*, 1991, 148(9):1246-8.
6. Roy A, "Recent Biological Studies on Suicide," *Suicide Life Threat Behav*, 1994, 24(1):10-4.

References

Fitzgibbon MC and Tormey WP, "Paediatric Reference Ranges for Urinary Catecholamines/Metabolites and Their Relevance in Neuroblastoma Diagnosis," *Ann Clin Biochem*, 1994, 31(Pt 1):1-11.

Javors MA, Bowden CL, and Maas JW, "3-Methoxy-4-Hydroxyphenylglycol, 5-Hydroxyindoleacetic Acid, and Homovanillic Acid in Human Cerebrospinal Fluid. Storage and Measurement by Reversed-Phase High Performance Liquid Chromatography and Coulometric Detection Using 3-Methoxy-4-Hydroxyphenylacetic Acid as an Internal Standard," *J Chromatogr*, 1984, 336(2):259-69.

2-Hour PP Glucose *see* Glucose, 2-Hour Postprandial *on page 136*

HP *see* Haptoglobin, Serum *on page 141*

Hp *see* Haptoglobin, Serum *on page 141*

hPL *see* Placental Lactogen, Human *on page 184*

5-HT *see* Serotonin *on page 198*

Human Chorionic Gonadotropin, Serum

CPT 84702

Related Information

Alpha$_1$-Fetoprotein, Serum *on page 72*
Placental Lactogen, Human *on page 184*
Pregnancy Test *on page 190*
Progesterone *on page 191*

Synonyms Beta Subunit, hCG; Chorionic Gonadotropin, Beta Subunit; hCG

Applies to GnRH; Inhibin A; Pregnancy Testing

Abstract A glycoprotein heterodimer, hCG derives from trophoblastic cells. Gonadotropin releasing hormone (GnRH) may stimulate its production. Physiologically, it stimulates progesterone secretion by the corpus luteum, which maintains secretory endometrium. In pregnancy, hCG promotes trophoblastic differentiation.

Patient Preparation Avoid radioisotope scan prior to collection of specimen if RIA is used for assay.

Specimen Serum; cerebrospinal fluid to manage intracranial germ cell tumors

Container Red top tube

Storage Instructions Serum stable 24 hours at 25°C and 4 days at 4°C. Freeze at -20°C for longer storage.[1]

Special Instructions For females, state date of last menstrual period. Length of gestation is relevant for prenatal screening. To monitor patients with testicular tumors, both α-fetoprotein and hCG should be measured, and LDH as well.

Reference Range Depends on application and methodology. <3 mIU/mL (SI: <3 IU/L) usually normal (nonpregnant). Greater than 300% differences in means of different methods has been documented. Concentration of hCG doubles each 1.5-2.5 days during the first 6 weeks of gestation, peaking at ~100,000 IU/L 60-70 days following implantation. Wide individual variation is seen, partly explained by maternal plasma volume increases. The reference range in gestation relates to maternal weight and gestational age; β-hCG >50,000 IU/L supports but does not guarantee the diagnosis of viable intrauterine pregnancy.

Critical Values In subjects with concentration <2000 IU/L, increase of serum hCG <66% in 2 days is suggestive of spontaneous abortion or ruptured ectopic gestation in appropriate clinical setting. Rate of increase diminishes with gestation. After the 14th week, hCG continues its rise in gestational trophoblastic disease but falls in normal pregnancy. Levels of hCG >100,000 IU/L can be found in the sera of patients with choriocarcinoma.

Use Work up and manage **germ cell neoplasms** including choriocarcinoma and embryonal carcinoma. High levels are found also with **gestational trophoblastic tumors** (hydatidiform mole, partial mole and (Continued)

Human Chorionic Gonadotropin, Serum
(Continued)

choriocarcinoma) and increases are found with multiple gestation pregnancy and with erythroblastosis fetalis. Some islet cell tumors may make hCG, as may some carcinomas of lung, stomach, colon, pancreas, liver, and breast. **Prenatal screening** for trisomy 21 (Down syndrome) utilizes hCG;[2] β subunit of hCG is elevated in maternal serum early and later in gestation.[3] In combination with serum estriol and serum AFP, the detection of Down syndrome is increased. Low levels of intact and β-hCG are found with trisomy 18.[3] Decreases occur in settings in which trophoblastic function is compromised such as **ectopic pregnancy** and **spontaneous abortion**.

Limitations Normal hCG levels do not rule out germ cell tumor. The same test method may not be suitable for use as a tumor marker and for pregnancy testing. Several reference preparations including World Health Organization sources may be used as standards, different methods calibrated against different materials, and differences in circulating forms of hCG make interlaboratory comparisons difficult. At least 50 commercial kits for serum have been available in the 1990s. Although overlap exists between inevitable abortion and ectopic pregnancy, the rate of change of hCG and progesterone concentrations distinguish normal intrauterine gestation from pathologic pregnancies (ectopic gestation and inevitable abortion).[4] About 40 kits for urinary hCG measurement have been available.

Methodology Chemiluminometric sandwich immunoassay is available.[4] Two site immunoradiometric assay (IRMA), radioimmunoassay (RIA); two site enzyme-linked immunosorbent assay (ELISA) methods have been especially successful commercially to assist the diagnosis of early pregnancy.[5,6] Time resolved europium-chelate fluorescence procedures may exceed RIA in sensitivity.[7] Two site fluorescent immunoassay is capable of measurement to the 1 mIU/mL.[8] hCG by RIA measures the immunologic activities of both hCG and its free β-subunit (sometimes called total beta assays).

Additional Information Human chorionic gonadotropin is a glycoprotein hormone normally produced by the developing placenta, and aberrantly produced by some germ cell neoplasms. It is composed of glycopeptide α- and β-subunits. The α-subunit, a 92-amino acid sequence, is essentially identical with that of luteinizing hormone, follicle stimulating hormone, and thyroid stimulating hormone. It is this shared structure which accounts for some false-positives in pregnancy tests not based on the β-subunit. The β-subunit, a 145 amino acid sequence, is unique to hCG, and specific assays based on the β subunit are not subject to hormonal cross reactivity. β-subunit specific assays are now sensitive enough to detect a normal pregnancy 6-14 days after implantation. hCG can be detected as low as 5 mIU/mL (SI: 5 IU/L).

About 10% of hCG molecules in the first trimester are "nicked" by enzymatic cleavage, rendering them inactive and unstable. Nicked molecules reach 20% in the third trimester and contribute to variability between assays. β core fragments also circulate.

Chorionic gonadotropin assays are sometimes used to support the diagnosis of **ectopic pregnancy**. Ectopic gestations typically secrete decreased amounts of hCG and progesterone compared to intrauterine pregnancies. Abnormally low hCG levels with abnormal rates of change[4] coupled with transvaginal ultrasound detect many ectopic pregnancies prior to rupture.[9] It is helpful to use hCG and progesterone sequentially every other day to detect a lack of rise in the levels. The rate of change of hCG can be calculated.[4] It has been demonstrated that viable and nonviable pregnancy can be distinguished by the ratio of serial hCG values separated by 48 hours. The relationship for various sampling intervals has been plotted on the accompanying chart by Leland B Baskin,[10] based on prior investigation by Kadar N et al and Romero R et al. The sampling interval is plotted on the horizontal axis and the ratio of the determined βhCG values for that interval is plotted on the vertical axis. If the intersection of the lines extending from those two points (the sampling interval and the βhCG ratio) is above the curve, it is likely a viable intrauterine pregnancy, and if below the line, it is a nonviable pregnancy.

The detection of fetal **trisomy 21 (Down syndrome)** is now well established using hCG. Midtrimester hCG elevation permits detection in up to 60% of cases, along with maternal AFP, unconjugated estriol, and maternal age. Measurement of the β subunit offers improved detection.[4] Detection of Down syndrome is enhanced with use of inhibin A.[3]

Decrease in hCG at midtrimester is found with **trisomy 18** (Edward's syndrome).

hCG levels are extremely useful in following those **germ cell neoplasms** which produce hCG, particularly trophoblastic neoplasms. Following evacuation of a trophoblastic lesion, serum β-hCG concentrations should return to normal in 6-8 weeks. Oral contraceptive use may delay this fall. Any other delay in the fall, or subsequent rise, is an

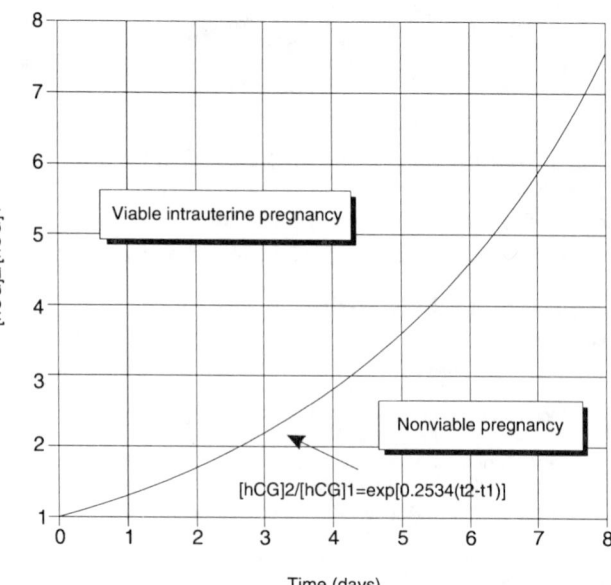

Serum hCG Concentration

[hCG]2/[hCG]1

Viable intrauterine pregnancy

Nonviable pregnancy

$$[hCG]2/[hCG]1 = \exp[0.2534(t2-t1)]$$

Time (days)

Minimum increase in viable IUP during 1st trimester:
The ratio of successive serum hCG concentrations during the first trimester of a viable intrauterine pregnancy based on an exponential increase of 66% in 2 days (0.2534 days^{-1} = ln(1.66)/2 days), (sensitivity~90%; specificity~87%).

Courtesy of Leland B. Baskin, MD, assistant professor, the University of Texas Southwestern Medical Center at Dallas, with permission.

From Kadar N, Caldwell BV, and Romero R, "A Method for Screening for Ectopic Pregnancy and Its Indications," *Obstet Gynecol*, 1981, 58:162-5. Romero R, Kadar N, Copel JA, et al, "The Value of Serial Human Chorionic Gonadotropin Testing as a Diagnostic Tool in Ectopic Pregnancy," *Am J Obstet Gynecol*, 1986, 155:392-4.

indication for further evaluation. CSF hCG is useful for diagnosis of certain intracranial germinal neoplasms.

In germ cell neoplasms in the male, β-hCG and α-fetoprotein are both useful tumor markers. They can be demonstrated histochemically in tissue to confirm diagnosis and can be followed in serum to evaluate recurrence. Prognostic factors for metastatic testicular germ cell neoplasms include pretreatment evaluation of concentrations of LDH and hCG.[11]

Some of the hCG methods available are only intended for pregnancy applications. Such assays do not necessarily detect degraded or more homogenous molecules found in trophoblastic diseases.[12]

hCG has high carbohydrate content, 30% of its molecular weight is due to sugars, 8% to 9% is the result of sialic acid. Removal of sialic acid residues from the β-subunit decreases biologic activity by 50%. Considerable understanding of the molecular structure and molecular biologic function has developed.

Footnotes

1. Hohnadel DC and Kaplan LA, "Hormones and Their Metabolites; β-hCG (β-Human Chorionic Gonadotropin)," *Clinical Chemistry: Theory, Analysis, and Correlation*, 2nd ed, Kaplan LA and Pesce AJ, eds, St Louis, MO: Mosby-Year Book Inc, 1989, 938-44.
2. Spencer K, "Screening for Down's Syndrome. The Role of Intact hCG and Free Subunit Measurement," *Scand J Clin Lab Invest Suppl*, 1993, 216:79-96.
3. Aitken DA, Wallace EM, Crossley JA, "Dimeric Inhibin A as a Marker for Down's Syndrome in Early Pregnancy," *N Engl J Med*, 1996, 334(19):1231-6.
4. Stewart BK, Nazar-Stewart V, and Toivola B, "Biochemical Discrimination of Pathologic Pregnancy From Early, Normal Intrauterine Gestation in Symptomatic Patients," *Am J Clin Pathol*, 1995, 103(4):386-90.
5. Bandi ZL, Schoen I, and DeLara M, "Enzyme-Linked Immunosorbent Urine Pregnancy Tests: Clinical Specificity Studies," *Am J Clin Pathol*, 1987, 87(2):236-42.
6. Braunstein GD, Kelley L, Farber S, et al, "Two Rapid, Sensitive, and Specific Immunoenzymatic Assays of Human Choriogonadotropin in Urine Evaluated," *Clin Chem*, 1986, 32(7):1413-4.
7. Lövgren T, Hemmilä I, Pettersson K, et al, "Time-Resolved Fluorometry in Immunoassays," *Alternative Immunoassays*, Collins WP, ed, New York, NY: John Wiley and Sons, 1985, 203-17.
8. Pettersson K, Siitari H, Hemmilä I, et al, "Time-Resolved Fluoroimmunoassay of Human Choriogonadotropin," *Clin Chem*, 1983, 29:60-4.
9. Churgay CA and Apgar BS, "Ectopic Pregnancy. An Update on Technologic Advances in Diagnosis and Treatment," *Prim Care*, 1993, 20(3):629-38.
10. Baskin LB, "Ectopic Pregnancy: Laboratory Detection and Monitoring, Contribution of hCG and Progesterone," *3rd Annual Progress in Clinical Pathology*, Dallas, TX: University of Texas Southwestern Medical Center, Sept 28-30, 1995.
11. Bosl GJ, "Prognostic Factors for Metastatic Testicular Germ Cell Tumours: The Memorial Sloan-Kettering Cancer Model," *Eur Urol*, 1993, 23(1):182-7.
12. Cole LA, Kohorn EI, and Kim GS, "Detecting and Monitoring Trophoblastic Disease. New Perspectives on Measuring Human Chorionic Gonadotropin Levels," *J Reprod Med*, 1994, 39(3):193-200.

References

Goldstein PP and Berkowitz RS, "Current Management of Complete and Partial Molar Pregnancy," *J Reprod Med*, 1994, 39(3):139-46.

Hellemans P, Gerris J, Joostens M, et al, "Serum hCG Decline Following Salpingotomy or Salpingectomy for Extrauterine Pregnancy," *Eur J Obstet Gynecol Reprod Biol*, 1994, 53(1):59-64.

Khazaeli MB, Buchina ES, Pattillo RA, et al, "Radioimmunoassay of Free Beta-Subunit of Human Chorionic Gonadotropin in Diagnosis of High-Risk and Low-Risk Gestational Trophoblastic Disease," *Am J Obstet Gynecol*, 1989, 160(2):444-9.

Klee GG, "Human Chorionic Gonadotropin," *Mayo Clin Proc*, 1994, 69(4):391-2.

Nomura F, Ohnishi K, and Tanabe Y, "Clinical Features and Prognosis of Hepatocellular Carcinoma With Reference to Serum Alpha-Fetoprotein Levels," *Cancer*, 1989, 64(8):1700-7.

Tyrey L, "Human Chorionic Gonadotropin Assays and Their Uses," *Obstet Gynecol Clin North Am*, 1988, 15(3):457-75.

Vaitukaitis JL, "Radioimmunoassay of Human Choriogonadotropin," *Clin Chem*, 1985, 31(10):1749-54.

Human Chorionic Gonadotropin, Urine *see* Pregnancy Test *on page 190*

Human Chorionic Somatomammotropin *see* Placental Lactogen, Human *on page 184*

Human Pancreatic Polypeptide *see* Pancreatic Polypeptide, Human *on page 177*

Human Placental Lactogen *see* Placental Lactogen, Human *on page 184*

HVA *see* Homovanillic Acid, Urine *on page 145*

Hydrocortisone, Serum *see* Cortisol, Blood *on page 112*

11-Hydroxyandrosterone *see* 17-Ketosteroids Fractionation, Urine *on page 152*

β-Hydroxybutyrate *see* Ketone Bodies, Blood *on page 152*

17-Hydroxycorticosteroids *see* Cortisol, Blood *on page 112*

17-Hydroxycorticosteroids, Urine
CPT 83491
Related Information
Cortisol, Blood *on page 112*
17-Ketogenic Steroids, Urine *on page 151*
Metyrapone Stimulation Test *on page 167*
Urine Collection, 24-Hour *on page 30*
Synonyms 17-OHCS; Porter-Silber Chromogens, Urine
Abstract These steroids are metabolites of cortisol and other adrenal cortical steroids. Two methods are used: Porter-Silber chromogens and 17-ketogenic steroids (Norymberski method). The former measures fewer metabolites.
Patient Preparation All drugs ideally should be withheld for several days prior to collection of urine, if possible, without doing harm to the patient. Avoid patient stress.
Specimen 24-hour urine
Container Plastic container with hydrochloric or acetic acid as preservative
Storage Instructions Refrigerate during collection, refrigerate or freeze after collection. Stable 45 days if refrigerated and acidified.
Reference Range Some variation exists between published ranges and two different methods may be used. See table for values of Porter-Silber chromogens. When 17-ketogenics are measured, the values are approximately doubled.

17-Hydroxycorticosteroids, Urine

Age	Conventional Units	SI Units
<8 y	<1.5 mg/24 h	< 4.1 µmol/d
8-12 y	<4.5 mg/24 h	<12.4 µmol/d
Adults male	4.5-12.0 mg/24 h	12.4-33.1 µmol/d
female	2.5-10.0 mg/24 h	6.9-27.6 µmol/d

Adults: 2-6 mg/g creatinine

Use Adrenal function test done in evaluation of glucocorticoid production; increased in ectopic ACTH syndrome, Cushing's syndrome, and stress; decreased in Addison's disease, adrenogenital syndrome, pituitary insufficiency.[1] Urinary metabolites of glucocorticoids can be measured as 17-ketogenic steroids and 17-hydroxycorticosteroids.
Limitations Subject to interferences and variability due to unreliable 24-hour urine collections. Serum or urine cortisol measurements are preferred. **Urinary free cortisol is a more sensitive and specific test for hypercortisolism.**[2]

17-OHCS (Porter-Silber) does not measure pregnanetriol; 17-ketogenic steroids do.

Methodology Porter-Silber color reaction or Norymberski method for 17-ketogenic steroids
Additional Information The Porter-Silber color reaction detects steroids with a dihydroxyacetone group at carbon 17, including major glucocorticoid metabolites. By pretreating with a strong reducing agent, one increases the number of metabolites detected (ie, 17-ketogenic steroids). Either 17-hydroxysteroid or 17-ketogenic steroid measurements can be used as an estimate of adrenal steroid production, either as baseline values or in stimulation or suppression tests.

Deoxycorticosterone (DOC), corticosterone (compound B) and aldosterone lack a 17-hydroxyl group and are not detected in 17-KG and 17-OHCS procedures.[2]
Footnotes
1. Zeiger MA, Nieman LK, Cutler GB, et al, "Primary Bilateral Adrenocortical Causes of Cushing's Syndrome," *Surgery*, 1991, 110(6):1106-15.
2. Flack MR, Oldfield EH, Cutler GB Jr, et al, "Urine Free Cortisol in the High-Dose Dexamethasone Suppression Test for the Differential Diagnosis of the Cushing Syndrome," *Ann Intern Med*, 1992, 116(3):211-7.
References
Speroff L, Glass RH, and Kase NG, *Clinical Gynecologic Endocrinology and Infertility*, 4th ed, Baltimore, MD: Williams & Wilkins, 1989.

16-Hydroxyestradiol *see* Estriol, Unconjugated, Pregnancy, Blood or Urine *on page 126*

11-Hydroxyetiocholanolone *see* 17-Ketosteroids Fractionation, Urine *on page 152*

5-Hydroxyindoleacetic Acid, Quantitative, Urine
CPT 83497
Related Information
Serotonin *on page 198*
Urine Collection, 24-Hour *on page 30*
Synonyms 5-HIAA, Quantitative, Urine
Applies to Serotonin, Metabolite
Abstract A serotonin metabolite, urinary excretion of 5-hydroxyindoleacetic acid (5-HIAA) occurs in the presence of carcinoid tumors. Carcinoid tumors are enterochromaffin neoplasms containing amine precursor uptake and decarboxylation cells (APUDomas). They occur in the multiple endocrine neoplasia syndrome (MEN) I or II but are often not a part of those entities.
Patient Preparation Avoid bananas, avocados, chocolate, plums, eggplant, tomatoes, plantain, pineapples, walnuts, acetaminophen, salicylates, phenacetin, cough syrup containing glyceryl guaiacolate, naproxen (Naprosyn®, Anaprox®), mephenesin, methocarbamol, imipramine, isoniazid, MAO inhibitors, methenamine, methyldopa, phenothiazines, for a 48-hour period or more prior to and during the collection. Drug interference relates to method; check with laboratory.
Specimen 24-hour urine
Container Check with laboratory. Glacial acetic, hydrochloric, or boric acids are often recommended as preservative.
Storage Instructions Stable 7 days if acidified and refrigerated.
Reference Range Approximately 1-9 mg/24 hours (SI: 5-48 µmol/day)
Critical Values >25 mg/24 hours indicative of carcinoid syndrome
Use Diagnose carcinoid tumors and syndrome; values >25 mg/24 hours (higher if the patient has malabsorption) are strong evidence for carcinoid.
Limitations 5-HIAA may be normal with nonmetastatic carcinoid tumor and may be normal even with the carcinoid syndrome, particularly in subjects without diarrhea. Some patients with the carcinoid syndrome excrete nonhydroxylated indolic acids, not measured as 5-HIAA. Midgut carcinoids are most apt to produce the carcinoid syndrome with 5-HIAA elevation. Patients with renal disease may have falsely low 5-HIAA levels in the urine. 5-HIAA is increased in untreated patients with malabsorption, who have increased urinary tryptophan metabolites. Such patients include those with celiac disease, tropical sprue, Whipple's disease, stasis syndrome, and cystic fibrosis. It is increased in those with chronic intestinal obstruction and with some noncarcinoid islet cell tumors. Poor correlation exists between 5-HIAA level and the clinical severity of the carcinoid syndrome. It is used as a prognostic factor in this disease.[1]
Contraindications False elevated results if foods containing serotonin or drugs producing metabolites that react with nitrosonaphthol, a reagent used in this determination, are ingested within 2 days prior to collection.
Methodology Colorimetry after extraction, spectrophotometric, gas chromatography (GC), high performance liquid chromatography (HPLC),[2] fluorescence polarization immunoassay (FPIA). A carbon fiber electrode technique allows *in vivo* monitoring of 5-HIAA from small brain nuclei.[3]
Additional Information 5-HIAA is the major urinary metabolite of serotonin, a ubiquitous bioactive amine. Serotonin, and consequently 5-HIAA, are produced in excess by most carcinoid tumors, especially
(Continued)

5-Hydroxyindoleacetic Acid, Quantitative, Urine
(Continued)

those producing the carcinoid syndrome of flushing, hepatomegaly, diarrhea, bronchospasm, and heart disease. Quantitation of urinary 5-HIAA is the best test for carcinoid, but scrupulous care must be taken that specimen collection and patient preparation have been correct. Carcinoid tumors may cause increased excretion of tryptophan, 5-hydroxytryptophan and histamine as well as serotonin. Serum serotonin assay may detect some carcinoids missed by 5-HIAA assay. It may be done by HPLC, RIA, or radioenzymatic assay, but it is not offered by many laboratories, even prestigious reference laboratories. Serotonin measured in blood platelets may be more sensitive than measurement of 5-HIAA or serum serotonin.[4] Of 75 patients with carcinoid tumors, 75% had increased urinary 5-HIAA excretion and 64% had increased serotonin excretion. Six patients with increased urinary serotonin had normal urinary 5-HIAA.

Footnotes
1. Agranovich AL, Anderson GH, Manji M, et al, "Carcinoid Tumour of the Gastrointestinal Tract: Prognostic Factors and Disease Outcome," *J Surg Oncol*, 1991, 47(1):45-52.
2. Stroomer AE, Overmars H, Abeling NG, et al, "Simultaneous Determination of Acidic 3,4-Dihydroxyphenylalanine Metabolites and 5-Hydroxyindole-3-Acetic Acid in Urine by High Performance Liquid Chromatography," *Clin Chem*, 1990, 36(10):1834-7.
3. Suaud-Chagny MF, Cespuglio R, Rivot JP, et al, "High Sensitivity Measurement of Brain Catechols and Indoles *In Vivo* Using Electrochemically Treated Carbon Fiber Electrodes," *J Neurosci Methods*, 1993, 48(3):241-50.
4. DeVries EG, Kerma IP, Slooff MJ, et al, "Recent Development in Diagnosis and Treatment of Metastatic Carcinoid Tumors," *Scand J Gastroenterol Suppl*, 1993, 200:87-93.

References
Deacon AC, "The Measurement of 5-Hydroxyindoleacetic Acid in Urine," *Ann Clin Biochem*, 1994, 31(Pt 3):215-32.

Farmer KL, "Additional Tests of Interest to the Dermatologist," *Dermatol Clin*, 1994, 12(1):191-9.

Lechago J, "Neuroendocrine Cells of the Gut and Their Disorders," *Gastrointestinal Pathology*, Goldman H, Appelman HD, and Kaufman N, eds, Baltimore, MD: Williams & Wilkins, 1990, 181-219.

Vinik AI, McLeod MK, Fig LM, et al, "Clinical Features, Diagnosis, and Localization of Carcinoid Tumors and Their Management," *Gastroenterol Clin North Am*, 1989, 18(4):865-96.

17-Hydroxyprogesterone, Blood or Amniotic Fluid
CPT 83498

Related Information
Androstenedione, Serum *on page 80*
17-Ketogenic Steroids, Urine *on page 151*
17-Ketosteroids, Total, Urine *on page 153*
Pregnanetriol, Urine *on page 191*
Progesterone *on page 191*

Synonyms 17-OHP

Replaces Urine 17-Ketogenic Steroids; Urine Pregnanetriol Assay

Abstract A C-21 steroid, 17-hydroxyprogesterone is produced by adrenal cortices, ovaries, testes, and placenta. It is a precursor of cortisol.

Patient Preparation No recent radioactive isotopes

Specimen Serum or plasma, amniotic fluid[1]

Container Red top tube or lavender top (EDTA) tube; check with laboratory.

Sampling Time Blood levels peak in the morning.

Storage Instructions Separate within 4 hours. Serum or plasma stable 7 days at 4°C to 25°C.

Reference Range Ranges vary between laboratories. These are examples. Adults: male: 50-200 ng/dL (SI: 1.5-6.0 nmol/L), female: follicular phase: 20-80 ng/dL (SI: 0.6-2.4 nmol/L), luteal phase: 100-300 ng/dL (SI: 3.0-9.0 nmol/L), postmenopausal: <50 ng/dL (SI: <1.5 nmol/L)

Critical Values The lack of required levels of adrenocortical steroids in the adrenogenital syndrome can be life-threatening. Early diagnosis and therapy are indicated.

Use Markedly elevated in patients with congenital adrenal hyperplasia (adrenogenital syndrome) due to 21-hydroxylase deficiency. Evaluate hirsutism and/or infertility, female hermaphroditism. Assess certain adrenal or ovarian tumors which may have endocrine activity.

Limitations Elevated, but less so, in 11-hydroxylase deficiency. Measurement of serum 11-desoxycortisol (substance S) can differentiate these abnormalities.

Methodology Radioimmunoassay (RIA), high performance liquid chromatography (HPLC). New methods include gas chromatography (GC) and mass spectrometry (MS).

Additional Information 17-Hydroxyprogesterone is the substrate for subsequent 21- and 11-hydroxylation, on the pathway to cortisol. The two critical enzymes, 21-hydroxylase and 11-beta-hydroxylase, participate in cortisol biosynthesis. If hydroxylation, at either position, cannot

take place because of enzyme deficiency, cortisol synthesis decreases, accompanied by increased ACTH. Congenital adrenal hyperplasia and adrenogenital syndrome result from lack of normal glucocorticoids and build-up of precursors (mostly virilizing). Lack of 21-hydroxylase is the most common cause of adrenogenital syndrome. The syndrome of 21-hydroxylase deficiency is often characterized by androgen excess (virilization) and mineralocorticoid deficiency. Mutations in the gene that encodes 21-hydroxylase have been described.[1]

Congenital adrenal hyperplasia caused by 21-hydroxylase deficiency is the most common cause of female hermaphroditism.[2] It is an autosomal recessive disease. Basal 17-hydroxyprogesterone levels can be normal in late-onset 21-hydroxylase deficiency presenting as hirsutism. Such patients are described as having a dramatically increased 17-hydroxyprogesterone response to ACTH. Patients with 21-hydroxylase deficiency have increased 17-ketosteroids, urine pregnanetriol, as well as, high 17-hydroxyprogesterone.

17-Hydroxyprogesterone may be measured on heelstick blood collected on filter paper for infant screening. Prenatal diagnosis of congenital adrenal hyperplasia is possible by HLA typing, by DNA analysis, or by hormone measurements from amniotic fluid, including 17-hydroxyprogesterone.[2] Some nonspecificity is seen when amniotic fluid analysis is used.[3] Congenital adrenal hyperplasia with adult onset is among causes of hirsutism and/or infertility.

Footnotes
1. White PC, Tasie-Luna MT, New MI, et al, "Mutations in Steroid 21-Hydroxylase (CYP21)," *Human Mutat*, 1994, 3(4):373-8.
2. Pang S, Pollack MS, Marshall RN, et al, "Prenatal Treatment of Congenital Adrenal Hyperplasia Due to 21-Hydroxylase Deficiency," *N Engl J Med*, 1990, 322(2):111-5.
3. Lee A and Ellis G, "Serum 17-Alpha-Hydroxyprogesterone in Infants and Children as Measured by a Direct Radioimmunoassay Kit," *Clin Biochem*, 1991, 24(6):505-11.

References
Check JH, Vaze MM, Epstein R, et al, "17-Hydroxyprogesterone Level as a Marker for Corpus Luteum Function in Aborters Versus Nonaborters," *Int J Fertil*, 1990, 35(2):112-5.

Honour JW and Rumsby G, "Problems in Diagnosis and Management of Congenital Adrenal Hyperplasia Due to 21-Hydroxylase Deficiency," *J Steroid Biochem Mol Biol*, 1993, 45(1-3):69-74.

Hydroxyproline, Total, Urine
CPT 83505

Related Information
Alkaline Phosphatase, Serum *on page 69*
Urine Collection, 24-Hour *on page 30*

Abstract Collagen has a very high content of proline and hydroxyproline. Urinary excretion of hydroxyproline reflects collagen catabolism and is high in periods of rapid bone turnover (eg, Paget's disease of bone). Elevated serum alkaline, phosphatase occurs with increased bone formation. Excretion of hydroxyproline provides an index of bone resorption or destruction.

Patient Preparation Avoid foods containing gelatin (cooked collagen) and meat prior to and during urine collection. These include gelatin desserts (Jello®), ice creams, candies. Patient must avoid aspirin-containing drugs. Hormonal agents affect quantitation.

Specimen 24-hour urine

Collection Add 30 mL of 6N HCl to container before the beginning of collection. Refrigerate during collection. A 2-hour collection after overnight fast may also be used.

Special Instructions Provide patient's age and sex to the laboratory.

Reference Range Adult male: 15-45 mg/24 hours (1-4 mg/2 hours) (7-20 μg/mg creatinine) (SI: 76-381 μmol/day). Adult female values are about one-half of the male ranges. Infants, children, and adolescents variably higher depending on growth spurts. Normal range is higher in infancy, childhood, and adolescence, especially during growth spurts. **Care must be taken to note the type of diet employed in establishing the reference range of a given laboratory.** Most reference values have been obtained on low-dose gelatin, not gelatin-free diets.

Use Evaluate collagen metabolism of bone, bone resorption, bone destruction. High in Paget's disease of bone, healing fracture, primary and secondary hyperparathyroidism. Congenital hydroxyprolinemias are extremely rare. Iminoglycinuria occurs with a frequency of about 1:16,000. A benign autosomal recessive disease, it represents a renal tubular defect. Excessive excretion of glycine, proline, and hydroxyproline occurs. Other hydroxyprolinurias also exist, also without established clinical entities. Measured in osteomalacia when serum alkaline phosphatase is normal, or with coexisting hepatic disease and secondary increase of alkaline phosphatase. Increased with elevated thyroid function probably because of increased bone turnover in this condition.[1]

Methodology Extraction/colorimetry; high performance liquid chromatography (HPLC)

Additional Information Increased urinary excretion of hydroxyproline occurs in osteoporosis, osteomalacia, rickets, with prolonged bedrest, pregnancy, and acromegaly. Hydroxyproline may be measured as a marker of metastasis to bone. Multiple myeloma may increase urinary hydroxyproline levels. Urinary hydroxyproline, like serum alkaline phosphatase, is useful in evaluation and response to treatment of Paget's disease of bone.[2]

Other new markers for the evaluation of bone turnover include assay for procollagen I fragments, osteocalcin, and a bone-specific isoenzyme of alkaline phosphatase.[3]

Footnotes

1. Krakauer JC and Kleerekoper M, "Borderline-Low Serum Thyrotropin Level Is Correlated With Increased Fasting Urinary Hydroxyproline Excretion," *Arch Intern Med*, 1992, 152(2):360-4.
2. Leavelle DE, *Mayo Medical Laboratories Interpretive Handbook*, Rochester, MN: Mayo Medical Laboratories, 1994.
3. Van Daele PL, Birkenhager JC, and Pols HA, "Biochemical Markers of Bone Turnover: An Update," *Neth J Med*, 1994, 44(2):65-72.

References

Delmas PD, "Biochemical Markers of Bone Turnover. I: Theoretical Considerations and Clinical Use in Osteoporosis," *Am J Med*, 1993, 95(5A):11S-6S.

Gilbertson TJ, Branden MN, Gruszczyk SB, et al, "Serum Total Hydroxyproline Assay Effects of Age, Sex, and Paget's Bone Disease," *J Clin Chem Clin Biochem*, 1983, 21:129-32.

5-Hydroxytryptamine, Blood *see Serotonin on page 198*

25-Hydroxy Vitamin D$_3$ *see Vitamin D$_3$, Serum on page 218*

Hyperlipoproteinemias *see Lipoprotein Electrophoresis on page 161*

Hyperphenylalaninemia Screen *see Phenylalanine, Blood on page 181*

ICSH *see Luteinizing Hormone, Blood or Urine on page 163*

IgE Allergen Specific *see Allergen Specific IgE Antibody on page 71*

IGF-I *see Somatomedin-C on page 201*

Immunoreactive Insulin *see Insulin, Blood on this page*

Immunoreactive PTH *see Parathyroid Hormone on page 178*

Inborn Errors of Metabolism Screen *see Amino Acid Screen, Plasma on page 74*

Inborn Errors of Metabolism Screen *see Amino Acid Screen, Qualitative, Urine on page 75*

Inhibin A *see Alpha$_1$-Fetoprotein, Serum on page 72*

Inhibin A *see Human Chorionic Gonadotropin, Serum on page 145*

Insulin Antibody, Serum

CPT 86337

Related Information

C-Peptide *on page 114*

Test Commonly Includes Antibodies to both beef and pork insulin

Abstract Development of IgG antibodies to insulin in diabetic subjects on exogenous insulin therapy may lead to need for larger insulin doses. IgE antibodies can also develop, leading to reactions such as urticaria or, rarely, anaphylaxis.

Patient Preparation Avoid radioisotopes prior to collection of specimen if RIA is used for assay.

Specimen Serum

Container Red top tube

Storage Instructions Serum stable for 7 days at 4°C.

Reference Range Method dependent. Results may be reported as percent binding of patient's serum to labeled insulin. Reference ranges are <3%.

Use Determine the presence of antibodies against heterologous insulins. The presence of insulin antibody points to exogenous insulin administration (eg, use of beef and pork insulins by diabetics) or to insulin autoimmune hypoglycemia. Insulin antibody may be found in factitious hypoglycemia.

Limitations Antibodies to insulin are frequently detected in diabetics, even those who use human insulin. These are usually of little significance; however, high levels may be associated with insulin resistance. There is no definite titer associated with insulin resistance, although 1:64 has been suggested.

Methodology Radioimmunoassay (RIA) or enzyme-linked immunosorbent assay (ELISA). Recent work suggests insulin autoantibodies measured by RIA are more related to IDDM than those measured by ELISA.[1]

Additional Information Insulin antibodies develop from impurities in animal insulins. Beef insulin is more allergenic than either pork or human insulins. Antibodies to insulin develop in insulin autoimmune hypoglycemia, a rare entity. In management of autoimmune disorders such as systemic lupus erythematosus (SLE), steroids are used and can induce

diabetes mellitus. Such steroid-induced diabetes is a widely recognized complication of therapy of SLE. When insulin is required, such diabetic patients may be subject to risk of immunologic complications, developing antibodies while on steroid therapy. A case is reported of insulin antibodies in a patient with SLE before treatment with steroids.[2]

Incidence of insulin allergy in the past has decreased from 5% to 1% due to efforts to reduce peptide contaminants in insulin preparations and the use of semisynthetic and recombinant human insulin preparations. Development of immunoglobulin G insulin antibodies which lead to insulin resistance is rare and tends to occur in patients with interrupted insulin therapy.[3]

Footnotes

1. Greenbaum CJ, Palmer JP, Kuglin B, et al, "Insulin Autoantibodies Measured by Radioimmunoassay Methodology Are More Related to Insulin-Dependent Diabetes Mellitus Than Those Measured by Enzyme-Linked Immunosorbent Assay: Results of the Fourth International Workshop on the Standardization of Insulin Autoantibody Measurement," *J Clin Endocrinol Metab*, 1992, 74(5):1040-4.
2. Varga J, Lopatin M, and Boden G, "Hypoglycemia Due to Anti-insulin Receptor Antibodies in Systemic Lupus Erythematosus," *J Rheumatol*, 1990, 17(9):1226-9.
3. Schernthaner G, "Immunogenicity and Allergic Potential of Animal and Human Insulins," *Diabetes Care*, 1993, 16(Suppl 3):155-65.

References

Despres JP and Marette A, "Relation of Components of Insulin Resistance Syndrome to Coronary Disease Risk," *Curr Opin Lipidol*, 1994, 5(4):274-89.

Taylor SI, Accili D, Haft CR, et al, "Mechanisms of Hormone Resistance: Lessons From Insulin-Resistant Patients," *Acta Paediatr Scand Suppl*, 1994, 399:95-104.

Insulin, Blood

CPT 83525

Related Information

C-Peptide *on page 114*
C-Reactive Protein *on page 387*
Glucose, Fasting *on page 137*
Glucose, Random *on page 138*
Glucose Tolerance Test *on page 139*

Synonyms Immunoreactive Insulin

Test Commonly Includes Glucose must be drawn simultaneously. Glucose for hypoglycemia work-up should not be done by reflectance meter.

Abstract The earliest molecule of insulin production is preproinsulin. The precursor of insulin is proinsulin. Proinsulin as well as insulin are secreted by islet beta cells in response to glucose ingestion. Causes of fasting hypoglycemia include islet cell tumor (insulinoma), exogenous insulin or oral hypoglycemic drugs, alcohol use, pituitary or adrenal insufficiency, bulky extrapancreatic tumor, and instances of very severe hepatic disease.

Patient Preparation If insulin is requested, the patient ideally should be fasting for 7 hours. Avoid radioisotopes prior to collection of specimen if RIA is used for assay.

Specimen Serum or plasma

Container Red top tube or green top (heparin) tube

Storage Instructions Stable 12 hours at room temperature and 1 week at 4°C.

Causes for Rejection Blood glucose >50 mg/dL

Reference Range Fasting level: up to 20-35 µIU/mL (SI: 144-243 pmol/L), with slight differences in upper limit of normal between laboratories (RIA methodology).

Possible Panic Range Fasting insulin levels >35 µIU/mL (SI: >250 pmol/L)

Use Suspect islet cell tumor when fasting glucose is <50 mg/dL (SI: <2.8 mmol/L), especially if there is patient or family history of multiple endocrine neoplasia (MEN). Work-up for fasting hypoglycemia: evaluate for insulin-producing neoplasm (islet cell tumor, insulinoma) or pancreatic islet cell hyperplasia. The diagnosis of insulinoma is established when serum insulin and C-peptide levels are significantly increased, drawn when symptoms of hypoglycemia are present and plasma glucose is low. Serum insulin is high in factitious hypoglycemia from exogenous insulin without elevation of serum C-peptide.

Limitations The assay fails to distinguish between endogenous and exogenous insulins. Insulin antibodies in diabetic subjects who have been treated with animal insulins may invalidate results of insulin assays. Many diabetics, particularly obese individuals, have been thought to have normal or high serum insulin, fasting and after glucose administration. However, a highly specific assay which does not cross react with proinsulin provides evidence that serum insulin concentrations fall in type II diabetics with glucose.[1] Proinsulin is increased in type II diabetics.

In work-up for insulinoma, factitious hypoglycemia must be considered. C-peptide is the result of cleavage of proinsulin within the β-cell; it is not present in pharmaceutical insulin, and serum C-peptide level is low with surreptitious injection of insulin. It is increased in insulinoma when
(Continued)

Insulin, Blood (Continued)

plasma glucose is <40 mg/dL (SI: <2.2 mmol/L). Insulin is taken up by the liver, but C-peptide is not; thus, C-peptide reflects beta-cell secretion.

Most insulin assays react immunologically with proinsulin related molecules, which exhibit little insulin-like activity on target tissues.

Methodology Radioimmunoassay (RIA), immunometric

Additional Information Relationship of fasting glucose to insulin is critical in work-up of insulinoma. Inappropriately elevated insulin is found in two conditions: insulinoma and exogenous administration of insulin. Criteria for insulinoma include hypoglycemia (plasma glucose <30 mg/dL; SI: <1.7 mmol/L) with hyperinsulinemia (>6 µIU/mL; SI: >43 pmol/L). About 33% of insulinoma patients have a normal serum insulin concentration; it needs to be shown that insulin is high for the patient's glucose value. A diagnosis of islet cell tumor also requires a decreased plasma glucose, <57 mg/dL (SI: <3.2 mmol/L) and insulin >20 µIU/mL (SI: >144 pmol/L) 2-3 hours after tolbutamide. Fraker and Norton require, for preoperative evaluation of patients with islet cell tumors:

- 72-hour fasting hypoglycemia (blood glucose <40 mg/dL; SI: <2.2 mmol/L) and hyperinsulinism (serum insulin >6 µIU/mL; SI: >43 pmol/L)
- high or normal C-peptide and high proinsulin level (>25%)
- insulin/glucose ratio >0.3[1]

Since release of insulin from an insulinoma may be erratic, it may be necessary to have the patient fast for up to 72 hours, drawing a specimen every 4 hours for glucose and insulin assay. Occasionally, only a single specimen in such a long fasting period will show an insulin/glucose ratio diagnostic of insulinoma. Care must be taken in selecting a laboratory whose insulin results are sensitive and reliable.

The most common cause of hyperinsulinemia is obesity. Stimulation and inhibition tests are helpful in differentiating whether hyperinsulinism is due to obesity or to tumors.

Increased serum insulin concentrations are found in Cushing's syndrome, in women on oral contraceptives, in subjects on exogenous corticosteroids, and in acromegaly. Adrenocortical steroids and growth hormone are insulin antagonists. Levodopa causes increased serum concentrations.

Insulin secretory reserve distinguishes between two apparently different syndromes: induced serum insulin peak <60 µIU/mL (SI: <431 pmol/L), with complications of diabetes developing, and insulin peaks ≥60 µIU/mL (SI: ≥431 pmol/L) without complications. If only one insulin is ordered, it should be a fasting specimen. Insulin concentrations can also be ordered with glucose tolerance tests, but in practice this is seldom necessary. Specimens so ordered are drawn each time a glucose specimen is drawn, unless otherwise specified. Obese patients may have insulin resistance and high fasting and postprandial insulin levels.

Boden provides a useful diagnostic summary.[2]

It has been shown that pancreatic secretion of insulin is pulsatile.[3]

Footnotes

1. Fraker DL and Norton JA, "The Role of Surgery in the Management of Islet Cell Tumors," *Gastroenterol Clin North Am*, 1989, 18(4):805-30.
2. Boden G, "Glucagonomas and Insulinomas," *Gastroenterol Clin North Am*, 1989, 18(4):831-45.
3. Chou HF, Ipp E, Bowsher RR, et al, "Sustained Pulsatile Insulin Secretion From Adenomatous Human Beta-Cells. Synchronous Cycling of Insulin, C-Peptide, and Proinsulin," *Diabetes*, 1991, 40(11):1453-8.

References

Clark PM and Hales CN, "How to Measure Plasma Insulin," *Diabetes Metab Rev*, 1994, 10(2):79-90.

McMahon MM, O'Brien PC, and Service FJ, "Diagnostic Interpretation of the Intravenous Tolbutamide Test for Insulinoma," *Mayo Clin Proc*, 1989, 64(12):1481-8.

Ostlund RE Jr, Staten M, Kohrt WM, et al, "The Ratio of Waist-to-Hip Circumference, Plasma Insulin Level, and Glucose Intolerance as Independent Predictors of the HDL₂ Cholesterol Level in Older Adults," *N Engl J Med*, 1990, 322(4):229-34.

Samaan NA, Ouais S, Ordonez NG, et al, "Multiple Endocrine Syndrome Type I: Clinical, Laboratory Findings, and Management in Five Families," *Cancer*, 1989, 64(3):741-52.

Sheppard BC, Norton JA, Doppman JL, et al, "Management of Islet Cell Tumors in Patients With Multiple Endocrine Neoplasia: A Prospective Study," *Surgery*, 1989, 106(6):1108-17.

Shuster LT, Go VL, Rizza RA, et al, "Potential Incretins," *Mayo Clin Proc*, 1988, 63(8):794-800.

Solcia E, Capella C, Fiocca R, et al, "The Gastroenteropancreatic Endocrine System and Related Tumors," *Gastroenterol Clin North Am*, 1989, 18(4):671-93.

Insulin-Connecting Peptide see C-Peptide on page 114

Insulin C-Peptide see C-Peptide on page 114

Insulin-Like Growth Factor I see Somatomedin-C on page 201

Interstitial Cell Stimulating Hormone see Luteinizing Hormone, Blood or Urine on page 163

Ion Gap see Anion Gap on page 81

Ionized Calcium see Calcium, Ionized on page 96

Iontophoresis see Chloride, Sweat on page 108

Iron and Total Iron Binding Capacity/Transferrin

CPT 83540 (iron); 83550 (iron binding capacity); 84466 (transferrin)

Related Information

Synonyms Fe and TIBC; Iron Binding Capacity; Iron Profile; TIBC; Total Iron Binding Capacity

Test Commonly Includes Serum iron, total iron binding capacity and/or transferrin, percent transferrin saturation

Patient Preparation Specimen should be drawn fasting in the morning (circadian rhythm affects iron; levels are lower in the evening). Sample should be drawn before patient is given therapeutic iron or blood transfusion. Iron determinations on patients who have had blood transfusions should be delayed several days.

Specimen Serum

Container Red top tube

Sampling Time Morning; marked daily variation occurs. Serum iron levels are 30% higher in the morning and blood levels should be determined on fasting AM samples.

Collection Blood should be drawn before other specimens which require anticoagulated tubes. Separate serum from cells as soon as possible.

Storage Instructions Stable 1 week at 4°C

Reference Range A variety of approaches to the estimation of serum iron, TIBC, and transferrin are in use. Expect normal ranges to vary between laboratories as they are in part method dependent. Iron: 50-160 µg/dL (SI: 9.0-28.8 µmol/L) for adult males; slightly lower (5% to 10%) values for adult females. **Iron binding capacity**: 250-350 µg/dL (SI: 45-63 µmol/L). **Percent saturation (transferrin saturation)**: 20% to 50%. **Transferrin**: 200-380 mg/dL (SI: 2.0-3.8 g/L). **TIBC is an approximation of transferrin**. Quantitative assays for transferrin are widely available. A mathematical relationship between TIBC and transferrin can be derived. Transferrin can be measured, while TIBC is calculated. TIBC (µg/dL) = transferrin (mg/dL) x 1.25.

Critical Values Transferrin saturation >62% predicts homozygous genotype for hemochromatosis in 92% of cases, but in women, >50% is recommended;[1] *vide infra*.

Use Differential diagnosis of anemia, especially with hypochromia and/or low MCV. The **percent saturation** sometimes is more helpful than is the iron result to estimate iron stores and iron deficiency anemia. Evaluate thalassemia and possible sideroblastic anemia; work up hemochromatosis, in which iron is increased and iron saturation is high. Decrease in iron level after performance of a Schilling test supports the diagnosis of vitamin B_{12} deficiency, *vide infra*. Evaluate iron poisoning (toxicity) and overload in renal dialysis patients or patients with transfusion dependent anemias. Use of TIBC in iron toxicity may be less useful than previously believed.[2,3] TIBC or transferrin is a useful index of nutritional status. See table for iron status indicators in various disease states.

Iron Status Indicators in Various Disease States

Disease	Ferritin	Transferrin	TIBC	Serum Iron	Iron Saturation
Uncomplicated iron deficiency	↓	↑	↑	↓	N/↓
Anemia of chronic disease	N/↑	N/↓	N/↓	↓	N/↓
Sideroblastic anemias	↑	N/↓	N/↓	N/↑	↑
Hemolytic anemias	↑	N/↓	N/↓	↑	↑
Hemochromatosis	↑	Slight ↓	Slight ↓	↑	↑↑
Protein depletion		N/↓	N/↓	N/↓	N/↓
Acute liver disease	↑	Var/↑	Var/↑	↑	↑

↑ = increase

↓ = decrease

N = normal

Var = variable

Uncomplicated iron deficiency: Serum transferrin (and TIBC) high, serum iron low, saturation low. Usual causes of depleted iron stores include blood loss, inadequate dietary iron. RBCs in moderately severe iron deficiency are hypochromic and microcytic. The red cell distribution width increases and MCV decreases. Stainable marrow iron is absent. Serum ferritin decrease is the earliest indicator of iron deficiency if inflammation is absent.

Anemia of chronic disease: Serum transferrin (and TIBC) low to normal, serum iron low, saturation low or normal. Transferrin decreases with many inflammatory diseases. With chronic disease there is a block in movement to and utilization of iron by marrow. This leads to low serum iron and decreased erythropoiesis. Examples include acute and chronic infections, malignancy, and renal failure.

Sideroblastic anemia: Serum transferrin (and TIBC) normal to low, serum iron normal to high, saturation high.

Hemolytic anemias: Serum transferrin (and TIBC) normal to low, serum iron high, saturation high.

Hemochromatosis: Serum transferrin (and TIBC) slightly low, serum iron high, saturation very high. Transferrin saturation >55% with serum ferritin >400 µg/L establishes the diagnosis[1] in the appropriate clinical setting. Liver biopsy can confirm iron overload and represents the "gold standard" when hepatic iron concentration is measured.[4] **Increased saturation** occurs with HLA-related (classical) hemochromatosis before ferritin is greatly increased, and also with iron overload (eg, cirrhosis and portacaval shunt), in hemolytic anemias, and with iron therapy. Sample contamination and the vagaries of fluctuation in serum iron levels can make percent saturation misleading on occasion.

Protein depletion: Serum transferrin (and TIBC) may be low, serum iron normal or low (if patient also is iron deficient). This may occur as a result of malnutrition, liver disease, renal disease (eg, nephrosis), or other entities.

Liver disease: Serum transferrin variable; with acute viral hepatitis, high along with serum iron and ferritin. With chronic liver disease (eg, cirrhosis), transferrin may be low. Patients who have cirrhosis and portacaval shunting have saturated TIBC/transferrin as well as high ferritin.

Chronic dialysis for renal failure: Monitor iron levels in patients undergoing dialysis. To follow treatment of iron overload with deferoxamine or with regimen of recombinant human erythropoietin and phlebotomy.[5]

Limitations Except for iron poisoning, a serum iron without TIBC or transferrin is of limited value. Ferritin levels are also useful for iron deficiency. Low iron level may not indicate iron deficiency in acute infection with leukocytosis. Low iron levels may be misleading in chronic infection, inflammation, and malignancy; high ferritin levels occur in many such states. TIBC and transferrin are increased in patients on oral contraceptives, with normal saturation. Gross hemolysis may interfere with serum iron. Some laboratories may have high coefficients of variability, suggesting unacceptable accuracy.[3]

Contraindications Parenteral iron before sample is drawn will cause misleading high iron results. Recent blood transfusion may have only a small positive effect on iron.

Methodology Ferrozine, bathophenanthroline (iron); nephelometry (transferrin); $MgCO_3$ column, other methods (TIBC); atomic absorption (iron, TIBC), anodal stripping; inductively coupled plasma atomic emission spectroscopy

Additional Information Serum iron is **increased** in hemosiderosis, hemolytic anemias especially thalassemia, sideroachrestic anemias, hepatitis, acute hepatic necrosis, hemochromatosis, and with inappropriate iron therapy. Iron may reach high levels with iron poisoning. Some patients who receive multiple transfusions (eg, some hemolytic anemias, thalassemia, renal dialysis patients) will have increased serum iron levels.

Serum iron is **decreased** with insufficient dietary iron, chronic blood loss (including the hemolytic anemias, paroxysmal nocturnal hemoglobinuria), inadequate absorption of iron, and impaired release of iron stores as in inflammation, infection, and chronic diseases. The combination of low iron, high TIBC and/or transferrin, and low saturation indicates iron deficiency. Without all of these findings together, iron deficiency is unproven. Low ferritin confirms the diagnosis of iron deficiency. **Detection of iron deficiency may lead to detection of adenocarcinoma of gastrointestinal tract, a point which cannot be overemphasized.**

In recovery from pernicious anemia, especially just after B_{12} dose, iron levels are low. In fact, the **drop in serum iron 1 to several days after the Schilling test flushing dose** of vitamin B_{12} may be more useful in diagnosis than the radioactivity of the 24-hour urine collection. Serum iron is reported to drop with acute infarct of myocardium. Changes in TIBC are parallel with changes in transferrin.

TIBC is increased in iron-deficiency, use of oral contraceptives, and in pregnancy.

TIBC decreased in hypoproteinemia from many causes including kwashiorkor and in a number of inflammatory states.

The serum **ferritin** is usually a more sensitive test than the serum iron or TIBC for iron deficiency and for iron overload. When all these tests are used together, as is often necessary, they usually can distinguish between iron deficiency anemia and the anemia of chronic disease. The best and most reliable evaluation of total body iron stores is by **bone marrow aspiration and biopsy**. The best evaluation of iron deficiency in childhood (unless lead toxicity is suspected) is **free erythrocyte porphyrins**.

With recombinant erythropoietin therapy serum iron, transferrin saturation, and ferritin levels decline due to rapid utilization by stimulated erythropoiesis with resultant decrease in storage iron.[5]

While iron is usually considered in relation to hematopoiesis and oxygen transport functions of red cells, it is also of prime import to the lympho-myeloid systems.[6] The immune response appears to be resistant to alterations in iron status that might impair other systems. It is suggested that cells of the immune system are adapted to have high priority access to iron when supply is low and high level protection against iron related toxicity when supply is in excess.[7]

Footnotes
1. Edwards CQ and Kushner JP, "Screening for Hemochromatosis," *N Engl J Med*, 1993, 328(22):1616-20.
2. Tenenbein M and Yatscoff RW, "The Total Iron-Binding Capacity in Iron Poisoning. Is It Useful?" *Am J Dis Child*, 1991, 145(4):437-9.
3. Thompson DF, "Reassessment of Measuring Total Iron Binding Capacity in Acute Iron Overdose," *Ann Pharmacother*, 1994, 28(1):63-6.
4. "Case Records of the Massachusetts General Hospital. Weekly Clinicopathological Exercises. Case 31-1994. A 25-Year-Old Man With Congestive Heart Failure and Atrial Fibrillation," *N Engl J Med*, 1994, 331(7):460-6.
5. McCarthy JT, Johnson WJ, Nixon DE, et al, "Transfusional Iron Overload in Patients Undergoing Dialysis: Treatment With Erythropoietin and Phlebotomy," *J Lab Clin Med*, 1989, 114(2):193-9.
6. deSousa M and Brock JH, *Iron in Immunity, Cancer and Inflammation*, New York, NY: John Wiley and Sons, 1989.
7. Kemp JD, "The Role of Iron and Iron Binding Proteins in Lymphocyte Physiology and Pathology," *J Clin Immunol*, 1993, 13(2):81-92.

References
Brown EB, "Iron Metabolism: A 40 Year Overview," *Am J Med*, 1989, 87(3N):35N-39N.
Burns ER, Goldberg SN, Lawrence C, et al, "Clinical Utility of Serum Test for Iron Deficiency in Hospitalized Patients," *Am J Clin Pathol*, 1990, 93(2):240-5.
Finch CA and Huebers H, "Perspectives in Iron Metabolism," *N Engl J Med*, 1982, 306:1520-8.
Oski FA, "Iron Deficiency in Infancy and Childhood," *N Engl J Med*, 1993, 329(3):190-3.

17-Ketogenic Steroids, Urine

CPT 83582

Related Information
Cortisol, Blood *on page 112*
Cortisol, Urine *on page 113*
17-Hydroxycorticosteroids, Urine *on page 147*
17-Hydroxyprogesterone, Blood or Amniotic Fluid *on page 148*
Urine Collection, 24-Hour *on page 30*

Synonyms 17-KGS

Test Commonly Includes Metabolic products of cortisol and 21-hydroxysteroids, including pregnanetriol

Abstract Derived from adrenal cortical steroids, 17-KGS determinations are now an obsolescent approach to laboratory investigation. It measures 17-ketosteroids (KS) after 17-OHCS, cortols, cortolones, and pregnanetriol are oxidized to 17-KS.[1] **Better tests are now available.** 17-KGS has little advantage over assays of 17-OHCS (17-hydroxycorticosteroids by Porter-Silber method).[1]

Specimen 24-hour urine

Collection 25 mL 50% acetic acid added as a preservative before urine is collected

Reference Range 5-23 mg/24 hours (Norymberski method)

Use Decreased with Addison's disease, hypopituitarism, cretinism; increased with Cushing's syndrome, stress, and in forms of the adrenogenital syndromes (11- and 21-hydroxylase deficiencies).
(Continued)

17-Ketogenic Steroids, Urine *(Continued)*

Limitations Pregnanetriol, which is measured, is not a cortisol metabolite. **Urine free cortisol is a more sensitive and specific test for hypercortisolism.**

Additional Information See listing 17-Hydroxycorticosteroids, Urine *on page 147.*

Footnotes
1. Orth DW, Kovacs WJ, and DeBold CR, "The Adrenal Cortex," *Williams Textbook of Endocrinology*, 8th ed, Wilson JD and Foster DW, eds, Philadelphia, PA: WB Saunders Co, 1992, 581.

References
Leavelle DE, *Mayo Medical Laboratories Interpretive Handbook*, Rochester, MN: Mayo Medical Laboratories, 1994.

Ketone Bodies, Blood

CPT 82009 (qualitative); 82010 (quantitative)

Related Information
Alcohol, Blood or Urine *on page 531*
Amino Acid Screen, Plasma *on page 74*
Ammonia, Blood *on page 75*
Anion Gap *on page 81*
Glucose, Fasting *on page 137*
Glucose, Quantitative, Urine *on page 635*
Glucose, Random *on page 138*
Glucose, Semiquantitative, Urine *on page 636*
HCO_3, Blood *on page 142*
Ketones, Urine *on page 639*
Lactic Acid, Blood *on page 156*
Magnesium, Serum *on page 164*
Magnesium, Urine *on page 165*
Osmolality, Calculated *on page 172*
Osmolality, Serum *on page 172*
pH, Blood *on page 180*
Phosphorus, Serum *on page 182*
Red Blood Cell Indices *on page 343*
Reducing Substances, Urine *on page 652*
Toxicology Drug Screen, Blood *on page 576*
Volatile Screen *on page 579*

Synonyms Ketones, Blood; Nitroprusside Reaction, Blood

Applies to Acetoacetate; Acetone; Beta-Hydroxybutyrate; β-Hydroxybutyrate

Abstract Carbohydrate deprivation and increased catabolism of fatty acids leads to increases in the ketone bodies (acetoacetate and acetone). β-hydroxybutyrate is also increased and is usually listed with the "ketone" bodies, although it is not a ketone. Blood β-hydroxybutyrate and acetoacetate are among tests indicated to assess an ill infant or child in whom an inborn error of metabolism is suspected.[1]

Specimen Serum

Container Red top tube

Collection Capillary tubes should be filled as much as possible using technique to avoid air bubbles. Free flowing heelstick. Avoid hemolysis.

Causes for Rejection Hemolysis

Special Instructions Placement of peripheral venous catheter on admission may be useful in selected cases, such as instances of ketoacidosis. Lactic acid, glucose, electrolytes, urea nitrogen, venous or arterial pH should also be measured in possible ketoacidosis, with alcohol level, CBC, and urinalysis if clinically indicated. Serum osmolality is often needed.

Reference Range Negative in normal nutritional states by semiquantitative screening tests (Ames Acetest® tablet).

Possible Panic Range Positivity in 1:32 dilution indicates severe ketosis.

Use Elevated in metabolic states that lead to lipolysis such as chronic starvation and diabetes mellitus. Diagnose ketonemia, ketoacidosis resulting from diabetes mellitus, alcoholism, stress, intestinal disorders including emesis, glycogen storage disease (von Gierke's), infantile organic acidemias, and other metabolic disorders. Determination of the presence of ketone bodies is useful when isopropanol ingestion is suspected.

Limitations False-negatives or falsely weak reactions may occur. Up to 33% of cases of diabetic ketoacidosis also have lactic acidosis. Acidosis shifts ketone bodies to β-hydroxybutyrate. However, β-hydroxybutyrate is not measured by nitroprusside, which reacts with both acetoacetic acid and acetone. The reagent is 5 to 20 times more sensitive to acetoacetic acid than to acetone and does not react with β-hydroxybutyrate. Thus, as ketoacidosis is treated, an apparent positive Acetest® is found while there is an actual reduction of total plasma ketone body concentration. Acidosis shifts equilibrium toward β-hydroxybutyrate (unmeasured), but treatment of ketoacidosis results in increased acetoacetate (measured) and thus a more positive "acetone" reaction, before ketone

bodies decrease. Ketostix® false-positives occur with large amounts of levodopa. Nonketotic coma in diabetes may be caused by hyperosmolarity.

Methodology Nitroprusside reaction (colorimetry). Usually, semiquantitative testing is done using Ames Acetest® tablets. Gas chromatography (GC) and enzymatic methods are used in some institutions, but fast laboratory response is usually needed.

Additional Information Strongly positive serum acetone without severe acidosis, with normal anion gap, bicarbonate, and plasma glucose suggests the possibility of rubbing alcohol intoxication. Look for dehydration with ketosis. Ketoacidosis in diabetes usually occurs with decreased plasma pH and bicarbonate, increased glucose and other abnormalities. As ketoacidosis and metabolic acidosis are treated, hypokalemia may become evident. A normal or low potassium on admission of a patient with ketoacidosis may indicate severe potassium depletion. Thus, potassium is especially important among the parameters to follow in treatment of ketoacidosis. Hypophosphatemia may evolve. Acetone may be elevated due to absolute or relative starvation, especially in children. A significant mortality rate exists; in children younger than 10 years of age, diabetic ketoacidosis is reported to account for 70% of diabetes related deaths.[2] A multipoint kinetic method allows determination of acetoacetate, β-hydroxybutyrate, lactate and pyruvate in a single cuvette.[3]

Footnotes
1. Lindor NM and Karnes PS, "Initial Assessment of Infants and Children With Suspected Inborn Errors of Metabolism," *Mayo Clin Proc*, 1995, 70(10):987-8.
2. Bonadio WA, Gutzeit MF, Losek JD, et al, "Outpatient Management of Diabetic Ketoacidosis," *Am J Dis Child*, 1988, 142(4):448-50.
3. Nuwayhid NF, Johnson GF, and Feld RD, "Multipoint Kinetic Method for Simultaneously Measuring the Combined Concentrations of Acetoacetate-Beta-Hydroxybutyrate and Lactate-Pyruvate," *Clin Chem*, 1989, 35(7):1526-31.

References
Burtis CA and Ashwood ER, *Tietz Textbook of Clinical Chemistry*, 2nd ed, Philadelphia, PA: WB Saunders Co, 1994, 971-4.
Hagay ZJ, "Diabetic Ketoacidosis in Pregnancy: Etiology, Pathophysiology, and Management," *Clin Obstet Gynecol*, 1994, 37(1):39-49.
Kaplan LA, "Ketones," *Clinical Chemistry - Theory, Analysis, and Correlation*, 2nd ed, Kaplan LA and Pesce AJ, eds, St Louis, MO: Mosby-Year Book Inc, 1989, 856-8.
Shaffer PA, "Antiketogenesis: Its Mechanism and Significance. 1932 (Classical Article)," *Medicine (Baltimore)*, 1990, 69(5):317-23.

Ketones, Blood *see* Ketone Bodies, Blood *on this page*

17-Ketosteroids Fractionation, Urine

CPT 83593

Related Information
17-Ketosteroids, Total, Urine *on next page*
Urine Collection, 24-Hour *on page 30*

Synonyms 17-KS Fractionation

Applies to Androsterone; Dehydroepiandrosterone; Etiocholanolone; 11-Hydroxyandrosterone; 11-Hydroxyetiocholanolone; 11-Ketoandrosterone; 11-Ketoetiocholanolone

Test Commonly Includes Quantitation of some or all of the following: androsterone, etiocholanolone, and dehydroepiandrosterone (DHEA); these are the three major metabolites of androgens in the urine. Such fractionation may also include 11-ketoandrosterone, 11-ketoetiocholanolone, 11-hydroxyandrosterone, 11-hydroxyetiocholanolone, pregnanediol, pregnanetriol, delta-5-pregnanetriol, and 11-ketopregnanetriol.

Abstract Metabolites of steroids from adrenal cortices (two-thirds) and from the testes (one-third).

Specimen 24-hour urine

Container Plastic urine container with acetic acid or hydrochloric acid preservative, as requested by the laboratory.

Collection Add preservative to the container prior to the start of collection.

Storage Instructions Adjust pH as required. Keep refrigerated.

Causes for Rejection Incomplete collection

Reference Range Normal ranges are usually provided by laboratories doing such fractionation. They are often stratified by age and sex. Typical values for adult males: androsterone: 1-6 mg/day, dehydroepiandrosterone: 0.1-3.0 mg/day; etiocholanolone: 2-5 mg/day; adult females: androsterone: 0.5-2.5 mg/day, dehydroepiandrosterone: 0.1-1.5 mg/day, etiocholanolone: 1.0-3.5 mg/day.

Use Used in evaluation of adrenal and gonadal abnormalities including the adrenogenital syndrome, differential diagnosis of adrenocortical hyperplasia and carcinoma; arrhenoblastoma, Stein-Leventhal syndrome.

Methodology Column chromatography or gas-liquid chromatography (GLC)

Additional Information Derksen et al[1] report the findings of lack of suppression of serum dehydroepiandrosterone sulfate concentrations and urinary 17-ketosteroid excretion in hirsute women with adrenal neoplasms.

Footnotes

1. Derksen J, Nagesser SK, Meinders AE, et al, "Interpretation of Virilizing Adrenal Tumors in Hirsute Women," *N Engl J Med*, 1994, 331(15):968-73.

References

Speroff L, Glass RH, and Kase NG, *Clinical Gynecologic Endocrinology and Infertility*, 4th ed, Baltimore, MD: Williams & Wilkins, 1989.

Weykamp CW, Penders TJ, Schmidt NA, et al, "Steroid Profile for Urine: Reference Values," *Clin Chem*, 1989, 35(12):2281-4.

17-Ketosteroids, Total, Urine

CPT 83586

Related Information

Dehydroepiandrosterone Sulfate *on page 120*

17-Hydroxyprogesterone, Blood or Amniotic Fluid *on page 148*

17-Ketosteroids Fractionation, Urine *on previous page*

Testosterone, Free and Total *on page 202*

Urine Collection, 24-Hour *on page 30*

Synonyms 17-KS

Abstract **An obsolete test that has been replaced by immunoassays for specific analytes.**

A ketone on the steroid nucleus is at C-17. Two precursors of 17-KS are DHEA (dehydroepiandrosterone) and DHEA-S (dehydroepiandrosterone sulfate). DHEA-S is the only substance in blood which can replace 17-KS in the work-up for hirsutism. 17-KS are metabolites of androstenedione, testosterone, and other compounds.

Patient Preparation ACTH will cause increases, as will stress.

Specimen 24-hour urine

Container Plastic urine container with hydrochloric acid or 33% acetic acid preservative, depending on laboratory. Some laboratories ask for pH adjustment following collection.

Collection Add preservative to container prior to the start of collection.

Storage Instructions Record total volume. Pour off proper aliquot and refrigerate.

Causes for Rejection Incomplete collection

Reference Range Adults: male: 8-20 mg/24 hours (SI: 28-69 µmol/day), female: 6-15 mg/24 hours (SI: 21-52 µmol/day) with decrease in advancing years; exact ranges vary somewhat between laboratories. Prepubertal children are much lower.

Use Assess adrenal androgens. 17-Ketosteroids are elevated in Cushing's syndrome, adrenogenital syndrome, some adrenal and gonadal tumors, pregnancy, and female pseudohermaphrodism.

Limitations Increased with obesity. Numerous drugs in common use cause spurious increase or decrease including carbamazepine, cephalothin, and tiaprofenic acid. Excretion of the 17-ketosteroids is variable over time. Although often used to evaluate androgenic status, this test essentially **does not detect the major androgens, testosterone and dihydrotestosterone.** If low androgens are anticipated, serum testosterone is the test of choice, not 17-KS.

Methodology Zimmermann reaction (colorimetry after extractions). Zimmermann reaction detects androsterone, dehydroepiandrosterone, etiocholanolone, 11-ketoetiocholanolone, dehydroepiandrosterone (DHEA), 11-ketoandrosterone, 11-beta-hydroxyandrosterone, and 11-beta-hydroxyetiocholanolone.

Additional Information In men, about one-third of 17-KS is of gonadal origin; in women and children, the adrenal is the predominant source. Cortisol, estrogens, pregnanediol, pregnanetriol, testosterone, and dihydrotestosterone are not 17-KS. The adrenogenital syndromes, virilizing entities, include adrenal tumors and congenital hyperplasias. The latter include partial 21-hydroxylase deficiency, complete 21-hydroxylase deficiency (salt-losing), and 11-beta-hydroxylase deficiency (mostly hypertensive). Other types of congenital adrenal hyperplasia exist as well. **With the availability of specific hormone and hormone metabolite tests, this assay is obsolete.**

References

Salway JG, ed, *Drug-Test Interaction Handbook*, New York, NY: Raven Press, 1990, 938-41.

Weykamp CW, Penders TJ, Schmidt NA, et al, "Steroid Profile for Urine: Reference Values," *Clin Chem*, 1989, 35(12):2281-4.

17-KGS *see* 17-Ketogenic Steroids, Urine *on page 151*

Kidney Profile

CPT 80007

Related Information

Anti-DNA *on page 365*

Antineutrophil Cytoplasmic Antibody *on page 367*

Antinuclear Antibody *on page 368*

C3 Complement, Serum *on page 373*

C4 Complement, Serum *on page 374*

Complement, Total, Serum *on page 386*

Complete Blood Count *on page 312*

Creatinine Clearance *on page 117*

Cryoglobulin, Qualitative, Serum *on page 388*

Glomerular Basement Membrane Antibody *on page 395*

Immunoglobulin A *on page 408*

Kidney Biopsy *on page 47*

Osmolality, Serum *on page 172*

Osmolality, Urine *on page 173*

Platelet Count *on page 340*

Streptozyme *on page 432*

Urinalysis *on page 658*

Synonyms Renal Panel; Renal Profile

Test Commonly Includes Urea nitrogen, creatinine, uric acid, glucose, electrolytes. Glomerular filtration rate/creatinine clearance are also useful to assess renal function.

Abstract A test grouping ordered on a regular basis by nephrologists caring for patients with renal diseases.

Specimen Serum

Container Red top tube

Collection See individual tests for specimen collection instructions.

Reference Range See normals under individual test listings for tests in profile or panel.

Use Evaluate renal diseases

Additional Information Electrolytes are needed to evaluate renal problems. The rationale for this test grouping is that patients who require frequent monitoring of renal function also require monitoring of serum electrolytes. Hyponatremia may indicate hyperglycemia. Many of these patients are diabetic and others are on intravenous glucose infusions, another reason to monitor glucose. Finally, interpretation and correction of potassium fluctuations are aided by current knowledge of glucose concentration.

Glomerular filtration rate (creatinine clearance) may be the most important test to monitor the effects of aging upon renal function.[1]

For further possible work-up, see Osmolality, Serum *on page 172*; Osmolality, Urine *on page 173*; Complement Total, Serum *on page 386*; C3 Complement, Serum *on page 373*; and C4 Complement, Serum *on page 374*. Patients with possible glomerulopathy, nephrotic syndrome, and/or glomerulonephritis may need some of the following tests, depending on the clinical picture: ANA; anti-DNA; streptozyme; cryoglobulins; platelet count (for nephrosis in anaphylactoid purpura, thrombotic thrombocytopenic purpura); IgA (for cases of IgA nephropathy); antiglomerular basement membrane antibody. Urinalyses are also needed.

Footnotes

1. Lindeman RD, "Changes in Renal Function With Aging. Implications for Treatment," *Drugs Aging*, 1992, 2(5):423-31.

References

Duarte CG and Preuss HG, "Assessment of Renal Function - Glomerular and Tubular," *Clin Lab Med*, 1993, 13(1):33-52.

17-KS *see* 17-Ketosteroids, Total, Urine *on this page*

K+, Serum or Plasma *see* Potassium, Serum or Plasma *on page 188*

17-KS Fractionation *see* 17-Ketosteroids Fractionation, Urine *on previous page*

K+, Urine *see* Potassium, Urine *on page 189*

Lactate, Blood *see* Lactic Acid, Blood *on page 156*

Lactate Dehydrogenase

CPT 83615

Related Information

Alanine Aminotransferase *on page 65*

Aspartate Aminotransferase *on page 84*

Body Fluid Lactate Dehydrogenase *on page 92*

Cardiac Enzymes/Isoenzymes *on page 102*

Creatine Kinase *on page 115*

Hemosiderin Stain, Urine *on page 637*

Lactate Dehydrogenase Isoenzymes *on next page*

Myoglobin, Blood *on page 167*

Troponin *on page 212*

Synonyms Lactic Acid Dehydrogenase; LD; LDH

Abstract This enzyme catalyzes the interconversion of lactate and pyruvate. It is found in all cells of the body and exists in five molecular forms (isoenzymes).

Specimen Serum

Container Red top tube, serum separator tube is acceptable. Green top (heparin) tube is also acceptable.

Storage Instructions Avoid hemolysis. Stable 2-3 days at room temperature.[1]

Causes for Rejection Hemolysis in collection of sample

(Continued)

Lactate Dehydrogenase *(Continued)*

Reference Range Normal ranges for serum LD vary among methods. They are higher in childhood. For adults, in most laboratories, the range is up to approximately 200 units/L. See table for approximate ranges.

Lactate Dehydrogenase

Age	units/L
0-2 y	125-275
2-3 y	166-232
3-4 y	112-221
4-5 y	108-206
5-6 y	104-205
6-7 y	100-204
7-8 y	95-203
8-12 y	90-201
12-14 y	90-199
14-16 y	Up to 168
16-17 y	Up to 161
17-43 y	90-156
≥43 y	90-176

Use Causes of **high LD: Neoplastic states** (especially with high alkaline phosphatase, very high total LD, and isomorphic pattern of LD isoenzymes); **hypoxic cardiorespiratory diseases; hemolytic anemia; megaloblastic anemias**, including pernicious anemia (levels may be >2000 units/L and LD isoenzymes reveal LD_1:LD_2 flip); **infectious mononucleosis; inflammation; hypothyroidism** (some cases); **myocardial infarct**: LD begins to rise about 12 hours after infarct and usually returns to normal after CK (CPK) and AST (SGOT) levels return to normal, isoenzymes usually most useful 48 hours from onset of infarct to reveal LD_1:LD_2 inversion; **pulmonary infarct** (rarely, triad of LD, bilirubin, AST increases occurs); other **lung diseases**.

Diseases of **liver**, including cirrhosis. Total LD in cirrhosis is usually not greatly increased. In acute viral hepatitis, LD is not greatly elevated and AST is usually three or more times higher (in relation to the upper limit of normal) than LD; **chronic alcoholism** is usually associated with some combination of elevated MCV (mean corpuscular volume), triglyceride, alkaline phosphatase, AST (SGOT), ALT (SGPT), GGT, and bilirubin and low folate.

Renal infarct - high LD, out of proportion to AST and alkaline phosphatase; **seizures, other CNS diseases**; acute **pancreatitis; collagen diseases**; excessive **destruction of cells; fracture**, other **trauma**, including head trauma, **muscle damage; muscular dystrophy; focal necrosis; shock, hypotension; intestinal obstruction**.

LD isoenzymes may be useful in the diagnosis of a number of the disease states mentioned above including myocardial infarction, neoplastic states, hemolytic anemia, megaloblastic anemias including pernicious anemia, infectious mononucleosis, some cases of hypothyroidism, diseases of the liver, renal infarct, and excessive destruction of cells, especially in hematopoietic neoplasms.

Other causes of increased LD include specimen tube artifact, such as serum contact with clot or exposure to heat. Chemistry profile with very high LD and no glucose may relate to unseparated serum and cells in a tube at room temperature or higher. Since LD is found in virtually every tissue in the body, the diagnostic value of an elevated level is limited.

Useful with protein in initial assessment of pleural effusion.[2]

Limitations Hemolysis elevates LD results, oxalate inhibits LD, ascorbic acid can decrease LD values. Bovine or porcine heparin therapy can cause increases of AST, ALT, and LD with elevated LD hepatic fractions.

Methodology Lactate to pyruvate monitored at 340 nm is predominant method but pyruvate to lactate is used. Pyruvate to lactate assay produces values about twice those of the lactate to pyruvate method. The temperature is usually 37°C but 30°C is also used.

Additional Information In infectious mononucleosis, LD is usually more elevated than AST, and there is usually an isomorphic pattern of LD isoenzymes. In **viral hepatitis**, by contrast, AST and ALT (the transaminases) are much more increased than is LD, about three or more times higher than total LD, and LD_5 is high. The differential diagnosis of acute infarct of myocardium includes pericarditis and angina, entities in which enzymes are usually not substantially increased. LD is useful in selected settings as a tumor marker,[3,4,5,6,7] but LD is not helpful as a screening test for cancer. Tumor burden in childhood non-Hodgkin's lymphoma is estimated by serum LDH concentration and disease stage.[8] (Other applications as a tumor marker are included in the subsequent listing.)

Footnotes

1. Moss DW, Henderson AR, and Kachmar JF, "Enzymes," *Textbook of Clinical Chemistry*, Tietz NW, ed, Philadelphia, PA: WB Saunders Co, 1986, 379-83.
2. Dev D and Basran GS, "Pleural Effusion: A Clinical Review," *Monaldi Arch Chest Dis*, 1994, 49(1):25-35.
3. Barlogie B, Smallwood L, Smith T, et al, "High Serum Levels of Lactic Dehydrogenase Identify a High-Grade Lymphoma-Like Myeloma," *Ann Intern Med*, 1989, 110(7):521-5.
4. Farley FA, Healey JH, Caparros-Sison B, et al, "Lactase Dehydrogenase as a Tumor Marker for Recurrent Disease in Ewing's Sarcoma," *Cancer*, 1987, 59(7):1245-8.
5. Ganz PA, Ma PY, Wang HJ, et al, "Evaluation of Three Biochemical Markers for Serially Monitoring the Therapy of Small-Cell Lung Cancer," *J Clin Oncol*, 1987, 5(3):472-9.
6. Hamrick RM III and Murgo AJ, "Lactate Dehydrogenase Values and Bone Scans as Predictors of Bone Marrow Involvement in Small-Cell Lung Cancer," *Arch Intern Med*, 1987, 147(6):1070-1.
7. Schwartz MK, "Lactic Dehydrogenase: An Old Enzyme Reborn as a Cancer Marker?" *Am J Clin Pathol*, 1991, 96(4):441-3.
8. Sandlund JT, Downing JR, and Crist WM, "Non-Hodgkin's Lymphoma in Childhood," *N Engl J Med*, 1996, 334(19):1238-48.

References

Adams JE 3rd, Abendscheim DR, and Jaffe AS, "Biochemical Markers of Myocardial Injury. Is MB Creatinine Kinase the Choice for the 1990's?" *Circulation*, 1993, 88(2):750-63.

Gulbis B, Unger P, Lenaers A, et al, "Mass Concentration of Creatine Kinase MB Isoenzyme and Lactate Dehydrogenase Isoenzyme 1 in Diagnosis of Perioperative Myocardial Infarction After Coronary Bypass Surgery," *Clin Chem*, 1990, 36(10):1784-8.

Hornykewyez S, Gabriel H, and Huber K, "Biochemical Markers of Myocardial Necrosis in Acute Myocardial Infarction and Thrombolysis," *Ann Hematol*, 1994, 69(4):S59-63.

Kagawa FT, Kirsch CM, Yenokida GG, et al, "Serum Lactate Dehydrogenase Activity in Patients With AIDS and *Pneumocystis carinii* Pneumonia: An Adjunct to Diagnosis," *Chest*, 1988, 94(5):1031-3.

Reis GJ, Kaufman HW, Horowitz GL, et al, "Usefulness of Lactate Dehydrogenase and Lactate Dehydrogenase Isoenzymes for Diagnosis of Acute Myocardial Infarction," *Am J Cardiol*, 1988, 61(10):754-8.

Schiele F, "Lactate Dehydrogenase," *Drug Effects on Laboratory Test Results Analytical Interferences and Pharmacological Effects*, Siest G and Galteau MM, eds, Littleton, MA: PSG Publishing Co Inc, 1988, 269-306.

Lactate Dehydrogenase, Cerebrospinal Fluid *see* Cerebrospinal Fluid LD *on page 106*

Lactate Dehydrogenase Isoenzymes

CPT 83625

Related Information

Cardiac Enzymes/Isoenzymes *on page 102*
Creatine Kinase Isoenzymes/Isoforms *on page 115*
Lactate Dehydrogenase *on previous page*
Myoglobin, Blood *on page 167*
Myoglobin, Qualitative, Urine *on page 644*
Troponin *on page 212*

Synonyms Lactic Acid Dehydrogenase Isoenzymes; LDH Isoenzymes; LD Isoenzymes

Replaces Alpha-Hydroxybutyric Dehydrogenase, Serum

Test Commonly Includes Total serum LD (LDH) and electrophoretic quantitation of isoenzymes

Abstract Changes of LD isoenzymes are periodically measured following onset of chest pain, to study the relationships of the anodic fractions and to provide important information for the differential diagnosis of acute infarct of myocardium ("LD_1/LD_2 flip"). The differential diagnosis of certain other diseases is enhanced as well with use of LD isoenzymes.

Specimen Serum

Container Red top tube

Sampling Time Cardiac enzymes and isoenzymes are best interpreted as a sequential series, at admission (or initial event) and at subsequent intervals. This applies particularly to CKMB, troponin I, and myoglobin. LDH isoenzymes are most useful for diagnosis of acute infarct which took place 24-72 hours earlier. Change in pattern over time is crucial to establish diagnosis.

Collection Avoid hemolysis

Causes for Rejection Specimen collected in oxalate, citrate, fluoride, or other anticoagulants

Special Instructions Normal total LD is not necessarily always a contraindication to isoenzymes. LD_1:LD_2 flip occurs in some sera in which total LD is within normal range.

Reference Range Method dependent. Normally LD separates electrophoretically into five bands, each an isoenzyme. One set of normal ranges, based on agarose: LD_1: 22% to 36%, LD_2: 35% to 46%, LD_3: 13% to 26%, LD_4: 3% to 10%, LD_5: 2% to 12%. LD_1 and LD_2 (anodal fractions) are associated with cardiac and RBC origin. LD_5 and LD_4 are associated with hepatic and skeletal muscle origin. LD_2 is greater than LD_1 normally. Thus, the LD_1:LD_2 ratio is normally 0.50-0.80. In myocardial damage, such as acute infarct of myocardium, there is flip or inversion of LD_1:LD_2 (LD_1 becoming greater than LD_2). (Some laboratories use an LD_1:LD_2 ratio >0.9 as indicative of a flip. This is method dependent; in other laboratories a moderate fraction of normal employees normally have LD 1:2 of 0.9.) LD_4 is normally less than LD_5, and the normal $LD_5:LD_4$ ratio is up to 0.8.

Possible Panic Range $LD_1:LD_2$ flip in a patient not in a coronary unit, not known to have pernicious anemia or hemolytic anemia.

Use Useful in the differential diagnosis of acute myocardial infarction, megaloblastic anemia (folate deficiency, pernicious anemia), hemolytic anemia, and very occasionally renal infarct. These entities are characterized by LD_1 increases, often with $LD_1:LD_2$ inversion.

The **isomorphic pattern** (total LD significantly high with no significant increase in percentage, of any fraction) is seen with neoplasia, cardiorespiratory diseases, hypothyroidism, infectious mononucleosis, and other inflammatory states, uremia, and necrosis.[1]

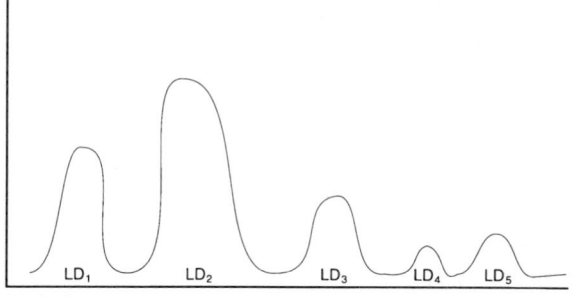

Normal pattern
Isomorphic pattern (if LDH significantly greater than reference range)

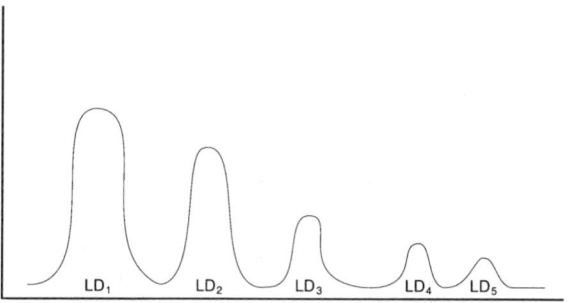

"LD_1 Flip" seen in acute myocardial infarct, hemolytic anemia, megaloblastic anemia, and occasionally in renal injury

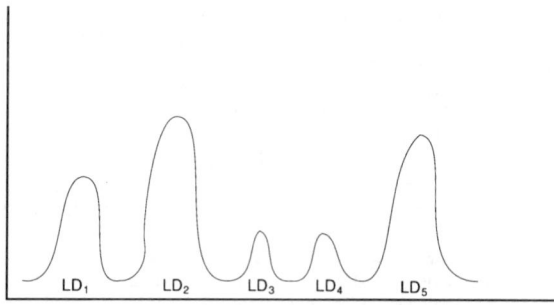

Elevated LD_5 with increased $LD_5:LD_4$ ratio; typically seen in liver disease, skeletal muscle injury, and pulmonary edema

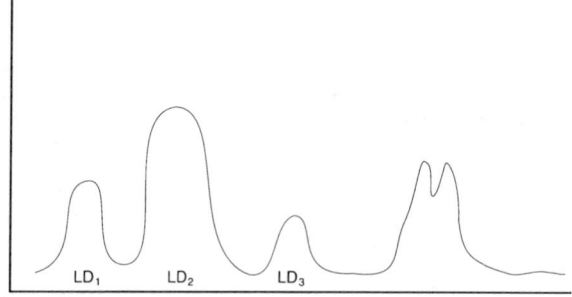

Macroenzyme complex (compare with others)

LD_5 **increases** are seen with striated muscle lesions (eg, trauma) and with liver diseases (eg, hepatic congestion, congestive heart failure, hepatitis, cirrhosis, alcoholism). LD_5 increase is probably more significant when the $LD_5:LD_4$ ratio is increased.

Although a modicum of controversy exists regarding the most suitable criteria for LD isoenzymes for the diagnosis of acute myocardial infarction, **almost all laboratories recognize abnormality when LD_1 equals or is greater than LD_2.** Alternatives to LD_1 greater than LD_2 have been proposed. Using an electrophoretic method (Helena), Rotenberg et al suggested the criterion of LD_1 >90 units/L.[2] **Such expression of LD_1 in absolute units may be helpful but, of course, may be misleading when total LD is substantially increased.** Others have modified this suggested normal range. Application of $LD_1:LD_4$ ratio and other ratios found the $LD_1:LD_4$ ratio to be a powerful diagnostic ratio for acute myocardial infarction,[3,4] but others have not used the $LD_1:LD_4$ ratio successfully.

In many laboratories, a few percent of normal individuals may have $LD_1:LD_2$ ratios as high as 0.81. A ratio of 0.82-0.99 is suspicious of myocardial injury. A ratio >1.0 is diagnostic of myocardial injury, if other clinical criteria are met, especially in the absence of increased MCV (ie, without megaloblastic anemia). In unstable angina, an increase of the $LD_1:LD_2$ ratio is described with normal total LD. However, progressively increasing $LD_1:LD_2$ ratio without complete inversion may have diagnostic significance for acute myocardial infarct.

Persistent $LD_1:LD_2$ flip following acute myocardial infarct may represent a marker for reinfarction[5]. Especially when acute myocardial infarction is complicated by shock, the isomorphic pattern may be found.[6] $LD_1:LD_2$ inversion commonly appears subsequent to the isomorphic pattern in instances of acute myocardial infarction.[1]

The appearance of an LD "flip" (when LD_1 is greater than LD_2) is extremely helpful in diagnosis of MI. **The presence of a LD "flip" a day following or with the detection of CK-MB is essentially diagnostic of MI, if baseline cardiac enzymes/isoenzymes are normal and if rises and falls are as anticipated for the diagnosis of acute MI.** While CK-MB peaks 12-24 hours after onset of infarction, LD isoenzymes usually become diagnostic at about 36-55 hours after onset and return to normal 3-14 days after onset. Each laboratory must define its own criteria for this important test.

Limitations Timing is important in diagnosis of acute myocardial infarct (MI). Patients often do not recall accurately when chest pain or cardiac symptoms first began.

In a small percentage of patients with acute myocardial infarction, the expected flip (reversal) of $LD_1:LD_2$ does not occur; in such patients there is often simply an increase in LD_1. LDH isoenzymes in the diagnosis of acute myocardial infarct are slowly being replaced by serum troponin measurements for this purpose.

Methodology Electrophoresis; immunochemical methods have been introduced including immunoprecipitation

Additional Information Patterns of LD isoenzymes in acute pulmonary edema include the isomorphic pattern and LD_5 increases.[7] Serum LD increases also in patients with bacterial pneumonia, in whom LD isoenzyme patterns are described.[8]

Macroenzymes, high molecular weight complexes, occur with LD as well as with CK and other enzymes. LD isoenzymes may complex to IgA or IgG. Such LD macroenzymes are characterized by abnormal position of isoenzyme bands, broadening or abnormal motility of a band, and otherwise unexplained increase of total serum LD. Some of these patients have abnormal ANA results and IgG complexes.[9] Some have abnormalities of light chains. Treatment with streptokinase was found to produce a LD-streptokinase complex which was seen as a band at the origin in electrophoresis.[10]

An isoenzyme band cathodal to LD_5 has been called LD_6. It is not an immunoglobulin complex. It has occurred in subjects with liver disease and is said to indicate a grave prognosis.[11]

The association between LD_1 and testicular seminoma has been widely recognized. Its relationship to nonseminomatous testicular tumors as well are described.[12] The ovarian equivalent of seminoma is dysgerminoma, which also may relate to LD_1 increases.[13,14] A variety of malignant tumors are characterized by total LD increases, sometimes with isomorphic patterns[1] or with LD_5 increases.[15] Increase $LD_5:LD_1$ ratio is suggestive of prostatic carcinoma or other cancers.[16]

In a series of 220 patients with carcinoma of breast, LD was the most common enzyme elevated. The nonspecificity of single enzyme elevation was discussed, but enzymes provide an inexpensive baseline for postoperative follow-up. Enzyme elevation defines a subgroup of patients deserving further evaluation.[17] In malignancy of various types, there is reported an abnormal isoenzyme of LD migrating between albumin and LD_1 on agarose gel electrophoresis.[18]

An inverted $LD_5:LD_4$ ratio is not to be confused with $LD_1:LD_2$ ratio, used to evaluate acute MI. There is evidence that when LD_5 sufficiently exceeds LD_4, liver disease might exist. Such liver disease might be primary or secondary (eg, congestive heart failure). Additional tests which may be useful, if clinically indicated, to work up such possible liver (Continued)

Lactate Dehydrogenase Isoenzymes (Continued)

disease or injury might include ALT (SGPT), GGT, serum protein electrophoresis, and prothrombin time. LD_5 is the striated muscle as well as the liver fraction. Although striated muscle problems are usually clinically obvious, occasionally the physician does not get a clinical history of the postictal state or of various withdrawal syndromes. In such situations a CK may be helpful.

LD with LD isoenzymes is useful as a tumor marker. Schwartz has outlined applications in adenocarcinoma of lung, colorectal carcinoma, malignant germ cell tumors, and in lymph nodes.[19] LD_3 may be useful in chronic granulocytic leukemia.[20] High serum LDH is described as a marker for drug resistance with high tumor volume in multiple myeloma.[21]

Footnotes

1. Jacobs DS, Robinson RA, Clark GM, et al, "Clinical Significance of the Isomorphic Pattern of the Isoenzymes of Serum Lactate Dehydrogenase," *Ann Clin Lab Sci*, 1977, 7:411-21.

2. Rotenberg Z, Davidson E, Weinberger I, et al, "The Efficiency of Lactate Dehydrogenase Isoenzyme Determination for the Diagnosis of Acute Myocardial Infarction," *Arch Pathol Lab Med*, 1988, 112(9):895-7.

3. Loughlin JF, Krijnen PM, Jablonsky G, et al, "Diagnostic Efficiency of Four Lactate Dehydrogenase Isoenzyme-1 Ratios in Serum After Myocardial Infarction," *Clin Chem*, 1988, 34(10):1960-5.

4. Galbraith LV, Leung FY, Jablonksy G, et al, "Time-Related Changes in the Diagnostic Utility of Total Lactate Dehydrogenase, Lactate Dehydrogenase Isoenzyme-1, and Two Lactate Dehydrogenase Isoenzyme-1 Ratios in Serum After Myocardial Infarction," *Clin Chem*, 1990, 36(7):1317-22.

5. Rotenberg Z, Weinberger I, Sagie A, et al, "Lactate Dehydrogenase Isoenzymes in Serum During Recent Acute Myocardial Infarction," *Clin Chem*, 1987, 33(8):1419-20.

6. Rotenberg Z, Weinberger I, Davidson E, et al, "Atypical Patterns of Lactate Dehydrogenase Isoenzymes in Acute Myocardial Infarction," *Clin Chem*, 1988, 34(6):1096-8.

7. Rotenberg Z, Weinberger I, Davidson E, et al, "Patterns of Lactate Dehydrogenase Isoenzymes in Serum of Patients With Acute Pulmonary Edema," *Clin Chem*, 1988, 34(9):1882-4.

8. Rotenberg Z, Weinberger I, Davidson E, et al, "Significance of Isolated Increases in Total Lactate Dehydrogenase and Its Isoenzymes in Serum of Patients With Bacterial Pneumonia," *Clin Chem*, 1988, 34(7):1503-5.

9. Gorus F, Aelbrecht W, and Van Camp B, "Circulating IgG-LD Complex, Dissociable by Addition of NAD^+," *Clin Chem*, 1982, 28:236-9.

10. Podlasek SJ, Dufour DR, and McPherson RA, "Alterations in Lactate Dehydrogenase Isoenzyme Patterns After Therapy With Streptokinase or Streptococcal Infection," *Clin Chem*, 1989, 35(8):1763-6.

11. Wolf PL, "Lactate Dehydrogenase-6. A Biochemical Sign of Serious Hepatic Circulatory Disturbance," *Arch Intern Med*, 1985, 145(8):1396-7.

12. Law TM, Motzer RJ, Bajorin DF, et al, "The Management of Patients With Advanced Germ Cell Tumors - Seminoma and Nonseminoma," *Urol Clin North Am*, 1994, 21(14):773-83.

13. Schwartz PE and Morris JM, "Serum Lactic Dehydrogenase: A Tumor Marker for Dysgerminoma," *Obstet Gynecol*, 1988, 72(3 Pt 2):511-5.

14. Yoshimura T, Takemori K, Okazaki T, et al, "Serum Lactic Dehydrogenase and Its Isoenzymes in Patients With Ovarian Dysgerminoma," *Int J Gynaecol Obstet*, 1988, 27(3):459-65.

15. Rotenberg Z, Weinberger I, Sagie A, et al, "Total Lactate Dehydrogenase and Its Isoenzymes in Serum of Patients With Non-Small-Cell Lung Cancer," *Clin Chem*, 1988, 34(4):668-70.

16. Manzo V, Sun T, and Lien YY, "Misdiagnosis of Acute Myocardial Infarction," *Ann Clin Lab Sci*, 1990, 20(5):324-8.

17. Clark CP 3d, Foreman ML, Peters GN, et al, "Efficacy of Preoperative Liver Function Tests and Ultrasound in Detecting Hepatic Metastasis in Carcinoma of the Breast," *Surg Gynecol Obstet*, 1988, 167(6):510-4.

18. Giannoulaki EE, Kalpaxis DL, Tentas C, et al, "Lactate Dehydrogenase Isoenzyme Pattern in Sera of Patients With Malignant Diseases," *Clin Chem*, 1989, 35(3):396-9.

19. Schwartz MK, "Lactic Dehydrogenase: An Old Enzyme Reborn as a Cancer Marker?" *Am J Clin Pathol*, 1991, 96(4):441-3.

20. Buchsbaum RM, Liu FJ, and Trujillo JM, "Serum Lactate Dehydrogenase-3 Isoenzyme in Chronic Granulocytic Leukemia," *Am J Clin Pathol*, 1991, 96(4):464-9.

21. Dimopoulos MA, Barlogie B, Smith TL, et al, "High Serum Lactate Dehydrogenase Level as a Marker for Drug Resistance and Short Survival in Multiple Myeloma," *Ann Intern Med*, 1991, 115(12):931-5.

References

Agency for Health Care Policy and Research, "Unstable Angina: Diagnosis and Management," *Clinical Practice Guideline*, Number 10, U.S. Department of Health and Human Services, 1994.

Jacobs DS, Clark GM, Beers AL, et al, "Automation of Interpretive Clinical Laboratory Reports: Isoenzymes of Serum Lactate Dehydrogenase," *Lab Med*, 1979, 10:636-9.

Kagawa FT, Kirsch CM, Yenokida GG, et al, "Serum Lactate Dehydrogenase Activity in Patients With AIDS and *Pneumocystis carinii* Pneumonia: An Adjunct to Diagnosis," *Chest*, 1988, 94(5):1031-3.

Kippenberger DJ, "Electrophoretic Evidence of a Patient With Only Three Lactate Dehydrogenase Isoenzymes," *Lab Med*, 1979, 10:153.

Rotenberg Z, Seip R, Wolfe LA, et al, "Flipped Patterns of Lactate Dehydrogenase Isoenzymes in Serum of Elite College Basketball Players," *Clin Chem*, 1988, 34(11):2351-4.

Wolf PL, "Lactate Dehydrogenase Isoenzymes in Myocardial Disease," *Clin Lab Med*, 1989, 9(4):655-65.

Wukich DK, Callaghan JJ, Graeber GM, et al, "Operative Treatment of Acute Hip Fractures: Its Effect on Serum Creatine Kinase, Lactate Dehydrogenase and Their Isoenzymes," *J Trauma*, 1989, 29(3):375-9.

Lactate Dehydrogenase, Variable see Body Fluid Lactate Dehydrogenase on page 92

Lactic Acid, Blood

CPT 83605

Related Information

Synonyms Blood Lactate; Lactate, Blood

Applies to Biotin; Metformin; Oxygen Transport; Phenformin

Abstract Hypoperfusion is the most common cause of lactic acidosis, and hyperlactacidemia may be the only marker of tissue hypoperfusion.[1]

Specimen Whole blood, arterial or venous, or plasma, *vide infra*

Container Gray top (sodium fluoride) tube; heparinized syringe, heparin-containing tube, anaerobic draw,[2] depending upon available instrumentation

Collection Avoid hand-clenching, and if possible use of a tourniquet. A tourniquet or a patient clenching and unclenching his/her hand will lead to build-up of potassium and lactic acid from the hand muscles.

Lactic acid is commonly needed with or as stat follow-up to venous or arterial pH. Serial determinations are often valuable.[1] **Send specimen on ice.**

Storage Instructions Centrifuge immediately and take off plasma (unless laboratory uses a whole blood method). Keep plasma on ice or at 2°C to 8°C, analyze promptly. A study of blood handling techniques and their effect on lactate concentration has been published.[3]

Causes for Rejection Specimen not received on ice

Turnaround Time Good agreement between whole blood and plasma lactate is reported. Use of whole blood enhances turnaround time.[2]

Special Instructions Keep tube on ice until delivered. Tube must be processed within 15 minutes of being drawn.

Reference Range Plasma values: venous: 4.5-19.8 mg/dL (SI: 0.5-2.2 mmol/L); arterial: 4.5-14.4 mg/dL (SI: 0.5-1.6 mmol/L)

Critical Values In general, an inverse relationship between hyperlactatemia and survival exists; high blood lactate serves as a prognostic indicator in ICU and ED patients. Lactate >36 mg/dL (4 mmol/L) is a strong predictor of need for hospital admission from Emergency Department (ED) as well as predictor of mortality.[2]

Possible Panic Range ≥45.0 mg/dL

Use Suspect lactic acidosis when unexplained high anion gap metabolic acidosis is encountered, especially if azotemia or ketoacidosis are not present; see listing Anion Gap on page 81. Evaluate metabolic acidosis, regional or diffuse tissue hypoperfusion, hypoxia, shock, oliguria, congestive heart failure, dehydration, complicated operative/postoperative state including cardiac surgery, extracorporeal membrane oxygenation, ketoacidosis or nonketotic acidosis in diabetes mellitus, patients with infections, inflammatory states, postictal state, certain myopathies, acute leukemia and other neoplasia, enzyme defects, glycogen storage disease (type I), thiamine deficiency, and hepatic failure. A spontaneous form of lactic acidosis occurs. Lactic acid provides a prognostic index in particular clinical settings, especially in critically ill patients in shock. Lactic acidosis in shock may be an indicator of lack of adequate systemic oxygenation and left ventricular function.[4] A relationship to renal disease also exists. With skin rash, seizures, alopecia, ataxia, keratoconjunctivitis, and lactic acidosis in children, consider defective biotin metabolism. Phenformin, ethanol, methanol, salicylate and ethylene glycol (antifreeze) poisoning may cause lactic acidosis. Acetaminophen toxicity causes lactic acidosis, sometimes with hypoglycemia. Cyanide, isoniazid, and propylene glycol are among the causes of lactic acidosis.[1] Lactic acidosis may be due to inborn errors of metabolism.

Lactic acid determination is generally indicated if anion gap is >20 mmol/L and if pH is <7.25 and the pCO_2 is not elevated. (Mizock uses pH 7.35 as a diagnostic criterion.[1])

Limitations Gross hemolysis depresses results. Intravenous injections or infusions which modify acid-base balance, may cause alterations in lactate levels. Epinephrine and exercise elevate lactate, as may I.V. sodium bicarbonate, glucose, and hyperventilation. False low values with a high LD (LDH) value. Normal L-lactate occurs with high D-lactate in D-lactic acidosis. Metabolic acidosis following bypass for obesity, related to altered gastrointestinal flora, is a feature of subjects who develop mental changes as well, in whom D-lactate is the causative anion.[1]

Contraindications Lack of acidosis is **not** a contraindication for this test.

Methodology Enzymatic; other methods include gas chromatography (GC); amperometric, enzymatic, substrate-specific electrode[2]

Additional Information Phosphorus is sometimes significantly abnormal in lactic acidosis. Creatinine is higher in ketoacidosis than in lactic acidosis, by interference produced by acetoacetic acid on creatinine. Causes of lactic acidosis (usually <45 mg/dL (SI: <5.0 mmol/L)) include carbohydrate infusions, exercise, diabetic ketosis, alcohol. Causes of lactic acidosis (>45 mg/dL) include shock (in which lactic acidosis may occur early, before fall in blood pressure, decrease in urine output), hypoxia (including congestive failure, severe anemia, hypotension) and malignancies. Severe lactic acidosis can develop in minutes. Lactic acidosis can accompany dehydration. Blood lactate concentration correlates negatively with survival in patients with acute myocardial infarction, with persistent elevation, >36 mg/dL (SI: >4.0 mmol/L) for more than 12 hours, being associated with poor prognosis. At a given bicarbonate level, the average pCO_2 is lower in lactic acidosis than in diabetic ketoacidosis.

The measurement of lactate levels may be indicated in the clinical setting of metabolic acidosis. Serum salicylate, ethanol level, and osmolality may be helpful. Spontaneous lactic acidosis may be fatal. Protocols are available for measurement of lactate in cord blood.[5]

Factors additional to anaerobic metabolism which affect lactate levels include glycolysis, catabolism, hepatic metabolism, and pyruvate dehydrogenase.[2] Unlike phenformin (which was removed from the market in the U.S. in 1977), metformin is relatively safe. It bears a risk of lactic acidosis of about three cases per 100,000 patient-years, and the risk is found predominantly in subjects whose renal function is impaired. Used in patients without hypoxia or renal impairment, metformin would not be anticipated to cause lactic acidosis.[6]

Lactate is increased with mesenteric ischemia, bacterial peritonitis and in half of a series of instances of intestinal obstruction.[7]

Footnotes

1. Mizock BA, "Lactic Acidosis," *Dis Mon*, 1989, 35(4):233-300.
2. Aduen J, Bernstein WK, Khastgir T, et al, "The Use and Clinical Importance of a Substrate-Specific Electrode for Rapid Determination of Blood Lactate Concentrations," *JAMA*, 1994, 272(21):1678-85.
3. Bishop PA, May M, Smith, JF, et al, "Influence of Blood Handling Techniques on Lactic Acid Concentrations," *Int J Sports Med*, 1992, 13(1):56-9.
4. Rady MY, "The Role of Central Venous Oximetry, Lactic Acid Concentration and Shock Index in the Evaluation of Chemical Shock: A Review," *Resuscitation* (Ireland), 1992, 24(1):55-60.
5. Prentice A, Vadgama P, Appleton DR, et al, "A Protocol for the Routine Measurement of Lactate and Pyruvate in Cord Blood," *Br J Obstet Gynaecol*, 1989, 96(7):861-6.
6. Crofford OB, "Metformin," *N Engl J Med*, 1995, 333(9):588-9.
7. Lange H and Jäckel R, "Usefulness of Plasma Lactate Concentration in the Diagnosis of Acute Abdominal Disease," *Eur J Surg*, 1994, 160(6-7):381-4.

References

Stacpoole PW, "Lactic Acidosis," *Endocrinol Metab Clin North Am*, 1993, 22(2):221-45.
Toffaletti J, "Physiology and Regulation. Ionized Calcium, Magnesium and Lactate Measurements in Critical Care Settings," *Am J Clin Pathol*, 1995, 104(4 Suppl 1):S88-94.

Lactic Acid, Body Fluid see Body Fluid on page 89

Lactic Acid, Cerebrospinal Fluid see Cerebrospinal Fluid Lactic Acid on page 106

Lactic Acid Dehydrogenase see Lactate Dehydrogenase on page 153

Lactic Acid Dehydrogenase, Fluid see Cerebrospinal Fluid LD on page 106

Lactic Acid Dehydrogenase Isoenzymes see Lactate Dehydrogenase Isoenzymes on page 154

Lactose Tolerance Test

CPT 82951 (3 specimens); 82952 (more than 3 specimens)

Related Information

d-Xylose Absorption Test on page 122
Reducing Substances, Stool on page 651
Urine Collection, 24-Hour on page 30

Synonyms Tolerance Test, Lactose

Applies to Breath Hydrogen

Test Commonly Includes Fasting, 30-, 60-, 120-, 180-, and 240-minute glucose measurements

Abstract Lactose intolerance provides an example of osmotic diarrhea from ingestion of solutes not absorbable by a given subject. The lactose tolerance test reflects lactase deficiency of enterocytes. **Since lactase deficiency can be inferred from effects of ingestion of milk, the**

lactose tolerance test is not often needed or done. If available, breath tests may be preferable.

Patient Preparation A trial of withdrawal from lactose-containing food is advocated before the lactose tolerance test. Such a trial may make the test unnecessary. Patient should fast for 8 hours before testing, usually overnight. No smoking or gum chewing allowed during test. Occurrence of any vomiting should be reported to the patient's physician. Patient is encouraged to drink a moderate amount of water during the test, one to two glasses. Patient should remain seated or in bed.

Aftercare Test may produce diarrhea and cramps.

Specimen Plasma or 24-hour urine

Container Gray top (sodium fluoride) tube, plastic 24-hour urine container

Collection Draw specimens in gray top tubes fasting and at 30 minutes, 1, 2, 3, and 4 hours after lactose load to be analyzed for glucose. (Samples can be taken fasting, 15 minutes, 30 minutes, 45 minutes, 1 hour, and 2 hours.) Record patient symptoms (especially cramps, nausea, watery diarrhea).

Special Instructions Lactose load: Adults: 50 g/m^2 body surface or 1 g/kg body weight should be consumed in 5-10 minutes. If severe lactase deficiency is suspected, the dose should be lowered. In infants and young children suspected of severe intolerance, a lower lactose dose should be used to avoid extreme reaction. Ingestion of 15 g lactose in 250 mL of water has been suggested in a recent report.[1]

Reference Range An increase in plasma glucose >30 mg/dL (SI: >1.7 mmol/L) is normal. An increase of plasma glucose <20 mg/dL (SI: <1.1 mmol/L) over the fasting level, with symptoms, is considered abnormal and is evidence for lactase deficiency. A flat curve can be defined as an increase <20 mg/dL (SI: <1.1 mmol/L) and is seen in most subjects with lactose deficiency who are not diabetic. Urine reference range: children: <1.5 mg/100 dL; adults: 12-40 mg/dL (SI: 0.7-2.2 mmol/L).

Breath hydrogen increase <10 ppm (0.9 x 10^{-6} g hydrogen/L air, or 0.45 µmol/L).[1] Less than 10 ppm H_2 gas in the exhaled breath is normal. Lactase deficient subjects usually have ≥50 ppm H_2 in exhaled air.

Use Work-up for distension, diarrhea and/or cramping after ingestion of milk. Diagnose idiopathic lactase deficiency, which is found in a majority of black and Oriental adults, as well as in 5% to 15% of adult Caucasians. It is also found in children. Evaluate lactose intolerance, malabsorption syndromes.

Limitations Lactose is an easily injured enteric enzyme and rate limiting for the absorption of lactose. Secondary lactose deficiency is common in infectious enteritis, bacterial overgrowth, immune defects, and inflammatory bowel disease, among other conditions. Up to 20% incidence of false-positives and negatives is reported. Since lactase-deficient patients have had normal tolerance curves, this test is of questionable value. May be abnormal with Crohn's disease, small bowel resections, jejunitis, sprue, *Giardia lamblia* infestation, Whipple's disease, and in cystic fibrosis of the pancreas.

Methodology Blood specimens are analyzed for glucose after an oral dose of lactose. Hydrogen breath analysis is an alternate method.

Additional Information Lactose is a disaccharide digested by lactase. It yields glucose and galactose. The latter is converted to glucose by the liver after its absorption. Glucose is measured and it is the increase or lack of increase over the fasting specimen that is used for interpretation.

The hydrogen breath test detects increases in expired H_2 after ingestion of lactose. Increased breath H_2 implies that the lactose is escaping absorption in the small bowel and arrives in the colon. Colonic organisms metabolize lactose and produce hydrogen gas.

Diabetic patients may have abnormal lactose tolerance curves due to abnormal carbohydrate metabolism and not necessarily due to lactose intolerance. Since 25% of normal individuals have flat glucose tolerance tests, it has been suggested that patients with flat lactose tolerance tests should also have a glucose tolerance test. Ethanol can prevent conversion of galactose to glucose by the liver; blood or urine galactose can be measured. A test strip has been described which may replace the lactose tolerance test, at least for some purposes, such as mass screening.

Footnotes

1. Suarez FL, Savaiano DA, and Levitt MD, "A Comparison of Symptoms After the Consumption of Milk or Lactose-Hydrolyzed Milk by People With Self-Reported Severe Lactose Intolerance," *N Engl J Med*, 1995, 333(1):1-4.

References

Arola H, "Diagnosis of Hypolactasia and Lactose Malabsorption," *Scand J Gastroenterol Suppl*, 1994, 202:26-35.
Brummer RJ, Karibe M, and Stockbrugger RW, "Lactose Malabsorption. Optimalization of Investigational Methods," *Scand J Gastroenterol*, 1993, 200(Suppl):65-9.
Malagelada JR, "Lactose Intolerance," *N Engl J Med*, 1995, 333(1):53-4.
Wright TL and Heyworth MF, "Maldigestion and Malabsorption," *Gastrointestinal Disease*, Sleisenger MH and Fordtran JS, eds, Philadelphia, PA: WB Saunders Co, 1989, 263-82.

LAP see Leucine Aminopeptidase on next page

L-Aspartate: 2-Oxoglutarate Aminotransferase see Aspartate Aminotransferase on page 84

LD see Lactate Dehydrogenase on page 153

LD, Body Fluid see Body Fluid on page 89

LD, Fluid see Body Fluid Lactate Dehydrogenase on page 92

LDH see Lactate Dehydrogenase on page 153

LDH Isoenzymes see Lactate Dehydrogenase Isoenzymes on page 154

LD Isoenzymes see Lactate Dehydrogenase Isoenzymes on page 154

LD Isoenzymes see Cardiac Enzymes/Isoenzymes on page 102

LDLC see Low Density Lipoprotein Cholesterol on page 162

LDLC/HDLC Ratio see Lipid Profile on next page

LDLC/HDLC Ratio see Low Density Lipoprotein Cholesterol on page 162

LD Variable see Body Fluid Lactate Dehydrogenase on page 92

Lecithin/Sphingomyelin Ratio see Amniotic Fluid Lecithin/Sphingomyelin Ratio and Phosphatidylglycerol on page 77

Leucine Aminopeptidase

CPT 83670

Related Information
Alkaline Phosphatase, Serum on page 69
Gamma Glutamyl Transferase on page 133
5' Nucleotidase on page 171

Synonyms Arylamidase; Arylamidase Naphthylamidase; LAP

Abstract A cellular peptidase used as a test of biliary excretory function. Not in widespread use.

Specimen Serum, ascitic fluid

Container Red top tube

Reference Range Depends on method. 45-55 units/L (fluorometric, rate); higher values in males. Little age-related change.

Use Like 5' nucleotidase and GGT, LAP is used to investigate the origin of increased serum alkaline phosphatase. LAP is not elevated in bone disease. Elevated levels are observed in biliary cirrhosis, other types of cirrhosis, obstructive jaundice, metastatic tumor and granulomas in liver, choledocholithiasis, other biliary and liver diseases. It is often increased in primary carcinomas of pancreas and in some patients with pancreatitis. LAP is found in high concentration in ascitic fluid in malignancy.

Limitations Increased in the last trimester of pregnancy. Seldom used at present.

Methodology Colorimetry and fluorometry

Additional Information Helpful in evaluation of the biliary tract. The tests of biliary function include total and direct bilirubin and alkaline phosphatase, as well as GGT, LAP, and 5' nucleotidase. LAP and 5' nucleotidase are comparable clinically. In the newborn, LAP activity is normal in hemolytic disease (Rh and ABO incompatibilities) and in physiological jaundice. LAP is normal in diseases of bone which cause increases of alkaline phosphatase.

L-Glyceric Acid, Urine see Oxalate, Urine on page 174

LH see Luteinizing Hormone, Blood or Urine on page 163

Liley Test see Amniotic Fluid Analysis for Erythroblastosis Fetalis (OD 450) on page 76

Lipase, Serum

CPT 83690

Related Information
Amylase, Serum on page 79
Amylase, Urine on page 79
Bilirubin, Total on page 86
Body Fluid Amylase on page 91
C-Reactive Protein on page 387

Synonyms Triacylglycerol Acylhydrolase

Applies to Body Fluid Lipase; Elastase, Serum

Abstract Lipase, a glycoprotein, is an enzyme produced by the pancreas. It is elevated in pancreatitis. **The new lipase methods are superior to total serum amylase in sensitivity and specificity for the diagnosis of acute pancreatitis, but both are useful.** Lipase levels are usually increased in both alcoholic and nonalcoholic forms of pancreatitis.

Specimen Serum; lipase (unlike amylase) is not applicable to urine. Lipase may be run on pleural or peritoneal fluid.

Container Red top tube

Storage Instructions Stable 1 week at 25°C, 3 weeks at 4°C.

Reference Range Method dependent but typically <200 units/L (triolein methods by titration or turbidimetry)

Use Diagnose acute and chronic pancreatitis. Since amylase levels are apt to return to normal range first, assay of serum lipase is especially helpful in subjects who appear several days after onset.

Limitations EDTA anticoagulant may interfere. Hemoglobin at ≤250 mg/dL may interfere, depending on method. Fifty-five percent of patients with primary biliary cirrhosis had raised serum lipase activity.[1] Lipase is increased in about 50% of the patients with chronic renal failure. About 75% of such patients have increased serum amylase as well.[2] Serum lipase concentrations increase with hemodialysis.[3] This increase is apparently due to heparin-induced lipolytic activity. Therefore, predialysis blood samples are recommended for lipase measurement. Both serum amylase and lipase may be elevated in the absence of acute pancreatitis,[4] an observation published relevant to chronic alcoholics[5] but applicable to others as well.

Methodology Turbidimetric (using triolein), spectrophotometric, fluorometric, titration, radioimmunoassay (RIA)

Additional Information Serum lipase is usually normal in those patients with elevated serum amylase, without pancreatitis, who have peptic ulcer, salivary adenitis, inflammatory bowel disease, intestinal obstruction, and macroamylasemia. Lipase activity is usually absent in urine, possibly from inactivation of the enzyme. Coexistence of increased serum amylase with normal amylase may be a helpful clue to the presence of macroamylasemia.[6] Lipase is elevated with amylase in acute pancreatitis, but the elevation of lipase is more prolonged.

Pancreatic isoamylase may be useful in mild elevations of total serum amylase. Electrolytes, serum calcium, glucose, and acetone are also often needed. Immunoreactive trypsin is technically more difficult than lipase and probably no better. The serum lipase/amylase ratio may help distinguish alcoholic from nonalcoholic pancreatitis. Ratios >2 (expressed as multiples of the upper limits of normal) suggest an alcoholic etiology.[7] Higher lipase:amylase ratios in patients with alcoholic pancreatitis were described as well by others.[8] Lipase isoforms or isoenzymes have been studied.[9]

An association of intracranial bleeding with increased concentrations of amylase and lipase, in individuals without pancreatitis, is recognized.[10]

Alanine aminotransferase (ALT) (SGPT) levels increased to three times baseline or greater provides evidence for gallstone-induced pancreatitis. The most common obstructive etiology of acute pancreatitis is gallstone disease. The most common toxin causing acute pancreatitis is ethyl alcohol, and over 85 drugs have been implicated. Causes include hypertriglyceridemia and hypercalcemia. Other causes are listed as well.[11]

Laboratory and other factors useful to project severity of pancreatitis are published. These include C-reactive protein.[11]

Serum trypsin is not widely available. **Serum elastase** provides no advantage over amylase or lipase.[12]

Footnotes
1. Fonseca V, Epstein O, Katrak A, et al, "Serum Immunoreactive Trypsin and Pancreatic Lipase in Primary Biliary Cirrhosis," J Clin Pathol, 1986, 39(6):638-40.
2. Royse VL, Jensen DM, and Corwin HL, "Pancreatic Enzymes in Chronic Renal Failure," Arch Intern Med, 1987, 147(3):537-9.
3. Vaziri ND, Chang D, Malekpour A, et al, "Pancreatic Enzymes in Patients With End-Stage Renal Disease Maintained on Hemodialysis," Am J Gastroenterol, 1988, 83(4):410-2.
4. Orebaugh SL, "Normal Amylase Levels in the Presentation of Acute Pancreatitis," Am J Emerg Med, 1994, 12:21-4.
5. Gumaste VV, Sereny G, Dave P, et al, "Serum Lipase Levels in Chronic Alcoholics," J Clin Gastroenterol, 1991, 13(4):407-10.
6. Andrews PA and Thomas PA, "Macroamylasaemia as a Cause of Persistently Raised Serum Amylase," Br J Surg, 1988, 75(10):1035.
7. Gumaste VV, Dave PB, Weissman D, et al, "Lipase/Amylase Ratio. A New Index That Distinguishes Acute Episodes of Alcoholic From Nonalcoholic Acute Pancreatitis," Gastroenterology, 1991, 101(6):1361-6.
8. Tenner SM and Steinberg W, "The Admission Serum Lipase:Amylase Ratio Differentiates Alcoholic From Nonalcoholic Acute Pancreatitis," Am J Gastroenterol, 1992, 87(12):1755-8.
9. Lott JA and LU CJ, "Lipase Isoforms and Amylase Isoenzymes: Assays and Application in the Diagnosis of Acute Pancreatitis," Clin Chem, 1991, 37(3):361-8.
10. Justice AD, Di Benedetto RJ, and Stanford E, "Significance of Elevated Pancreatic Enzymes in Intracranial Bleeding," South Med J, 1994, 87(9):889-93.
11. Steinberg W and Tenner S, "Acute Pancreatitis," N Engl J Med, 1994, 330(17):1198-210.
12. Gumaste VV, "Diagnostic Tests for Acute Pancreatitis," Gastroenterologist, 1994, 2(2):119-30.

References
Marshall JB, "Acute Pancreatitis. A Review With an Emphasis on New Developments," Arch Intern Med, 1993, 153(10):1185-98.
Tietz NW and Shuey DF, "Lipase in Serum - The Elusive Enzyme: An Overview," Clin Chem, 1993, 39(5):746-56.
Ventrucci M, "Update on Laboratory Diagnosis and Prognosis of Acute Pancreatitis," Dig Dis, 1993, 11(3):189-96.

Lipid Profile

CPT 80061

Related Information

Apolipoprotein A and B *on page 82*
Apolipoprotein E *on page 82*
Cholesterol, Serum *on page 110*
High Density Lipoprotein Cholesterol *on page 143*
Lipoprotein (a) *on next page*
Lipoprotein Electrophoresis *on page 161*
Low Density Lipoprotein Cholesterol *on page 162*
Triglycerides *on page 209*

Synonyms Coronary Heart Disease Risk Index; Lipoprotein Analysis; Risk Index for Coronary Arterial Disease

Applies to Apoproteins; LDLC/HDLC Ratio

Test Commonly Includes Fasting triglycerides, total cholesterol, high density lipoprotein cholesterol (HDLC), low density lipoprotein cholesterol (LDLC), estimate (by calculation) of VLDL cholesterol (if triglycerides are <400 mg/dL)

Abstract A panel of tests involving serum lipids used to evaluate coronary heart disease risk. Lipid profiles usually include fasting serum cholesterol, triglycerides, HDL, and calculated LDL.

Patient Preparation Patient should be on stable diet ideally for 2-3 weeks prior to collection of blood and should fast for at least 10 hours before collection of the specimen. There is inconclusive evidence for 72 hours of abstinence from alcohol before sampling for lipid profile. See Preparation in the listing Cholesterol, Serum *on page 110.*

Specimen Serum

Container Red top tube

Collection Lipid profiles are best avoided following acute myocardial infarct, for up to 3 months. Although cholesterol can be measured in the first 24 hours, it may decrease to 47% of preinfarct concentrations within 5 days after infarct.[1]

Storage Instructions Lipoproteins are labile. Even stored at 4°C, analysis should not be delayed more than a few days.

Reference Range Reference values for blood lipids have been published as extensive tables, providing percentile distributions by age groups.[2] See tables 1-8.

Use The role of lipid profiles is not only to evaluate hyperlipidemia as an index to coronary artery disease, but as well to identify individuals at risk and to lower morbidity and mortality from dyslipidemia. Investigation of serum lipids is indicated in those with coronary and other arterial disease, especially when it is premature, and/or in those with family history of atherosclerosis and/or hyperlipidemia, angina pectoris, peripheral vascular disease, cerebrovascular disease, or sudden cardiac death before age 55.[3] The expression "premature coronary arterial disease" has been mostly used to include those younger than 40 years of age. Patients with xanthomas should be worked up with lipid profiles, but not those with xanthofibromas in the sense of dermatofibromas. Those whose fasting serum is lipemic should have a lipid profile, but the serum of a subject with high cholesterol but normal triglyceride is not milky in appearance. The patient with high cholesterol (>240 mg/dL) should have a lipid profile. Patients with cholesterol levels between 200-240 mg/dL plus two other coronary heart disease risk factors should also have a lipid profile.[4] In addition to application in screening programs for evaluation of risk factors for coronary arterial disease, lipid profiling may lead to detection of some cases of hypothyroidism. If a patient has low LDLC, but very low HDLC, he/she may still be in jeopardy (Castelli of the Framingham study); therefore, LDLC/HDLC ratios are useful. **Primary hyperlipoproteinemia** includes hypercholesterolemia, a direct risk factor for coronary heart disease. **Secondary hyperlipoproteinemias** include increases of lipoproteins secondary to hypothyroidism, nephrosis, renal failure, obesity, diabetes mellitus, alcoholism, primary biliary cirrhosis, and other types of cholestasis. **Decreased** lipids are found with some cases of malabsorption, malnutrition, advanced liver disease. In abetalipoproteinemia, cholesterol is <70 mg/dL (SI: <1.81 mmol/L).

Limitations Patients with obstructive liver disease may develop lipoprotein abnormalities. Serum lipid factors have not been demonstrated to strongly influence recurrent stenosis following coronary angioplasty, the pathogenesis of which is presently not well understood. An association of low HDLC and tendency for restenosis is perceived following percutaneous transluminal coronary angioplasty.[5]

Contraindications Patient on antihyperlipidemic drugs, endocrine imbalance, unstable weight, abnormal diet. LDLC should not be calculated if triglyceride is >400 mg/dL (SI: >4.52 mmol/L). Direct measurement of LDLC avoids this limitation.

Table 1. Selected Reference Values for Plasma Total Cholesterol (mg/dL) in White Male Subjects

Age	No.	Mean	Percentiles			
			5	75	90	95
0-19 y	5749	155	115	170	185	200
20-24 y	882	165	125	185	205	220
25-29 y	2042	180	135	200	225	245
30-34 y	2444	190	140	215	240	255
35-39 y	2320	200	145	225	250	270
40-44 y	2428	205	150	230	250	270
45-69 y	7710	215	160	235	260	275
70+ y	850	205	150	230	250	270

Table 2. Selected Reference Values for Plasma Total Cholesterol (mg/dL) in White Female Subjects

Age	No.	Mean	Percentiles			
			5	75	90	95
0-19 y	5470	160	120	175	190	200
20-24 y	1566	170	125	190	215	230
25-34 y	4340	175	130	195	220	235
35-39 y	2012	185	140	205	230	245
40-44 y	2050	195	145	215	235	255
45-49 y	2149	205	150	225	250	270
50-54 y	1992	220	165	240	265	285
55+ y	4478	230	170	250	275	295

Table 3. Selected Reference Values for Plasma Low-Density Lipoprotein Cholesterol (mg/dL) in White Male Subjects

Age	No.	Mean	Percentiles			
			5	75	90	95
5-19 y	713	95	65	105	120	130
20-24 y	118	105	65	120	140	145
25-29 y	253	115	70	140	155	165
30-34 y	403	125	80	145	165	185
35-39 y	371	135	80	155	175	190
40-44 y	385	135	85	155	175	185
45-69 y	1162	145	90	165	190	205
70+ y	119	145	90	165	180	185

Table 4. Selected Reference Values for Plasma Low-Density Lipoprotein Cholesterol (mg/dL) in White Female Subjects

Age	No.	Mean	Percentiles			
			5	75	90	95
5-19 y	652	100	65	110	125	140
20-24 y	199	105	55	120	140	160
25-34 y	646	110	70	125	145	160
35-39 y	299	120	75	140	160	170
40-44 y	318	125	75	145	165	175
45-49 y	326	130	80	150	175	185
50-54 y	256	140	90	160	185	200
55+ y	668	150	95	170	195	215

Table 5. Selected Reference Values for Plasma High-Density Lipoprotein Cholesterol (mg/dL) in White Male Subjects

Age	No.	Mean	Percentiles		
			5	10	95
5-14 y	438	55	35	40	75
15-19 y	299	45	30	35	65
20-24 y	118	45	30	30	65
25-29 y	253	45	30	30	65
30-34 y	403	45	30	30	65
35-39 y	371	45	30	30	60
40-44 y	383	45	25	30	65
45-69 y	1162	50	30	30	70
70+ y	119	50	30	35	75

(Continued)

Lipid Profile (Continued)

Table 6. Selected Reference Values for Plasma High-Density Lipoprotein Cholesterol (mg/dL) in White Female Subjects

Age	No.	Mean	Percentiles		
			5	10	95
5-19 y	666	55	35	40	70
20-24 y	199	55	35	35	80
25-34 y	649	55	35	40	80
35-39 y	298	55	35	40	80
40-44 y	318	60	35	40	90
45-49 y	328	60	35	40	85
50-54 y	256	60	35	40	90
55+ y	668	60	35	40	95

Table 7. Selected Reference Values for Plasma Triglycerides (mg/dL) in White Male Subjects

Age	No.	Mean	Percentiles		
			5	90	95
0-9 y	1491	55	30	85	100
10-14 y	2278	65	30	100	125
15-19 y	1980	80	35	120	150
20-24 y	882	100	45	165	200
25-29 y	2042	115	45	200	250
30-34 y	2444	130	50	215	265
35-39 y	2320	145	55	250	320
40-54 y	6862	150	55	250	320
55-64 y	2526	140	60	235	290
65+ y	1600	135	55	210	260

Table 8. Selected Reference Values for Plasma Triglycerides (mg/dL) in White Female Subjects

Age	No.	Mean	Percentiles		
			5	90	95
0-9 y	1304	60	35	95	110
10-19 y	4166	75	40	115	130
20-34 y	5906	90	40	145	170
35-39 y	2012	95	40	160	195
40-44 y	2050	105	45	170	210
45-49 y	2149	110	45	185	230
50-54 y	1992	120	55	190	240
55-64 y	2768	125	55	200	250
65+ y	1710	130	60	205	240

Methodology See individual listings for cholesterol, triglycerides, and lipoproteins. LDLC is calculated as follows: LDLC = total cholesterol - (VLDLC + HDLC). Very low density lipoprotein cholesterol (VLDLC) is estimated as follows: VLDLC = triglycerides/5. Lipoprotein electrophoresis has a very limited role. Ultracentrifugation is not available to many laboratories. Direct measurement of LDLC is currently available.

Additional Information Several other factors are well-documented as **risk factors** in developing coronary heart disease and are known to be additive in effect to hyperlipidemia. These include "rich" diet - habitually high saturated fat, cholesterol, and calories in relation to energy expenditure; cigarette smoking; hypertension; obesity (>30% excess body weight); sedentary lifestyle; glucose intolerance/diabetes mellitus; and left ventricular hypertrophy. Uncontrollable risk factors include genetic background, age, and male gender.

In contemporary medical practice, lipid analyses are presently very predominantly limited to cholesterol, triglyceride, HDL, and calculated LDL. **Apolipoproteins** can be measured but their major applications have so far been limited. Thirteen genetically determined lipoprotein apoproteins are presently recognized. Apoproteins AI and B are thought to have potential for atherosclerotic heart disease risk prediction. A ratio of apoprotein AI to apoprotein B may prove to be a useful predictor of cardiovascular risk - the lower the ratio, the higher the risk. However, lack of interlaboratory agreement and standardization, and the use of different methods are among the barriers to more widespread application of apoproteins. More work is needed.[3] Characteristics of apolipoproteins are outlined. Apolipoproteins act as acute phase reactants and should not be measured in ill subjects. Variations in serum lipid and lipoprotein concentrations have been described.[1]

Nonsmoking men without hypertension with cholesterol >245 mg/dL (>6.37 mmol/L) had a fourfold risk of fatal coronary arterial disease when compared to those whose cholesterol was <180 mg/dL (<4.7 mmol/L), in the multiple risk factor intervention trial (MRFIT).[3]

Most antihypertensive drugs with the exception of calcium antagonists, have an affect on lipids.[6]

Footnotes

1. Rosenson RS, "Myocardial Injury: The Acute Phase Response and Lipoprotein Metabolism," *J Am Coll Cardiol*, 1993, 22(3):933-40.
2. Rifkind BM and Segal P, "Lipid Research Clinics Program Reference Values for Hyperlipidemia and Hypolipidemia," *JAMA*, 1983, 250:1869-72.
3. Hostetter AL, "Screening for Dyslipidemia. Practice Parameter," *Am J Clin Pathol*, 1995, 103(4):380-5.
4. "Report of the National Cholesterol Treatment Program Expert Panel on Detection, Evaluation, and Treatment of High Blood Cholesterol in Adults," *Arch Intern Med*, 1988, 148(1):36-64.
5. Roth A, Eshchar Y, Keren G , et al, "Serum Lipids and Restenosis After Successful Percutaneous Transluminal Coronary Angioplasty. Ichilov Magnesium Study Group," *Am J Cardiol*, 1994, 73(16):1154-8.
6. Kasiske BL, Ma JZ, Kalil RS, et al, "Effects of Antihypertensive Therapy on Serum Lipids," *Ann Intern Med*, 1995, 122(2):133-41.

References

Austin GE, Hollman J, Lynn MJ, et al, "Serum Lipoprotein Levels Fail to Predict Postangioplasty Recurrent Coronary Artery Stenosis," *Cleve Clin J Med*, 1989, 56(5):509-14.

Brown WV, "Lipoprotein Disorders in Diabetes Mellitus," *Med Clin North Am*, 1994, 78(1):143-61.

Fraser GE, "Diet and Coronary Heart Disease: Beyond Dietary Fats and Low-Density-Lipoprotein Cholesterol," *Am J Clin Nutr*, 1994, 59(5 Suppl):1117S-23S.

Gaziano JM, Buring JE, Breslow JL, et al, "Moderate Alcohol Intake, Increased Levels of High-Density Lipoprotein and Its Subfractions, and Decreased Risk of Myocardial Infarction," *N Engl J Med*, 1993, 329(25):1829-34.

Mount JN, Kearney EM, Rosseneu M, et al, "Immunoturbidimetric Assays for Serum Apolipoproteins A1 and B Using Cobas Bio Centrifugal Analyzer," *J Clin Pathol*, 1988, 41(4):471-4.

Rosenson RS, "Low Levels of High Density Lipoprotein Cholesterol (Hypoalphalipoproteinemia). An Approach to Management," *Arch Intern Med*, 1993, 153(13):1528-38.

Schectman G and Sasse E, "Variability of Lipid Measurements: Relevance for the Clinician," *Clin Chem*, 1993, 39(7):1495-503.

Segrest JP and Anantharamaiah GM, "Pathogenesis of Atherosclerosis," *Curr Opin Cardiol*, 1994, 9(4):404-10.

Slyper AH, "Low-Density Lipoprotein Density and Atherosclerosis. Unraveling the Connection," *JAMA*, 1994, 272(4):305-8.

Stern MP, Patterson JK, Haffner SM, "Lack of Awareness and Treatment of Hyperlipidemia in Type II Diabetes in a Community Survey," *JAMA*, 1989, 262(3):360-4.

Tasaki H, Nakashima Y, Nandate H, et al, "Comparison of Serum Lipid Values in Variant Angina Pectoris and Fixed Coronary Artery Disease With Normal Subjects," *Am J Cardiol*, 1989, 63(20):1441-5.

Lipoprotein (a)

CPT 84999

Related Information

Apolipoprotein A and B *on page 82*

Apolipoprotein E *on page 82*

Lipid Profile *on previous page*

Low Density Lipoprotein Cholesterol *on page 162*

Synonyms Lp(a)

Abstract This is a plasma lipoprotein with a lipid composition very similar to low density lipoprotein (LDL). The apolipoprotein, however, is composed of two proteins linked by disulfide bonds. The plasma level of Lp(a) is correlated in some but not all studies with the occurrence of coronary heart disease (CHD) in hyperlipidemic subjects.

Specimen Plasma or serum

Container Lavender top (EDTA) tube, red top tube

Storage Instructions Spin at low temperature. Stable at 4°C for 1 week and frozen for months.

Reference Range 10-30 mg/dL (ELISA).[1] Range is method dependent. Some other methods have higher expected ranges. These values are for Caucasians. African-American values are an average of 1.7-fold higher.

Critical Values Plasma levels >30 mg/dL are reported to be associated with a two- to threefold increased risk of coronary artery disease (CAD), but *vide infra*.

Use The value of screening for Lp(a) is controversial. Routine screening cannot be recommended at this time.

Limitations Correlation with CAD was not found in subjects with noninsulin-dependent diabetes mellitus[2] or with risk of future myocardial infarct among predominantly middle-aged white males.[3,4] No evidence of significant association between baseline Lp(a) concentration and future risk of stroke was identified.[5] Lp(a) has not been extensively studied in women.

Methodology Enzyme-linked immunosorbent assay (ELISA), rate and endpoint nephelometry, electroimmunodiffusion. Measurements are not well standardized.

Additional Information The two proteins that make up the apoprotein are B-100 (a major apoprotein of LDL) and a second which has a very high homology with plasminogen. There is significant variation in concentration of this lipoprotein among individuals, but within any individual it tends to remain relatively constant for long periods. At least six isoforms of apo Lp(a) exist and the molecular mass varies from 400,000-700,000. These isoforms react differently in most immunochemical tests, which accounts for the wide range of expected values. Further study of the separate isoforms may be needed. High Lp(a) values in hyperlipidemic subjects were clearly an independent risk factor for CAD and possible cerebral infarction in a number of studies. The association is not as clear in normolipidemic subjects. There is evidence to suggest that Lp(a) competes for some of the physiologic functions of plasminogen in the coagulation and fibrinolytic cascade in vitro.[6] When Lp(a) binds to fibrin, fibrinogen, heparin, or cells, it blocks activation of plasminogen by tissue plasminogen activator.[7] These effects are antifibrinolytic. High plasma concentrations of Lp(a) may also have a thrombogenic potential.[6]

Recent review of literature suggests that quantitation of apo B and Lp(a) may be indicated in subgroups or persons with a history of premature coronary artery disease or family histories of coronary artery disease. Use of apo B or Lp(a) quantitation for screening was not supported by literature review.[8]

Footnotes
1. Labeur C, Michiels G, Bury J, et al, "Lipoprotein (a) Quantified by an Enzyme-Linked Immunosorbent Assay With Monoclonal Antibodies," Clin Chem, 1989, 35(7):1380-4.
2. O'Brien T, Nguyen TT, Harrison JM, et al, "Lipids and Lp (a) Lipoprotein Levels and Coronary Artery Disease in Subjects With Noninsulin-Dependent Diabetes Mellitus," Mayo Clin Proc, 1994, 69(5):430-5.
3. Ridker PM, Hennekens CH, and Stampfer MJ, "A Prospective Study of Lipoprotein (a) and the Risk of Myocardial Infarction," JAMA, 1993, 270(18):2195-9.
4. Barnathan ES, "Has Lipoprotein 'Little' (a) Shrunk?" JAMA, 1993, 270(18):2224-5.
5. Ridker PM, Stampfer MJ, and Hennekens CH, "Plasma Concentration of Lipoprotein (a) and the Risk of Future Stroke," JAMA, 1995, 273(16):1269-73.
6. Karmansky I and Gruener N, "Structure and Possible Biologic Roles of Lp(a)," Clin Biochem, 1994, 27(3):151-62.
7. Edelberg J and Pizzo SV, "Lipoprotein (a) Regulates Plasmin Generation and Inhibition," Chem Phys Lipids, 1994, 67-8, 363-8.
8. Rader DJ, Hoeg JM, and Brewer HB Jr, "Quantitation of Plasma Apolipoproteins in Primary and Secondary Prevention of Coronary Artery Disease," Ann Intern Med, 1994, 120(12):1012-25.

References
Gurewich V and Mittleman M, "Lipoprotein (a) in Coronary Heart Disease. Is It a Risk Factor After All?" JAMA, 1994, 271(13):1025-6.
Scanu AM, "Lipoprotein (a): Its Inheritance and Molecular Basis of Its Atherothrombotic Role," Mol Cell Biochem, 1992, 113(2):127-31.
Schaefer EJ, Lamon-Fava S, Jenner JL, et al, "Lipoprotein (a) Levels and Risk of Coronary Heart Disease in Men. The Lipid Research Clinics Coronary Primary Prevention Trial," JAMA, 1994, 271(13):999-1003.

Lipoprotein Analysis see Lipid Profile on page 159

Lipoprotein Electrophoresis
CPT 83715

Related Information
Apolipoprotein A and B on page 82
Apolipoprotein E on page 82
Cholesterol, Serum on page 110
High Density Lipoprotein Cholesterol on page 143
Lipid Profile on page 159
Low Density Lipoprotein Cholesterol on next page
Triglycerides on page 209

Synonyms Lipoprotein Phenotyping

Applies to Hyperlipoproteinemias; Lipoprotein X

Test Commonly Includes Separation of lipoprotein patterns and classification by electrophoresis. Serum triglyceride and cholesterol determination should also be ordered if this study is requested.

Abstract This procedure separates some of the lipid fractions based on electrophoretic mobility. **It is outdated and not very useful**.

Patient Preparation Patient should be on a stable diet for 2-3 weeks and should be fasting for 12-14 hours.

Specimen Serum

Container Red top tube

Causes for Rejection Patient not fasting for 12 hours

Reference Range Quantitation not available from this procedure. Visual estimates of stain density in comparison to normal patterns are usually done.

Use Evaluate hyperlipidemia to determine abnormal lipoprotein distribution and concentration in the serum (eg, work up Tangier disease)

Limitations Does not directly provide cholesterol or HDL cholesterol quantitation. Patients with different Fredrickson phenotypes on lipoprotein electrophoresis were found within given families, and the same patient did not always fall within the same phenotype on repeat analyses. **Examination of the fasting specimen following overnight refrigeration, with quantitation of cholesterol and triglyceride, often**

provides the same or better information than lipoprotein electrophoresis. Development of quantitative methods for HDLC further diminished the status of the lipoprotein electrophoresis. **Few laboratories provide the assay any longer.**

Methodology Electrophoresis provides phenotypes as a classification of hyperlipoproteinemias. **Analytical ultracentrifugation** provides flotation rate, expressed as Svedberg units: smaller molecules are more dense and contain more protein and less lipid and sediment more rapidly.

Additional Information The lipid profile has generally replaced this test. Attempts to predict high density lipoprotein cholesterol from lipoprotein electrophoretic patterns have been unsuccessful. Lipoprotein electrophoresis may still be used to establish the diagnosis of type III broad beta disease with cholesterol quantitation with subsequent ultracentrifugation to detect abnormal betalipoprotein. **Familial dysbetalipoproteinemia** occurs with **palmar or tuberous xanthomas** and with **substantially elevated cholesterol levels.** Phenotyping of Apo E supports this diagnosis. See listing Apolipoprotein E on page 82. In hyperalphalipoproteinemia, cholesterol is increased as alphalipoprotein cholesterol as in familial hyperalphalipoproteinemia and also as a secondary entity. Lipoprotein electrophoresis provides a classification based on electrophoretic mobility as the designations prebeta, beta, and alpha fractions. See table.

Lipoprotein Electrophoresis

Electrophoresis	Composition
Chylomicrons	About 90% triglyceride
Prebeta (very low density lipoprotein) (VLDL)	**Triglyceride,** phospholipid, cholesterol, protein
Beta (low density lipoprotein) (LDL)	**Cholesterol,** protein, phospholipid, triglyceride
Alpha (high density lipoprotein) (HDL)	**Protein, phospholipid,** cholesterol, triglyceride

Lipoprotein Phenotyping see Lipoprotein Electrophoresis on this page

Lipoprotein X see Lipoprotein Electrophoresis on this page

Liver Battery see Liver Profile on this page

Liver Iron Concentration see Ferritin, Serum on page 127

Liver Panel see Liver Profile on this page

Liver Profile
CPT 80058

Related Information
Acetaminophen, Serum on page 530
Alanine Aminotransferase on page 65
Albumin, Serum on page 66
Alcohol, Blood or Urine on page 531
Alpha₁-Antitrypsin Phenotyping on page 362
Alpha₁-Antitrypsin, Serum on page 363
Amiodarone, Serum on page 532
Antimitochondrial Antibody on page 366
Aspartate Aminotransferase on page 84
Bilirubin, Total on page 86
Echinococcosis Serological Test on page 390
Ferritin, Serum on page 127
Gamma Glutamyl Transferase on page 133
Hepatitis B Core Antibody on page 396
Hepatitis B DNA Detection on page 513
Hepatitis Be Antibody on page 397
Hepatitis Be Antigen on page 397
Hepatitis B Surface Antibody on page 398
Hepatitis B Surface Antigen on page 399
Hepatitis C RNA Detection on page 513
Hepatitis C Serology on page 399
Iron and Total Iron Binding Capacity/Transferrin on page 150
Liver Biopsy on page 48
Liver/Kidney Microsomal Type 1 Antibodies on page 415
Prothrombin Time on page 262
Smooth Muscle Antibody on page 431

Synonyms Liver Battery; Liver Panel

Applies to Acetaminophen

Test Commonly Includes Liver profile most often includes total bilirubin, conjugated bilirubin, alkaline phosphatase, LD (LDH), AST (SGOT), with ALT (SGPT), GGT (GGTP). It may also include serum protein electrophoresis, prothrombin time, and hepatitis serological tests (Continued)

Liver Profile (Continued)

when indicated. Alpha$_1$-antitrypsin phenotype and quantitation on occasion explains cases otherwise difficult to classify but is rarely if ever included in liver profiles.

Abstract Characterization of liver disease requires intelligent correlation of the medical history, physical examination, and laboratory test results.[1]

Specimen Serum

Container Red top tube

Storage Instructions Protect bilirubin specimens from light.

Causes for Rejection Hemolysis interferes with certain tests (see individual listings).

Special Instructions The specimen should be handled with extra precaution, especially if there is a greater than usual possibility of hepatitis. Prothrombin time tube should be spun down immediately, plasma separated from cells, placed in special plastic tube, kept refrigerated, and analyzed within 4 hours.

Use Evaluate liver disease, biliary disease, hepatoma, autoimmune hepatitis, cirrhosis, including biliary cirrhosis; investigate otherwise unexplained increases in such tests as AST, ALT, alkaline phosphatase, or prolongation of the prothrombin time; work up possible alcoholism.

A number of useful tests include those to work up **pancreatitis**, such as serum and urine amylase and serum lipase. Other tests which may be helpful in evaluation of liver disease include immunoglobulins IgG, IgA, IgM; ANA; antimitochondrial antibody; smooth muscle antibody; LD isoenzymes; alpha-fetoprotein, and 2-hour urine urobilinogen. Ammonia is useful in selected cases, **(eg, Reye's syndrome)**.

Use of blood alcohol determinations for investigation of liver disease has been advocated, because the test is cheap and simple. Other tests useful in **alcoholism** include MCV and folate levels, triglycerides as well as GGT, AST, and bilirubin. Prothrombin time is often helpful. Liver disease related to **alpha$_1$-antitrypsin** deficiency must be considered.

Limitations Many physicians prefer to order tests individually, as clinically indicated. Among the problems with such profiles, tests appropriate for specific clinical indications may not be included. Few physicians recall accurately the content of a liver profile offered by a specific clinical laboratory.

Repeat testing on initial abnormalities is important.[2]

Additional Information Liver profile interpretation can be considered as follows:

Cholestasis and biliary tract: alkaline phosphatase, GGT, total bilirubin, conjugated bilirubin, eosinophil count, urine bile (as part of urinalysis) are used. In extrahepatic biliary obstruction the serum alkaline phosphatase is increased two to three times or more while AST remains <300 units/L. Very high alkaline phosphatase levels may be found with intrahepatic cholestasis, such that alkaline phosphatase which is high out of proportion to the severity of jaundice, may indicate an intrahepatic disease.[1] Viral, alcoholic, or drug-related cholestatic hepatitis may give rise to chemistry tests indistinguishable from those of extrahepatic obstruction.[1]

Liver excretory function: urine urobilinogen, total bilirubin, conjugated bilirubin.

Hepatoma (carcinoma, liver) and other tumors: alkaline phosphatase, GGT, total LD, CEA, HB$_s$Ag (hepatitis B surface antigen). Alpha$_1$-fetoprotein may increase moderately in nonmalignant liver diseases; rising or high levels may indicate hepatoma.[1] Such clinical laboratory tests do not prove tumor without imaging and biopsy.

Hepatocellular disease: AST, ALT (more specific than AST), LD, LD$_4$, LD$_5$ (fractions related to liver in LD isoenzymes), liver biopsy, HB$_s$Ag (hepatitis B surface antigen), anti-HB$_s$ (antibody to hepatitis B surface antigen), anti-HB$_c$ (antibody to hepatitis B core antigen), HB$_e$Ag (hepatitis B "e" antigen), anti-HB$_e$ (antibody to hepatitis B$_e$ antigen), anti-HAV, IgM (antibody to hepatitis A virus, IgM), hepatitis C serology.

Liver metabolic function: Serum ammonia may increase in liver necrosis and cirrhosis as well as in Reye's syndrome.

Hemochromatosis: Mild abnormalities in liver profile tests (AST, ALT, ALP) may occur in hemochromatosis.[2] Iron, IBC, and/or ferritin are indicated.

Immunologic stimulation: Protein electrophoresis: features suggestive of cirrhosis but not always present in that disease include low albumin, low alpha$_2$, polyclonal or oligoclonal gammopathy, and beta/gamma bridging. Many but not all cases of conventional hepatic cirrhosis are accompanied by polyclonal gammopathy, sometimes with beta/gamma bridging. Oligoclonal gammopathy is found in <50% of cases of autoimmune hepatitis. HLA phenotypes may be relevant.

Immunoglobulins: IgM: very helpful in primary biliary cirrhosis; high in acute and chronic hepatitis, cholangitis, and autoimmune hepatitis. Alpha$_1$-globulin tends to fall with serum albumin. Both alpha and beta globulins may decrease in hepatocellular failure.

Antibodies: ANA: A portion of cases of autoimmune hepatitis have positive ANA. **Antimitochondrial antibody:** Extremely useful in primary biliary cirrhosis; high more often in cholangitis than in cholecystitis. **Smooth muscle antibody:** Hepatitis and conventional as well as biliary cirrhosis; especially useful for autoimmune hepatitis. Antibodies usually negative in drug jaundice and nonfebrile extrahepatic obstruction. In intrahepatic or extrahepatic biliary obstructive disease, the tests listed under Cholestasis and Biliary Tract are more abnormal than those listed under Hepatocellular Disease. Anti-LKM1 may be helpful.

In **viral hepatitis**, AST is usually three to five times or more higher (as multiples of the upper limit of normal) than LD; in cases which clinically resemble hepatitis, but in which LD equals or exceeds AST, LD isoenzymes may be useful. LD$_4$ and LD$_5$ are the hepatic fractions. An isomorphic pattern, if detected, may suggest infectious mononucleosis, CMV infection, neoplasm, or cirrhosis/alcoholism, depending on clinical setting. Appropriate positive serological tests support a diagnosis of viral hepatitis, while negative ones provide support for drug-induced hepatitis. Resolution of liver disease with removal of the offending agent enhances the latter diagnosis. An excellent review of drug-induced hepatotoxicity has recently been published.[3]

Hepatic functional reserve: Both albumin and prothrombin time are useful in evaluation of the liver, but they are nonspecific. Abnormalities in hepatic function leading to decreased and abnormal coagulation factors has been reviewed.[4] Albumin reflects hepatic synthesis and nutritional status but is lost in a variety of gastrointestinal and renal diseases.

With hypoceruloplasminemia, hypocupremia, and hypercupremia, a diagnosis of Wilson's disease is expedited, but liver biopsy for microscopy including rhodamine and orcein stains and tissue copper analysis are recently reviewed.[5]

An estimated 15 to 20 million Americans are alcoholics. Alcoholism causes malnutrition including deficiencies of vitamins including thiamine and vitamin A as well as folate. It leads to hyperlacticacidemia, hyperuricemia, ketosis, and hyperlipidemia. Alcoholics are vulnerable to a wide variety of substances, solvents and medications including acetaminophen. Alcoholism may lead to a variety of complications including cirrhosis, gastritis, malnutrition, pancreatitis, and cardiomyopathy.[6]

Liver biopsy remains a vital diagnostic modality. Its interpretation commonly requires and is supported by clinical laboratory investigation. Results of testing must be provided to the histopathologist who works up and holds responsibility for interpretation of the liver biopsy. See listing Liver Biopsy *on page 48.*

Footnotes

1. Frank BB and Members of the Patient Care Committee of the American Gastroenterological Association, "Clinical Evaluation of Jaundice - A Guideline of the Patient Care Committee of the American Gastroenterological Association," *JAMA*, 1989, 262(21):3031-4.
2. Lin E and Adams PC, "Biochemical Liver Profile in Hemochromatosis. A Survey of 100 Patients," *J Clin Gastroenterol*, 1991, 13(3):316-20.
3. Lee WM, "Drug-Induced Hepatotoxicity," *N Engl J Med*, 1995, 333(17):1118-27.
4. Mammen EF, "Coagulation Abnormalities in Liver Disease," *Hematol Oncol Clin North Am*, 1992, 6(6):1247-57.
5. Ludwig J, Moyer TP, and Rakela J, "The Liver Biopsy Diagnosis of Wilson's Disease. Methods in Pathology," *Am J Clin Pathol*, 1994, 102(4):443-6.
6. Lieber CS, "Medical Disorders of Alcoholism," *N Engl J Med*, 1995, 333(16):1058-65.

References

Burgart LJ, Batts KP, Ludwig J, et al, "Recent-Onset Autoimmune Hepatitis - Biopsy Findings and Clinical Correlations," *Am J Surg Pathol*, 1995, 19(6):699-708.
Lee WM, "Acute Liver Failure," *N Engl J Med*, 1993, 329(25):1862-72.
Rosalki SB and Dooley JS, "Liver Function Profiles and Their Interpretation," *Br J Hosp Med*, 1994, 51(4):181-6.

Low Density Lipoprotein Cholesterol

CPT 83721

Related Information

Apolipoprotein A and B *on page 82*
Cholesterol, Serum *on page 110*
Lipid Profile *on page 159*
Lipoprotein (a) *on page 160*
Lipoprotein Electrophoresis *on previous page*
Triglycerides *on page 209*

Synonyms Beta Lipoproteins; LDLC

Applies to LDLC/HDLC Ratio

Abstract The concentration of cholesterol in this lipoprotein is positively correlated with coronary heart disease risk (see table).

Patient Preparation See Preparation in the listing Cholesterol, Serum *on page 110.*

Specimen Serum

Container Red top tube

Sampling Time 12- to 14-hour fast before drawing

Reference Range Up to approximately 130 mg/dL (SI: ≤3.36 mmol/L).

Critical Values >160 mg/dL

Use An association exists between increased LDLC and total prediction of risk of coronary arterial atherosclerosis. High LDLC is a direct risk factor for coronary atherosclerosis. Screening early in life has been suggested.[1]

Limitations If triglyceride is >400 mg/dL, LDL cannot be calculated accurately by the Friedewald formula. See notes in methodology. For reliable LDLC levels by calculation, accurate HDLC, cholesterol, and triglyceride methods are necessary; vide infra.

Methodology Usually a calculation (see Additional Information) rather than a direct measurement. LDL can be separated in the analytical ultracentrifuge (vide infra), but that instrument is expensive, time consuming, and not very cost effective or practical for hospital laboratories. An immunoprecipitation method has recently been described,[2] a direct assay for LDLC. It is more precise.

Additional Information LDL carries cholesterol in plasma. LDL is the major transport protein for cholesterol. LDL is derived using the Friedewald formula. The current formula when expressed in mg/dL: LDLC = total cholesterol - (HDLC + 0.20 x triglycerides [mg/dL]); or when concentrations are expressed in mmol/L: LDLC = total cholesterol - (HDLC + 0.46 x triglyceride).[3,4] This formula is not valid for specimens with chylomicrons present or triglyceride levels >400 mg/dL (SI: >4.52 mmol/L). Direct LDLC avoids this limitation. LDLC/HDLC ratio provides a better signal for risk than either single result. Pseudocholinesterase/HDLC ratio has been studied. The National Cholesterol Education Program (NCEP) has defined a classification based on LDLC,[5] vide infra. However, Palumbo perceives some NCEP recommendations as only arbitrarily acceptable.[6]

Human low density lipoproteins comprise a spectrum of particles that have been characterized by size, chemical composition, metabolic behavior, and atherogenicity. LDL has been subfractionated into three fractions: buoyant, intermediate, and small dense (LDL1-LDL3).[7] There is speculation that oxidized LDL is taken up by macrophages forming the foam cells of atherosclerotic plaques.[8,9] Tissue pathway factor pathway inhibitor (FFPI), a potent inhibitor of extrinsic coagulation is associated with and regulated by LDL.[10] Phenolic substances in red wine inhibit LDL oxidation[11] possibly explaining why red wine appears to be protection against atherosclerosis in epidemiologic studies in France. Interestingly, at least one study has shown that LDL proteins from diabetics have in vivo modifications in protein and lipid moiety, that are able to induce massive cholesterol accumulation in cultured aortic intimal cells.[12]

NCEP CLASSIFICATION BASED ON LDL CHOLESTEROL[5]
- Desirable LDL cholesterol: <130 mg/dL (SI: <3.36 mmol/L)
- Borderline high-risk LDL cholesterol: 130-159 mg/dL (SI: 3.36-4.11 mmol/L)
- High-risk LDL cholesterol: ≥160 mg/dL (SI: ≥4.14 mmol/L)

The LDL cholesterol level is part of the basis for decisions relevant to initiation of dietary or drug therapy.

Patients with LDL cholesterol levels ≥160 mg/dL (SI: ≥4.14 mmol/L) are considered at high risk for CHD. These patients should be given cholesterol-lowering treatment.

Patients with borderline high-risk LDL cholesterol levels, 130-159 mg/dL (SI: 3.36-4.11 mmol/L), should also be treated to lower their cholesterol if they have definite CHD or two other CHD risk factors (see listing Cholesterol, Serum on page 110 for additional definition of risk factors).

Footnotes
1. Webber LS, Srinivasan SR, Wattigney WA, et al, "Tracking of Serum Lipids and Lipoproteins From Childhood to Adulthood, The Bogalusa Heart Study," Am J Epidemiol, 1991, 133(9):884-99.
2. Jialal I, Hirany SV, Devaraj S, et al, "Comparison of an Immunoprecipitation Method for Direct Measurement of LDL-Cholesterol With Beta-Quantification (Ultracentrifugation)," Am J Clin Pathol, 1995, 104(1):76-81.
3. Warnick GR, Knopp RH, Fitzpatrick V, et al, "Estimating Low Density Lipoprotein Cholesterol by the Friedewald Equation Is Adequate for Classifying Patients on the Basis of Nationally Recommended Cutpoints," Clin Chem, 1990, 36(1):15-9.
4. Rifai N, Warnick GR, McNamara JR, et al, "Measurement of Low Density Lipoprotein in Serum: A Status Report," Clin Chem, 1992, 38(1):150-60.
5. "National Cholesterol Education Program, Adult Treatment Panel Report 1987," National Cholesterol Education Program, National Heart, Lung, and Blood Institute, National Institutes of Health, 1987, C-200, Bethesda, MD.
6. Palumbo PJ, "National Cholesterol Education Program: Does the Emperor Have Any Clothes?" Mayo Clin Proc, 1988, 63(1):88-90.
7. Watson TD, Caslake MJ, Freeman DJ, et al, "Determinants of LDL Subfraction Distribution and Concentrations in Young Normolipemic Subjects," Arterioscler Thromb, 1994, 14(6):902-10.
8. Young SG and Parthasarathy S, "Why are Low-Density Lipoproteins Atherogenic?" West J Med, 1994, 160(2):153-64.
9. Kanazawa T, Osanai T, Uemura T, et al, "Evaluation of Oxidized Low-Density Lipoprotein and Large Molecular Size Low-Density Lipoproteins in Atherosclerosis," Pathobiology, 1993, 61(3-4):200-10.
10. Hansen JB, Huseby NE, Sandset PM, et al, "Tissue-Factor Pathway Inhibitor and Lipoproteins. Evidence for Association With and Regulation by LDL in Human Plasma," Arterioscler Thromb, 1994, 14(2):223-9.
11. "Inhibition of LDL Oxidation by Phenolic Substances in Red Wine: A Clue to the French Paradox," Nutr Rev, 1993, 51(6):185-7.
12. Solenin IA, Tehton VV, and Ohekhov AN, "Characterization of Chemical Composition of Native and Modified Low Density Lipoprotein Occurring in the Blood of Diabetic Patients," Int Angiol, 1994, 13(1):78-83.

References
Austin MA, Breslow JL, Hennekens CH, et al, "Low-Density Lipoprotein Subclass Patterns and Risk of Myocardial Infarction," JAMA, 1988, 260(13):1917-21.
Garber AM, "Where to Draw the Line Against Cholesterol," Ann Intern Med, 1989, 111(8):625-7.
Goodman DS, Hulley SB, Clark LT, et al, "Report of the National Cholesterol Education Program Expert Panel on Detection, Evaluation, and Treatment of High Blood Cholesterol in Adults," Arch Intern Med, 1988, 148(1):36-69.
Grundy SM, Goodman DS, Rifkind BM, et al, "The Place of HDL in Cholesterol Management: A Perspective From the National Cholesterol Education Program," Arch Intern Med, 1989, 149(3):505-10.
Hostetter AL, "Screening for Dyslipidemia, Practice Parameter," Am J Clin Pathol, 1995, 103(4):380-5.
Rifkind BM and Segal P, "Lipid Research Clinics Program Reference Values for Hyperlipidemia and Hypolipidemia," JAMA, 1983, 250:1869-72.
Steinberg D, Parthasarathy S, Carew TE, et al, "Beyond Cholesterol. Modifications of Low-Density Lipoprotein That Increase Its Atherogenicity," N Engl J Med, 1989, 320(14):915-24.

Lp(a) see Lipoprotein (a) on page 160

L/S Ratio see Amniotic Fluid Lecithin/Sphingomyelin Ratio and Phosphatidylglycerol on page 77

Luteinizing Hormone, Blood or Urine

CPT 83002

Related Information
Adrenocorticotropic Hormone on page 63
Ataxia-Telangiectasia, Chromosome Breakage Study on page 274
Clomiphene Test on page 112
Estradiol, Serum on page 125
Estrogens, Nonpregnant, Urine on page 126
Follicle Stimulating Hormone on page 129
Prolactin on page 192
Testosterone, Free and Total on page 202
Urine Collection, 24-Hour on page 30

Synonyms Follitropin; ICSH; Interstitial Cell Stimulating Hormone; LH; Pituitary Gonadotropins

Test Commonly Includes Usually measured with FSH

Abstract Levels of LH and FSH are used to assess the level of anterior pituitary gonadotropic function, sexual differentiation, fertility, and pseudohermaphroditism.

Patient Preparation Avoid radioisotope administration to patient prior to collection of specimen if RIA is used for assay.

Specimen Serum or 24-hour urine

Container Red top tube; plastic urine container containing boric acid

Storage Instructions Separate serum from cells. Stable 14 days at 4°C to 25°C.

Special Instructions In females, date of last menstrual period should be supplied. It is important to measure both FSH and LH.

Reference Range There is a large variation in reference ranges among laboratories but these are typical for urine values: Adults: male: 7-24 mIU/mL (SI: 7-24 IU/L), female: 6-30 mIU/mL (SI: 6-30 IU/L) (baseline), midcycle peak for follicular or luteal phase: over four times baseline. Low levels are found in hypogonadotropic states. High values are found following menopause, ovarian failure, and with castration. Lower values are observed in children up to the midteens. Use values supplied by laboratory performing the assay.

Use Excessive FSH and LH, gonadotropins, are found in anorchia, gonadal failure, complete testicular feminization syndrome, and menopause. FSH and LH are pituitary products, useful to distinguish primary gonadal failure from secondary (hypothalamic/pituitary) causes of gonadal failure, menstrual disturbances, and amenorrhea. Useful in infertility evaluation of women and testicular dysfunction in men. FSH is commonly used together with LH, which also is a gonadotropin. Both are low with primary pituitary or hypothalamic failure. When one is high and the other low, a gonadotropin-producing pituitary tumor is likely.

LH stimulates ovarian theca cells which produce androgen precursors that undergo aromatization to estradiol. Subsequently, LH promotes follicular maturation and ovulation then corpus luteum formation and progesterone secretion.[1] Elevated basal LH with high LH/FSH ratio, >2, with some increase of ovarian androgen, in an essentially nonovulatory adult female is presumptive evidence of Stein-Leventhal syndrome in the appropriate clinical setting. High concentrations of LH (during the follicular phase) in patients with polycystic ovary syndrome interfere with conception and may contribute to early pregnancy loss in these patients.[2]

LH acts upon and is used to assess Leydig cell function in males. It regulates male sexual differentiation, androgenization, and sexual function.[1] In males, LH has been called interstitial cell stimulating hormone (ICSH) because of its effect on testosterone production by Leydig cells, necessary for normal maturation of spermatozoa.

Urinary LH and FSH are used in children who have precocious puberty, in many of whom FSH and LH levels overlap the normal range. An (Continued)

Luteinizing Hormone, Blood or Urine (Continued)

advantage of 24-hour urine collections is that they overcome problems of pulsatile secretion spikes.

FSH, LH and testosterone are low in Kallmann's syndrome. Isolated LH deficiency is a variant of Kallmann's syndrome. Patients who have growth hormone deficiency have FSH and/or LH deficiency as well.

Limitations Secretion of both LH and FSH are pulsatile, in response to the normal intermittent release of gonadotropin releasing hormone (GnRH). While both are pulsatile, LH exhibits a circadian rhythm while FSH does not.[3] In addition, in females both FSH and LH vary over the course of the menstrual cycle, with peaks at time of ovulation. Thus, interpretation of a single determination may be difficult. Only 75% of patients with polycystic ovary syndrome have increase of LH. Increased LH with normal or low FSH may occur with obesity, hyperthyroidism, and in liver disease. The extreme chemical similarity of LH and hCG may cause technical problems of cross reactivity. Monoclonal assays have provided improvement. Use of multiple or pooled blood samples or urine (24-hour) is recommended. Problems of secretion spikes are minimized with 24-hour urine collections. Normal LH and FSH (RIA) levels can occur in hypoestrogenic patients. The glycoprotein hormones can be heterogeneous inactive molecules which may circulate and cross react with reagent antibodies in the radioimmunoassay to give a false value. FSH and LH within normal range can occur with CNS/pituitary failure.

Gonadal resistance to LH caused by mutations to the LH receptor gene are described.[1]

Methodology Radioimmunoassay (RIA), immunoradiometric assay (IRMA), radioreceptor assay,[4] dissociation enhanced lanthanide fluoroimmunoassay (DELFIA),[5] chemiluminescence immunoassay (CIA),[6] immunofluorometric assay

Additional Information FSH and LH are glycoprotein pituitary hormones which have unique β-subunits, and α-subunits in common with TSH and hCG. They are under complex regulation by hypothalamic GnRH and by gonadal sex hormones, estrogen and progesterone in females, and testosterone.

On the simplest level, FSH and LH are high in conditions in which sex hormones cannot be elaborated, and low in conditions of primary pituitary dysfunction.

Footnotes

1. Latronico AC, Anasti J, Arnhold IJ, et al, "Brief Report: Testicular and Ovarian Resistance to Luteinizing Hormone Caused by Inactivating Mutations of the Luteinizing Hormone-Receptor Gene," *N Engl J Med*, 1996, 334(8):507-12.
2. Homburg R, Armar NA, Eshel A, et al, "Influence of Serum Luteinizing Hormone Concentrations on Ovulation, Conception, and Early Pregnancy Loss in Polycystic Ovary Syndrome," *Br Med J (Clin Res Ed)*, 1988, 297(6655):1024-6.
3. Dunkel L, Alfthan H, Stenman UH, et al, "Developmental Changes in 24-Hour Profiles of Luteinizing Hormone and Follicle-Stimulating Hormone From Prepuberty to Midstages of Puberty in Boys," *J Clin Endocrinol Metab*, 1992, 74(4):890-7.
4. Whitcomb RW and Schneyer AL, "Development and Validation of a Radioligand Receptor Assay for Measurement of Luteinizing Hormone in Human Serum," *J Clin Endocrinol Metab*, 1990, 71(3):591-5.
5. Menjivar M, Ortiz G, Cardenas M, et al, "Comparison of the DELFIA and RIA Methods for Measuring Luteinizing and Follicle Stimulating Hormones in Serum," *Rev Invest Clin*, 1993, 45(6):579-84.
6. Rojanasakul A, Udomsubpayakul U, and Chinsomboon S, "Chemiluminescence Immunoassay Versus Radioimmunoassay for the Measurement of Reproductive Hormones," *Int J Gynaecol Obstet*, 1994, 45(2):141-6.

References

Apter D, Cacciatore B, Alfthan H, et al, "Serum Luteinizing Hormone Concentrations Increase 100-Fold in Females From 7 Years to Adulthood, as Measured by Time-Resolved Immunofluorometric Assay," *J Clin Endocrinol Metab*, 1989, 68(1):53-7.
Kossoy LR, Hill GA, Parker RA, et al, "Luteinizing Hormone and Ovulation Timing in a Therapeutic Donor Insemination Program Using Frozen Semen," *Am J Obstet Gynecol*, 1989, 160(5 Pt 1):1169-72.
Nippoldt TB, Reame NE, Kelch RP, et al, "The Roles of Estradiol and Progesterone in Decreasing Luteinizing Hormone Pulse Frequency in the Luteal Phase of the Menstrual Cycle," *J Clin Endocrinol Metab*, 1989, 69(1):67-76.
Vance ML, "Hypopituitarism," *N Engl J Med*, 1994, 330(23):1651-62.

Magnesium-loading Test see Magnesium, Urine on next page

Magnesium Retention Test see Magnesium, Urine on next page

Magnesium, Serum

CPT 83735

Related Information

Aminoglycosides on page 531
Amphotericin B on page 535
Calcium, Serum on page 97
Cyclosporine on page 545
Digoxin on page 546
Ketone Bodies, Blood on page 152
Kidney Stone Analysis on page 640
Magnesium, Urine on next page
Oxalate, Urine on page 174

Potassium, Serum or Plasma on page 188
Vitamin D$_3$, Serum on page 218

Synonyms Mg, Serum

Abstract Magnesium (Mg) is one of the major inorganic cations; the others are sodium, potassium, and calcium. Intracellular magnesium concentrations are much higher than extracellular (serum) values, but measurement of serum magnesium is still relevant. Most intracellular magnesium is complexed. The clinical importance of hypomagnesemia in the critically ill is still being developed. Urinary magnesium declines before serum magnesium. Cardiovascular benefits of doses of magnesium following myocardial infarct may need further study.

Specimen Serum

Container Red top tube

Collection Draw without venous stasis, separate serum from red cells as soon as possible.

Storage Instructions Refrigerate. Serum separated from cells is stable at 2°C to 6°C for several days.

Causes for Rejection Hemolysis

Reference Range 1.5-2.3 mg/dL (SI: 0.60-0.95 mmol/L), not entirely consistent among published papers, laboratories, and geographic areas. Four sets of units are in use to express concentration of magnesium: 1.0 mEq/L = 1.22 mg/dL = 0.5 mmol/L = 12.2 mg/L. Magnesium, like calcium, is partly protein bound. Slightly low values in the presence of hypoalbuminemia or hypoproteinemia should not, therefore, be of major concern. A 1996 paper provides a range of 1.8-2.2 mg/dL.[1]

Critical Values In patients with acute myocardial infarct, serum magnesium <2.0 mg/dL (SI: <0.82 mmol/L) may increase the risk of ventricular arrhythmia in the presence of hypokalemia.

Possible Panic Range Symptoms appear at <1.2 mg/dL (SI: <0.5 mmol/L); serum concentrations at <1.2 mg/dL are regarded as severe depletion. Slightly low levels should be repeated on a new specimen. Hospital diet often improves magnesium levels, especially in those who have not been on a normal diet. Toxic symptoms appear >4.9 mg/dL (SI: >2.0 mmol/L). Possible death from respiratory failure >14.6 mg/dL (SI: >6.0 mmol/L).

Use Magnesium deficiency produces neuromuscular spasm, fasciculations, hyperactivity and may cause weakness, dizziness, tremors, tetany, and convulsions. Coronary arterial spasm, hypertension and development of kidney stones may relate to hypomagnesemia. Magnesium deficiency may be associated with and may cause cardiac arrhythmias. An association with acute infarct and sudden death exists. Magnesium depletion induces vitamin D resistance.[1] Hypomagnesemia is associated with hypocalcemia, hypokalemia, long-term hyperalimentation, intravenous therapy, diabetes mellitus, especially during treatment of ketoacidosis; alcoholism and other types of malnutrition; short bowel syndrome; malabsorption and chronic diarrhea; hyperparathyroidism; dialysis; pregnancy; and hyperaldosteronism. Renal loss of magnesium occurs with cisplatin therapy. Alfrey also adds amphotericin toxicity to the causes of hypomagnesemia.

Increased magnesium levels relate mostly to patients in renal failure. Marked increases may be found in such patients who take magnesium salts (eg, as antacids which contain magnesium). Increased serum magnesium is also found with Addison's disease and in pregnant patients with severe pre-eclampsia or eclampsia who are receiving magnesium sulfate as an anticonvulsant. Hypermagnesemia may occur in patients using magnesium-containing cathartics.[2] High magnesium levels are manifested by decreased reflexes, somnolence, and heart block.

Indications for measurement of serum magnesium include the presence of unexplained hypocalcemia, instances in which hypokalemia is unresponsive to potassium supplementation, and in patients who have cardiac disorders in which hypomagnesemia may be especially hazardous such as congestive failure, myocardial infarct, ventricular ectopy, digitalis use, or left ventricular hypertrophy. Serum magnesium is indicated only selectively in patients on diuretics: those on high dose thiazides, loop diuretics such as furosemide, or hydrochlorothiazide in doses >50 mg/day.

Because an association between aminoglycoside therapy and severe hypomagnesemia is described, a recommendation is published to measure serum magnesium in subjects receiving aminoglycosides. Recommendations also exist to measure it in patients on cyclosporine,[3] cisplatin.

Limitations Hemolysis will yield elevated results as levels in erythrocytes are two to three times higher than serum. Bilirubin may cause falsely low values. Serum magnesium concentrations may not adequately reflect magnesium status. Magnesium deficiency sufficiently severe to lead to hypocalcemia and cardiac arrhythmias may exist in the presence of normal levels of serum magnesium.[1]

Methodology Spectrophotometry using calmagite dye, methylthymol blue; atomic absorption spectrophotometry. These methods were found to correlate, although a slight bias to higher values was reported with the Du Pont aca®, for levels >2.4 mg/dL (SI: >1.0 mmol/L). Ion-selective electrodes have recently become available. Inductively coupled plasma emission spectroscopy is in current use.[1]

Additional Information Magnesium is the second most abundant intracellular ion. Ionized magnesium (Mg^{2+}) is the physiologically active form with the protein bound and chelated magnesium forming a pool. Approximately 50% of the total body magnesium is present in soft tissues with the other half stored in bone. Less than 1% of the total body magnesium is present in serum.[4]

Only about 1% of intracellular magnesium is present in the free ionized form (Mg^{2+}). Free Mg^{2+} levels are carefully controlled within the cell. Total cellular magnesium is maintained at the expense of extracellular and bone magnesium.[5]

Parathormone enhances tubular reabsorption of magnesium. Measure magnesium in patients with hypocalcemia, of whom 23%, without renal failure, were found in one study to have hypomagnesemia. Magnesium-containing drugs can cause toxic levels in patients with impaired renal function. A causal relation between decreased Mg^{2+} content of cardiac muscle/coronary arteries and nonocclusive sudden-death ischemic heart disease has been proposed. Serum magnesium constitutes only a small fraction of total body stores and may not predict magnesium status correctly.[1,6] Magnesium acts as a metallic cofactor in over 300 enzymatic reactions.[7] A positive correlation between normomagnesemia and successful resuscitation is reported. Serum magnesium has prognostic importance in congestive heart failure.[8] Magnesium-depleted ICU patients have higher mortality rates than magnesium-repleted patients.[9]

Footnotes
1. Fleming CR, George L, Stoner GL, et al, "The Importance of Urinary Magnesium Values in Patients With Gut Failure," *Mayo Clin Proc*, 1996, 71(1):21-4.
2. Gerard SK, Hernandez C, and Khayam-Bashi H, "Extreme Hypermagnesemia Caused by an Overdose of Magnesium-Containing Cathartics," *Ann Emerg Med*, 1988, 17(7):728-31.
3. Chernow B, Bamberger S, Stoiko M, et al, "Hypomagnesemia in Patients in Postoperative Intensive Care," *Chest*, 1989, 95(2):391-7.
4. Elin RJ, "Magnesium: The Fifth But Forgotten Electrolyte," *Am J Clin Pathol*, 1994, 102(5):616-22.
5. Quamme GA, "Magnesium Homeostasis and Renal Magnesium Handling," *Miner Electrolyte Metab*, 1993, 19(4-5):218-25.
6. Elin RJ, "Assessment of Magnesium Status," *Clin Chem*, 1987, 33(11):1965-70.
7. Reinhart RA, "Clinical Correlates of the Molecular and Cellular Actions of Magnesium on the Cardiovascular System," *Am Heart J*, 1991, 121(5):1513-21.
8. Gottlieb SS, Baruch L, Kukin ML, et al, "Prognostic Importance of the Serum Magnesium Concentration in Patients With Congestive Heart Failure," *J Am Coll Cardiol*, 1990, 16(4):827-31.
9. Olerich MA and Rude RK, "Should We Supplement Magnesium in Critically Ill Patients?" *New Horiz*, 1994, 2(2):186-92.

References
Castelbaum AR, Donofrio PD, Walker FO, et al, "Laxative Abuse Causing Hypermagnesemia, Quadriparesis, and Neuromuscular Junction Defect," *Neurology*, 1989, 39(5):746-7.
Gottlieb SS, "Importance of Magnesium in Congestive Heart Failure," *Am J Cardiol*, 1989, 63(14):39G-42G.
Gren J and Woolf A, "Hypermagnesemia Associated With Catharsis in a Salicylate-Intoxicated Patient With Anorexia Nervosa," *Ann Emerg Med*, 1989, 18(2):200-3.
Lum G, "Hypomagnesemia in Acute and Chronic Care Patient Populations," *Am J Clin Pathol*, 1992, 97(6):827-30.
McLean RM, "Magnesium and Its Therapeutic Uses: A Review," *Am J Med*, 1994, 96(1):63-76.
Quamme GA, "Laboratory Evaluation of Magnesium Status: Renal Function and Free Intracellular Magnesium Concentration," *Clin Lab Med*, 1993, 13(1):209-23.
Ryan MF, "The Role of Magnesium in Clinical Biochemistry: An Overview," *Ann Clin Biochem*, 1991, 28(Pt 1):19-26.
Toffaletti J, "Physiology and Regulation. Ionized Calcium, Magnesium, and Lactate Measurements in Critical Care Settings," *Am J Clin Pathol*, 1995, 104(4 Suppl):S88-94.
Weber CA and Santiago RM, "Hypermagnesemia. A Potential Complication During Treatment of Theophylline Intoxication With Oral Activated Charcoal and Magnesium-Containing Cathartics," *Chest*, 1989, 95(1):56-9.

Magnesium, Urine

CPT 83735

Related Information

Aminoglycosides *on page 531*
Amphotericin B *on page 535*
Calcium, Serum *on page 97*
Calcium, Urine *on page 99*
Cyclosporine *on page 545*
Digoxin *on page 546*
Ketone Bodies, Blood *on page 152*
Kidney Stone Analysis *on page 640*
Magnesium, Serum *on previous page*
Oxalate, Urine *on page 174*
Potassium, Serum or Plasma *on page 188*
Urine Collection, 24-Hour *on page 30*
Vitamin D$_3$, Serum *on page 218*

Synonyms Mg, Urine

Applies to Magnesium-loading Test; Magnesium Retention Test

Abstract Urine magnesium collections are used to evaluate urine magnesium loss and balance. Magnesium excretion controls magnesium balance. Urinary magnesium diminishes before serum magnesium does and provides earlier indication of evolving deficiency. Magnesium deficiency sufficiently severe to lead to hypocalcemia and cardiac arrhythmias can exist in the presence of normal serum magnesium concentrations.[1]

Patient Preparation Patient should be instructed to use a plastic bedpan; *vide infra.*

Specimen 24-hour urine

Container Plastic acid-washed urine container; addition of an acidifying agent such as hydrochloric acid as preservative is desirable; check with laboratory.

Collection Since a circadian rhythm exists for magnesium excretion, 24-hour collections are indicated.

Storage Instructions Refrigerate

Causes for Rejection Specimen allowed to contact metal.

Reference Range 7.3-12.2 mg/dL (SI: 3-5 mmol/day). Some laboratories report in mg/24 hours. The mean in control subjects was 127 mg/24 hours in a 1996 paper. See information regarding units in the listing Magnesium, Serum *on page 164*. Values are slightly higher in males.

Use Urinary collection is valuable to detect magnesium deficiency due to medication, gut failure, Crohn's disease, or abnormal renal function.[1,2] Magnesium urinary excretion is enhanced by increasing blood alcohol levels, diuretics, Bartter's syndrome, corticosteroids, cis-platinum therapy, and aldosterone. Renal magnesium wasting occurs in renal transplant recipients who are on cyclosporine and prednisone. Renal conservation of magnesium is diminished by hypercalciuria, salt-losing conditions, and the syndrome of inappropriate secretion of antidiuretic hormone. Although urinary magnesium analyses have been advocated before and after therapeutic magnesium administration to further investigate the significance of an apparent low serum concentration,[3] in fact significantly diminished urinary magnesium concentration is found in some subjects whose serum magnesium is within normal limits.[1]

Limitations A lack of uniformity exists among references regarding boundaries of reference range for urine magnesium. Lack of consistent normal ranges for serum magnesium between published papers, laboratories, and geographic areas is also evident.

Methodology Atomic absorption (AA), inductively coupled plasma emission spectroscopy

Additional Information Regulation of magnesium balance is via intestinal absorption (dietary source) and renal excretion. Magnesium is filtered at the glomerulus and reabsorbed along various tubular segments. The loop of Henle plays the major role in determining magnesium resorption and urinary magnesium excretion.[4]

Hypercalcemia, hypophosphatemia, and acidosis are among inhibitors of tubular reabsorption of magnesium. A magnesium retention test is described to assess magnesium deficit in bone, but problems exist.[2] The most widely accepted criterion used to ascertain the magnitude of magnesium deficiency is the magnesium-loading test.[1]

Footnotes
1. Fleming CR, George L, Stoner GL, et al, "The Importance of Urinary Magnesium Values in Patients With Gut Failure," *Mayo Clin Proc*, 1996, 71(1):21-4.
2. Elin RJ, "Magnesium: The Fifth but Forgotten Electrolyte," *Am J Clin Pathol*, 1994, 102(5):616-22.
3. Chernow B, Bamberger S, Stoiko M, et al, "Hypomagnesemia in Patients in Postoperative Intensive Care," *Chest*, 1989, 95(2):391-7.
4. Quamme GA, "Magnesium Homeostasis and Renal Magnesium Handling," *Miner Electrolyte Metab*, 1993, 19(4-5):218-25.

References
Dorup I, "Magnesium and Potassium Deficiency. Its Diagnosis, Occurrence and Treatment in Diuretic Therapy and Its Consequences for Growth, Protein Synthesis and Growth Factors," *Acta Physiol Scand*, 1994, 618(Suppl):1-55.
Nicoll GW, Struthers AD, and Fraser CG, "Biological Variation of Urinary Magnesium," *Clin Chem*, 1991, 37(10 Pt 1):1794-5.
Roelofsen JM, Berkel GM, Uttendorfsky OT, et al, "Urinary Excretion Rates of Calcium and Magnesium in Normal and Complicated Pregnancies," *Eur J Obstet Gynecol Reprod Biol*, 1988, 27(3):227-36.

Metabolic Screen for Amino Acids *see* Amino Acid Screen, Plasma *on page 74*

Metabolic Screen for Amino Acids *see* Amino Acid Screen, Qualitative, Urine *on page 75*

Metanephrines

CPT 83835

Related Information

Catecholamines, Fractionation, Plasma *on page 103*
Catecholamines, Fractionation, Urine *on page 104*
Homovanillic Acid, Urine *on page 145*
Multiple Endocrine Neoplasia/Familial Medullary Thyroid Carcinoma *on page 519*
(Continued)

Metanephrines *(Continued)*

Urine Collection, 24-Hour *on page 30*
Vanillylmandelic Acid, Urine *on page 216*

Synonyms Total Metanephrines

Applies to Catecholamines; Epinephrine; Norepinephrine

Replaces Catecholamines, Plasma

Test Commonly Includes Metanephrine and normetanephrine

Abstract The immediate metabolites of epinephrine and norepinephrine are known as metanephrines. They are catecholamine metabolites. Increases in catecholamine production by the adrenal medulla and, therefore, increased urinary excretion of metanephrines occur in the presence of pheochromocytoma. Plasma metanephrines are more sensitive than urinary metanephrines for pheochromocytoma.[1]

Patient Preparation Methylxanthine-containing food products are avoided after midnight, and patients should refrain from smoking after midnight. See Limitations.

Urine: Consult the laboratory which will do the assay. Emotional and physical stress may interfere through stimulation of endogenous catecholamines.[2] Drugs may interfere including alpha$_2$-agonists, calcium channel blockers, converting enzyme inhibitors, bromocriptine, phenothiazines, tricyclic antidepressants, and levodopa.[2] Endogenous and exogenous catecholamines and therapy with methyldopa, monoamine oxidase inhibitors increase metanephrine excretion.[2]

Blood: Following rest for 20 minutes, blood is collected from an antecubital vein through an indwelling catheter; arterial blood can be used.[1]

Specimen 24-hour urine, plasma

Container Plastic urine container; green top (heparin) tube, prechilled

Collection Urine: Specimens for catecholamines, VMA, and metanephrines should be obtained while the patient is resting, not on medications, and without recent exposure to imaging contrast materials.[2] The likelihood of detection of pheochromocytoma is enhanced if the collection period is initiated by or includes a crisis. If crises occur less often than once a day, the patient may bring in specimen initiated by a crisis. Acidify to pH 4 after collection is complete with hydrochloric acid. 30 mL 6M HCl was used by the NIH study.[1]

Blood: Collect blood into precooled tubes containing heparin; centrifuge within 30 minutes.[1]

Storage Instructions Keep urine collection cold. Freeze plasma until assay.

Reference Range Urine: Mean 0.6 mg/24 hours (SI: 3 μmol/24 hours), up to 1.0 mg/24 hours (SI: 5.0 μmol/day) or <1.2 μg/mg creatinine, with some variation between laboratories. **Blood:** See Lenders et al.[1]

Critical Values >2.2 μg/mg creatinine indicative of pheochromocytoma

Possible Panic Range Median urinary excretion in pheochromocytoma patients 24.2 μmol/day, range 2.1-24.2 μmol/day

Use Evaluation for the presence of abnormal catecholamine production. An established method, useful in the diagnosis of pheochromocytoma, secreting paraganglioma, neuroblastoma, and ganglioneuroblastoma.

Limitations Urine: False-negative **urinary** results occur (eg, interference by methylglucamine in x-ray contrast medium).[2] False-positive **urinary** results occur; results should be confirmed by other means, such as urine catecholamines and VMA. False-positives can be caused by stress and drugs. Interfering substances partly depend on analytical methods. Drugs causing interference include phenacetin and antihypertensive drugs (eg, alpha-adrenergic receptor blocking agents). Propranolol interferes with a spectrophotometric assay. A valuable table of causes of interference with urinary biochemical diagnosis of pheochromocytoma has been published.[2]

Blood: Acetaminophen interferes with the plasma assay and should be avoided for several days.[1] A few patients with secondary hypertension or cardiac failure had increased plasma metanephrines. False-positive plasma assays may occur in patients with chronic renal disease.

Methodology Colorimetry, fluorometry, gas chromatography (GC), and liquid chromatography (LC) techniques (particularly, HPLC). Liquid chromatography with electrochemical detection for plasma assay.[1]

Additional Information Metanephrine and normetanephrine are metabolic products of epinephrine and norepinephrine, the adrenal medullary hormones secreted by pheochromocytomas. Because secretion is usually episodic, plasma catecholamine drawn during an asymptomatic period may be normal, while total urinary metanephrines collected over 24 hours would be abnormal. On the other hand, a tumor could be intermittently active, but secrete over a full 24-hour period total metanephrines that are within reference ranges. Analyses of 24-hour urine specimens are preferable to spot (random) urine samples for catecholamines, VMA, and metanephrines.

Assay of total metanephrines has provided the highest number of true positive results for pheochromocytoma. It has become the first choice as a screening test. Urinary metanephrine has been positive in 98% to 99%, VMA in about 90% of patients with pheochromocytoma.

When only a spot urine sample is available or the 24-hour urine collection is incomplete, simultaneous measurement of urine creatinine permits expression of the metanephrine/creatinine ratio. Some clinicians use >2.2 μg metanephrines/mg creatinine to distinguish pheochromocytoma from normal with this ratio. Reference intervals for 24-hour urinary metanephrines in hypertensives have been published.[3] Pheochromocytomas cause hypertension that is classically paroxysmal. They may cause sudden headache, pallor, perspiration, and palpitation. Rarely, hypotension presents as the initial manifestation.[2]

Use of HPLC methods for plasma and urinary catecholamine estimation, may render measurement of urinary metabolites obsolete for the diagnosis of pheochromocytoma and paraganglioma.[4]

Other tests for neuroblastoma include HVA, VMA, and CEA.

Footnotes

1. Lenders JW, Keiser HR, Goldstein DS, et al, "Plasma Metanephrines in the Diagnosis of Pheochromocytoma," *Ann Intern Med*, 1995, 123(2):101-9.
2. Sheps SG, Jiang N-S, Klee GG, et al, "Recent Developments in the Diagnosis and Treatment of Pheochromocytoma," *Mayo Clin Proc*, 1990, 65(1):88-95.
3. Kairisto V, Koskinen P, Mattila K, et al, "Reference Intervals for 24-Hour Urinary Normetanephrine, Metanephrine, and 3-Methoxy-4-Hydroxymandelic Acid in Hypertensive Patients," *Clin Chem*, 1992, 38(3):416-20.
4. Fonseca V and Bouloux PM, "Pheochromocytoma and Paraganglioma," *Baillieres Clin Endocrinol Metab*, 1993, 7(2):509-44.

References

Jessurun CR, Adam K, Moise KJ Jr, et al, "Pheochromocytoma-Induced Myocardial Infarction in Pregnancy. A Case Report and Literature Review," *Tex Heart Inst J*, 1993, 20(2):120-2.
Krakoff LR, "Searching for Pheochromocytoma: A New and Better Test?" *Ann Intern Med*, 1995, 123(2):150-1.
Rosano TG, Swift TA, and Hayes LW, "Advances in Catecholamine and Metabolite Measurements for Diagnosis of Pheochromocytoma," *Clin Chem*, 1991, 37(10 Pt 2):1854-67.

Metformin *see Lactic Acid, Blood on page 156*

MetHb *see Methemoglobin on this page*

Methemoglobin

CPT 83045 (qualitative); 83050 (quantitative)

Related Information

Blood Gases, Arterial *on page 87*
Carboxyhemoglobin *on page 541*
Hemoglobin Electrophoresis *on page 324*

Synonyms MetHb

Applies to Cytochrome b$_5$ Reductase (NADH-metHb Reductase)

Abstract This pigment is hemoglobin in which the iron has been oxidized from the normal ferrous to the ferric (trivalent) state. It cannot bind oxygen to act as an oxygen carrier.

Specimen Whole blood

Container Green top (heparin) tube

Storage Instructions Keep tube on ice. pH dependent. Should be run within 8 hours, or false-negatives may occur. Run as promptly as possible after draw. Studies have shown up to 10% drop in 4 hours, up to 16% drop in 8 hours, in samples kept on ice. Such studies have not been extensive. May be drawn into sodium fluoride-containing tubes and immediately frozen at 0°C to -4°C prior to analysis.

Reference Range Up to 1.5% of total hemoglobin. Smokers have a slightly higher percent metHb than do nonsmokers.

Possible Panic Range Headache and other symptoms occur at levels >30%. Methemoglobinemia can be fatal, particularly >70% saturation levels.

Use Evaluate cyanosis, especially in the presence of normal arterial gases, cyanosis unresponsive to oxygen administration or a distinctive brown color to arterial blood; evaluate polycythemia and hemoglobinopathies; work up dyspnea and headache; work up "poppers" and "sniffers"; evaluate drug or chemical toxicity, since most instances of methemoglobinemia are so acquired; monitor patients on high dose nitrate therapy; measurement in CSF may detect small cerebral and subdural hematomas.[1]

Limitations Sulfhemoglobin, methylene blue, and Evans blue dye may interfere. MetHb exhibits pH sensitivity.

Methodology Spectrophotometry; Hb M variants are best detected by electrophoresis because spectrophotometry is unreliable due to their abnormal ferrihemoglobin spectra.

Additional Information Methemoglobin (metHb) is an inactive, oxidized form of hemoglobin which does not contribute to the oxygen-carrying capacity of blood. Concentrations of metHb of over 10% to 15% of hemoglobin will cause cyanosis. Sulfhemoglobin will interfere with metHb determined by the above method. Methemoglobinemia may be hereditary or acquired. Polycythemia is occasionally present as a compensatory mechanism. Elevations of metHb lead to dyspnea, cyanosis, and headache, and can be lethal. Most instances of methemoglobinemia are acquired, from drugs and chemicals. Nitro and amino groups are especially involved, eg, aniline and derivatives, nitrites, nitroglycerin, nitrate salts in burn patients, dapsone (perhaps the most common cause of drug-induced methemoglobinemia), phenacetin, acetophenetidin, and some sulfonamides, chlorates, quinones, large doses of ferrous sulfate, and many other drugs and some intestinal bacteria.[1] The aniline ring is found in many medications including virtually all local anesthetic agents. Recently, methemoglobinemia was recognized from topically applied anesthetic spray.[2] Well water containing nitrate is the most common cause of methemoglobinemia in the newborn. Methemoglobinemia has been reported after exposure to automobile exhaust fumes.[3]

Hereditary methemoglobinemia is uncommon. It may be due to a deficiency of red cell NADH-methemoglobin reductase (diaphorase, also termed cytochrome b_5 reductase), which is inherited as an autosomal recessive trait. Homozygotes have metHb levels of 15% to 20%. Heterozygotes are apt to develop toxic methemoglobinemia when exposed to substances which can act as oxidants to hemoglobin iron. Each group carries decreased methemoglobin reductase.[2] It may also be the result of presence of certain hemoglobinopathies, members of the Hb M family including Hb M Saskatoon, Boston, Iwate, Hyde Park, and Milwaukee. These have autosomal dominant mode of inheritance and may be associated with clinical cyanosis. Hb Seattle and other hemoglobinopathies also show increase in the in vitro rate of metHb formation.[4] A recently identified new hemoglobin variant, Hb Warsaw, is also characterized by elevated blood levels of metHb.[5]

A study of postmortem metHb levels showed a range of 0.8% to 57% in individuals who, clinically, should have had normal antemortem concentrations. There was no correlation with antemortem circumstances, autopsy findings, or interval of time from death to autopsy.[6]

Footnotes
1. Trbojevic-Cepe M, Vogrinc Z, and Brinar V, "Diagnostic Significance of Methemoglobin Determination in Colorless Cerebrospinal Fluid," *Clin Chem*, 1992, 38(8 Pt 1):1404-8.
2. Dinneen SF, Mohr DN, and Fairbanks VF, "Methemoglobinemia From Topically Applied Anesthetic Spray," *Mayo Clin Proc*, 1994, 69(9):886-8.
3. Laney RF and Hoffman RS, "Methemoglobinemia Secondary to Automobile Exhaust Fumes," *Am J Emerg Med*, 1992, 10(5):426-8.
4. Beutler E, "Hemoglobinopathies Producing Cyanosis," *Hematology*, 4th ed, Chapter 78, Williams WJ, Beutler E, Ersler AJ, et al, eds, New York, NY: McGraw-Hill Inc, 1990, 746-51.
5. Honig GR, Telfer MC, Rosenblum BB, et al, "Hb Warsaw (β42 Phe → Val): An Unstable Hemoglobin With Decreased Oxygen Affinity. I. Hematologic and Clinical Expression," *Am J Hematol*, 1989, 32(1):36-41.
6. Reay DT, Insalaco SJ, and Eisele JW, "Postmortem Methemoglobin Concentrations and Their Significance," *J Forensic Sci*, 1984, 29(4):1160-3.

References
Dean BS, Lopez G, and Krenzelok EP, "Environmentally-Induced Methemoglobinemia in an Infant," *J Toxicol Clin Toxicol*, 1992, 30(1):127-33.
Johnson WS, Hall AH, and Rumack BH, "Cyanide Poisoning Successfully Treated Without Therapeutic Methemoglobin Levels," *Am J Emerg Med*, 1989, 7(4):437-40.
Mansouri A and Lurie AA, "Concise Review: Methemoglobinemia," *Am J Hematol*, 1993, 42(1):7-12.
"From the Centers for Disease Control and Prevention. Prilocaine-Induced Methemoglobinemia - Wisconsin, 1993," *JAMA*, 1994, 272(18):1403-4.
Williamson D, "The Unstable Haemoglobins," *Blood Rev*, 1993, 7(3):146-63.

3-Methoxy-4-Hydroxymandelic Acid *see* Vanillylmandelic Acid, Urine *on page 216*

Methylimidazoleacetic Acid *see* Histamine *on page 144*

Metyrapone Stimulation Test
CPT 80436

Related Information
Adrenocorticotropic Hormone *on page 63*
Cortisol, Blood *on page 112*
Cortisol, Urine *on page 113*
Cosyntropin Test *on page 114*
17-Hydroxycorticosteroids, Urine *on page 147*
Prolactin *on page 192*
Urine Collection, 24-Hour *on page 30*

Applies to 11-Deoxycortisol; Dexamethasone Suppression Test

Test Commonly Includes 8 AM serum 11-deoxycortisol and cortisol after oral metyrapone

Abstract Metyrapone is a 11-β-hydroxylase inhibitor and inhibits the conversion of 11-deoxycortisol to cortisol. Serum 11-deoxycortisol will increase and serum cortisol decrease if normal pituitary stimulation of the adrenal with ACTH occurs.

The differential diagnosis of Cushing's syndrome includes corticotropin-independent and corticotropin-dependent categories; see listing Adrenocorticotropic Hormone *on page 63*. The corticotropin dependent type includes **pituitary Cushing's disease** and **ectopic Cushing's syndrome**. The latter is caused by ectopic ACTH production in small cell

carcinomas of lung, bronchial carcinoids, and medullary carcinomas of thyroid, and by a few other neuroendocrine neoplasms.

Patient Preparation Other measures, possibly including the cosyntropin test, should be done first (ie, the patient's adrenals must be known to be able to respond to ACTH). If response to exogenous ACTH has not been demonstrated, then an attempt to produce release of endogenous ACTH may carry risk to the patient. No recent administration of radioisotopes. Metyrapone is given at 11 PM the night before the specimen is collected. Dose ranges (by patient weight) from 2-3 g.

Specimen Serum, 24-hour urine collections

Container Red top tube

Sampling Time 8 AM, morning after oral metyrapone

Storage Instructions For 11-deoxycortisol, separate as soon as possible. Freeze serum if assay is not performed within 24 hours.

Reference Range Serum: 11-deoxycortisol increased to >7 µg/dL (SI: >202 nmol/L); cortisol <3 µg/dL (SI: <83 nmol/L)

Use Differential diagnosis of Cushing's syndrome, pituitary adenoma (Cushing's disease), and ectopic ACTH syndrome (differential diagnosis of pituitary and ectopic types of corticotropin-dependent Cushing's syndrome). Ectopic ACTH syndrome was not extensively studied in the key paper reporting this evaluation. The authors of this study did not encourage dexamethasone or metyrapone testing for this differential diagnosis. Later reports suggest that ectopic sources for ACTH versus pituitary sources in Cushing's syndrome can be differentiated by this test.[1] Subsequently, others evaluated the metyrapone and dexamethasone suppression tests to resolve the differential diagnosis between ACTH-producing microadenoma and ectopic ACTH dependent Cushing's syndrome. For the metyrapone test, urine 17-hydroxysteroid excretion by Porter-Silber reaction and plasma 11-deoxycortisol were studied. For dexamethasone suppression, urine hydroxysteroid and free cortisol were measured.[2] Although they confirm that each of these two tests is useful, and both together are better, others express concern about possible patient selection bias and the mathematical approach to diagnosis.[3]

Limitations Significant problems are addressed in current literature.[4]

Contraindications Should not be used in patients with possible adrenal insufficiency.

Methodology Radioimmunoassay (RIA)

Additional Information Metyrapone inhibits conversion of 11-deoxycortisol to cortisol. The decrease in cortisol levels causes increased secretion of ACTH. ACTH stimulates adrenocortical secretion of 11-deoxycortisol, precursor to cortisol. Thus, giving metyrapone tests pituitary ACTH reserve and the integrity of the adrenal cortical-pituitary feedback loop. Serum 11-deoxycortisol increases in patients with pituitary adenoma (Cushing's disease) and does not rise in patients with adrenal cortical tumor, in whom pituitary corticotropin suppression is anticipated. In adrenogenital syndrome with 21-hydroxylase deficiency (the most common form) 11-deoxycortisol is low, but in 11-hydroxylase deficiency it is high. It may also be high in adrenal carcinoma. A 3-day metyrapone test protocol is also available. The reader is urged to review footnotes 2, 3, and 4 for relevant further information.

Footnotes
1. Blunt SB, Sandler LM, Burrin JM, et al, "An Evaluation of the Distinction of Ectopic and Pituitary ACTH Dependent Cushing's Syndrome by Clinical Features, Biochemical Tests, and Radiological Findings," *Q J Med*, 1990, 77(283):1113-33.
2. Avgerinos PC, Yanovski JA, Oldfield EH, et al, "The Metyrapone and Dexamethasone Suppression Tests for the Differential Diagnosis of the Adrenocorticotropin-Dependent Cushing's Syndrome: A Comparison," *Ann Intern Med*, 1994, 121(5):318-27.
3. Orth DN, "The Cushing Syndrome: Quest for the Holy Grail," *Ann Intern Med*, 1994, 121(5):377.
4. Orth DN, "Cushing's Syndrome," *N Engl J Med*, 1995, 332(12):791-803.

References
Orth D, Kovacs D, and DeBold C, "The Adrenal Cortex," *Williams Textbook of Endocrinology*, 8th ed, Wilson J and Foster D, eds, Philadelphia, PA: WB Saunders Co, 1992.
von Bardeleben U, Stalla GK, Muller OA, et al, "Blunting of ACTH Response to Human CRH in Depressed Patients Is Avoided by Metyrapone Pretreatment," *Biol Psychiatry*, 1988, 24(7):782-6.

Mg, Serum *see* Magnesium, Serum *on page 164*

Mg, Urine *see* Magnesium, Urine *on page 165*

Microbilirubin *see* Bilirubin, Neonatal *on page 86*

Murphy-Pattee *replaced by* Thyroxine *on page 206*

Myocardial Infarct Panel *see* Cardiac Enzymes/Isoenzymes *on page 102*

Myoglobin, Blood
CPT 83874

Related Information
Cardiac Enzymes/Isoenzymes *on page 102*
Creatine Kinase *on page 115*
Creatine Kinase Isoenzymes/Isoforms *on page 115*
(Continued)

Myoglobin, Blood *(Continued)*

Haptoglobin, Serum *on page 141*
Lactate Dehydrogenase *on page 153*
Lactate Dehydrogenase Isoenzymes *on page 154*
Muscle Biopsy *on page 53*
Myoglobin, Qualitative, Urine *on page 644*
Troponin *on page 212*

Applies to Carbonic Anhydrase III

Abstract Myoglobin is a low molecular weight (17,900 d) cytoplasmic heme protein (oxygen-binding) which is found in cardiac and striated muscle. An increase in its concentration is a useful marker for early detection of recent myocardial infarct. Only a narrow window at presentation is available for assay. **False-positives and false-negatives are seen.**

Patient Preparation No recent administration of radioactive substances if RIA method is used.

Specimen Serum

Container Red top tube

Sampling Time Use of two to three samples at 1- to 2-hour intervals is advocated at presentation.[1,2] Optimal sensitivity was at 2 hours following onset.[2]

Storage Instructions Serum may be stored at 4°C for 2 years or frozen at -20°C.[2]

Reference Range Approximate range: 5-70 µg/L (SI: 5-70 µg/L) (immunonephelometric assay). Varies with method. Level may be up to 25% higher in men.

Use Diagnose skeletal or acute myocardial muscle injury. Serum myoglobin is detectable earlier than is CK or CK-MB increase in patients with acute myocardial infarction.[1,2,3] Serum myoglobin has been found also in 50% of patients with acute coronary insufficiency. Myoglobin concentrations correlate with size of infarct.[1] Used to diagnose rhabdomyolysis. Myoglobin appears with trauma, ischemia, malignant hyperthermia, exertion, dermatomyositis, polymyositis, and muscular dystrophy. Serum myoglobin levels are claimed to have their greatest utility as a negative indicator (ie, if not elevated in 1-3 hours after onset of chest pain, a myocardial infarct is unlikely).

Limitations Increased myoglobin levels occur after intramuscular injections, other muscle injury and shock. Increased myoglobin has been reported after high voltage electrical accident. Many laboratories prefer CK isoenzymes (CK-MB does not rise after intramuscular injection) and do not provide plasma myoglobin levels. Better specificity is seen with CK-MB.[2] Recent technical improvements in the assay will allow more widespread use of the test. As an index of myocardial infarct, myoglobin returns rapidly to baseline levels.[4] **Rising serum myoglobin concentrations may be missed if there is delay in seeking medical attention following the onset of chest pain.** Myoglobin is released following open heart surgery and false-positives occur with renal failure. It is not tightly bound to protein and is rapidly excreted.[5] In patients with massive myoglobinemia, blood myoglobin may rapidly fall independent of renal function or therapeutic manipulation.[5]

Contraindications Administration of radioactive material before test if RIA method is used.

Methodology Radioimmunoassay (RIA), fluorometric immunoassay, immunoturbidimetry, dual-label time-resolved fluoroimmunoassay, nephelometry

Additional Information Serum myoglobin is rapidly cleared by the kidneys. Elevated levels may be associated with cocaine use.[6] It is increased in cardiac surgery, thrombolytic therapy,[7,8] myocardial infarction,[9] exercise, shock, renal failure, progressive muscular dystrophy, and rhabdomyolysis from any cause. Its **main advantage** is as a sensitive (99% to 100%) marker for **early myocardial injury** because it is released earlier from necrotic cells than CK, allowing for earlier detection of myocardial infarction.[9] Levels rise as early as 1 hour after infarct and peak within 4-12 hours.[10] Repeat myoglobin that has doubled within 1-2 hours after presentation, even if still within the normal range, may signify an acute myocardial infarct.[11]

Because myoglobin is not specific to myocardial muscle, the issue of specificity arises in cases of acute myocardial injury associated with muscle trauma, where a distinction cannot be made as to the origin of myoglobin. If one measures **carbonic anhydrase III**, an 18,000-d cytoplasmic protein present in skeletal muscle but **not** in cardiac muscle, the separation can be made.[5] Simultaneous assay of both proteins shows that in skeletal muscle injury the ratio of myoglobin to carbonic anhydrase III is constant; while in patients with AMI, the ratio shows a temporal pattern similar to myoglobin alone. Serum troponin I concentrations have recently been shown to present significant advantages (see Troponin *on page 212*) because of high specificity.

Footnotes

1. Woo J, Lacbawan FL, Sunheimer R, et al, "Is Myoglobin Useful in the Diagnosis of Acute Myocardial Infarction in the Emergency Department Setting?" *Am J Clin Pathol*, 1995, 103(6):725-9.
2. Montague C and Kircher T, "Myoglobin in the Early Evaluation of Acute Chest Pain," *Am J Clin Pathol*, 1995, 104(4):472-6.
3. Keffer JH, "Myocardial Markers of Injury. Evolution and Insights," *Am J Clin Pathol*, 1996, 105:304-20.
4. Isakov A, Shapira I, Burke M, et al, "Serum Myoglobin Levels in Patients With Ischemic Myocardial Insult," *Arch Intern Med*, 1988, 148(8):1762-5.
5. Wakabayashi Y and Kikuno T, Ohwada T, et al, "Rapid Fall in Blood Myoglobin in Massive Rhabdomyolysis and Acute Renal Failure," *Intensive Care Med*, 1994, 20(2):109-12.
6. Pogue VA and Nurse HM, "Cocaine-Associated Acute Myoglobinuric Renal Failure," *Am J Med*, 1989, 86(2):183-6.
7. McCullough DA, Harrison PG, Forshall JM, et al, "Serum Myoglobin and Creatine Kinase Enzymes in Acute Myocardial Infarction Treated With Anistreplase," *J Clin Pathol*, 1992, 45(5):405-7.
8. Laperche T, Steg PG, Benessiano J, et al, "Patterns of Myoglobin and MM Creatine Kinase Isoforms Release Early After Intravenous Thrombolysis of Direct Percutaneous Transluminal Coronary Angioplasty for Acute Myocardial Infarction, and Implications for the Early Noninvasive Diagnosis of Reperfusion," *Am J Cardiol*, 1992, 70(13):1129-34.
9. Apple FS, "Acute Myocardial Infarction and Coronary Reperfusion. Serum Cardiac Markers for the 1990's," *Am J Clin Pathol*, 1992, 97(2):217-26.
10. Van Blerk M, Maes V, Huyghens L, et al, "Analytical and Clinical Evaluation of Creatine Kinase MB Mass Assay by IMx: Comparison With MB Isoenzyme Activity and Serum Myoglobin for Early Diagnosis of Myocardial Infarction," *Clin Chem*, 1992, 38(12):2380-6.
11. Tucker JF, Collins RA, Anderson AJ, et al, "Value of Serial Myoglobin Levels in the Early Diagnosis of Patients Admitted for Acute Myocardial Infarction," *Ann Emerg Med*, 1994, 24(4):704-8.

References

Brogan GX Jr, Friedman S, McCuskey C, et al, "Evaluation of a New Rapid Quantitative Immunoassay for Serum Myoglobin Versus CK-MB for Ruling Out Acute Myocardial Infarction in the Emergency Department," *Ann Emerg Med*, 1994, 24(4):665-71.
Castaldo AM, Ercolini F, Forino F, et al, "Plasma Myoglobin in the Early Diagnosis of Acute Myocardial Infarction," *Eur J Clin Chem Clin Biochem*, 1994, 32(5):349-53.
Delanghe J, Chapelle JP, el Allaf M, et al, "Quantitative Turbidimetric Assay for Determining Myoglobin Evaluated," *Clin J Clin Biochem*, 1991, 28(Pt 5):474-9.
Kasik JW, Leuschen MP, Bolam DL, et al, "Rhabdomyolysis and Myoglobinemia in Neonates," *Pediatrics*, 1985, 76(2):255-8.
Klootwijk P, Cobbaert C, Fioretti P, et al, "Noninvasive Assessment of Reperfusion and Reocclusion After Thrombolysis in Acute Myocardial Infarction," *Am J Cardiol*, 1993, 72(19):75G-84G.
Lee HS, Cross SJ, Garthwaite P, et al, "Comparison of the Value of Novel Rapid Measurement of Myoglobin, Creatine Kinase, and Creatine Kinase-MB With the Electrocardiogram for the Diagnosis of Acute Myocardial Infarction," *Br Heart J*, 1994, 71(4):311-5.
Mair J, Smidt J, Artner-Dworzak E, et al, "Rapid Diagnosis of Myocardial Infarction by Immunoturbidimetric Myoglobin Measurement," *Lancet*, 1991, 337(8753):1343-4.
Miyata M, Abe S, Arima S, et al, "Rapid Diagnosis of Coronary Reperfusion by Measurement of Myoglobin Level Every 15 Min in Acute Myocardial Infarction," *J Am Coll Cardiol*, 1994, 23(5):1009-15.
Seguin J, Saussine M, Ferriere M, et al, "Comparison of Myoglobin and Creatine Kinase MB Levels in the Evaluation of Myocardial Injury After Cardiac Operations," *J Thorac Cardiovasc Surg*, 1988, 95(2):294-7.
Serrano S, Chueca P, Carrasco E, et al, "Predictive Value of Myoglobin in Early Diagnosis of Acute Myocardial Infarction," *Ann Emerg Med*, 1990, 19(8):953.
Silva DP Jr, Landt Y, Porter SE, et al, "Development and Application of Monoclonal Antibodies to Human Cardiac Myoglobin in A Rapid Fluorescence Immunoassay," *Clin Chem*, 1991, 37(8):1356-64.
Vrenna L, Castaldo AM, Castaldo P, et al, "Comparison Between Nephelometric and RIA Methods for Serum Myoglobin, and Efficiency of Myoglobin Assay for Early Diagnosis of Myocardial Infarction," *Clin Chem*, 1992, 38(5):789-90.

Na+ *see* Sodium, Blood *on page 199*

NAG *see* Beta-Hexosaminidase, Serum *on page 85*

Naproxen *see* Porphyrins, Quantitative, Urine *on page 186*

Na, Urine *see* Sodium, Urine *on page 199*

Nephrogenous Cyclic AMP *see* Cyclic AMP, Plasma *on page 119*

Nephrogenous Cyclic AMP *see* Cyclic AMP, Urine *on page 119*

Neurofibrillary Tangles *see* Apolipoprotein E *on page 82*

Neuron-Specific Enolase, Serum

CPT 83520

Synonyms NSE; S-NSE

Abstract The gamma-gamma isoenzyme of enolase is found only in neuronal tissue (including cells of neuroendocrine origin). Serum levels may be elevated in processes characterized by nerve cell or neuroendocrine cell destruction, including neoplasms of neural or neuroendocrine origin. Serum levels may be useful as a marker for small cell carcinoma of lung, for staging of such tumors, and for monitoring for relapse after therapy.

Specimen Serum

Container Red top tube

Collection Must avoid hemolysis. Place blood on ice immediately after collecting.

Storage Instructions Centrifuge within 30-45 minutes. Maintain at 4°C and analyze same day or freeze at -70°C until assayed.

Causes for Rejection Specimen with hemolysis (RBCs contain γγ-enolase)

Turnaround Time Approximately 1 week, as this analysis will be performed by a reference laboratory in most situations

Reference Range 0-9 ng/mL (RIA method);[1] 1-6 ng/mL (EIA method);[3] method and laboratory variable

Use May have a role in evaluation of neoplasms of neural or neuroectodermal derivation (eg, small cell carcinoma of lung, neuroblastoma, and others); monitoring therapy and detection of relapse; not of use in screening for early stages of such neoplasms

Methodology Radioimmunoassay (RIA), enzyme immunoassay (EIA), immunobioluminescence assay

Additional Information Enolase, one of the enzymes of the glycolytic pathway, exists in the serum as a number of isomeric variants. The enzyme exists as an intracytoplasmic dimer accounting for up to 3% of soluble protein in some tissues. There are three distinct subunits, α, β, and γ, five isoenzymes have been identified, αα, ββ, γγ, αβ, and αγ. β-enolase (ββ isomer) is found in muscle, hybrid forms (αα, αβ) are found in megakaryocytes and platelets. The gamma-gamma isoenzyme appears to be found largely in neural tissue. This enzyme is released into the CSF when neural tissue is injured. Neoplasms derived from neural or neuroendocrine tissue may release NSE into the blood. The test may have value in prediction of response to therapy. In a group of 13 patients with small cell carcinoma of lung, very high levels of NSE (≥100 ng/mL, mean of 490 ng/mL) were found in seven of eight responders. Levels <100 ng/mL (mean 28 ng/mL) were found in the remaining six patients, only two of whom were responders. These values are from samples obtained during the first 3-day course of chemotherapy. There is evidence that the level of serum neuron-specific enolase correlates with tumor burden.[1] Increase occurs more commonly and is at higher levels in advanced stage than in limited stage disease.

Serum NSE levels are increased in cases of neuroblastoma but also in other certain childhood tumors. Levels >100 ng/mL in children are, however, highly suggestive of advanced neuroblastoma. Use of NSE to monitor treated neuroblastoma patients has not been found to be a sensitive index of residual tumor. NSE levels may also be increased in some patients with seminoma[2] and some patients with uremia who have been on dialysis. The specificity of serum neuron-specific enolase may not yet be clearly established. In immunocytochemistry, its specificity leaves a great deal to be desired. Levels of this enzyme in spinal fluid seems to correlate with levels of S-100 protein and myelin basic protein in patients with neurological lesions.[3]

The time course of plasma NSE appears to be correlated with clinical findings and clinical outcome during the first 72 hours of a cerebral infarct or cerebral hypoxia-ischemia event.[4]

Footnotes
1. Anastasiades KD, Mullins RE, and Conn RB, "Neuron-Specific Enolase. Assessment by ELISA in Patients With Small Cell Carcinoma of the Lung," *Am J Clin Pathol*, 1987, 87(2):245-9.
2. Kuzmits R, Schernthaner G, and Krisch K, "Serum Neuron-Specific Enolase. A Marker for Response to Therapy in Seminoma," *Cancer*, 1987, 60(5):1017-21.
3. van Engelen BG, Lamers KJ, Gabreels FJ, et al, "Age-Related Changes of Neuron-Specific Enolase, S-100 Protein, and Myelin Basic Protein Concentrations in Cerebrospinal Fluid," *Clin Chem*, 1992, 38(6):813-6.
4. Schaarschmidt H, Prange HW, and Reiber H, "Neuron-Specific Enolase Concentrations in Blood as a Prognostic Parameter in Cerebrovascular Diseases," *Stroke*, 1994, 25(3):558-65.

References
Chen CA, Wu CC, Juang GT, et al, "Serum Neuron Specific Enolase Levels in Patients With Small Cell Carcinoma of the Uterine Cervix," *J Formos Med Assoc*, 1994, 93(1):81-3.
Kaiser E, Kuzmits R, Pregnant P, et al, "Clinical Biochemistry of Neuron Specific Enolase," *Clin Chim Acta*, 1989, 183(1):13-31.
Prados MC, Alvarez-Sala R, Blasco R, et al, "The Clinical Value of Neuron-Specific Enolase as a Tumor Marker in Bronchoalveolar Lavage," *Cancer*, 1994, 74(5):1552-5.
Virji MA, Mercer DW, and Herberman RB, "Tumor Markers in Cancer Diagnosis and Prognosis," *CA Cancer J Clin*, 1988, 38:105-26.

Newborn Screen for Phenylketonuria

CPT 84030

Related Information
Newborn Screen for T$_4$ *on next page*
Phenylalanine, Blood *on page 181*
Phenylalanine Test, Urine *on page 647*

Synonyms Phenylketonuria, Newborn Screen; PKU, Neonatal

Applies to Phenylalanine Hydroxylase Activity

Test Commonly Includes Phenylalanine screen using filter paper collection. Sample for newborn screen for congenital hypothyroidism is usually obtained at the same time.

Abstract Autosomal recessive aminoacidopathy due to phenylalanine hydroxylase or biopterin (folic acid constituent) cofactor deficiencies.

Detection by low cost dried blood spot screening can result in early treatment, intended to prevent mental retardation.

Patient Preparation Newborns should have milk (protein) feeding ideally for 48 hours before testing; sample as late as possible prior to discharge from hospital. Blood should be obtained 2-4 days after birth. Collection is recommended at 4-10 days for low birth weight infants.

Specimen Whole blood, serum or plasma

Container Newborns: PKU test card; screening: filter paper sheet. Pediatrics: Small red top tube, gray top (sodium fluoride) tube or green top (heparin) tube; check with the laboratory.

Sampling Time Just before infant is discharged from the nursery

Collection Test card must be labeled with patient's name, date, time, date of birth, and time of first milk feeding. In order to obtain accurate test results for PKU, blood collection should preferably be made when the infant is 48-120 hours of age and has been on a protein feeding for at least 24 hours. Do not oversaturate filter paper. Do not fill circles on one side and then fill circles on reverse side. Do not collect blood with a capillary tube to apply to filter paper. Include information regarding blood transfusions and antibiotics or other medications administered to the infant, which may influence screening test results.

Storage Instructions Newborns: Air dry specimens at room temperature in a horizontal position for at least 2 hours. Do not use hermetically sealed envelopes. Pediatrics: Separate serum and transfer to a plastic vial containing 10 mg NaF. (Check with the laboratory for other possible specimen requirements.) Separate within 4 hours of collection. Serum or plasma is stable 5 days at 4°C. Care in handling the filter paper specimens is essential, because exposure to extreme heat or light or touching the filter paper portion of the form can cause erroneous test results. Specimens containing contaminants, such as alcohol or other liquids, or antibiotics may not be satisfactory for testing. (See following discussion.) The phenylalanine in filter paper dried blood spots is stable for years when not exposed to environmental extremes.

Causes for Rejection Filter paper not thoroughly saturated, inadequate specimen identification, specimens which are respotted (several drops of blood applied to the same circle), specimens which are QNS (quantity not sufficient). **Cord blood cannot be sued. Phenylalanine is not significantly increased at birth.** Blood should **not** be drawn before milk diet of at least 24 hours prior to sampling, but need to sample before discharge from the nursery may take priority if outpatient sampling is not assured.

Reference Range Phenylalanine: ≤2 mg/dL (SI: ≤121 µmol/L) by Guthrie bacterial inhibition assay; <4 mg/dL (SI: <242 µmol/L) by fluorometry in some laboratories.

Possible Panic Range Phenylalanine: ≥4 mg/dL (SI: ≥242 µmol/L) by Guthrie bacterial inhibition assay. Specific diagnosis after identification of a candidate case (by screening program) requires that plasma levels of phenylalanine be >2 mg/dL (SI: >121 µmol/L) on 2 consecutive days.

Use Screen for PKU in newborns (mandatory in many areas); prevent mental retardation by early diagnosis. Siblings of children with PKU, PHP (persistent hyperphenylalaninemias) deserve special priority.[1]

Limitations When a baby is discharged early (before 72 hours of age), many states, hospitals, and physicians prefer to take a sample early, rather than risk no sample at all.[1] Early sampling for **PKU** risks some false-negative results. Essentially all phenylketonurics may be positive within the first 24 hours if a cutoff of 2 mg/dL is used.[2] Subclassification of phenylalanine hydroxylase deficiency can be made based on blood phenylalanine levels.[3] Identification of non-PKU forms of hyperphenylalaninemia (see following information) requires additional testing for tetrahydrobiopterin pathway enzyme defects. **Not all individuals with increased blood phenylalanine have phenylketonuria.** When an infant is tested for PKU before 24 hours of age, there is a 16% chance of missing a postive case. When screened between 24 and 72 hours of age, there is a 4% chance of missing a positive.[2] If screening (PKU) occurs before 24 hours of life, rescreening should be done. Sick and/or premature infants should be screened (PKU) by age 7 days independent of feeding history or antibiotic therapy.[1]

Any inadequate specimen must be repeated.

Screening must be integrated with follow-up, confirmation of diagnosis, and treatment. Problems have included failure to screen all neonates and imperfect compliance with follow-up screening.

Methodology Guthrie method is widely used for neonatal PKU testing. Phenylalanine can also be quantitated by fluorometry. False-positive PKU tests due to antibiotic usage, in particular ampicillin, have been noted and methods for their avoidance (use of penicillinase in test agar or fixing with formic acid vapors) have been reported.[4,5,6]

Additional Information Successful detection of phenylketonuria by screening newborns for hyperphenylalaninemia has as its goal the identification of infants subject to central nervous system damage (in particular mental retardation) due to excessive levels of phenylalanine. (Continued)

Newborn Screen for Phenylketonuria (Continued)

Once identified, harmful CNS effects can be largely avoided by dietary measures, notably a semisynthetic diet low in phenylalanine. In young PKU patients, the tolerance for dietary phenylalanine (to maintain nontoxic plasma levels) is about 250-550 mg/day. Widespread institution of PKU screening programs, worldwide, is an outstanding public health triumph of the 20th century. Incidence is 1:10,000 to 1:25,000 in the United States. For African-Americans in Maryland, the reported incidence is 1;50,000.

Scriver and Clow indicate that an adequate sample is obtained from a term neonate at least 24 hours after milk feeding is started and as close to hospital discharge as possible. For the premature infant, they define an adequate sample as one obtained between the fifth and seventh days of life.[7]

The standard is established that all infants be tested for PKU and congenital hypothyroidism (see listing Newborn Screen for T$_4$ on **page 170) prior to discharge.**

Presence of hyperphenylalaninemia implies a disorder of phenylalanine hydroxylation (to tyrosine). PKU due to phenylalanine hydroxylase (PAH) deficiency is the common example. However, in addition to PAH, hydroxylation requires oxygen and tetrahydrobiopterin (BH$_4$) as a cofactor. A defect in the metabolism of BH$_4$ that results in BH$_4$ deficiency will impair hydroxylation and result in increased plasma phenylalanine concentrations. In the past 15 years, three types of inborn errors of BH$_4$ metabolism ("atypical PKU") have been identified. Defects in BH$_4$ synthesis are guanosine triphosphate cyclohydrolase I deficiency and pyruvoyl tetrahydropterin synthase deficiency. The third type of defect involves the regeneration of BH$_4$ catalyzed by the enzyme dihydropteridine reductase. Experience with treatment of PKU over the past 25 years has shown that some 3% (variable between different populations) fail to respond. These are largely cases of BH$_4$ cofactor deficiency> There are important differences in therapy between classical PKU and the various BH$_4$ cofactor deficiencies. "PKU positive" cases (identified as the result of phenylalanine screening tests) should be additionally tested for BH$_4$ deficiency.

To maintain intellectual function, the importance of long-term (eg, beyond 10 years) dietary control of the blood phenylalanine level has been recently re-emphasized. Significant phenylalanine hydroxylation in vivo in PKU homozygotes has been demonstrated. Such findings suggest significant alternative pathway activity such as tyrosine hydroxylase. Promotion of such latent hydroxylating capabilities may eventually lead to therapies which will complement phenylalanine restriction.

Spuriously high blood phenylalanine levels (false-positives) may occur with Guthrie test screening due to uninterpretable "clear zone" effect, the result of antibiotics (usually ampicillin). Because of an increase in the number of cases and amounts of the awards in litigation involving PKU screening (usually false-negative cases), vagaries of PKU testing, while uncommon, are of considerable import and generate comment and innovation.

Intrauterine fetal injury results from exposure of the developing fetus to increased intrapartum maternal plasma phenylalanine levels. There is a high incidence of resultant fetal damage including microcephaly, intrauterine growth retardation, mental retardation, and congenital heart disease, as a result of maternal hyperphenylalaninemia. Dietary management of mothers identified by newborn screening programs has as its goal the maintenance of near normal maternal phenylalanine levels throughout pregnancy. In order to retain the achievements of over three decades of early detection and treatment of PKU, increasing attention is being turned to control of maternal hyperphenylalaninemia. The risk of maternal phenylketonuria and hyperphenylalaninemia syndrome is increasing. There is a nearly 100% risk of recurrence if treatment is not given. A number of suggestions have been made to deal with the grwoing problem of maternal PKU including use of genetic registers. High performance liquid chromatography and polymerase chain reaction based tests have been suggested to screen for carriers of PKU.[8,9]

A Japanese study reports a cost to benefit ratio of 1:2.5 for PKU testing.[10]

Footnotes

1. American Academy of Pediatrics, Committee on Genetics, "Newborn Screening Fact Sheets: Congenital Hypothyroidism," Pediatrics, 1989, 83(3):454-6, 461-2.
2. Doherty LB, Rohr FJ, and Levy HL, "Detection of Phenylketonuria in the Very Early Newborn Blood Specimen," Pediatrics, 1991, 87(2):240-4.
3. Matalon R and Michals K, "Phenylketonuria: Screening, Treatment, and Maternal PKU," Clin Biochem, 1991, 24(4):337-42.
4. Mabry CC, Reid MC, and Kuhn RJ, "A Source of Error in Phenylketonuria Screening," Am J Clin Pathol, 1988, 90(3):279-83.
5. Wilcken B, Brown AR, Liu A, et al, "Eliminating Some Possible Errors in Phenylketonuria Screening," Am J Clin Pathol, 1989, 92(3):396.
6. Kremensky I and Kalaydjieva L, "Avoiding Sources of Error in PKU Screening," Am J Clin Pathol, 1989, 92(3):396-7.
7. Scriver CR and Clow CL, "Phenylketonuria: Epitome of Human Biochemical Genetics," N Engl J Med, 1989, 303:1336-42, 1394-400.

8. Hilton MA, Sharpe JN, Hicks LG, et al, "A Simple Method for Detection of Heterozygous Carriers of the Gene for Classic Phenylketonuria," J Pediatr, 1986, 109(4):601-4.
9. Eisnesmith RC, Goltsov AA, and Woo SLC, "A Simple, Rapid, and Highly Informative PCR-Based Procedure for Prenatal Diagnosis and Carrier Screening of Phenylketonuria," Prenat Diagn, 1994, 14:1113-8.
10. Hisashige A, "Health Economic Analysis of Neonatal Screening Program in Japan," Int J Technol Assess Health Care, 1994, 10(3):382-91.

References

Koch R, Levy HL, Matalon R, et al, "The North American Collaborative Study of Maternal Phenylketonuria. Status Report 1993," Am J Dis Child, 1993, 147(11):1224-30.

Levy HL, Lobbregt D, Sansaricq C, et al, "Comparison of Phenylketonuric and Nonphenylketonuric Sibs From Untreated Pregnancies in a Mother With Phenylketonuria," Am J Med Genet, 1992, 44(4):439-42.

Mabry CC, "Phenylketonuria: Contemporary Screening and Diagnosis," Ann Clin Lab Sci, 1990, 20(6):393-7.

Michals K, Azen C, Acosta P, et al, "Blood Phenylalanine Levels and Intelligence of 10-Year-Old Children With PKU in the National Collaborative Study," J Am Diet Assoc, 1988, 88(10):1226-9.

Scriver CR, "Whatever Happened to PKU?" Clin Biochem, 1995, 28(2):137-44.

Waisbren SE, Mahon BE, Schnell RR, et al, "Predictors of Intelligence Quotient and Intelligence Quotient Change in Persons Treated for Phenylketonuria Early in Life," Pediatrics, 1987, 79(3):351-5.

Wilcken B, Brown AR, Liu A, et al, "Eliminating Some Possible Errors in Phenylketonuria Screening," Am J Clin Pathol, 1989, 92(3):396.

Newborn Screen for T$_4$

CPT 84437

Related Information

Galactose Screening Tests for Galactosemia on page 132
Newborn Screen for Phenylketonuria on previous page
Phenylalanine, Blood on page 181
Thyroglobulin, Serum on page 203
Thyroid Stimulating Hormone Screen, Filter Paper on page 205

Synonyms T$_4$ Neonatal; Thyroid Screen for Newborns

Abstract Newborns with congenital hypothyroidism, characterized by low serum T$_4$ and high TSH, must be identified early. Screening for congenital hypothyroidism now occurs in all 50 states. The importance of newborn screening for hypothyroid case detection and early initiation of treatment has led to filter paper screening programs of T$_4$ and/or TSH in many countries of the world. If hypothyroidism is undetected, growth and mental retardation occur, and in rare instances, death.

Specimen Whole blood. Unlike PKU testing, cord blood is satisfactory. Heel blood at discharge is also acceptable.

Container Special filter paper collection card

Sampling Time T$_4$ peaks at 24 hours

Collection Obtain heelstick whole blood sample and thoroughly saturate circles on the filter paper. Label the card with the patient's name, age, and physician. Prompt collection and processing of infants' blood samples is crucial to early detection of these disorders. Steps for collection: Warm the foot and/or massage the leg. Clean the puncture site with an alcohol swab, then dry with a sterile sponge to remove alcohol. Puncture the infant's heel with a sterile lancet <2.5 mm. Wipe away the first drop of blood. Touch the filter paper to the drops and allow them to flow onto the filter paper and diffuse through the circles. Apply a sterile covering to the site.

Causes for Rejection Filter paper not thoroughly saturated, radioactive tracer given to baby before the sample is obtained, specimens which are QNS (quantity not sufficient), exposure of card to extreme heat or light or touching the filter paper portion of the form can cause erroneous test results

Special Instructions The T$_4$ specimen is usually collected at the same time the PKU specimen is obtained. Optimal collection time is 3-7 days after birth, when the baby has been on protein feeding for 24 hours (ie, usually just before discharge); 4-10 days after birth recommended for low birth weight infants. With early release (less than 24 hours postdelivery), babies must be brought back to the physician's office for thyroid screening

Reference Range T$_4$ results in infancy are higher than adult ranges. Thyroxine levels are lower in prematures. Peak occurs at about 24 hours; then T$_4$ decreases. Newborns that have a low T$_4$ are tested for TSH. For infants 1-2 weeks old: 10-17 µg/dL.

Possible Panic Range Low result for T$_4$; high TSH. Abnormal value for infants 7 days old or younger: T$_4$ ≤6.5 µg/dL (SI: ≤84 nmol/L); for infants 8 days old and older: T$_4$ ≤5.0 µg/dL (SI: ≤64 nmol/L). See report of individual laboratory.

Use Screen for congenital hypothyroidism

Limitations Congenital thyroglobulin deficiency will result in low T$_4$ values even though the patient is euthyroid. TSH is low in TBG deficiency but T$_3$ uptake is high.[1] TSH is more sensitive for primary hypothyroidism. The risk of a false-negative result is increased when subjects with incomplete absence of thyroid parenchyma are screened only by T$_4$.

Methodology Radioimmunoassay (RIA). Thyroxine value may be determined from filter paper discs saturated with whole blood. Some laboratories do TSH to screen for congenital hypothyroidism, others do a T_4 as is done for adults, and most use the filter paper disc method.

Additional Information There is evidence that growth becomes thyroid hormone dependent immediately after birth. Decreased growth rate, short stature, and abnormal epiphyseal maturation are clinical features of thyroid deficiency. While height may be normal at birth, growth velocity is decreased during the first weeks of life, increasing after the start of therapy.[2] Patients who are not detected and who do not receive early therapy will develop mental retardation, variable growth failure, metabolic changes of hypothyroidism, deafness, and neurologic abnormalities. There is a higher incidence of detection from screening programs than from clinical surveillance since clinical signs in the great majority of cases are minimal at birth. Timing of sampling, retesting, and hazards of screening are important considerations.[3] Transient hypothyroxinemia and transient hyperthyroxinemia occur.[1]

If low values are obtained, the patient must have confirmatory tests run: T_4, TSH, sometimes T_3 uptake, and possibly TBG assessment. For rescreening, combined T_4 and TSH is recommended, when the initial T_4 is low.[3] Excessive quantities of TBG result in increased T_4, while deficiency in TBG has the opposite effect. Extrathyroidal conditions resulting in depressed T_4 levels include low birth weight (LBW). In normal as well as LBW infants, the T_4 will be lower, between 5 and 9 days, compared to 3-5 days after birth. The incidence of permanent abnormalities leading to hypothyroidism is approximately 1:3600-5000 live births (as determined by screening tests in the United States).[3] The incidence of congenital hypothyroidism in Bohemia/Moravia since 1985 is 1:5700 of live newborn infants.[4] In a Netherlands study, the incidence of total organification defect (an autosomal process) was about 1 in 60,000 neonates.[5] **Seven million newborns are screened annually for hypothyroidism. Three hundred and sixty are spared delayed growth and severe mental retardation while 1200 more babies avoid subnormal intelligence with early diagnosis.**[6]

Footnotes
1. Howanitz JH, Howanitz PJ, and Henry JB, "Evaluation of Endocrine Function," *Todd-Sanford-Davidsohn Clinical Diagnosis and Management by Laboratory Methods*, 18th ed, Henry JB, ed, Philadelphia, PA: WB Saunders Co, 1991, 308-20.
2. Leger J and Czernichow P, "Congenital Hypothyroidism: Decreased Growth Velocity in the First Week of Life," *Biol Neonate*, 1989, 55(4-5):218-23.
3. American Academy of Pediatrics, Committee on Genetics, "Newborn Screening Fact Sheets," *Pediatrics*, 1989, 83(3):449-64.
4. Hnikova O, Kracmar P, Zelenka Z, et al, "Screening of Congenital Hypothyroidism in Newborns in Bohemia and Moravia," *Endocrinol Exp*, 1989, 23(2):117-23.
5. Vulsma T, Gons MH, and de Vijlder JJM, "Maternal-Fetal Transfer of Thyroxine in Congenital Hypothyroidism Due to a Total Organification Defect or Thyroid Agenesis," *N Engl J Med*, 1989, 321(1):13-6.
6. Willi SM and Moshang T Jr, "Diagnostic Dilemmas. Results of Screening Tests for Congenital Hypothyroidism," *Pediatr Clin North Am*, 1991, 38(3):555-66.

References
Burrow GN, Fisher DA, and Larsen PR, "Maternal and Fetal Thyroid Function," *N Engl J Med*, 1994, 331(16):1072-8.
Fisher DA, "Euthyroid Low Thyroxine (T_4) and Triiodothyronine (T_3) States in Premature and Sick Neonates," *Pediatr Clin North Am*, 1990, 37(6):1297-312.
Gravdal JA, Meenan A, and Dyson AE, "Congenital Hypothyroidism," *J Fam Pract*, 1989, 29(1):47-50.
Gruters A, "Congenital Hypothyroidism," *Pediatr Ann*, 1992, 21(1):15, 18-21, 24-8.
La Franchi SH, Hanna CE, Krainz PL, et al, "Screening for Congenital Hypothyroidism With Specimen Collection at Two Time Periods: Results of the Northwest Regional Screening Program," *Pediatrics*, 1985, 76(5):734-40.

NH₃, Blood see Ammonia, Blood on page 75

NH$_3$, Blood see Ammonia, Blood *on page 75*

Nitroprusside Reaction, Blood see Ketone Bodies, Blood *on page 152*

Nitroprusside Screening see Cystine, Urine *on page 120*

Norepinephrine see Metanephrines *on page 165*

Norepinephrine, Urine see Catecholamines, Fractionation, Urine *on page 104*

NSE see Neuron-Specific Enolase, Serum *on page 168*

5'NT see 5' Nucleotidase *on this page*

5' Nucleotidase

CPT 83915

Related Information
Alkaline Phosphatase, Serum *on page 69*
Gamma Glutamyl Transferase *on page 133*
Leucine Aminopeptidase *on page 158*
Synovial Fluid Analysis *on page 656*

Synonyms Ecto-5'NT; 5'NT

Replaces BSP

Abstract A plasma membrane enzyme relevant to the biliary tract. The test is not widely available.

Patient Preparation A fasting specimen is preferred.

Specimen Serum, synovial fluid

Container Red top tube

Storage Instructions Stable 4 days at 4°C or 3 months at -20°C. Unstable at room temperature.

Reference Range Varies with laboratory. Serum: 5-10 units/L (kinetic).

Use Like GGT and LAP, 5' nucleotidase is used to investigate the origin of increased serum alkaline phosphatase. It is a liver-related enzyme used to work up cholestatic/biliary obstruction. It parallels the increases of alkaline phosphatase and leucine aminopeptidase in hepatobiliary diseases, but is not usually elevated in skeletal disorders such as Paget's disease of bone. It is useful in pregnancy. It is increased with metastatic neoplasia in the liver, primary biliary cirrhosis, and biliary obstruction secondary to calculi or tumor. *Vide infra*.

Limitations Some feel that 5' nucleotidase and leucine aminopeptidase offer little which is not provided by GGT.

Methodology Varies widely. Activity is generally measured by hydrolyzing a particular nucleotide such as 5'-AMP, 5'-CMP, or 5'-IMP. Detection methods include detecting inorganic phosphate measured by a molybdate color reaction, detecting nucleoside reaction products after separation by high performance liquid chromatography, coupled reactions to detect ammonia, NADH, or urate, or radioligand release.[1] A method for measuring 5'NT cytosolic activity uses coupled reactions utilizing cytidine monophosphate as substrate, cytidine deaminase, and uridine nucleosidase, measuring ultraviolet differential absorption between CMP and uracil, the latter one of the end products of the coupled reactions.[2]

Additional Information 5' Nucleotidase comprises a group of widely distributed enzymes that are found in both prokaryotic and eukaryotic organisms. It is located predominantly on plasma membranes in mammalian cells. In lymphocytes, hepatocytes, and placental cells, 5'NT is located on the external surface of the cell membrane and may be classified as an ectoenzyme "ecto-5'NT". 5'NT is probably a metalloprotein with zinc as the likely native constituent metal. Human erythrocytes contain at least two cytosolic 5'NT activities; several isoenzymes of erythrocyte pyrimidine 5'NT have been characterized. Primary function of ecto-5'NT is conversion of impermeable extracellular nucleotides to corresponding nucleotides which are permeable, and may be utilized as metabolic substrates or modulators (eg, adenosine).[1] ·

Isoforms of 5'NT with α_1-electrophoretic mobility vary inversely with serum bile acid concentrations. They increase in serum after surgical correction of biliary obstruction.[3] In rabbits myocardial activity of 5'NT is associated with improved postischemic recovery of ventricular functions.[4] Patients with multiple myeloma have increased numbers of plasma cells with cytoplasmic 5'NT activity when compared to control patients or patients with monoclonal gammopathy of undetermined significance.[5] Such determinations of plasma cell 5'NT activity are not currently used to study myeloma. 5'NT activity is increased in synovial fluid of patients with calcium pyrophosphate dehydrate deposition. Synovial fluid 5'NT activity is greater in patients with osteoarthritis compared to those with gout, pseudogout, or rheumatoid arthritis.[6] 5'NT activity has been shown to be increased in the myofiber interstitium in polymyositis.[7] Prostate epithelium in benign prostatic hyperplasia appears to express high levels of 5'NT activity compared with prostatic carcinomas.[8]

5' Nucleotidase did not change between the first and third trimesters of pregnancy in a study of 219 pregnant women.[9]

In patients receiving antiepileptic drugs, the frequency of enzyme elevation was similar to that of alkaline phosphatase but lower than that of GGT.[10]

Footnotes
1. Sunderman FW Jr, "The Clinical Biochemistry of 5'-Nucleotidase," *Ann Clin Lab Sci*, 1990, 20(2):123-39.
2. Amici A, Natalini P, Ruggieri S, et al, "A Spectrophotometric Method for the Assay of Pyrimidine 5'-Nucleotidase in Human Erythrocytes," *Br J Haematol*, 1989, 73(3):392-5.
3. Novo FJ and Tutor JC, "Changes in Alkaline Phosphatase and 5'-Nucleotidase Multiple Forms After Surgical Management of Biliary Obstruction," *Clin Chem*, 1992, 38(7):1340-2.
4. Grosso MA, Banerjee A, St Cyr JA, et al, "Cardiac 5'-Nucleotidase Activity Increases With Age and Inversely Relates to Recovery from Ischemia," *J Thorac Cardiovasc Surg*, 1992, 103(2):206-9.
5. Majumdar G, Heard SE, and Singh AK, "Use of Cytoplasmic 5' Nucleotidase for Differentiating Malignant From Benign Monoclonal Gammopathies," *J Clin Pathol*, 1990, 43(11):891-2.
6. Wortmann RL, Veum JA, and Rachow JW, "Synovial Fluid 5'-Nucleotidase Activity - Relationship to Other Purine Catabolic Enzymes and to Arthropathies Associated With Calcium Crystal Deposition," *Arthritis Rheum*, 1991, 34(8):1014-20.
7. Hilton DA, Eagles ME, and Fletcher A, "Histochemical Demonstration of 5'-Nucleotidase Activity in Inflammatory Muscle Disease," *Arch Pathol Lab Med*, 1991, 115(4):362-4.
8. Rackley RR, Lewis TJ, Preston EM, et al, "5'-Nucleotidase Activity in Prostatic Carcinoma and Benign Prostatic Hyperplasia," *Cancer Res*, 1989, 49(13):3702-7.
9. Alvi MH, Amer NA, and Sumerin I, "Serum 5' Nucleotidase and Serum Sialic Acid in Pregnancy," *Obstet Gynecol*, 1988, 72(2):171-4.
10. Fortman CS and Witte DL, "Serum 5' Nucleotidase in Patients Receiving Antiepileptic Drugs," *Am J Clin Pathol*, 1985, 84(2):197-201.

Nutritional Status *see* Albumin, Serum *on page 66*

O₂ Capacity *see* Oxygen Saturation, Blood *on page 175*

O₂ Content *see* Oxygen Saturation, Blood *on page 175*

OD 450 Method *see* Amniotic Fluid Analysis for Erythroblastosis Fetalis (OD 450) *on page 76*

OGTT *see* Glucose Tolerance Test *on page 139*

1,25-(OH)₂ D₃ *see* Vitamin D₃, Serum *on page 218*

17-OHCS *see* 17-Hydroxycorticosteroids, Urine *on page 147*

25-(OH) D₃ *see* Vitamin D₃, Serum *on page 218*

17-OHP *see* 17-Hydroxyprogesterone, Blood or Amniotic Fluid *on page 148*

***o*-Phosphoric-Monoester Phosphohydrolase** *see* Acid Phosphatase *on page 62*

Oral Glucose Tolerance Test *see* Glucose Tolerance Test *on page 139*

Organic Acids, Urine *see* Amino Acid Screen, Plasma *on page 74*

Osmolal Gap *see* Osmolality, Calculated *on this page*

Osmolal Gap *see* Osmolality, Serum *on this page*

Osmolal Gap *see* Sodium, Blood *on page 199*

Osmolal Gap, Urine *see* Osmolality, Urine *on next page*

Osmolality, Calculated

CPT 83930

Related Information

Alcohol, Blood or Urine *on page 531*
Anion Gap *on page 81*
Creatinine, Serum *on page 118*
Electrolytes, Serum or Plasma *on page 123*
Ethylene Glycol *on page 550*
HCO₃, Blood *on page 142*
Ketone Bodies, Blood *on page 152*
Ketones, Urine *on page 639*
Lactic Acid, Blood *on page 156*
Osmolality, Serum *on this page*
pH, Blood *on page 180*
Sodium, Blood *on page 199*
Urea Nitrogen, Blood *on page 213*
Urinalysis *on page 658*

Applies to Holmes Formula; Osmolal Gap; Weisberg Formula

Test Commonly Includes Sodium, urea nitrogen (BUN), glucose

Abstract The **osmolal gap**, the difference between measured serum osmolality and calculated serum osmolality, is useful for demonstration of the presence of osmotically active molecules within serum not attributable to electrolytes, glucose, or serum urea nitrogen. Use of osmolal gap may point to the presence of ethanol, other osmotically active alcohols,[1] or glycols. Calculated osmolality is not very useful by itself.

Patient Preparation Patient ideally should be fasting for 8 hours, a setting not usually possible when the need for investigation of osmolality arises.

Specimen Serum or plasma

Container Red top tube, green top (heparin) tube

Collection Keep one green top tube on ice, should a pH be needed.

Causes for Rejection Gross hemolysis

Reference Range Calculated osmolality: 275-295 mOsm/kg H₂O (SI: 275-295 mmol/kg H₂O). The normal **serum osmolal gap** is about 9-15 mOsm/kg H₂O (SI: 9-15 mmol/kg H₂O). **Measured osmolality** is usually greater than the calculated value. Osmolality may be calculated by the **Holmes formula:** $(1.86 \times sodium) + (glucose/18) + (BUN/2.8)$, expressing sodium, glucose, and BUN in conventional units. It may be rounded off as: $(2 \times sodium) + (glucose/18) + (BUN/2.8)$. **Dr Weisberg's formula:** calculated osmolality = $(2 \times sodium) + (glucose/20) + (BUN/3)$. Still another formula in use is: $(1.86 \times sodium) + (glucose/18) + (BUN/2.8) + 9$. With the latter formula, the gap should be near zero.

Possible Panic Range A gap >20 mOsm/kg H₂O (SI: >20 mmol/kg H₂O)

Use Screen, monitor electrolyte status, renal function. **Elevated osmolal gap** with decreased calculated value is found in shock, and in hyperglobulinemia and hyperlipidemia; in hyperproteinemia and hyperlipidemia water is being displaced, and serum sodium is decreased, but measured osmolality remains normal.[2] Increased osmolal gap occurs with chronic renal failure, as well as with methanol or ethanol ingestion, ketosis including diabetic ketoacidosis, mannitol therapy, and ethylene glycol toxicity. **High anion gap metabolic acidosis with large osmolal gap** is

in keeping with ethylene glycol or methyl alcohol toxicity.[3] See listing Anion Gap *on page 81*. Writing in a surgical journal, Baker describes increased gaps in two settings, acute and chronic surgical illness, the latter accompanied by decreased serum water content. The former relates to the sick cell syndrome.[2]

The osmole gap may also be helpful for confirming pseudohyponatremia and as a prognostic indicator in circulatory shock.[4]

Methodology The tests above can be done on a variety of instruments, that have in common the items necessary to calculate osmolality and to follow many of the patients seen in hospital practice, with other tests ordered as clinically indicated.

Additional Information Look for crystalluria in the urinary sediment to further investigate ethylene glycol toxicity. Calcium oxalate and/or hippurate crystals would support this impression, as would the documentation of severe high anion gap metabolic acidosis.[5] Elevated osmolal gap with normal blood pH and ketosis occurs with isopropyl alcohol intoxication.

Footnotes

1. Snyder H, Williams D, Zink B, et al, "Accuracy of Blood Ethanol Determination Using Serum Osmolality," *J Emerg Med*, 1992, 10(2):129-33.
2. Baker RJ, "Biochemical Gaps: Osmolal and Anion," *Curr Surg*, 1987, 44(5):378-81.
3. Light RT, Nelson KM, and Eckfeldt JH, "Ethylene Glycol Poisoning," *JAMA*, 1981, 246:1769.
4. Kruse JA and Cadnapaphornchai P, "The Serum Osmole Gap," *J Crit Care*, 1994, 9(3):185-97.
5. Terlinsky AS, Grochowski J, Geoly KL, et al, "Identification of Atypical Calcium Oxalate Crystalluria Following Ethylene Glycol Ingestion," *Am J Clin Pathol*, 1981, 76:223-6.

References

Emmett M and Narins RG, "Clinical Use of the Anion Gap," *Medicine (Baltimore)*, 1977, 56:38-54.
Halperin ML, Margolis BL, Robinson LA, et al, "The Urine Osmolal Gap: A Clue to Estimate Urine Ammonium in "Hybrid" Types of Metabolic Acidosis," *Clin Invest Med*, 1988, 11(3):198-202.
Hertford JA, McKenna JP, and Chamovitz BN, "Metabolic Acidosis With an Elevated Anion Gap," *Am Fam Physician*, 1989, 39(4):159-68.
Hirasawa H, Odaka M, Sugai T, et al, "Prognostic Value of Serum Osmolality Gap in Patients With Multiple Organ Failure Treated With Hemopurification," *Artif Organs*, 1988, 12(5):382-7.
Norris SH, "Quiz of the Month. Severe Acidosis and an Osmolar Gap in an Alcoholic," *Am J Nephrol*, 1989, 9(2):144, 175-6.
Oster JR, Perez GO, and Materson BJ, "Use of the Anion Gap in Clinical Medicine," *South Med J*, 1988, 81(2):229-37.
Sklar AH and Linas SL, "The Osmolal Gap in Renal Failure," *Ann Intern Med*, 1983, 98:481-2.
Sweeney TE and Beuchat CA, "Limitations of Methods of Osmometry: Measuring the Osmolality of Biological Fluids," *Am J Physiol*, 1993, 264(3 Pt 2):R469-80.
Weisberg HF, "Unraveling the Laboratory Model of a Syndrome: The Osmolality Model," *Clinician and Chemist. The Relationship of the Laboratory to the Physician*, Young DS, Hicks J, Nipper H, et al, eds, Washington, DC: American Association of Clinical Chemistry, 1979, 200-43.

Osmolality, Serum

CPT 83930

Related Information

Alcohol, Blood or Urine *on page 531*
Drugs of Abuse Testing, Urine *on page 548*
Electrolytes, Serum or Plasma *on page 123*
Ethylene Glycol *on page 550*
Ketone Bodies, Blood *on page 152*
Ketones, Urine *on page 639*
Kidney Profile *on page 153*
Lactic Acid, Blood *on page 156*
Osmolality, Calculated *on this page*
Volatile Screen *on page 579*

Synonyms Serum Osmolality

Applies to Osmolal Gap

Replaces Osmolarity

Abstract The osmolality of a solution is defined as the number of molecules or ions (particles) in a liter of solution. Osmolality is independent of particle size or charge. Nonpolar solutions yield one molecule (eg, glucose) while polar solutions yield multiples of the number of ions solubilized (eg, sodium chloride yields two ions while magnesium chloride yields three ions).

Specimen Serum

Container Red top tube

Collection Pediatrics: Blood drawn from heelstick

Storage Instructions Refrigerate or freeze serum if not run within 4 hours.

Reference Range 275-295 mOsm/kg H₂O (SI: 275-295 mmol/kg H₂O)

Possible Panic Range <265 mOsm/kg H₂O (SI: <265 mmol/kg H₂O), >320 mOsm/kg H₂O (SI: >320 mmol/kg H₂O). Result of 385 mOsm/kg H₂O (SI: 385 mmol/kg H₂O) relates to stupor in hyperglycemia. Values 400-420 mOsm/kg H₂O (SI: 400-420 mmol/kg H₂O) can relate to grand mal seizures. Values >420 mOsm/kg H₂O (SI: >420 mmol/kg H₂O) may be lethal.

Use Evaluate electrolyte and water balance, hyperosmolar status and hydration status, dehydration, acid-base balance, seizures; evaluate antidiuretic hormone function, liver disease, hyperosmolar coma. Osmolality measures the concentration of particles in solution. Freezing point depression serum osmolality with calculated osmolal gap, is useful in screening for and approximating the serum concentrations of certain low molecular weight toxins, such as ethanol, ethylene glycol, isopropanol, and methanol,[1] especially as a rapid approximation for emergent situations. See Limitations.

High serum osmolality may result from hypernatremia, dehydration, hyperglycemia, mannitol therapy, azotemia, ingestion of ethanol, methanol, ethylene glycol. Thus, osmolality has a role in toxicology and in coma evaluation. Very low birth weight infants may have elevated serum osmolality for the first week of life.[2]

Low serum osmolality may be secondary to overhydration, hyponatremia, syndrome of inappropriate antidiuretic hormone secretion (SIADH) with carcinoma of lung and other entities.

Causes of hyperosmolality, hypo-osmolality, and of factors affecting ADH are published.[3] Serum osmolality measurements do not measure the fraction of serum that is water. Osmolality measurement by freezing point depression is also indifferent to permeability of solutes to cell membranes.[4]

Limitations When vapor pressure osmometry is used, volatile solutes (eg, alcohols and glycols) may remain in the vapor phase and not be detected.[1]

Methodology Freezing point depression (more often used) or vapor pressure elevation

Additional Information Measured osmolality is usually more than calculated osmolality. If measured osmolality is more than 15 mOsm/kg H_2O (SI: >15 mmol/kg H_2O) greater than calculated, consider methanol, ethylene glycol, or ethanol ingestion or other toxicity; shock; or trauma. Elevated serum osmolality with normal sodium suggests possible hyperglycemia, uremia, or alcoholism.[3] Both serum and urine values and calculated osmolality (see Osmolality, Calculated *on page 172*) are sometimes needed. Although lactic acidosis theoretically should not contribute to the osmolal gap, increases in the osmolal gap in lactic acidosis have been reported.[5] Drugs including thiazide diuretics, steroids, cimetidine, and others have been implicated in the development of hyperosmolar hyperglycemic nonketotic coma.[6] Elevations of endogenous glycerol acetone and acetone metabolite levels are reported to be a possible cause for an increased osmolal gap in an alcoholic patient.[7] Slight elevation of serum osmolality over expected values have been reported in the elderly.[8,9] After overnight dehydration, urine/serum ratio is usually ≥3.[3] Work-up of diabetes insipidus has been discussed by Bartter and Delea.[10]

Footnotes

1. Eisen TF, Lacouture PG, and Woolf A, "Serum Osmolality in Alcohol Ingestions: Differences in Availability Among Laboratories of Teaching Hospital, Nonteaching Hospital, and Commercial Facilities," *Am J Emerg Med*, 1989, 7(3):256-9.
2. Giacoia GP, Miranda R, and West KI, "Measured vs Calculated Plasma Osmolality in Infants With Very Low Birth Weights," *Am J Dis Child*, 1992, 146(6):712-7.
3. Weisberg HF, "Unraveling the Laboratory Model of a Syndrome: The Osmolality Model," *Clinician and Chemist. The Relationship of the Laboratory to the Physician*, Young DS, Hicks J, Nipper H, et al, eds, Washington, DC: American Association of Clinical Chemistry, 1979, 200-43.
4. Gennari FJ, "Current Concepts, Serum Osmolality, Uses and Limitations," *N Engl J Med*, 1984, 310(2):102-5.
5. Schelling JR, Howard RL, Winter SD, et al, "Increased Osmolal Gap in Alcoholic Ketoacidosis and Lactic Acidosis," *Ann Intern Med*, 1990, 113(8):580-2.
6. Pope DW and Dansky D, "Hyperosmolar Hyperglycemic Nonketotic Coma," *Emerg Med Clin North Am*, 1989, 7(4):849-57.
7. Braden GL, Strayhorn CH, Germain MJ, et al, "Increased Osmolal Gap in Alcoholic Acidosis," *Arch Intern Med*, 1993, 153(20):2377-80.
8. McLean KA, O'Neill PA, Davies I, et al, "Influence of Age on Plasma Osmolality: A Community Study," *Age Ageing*, 1992, 21(1):56-60.
9. O'Neill PA, Faragher EB, Davies I, et al, "Reduced Survival With Increasing Plasma Osmolality in Elderly Continuing-Care Patients," *Age Ageing*, 1990, 19(1):68-71.
10. Bartter FC and Delea CS, "Diabetes Insipidus: Its Nature and Diagnosis," *Lab Management*, Jan 1982, 23-8.

References

Aabakken L, Johansen KS, Rydningen EB, et al, "Osmolal and Anion Gaps in Patients Admitted to an Emergency Medical Department," *Hum Exp Toxicol*, 1994, 13(2):131-4.

Baker RJ, "Biochemical Gaps: Osmolal and Anion," *Curr Surg*, 1987, 44(5):378-81.

Demedts P, Theunis L, Wauters A, et al, "Excess Serum Osmolality Gap After Ingestion of Methanol: A Methodology-Associated Phenomenon?" *Clin Chem*, 1994, 40(8):1587-90.

Galvan LA and Watts MT, "Generation of an Osmolality Gap-Ethanol Nomogram From Routine Laboratory Data," *Ann Emerg Med*, 1992, 21(11):1343-8.

Fraser CL and Arieff AI, "Fatal Central Diabetes Mellitus and Insipidus Resulting From Untreated Hyponatremia: A New Syndrome," *Ann Intern Med*, 1990, 112(2):113-9.

Leech S and Penney MD, "Correlation of Specific Gravity and Osmolality of Urine in Neonates and Adults," *Arch Dis Child*, 1987, 62(7):671-3.

Maffly RH, "Renal Function and Disorders of Water, Sodium, and Potassium Balance," *Scientific American Medicine*, Section 10, Chapter 1, Rubenstein E and Federman DD, eds, New York, NY: Scientific American Inc, 1990, 2-34.

Nose H, Mack GW, Shi XR, et al, "Role of Osmolality and Plasma Volume During Rehydration in Humans," *J Appl Physiol*, 1988, 65(1):325-31.

Penney MD and Walters G, "Are Osmolality Measurements Clinically Useful?" *Ann Clin Biochem*, 1987, 24(Pt 6):566-71.

Snyder H, Williams D, Zink B, et al, "Accuracy of Blood Ethanol Determination Using Serum Osmolality," *J Emerg Med*, 1992, 10(2):129-33.

Sweeny TE and Beuchat CA, "Limitations of Methods of Osmometry: Measuring the Osmolality of Biological Fluids," *Am J Physiol*, 1993, 264(3 Pt 2):R469-80.

Worthley LI, Guerin M, and Pain RW, "For Calculating Osmolality, the Simplest Formula Is the Best," *Anaesth Intensive Care*, 1987, 15(2):199-202.

Osmolality, Urine

CPT 83935

Related Information

Concentration Test, Urine *on page 633*
Electrolytes, Urine *on page 124*
Glucose, Quantitative, Urine *on page 635*
Glucose, Semiquantitative, Urine *on page 636*
Kidney Profile *on page 153*
Protein, Quantitative, Urine *on page 649*
Protein, Semiquantitative, Urine *on page 650*
Sodium, Urine *on page 199*
Specific Gravity, Urine *on page 653*
Urinalysis *on page 658*
Urine Collection, 24-Hour *on page 30*

Synonyms Urine Osmolality

Applies to Osmolal Gap, Urine; U/P Ratio; Urine Osmolar Gap

Abstract Osmolality is a definitive measure of urine concentration.

Specimen Random or timed urine

Storage Instructions Refrigerate

Reference Range Random urine: neonates: 75-300 mOsm/kg H_2O (SI: 75-300 mmol/kg H_2O); children and adults: 250-900 mOsm/kg H_2O (SI: 250-900 mmol/kg H_2O). Normal range of serum sodium (mmol/L) to osmolality (mOsm/kg) ratio is 0.43-0.50.[1] Patients with normal renal function after 14-hour restriction of fluids should be able to concentrate to >800 mOsm/kg H_2O (SI: >800 mmol/kg H_2O).

Critical Values <400 mOsm/kg H_2O (SI: <400 mmol/kg H_2O) is interpreted by Weisberg as severe renal impairment.[2] Prolonged dehydration may be dangerous for some patients.

Possible Panic Range <100 mOsm/kg H_2O (SI: <100 mmol/kg H_2O) in overhydration, >800 mOsm/kg H_2O (SI: >800 mmol/kg H_2O) in dehydration

Use Evaluate concentrating ability of the kidneys (eg, in acute and chronic renal failure); evaluate electrolyte and water balance; used in work-up for renal disease, syndrome of inappropriate antidiuretic hormone secretion (SIADH), and diabetes insipidus; may be used with urinalysis when patient has had radiopaque substances, has glycosuria or proteinuria;[2] evaluate dehydration, amyloidosis; estimate urinary ammonium concentrations using the urine osmolal gap and detect increased osmolality due to the presence of unusual molecules.[3] Osmolality is desirable in examination of neonatal urine when protein or glucose are present.[4]

Limitations Serum osmolality is often needed to interpret urine osmolality.

Methodology Freezing point depression

Additional Information Osmolality is a better measurement of urine concentration than specific gravity. Osmolality is a measure of renal tubular concentration, depending on the state of hydration. Simultaneous determination of urine and serum osmolalities facilitates interpretation of results. High **urinary/plasma ratio** is seen in concentrated urine. Normal ranges for the U/P ratio are given by Weisberg as approximately 0.2-4.7, and >3.0 with overnight dehydration.[2] With poor concentrating ability the ratio is low but still ≥1.0. In SIADH urine sodium and urine osmolality are high for plasma osmolality.[5] The ability of the kidney to produce a concentrated urine decreases with age.[6]

Neonatal urine osmolality is discussed in a 1987 paper. Specifically derived regression equations are advocated to predict urine osmolality from specific gravity measurements.[4] Low birthweight infants have been reported to have increased serum osmolality with normal urine osmolality.[7]

The urine osmolal gap is described as the sum of urinary concentrations of sodium, potassium, bicarbonate, chloride, glucose, and urea compared to measured urine osmolality. The gap is normally 80-100 mOsm/kg H_2O (SI: 80-100 mmol/kg H_2O) greater for measured than for calculated. Determination of the urine osmolal gap is used to characterize metabolic acidosis. High urine osmolal gap can be used semiquantitatively.[8]

Footnotes

1. Preuss HG, Podlasek SJ, and Henry JB, "Evaluation of Renal Function and Water, Electrolyte, and Acid Base Balance," *Todd-Sanford-Davidsohn Clinical Diagnosis and Management by Laboratory Methods*, 18th ed, Henry JB, ed, Philadelphia, PA: WB Saunders Co, 1991, 118-39.
2. Weisberg HF, "Unraveling the Laboratory Model of a Syndrome: The Osmolality Model," *Clinician and Chemist. The Relationship of the Laboratory to the Physician*, Young DS, Hicks J, Nipper H, et al, eds, Washington, DC: American Association of Clinical Chemistry, 1979, 200-43.

(Continued)

Osmolality, Urine *(Continued)*

3. Kamel KS, Ethier JH, Richardson RM, et al, "Urine Electrolytes and Osmolality: When and How to Use Them," *Am J Nephrol*, 1990, 10(2):89-102.
4. Leech S and Penney MD, "Correlation of Specific Gravity and Osmolality of Urine in Neonates and Adults," *Arch Dis Child*, 1987, 62(7):671-3.
5. Kovacs L and Robertson GL, "Syndrome of Inappropriate Antidiuretics," *Endocrinol Metab Clin North Am*, 1992, 21(4):859-75.
6. O'Neill PA and McLean KA, "Water Homeostasis and Aging," *Med Lab Sci*, 1992, 49:291-8.
7. Giacoia GP, Miranda R, and West KI, "Measured vs Calculated Plasma Osmolality in Infants With Very Low Birth Weights," *Am J Dis Child*, 1992, 146(6):712-7.
8. Halperin ML, Margolis BL, Robinson LA, et al, "The Urine Osmolal Gap: A Clue to Estimate Urine Ammonium in "Hybrid" Types of Metabolic Acidosis," *Clin Invest Med*, 1988, 11(3):198-202.

References

Davis BB and Zenser TV, "Evaluation of Renal Concentrating and Diluting Ability," *Clin Lab Med*, 1993, 13(1):131-4.
Fraser CL and Arieff AI, "Fatal Central Diabetes Mellitus and Insipidus Resulting From Untreated Hyponatremia: A New Syndrome," *Ann Intern Med*, 1990, 112(2):113-9.

Osmolarity *replaced by* Osmolality, Serum *on page 172*

Osteocalcin, Serum

Related Information

Alkaline Phosphatase Isoenzymes *on page 69*
Alkaline Phosphatase, Serum *on page 69*
Aluminum, Bone *on page 586*
Calcium, Serum *on page 97*
Parathyroid Hormone *on page 178*
Vitamin D₃, Serum *on page 218*

Synonyms BGP; Bone GLA Protein

Abstract An important bone protein, a portion of the organic matrix synthesized by osteoblasts, and a sensitive marker for bone metabolism. Increased serum levels reflect osteoblastic synthesis.

Patient Preparation Avoid radioactive scans and other tracers prior to specimen collection.

Specimen Serum

Container Red top tube

Sampling Time Circadian rhythms: peak at night, nadir in morning; fasting specimen drawn in the morning is best.

Storage Instructions Stable frozen.

Special Instructions Usually sent to reference laboratory.

Reference Range Adults: male: 3.0-13.0 ng/mL; female: premenopausal: 0.4-8.0 ng/mL, postmenopausal: 3.0-12.0 ng/mL. Values vary between laboratories due to difference in antibody.

Use Select patients for and monitor calcitonin or estrogen therapy for osteoporosis; a marker for increase in bone formation and bone turnover, eg, as in renal osteodystrophy. Correlation with results of bone histomorphometry makes this a useful, cost effective assay.

Methodology Radioimmunoassay (RIA)

Additional Information Changes in serum osteocalcin generally parallel collagen synthesis and changes in serum alkaline phosphatase activity. It is decreased in patients with osteoporosis or Paget's disease of bone treated with drugs such as calcitonin. It is increased in subjects with osteoporosis.

References

Antoniazzi F, Radetti G, Zamboni G, et al, "Effects of 1,25-Dihydroxyvitamin D3 and Growth Hormone Therapy on Serum Osteocalcin Levels in Children With Growth Hormone Deficiency," *Bone Miner*, 1993, 21(2):151-6.
Diaz Diego EM, Guerrero R, and de la Piedra C, "Six Osteocalcin Assays Compared," *Clin Chem*, 1994, 40(11 Pt 1):2071-7.
Franck H, Ittel TH, Tasch O, et al, "Osteocalcin in Patients with Rheumatoid Arthritis. A One-Year Followup Study," *J Rheumatol*, 1994, 21(7):1256-9.
Joffe I, Heaf JG, and Hyldstrup L, "Osteocalcin: A Non-Invasive Index of Metabolic Bone Disease in Patients Treated by CAPD," *Kidney Int*, 1994, 46(3):838-46.
Kaddam IM, Iqbal SJ, Holland S, et al, "Comparison of Serum Osteocalcin With Total and Bone Specific Alkaline Phosphatase and Urinary Hydroxyproline:Creatinine Ratio in Patients With Paget's Disease of Bone," *Ann Clin Biochem*, 1994, 31(Pt 4):327-30.
Kao PC, Riggs BL, and Schryver PG, "Development and Evaluation of an Osteocalcin Chemiluminoimmunoassay," *Clin Chem*, 1994, 39(7):1369-74.
Leavelle DE, *Mayo Medical Laboratories Interpretive Handbook*, Rochester, MN: Mayo Medical Laboratories, 1994.
Minisola S, Carnevale V, Pacitti MT, et al, "Serum Osteocalcin in Metabolic Bone Diseases: What Is Its Real Significance?" *J Endocrinol Invest*, 1993, 16(4):277-9.
Minisola S, Piccioni AL, Rosso R, et al, "Reduced Serum Levels of Carboxy-Terminal Propeptide of Human Type I Procollagen in a Family With Type I-A Osteogenesis Imperfecta," *Metabolism*, 1994, 43(10):1261-5.
Namgung R, Tsang RC, Specker BL, et al, "Reduced Serum Osteocalcin and 1,25-Dihydroxyvitamin D Concentrations and Low Bone Mineral Content in Small for Gestational Age Infants: Evidence of Decreased Bone Formation Rates," *J Pediatr*, 1993, 122(2):269-75.
Overgaard K, "Effect of Intranasal Salmon Calcitonin Therapy on Bone Mass and Bone Turnover in Early Postmenopausal Women: A Dose-Response Study," *Calcif Tissue Int*, 1994, 55(2):82-6.
Rosenquist C, Bonde M, Fledelius C, et al, "A Simple Enzyme-Linked Immunosorbent Assay of Human Osteocalcin," *Clin Chem*, 1994, 40(7 Pt 1):1258-64.

OVX1 *see* CA 125 *on page 94*

Oxalate, Urine

CPT 83945

Related Information

Ascorbic Acid, Blood *on page 84*
Ethylene Glycol *on page 550*
Kidney Stone Analysis *on page 640*
Magnesium, Serum *on page 164*
Magnesium, Urine *on page 165*
Urinalysis *on page 658*
Urine Collection, 24-Hour *on page 30*

Synonyms Calcium Oxalate, Urine; Urine Oxalate

Applies to Glycolic Acid, Urine; Glyoxylic Acid, Urine; L-Glyceric Acid, Urine; Vitamin C

Abstract Calcium oxalate stones are common in the urinary tract. Oxalate excretion is a predictor of oxalate nephrolithiasis.

Patient Preparation Avoid vitamin C for 24 hours before collection. Pyridoxine is said to diminish oxaluria. The patient should be ambulatory, preferably at home, on usual fluid and food intake, to best interpret risk factors for nephrolithiasis.

Specimen 24-hour urine; first morning urine may give oxalate concentrations similar to 24-hour collections.[1] Total amount of oxalate excreted might be estimated using first morning urinary oxalate concentration and an estimate of daily urine output.

Container Acid-washed plastic container with 20 mL of 6N HCl added prior to collection (depending upon laboratory). Acid prevents oxalate crystallization and conversion of ascorbate to oxalate. No metal cap.

Collection Instruct the patient to void at 8 AM and discard the specimen. Then collect all urine including the final specimen voided at the end of the 24-hour collection period (ie, 8 AM the next morning). Many laboratories request addition of acid to container before urine collection is started. HCl is used to avoid oxalate crystallization and conversion of ascorbate to oxalate. Twenty-four hour urine volume must be recorded.

Reference Range 20-60 mg/24 hours (SI: 0.23-0.68 mmol/day).[2] Greater excretion of oxalic acid in men is recognized in healthy subjects as well as in stone formers. The differences were unexplained on the basis of body surface. A relationship with age was not found.[3]

Use Patients who form calcium oxalate kidney stones appear to absorb and excrete a higher fraction of dietary oxalate in urine than do normals. Hyperoxaluria is not uncommon in subjects with malabsorption. Twenty-four hour urine collections for oxalate are indicated in patients with surgical loss of distal small intestine, especially those with Crohn's disease. The incidence of nephrolithiasis in patients who have inflammatory bowel disease is 2.6% to 10%.[4] Hyperoxaluria is regularly present after jejunoileal bypass for morbid obesity; such patients may develop nephrolithiasis.

Limitations Interference by ascorbate is a major impediment in developing a simple assay. Urine specimens containing significant amounts of ascorbic acid (10-325 µg/dL) experience interference in two forms. First, ascorbic acid is converted nonenzymatically to oxalate at alkaline pH or if urine is not acidified after bicarbonate administration.[5] Second, ascorbate inhibits oxalate oxidase (enzymatic method) and markedly decreases recovery of oxalates.[6,7] Methods to eliminate ascorbate meet with varied success depending upon the urine ascorbate concentration.[7]

Methodology Colorimetry following anion exchange resin; atomic absorption (AA) after precipitation with calcium; enzymatic, oxalate oxidase; high performance liquid chromatography (HPLC). A method for routine clinical urinary oxalate has been reported.[8]

Additional Information Oxaluria is characteristic of ethylene glycol intoxication. Oxalic acid excretion is increased with methoxyflurane. Serum calcium and urinary calcium excretion are also often needed; calcium oxalate renal stones are common.

Hyperoxaluria may occur with high intake of animal protein, purines, gelatin, calcium, strawberries, pepper, rhubarb, beans, beets, spinach, tomatoes, chocolate, cocoa, and tea.[9] Hyperoxaluria is described with pyridoxine deficiency. Urinary oxalate derives from the metabolism of glycine and ascorbic acid more than from dietary ingestion. Oxalate excretion was increased in vegetarians, despite low animal protein ingestion.[10] Dietary intake of animal protein is also directly associated with the risk of stone formation. Limited calcium supplementation does not appear to increase the risk of nephrolithiasis in men. Calcium taken orally with oxalate loads decreases urinary oxalate excretion in patients with ileal disease. Calcium supplements taken with meals are less likely to lead to nephrolithiasis.[11]

Vitamin C increases oxalate excretion and may be a risk factor for calcium oxalate nephrolithiasis in individuals consuming "megadose" vitamin C. Such ingestion can usually be determined by history. If a vitamin C using stone former is found to have high urine oxalate excretion, the habit should be stopped. If oxalate excretion drops to normal, additional therapy to prevent stones may not be required.

Hyperoxaluria can result from intestinal hyperabsorption related to low calcium intake or high calcium enteric binding to compounds such as phytates. Conversely, increased dietary calcium may reduce the absorption of oxalate in patients with recurrent oxalate kidney stones.[9] Unabsorbed fat can bind calcium. Increased urinary uric acid excretion is frequently found in subjects who have calcium oxalate nephrolithiasis. Calcium nephrolithiasis in patients with hyperuricosuria has been related to urate-induced crystallization of calcium oxalate.[12] Urinary oxalate concentrations have been found to be increased in very low birth weight infants receiving parenteral amino acid solutions.[13]

Rare genetic disorders which increase endogenous oxalate production; there are two types of primary hyperoxaluria. They are characterized by elevated urinary oxalate excretion and recurrent oxalate nephrocalcinosis. In type I, a defect in glyoxalate metabolism is found, leading to increased oxalate synthesis. Excessive quantities of urinary glyoxylic and glycolic acid excretion occur. Type II is rare; it is characterized by excessive urinary excretion of oxalic and L-glyceric acids with normal excretion of glycolic acid.[14] Type I causes renal failure and systemic oxalosis, but type II rarely does so.[15]

Glycine irrigation during transurethral prostatic resections does not raise the urinary oxalate level during the postoperative period. This suggests that post-transurethral forced diuresis may not be indicated solely for bladder irrigation with glycine.[16]

The importance of magnesium supplements to prevent calcium oxalate nephrolithiasis in subjects with gastrointestinal disease has been recently addressed.[17] See listings Magnesium, Serum *on page 164* and Magnesium, Urine *on page 165*.

Footnotes

1. Balchin ZEC, Moss PA, and Fraser CG, "Biological Variation of Urinary Oxalate in Different Specimens Types," *Ann Clin Biochem*, 1991, 28(Pt 6):622-3.
2. Wilson DM and Liedtke RR, "Modified Enzyme-Based Colorimetric Assay of Urinary and Plasma Oxalate With Improved Sensitivity and No Ascorbate Interference: Reference Values and Sample Handling Procedures," *Clin Chem*, 1991, 37(7):1229-35.
3. Hesse A, Klocke K, Classen A, et al, "Age and Sex as Factors in Oxalic Acid Excretion in Healthy Persons and Calcium Oxalate Stone Patients," *Contrib Nephrol*, 1987, 58:16-20.
4. Earnest DL, "Enteric Hyperoxaluria," *Adv Intern Med*, 1979, 24:407-27.
5. Lemann J Jr, Hornick LJ, Pleuss JA, et al, "Oxalate Is Overestimated in Alkaline Urines Collected During Administration of Bicarbonate With No Specimen pH Adjustment," *Clin Chem*, 1989, 35(10):2107-10.
6. Li MG and Madappally MM, "Rapid Enzymatic Determination of Urinary Oxalate," *Clin Chem*, 1989, 35(12):2330-3.
7. Inamdar KV, Raghavan KG, and Pradhan DS, "Five Treatment Procedures Evaluated for the Elimination of Ascorbate Interference in the Enzymatic Determination of Urinary Oxalate," *Clin Chem*, 1991, 37(6):864-8.
8. Mazzuchin A, Michelutti L, and Falter H, "Modifications to Commercial Oxalate Oxidase Based Determination of Urinary Oxalate: A Method Suitable for Routine Clinical Analysis," *Clin Biochem*, 1990, 23(2):173-7.
9. Massey LK, Roman-Smith H, and Sutton RA, "Effect of Dietary Oxalate and Calcium on Urinary Oxalate and Risk of Formation of Calcium Oxalate Kidney Stones," *J Am Diet Assoc*, 1993, 93(8):901-6.
10. Marangella M, Bianco I, Martini C, et al, "Effect of Animal and Vegetable Protein Intake on Oxalate Excretion in Idiopathic Calcium Stone Disease," *Br J Urol*, 1989, 63(4):348-51.
11. Curhan GC, Willett WC, Rimm EB, et al, "A Prospective Study of Dietary Calcium and Other Nutrients and the Risk of Symptomatic Kidney Stones," *N Engl J Med*, 1993, 328(12):833-8.
12. Pak CY and Peterson R, "Successful Treatment of Hyperuricosuric Calcium Oxalate Nephrolithiasis With Potassium Citrate," *Arch Intern Med*, 1986, 146(5):863-7.
13. Campfield T and Braden G, "Urinary Oxalate Excretion by Very Low Birth Weight Infants Receiving Parenteral Nutrition," *Pediatrics*, 1989, 84(5):860-3.
14. Yendt ER and Cohanim M, "Response to Physiologic Dose of Pyridoxine in Type 1 Primary Hyperoxaluria," *N Engl J Med*, 1985, 312(15):953-7.
15. Marangella M, Petrarulo M, Cosseddu D, et al, "End-Stage Renal Failure in Primary Hyperoxaluria Type 2," *N Engl J Med*, 1994, 330(23):1690.
16. Hahn RG, "Glycine Irrigation and Urinary Oxalate Excretion," *Br J Urol*, 1989, 64(3):287-9.
17. Fleming CR, George L, Stoner GL, et al, "The Importance of Urinary Magnesium Values in Patients With Gut Failure," *Mayo Clin Proc*, 1996, 71(1):21-4.

References

Allen LC, Kadijevic L, and Romaschin AD, "An Enzymatic Method for Oxalate Automated With the Cobas Fara Centrifugal Analyzer," *Clin Chem*, 1989, 35(10):2098-100.
Barratt TM, Kasidas GP, Murdoch I, et al, "Urinary Oxalate and Glycolate Excretion and Plasma Oxalate Concentration," *Arch Dis Child*, 1991, 66(4):501-3.
Cowley DM, McWhinney BC, Brown JM, et al, "Effect of Citrate on the Urinary Excretion of Calcium and Oxalate: Relevance to Calcium Oxalate Nephrolithiasis," *Clin Chem*, 1989, 35(1):23-8.
Goldfarb S, "Diet and Nephrolithiasis," *Annu Rev Med*, 1994, 45:235-43.
Milliner DS, Eickholt JT, Bergstralh EJ, et al, "Results of Long-Term Treatment With Orthophosphate and Pyridoxine in Patients With Primary Hyperoxaluria," *N Engl J Med*, 1994, 331(23):1553-8.
Petrarulo M, Marangella M, Bianco O, et al, "Preventing Ascorbate Interference in Ion-Chromatographic Determinations of Urinary Oxalate: Four Methods Compared," *Clin Chem*, 1990, 36(9):1642-5.
Ryall RL, Harnett RM, Hibberd CM, et al, "Urinary Risk Factors in Calcium Oxalate Stone Disease: Comparison of Men and Women," *Br J Urol*, 1987, 60(6):480-8.
Sharma S, Nath R, and Thind SK, "Recent Advances in Measurement of Oxalate in Biological Materials," *Scanning Microsc*, 1993, 7(1):431-41.

2-Oxoglutarate Aminotransferase *see Alanine Aminotransferase on page 65*

Oxygen Content *see Blood Gases, Arterial on page 87*

Oxygen-Hemoglobin Dissociation Curve (ODC) *see Oxygen Saturation, Blood on this page*

Oxygen-Hemoglobin Dissociation Curve (ODC) *see P-50 Blood Gas on next page*

Oxygen Saturation *see Blood Gases, Arterial on page 87*

Oxygen Saturation, Blood

CPT 82810

Related Information

Blood Gases, Arterial *on page 87*
Hemoglobin *on page 323*
P-50 Blood Gas *on next page*
pH, Blood *on page 180*

Synonyms Hemoglobin Saturation, Percent; saO_2; sO_2

Applies to 2,3-DPG; O_2 Capacity; O_2 Content; Oxygen-Hemoglobin Dissociation Curve (ODC); Transcutaneous Pulse Oximetry

Test Commonly Includes A part of blood gas determination in many laboratories.

Abstract The partial pressure of oxygen physically dissolved in plasma determines the oxygen bound to hemoglobin compared to the amount bound if the hemoglobin was totally saturated. It is oxygen content divided by oxygen capacity and is expressed as percent saturation (sO_2).

Specimen Whole blood, arterial

Container Heparinized syringe, capillary tubes, or green top (heparin) tube

Collection Draw specimen into heparinized syringe, avoid air bubbles, and stopper tightly, knotting scalp vein infusion set tubing, fitting shank of syringe with a special closure or other means of insuring an airtight fit. Place heparinized specimen on ice. Take to the laboratory immediately.

Causes for Rejection Specimens received with clots or air bubbles in the syringe, specimens not on ice, specimens not tightly stoppered must be rejected.

Special Instructions If capillaries are used to collect the specimen, warm skin 10-15 minutes prior to puncture, obtain free flow of blood with a sufficiently deep puncture ("arterialized capillary blood"), fill heparinized capillaries completely full (enough capillaries to provide at least 0.5 mL whole blood), cap and mix.

Reference Range Children and adults: sO_2 95% to 99%. Arterial pO_2 of 80 mm Hg, sO_2 of 95% are normal for the aged. Arterial pO_2 of 100 mm Hg, sO_2 of 97% are normal for the young.

Possible Panic Range Arterial pO_2 of 20 mm Hg, sO_2 of 35% are critically low, life-endangering levels; the same values from mixed venous blood indicate tissue hypoxia. Arterial pO_2 of 40 mm Hg, sO_2 of 75% are panic values that correlate with cyanosis, but these values are normal for mixed venous blood.

Use Evaluate the extent of oxygenation of hemoglobin and adequacy of tissue oxygenation, together with pO_2. Allows evaluation of oxygenation and oxyhemoglobin dissociation of blood with use of the oxygen dissociation curve (ODC). The dissociation curve expresses relationships between pO_2 and oxyhemoglobin saturation. Diagnose hypoxia; monitor respiratory function during mechanical ventilation.[1] Central venous oxygen saturation may also be used in detection of blood loss in cases of acute injury.[2]

Limitations Accuracy and precision may be affected by the presence of other pigments in the blood, including especially other heme derivatives (eg, carboxyhemoglobin), low hemoglobin concentrations, plasma turbidity (ie, as with lipemia), and presence of cell fragments. Interpretation is more meaningful if the nature of patient's inspired gas is recorded (ie, room air or mixture of gases with a controlled oxygen content).

Contraindications Contraindications of arterial puncture

Methodology Spectrophotometric analysis of hemolysate with current automated analyzers directly measuring sO_2. Alternatively, a calculated sO_2 may be derived from the Hill equation using measured pH and pO_2. In the latter method, blood is analyzed at two wavelengths, one with a large difference in absorbance between oxygenated and deoxygenated hemoglobin, the other at the isobestic point (molar absorbance identical for the oxygenated and deoxygenated forms).[3] Transcutaneous pulse oximetry measures the absorption of different wavelengths of light passed through living tissue. See following discussion and footnotes.

Additional Information The terms "O_2 content," "O_2 capacity," and "O_2 saturation" refer to various definitions of the amount of oxygen carried in the blood. **Oxygen content** is the total amount of oxygen present (bound to hemoglobin and dissolved in plasma) in the blood. Normally hemoglobin exists in blood in the oxygen-bound state (oxyhemoglobin) and in some unoxygenated forms (reduced hemoglobin, methemoglobin, carboxyhemoglobin, and sulfhemoglobin). Inactive forms account for about 4% of the total hemoglobin. **Oxygen capacity** is the amount of O_2 that would bind to hemoglobin if all the hemoglobin were oxygenated. (Continued)

Oxygen Saturation, Blood *(Continued)*

Oxygen saturation is the ratio (in %) of oxyhemoglobin to the total amount of hemoglobin present.

The large pool of hemoglobin allows blood to transport 65 times the amount of oxygen dissolved in plasma. This relationship is dependent upon (primarily) pH (and thereby CO_2 parameters that contribute to the control of pH), temperature, the concentration of 2,3-diphosphoglycerate (2,3-DPG), and the molecular species of hemoglobin. When graphed, the relationship results in a sigmoid (S-shaped) oxygen-hemoglobin dissociation curve (ODC). The oxygen saturation (in %) is represented on the Y axis, the partial pressure of oxygen (in mm Hg) on the X axis with the curve shifted to the right or left (isobars) by changes in pH or other parameters. This is a biochemically fixed relation such that if any two of the three determinants, pH, pO_2, or O_2 saturation are known, the other may be predicted. With the ODC in hand one can verify the accuracy of laboratory performance by assuring that the three reported values are consistent with each other as defined by the ODC (assuming normal molecular species of hemoglobin, concentration of 2,3-DPG, and constant temperature).

Red cell 2,3-DPG concentration plays an important role in regulation of hemoglobin's affinity for oxygen. 2,3-DPG binds to the β chains of oxyhemoglobin and results in displacement of O_2 by the following equation:[4] Hgb O_2 + 2,3-DPG = Hgb-2,3-DPG + O_2. An increase in 2,3-DPG will cause a shift of the reaction to the right. Greater affinity of fetal hemoglobin for oxygen has been ascribed to the poor binding of 2,3-DPG by the γ chains of fetal hemoglobin. Increased erythrocyte 2,3-DPG concentrations decrease intracellular pH resulting in a further reduction in oxygen affinity. 2,3-DPG is increased with hypoxia.

Red cells of newborns contain approximately 80% hemoglobin F. Hemoglobin F has a slightly lower oxygen affinity compared to hemoglobin A (normal adult hemoglobin) and binds 2,3-DPG less strongly than hemoglobin A. Following birth, O_2 affinity decreases as red cell 2,3-DPG concentrations rise (20% during the first week of life). At 1-4 weeks, healthy prematures have P-50 values approaching those of normal adults.[5]

Decreased oxygen saturation relates to impaired cardiorespiratory function at the macro-organ level of heart and/or lungs (due to a variety of diseases) or at the intracellular chemical respiratory level (a number of pathologic mechanisms resulting in methemoglobinemia). The four mechanisms of abnormal gas exchange are hypoventilation, ventilation-perfusion disturbance, diffusion defect, and venous admixture. The hypoxemia accompanying right-to-left shunting in cardiac diseases (venous admixture) is preferentially evaluated with oxygen saturation. O_2 saturation provides a more direct indication of the size of the shunt than the pO_2 value.[6] Decreased central venous oxygen saturation was found to correlate better with estimated blood loss volumes in 26 trauma patients than vital signs including heart rate, blood pressure, central venous pressure, pulse pressure, and urine output. In this series of trauma patients, all had normal vital signs upon admission and a significant percentage of these patients had serious injuries and ongoing blood loss that required immediate attention.[2]

In some clinical situations, measurement of pO_2 alone may give misleading information as to sufficiency of the blood's oxygen-carrying ability. Partial pressure of oxygen may be normal or even increased while O_2 saturation may be decreased as the result of an abnormal heme compound (eg, carboxyhemoglobin as in cases of carbon monoxide poisoning).[7] Oxygen saturation is preferably measured directly (spectrophotometrically) and not derived from the pH and pO_2 values by use of the ODC relationships. Derived sO_2 values would give false normal results in the above example.

Arterial oxygen desaturation occurs after sedation for peritoneoscopy with resultant hypoxemia, hypercarbia, and acidosis.[8]

There is growing use of **transcutaneous pulse oximetry** to determine oxygen saturation, particularly in premature and in critically ill newborns and children. This noninvasive technique avoids the rigors of arterial puncture, necessity of subsequent proper sample handling, and can provide continual monitoring. This technique has generally been found reliable and useful in monitoring adequacy of oxygenation, effectiveness of resuscitative efforts, detection of development of prolonged periods of decreased sO_2 in neonates, and monitoring preterm infant's response to physical therapy.[1,9,10,11,12,13] Pulse oximetry has also been applied to detection of hyperoxemia in newborns but has low specificity.[14] Limitations of pulse oximetry have included overestimation of sO_2 at values 65% and less,[12,15] and variation from *in vitro* determined sO_2 in samples with >50% fetal hemoglobin as compared with samples having under 25% fetal hemoglobin.[11] A study of pulse oximeter determined oxygen saturation in pregnant patients and their newborns has found that sO_2 in neonates is commonly 90% or less within 10 minutes after birth and may not always be indicative of pathologic hypoxia.[16] Specialized devices (eg, balloon-tipped, thermodilution, fiberoptic, pulmonary arterial catheter) have been developed for the intraoperative monitoring of mixed venous oxygen saturation.[17]

Footnotes

1. Shannon DC, "Rational Monitoring of Respiratory Function During Mechanical Ventilation of Infants and Children," *Intensive Care Med*, 1989, 15(Suppl 1):S13-6.
2. Scalea TM, Hartnett RW, Duncan AO, et al, "Central Venous Oxygen Saturation: A Useful Clinical Tool in Trauma Patients," *J Trauma*, 1990, 30(12):1539-43.
3. Bruegger BB and Sherwin JE, "Blood Gas Analysis and Oxygen Saturation," *Methods in Clinical Chemistry*, Chapter 8, Pesce AJ and Kaplan LA, eds, St Louis, MO: Mosby-Year Book Inc, 1987, 54-66.
4. Ganong WF, *Review of Medical Physiology*, 15th ed, Norwalk, CT: Appleton & Lange, 1991, 616-22.
5. Bunn HF and Forget BG, "Oxygen and Carbon Dioxide Transport," *Hemoglobin: Molecular, Genetic and Clinical Aspects*, Chapter 5, Philadelphia, PA: WB Saunders Co, 1986, 91-125.
6. Siggaard-Andersen O, "Hydrogen Ions and Blood Gases," *Chemical Diagnosis of Disease*, Brown SS, Mitchell FL, and Young DS, eds, New York, NY: Elsevier/North Holland Biomedical Press, 1979, 219-38.
7. Browning RJ, "Pulmonary Disease: Putting Blood Gas Tests to Work," *Diagn Med*, 1982, 5:54-63.
8. Brady CE III, Harkleroad LE, and Pierson WP, "Alterations in Oxygen Saturation and Ventilation After Intravenous Sedation for Peritoneoscopy," *Arch Intern Med*, 1989, 149(5):1029-32.
9. Deckardt R, Schneider KT, and Graeff H, "Monitoring Arterial Oxygen Saturation in the Neonate," *J Perinat Med*, 1987, 15(4):357-60.
10. House JT, Schultetus RR, and Gravenstein N, "Continuous Neonatal Evaluation in the Delivery Room by Pulse Oximetry," *J Clin Monit*, 1987, 3(2):96-100.
11. Jennis MS and Peabody JL, "Pulse Oximetry: An Alternative Method for the Assessment of Oxygenation in Newborn Infants," *Pediatrics*, 1987, 79(4):524-8.
12. Lewallen PK, Mammel MC, Coleman JM, et al, "Neonatal Transcutaneous Arterial Oxygen Saturation Monitoring," *J Perinatol*, 1987, 7(1):8-10.
13. Kelly MK, Palisano RJ, and Wolfson MR, "Effects of a Developmental Physical Therapy Program on Oxygen Saturation and Heart Rate in Preterm Infants," *Phys Ther*, 1989, 69(6):467-74.
14. Bucher HU, Fanconi S, Baeckert P, et al, "Hyperoxemia in Newborn Infants: Detection by Pulse Oximetry," *Pediatrics*, 1989, 84(2):226-30.
15. Fanconi S, "Pulse Oximetry and Transcutaneous Oxygen Tension for Detection of Hypoxemia in Critically Ill Infants and Children," *Adv Exp Med Biol*, 1987, 220:159-64.
16. Porter KB, Goldhamer R, Mankad A, et al, "Evaluation of Arterial Oxygen Saturation in Pregnant Patients and Their Newborns," *Obstet Gynecol*, 1988, 71(3 Pt 1):354-7.
17. Thys DM, Cohen E, and Eisenkraft JB, "Mixed Venous Oxygen Saturation During Thoracic Anesthesia," *Anesthesiology*, 1988, 69(6):1005-9.

References

Burtis CA and Ashwood ER, *Tietz Textbook of Clinical Chemistry*, 2nd ed, Philadelphia, PA: WB Saunders Co, 1994, 1388.

Chripko D, Bevan JC, Archer DP, et al, "Decreases in Arterial Oxygen Saturation in Paediatric Outpatients During Transfer to the Postanaesthetic Recovery Room," *Can J Anaesth*, 1989, 36(2):128-32.

Grebstad JA, Svendsen L, and Gulsvik A, "Precision of Arterial Blood Gases and Cutaneous Oxygen Saturation in Healthy Nonsmokers," *Scand J Clin Lab Invest*, 1989, 49(3):265-8.

Kwant B, Oeseburg B, and Zijistra WG, "Reliability of the Determination of Whole-Blood Oxygen Affinity by Means of Blood-Gas Analyzers and Multiwavelength Oximeters," *Clin Chem*, 1989, 35(5):773-7.

Porter KB, "Evaluation of Arterial Oxygen Saturation of the Newborn in the Labor and Delivery Suite," *J Perinatol*, 1987, 7(4):337-9.

Oxygen Transport *see* Lactic Acid, Blood *on page 156*

P-5'-P *see* Vitamin B_6 *on page 217*

P-50 Blood Gas

CPT 82820

Related Information

Carboxyhemoglobin *on page 541*

Hemoglobin *on page 323*

Hemoglobin Electrophoresis *on page 324*

Oxygen Saturation, Blood *on previous page*

Synonyms Blood Gas P-50; pO_2 (0.5); pO_2 at Half Saturation

Applies to 2,3-DPG; Hill Plots; Oxygen-Hemoglobin Dissociation Curve (ODC)

Abstract P-50 is that pO_2 (partial pressure of oxygen) at which hemoglobin is 50% saturated.

Specimen Arterial whole blood

Container Heparinized syringe

Collection Avoid contact with air, insert needle into cork or hard rubber block, place on ice, and deliver to the laboratory immediately.

Causes for Rejection Specimen clotted, air bubbles in syringe, needle not tightly capped

Reference Range Adults: pO_2 of approximately 27 mm Hg; range: 25-29 mm Hg (corrected to pH 7.4)

Use The oxygen-dissociation curve (ODC) is a representation of percent oxygen saturation versus pO_2. Hill plots are logarithmic curves representing an empirical expression for the equilibrium of hemoglobin or myoglobin with oxygen. Determination of P-50 value assumes that a tightly maintained physiologic relation between pO_2 and oxygen saturation exists and by implication that hemoglobin function (and thereby presumably structure as far as oxygen transport is concerned) is normal. This assumption does not necessarily apply to all hemoglobin types.

Methodology The oxygen dissociation curve may be measured by discontinuous methods in which individual points of pO_2 are obtained with an oxygen electrode for a given saturation. Continuous methods utilize special cuvettes in which O_2 is generated at a constant rate. pO_2 is continuously measured as the oxygen content is increased. A review of instrumentation (including continuous technique) by Hedlund is informative.[1] Continuous oxygen saturation may be monitored *in vivo* by the use of pulse oximetry.[2] Single point methods have been described.[3,4] The reliability of such methods (using usually commonly available blood-gas analyzer/oximeter combinations) has been assessed.[5] The methods have been found suitable for detection of clinically significant abnormalities in O_2 affinity such as occur in patients with abnormal hemoglobins and CO poisoning. These procedures, however, did not provide truly accurate P_{50} and Hill values. They were unable to discriminate between high and low values for P_{50} within the normal range.[5] Empirical equations and the use of a nomogram have been described that make possible calculation of P-50 from known values of pCO_2, pH, 2,3-DPG, and temperature present in physiological and pathological conditions.[6]

Additional Information The **oxygen-hemoglobin dissociation curve (ODC)** is a graphical representation of the percent saturation of hemoglobin by exposure of blood to differing partial pressures of oxygen. The relation of oxygen saturation to pO_2 is dependent upon (primarily) pH (and thereby CO_2 parameters that contribute to the control of pH), temperature, 2,3-DPG (diphosphoglycerate) and the molecular species of hemoglobin. In the normal adult, the curve has a characteristic sigmoid configuration relating to the interaction of the components of the hemoglobin tetramer ("heme-heme interaction") and to the acceptance by the tetramer of DPG as oxygen is progressively bound or released. In effect, conformational changes occur on the molecular level (there is actually a physical change in the globin chain configuration and chain-to-chain positions with oxygenation/deoxygenation). The "normal" situation is taken at pH 7.4, temperature 37°C under which conditions a pO_2 of approximately 27 mm Hg results in 50% saturation of hemoglobin with oxygen. The P-50 value then is one point on the ODC (that pO_2 necessary to produce half saturation) reflecting the affinity of hemoglobin for oxygen. When the P-50 (and ODC curve) is shifted to the right, there will be less oxygen loaded on to hemoglobin at any given pO_2. This occurs with increased acidity (decreased pH) and with increased CO_2 content, ionic concentration, or temperature. With a "shift to the left" (as occurs with alkalosis or decrease in temperature), there is increased oxygen affinity (more oxygen loaded - higher oxygen saturation at any given pO_2). These characteristics have important implications to the availability of oxygen at the tissue level. The following is a summary:

$$\uparrow \begin{matrix} RBC \\ 2,3\text{-}DPG \end{matrix} \rightarrow \uparrow P\text{-}50 \begin{cases} \uparrow pO_2 \text{ necessary to} \rightarrow 50\% \text{ saturation Hgb with } O_2 \\ \\ \downarrow O_2 \text{ affinity, } \uparrow \text{ tissue availability} \end{cases}$$

$$\downarrow \begin{matrix} RBC \\ 2,3\text{-}DPG \end{matrix} \rightarrow \downarrow P\text{-}50 \begin{cases} \downarrow pO_2 \text{ necessary to} \rightarrow 50\% \text{ saturation Hgb with } O_2 \\ \\ \uparrow O_2 \text{ affinity, } \downarrow \text{ tissue availability} \end{cases}$$

Some hemoglobinopathies are characterized by an abnormal P-50 value, ODC right or left shifted, reflecting altered affinity for oxygen. A variety of molecular bases for 70 different hemoglobins with high oxygen affinities have been grouped by Perutz into eight classes.[7] Low oxygen affinity hemoglobins (28) fall into four classes based on molecular mechanism. Fairbanks lists 13 α-chain and 59 β-chain hemoglobin variants with increased oxygen affinity, not all of which have polycythemia or cyanosis.[8] Five α-chain and 22 β-chain variants have decreased O_2 affinity, some with cyanosis, and/or hemolysis and/or "anemia." The "anemia" may reflect a condition defined by a laboratory result rather than a physiologic deficiency, as the lowered affinity should allow a decreased mass of circulating hemoglobin to deliver a sufficient amount of oxygen. Hb Seattle, among many others, appears to be such an example.[9] A laboratory study of the ODC is important in cases of suspect hemoglobinopathy as some (eg, Hb Malmo[10]) have normal electrophoretic patterns using routine techniques.

Shifts in oxygen/hemoglobin relationships that favor survival appear to occur in ischemic heart disease,[11] but it is not clear if increased oxygen affinity is etiologic in occasional examples of myocardial ischemia and necrosis.[12] Interrelations between oxygen delivery, P-50, and oxygen consumption have been investigated in patients with acute myocardial infarct.[13] Oxygen consumption in nonsurvivors increased compared to survivors and was partially explained by an increased P-50. The authors noted that finding increased oxygen consumption in a patient with myocardial infarct should be interpreted with caution, as it may imply a precarious oxygen transport/requirement balance in peripheral tissue.

Sodium bicarbonate, which is used to treat acidosis, has been found in one study[14] to decrease the P-50, decrease arterial pO_2 by 10 mm Hg, and increase blood lactate concentrations. P-50 has been found to decrease with use of some radiologic contrast agents.[15] Slight decrease in P-50 has also been reported in the critically ill.[16] Phosphates may increase the P-50.[17]

While normal pregnancy is associated with an increase in P-50, a significant decrease occurs in pre-eclampsia. This appears to be due in part to an increase in COHb present in pre-eclamptic pregnant women.[18]

Footnotes

1. Hedlund B, "Measurement of the Oxygen Dissociation Curve in the Clinical Laboratory," *Hemoglobinopathies and Thalassemias*, Fairbanks VF, ed, New York, NY: Thieme-Stratton Inc, 1980, 75-80.
2. Dodson SR, Hensley FA Jr, Martin DE, et al, "Continuous Oxygen Saturation Monitoring During Cardiac Catheterization in Adults," *Chest*, 1988, 94(1):28-31.
3. Pruden EL, Siggaard-Anderson O, and Tietz NW, "Blood Gases and pH," *Fundamentals of Clinical Chemistry*, 3rd ed, Chapter 19, Section 2, Philadelphia, PA: WB Saunders Co, 1987, 624-45.
4. Lichtman MA, Murphy MS, and Adamson JW, "Detection of Mutant Hemoglobins With Altered Affinity for Oxygen. A Simplified Technique," *Ann Intern Med*, 1976, 84:517-20.
5. Kwant G, Oeseburg B, and Zijlstra WG, "Reliability of the Determination of Whole-Blood Oxygen Affinity by Means of Blood-Gas Analyzers and Multiwavelength Oximeters," *Clin Chem*, 1989, 35(5):773-7.
6. Samaja M, Melotti D, Rovida E, et al, "Effect of Temperature on the P-50 Value for Human Blood," *Clin Chem*, 1983, 29:110-4.
7. Perutz MF, "Molecular Anatomy, Physiology, and Pathology of Hemoglobin," *The Molecular Basis of Blood Diseases*, Chapter 5, Stamatoyannopoulos G, Nienhuis AW, Leder P, et al, eds, Philadelphia, PA: WB Saunders Co, 1987, 127-78.
8. Fairbanks VF, *Hemoglobinopathies and Thalassemias*, New York, NY: Thieme-Stratton Inc, 1980, 285-7.
9. Honig GR and Adams JG 3d, *Human Hemoglobin Genetics*, Chapter 6, New York, NY: Springer-Vehlay, Wien, 1986, 163-213, 292-349.
10. Fairbanks VF, Maldonado JE, Charache S, et al, "Familial Erythrocytosis Due to Electrophoretically Undetectable Hemoglobin With Impaired Oxygen Dissociation (Hemoglobin Malmo $\alpha_2 \beta_2^{97gln}$)," *Mayo Clin Proc*, 1971, 46:721-7.
11. Nevins MA, "Oxyhemoglobin Equilibrium in Ischemic Heart Disease," *JAMA*, 1974, 229:804-8.
12. Eliot RS and Bratt G, "The Paradox of Myocardial Ischemia and Necrosis in Young Women With Normal Coronary Arteriograms: Relation to Abnormal Hemoglobin-Oxygen Dissociation," *Am J Cardiol*, 1969, 23:633-8.
13. Sumimoto T, Takayama Y, Iwasaka T, et al, "Oxygen Delivery, Oxygen Consumption and Hemoglobin-Oxygen Affinity in Acute Myocardial Infarction," *Am J Cardiol*, 1989, 64(16):975-9.
14. Bersin RM, Chatterjee K, and Arieff AI, "Metabolic and Hemodynamic Consequences of Sodium Bicarbonate Administration in Patients With Heart Disease," *Am J Med*, 1989, 87(1):7-14.
15. Kim SJ, Salem MR, Joseph NJ, et al, "Contrast Media Adversely Affect Oxyhemoglobin Dissociation," *Anesth Analg*, 1990, 71(1):73-6.
16. Myburgh JA, Webb RK, and Worthley LIG, "The P50 Is Reduced in Critically Ill Patients," *Intensive Care Med*, 1991, 17(6):355-8.
17. Clerbaux T, Reynaert M, Willems E, et al, "Effect of Phosphate on Oxygen-Hemoglobin Affinity, Diphosphoglycerate and Blood Gases During Recovery From Diabetic Ketoacidosis," *Intensive Care Med*, 1989, 15(8):495-8.
18. Kambam JR, Entman S, Mouton S, et al, "Effect of Pre-eclampsia on Carboxyhemoglobin Levels: A Mechanism for a Decrease in P-50," *Anesthesiology*, 1988, 68(3):433-4.

References

Brown EG, Krouskop RW, McDonnell FE, et al, "A Technique to Continuously Measure Arteriovenous Oxygen Content Difference and P-50 In Vivo," *J Appl Physiol*, 1985, 58(4):1383-9.
Burtis CA and Ashwood ER, *Tietz Textbook of Clinical Chemistry*, 2nd ed, Philadelphia, PA: WB Saunders Co, 1994, 1391-2.
Konzuki H, Enoki Y, Sakata S, et al, "A Simple Microtonometric Method for Whole Blood Oxygen Dissociation Curve and a Critical Evaluation of the "Single Point" Procedure for Blood P-50," *Jpn J Physiol*, 1983, 33:987-94.
Ostrander LE, Paloski WH, Barie PS, et al, "A Computer Algorithm to Calculate P-50 From a Single Blood Sample," *IEEE Trans Biomed Eng*, 1983, 30:250-4.

Paigen Test (*E. coli* Bacteriophage Resistance to Lysis Assay)

see Galactose Screening Tests for Galactosemia *on page 132*

Pancreatic Polypeptide, Human

CPT 83519

Synonyms Human Pancreatic Polypeptide; PP

Abstract Pancreatic polypeptide is a hormone of unknown physiologic function produced by pancreatic endocrine cells. Its release is stimulated by ingestion of food, and it is often, but not uniformly, increased in cases of neoplasms of the APUD system, for which it may serve as a marker. Pancreatic polypeptide has never enjoyed clinical utility.

Patient Preparation Avoid recent radioactive scan. Fasting, then sampled after food stimulation.

Specimen Plasma

Container Lavender top (EDTA) tube; check with laboratory. Reference laboratories provide specific instructions.

Reference Range 50-300 pg/mL (SI: 50-300 mmol/L), fasting. Basal levels increase with age.

Critical Values Fasting level >300 pg/mL (SI: >300 mmol/L) is suspicious of tumor-producing pancreatic polypeptide ("PPoma").

Use Increased in some pancreatic APUD tumors. High levels may occur as a part of multiple endocrine adenomatosis type 1.[1] About 50% of patients with endocrine pancreatic tumors have elevated levels. Assay of
(Continued)

Pancreatic Polypeptide, Human (Continued)

PP is useful for diagnosis of such tumors and to follow patients with them. It is described as an adjunctive marker for many pancreatic endocrine tumors.[2]

Limitations Levels of this polypeptide may be increased in a wide variety of settings other than PPoma, including renal failure, diabetes, hypoglycemia, and the postprandial state.[2] It has low sensitivity.[3,4] There usually are no characteristic clinical features of PPoma recognized.

Methodology Radioimmunoassay (RIA)

Additional Information An atropine suppression test is used to distinguish tumor-related secretion of the peptide from normal. Release of the polypeptide from normal cells is under cholinergic control, inhibited by atropine, while autonomous secretion from a PPoma is anticipated.[2] Pancreatic endocrine tumors often secrete more than a single peptide. The peptides associated with such tumors include vasoactive intestinal polypeptide, gastrin, glucagon, somatostatin, and neurotensin.[2] Prediction of autonomic neuropathy in insulin-dependent diabetic patients; such patients, who are predisposed to the development of autonomic neuropathy may demonstrate a decreased pancreatic polypeptide (and epinephrine) response to insulin-induced hypoglycemia.[5] PP may be a glucoregulatory hormone.[6] Its release appears to be dependent upon intraluminal starch digestion.[7] The cholinergic system appears to be crucial and superimposed upon cholecystokinin in stimulating pancreatic polypeptide release.[8]

See listing Vasoactive Intestinal Polypeptide *on page 216*.

Footnotes
1. Gelston AL, Delisle MB, and Patel YC, "Multiple Endocrine Adenomatosis Type I. Occurrence in Octogenarian With High Levels of Circulating Pancreatic Polypeptide," *JAMA*, 1982, 247:665-6.
2. Adrian TE, Uttenthal LO, Williams SJ, et al, "Secretion of Pancreatic Polypeptide in Patients With Pancreatic Endocrine Tumors," *N Engl J Med*, 1986, 315(5):287-91.
3. Langstein HN, Norton JA, Chiang H-CV, et al, "The Utility of Circulating Levels of Human Pancreatic Polypeptide as a Marker for Islet Cell Tumors," *Surgery*, 1990, 108(6):1109-16.
4. Chiang H-CV, O'Dorisio TM, Huang SC, et al, "Multiple Hormone Elevations in Zollinger-Ellison Syndrome - Prospective Study of Clinical Significance and of the Development of a Second Symptomatic Pancreatic Endocrine Tumor Syndrome," *Gastroenterology*, 1990, 99(6):1565-75.
5. Kennedy FP, Go VL, Cryer PE, et al, "Subnormal Pancreatic Polypeptide and Epinephrine Responses to Insulin-Induced Hypoglycemia Identify Patients With Insulin-Dependent Diabetes Mellitus Predisposed to Develop Overt Autonomic Neuropathy," *Ann Intern Med*, 1988, 108(1):54-8.
6. Seymour NE, Brunicardi FC, Chaiken RL, et al, "Reversal of Abnormal Glucose Production After Pancreatic Resection by Pancreatic Polypeptide Administration in Man," *Surgery*, 1988, 104(2):119-29.
7. Layer P, Go VL, and DiMagno EP, "Carbohydrate Digestion and Release of Pancreatic Polypeptide in Health and Diabetes Mellitus," *Gut*, 1989, 30(9):1279-84.
8. Meier R, Hildebrand P, Thumshirn M, et al, "Effect of Loxiglumide, a Cholecystokinin Antagonist, on Pancreatic Polypeptide Release in Humans," *Gastroenterology*, 1990, 99(6):1757-62.

References
Bank S and Chow KW, "Diagnostic Tests in Chronic Pancreatitis," *Gastroenterologist*, 1994, 2(3):224-32.
Brunicardi FC, Druck P, Sun YS, et al, "Regulation of Pancreatic Polypeptide Secretion in the Isolated Perfused Human Pancreas," *Am J Surg*, 1988, 155(1):63-9.
Feldman M, Samson WK, and O'Dorisio TM, "Apomorphine-Induced Nausea in Humans: Release of Vasopressin and Pancreatic Polypeptide," *Gastroenterology*, 1988, 95(3):721-6.
Green DW, Gomez G, and Greeley GH Jr, "Gastrointestinal Peptides," *Gastroenterol Clin North Am*, 1989, 18(4):695-733.
Hazelwood RL, "The Pancreatic Polypeptide (PP-Fold) Family: Gastrointestinal, Vascular, and Feeding Behavioral Implications," *Proc Soc Exp Biol Med*, 1993, 202(1):44-63.
Inoue K, Tobe T, Suzuki T, et al, "Plasma Cholecystokinin and Pancreatic Polypeptide Response After Radical Pancreatoduodenectomy With Billroth I and Billroth II Type of Reconstruction," *Ann Surg*, 1987, 206(2):148-54.
Medeiros MS and Turner AJ, "Post-Secretory Processing of Regulatory Peptides: The Pancreatic Polypeptide Family as a Model Example," *Biochimie*, 1994, 76(3-4):283-7.

PAP *see* Acid Phosphatase *on page 62*

Paracentesis Fluid Analysis *see* Body Fluid *on page 89*

Parathormone *see* Parathyroid Hormone *on this page*

Parathyroid Hormone

CPT 83970

Related Information

Calcium, Ionized *on page 96*
Calcium, Serum *on page 97*
Calcium, Urine *on page 99*
Cyclic AMP, Plasma *on page 119*
Cyclic AMP, Urine *on page 119*
Kidney Stone Analysis *on page 640*
Osteocalcin, Serum *on page 174*
Phosphorus, Serum *on page 182*
Phosphorus, Urine *on page 183*

Synonyms Immunoreactive PTH; Parathormone; PTH

Applies to Parathyroid Hormone, C-Terminal; Parathyroid Hormone, Intact; Parathyroid Hormone, N-Terminal; Parathyroid Hormone Related Protein; PRP; PTH-Related Protein

Test Commonly Includes Serum calcium is needed for interpretation. Serum phosphorus and creatinine are relevant.

Abstract Parathormone is among the first approaches in evaluation of hypercalcemia. It is used to investigate parathyroid function and calcium metabolism. It is needed to resolve the differential diagnosis of the two most common causes of hypercalcemia: primary hyperparathyroidism and malignancy.

Patient Preparation Patient should be fasting. Recent injection of radioisotope may interfere, depending on assay system used.

Specimen Serum

Container Red top tube

Sampling Time Diurnal rhythm exists. Nadir is in the morning. Morning draw is recommended.

Collection Centrifuge promptly. Freeze immediately. Consult reference laboratory for specific instructions regarding exact PTH moiety being analyzed.

Reference Range Typical reference range (immunochemiluminometric assay (ICMA)) for PTH, intact: 10-50 pg/mL (SI: 1.1-5.3 pmol/L), N-terminal: 8-24 pg/mL (SI: 0.8-2.5 pmol/L), C-terminal: 0-340 pg/mL (SI: 0-35.8 pmol/L); hypoparathyroid patients: <9 pg/mL (SI: <1.0 pmol/L); hyperparathyroidism patients: >47 pg/mL (SI: >5.0 pmol/L)

Use Evaluate hypercalcemia, differential diagnosis of primary hyperparathyroidism. When the serum PTH concentration is inappropriately high for the level of hypercalcemia, the differential diagnosis includes primary hyperparathyroidism, hypocalciuric familial benign hypercalcemia, lithium-induced hypercalcemia and rarely, ectopic parathormone-producing neoplasms.[1] In hyperparathyroidism PTH correlates with bone disease. PTH aids in distinction of hyperparathyroidism from nonparathyroid causes of hypercalcemia, such as neoplasia, vitamin D intoxication, and Graves' disease. Monitor therapy of secondary hyperparathyroidism in chronic renal failure; work up hypoparathyroidism, osteomalacia.

Limitations PTH is an 84-amino acid peptide that circulates in at least four molecular forms. Intact PTH possesses the greatest degree of activity and is present in the lowest plasma concentration. C-terminal peptide is inactive and is present in the highest concentration due to its long half-life. Older polyclonal assays measure more than one form of parathyroid hormone leading to substantial imprecision. Currently, two-site assays are able to detect intact parathyroid hormone in the presence of excess amounts of inactive C-terminal fragments.[2] PTH measurements should always be interpreted in conjunction with a total calcium level. Ionized calcium, additionally, may be helpful. All PTH fragments accumulate in renal failure to a greater extent if hyperparathyroidism is present.

PTH may be increased with hypercalcemia of malignancy, but in the bulk of the cases a PTH-like factor, PTH-related protein (PRP), is involved.[2,3] PRP shows considerable homology with the N-terminus of parathyroid hormone; eight of the first 13 amino acids are identical.[4] Some patients with hyperparathyroidism have had normal serum PTH concentrations.

Patients with primary hyperparathyroidism may not have a synchronized circadian rhythm. If primary hyperparathyroidism is a differential consideration, then measurement after 10 AM might be desirable.[5]

Methodology Immunochemiluminometric (ICMA);[6] bioassay of functional aminoterminal PTH; radioimmunoassay (RIA); immunoradiometric assay (IRMA). See article by Wood PJ for a review of the state of detection of intact PTH. A rapid (modified immunoradiometric) parathyroid hormone assay has been described which may be utilized during surgery.[7,8]

Additional Information No single assay previously has been suitable for evaluation of all suspected parathyroid disorders. Wood reports that utilization of two-site intact parathyroid hormone assays justifies the introduction of a national external quality assessment scheme in the UK.[2] Intact two-site PTH assays are direct measurements of parathyroid gland function, and are independent of renal disease. Such assays allow for excellent differentiation of hypoparathyroidism (low PTH, low calcium), primary hyperparathyroidism (high-normal to elevated PTH, high calcium), and nonparathyroid causes of hypercalcemia (Low or low-normal PTH, high calcium). In patients with chronic renal disease, these assays are also helpful for distinguishing patients with osteomalacia or aplasia (normal to slightly elevated PTH levels) from those with osteitis fibrosa (markedly elevated PTH levels). Consultation with reference laboratories regarding the specific performance of assays in various clinical states is desirable.

In a series of 61 cases of primary hyperparathyroidism, calcium varied from 10.8-16.6 mg/dL (SI: 2.69-4.14 mmol/L) with poor correlation between calcium and PTH levels. Forty percent had increased alkaline phosphatase; 33% had hypercalciuria. See chart.

Correlation of Clinical Diagnosis With Parathyroid Hormone and Calcium Levels

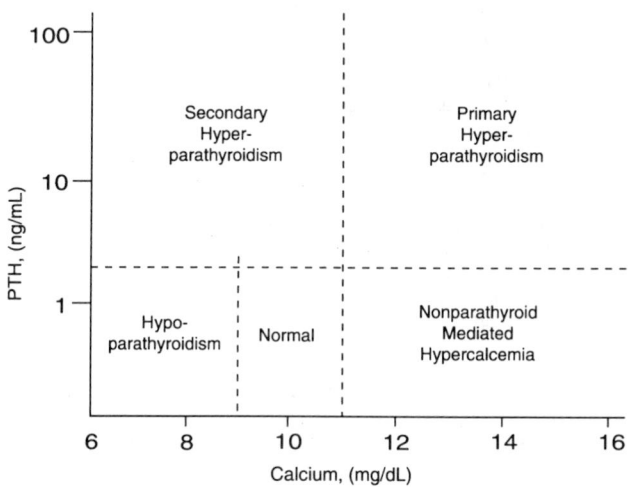

Following parathyroid surgery for hyperparathyroidism, 42% of patients in a European series had increased serum PTH with low phosphorus levels.[9]

Parathyroid carcinoma should be considered when a patient presents with features of hyperparathyroidism, a palpable neck mass, both bone disease and nephrolithiasis, and marked increases of both serum calcium and PTH levels.[10]

When a nonparathyroid tumor is associated with hypercalcemia, decreased serum phosphorus and increased concentrations of parathyroid hormone related peptide, the neoplasm is most often squamous cell bronchogenic carcinoma. This clinical syndrome, recently called **ectopic hyperparathyroidism**, is now named **humoral hypercalcemia of malignancy**.[11] Parathyroid hormone-related peptide is now considered to be the major mediator of humoral hypercalcemia of malignancy.[12]

Familial benign hypercalcemia is a rare autosomal dominant entity which may be confused with primary hyperparathyroidism. Hypercalcemia begins in the first two decades. Although there is moderate hypercalcemia, hypercalciuria is not found. Serum calcium is elevated out of proportion to the concentration of PTH. Subtotal parathyroidectomy fails to eliminate hypercalcemia.

Hormonal control of normal skeletal growth, modeling, and remodeling including interactions with parathyroid hormone is reviewed.[13]

Footnotes
1. Kreisberg RA, "Clinical Problem-Solving. Stopping Short of Certainty," *N Engl J Med*, 1994, 331(1):42-5.
2. Wood PJ, "The Measurement of Parathyroid Hormone," *Ann Clin Biochem*, 1992, 29(Pt 1):11-21.
3. Pandian MR, Morgan CH, Carlton E, et al, "Modified Immunoradiometric Assay of Parathyroid Hormone-Related Protein: Clinical Application in the Differential Diagnosis of Hypercalcemia," *Clin Chem*, 1992, 38(2):282-8.
4. Lufkin EG, Kao PC, and Heath H III, "Parathyroid Hormone Radioimmunoassays in the Differential Diagnosis of Hypercalcemia Due to Primary Hyperparathyroidism or Malignancy," *Ann Intern Med*, 1987, 106(4):559-60.
5. Wood PJ, "Investigation of Calcium Disorders," *JIFCC*, 1994, 6(5):181-5.
6. Leavelle DE, *Interpretive Handbook*, Rochester, MN: Mayo Medical Laboratories, 1994.
7. Ryan MF, Jones SR, and Barnes AD, "Clinical Evaluation of a Rapid Parathyroid Hormone Assay," *Ann Clin Biochem*, 1992, 29(Pt 1):48-51.
8. Ryan MF, Jones SR, and Barnes AD, "Modification to a Commercial Immunoradiometric Assay Permitting Intraoperative Monitoring of Parathyroid Hormone Levels," *Ann Clin Biochem*, 1990, 27(Pt 1):65-8.
9. Mulder H, Koster J, Hackeng WH, et al, "Normocalcaemic Hyperparathyroidism After Parathyroidectomy: A Retrospective Study," *Scand J Clin Lab Invest*, 1993, 53(6):607-10.
10. Wynne AG, van Heerden J, Carney JA, et al, "Parathyroid Carcinoma: Clinical and Pathologic Features in 43 Patients," *Medicine (Baltimore)*, 1992, 71(4):197-205.
11. Wysolmerski JJ and Broadus AE, "Hypercalcemia of Malignancy: The Central Role of Parathyroid Hormone-Related Protein," *Annu Rev Med*, 1994, 45:189-200.
12. Law F, Ferrari S, Rizzoli R, et al, "Parathyroid Hormone-Related Protein and Calcium Phosphate Metabolism," *Pediatr Nephrol*, 1993, 7(6):827-33.
13. Avioli LV, "Hormonal Alterations and Osteoporotic Syndromes," *J Bone Miner Res*, 1993, 8(Suppl 2):S511-4.

References
Bourke E and Delaney V, "Assessment of Hypocalcemia and Hypercalcemia," *Clin Lab Med*, 1993, 13(1):157-81.
Budayr AA, Nissenson RA, Klein RF, et al, "Increased Serum Levels of a Parathyroid Hormone-Like Protein in Malignancy-Associated Hypercalcemia," *Ann Intern Med*, 1989, 111(10):807-12.
Delellis RA, "Tumors of the Parathyroid Gland," *Atlas of Tumor Pathology*, Third Series, Fascicle 6, Bethesda, MD: Armed Forces Institute of Pathology under the auspices of Universities Associated for Research and Education in Pathology, Inc, 1993.
Firek AF, Kao PC, and Heath H 3d, "Plasma Intact Parathyroid Hormone (PTH) and PTH-Related Peptide in Familial Benign Hypercalcemia: Greater Responsiveness to

Endogenous PTH Than in Primary Hyperparathyroidism," *J Clin Endocrinol Metab*, 1991, 72(3):541-6.
Flentje D, Schmidt-Gayk H, Fischer S, et al, "Intact Parathyroid Hormone in Primary Hyperparathyroidism," *Br J Surg*, 1990, 77(2):168-72.
Hage DS, Taylor B, and Kao PC, "Intact Parathyroid Hormone: Performance and Clinical Utility of an Automated Assay Based on High-Performance Immunoaffinity Chromatography and Chemiluminescence Detection," *Clin Chem*, 1992, 38(8 Pt 1):1494-1500.
Kao PC, van Heerden J, Grant CS, et al, "Clinical Performance of Parathyroid Hormone Immunometric Assays," *Mayo Clin Proc*, 1992, 67(7):637-45.
Lobaugh B, Neelon FA, Oyama H, et al, "Circadian Rhythms for Calcium, Inorganic Phosphorus, and Parathyroid Hormone in Primary Hyperparathyroidism: Functional and Practical Considerations," *Surgery*, 1989, 106(6):1009-16.
Mallette LE, Khouri K, Zengotita H, et al, "Lithium Treatment Increases Intact and Midregion Parathyroid Hormone and Parathyroid Volume," *J Clin Endocrinol Metab*, 1989, 68(3):654-60.
Quarles LD, Lobaugh B, and Murphy G, "Intact Parathyroid Hormone Overestimates the Presence and Severity of Parathyroid-Mediated Osseous Abnormalities in Uremia," *J Clin Endocrinol Metab*, 1992, 75(1):145-50.
Ross DS and Nussbaum SR, "Reciprocal Changes in Parathyroid Hormone and Thyroid Function After Radioiodine Treatment of Hyperthyroidism," *J Clin Endocrinol Metab*, 1989, 68(6):1216-9.
Rudnicki M, "Increasing Parathyroid Hormone Concentrations in Primary Hyperparathyroidism," *J Intern Med*, 1992, 232(5):421-5.
Samaan NA, Ouais S, Ordonez NG, et al, "Multiple Endocrine Syndrome Type I: Clinical, Laboratory Findings, and Management in Five Families," *Cancer*, 1989, 64(3):741-52.
Silverberg SJ, Shane E, de la Cruz L, et al, "Abnormalities in Parathyroid Hormone Secretion and 1,25-Dihydroxyvitamin D_3 Formation in Women With Osteoporosis," *N Engl J Med*, 1989, 320(5):277-81.
Solal ME, Sebert JL, Boudailliez B, et al, "Comparison of Intact, Midregion, and Carboxy Terminal Assays of Parathyroid Hormone for the Diagnosis of Bone Disease in Hemodialyzed Patients," *J Clin Endocrinol Metab*, 1991, 73(3):516-24.
Woodhead JS, "The Measurement of Circulating Parathyroid Hormone," *Clin Biochem*, 1990, 23(1):17-21.
Young DS, *Effects of Drugs on Clinical Laboratory Tests*, 4th ed, Washington, DC: AACC Press, 1996.

Parathyroid Hormone, C-Terminal *see* Parathyroid Hormone *on previous page*

Parathyroid Hormone, Intact *see* Parathyroid Hormone *on previous page*

Parathyroid Hormone, N-Terminal *see* Parathyroid Hormone *on previous page*

Parathyroid Hormone-Related Protein *see* Calcium, Serum *on page 97*

Parathyroid Hormone Related Protein *see* Parathyroid Hormone *on previous page*

Pbg-D *see* Porphobilinogen Deaminase, Erythrocyte *on page 185*

PBI *replaced by* Thyroxine *on page 206*

PChE *see* Pseudocholinesterase, Serum *on page 196*

pCO₂ *see* Blood Gases, Arterial *on page 87*

pCO₂, Blood
CPT 82803

Related Information
Arterial Blood Collection *on page 24*
Blood Gases, Arterial *on page 87*
Blood Gases, Capillary *on page 89*
Carbon Dioxide, Blood *on page 100*
HCO_3, Blood *on page 142*
pH, Blood *on next page*
Venous Blood Collection *on page 30*

Applies to Acid-Base Status

Test Commonly Includes Test is part of blood gas panels and often, electrolyte panels

Abstract Disturbances of respiration primarily affect pCO_2, while metabolic disturbances are reflected by bicarbonate levels.

Specimen Whole blood (arterial, venous, or capillary)

Collection See Blood Gases, Capillary *on page 89* listing. Deliver immediately to the laboratory. When pCO_2 is drawn as a venous specimen, avoid a tourniquet if possible. Especially, **avoid fist clenching**. It is often collected with venous pH; see Collection in the listing pH, Blood *on page 180* and also see listings Arterial Blood Collection *on page 24* and Venous Blood Collection *on page 30*.

Storage Instructions Must be analyzed within 1 hour. *In vitro* changes in blood gas parameters:[1] pO_2, 37°C: 33 mm Hg/10 minutes, 4°C: 3 mm Hg/10 minutes; pCO_2, 37°C: 1 mm Hg/10 minutes, 4°C: 0.1 mm Hg/10 minutes.

Causes for Rejection Specimen with clots, air bubbles, not received on ice, needle not tightly stoppered

Turnaround Time Usually 30 minutes or less

Reference Range Newborns, infants, and children up to approximately 2 years of age, with **arterialized capillary blood** (heel, fingertip, big toe) or arterial blood; 27-40 mm Hg; children older than 2 years of age and adults: **arterial:** 40-52 mm Hg, **venous:** 35-48 mm Hg

Possible Panic Range <20 mm Hg, >70 mm Hg

(Continued)

pCO$_2$, Blood (Continued)

Use Alveolar ventilation varies inversely as arterial pCO$_2$; therefore, pCO$_2$ is an indication of adequacy of CO$_2$ elimination by the lungs. **Respiratory alkalosis** (hyperventilation) results in low pCO$_2$ with elevated pH. **Respiratory acidosis** (hypoventilation) results in high pCO$_2$ with lowered pH.

Limitations Venous and arterial values are sensitive to sampling technique.

Methodology pCO$_2$ electrode. This is a modified pH electrode which is present in a carbonate-bicarbonate buffer system. A plastic membrane (permeable to CO$_2$) is positioned between the blood sample and the electrode's surrounding buffer. CO$_2$ from the sample diffuses into the buffer; any pH change is detected by the electrode, and the resultant voltage change is read as pCO$_2$.

Additional Information Respiratory compensation for metabolic acidosis and alkalosis involves adjustment of the pCO$_2$ level by hypoventilation (as in cases of metabolic alkalosis with resultant rise in pCO$_2$) or by hyperventilation (as in cases of metabolic acidosis with decreasing pCO$_2$). Helpful background is provided in the references listed. As CO$_2$ is highly soluble, there is a quickly attained equilibrium between arterial carbon dioxide tension **(PaCO$_2$)** and alveolar carbon dioxide tension. The arterial CO$_2$ measurement, then also determines the status of ventilation. PaCO$_2$ has a reverse relationship to alveolar ventilation.[1]

The expression "**hypercapnia**" indicates the presence of excessive carbon dioxide in the blood. Disorders associated with hypercapnia include central depression, abnormal neuromuscular function, chest wall abnormality, upper or lower respiratory tract disease, or hypercapnia secondary to cardiac disease.[2] Arterial pCO$_2$ may be an indicator of systemic perfusion during cardiopulmonary resuscitation.[3] Increased venous-arterial pCO$_2$ gradients do not appear to be a reliable indicator of inadequate tissue perfusion during cardiopulmonary bypass.[4] Transcutaneous measurements of pCO$_2$ may be a convenient means of monitoring the neonate in intensive care units. Acidosis does affect the ability to correlate transcutaneous and arterial pCO$_2$ values.[5]

Regulation of cerebral blood flow and volume appears to rely heavily upon changes in arterial pCO$_2$.[6]

Footnotes

1. Bruegger BB and Sherwin JE, "Blood Gas Analysis and Oxygen Saturation," *Methods in Clinical Chemistry*, Chapter 8, Pesce AJ and Kaplan LA, eds, St Louis, MO: Mosby-Year Book Inc, 1987, 54-66.
2. Weinberger SE, Schwartzstein RM, and Weiss JW, "Hypercapnia," *N Engl J Med*, 1989, 321(18):1223-31.
3. Gazmuri RJ, von Planta M, Weil MH, et al, "Arterial PCO$_2$ as an Indicator of Systemic Perfusion During Cardiopulmonary Resuscitation," *Crit Care Med*, 1989, 17(3):237-40.
4. Ariza M, Gothard JW, Macnaughton P, et al, "Blood Lactate and Mixed Venous-Arterial pCO$_2$ Gradient as Indices of Poor Peripheral Perfusion Following Cardiopulmonary Bypass Surgery," *Intensive Care Med*, 1991, 17(6):320-4.
5. Hand IL, Shepard EK, Krauss AN, et al, "Discrepancies Between Transcutaneous and End-Tidal Carbon Dioxide Monitoring in the Critically Ill Neonate With Respiratory Distress Syndrome," *Crit Care Med*, 1989, 17(6):556-9.
6. Madden JA, "The Effect of Carbon Dioxide on Cerebral Arteries," *Pharmacol Ther*, 1993, 59(2):229-50.

References

Barrett CR Jr, "Pulmonary Physiologic Testing: Arterial Blood Gases," *The Laboratory in Clinical Medicine: Interpretation and Application*, Halsted JA and Halsted CH, eds, Philadelphia, PA: WB Saunders Co, 1981, 370-9.

Burnett RW and Itano M, "An Interlaboratory Study of Blood-Gas Analysis: Dependence of pO$_2$ and pCO$_2$ Results on Atmospheric Pressure," *Clin Chem*, 1989, 35(8):1779-81.

Gay PC and Edmonds LC, "Severe Hypercapnia After Low-Flow Oxygen Therapy in Patients With Neuromuscular Disease and Diaphragmatic Dysfunction," *Mayo Clin Proc*, 1995, 70(4):327-30.

Hansen JE, Casaburi R, Crapo RO, et al, "Assessing Precision and Accuracy in Blood Gas Proficiency Testing," *Am Rev Respir Dis*, 1990, 141(5 Pt 1):1190-3.

Meyerhoff ME, "New *In Vitro* Analytical Approaches for Clinical Chemistry Measurements in Critical Care," *Clin Chem*, 1990, 36(8 Pt 2):1567-72.

Narins RG and Emmett M, "Simple and Mixed Acid-Base Disorders: A Practical Approach," *Medicine (Baltimore)*, 1980, 59:161-87.

Preuss HG, "Fundamentals of Clinical Acid-Base Evaluation," *Clin Lab Med*, 1993, 13(1):103-16.

Tobin MJ and Jubran A, "Oxygen Takes the Breath Away: Old Sting, New Setting," *Mayo Clin Proc*, 1995, 70(4):403-4 (editorial).

Pentagastrin Stimulation Test *see* Gastric Analysis *on page 133*

Pentagastrin Stimulation Test *see* Calcitonin *on page 96*

Peptavlon® Stimulation Test *see* Gastric Analysis *on page 133*

Pericardial Fluid Analysis *see* Body Fluid *on page 89*

Peritoneal Fluid Analysis *see* Body Fluid *on page 89*

Peritoneal Fluid pH *see* Body Fluid pH *on page 92*

pH *see* Blood Gases, Arterial *on page 87*

pH, Blood

CPT 82800

Related Information

Anion Gap *on page 81*
Arterial Blood Collection *on page 24*
Blood Gases, Arterial *on page 87*
Blood Gases, Capillary *on page 89*
Blood Gases, Venous *on page 89*
Carbon Dioxide, Blood *on page 100*
Delta Base, Blood *on page 121*
Glucose, Fasting *on page 137*
Ketone Bodies, Blood *on page 152*
Lactic Acid, Blood *on page 156*
Osmolality, Calculated *on page 172*
Oxygen Saturation, Blood *on page 175*
pCO$_2$, Blood *on previous page*
pH, Urine *on page 648*
Salicylate *on page 573*
Venous Blood Collection *on page 30*

Synonyms Blood pH

Abstract Blood pH is used to indicate the presence of acidemia or alkalemia.

Specimen Whole blood (arterial, venous, or capillary)

Container Green top (heparin) tube or heparinized syringe

Collection For venous sample, it is best to collect without tourniquet if possible. **Do not allow patient to clench/unclench his/her hand.** This builds up lactic acid. Draw specimen into air-free heparinized syringe with needle quickly stoppered, making sure that no air bubbles remain. Capillary tubes should be filled as much as possible, metal flea inserted, capped, and mixed well with magnet. All specimens should be on ice and brought to the laboratory immediately. For capillary collection, the skin area to be punctured should be warmed 10-15 minutes. The puncture should be deep enough to allow a free flow of blood. See listings Arterial Blood Collection *on page 24* and Venous Blood Collection *on page 30*.

Storage Instructions Keep on ice in a syringe. pH changes 0.01/10 minutes at 37°C and 0.001/10 minutes at 4°C.[1]

Causes for Rejection Specimen with clots, air bubbles, not iced, needle not tightly stoppered

Turnaround Time Stability of iced green top tube for pH is not in excess of 4 hours. Usually reported in less than 30 minutes.

Reference Range Pediatrics: newborns, with **arterialized capillary blood** (heel, fingertip, big toe) or arterial blood; 7.32-7.49; 2 months to 2 years, arterialized capillary or arterial blood: 7.34-7.46; children and adults: **arterial:** 7.35-7.45, **venous:** 7.32-7.43. **Blood pH can be measured from either arterial or venous blood samples, usually with only very small differences in normal range.** Such differences are partly addressed in the listing Blood Gases, Venous *on page 89*.

Possible Panic Range <7.20, >7.60. Occasionally, patients with acidosis as severe as pH 6.80 survive. Many of these present with diabetic ketoacidosis, for which effective therapy is available.

Use Diagnose acidosis (eg, ketoacidosis), alkalosis (eg, emesis with loss of gastric juice); evaluate acid-base balance, significance of serum or plasma potassium levels; work up hypokalemia; use of oxyhemoglobin dissociation curves. May be useful for assessment of birth asphyxia in the depressed newborn. **Increased** with uncompensated metabolic and respiratory alkalosis, **decreased** with uncompensated metabolic and respiratory acidosis.

Limitations pH values are sensitive to sampling technique. Concurrent metabolic acidosis and respiratory alkalosis may result in normal pH[1], pCO$_2$, HCO$_3$, and anion gap, but abnormality might be detected by potassium level and blood volume measurement. Organic acidemias of infancy are beyond the scope of this manual.

Methodology Glass pH electrode

Additional Information pH should be judged in relation to other parameters such as pCO$_2$, HCO$_3$, Na$^+$, K$^+$, Cl$^-$, glucose, ketone bodies, phosphorus, and lactic acid, BUN, creatinine, and osmolality of serum and urine. A small amount of information about some acid base disorders is provided in the listing Anion Gap *on page 81* and the references which are included. The osmolal gap is addressed in the listing Osmolality, Calculated *on page 172*.

Causes of metabolic acidosis with normal and with increased anion gap are provided in the reference by Narins and Emmett. See Anion Gap listing as well.

Methanol, ethylene glycol, paraldehyde, salicylate toxicity, diabetic ketoacidosis, alcoholic ketoacidosis, lactic acidosis, renal failure, and starvation are causes of **high anion gap metabolic acidosis.**

Additional to electrolytes and other tests listed above, relevant laboratory findings in acidemia may also include ketones, ethanol concentration, uric acid, albumin, CBC, urinalysis with examination for oxalate crystals, and salicylate concentration.

Hypoproteinemia causes a metabolic alkalosis.[2]

Umbilical artery pH may be useful in the assessment of birth asphyxia[3,4] of the depressed neonate. Others contend that infants must be severely depressed with Apgar scores ≤3 at 1 and 5 minutes to be reflected in a decreased serum pH.[5] Blood may be obtained from a clamped umbilical segment up to 1 hour after delivery.[6]

In hypotensive patients, tissue hypoxia may be assessed by measurements of arterial pH, mixed venous pH, and bicarbonate concentrations.[7] Such measurements do not appear to reliably assess tissue hypoxia in patients with fulminant hepatic failure.[8] For such patients, oxygen flux (the difference between arterial and venous oxygen) remains the best way to detect the presence of covert tissue hypoxia.

Footnotes

1. Bruegger BB and Sherwin JE, "Blood Gas Analysis and Oxygen Saturation," *Methods in Clinical Chemistry*, Chapter 8, Pesce AJ and Kaplan LA, eds, St Louis, MO: Mosby-Year Book Inc, 1987, 54-66.
2. McAuliffe JJ, Lind LJ, Leith DE, et al, "Hypoproteinemic Alkalosis," *Am J Med*, 1986, 81(1):86-90.
3. Goldaber KG and Gilstrap LC 3d, "Correlations Between Obstetric Clinical Events and Umbilical Cord Blood Acid-Base and Blood Gas Values," *Clin Obstet Gynecol*, 1993, 36(1):47-59.
4. Blackstone J and Young BK, "Umbilical Cord Blood Acid-Base Values and Other Descriptors of Fetal Condition," *Clin Obstet Gynecol*, 1993, 36(1):33-46.
5. Gilstrap LC 3d, Leveno KJ, Burris J, et al, "Diagnosis of Birth Asphyxia on the Basis of Fetal pH, Apgar Score, and Newborn Cerebral Dysfunction," *Am J Obstet Gynecol*, 1989, 161(3):825-30.
6. Duerbeck NB, Chaffin DG, and Seeds JW, "A Practical Approach to Umbilical Artery pH and Blood Gas Determinations," *Obstet Gynecol*, 1992, 79(6):959-62.
7. Adrogué HJ, Rashad MN, Gorin AB, et al, "Assessing Acid-Base Status in Circulatory Failure: Differences Between Arterial and Central Venous Blood," *N Engl J Med*, 1989, 320(20):1312-6.
8. Wendon JA, Harrison PM, Keays R, et al, "Arterial-Venous pH Differences and Tissue Hypoxia in Patients With Fulminant Hepatic Failure," *Crit Care Med*, 1991, 19:(11)1362-4.

References

Adrogué HJ, Wilson H, Boyd AE III, et al, "Plasma Acid-Base Patterns in Diabetic Ketoacidosis," *N Engl J Med*, 1982, 307:1603-10.
Narins RG and Emmett M, "Simple and Mixed Acid-Base Disorders: A Practical Approach," *Medicine*, 1980, 59:161-87.
Nicolaides KH, Economides DL, and Soothill PW, "Blood Gases, pH, and Lactate in Appropriate- and Small-for-Gestational-Age Fetuses," *Am J Obstet Gynecol*, 1989, 161(4):996-1001.
Preuss HG, "Fundamentals of Clinical Acid-Base Evaluation," *Clin Lab Med*, 1993, 13(1):103-16.
Shapiro BA, "pH and Blood Gas Measurements: Discerning Innovation From Sophistication," *Crit Care Med*, 1989, 17(9):966.
Shapiro BA, Cane RD, Chomka CM, et al, "Preliminary Evaluation of an Intra-Arterial Blood Gas System in Dogs and Humans," *Crit Care Med*, 1989, 17(5):455-60.
Thorp JA, Sampson JE, Parisi VM, et al, "Routine Umbilical Cord Blood Gas Determinations?" *Am J Obstet Gynecol*, 1989, 161(3):600-5.
Wang F, Butler T, Rabbani GH, et al, "The Acidosis of Cholera: Contributions of Hyperproteinemia, Lactic Acidemia, and Hyperphosphatemia to an Increased Serum Anion Gap," *N Engl J Med*, 1986, 315(25):1591-5.

pH Body Fluid *see* Body Fluid pH *on page 92*

Phenformin *see* Lactic Acid, Blood *on page 156*

Phenylalanine, Blood

CPT 84030 (Guthrie)

Related Information

Amino Acid Screen, Plasma *on page 74*
Amino Acid Screen, Qualitative, Urine *on page 75*
Newborn Screen for Phenylketonuria *on page 169*
Newborn Screen for T$_4$ *on page 170*
Phenylalanine Test, Urine *on page 647*

Synonyms Guthrie Test; Hyperphenylalaninemia Screen; Phenylalanine Screening Test, Blood; Phenylketonuria Test; PKU Test

Abstract Autosomal recessive aminoacidopathy due to phenylalanine hydroxylase or biopterin (folic acid constituent) cofactor deficiencies. Detection by low cost dried blood spot screening can result in early treatment, intended to prevent mental retardation. Clinical diversity relates to genetic heterogeneity.

Patient Preparation Newborn should have milk (protein) feeding ideally for 48 hours before testing; sample as late as possible prior to discharge from hospital. Collection is recommended at 4-10 days for low birth weight infants.

Specimen Whole blood, serum or plasma

Container Newborns: PKU test card; screening: filter paper sheet. Pediatrics: Small red top tube, gray top (sodium fluoride) tube or green top (heparin) tube; check with laboratory

Sampling Time With newborn, just before infant is discharged from the nursery

Collection Test card must be labeled with patient's name, date, time, date of birth and time of first milk feeding. In order to obtain accurate tests results for PKU, blood collection should preferably be made when the infant is 48-120 hours of age and has been on a protein feeding for at least 24 hours. Do not oversaturate filter paper. Do not fill circles on one side and then fill circles on reverse side. Do not collect blood with a capillary tube to apply to filter paper. Include information regarding blood transfusions and antibiotics or other medications administered to the infant, which may influence screening test results.

Storage Instructions Newborns: Air dry specimens at room temperature in a horizontal position for at least 2 hours. Do not use hermetically sealed envelopes. Pediatrics: Separate serum and transfer to plastic vial containing 10 mg NaF. (Check with laboratory for other possible specimen requirements.) Separate within 4 hours of collection. Serum or plasma is stable 5 days at 4°C. Care in handling the filter paper specimens is essential, because exposure to extreme heat or light or touching the filter paper portion of the form can cause erroneous test results. Specimens containing contaminants, such as alcohol or other liquids, or antibiotics may not be satisfactory for testing. (See following discussion.) The phenylalanine in filter paper dried blood spots is stable for years when not exposed to environmental extremes.

Causes for Rejection Filter paper not thoroughly saturated, inadequate specimen identification, specimens which are respotted (several drops of blood applied to the same circle), specimens which are QNS (quantity not sufficient). **Cord blood cannot be used. Phenylalanine is not significantly increased at birth.** Blood should not be drawn before milk diet of at least 24 hours prior to sampling, but need to sample before discharge from the nursery may take priority if outpatient sampling is not assured.

Reference Range ≤2 mg/dL (SI: ≤121 μmol/L) by Guthrie bacterial-inhibition assay; <4 mg/dL (SI: <242 μmol/L) by fluorometry in some laboratories. Positive tests by Guthrie assay should be confirmed by a chemical method (fluorometry or chromatography).

Possible Panic Range ≥4 mg/dL (SI: ≥242 μmol/L) by Guthrie bacterial-inhibition assay. Specific diagnosis after identification of a candidate case (by screening program) requires that plasma levels of phenylalanine be >2 mg/dL (SI: >121 μmol/L) on 2 consecutive days.

Use Evaluate patients for phenylketonuria, monitor therapy with phenylalanine restricted diet

Limitations Cases have been missed because blood phenylalanine was not increased, even after the third day of life.[1] Identification of non-PKU forms of hyperphenylalaninemia (see following information) requires additional testing for tetrahydrobiopterin pathway enzyme defects. **Not all individuals with increased blood phenylalanine have phenylketonuria.** When the infant is tested for PKU before 24 hours of age, there is a 16% chance of missing a positive case. When screened between 24 and 48 hours of birth, there is a 2.2% chance of missing a positive, between 48 and 72 hours, 0.3% chance.

Methodology Guthrie testing (microbiologic inhibition assay) (semiquantitative), chromatography, fluorometry, polymerase chain reaction (PCR)

Additional Information Successful detection of phenylketonuria by screening newborns for hyperphenylalaninemia has as its goal the identification of infants subject to central nervous system damage (in particular mental retardation) due to excessive levels of phenylalanine. Once identified, harmful CNS effects can be largely avoided by dietary measures, notably a semisynthetic diet low in phenylalanine. In young PKU patients, the tolerance for dietary phenylalanine (to maintain nontoxic plasma levels) is about 250-550 mg/day. Widespread institution of PKU screening programs, worldwide, is an outstanding public health triumph of the 20th century. Incidence is 1:10,000 to 1:25,000 in the United States. For blacks in Maryland the reported incidence is 1:50,000.[2]

State laws require PKU testing of infants within 28 days or less; in some states, prior to hospital discharge regardless of age. Disease caused by lack of phenylalanine hydroxylase leads to mental retardation if not treated. A second screening should be considered but is not universally mandated in infants whose first test occurred within the first 24 hours of life. Screening generally includes testing for hypothyroidism and in some areas for galactosemia and maple syrup disease as well as for phenylketonuria. Every effort must be made to assure that immediate diagnosis and treatment is provided for infants with abnormal results.

Presence of hyperphenylalaninemia implies a disorder of phenylalanine hydroxylation (to tyrosine). PKU due to phenylalanine hydroxylase (PAH) deficiency is the common example. However, in addition to PAH, hydroxylation requires oxygen and tetrahydrobiopterin (BH$_4$) as a cofactor. A defect in the metabolism of BH$_4$ that results in BH$_4$ deficiency will impair hydroxylation and result in increased plasma phenylalanine concentrations. In the past 15 years three types of inborn errors of BH$_4$ metabolism ("atypical PKU") have been identified. Defects in BH$_4$ synthesis are guanosine triphosphate cyclohydrolase I deficiency and pyruvoyl (Continued)

Phenylalanine, Blood (Continued)

tetrahydropterin synthase deficiency. The third type of defect involves the regeneration of BH_4 catalyzed by the enzyme dihydropteridine reductase. Experience with treatment of PKU over the past 25 years has shown that some 3% (variable between different populations) fail to respond.[3] These are largely cases of BH_4 cofactor deficiency. There are important differences in therapy between classical PKU and the various BH_4 cofactor deficiencies. "PKU positive" cases (identified as the result of phenylalanine screening tests) should be additionally tested for BH_4 deficiency. Clinical features; urine, blood, and enzyme analyses; prenatal diagnosis; and therapy of BH_4 deficiencies have been reviewed.[3]

Classical PKU is an autosomal recessive disorder. Relatives (eg, siblings) of a PKU homozygote or heterozygote have a 50% to 66.7% probability of being heterozygous for PKU. High performance liquid chromatography and PCR-based methods have been proposed as screening tests for PKU heterozygotes.[4]

To maintain intellectual function, the importance of long-term (eg, beyond 10 years) dietary control of the blood phenylalanine level has been recently re-emphasized.[5,6] Significant phenylalanine hydroxylation in vivo in PKU homozygotes has been demonstrated.[7] Such findings suggest significant alternative pathway activity such as tyrosine hydroxylase. Promotion of such latent hydroxylating pathways may eventually lead to therapies which will complement phenylalanine restriction.

Spuriously high blood phenylalanine levels (false-positives) may occur with Guthrie test screening due to uninterpretable "clear zone" effect, the result of antibiotics (usually ampicillin). Because of an increase in the number of cases and amounts of the awards in litigation involving PKU screening (usually false-negative cases), vagaries of PKU testing, while uncommon, are of considerable import and generate comment and innovation.[8,9,10]

Consult references (below) by Scriver et al and by Güttler et al for review of the genetic/molecular biology of the hyperphenylalaninemias. Clinical heterogeneity of PKU relates to the existence of multiple different mutations in the PAH gene and to combinations of mutations. Such genetic considerations have important implications for therapy and its outcome.

Intrauterine fetal injury results from exposure of the developing fetus to increased intrapartum maternal plasma phenylalanine levels. There is a high incidence of resultant fetal damage including microcephaly, intrauterine growth retardation, mental retardation, and congenital heart disease, as a result of maternal hyperphenylalaninemia.[11] Dietary management of mothers identified by newborn screening programs has as its goal the maintenance of near normal maternal phenylalanine levels throughout pregnancy.[12] In order to retain the achievements of over three decades of early detection and treatment of PKU, increasing attention is being turned to control of maternal hyperphenylalaninemia. The risk of maternal phenylketonuria and hyperphenylalaninemia syndrome is increasing. There is a nearly 100% risk of recurrence if treatment is not given. A number of suggestions have been made to deal with the growing problem of maternal PKU including use of genetic registers.[13]

Footnotes

1. Committee on Genetics. American Academy of Pediatrics, "New Issues in Newborn Screening for Phenylketonuria and Congenital Hypothyroidism," Pediatrics, 1982, 69:104-6.
2. Hofman KJ, Steel G, Kazazian HH, et al, "Phenylketonuria in U.S. Blacks: Molecular Analysis of the Phenylalanine Hydroxylase Gene," Am J Hum Genet, 1991, 48(4):791-8.
3. Matalon R, Michals K, Blau N, et al, "Hyperphenylalaninemia Due to Inherited Deficiencies of Tetrahydrobiopterin," Advanced Pediatrics, eds, Barness LA, DeViro DC, Morrow G, et al, Chicago, IL: Year Book Medical Publishers, 1989, 36:67-89.
4. Eisensmith RC, Goltsov AA, and Woo SLC, "A Simple, Rapid, and Highly Informative PCR-Based Procedure for Prenatal Diagnosis and Carrier Screening of Phenylketonuria," Prenat Diagn, 1994, 14(12):1113-8.
5. Waisbren SE, Mahon BE, Schnell RR, et al, "Predictors of Intelligence Quotient and Intelligence Quotient Change in Persons Treated for Phenylketonuria Early in Life," Pediatrics, 1987, 79(3):351-5.
6. Michals K, Azen C, Acosta P, et al, "Blood Phenylalanine Levels and Intelligence of 10-Year-Old Children With PKU in the National Collaborative Study," J Am Diet Assoc, 1988, 88(10):1226-9.
7. Thompson GN and Halliday D, "Significant Phenylalanine Hydroxylation In Vivo in Patients With Classical Phenylketonuria," J Clin Invest, 1990, 86(1):317-22.
8. Mabry CC, Reid MC, and Kuhn RJ, "A Source of Error in Phenylketonuria Screening," Am J Clin Pathol, 1988, 90(3):279-83.
9. Clemens PC and Plettner C, "Phenylketonuria Screening: Avoiding a Source of Error by Simplifying the Procedure," Am J Clin Pathol, 1989, 91(6):747.
10. Wilcken B, Brown AR, Liu A, et al, "Eliminating Some Possible Errors in Phenylketonuria Screening," Am J Clin Pathol, 1989, 92(3):396.
11. Brenton DP, "Cardiac Defects in the Children of Mothers With High Concentrations of Plasma Phenylalanine," Br Heart J, 1990, 63(3):143-4.
12. Thompson GN, Francis DEM, Kirby DM, et al, "Pregnancy in Phenylketonuria: Dietary Treatment Aimed at Normalising Maternal Plasma Phenylalanine Concentration," Arch Dis Child, 1991, 66(11):1346-9.
13. Luder AS and Greene CL, "Maternal Phenylketonuria and Hyperphenylalaninemia: Implications for Medical Practice in the United States," Am J Obstet Gynecol, 1989, 161(5):1102-5.

References

"American Academy of Pediatrics, Committee on Genetics, Newborn Screening Fact Sheets: Phenylketonuria," Pediatrics, 1989, 83(3):461-2.

Atherton ND, "HPLC Measurement of Phenylalanine by Direct Injection of Plasma Onto an Internal-Surface Reverse-Phase Silica Support," Clin Chem, 1989, 35(6):975-8.

Eisensmith RC, Goltsov AA, and Woo SL, "A Simple, Rapid, and Highly Informative PCR-Based Procedure for Prenatal Diagnosis and Carrier Screening of Phenylketonuria," Prenat Diagn, 1994, 14(12):1113-8.

Gerasimova NS, Steklova IV, and Tuuminen T, "Fluorometric Method for Phenylalanine Microplate Assay Adapted for Phenylketonuria Screening," Clin Chem, 1989, 35(10):2112-5.

Güttler F and Guldberg P, "Mutations in the Phenylalanine Hydroxylase Gene: Genetic Determinants for the Phenotypic Variability of Hyperphenylalaninemia," Acta Paediatr Suppl, 1994, 407:49-56.

"Phenylketonuria - Past, Present, Future," Proceedings of a Symposium Held in Elsinore, Denmark, May 23-25, 1994, Acta Paediatr Scand Suppl, 407:1-129.

Scriver CR, "Whatever Happened to PKU?" Clin Biochem, 1995, 28(2):137-44.

Scriver CR, Kaufman S, Eisensmith RC, et al, "The Hyperphenylalaninemias," The Metabolic and Molecular Bases of Inherited Disease, 7th ed, Vol 1, Chapter 27, Scriver CR, Beaudet AL, Sly WS, et al, eds, New York, NY: McGraw-Hill Inc, 1995, 1015-75.

Tessari P, Inchiostro S, Vettore M, et al, "A Fast High-Performance Liquid Chromatographic Method for the Measurement of Plasma Concentration and Specific Activity of Phenylalanine," Clin Biochem, 1991, 24(5):425-8.

Phenylalanine Hydroxylase Activity see Newborn Screen for Phenylketonuria on page 169

Phenylalanine Screening Test, Blood see Phenylalanine, Blood on previous page

Phenylketonuria, Newborn Screen see Newborn Screen for Phenylketonuria on page 169

Phenylketonuria Test see Phenylalanine, Blood on previous page

Phosphatase, Acid see Acid Phosphatase on page 62

Phosphatase, Alkaline see Alkaline Phosphatase, Serum on page 69

Phosphate, Blood see Phosphorus, Serum on this page

Phosphatidylglycerol see Amniotic Fluid Lecithin/Sphingomyelin Ratio and Phosphatidylglycerol on page 77

Phosphatidylinositol see Amniotic Fluid Lecithin/Sphingomyelin Ratio and Phosphatidylglycerol on page 77

Phospholipid Profile, Amniotic Fluid see Amniotic Fluid Lecithin/Sphingomyelin Ratio and Phosphatidylglycerol on page 77

Phosphorus, Serum

CPT 84100

Related Information

Alcohol, Blood or Urine on page 531
Calcium, Serum on page 97
Ketone Bodies, Blood on page 152
Kidney Stone Analysis on page 640
Lactic Acid, Blood on page 156
Parathyroid Hormone on page 178
Vitamin D_3, Serum on page 218

Synonyms Phosphate, Blood

Abstract Phosphorus plays a pivotal role in cell physiology. Its metabolism is regulated principally by the renal tubules. With exclusion of factitious types of hyperphosphatemia, causes of increased phosphate include diminished glomerular filtration, increased absorption in the renal tubules, and/or increased exogenous or endogenous phosphate loads. Hypophosphatemia and its complications are outlined. Abnormalities of phosphate concentration can jeopardize life.

Patient Preparation Ideally, patient should be fasting. Phosphate levels are lower following meals.

Specimen Serum

Container Red top tube

Collection Pediatrics: Blood drawn from heelstick for capillary

Storage Instructions Serum should be promptly separated from the clot to avoid false elevations. Avoid overheating.

Causes for Rejection Observable hemolysis

Reference Range Both low and high ends of the normal range are higher in children than in adults. Children: approximately 4.0-6.0 mg/dL (SI: 1.29-1.94 mmol/L). Adults: 2.5-4.5 mg/dL (SI: 0.81-1.45 mmol/L). Some variation exists among authorities.

Possible Panic Range <1.0 mg/dL is critical

Use Causes of **high phosphorus:** Youth; exercise; dehydration and hypovolemia; high phosphorus content enema; acromegaly; hypoparathyroidism; pseudohypoparathyroidism; bone metastases; hypervitaminosis D; sarcoidosis; milk-alkali syndrome; liver disease, such as portal cirrhosis; catastrophic events such as cardiac resuscitation, pulmonary embolism, renal failure; diabetes mellitus with ketosis; serum artifact - sample not refrigerated; overheated, hemolyzed sample, or serum allowed to remain too long on the clot. Thrombocytosis causes elevated serum concentrations, but plasma phosphate remains unaltered.[1]

Although phosphate accumulation occurs as renal disease progresses, hyperphosphatemia is not a feature of early renal failure;[2] it does not usually develop before renal function has diminished to about 25% of normal.[3] Osteitis fibrosa in uremic subjects, from excessive bone turnover, relates to hyperphosphatasia. The role of hyperphosphatemia in promotion of such secondary hyperparathyroidism is established.[4] A relationship to osteomalacia in hemodialysis patients exists.[4]

Causes of **low phosphorus:** (Hypophosphatemia may occur with or without phosphate depletion. Serum levels vary as much as 2.0 mg/dL (SI: 0.65 mmol/L) during the day.)

Very severely malnourished subjects may have low phosphate levels, but even in starvation, phosphorus levels usually are normal. Antacids, diuretics, and long-term steroids are among the common agents bearing a relationship to severe hypophosphatemia.[5] Recent carbohydrate ingestion decreases phosphorus, as does intravenous glucose administration; cases of hypophosphatemia relate to I.V. carbohydrate,[5] dialysis, hyperalimentation, prolonged intravenous administration of phosphate-free fluids, metabolic states involving glucose, potassium, and pH. Depletion of phosphate occurs in diabetic ketoacidosis. Like potassium, phosphorus returns to the cell with therapy of diabetic ketoacidosis, and serum levels may diminish significantly during treatment. Osmotic diuresis induced by glycosuria in poorly controlled diabetes may lead to urinary phosphate losses with negative phosphorus balance. Phosphate levels may prove useful in initiation of insulin therapy, in diabetic ketoacidosis and other situations of insulin lack; with hyperglucagonemia, corticosteroid and epinephrine use, and in respiratory alkalosis. Association of hypophosphatemia with impaired glucose metabolism is recognized. Alcoholism and other hepatic disorders are found very frequently among patients with low phosphate. Alcoholic ketosis and alcohol withdrawal are among causes of hypophosphatemia. There is a slight decrease in serum phosphorus in the last trimester of pregnancy.

Primary hyperparathyroidism and other causes of calcium elevation, including ectopic hyperparathyroidism (pseudohyperparathyroidism).

Patients with sepsis, including Legionnaires' disease and other respiratory infections. Twenty-two percent of instances of respiratory infections had serum phosphorous ≤2.4 mg/dL. Halevy and Bulvik report gram-negative septicemia as a common cause of severe hypophosphatemia among 55,000 chemistry profiles of hospitalized patients they studied.[5] (Hypophosphatemia impairs bactericidal activity).

Vitamin D deficiency; osteomalacia, inherited and sporadic forms of hypophosphatemic rickets. In work-up for osteomalacia, look for decreased calcium and phosphorus and increased alkaline phosphatase. Biopsy, however, can be abnormal even when these biochemical parameters are within normal limits.

Renal tubular disorders (Fanconi syndrome, renal tubular acidosis); use of antacids that bind phosphorus (look for hypercalciuria, low urinary phosphorus, high alkaline phosphatase); dialysis; vomiting; saline or lactate I.V.; steatorrhea, malabsorption, severe diarrhea, nasogastric suction; hypokalemia; negative nitrogen balance; decreased dietary phosphate intake; recovery from severe burn injury; salicylate poisoning; acute gout; tumor-related: described as including hemangiopericytomas (uncommon pathologic entities) and neurofibromatosis; transfusion of blood; arteriography.

The signs and symptoms of phosphate depletion may include neuromuscular, neuropsychiatric, gastrointestinal, skeletal, and cardiopulmonary systems. Manifestations usually are accompanied by serum levels <1.0 mg/dL (SI: <0.32 mmol/L).

Tumor-induced osteomalacia (oncogenic osteomalacia) is a rare entity in which hypophosphatemia, hyperphosphaturia, low 1,25-dihyroxy-vitamin D and rickets or osteomalacia are reversed with removal of the tumor.[6]

Severe hypophosphatemia is most common in elderly patients and is often found in postoperative subjects.[5]

Complications of hypophosphatemia: Effect on RBC 2,3-diphosphoglycerate and oxygen dissociation. Depression of myocardial function (contractility), decreased cardiac output; respiratory failure and respiratory muscle weakness; increased incidence of sepsis, impairment of bactericidal activities.[7] CNS consequences: polyradiculopathy, paresthesias, tremor, ataxia, weakness, slurred speech, stupor, coma, seizure; joint stiffness; myopathy; renal stones; hypercalciuria secondary to renal phosphate leak; insulin resistance, glucose intolerance. Rhabdomyolysis may complicate marked hypophosphatemia. A mortality rate of 20% is described in patients whose phosphorus concentration was 1.1-1.5 mg/dL (SI: 0.36-0.48 mmol/L).[5]

Limitations Ninety-seven percent of hyperparathyroid subjects with normal renal function have <3.3 mg/dL serum phosphate, 80% <3.0 mg/dL and 40% <2.5 mg/dL.[8] Collection of multiple data points throughout the day may help to establish the diagnosis of primary hyperparathyroidism in patients with borderline serum biochemistries.[9] Thus, some

hyperparathyroid patients have serum phosphorus levels within normal limits. Hemolysis, glassware contaminated with detergents, hyperbilirubinemia, or dysproteinemia may cause increased results. Spurious hyperphosphatemia may be due to increased serum triglycerides. Phosphorus measurement on the Du Pont aca® was reported to be low with I.V. mannitol administration. Falsely elevated serum phosphate concentrations have been reported in patients with multiple myeloma using a molybdate colorimetric assay on the Hitachi® 717.[10] Drug effects have been summarized.[11]

Contraindications Sampling not long after a phosphorus-containing enema can provide startlingly high phosphate levels.

Methodology Phosphomolybdate - colorimetric; modified molybdate - enzymatic, colorimetric[10]

Additional Information Increasing dietary intake of potassium has been reported to increase serum phosphate concentrations apparently by decreasing renal excretion of phosphate.[12] During the last trimester of pregnancy, there is a sixfold increase in calcium and phosphorus accumulation as the fetus triples its weight. Plasma phosphorus concentrations may provide a useful means to assess response to phosphate supplements in the premature infant.[13] Control of serum phosphorus in dialysis patients is a complex topic which includes nutritional needs with protein intake.[14]

Footnotes

1. Lutomski DM and Bower RH, "The Effect of Thrombocytosis on Serum Potassium and Phosphorus Concentrations," *Am J Med Sci*, 1994, 307(4):255-8.
2. Hakim RM and Lazarus JM, "Biochemical Parameters in Chronic Renal Failure," *Am J Kidney Dis*, 1988, 11(3):238-47.
3. Coburn JW and Salusky IB, "Control of Serum Phosphorus in Uremia," *N Engl J Med*, 1989, 320(17):1140-2.
4. Delmez JA, Fallon MD, Harter HR, et al, "Does Strict Phosphorus Control Precipitate Renal Osteomalacia?" *J Clin Endocrinol Metab*, 1986, 62(4):747-52.
5. Halevy J and Bulvik S, "Severe Hypophosphatemia in Hospitalized Patients," *Arch Intern Med*, 1988, 148(1):153-5.
6. Cai Q, Hodgson SF, Kao PC, et al, "Brief Report: Inhibition of Renal Phosphate Transport by a Tumor Product in a Patient With Oncogenic Osteomalacia," *N Engl J Med*, 1994, 330(23):1645-9.
7. Knochel JP, "The Pathophysiology and Clinical Characteristics of Severe Hypophosphatemia," *Arch Intern Med*, 1977, 137:203-20.
8. Kao PC, "Parathyroid Hormone Assay," *Mayo Clin Proc*, 1982, 57:596-7.
9. Lobaugh B, Neelon FA, Oyama H, et al, "Circadian Rhythms for Calcium, Inorganic Phosphorus, and Parathyroid Hormone in Primary Hyperparathyroidism: Functional and Practical Considerations," *Surgery*, 1989, 106(6):1009-16.
10. Bakker AJ, Bosma H, and Christen PJ, "Influence of Monoclonal Immunoglobulins in Three Different Methods for Inorganic Phosphorus," *Ann Clin Biochem*, 1990, 27(Pt 3):227-31.
11. Hitz J, Jaudon MC, and Galli A, "Phosphates," *Drug Effects on Laboratory Test Results Analytical Interferences and Pharmacological Effects*, Siest G and Galteau MM, eds, Littleton, MA: PSG Publishing Co Inc, 1988, 330-43.
12. Sebastian A, Hernandez RE, Portale AA, et al, "Dietary Potassium Influences Kidney Maintenance of Serum Phosphorus Concentration," *Kidney Int*, 1990, 37(5):1341-9.
13. Mayne PD and Kovar IZ, "Calcium and Phosphorus Metabolism in the Premature Infant," *Ann Clin Biochem*, 1991, 28(Pt 2):131-42.
14. Delmez JA and Slatopolsky E, "Hyperphosphatemia: Its Consequences and Treatment in Patients With Chronic Renal Disease," *Am J Kidney Dis*, 1992, 19(4):303-17.

References

Bourke E and Yanagawa M, "Assessment of Hyperphosphatemia and Hypophosphatemia," *Clin Lab Med*, 1993, 13(1):183-207.
DeVizia B and Mansi A, "Calcium and Phosphorus Metabolism in Full-Term Infants," *Monatsschr Kinderheilkd*, 1992, 140(9 Suppl 1):S8-12.
Econs MJ and Drezner MK, "Tumor-Induced Osteomalacia - Unveiling a New Hormone," *N Engl J Med*, 1994, 330(23):1679-81 (editorial).
Gravelyn TR, Brophy N, Siegert C, et al, "Hypophosphatemia-Associated Respiratory Muscle Weakness in a General Inpatient Population," *Am J Med*, 1988, 84(5):870-6.
Hanukoglu A, Chalew SA, Sun CJ, et al, "Surgically Curable Hypophosphatemic Rickets. Diagnosis and Management," *Clin Pediatr (Phila)*, 1989, 28(7):321-5.
Hodgson SF and Hurley DL, "Acquired Hypophosphatemia," *Endocrinol Metab Clin North Am*, 1993, 22(2):397-409.
Laaban J-P, Waked M, Laromiguiere M, et al, "Hypophosphatemia Complicating Management of Acute Severe Asthma," *Ann Intern Med*, 1990, 112(1):68-9.
Loghman-Adham M, "Role of Phosphate Retention in the Progression of Renal Failure," *J Lab Clin Med*, 1993, 122(1):16-26.
Root AW and Diamond FB Jr, "Disorders of Calcium and Phosphorus Metabolism in Adolescents," *Endocrinol Metab Clin North Am*, 1993, 22(3):573-92.
Tieder M, Modai D, Samuel R, et al, "Hereditary Hypophosphatemic Rickets With Hypercalciuria," *N Engl J Med*, 1985, 312(10):611-7.

Phosphorus, Urine

CPT 84105

Related Information

Synonyms Urine Phosphorus

Test Commonly Includes Phosphorus on random or timed urine specimen

(Continued)

Phosphorus, Urine *(Continued)*

Abstract Urinary phosphorus helps in evaluating calcium/phosphorus balance.

Specimen Timed or random urine. Diurnal variation exists.

Collection For 24-hour urine collection: Instruct the patient to void at 8 AM and discard the specimen. Then collect all urine including the final specimen voided at the end of the 24-hour collection period (ie, 8 AM the next morning). Container must be labeled with patient's name, date and time collection started and date and time collection finished.

Storage Instructions Refrigerate. Laboratory adjusts final pH of urine aliquot to 6.

Reference Range Adults: 0.9-1.3 g/24 hours (SI: 29-42 mmol/day), dependent on dietary intake

Use Evaluate calcium/phosphorus balance. **High** urinary phosphorus (ie, increased renal losses) occurs in primary hyperparathyroidism, vitamin D deficiency, renal tubular acidosis, diuretic use. Phosphates are among the substances which may be lost in the Fanconi syndrome. Renal loss of phosphate may itself lead to rickets or osteomalacia. **Low** in hypoparathyroidism, pseudohypoparathyroidism, and vitamin D intoxication.

Effects on Phosphorus Transport

Atrial natriuretic peptide	↓
Calcitonin	↓
Glucocorticoid	↑
Growth hormone	↑
Insulin-like growth factor-I	↑
Metabolic acidosis (chronic)	↓
Metabolic alkalosis	↑
Parathyroid hormone	↓
Parathyroid hormone-related peptide (HHM factor)	↓
Phosphorus supply	↑ or ↓
Vasopressin	↓
Vitamin D	↑
Volume expansion	↓

From Hruska KA, "Phosphate Balance and Metabolism," *The Principles and Practice of Nephrology*, Chapter 19, Jacobson HR, Striker GE, and Klahr S, eds, Philadelphia, PA: Mosby-Year Book Inc, 1991, 122, with permission.

Evaluate nephrolithiasis. Hypophosphatemia with normal serum calcium, high alkaline phosphatase, hypercalciuria, low urinary phosphorus occurs with osteomalacia from excessive antacid ingestion. Observations of renal phosphate excretion have led to the classical theory of a maximal transport capacity (T_m). By this model, phosphate is reabsorbed to a maximum rate after which phosphate appears in the urine once the T_m is exceeded. Mechanisms and effectors of reabsorption are described.[1] The table lists some important effectors of phosphate transport in the proximal nephron. Largely, however, urine phosphate simply reflects phosphate intake in patients not on phosphate-binding medications.

Methodology Enzymatic, colorimetric[2]

Additional Information Children with thalassemia may have normal phosphorus absorption but high renal phosphaturia, leading to a deficiency of phosphorus. Increasing dietary intake of potassium has been reported to increase serum phosphate concentrations apparently by decreasing renal excretion of phosphate.[3] During the last trimester of pregnancy, there is a sixfold increase in calcium and phosphorus accumulation as the fetus triples its weight. Plasma phosphorus concentrations and increased urinary phosphate may provide a useful means to assess response to phosphate supplements in the premature infant.[4]

Tumor-induced osteomalacia (oncogenic osteomalacia) is a rare entity in which hypophosphatemia, hyperphosphaturia, low 1,25-dihydroxy vitamin D, and rickets or osteomalacia can be reversed with removal of the tumor.[5]

Footnotes

1. Hruska KA, "Phosphate Balance and Metabolism," *The Principles and Practice of Nephrology*, Chapter 19, Jacobson HR, Striker GE, and Klahr S, eds, Philadelphia, PA: BC Decker Inc, 1991, 122.
2. Berti G, Fossati P, Tarenghi G, et al, "Enzymatic Colorimetric Method for the Determination of Inorganic Phosphorus in Serum and Urine," *J Clin Chem Clin Biochem*, 1988, 26(6):399-404.
3. Sebastian A, Hernandez RE, Portale AA, et al, "Dietary Potassium Influences Kidney Maintenance of Serum Phosphorus Concentration," *Kidney Int*, 1990, 37(5):1341-9.
4. Mayne PD and Kovar IZ, "Calcium and Phosphorus Metabolism in the Premature Infant," *Ann Clin Biochem*, 1991, 28(Pt 2):131-42.
5. Cai Q, Hodgson SF, Kai PC, et al, "Brief Report: Inhibition of Renal Phosphate Transport by a Tumor Product in a Patient With Oncogenic Osteomalacia," *N Engl J Med*, 1994, 330(23):1645-9.

References

Bakker AJ, Bosma H, and Christen PJ, "Influence of Monoclonal Immunoglobulins in Three Different Methods for Inorganic Phosphorus," *Ann Clin Biochem*, 1990, 27(Pt 3):227-31.

Juan D, "The Causes and Consequences of Hypophosphatemia," *Surg Gynecol Obstet*, 1981, 153:589-97.

Somell A and Alveryd A, "Diurnal Variations in the Urinary Excretion of Calcium and Phosphate in Hyperparathyroidism," *Acta Chir Scand*, 1976, 142:357-9.

Weintraub Z, Iancu TC, Sheinfeld M, et al, "Urinary and Blood Levels of Adenosine 3', 5'-Monophosphate, Phosphorus, and Calcium in Infants," *Biol Neonate*, 1989, 55(4-5):233-7.

PIIINP *see* CA 125 *on page 94*

Pituitary Gonadotropins *see* Luteinizing Hormone, Blood or Urine *on page 163*

PKU, Neonatal *see* Newborn Screen for Phenylketonuria *on page 169*

PKU Test *see* Phenylalanine, Blood *on page 181*

Placental Alkaline Phosphatase *see* CA 125 *on page 94*

Placental Lactogen, Human

CPT 83632

Related Information

Human Chorionic Gonadotropin, Serum *on page 145*

Synonyms Chorionic Somatomammotropin; hCS; hPL; Human Chorionic Somatomammotropin; Human Placental Lactogen

Abstract Related to the functional placental mass, hPL is an adjunctive rather than a definitive test. This test is seldom used.

Patient Preparation Avoid recent radioactive scan if RIA is the method in use.

Specimen Serum or plasma

Container Red top tube, lavender top (EDTA) tube, or green top (heparin) tube

Storage Instructions Freeze serum or plasma immediately.

Reference Range Varies with duration of gestation. Levels rise with advancing gestation to plateau at about 37 weeks. May reach 10 µg/mL (SI: 463 nmol/L).

Critical Values Maternal serum hPL <4 µg/mL (SI: <185 nmol/L) after 30 weeks gestation; imperfect correlation exists with adverse outcome

Use Evaluate antepartum placental function: the maternal serum concentration correlates with placental weight; used as an index of fetal well-being, hPL tends to be low with intrauterine growth retardation

Limitations Single results are not as useful as a series over time. Test is not as useful as hCG in following course of trophoblastic neoplasia. Role of hPL in monitoring fetal well-being is controversial. Normal levels do not provide assurance of lack of complications. Low levels at term are especially difficult to interpret, since these have been reported in normal pregnancy. Intrauterine growth retardation is not always caused by placental disease.

Methodology Radioimmunoassay (RIA), turbidimetric latex immunoassay[1]

Additional Information Human placental lactogen (chorionic somatomammotropin) is a growth-promoting hormone of placental origin, similar to chorionic gonadotropin. Placental lactogen appears to act through distinct PL receptors to regulate and coordinate growth and metabolism in the fetus and metabolism in the mother. Growth effects upon the fetus appear to be predominant in the first half of pregnancy. Metabolic effects appear to predominate in the last half of pregnancy.[2,3] It has been proposed that a major role of hPL is to provide optimum metabolic conditions for procurement of nutrients and use of these nutrients by the fetus, especially in the last half of pregnancy. **A poor correlation of maternal serum concentrations with "fetal well-being" during the last half of pregnancy exists.**

Immediately after its discovery, hPL was recommended to evaluate placental function and fetal well-being in pregnancies at risk, and prognosticate the inevitability of abortion (low levels or falling levels indicate poor prognosis). It was also recommended as a marker for trophoblastic neoplasia (elevated). These roles are controversial. Measurement of hPL has been suggested as a method for assessing gestational age.[4] hPL has been detected in some patients with nongerm cell neoplasms.[5]

High hPL may be found in instances of Rh isoimmunization and in multiple gestation, in each of which large placentas occur.[6] It is largely discarded in clinical practice of obstetrics.[7]

In twin pregnancy, hPL is described as an indicator of intrauterine growth retardation.[8]

Footnotes

1. Collet-Cassart D, Limet JN, Van Krieken L, et al, "Turbidimetric Latex Immunoassay of Placental Lactogen on Microtiter Plates," *Clin Chem*, 1989, 35(1):141-3.
2. Handwerger S, "Clinical Counterpoint: The Physiology of Placental Lactogen in Human Pregnancy," *Endocr Rev*, 1991, 12:329-36.

3. Parsons JA, Brelje TC, and Sorenson RL, "Adaptation of Islets of Langerhans to Pregnancy: Increased Islet Cell Proliferation and Insulin Secretion Correlates With the Onset of Placental Lactogen Secretion," *Endocrinology*, 1992, 130(3):1459-66.
4. Whittaker PG, Lind T, and Lawson JY, "A Prospective Study to Compare Serum Human Placental Lactogen and Menstrual Dates for Determining Gestational Age," *Am J Obstet Gynecol*, 1987, 156(1):178-82.
5. Heyderman E, Chapman DV, Richardson TC, et al, "Human Chorionic Gonadotropin and Human Placental Lactogen in Extragonadal Tumors, An Immunoperoxidase Study of Ten Non-Germ Cell Neoplasms," *Cancer*, 1985, 56(11):2674-82.
6. Ray DA, "Biochemical Fetal Assessment," *Clin Obstet Gynecol*, 1987, 30(4):887-98.
7. Catanzarite VA, Perkins RP, and Pernoll ML, "Assessment of Fetal Well-Being," *Current Obstetric & Gynecologic Diagnosis & Treatment 1987*, Pernoll ML and Benson RC, eds, Norwalk, CT: Appleton & Lange, 1987, 279-302.
8. Trapp M, Kato K, Bohnet HG, et al, "Human Placental Lactogen and Unconjugated Estriol Concentrations in Twin Pregnancy: Monitoring of Fetal Development in Intrauterine Growth Retardation and Single Intrauterine Fetal Death," *Am J Obstet Gynecol*, 1986, 155(5):1027-31.

References

Halmesmaki E, Autti I, Granstrom ML, et al, "Alpha-Fetoprotein, Human Placental Lactogen, and Pregnancy-Specific Beta 1-Glycoprotein in Pregnant Women Who Drink: Relation to Fetal Alcohol Syndrome," *Am J Obstet Gynecol*, 1986, 155(3):598-602.

Hill DJ, Freemark M, Strain AJ, et al, "Placental Lactogen and Growth Hormone Receptors in Human Fetal Tissues: Relationship to Fetal Plasma Human Placental Lactogen Concentrations and Fetal Growth," *J Clin Endocrinol Metab*, 1988, 66(6):1283-90.

Southard JN and Talamantes F, "High Molecular Weight Forms of Placental Lactogen: Evidence for Lactogen-Macroglobulin Complexes in Rodents and Humans," *Endocrinology*, 1989, 125(2):791-800.

Stewart MO, Whittaker PG, Persson B, et al, "A Longitudinal Study of Circulating Progesterone, Oestradiol, hCG, and hPL During Pregnancy in Type I Diabetic Mothers," *Br J Obstet Gynaecol*, 1989, 96(4):415-23.

Walker WH, Fitzpatrick SL, Barrera-Saldana HA, et al, "The Human Placental Lactogen Genes: Structure, Function, Evolution, and Transcriptional Regulation," *Endocr Rev*, 1991, 12(4):316-28.

Plasma Cholinesterase *see* Pseudocholinesterase, Serum *on page 196*

Plasma Electrolytes *see* Electrolytes, Serum or Plasma *on page 123*

Plasma Neuropeptide Y *see* Catecholamines, Fractionation, Plasma *on page 103*

Plasma Renin Activity *see* Renin, Plasma *on page 197*

Pleural Fluid Analysis *see* Body Fluid *on page 89*

Pleural Fluid pH *see* Body Fluid pH *on page 92*

pO$_2$ *see* Blood Gases, Arterial *on page 87*

pO$_2$ (0.5) *see* P-50 Blood Gas *on page 176*

pO$_2$ at Half Saturation *see* P-50 Blood Gas *on page 176*

Porphobilinogen *see* Porphyrins, Quantitative, Urine *on next page*

Porphobilinogen *see* Porphobilinogen Deaminase, Erythrocyte *on this page*

Porphobilinogen Deaminase, Erythrocyte

CPT 84999

Related Information

Porphobilinogen, Qualitative, Urine *on this page*
Porphyrins, Quantitative, Urine *on next page*

Synonyms Erythrocyte Porphobilinogen Deaminase; Erythrocyte Uroporphyrinogen I Synthase; Pbg-D; Uroporphyrinogen-Cosynthetase; Uroporphyrinogen I Synthase

Applies to Porphobilinogen; Porphobilinogen Deaminase Red Blood Cell

Abstract The enzymatic defect of acute intermittent porphyria (AIP) is a partial deficiency of uroporphyrin I synthase in erythrocytes and other cells.[1,2] Inheritance of AIP is autosomal dominant with low penetrance. This assay is described as the most reliable test for diagnosis of AIP.[2]

Patient Preparation Patient should fast for 12-14 hours, abstain from alcohol and ideally be off medications for 2 weeks.

Specimen Whole blood (done on erythrocytes)

Container Green top (heparin) tube, lavender top (EDTA) tube

Storage Instructions If test can be done promptly, a red cell hemolysate is prepared directly from whole blood. The whole blood sample can be stored for 1 week at 4°C. If there will be a delay of over a week, centrifuge heparinized specimen. After plasma and buffy layer are removed, wash red cells three times with cold isotonic saline. Pack by centrifugation. Freeze in dry ice-acetone.[1] Store at -20°C. There is loss of activity at 4°C, more at room temperature as red cells age. The test is done on a red cell hemolysate.

Turnaround Time Usually sent to reference laboratories

Special Instructions Hemoglobin and reticulocyte count should also be ordered.

Reference Range ≥7.0 nmol/second/L red cells.

Method of Ford and associates:[2] red cell lysates: women: 5.3-9.2 nmol/second/L red cells, men: 3.4-8.5 nmol/second/L red cells.

ELISA assay: >110 µg/g hemoglobin.

Varies among methods and among laboratories. Patients with acute intermittent porphyria have levels about half normal; *vide infra*. Hemoglobin determination is done on the hemolysate for calculation of activity on a per gram of hemoglobin basis.

Critical Values Indeterminate: 3.5-3.9 nmol/second/L; diminished: <3.5 nmol/second/L

Use Evaluate subjects with episodes of abdominal pain, especially when such episodes are recurrent, and with tachycardia. Uroporphyrin-1-synthase is low in the latent or carrier state of acute intermittent porphyria, normal in the other hereditary porphyrias. It is thought to provide support in the differential diagnosis of acute intermittent porphyria from other neurological porphyrias,[1] following the first steps of PBG and ALA.

Limitations Only a minority of carriers of the defective enzyme will experience clinical AIP.[3] A small overlap with normals exists. Repeat assay at a later time is indicated to confirm carrier status. Qualitative and quantitative urinary porphobilinogen and family studies are also useful. Indeterminate or normal values for this enzyme may occur in some patients with acute intermittent porphyria. Interpretation is difficult at the low end of the normal range. Red cell uroporphyrin-1-synthase activity varies with cell age. Younger red cells (newborn subjects) or other settings in which younger red cells are found, with reticulocytosis ≥5%, may lead to increased activity of this assay, which therefore may be high in various anemias, and may also mask the diagnosis of acute intermittent porphyria.

Methodology Fluorometric assay; ELISA assay;[2] single strand conformation polymorphism analysis;[2] method at Mayo Medical Laboratories is described.[4]

Additional Information More than 40 mutations causing AIP are described.[2] This is the enzyme which converts porphobilinogen to uroporphyrinogen I. Uroporphyrin I synthase is a method of detection of asymptomatic carriers of acute intermittent porphyria. Another is quantitation of urine porphobilinogen. Both are recommended. Uroporphyrin-1-synthase is normal or increased with lead poisoning, because of anemia in plumbism.[5] In acute intermittent porphyria excessive excretion of porphobilinogen and delta aminolevulinic acid occurs during acute attacks, but excretion may be normal between them. Red blood cell porphobilinogen deaminase (uroporphyrinogen I synthase) activity, measured by a spectrofluorometric assay on erythrocytes, defines most patients with acute intermittent porphyria, while 55 of 56 subjects with other porphyrias were reported as having normal activity. This assay identified a number of latent carriers but not all patients with assumed acute intermittent porphyria.[6] Either Pbg-D or ALA-D (aminolevulinic acid dehydratase) in red cells is expected to be decreased in subjects with AIP.[4]

Footnotes

1. Forman DT, "Erythrocyte Uroporphyrinogen I Synthase Activity as an Indicator of Acute Porphyria," *Ann Clin Lab Sci*, 1989, 19(2):128-32.
2. Schreiber WE, Jamani A, and Armstrong JG, "Acute Intermittent Porphyria in a Native North American Family - Biochemical and Molecular Analysis," *Am J Clin Pathol*, 1995, 103(6):730-4.
3. Nuttall KL, "Porphyrins and Disorders of Porphyrin Metabolism," *Tietz Textbook of Clinical Chemistry*, 2nd ed, Burtis CA and Ashwood ER, eds, Philadelphia, PA: WB Saunders Co, 1994, 2073-106.
4. Leavelle DE, *Mayo Medical Laboratories Interpretive Handbook*, Rochester, MN: Mayo Medical Laboratories, 1994.
5. Bird TD, Wallace DM, and Labbe RF, "The Porphyria, Plumbism, Pottery Puzzle," *JAMA*, 1982, 247:813-4.
6. Pierach CA, Weimer MK, Cardinal RA, et al, "Red Blood Cell Porphobilinogen Deaminase in the Evaluation of Acute Intermittent Porphyria," *JAMA*, 1987, 257(1):60-1.

Porphobilinogen Deaminase Red Blood Cell *see* Porphobilinogen Deaminase, Erythrocyte *on this page*

Porphobilinogen, Qualitative, Urine

CPT 84106

Related Information

Delta Aminolevulinic Acid, Urine *on page 121*
Lead, Blood *on page 556*
Porphobilinogen Deaminase, Erythrocyte *on this page*
Porphyrins, Quantitative, Urine *on next page*
Protoporphyrin, Free Erythrocyte *on page 195*
Urobilinogen, 2-Hour Urine *on page 660*

Synonyms Watson-Schwartz Test

Applies to Hoesch Test; Porphyrins, Fecal

Test Commonly Includes Qualitative screen for urobilinogen and porphobilinogen

Abstract Porphobilinogen (PBG) and delta aminolevulinic acid (ALA) are early porphyrin precursors, which are excreted. Acute intermittent porphyria (AIP) can be fatal. Urine delta ALA and/or PBG is/are increased in acute neurological porphyrias during attacks. These include (Continued)

Porphobilinogen, Qualitative, Urine *(Continued)*

acute intermittent porphyria, hereditary coproporphyria, and variegate porphyria.

Specimen Random urine

Container Any clean dark container, no preservative

Sampling Time PBG levels in the urine should be measured during acute attacks of abdominal pain, extremity pain or paresthesias, tachycardia, hypertension, nausea and vomiting, neurologic abnormalities, and in the investigation of dark urine.

Collection Keep refrigerated during collection and thereafter. Prevent exposure to light. Some authorities suggest collecting in a dark bottle with 5 g sodium bicarbonate, as well as keeping under refrigeration.

Storage Instructions Specimen may be stored for a brief period in refrigerator, but must be analyzed promptly. Adjust to pH 6-7 with sodium bicarbonate. Stabilized specimen is stable 12 hours at 25°C and 7 days at 4°C.

Reference Range Negative

Use PBG is a screen for **acute intermittent porphyria (AIP)**, which is characterized by urinary excretion of PBG and delta ALA during acute attacks. The Watson-Schwartz test may detect some patients in latent periods who have AIP. Increased urinary excretion of PBG may also be caused by acute attacks of **variegate porphyria** or of **hereditary coproporphyria**, and rarely in lead poisoning. In lead poisoning, urinary ALA measurement is more useful.

Limitations False-negatives may occur. The major drawback of the Watson-Schwartz and Hoesch tests is the need for subjective interpretation of the visual endpoint.[1] Schreiber et al have described an anion-exchange resin. Columns were prepared by packing polybenzimidazole resin.[1] Positive results must be confirmed by other methods, including quantitative tests for PBG and for ALA. A quantitative method using a condensation reaction with *p*-dimethylaminobenzaldehyde, with spectrophotometric analysis, is widely used. (Normal 0-2.0 mg/day or 0-8.8 mmol/day.)

May be negative in the patient with asymptomatic (latent) phase of AIP, in whom uroporphyrinogen I synthase may detect the presence of AIP; see listing Porphobilinogen Deaminase, Erythrocyte *on page 185* for this assay.

The intoxication porphyrinurias (including lead poisoning) are better detected by delta aminolevulinic acid and other tests.

Fecal porphyrins are elevated with the neurocutaneous porphyrias. Fecal porphyrins are useful in hereditary coproporphyria and variegate porphyria and to distinguish these from AIP. In variegate porphyria and erythropoietic protoporphyria, increased fecal protoporphyrins are anticipated.

Methodology Watson-Schwartz test, Ehrlich's reagent. A variant of the Watson-Schwartz test, the newer **Hoesch test** does not react with urobilinogen, an advantage. In both tests, there is a chemical interference (decrease in results) if indolic compounds (indole, indican, 5-HIAA) are present in large amounts.

Polybenzimidazole (PBI) resin columns:[1] A Dowex 2 resin is used to adsorb alkaline PBG, then acid elution of the PBG, followed by reaction with Ehrlich's reagent, and reading by spectrophotometry. The sensitivity is greatly increased.[2] Others have quantified the eluate by HPLC.[3]

Additional Information Acute attacks of AIP are precipitated by drugs, including barbiturates, sulfa drugs, heavy metals, hydantoins, hormones, infection, and diet. The most common symptom of AIP is abdominal pain. The most common sign is tachycardia.[4] Such autonomic attacks include emesis, fever, leukocytosis, and neurologic findings. Subjects with the porphyrias may pass urine the color of port wine. The term porphyria derives from the Greek "porphyria," an expression for the color purple.[4]

Quantitative urine PBG will pick up many but not all patients with acute intermittent porphyria in the latent period.

The Watson-Schwartz test is negative with cutanea tarda porphyria and in Günther's disease, congenital erythropoietic porphyria.

Footnotes

1. Schreiber WE, Jamani A, and Pudek MR, "Screening Tests for Porphobilinogen Are Insensitive. The Problem and Its Solution," *Am J Clin Pathol*, 1989, 92(5):644-9.
2. Buttery JE, Chamberlain BR, and Beng CG, "A Sensitive Method of Screening for Urinary Porphobilinogen," *Clin Chem*, 1989, 35(12):2311-2.
3. Jamani A, Pudek M, and Schreiber WE, "Liquid-Chromatographic Assay of Urinary Porphobilinogen," *Clin Chem*, 1989, 35(3):471-5.
4. Bloomer JR and Bonkovsky HL, "The Porphyrias," *Dis Mon*, 1989, 35(1):1-54.

References

Buttery JE, Carrera AM, and Pannall PR, "Analytical Sensitivity and Specificity of Two Screening Methods for Urinary Porphobilinogen," *Ann Clin Biochem*, 1990, 27(Pt 2):165-6.

Buttery JE, Chamberlain BR, and Beng CG, "Assessment of Two Anion-Exchange Resins for Direct Use in the Screening Method for Urinary Porphobilinogen," *Clin Chem*, 1990, 36(3):584.

Buttery JE and Stuart S, "Measurement of Porphobilinogen in Urine by a Simple Resin Method With Use of A Surrogate Standard," *Clin Chem*, 1991, 37(12):2133-6.

Desnick RJ, "The Porphyrias," *Harrison's Principles of Internal Medicine*, 13th ed, Vol 2, Isselbacher KJ, Braunwald E, Wilson JD, et al, eds, New York, NY: McGraw-Hill Inc, 1994, 2073-9.

Galbraith RA, Sassa S, and Kappas A, "A Comparison of the Utility of Dowex Resin and Polybenzimidazole Aurorez Resin in the Determination of Urinary Porphobilinogen Concentrations," *Clin Chim Acta*, 1987, 164(2):235-9.

Hindmarsh JT, "Variable Phenotypic Expression of Genotypic Abnormalities in the Porphyrias," *Clin Chim Acta*, 1993, 217(1):29-38.

Holman JR and Green JB, "Acute Intermittent Porphyria. More Than Just Abdominal Pain," *Postgrad Med*, 1989, 86(5):295-8.

Lip GY, McColl KE, and Moore MR, "The Acute Porphyrias," *Br J Clin Pract*, 1993, 47(1):38-43.

Meola T and Lim HW, "The Porphyrias," *Dermatol Clin*, 1993, 11(3):583-96.

Moore MR, "Biochemistry of Porphyria," *Int J Biochem*, 1993, 25(10):1353-68.

Nuttall KL, "Porphyrins and Disorders of Porphyrin Metabolism," *Tietz Textbook of Clinical Chemistry*, 2nd ed, Burtis CA and Ashwood ER, eds, Philadelphia, PA: WB Saunders Co, 1994, 2073-106.

Tefferi A, Colgan JP, and Solberg LA Jr, "Acute Porphyrias: Diagnosis and Management," *Mayo Clin Proc*, 1994, 69(10):991-5.

Tefferi A, Solberg LA Jr, and Ellefson, "Porphyrias: Clinical Evaluation and Interpretation of Laboratory Tests," *Mayo Clin Proc*, 1994, 69(3):289-90.

Vavra JD and Avioli LV, "Intermittent Acute Porphyria," *Arch Intern Med*, 1982, 142(8):1527-9.

Porphyrins, Erythrocytes see Porphyrins, Quantitative, Urine *on this page*

Porphyrins, Fecal see Porphobilinogen, Qualitative, Urine *on previous page*

Porphyrins, Feces see Porphyrins, Quantitative, Urine *on this page*

Porphyrins, Plasma see Porphyrins, Quantitative, Urine *on this page*

Porphyrins, Quantitative, Urine

CPT 84120

Related Information

Delta Aminolevulinic Acid, Urine *on page 121*
Iron and Total Iron Binding Capacity/Transferrin *on page 150*
Lead, Blood *on page 556*
Lead, Urine *on page 557*
Phlebotomy, Therapeutic *on page 614*
Porphobilinogen Deaminase, Erythrocyte *on previous page*
Porphobilinogen, Qualitative, Urine *on previous page*
Protoporphyrin, Free Erythrocyte *on page 195*
Urine Collection, 24-Hour *on page 30*
Uroporphyrinogen III Synthase, Erythrocyte *on page 215*

Synonyms Coproporphyrins; Porphobilinogen; Uroporphyrins

Applies to Naproxen; Porphyrins, Erythrocytes; Porphyrins, Feces; Porphyrins, Plasma; Uroporphyrinogen Decarboxylase

Test Commonly Includes Uroporphyrins (octacarboxylporphyrins), heptacarboxylporphyrins, hexacarboxylporphyrins, pentacarboxylporphyrins, coproporphyrins (tetracarboxylporphrins)[1]

Abstract Porphyrins are byproducts of porphyrinogens. Accumulations of either cause porphyrias, which are hereditary enzyme disorders. They affect the heme biosynthetic pathway and are characterized by increased excretion of porphyrins, porphyrinogens, or their precursors. Such precursors include delta aminolevulinic acid and porphobilinogen. These are water soluble and appear in the urine, in common with coproporphyrin and uroporphyrin. The disease entities relate to specific enzyme defects. Most are inherited as autosomal dominant with low disease penetrance.

Patient Preparation Avoid alcohol and excessive fluid intake during collection. Phenothiazines may cause misleading porphobilinogen results.

Specimen 24-hour urine

Container Clean, dark container. Must be kept covered.

Collection Check with laboratory; 5 g sodium bicarbonate is usually added to container before collection. Instruct the patient to void at 8 AM and discard the specimen. Then collect all urine including the final specimen voided at the end of the 24-hour collection period (ie, 8 AM next morning). Specimen should be kept cool during collection. Container must be labeled with patient's name, date and time collection started, and date and time collection finished. Transport specimen immediately to the laboratory upon completion of collection. Adjust to pH 6-7 with sodium bicarbonate.

Storage Instructions Refrigerate during collection. **Protect specimen from light.**

Causes for Rejection Sodium phosphate is undesirable as a preservative.

Reference Range Total porphyrins: <320 nmol/L; see also literature from individual laboratory

Use Evaluate patients for porphyrias. Early precursors are delta aminolevulinic acid and porphobilinogen.

In **congenital erythropoietic porphyria**, a decrease of red cell uroporphyrinogen III synthase of red cells occurs. Severe hemolysis and photosensitivity are found; see listing Uroporphyrinogen III Synthase, Erythrocyte *on page 215.*

In **acute intermittent porphyria**, porphobilinogen and delta aminolevulinic acid are elevated in acute attacks, and mild increases of urinary uroporphyrin and coproporphyrin may be found. Porphobilinogen is increased in many but not all patients with acute intermittent porphyria in latent periods. Quantitative porphobilinogen is a better test than delta aminolevulinic acid overall for acute intermittent porphyria, but both are used (as well as the Watson-Schwartz test).[2] Porphobilinogen deaminase activity can be measured; see listing Porphobilinogen Deaminase, Erythrocyte *on page 185.*

Coproporphyrin and porphobilinogen excretion in urine are markedly increased during acute attacks of **hereditary coproporphyria**, increase of urinary uroporphyrin may be found, and increased fecal coproporphyrin III is described. Urinary ALA and PBG are increased with acute attacks.

In **variegate porphyria (VP)** in acute attacks, results are similar to those of acute intermittent porphyria. Porphobilinogen and ALA are increased with acute attacks but are prone to become normal between attacks. Urine coproporphyrin exceeds uroporphyrin excretion during acute attacks. Fluorescence emission in plasma is used to distinguish VP from PCT.[3]

Chemical porphyrias occur. Porphyrinogenic chemicals include certain halogenated hydrocarbons which cause the excretion of increased uroporphyrin.

In **lead poisoning** elevation of delta aminolevulinic acid greater than that of porphobilinogen occurs and porphobilinogen may be normal. Urinary coproporphyrin characteristically is increased. Free erythrocyte protoporphyrin is increased. (See listing Lead, Blood *on page 556.*) Toxins such as lead interfere with heme synthesis and cause porphyrinuria.

Increased urine excretion of uroporphyrinogen, uroporphyrin, and coproporphyrin occurs in **porphyria cutanea tarda (PCT)**. Uroporphyrinogen decarboxylase is decreased. It is done on red cells; whole blood is collected. It is normal in acquired PCT and in some inherited cases.[1] It is found in middle-aged men who like ethanol, young women on oral contraceptives, selective hydrocarbon exposure, and in subjects on dialysis. These patients do not excrete increased porphobilinogen, but may have slight elevations of delta aminolevulinic acid. Iron overload is found with the acquired form, for which treatment includes repeated phlebotomies.

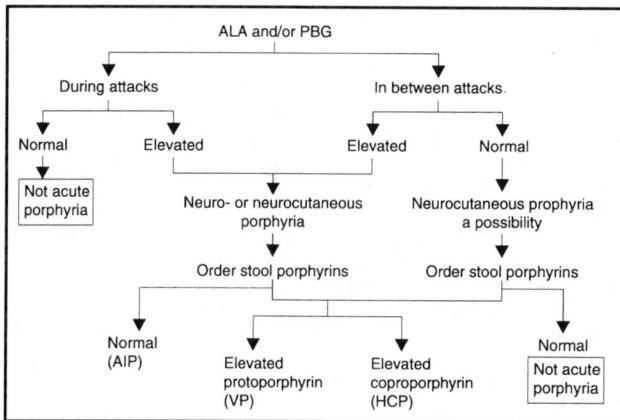

Interpretation of urine studies, as the cause of symptoms, during evaluation of acute porphyria. AIP = acute intermittent porphyria; ALA = Δ- aminolevulinic acid; HCP = hereditary coproporphyria; PBG = porphobilinogen; VP = variegate porphyria.
From Tefferi A, Solberg LA, and Ellefson RD, "Porphyrias: Clinical Evaluation and Interpretation of Laboratory Tests," *Mayo Clin Proc*, 1994, 69:289-90 with permission.

Limitations Increased porphobilinogen may occur in patients on oral contraceptives. This test and delta aminolevulinic acid will not detect protoporphyria. Coproporphyrinuria alone lacks specificity and sensitivity for lead screening. Erythrocyte uroporphyrinogen I synthase is decreased in latent acute intermittent porphyria, and is needed in patients with possible latent acute intermittent porphyria. Quantitative porphobilinogen is of value in active and in many cases of latent acute intermittent porphyria, but will miss some of the latter when compared to red cell uroporphyrinogen I synthase.

Porphyrias: Overview

Disorder	Inheritance	Age of Clinical Onset	Primary Organ Involvement	Useful Tests	Primary Symptoms
Congenital erythropoietic porphyria	Autosomal recessive	Birth – 5 y	Erythroid cells	Urinary porphyrins Fecal porphyrins Uroporphyrinogen III synthase, erythrocytes *see page 215*	Severe photosensitivity
(Günther's disease)	Rare			Fluorescence of a diaper under Wood's light	Red urine Stains diapers Hemolytic anemia
Acute intermittent porphyria	Autosomal dominant	Adults	Hepatic, probably erythroid cells	Urine porphobilinogen Porphobilinogen deaminase, erythrocyte *see page 185* Urine porphyrins Urinary delta aminolevulinic acid Erythrocyte uroporphyrinogen 1 synthase Fecal porphyrins	Mild to severe neurologic/visceral (autonomic) symptoms
Precipitating causes include barbiturates, hydantoins, sulfonamides	Most common acute hepatic porphyria in U.S.				Acute attacks
Hereditary coproporphyria	Autosomal dominant	Adults	Hepatic, possibly erythroid cells	Urine PBG and ALA in acute attacks Urine porphyrins including coproporphyrin Fecal porphyrins Plasma porphyrins	Similar to variegate porphyria Acute attacks
Variegate porphyria	Autosomal dominant	Adults	Hepatic, possibly erythroid cells	Urine PBG and ALA in acute attacks Urine porphyrins Fecal porphyrins Plasma porphyrins Erythrocyte uroporphyrinogen-1-synthase	Mild to severe photosensitivity and neurologic-visceral symptoms Acute attacks
Porphyria cutanea tarda	Autosomal dominant, type II (inherited type); sporadic type also known Most common porphyria in U.S.	Adults	Hepatic, possibly erythroid cells; photosensitivity	Urine porphyrins Plasma porphyrins Uroporphyrinogen decarboxylase, type II (RBCs)	Similar to variegate porphyria Photosensitization Liver damage
Protoporphyria	Autosomal dominant	Usually childhood	Erythroid cells, probably liver	Protoporphyrin, free erythrocyte *see page 195*	Photosensitization Liver damage
Acquired (intoxication) porphyria	Acquired	Children and adults	Hepatic, erythroid cells	Erythrocyte porphyrins Urinary delta aminolevulinic acid Urine porphobilinogen Urine porphyrins Fecal porphyrins	Mild photosensitivity

(Continued)

Increased urine porphyrin excretion may be secondary to other diseases (eg, hepatobiliary diseases), especially coproporphyrin excretion. These are secondary porphyrinurias. They lack increased urinary porphobilinogen or Δ-ALA, with the important exception of lead poisoning.[4]

Methodology High performance liquid chromatography (HPLC) is the method of choice; chromatography, fluorometry are also used.

Additional Information Heme is a component not only of hemoglobin, but of enzymes such as the cytochrome P-450 system. It includes a tetrapyrole ring (protoporphyrin IX) and iron.

The table provides an abbreviated overview of the porphyrias. Porphyrin fractionation of plasma can be done. Increases of urine porphyrins are found with congenital erythropoietic porphyria, acute intermittent porphyria, hereditary coproporphyria, variegate porphyria, and porphyria cutanea tarda.

Fecal porphyrin examination for hereditary coproporphyria, variegate porphyria, and protoporphyria can be used for adult patients. Stool examination for coproporphyrin and protoporphyrin is recommended for diagnosis of variegate porphyria.[5]

Neurologic dysfunction occurs in the **hepatic porphyrias**, the types of porphyria in which acute attacks develop: acute intermittent porphyria, variegate porphyria, hereditary coproporphyria, and ALA dehydrase deficiency. Abdominal pain, caused by autonomic neuropathy, occurs with acute attacks (eg, acute intermittent porphyria). It is the most common symptom of acute intermittent porphyria.[4]

The acute porphyrias include acute intermittent porphyria (AIP), variegate porphyria, and hereditary coproporphyria. Attacks may be life-threatening.[6] Symptoms may include colicky abdominal pain, fever, vomiting, neuritis, and psychosis.

The non-acute porphyrias include cutaneous hepatic porphyria, erythropoietic protoporphyria, and congenital porphyria. Dermatological symptoms are caused by circulating porphyrins which cause photosensitivity.[6]

Hepatic complications are found with **porphyria cutanea tarda** and **protoporphyria**. Fluorescence is demonstrable in liver biopsies from patients with the former, as well as siderosis. Crystalline deposits may be found in protoporphyria.[4] The amount of porphobilinogen excreted in acute intermittent porphyria is usually greater than the excretion of delta aminolevulinic acid (Δ-ALA). When there is more Δ-ALA, another diagnosis should be considered, including lead poisoning, another type of porphyria, or hereditary tyrosinemia.[4] See also listing Protoporphyrin, Free Erythrocyte on page 195, which pertains to lead poisoning, and erythropoietic protoporphyria. The differential diagnosis of lead poisoning is relevant,[7] vide supra. Drugs can cause confusion. Naproxen is reported to cause a reaction clinically and histopathologically similar to porphyria cutanea tarda.[8]

This is a complex group of diseases, of which most are uncommon. Some are extremely rare (eg, hepatoerythropoietic porphyria). Larger sources are recommended for more comprehensive review.[3,9,10,11,12]

Footnotes
1. Leavelle DE, Mayo Medical Laboratories Interpretive Handbook, Rochester, MN: Mayo Medical Laboratories, 1994.
2. Tschudy DP, "Porphyrins," Chemical Diagnosis of Disease, Brown SS, Mitchell FL, and Young DS, eds, Amsterdam, Holland: Elsevier/North Holland Biomedical Press, 1979, 1039-58.
3. Desnick RJ, "The Porphyrias," Harrison's Principles of Internal Medicine, 13th ed, Vol 2, Isselbacher KJ, Braunwald E, Wilson JD, et al, eds, New York, NY: McGraw-Hill Inc, 1994, 2073-9.
4. Bloomer JR and Bonkovsky HL, "The Porphyrias," Dis Mon, 1989, 35(1):1-54.
5. Muhlbauer JE, Pathak MA, Tishler PV, et al, "Variegate Porphyria in New England," JAMA, 1982, 247:3095-102.
6. Moore MR, "Biochemistry of Porphyria," Int J Biochem, 1993, 25(10):1353-68.
7. Bird TD, Wallace DM, and Labbe RF, "The Porphyria, Plumbism, Pottery Puzzle," JAMA, 1982, 247:813-4.
8. Fitzpatrick JE, "New Histopathologic Findings in Drug Eruptions," Dermatol Clin, 1992, 10(1):19-36.
9. Bickers DR, "Photosensitivity and Other Reactions to Light," Harrison's Principles of Internal Medicine, 13th ed, Vol 2, Isselbacher KJ, Braunwald E, Wilson JD, et al, eds, New York, NY: McGraw-Hill Inc, 1994, 307-12.
10. Nuttall KL, "Porphyrins and Disorders of Porphyrin Metabolism," Tietz Textbook of Clinical Chemistry, 2nd ed, Burtis CA and Ashwood ER, eds, Philadelphia, PA: WB Saunders Co, 1994, 2073-106.
11. Tefferi A, Colgan JP, and Solberg LA, "Acute Porphyrias: Diagnosis and Management," Mayo Clin Proc, 1994, 69(10):991-5.
12. Tefferi A, Solberg LA Jr, and Ellefson RD, "Porphyrias: Clinical Evaluation and Interpretation of Laboratory Tests," Mayo Clin Proc, 1994, 69(3):289-90.

References
Ayala F and Santoianni P, "Drug-Induced Cutaneous Porphyria," Clin Dermatol, 1993, 11(4):535-9.
"Case Records of the Massachusetts General Hospital. Weekly Clinicopathological Exercises. Case 39-1984. A 29-Year-Old Woman With Abdominal Pain, Myalgia, and Muscle Weakness," N Engl J Med, 1984, 311(13):839-47.
Edwards CQ, Griffen LM, Goldgar DE, et al, "HLA-Linked Hemochromatosis Alleles in Sporadic Porphyria Cutanea Tarda," Gastroenterology, 1989, 97(4):972-81.
Elder GH, Urquhart AJ, De Salamanca RE, et al, "Immunoreactive Uroporphyrinogen Decarboxylase in the Liver in Porphyria Cutanea Tarda," Lancet, 1985, 2(8449):229-33.
Hift RJ, Meissner PN, Todd G, et al, "Homozygous Variegate Porphyria: An Evolving Clinical Syndrome," Postgrad Med J, 1993, 69(816):781-6.
Hindmarsh JT, "Variable Phenotypic Expression of Genotypic Abnormalities in the Porphyrias," Clin Chim Acta, 1993, 217(1):29-38.
Lip GY, McColl KE, and Moore MR, "The Acute Porphyrias," Br J Clin Pract, 1993, 47(1):38-43.
Meola T and Lim HW, "The Porphyrias," Dermatol Clin, 1993, 11(3):583-96.
Milo R, Neuman M, Klein C, et al, "Acute Intermittent Porphyria in Pregnancy," Obstet Gynecol, 1989, 73(3 Pt 2):450-2.
Pierach CA and Ippen H, "A Porphyrin-Soaked Diaper," N Engl J Med, 1994, 330(23):1690.
Todd DJ, "Erythropoietic Protoporphyria," Br J Dermatol, 1994, 131(6):751-66.
Westerlund J, Pudek M, and Schreiber WE, "A Rapid and Accurate Spectrofluorometric Method for Quantification and Screening of Urinary Porphyrins," Clin Chem, 1988, 34(2):345-51.

Porter-Silber Chromogens, Urine see 17-Hydroxycorticosteroids, Urine on page 147

Postprandial Glucose see Glucose, 2-Hour Postprandial on page 136

Potassium, Arterial see Potassium, Serum or Plasma on this page

Potassium, Serum or Plasma

CPT 84132

Related Information
Aldosterone, Blood on page 67
Aldosterone, Urine on page 68
Calcium, Serum on page 97
Chloride, Serum on page 108
Chloride, Urine on page 109
Concentration Test, Urine on page 633
Electrolytes, Serum or Plasma on page 123
Magnesium, Serum on page 164
Magnesium, Urine on page 165
Renin, Plasma on page 197
Salicylate on page 573
Venous Blood Collection on page 30

Synonyms K⁺, Serum or Plasma

Applies to Potassium, Arterial

Abstract The major intracellular cation, K⁺ is very commonly measured as one of the serum or plasma electrolytes and as a urinary electrolyte as well. **Causes of hyperkalemia** include drugs such as spironolactone, triamterene, and excessive theophylline.

Causes of hypokalemia include diarrhea, diuretics, emesis, metabolic alkalosis, Cushing's syndrome, primary aldosteronism, and with renal tubular abnormalities.

Specimen Serum, plasma

Container Red top tube or green top (heparin) tube

Collection Avoid very small needles if possible. Avoid stasis, use of tourniquet if possible and **avoid hand clenching**. Fist clenching increases K⁺. If a tourniquet must be used, sample blood 1-2 minutes after the hand is relaxed and the tourniquet removed. Avoid potassium-containing tubes such as potassium oxalate. Potassium can be reported from arterial as well as from venous blood. If arterial puncture is done for pO₂, plasma can be tested for Na⁺, K⁺, and Cl⁻ so long as lithium and not potassium heparinate anticoagulant is used.

Storage Instructions Remove plasma or serum from red cells within 4 hours before specimen is refrigerated. Storage of unspun blood at 4°C causes serum and plasma K⁺ to increase.

Causes for Rejection Hemolyzed specimen, serum specimen not removed from clot in patient with high platelet count. Such specimens may be analyzed but the likelihood of a falsely high potassium level must be recognized and stated in report. Preferably, hemolyzed samples should be rejected.

Reference Range Plasma: 3.5-5.0 mmol/L (SI: 3.5-5.0 mmol/L). Add **approximately** 0.1 to normal ranges if serum is sampled rather than plasma. Pediatric ranges are sometimes reported as slightly higher than adult levels. Differences may well relate to the amount of hemolysis in specimens used to establish normal ranges. In daily practice some degree of hemolysis may occur in neonatal and pediatric specimens. Although grossly hemolyzed specimens are usually rejected, the acceptability of samples with slight hemolysis is debatable. Even slight hemolysis can dramatically increase K⁺ results; red cells have an intracellular K⁺ concentration of 100-120 mmol/L or more.

Possible Panic Range Newborns: <2.5 mmol/L (SI: <2.5 mmol/L), >7.0 mmol/L (SI: >7.0 mmol/L); adults: <2.5 mmol/L (SI: <2.5 mmol/L), >6.5 mmol/L (SI: >6.5 mmol/L). With unanticipated high or low K⁺, ECG may be indicated. If potassium is high and serum was used, examine peripheral blood smear for thrombocytosis and/or leukocytosis; obtain platelet and white count if indicated, vide infra.

Use Evaluate electrolyte balance; K⁺ level should be followed especially in elderly patients, those on intravenous hyperalimentation, in patients on diuretic therapy and in cases of renal disease, particularly patients on hemodialysis. As one of the major electrolytes, serum K^+ concentrations are a part of regular assessment of acid-base balance, management of intravenous therapy, and evaluation of patients with hypertension.

Evaluate muscular weakness and irritability, mental confusion, weakness; manage leukemia, diseases of gastrointestinal tract including laxative abuse, hepatic encephalopathy, fistulas and tube drainage; evaluate and prevent cardiac arrhythmias;[1,2] evaluate alcoholism with delirium tremens; detect, diagnose, and manage mineralocorticoid excess (primary aldosteronism, Cushing's syndrome, tumors with ectopic ACTH production, some cases of congenital adrenal hyperplasia), heat stroke, licorice ingestion mineralocorticoid effect.

Hypokalemia (low potassium) has been found in 80% to 90% of hypertensive patients with primary aldosteronism. This uncommon entity is a curable cause of hypertension. Serum/plasma levels are lower in patients whose primary aldosteronism is caused by adenomas than in those with nonadenomatous hyperplasia. Twenty percent of the latter group had serum levels within normal range.[3] Low K^+ occurs with endogenous or exogenous increase in other corticosteroids, including that in Cushing's syndrome as well as with dietary or parenteral deprivation of K^+ (eg, parenteral therapy without adequate K^+ replacement). Hypokalemia occurs with vomiting, diarrhea, fistulas, laxatives, diuretics, burns, excessive perspiration, acid/base abnormalities, Bartter's syndrome, malnutrition, ureterosigmoidostomy, colorectal villous tumor, some cases of alcoholism and folic acid deficiency, in renal tubular disorders, as well as in other entities.

Hyperkalemia (high potassium) reflects generally inadequate renal excretion, mobilization of potassium from the tissues, or excessive intake or administration. Hyperkalemia occurs with trauma,[4] with administration of K^+ salts of some drugs, ACE inhibitors, Addison's disease, acidosis including ketoacidosis as in diabetes mellitus, insulin lack, with increased osmolality (eg, glucose, mannitol), and in other entities as well as in renal diseases with azotemia, with malignant hyperthermia, and with renal tubular acidosis. Increased K^+ can occur with potassium-sparing diuretics, nonsteroidal anti-inflammatory drugs, especially in the presence of renal disease. Systemic heparin therapy can suppress aldosterone release and increase K^+, especially in the presence of other factors. Hyperkalemia is reported with high-dose trimethoprim-sulfamethoxazole therapy.[5] Other factors which may cause hyperkalemia include dehydration, exercise, pregnancy, standing posture, and hyperventilation.[6] **Artifact causing hyperkalemia includes hemolysis from collection, storage, or processing.**

Drug effects are summarized.[7]

Limitations Inadequate sodium intake may mask the hypokalemia of aldosteronism; sodium loading in that setting may make hypokalemia recognizable. Heparinized plasma is probably the specimen of choice for K^+, because clotting causes cytolysis and may elevate serum values, usually but not always only slightly.

Be wary of potentially falsely high K^+ concentrations in blood samples that have sat unattended for several hours. Such samples may have falsely elevated K^+ in the absence of visible hemolysis ("pocket syndrome"). If doubt exists, repeat measurements on a fresh specimen.

While acute hypokalemia is reflected largely by serum/plasma K^+ concentration, chronic hypokalemia is more apt to be accompanied by reduction of total body stores, as well as serum/plasma concentrations.

Methodology Flame emission photometry or ion-selective electrode (ISE)

Additional Information Low K^+ is much more significant with a low pH than with a high pH. When pH increases by 0.1, K^+ decreases approximately 0.6 mmol/L. With low pH, as in ketoacidosis, as therapeutic adjustment towards normal is made, plasma/serum K^+ concentrations will decrease. Phosphorus concentrations tend to follow potassium downwards during therapy of diabetic ketoacidosis; both are largely intracellular. With insulin therapy (and increased utilization of carbohydrate), potassium moves into cells and serum/plasma concentrations fall. Hyperalimentation may have a similar effect. Hypokalemia has been reported in slightly >50% of a series of 32 patients with acute myelogenous leukemia, but thrombocytosis can increase serum K^+ levels, *vide supra*.

Thiazide/chlorthalidone therapy may cause hyperuricemia and hypercalcemia as well as hypokalemia.

The watery diarrhea-hypokalemia-achlorhydria (WDHA) syndrome most often is related to vasoactive intestinal polypeptide (VIP).

Consider magnesium status in patients who have hypokalemia.[8]

Since platelets release K^+ during coagulation, samples from patients who have thrombocytosis (eg, some cases of polycythemia vera and other myeloproliferative diseases) yield spuriously elevated K^+ concentrations. This "pseudohyperkalemia" may also occur in cases of leukemia

with high WBC count (notably chronic myelogenous leukemia) as potassium is released from WBCs and platelets during clot formation. For such patients it is best to assay K^+ on a heparinized sample. Pseudohyperkalemia in serum specimens may be due to increased platelets.[9] Serum potassium increases with the platelet count in normal subjects and in those with thrombocytosis, and such pseudohyperkalemia increment is an artifact.[10] Plasma concentrations are not affected.

A discussion of the relation between lactic acidosis, ketoacidosis, and elevated serum K^+ levels is provided in a paper by Fulop.[11]

Footnotes

1. Clausen TG, Brocks K, and Ibsen H, "Hypokalemia and Ventricular Arrhythmias in Acute Myocardial Infarction," *Acta Med Scand*, 1988, 224(6):531-7.
2. Borra S, Shaker R, and Kleinfeld M, "Hyperkalemia in an Adult Hospitalized Population," *Mt Sinai J Med*, 1988, 55(3):226-9.
3. Blumenfeld JD, Sealey JE, Schlussel Y, et al, "Diagnosis and Treatment of Primary Hyperaldosteronism," *Ann Intern Med*, 1994, 121(11):877-85.
4. Vanek VW, Seballos RM, Chong D, et al, "Serum Potassium Concentrations in Trauma Patients," *South Med J*, 1994, 87(1):41-6.
5. Greenberg S, Reiser IW, and Chou SY, "Hyperkalemia With High-Dose Trimethoprim-Sulfamethoxazole Therapy," *Am J Kidney Dis*, 1993, 22(4):603-6.
6. Gambino R, "Nondisease Factors That Affect Potassium Levels," *Lab Rep*, 1995, 17(10):69-71.
7. Hitz J and Trivin F, "Potassium," *Drug Effects on Laboratory Test Results Analytical Interferences and Pharmacological Effects*, Siest G and Galteau MM, eds, Littleton, MA: PSG Publishing Co Inc, 1988, 362-74.
8. Ryan MP, "Interrelationships of Magnesium and Potassium Homeostasis," *Miner Electrolyte Metab*, 1993, 19(4-5):290-5.
9. Ralston SH, Lough M, and Sturrock RD, "Rheumatoid Arthritis: An Unrecognized Cause of Pseudohyperkalaemia," *Br Med J (Clin Res Ed)*, 1988, 297(6647):523-4.
10. Graber M, Subramani K, Corish D, et al, "Thrombocytosis Elevates Serum Potassium," *Am J Kidney Dis*, 1988, 12(2):116-20.
11. Fulop M, "Hyperkalemia in Diabetic Ketoacidosis," *Am J Med Sci*, 1990, 299(3):164-9.

References

Agarwal R, Afzalpurkar R, and Fordtran JS, "Pathophysiology of Potassium Absorption and Secretion by the Human Intestine," *Gastroenterology*, 1994, 107(2):548-71.
Alpern RJ and Toto RD, "Hypokalemic Nephropathy - A Clue to Cystogenesis?" *N Engl J Med*, 1990, 322(6):398-9.
Brem AS, "Disorders of Potassium Homeostasis," *Pediatr Clin North Am*, 1990, 37(2):419-27.
Corr LA, Grounds RM, Beacham JL, et al, "Effects of Circulating Endogenous Catecholamines on Plasma Glucose, Potassium, and Magnesium," *Clin Sci*, 1990, 78(2):185-91.
Gambino R, "Hypokalemia and Heat Stress - Men vs Women. A Closer Look at the Untold Medical Story Behind the Headlines of the Citadel Incident," *Lab Med*, 1995, 17(9):61-4.
Gitelman HJ, "Unresolved Issues in the Pathogenesis of Bartter's Syndrome and Its Variants," *Curr Opin Nephrol Hypertens*, 1994, 3(4):471-4.
Higham PD, Adams PC, Murray A, et al, "Plasma Potassium, Serum Magnesium, and Ventricular Fibrillation: A Prospective Study," *Q J Med*, 1993, 86(9):609-17.
Hitz J and Trivin F, "Potassium," *Drug Effects on Laboratory Test Results Analytical Interferences and Pharmacological Effects*, Siest G and Galteau MM, eds, Littleton, MA: PSG Publishing Co Inc, 1988, 362-74.
Krishna GG, "Role of Potassium in the Pathogenesis of Hypertension," *Am J Med Sci*, 1994, 307(Suppl 1):S21-5.
Latta K, Hisano S, and Chan JC, "Perturbations in Potassium Balance," *Clin Lab Med*, 1993, 13(1):149-56.
Maffly RH, "Renal Function and Disorders of Water, Sodium, and Potassium Balance," *Scientific American Medicine*, Section 10, Chapter 1, Rubenstein E and Federman DD, eds, New York, NY: Scientific American Inc, 1990, 2-34.
Pierson RN Jr and Wang J, "Body Composition Denominators for Measurements of Metabolism: What Measurements Can Be Believed?" *Mayo Clin Proc*, 1988, 63(9):947-9.
Quamme GA, "Laboratory Evaluation of Magnesium Status. Renal Function and Free Intracellular Magnesium Concentration," *Clin Lab Med*, 1993, 13(1):209-23.
Solomon R, Weinberg MS, and Dubey A, "The Diurnal Rhythm of Plasma Potassium: Relationship to Diuretic Therapy," *J Cardiovasc Pharmacol*, 1991, 17(5):854-9.
Torres VE, Young WF Jr, Offord KP, et al, "Association of Hypokalemia, Aldosteronism, and Renal Cysts," *N Engl J Med*, 1990, 322(6):345-51.
Wong KC, Schafer PG, and Schultz JR, "Hypokalemia and Anesthetic Implications," *Anesth Analg*, 1993, 77(6):1238-60.
Young WF Jr, Hogan MJ, Klee GG, et al, "Primary Aldosteronism: Diagnosis and Treatment," *Mayo Clin Proc*, 1990, 65(1):96-110.

Potassium, Urine

CPT 84133

Related Information

Aldosterone, Blood *on page 67*
Chloride, Urine *on page 109*
Electrolytes, Urine *on page 124*
Kidney Stone Analysis *on page 640*
Renin, Plasma *on page 197*
Urine Collection, 24-Hour *on page 30*

Synonyms K^+, Urine; Urine K^+

Abstract Urine potassium studies provide explanation for disturbances of serum or plasma values.

Specimen Random or timed urine (ie, 8-, 12-, or 24-hour)

Container No preservative

Storage Instructions Refrigerate

Reference Range 26-123 mmol/24 hours (SI: 26-123 mmol/day), markedly intake dependent. If significantly decreased serum or plasma K^+ has existed for days or more, urine K^+ excretion should be low: ≤15 mmol/L (SI: ≤15 mmol/L), or ≤30 mmol/24 hours (SI: ≤30 mmol/day). There is significant diurnal variation, output greater at night.[1]

(Continued)

Potassium, Urine (Continued)

Use Evaluate electrolyte balance, acid-base balance; evaluate hypokalemia; Carroll and Oh point out that urinary loss of 40 mmol/24 hours (SI: 40 mmol/day) in the presence of hypokalemia <3 mmol/L is excessive.[2] In the presence of such hypokalemia, urine excretion is helpful to separate renal from nonrenal losses. Excretion <20 mmol/24 hours (SI: <20 mmol/day) is evidence that hypokalemia is not from renal loss.[1] Renal loss >50 mmol/L in a hypokalemic, hypertensive patient not on a diuretic may indicate primary or secondary aldosteronism. The kidneys do not respond quickly to potassium deprivation. There is renal wastage of K[+] in secondary aldosteronism. Glucocorticoids, including endogenous steroids in Cushing's syndrome, are among the causes of kaliuresis. A 24-hour urine collection for potassium represents an appropriate screening test for hyperaldosteronism, preferably following K[+] repletion to achieve serum level >3 mmol/L.[3]

Methodology Flame emission photometry, ion-selective electrode (ISE)

Additional Information Urinary K[+] may be elevated with dietary (food and/or medicinal) increase, hyperaldosteronism, renal tubular acidosis, onset of alkalosis, and with other disorders. Time relationships are important in interpretation. K[+] will decrease in Addison's disease and in renal disease with decreased urine flow (nephrosclerosis, pyelonephritis, glomerulonephritis).

Footnotes

1. Moore-Ede MC, Czeisler CA, and Richardson GS, "Circadian Timekeeping in Health and Disease, Part 2. Clinical Implications of Circadian Rhythmicity," *N Engl J Med*, 1983, 309:530-6.
2. Carroll HJ and Oh MS, *Water Electrolyte and Acid-Base Metabolism: Diagnosis and Management*, Philadelphia, PA: JB Lippincott Co, 1978.
3. "Case Records of the Massachusetts General Hospital. Weekly Clinicopathological Exercises. Case 24-1992. A 52-Year-Old Man With Hypertension, Hypokalemia, and an Adrenal Mass," *N Engl J Med*, 1992, 326(24):1617-23.

References

Epstein M and Oster JR, "Disorders of Potassium Homeostasis," *The Laboratory in Clinical Medicine: Interpretation and Application*, 2nd ed, Halsted JA and Halsted CH, eds, Philadelphia, PA: WB Saunders Co, 1981, 296-303.

White PC, "Disorders of Aldosterone Biosynthesis and Action," *N Engl J Med*, 1994, 331(4):250-8.

PP *see* Pancreatic Polypeptide, Human *on page 177*

PP, 2-Hour *see* Glucose, 2-Hour Postprandial *on page 136*

PRA *see* Renin, Plasma *on page 197*

Pregnancy Test

CPT 81025 (color comparison); 84703 (qualitative)

Related Information

Human Chorionic Gonadotropin, Serum *on page 145*
Progesterone *on next page*

Synonyms Beta-Subunit Human Chorionic Gonadotropin Urine or Serum; hCG, Slide Test, Stat; hCG, Urine; Human Chorionic Gonadotropin, Urine

Abstract Urinary human chorionic gonadotropin (β-hCG) is used as a indication of pregnancy or hCG-producing tumors.

Specimen Urine or serum; first voided morning specimen is preferred if urine is tested (to obtain most concentrated specimen).

Container Urine container or red top tube

Storage Instructions Urine stable 4 hours at 25°C and 3 days at 4°C. Serum should be frozen at -20°C if not run within 48 hours.

Causes for Rejection Urine specimen grossly contaminated, low urinary specific gravity, proteinuria (applicable to certain tests), gross lipemia or turbidity

Special Instructions Centrifuge turbid urine specimens prior to testing.

Reference Range Normal males and nonpregnant females: negative; normal pregnant females: positive. Sensitivity and specificity of β-subunit two point RIA or EIA tests may allow early diagnosis of pregnancy, within 6 days after conception. Presently, qualitative tests are positive when intact hCG exceeds 25 IU/L (first international reference preparation, IRP, from World Health Organization).

Use Diagnose pregnancy; screen for women at risk of being pregnant prior to performance of x-ray, sterilization, menstrual regulation, and curettage procedures and/or prior to the initiation of gestation/embryo/fetal potentially injurious medication; detect and/or evaluate incomplete/complete abortions; detect ectopic gestation. A sensitive and quantitative test for the presence of hCG is preferable to rule out or follow gestational trophoblastic neoplasia or ectopic hCG-producing tumor.

Limitations Results may be negative in early pregnancy or with low specific gravity. In early pregnancy, incomplete abortion, recent complete abortion, ectopic pregnancy (in which hCG level is low), slide test end points may be difficult to interpret. Methods using covalent bonded latex particles and tests producing macroagglutination are more reliably interpreted.

Methodology Slide or tube agglutination-inhibition tests (urine) are largely replaced by enzyme immunoassay; β-subunit hCG by radioimmunoassay (serum or urine); immunoradiometric (IRMA) (eg, Tandem® hCG which incorporates two monoclonal antibodies, each with immunospecificity for different sites on the hCG molecule, one coated on a plastic bead on which the solid phase develops). Enzyme immunoassay, including sensitive (to 20-40 mIU/mL level of hCG, SI: 20-40 IU/L) two-point urine or serum qualitative/quantitative membrane based tests of which Tandem® ICON® is most well known.

Additional Information Pregnancy testing is usually performed on urine. It is based on the the detection of human chorionic gonadotropin (hCG). Concentrations of hCG in the urine approach those seen in serum. In normal pregnancy, hCG levels rise at implantation and peak at 8-12 weeks. Although newer urine pregnancy tests are quite sensitive, false-negatives can occur early in gestation. In such cases, if ectopic pregnancy is suspected, serial serum hCG and progesterone assays may be of value; see these listings.

Early in the first trimester of pregnancy (1-2 weeks) serum hCG concentrations are from 50-500 mIU/mL (SI: 50-500 IU/L). Current generation sensitive tests can detect pregnancy shortly (2-3 days) after implantation of the ovum. By 3-4 weeks of gestation, hCG is at the 500-10,000 mIU/mL level (SI: 500-10,000 IU/L). Serum hCG level peaks during the second to third month of gestation (30,000-100,000 mIU/mL) (SI: 30,000-100,000 IU/L). Use of serum for pregnancy testing may provide greater sensitivity, of special value in cases of early pregnancy, and is of greater value in serial testing for follow-up of an abnormal gestation (eg, ectopic pregnancy or a gestational trophoblastic neoplasm). If serum (or urine) hCG concentrations do not appear to correlate with the anticipated clinical situation, periodic repeat hCG and progesterone determinations may be helpful. If there is demise of the developing embryo/fetus (eg, ectopic pregnancy), hCG and progesterone concentrations will fall. Because of slow clearance from the serum, hCG may be detected in serum/urine for as long as 4 weeks following abortion.

Currently, the tests most commonly used to screen for pregnancy are two-point EIA "concentration" methods. A variety of different forms are commercially available. An antibody (frequently monoclonal) is immobilized on a membrane or other solid phase and the sample hCG is "concentrated" in a small central area of the surface (a membrane, bead, paddle, tube, or dipstick). Color development occurs within minutes of addition of enzyme tagged monoclonal anti-β-hCG. These tests are sensitive, specific, and fast. They have largely supplanted slide/tube screening procedures.

A study of specificity (six commercially available ELISA urine pregnancy tests) utilizing specimens from men and postmenopausal females found variable performance by the different methods, not explained by review of the medical records. Test systems with provision for a negative reference area gave fewer false-positive results (had greater specificity).[1] Correlation was found between mucous content of the postmenopausal female group's urine samples and the incidence of false-positive hCG results.

One year of routine use of Tandem® ICON® system for urine pregnancy testing (University of Texas) did not result in a report of known false-positive results. Stability of color development after addition of color reagents and presence or absence of a built in positive control could influence choice of a test system for routine use.

Serum progesterone levels used with β-hCG levels may assist in differentiating normal intrauterine from abnormal intrauterine or **ectopic pregnancy** (cutoff: 15 ng/mL) (SI: 48 nmol/L). β-hCG and progesterone levels are lower in abnormal pregnancies. Less overlap occurs, however, between progesterone (as compared to β-hCG) values in normal versus ectopic and abnormal pregnancies.[2] When a positive pregnancy test is obtained, differential considerations should include the possibility of simultaneous intrauterine and extrauterine gestations[3] (albeit unlikely) and the possibility of passively acquired hCG as in an individual recently transfused with fresh frozen plasma prepared from pregnant donors.[4] When an embryo is large enough to produce in excess of 1600 IU/L hCG (first IRP) one may anticipate that in normal gestation the sac should be visible on transvaginal ultrasonography, **depending upon methods**.[5]

A number of commercially successful home pregnancy tests have been introduced. They have been found to vary widely in performance (optimal accuracy, sensitivity, specificity, human factor useability).[6] A study of the use of such home pregnancy test kits has resulted in the suggestion that pharmacists have an opportunity in taking a more active role in promoting the appropriate use of such self-testing products.[7]

Footnotes

1. Bandi ZL, Schoen I, and DeLara M, "Enzyme-Linked Immunosorbent Urine Pregnancy Tests: Clinical Specificity Studies," *Am J Clin Pathol*, 1987, 87(2):236-42.
2. Riss PA, Radivojevic K, and Bieglmayer C, "Serum Progesterone and Human Chorionic Gonadotropin in Very Early Pregnancy: Implications for Clinical Management," *Eur J Obstet Gynecol Reprod Biol*, 1989, 32(2):71-7.
3. Boutiette LA and Anderson GV Jr, "Heterotopic Pregnancy," *J Emerg Med*, 1989, 7(1):33-5.

4. Kruskall MS, Owings DV, Donovan LM et al, "Passive Transfusion of Human Chorionic Gonadotropin From Plasma Donated During Pregnancy," *Vox Sang*, 1989, 56(2):71-4.
5. Klee GG, "Human Chorionic Gonadotropin," *Mayo Clin Proc*, 1994, 69(4):391-2.
6. Latman NS and Bruot BC, "Evaluation of Home Pregnancy Test Kits," *Biomed Instrum Technol*, 1989, 23(2):144-9.
7. Coons SJ, "A Look at the Purchase and Use of Home Pregnancy Test Kits," *Am Pharm*, 1989, NS29(4):46-8.

References

Aziz K, "Sensitivity and Specificity of Pregnancy Tests," *Am Clin Lab*, 1989, 8:12, 15-6.
Christensen H, Thyssen HH, Schebye O, et al, "Three Highly Sensitive "Bedside" Serum and Urine Tests for Pregnancy Compared," *Clin Chem*, 1990, 36(9):1686-8.
Fields SA and Toffler WL, "Pregnancy Testing - Home and Office," *West J Med*, 1991, 154(3):327-8.
Norman RJ, "Analytical and Clinical Sensitivity and Specificity in Pregnancy Testing," *Am J Obstet Gynecol*, 1989, 161(3):835-6.
Norman RJ, Gilmore TA, and McLoughlin JW, "Simple Quantitative Measurement of Serum Choriogonadotropin Compared With Immunoradiometric, Immunoenzymometric, and Chemiluminescent Assays," *Clin Chem*, 1992, 38(1):144-7.
Taylor CA Jr, Overstreet JW, Samuels SJ, et al, "Prospective Assessment of Early Fetal Loss Using An Immunoenzymometric Screening Assay for Detection of Urinary Human Chorionic Gonadotropin," *Fertil Steril*, 1992, 57(6):1220-4.
Tyrey L, "Human Chorionic Gonadotropin Assays and Their Uses," *Obstet Gynecol Clin North Am*, 1988, 15(3):457-75.
Wyte CD, "Diagnostic Modalities in the Pregnant Patient," *Emerg Med Clin North Am*, 1994, 12(1):9-43.

Pregnancy Testing *see* Human Chorionic Gonadotropin, Serum *on page 145*

Pregnanetriol, Urine

CPT 84138

Related Information

17-Hydroxyprogesterone, Blood or Amniotic Fluid *on page 148*
Urine Collection, 24-Hour *on page 30*

Test Commonly Includes May be included with 17-ketogenic steroids

Abstract Used to evaluate adrenal cortical function. A urinary metabolite of 17-hydroxyprogesterone, urine pregnanetriol is increased in congenital adrenal hyperplasia caused most often by 21-hydroxylase deficiency.

Patient Preparation Avoid muscular exercise before and during collection.

Specimen 24-hour urine

Collection Preserve with boric acid.

Reference Range Varies with age. Up to 2.5 mg/24 hours (SI: 7.5 µmol/day) for adults, less in children; it slightly increases in third trimester of pregnancy.

Use Increased in congenital adrenal hyperplasia, in the most common form of the adrenogenital syndrome, 21-hydroxylase deficiency. May be increased with certain tumors of ovary and adrenal cortices and in the Stein-Leventhal syndrome.

Limitations 17-hydroxyprogesterone is used more often for evaluation of congenital adrenal hyperplasia.

Methodology Extraction/gas-liquid chromatography (GLC), spectrophotometry

Additional Information Muscular exercise may increase urinary pregnanetriol. Pregnanetriol is a major metabolite of 17-hydroxyprogesterone. Increased urinary 17-ketosteroids are usually found in 21-hydroxylase deficiency, with increased serum 17-hydroxyprogesterone. Pregnanetriol is not a ketosteroid; it is a ketogenic steroid.

References

Shackleton CH, Irias J, McDonald C, et al, "Late-Onset 21-Hydroxylase Deficiency: Reliable Diagnosis by Steroid Analysis of Random Urine Collections," *Steroids*, 1986, 48(3-4):239-50.
Weykamp CW, Penders TJ, Schmidt NA, et al, "Steroid Profile for Urine: Reference Values," *Clin Chem*, 1989, 35(12):2281-4.

Pressor Amines *see* Catecholamines, Fractionation, Plasma *on page 103*

Progesterone

CPT 84144

Related Information

Estrogens, Nonpregnant, Urine *on page 126*
Human Chorionic Gonadotropin, Serum *on page 145*
17-Hydroxyprogesterone, Blood or Amniotic Fluid *on page 148*
Pregnancy Test *on previous page*

Abstract A C-21 steroid, progesterone is made by the corpus luteum. Its major source in pregnancy is the placenta.

Patient Preparation Recent injection of radioisotope may interfere, depending on the assay system in use.

Specimen Serum

Container Red top tube

Storage Instructions Serum stable 4 days at 4°C and 3 months at -20°C.

Turnaround Time Approximately 5 hours by radioimmunoassay (RIA)

Special Instructions Patient's LMP (last menstrual period) and trimester of pregnancy are relevant.

Reference Range Ovarian production of progesterone is low during the first (follicular) phase of the menstrual cycle. After the LH surge at the time of ovulation, progesterone levels rise for 4-5 days, and then fall. First trimester progesterone levels in pregnancy >20 ng/mL provide a degree of evidence to project a normal gestation. Gestational serum progesterone ≥25 ng/mL (79.5 mmol/L) excludes most abnormal pregnancies. A rapid rise in the saliva estriol:progesterone ratio precedes the spontaneous onset of labor at term.[1]

With sensitive techniques, serum progesterone concentrations are <1 ng/mL prior to ovulation. After luteinizing hormone (LH) surge, serum concentrations rise to as high as 20 ng/mL. Serum concentrations then decrease prior to onset of menses. In adult males and prepubertal females, serum concentrations are <1 ng/mL.

Critical Values Levels <10 ng/mL are likely to be associated with abnormal pregnancy outcome (75% sensitivity, 78% specificity).[2]

Possible Panic Range Gestational level ≤5-10 ng/mL (≤15.9-31.8 mmol/L) indicates risk for pathologic pregnancy and levels ≤5 ng/mL (≤15.9 mmol/L) provide indication of nonviability.[3] These figures include subjects with failing intrauterine pregnancies as well as cases of ectopic gestation. Others use a progesterone cutoff of 8 ng/mL with rate of change of hCG concentration to distinguish ectopic pregnancy and inevitable abortion from normal intrauterine gestation.[4]

Use A female sex hormone, serum progesterone is used to confirm the occurrence of ovulation and to assess corpus luteum function. A series of measurements can help define the day of ovulation.[5] Diagnose inadequate luteal phase[6] and luteal phase defects;[7] investigate deficient progesterone production as a possible but unproven cause of habitual abortion. The test is useful for monitoring patients having ovulation during induction with hCG, hMG, FSH/LHRH, or clomiphene. The diagnosis of unruptured ectopic pregnancy often requires laboratory support in addition to appropriate imaging studies. Its measurement may be useful to identify patients at risk for ectopic gestation. A single measurement should be considered a screening test for ectopic pregnancy. The listing Pregnancy Test *on page 190* supplements information relevant to the role of progesterone in the evaluation of pregnancy.

Limitations Progesterone assay is not available quickly in many areas of the U.S. Beta hCG titers are a more popular analyte for pregnancy screening.

Methodology Radioimmunoassay (RIA), competitive binding radioimmunoassay.[4] A direct enzyme immunoassay for the measurement of salivary progesterone levels has been shown to be acceptable to patients and allows for a more comprehensive evaluation of ovarian function than can be obtained from a limited number of serum levels.[8] Direct time-resolved fluorescence immunoassay is available.[9] A competitive chemiluminescent immunoassay is in use.

Additional Information Progesterone and 17-α-hydroxyprogesterone are weak androgens. Progesterone is increased in congenital adrenal hyperplasia due to 21-hydroxylase, 17-hydroxylase, and 11-β-hydroxylase deficiencies. It is decreased in threatened abortion, primary or secondary hypogonadism, and short luteal phase syndrome. Serum progesterone measurements may be helpful in the detection of abnormal gestational development (eg, ectopic pregnancy, inevitable abortion). Discriminatory levels of progesterone fail to include all abnormal gestations, but serial progesterone concentrations may predict gestational complications as does the human chorionic gonadotropin rate of change[4] or doubling time.[10] Measurement of progesterone with such hCG assays may be expected to provide independent predictive values for complications of gestation. Done serially, they can be helpful to recognize instances of ectopic pregnancy and spontaneous abortion.

Progesterone levels decrease as pregnancy fails.

Footnotes

1. Darne J, McGarrigle HH, and Lachelin GC, "Saliva Oestriol, Oestradiol, Oestrone and Progesterone Levels in Pregnancy: Spontaneous Labour at Term Is Preceded by a Rise in the Saliva Oestriol:Progesterone Ratio," *Br J Obstet Gynaecol*, 1987, 94(3):227-35.
2. Daily CA, Laurent SL, and Nunley WC Jr, "The Prognostic Value of Serum Progesterone and Quantitative β-Human Chorionic Gonadotropin in Early Human Pregnancy," *Am J Obstet Gynecol*, 1994, 171(2):380-4.
3. Carson SA, and Buster JE, "Ectopic Pregnancy," *N Engl J Med*, 1993, 329(16):1174-81.
4. Stewart BK, Nazar-Stewart V, and Toivola B, "Biochemical Discrimination of Pathologic Pregnancy From Early, Normal Intrauterine Gestation in Symptomatic Patients," *Am J Clin Pathol*, 1995, 103(4):386-90.
5. Daya S, "Optimal Time in the Menstrual Cycle for Serum Progesterone Measurement to Diagnose Luteal Phase Defects," *Am J Obstet Gynecol*, 1989, 161(4):1009-11.
6. Soules MR, Clifton DK, Cohen NL, et al, "Luteal Phase Deficiency: Abnormal Gonadotropin and Progesterone Secretion Patterns," *J Clin Endocrinol Metab*, 1989, 69(4):813-20.
7. Bopp B and Shoupe D, "Luteal Phase Defects," *J Reprod Med*, 1993, 38(5):348-56.
8. Finn MM, Gosling JP, Tallon DF, et al, "Normal Salivary Progesterone Levels Throughout the Ovarian Cycle as Determined by a Direct Enzyme Immunoassay," *Fertil Steril*, 1988, 50(6):882-7.

(Continued)

Progesterone *(Continued)*

9. Kakabakos SE and Khosravi MJ, "Direct Time-Resolved Fluorescence Immunoassay of Progesterone in Serum Involving the Biotin-Streptavidin System and the Immobilized-Antibody Approach," *Clin Chem*, 1992, 38(5):725-30.
10. Cowan BD, "Ectopic Pregnancy," *Curr Opin Obstet Gynecol*, 1993, 5(3):328-32.

References

Carson SA and Buster JE, "Ectopic Pregnancy," *N Engl J Med*, 1994, 330(10):713-4 (letter).

Hilborn S and Krahn J, "Effect of Time of Exposure of Serum to Gel-Barrier Tubes on Results for Progesterone and Some Other Endocrine Tests," *Clin Chem*, 1987, 33(1):203-4.

Nippoldt TB, Reame NE, Kelch RP, et al, "The Roles of Estradiol and Progesterone in Decreasing Luteinizing Hormone Pulse Frequency in the Luteal Phase of the Menstrual Cycle," *J Clin Endocrinol Metab*, 1989, 69(1):67-76.

Stewart MO, Whittaker PG, Persson B, et al, "A Longitudinal Study of Circulating Progesterone, Oestradiol, hCG, and hPL During Pregnancy in Type 1 Diabetic Mothers," *Br J Obstet Gynaecol*, 1989, 96(4):415-23.

Proinsulin C-Peptide *see* C-Peptide *on page 114*

Prolactin

CPT 84146

Related Information

Dehydroepiandrosterone Sulfate *on page 120*
Estradiol, Serum *on page 125*
Follicle Stimulating Hormone *on page 129*
Luteinizing Hormone, Blood or Urine *on page 163*
Metyrapone Stimulation Test *on page 167*

Abstract The most common causes of hyperprolactinemia are **prolactinoma** (a prolactin-secreting adenoma of pituitary) and **idiopathic hyperprolactinemia**. Hyperprolactinemia occurs not only with prolactin-secreting tumors but with interference with the transport of dopamine (the inhibitory hormone) to the pituitary and with neuroleptic therapy. Its characteristics include amenorrhea, infertility, and galactorrhea in women; diminished libido and impotence in men.

Patient Preparation Patient should be fasting. Recently administered radioisotopes may interfere if RIA is used for assay. Phenothiazines may cause hyperprolactinemia. Prolactin secretion is inhibited by levodopa, dopamine, bromocriptine, pergolide mesylate, and thyroid hormones and is influenced by estrogens and antihypertensives.

Specimen Serum

Container Red top tube

Collection Venipuncture itself can occasionally elevate prolactin level. Draw between 8 AM and 10 AM. Draw in chilled tube. Keep specimen on ice.

Storage Instructions Separate serum in refrigerated centrifuge and freeze. Stable 3 months at -20°C.

Reference Range Normal range is given by one source as <20 ng/mL (SI: <20 µg/L) in nonlactating subjects. Normal ranges for prolactin are not interchangeable between all laboratories. Prolactin deficiency should be confirmed by lack of TRH response.

Critical Values Although levels >200 ng/mL (SI: >200 µg/L) indicate prolactin-secreting tumor in a nonlactating woman, lower levels are found in instances of prolactinoma.

Use Prolactin level, for **hyperprolactinemia**, is the first test for work-up of galactorrhea (inappropriate lactation). About 75% of patients with galactorrhea and amenorrhea have hyperprolactinemia. A premenopausal female having amenorrhea and galactorrhea is suspect of pituitary prolactinoma and is considered a candidate for radiologic evaluation of the pituitary as well as serum prolactin concentrations. Prolactin level is a test for pituitary and hypothalamic lesions as well as for detection of prolactin-secreting pituitary tumors (microadenomas, macroadenomas) (Forbes-Albright syndrome) with or without galactorrhea. Postpartum hyperprolactinemia is the Chiari-Frommel syndrome. Hirsutism occurs in occasional patients with prolactinomas, but there does not seem to be a relationship to virilization. Work up infertility, amenorrhea, and oligomenorrhea. Of women with amenorrhea, 15% to 25% may have hyperprolactinemia. In males, hyperprolactinemia may present with impotence, gynecomastia, and hypogonadism.

A transient increase of prolactin occurs often with generalized seizures. A sample can be drawn about 15-30 minutes after the episode and the baseline sampled after an hour.

Sequelae of hyperprolactinemia include amenorrhea, anovulation, and estrogen deficiency with secondarily decreased bone density. Both 17-KS and dehydroepiandrosterone sulfate are increased with hyperprolactinemia. Elevations are reported in some patients with renal cell carcinoma or with bronchogenic carcinoma.

The only result of **prolactin deficiency** is the absence of postpartum lactation.

Limitations Normal prolactin level does not rule out pituitary tumor. High values do not always indicate prolactinoma. Prolactin secretion is episodic and is influenced by stress and by low glucose levels. Drugs can increase prolactin secretion: *vide infra.*

Methodology Immunoassay,[1] radioimmunoassay (RIA)

Additional Information Prolactin is increased in patients on estrogens, antihypertensives, phenothiazines, tricyclic antidepressants, haloperidol, methyldopa, butyrophenones, cimetidine, metoclopramide, or reserpine, and in patients with hypothyroidism. Verapamil has been reported to have induced hyperprolactinemia and galactorrhea.[2] Other pathologic increases in serum prolactin include abuse of opiates, renal insufficiency, cirrhosis, hypothyroidism adrenal insufficiency, and neurogenic stimulation.[3]

Antipsychotic drugs may elevate serum prolactin. Antipsychotics block dopamine, thereby elevating serum prolactin levels. Hyperprolactinemia is present in many patients receiving neuroleptics with an occasional patient developing amenorrhea, galactorrhea, and/or decreased libido. Amoxapine, a dibenzoxazepine type of tricyclic with antidepressant and antipsychotic characteristics, has been found to cause galactorrhea and oligomenorrhea with hyperprolactinemia. Amoxapine may have a dopamine blocking action. The prolactin level may rise significantly but only briefly. Point prolactin level determinations during therapy may be within normal range while total integrated 24-hour secretion is significantly increased. It has been recommended that patients who develop amenorrhea and/or galactorrhea during neuroleptic therapy should be observed regularly for possible emergence of a pituitary tumor.

Levels rise during pregnancy and are elevated during lactation, in postpartum subjects, and following bilateral oophorectomy. Destructive pituitary diseases cause low levels. Hypothalamic lesions may be associated with increased values. Many pituitary tumors which previously were classified as chromophobe adenomas are now recognizable as prolactinomas.

Patients with hyperprolactinemia may have multiple endocrine neoplasia syndrome, MEN-1.

Baseline work-up recommendations include FSH, LH, thyroxine, AM and PM cortisols, and testosterone.[2]

Provocative tests used in work-up of hyperprolactinemia include metyrapone stimulation of ACTH[2] and TRH provocative test.[4]

Persistent elevations of plasma prolactin levels may be observed with, and after withdrawal from, chronic cocaine abuse, and may reflect a cocaine-induced derangement in the neural dopaminergic regulatory systems.[5]

Women with apparently normal ovarian function have been found with hyperprolactinemia. Many have been found to have **big big prolactin, BBPRL**. Presently it is thought to be a poorly understood scientific curiosity,[6] and a genetic basis is likely.[7] Prolactin has molecular heterogeneity.[8]

Serum prolactin concentrations may be used as a guide to therapy in prolactinomas. True prolactinomas characterized by pituitary lesions with <100 µg/L are thought to be best treated with doxamine agonists such as bromocriptine.[9] A number of therapeutic agents appear to be available for medical treatment of prolactinomas.[10] Untreated macroprolactinomas can cause visual impairment or hypopituitarism. Rare cases of prolactin-secreting pituitary carcinoma have been described.[11]

Footnotes

1. Babiel R, Willnow P, Baer M, et al, "A New Enzyme Immunoassay for Prolactin in Serum or Plasma," *Clin Chem*, 1990, 36(1):76-80.
2. Gluskin LE, Strasberg B, and Shah JH, "Verapamil-Induced Hyperprolactinemia and Galactorrhea," *Ann Intern Med*, 1981, 95:66-7.
3. Molitch ME, "Pathologic Hyperprolactinemia," *Endocrinol Metab Clin North Am*, 1992, 21(4):877-901.
4. Randall RV, Laws ER Jr, Abboud CF, et al, "Transsphenoidal Microsurgical Treatment of Prolactin-Producing Pituitary Adenomas. Results in 100 Patients," *Mayo Clin Proc*, 1983, 58:108-21.
5. Mendelson JH, Teoh SK, Lange U, et al, "Anterior Pituitary, Adrenal, and Gonadal Hormones During Cocaine Withdrawal," *Am J Psychiatry*, 1988, 145(9):1094-8.
6. Fraser IS, Lun ZG, Zhou JP, et al, "Detailed Assessment of Big Big Prolactin in Women With Hyperprolactinemia and Normal Ovarian Function," *J Clin Endocrinol Metab*, 1989, 69(3):585.
7. Larrea F, Escorza A, Valero A, et al, "Heterogeneity of Serum Prolactin Throughout the Menstrual Cycle and Pregnancy in Hyperprolactinemic Women With Normal Ovarian Function," *J Clin Endocrinol Metab*, 1989, 68(5):982.
8. Smith CR and Norman MR, "Prolactin and Growth Hormone: Molecular Heterogeneity and Measurement in Serum," *Ann Clin Biochem*, 1990, 27(Pt 6):542-50.
9. Besser M, "Criteria for Medical as Opposed to Surgical Treatment of Prolactinomas," *Acta Endocrinol*, 1993, 129(Suppl 1):27-30.
10. Sarapura V and Schlaff WD, "Recent Advances in the Understanding of the Pathophysiology and Treatment of Hyperprolactinemia," *Curr Opin Obstet Gynecol*, 1993, 5(3):360-7.
11. Gollard R, Kosty M, Cheney C, et al, "Prolactin-Secreting Pituitary Carcinoma With Implants in the Cheek Pouch and Metastases to the Ovaries," *Cancer*, 1995, 76:1814-20.

References

Baskin HJ, "Endocrinologic Evaluation of Impotence," *South Med J*, 1989, 82(4):446-9.
Fujimoto VY, Clifton DK, Cohen NL, et al, "Variability of Serum Prolactin and Progesterone Levels in Normal Women: The Relevance of Single Hormone Measurements in the Clinical Setting," *Obstet Gynecol*, 1990, 76(1):71-8.

Kelly PA, Djiane J, Postel-Vinay MC, et al, "The Prolactin/Growth Hormone Receptor Family," *Endocr Rev*, 1991, 12(3):235-51.

Schlechte J, Dolan K, Sherman B, et al, "The Natural History of Untreated Hyperprolactinemia: A Prospective Analysis," *J Clin Endocrinol Metab*, 1989, 68(2):412-8.

Schulster D, Gaines-Das RE, and Jeffcoate SL, "International Standards for Human Prolactin: Calibration by International Collaborative Study," *J Endocrinol*, 1989, 121(1):157-66.

Serri O, "Progress in the Management of Hyperprolactinemia,"' *N Engl J Med*, 1994, 331(14):942-4.

Smith CR, Butler J, Hashim I, et al, "Serum Prolactin Bioactivity and Immunoactivity in Hyperprolactinaemic States," *Ann Clin Biochem*, 1990, 27(Pt 1):3-8.

Tippet PD, Simon JA, Rifka SM, et al, "Luteal Phase Hyperprolactinemia During Ovulation Induction With Human Menopausal Gonadotropins: Incidence, Recurrence, and Effect on Pregnancy Rates," *Obstet Gynecol*, 1989, 73(4):613.

Vance ML, "Hypopituitarism," *N Engl J Med*, 1994, 330(23):1651-62.

Veldhuis JD, Evans WS, and Stumpf PG, "Mechanisms That Subserve Estradiol's Induction of Increased Prolactin Concentrations: Evidence of Amplitude Modulation of Spontaneous Prolactin Secretory Bursts," *Am J Obstet Gynecol*, 1989, 161(5):1149-58.

Prostate Specific Antigen, Serum

CPT 84153

Related Information

Acid Phosphatase *on page 62*

Immunoperoxidase Procedures *on page 43*

Synonyms PSA

Applies to Finasteride; PSA Density; PSA Velocity

Abstract The best, most accurate and the most useful marker for adenocarcinoma of prostate, PSA is increased in most men with clinically significant prostate cancer, but it may be increased in benign entities and within normal range even with advanced prostatic adenocarcinoma.[1] It increases rates of **detection** of prostatic adenocarcinoma, but some of the carcinomas it detects are biologically insignificant.[2] It is best when followed by digital rectal examination,[3] to which it is complementary. Serially measured, PSA is extremely useful in monitoring presurgical, as well as postsurgical patients. PSA level, PSA density, ratio of total to free PSA, and needle biopsy histopathologic observations represent predictors of extent of tumor. Ultimately, it is clinical outcome which is most important. PSA is proving to be an indispensable predictor for recurrent adenocarcinoma in postsurgical patients and those treated with radiation therapy.[4,5,6] It is an important aid in selection of adjunctive therapy.[7,8]

Patient Preparation Fasting specimen is preferred. The practice of sampling at least 4 weeks following digital rectal examination and needle biopsy is published;[2] *vide infra*. Avoid recent exposure to radioactivity if RIA is used.

Specimen Serum

Container Red top tube

Sampling Time Recent prostatic manipulation probably should be avoided; *vide supra*. PSA has little diurnal variation[9]. Although it is often sampled together with prostatic acid phosphatase (PAP), the latter has fallen into disrepute.

Collection Rectal examination within 48 hours of specimen collection may cause elevation of results; mixed recommendations are published.[10,11]

Storage Instructions PSA is stable in serum for 48 hours if refrigerated. For longer periods, store at -20°C or colder.[9] No special treatment of serum is required. Ship to a reference laboratory in a plastic vial on dry ice.

Special Instructions Individual patients should be followed with the same assay consistently. When a decision is made to follow patients without immediate therapy, serial assays are recommended to ascertain rate of change of PSA. This is called **PSA velocity**.[2]

Reference Range Male: <4 ng/mL; female <0.5 ng/mL (immunoassay method); *vide infra*. Age adjusted reference ranges have been advocated; PSA results increase moderately with age; *vide infra*. Use of upper limit of 4.5 ng/mL for men 60-69 years of age and 6.5 ng/mL for those 70 years and older would decrease sensitivity from 86% to 77% but would enhance specificity from 56% to 67%. It would decrease the numbers of biopsies.[12]

Use Prostate specific antigen is a kallikrein-like serine protease that is produced exclusively by epithelial cells of prostatic tissue. It is present at high concentrations in seminal fluid and functions in the liquefaction of seminal coagulum.[13] Preoperative PSA serum levels correlate (but imperfectly) with extent of disease in patients with prostate cancer. **PSA density** is obtained by division of serum PSA result by prostatic weight utilizing transrectal ultrasound **(TRUS)** volumetric measurements. PSA density is not definitive; it is increased with prostatitis[14] but may be useful in patient selection for radical prostatectomy.[15] With PSA assay and histopathologic interpretation from prostate needle biopsy, correlation of **extent of tumor** can be improved. (Of these, TRUS has not consistently been found to predict tumor extent.)[2] PSA is useful in detection of

residual tumor and disease progression in postoperative stage of prostate cancer.[16] PSA has several advantages over prostatic acid phosphatase (PAP). It is more stable and does not have a significant diurnal variation. It has been shown to be elevated in 95% of newly diagnosed cases of prostatic carcinoma (vs 60% for PAP) and in 97% of recurrent cases (PAP 66%).[17] PSA relates to increasing Gleason score[18] and outcome. (Unfortunately, Gleason scores are themselves problematical.) PSA is successfully widely used in screening selected populations of patients with or without symptoms indicative of prostate cancer,[19] but the value of prostate cancer screening remains controversial in terms of patient morbidity and longevity; ie, outcome.[11,20,21] It detects incidental, as well as, aggressive neoplasms. Some of the former are biologically indolent, posing no threat to the life of the patient.[2] Sensitivity for aggressive carcinoma of prostate was 87% for tumors occurring within the first 4 years.[21,22] PSA lacks sufficient sensitivity and specificity to be used alone as a screening test for prostatic carcinoma. In conjunction with digital rectal examination and TRUS, PSA greatly increases prostatic carcinoma detection rates.[23]

A PSA assay is indicated prior to initiation of finasteride therapy for benign hyperplasia of prostate, since this drug causes an approximately 50% decrease in serum PSA concentration.

Limitations Approximately 25% to 46% of men with benign prostatic hyperplasia have an elevated serum PSA concentration. One-third of men with PSA >4 ng/mL will have carcinoma on prostate biopsy but two-thirds will not.[3] Between 20% and 40% of patients with organ-confined prostatic carcinoma have serum PSA concentrations within the reference range.[13] PSA is not acceptable used alone for staging[23] and alone should not be used to select candidates for radical prostatectomy. Physiologic fluctuation ≤30% is described. PSA is not specific for prostatic adenocarcinoma, but serum levels are specific for prostatic tissue. Elevations may also be associated with urethral instrumentation, prostatitis, TUR, prostatic needle biopsy, urinary retention, or prostatic ischemia or infarct.[24] Used in preoperative patients, PSA does not sharply distinguish intracapsular from extracapsular carcinoma. Despite wide availability of screening tests to detect prostatic carcinoma, no trial has proven significant overall prolongation of survival.[25] Digital rectal examination is claimed not to alter levels significantly, but *vide supra*.[26,27,28] It is now known that 50% to 90% of serum PSA is bound to an inhibitor called α_1-antichymotrypsin. The antibodies used in assays have different affinities for bound and free PSA. An effort has been made to provide a calibration with 90% bound and 10% free PSA, which should be appropriate for the vast majority of men. When following patient values, it is most important to continue use of the same assay.[29]

Methodology Radioimmunoassay (RIA), immunofluorometric assay,[30] monoclonal two-site immunoradiometric assay.[31] An ultrasensitive RIA has been developed.[32] All methods have not measured precisely the same substances.[33] The Abbott IMx, Hybriditech Tandem-E, Hybriditech Tandem-R, and Tosoh AIA-Pack have been evaluated recently.[34]

Additional Information The PSA-alpha$_1$-antichymotrypsin (PSA-ACT) complex is the predominant molecular form of serum PSA with the free noncomplexed form of serum PSA constituting a minor fraction.[35] It has been suggested that assays measuring the PSA-ACT complex only may improve the differentiation between prostatic carcinoma and benign prostatic hyperplasia.[36] The ratio of free to complexed PSA can be determined and may be relevant. A lower proportion of free PSA is found in patients with prostate carcinoma (<10% free suggests carcinoma).

Three to 6 months after radical prostatectomy, PSA is reported to provide a sensitive indicator of persistent disease. Six months following introduction of antiandrogen therapy, PSA is reported as capable of distinguishing patients with favorable response from those in whom limited response is anticipated.[37]

Patients with stage C prostatic carcinoma who were most likely to benefit from postoperative radiation therapy are those with initially undetectable postoperative serum PSA concentrations.[38] Use of age-specific reference ranges may make PSA density superfluous.[11] Use of age-specific reference ranges for PSA has been claimed to provide greater sensitivity in patients younger than the age of 60 and greater specificity in older patients.[11,39]

PSA velocity is an expression used to indicate rate of change of PSA. It may provide an index capable of earlier detection of adenocarcinoma of prostate with distinction from benign hyperplasia and normal and may support clinical decisions following radical prostatectomy.[40] PSA increase of 0.8 ng/mL/year in a man whose PSA is within reference range, with a minimum of three assays, is described as an indication for further investigation.[11] Such measurements should be based on two-year intervals.[41]

Prostatic specific antigen is a reliable immunocytochemical marker for primary and metastatic adenocarcinoma of prostate, reacting with at least some cells in almost all adequate biopsies.

(Continued)

Prostate Specific Antigen, Serum *(Continued)*

Footnotes

1. Leibman BD, Dillioglugil O, Wheeler TM, et al, "Distant Metastasis After Radical Prostatectomy in Patients Without an Elevated Serum Prostate Specific Antigen Level," *Cancer*, 1995, 76:2530-4.
2. Epstein JI, Walsh PC, Carmichael M, et al, "Pathologic and Clinical Findings to Predict Tumor Extent of Nonpalpable (Stage T1c) Prostate Cancer," *JAMA*, 1994, 271(5):368-74.
3. Woolf SH, "Screening for Prostate Cancer With Prostate-Specific Antigen. An Examination of the Evidence," *N Engl J Med*, 1995, 333(21):1401-5.
4. Chauvet B, Félix-Faure C, Lupsascka N, et al, "Prostate-Specific Antigen Decline: A Major Prognostic Factor for Prostate Cancer Treated With Radiation Therapy," *J Clin Oncol*, 1994, 12(7):1402-7.
5. Ruckle HC, Klee GG, and Oesterling JE, "Prostate-Specific Antigen: Concepts for Staging Prostate Cancer and Monitoring Response to Therapy," *Mayo Clin Proc*, 1994, 69(1):69-79.
6. Fowler JE Jr, Pandey P, Braswell NT, et al, "Prostate Specific Antigen Progression Rates After Radical Prostatectomy or Radiation Therapy for Localized Prostate Cancer," *Surgery*, 1994, 116(2):302-6.
7. Schild ST, Wong WW, Grado GL, et al, "Radiotherapy for Isolated Increases in Serum Prostate-Specific Antigen Levels After Radical Prostatectomy," *Mayo Clin Proc*, 1994, 69(7):613-9.
8. Zietman AL, "When Should Radiation Therapy Follow Radical Prostatectomy in the Management of Prostatic Cancer?" *Mayo Clin Proc*, 1994, 69(7):700-1.
9. Schifman RB, Ahmann FR, Elvick A, et al, "Analytical and Physiological Characteristics of Prostate-Specific Antigen and Prostatic Acid Phosphatase in Serum Compared," *Clin Chem*, 1987, 33(11):2086-8.
10. The Internal Medicine Clinic Research Consortium, "Effect of Digital Rectal Examination on Serum Prostate-Specific Antigen in a Primary Care Setting," *Arch Intern Med*, 1995, 155(4):389-92.
11. Ruckle HC, Klee GG, and Oesterling JE, "Prostate-Specific Antigen: Critical Issues for the Practicing Physician," *Mayo Clin Proc*, 1994, 69(1):59-68.
12. Oesterling JE, Jacobsen SJ, and Cooner WH, "The Use of Age-Specific Reference Ranges for Serum Prostate-Specific Antigen in Men 60 Years Old or Older," *J Urol*, 1995, 153(4):1160-3.
13. Oesterling JE, "Prostate-Specific Antigen and Diagnosing Early Malignancies of the Prostate," *J Cell Biochem Suppl*, 1992, 16H:31-43.
14. Bare R, Hart L, and McCullough DL, "Correlation of Prostate-Specific Antigen and Prostate-Specific Antigen Density With Outcome of Prostate Biopsy," *Urology*, 1994, 43(2):191-6.
15. Seaman EK, Whang IS, Cooner W, et al, "Predictive Value of Prostate-Specific Antigen Density for the Presence of Micrometastatic Carcinoma of the Prostate," *Urology*, 1994, 43(5):645-8.
16. Carter HB, Partin AW, Epstein JI, et al, "The Relationship of Prostate Specific Antigen Levels and Residual Tumor Volume in Stage A Prostate Cancer," *J Urol*, 1990, 144(5):1167-70.
17. Rainwater LM, Morgan WR, Klee GG, et al, "Prostate-Specific Antigen Testing in Untreated and Treated Prostatic Adenocarcinoma," *Mayo Clin Proc*, 1990, 65(8):1118-26.
18. Stamey TA and Kabalin JN, "Prostate Specific Antigen in the Diagnosis and Treatment of Adenocarcinoma of the Prostate. Untreated Patients," *J Urol*, 1989, 141(5):1070-5.
19. Armbruster DA, "Prostate-Specific Antigen: Biochemistry, Analytical Methods, and Clinical Application," *Clin Chem*, 1993, 39(2):181-95.
20. Chodak GW, "Screening for Prostate Cancer. The Debate Continues," *JAMA*, 1994, 272(10):773-80.
21. Krahn MD, Mahoney JE, Eckman MH, et al, "Screening for Prostate Cancer. A Decision Analytic View," *JAMA*, 1994, 272(10):773-80.
22. Lange PH, "New Information About Prostate-Specific Antigen and the Paradoxes of Prostate Cancer," *JAMA*, 1995, 273(4):336-7.
23. Crawford ED and De Antoni EP, "PSA as a Screening Test for Prostate Cancer," *Urol Clin North Am*, 1993, 20(4):637-46.
24. Brawer MK and Lange PH, "Prostate-Specific Antigen in Management of Prostatic Carcinoma," *Urology*, 1989, 33(5 Suppl):11-6.
25. Small EJ, "Prostate Cancer: Who to Screen and What the Results Mean," *Geriatrics*, 1993, 48(12):28-30, 35-8.
26. Thomson RD and Clejan S, "Digital Rectal Examination-Associated Alterations in Serum Prostate-Specific Antigen," *Am J Clin Pathol*, 1992, 97(4):528-34.
27. Yuan JJ, Coplen DE, Petros JA, et al, "Effects of Rectal Examination, Prostatic Massage, Ultrasonography and Needle Biopsy on Serum Prostate Specific Antigen Levels," *J Urol*, 1992, 147(3 Pt 2):810-4.
28. Catalona WJ, Smith DS, Ratliff TL, et al, "Measurement of Prostate-Specific Antigen in Serum as a Screening Test for Prostate Cancer," *N Engl J Med*, 1991, 324(17):1156-61.
29. Catalona WJ, Smith DS, Wolfert RL, et al, "Evaluation of Percentage of Free Serum Prostate Specific Antigen to Improve Specificity of Prostate Cancer Screening," *JAMA*, 1995, 274(15):1214-20.
30. Jacobsen SJ, Klee GG, Lilja H, et al, "Stability of Serum Prostate-Specific Antigen Determination Across Laboratory, Assay, and Storage Time," *Urology*, 1995, 45(3):447-53.
31. Lindstedt G, Jacobsson A, Lundberg PA, et al, "Determination of Prostate-Specific Antigen in Serum by Immunoradiometric Assay," *Clin Chem*, 1990, 36(1):53-8.
32. Graves HC, Wehner N, and Stamey TA, "Ultrasensitive Radioimmunoassay of Prostate-Specific Antigen," *Clin Chem*, 1992, 38(5):735-42.
33. Gambino R, "Standardization of Prostate-Specific Antigen (PSA) Tests," *Lab Rep*, 1994, 16(10):75-7.
34. Garg UC, Howanitz JH, Nakamura RM, et al, "Production, Analysis, and Characterization of Reference Materials for Prostate-Specific Antigen," *Arch Pathol Lab Med*, 1995, 119(12):1104-8.
35. Lilja H, "Significance of Different Molecular Forms of Serum PSA. The Free, Noncomplexed Form of PSA Versus That Complexed to Alpha₁-Antichymotrypsin," *Urol Clin North Am*, 1993, 20(4):681-6.
36. Wu JT, "Assay for Prostate Specific Antigen (PSA): Problems and Possible Solutions," *J Clin Lab Anal*, 1994, 8(1):51-62.
37. Zietman AL, Shipley WU, and Willett CG, "Residual Disease After Radical Surgery or Radiation Therapy for Prostate Cancer. Clinical Significance and Therapeutic Implications," *Cancer*, 1993, 71(3 Suppl):959-69.
38. McCarthy JF, Catalona WJ, and Hudson MA, "Effect of Radiation Therapy on Detectable Serum Prostate Specific Antigen Levels Following Radical Prostatectomy: Early Versus Delayed Treatment," *J Urol*, 1994, 151(6):1575-8.
39. Cooner WH, "Prostate-Specific Antigen and Transrectal Ultrasound of the Prostate in Detection of Prostate Cancer," *Clin Invest Med*, 1993, 16(6):471-4.
40. Partin AW, Pearson JD, Landis PK, et al, "Evaluation of Serum Prostate-Specific Antigen Velocity After Radical Prostatectomy to Distinguish Local Recurrence From Distant Metastases," *Urology*, 1994, 43(5):649-59.
41. Carter HB, Pearson JD, Waclawiw Z, et al, "Prostate-Specific Antigen Variability in Men Without Prostate Cancer: Effect of Sampling Interval on Prostate-Specific Antigen Velocity," *Urology*, 1995, 45(14):591-6.

References

Babaian RJ, Mettlin C, Kane R, et al, "The Relationship of Prostate-Specific Antigen to Digital Rectal Examination and Transrectal Ultrasonography. Findings of the American Cancer Society National Prostate Cancer Detection Project," *Cancer*, 1992, 69(5):1195-200.

Benson MC, Whang IS, Olsson CA, et al, "The Use of Prostate Specific Antigen Density to Enhance the Predictive Value of Intermediate Levels of Serum Prostate Specific Antigen," *J Urol*, 1992, 147(3 Pt 2):817-21.

Catalona WJ, "Management of Cancer of the Prostate," *N Engl J Med*, 1994, 331(15):996-1004.

Clinton JJ, "From the Agency for Health Care Policy and Research," *JAMA*, 1994, 271(15):1151.

Cohen RJ, Haffejee Z, Steele GS, et al, "Advanced Prostate Cancer With Normal Serum Prostate-Specific Antigen Values," *Arch Pathol Lab Med*, 1994, 118(11):1123-6.

Drago JR and York JP, "Prostate-Specific Antigen, Digital Rectal Examination, and Transrectal Ultrasound in Predicting the Probability of Cancer," *J Surg Oncol*, 1992, 49(3):172-5.

"Effect of Digital Rectal Examination on Serum Prostate-Specific Antigen in a Primary Care Setting, the Internal Medicine Clinic Research Consortium, " *Arch Intern Med*, 1995, 155(4):389-92.

Epstein JL, "Prostate Biopsy Interpretation," 1989, NY: Raven Press.

Gann PH, Hennekens CH, and Stampfer MJ, "A Prospective Evaluation of Plasma Prostate-Specific Antigen for Detection of Prostate Cancer," *JAMA*, 1995, 273(4):289-94.

Gillenwater JY, "Digital Rectal Examination-Associated Alterations in Serum Prostate-Specific Antigen," *Am J Clin Pathol*, 1992, 97(4):466-7.

Glenski WJ, Malek RS, Myrtle JF, et al, "Sustained, Substantially Increased Concentration of Prostate-Specific Antigen in the Absence of Prostatic Malignant Disease: An Unusual Clinical Scenario," *Mayo Clin Proc*, 1992, 67(3):249-52.

Grignon DJ and Hammond EH, "College of American Pathologists Conference XXVI on Clinical Relevance of Prognostic Markers in Solid Tumors. Report of the Prostate Cancer Working Group," *Arch Pathol Lab Med*, 1995, 119(12):1122-6.

Grob BM, Haley C, Schellhammer PF, et al, "The Detection of Prostate Specific Antigen, MHS-5, and Other Markers in Invasive Prostate Cancer and Seminal Vesicle," *J Urol*, 1992, 147(5):1435-8.

Hortin GL, Bahnson RR, Daft M, et al, "Differences in Values Obtained With 2 Assays of Prostate Specific Antigen," *J Urol*, 1988, 139(4):762-5.

Howanitz JH, "Immunoassay for Measuring Prostate-Specific Antigen," *Lab Med*, 1996, 27(4):255-8.

Killian CS, Emrich LJ, Vargas FP, et al, "Relative Reliability of Five Serially Measured Markers for Prognosis of Progression in Prostate Cancer," *J Natl Cancer Inst*, 1986, 76(2):179-85.

Leibman BD, Dillioglugil O, Wheeler TM, et al, "Distant Metastasis After Radical Prostatectomy in Patients Without an Elevated Serum Prostate Specific Antigen Level," *Cancer*, 1995, 76:2530-4.

Littrup PJ, Kane RA, Williams CR, et al, "Determination of Prostate Volume With Transrectal US for Cancer Screening. Part I. Comparison With Prostate-Specific Antigen Assays," *Radiology*, 1991, 178(2):537-42.

Pollack A, Zagars GK, and Kavadi VS, "Prostate Specific Antigen Doubling Time and Disease Relapse After Radiotherapy for Prostate Cancer," *Cancer*, 1994, 74(2):670-8.

Porter JR, and Brawer MK, "Prostatic Intraepithelial Neoplasia and Prostate-Specific Antigen," *World J Urol*, 1993, 11(4):196-200.

Sershon PD, Barry MJ, and Oesterling JE, "Serum Prostate-Specific Antigen Discriminates Weakly Between Men With Benign Prostatic Hyperplasia and Patients With Organ-Confined Prostate Cancer," *Eur Urol*, 1994, 25(4):281-7.

Smith EM and Resnick MI, "Prostate Specific Antigen: Clinical Applications and New Developments," *The Kidney*, 1993, 25(5):1-6.

Vessella RL and Lange PH, "Issues in the Assessment of PSA Immunoassays," *Urol Clin North Am*, 1993, 20(4):607-19.

Prostatic Acid Phosphatase *see* Acid Phosphatase *on page 62*

Protein, Body Fluids *see* Body Fluid *on page 89*

Protein, Body Fluids *see* Body Fluid Lactate Dehydrogenase *on page 92*

Protein, Total, Serum

CPT 84155

Related Information

Albumin, Serum *on page 66*
Cerebrospinal Fluid Protein Electrophoresis *on page 381*
Immunoelectrophoresis, Serum or Urine *on page 408*
Immunofixation Electrophoresis *on page 408*
Immunoglobulin A *on page 408*
Immunoglobulin G *on page 409*
Immunoglobulin G Subclasses *on page 410*
Immunoglobulin M *on page 410*
Protein Electrophoresis, Serum *on page 424*
Protein, Quantitative, Urine *on page 649*

Synonyms Total Protein, Serum

Applies to Globulin

Test Commonly Includes Total protein, albumin, A/G ratio

Abstract Used to evaluate protein nutritional status and protein altering diseases

Specimen Serum

Container Red top tube

Collection Pediatrics: Blood drawn from heelstick for capillary.

Storage Instructions Separate serum from cells. Refrigerate.

Reference Range Adults: 6.0-8.0 g/dL (SI: 60-80 g/L) in later childhood and adults. Lower ranges occur in early childhood. Ambulatory values are slightly higher than are those found in recumbency. If normal ranges are set for inpatients, then many outpatients appear to be a little above the upper limit.

Use Evaluate nutritional status; investigate edema.

In the entities which follow, the diseases listed are sometimes increased or decreased as indicated, but are not always so.

Causes of **high total protein:** dehydration; some cases of chronic liver disease, including autoimmune hepatitis and cirrhosis; neoplasms, especially myeloma; macroglobulinemia of Waldenström; tropical diseases (eg, kala-azar, leprosy, and others); granulomatous diseases, such as sarcoidosis; diseases in which total protein is sometimes high include collagen disease (eg, lupus erythematosus (SLE), and other instances of chronic infection/inflammation).

Causes of **low total protein:** pregnancy; intravenous fluids; cirrhosis or other liver disease, including chronic alcoholism; prolonged immobilization; heart failure; nephrotic syndromes; glomerulonephritis; neoplasia; protein losing enteropathies; Crohn's disease and chronic ulcerative colitis; starvation, malabsorption, or malnutrition; hyperthyroidism; burns; severe skin disease; and other chronic diseases.

Very low total protein (<4.0 g/dL (SI: <40 g/L)) and low albumin cause edema (eg, nephrotic syndromes).

Limitations Venous stasis during venipuncture can lead to increased values. Hyperviscosity was reported to cause error in total protein through a discrete laboratory sampler-dilutor.[1] Hemolysis can falsely elevate total protein. Clinical interpretation is greatly enhanced by examination of the fractions composing total protein, when such separation is clinically indicated (ie, serum protein electrophoresis, quantitative immunodiffusion or other methods for IgG, IgA, IgM, immunofixation, immunoelectrophoresis).

Methodology Biuret for total protein, refractometry, BCG for albumin[2,3]

Additional Information Total protein and albumin normally decrease by 5% to 10% upon recumbency, as in hospitalization. "Globulin" may be provided as a calculation, total protein - albumin = globulin. Such a result is a screening test much less definitive than other methods. Total protein and albumin are commonly measured on chemistry profiling instruments.

Following an acute phase stimulus such as infection or trauma, many liver derived plasma proteins increase in concentration, while albumin decreases. Thus, while the total serum protein concentration may remain the same in acute phase reactions, the composition of the serum proteins is altered.[4]

Drug effects are summarized.[5]

Footnotes

1. Chan KM and Ladenson JH, "Sample Viscosity Can Be a Source of Analytical Error When Discrete Sampler-Dilutors Are Used," *Clin Chem*, 1981, 27:1896-8.
2. Dawnay AB, Hirst AD, Perry DE, et al, "A Critical Assessment of Current Analytical Methods for the Routine Assay of Serum Total Protein and Recommendations for Their Improvement," *Ann Clin Biochem*, 1991, 28(Pt 6):556-67.
3. Camara PD, Wright C, Dextraze P, et al, "Comparison of a Commercial Method for Total Protein With a Candidate Reference Method," *Ann Clin Lab Sci*, 1991, 21(5):335-9.
4. Steel DM and Whitehead AS, "The Major Acute Phase Reactants: C-Reactive Protein, Serum Amyloid P Component and Serum Amyloid A Protein," *Immunol Today*, 1994, 15(2):81-8.
5. Herbeth B, Diemert MC, and Galli A, "Total Proteins," *Drug Effects on Laboratory Test Results Analytical Interferences and Pharmacological Effects*, Siest G and Galteau MM, eds, Littleton, MA: PSG Publishing Co Inc, 1988, 375-90.

References

Burtis CA and Ashwood ER, *Tietz Textbook of Clinical Chemistry*, 2nd ed, Philadelphia, PA: WB Saunders Co, 1994, 695-700.

Protoporphyrin, Free Erythrocyte

CPT 84202 (quantitative); 84203 (screen)

Related Information

Delta Aminolevulinic Acid, Urine *on page 121*
Hemoglobin *on page 323*
Iron and Total Iron Binding Capacity/Transferrin *on page 150*
Lead, Blood *on page 556*
Lead, Urine *on page 557*
Porphobilinogen, Qualitative, Urine *on page 185*
Porphyrins, Quantitative, Urine *on page 186*
Protoporphyrin, Zinc, Blood *on next page*

Synonyms FEP; Free Erythrocyte Protoporphyrin; Protoporphyrins, Fractionation, Erythrocytes; RBC Protoporphyrin

Abstract Free erythrocyte protoporphyrin expresses the amount of nonheme protoporphyrin in red cells. Unless lead toxicity is suspected, it is useful for evaluation of iron deficiency in childhood and its differential diagnosis; molecules accumulate with slowing of hemoglobin synthesis

with iron deficiency. Erythropoietic protoporphyria is an erythropoietic porphyria for which red cell protoporphyrin is tested. It is a deficiency of ferrocholarase.

Specimen Whole blood (test done on washed erythrocytes)

Container Lavender top (EDTA) tube (preferred) or green top (heparin) tube

Collection Pediatrics: Blood drawn from heelstick for capillary.

Storage Instructions Stable 3 weeks at 4°C. Do not freeze.

Special Instructions Current hematocrit must be measured or specified.

Reference Range Depends on method; ascertain ranges for individual testing laboratory. The FEP is considered unreliable in infants younger than 6 months of age.[1] Pediatric upper limit is 50 μg/dL (SI: 0.89 μmol/L) RBC. Higher levels prevail through infancy. Adults: male: <30 μg/dL (SI: <0.53 μmol/L), female: <40 μg/dL (SI: <0.71 μmol/L) by hematofluorometer; 11-45 μg/dL (SI: 0.20-0.80 μmol/L) for adult men and 19-52 μg/dL (SI: 0.34-0.92 μmol/L) for adult women by Piomelli. FEP is expressed as μg/dL blood.[2]

Possible Panic Range >190 μg/dL (SI: >3.38 μmol/L)

Use Differential diagnosis of disorders of heme production versus diseases of globin synthesis.[3] FEP is increased in lead poisoning, erythropoietic protoporphyria, in iron deficiency,[4,5,6,7] as well as in anemia of chronic disease and with some sideroblastic anemias.[3] With lead poisoning and iron deficiency, photosensitivity is not found. FEP levels are also reported increased in entities characterized by marked increase in erythropoiesis, such as severe hemolytic anemias. Thus, FEP is useful in work-up of the microcytic anemias. FEP is not increased in acute intermittent porphyria.[8,9,10] FEP is reported normal with presumed alpha thalassemia trait, hemoglobin H, beta thalassemia trait, and hemoglobin E.

Limitations Fluorescent substances in plasma may interfere with hematofluorometer results. Elevated FEPs should be verified by retesting washed RBCs or by microextraction. Skin contamination may lead to false elevations. Both this test and blood lead are needed for full evaluation.

Methodology Hematofluorometer, extraction method, and high performance liquid chromatography (HPLC). The hematofluorometer measures porphyrins unbound in erythrocytes. With iron deficiency and diminished heme synthesis, free porphyrin accumulates in the red blood cell.

Additional Information "Free" protoporphyrin is not complexed, nonheme protoporphyrin. **Lead poisoning** is characterized by elevated plasma and urine delta aminolevulinic acid and increased urinary coproporphyrin. Urinary porphobilinogen and uroporphyrin are normal to slightly increased. Free erythrocyte protoporphyrin is a sensitive test for lead toxicity or chronic exposure,[10] **although, a careful study based on receiver operator curves showed that erythrocyte protoporphyrin levels should not be used as a screening test for lead poisoning in children.** The diagnosis of lead exposure or poisoning includes consideration of environmental exposure, as well as symptoms and abnormal erythrocyte protoporphyrin. FEP is given as 92-288 μg/dL (SI: 1.63-5.12 μmol/L) RBC in level II increased lead absorption, with higher FEP results in level III. Increased lead absorption is reported in the presence of iron deficiency.[11] Increased erythrocyte protoporphyrin exists as free protoporphyrin in protoporphyria, not as a zinc chelate, in contrast to lead poisoning and iron deficiency.[12] Zinc protoporphyrin and metal free protoporphyrin can be distinguished from each other by spectrophotofluorometry.

Ferrocholarase activity can be assayed using red blood cells and fibroblasts.

Footnotes

1. Benjamin JT, Dickens MD, Ford RF, et al, "Normative Data of Hemoglobin Concentration and Free Erythrocyte Protoporphyrin in a Private Pediatric Practice," *Clin Pediatr (Phila)*, 1986, 25(4):206-8.
2. Marsh WL Jr, Nelson DP, and Koenig HM, "Free Erythrocyte Protoporphyrin (FEP) I. Normal Values for Adults and Evaluation of the Hematofluorometer," *Am J Clin Pathol*, 1983, 79:655-60.
3. Marsh WL Jr, Nelson DP, and Koenig HM, "Free Erythrocyte Protoporphyrin (FEP) II. The FEP Test Is Clinically Useful in Classifying Microcytic RBC Disorders in Adults," *Am J Clin Pathol*, 1983, 79:661-6.
4. Benjamin JT, Dickens MD, Ford RF, et al, "Normative Data of Hemoglobin Concentration and Free Erythrocyte Protoporphyrin in A Private Pediatric Practice: A 1990 Update," *Clin Pediatr (Phila)*, 1991, 30(2):74-6.
5. Parsons PJ, Stanton NV, Gunter EW, et al, "An Interlaboratory Comparison of Control Materials for Use With Hematofluorometers," *Clin Chem*, 1989, 35(10):2059-65.
6. Brown RG, "Determining the Cause of Anemia. General Approach, With Emphasis on Microcytic Hypochromic Anemias," *Postgrad Med*, 1991, 89(6):161-4, 167-70.
7. Beaton GH, Corey PN, and Steele C, "Conceptual and Methodological Issues Regarding the Epidemiology of Iron Deficiency and Their Implications for Studies of the Functional Consequences of Iron Deficiency," *Am J Clin Nutr*, 1989, 50(3 Suppl):575-88.
8. Turk DS, Schonfeld DJ, Cullen M, et al, "Sensitivity of Erythrocyte Protoporphyrin as a Screening Test for Lead Poisoning," *N Engl J Med*, 1992, 326(2):137-8.
9. McElvaine MD, Orbach HG, Binder S, et al, "Evaluation of the Erythrocyte Protoporphyrin Test as a Screen for Elevated Blood Lead Levels," *J Pediatr*, 1991, 119(4):548-50.

(Continued)

Protoporphyrin, Free Erythrocyte (Continued)

10. DeBaun MR and Sox HC Jr, "Setting the Optimal Erythrocyte Protoporphyrin Screening Decision Threshold for Lead Poisoning: A Decision Analytic Approach," *Pediatrics*, 1991, 88(1):121-31.
11. Carraccio CL, Bergman GE, and Daley BP, "Combined Iron Deficiency and Lead Poisoning in Children. Effect on FEP Levels," *Clin Pediatr*, 1987, 26(12):644-7.
12. Bloomer JR and Bonkovsky HL, "The Porphyrias," *Dis Mon*, 1989, 35(1):1-54.

References

Bird TD, Wallace DM, and Labbe RF, "The Porphyria, Plumbism, Pottery Puzzle," *JAMA*, 1982, 247:813-4.

McCabe ER, "The Metabolic Encephalopathies," *Principles and Practice of Pediatrics*, 2nd ed, Oski FA, DeAngelis CD, Feigin RD, et al, eds, Philadelphia, PA: JB Lippincott Co, 1994.

Zanella A, Gridelli L, Berzuini A, et al, "Sensitivity and Predictive Value of Serum Ferritin and Free Erythrocyte Protoporphyrin for Iron Deficiency," *J Lab Clin Med*, 1989, 113(1):73-8.

Protoporphyrins, Fractionation, Erythrocytes

see Protoporphyrin, Free Erythrocyte on previous page

Protoporphyrin, Zinc, Blood

CPT 84202

Related Information

Delta Aminolevulinic Acid, Urine on page 121
Ferritin, Serum on page 127
Iron and Total Iron Binding Capacity/Transferrin on page 150
Lead, Blood on page 556
Protoporphyrin, Free Erythrocyte on previous page
Transferrin on page 209

Synonyms Zinc Protoporphyrin; ZPP

Abstract Zinc protoporphyrin measurement may in some cases, be a useful adjunct in the diagnosis of nonanemic iron deficiency[1] but is not useful in screening programs for lead intoxication.[2] Its determination lends itself to office equipment.

Specimen Whole blood

Container Lavender top (EDTA) tube, green top (heparin) tube

Collection Routine venipuncture

Storage Instructions Do not centrifuge. Refrigerate and protect from light. Stable 1 week at 4°C.

Causes for Rejection Hemolysis, icterus

Reference Range 20-40 µg/dL whole blood (SI: 0.27-1.23 µmol/L). Results may be obtained as ZPP/heme ratio; reference range: 30-80 µmol/mol heme

Critical Values >100 µg/dL (SI: >1.6 µmol/L)

Use Evaluate iron deficiency, especially nonanemic iron deficiency. ZPP is superior to hemoglobin in identifying female blood donors with nonanemic iron deficiency.[1]

Limitations Zinc protoporphyrin is increased in lead poisoning but not with thalassemia. ZPP should **not** be used to screen or diagnose lead poisoning.[2,3]

Methodology Hematofluorometry (front-face); if washed erythrocytes are used, the assay becomes more specific and sensitive[4]

Additional Information Zinc protoporphyrin levels increase as blood lead levels increase. Various authorities caution using ZPP as a screening test for lead poisoning. The Centers for Disease Control has lowered the cutoff level for lead intoxication in children younger than 6 years of age to **10 µg/dL (SI: 0.48 µmol/L)**, and this level is so low that **ZPP is not useful** in this context because it is insensitive to such a lead level. Therefore, it is mandatory to measure lead levels in any screening program, rather than ZPP. ZPP appears only in new RBCs and remains for the life of the RBC; therefore, ZPP does not increase until several weeks after the onset of lead exposure and remains high long after exposure to lead. It is a reasonable indicator of total body burden of lead and remains a useful adjunct to the diagnosis of iron deficiency, particularly in nonanemic or questionably anemic patients. It reflects iron depletion in the bone marrow.

Footnotes

1. Jensen BM, Sando SH, Grandjean P, et al, "Protoporphyrin for Iron Deficiency in Nonanemic Female Blood Donors," *Clin Chem*, 1990, 36(6):846-8.
2. Turk DS, Schonfeld DJ, Cullen M, et al, "Sensitivity of Erythrocyte Protoporphyrin as a Screening Test for Lead Poisoning," *N Engl J Med*, 1992, 326(2):137-8.
3. Rolfe PB, Marcinak JF, Nice AJ, et al, "Use of Zinc Protoporphyrin Measured by the Protofluor-Z Hematofluorometer in Screening Children for Elevated Blood Lead Levels," *Am J Dis Child*, 1993, 147(1):66-8.
4. Hastka J, Lasserre JJ, Schwarzbeck A, et al, "Washing Erythrocytes to Remove Interferents in Measurement of Zinc Protoporphyrin by Front-Face Hematofluorometry," *Clin Chem*, 1992, 38(11):2184-9.

References

Cone DC, "Lead Screening and Follow-Up in an Urban Pediatric Clinic," *N Y State J Med*, 1992, 92(8):338-42.

Hastka J, Lasserre JJ, Schwarzbeck A, et al, "Zinc Protoporphyrin in Anemia of Chronic Disorders," *Blood*, 1993, 81(5):1200-4.

Labbe RF, "Clinical Utility of Zinc Protoporphyrin," *Clin Chem*, 1992, 38(11):2167-8.

McCabe ER, "The Metabolic Encephalopathies," *Principles and Practice of Pediatrics*, 2nd ed, Oski FA, DeAngelis CD, Feigin RD, et al, eds, Philadelphia, PA: JB Lippincott Co, 1994.

Zwennis WC, Franssen AC, and Wijnans MJ, "Use of Zinc Protoporphyrin in Screening Individuals for Exposure to Lead," *Clin Chem*, 1990, 36(8 Pt 1):1456-9.

PRP see Parathyroid Hormone on page 178

PSA see Prostate Specific Antigen, Serum on page 193

PSA Density see Prostate Specific Antigen, Serum on page 193

PSA Velocity see Prostate Specific Antigen, Serum on page 193

Pseudocholinesterase Inhibition see Dibucaine Number on page 122

Pseudocholinesterase, Serum

CPT 82480

Related Information

Acetylcholinesterase, Red Cell on page 62
Dibucaine Number on page 122

Synonyms Acetylcholinesterase; Cholinesterase II; Cholinesterase, Serum; PChE; Plasma Cholinesterase

Abstract Two types of cholinesterase are found in blood: **"true" cholinesterase (acetylcholinesterase)** in red cells, lung, and brain, while **"pseudocholinesterase"** (acylcholine acylhydrolase) **(PChE)** is found in serum (plasma). PChE, a sialated glycoprotein, is synthesized in the liver. Organophosphorus-containing insecticides inhibit RBC cholinesterase and depress serum pseudocholinesterase.

Specimen Serum

Container Red top tube

Storage Instructions Cholinesterase is stable in separated serum for 80 days at room temperature and 3 years at -20°C. However, specimens submitted to evaluate possible pesticide toxicity should be collected on ice, separated in a refrigerated centrifuge, and frozen until analyzed.[1]

Reference Range Low in infancy, then increasing in early childhood. Ranges vary between methods and laboratories. Typical values: 7-19 units/mL (Du Pont)

Critical Values Intermediate levels are found in heterozygotes.

Possible Panic Range Less than lower limit of normal

Use Screen preoperative patients for inherited succinylcholine (suxamethonium) anesthetic sensitivity, genetic or secondary to insecticide exposure, in appropriate circumstances. The diagnosis of the cholinergic syndrome is based on clinical findings as well as PChE activity. Prevent or evaluate prolonged anesthetic effect, prolonged apnea, after surgery. Very small amounts (0.04-0.06 mg/kg) of succinylcholine are needed to obtain 90% of neuromuscular blockade in patients with an abnormal allele who have low levels of plasma cholinesterase activity.[2]

Monitor and diagnose organophosphorous or carbamate insecticide exposure and poisoning, in which pseudocholinesterase level is decreased; establish patient's baseline value before exposure. Indications include pesticide exposure for patients with miosis, blurred vision, muscle weakness, twitching, and fasciculation, bradycardia, nausea, diarrhea, vomiting, salivation, sweating, respiratory failure, pulmonary edema, ventricular arrhythmias, and convulsions. The value of assessment of risk status in persons exposed to organophosphate insecticides on the basis of plasma cholinesterase levels alone has been called into question.[3] Are normal levels indicative of no exposure or of a genetic variant with or without exposure? Interpretive problems exist with low or high values.[3]

Family studies may be done when an individual with a genetically abnormal type is documented by serum pseudocholinesterase deficiency and, ideally, confirmed by phenotyping.

Limitations Serum pseudocholinesterase may be decreased in patients on estrogens and oral contraceptives.[1] Fluoride interferes. Pseudocholinesterase is also low in some instances of liver disease, including decompensated cirrhosis, hepatitis, metastatic carcinoma, CHF, and in malnutrition, but not sufficiently consistently enough to be a useful clinical test for such disorders. Genetic atypical enzyme does not explain every instance of prolonged postsurgical apnea (ie, normal serum PChE does not entirely assure lack of sensitivity to succinylcholine). Red cell cholinesterase is more useful for chronic insecticide exposure. Carbamate-poisoned persons can appear to have near normal or normal levels of pseudocholinesterase. PChE is elevated in obese and diabetic individuals.[4]

Contraindications Not useful to screen for toxicity from chlorinated insecticides.

Methodology Colorimetry, kinetic enzyme utilizing different substrates, fluorometry[5]

Additional Information Low serum cholinesterase activity may relate to exposure to insecticides or to one of a number of variant genotypes.

Dibucaine and fluoride numbers are useful to phenotype such homozygous and heterozygous individuals, who are genetically sensitive to succinylcholine.

One patient in 1500 is susceptible to succinyldicholine anesthetic mishap.

Plasmapheresis has been noted to decrease the level of plasma cholinesterase. Patients with abnormally low cholinesterase activity after transfusion of blood or plasma will experience temporary augmentation of enzyme level. In estimating the duration of this enhanced activity, measures of plasma cholinesterase half-life have been utilized. The true half-life value is, however, uncertain. A half-life value determined by measuring the rate of disappearance after intravenous injection of human cholinesterase has provided an average value of 11 days.[6]

A low level of activity of pseudocholinesterase has been demonstrated in cerebrospinal fluid, at about 1/20 to 1/100 the activity present in the corresponding plasma. With clinical conditions characterized by bleeding into the CSF, pseudocholinesterase activity increases 25% to 50% that of plasma.[7]

Patients with a variety of carcinomas have been reported to accumulate an embryonic type of cholinesterase activity in their sera. Such novel cholinesterase activity was found only in the sera of patients undergoing antitumor therapy (eg, chemotherapy or radiation therapy and/or hormone therapy).[8]

Increase in acetylcholinesterase activity, notably, in an acetylcholinesterase to butyrylcholine esterase ratio (histochemical study, not as measured in serum) has provided discriminatory diagnostic value in some cases of Hirschsprung's disease.[9]

Footnotes

1. Ladenson JH, "Nonanalytical Sources of Variation in Clinical Chemistry Results," *Gradwohl's Clinical Laboratory Methods and Diagnosis*, 8th ed, Sonnenwirth AC and Jarett L, eds, St Louis, MO: Mosby-Year Book Inc, 1980, 160.
2. Hickey DR, O'Connor JP, and Donati F, "Comparison of Atracurium and Succinylcholine for Electroconvulsive Therapy in a Patient With Atypical Plasma Cholinesterase," *Can J Anaesth*, 1987, 34(3 Pt 1):280-3.
3. Alexiou NG, Williams JF, Yeung HW, et al, "Paradoxical Elevation of Plasma Cholinesterase," *Am J Prev Med*, 1986, 2(4):235-8.
4. Kutty KM and Payne RH, "Serum Pseudocholinesterase and Very-Low-Density Lipoprotein Metabolism," *J Clin Lab Anal*, 1994, 8(4):247-50.
5. Kusu F, Tsuneta T, and Takamura K, "Fluorometric Determination of Pseudocholinesterase Activity in Postmortem Blood Samples," *J Forensic Sci*, 1990, 35(6):1330-4.
6. Ostergaard D, Viby-Mogensen J, Hanel HK, et al, "Half-Life of Plasma Cholinesterase," *Acta Anaesthesiol Scand*, 1988, 32(3):266-9.
7. Kambam JR, Horton B, Parris WC, et al, "Pseudocholinesterase Activity in Human Cerebrospinal Fluid," *Anesth Analg*, 1989, 68(4):486-8.
8. Zakut H, Even L, Birkenfeld S, et al, "Modified Properties of Serum Cholinesterases in Primary Carcinomas," *Cancer*, 1988, 61(4):727-37.
9. Causse E, Vaysse P, Fabre J, et al, "The Diagnostic Value of Acetylcholinesterase/Butyrylcholinesterase Ratio in Hirschsprung's Disease," *Am J Clin Pathol*, 1987, 88(4):477-80.

References

Bardin PG, van Eeden SF, Moolman JA, et al, "Organophosphate and Carbamate Poisoning," *Arch Intern Med*, 1994, 154(13):1433-41.
Burgess JL, Bernstein JN, and Hurlbut K, "Aldicarb Poisoning. A Case Report With Prolonged Cholinesterase Inhibition and Improvement After Pralidoxime Therapy," *Arch Intern Med*, 1994, 154(2):221-4.
Hoffman RS, Henry GC, Howland MA, et al, "Association Between Life-Threatening Cocaine Toxicity and Plasma Cholinesterase Activity," *Ann Emerg Med*, 1992, 21(3):247-53.
Marrs TC, "Organophosphate Poisoning," *Pharmacol Ther*, 1993, 58(1):51-66.
Newman MA and Que Hee SS, "Interconversion and Comparison of Three Methods for Acetyl Cholinesterase in Serum," *Clin Chem*, 1984, 30(2):308-10.
Pantuck EJ, "Plasma Cholinesterase: Gene and Variations," *Anesth Analg*, 1993, 77(2):380-6.
Wu AH, "Diagnostic Enzymology," *Clinical Laboratory Medicine*, McClatchey KD, ed, Baltimore, MD: Williams and Wilkins, 1994, 259-86.

PTH *see* Parathyroid Hormone *on page 178*

PTH-Related Protein *see* Parathyroid Hormone *on page 178*

Pulmonary Surfactant *see* Amniotic Fluid Pulmonary Surfactant *on page 78*

Pyridoxal-5-Phosphate *see* Vitamin B$_6$ *on page 217*

Pyridoxine *see* Vitamin B$_6$ *on page 217*

Quantitative Fecal Fat, 72-Hour Collection *see* Fecal Fat, Quantitative, 72-Hour Collection *on page 127*

Radioallergosorbent Test (RAST®) *see* Allergen Specific IgE Antibody *on page 71*

Rapid ACTH Test *see* Cosyntropin Test *on page 114*

RBC Galactokinase *see* Galactokinase, Blood *on page 131*

RBC Protoporphyrin *see* Protoporphyrin, Free Erythrocyte *on page 195*

Renal Panel *see* Kidney Profile *on page 153*

Renal Profile *see* Kidney Profile *on page 153*

Renin, Plasma

CPT 84244

Related Information
Aldosterone, Blood *on page 67*
Aldosterone, Urine *on page 68*
Electrolytes, Urine *on page 124*
Potassium, Serum or Plasma *on page 188*
Potassium, Urine *on page 189*

Synonyms Plasma Renin Activity; PRA

Applies to Angiotensin; Captopril Test; RVR Ratio

Test Commonly Includes Fasting supine or upright specimens, catheterization studies

Abstract The juxtaglomerular apparatus which surrounds the renal afferent arterioles produces renin, a proteolytic enzyme. Renin converts angiotensinogen to angiotensin I. Angiotensin I is in turn converted to angiotensin II, the biologically active metabolite. Angiotensin II stimulates the release of aldosterone from the adrenal cortex and has direct vasopressor effects. Primary aldosteronism may be considered "low-renin aldosteronism." Its characteristics include hypertension and hypokalemia. In secondary aldosteronism, stimulation is extra-adrenal.

Patient Preparation Antihypertensive drugs, steroids, cyclic progestogens, estrogens, diuretics, and licorice should be terminated at least 2 weeks and preferably 4 weeks before a renin-aldosterone work-up is to begin. A special sodium diet may be ordered for 3 days only. A normal sodium diet is requested for 2-4 weeks unless renin activity is to be measured following salt depletion for aldosteronism. Upright posture, administration of diuretics and low-sodium diets stimulate renin release. Renins are commonly drawn at the end of a 24-hour collection of urine for sodium and creatinine and after several days of stable sodium intake controlled by the physician.

No recent administration of radioactivity; no recent radioactive tracers; no caffeine before or during collection. There are special instructions for preparation for sodium depletion renins, renal venous renin ratio, and primary aldosteronism work-up. There are special diet instructions, sodium intake requirements. Check with the laboratory for particular patient preparation instructions.

Specimen Plasma, peripheral venous blood, bilateral renal vein samples

Container Lavender top (EDTA) tube

Sampling Time Normally, higher levels are found in upright subjects drawn in the morning.

Collection Draw specimen into a prechilled syringe. Place in chilled lavender top tubes (with the rubber stopper off). Recap, mix, and immediately place on ice and deliver to the laboratory. **Posture of the patient must be recorded.**

Storage Instructions Place in an ice-water bath. After the specimen is well cooled, centrifuge at 4°C. Separate plasma immediately and freeze in a plastic container.

Causes for Rejection Clotted sample, patient preparation incorrect for the sample desired

Special Instructions Request should provide posture and dietary status.

Reference Range Adults, upright (normal sodium diet): 1-6 ng/mL/hour (SI: 0.77-4.6 nmol/L/hour). Depends upon sodium depletion, age, posture. Results depend on whether or not there has been stimulation (eg, furosemide). Values from right and left renal veins should normally be equal. In arterial constriction, a ratio >1.5 is considered abnormal.

Critical Values More than 90% of patients with aldosterone-producing adenomas had PRA <1.0 ng/mL per hour.[1]

Use Renin is useful in the differential diagnosis of hypertension with hypokalemia. Renin is suppressed by high aldosterone levels in most patients with primary aldosteronism. Evaluate hypokalemia; diagnosis of primary aldosteronism is considered in the hypertensive patient with hypokalemia (≤3.6 mEq/L) who excretes ≥40 mmol/L potassium in a 24-hour urine collection without diuretics.[1] The patient with primary aldosteronism is characterized by hypokalemia, low plasma renin, and high serum and urine aldosterone. The suppressed renin which characterizes primary aldosteronism fails to increase appropriately with volume depletion (eg, upright posture, volume/sodium depletion). Such patients are not edematous.[2] Subjects with secondary aldosteronism may have elevated renin, in contrast to those with primary aldosteronism. Secondary aldosteronism occurs with the accelerated phase of hypertension, with an edema disorder and in pregnancy.[2]

Evaluate renovascular hypertension.

Renin-producing tumors occur but are extremely rare (juxtaglomerular cell tumor). Patients with them resemble subjects with renovascular hypertension chemically. Hyporeninemic hypoaldosteronism causes renal salt wasting, hyperkalemia, and metabolic acidosis. Idiopathic hyperaldosteronism (bilateral hyperplasia of zona glomerulosa) is a less (Continued)

Renin, Plasma *(Continued)*

common cause of primary aldosteronism than aldosterone-producing adenoma.[3] A few have unilateral nodular adrenal hyperplasia.[4]

Limitations Disease entities besides primary aldosteronism cause hypertension with low renin levels. Salt-restricted diets increase supine renin levels by a factor of 2; upright renin levels by a factor of 6. Renin increases in pregnancy, with patients on oral contraceptives and with salt loss, Addison's disease, and certain types of renal diseases. Diabetes mellitus can affect PRA. Random samples may be difficult to interpret unless medications and state of sodium balance are defined. Specimen must be collected with scrupulous attention to technical detail. Drugs may alter results. Thus, PRA is used less often as an approach to screening for renovascular hypertension.[5] Antihypertensive drugs affect PRA. Diuretics, direct vasodilators, angiotensin-converting enzyme inhibitors stimulate; β-adrenergic antagonists and central sympathetic drugs suppress.

Contraindications Random drawing of sample for renin activity rarely yields clinically meaningful information.

Methodology Radioimmunoassay (RIA). A kinetic assay in which enzymatic activity of renin is measured **indirectly** by the formation of angiotensin I from angiotensinogen.[6]

Additional Information A renin-aldosterone axis involves angiotensin. It regulates sodium and potassium balance, blood volume, and blood pressure. Renal reabsorption of sodium affects plasma volume. Low plasma volume, blood pressure, and low sodium induce renin release. Renin causes increased aldosterone through stimulation of angiotensin. Potassium loss suppresses renin release through aldosterone secretion. Aldosterone retains sodium, increasing plasma volume, elevating blood pressure, and causing potassium loss.

Adrenal vein sampling for aldosterone is useful; an increase on the side bearing the aldosteronoma supports diagnosis as well as location. The hypokalemia of Bartter's syndrome (a renal tubular nephropathy) is associated with edema, alkalosis, increased renin and aldosterone. Such patients are not edematous and have normal blood pressure.[2] Chapman et al have shown that the renin-angiotension-aldosterone system affects hypertension in polycystic kidney disease and that use of angiotensin converting enzyme inhibitors can ameliorate the effect of increased renin levels.[7]

A captopril test exists for screening for renovascular hypertension.[5]

Bilateral renal vein renin can provide an RVR ratio (affected/nonaffected side) to predict blood pressure response to revascularization.[5]

The evaluation and differential diagnosis of aldosteronism includes considerable clinical and biochemical diversity. Ratio of plasma aldosterone to PRA is addressed with its relevance to differential diagnosis.[1] See listings Aldosterone, Blood *on page 67* and Aldosterone, Urine *on page 68.*

Footnotes

1. Blumenfeld JD, Sealey JE, Schlussel Y, et al, "Diagnosis and Treatment of Primary Hyperaldosteronism," *Ann Intern Med*, 1994, 121(11):877-85.
2. Williams GH and Dluhy RG, "Diseases of the Adrenal Cortex," *Harrison's Principles of Internal Medicine*, 13th ed, Vol 2, Isselbacher KJ, Braunwald E, Wilson JD, et al, eds, New York, NY: McGraw-Hill Inc, 1994, 1953-76.
3. Bortolotto LA, Silva HB, Lopes HF, et al, "Primary Hyperaldosteronism and Adrenal Tumors. Clinico-Surgical Experience with 9 Patients," *Arq Bras Cardiol*, 1994, 62(3):165-9.
4. White PC, "Disorders of Aldosterone Biosynthesis and Action," *N Engl J Med*, 1994, 331(4):250-8.
5. Canzanello VJ and Textor SC, "Noninvasive Diagnosis of Renovascular Disease," *Mayo Clin Proc*, 1994, 69(12):1172-81.
6. Sealey JE, "Plasma Renin Activity and Plasma Prorenin Assays," *Clin Chem*, 1991, 37(10 Pt 2):1811-9.
7. Chapman AB, Johnson A, Gabow PA, et al, "The Renin-Angiotensin-Aldosterone System and Autosomal Dominant Polycystic Kidney Disease," *N Engl J Med*, 1990, 323(16):1091-6.

References

Scammell AM and Diver MJ, "Plasma Aldosterone and Renin Activity," *Arch Dis Child*, 1989, 64(1):139-41.
Torres VE, Young WF Jr, Offord KP, et al, "Association of Hypokalemia, Aldosteronism, and Renal Cysts," *N Engl J Med*, 1990, 322(6):345-51.

Resin Triiodothyronine Uptake *see* T$_3$ Uptake *on page 201*

Resin Uptake Ratio *see* T$_3$ Uptake *on page 201*

Retinoids *see* Vitamin A, Serum *on page 217*

Retinol, Serum *see* Vitamin A, Serum *on page 217*

Rheumatoid Factor, Body Fluid *see* Body Fluid *on page 89*

Risk Index for Coronary Arterial Disease *see* Lipid Profile *on page 159*

RVR Ratio *see* Renin, Plasma *on previous page*

saO$_2$ *see* Oxygen Saturation, Blood *on page 175*

Saturated Phosphatidylcholine (SPC) *see* Amniotic Fluid Lecithin/Sphingomyelin Ratio and Phosphatidylglycerol *on page 77*

Secretin *see* Vasoactive Intestinal Polypeptide *on page 216*

Secretin Test *see* Gastrin, Serum *on page 135*

S-Epo *see* Erythropoietin, Serum *on page 124*

Serotonin

CPT 84260

Related Information
5-Hydroxyindoleacetic Acid, Quantitative, Urine *on page 147*

Synonyms 5-HT; 5-Hydroxytryptamine, Blood

Applies to Serotonin, Cerebrospinal Fluid

Abstract Serotonin (5-hydroxytryptamine [5-HT]) is synthesized from tryptophan. Serotonin's major metabolite, 5-HIAA, is measured more commonly than 5-HT (parent compound). This test is rarely utilized.

Patient Preparation Monoamine oxidase inhibitor drugs should be discontinued for at least 1 week prior to sampling, since they tend to increase the level of serotonin. Avoid application of radioisotopes (eg, scans) before collection of specimen if RIA is used for assay. Some methods require a low indole diet for several days. Avoid eggplant, avocado, bananas, tomatoes, pineapple, walnuts, and red plums.

Specimen Whole blood, cerebrospinal fluid

Container Tube with EDTA, sometimes with ascorbic acid. Check with laboratory if the assay is available at all.

Collection Draw in chilled tubes. Keep on ice.

Storage Instructions Place whole blood in plastic bottle containing 10 mg EDTA and 75 mg ascorbic acid. Freeze within 4 hours of collection. Stable 7 days at -20°C.

Reference Range 10-30 μg/dL (SI: 570-1700 nmol/L). Values vary among laboratories and are method dependent. In serum, serotonin (5-hydroxytryptamine) levels in females were about 1.3-fold that of males. By RIA, a study provided ranges: male: 7-12 μg/dL (SI: 380-680 nmol/L), female: 9-16 μg/dL (SI: 520-900 nmol/L).[1]

Use Diagnose carcinoid syndrome only in unusual circumstances. The classical syndrome includes flushing and vasomotor instability, diarrhea, hepatomegaly, and endocardial lesions. Ectopic production may occur from oat cell carcinomas of lung, islet cell tumors of pancreas, and medullary carcinoma of thyroid. Carcinoid tumors occur in multiple endocrine neoplasia, types I and II.

Limitations Serotonin assays are not widely available and only rarely used. It may be useful to measure when normal or borderline increases of 5-HIAA are seen in a patient with clinical evidence of carcinoid syndrome. **Urinary 5-HIAA is more sensitive and specific for diagnosis of carcinoid tumors.** Engbaek and Voldby indicate that 5-methoxytryptamine and tryptamine cross react with their RIA method.[1]

Methodology Fluorometry, radioimmunoassay (RIA), gas chromatography (GC), liquid chromatography with electrochemical detection, radioenzymatic assay

Additional Information Serotonin is produced by cells of the APUD system, including the enterochromaffin (Kulchitsky) cells distributed through the mucosa of the gastrointestinal tract. Most serotonin in blood is usually concentrated in platelets, which release it during platelet aggregation. Serotonin may be measured to confirm the diagnosis of carcinoid syndrome if a problem emerges with conventional investigation. The carcinoid syndrome is usually caused by primary carcinoids of the ileum, but the syndrome is occasionally caused by primary carcinoids of the stomach. Other organs give rise to carcinoids including pancreas, duodenum, bronchus, and ovary. Many patients with the carcinoid syndrome have hepatic metastases. A role of serotonin in psychiatric disorders has been suggested.[2] A urinary serotonin assay is described but also is not widely available.[3]

Footnotes

1. Engbaek F and Voldby B, "Radioimmunoassay of Serotonin (5-Hydroxytryptamine) in Cerebrospinal Fluid, Plasma, and Serum," *Clin Chem*, 1982, 624-8.
2. Meltzer HY, "The Role of Serotonin in Schizophrenia and the Place of Serotonin-Dopamine Antagonist Antipsychotics," *J Clin Psychopharmacol*, 1995, 15(1 Suppl 1):2S-3S.
3. Feldman JM, "Urinary Serotonin in the Diagnosis of Carcinoid Tumors," *Clin Chem*, 1986, 32(5):840-4.

References

Fuller RW, "Basic Advances in Serotonin Pharmacology," *J Clin Psychiatry*, 1992, 53(Suppl):36-45.

Serotonin, Cerebrospinal Fluid *see* Serotonin *on this page*

Serotonin, Metabolite *see* 5-Hydroxyindoleacetic Acid, Quantitative, Urine *on page 147*

Serum-Ascites Albumin Gradient *see* Body Fluid *on page 89*

Serum Electrolytes *see* Electrolytes, Serum or Plasma *on page 123*

Serum Osmolality *see* Osmolality, Serum *on page 172*

Sex Hormone Binding Globulin see Testosterone, Free and Total on page 202

SGOT see Aspartate Aminotransferase on page 84

SGPT see Alanine Aminotransferase on page 65

Shake Test see Amniotic Fluid Pulmonary Surfactant on page 78

SHBG see Testosterone, Free and Total on page 202

Siderophilin see Transferrin on page 209

Sm-C see Somatomedin-C on page 201

S-NSE see Neuron-Specific Enolase, Serum on page 168

sO₂ see Oxygen Saturation, Blood on page 175

Sodium, Arterial Blood see Sodium, Blood on this page

Sodium, Blood

CPT 84295

Related Information

Anion Gap on page 81
Chloride, Serum on page 108
Chloride, Urine on page 109
Concentration Test, Urine on page 633
Electrolytes, Serum or Plasma on page 123
Lithium on page 558
Osmolality, Calculated on page 172
Sodium, Urine on this page
Urea Nitrogen, Blood on page 213
Uric Acid, Serum on page 213

Synonyms Na+

Applies to Osmolal Gap; Sodium, Arterial Blood; Sodium, Corrected

Abstract Sodium with its accompanying anions is the most important extracellular osmotically active solute.[1] The major cation of extracellular fluid, Na+ is extremely important in maintenance of water and osmotic pressure equilibrium in the extracellular compartment.

Specimen Serum or plasma

Container Red top tube or green top (lithium heparin) tube

Collection Pediatrics: Blood drawn from heelstick for capillary sample. Na+, with K+ and Cl-, can be reported from arterial or venous blood. If an arterial puncture is done for pO₂, lithium heparin anticoagulant must be used.

Reference Range Adults: 135-145 mmol/L

Possible Panic Range <120 mmol/L, >160 mmol/L

Use Evaluation of electrolytes, acid-base balance, water balance, water intoxication, dehydration

Hypernatremia occurs from loss of water or from Na retention.[1] It is found in dehydration and with diuretic use. Increased insensible water loss with fever, burns, hyperpnea, sweating, and ambient temperature causes hypernatremia. Nasogastric protein feeding with insufficient fluids may cause hypernatremia, as can vomiting and diarrhea. Hypernatremia without obvious cause may relate to Cushing's syndrome, central or nephrogenic diabetes insipidus with insufficient fluids, primary aldosteronism, and other diseases. Often, patients who have primary aldosteronism have mild hypernatremia.[1] Severe hypernatremia may be associated with volume contraction, lactic acidosis, and azotemia. Increased hematocrit may provide evidence of dehydration. The corrected serum Na+ is often high in nonketotic hyperosmolar coma. (A corrected Na+ is calculated by increasing Na+ by 1.3-1.6 mmol/L for each 100 mg/dL increment in serum or plasma glucose.) 100 mg = 5.56 mmol/L. The corrected serum Na+ level should be calculated in nonketotic hyperosmolar coma. **Apparent mild hyponatremia with very high glucose may actually mean hypernatremia.**[2] Infusion of hypertonic saline or sodium bicarbonate or ingestion of Na+ may cause sodium retention.

Hyponatremia occurs with nephrotic syndrome, cachexia, hypoproteinemia, intravenous glucose (salt-free) infusion, congestive heart failure, mineralocorticoid deficiency, and cystic fibrosis. Mineralocorticoid deficiency leads to hyponatremia, hypovolemia, and hypokalemia through inadequate Na+ and water resorption and diminished potassium excretion.[3] Serum sodium is a factor predictive of cardiovascular mortality in patients with severe congestive heart failure.[2] **Hyponatremia** without congestive heart failure or dehydration may occur with hypothyroidism, the syndrome of inappropriate secretion of antidiuretic hormone (SIADH), renal failure, or renal sodium loss.

The differential diagnosis of hyponatremia includes Addison's disease, hypopituitarism, liver disease including cirrhosis, hypertriglyceridemia, and psychogenic polydipsia. Diuretics and other drugs may cause hyponatremia. Sodium decreasing to levels <115 mmol/L can lead to significant neurological dysfunction with cerebral edema and increased intracranial pressure.

The differential diagnosis of hyponatremia includes determination of urine sodium and osmolality and serum urea nitrogen (BUN). BUN is often normal or decreased in SIADH, but is increased in states in which hyponatremia is related to volume depletion. (Extracellular volume is normal or increased in SIADH.) Hyperlipidemia, hyperproteinemia, and hyperglycemia must be considered; vide infra.

Limitations Care should be taken that one is not dealing with "pseudohyponatremia;" vide infra.

Methodology Flame emission photometry, ion-selective electrode (ISE)

Additional Information The ratio of serum sodium to osmolality is normally 0.43-0.50; a decreased ratio is found in uremia and other states in which there are increased substances with osmotic activity.

See Urea Nitrogen, Blood on page 213 regarding hyponatremia with sodium <128 mmol/L, hypo-osmolality, low BUN, and the syndrome of inappropriate secretion of antidiuretic hormone.

A number of situations result in "pseudohyponatremia." In these circumstances, treatment may be undesirable. With pseudohyponatremia serum sodium is decreased but the serum is not hypotonic (serum osmolality is normal or even increased). This may occur as the result of other molecules replacing water in relation to sodium. The water content is effectively lowered - sodium is "diluted." In severe hypertriglyceridemia or paraprotein-related marked increase in protein, the concentration of sodium in relation to water is normal but the analytic result is determined as mmol/L of serum. Osmolality in this situation is determined as the amount of particles per kg of water and will be normal. It has been shown that analyses by sodium electrode of the direct potentiometric type (requires no dilution) are not artifactually low in patients with hyperlipidemia.[4] If large amounts of solute, such as glucose or mannitol, are present, movement of intracellular water into the extracellular space may produce dilutional hyponatremia. In this case, sodium concentration in relation to water is actually low. "Osmolal gap" however exists between measured and calculated serum osmolality. Other substances capable of increasing serum osmolality (eg, ethanol) may also cause increase in the osmolal gap.

Yet another cause of pseudohyponatremia is increased serum viscosity due to increased globulin proteins, occurring particularly in Waldenström's macroglobulinemia. Analyzers may aspirate too little sample when viscosity is so high, leading to a factitious low sodium concentration.

Studying a geriatric group, hyponatremia on admission to hospital bears association with poor prognosis.[5]

Hyponatremia may manifest lethal neurological complications (water intoxication with brain edema).

Drug effects are summarized.[6]

Footnotes

1. Gregoire JR, "Adjustment of the Osmostat in Primary Aldosteronism," Mayo Clin Proc, 1994, 69(11):1108-10.
2. Daugirdas JT, Kronfol NO, Tzamaloukas AH, et al, "Hyperosmolar Coma: Cellular Dehydration and the Serum Sodium Concentration," Ann Intern Med, 1989, 110(11):855-7.
3. White PC, "Disorders of Aldosterone Biosynthesis and Action," N Engl J Med, 1994, 331(4):250-8.
4. Aw TC and Kiechle FL, "Pseudohyponatremia," Am J Emerg Med, 1985, 3(3):236-9.
5. Terzian C, Frye EB, and Piotrowski ZH, "Admission Hyponatremia in the Elderly: Factors Influencing Prognosis," J Gen Intern Med, 1994, 9(2):89-91.
6. Hitz J and Trivin F, "Sodium," Drug Effects on Laboratory Test Results Analytical Interferences and Pharmacological Effects, Siest G and Galteau MM, eds, Littleton, MA: PSG Publishing Co Inc, 1988, 391-404.

References

DeVita MV and Michelis MF, "Perturbations in Sodium Balance: Hyponatremia and Hypernatremia," Clin Lab Med, 1993, 13(1):135-48.
Epstein M and Oster JR, "Disorders of Hyponatremia and Hypernatermia," The Laboratory in Clinical Medicine. Interpretation and Application, 2nd ed, Halsted JA and Halsted CH, eds, Philadelphia, PA: WB Saunders Co, 1981, 289-95
Leehey DJ, Daugirdas JT, Manahan FJ, et al, "Prolonged Hypernatremia Associated With Azotemia and Hyponatruria," Am J Med, 1989, 86(4):494-6.
Maffly RH, "Renal Function and Disorders of Water, Sodium, and Potassium Balance," Scientific American Medicine, Section 10, Chapter 1, Rubenstein E and Federman DD, eds, New York, NY: Scientific American Inc, 1990, 2-34.
Oh MS and Carroll HJ, "Disorders of Sodium Metabolism: Hypernatremia and Hyponatremia," Crit Care Med, 1992, 20(1):94-103.
Votey SR, Peters AL, and Hoffman JR, "Disorders of Water Metabolism: Hyponatremia and Hypernatremia," Emerg Med Clin North Am, 1989, 7(4):749-69.

Sodium, Corrected see Sodium, Blood on this page

Sodium, Sweat see Chloride, Sweat on page 108

Sodium, Urine

CPT 84300

Related Information

Chloride, Urine on page 109
Electrolytes, Urine on page 124
Kidney Stone Analysis on page 640
Osmolality, Urine on page 173
Sodium, Blood on this page
(Continued)

Sodium, Urine *(Continued)*

Urine Collection, 24-Hour *on page 30*

Synonyms Na, Urine; Urine Na

Abstract Urinary sodium excretion normally relates to intake. Body sodium stores are based upon intake and renal excretion.

Specimen Timed or random urine

Container Plain urine container

Reference Range 24-hour urine: 27-287 mmol/day, varies markedly with dietary intake of sodium. There is diurnal variation (output is lower at night). A European study provides average sodium excretion: male: 162 mmol/day, range: 143-208 mmol/day; female: 134 mmol/day, range: 119-165 mmol/day; within person CV: male: 30%, female: 34%.[1]

Use Work up volume depletion, acute renal failure, acute oliguria, and differential diagnosis of hyponatremia.[2] Division of hyponatremia into hypervolemia or not, edema or not, and urinary Na^+ less than or greater than 10 mmol/L provides a classification of hyponatremia.[3] History of diuretics, other drug intake, setting of osmotic diuresis or not, serum/plasma electrolytes, and other factors are needed.

Limitations It is often advantageous to request urine potassium and creatinine along with sodium measurement. High urine sodium does not necessarily indicate that total body sodium is increased (eg, salt-losing nephritis). This area is complex; the reader is referred to the footnotes and references.

Methodology Flame emission photometry or ion-selective electrode (ISE)

Additional Information In cases of hyponatremia, random urine Na^+ <10 mmol/L commonly indicates extrarenal depletion: dehydration (gastrointestinal or sweat loss), congestive heart failure, liver disease or nephrotic syndromes. With renal or adrenal diseases, urinary Na^+ concentration is usually >20 mmol/L.

Random urine Na^+ >10 mmol/L may indicate diuretics, emesis, intrinsic renal diseases, Addison's disease, hypothyroidism, or syndrome of inappropriate antidiuretic hormone (SIADH).[3] In hypothyroidism and in SIADH, Na^+ and Cl^- may be >40 mmol/L.[4] (Depending on intake, such results also can be found in normal individuals.) In SIADH, random urinary sodium usually is >20 mmol/L. SIADH has been found in 7% of patients with small cell lung cancer.[5] Such patients have hyponatremia,

Evaluation and Treatment of **Hyponatremic** Patient

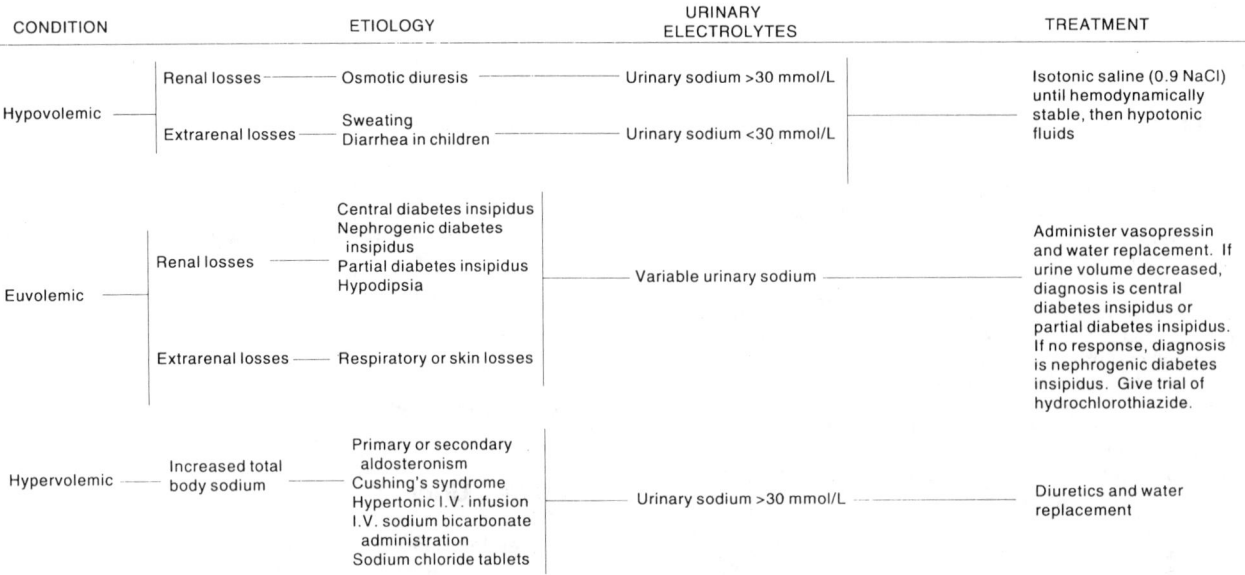

CONDITION	CLINICAL PRESENTATION	URINARY ELECTROLYTES	ETIOLOGY	TREATMENT
Hypovolemic	Orthostatic hypotension Tachycardia Azotemia	Urinary sodium >30 mmol/L	Diuretics, RTA, mineralocorticoid deficiency, salt-wasting nephritis	0.9 NaCl I.V.
		Urinary sodium <30 mmol/L	Extrarenal losses: vomiting, diarrhea, burns, sequestration	
Euvolemic	No evidence of volume depletion or overload. Subclinical increase in TBW may be present.	Urinary sodium >20 mmol/L	Hypothyroidism	Thyroid replacement
			Glucocorticoid deficiency	I.V. glucocorticoids
			SIADH, drugs, acute water intoxication	Fluid restriction
Hypervolemic	Volume excess Edema	Urinary sodium >30 mmol/L	Acute and chronic renal failure	Fluid restriction; treat renal failure
		Urinary sodium <10 mmol/L	Cirrhosis Cardiac failure Nephrotic syndrome	Fluid restriction; sodium restriction; treat underlying disorders

From Devita MV and Michelis MF, "Perturbations in Sodium Balance: Hyponatremia and Hypernatremia," *Clinics in Laboratory Medicine*, Vol 13, Preuss HG, ed, Philadelphia, PA: WB Saunders Co, 1993, 135-48, with permission.

Evaluation and Treatment of the **Hypernatremic** Patient

CONDITION	ETIOLOGY		URINARY ELECTROLYTES	TREATMENT
Hypovolemic	Renal losses	Osmotic diuresis	Urinary sodium >30 mmol/L	Isotonic saline (0.9 NaCl) until hemodynamically stable, then hypotonic fluids
	Extrarenal losses	Sweating Diarrhea in children	Urinary sodium <30 mmol/L	
Euvolemic	Renal losses	Central diabetes insipidus Nephrogenic diabetes insipidus Partial diabetes insipidus Hypodipsia	Variable urinary sodium	Administer vasopressin and water replacement. If urine volume decreased, diagnosis is central diabetes insipidus or partial diabetes insipidus. If no response, diagnosis is nephrogenic diabetes insipidus. Give trial of hydrochlorothiazide.
	Extrarenal losses	Respiratory or skin losses		
Hypervolemic	Increased total body sodium	Primary or secondary aldosteronism Cushing's syndrome Hypertonic I.V. infusion I.V. sodium bicarbonate administration Sodium chloride tablets	Urinary sodium >30 mmol/L	Diuretics and water replacement

From Devita MV and Michelis MF, "Perturbations in Sodium Balance: Hyponatremia and Hypernatremia", *Clinics in Laboratory Medicine*, Vol 13, Preuss HG, ed, Philadelphia, PA: WB Saunders Co, 1993, 135-48, with permission.

often severe, with hypo-osmolar serum, absence of clinical evidence of volume depletion, high urinary sodium excretion with urine osmolality greater than that of serum. Urine may not be maximally concentrated in some patients but it should not have osmolarity less than that of serum. Acute and subacute diseases of the CNS, TB, and other chronic pulmonary diseases may also cause SIADH. SIADH may also be caused by other entities including acute intermittent porphyria, LE, malignant tumors additional to small cell lung carcinoma, and a number of drugs.

The classification as presented here is overly abbreviated for clinical application. Pitfalls exist (eg, increase of Na⁺ necessary to balance excretion of penicillin).[4]

Urine Na⁺ >40 mmol/L in oliguria is found in acute tubular necrosis.[4,6]

Low Na⁺ excretion may be found with early obstructive uropathy and with the oliguria of acute glomerulonephritis[4] and in some patients with x-ray contrast acute renal failure.

It is important to know the urinary sodium concentration in patients with unexplained hyperchloremic metabolic acidosis when the diagnosis of distal renal tubular acidosis is being considered.[7]

Footnotes
1. Knuiman JT, Hautvast JG, van der Heijden L, et al, "A Multicentre Study on Within-Person Variability in the Urinary Excretion of Sodium, Potassium, Calcium, Magnesium, and Creatinine in 8 European Centres," *Hum Nutr Clin Nutr*, 1986, 40(5):343-8.
2. Harrington JT and Cohen JJ, "Measurement of Urinary Electrolytes - Indications and Limitations," *N Engl J Med*, 1975, 293:1241-3.
3. DeVita MV and Michelis MF, "Perturbations in Sodium Balance: Hyponatremia and Hypernatremia," *Clin Lab Med*, 1993, 13(1):135-48.
4. Sherman RA and Eisinger RP, "The Use (and Misuse) of Urinary Sodium and Chloride Measurements," *JAMA*, 1982, 247:3121-4.
5. Hainsworth JD, Workman R, and Greco FA, "Management of the Syndrome of Inappropriate Antidiuretic Hormone Secretion in Small Cell Lung Cancer," *Cancer*, 1983, 51:161-5.
6. Schrier RW, "Acute Renal Failure," *JAMA*, 1982, 247:2518-22, 2524.
7. Batlle DC, von Riotte A, and Schlueter W, "Urinary Sodium in the Evaluation of Hyperchloremic Metabolic Acidosis," *N Engl J Med*, 1987, 316(3):140-4.

References
Brown MA, Gallery ED, Ross MR, et al, "Sodium Excretion in Normal and Hypertensive Pregnancy: A Prospective Study," *Am J Obstet Gynecol*, 1988, 159(2):297-307.

Intersalt Cooperative Research Group, "Intersalt: An International Study of Electrolyte Excretion and Blood Pressure. Results for 24-Hour Urinary Sodium and Potassium Excretion," *BMJ*, 1988, 297(6644):319-28.

Kamel KS, Ethier JH, Richardson RM, et al, "Urine Electrolytes and Osmolality: When and How to Use Them," *Am J Nephrol*, 1990, 10(2):89-102.

Levinsky NG, "Fluids and Electrolytes," *Harrison's Principles of Internal Medicine*, Isselbacher KJ, Braunwald E, Wilson JD, et al, eds, New York, NY: McGraw-Hill Inc, 1994, 242-53.

Preuss HG, Podlasek SJ, and Henry JB, "Evaluation of Renal Function and Water, Electrolyte, and Acid-Base Balance," *Todd-Sanford-Davidsohn Clinical Diagnosis and Management by Laboratory Methods*, 18th ed, Henry JB, ed, Philadelphia, PA: WB Saunders Co, 1991, 118-39.

Robillard JE, Smith FG, and Segai JL, et al, "Mechanisms Regulating Renal Sodium Excretion During Development," *Pediatr Nephrol*, 1992, 6(2):205-13.

Somatomedin-C

CPT 84305

Related Information
Growth Hormone *on page 141*

Synonyms IGF-I; Insulin-Like Growth Factor I; Sm-C; Sulfation Factor

Abstract Secreted by the anterior pituitary, growth hormone (GH) stimulates growth through stimulation of synthesis of somatomedins. Somatomedins are GH-dependent peptides. Two peptides have a somatomedinic effect: IGF-I (Sm-C) and IGF-II. The former is used in evaluation of growth disorders,[1] and is generally a better test than is assay for growth hormone. IGF-II increases in tumor-related hypoglycemia but not in acromegaly.

Patient Preparation Overnight fast is preferable, no recent administration of radioactivity if assay is to be done by RIA.

Specimen Plasma

Container Lavender top (EDTA) tube; check with the laboratory.

Storage Instructions Separate plasma immediately by centrifuging at 4°C. Freeze plasma in a plastic tube.

Reference Range GH and Sm-C are elevated during normal puberty. Values vary with age, sex, and among laboratories. Adults: 130-450 ng/mL. Its values decline with age. Range is lower in males. It is increased with puberty and pregnancy.[2]

Use An excellent test for acromegaly, in which Sm-C and GH are increased; evaluate hypopituitarism and hypothalamic lesions in children (diagnosis of dwarfism and response to therapy). IGF-I (Sm-C) is the assay of choice for the diagnoses of acromegaly since it has little variation in blood levels throughout the day, unlike GH. Normal somatomedin results are evidence against growth hormone deficiency but IGF-1 is not consistently valid to screen for growth hormone deficiency.[2] Low levels occur in Laron dwarfism, an entity in which GH is increased.

Limitations Malnutrition will cause low somatomedin-C levels in spite of normal amounts of circulating growth hormone. The Sm-C level does not

distinguish pituitary dwarfism from constitutional delay of growth and development.[3] Chloridine stimulation can distinguish between the two.

Methodology Radioimmunoassay (RIA) following dissociation from binding protein and chromatography; immunoradiometric assay (IRMA)

Additional Information Somatomedin-C is a polypeptide hormone produced by the liver and other tissues, with effect on growth promoting activity and glucose metabolism (insulin-like activity). Somatomedin-C is carried in blood bound to a carrier protein which prolongs its half-life. Its level is, therefore, more constant than that of growth hormones.

Low values are described with the extremes of age (first 5-6 years and advanced age), hypopituitarism, malnutrition, diabetes mellitus, hypothyroidism, maternal deprivation syndrome, pubertal delay, cirrhosis, hepatoma, Laron dwarfism, and some cases of short stature and normal GH response to pharmacologic tests.[1] Low values may be found with nonfunctioning pituitary tumors, with constitutional delay of growth and development, and with anorexia nervosa.[3]

High values occur with adolescence, true precocious puberty, pregnancy, obesity, pituitary gigantism, **acromegaly**, and diabetic retinopathy.[1]

Since Sm-C is decreased with malnutrition, its concentration provides a useful index with which to monitor therapy for food deprivation.[4]

Provocative testing is done for assays of growth hormone; Sm-C provides another approach for evaluation of pituitary GH secretion.

Footnotes
1. Cacciari E and Cicognani A, "Somatomedin-C in Pediatric Pathophysiology," *Pediatrician*, 1987, 14(3):146-53.
2. Vance ML, "Hypopituitarism," *N Engl J Med*, 1994, 330(23):1651-62.
3. Kao PC, Abboud CF, and Zimmerman D, "Somatomedin-C: An Index of Growth Hormone Activity," *Mayo Clin Proc*, 1986, 61(11):908-9.
4. Isley WL, Newton G, Dev J, et al, "Somatomedin C in Rheumatoid Arthritis," *N Engl J Med*, 1985, 312(18):1197.

References
Daughaday WH, Hall K, Salmon WD Jr, et al, "On the Nomenclature of the Somatomedins and Insulin-Like Growth Factors," *J Clin Endocrinol Metab*, 1987, 65(5):1075-6.

Pintor C, Cella SG, and Baumann G, "Correction and Withdrawal of Conclusion - A Child With Phenotypic Laron Dwarfism and Normal Somatomedin Levels," *N Engl J Med*, 1992, 323(21):1485.

Pintor C, Loche S, Cella SG, et al, "A Child With Phenotypic Laron Dwarfism and Normal Somatomedin Levels," *N Engl J Med*, 1989, 320(6):376-9.

Rappaport R, Prevot C, and Brauner R, "Somatomedin-C and Growth in Children With Precocious Puberty: A Study of the Effect of the Level of Growth Hormone Secretion," *J Clin Endocrinol Metab*, 1987, 65(6):1112-7.

Somatomedins see Growth Hormone *on page 141*

Somatotropin see Growth Hormone *on page 141*

Spectral Analysis, Amniotic Fluid see Amniotic Fluid Analysis for Erythroblastosis Fetalis (OD 450) *on page 76*

Spinal Fluid Glucose see Cerebrospinal Fluid Glucose *on page 105*

Spinal Fluid Glutamine see Cerebrospinal Fluid Glutamine *on page 105*

Spinal Fluid Lactic Acid see Cerebrospinal Fluid Lactic Acid *on page 106*

Spinal Fluid LDH see Cerebrospinal Fluid LD *on page 106*

Stool Fat, Quantitative see Fecal Fat, Quantitative, 72-Hour Collection *on page 127*

sTSH see Thyroid Stimulating Hormone *on page 204*

Sugar, Fasting see Glucose, Fasting *on page 137*

Sulfation Factor see Somatomedin-C *on this page*

Sweat, Chloride see Chloride, Sweat *on page 108*

Synthetic α 1-24-ACTH Stimulation Test see Cosyntropin Test *on page 114*

T₃ Resin Uptake see T₃ Uptake *on this page*

T₃RU see T₃ Uptake *on this page*

T₃, Total see Triiodothyronine *on page 211*

T₃U see T₃ Uptake *on this page*

T₃ Uptake

CPT 84479

Related Information
Free Thyroxine Index *on page 129*
Thyroid Antimicrosomal Antibody *on page 433*
Thyroid Stimulating Hormone *on page 204*
Thyrotropin Receptor Antibody *on page 434*
Thyroxine *on page 206*
(Continued)

T₃ Uptake (Continued)

Thyroxine Binding Globulin *on page 207*

Synonyms Resin Triiodothyronine Uptake; Resin Uptake Ratio; T₃ Resin Uptake; T₃RU; T₃U

Applies to Thyroid Binding Ratio (THBR)

Test Commonly Includes T₃ uptake with T₄ or equivalent are part of the thyroid profile done very widely by most laboratories.

Abstract An indirect measure of thyroid binding globulin (measures unsaturated binding sites on the thyroid binding proteins). T₃ uptake does **not** measure serum T₃ levels. The first T₃ uptake had been described by Hamolsky et al by 1957, using red blood cells. Radioactive T₃ was used in preference to T₄ because of lesser affinity of TBG for T₃ compared to T₄. Such red cells were subsequently replaced by resins. The use of T₃ uptake is limited to testing with T₄ (thyroxine) to calculate the free thyroxine index (FTI). In some clinical circumstances, both FTI and sTSH are desirable.

Patient Preparation Avoid recent isotope scan before collection of specimen.

Specimen Serum is preferred, plasma may also be used.

Container Red top tube; lavender top (EDTA) tube or green top (heparin) tube is also acceptable.

Storage Instructions Separate within 48 hours. Store at 2°C to 8°C.

Reference Range Varies with different laboratories. A range of 24% to 34% is frequently used. The T₃ uptake can be expressed in several ways. The Committee on Nomenclature of the American Thyroid Association recommends that raw uptake results be normalized by dividing the raw T₃ uptake by the T₃ uptake of normal pooled serum to form the Thyroid Binding Ratio (THBR). The THBR in all laboratories will have a reference range centered on 1.00 and is usually given as 0.90-1.10.[1] See also table in listing Thyroxine Binding Globulin *on page 207*.

Use Thyroid function test for the diagnosis of hypothyroidism or hyperthyroidism, used with T₄ or equivalent to provide free thyroxine index (free T₄ index, FT₄I). An indirect measure of binding protein, the T₃ uptake reflects available binding sites (ie, reflects TBG). T₃ uptake is **not** a measurement of serum T₃. It should never be used alone; rather, its usual application is in conjunction with total T₄ measurement. THBR is preferred and should be used instead of T₃U. See table for typical examples of use.

Thyroid Function Tests

Clinical Condition	T₄	T₃U	FT₄I
Normal	Normal	Normal	Normal
Hyperthyroid	Increased	Increased	Increased
Hypothyroid	Decreased	Decreased	Decreased
Increased TBG (eg, pregnancy)	Increased	Decreased	Normal
Decreased TBG (eg, nephrotic syndrome)	Decreased	Increased	Normal

Limitations An **increase** in T₃U occurs in hyperthyroidism; in situations where drugs displace T₄ from TBG such as high doses of salicylates, phenytoin, phenylbutazone, etc; and in cases where the TBG concentration decreases such as in nephrotic syndrome, malnutrition, active acromegaly, etc. Nicotinic acid increases T₃ resin uptake ratios. A **decrease** in T₃U occurs in hypothyroidism and in cases where an increase in TBG occurs, such as estrogen administration (as contraceptive, during menopause, or treatment of osteoporosis), during pregnancy, and in conjunction with perphenazine.

Alterations in binding capacity of TBG are described with major illness and with high doses of salicylates and corticosteroids, and with use of heroin, methadone, phenytoin, and perphenazine. Alterations occur with malnutrition, such as in metastatic malignancy, and are found in patients with abnormal serum protein patterns (eg, nephrotic syndromes, cirrhosis). Other states in which changes in TBG occur include infancy, acromegaly, molar and ordinary pregnancy, oral contraceptives, and with exogenous hormones including androgens, anabolic steroids, and estrogens. Hereditary increase and decrease of TBG occurs. Most authorities have abandoned this test in favor of more specific, sensitive tests such as FT₄, TSH, and FT₃.

Contraindications T₃ uptake cannot be run after administration of therapeutic or diagnostic radioactive material. This test should not be ordered alone; it is only useful with T₄ type tests.

Methodology Resin sponge uptake, charcoal bead uptake, related methods, based on *in vitro* competition for thyroid hormone between thyroid binding globulin and the added inert receptor. For THBR, divide raw T₃ by T₃U for normal or reference serum.

Additional Information When T₃ uptake is reported as a range, for example, such that 23% and less signifies low, and 34% and more indicates high, then the index may be calculated as follows:

FT₄I = % T₃U (patient) / % T₃U (reference serum) x T₄ (µg/dL)

The FT₄I range usually approximates the range for total T₄. In the presence of thyroid binding globulin abnormalities, the free thyroxine index is a useful laboratory parameter regarding clinical thyroid status.

Footnotes

1. Burtis CA and Ashwood ER, *Tietz Textbook of Clinical Chemistry*, Philadelphia, PA: WB Saunders Co, 1994, 1724.

References

Feldkamp CS and Carey JL, "An Algorithmic Approach to Thyroid Function Testing in a Managed Care Setting. 3-Year Experience," *Am J Clin Pathol*, 1996, 105(1):11-6.

Franklyn JA, "The Management of Hyperthyroidism," *N Engl J Med*, 1994, 330(24):1731-8.

Gruhn JG, Barsano CP, and Kumar Y, "The Development of Tests of Thyroid Function," *Arch Pathol Lab Med*, 1987, 111(1):84-100.

Helfand M and Crapo LM, "Screening for Thyroid Disease," *Ann Intern Med*, 1990, 112(11):840-9.

Larsen PR and Ingbar SH, "The Thyroid Gland," *Williams Textbook of Endocrinology*, 8th ed, Philadelphia, PA: WB Saunders Co, 1992, 357-458.

Surks MI, "Guidelines for Thyroid Testing," *Lab Med*, 1993, 24(5):270-4.

T₄ *see* Thyroxine *on page 206*

T₄-Binding Globulin *see* Thyroxine Binding Globulin *on page 207*

T₄ by EIA *see* Thyroxine *on page 206*

T₄ CPB *replaced by* Thyroxine *on page 206*

T₄, Free *see* Thyroxine, Free *on page 208*

T₄ Neonatal *see* Newborn Screen for T₄ *on page 170*

T₄ (RIA) *see* Thyroxine *on page 206*

TAG-72 *see* CA 19-9 *on page 93*

TAG 72 *see* CA 125 *on page 94*

Tau Protein *see* Transferrin *on page 209*

TBG *see* Thyroxine Binding Globulin *on page 207*

tCO₂ *see* Carbon Dioxide, Blood *on page 100*

Testosterone, Free and Total

CPT 84402 (free); 84403 (total)

Related Information

Adrenocorticotropic Hormone *on page 63*
Androstenedione, Serum *on page 80*
Cortisol, Blood *on page 112*
Dehydroepiandrosterone Sulfate *on page 120*
Follicle Stimulating Hormone *on page 129*
17-Ketosteroids, Total, Urine *on page 153*
Luteinizing Hormone, Blood or Urine *on page 163*

Synonyms Free Testosterone

Applies to Dexamethasone Suppression Test; Sex Hormone Binding Globulin; SHBG

Abstract Testosterone is the major androgen responsible for sexual differentiation and male secondary sex characteristics. It is carried in the blood by sex hormone binding globulin (SHBG). The major use of these assays is in the evaluation of hirsute women. The association of chronic anovulation with hyperandrogenism, caused by the polycystic ovary syndrome, is a commonplace clinical entity.[1]

Testosterone assay is a good laboratory screening test for testicular failure.

Patient Preparation Avoid recent administration of radioactive isotopes if assay is to be done by RIA.

Specimen Serum or plasma

Container Red top tube, green top (heparin) tube, or lavender top (EDTA) tube

Storage Instructions Separate serum or plasma and freeze.

Reference Range Free: adults: male: 9-30 ng/dL (SI: 0.3-1.0 nmol/L), female: 0.3-1.9 ng/dL (SI: 0.01-0.06 nmol/L). **Total**: adults: male: 300-1200 ng/dL (SI: 10.4-41.6 nmol/L), female: 20-80 ng/dL (SI: 0.7-2.8 nmol/L). Values in children are lower. Values in normal elderly men diminish moderately.

Critical Values The testosterone concentration with moderate hyperandrogenemia of a benign ovarian cause of hirsutism is in the range of 85-150 ng/dL (3-5 nmol/L).

Possible Panic Range Testosterone concentrations in women >200 ng/dL (7 nmol/L) may indicate androgenic tumors of ovary or adrenal, especially in the presence of a brief history or severe hirsutism.

Use An indicator of LH secretion and Leydig cell function, testosterone assay is used to evaluate gonadal and adrenal function. It is helpful in the diagnosis of hypogonadism, hypopituitarism, Klinefelter syndrome and impotence (low values), and hirsutism, anovulation, amenorrhea, and virilization in females due to Stein-Leventhal syndrome, masculinizing tumors of ovary such as Sertoli-Leydig cell tumor, tumors of the adrenal cortices, and congenital adrenal hyperplasia (high values). The most common cause of anovulation and hirsutism in females is polycystic ovary syndrome.[1] Adrenal causes are uncommon. Hyperandrogenism (including hirsutism, acne, alopecia) is investigated with testosterone and androstenedione. Moderately increased concentrations are anticipated. LH is often increased but may be normal. FSH is normal to low.[1]

Testosterone is used in investigation of male precocious puberty. Male pseudohermaphroditism includes defective testosterone synthesis, androgen insensitivity syndromes, 5-α-reductase deficiency, and testicular dysgenesis.

Limitations Total serum testosterone may be normal in women with hirsutism, who may have abnormal free testosterone. Plasma testosterone level may be elevated in patients using cimetidine. In Klinefelter syndrome, testosterone can be at the low end of the reference range or lower. Even when it is almost normal, LH levels are increased.

Methodology Radioimmunoassay (RIA), immunoassay (nonisotopic). Testosterone can be measured in saliva to provide an index of free testosterone.[2] Free testosterone generally done after ultrafiltration or equilibrium dialysis by RIA.

Additional Information The differential diagnosis of polycystic ovary syndrome includes hyperprolactinemia, acromegaly, and congenital adrenal hyperplasia. The 17-α-hydroxyprogesterone response to corticotropin serves to distinguish congenital adrenal hyperplasia due to 21-hydroxylase deficiency. In males, testosterone may be normal or decreased in hypopituitarism, including selective gonadotropin deficiency (eg, Kallmann's syndrome). It may be decreased with hepatic cirrhosis, estrogen therapy, and with severe obesity. Low testosterone and high LH are encountered with renal failure and in malnutrition. It is decreased with excessive alcohol intake. Testosterone is usually increased in precocious puberty, related to idiopathic or CNS lesion. It may also be elevated due to adrenal tumors or congenital adrenal hyperplasia. Adrenal neoplasm is unlikely in hirsute women when testosterone and dehydroepiandrosterone sulfate are normal. Increased DHEA and testosterone in hirsute women should be further investigated with dexamethasone suppression testing. After dexamethasone suppression, idiopathically caused hirsutism will show a decrease in male hormone levels and adrenal carcinoma will not.[3]

Testosterone exists in serum both free (40%) and bound (60%) to albumin and to sex hormone binding globulin (SHBG) (testosterone binding globulin). Unbound (free) testosterone is the active moiety. Free and total testosterone can be measured. Usual testosterone assays measure both bound and unbound levels. In certain settings, total testosterone can be normal while free testosterone is increased, or the reverse. Free testosterone measured by analog RIA is reported to have greater diagnostic efficiency than total testosterone.[4]

The major androgens of normal females include dehydroepiandrosterone (DHEA) and androstenedione, both weak androgens. Each derives from adrenal glands as well as gonads, and can be converted to testosterone. About half of testosterone in the female derives from peripheral conversion of androstenedione.

LH stimulates androgen production. ACTH and TSH deficiencies are the more likely causes of secondary testicular failure than is an LH decrease. Low or normal LH with low testosterone is evidence of pituitary failure.[5]

Footnotes
1. Franks S, "Polycystic Ovary Syndrome," *N Engl J Med*, 1995, 333(13):853-61.
2. Navarro MA, Juan L, Bonnin MR, et al, "Salivary Testosterone: Relationship to Total and Free Testosterone in Serum," *Clin Chem*, 1986, 32(1 Pt 1):231-2.
3. Derksen J, Nagesser SK, Meinders AE, et al, "Identification of Virilizing Adrenal Tumors in Hirsute Women," *N Engl J Med*, 1994, 331(15):968-73.
4. Wilke TJ and Utley DJ, "Total Testosterone, Free-Androgen Index, Calculated Free Testosterone, and Free Testosterone by Analog RIA Compared in Hirsute Women and in Otherwise Normal Women With Altered Binding of Sex-Hormone-Binding Globulin," *Clin Chem*, 1987, 33(8):1372-5.
5. Vance ML, "Hypopituitarism," *N Engl J Med*, 1994, 330(23):1651-62.

References
Henry JB, "Evaluation of Endocrine Function," *Todd-Sanford-Davidsohn Clinical Diagnosis and Management by Laboratory Methods*, 18th ed, Henry JB, ed, Philadelphia, PA: WB Saunders Co, 1991, 343-5.
Rittmaster RS, "Clinical Relevance of Testosterone and Dihydrotestosterone Metabolism in Women," *Am J Med*, 1995, 98(1A):17S-21S.
Ruutiainen K, Sannikka E, Santti R, et al, "Salivary Testosterone in Hirsutism: Correlations With Serum Testosterone and the Degree of Hair Growth," *J Clin Endocrinol Metab*, 1987, 64(5):1015-20.
Swinkels LM, van Hoof HJ, Ross HA, et al, "Low Ratio of Androstenedione to Testosterone in Plasma and Saliva of Hirsute Women," *Clin Chem*, 1992, 38(9):1819-23.
Wheeler JE and Rudy FR, "The Testis, Paratesticular Structures, and Male External Genitalia," *Principles and Practice of Surgical Pathology*, 2nd ed, Vol 2, Silverberg SG, ed, New York, NY: Churchill Livingstone, 1990, 1531-85.

Tetraiodothyronine *see* Thyroxine *on page 206*

Tg *see* Thyroglobulin, Serum *on this page*

TG *see* Triglycerides *on page 209*

Thoracentesis Fluid Analysis *see* Body Fluid *on page 89*

Thoracentesis Fluid pH *see* Body Fluid pH *on page 92*

Thymol Turbidity *replaced by* Alanine Aminotransferase *on page 65*

Thymol Turbidity *replaced by* Aspartate Aminotransferase *on page 84*

Thyrocalcitonin *see* Calcitonin *on page 96*

Thyroglobulin, Serum
CPT 84432
Related Information
Newborn Screen for T_4 on page 170
Synonyms Tg
Abstract Thyroglobulin is a secretory product of thyroid follicular epithelium, a high molecular weight (660,000 daltons) iodinated glycoprotein. Its only origin is the thyroid gland. It is the storage form of the thyroid hormones, T_4, and T_3. Its major clinical use is in the management (not diagnosis) of differentiated thyroid carcinomas.
Patient Preparation Avoid scans and other recent prior administration of radioisotopes before collection of specimen if RIA is used for assay. Do not draw a specimen for this test soon after needle biopsy, thyroid surgery, or radioiodine therapy. Levels >15 ng/mL are more significant when the patient has not been on thyroid hormone replacement therapy after thyroidectomy.
Specimen Serum
Container Red top tube
Storage Instructions Freeze serum.
Causes for Rejection Plasma collected
Special Instructions This is **not** thyroxine binding globulin (TBG).
Reference Range Approximately 3-42 ng/mL. Detectable in most healthy adults; moderately elevated (several fold) in the last trimester of gestation and in neonates. In athyroidic patient, <5 ng/mL.
Critical Values Thyroglobulin levels >50.0 ng/mL are associated with tumor recurrence in patients who lack thyroid tissue.
Possible Panic Range Ranges for the individual laboratory must be obtained.
Use Thyroglobulin is elevated in several thyroid disorders: endemic goiter, untreated Graves' disease, thyroiditis, and differentiated thyroid carcinomas.

Those thyroid cancer patients who have no remaining thyroid tissue, following surgery and/or irradiation, would not be expected to have a source of thyroglobulin. Thyroglobulin then is **a tumor marker useful to assess the presence of residual papillary-follicular carcinoma of thyroid**,[1] following resection, including tumors which fail to concentrate radioiodine. High values are found with many instances of tumor dissemination. Thus, thyroglobulin assays are used to monitor postoperative thyroid carcinoma patients. Such assays are best used in concert with total body scans. Possibly it will be useful in patients with bone metastases in whom the primary site is unknown.

Thyroglobulin is elevated in patients with thyroiditis and thyrotoxicosis. Low or undetectable levels are a clue to thyrotoxicosis factitia (surreptitious use of thyroid hormone). The assay may be useful to support a diagnosis of subacute thyroiditis and may be used to monitor response to treatment of nodular or diffuse nontoxic goiter. The absence of thyroglobulin from the serum of neonates suggests congenital athyreosis.[2] Thyroglobulin may prove useful as an indicator of T_4 therapy in patients with solitary nodules.[3]

Limitations Thyroglobulin is useful in the management but not diagnosis of differentiated thyroid carcinomas. Thyroglobulin is not valid as a tumor marker for anaplastic or medullary carcinoma of thyroid. High values are reported with surgery or irradiation to the thyroid, with thyroiditis, T_4 binding globulin deficiency, with administration of TRH, TSH, iodine, and of anticancer drugs. High levels of thyroglobulin occur in goiter and in many types of hyperthyroidism. Normal levels are found in patients with small thyroid carcinomas. Low values occur with thyroid hormone administration. This is not a screening test for thyroid cancer. RIA methods are subject to interference in serums containing autoantibodies (eg, most patients with Hashimoto's thyroiditis). Newer methods, using IRMA technology, can reliably measure thyroglobulin in the presence of antithyroglobulin autoantibodies,[4,5] an adjunct to ^{131}I scanning in care of the thyroid cancer patient.[6] Thyroglobulin is decreased with fasting.[7]
Methodology Radioimmunoassay (RIA), immunoradiometric assay (IRMA), sandwich enzyme immunoassay (EIA)
Additional Information Since functioning metastatic thyroid carcinoma causing hyperthyroidism is extremely uncommon, serial thyroglobulin
(Continued)

Thyroglobulin, Serum (Continued)

assays provide a means of following such patients.[1] Serial thyroglobulin determinations may be helpful for detecting metastases which do not accumulate radioiodine.[8]

Footnotes

1. Black EG and Sheppard MC, "Serum Thyroglobulin Measurements in Thyroid Cancer: Evaluation of "False"-Positive Results," *Clin Endocrinol*, 1991, 35(6):519-20.
2. DiGeorge AM, "The Endocrine System," *Nelson Textbook of Pediatrics*, 14th ed, Behrman RE, Kliegman RM, and Nelson WE, eds, Philadelphia, PA: WB Saunders Co, 1992, 1414-28.
3. Morita T, Tamai H, Ohshima A, et al, "Changes in Serum Thyroid Hormone, Thyrotropin and Thyroglobulin Concentrations During Thyroxine Therapy in Patients With Solitary Thyroid Nodules," *J Clin Endocrinol Metab*, 1989, 69(2):227-30.
4. Piechaczyk M, Baldet L, Pau B, et al, "Novel Immunoradiometric Assay of Thyroglobulin in Serum With Use of Monoclonal Antibodies Selected for Lack of Cross-Reactivity With Autoantibodies," *Clin Chem*, 1989, 35(3):422-4.
5. Wilson R, McKillop JH, Jenkins C, et al, "Serum Thyroglobulin - Its Measurement and Clinical Use," *Ann Clin Biochem*, 1989, 26(Pt 5):401-6.
6. Aiello DP and Manni A, "Thyroglobulin Measurement vs Iodine-131 Total Body Scan for Follow-Up of Well-Differentiated Thyroid Cancer," *Arch Intern Med*, 1990, 150(2):437-9.
7. Unger J, "Fasting Induces a Decrease in Serum Thyroglobulin in Normal Subjects," *J Clin Endocrinol Metab*, 1988, 67(6):1309-11.
8. Botsch H, Glatz J, Shulz E, et al, "Long-Term Follow-Up Using Serial Serum Thyroglobulin Determinations in Patients With Differentiated Thyroid Carcinoma," *Cancer*, 1983, 52:1856-9.

References

Associated Regional and University Pathologists, Inc, "Thyroglobulin," Salt Lake City, UT, 1995.
Grant S, Luttrell B, Reeve T, et al, "Thyroglobulin May Be Undetectable in the Serum of Patients With Metastatic Disease Secondary to Differentiated Thyroid Carcinoma," *Cancer*, 1984, 54(8):1625-8.
Lubin E, Mechlis-Frish S, Zatz S, et al, "Serum Thyroglobulin and Iodine-131 Whole-Body Scan in the Diagnosis and Assessment of Treatment for Metastatic Differentiated Thyroid Carcinoma," *J Nucl Med*, 1994, 35(2):257-62.
Sheppard MC, "Serum Thyroglobulin and Thyroid Cancer," *Q J Med*, 1986, 59(229):429-33.
Wilson JD and Foster DW, eds, *Williams Textbook of Endocrinology*, 8th ed, Philadelphia, PA: WB Saunders Co, 1992.

Thyroid Binding Ratio (THBR) see T_3 Uptake *on page 201*

Thyroid Screen for Newborns see Newborn Screen for T_4 *on page 170*

Thyroid Stimulating Hormone

CPT 84443

Related Information

Adrenocorticotropic Hormone *on page 63*
Amiodarone, Serum *on page 532*
Free Thyroxine Index *on page 129*
Lithium *on page 558*
T_3 Uptake *on page 201*
Thyroid Antimicrosomal Antibody *on page 433*
Thyrotropin Receptor Antibody *on page 434*
Thyroxine *on page 206*
Triiodothyronine *on page 211*

Synonyms sTSH; Thyrotropin; TSH; Ultrasensitive TSH

Applies to TRH Stimulation Test

Abstract Produced by the anterior pituitary gland, thyroid stimulating hormone (TSH) stimulates secretion of T_4 (thyroxine) and T_3 (triiodothyronine). TSH secretion is physiologically regulated by T_3 and T_4 (feedback inhibition) and is stimulated by TRH (thyrotropin releasing hormone) from the hypothalamus. TSH assay was originally used to diagnose or confirm primary hypothyroidism. The new sensitive assays (sTSH) permit recognition of hyperthyroidism as well. Thus, they have altered diagnostic thyroid testing strategies.[1] Sensitive TSH has become the best single thyroid test.[2] Not bound to carrier proteins, sTSH is not plagued with problems of estrogen administration, hepatic or renal disorders which characterize other important thyroid tests. Thyroid tests are interpreted in clinical context, including history, physical examination, T_4, FT_4, and T_3 concentrations as needed.

Patient Preparation Avoid radioisotope administration before collection of specimen if RIA is used for assay.

Specimen Serum

Container Red top tube

Sampling Time A diurnal rhythm exists. Peak levels occur at about 11 PM. TSH release is pulsatile.

Storage Instructions Separate serum within 4 hours and refrigerate. Stable 4 days at 4°C.

Reference Range Dependent on method. Neonates: <20 mIU/L by third day of life. Using one of the newer ultrasensitive assays (chemiluminometric two-site assay), Mayo Medical Laboratories has published age-stratified ranges, of which the lower limit is 0.4 mIU/L and the upper limit up to 10.0 mIU/L (for those 80 years of age and older). Values 0.1-0.3 mIU/L are equivocal in sensitive TSH assays.[3] Adults (20-55 years): 0.4-4.2 mIU/L.

Critical Values <0.1 mIU/L provides indication of primary hyperthyroidism or exogenous thyrotoxicosis. Risk exists for atrial fibrillation at TSH levels <0.1, but the degree of risk (atrial fibrillation[3] is a major risk factor for stroke) is controversial.

Use This has become the primary thyroid function test for stable ambulatory subjects who lack pituitary or neuropsychiatric illness.[1] Investigation of low T_4 result; the differential diagnosis of primary hypothyroidism from normal, and the differential diagnosis of primary hypothyroidism from pituitary/hypothalamic hypothyroidism. **TSH is high in primary hypothyroidism.** Among those age 60 and older, low sTSH (≤0.1 mIU/L) is a risk factor for atrial fibrillation.[4] (Atrial fibrillation is a risk factor for arterial embolization.) **Low TSH occurs in hyperthyroidism.** When TSH is low and T_4 or FT_4 is normal, high T_3 confirms triiodothyronine toxicosis; see listing Triiodothyronine *on page 211*.

Evaluation of therapy in hypothyroid patients, receiving various thyroid hormone preparations: low values are found in states of excessive thyroid replacement. Normal result on a new sensitive TSH assay is acceptable evidence of adequate thyroid replacement.

Follow-up of patients who have had hyperthyroidism treated with radioiodine or surgery, and for low T_4 newborn screen results. Therapeutic levothyroxine can be titrated with sTSH assays.[5]

The prevalence of hypothyroidism is increased in those with hypercholesterolemia.[6]

TSH had been used in the **TRH stimulation test** for borderline thyrotoxicosis. Such testing was not often needed[7] even before the introduction of sensitive immunoassays for serum thyrotropin, and is now mostly, but not completely, obviated.

The new highly sensitive TSH assays, among other roles, are used to screen for thyroid disease. A result within the accepted reference range provides strong evidence for euthyroidism. A simple algorithm for thyroid testing can be found in the chart, used by the Mayo Clinic Laboratory.[1]

Limitations TSH is decreased by glucocorticoids, levodopa, dopamine, and may be affected by stress and by severe nonthyroidal illness, and these remain limitations even for the new, sensitive TSH assays. Causes of transient increase in TSH include lithium, methimazole, propylthiouracil, and in certain patients, iodine, amiodarone, and radiologic contrast media.[3] Effects of drugs upon thyroid testing and physiology have recently been reviewed.[8] A table relevant to drugs and thyroid is included in the listing Thyroxine Binding Globulin *on page 207*. TSH suppression in hypothyroidism with severe illness has been reported with TSH increase with recovery.[9] Normal TSH levels in the presence of hypothyroidism have been reported with head injury. TSH is not elevated in secondary hypothyroidism (that due to hypopituitarism) nor in hypothalamic hypothyroidism.

Suppressed TSH may be found early in pregnancy.[3] The diagnosis of hyperthyroidism in pregnancy may require assay of free thyroid hormones and a TRH test.[10]

Rare pituitary neoplasms can cause hyperthyroidism by production of TSH.

Probably no single test, even the sensitive immunoassays, can be expected to adequately reflect thyroid status under all circumstances. Among possible problems are the recovery phase of nonthyroidal illness, states of resistance to thyroid hormone, thyrotropin-producing tumors, thyroid status in acute psychiatric illness, early in thyrotoxicosis and in subacute thyroiditis.[11]

Methodology Immunoassays including radioimmunoassay (RIA), immunochemiluminometric (ICMA) assays (chemiluminescent markers), sandwich immunoradiometric assays (IRMA), fluorometric enzyme immunoassay with use of monoclonal antibodies, microparticle enzyme immunoassay (MEIA) on IMx (Abbott Laboratories)

Additional Information Unsuspected **increase** in the level of serum TSH is not uncommon in elderly subjects. TSH is the single most sensitive test for primary hypothyroidism. Elevated sTSH in apparently euthyroid individuals can be followed by FT_4 and assay for antimicrosomal antibodies. If positive for antimicrosomal antibodies, such patients are at risk for subsequent evolution of hypothyroidism, especially if FT_4 is marginally decreased. Such risk is between 5% and 26% annually.[1] If there is clear evidence for hypothyroidism and the TSH is not elevated, hypopituitarism should be considered (secondary hypothyroidism).

TSH levels have been **elevated** or inappropriately detectable for high thyroid hormone levels in some patients with thyrotropin-secreting pituitary adenomas. Delay in diagnosis of these tumors may progress to visual compromise. The effects of such neoplasms can be misdiagnosed as those of primary hyperthyroidism.[12] A thyroid testing cascade, in use at the Mayo Clinic, would follow decrease of sTSH with FT_4. If FT_4 is normal, T_3 is assayed.[1] The most common cause of low sTSH among outpatients is excessive replacement of thyroid hormone.[3]

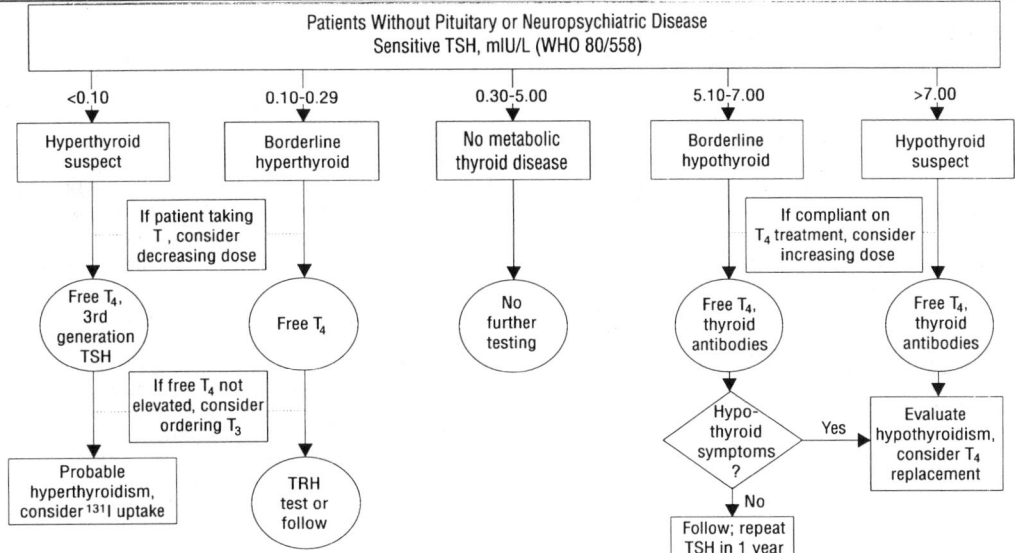

Strategy for use of sensitive thyrotropin (TSH) for thyroid function testing. T_3 = triiodithyronine; T_4 = thyroxine; TRH = thyrotropin releasing hormone; WHO = World Health Organization.
From Klee GG and Hay ID, "Role of Thyrotropin Measurements in the Diagnosis and Management of Thyroid Disease," *Clin Lab Med*, 1993, 13:673-82, with permission.

Until the late 1980s, TSH assays were not sufficiently sensitive to distinguish hyperthyroidism from euthyroid (normal) subjects. The new generation of ultrasensitive TSH immunoassays have provided a far more effective diagnostic separation of thyrotoxicosis from euthyroidism. They may well be the best possible screening test. However, Gambino has been among those finding it difficult to accept a single screening test without a confirmatory test[13] (eg, hemoglobin and hematocrit are generally ordered together).

See table, Drugs That Influence Thyroid Function in the listing Thyroxine Binding Globulin *on page 208.*

Footnotes

1. Klee GG and Hay ID, "Biochemical Thyroid Function Testing," *Mayo Clin Proc*, 1994, 69(5):469-70.
2. Utiger RD, "Subclinical Hyperthyroidism - Just a Low Serum Thyrotropin Concentration, or Something More?" *N Engl J Med*, 1994, 331(19):1302-3 (editorial).
3. Smith SA, "Commonly Asked Questions About Thyroid Function," *Mayo Clin Proc*, 1995, 70(6):573-7.
4. Sawin CT, Geller A, Wolf PA, et al, "Low Serum Thyrotropin Concentrations as a Risk Factor for Atrial Fibrillation in Older Patients," *N Engl J Med*, 1994, 331(19):1249-52.
5. Cooper DS, "Thyroid Hormone, Osteoporosis, and Estrogen," *JAMA*, 1994, 271(16):1283-4.
6. Oettgen P, Ginsburg GS, Horowitz GL, et al, "Frequency of Hypothyroidism in Adults With Serum Total Cholesterol Levels 200 mg/dL," *Am J Cardiol*, 1994, 73(13):955-7.
7. Nicoloff JT and Spencer CA, "Clinical Review 12: The Use and Misuse of the Sensitive Thyrotropin Assays," *J Clin Endocrinol Metab*, 1990, 71(3):553-8.
8. Surks MI and Sievert R, "Drugs and Thyroid Function," *N Engl J Med*, 1995, 333(25):1688-94.
9. Spencer CA, "Clinical Utility and Cost-Effectiveness of Sensitive Thyrotropin Assays in Ambulatory and Hospitalized Patients," *Mayo Clin Proc*, 1988, 63(12):1214-22.
10. Toft AD, "Use of Sensitive Immunoradiometric Assay for Thyrotropin in Clinical Practice," *Mayo Clin Proc*, 1988, 63(10):1035-42.
11. Ehrmann DA and Sarne DH, "Serum Thyrotropin and the Assessment of Thyroid Status," *Ann Intern Med*, 1989, 110(3):179-81.
12. Gesundheit N, Petrick PA, Nissim M, et al, "Thyrotropin-Secreting Pituitary Adenomas: Clinical and Biochemical Heterogeneity - Case Reports and Follow-Up of Nine Patients," *Ann Intern Med*, 1989, 111(10):827-35.
13. Gambino R, "TSH and Thyroid Status," *Lab Report for Physicians*, 1989, 11:33-5.

References

Bahn RS and Heufelder AE, "Pathogenesis of Graves' Ophthalmopathy," *N Engl J Med*, 1993, 329(20):1468-75.
Brennan MD, Klee GG, Preissner CM, et al, "Heterophilic Serum Antibodies: A Cause for Falsely Elevated Serum Thyrotropin Levels," *Mayo Clin Proc*, 1987, 62(10):894-98.
Clark PM, Clark JD, Holder R, et al, "Pulsatile Secretion of TSH in Healthy Subjects," *Ann Clin Biochem*, 1987, 24(Pt 5):470-6.
Gorman CA, "Symposium on Sensitivity TSH Assays - Introduction: Thyroid Function Testing: A New Era," *Mayo Clin Proc*, 1988, 63(10):1026-7.
Greenspan SL, Klibanski A, Schoenfeld D, et al, "Pulsatile Secretion of Thyrotropin in Man," *J Clin Endocrinol Metab*, 1986, 63(3):661-8.
Hamblin PS, Dyer SA, Mohr VS, et al, "Relationship Between Thyrotropin and Thyroxine Changes During Recovery From Severe Hypothyroxinemia of Critical Illness," *J Clin Endocrinol Metab*, 1986, 62(4):717-22.
Howanitz JH, "Review of the Influence of Polypeptide Hormone Forms on Immunoassay Results," *Arch Pathol Lab Med*, 1993, 117(4):369-72.
Howanitz JH, Howanitz PJ, and Henry JB, "Evaluation of Endocrine Function," *Clinical Diagnosis and Management by Laboratory Methods*, 18th ed, Henry JB, ed, Philadelphia, PA: WB Saunders Co, 1991, 308-20.
Jackson JA, Verdonk CA, Spiekerman AM, et al, "Euthyroid Hyperthyroxinemia and Inappropriate Secretion of Thyrotropin. Recognition and Diagnosis," *Arch Intern Med*, 1987, 147(7):1311-3.
Klee GG and Hay ID, "Sensitive Thyrotropin Assays: Analytic and Clinical Performance Criteria," *Mayo Clin Proc*, 1988, 63(11):1123-32.

Martinez M, Derksen D, and Kapsner P, "Making Sense of Hypothyroidism. An Approach to Testing and Treatment," *Postgrad Med*, 1993, 93(6):135-8, 141-5.
McDermott MT and Ridgway EC, "Thyroid Hormone Resistance Syndromes," *Am J Med*, 1993, 94(4):424-32.
Ridgway EC, "Thyrotropin Radioimmunoassays: Birth, Life, and Demise," *Mayo Clin Proc*, 1988, 63(10):1028-34.
Rosenthal MJ, Hunt WC, Garry PJ, et al, "Thyroid Failure in the Elderly - Microsomal Antibodies as Discriminant for Therapy," *JAMA*, 1987, 258(2):209-13.
Sawin CT, Geller A, Hershman JM, et al, "The Aging Thyroid: The Use of Thyroid Hormone in Older Persons," *JAMA*, 1989, 261(18):2653-5.
Spencer CA, "Clinical Utility and Cost-Effectiveness of Sensitive Thyrotropin Assays in Ambulatory and Hospitalized Patients," *Mayo Clin Proc*, 1988, 63(12):1214-22.
Surks MI, "Guidelines for Thyroid Testing," *Lab Med*, 1993, 24(5):270-4.

Thyroid Stimulating Hormone Screen, Filter Paper

CPT 84443

Related Information

Newborn Screen for T_4 *on page 170*

Synonyms TSH, Filter Paper

Abstract The importance of newborn screening for hypothyroid case detection and early initiation of treatment has led to filter paper screening programs of T_4 and/or TSH in many countries of the world. If hypothyroidism is undetected, growth and mental retardation occur, and in rare instances, death.

Patient Preparation After cleansing infant's heel, puncture to obtain free-flowing blood for spotting on collection card. Spot blood directly on card, using no pipets or blood collection equipment. Avoid radioisotope administration before collection of specimen if RIA is used for assay.

Specimen Whole blood, soaked through special collection paper

Container Special filter paper collection card

Sampling Time Test newborn at 7-10 days.

Collection Cord blood can be used, or sample can be collected at 3-5 days after birth. Using a large drop of blood, soak through the special collection paper at a minimum of one spot.

Causes for Rejection Blood not soaked through collection card, recently administered radioisotope if RIA is used for assay

Reference Range TSH peaks just after birth to two to three times "normal", then declines.[1] "Normal" after immediate postpartum period is <7 µIU/mL (SI: <7 mIU/L). Adult levels are reached by 10 days of age. Adults: 0.4-4.2 mIU/L.

Possible Panic Range Elevated TSH with low T_4, or high TSH with normal T_4

Use Follow-up testing after, with, or instead of T_4 filter paper test for congenital hypothyroidism.

Methodology Enzyme immunoassay (EIA), radioimmunoassay (RIA)

Additional Information The incidence of congenital hypothyroidism in the United States (on the basis of screening programs) is from 1:3600 to 1:5000. The incidence is significantly less in black populations. Without screening the diagnosis is likely to be missed because signs are usually minimal just after birth. Without detection and treatment mental and (Continued)

Thyroid Stimulating Hormone Screen, Filter Paper (Continued)

physical disability results including retardation, poor growth, low metabolic rate, constipation, bradycardia, and myxedema. Screening for congenital hypothyroidism is now performed by all states of the USA. Second screening at 2-6 weeks of age may be required to detect all cases. Combined screening for low T_4 and high TSH has greater specificity than the use of either test alone. Measurement of TSH is the best confirmatory test for primary hypothyroidism, in which it is elevated. Neonatal TSH screening can also find newborns with congenital hyperthyroidism.[2]

Footnotes
1. Howanitz JH, Howanitz PJ, and Henry JB, "Evaluation of Endocrine Function," *Todd-Sanford-Davidsohn Clinical Diagnosis and Management by Laboratory Methods*, 18th ed, Henry JB, ed, Philadelphia, PA: WB Saunders Co, 1991, 308-20.
2. Kopp P, van Sande J, Parma J, et al, "Brief Report: Congenital Hyperthyroidism Caused by a Mutation in the Thyrotropin-Receptor Gene," *N Engl J Med*, 1995, 332(3):150-4.

References
American Academy of Pediatrics Committee on Genetics, "Newborn Screening Fact Sheets: Congenital Hypothyroidism," *Pediatrics*, 1989, 83:454-6 and 461-2.

Burrow GN, Fisher DA, and Larsen PR, "Maternal and Fetal Thyroid Function," *N Engl J Med*, 1994, 331(16):1072-8.

LaFranchi S, "Diagnosis and Treatment of Hypothyroidism in Children," *Compr Ther*, 1987, 13(10):20-30.

Meites S, *Pediatric Clinical Chemistry: Reference (Normal) Values*, 3rd ed, Washington, DC: American Association of Clinical Chemistry Press, 1989, 250-2.

Surks MI, "Guidelines for Thyroid Testing," *Lab Med*, 1993, 24(5):270-4.

Thorpe-Beeston JG, Nicolaides KH, and McGregor AM, "Fetal Thyroid Function," *Thyroid*, 1992, 2(3):207-17.

Thyrotropin see Thyroid Stimulating Hormone on page 204

Thyroxine

CPT 84436

Related Information
Adrenocorticotropic Hormone on page 63
Amiodarone, Serum on page 532
Free Thyroxine Index on page 129
Lithium on page 558
T_3 Uptake on page 201
Thyroid Antimicrosomal Antibody on page 433
Thyroid Stimulating Hormone on page 204
Thyrotropin Receptor Antibody on page 434
Thyroxine Binding Globulin on next page
Thyroxine, Free on page 208
Triiodothyronine on page 211

Synonyms T_4; T_4 by EIA; T_4 (RIA); Tetraiodothyronine; Thyroxine by RIA

Applies to Free Thyroid Index; Thyroxine-Binding Protein Electrophoresis

Replaces T_4 CPB; Murphy-Pattee; PBI

Abstract Thyroxine (T_4) is the major secretory product of the thyroid gland. It is carried through the blood bound (in equilibrium) to thyroxine binding globulin (TBG) (>99.9%), prealbumin, and albumin. T_4 secretion is stimulated by thyrotropin (thyroid stimulating hormone) (TSH). Alterations in thyroid binding proteins occur in patients with nonthyroidal illness, leading to a need for sensitive TSH (sTSH) and/or other investigation.

Thyroxine physiologically is converted to triiodothyronine (T_3), the active hormone.

Patient Preparation Avoid radioisotope administration prior to collection of specimen if testing is by RIA.

Specimen Serum

Container Red top tube

Storage Instructions Separate serum within 48 hours and refrigerate. Separated serum stable 1 week at 25°C.

Reference Range Pediatrics: cord T_4 and values in the first few weeks are much higher, falling over the first months and years; 10 years and older: approximately 5.8-11.0 µg/dL (SI: 75-142 nmol/L), varying somewhat between laboratories. Borderline low is ≤4.5-5.7 µg/dL (SI: ≤58-73 nmol/L); low is ≤4.4 µg/dL (SI: ≤57 nmol/L); results <2.5 µg/dL (SI: <32 nmol/L) are strong evidence for hypothyroidism.[1]

Approximate adult normal range is 4.0-12.0 µg/dL (SI: 51-154 nmol/L) with some variation between sources. Normal range is increased in women on birth control pills, owing to increased TBG. Free thyroxine index will still be within the normal range. Normal range in pregnancy: approximately 5.5-16.0 µg/dL (SI: 71-206 nmol/L).

Possible Panic Range At values <2.0 µg/dL (SI: <26 nmol/L), myxedema coma is possible. At values >20 µg/dL (SI: >257 nmol/L), thyroid storm is possible.

Use Following detection of abnormality of sTSH, laboratory testing may include T_4 or FT_4. Thyroxine remains a good general thyroid function

screening test. The free thyroxine index is calculated as T_4 x T_3 uptake. Those most likely to benefit from thyroid testing include the elderly, women in the postpartum state 4-8 weeks following delivery, patients with autoimmune disorders, and those with family history of thyroid disease.[2] **Decreased** in hypothyroidism, in genetically decreased TBG, and in third stage of (painful) subacute thyroiditis; **increased** with hyperthyroidism, with subacute thyroiditis in its first stage, with thyrotoxicosis due to Graves' disease, with increased TBG (pregnancy, genetically increased TBG, acute intermittent porphyria, primary biliary cirrhosis), thyrotoxicosis factitia, and occasionally in euthyroid patients with familial dysalbuminemic hyperthyroxinemia. Used to diagnose T_4 thyrotoxicosis.

Primary hypothyroidism (hypometabolism) is caused by Hashimoto's thyroiditis, idiopathic myxedema, prior radioactive iodine therapy for hyperthyroidism, prior thyroid surgery, endemic goiter, use of lithium carbonate, and other entities. Congenital causes include enzyme blocks and agenesis. Causes of **secondary hypothyroidism** include primary pituitary disease (eg, postpartum pituitary necrosis (Sheehan's syndrome) and pituitary tumors). The expression "myxedema" indicates advanced clinical hypothyroidism, with dermal mucopolysaccharide deposits. A diagnosis of primary hypothyroidism should be confirmed by a sTSH assay.

Graves' disease is classical thyrotoxicosis (hypermetabolism), an immune or autoimmune disorder. Other causes of **hyperthyroidism** include toxic multinodular or uninodular goiter, phases of thyroiditis, and a number of uncommon to rare entities which cause increased T_4.[3]

T_4, sTSH, FT_4, and other tests are used to investigate goiter, an expression for thyroid enlargement, which may be found with hypothyroidism, euthyroidism, or hyperthyroidism.

Limitations T_4 may be increased with excess intake of iodine or or with surreptitious use of thyroxine. T_4 levels may be abnormal in the presence of systemic nonthyroidal disease. Alterations in binding capacity or quantity of TBG may increase or decrease total thyroxine without causing symptoms. A cause of elevated T_4 in nonthyroidal disease is said to be liver disease.

Serum thyroxine and free thyroxine (FT_4) are increased in familial dysalbuminemic hyperthyroxinemia, a euthyroid syndrome in which an abnormal binding site has affinity for thyroxine. The T_3 is usually normal in this entity, as is T_3 uptake. Thus, T_3 uptake is commonly ordered with T_4 and presented as thyroxine binding ratio (THBR). **Thyroxine-binding protein electrophoresis** on polyacrylamide gel can be used to characterize such proteins.[2]

T_4 is less sensitive than sTSH in the diagnosis of early primary hypothyroidism or hyperthyroidism.

Euthyroid hyperthyroxinemia is an expression used as a collective term for nonthyroidal diseases and states which increase thyroxine levels with normal thyroid tissue and metabolism. In addition to congenital or acquired thyroid hormone binding globulin changes (excessive thyroid binding globulin, familial dysalbuminemic hyperthyroxinemia, and others[2]) and drug related phenomena, peripheral resistance to thyroid hormones and increases related to medical and acute psychiatric illness are described. Hyperemesis gravidarum and hyponatremia may cause euthyroid hyperthyroxinemia.

Anti-T_4 antibodies may exist, interfering with T_4 and free T_4 determinations.

Methodology Radioimmunoassay (RIA), enzyme-linked immunosorbent assay (ELISA), fluorescence polarization immunoassay (FPIA), chemiluminescence assay (CIA)

Additional Information The combination of the serum T_4 and T_3 uptake (an estimate of FT_4I) as an assessment of TBG, helps to determine whether an abnormal T_4 value is due to alterations in serum thyroxine binding globulin or to changes of thyroid hormone levels. The **free thyroid index** is T_4 x resin uptake ratio (RU). It is used presently as spinoff (reflex testing) to evaluate selected results from sTSH screening.[4] Deviations of both tests in the same direction usually indicate that an abnormal T_4 is due to abnormalities in thyroid hormone. Deviations of the two tests in opposite directions provide evidence that an abnormal T_4 may relate to alterations in TBG.

Causes of increased TBG binding include neonatal state, molar and conventional pregnancy, estrogens, oral contraceptives, heroin, methadone, 5-fluorouracil, clofibrate, infectious hepatitis, chronic active hepatitis, and primary biliary cirrhosis, acute intermittent porphyria, lymphoma, and hereditary TBG increase.

Causes of decreased TBG binding include abnormal protein states. These include nephrotic syndrome, androgens, anabolic steroids, prednisone, acromegaly, liver or other systemic illness, severe stress, and hereditary TBG deficiency. Salicylates, T_3, and diphenylhydantoin may lower T_4 significantly, and nicotinic acid appears to do so.[5] Amiodarone

Thyroid Tests With Disease and Varying TBG

Diagnosis	T_4	FT_4 (or FT_4I)	TSH
Normal	Normal	Normal	Normal
Hyperthyroid	Increased	Increased	Decreased
Hypothyroid	Decreased	Decreased	Increased
Increased TBG	Increased	Normal	Normal
Decreased TBG	Decreased	Normal	Normal

may cause increased thyroxine levels and can cause hypothyroidism or hyperthyroidism.

Lithium carbonate may cause goiter with or without hypothyroidism.

Carbamazepine (Tegretol®) is reported to cause decreased values in thyroid function tests.

This brief review must point out that clinical interpretation of patients' signs and symptoms has primary significance. Definitive treatment based on insufficient laboratory tests is condemned.

The sensitive TSH assay is advocated as a single screening test for thyroid disease. Such proposals are controversial;[6] others find it difficult to accept one test as adequate for screening[7] and warn that a single test cannot adequately, in all settings, reflect thyroid status.[8] An inverse relationship exists between thyroxine and TSH. While the former represents thyroid hormone concentration, the latter is a test of thyroid regulation.

Relationships of drugs to thyroid testing and physiology have recently been updated.[9] See table in listing Thyroxine Binding Globulin *on page 208.*

Footnotes
1. Larsen RP and Ingbar SH, "The Thyroid," *Williams Textbook of Endocrinology*, 8th ed, Wilson J and Foster N, eds, Philadelphia, PA: WB Saunders Co, 1992, 357-488.
2. Smith SA, "Commonly Asked Questions About Thyroid Function," *Mayo Clin Proc*, 1995, 70(6):573-7.
3. Franklyn JA, "The Management of Hyperthyroidism," *N Engl J Med*, 1994, 330(24):1731-8.
4. Feldkamp CS and Carey JL, "An Algorithmic Approach to Thyroid Function Testing in a Managed Care Setting. 3-Year Experience," *Am J Clin Pathol*, 1996, 105(1):11-6.
5. Shakir KM, Kroll S, Aprill BS, et al, "Nicotinic Acid Decreases Serum Thyroid Hormone Levels While Maintaining a Euthyroid State," *Mayo Clin Proc*, 1995, 70(6):556-8.
6. Helfand M and Schmittner J, "Screening for Thyroid Dysfunction: Which Test Is Best?" *JAMA*, 1993, 270(19):2297-8.
7. Gambino R, "TSH and Thyroid Status," *Lab Report for Physicians*, 1989, 11:33-5.
8. Ehrmann DA and Sarne DH, "Serum Thyrotropin and the Assessment of Thyroid Status," *Ann Intern Med*, 1989, 110(3):179-81.
9. Surks MI and Sievert R, "Drugs and Thyroid Function," *N Engl J Med*, 1995, 333(25):1688-94.

References
Brent GA, "The Molecular Basis of Thyroid Hormone Action," *N Engl J Med*, 1994, 331(13):847-53.
Franklyn JA, Davis JR, Ramsden DB, et al, "Phenytoin and Thyroid Hormone Action," *J Endocrinol*, 1985, 104(2):201-4.
Griffin JE, "Hypothyroidism in the Elderly," *Am J Med Sci*, 1990, 299(5):334-45.
Gruhn JG, Barsano CP, and Kumar Y, "The Development of Tests of Thyroid Function," *Arch Pathol Lab Med*, 1987, 111(1):84-100.
Miller MJ, Pan C, and Barzel US, "The Prevalence of Subclinical Hypothyroidism in Adults With Low-Normal Blood Thyroxine Levels," *N Y State J Med*, 1990, 90(11):541-4.
Rallison ML, Dobyns BM, Meikle AW, et al, "Natural History of Thyroid Abnormalities: Prevalence, Incidence, and Regression of Thyroid Diseases in Adolescents and Young Adults," *Am J Med*, 1991, 91(4):363-70.
Ruiz M, Rajatanavin R, Young RA, et al, "Familial Dysalbuminemic Hyperthyroxinemia: A Syndrome That Can Be Confused With Thyrotoxicosis," *N Engl J Med*, 1982, 306:635-9.
Staub JJ, Althaus BU, Engler H, et al, "Spectrum of Subclinical and Overt Hypothyroidism: Effect on Thyrotropin, Prolactin, and Thyroid Reserve, and Metabolic Impact on Peripheral Target Tissues," *Am J Med*, 1992, 92(6):631-42.
Surks MI, "Guidelines for Thyroid Testing," *Lab Med*, 1993, 24(5):270-4.
Toft AD, "Thyroxine Therapy," *N Engl J Med*, 1994, 331(3):174-80.
Tomer Y and Davies TF, "Infection, Thyroid Disease, and Autoimmunity," *Endocr Rev*, 1993, 14(1):107-20.
Woeber KA, "Thyrotoxicosis and the Heart," *N Engl J Med*, 1992, 327(2):94-8.
Wolf PG and Meek JC, "Practical Approach to the Treatment of Hypothyroidism," *Am Fam Physician*, 1992, 45(2):722-31.

Thyroxine Binding Globulin
CPT 84442

Related Information
Free Thyroxine Index *on page 129*
T_3 Uptake *on page 201*
Thyroxine *on previous page*
Thyroxine, Free *on next page*

Synonyms T_4-Binding Globulin; TBG

Applies to Free Thyroxine Index, Calculated

Abstract Serum thyroid binding proteins include albumin, transthyretin (thyroid binding prealbumin), and, most important, thyroxine binding globulin. Familial TBG abnormalities may cause abnormalities in thyroid tests in essentially euthyroid subjects. TBG normally binds approximately 70% of total T_4 and a larger fraction of serum T_3[1]; affected euthyroid persons have low T_4.[2] T_3 and T_4 circulate almost entirely bound to the three thyroid hormone binding proteins. TBG is a glycoprotein. Its abnormalities are not clinical diseases (ie, they do not themselves require treatment). **This test is not for thyroglobulin.**

Patient Preparation No recent administration of radioactive isotopes or *in vivo* uptakes if method is by RIA.

Specimen Serum

Container Red top tube

Reference Range Adults: 1.2-2.5 mg/dL; 0-1 week: 3-8 mg/dL; 1-12 months: 3-6 mg/dL. Adult normals are reached about age 14.

Use Determine binding capacity for T_4 to distinguish between hyperthyroidism causing high T_4, and euthyroid individuals with increased binding by TBG who have increased T_4 and normal levels of free hormones. Document cases of hereditary deficiency or increase of TBG. In work-up of thyroid disease, in patients with low T_4, high T_3 uptake or the reverse, who clinically seem eumetabolic and have normal FTI, measurement of TBG is only occasionally needed. Some such patients may have hereditary anomalies of TBG. The most common explanation for increased TBG is increased endogenous or exogenous estrogens.[1] TBG is also increased by tamoxifen, pregnancy, perphenazine, and in some cases of liver disease, including hepatitis. TBG is increased in about 50% of individuals who have prolonged history of heroin use or who are treated with methadone.[1] Decreased TBG is found with some instances of chronic liver disease, nephrosis, and systemic disease, and with large amounts of glucocorticoids and in acromegaly. Individuals on androgens or anabolic steroids remain euthyroid in spite of decreased TBG and T_4 concentrations.[1] Increased TBG is found in certain genetically determined states. More information is provided in the article by Surks and Sievert. Although alterations of TBG are usually resolved by the thyroid profile, TBG must occasionally be directly measured.

Kindreds are described with elevated TBG and hyperthyroxinemia as a harmless genetic abnormality. They have normal levels of TSH and free T_4 and decreased T_3 uptake. Structural variants of TBG are inherited as X-chromosome linked traits, most inherited structural abnormalities in TBG cause decreased affinity for thyroid hormone.[1] Six families have been described with complete TBG deficiency. Such kindreds appear to have no gross structural defects in the TBG gene.[3]

A recent paper describes the effects of nicotinic acid on serum T_4, free T_4 index, and thyroxine-binding globulin (decreases), evaluating effects of nicotinic acid while maintaining a euthyroid state. Triiodothyronine (T_3) resin uptake ratios are increased.[4]

Limitations TBG is normal in **familial dysalbuminemic hyperthyroxinemia**, an entity which can be incorrectly identified as thyrotoxicosis.[5] Low T_3 uptake and normal **calculated free T_4 index** or thyroxine binding ratio often make measurement of TBG by RIA unnecessary.

Methodology Double antibody precipitation,[1] radioimmunoassay (RIA)

Additional Information The usual thyroid function studies (eg, free T_4 and TSH) should be performed before considering this test. The major indication for TBG testing is in diagnosis of **hereditary deficiency of TBG**. A euthyroid subject with a structural abnormality such as TBG-San Diego can be expected to have low total T_4 and free T_4 (FT_4) index but normal TSH.[1] Serum TBG concentration is increased in adults with late-stage HIV infections[6] and in children with HIV infections.[7] It is unchanged in long-term fasting (protein sparing)[8] and decreased with nicotinic acid therapy.[9]

Footnotes
1. Surks MI and Sievert R, "Drugs and Thyroid Function," *N Engl J Med*, 1995, 333(25):1688-94.
2. Sarne DH, Refetoff S, Nelson JC, et al, "A New Inherited Abnormality of Thyroxine-Binding Globulin (TBG-San Diego) With Decreased Affinity for Thyroxine and Triiodothyronine," *J Clin Endocrinol Metab*, 1989, 68(1):114-9.
3. Mori Y, Refetoff S, Flink IL, et al, "Detection of the Thyroxine-Binding Globulin (TBG) Gene in Six Unrelated Families With Complete TBG Deficiency," *J Clin Endocrinol Metab*, 1988, 67(4):727-33.
4. Shakir KM, Kroll S, Aprill BS, et al, "Nicotinic Acid Decreases Serum Thyroid Hormone Levels While Maintaining a Euthyroid State," *Mayo Clin Proc*, 1995, 70(6):556-8.
5. Ruiz M, Rajatanavin R, Young RA, et al, "Familial Dysalbuminemic Hyperthyroxinemia: A Syndrome That Can Be Confused With Thyrotoxicosis," *N Engl J Med*, 1982, 306:635-9.
6. Lambert M, Zech F, De Nayer P, et al, "Elevation of Serum Thyroxine-Binding Globulin (but Not of Cortisol-Binding Globulin and Sex Hormone-Binding Globulin) Associated With the Progression of Human Immunodeficiency Virus Infection," *Am J Med*, 1990, 89(6):748-51.
7. Laue L, Pizzo PA, Butler K, et al, "Growth and Neuroendocrine Dysfunction in Children With Acquired Immunodeficiency Syndrome," *J Pediatr*, 1990, 117(4):541-5.
8. Marine N, Hershman JM, Maxwell MH, et al, "Dietary Restriction on Serum Thyroid Hormone Levels," *Am J Med Sci*, 1991, 301(5):310-3.
9. O'Brien T, Silverberg JD, and Nguyen TT, "Nicotinic Acid-Induced Toxicity Associated With Cytopenia and Decreased Levels of Thyroxine-Binding Globulin," *Mayo Clin Proc*, 1992, 67(5):465-8.

(Continued)

Thyroxine Binding Globulin *(Continued)*

Drugs That Influence Thyroid Function*

Drugs That Decrease TSH Function
Dopamine
Glucocorticoids
Octreotide
Drugs That Alter Thyroid Hormone Secretion
Decreased thyroid hormone secretion
Lithium
Iodide
Amiodarone
Aminoglutethimide
Increased thyroid hormone secretion
Iodide
Amiodarone
Drugs That Decrease T_4 Absorption
Colestipol
Cholestyramine
Aluminum hydroxide
Ferrous sulfate
Sucralfate
Drugs That Alter T_4 and T_3 Transport in Serum
Increased serum TBG concentration
Estrogens
Tamoxifen
Heroin
Methadone
Mitotane
Fluorouracil
Decreased serum TBG concentration
Androgens
Anabolic steroids (eg, danazol)
Slow-release nicotinic acid
Glucocorticoids
Displacement from protein binding sites
Furosemide
Fenclofanac
Mefenamic acid
Salicylates
Drugs That Alter T_4 and T_3 Metabolism
Increased hepatic metabolism
Phenobarbital
Rifampin
Phenytoin
Carbamazepine
Decreased T_4 5'-deiodinase activity
Propylthiouracil
Amiodarone
Beta-adrenergic-antagonist drugs
Glucocorticoids
Cytokines
Interferon alfa
Interleukin-2

*TSH denotes thyrotropin, thyroxine (T_4), triiodothyronine (T_3), and thyroxine binding globulin (TBG).

From Surks MI and Sievert R, "Drugs and Thyroid Function," *N Engl J Med*, 1995, 333(25):1691, with permission.

References

Langsteger W, Stockigt JR, Docter R, et al, "Familial Dysalbuminaemic Hyperthyroxinaemia and Inherited Partial TBG Deficiency: First Report," *Clin Endocrinol*, 1994, 40(6):751-8.

Larsen PR, "The Thyroid," *Cecil Textbook of Medicine*, Wyngarden JB, Smith LH, and Bennett JC, eds, Philadelphia, PA: WB Saunders Co, 1992, 1248-71.

Nelson JC and Tomei RT, "Dependence of the Thyroxine/Thyroxine-Binding Globulin (TBG) Ratio and the Free Thyroxine Index on TBG Concentrations," *Clin Chem*, 1989, 35(4):541-4.

Refetoff S, "Inherited Thyroxine-Binding Globulin Abnormalities in Man," *Endocr Rev*, 1989, 10(3):275-93.

Surks MI, "Guidelines for Thyroid Testing," *Lab Med*, 1993, 24(5):270-4.

Thyroxine-Binding Protein Electrophoresis *see Thyroxine on page 206*

Thyroxine by RIA *see Thyroxine on page 206*

Thyroxine, Free

CPT 84439

Related Information

Free Thyroxine Index *on page 129*

Thyroid Antimicrosomal Antibody *on page 433*
Thyrotropin Receptor Antibody *on page 434*
Thyroxine *on page 206*
Thyroxine Binding Globulin *on previous page*
Triiodothyronine *on page 211*

Synonyms Free T_4; Free Thyroxine; FT_4; T_4, Free; Unbound T_4

Abstract Free T_4 is a very small fraction of total thyroxine (0.04%); it is the metabolically active fraction. Impetus for development of free T_4 emerged with recognition of euthyroid sick syndrome and euthyroid hyperthyroxinemia syndrome, settings in which conventional tests such as T_4 (total) and FTI fail to reliably reflect the patient's clinical thyroid status.[1]

Patient Preparation Recent injection of radioisotope may interfere, depending on assay system in use.

Specimen Serum

Container Red top tube

Storage Instructions Separate serum within 48 hours. Stable 2 weeks at 4°C.

Reference Range Approximately 0.7-1.8 ng/dL (SI: 9-23 pmol/L);[2] this example of a normal range is placed to permit comparison with the units in which conventional T_4 by RIA is expressed. Actual normal range varies somewhat between laboratories. Not increased in normal pregnancy.

Use A sensitive test for thyroid function, increased with hyperthyroidism.[2] Free T_4 is indicated when binding globulin (TBG) problems are perceived, or when conventional test results are borderline or seem inconsistent with clinical observations. Free thyroxine is normal in subjects with high thyroxine binding globulin hormone binding who are euthyroid (ie, free thyroxine should be normal in nonthyroidal diseases). It should be normal in familial dysalbuminemic hyperthyroxinemia. FT_4 is used to assess the severity of hyperthyroidism (eg, when sTSH is suppressed). FT_4 or thyroxine clarifies patient status in situations such as secondary hypothyroidism related to pituitary damage. When sTSH, used as the primary screening test is suppressed and FT_4 is normal, measurement of serum T_3 is indicated.[3] A diagnostic strategy for diagnostic work up of thyroid disease using TSH and FT_4 can be found in the listing Thyroid Stimulating Hormone *on page 204.*

Limitations FT_4 may be increased with radiologic contrast agents, propranolol, amiodarone, and heparin. It may be decreased with carbamazepine (Tegretol®). Free T_4 is a small part of total T_4 (0.04%). Free T_4 will not detect T_3 thyrotoxicosis. Increased free T_4 levels may occur in subjects with nonthyroid diseases. Such elevations are described as transient.[4] Low values are reported in patients with nonthyroidal illness. Discrepancies in free T_4 levels between methods are recognized.[1] Free T_4 is influenced by albumin concentration, requiring a number of follow-up tests. Reliability problems continue to be discussed with the newer methods.[5] Results of kits intended to serve in place of equilibrium dialysis technique may differ from the reference method. Concentrations of sTSH become abnormal before FT_4 levels do so early in primary hypo- and hyperthyroidism.

Methodology Equilibrium dialysis is the reference method; radioimmunoassay (RIA)

Additional Information The **free thyroxine index (FTI** or FTI-2) is a calculation derived from T_3 uptake and T_4 RIA, which are tests which remain in widespread use. Generally, the FTI and the free T_4 provide comparable information, but this is a complex topic. Costs of each should be compared. FT_4 is increased with levothyroxine therapy. **A free T_3** test exists as well. It is briefly discussed in the listing Triiodothyronine *on page 211.* Relationships of drugs to thyroid testing and physiology have recently been updated.[6] See table in listing Thyroxine Binding Globulin *on page 208.*

Footnotes

1. Gruhn JG, Barsano CP, and Kumar Y, "The Development of Tests of Thyroid Function," *Arch Pathol Lab Med*, 1987, 111(1):84-100.
2. Gupta MK, Salazar R, and Schumacher OP, "A Solid-Phase Radioimmunoassay for the Measurement of Free Thyroxine. A New Screening Test for Thyroid Function?" *Am J Clin Pathol*, 1983, 79:334-40.
3. Klee GG and Hay ID, "Biochemical Thyroid Function Testing," *Mayo Clin Proc*, 1994, 69(5):469-70.
4. Cooke RR and Pratt R, "Thyroid Function Tests in Acutely Ill Patients. Comparison of Analogue Based Free Thyroid Hormone Assays With Free Thyroxine Index," *Pathology*, 1986, 18(1):94-7.
5. Bethune JE, "Interpretation of Thyroid Function Tests," *Dis Mon*, 1989, 35(8):541-95.
6. Surks MI and Sievert R, "Drugs and Thyroid Function," *N Engl J Med*, 1995, 333(25):1688-94.

References

Kaptein EM, "Clinical Application of Free Thyroxine Determinations," *Clin Lab Med*, 1993, 13(3):653-72.

Surks MI, "Guidelines for Thyroid Testing," *Lab Med*, 1993, 24(5):270-4.

Utiger RD, "Subclinical Hyperthyroidism - Just a Low Serum Thyrotropin Concentration, or Something More?" *N Engl J Med*, 1994, 331(19):1302-3

Wilkins TA, "Free Thyroxine Assays: Analogue Methods," *Lancet*, 1985, 2(8460):884.

TIBC *see* Iron and Total Iron Binding Capacity/Transferrin *on page 150*

Tissue Polypeptide Antigen *see* CA 19-9 *on page 93*

Tocopherol *see* Vitamin E, Serum *on page 219*

α-Tocopherol *see* Vitamin E, Serum *on page 219*

Tolbutamide Test *see* Glucose, Fasting *on page 137*

Tolerance Test, Lactose *see* Lactose Tolerance Test *on page 157*

Total Bilirubin *see* Bilirubin, Total *on page 86*

Total Bilirubin, Neonatal *see* Bilirubin, Neonatal *on page 86*

Total Calcium, Serum *see* Calcium, Serum *on page 97*

Total Iron Binding Capacity *see* Iron and Total Iron Binding Capacity/Transferrin *on page 150*

Total Metanephrines *see* Metanephrines *on page 165*

Total Protein, Serum *see* Protein, Total, Serum *on page 194*

Total T₃ *see* Triiodothyronine *on page 211*

Total Urinary Catecholamines *replaced by* Catecholamines, Fractionation, Urine *on page 104*

Total Urinary Estrogens *see* Estrogens, Nonpregnant, Urine *on page 126*

TPA *see* CA 19-9 *on page 93*

Transaminase *see* Alanine Aminotransferase *on page 65*

Transaminase *see* Aspartate Aminotransferase *on page 84*

Transcutaneous Pulse Oximetry *see* Oxygen Saturation, Blood *on page 175*

Transferrin

CPT 84466

Related Information
Ferritin, Serum *on page 127*
Iron and Total Iron Binding Capacity/Transferrin *on page 150*
Protoporphyrin, Zinc, Blood *on page 196*

Synonyms Siderophilin; Tau Protein; TRF

Applies to Transferrin Index; Transferrin Receptors

Abstract Transferrin is an iron transport protein which binds iron released during hemoglobin catabolism as well as iron absorbed through the intestine, and transports it to the liver and reticuloendothelial system for storage.

Patient Preparation Fasting specimen is preferred.

Specimen Serum

Container Red top tube

Sampling Time Morning

Collection See Iron and Total Iron Binding Capacity/Transferrin *on page 150.*

Causes for Rejection Hemolysis

Reference Range Approximately 200-380 mg/dL (SI: 2.0-3.8 g/L), with some variation between laboratories

Use Increased in iron deficiency anemia. It is decreased in chronic inflammatory states, hereditary atransferrinemia, some instances of acquired liver disease, neoplasia, and renal disease. Transferrin is an index of nutritional status. Transferrin (tau protein) can be used as a marker for the presence of CSF in patients presenting with a nasal discharge of clear fluid.

Screening for hereditary hemochromatosis is addressed in the listing Iron and Total Iron Binding Capacity/Transferrin *on page 150.*

Limitations Increased in patients on oral contraceptives and in late pregnancy. May not be elevated in iron-deficient states in which there is severe protein malnutrition (eg, kwashiorkor) or chronic inflammation.

Methodology Radial immunodiffusion (RID), rate nephelometry, nephelometric scattering, immunoturbidity. The latter three immunochemical methods have shown good agreement in calibrator crossover and patient studies.[1]

Additional Information Transferrin is responsible for 50% to 70% of the iron binding capacity of serum. Since other proteins may bind iron, transferrin is not identical to TIBC. Transferrin is an iron transport protein receiving and binding iron for delivery to receptors at recipient cells. The human transferrin gene, responsible for production of this single chain, 77,000 dalton polypeptide resides on chromosome 3, band q 21-25. Transferrin has two iron-binding sites and is largely, but not exclusively, synthesized by the liver. There are over 20 genetic variants, largely single amino acid substitutions. Transferrin levels rise with iron deficiency and fall in cases of iron overload. Transferrin is normally only about one-third saturated and is responsible for circadian variation in serum iron (peak in AM) due to variable activity of the reticuloendothelial system. Transferrin saturation calculated as serum iron/TIBC may be used to screen for iron overload. **Transferrin index** calculated as serum iron/transferrin has been suggested as a better screen for iron overload.[2,3]

If used to screen for hemochromatosis,[3] repeat fasting transferrin and serum ferritin concentration are recommended as the next step.[4]

Recent studies have indicated that plasma **transferrin receptor concentrations** have a constant relationship to tissue receptors and reflect the rate of erythropoiesis except in iron deficiency.[5] Serum transferrin receptor concentrations appear to be independent of inflammation or liver disease,[6] unlike transferrin. Decreased binding of transferrin to erythroblasts[7] may lead to impaired iron uptake and may be a mechanism for the anemia of chronic disease. Decreased serum transferrin concentration may be associated with a poor progression-free survival in children with Hodgkin's disease.[8]

Footnotes
1. Christenson RH, Finley PR, and Silverman LM, "Immunochemical Assays for IgG, IgA, IgM and Transferrin Compared," *Clin Biochem,* 1989, 22(4):271-6.
2. Beilby J, Olynyk J, Ching S, et al, "Transferrin Index: An Alternative Method for Calculating the Iron Saturation of Transferrin," *Clin Chem,* 1992, 38(10):2078-81.
3. Olynyk JK and Bacon BR, "Hereditary Hemochromatosis. Detecting and Correcting Iron Overload," *Postgrad Med,* 1994, 96(5):151-8, 161, 165.
4. Phatak PD and Cappuccio JD, "Management of Hereditary Hemochromatosis," *Blood Rev,* 1994, 8(4):193-8.
5. Huebers HA, Beguin Y, Pootrakul P, et al, "Intact Transferrin Receptors in Human Plasma and Their Relation to Erythropoiesis," *Blood,* 1990, 75(1):102-7.
6. Ferguson BJ, Skikne BS, Simpson KM, et al, "Serum Transferrin Receptor Distinguishes the Anemia of Chronic Disease From Iron Deficiency Anemia," *J Lab Clin Med,* 1992, 119(4):385-90.
7. Vreugdenhil G, Kroos MJ, van Eijk HG, et al, "Impaired Iron Uptake and Transferrin Binding by Erythroblasts in the Anaemia of Rheumatoid Arthritis," *Br J Rheumatol,* 1990, 29(5):335-9.
8. Hann HW, Lange B, Stahlhut MW, et al, "Prognostic Importance of Serum Transferrin and Ferritin in Childhood Hodgkin's Disease," *Cancer,* 1990, 66(2):313-6.

References
Cook JD, Skikne BS, and Baynes RD, "Iron Deficiency: The Global Perspective," *Adv Exp Med Biol,* 1994, 356:219-28.
Keir G, Zeman A, Brookes G, et al, "Immunoblotting of Transferrin in the Identification of Cerebrospinal Fluid Otorrhoea and Rhinorrhoea," *Ann Clin Biochem,* 1992, 29(Pt 2):210-3.
Macdougall IC, "Monitoring of Iron Status and Iron Supplementation in Patients Treated With Erythropoietin," *Curr Opin Nephrol Hypertens,* 1994, 3(6):620-5.
Sempos CT, Looker AC, Gillum RF, et al, "Body Iron Stores and the Risk of Coronary Heart Disease," *N Engl J Med,* 1994, 330(16):1119-24.

Transferrin Index *see* Transferrin *on this page*

Transferrin Receptor *see* Ferritin, Serum *on page 127*

Transferrin Receptors *see* Transferrin *on this page*

TRF *see* Transferrin *on this page*

TRH Stimulation Test *see* Thyroid Stimulating Hormone *on page 204*

Triacylglycerol Acylhydrolase *see* Lipase, Serum *on page 158*

Triacylglycerols *see* Triglycerides *on this page*

Triglycerides

CPT 84478

Related Information
Apolipoprotein A and B *on page 82*
Cholesterol, Serum *on page 110*
High Density Lipoprotein Cholesterol *on page 143*
Lipid Profile *on page 159*
Lipoprotein Electrophoresis *on page 161*
Low Density Lipoprotein Cholesterol *on page 162*

Synonyms TG; Triacylglycerols

Applies to Chylomicrons; VLDL

Test Commonly Includes Triglycerides are included in the lipid profiles (lipoprotein analyses) of most laboratories.

Abstract Triglycerides (TG) are a family of complex lipids composed of glycerol esterified with three fatty acids (saturated or unsaturated) of the same or different lengths. Triglycerides are not soluble in blood and are therefore transported as chylomicrons (TG from exogenous source) or as VLDL (TG from endogenous source). Triglycerides constitute 95% of tissue storage fat.

Patient Preparation The patient should be fasting for 12-14 hours and should be on a stable diet 3 weeks prior to collection of blood. Avoid alcohol for 3 days. See Preparation in listing Cholesterol, Serum *on page 110.*

Specimen Serum

Container Red top tube; lavender top (EDTA) tube is used by some outstanding laboratories

Causes for Rejection Specimen collected in a glycerinated tube, nonfasting specimen

(Continued)

Triglycerides *(Continued)*

Reference Range See tables. These tables are based on plasma triglycerides. Triglyceride values increase with aging. With cholesterol values within normal ranges, triglyceride levels <250 mg/dL (SI: <2.82 mmol/L) (90th percentile) are not thought to be related to risk; *vide infra*.

Reference Values for Plasma Triglycerides for White Males* (mg/L)

Age	Percentiles			
	5	50	90	95
0-9 y	300	550	850	1000
10-14 y	300	650	1000	1250
15-19 y	350	800	1200	1500
20-24 y	450	1000	1650	2000
25-29 y	450	1150	2000	2500
30-34 y	500	1300	2150	2650
35-39 y	550	1450	2500	3200
40-54 y	550	1500	2500	3200
55-64 y	600	1400	2350	2900
65+ y	550	1350	2100	2600

*From the LRC Prevalence Study (North America).

Reference Values for Plasma Triglycerides for White Females* (mg/L)

Age	Percentiles			
	5	50	90	95
0-9 y	350	600	950	1100
10-19 y	400	750	1150	1300
20-34 y	400	900	1450	1700
35-39 y	400	950	1600	1950
40-44 y	450	1050	1700	2100
45-49 y	450	1100	1850	2300
50-54 y	550	1200	1900	2400
55-64 y	550	1250	2000	2500
65+ y	600	1300	2050	2400

*From the LRC Prevalence Study (North America).

Reference Values for Plasma Triglycerides for Black Males* (mg/L)

Age	Percentiles†			
	5	50	90	95
0-9 y	310	470	750	880
10-19 y	310	530	880	1020
20-29 y	–	710	1250	–
30-39 y	420	910	1660	2240
40-49 y	520	970	2150	2940
50-59 y	–	1050	–	–
60+ y	–	960	–	–

†5th and 95th percentiles not given if n <100; 90th percentile not given if n <75.

*From the LRC Prevalence Study (North America).

Reference Values for Plasma Triglycerides for Black Females* (mg/L)

Age	Percentiles†			
	5	50	90	95
0-9 y	330	500	830	940
10-19 y	360	600	950	1100
20-29 y	380	680	1180	1370
30-39 y	380	740	1290	1500
40-49 y	430	840	1530	1880
50-59 y	–	940	1760	–
60+ y	–	1060	–	–

†5th and 95th percentiles not given if n <100; 90th percentile not given if n <75.

*From the LRC Prevalence Study (North America).

Use Evaluate turbid samples of blood, plasma, and serum; work-up of chylomicronemia; evaluate hyperlipidemia; occasional cases of diabetes mellitus and/or pancreatitis are detected by hypertriglyceridemia. High levels may occur with hypothyroidism, nephrotic syndromes, carbohydrate-sensitive hypertriglyceridemia, glycogen storage disease, and in hyperlipoproteinemias type I, IIb, III, IV, and V. Some alcoholics have hypertriglyceridemia which disappears with abstinence. Extremely high triglyceride levels may occur with alcohol abuse. Triglyceride is needed for calculation of LDLC (low density lipoprotein cholesterol) concentration. Disturbances in triglyceride metabolism relate to diabetes and are an interactive risk factor for atherosclerotic disease.[1] Although the role of hypertriglyceridemia as a risk factor for coronary arterial disease has been somewhat controversial, men and women with low serum HDL cholesterol and high serum triglyceride concentrations have a higher relative risk of coronary artery disease (*vide infra*). The combination of low HDL and high TG is important to project outcome following coronary bypass.[2] In familial combined hyperlipidemia, hypertriglyceridemia may be found before hypercholesterolemia. Many knowledgeable authorities favor screening with lipid profiles, including triglycerides, for reasons discussed elsewhere in this listing and in other listings. In exogenous hypertriglyceridemia, chylomicrons float as a layer in the tube of refrigerated, stored serum. Triglyceride determination is needed with cholesterol and HDLC to calculate LDLC:

Friedewald estimation = LDLC = cholesterol - HDLC - (TG/5).

This formula is valid when TG levels are <400 mg/dL (<10.4 mmol/L) without chylomicrons or floating beta VLDL.

Limitations If triglyceride is >400 mg/dL, LDL cannot be calculated accurately by the Friedewald formula.[3] Correction for free serum glycerol in critically ill patients or patients on hyperalimentation with glycerol-based solutions may be necessary in some enzymatic methods.[4] The most common cause of triglyceride increase is inadequate patient fasting, which is a cause for rejection of the specimen.

Methodology Enzymatic, colorimetric. A method for direct measurement of LDLC is now available. In this procedure, HDL and VLDL are separated from LDL by a filter which traps antibody coated latex beads.

Additional Information Classic research from the Framingham studies in the 1970s identified major risk factors for coronary artery disease as hypertension, high serum cholesterol concentrations, and cigarette smoking. New analyses from the Framingham heart study demonstrate that men and women with high serum triglyceride concentrations (>151 mg/dL, SI: >1.7 mmol/L) and low serum HDL concentrations have a significantly higher rate of coronary artery disease. This high risk group (high serum triglycerides, low serum HDL) appears independent of the major risk factors including low serum HDL concentrations.[5] The Helsinki Heart Study reported a 5 year randomized coronary prevention trial among dyslipemic, middle-aged men.[6] This study found a relative risk of 3.8 for those men with an **HDL cholesterol/LDL cholesterol** ratio of 5 and serum triglycerides >203 mg/dL (>2.3 mmol/L). Men with HDL cholesterol/LDL cholesterol ratios >5 and serum triglyceride concentrations <2.3 mmol/L had a relative risk of 1.2. A similar European study[7] reported similar findings. Clearly, serum triglyceride concentration is a factor interacting with effects of cholesterol and HDL cholesterol. Variations in apolipoprotein A-I and triglyceride concentrations account for 66% of the population variance in serum HDL cholesterol concentrations.[8] Fundamental relationships observed between HDL cholesterol, apolipoprotein A-I, and triglyceride were unaltered by levels of factors under personal volition such as obesity, physical activity/inactivity, and smoking.[8] Triglycerides commonly increase with obesity and may increase with chronic renal or liver disease. A positive association exists between diabetes mellitus and hypertriglyceridemia. Extremely high triglyceride levels suggest the possibility of pancreatitis. **Chylomicronemia**, although associated with pancreatitis, is not accompanied by increased atherogenesis. Chylomicrons are not seen in normal fasting serum, but are found in the sera of normal subjects following a fatty meal as exogenous triglycerides. Left refrigerated, chylomicrons float to the surface of a sample overnight; VLDL remains in suspension. Triglyceride physiologically is carried mostly as very low density lipoproteins (VLDL). The triglyceride in VLDL is endogenous from hepatic synthesis.

When turbidity of blood, serum, or plasma is seen, triglyceride is often >350 mg/dL. **Fasting chylomicronemia** occurs with, but is not limited to, deficiency of apo-CII (apolipoprotein work-up). It occurs also with deficiency of **lipoprotein lipase**.

A positive association exists between gout and hypertriglyceridemia.

Hypertriglyceridemia is found in glycogen storage **disease-Ia** with other abnormalities.[9]

Drug effects have been summarized.[10] Some women on estrogens and high estrogen oral contraceptives have an increase of triglyceride. Increases occur with pregnancy, similar to those with oral contraceptives. Hypertriglyceridemia is associated with use of thiazide diuretics and beta-adrenergic blocking agents.

Footnotes

1. Rifkind BM and Segal P, "Lipid Research Clinics Program Reference Values for Hyperlipidemia and Hypolipidemia," *JAMA*, 1983, 250:1869-72.

2. Lindén T, Bondjers G, Karlsson T, et al, "Serum Triglycerides and HDL Cholesterol - Major Predictors of Long-Term Survival After Coronary Surgery," *Eur Heart J*, 1994, 15(6):747-52.
3. Friedewald WT, Levy RI, and Fredrickson DS, "Estimation of the Concentration of Low-Density Lipoprotein Cholesterol in Plasma, Without Use of the Preparative Ultracentrifuge," *Clin Chem*, 1972, 18:499-502.
4. Jessen RH, Dass CJ, and Eckfeldt JH, "Do Enzymatic Analyses of Serum Triglycerides Really Need Blanking for Free Glycerol?" *Clin Chem*, 1990, 36(7):1372-5.
5. Castelli WP, "Epidemiology of Triglycerides: A View from Framingham," *Am J Cardiol*, 1992, 70(19):3H-9H.
6. Manninen V, Tenkanen L, Koskinen P, et al, "Joint Effects of Serum Triglyceride and LDL Cholesterol and HDL Cholesterol Concentrations on Coronary Heart Disease Risk in the Helsinki Heart Study - Implications for Treatment," *Circulation*, 1992, 85(1):37-45.
7. Assmann G and Schulte H, "Role of Triglycerides in Coronary Artery Disease: Lessons From the Prospective Cardiovascular Münster Study," *Am J Cardiol*, 1992, 70(19):10H-13H.
8. Patsch W, Sharrett AR, Sorlie PD, et al, "The Relation of High Density Lipoprotein Cholesterol and Its Subfractions to Apolipoprotein A-I and Fasting Triglycerides: The Role of Environmental Factors - The Atherosclerosis Risk in Communities (ARIC) Study," *Am J Epidemiol*, 1992, 136(5):546-57.
9. Talente GM, Coleman RA, Alter C, et al, "Glycogen Storage Disease in Adults," *Ann Intern Med*, 1994, 120(3):218-26.
10. Steinmetz J, Jouanel P, and Thuillier Y, "Triglycerides," *Drug Effects on Laboratory Test Results Analytical Interferences and Pharmacological Effects*, Siest G and Galteau MM, eds, Littleton, MA: PSG Publishing Co Inc, 1988, 405-22.

References
Criqui MH, Heiss G, Cohn R, et al, "Plasma Triglyceride Level and Mortality From Coronary Heart Disease," *N Engl J Med*, 1993, 328(17):1220-5.

Hostetter AL, "Screening for Dyslipidemia, Practice Parameter" *Am J Clin Pathol*, 1995, 103(4):380-5.

Kihara S, Matsuzawa Y, Kubo M, et al, "Autoimmune Hyperchylomicronemia," *N Engl J Med*, 1989, 320(19):1255-9.

Maeda I, Hayashi S, Fushimi R, et al, "Error Detection of High Concentrations of Endogenous Free Glycerol in Determination of Serum Triglyceride With the TBA-80S Automated Discrete Analyzer," *Clin Chem*, 1992, 38(7):1376-7.

McQueen MJ, Henderson AR, Patten RL, et al, "Results of a Province-Wide Quality Assurance Program Assessing the Accuracy of Cholesterol, Triglycerides, and High-Density Lipoprotein Cholesterol Measurements and Calculated Low-Density Lipoprotein Cholesterol in Ontario, Using Fresh Human Serum," *Arch Pathol Lab Med*, 1991, 115(12):1217-22.

O'Meara NM, Lewis GF, Cabana VG, et al, "Role of Basal Triglyceride and High Density Lipoprotein in Determination of Postprandial Lipid and Lipoprotein Responses," *J Clin Endocrinol Metab*, 1992, 75(2):465-71.

Peterson CM, Jovanovic-Peterson L, Mills JL, et al, "The Diabetes in Early Pregnancy Study: Changes in Cholesterol, Triglycerides, Body Weight, and Blood Pressure," *Am J Obstet Gynecol*, 1992, 166(2):513-8.

Sady SP, Thompson PD, Cullinane EM, et al, "Prolonged Exercise Augments Plasma Triglyceride Clearance," *JAMA*, 1986, 256(18):2552-5.

Uiterwaal CS, Grobbee DE, Witteman JC, et al, "Postprandial Triglyceride Response in Young Adult Men and Familial Risk for Coronary Atherosclerosis," *Ann Intern Med*, 1994, 121(8):576-83.

Yeshurun D and Gotto AM Jr, "Hyperlipidemia: Perspectives in Diagnosis and Treatment," *South Med J*, 1995, 88(4):379-91.

Triiodothyronine

CPT 84480

Related Information

Free Thyroxine Index *on page 129*
Thyroid Stimulating Hormone *on page 204*
Thyroxine *on page 206*
Thyroxine, Free *on page 208*

Synonyms T_3, Total; Total T_3; Triiodothyronine, Total

Abstract T_3 (triiodothyronine) is a thyroid hormone produced mainly from the peripheral conversion of T_4 (a prohormone). T_3 has a greater biological activity than T_4 and binds to TBG less tightly than T_4. When total or free thyroxine (T_4 or FT_4) are normal and TSH is low, high T_3 confirms triiodothyronine toxicosis.

Patient Preparation Avoid radioisotope administration prior to collection of specimen if RIA is used for assay. T_3 may be decreased with radiologic contrast agents, propranolol, and amiodarone.

Specimen Serum

Container Red top tube

Storage Instructions Separate serum within 48 hours. Stable up to 2 weeks at 25°C.

Reference Range Values in infancy and childhood are higher than in adults. Adults: Approximately 80-200 ng/dL (SI: 1.2-3.1 nmol/L) with some variation between laboratories. A computer-based method to validate reference ranges lists a normal range of 50-140 ng/dL (SI: 0.7-2.1 nmol/L).[1] Increase occurs in pregnancy.

Use This thyroid function test is indicated in patients with decreased sTSH and normal free thyroxine and/or thyroxine levels. It measures T_3, useful in evaluation of hyperthyroid states, particularly in the diagnosis of T_3 thyrotoxicosis, in which T_3 is increased and T_4 is within normal limits. (See diagnostic diagram in the listing Thyroid Stimulating Hormone *on page 204*.) T_3 toxicosis is occasionally found in Graves' disease. It occurs with a single toxic nodule, multinodular thyrotoxicosis, and following treatment with T_3 (Cytomel®).[2] It is increased in and helpful for confirmation of the diagnosis of conventional hyperthyroidism, in which commonly both serum T_3 and T_4 concentrations are increased. T_3 is needed in patients with clinical evidence for hyperthyroidism when the T_4

is normal and the patient is clinically hyperthyroid ("T_3 thyrotoxicosis"). It is normal to slightly increased with familial dysalbuminemic hyperthyroxinemia. Recommended for patients with supraventricular tachycardia, for patients with fatigue and weight loss not otherwise explained, or for those with proximal myopathy, in whom T_4 concentrations are not elevated.

Limitations T_3 is decreased with nonthyroidal chronic diseases and influenced by the state of nutrition. It may be normal with thyrotoxicosis (thyroxine thyrotoxicosis).[3,4] Variations in TBG and other binding proteins can affect T_3. It is decreased with nicotinic acid.[5] Increases may be found with use of oral contraceptives, pregnancy, and other binding protein abnormalities outlined in the listing Thyroxine *on page 206*. Fasting causes T_3 and TSH to decrease.[6]

Contraindications T_3 is not reliable for evaluation of hypothyroidism.

Methodology Radioimmunoassay (RIA), immunochemiluminometric assay, fluorescence polarization immunoassay (FPIA), fluorometric immunoassay

Additional Information Thyroid hormones exist in human plasma as free and bound forms (ie, free T_3 and free T_4, as well as bound T_3 and bound T_4). Less than 1% of total serum T_3 is in the free form. Serum concentrations of the free forms of T_3 and T_4 are regulated by feedback systems and appear to parallel rates of cellular uptake. Thus, the free hormone fraction determines the thyroid status of the individual. Essentially, bound fractions are unavailable to exert metabolic effects. Proteins that bind T_3 include thyroxine binding globulin, transthyretin, and albumin. As the serum concentrations of the binding proteins rise so does the total T_3, while the free T_3 fraction may be unchanged. An example of when this occurs is in pregnancy. T_3 has a higher metabolic potency relative to T_4. As approximately 33% of T_4 is converted to T_3, T_4 appears to have little intrinsic metabolic activity in humans. See table for comparison of T_3 with T_4.

Comparison of T_3 and T_4 in Humans

	T_3	T_4
Serum concentration		
total (µg/dL)	0.14	8.0
free (ng/dL)	0.4	1.6
Fraction of total serum hormone that is in the free form (%)	0.3	0.02
Distribution volume (L)	35	10
Fraction intracellular (%)	64	10-20
Half-life (days)	1	7
Production rate (µg/day)	33	80
Fraction directly from thyroid (%)	20	100
Relative metabolic potency	1	0.3

From Larsen PR, "The Thyroid," *Cecil Textbook of Medicine*, Vol 2, Wyngarden JB, Smith LH, and Bennett JC, eds, Philadelphia, PA: WB Saunders Co, 1992, 1250, with permission.

Increased T_3 often occurs in hyperthyroidism, but in approximately 5% of cases only T_3 is elevated, "T_3 toxicosis." Do not confuse T_3 with T_3 uptake; these are two different tests. The latter is done very commonly as part of the usual thyroid profile. **Free T_3** may be assayed by an RIA procedure.

Decreased serum T_3 concentrations are reported in individuals with increased serum tumor necrosis factor.[7]

Footnotes

1. Luttrell B and Watters S, "Computerized Method for Validating Laboratory Reference Ranges for Triiodothyronine and Thyroxine Immunoassays," *Clin Chem*, 1991, 37(3):438-42.
2. Bethune JE, "Interpretation of Thyroid Function Tests," *Dis Mon*, 1989, 35(8):541-95.
3. Blank MS and Tucci JR, "A Case of Thyroxine Thyrotoxicosis," *Arch Intern Med*, 1987, 147(5):863-4.
4. Woeber KA, "Thyrotoxicosis and the Heart," *N Engl J Med*, 1992, 327(2):94-8.
5. Shakir KM, Kroll S, Aprill BS, et al, "Nicotinic Acid Decreases Serum Thyroid Hormone Levels While Maintaining a Euthyroid State," *Mayo Clin Proc*, 1995, 70(6):556-8.
6. Unger J, "Fasting Induces a Decrease in Serum Thyroglobulin in Normal Subjects," *J Clin Endocrinol Metab*, 1988, 67(6):1309-11.
7. Mooradian AD, Reed RL, Osterweil D, et al, "Decreased Serum Triiodothyronine Is Associated With Increased Concentrations of Tumor Necrosis Factor," *J Clin Endocrinol Metab*, 1990, 71(5):1239-42.

References
Austin D and Toivola B, "Laboratory Evaluation of an Immunochemiluminometric Assay of Triiodothyronine in Serum," *Clin Chem*, 1990, 36(2):334-7.

Camara PD, Velletri K, Krupski M, et al, "Evaluation of the Boehringer Mannheim ES 300 Immunoassay Analyzer and Comparison With Enzyme Immunoassay, Fluorescence Polarization Immunoassay, and Radioimmunoassay Methods," *Clin Biochem*, 1992, 25(4):251-4.

Franklyn JA, "The Management of Hyperthyroidism," *N Engl J Med*, 1994, 330(24):1731-8.

Larsen PR, "The Thyroid," *Cecil Textbook of Medicine*, 19th ed, Vol 2, Wyngarden JB, Smith LH, and Bennett JC, eds, Philadelphia, PA: WB Saunders Co, 1992, 1248-71.

(Continued)

Triiodothyronine *(Continued)*

Papanastasiou-Diamandi A, Shankaran P, and Khosravi MJ, "Immunoassay of Triiodo-thyronine in Serum by Time-Resolved Fluorometric Measurement of Europium-Chelate Complexes in Solution," *Clin Biochem*, 1992, 25(4):255-61.

Price A, Griffiths H, Kennedy L, et al, "Comparison of Methods for the Determination of Unbound Triiodothyronine in Pregnancy," *Clin Endocrinol (Oxf)*, 1992, 37(1):41-4.

Runnels BL, Garry PJ, Hunt WC, et al, "Thyroid Function in a Healthy Elderly Population: Implications for Clinical Evaluation," *J Gerontol*, 1991, 46(1):B39-44.

Surks MI, "Guidelines for Thyroid Testing," *Lab Med*, 1993, 24(5):270-4.

Takamatsu J, Kuma K, and Mozai T, "Serum Triiodothyronine to Thyroxine Ratio: A Newly Recognized Predictor of the Outcome of Hyperthyroidism Due to Graves' Disease," *J Clin Endocrinol Metab*, 1986, 62(5):980-3.

Utiger RD, "Altered Thyroid Function in Nonthyroidal Illness and Surgery. To Treat or Not to Treat?" *N Engl J Med*, 1995, 333(23):1562-3.

Triiodothyronine, Total *see* Triiodothyronine *on previous page*

Troponin

CPT 83520

Related Information

Cardiac Enzymes/Isoenzymes *on page 102*
Creatine Kinase *on page 115*
Creatine Kinase Isoenzymes/Isoforms *on page 115*
Lactate Dehydrogenase *on page 153*
Lactate Dehydrogenase Isoenzymes *on page 154*
Myoglobin, Blood *on page 167*
Myoglobin, Qualitative, Urine *on page 644*

Synonyms Cardiac Troponin; cTnI (Troponin I); cTnT (Troponin T)

Applies to Troponin C; Troponin I; Troponin T

Abstract Cardiac **troponin I (cTnI)** and **troponin T (cTnT)** are very useful in the diagnosis of acute myocardial injury because some of their isoforms show a high degree of cardiac specificity.[1] CTnT, however, may be increased in patients with chronic renal failure, acute trauma involving muscle, rhabdomyolysis, polymyositis, or dermatomyositis, a nonspecificity not shared by cTnI. Cardiac cTnI is alone among markers for myocardial injury which is not expressed in a regenerative phase of striated (skeletal) muscle. Use of troponin I should provide simpler, more cost-effective care than routine application of echocardiography[2] or the use of several other cardiac enzyme markers.

Specimen Serum

Container Red top tube

Sampling Time Serial sampling, tracking sequential increases and decreases in analyte concentration is optimal for troponin as it is for CK, CK-MB, LDH, and LDH isoenzymes to document or rule out AMI. Sequences at 0, 4, 8, and 12 hours may be useful to rule out AMI.

Storage Instructions Serum stable 4 days at 4°C.

Causes for Rejection Specimen hemolyzed

Reference Range Depends on method. Troponin I: <0.35 ng/mL; troponin T: <0.2 µg/L (SI: <0.2 µg/L)[3]

Critical Values cTnI: >1.5 ng/mL

Use Diagnose AMI and minor myocardial cell damage from a few hours after onset of symptoms to as long as 5-7 days. The sensitivity of troponin T for detecting AMI was 100% 10-190 hours after onset; sensitivity on the seventh day after admission was 84%.[4] In another study, CK-MB was more sensitive during the first 4 hours after onset of chest pain, but thereafter the sensitivities of troponin I and CK-MB were similar up to 48 hours.[5] Troponin I remains increased longer than CK-MB and is more cardiac specific.[4,5] Its superior specificity over CK-MB in detection of perioperative myocardial injury or AMI is documented. Troponin I may be warranted following even minor trauma, when the differential diagnosis includes AMI.

Limitations Chemical markers do not signal an infarct beginning to take place at the moment of sampling. A single determination may be misleading. A bedside assay for cardiac troponin T is qualitative. For instance, it may not detect reinfarction.[6]

Troponin T occurs with angina at rest in some subjects, diminishing its specificity for diagnosis of AMI. cTnT may be increased in patients with renal failure, muscle injury, disease or rhabdomyolysis, nonspecificity not shared by cTnI.

Methodology Enzyme immunoassay (EIA), one-step[7]; double monoclonal sandwich enzyme immunoassay (EIA)[5]

Additional Information The contractile proteins of the myofibril include the regulatory protein, troponin. Troponin is a complex of three proteins, troponin C (the calcium-binding subunit, molecular weight 18 kD), troponin I (the actomyosin-adenosine triphosphatase-inhibiting subunit, molecular weight 26.5 kD), and troponin T (the tropomyosin-binding subunit, molecular weight 39 kD).[1] The distribution of these isoforms varies between cardiac muscle and slow- and fast-twitch skeletal muscle. Their importance lies in the fact that some isoforms show a high degree of cardiac specificity. An enzyme immunoassay for cardiac troponin T showed a cross reactivity with troponin T extracted from mixed skeletal muscle fibers <2%.[8] The measurement of either troponin I or troponin T is becoming the most important addition to the clinical assessment of myocardial injury.

Antman et al evaluated cardiac troponin T as a bedside assay for AMI. They found it rapid and sensitive.[6] However, they did not compare it to quantitative laboratory assay for troponin I or several other useful markers.[9]

Troponin I assays have excellent diagnostic accuracy of AMI following noncardiac surgery. The assay avoids many of the false-positives seen with use of CK-MB.[2] Troponin I assays may be performed rapidly to provide suitable emergency room application. Keffer predicts wide application of cTnI, CK-MB, and myoglobin.[10] A study of prediction of coronary arterial reperfusion 90 minutes following thrombolytic therapy found serial cardiac troponin I more accurate than CK-MB and myoglobin, but larger studies are needed.[11]

Footnotes

1. Apple FS, "Acute Myocardial Infarction and Coronary Reperfusion. Serum Cardiac Markers for the 1990s," *Clin Chem*, 1992, 97(2):217-26.

2. Adams JE 3rd, Sicard GA, Allen BT, et al, "Diagnosis of Perioperative Myocardial Infarction With Measurement of Cardiac Troponin I," *N Engl J Med*, 1994, 330(10):670-4.

3. Collinson PO, Moseley D, Stubbs PJ, et al, "Troponin T for the Differential Diagnosis of Ischaemic Myocardial Damage," *Ann Clin Biochem*, 1993, 30(Pt 1):11-6.

4. Mair J, Artner-Dworzak E, Lechleitner P, et al, "Cardiac Troponin T in Diagnosis of Acute Myocardial Infarction," *Clin Chem*, 1991, 37(6):845-52.

5. Bodor GS, Porter S, Landt Y, et al, "Development of Monoclonal Antibodies for An Assay of Cardiac Troponin I and Preliminary Results in Suspected Cases of Myocardial Infarction," *Clin Chem*, 1992, 38(11):2203-14.

6. Antman EM, Grudzien C, and Sacks DB, "Evaluation of a Rapid Bedside Assay for Detection of Serum Cardiac Troponin T," *JAMA*, 1995, 273(16):1279-82.

7. Katus HA, Looser S, Hallermayer K, et al, "Development and *in vitro* Characterization of A New Immunoassay of Cardiac Troponin T," *Clin Chem*, 1992, 38(3):386-93.

8. Katus HA, Remppis A, Neumann FJ, et al, "Diagnostic Efficiency of Troponin T Measurements in Acute Myocardial Infarction," *Circulation*, 1991, 83(3):902-12.

9. Borzak S, "Bedside Serum Cardiac Troponin T Analysis Was Sensitive for Myocardial Infarction," *ACP J Club*, 1995, 123(3):72.

10. Keffer JH, "Myocardial Markers of Injury," *Am J Clin Pathol*, 1996, 105:305-20.

11. Apple FS, Henry TD, Berger CR, et al, "Early Monitoring of Serum Cardiac Troponin I for Assessment of Coronary Reperfusion Following Thrombolytic Therapy," *Am J Clin Pathol*, 1996, 105(1):6-10.

References

Anderson PA, Malouf NN, Oakeley AE, et al, "Troponin T Isoform Expression in Humans. A Comparison Among Normal and Failing Adult Heart, Fetal Heart, and Adult and Fetal Skeletal Muscle," *Circ Res*, 1991, 69(5):1226-33.

Cummins B, Russell GJ, Chandler ST, et al, "Uptake of Radioiodinated Cardiac Specific Troponin I Antibodies in Myocardial Infarction," *Cardiovasc Res*, 1990, 24(4):317-27.

Donnelly R and Hillis WS, "Cardiac Troponin T," *Lancet*, 1993, 341(8842):410-1.

Gambino R, "Cardiac Troponin I and Glycogen Phosphorylase BB," *Lab Rep*, 1995, 17(9):65-6.

Gerhardt W, Katus H, Ravkilde J, et al, "S-Troponin T in Suspected Ischemic Myocardial Injury Compared With Mass and Catalytic Concentrations of S-Creatine Kinase Isoenzyme MB," *Clin Chem*, 1991, 37(8):1405-11.

Goldman L, "Assessment of Perioperative Cardiac Risk," *N Engl J Med*, 1994, 330(10):707-9.

Hamm CW, "New Serum Markers for Acute Myocardial Infarction," *N Engl J Med*, 1994, 331(9):561-6.

Hamm CW, Ravkilde J, Gerhardt W, et al, "The Prognostic Value of Serum Troponin T in Unstable Angina," *N Engl J Med*, 1992, 327(3):192-4.

Keffer JH, "The Revolution in Biochemical Assessment of Ischemic Myocardial Injury," presented at *Third Annual Progress in Clinical Pathology*, Sept 1995, University of Texas Southwestern Medical Center, Dallas, TX.

Parmacek MS and Leiden JM, "Structure, Function, and Regulation of Troponin C," *Circulation*, 1991, 84(3):991-1003.

"Troponin T and Myocardial Damage," *Lancet*, 1991, 338(8758):23-4.

Voss EM, Sharkey SW, Gernert AE, et al, "Human and Canine Cardiac Troponin T and Creatine Kinase-MB Distribution in Normal and Diseased Myocardium, Infarct Sizing Using Serum Profiles," *Arch Pathol Lab Med*, 1995, 119(9):799-806.

Zabel M, Koster W, and Hohnloser SH, "Usefulness of CKMB and Troponin T Determinations in Patients With Acute Myocardial Infarction Complicated by Ventricular Fibrillation," *Clin Cardiol*, 1993, 16(1):23-5.

Troponin C *see* Troponin *on this page*

Troponin I *see* Troponin *on this page*

Troponin T *see* Troponin *on this page*

True Cholinesterase *see* Acetylcholinesterase, Red Cell *on page 62*

Trypsin Activity, Stool *see* Chloride, Sweat *on page 108*

Trypsin, Immunoreactive *see* Amylase, Urine *on page 79*

Trypsinogen, Immunoreactive *see* Chloride, Sweat *on page 108*

TSH *see* Thyroid Stimulating Hormone *on page 204*

TSH, Filter Paper *see* Thyroid Stimulating Hormone Screen, Filter Paper *on page 205*

Tubeless Gastric Analysis *replaced by* Gastric Analysis *on page 133*

UDP Galactose-4-Epimerase Deficiency *see* Galactose-1-Phosphate Uridyl Transferase, Erythrocyte *on page 131*

U-III-S see Uroporphyrinogen III Synthase, Erythrocyte *on page 215*

Ultrasensitive TSH see Thyroid Stimulating Hormone *on page 204*

Unbound T$_4$ see Thyroxine, Free *on page 208*

Unconjugated Estriol, Pregnancy see Estriol, Unconjugated, Pregnancy, Blood or Urine *on page 126*

U/P Ratio see Osmolality, Urine *on page 173*

Urate see Uric Acid, Serum *on this page*

Urate, Urine see Uric Acid, Urine *on page 215*

Urea Clearance replaced by Creatinine Clearance *on page 117*

Urea Nitrogen, Blood

CPT 84520

Related Information
BUN/Creatinine Ratio *on page 92*
Creatinine Clearance *on page 117*
Creatinine, Serum *on page 118*
Kidney Biopsy *on page 47*
Kidney Stone Analysis *on page 640*
Osmolality, Calculated *on page 172*
Sodium, Blood *on page 199*

Synonyms Blood Urea Nitrogen; BUN

Applies to Dialysis; Urea Reduction Ratio

Abstract The end product of protein metabolism, urea is synthesized by the liver. Easily filtered by renal glomeruli, it is partially reabsorbed by the renal tubules. Urea nitrogen reflects the ratio between urea **production** and **clearance**. Increased urea nitrogen may be due to increased production or decreased excretion. Although many use the expression "BUN," (for blood urea nitrogen), most laboratories use serum, occasionally plasma, but never whole blood.

Specimen Serum, plasma

Container Red top tube. Avoid fluoride and sodium citrate tubes if urease reaction is used and ammonium heparin tubes when conductimetric method is used. EDTA is suitable as well as lithium heparin for young children.

Collection Pediatrics: Blood drawn from heelstick for capillary (lithium heparin tube)

Storage Instructions Stable 1 day at room temperature, 3 days at 4°C to 8°C, and 3 months at -20°C.

Reference Range Birth to 1 year: 4-16 mg/dL (SI: 1.4-5.7 mmol/L); 1-40 years: 5-20 mg/dL (SI: 1.8-7.1 mmol/L); gradual slight increase subsequently occurs over 40 years of age.

Possible Panic Range BUN >100 mg/dL (SI: >35.7 mmol/L) has been used in the definition of uremia.[2]

Use Useful to assess renal function, especially with serum creatinine. **High BUN** occurs in chronic glomerulonephritis, pyelonephritis, and other causes of chronic renal disease; with acute renal failure, decreased renal perfusion (prerenal azotemia) as in shock. With urinary tract obstruction BUN increases (postrenal azotemia), for example as caused by neoplastic infiltration of the ureters, hyperplasia, or carcinoma of prostate. BUN is useful to follow hemodialysis and other therapy. (A highly diffusible molecule, urea falls rapidly with dialysis.) "Uremia" was defined by Luke as an expression of a constellation of signs and symptoms in patients with severe azotemia secondary to acute or chronic renal failure.[2] Causes of increased BUN include severe congestive heart failure, increased protein catabolism, tetracyclines with diuretic use, hyperalimentation, ketoacidosis, and dehydration as in diabetes mellitus, but even moderate dehydration can cause BUN to increase. It is dependent on renal blood flow and urine flow rates. Corticosteroids tend to increase BUN by causing increased protein catabolism. Bleeding from the gastrointestinal tract is an important cause of high urea nitrogen, commonly accompanied by elevation of BUN/creatinine ratio. Nephrotoxic drugs must be considered.

Borderline high values may occur after recent ingestion of high protein meal and muscle wasting may cause an elevation as well.

Low BUN occurs in late normal pregnancy, decreased protein intake, with intravenous fluids, with some antibiotics, and in severe liver damage. BUN has a role in assessment of nutritional support.

The BUN is especially important when creatinine values are misleading (eg, with certain cephalosporins).

As described by DeCaux et al in 1980, in the syndrome of inappropriate secretion of antidiuretic hormone (SIADH), findings include hyponatremia with serum or plasma Na$^+$ ≤128 mmol/L, serum hypo-osmolality, <260 mOsm/kg, with urine osmolality >300 mOsm/kg (SI: >300 mmol/kg) with low BUN. Such findings occur in situations in which patients are overhydrated. Clinical findings included absence of edema or evidence of heart, liver, thyroid, renal or adrenal disease.[3] Hypouricemia, with uric acid levels in 16 of 17 patients <4 mg/dL (SI: <238 µmol/L), is reported with the syndrome of inappropriate secretion of antidiuretic hormone.[4] (SIADH can be seen with higher serum sodiums and lower osmolalities. Urine osmolality is greater than serum osmolality in SIADH. DeCaux in 1982 presented criteria modified from the 1980 paper.[5])

BUN is needed to assess calculated osmolality. Osmolality (mOsm/kg H$_2$O) may be calculated as follows: Osmolality = [Na$^+$ (mmol/L) x 2] + urea N (mg/dL)/2.8 + glucose (mg/dL)/18.

Limitations Creatinine is usually more specific for glomerular function but may be less sensitive to some types of early renal disease. Uremia and other types of renal dysfunction are best evaluated with creatinine as well as urea nitrogen. In both prerenal and postrenal azotemia, for instance, BUN is apt to be increased somewhat more than is creatinine. However, in a series of dehydrated children with gastroenteritis who had metabolic acidosis and increased anion gap, 88% had BUN concentration ≤18 mg/dL (SI: ≤6.4 mmol/L). The authors found bicarbonate and anion gap more sensitive indices in this setting.[6] In chronic progressive renal disease, about 75% of renal parenchyma must be damaged or destroyed before azotemia develops. BUN lacks sensitivity and specificity, but still remains a useful test.

Methodology Diacetyl monoxime; urease, Berthelot reaction; rate conductivity

Additional Information Although creatinine is generally considered a more specific test to evaluate renal function, BUN and creatinine are commonly used together. Luke points out that clinical renal failure is variable between individual patients.[2]

BUN before and following dialysis and between dialysis treatments is among the determinants of patients so treated. The **urea reduction ratio** (percent reduction in concentration of BUN during a dialysis treatment) is not as powerful as serum albumin as a predictor of death. Its calculation: 100 x (1-[C_t/C_o]); C_t is the BUN 5 minutes following the end of dialysis, C_o is predialysis BUN. This ratio bears relationship to blood clearance by dialysis, length of dialysis, and volume of distribution of urea in the patient. The ratio represents quantitation of an individual's urea clearance during a single dialysis.[7]

BUN concentrations are used to evaluate patients with lymphoma at risk for tumor lysis after chemotherapy.[8]

Drug effects have been summarized.[9]

Footnotes
1. Burtis CA and Ashwood ER, *Tietz Textbook of Clinical Chemistry*, 2nd ed, Philadelphia, PA: WB Saunders Co, 1994, 1527-44.
2. Luke RG, "Uremia and the BUN," *N Engl J Med*, 1981, 305:1213-5.
3. DeCaux G, Genette F, and Mockel J, "Hypouremia in the Syndrome of Inappropriate Secretion of Antidiuretic Hormone," *Ann Intern Med*, 1980, 93:716-7.
4. Beck LH, "Hypouricemia in the Syndrome of Inappropriate Secretion of Antidiuretic Hormone," *N Engl J Med*, 1979, 301:528-30.
5. DeCaux G, Unger J, Brimioulle S, et al, "Hyponatremia in the Syndrome of Inappropriate Secretion of Antidiuretic Hormone. Rapid Correction With Urea, Sodium Chloride, and Water Restriction Therapy," *JAMA*, 1982, 247:471-4.
6. Bonadio WA, Hennes HH, Machi J, et al, "Efficacy of Measuring BUN in Assessing Children With Dehydration Due to Gastroenteritis," *Ann Emerg Med*, 1989, 18(7):755-7.
7. Owen WF Jr, Lew NL, Liu Y, et al, "The Urea Reduction Ratio and Serum Albumin Concentration as Predictors of Mortality in Patients Undergoing Hemodialysis," *N Engl J Med*, 1993, 329(14):1001-6.
8. Hande KR and Garrow GC, "Acute Tumor Lysis Syndrome in Patients With High-Grade Non-Hodgkin's Lymphoma," *Am J Med*, 1993, 94(2):133-9.
9. Artur Y and Galimany R, "Urea," *Drug Effects on Laboratory Test Results Analytical Interferences and Pharmacological Effects*, Siest G and Galteau MM, eds, Littleton, MA: PSG Publishing Co Inc, 1988, 439-53.

References
Abuelo JG, "Benign Azotemia of Long-Term Hemodialysis: Increase in Blood Urea Nitrogen and Serum Creatinine Concentrations After the Initiation of Dialysis," *Am J Med*, 1989, 86(6 Pt 1):738-9.
Bidani A and Churchill PC, "Acute Renal Failure," *Dis Mon*, 1989, 35(2):57-132.
Comtois R, Bertrand S, Beauregard H, et al, "Low Serum Urea Level in Dehydrated Patients With Central Diabetes Insipidus," *Can Med Assoc J*, 1988, 139(10):965-8.
Mair B, "Q & A Column," *CAP Today*, Oct 1995, 72.

Urea Nitrogen Clearance replaced by Creatinine Clearance *on page 117*

Urea Nitrogen/Creatinine Ratio see BUN/Creatinine Ratio *on page 92*

Urea Reduction Ratio see Urea Nitrogen, Blood *on this page*

Urg-III-S see Uroporphyrinogen III Synthase, Erythrocyte *on page 215*

Uric Acid, Serum

CPT 84550

Related Information
Alcohol, Blood or Urine *on page 531*
Ammonia, Blood *on page 75*
Complete Blood Count *on page 312*
(Continued)

Uric Acid, Serum *(Continued)*

Synonyms Urate

Abstract Uric acid, the end product of purine metabolism, is increased in a variety of clinicopathologic entities in addition to gout.

Patient Preparation Ideally, patient should be fasting. Diurnal variations occur. Uric acid concentration is usually higher in the morning and lower in the evening.

Specimen Serum

Container Red top tube

Collection Separate serum. Do not collect in lavender top (EDTA) tube or gray top (sodium fluoride) tube for urease method.

Storage Instructions Urate is stable in serum for 3 days at 25°C, 3-7 days at 4°C, and 6-12 months at -20°C.[1]

Reference Range An increase occurs during childhood. Adults: male: 3.4-7.0 mg/dL (SI: 202-416 µmol/L), female: 2.4-6.0 mg/dL (SI: 143-357 µmol/L). Values >7.0 mg/dL (SI: >416 µmol/L) are sometimes arbitrarily regarded as hyperuricemia, but there is no sharp line between normals on the one hand, and the serum uric acid of those with clinical gout. Normal ranges cannot be adjusted for purine ingestion, but high purine diet increases uric acid. Uric acid may be increased with body size, exercise, and stress.

Possible Panic Range "Severe hyperuricemia" has been classified as uric acid >12.0 mg/dL (SI: >714 µmol/L).

Use An increased uric acid level does not necessarily translate to a diagnosis of gout; only about 10% to 15% of instances of hyperuricemia are caused by gout. The overlap between uric acid levels in those with and without gout is shown in a study in which the lowest level in a gouty subject was 6 mg/dL (SI: 357 µmol/L), while the highest uric acid in a nongouty person was 9.5 mg/dL (SI: 565 µmol/L).[2] Gouty tophi form in cooler portions of the body.

Elevations of uric acid occur in renal diseases with renal failure[3] and prerenal azotemia (eg, dehydration) as well as gout. Other drugs causing increased uric acid concentration include diuretics,[3] pyrazinamide, ethambutol, nicotinic acid, and aspirin in low doses.

Excessive cell destruction: neoplasia, even before as well as following chemotherapy and radiation therapy, especially lymphoma and leukemia; hemolytic anemia, resolving pneumonia and other inflammation; polycythemia, myeloma, pernicious anemia, infectious mononucleosis, congestive heart failure, large myocardial infarct.

Endocrine: hypothyroidism, hypoparathyroidism, hyperparathyroidism, pseudohypoparathyroidism; diabetes insipidus of nephrogenic type, Addison's disease.

Lead poisoning (saturnine gout) from paint, batteries, and moonshine. A causal relationship between plumbism and gout was recognized before 1876. Gout as a common complication of subclinical lead poisoning is described among the Roman aristocracy.[4]

Acidosis: lactic acidosis, diabetic ketoacidosis, recent and/or prolonged alcohol ingestion, alcoholic ketosis. Shock and hypoxia relate to hyperuricemia. Attention has been directed at the cause of hyperuricemia in the intensive care unit; severely increased uric acid levels in acutely ill patients is explained by degradation of ATP with degradation of accumulated nucleotides to purine metabolites, uric acid among them. Such ATP degradation may occur with strenuous exercise and the adult respiratory distress syndrome. With metabolism of ethanol to acetyl CoA, the degradation of ATP explains the hyperuricemia of alcohol use. Hyperuricemia becomes then a marker for cell injury crisis.[5] Hypouricemia is found as well in the ICU; *vide infra.*

Toxemia of pregnancy, diet, weight loss, fasting, or starvation. Decreased urate clearance: cyclosporine-induced hyperuricemia.[6]

Triglyceride increase bears an association with hyperuricemia, as do diabetes mellitus and obesity. Hyperuricemia bears an association with obesity, hypertension, and statistical association with myocardial infarct.

Hereditary gout: Lesch-Nyhan syndrome (X-linked) with choreoathetosis, spasticity, self-mutilation, and high uric acid and increased urate:creatinine ratio. Gout with partial absence HPRT. Increased 5-phosphoribosyl-1-pyrophosphate synthetase. Glycogen storage disease type 1a.[5]

Only a minority of individuals with hyperuricemia develop gout.

Three types of kidney disease are caused by precipitation: acute uric acid nephropathy, nephrolithiasis, and chronic urate nephropathy.[7]

Hyperuricemia in early essential hypertension correlates with renal vascular resistance and inversely with renal blood flow. Increased serum uric acid may indicate renal involvement.[8,9]

Low uric acid: Drugs: Drugs apparently bearing a relationship to low serum uric acid levels included aspirin (high doses), x-ray contrast agents, glyceryl guaiacolate or allopurinol. Corticosteroids and probenecid cause low uric acid. Massive doses of vitamin C are uricosuric.

Poor dietary intake of purines and protein; tea, coffee.

Renal tubular defects, Fanconi syndrome, late in Wilson's disease, outdated tetracycline, cystinosis, galactosemia, heavy metal poisoning, malignant neoplasms, hypereosinophilic syndrome.

Xanthinuria (deficiency of xanthine oxidase).

Hypouricemia is reported with acute intermittent porphyria, severe liver disease (especially obstructive biliary disease), and as an isolated defect in the tubular transport of uric acid.

With increased renal clearance of urate, hypercalciuria, and decreased bone density, diabetes,[10] and in SIADH.

With hyponatremia, serum hypo-osmolarity: Beck has described low uric acid with the syndrome of inappropriate secretion of antidiuretic hormone (SIADH): 16 of 17 patients with this syndrome were hypouricemic, with serum urate ≤4.0 mg/dL (SI: ≤238 µmol/L). All 13 patients with other causes of hyponatremia had serum urate ≥5.0 mg/dL (SI: ≥297 µmol/L).[11] Volume expansion, as with SIADH, causes decreased uric acid. The combination of low uric and low Na$^+$ may also be found in instances of liver disease and was anticipated with ticrynafen.

Azlocillin is reported to cause a decrease of serum uric acid levels.[12] Drug effects on uric acid metabolism are published in tabular form.[13,14]

In hospital patients, hypouricemia was most common in patients in intensive care. Hypouricemia was found in oncology patients, especially with hematologic malignant disease, with diabetics on insulin therapy, and with SIADH.[15]

Idiopathic hypouricemia commonly is transient. Familial hypouricemia has been described.

Limitations Positive interferences may be caused by ascorbic acid, caffeine, and theophylline. Uncommonly, gout may occur without hyperuricemia.[16]

Hyperuricosuria rather than hyperuricemia may be the only clue to the diagnosis of purine overproduction in children who have enzymatic defects or who develop hyperuricemia in the course of treatment of malignancies. This is due to a high uric acid clearance which occurs prior to puberty.[17]

Methodology Phosphotungstate, uricase, high performance liquid chromatography (HPLC)

Additional Information Drug effects have been summarized.[18]

Footnotes

1. Tammes AR, "Uric Acid," *Quality Assurance Service*, CAP Computer Center, 1986.
2. Seegmiller JE, Laster L, and Howell RR, "Biochemistry of Uric Acid and Its Relation to Gout," *N Engl J Med*, 1983, 712-6.
3. Langford HG, Blaufox MD, Borhani NO, et al, "Is Thiazide-Produced Uric Acid Elevation Harmful?" *Arch Intern Med*, 1987, 147(4):645-9.
4. Nriagu JO, "Saturnine Gout Among Roman Aristocrats," *N Engl J Med*, 1983, 308:660-3.
5. Talente GM, Coleman RA, Alter C, et al, "Glycogen Storage Disease in Adults," *Ann Intern Med*, 1994, 120(3):218-26.
6. Lin HY, Rocher LL, McQuillan MA, et al, "Cyclosporine-Induced Hyperuricemia and Gout," *N Engl J Med*, 1989, 321(5):287-92.
7. Dykman D and Simon EE, "Hyperuricemia and Uric Acid Nephropathy," *Arch Intern Med*, 1987, 147(1):1341-5.
8. Larson AW and Strong CG, "Initial Assessment of the Patient With Hypertension," *Mayo Clin Proc*, 1989, 64(12):1533-42.
9. Nunez BD, Frohlich ED, Garavaglia GE, et al, "Serum Uric Acid in Renovascular Hypertension: Reduction Following Surgical Correction," *Am J Med Sci*, 1987, 294(6):419-22.
10. Shichiri M, Iwamoto H, and Shiigai T, "Diabetic Renal Hypouricemia," *Arch Intern Med*, 1987, 147(2):225-8.
11. Beck LH, "Hypouricemia in the Syndrome of Inappropriate Secretion of Antidiuretic Hormone," *N Engl J Med*, 1979, 301:528-30.
12. Ernst JA and Sy ER, "Effect of Azlocillin on Uric Acid Levels in Serum," *Antimicrob Agents Chemother*, 1983, 24:609-10.
13. German DC and Holmes EW, "Gout and Hyperuricemia: Diagnosis and Management," *Hosp Pract (Off Ed)*, 1986, 21(11):119-26, 131-2.
14. German DC and Holmes EW, "Hyperuricemia and Gout," *Med Clin North Am*, 1986, 70(2):419-36.
15. Crook M, "Hypouricaemia in a Hospital Population," *Scand J Clin Lab Invest*, 1993, 53(8):883-5.
16. McCarty DJ, "Gout Without Hyperuricemia," *JAMA*, 1994, 271(4):302-3.
17. Pascual E, "Hyperuricemia and Gout," *Curr Opin Rheumatol*, 1994, 6(4):454-8.
18. Zhiri A and Jouanel P, "Urates," *Drug Effects on Laboratory Test Results Analytical Interferences and Pharmacological Effects*, Siest G and Galteau MM, eds, Littleton, MA: PSG Publishing Co Inc, 1988, 423-38.

References

Conger JD, "Acute Uric Acid Nephropathy," *Med Clin North Am*, 1990, 74(4):859-71.
Devgun MS and Dhillon HS, "Importance of Diurnal Variations on Clinical Value and Interpretation of Serum Urate Measurements," *J Clin Pathol*, 1992, 45(2):110-3.

Fievet P, Pleskov L, Desailly I, et al, "Plasma Renin Activity, Blood Uric Acid, and Plasma Volume in Pregnancy-Induced Hypertension," *Nephron*, 1985, 40(4):429-32.

Fox IH, Palella TD, and Kelley WN, "Hyperuricemia: A Marker for Cell Energy Crisis," *N Engl J Med*, 1987, 317(2):111-2.

Gores PF, Fryd DS, Sutherland DER, et al, "Hyperuricemia after Renal Transplantation," *Am J Surg*, 1988, 156(5):397-400.

Hande KR and Garrow GC, "Acute Tumor Lysis Syndrome in Patients With High-Grade Non-Hodgkin's Lymphoma," *Am J Med*, 1993, 94(2):133-9.

Joseph J and McGrath H, "Gout or Pseudogout: How to Differentiate Crystal-Induced Arthropathies," *Geriatrics*, 1995, 50(4):33-9.

Lieber CS, "Medical Disorders of Alcoholism," *N Engl J Med*, 1995, 333(16):1058-65.

Lindor NM and Karnes PS, "Initial Assessment of Infants and Children With Suspected Inborn Errors of Metabolism," *Mayo Clin Proc*, 1995, 70(10):987-8.

Mejías E, Navas J, Lluberes R, et al, "Hyperuricemia, Gout, and Autosomal Dominant Polycystic Kidney Disease," *Am J Med Sci*, 1989, 297(3):145-8.

Menon RK, Mikhailidis DP, Bell JL, et al, "Warfarin Administration Increases Uric Acid Concentrations in Plasma," *Clin Chem*, 1986, 32(8):1557-9.

O'Connor JP and Emmerson BT, "The Treatment of Hyperuricaemia and Gout," *Aust Fam Physician*, 1985, 14(3):193-8.

Uric Acid, Urine

CPT 84560

Related Information
Calcium, Urine *on page 99*
Creatinine, 12- or 24-Hour Urine *on page 117*
Kidney Stone Analysis *on page 640*
Lead, Urine *on page 557*
Uric Acid, Serum *on page 213*
Urine Collection, 24-Hour *on page 30*

Synonyms Urate, Urine

Abstract Uric acid concentration is the product of *de novo* synthesis and dietary sources. Seventy-five per cent of urate is eliminated through the kidney and 25% through the intestine. Renal excretion of urate involves reabsorption by the proximal tubules, secretion by the distal portion of the proximal tubules, and further reabsorption by the distal tubules.

Patient Preparation Twenty-four hour uric acid excretion is most often measured in patients with nephrolithiasis, in whom it is desirable to know the excretion of uric acid and other substances while the patient is on a **usual** diet. A number of drugs affect uric acid excretion including aspirin, other anti-inflammatory preparations, x-ray contrast agents, vitamin C, and warfarin. Diuretics decrease uric acid excretion.

Specimen 24-hour urine

Container To prevent precipitation in acid urine, add 10 mL of sodium hydroxide solution (12.5M) to specimen container prior to collection.

Storage Instructions Do not refrigerate. Stable about 3 days.

Reference Range Approximately 250-750 mg/24 hours (SI: 1.5-4.5 mmol/day) for women. Range for men may extend to 800 mg/24 hours (SI: 4.8 mmol/day). Increases on purine-rich diet.

Use Hyperuricosuria is associated with renal calculus formation. Identify overexcretors to determine risk of stone formation; identify genetic defects, influence of overexcretion on therapy of gout. Uric acid nephrolithiasis occurs in primary gout or in secondary hyperuricemia (eg, malignant diseases). Uric acid nephrolithiasis may complicate ulcerative colitis, Crohn's disease, and surgical jejunoileal bypass. Most subjects with uric acid stones do not have gout. Evaluate uric acid metabolism in gout.

Methodology Phosphotungstate, uricase, high performance liquid chromatography (HPLC)

Additional Information Even mild renal failure decreases uric acid excretion. Uric acid excretion is decreased with hypertension.

A young patient with acute gouty arthritis, uric acid stones, and any patient who excretes >1000 mg uric acid/24 hours (SI: >5.9 mmol/day), should be screened for hypoxanthine-quanine phosphoribosyl-transferase (HPRT) deficiency.[1] The uric acid/creatinine ratio has been used as a screen for Lesch-Nyhan syndrome (HPRTase deficiency). Normal control patients 0.21-0.59; partial enzyme deficient group 0.62-2.00; complete enzyme deficiency 1.98-5.35.

The ratio of uric acid to creatinine in morning samples of urine has been used as a screening test for detection of the Lesch-Nyhan syndrome, which is associated with virtually complete absence of activity of the enzyme hypoxanthine-guanine phosphoribosyltransferase. This ratio has also been applied to 24-hour urine samples from adult patients with gout for detection of partial deficiency of the same enzyme. Patients with gout exhibit uric acid:creatinine ratios of 0.15-0.73, whereas those patients with hyperuricemia associated with another disorder such as leukemia or glycogen storage disease have ratios of 0.25-1.77. The ratio is 0.27-0.58 for patients with nongouty arthritis. Patients with complete hypoxanthine-guanine phosphoribosyltransferase deficiency are reported to have urinary uric acid-to-creatinine ratios of 1.98-5.35, as compared to 0.62-2.00 for patients with gout accompanied by partial enzyme deficiency.

The ratio of uric acid to creatinine concentration on a random urine specimen has also been shown to be >1.0 in patients with acute renal failure secondary to acute uric acid nephropathy, but <1.0 in patients with acute renal failure resulting from other causes.

Risk for uric acid stone formation correlates with the degree of uric acid supersaturation in the urine, depending upon the degree of uric acid concentration and urinary pH.[2]

Footnotes
1. Wilson JM, Young AB, and Kelley WN, "Hypoxanthine-Guanine Phosphoribosyltransferase Deficiency. The Molecular Basis of the Clinical Syndromes," *N Engl J Med*, 1983, 309:900-10.
2. Halabe A and Sperling O, "Uric Acid Nephrolithiasis," *Miner Electrolyte Metab*, 1994, 20(6):424-31.

References
Dykman D and Simon EE, "Hyperuricemia and Uric Acid Nephropathy," *Arch Intern Med*, 1987, 147(7):1341-5.

Preminger GM, "Renal Calculi: Pathogenesis, Diagnosis, and Medical Therapy," *Semin Nephrol*, 1992, 12(2):200-16.

Urinary Free Cortisol *see* Cortisol, Urine *on page 113*

Urine 17-Ketogenic Steroids *replaced by* 17-Hydroxyprogesterone, Blood or Amniotic Fluid *on page 148*

Urine Cl *see* Chloride, Urine *on page 109*

Urine Cortisol *see* Cortisol, Urine *on page 113*

Urine Creatinine *see* Creatinine, 12- or 24-Hour Urine *on page 117*

Urine Electrolytes *see* Electrolytes, Urine *on page 124*

Urine K+ *see* Potassium, Urine *on page 189*

Urine Na *see* Sodium, Urine *on page 199*

Urine Osmolality *see* Osmolality, Urine *on page 173*

Urine Osmolar Gap *see* Osmolality, Urine *on page 173*

Urine Oxalate *see* Oxalate, Urine *on page 174*

Urine Phosphorus *see* Phosphorus, Urine *on page 183*

Urine Pregnanetriol Assay *replaced by* 17-Hydroxyprogesterone, Blood or Amniotic Fluid *on page 148*

Uroporphyrinogen-Cosynthetase *see* Porphobilinogen Deaminase, Erythrocyte *on page 185*

Uroporphyrinogen Decarboxylase *see* Porphyrins, Quantitative, Urine *on page 186*

Uroporphyrinogen III Co-synthase *see* Uroporphyrinogen III Synthase, Erythrocyte *on this page*

Uroporphyrinogen III Synthase, Erythrocyte

CPT 84311

Related Information
Porphyrins, Quantitative, Urine *on page 186*

Synonyms U-III-S; Urg-III-S; Uroporphyrinogen III Co-synthase

Abstract Congenital erythropoietic porphyria (Günther's disease) is caused by an autosomal recessive trait. Decreased enzyme activity is found in red blood cells. This enzyme catalyzes conversion of hydroxymethylbilane to uroporphyrinogen and produces the type III isomer.[1]

Patient Preparation Avoid medications for 1 week before test; fasting state for 12 hours before test; abstinence from ethanol for 24 hours before test.[2]

Specimen Blood, amniotic fluid

Container Green top (heparin) tube

Collection Place on wet ice immediately.[2] See instructions of reference laboratory.

Storage Instructions Maintain low temperatures; follow recommendations of laboratory which will perform the test.

Reference Range ≥40 relative units

Critical Values ≤10 relative units (congenital erythropoietic porphyria)[3]

Use Diagnose congenital erythropoietic porphyria (erythropoietic uroporphyria); investigate dark red urine, red to brown stained diapers, hemolytic anemia, splenomegaly, photosensitivity, mostly in neonates; investigate stained teeth, hirsutism, scarring of sun-exposed skin

Methodology Incubation of washed red cells[3]

Additional Information Teeth and fluid from vesicles are recognized by red fluorescence with ultraviolet light.

Footnotes
1. Nuttall KL, "Porphyrins and Disorders of Porphyrin Metabolism," *Tietz Textbook of Clinical Chemistry*, 2nd ed, Burtis CA and Ashwood ER, Philadelphia, PA: WB Saunders Co, 1994, 2073-106.
2. Kisabeth RM, *Mayo 1996 Test Catalogue*, Rochester, MN: Mayo Medical Laboratories, 1996.
3. Leavelle DE, *Mayo Medical Laboratories Interpretive Handbook*, Rochester, MN: Mayo Medical Laboratories, 1994.

References
Desnick RJ, "The Porphyrias," *Harrison's Principles of Internal Medicine*, Isselbacher KJ, Braunwald E, Wilson JD, et al, New York, NY: McGraw-Hill Inc, 1994, 2073-9.

Uroporphyrinogen I Synthase *see* Porphobilinogen Deaminase, Erythrocyte *on page 185*

Uroporphyrins *see* Porphyrins, Quantitative, Urine *on page 186*

Vanillylmandelic Acid, Urine

CPT 84585

Related Information

Catecholamines, Fractionation, Plasma *on page 103*
Catecholamines, Fractionation, Urine *on page 104*
Homovanillic Acid, Urine *on page 145*
Metanephrines *on page 165*
Urine Collection, 24-Hour *on page 30*

Synonyms 3-Methoxy-4-Hydroxymandelic Acid; VMA

Abstract Vanillylmandelic acid is a major metabolite of both epinephrine and norepinephrine, the result of the actions of both carboxy-o-methyl transferase and monoamine oxidase. It is significantly elevated in conditions with overproduction of catecholamines, notably pheochromocytoma. Plasma and urine assays for catecholamines and their metabolites (VMA, HVA, and metanephrines) are useful screens for pheochromocytoma. VMA and homovanillic acid screen for neuroblastoma. VMA is inferior to other tests in evaluation for pheochromocytoma.[1]

Patient Preparation Interfering substances relate to methodology. Drug and diet recommendations from the laboratory used are desirable. Many laboratories restrict foods, such as coffee, tea, bananas, and other foods. Some ask for no drug use (except for digitalis) for 2 weeks before the test. Aspirin, pyridoxine, levodopa, amoxicillin, carbidopa, reserpine, and disulfiram commonly interfere. Monoamine oxidase inhibitors decrease VMA excretion. See Limitations.

Specimen A small urine collection for pediatrics, up to 24-hour urine for adults

Container Plastic container with hydrochloric or acetic acid preservative added before collection, according to the protocol of the laboratory which will perform the test. Adjust to pH 2-4 after collection, according to procedures of the laboratory doing the analysis.

Collection Patient should be at rest during the collection, if possible taking no medication and without recent exposure to radiographic materials.

Storage Instructions Refrigerate. Stable up to 2 weeks.

Special Instructions For neuroblastoma, both HVA (homovanillic acid) and VMA should be collected. Metanephrines have been recommended as a first test for pheochromocytoma.[2]

Reference Range Adult normal range is usually up to approximately 7-9 mg/24 hours (SI: 35-45 µmol/day). See table.

Vanillylmandelic Acid, Urine

24-hour collection	mg/24 h	SI: µmol/d
0-1 y	Up to 1.8	Up to 9
1-4 y	Up to 3	Up to 15
4-15 y	Up to 4	Up to 20
15 y - adults	7-9	35-45
24- or 12-hour collection	**µg/mg creatinine**	
<1 y	15-27	
1-5 y	11-13	
6-15 y	Up to 7	
15 y - adults	Up to 4.5	
Adults	Up to 7	
24-hour collection	**µg/g body weight/24 h**	
<1 mo	Up to 180	
1 mo - 2 y	Up to 230	
>2 y	Up to 150	

Use Diagnose pheochromocytoma; evaluate hypertension; diagnose and follow up neuroblastoma, ganglioneuroma, and ganglioneuroblastoma. Most neuroblastoma patients excrete excess HVA in 24-hour collections. If VMA and HVA are both used in work-up, up to 80% of all cases will be detected.

Limitations MAO inhibitors may produce false low value; coffee, vanilla, and chocolate should be omitted before testing; VMA in a random specimen may yield a false-negative; 24-hour collections are preferred for adults. Normal VMA values are reported in patients with pheochromocytoma whose tumors secrete only epinephrine. VMA lacks diagnostic sensitivity.[3] Its specificity is limited as well for pheochromocytoma; urinary VMA falls somewhat short.[4] Some neuroblastoma patients are positive for urinary homovanillic acid abnormality but do not excrete increased VMA.[5] Twenty percent to 32% of patients with neuroblastoma

do **not** have elevation of VMA. Many will have other laboratory abnormalities such as increased metanephrines, homovanillic acid (HVA), or dopamine.

Methodology High performance liquid chromatography (HPLC), spectrophotometric following extraction

Additional Information Creatinine is measured concomitantly in a 24-hour urine specimen to ensure adequate collection and to calculate the excretion ratio of VMA/creatinine and metanephrine/creatinine (see table). Ninety-five percent of patients with neuroblastoma have an increase in VMA or HVA, or both. Interpretation of all results should be tempered by knowledge of influences causing false-negatives and false-positives (eg, stress, drugs, compounds that interfere with the assays).[2] The status of a mass screening program in Japan is reported. Virtually all 387 cases detected were at an early stage and 97% are expected to be cured.[6]

Footnotes

1. Lenders JW, Keiser HR, Goldstein DS, et al, "Plasma Metanephrines in the Diagnosis of Pheochromocytoma," *Ann Intern Med*, 1995, 123:101-9.
2. Sheps SG, Jiang N-S, Klee GG, et al, "Recent Developments in the Diagnosis and Treatment of Pheochromocytoma," *Mayo Clin Proc*, 1990, 65(1):88-95.
3. Gerlo EA and Sevens C, "Urinary and Plasma Catecholamines and Urinary Catecholamine Metabolites in Pheochromocytoma: Diagnostic Value in 19 Cases," *Clin Chem*, 1994, 40(2):250-6.
4. Krakoff LR, "Searching for Pheochromocytoma: A New and Better Test?" *Ann Intern Med*, 1995, 123(2):150-1.
5. Rothstein A, "Determination of Urinary Homovanillic Acid Using the Nitrosonaphthol Reaction," *Am J Clin Pathol*, 1987, 87(5):644-8.
6. Sawada T, Sugimoto T, Kawakatsu H, et al, "Mass Screening for Neuroblastoma in Japan," *Pediatr Hematol Oncol*, 1991, 8(2):93-109.

References

Bell S, Parker L, Craft AW, et al, "False Positive Results in a Neuroblastoma Screening Programme," *Med Pediatr Oncol*, 1994, 22(3):181-6.
Hanai J, Kawai T, Sato Y, et al, "Simple Liquid-Chromatographic Measurement of Vanillylmandelic Acid and Homovanillic Acid in Urine on Filter Paper for Mass Screening of Neuroblastoma in Infants," *Clin Chem*, 1987, 33(11):2043-6.
Knight JA and Wu JT, "Catecholamines and Their Metabolites: Clinical and Laboratory Aspects," *Lab Med*, 1987, 18:153-8.
Leavelle DE, *Mayo Medical Laboratories Interpretive Handbook*, Rochester, MN: Mayo Medical Laboratories, 1996.
Tuchman M, Auray-Blais C, Ramnaraine ML, et al, "Determination of Urinary Homovanillic and Vanillylmandelic Acids From Dried Filter Paper Samples: Assessment of Potential Methods for Neuroblastoma Screening," *Clin Biochem*, 1987, 20(3):173-7.

Vasoactive Intestinal Polypeptide

CPT 84586

Related Information

Glucagon, Plasma *on page 136*

Synonyms VIP

Applies to Glucagon; Secretin

Abstract VIP is a 28 amino acid polypeptide produced by neuroendocrine cells in the gut and elsewhere. It has apparent paracrine activity on the gut, which relates to and is thought to be the major mediator of the symptoms of WDHA (watery diarrhea hypokalemia achlorhydria) syndrome or WDHH (watery diarrhea hypokalemia hypochlorhydria). The major entity which causes high VIP is a group of neural crest neoplasms (VIPomas). VIP mediates water transport, stimulates chloride secretion, and inhibits sodium absorption in the intestines.

Patient Preparation Avoid recent administration of radioactive isotopes. Patient must be completely fasting for 10-12 hours. Not even water may be taken. No antacids for 24 hours prior to collection. All medications should be discontinued for 24-48 hours prior to collection.

Specimen Plasma

Sampling Time 6 AM to 8 AM

Collection Collect specimen in lavender top (EDTA) tube and transfer to red top tube containing 500 µL of 10,000 KIU/mL Trasylol®.

Storage Instructions Mix, centrifuge, and pour off plasma into transport tube supplied by reference laboratory. Transport frozen on dry ice.

Reference Range <76 ng/L.[1] Levels vary considerably between laboratories.

Use Hypersecretion of VIP is observed in "pancreatic cholera syndrome," also called Verner-Morrison syndrome, the watery diarrhea hypokalemia achlorhydria (WDHA) syndrome, or watery diarrhea hypokalemia hypochlorhydria (WDHH). It is characterized by insidious hypermotility, acid-base and electrolyte disturbances, dehydration, and weakness; these symptoms can be reproduced by VIP. Diagnosis is often delayed. VIP can be secreted by pancreatic or ectopic islet cell tumors and in islet-cell hyperplasia. It may be overproduced with neuroblastoma.

Limitations Not all patients with the syndrome have increased VIP. Increased VIP can be found in healthy controls and in laxative abusers.[2]

Methodology Radioimmunoassay (RIA), immunoassay

Additional Information Other features of some cases of VIPoma have included hypercalcemia, flushing, and glucose intolerance.[2] A study of islet cell tumors in patients with multiple endocrine neoplasia (MEN) included vasoactive intestinal polypeptide tumor (VIPoma) as well as

Zollinger-Ellison syndrome and insulinoma.[3] A VIP-producing tumor causing the pancreatic cholera syndrome was reported as a well differentiated mucinous adenocarcinoma which contained cells reactive for pancreatic peptide and VIP on immunocytochemistry.[4] Bronchial tumor, pheochromocytoma, ganglion-neuroma, ganglioneuroblastoma, and medullary thyroid carcinoma have been reported with the syndrome.

The severe watery diarrhea is a secretory diarrhea. Peak output can exceed 3 L a day. The diarrhea is electrolyte rich; potassium loss can be 300 mmol/day and there is acidosis from bicarbonate loss. Eighty percent of such patients have islet cell tumors, of which nearly 50% are malignant. Others have islet cell hyperplasia. The entity can lead to chronic renal failure.[5] Normal levels of VIP have been reported in ulcerative colitis, Crohn's disease, cirrhosis, ascites, and diabetes.

VIP is found to be present in normal human lung tissue. Serum VIP concentrations may be negatively correlated with airway resistance in asthma.[6]

A review of neuroendocrine gastrointestinal tumors was published recently.[7]

Footnotes

1. Koch Tr, Michener SR, and Go VL, "Plasma Vasoactive Intestinal Polypeptide Concentration Determination in Patients With Diarrhea," *Gastroenterology*, 1991, 100(1):99-106.
2. Krejs GJ, "Noninsulin-Secreting Tumors of the Pancreatic Islets," *Williams Textbook of Endocrinology*, 8th ed, Wilson JD and Foster DW, eds, Philadelphia, PA: WB Saunders Co, 1992, 1567-76.
3. Sheppard BC, Norton JA, Doppman JL, et al, "Management of Islet Cell Tumors in Patients With Multiple Endocrine Neoplasia: A Prospective Study," *Surgery*, 1989, 106(6):1108-18.
4. Rood RP, DeLellis RA, Dayal Y, et al, "Pancreatic Cholera Syndrome Due to a Vasoactive Intestinal Polypeptide-Producing Tumor: Further Insights Into the Pathophysiology," *Gastroenterology*, 1988, 94(3):813-8.
5. Grier JF, "WDHA (Watery Diarrhea, Hypokalemia, Achlorhydria) Syndrome: Clinical Features, Diagnosis, and Treatment," *South Med J*, 1995, 88(1):22-4.
6. Liu A, Li PS, and Zhang ZJ, "A Clinical Study on the Effect of Non-Adrenergic Non-Cholinergic Nerves in Asthma," *Chung-Hua Nei Ko Tsa Chih*, *Chin J Intern Med*, 1993, 32(4):223-5.
7. Delcore R and Friesen SR, "Gastrointestinal Neuroendocrine Tumors," *J Am Coll Surg*, 1994, 178(2):187-211.

References

Brunt LM, Mazoujian G, O'Dorisio TM, et al, "Stimulation of Vasoactive Intestinal Peptide and Neurotensin Secretion by Pentagastrin in a Patient With VIPoma Syndrome," *Surgery*, 1994, 115(3):362-9.

Deveney CW and Way LW, "Regulatory Peptides of the Gut," *Basic and Clinical Endocrinology*, 3rd ed, Greenspan FS and Forsham PH, eds, Los Altos, CA: Lange Medical Publications, 1991, 569-91.

Fraker DL and Norton JA, "The Role of Surgery in the Management of Islet Cell Tumors," *Gastroenterol Clin North Am*, 1989, 18(4):805-30.

Green DW, Gomez G, and Greeley GH Jr, "Gastrointestinal Peptides," *Gastroenterol Clin North Am*, 1989, 18(4):695-733.

Virgolini I, Radere M, Kurtaran A, et al, "Vasoactive Intestinal Peptide-Receptor Imaging for the Localization of Intestinal Adenocarcinomas and Endocrine Tumors," *N Engl J Med*, 1994, 331(17):1116-21.

Venous Blood Gases *see* Blood Gases, Venous *on page 89*

VIP *see* Vasoactive Intestinal Polypeptide *on previous page*

Vitamin A, Serum

CPT 84590

Related Information

Carotene, Serum *on page 103*

Vitamin E, Serum *on page 219*

Applies to Retinoids; Retinol, Serum

Test Commonly Includes Vitamin A and beta-carotene determination

Abstract Dietary vitamin A is derived from animal sources as well as supplements. Carotenoids including beta-carotene are synthesized from plants and are partly converted to retinol. The present recommended daily allowance for women is 800 retinol equivalents (about 2700 IU vitamin A) daily. The expression "vitamin A" refers to retinoids which have the biologic activity of retinol.[1] Vitamin A is a fat-soluble essential vitamin which is necessary for the integrity of epithelial cells. It also plays an important role in the visual cycle and is required for normal growth, development, and reproduction.

Patient Preparation Patient must fast a minimum of 8 hours.

Specimen Serum

Container Red top tube

Collection Draw in chilled tube. Protect from light. Keep specimen on ice.

Storage Instructions Separate serum in a 4°C centrifuge and freeze in a plastic vial immediately. Stable 2 years frozen. Stable 4 weeks at 4°C, although freezing is preferred. Protect from light.

Reference Range Vitamin A: 30-95 µg/dL (SI: 1.05-3.32 µmol/L); normal range may be slightly less in early childhood. Beta-carotene: 50-200 µg/dL (SI: 0.93-3.72 µmol/L). Retinyl esters: 3-5 µg/dL.

Critical Values <0.10 may provide evidence of marked deficiency.

Possible Panic Range Toxicity is best assessed by measuring plasma retinyl esters.

Use Differential diagnosis of hypervitaminosis A. A combination of a low serum carotene level and a low vitamin A suggests inadequate vitamin A nutrition. Probucol (Lorelco®) may interfere.

Limitations Serum levels do not correlate well with liver stores because of homeostatic control exerted by the liver. Increased in patients on oral contraceptives.

Methodology Fluorescence or UV/VIS spectroscopy, high performance liquid chromatography (HPLC), electrochemical

Additional Information Decreased levels of vitamin A are commonly due to dietary deficiency[2], or may occur in conditions of deficient pancreatic digestive enzymes, impaired intestinal absorption and zinc deficiency resulting in decreased retinol-binding protein (RBP) levels, or deficient bile. Vitamin A deficiency is found with prolonged ethanol consumption.[3] Hypovitaminosis A may lead to impaired skeletal growth, blindness, xerophthalmia, increased susceptibility to respiratory infections, and keratomalacia. Night blindness is the most common result.

Hypervitaminosis A may be due to increased intake, or conditions causing impaired disposal such as myxedema, diabetes mellitus, or renal disease. The toxic effects of increased vitamin A include elevation of intracranial pressure, skin desquamation, hair loss, joint pain, headache, nausea, fever, vertigo, and visual disorientation. Chronic hypervitaminosis A may cause anorexia, dry skin, alopecia, hepatomegaly, and fatigue. Toxicity is best assessed by measuring retinyl esters which normally comprise 5% of total vitamin A, but may comprise >30% of total vitamin A in toxicity (taking >50,000 IU/day). Toxicity appears when vitamin A levels exceed the capacity of retinol binding protein (RBP) to bind to it.

Retinoids can be teratogenic.[1]

Vitamin A deficiency may occur when diseases or conditions impair the conversion of carotene to vitamin A or reduce the levels of RBP. Children with hypovitaminosis A have increased morbidity with measles.[4,5] Depressed immune response to tetanus in children with vitamin A deficiency is recognized.[6] Serum vitamin A levels may be decreased during periods of infection.[7,8]

Prospective data will be available in several years relevant to vitamin A intake, other substances and cancer risk.[9]

Exaggerated, unsubstantiated claims do not exclude potential benefits of antioxidants, but skepticism remains.[10] See listing Carotene, Serum *on page 103*.

Footnotes

1. Rothman KJ, Moore LL, Singer MR, et al, "Teratogenicity of High Vitamin A Intake," *N Engl J Med*, 1995, 333(21):1369-73.
2. Usha N, Sankaranarayanan A, Walia BN, et al, "Early Detection of Vitamin A Deficiency in Children With Persistent Diarrhoea," *Lancet*, 1990, 335(8686):422.
3. Lieber CS, "Medical Disorders of Alcoholism," *N Engl J Med*, 1995, 333(16):1058-65.
4. Division of Field Epidemiology, Centers for Disease Control, "Vitamin A Levels and Severity of Measles. New York City," *Am J Dis Child*, 1992, 146(2):182-6.
5. Hussey GD and Klein M, "A Randomized, Controlled Trial of Vitamin A in Children With Severe Measles," *N Engl J Med*, 1990, 323(3):160-4.
6. Semba RD, Muhilal S, Scott AL, et al, "Depressed Immune Response to Tetanus in Children With Vitamin A Deficiency," *J Nutr*, 1992, 122(1):101-7.
7. Velasquez-Melendez G, Okani ET, Kiertsman B, et al, "Plasma Levels of Vitamin A, Carotenoids, and Retinol Binding Protein in Children With Acute Respiratory Infections and Diarrheal Diseases," *Rev Saude Publica*, 1994, 28(5):357-64.
8. Velasquez-Melendez G, Okani ET, Kiertsman B, et al, "Vitamin A Status in Children With Pneumonia," *Eur J Clin Nutr*, 1995, 49(5):379-84.
9. Willett WC and Hunter DJ, "Vitamin A and Cancers of the Breast, Large Bowel, and Prostate: Epidemiologic Evidence," *Nutr Rev*, 1994, 52(2 Pt 2):S53-9.
10. "The Effect of Vitamin E and Beta Carotene on the Incidence of Lung Cancer and Other Cancers in Male Smokers. The Alpha-Tocopherol, Beta Carotene Cancer Prevention Study Group," *N Engl J Med*, 1994, 330(15):1029-35.

References

Bloem MW, Wedel M, Egger RJ, et al, "Mild Vitamin A Deficiency and Risk of Respiratory Tract Diseases and Diarrhea in Preschool and School Children in Northeastern Thailand," *Am J Epidemiol*, 1990, 131(2):332-9.

Burtis CA and Ashwood ER, *Tietz Textbook of Clinical Chemistry*, 2nd ed, Philadelphia, PA: WB Saunders Co, 1994, 1278-83.

"Detecting Vitamin A Deficiency Early," *Lancet*, 1992, 339(8808):1514-5.

Jakob E and Elmadfa I, "Rapid HPLC Assay for the Assessment of Vitamin K₁, A, E, and Beta-Carotene Status in Children (7-19 Years)," *Int J for Vitamin & Nutrition Research*, 1995, 65(1):31-5.

Oakley GP Jr and Erickson JD, "Vitamin A and Birth Defects - Continuing Caution is Needed," *N Engl J Med*, 1995, 333(21):1414-5.

Sommer A, "Vitamin A Deficiency and Childhood Mortality," *Lancet*, 1992, 340(8817):488-9.

Suan EP, Bedrossian EH Jr, Eagle RC Jr, et al, "Corneal Perforation in Patients With Vitamin A Deficiency in the United States," *Arch Ophthalmol*, 1990, 108(3):350-3.

Vitamin B₆

CPT 84207

Synonyms P-5'-P; Pyridoxal-5-Phosphate; Pyridoxine

Abstract Vitamin B₆, a water soluble vitamin, acts as a coenzyme (pyridoxal-5-phosphate) in protein, carbohydrate, and lipid metabolism, as well as in heme synthesis.

Patient Preparation Avoid radioisotope scan prior to collection of specimen if RIA is used for assay.

Specimen Plasma

(Continued)

Vitamin B$_6$ *(Continued)*

Container Lavender top (EDTA) tube

Collection Transport specimen **immediately** to the laboratory following collection. Avoid exposing specimen to light.

Storage Instructions Separate plasma or serum and freeze **immediately**. Avoid exposure to light. Stable 10 days at -80°C; 50% loss in 7 days at -20°C.

Causes for Rejection Specimen more than 30 minutes in transit to the laboratory.

Special Instructions Communicate with laboratory before this test is ordered; it is not always routinely available. Scheduling and/or use of a reference laboratory may be required.

Reference Range 5-30 ng/mL (SI: 20-121 nmol/L) (varies considerably with method).

Critical Values <5 ng/mL (SI: <20 nmol/L) indicates deficiency

Use Detect vitamin B$_6$ deficiency

Limitations Evaluation is complicated by an unusually high requirement for vitamin B$_6$ in some individuals.

Methodology Enzyme assay, high performance liquid chromatography (HPLC) with fluorometric detection, immunoradiometric assay (IRMA)

Additional Information The family of "vitamin B$_6$" compounds includes pyridoxine as well as B$_6$ activity contributed by aldehyde (pyridoxal) and amine (pyridoxamine) derivatives, pyridoxine being the alcohol form of the 3-hydroxy-2-methylpyridine basic structure. In biologic material the B$_6$ compounds exist largely as phosphorylated derivatives. The vitamin is synthesized by plants and many microorganisms but not by the higher animals. It is widely available in natural diets, being present in fish, chicken, some fruits and vegetables, and wheat germ. It is partially destroyed by cooking and food processing. Vitamin B$_6$ is water soluble and is absorbed largely from the jejunum. A series of phosphorylase, oxidase, and kinase enzymes provide for extensive *in vivo* interconversion of pyridoxine and its derivatives.

Most B$_6$-dependent enzymes utilize pyridoxal-5-phosphate (the aldehyde form) in a coenzyme role. Critical amino acid/protein metabolic pathways (eg, transamination and decarboxylation reactions) are dependent upon B$_6$ enzymes. Glycogen phosphorylase requires B$_6$ as does delta aminolevulinic acid synthetase, and pyridoxal phosphate is required for DNA synthesis. With dietary deficiency, conservation of pyridoxal phosphate-dependent enzymes occurs with redistribution of available coenzyme and maintenance of more essential functions, thus rendering some clinical deficiency states difficult to define.

Deficiency of this vitamin has been implicated in a wide variety of clinical conditions. Important in neonatology is the syndrome of jittery characteristics, colic, irritability, easy startling and seizures due to B$_6$ deficiency following ingestion of formula rendered B$_6$ depleted by excessive heating. B$_6$ may be decreased with malabsorption and inflammatory disease of the small bowel and in some cases of jejunoileal bypass.

Pyridoxine is required for heme synthesis. With deficiency, a hypochromic form of sideroblastic anemia may occur, characterized by the presence of ring sideroblasts (iron positive granules deposited about the nuclei of red cell precursors). Occasionally the anemia may have megaloblastic characteristics. Most cases are the result of a block in the conversion of pyridoxine to pyridoxal phosphate, which inhibits the production of delta aminolevulinic acid and thus the production of heme. This form of sideroblastic anemia responds to large doses (>2 g) of pyridoxal phosphate per day. Inherited abnormalities of apoenzymes that bind with pyridoxal phosphate are responsible for newborn conditions characterized by mental retardation, skeletal deformities, thrombotic conditions, osteoporosis, and visual defects. Some are associated with increased urinary amino acids (eg, homocystinuria, hypermethioninemia, cystathioninuria). Some can be controlled with large doses of vitamin B$_6$.

In adults, elevated serum homocysteine levels due to vitamin B$_6$ deficiency may promote atherogenesis with resultant arteriosclerotic and thromboembolic cerebral, coronary, and/or peripheral vascular events.[1] With B$_6$ deficiency the activity of cystathionine β-synthase (which functions in amino acid metabolism) is inhibited. Pyridoxal-5′-phosphate is a cofactor for this enzyme. The influence of B$_6$ on serum cholesterol levels and platelet aggregation is controversial. Decreased plasma pyridoxal phosphate levels have been found in patients with acute MI.[2] Therapy with vitamin B$_6$ and folic acid apparently normalizes homocysteine metabolism in essentially all patients with cardiovascular disease and mild hyperhomocysteinemia.[3] Metabolic evidence of B$_6$, as well as B$_{12}$/ folate deficiency, in the presence of normal serum levels may be common in the elderly.[4] There is evidence against increased need for vitamin B$_6$ by athletes.[5]

Penicillamine, levodopa, disulfiram, oral contraceptive agents, theophylline, phenelzine,[6] and the antituberculous drugs isoniazid, cycloserine, and pyrazinoic acid may cause B$_6$ depletion in some cases with apparently associated sideroblastic anemia. B$_6$ supplements may be necessary.

B$_6$ may be decreased with pregnancy, lactation, alcoholism, diabetes mellitus, and in an uncommon B$_6$ dependency state, vitamin B$_6$ responsive neonatal convulsions. The effects of megadose vitamin B$_6$ consumption are controversial. There is evidence of significant neurotoxicity associated with pyridoxine megavitaminosis; tingling, numbness, clumsiness, gait disturbances, pseudoathetosis, with doses >2 g/day.[7]

Vitamin B$_6$ deficiency impairs immune function by inhibiting interleukin-2 production and lymphocyte proliferation.[8]

Pais et al report that children with leukemia had lower pyridoxal-5 phosphate levels than age-matched control children.[9]

Footnotes

1. Robinson K, Mayer E, and Jacobsen DW, "Homocysteine and Coronary Artery Disease," *Cleve Clin J Med*, 1994, 61(6):438-50
2. Kok FJ, Schrijver J, Hofman A, et al, "Low Vitamin B$_6$ Status in Patients With Acute Myocardial Infarction," *Am J Cardiol*, 1989, 63(9):513-6.
3. van den Berg M, Franken DG, Boers GH, et al, "Combined Vitamin B$_6$ Plus Folic Acid Therapy in Young Patients With Arteriosclerosis and Hyperhomocysteinemia," *J Vasc Surg*, 1994, 20(6):933-40.
4. Naurath HJ, Joosten E, Riezler R, et al, "Effects of Vitamin B$_{12}$, Folate, and Vitamin B$_6$ Supplements in Elderly People With Normal Serum Vitamin Concentrations," *Lancet*, 1995, 346(8967):85-9.
5. Dreon DM and Butterfield GE, "Vitamin B$_6$ Utilization in Active and Inactive Young Men," *Am J Clin Nutr*, 1986, 43(5):816-24.
6. Malcolm DE, Yu PH, Bowen RC, et al, "Phenelzine Reduces Plasma Vitamin B$_6$," *J Psychiatr Neurosci*, 1994, 19(5):332-4.
7. Schaumburg H, Kaplan J, Windebank A, et al, "Sensory Neuropathy From Pyridoxine Abuse," *N Engl J Med*, 1983, 309:445-8.
8. Rosenburg, IH, "Vitamin B$_6$ and Immune Function in the Elderly and HIV-Seropositive Subjects," *Nutr Rev*, 1992, 50(5):145-7.
9. Pais RC, Vanous E, Hollins B, et al, "Abnormal Vitamin B$_6$ Status in Childhood Leukemia," *Cancer*, 1990, 66(11):2421-8.

References

Borschel MW, Kirksey A, and Hannemann RE, "Effects of Vitamin B$_6$ Intake on Nutriture and Growth of Young Infants," *Am J Clin Nutr*, 1986, 43(1):7-15.

McCormick DB and Greene HL, "Vitamins," *Tietz Textbook of Clinical Chemistry*, 2nd ed, Chapter 27, Burtis CA and Ashwood ER, eds, Philadelphia, PA: WB Saunders Co, 1993, 1300-4.

Vitamin C *see* Ascorbic Acid, Blood *on page 84*

Vitamin C *see* Oxalate, Urine *on page 174*

Vitamin D$_1$ *see* Vitamin D$_3$, Serum *on this page*

Vitamin D$_3$, Serum

CPT 82306 (calcifediol); 82307 (calciferol)

Related Information

Aluminum, Bone *on page 586*

Calcium, Serum *on page 97*

Calcium, Urine *on page 99*

Fecal Fat, Quantitative, 72-Hour Collection *on page 127*

Kidney Stone Analysis *on page 640*

Magnesium, Serum *on page 164*

Magnesium, Urine *on page 165*

Osteocalcin, Serum *on page 174*

Phosphorus, Serum *on page 182*

Synonyms Cholecalciferol

Applies to Calcitriol; 1,25-Dihydroxy Vitamin D$_3$; Ergocalciferol (Vitamin D$_2$); 25-Hydroxy Vitamin D$_3$; 1,25-(OH)$_2$ D$_3$; 25-(OH) D$_3$; Vitamin D$_1$

Test Commonly Includes The expression "vitamin D" includes a group of sterols. Vitamin D$_3$ (cholecalciferol) is hydroxylated in the liver to produce 25-hydroxy vitamin D$_3$, 25-OHD$_3$. This is the major metabolite. 1,25-dihydroxy vitamin D$_3$ has vastly more activity; it is formed by another hydroxylation step.

Abstract With parathyroid hormone and calcitonin, 1,25-dihydroxy vitamin D$_3$ (essentially, the hormonal form) acts upon bone, parathyroid glands, kidneys, and intestine. It regulates calcium metabolism, osteoblast function, and parathormone release. It exerts effects or is involved in a wide range of tissues additional to its role in mineral homeostasis.

Patient Preparation Fasting specimen is preferred. Avoid radioisotope administration if RIA is used as the assay.

Specimen Serum, plasma

Container Red top tube, green top (heparin) tube

Storage Instructions Stable 3 days at 4°C to 25°C. Processed serum stable for months at -20°C, tolerates freeze-thaw cycles.[1]

Causes for Rejection Administration of radioisotopes if RIA is used for assay

Reference Range 25-hydroxy vitamin D$_3$: 10-60 ng/mL (SI: 25-150 nmol/L); **1,25-dihydroxy vitamin D$_3$**: 15-65 pg/mL (SI: 42-164 pmol/L). The normal range is method dependent and varies with diet, clothing, season, and UV light exposure. Some variation in ranges is found among laboratories.[2] Reference ranges are not well established.

Use Evaluate vitamin D deficiency as cause of osteopenia; both postmenopausal osteoporosis and senile osteoporosis are linked to vitamin D disturbances.[3] Its role includes investigation of the differential diagnosis of disorders of calcium and phosphorus metabolism; investigate diseases of bone including osteopenia, osteomalacia, and rickets; work up malabsorption. **Measurement of 25-hydroxy vitamin D_3 is the best indicator of vitamin D status, vitamin D toxicity, and nutrition.**

Hypervitaminosis D from excessive vitamin D_3 added to milk was characterized by increased serum 25-hydroxy vitamin D_3 (25-(OH) D_3) concentration; most patients had hypercalcemia. Vitamin D intoxication usually is from inappropriate use. Multivitamins may include vitamin D_2 or vitamin D_3. Exposure to sunlight can raise serum 25-(OH) D_3 levels to 79 ng/mL (197 mmol/L), but sunlight alone cannot cause vitamin D intoxication.[2]

Limitations **Values of vitamin D vary** with exposure to sunlight (in which increased levels of vitamin D_3 result from synthesis in the skin from 7-dehydrocholesterol, in a reaction catalyzed by UV light). Vitamin D_2 (ergocalciferol) metabolically similar to vitamin D_3, derives only from diet;[3] it is the form added to milk and infant formulas. There are also variations during the menstrual cycle, particularly at the time of ovulation. **Many assays detect inactive 24-hydroxy metabolites in addition to active metabolites.**

Total 1,25-$(OH)_2$ D_3 concentrations are often not increased with vitamin D toxicity. (It is 25-hydroxy vitamin D_3 (25-(OH) D_3) that should be measured to evaluate toxicity.) Free 1,25-dihydroxy vitamin D_3 may be useful.[4]

Methodology Competitive binding assay, radioimmunoassay (RIA), high performance liquid chromatography (HPLC)

Additional Information Vitamin D_3 **(cholecalciferol)** and **vitamin D_2 (ergocalciferol)** are hydroxylated in the liver to the 25-hydroxy form, and then to the active 1,25-dihydroxy form in the kidney. Functional abnormalities can result from failures of absorption or either hydroxylation step. In type II vitamin D-dependent rickets, there is end-organ unresponsiveness to 1,25-dihydroxy vitamin D_3. Long use of anticonvulsive drugs may lead to decreased levels of 25-hydroxy vitamin D_3, through induced increased hepatic metabolism, but this may not be clinically significant.

Vitamin D has a major action on intestinal absorption of calcium, bone calcium balance, and renal excretion of calcium. Thus, assessment of serum vitamin D levels is useful in the differential diagnosis of hypocalcemia, hypercalcemia, and hypophosphatemia. Specific measurement of both monohydroxy and dihydroxy forms can help pinpoint absorptive, hepatic, or renal abnormalities of vitamin D metabolism.

1,25-dihydroxy vitamin D_3 is increased in sarcoidosis and hyperparathyroidism. It may be elevated in cases of hypercalcemia associated with malignant lymphoma. It is decreased in rickets, type I vitamin D-resistant rickets, hypoparathyroidism, pseudohypoparathyroidism, renal osteodystrophy, and psoriasis.[5]

Dietary intake of phosphorus is a determinant of 1,25-dihydroxy D_3 production. Increases of 1,25-dihydroxy D relating to hypocalcemia are thought to be mediated through increased output of parathyroid hormone. Vitamin D is also influenced by thyroid status, estrogens, calcitonin, growth hormone, prolactin, insulin, and glucocorticoids. The vitamin D endocrine system is linked to vitamin D-resistant rickets as well as classic vitamin D-deficient rickets and hypophosphatemic oncogenic rickets.

Because of the complex, multifactorial control of calcium balance, it is often useful to measure parathyroid hormone when vitamin D is needed.

Tumor-induced (oncogenic) osteomalacia is a rare entity characterized by hypophosphatemia, hyperphosphaturia, low 1,25-dihydroxy vitamin D_3 levels, and osteomalacia. Tumor removal leads resolution of such abnormalities.[6]

Vitamin D_2 is a commercially manufactured D vitamin derived from plants used in vitamin preparations. It represents a fraction of the body's total vitamin D stores. Vitamin D_1 (24,25-dihydroxy - also called calcidiol) is the major renal metabolite but has no physiological role.

Magnesium depletion induces vitamin D resistance secondary to impaired skeletal response to calcitriol.[7]

Footnotes
1. Lissner D, Mason R, and Posen S, "Stability of Vitamin D Metabolites in Human Blood Serum and Plasma," *Clin Chem*, 1981, 27:773-4.
2. Jacobus CH, Holick MF, Shao Q, et al, "Hypervitaminosis D Associated With Drinking Milk," *N Engl J Med*, 1992, 326(18):1213-5.
3. Reichel H, Koeffler HP, and Norman AW, "The Role of the Vitamin D Endocrine System in Health and Disease," *N Engl J Med*, 1989, 320(15):980-91.
4. Pettifor JM, Bikle DD, Cavaleros M, et al, "Serum Levels of Free 1,25-Dihydroxy Vitamin D in Vitamin D Toxicity," *Ann Intern Med*, 1995, 122(7):511-3.
5. Morimoto S and Yoshikawa K, "Psoriasis and Vitamin D_3. A Review of Our Experience," *Arch Dermatol*, 1989, 125(2):231-4.
6. Cai Q, Hodgson SF, Kao PC, et al, "Brief Report: Inhibition of Renal Phosphate Transport By a Tumor Product in a Patient With Oncogenic Osteomalacia," *N Engl J Med*, 1994, 330(23):1645-9.
7. Fleming CR, George L, Stoner GL, et al, "The Importance of Urinary Magnesium Values in Patients With Gut Failure," *Mayo Clin Proc*, 1996, 71(1):21-4.

References
Brommage R and DeLuca HF, "Evidence That 1,25-Dihydroxy Vitamin D_3 Is the Physiologically Active Metabolite of Vitamin D_3," *Endocr Rev*, 1985, 6(4):491-511.
Burtis CA and Ashwood ER, *Tietz Textbook of Clinical Chemistry*, 2nd ed, Philadelphia, PA: WB Saunders Co, 1994, 1922-33.
DeLuca HF, "New Concepts of Vitamin D Functions," *Ann N Y Acad Sci*, 1992, 669:59-69.
Econs MJ and Drezner MK, "Tumor-Induced Osteomalacia - Unveiling a New Hormone," *N Engl J Med*, 1994, 330(23):1679-81.
Fournier A, Moriniere P, Boudaillez B, et al, "1,25-(OH) Vitamin D Deficiency and Renal Osteodystrophy: Should its Well-Accepted Pathogenetic Role in Secondary Hyperparathyroidism Lead to its Systematic Preventive Therapeutic Use?" *Nephrol Dial Transplant*, 1987, 2(6):498-503.
Garabédian M, Jacqz E, Guillozo H, et al, "Elevated Plasma 1,25-Dihydroxy Vitamin D Concentrations in Infants With Hypercalcemia and an Elfin Facies," *N Engl J Med*, 1985, 312(15):948-52.
Krall EA, Sahyoun N, Tannenbaum S, et al, "Effect of Vitamin D Intake on Seasonal Variations in Parathyroid Hormone Secretion in Postmenopausal Women," *N Engl J Med*, 1989, 321(26):1777-83.
Kumar R, "The Metabolism and Mechanism of Action of 1,25-Dihydroxy Vitamin D_3," *Kidney Int*, 1986, 30(6):793-803.
Leavelle DE, *Mayo Medical Laboratories Interpretive Handbook*, Rochester, MN: Mayo Medical Laboratories, 1994.
Lyles KW, Halsey DL, Friedman NE, et al, "Correlations of Serum Concentrations of 1,25-Dihydroxy Vitamin D, Phosphorus, and Parathyroid Hormone in Tumoral Calcinosis," *J Clin Endocrinol Metab*, 1988, 67(1):88-92.
Silverberg SJ, Shane E, de la Cruz L, et al, "Abnormalities in Parathyroid Hormone Secretion and 1,25-Dihydroxy Vitamin D_3 Formation in Women With Osteoporosis," *N Engl J Med*, 1989, 320(5):277-81.
Singer FR and Adams JS, "Abnormal Calcium Homeostasis in Sarcoidosis," *N Engl J Med*, 1986, 315(12):755-7.

Vitamin E, Serum
CPT 84446

Related Information
Carotene, Serum *on page 103*
Vitamin A, Serum *on page 217*

Synonyms Alpha Tocopherol; Tocopherol; α-Tocopherol

Abstract Vitamin E is a lipid soluble vitamin that acts as antioxidant, preventing damage to membranes by free radicals.

Specimen Serum, plasma

Container Red top tube, green top (heparin) tube

Storage Instructions Separate serum or plasma within 2 hours. Protect from light. Serum or plasma is stable 2 weeks at 25°C, 14 days at 4°C, and 1 year at -20°C.[1]

Reference Range 0.8-1.5 mg/dL (SI: 19-35 µmol/L), varies with method and age (ranges for premature babies, neonates, children, and adults can be stratified.)

Use Evaluate vitamin E deficiency in hemolytic disease in premature infants and neuromuscular disease in infants (and adults) with chronic cholestasis; evaluate patients on long-term parenteral nutrition; evaluate patients with malignancy or malabsorption (eg, patients with cystic fibrosis, cases of intestinal bypass surgery); investigate brown-bowel syndrome

Methodology High performance liquid chromatography (HPLC), fluorometry after solvent extraction, colorimetry

Additional Information Vitamin E (α-tocopherol) is an antioxidant so widely distributed in foodstuffs that deficiency rarely occurs from diet. However, vitamin E is fat soluble, and malabsorption and deficiency may develop in cases of chronic intraluminal intestinal bile deficiency. This has been particularly noted in premature infants and children with biliary atresia or cystic fibrosis (chronic intrahepatic cholestasis).[2] Clinically, this may lead to a hemolytic anemia, due to increased erythrocyte fragility, or to a slowly progressive neurologic disorder characterized by ataxia, areflexia, gaze disturbances, and loss of proprioception and vibratory sensation. A similar syndrome has been reported in adults with malabsorption. The syndrome may respond to treatment with parenteral vitamin E.

Early treatment with vitamin E may delay or prevent the neuropathy with ataxia that develops during the course of abetalipoproteinuria. Vitamin E therapy, in some cases, may have a favorable effect on moderate and severe cases of the retinopathy of prematurity[3] and the retinopathy of abetalipoproteinemia. While lipid malabsorption syndrome (with steatorrhea and malabsorption of vitamin E) may be etiologically related to ataxic spinocerebellar neurologic degenerative disease, there are reports of familial and sporadic vitamin E deficiency with neurologic impairment in the absence of fat malabsorption or demonstrated plasma lipoprotein level abnormality.[4,5,6] Vitamin E is transported into plasma lipoproteins. A recently described hepatic tocophenol binding protein appears to be deficient in some individuals who are vitamin E deficient.[6] The importance of not overlooking a treatable cause of neurologic degenerative disease has been emphasized.[7]

As an antioxidant, vitamin E assists the prevention of peroxidation of unsaturated fatty acids. Deficiency may result in accumulation of
(Continued)

Vitamin E, Serum *(Continued)*

oxidized lipids which may polymerize with polysaccharides to form ceroid/lipofuscin pigment. This PAS positive material deposits in tissue as intracytoplasmic pigment granules. In three patients with "brown-bowel syndrome," vitamin E levels were found to be "extremely low" (0.1-0.2 mg/dL (SI: 2-5 µmol/L)).[8]

There continues to be interest in correlating plasma vitamin E levels with a variety of plasma constituents, with some positive and some negative results. Significance and/or validity of some associations is uncertain. Notably, abnormal serum levels of vitamin E have not been shown to relate significantly to clinical patency of ductus arteriosus,[9] sickle cell anemia,[10] moderate freshwater fish consumption,[11] insulin-dependent diabetics,[12] and risk of cancer.[13,14,15] Plasma vitamin E level, in one study, showed a positive correlation with serum cholesterol, non-HDL cholesterol, triglycerides, and apolipoprotein B.[16] Vitamin E is reported to reduce the risk of coronary heart disease in men[17] and women.[18] It has been proposed that nutritional indices such as vitamin E/phospholipids and vitamin E/total lipids are better indicators of vitamin E status than single plasma or serum vitamin concentrations.[19]

Footnotes

1. Tietz NW, *Clinical Guide to Laboratory Tests*, 3rd ed, Philadelphia, PA: WB Saunders Co, 1995, 646.

2. Issa S, Rotthauwe HW, and Burmeister W, "25-Hydroxyvitamin D and Vitamin E Absorption in Healthy Children and Children With Chronic Intrahepatic Cholestasis," *Eur J Pediatr*, 1989, 148(7):605-9.

3. Johnson L, Quinn GE, Abbasi S, et al, "Effect of Sustained Pharmacologic Vitamin E Levels on Incidence and Severity of Retinopathy of Prematurity: A Controlled Clinical Trial," *J Pediatr*, 1989, 114(5):827-38.

4. Harding AE, Matthews S, Jones S, et al, "Spinocerebellar Degeneration Associated With a Selective Defect of Vitamin E Absorption," *N Engl J Med*, 1985, 313(1):32-5.

5. Sokol RJ, Kayden HJ, Bettis DB, et al, "Isolated Vitamin E Deficiency in the Absence of Fat Malabsorption - Familial and Sporadic Cases: Characterization and Investigation of Causes," *J Lab Clin Med*, 1988, 111(5):548-59.

6. Traber MG, "Determinants of Plasma Vitamin E Concentrations," *Free Radic Biol Med*, 1994, 16(2):229-39.

7. Harding AE, Macevilly CJ, and Muller DPR, "Serum Vitamin E Concentrations in Degenerative Ataxias," *J Neurol Neurosurg Psychiatry*, 1989, 52(1):132.

8. Michowitz M, Noy S, Chayen D, et al, "Brown-Bowel Syndrome," *Am J Surg*, 1989, 55(9):566-9.

9. Rudolph N, Schiller MS, and Wong SL, "Vitamin E and Selenium in Preterm Infants: Lack of Effect on Clinical Patency of Ductus Arteriosus," *Int J Vitam Nutr Res*, 1989, 59(2):140-6.

10. Broxson EH Jr, Sokol RJ, and Githens JH, "Normal Vitamin E Status in Sickle Hemoglobinopathies in Colorado," *Am J Clin Nutr*, 1989, 50(3):497-503.

11. Hänninen OO, Agren JJ, Laitinen MV, et al, "Dose-Response Relationships in Blood Lipids During Moderate Freshwater Fish Diet," *Ann Med*, 1989, 21:203-7.

12. Basu TK, Tze WJ, and Leichter J, "Serum Vitamin A and Retinol-Binding Protein in Patients With Insulin-Dependent Diabetes Mellitus," *Am J Clin Nutr*, 1989, 50(2):329-31.

13. Connett JE, Kuller LH, Kjelsberg MO, et al, "Relationship Between Carotenoids and Cancer. The Multiple Risk Factor Intervention Trial (MRFIT) Study," *Cancer*, 1989, 64(1):126-34.

14. "The Effect of Vitamin E and Beta Carotene on the Incidence of Lung Cancer and Other Cancers in Male Smokers. The Alpha-Tocopherol, Beta Carotene Cancer Prevention Study Group," *N Engl J Med*, 1994, 330(15):1029-35.

15. Greenberg ER, Baron JA, Tosteson TD, et al, "A Clinical Trial of Antioxidant Vitamins to Prevent Colorectal Adenoma," *N Engl J Med*, 1994, 331(3):141-7.

16. Rubba P, Mancini M, Fidanza F, et al, "Plasma Vitamin E, Apolipoprotein B and HDL Cholesterol in Middle-Aged Men From Southern Italy," *Atherosclerosis*, 1989, 77(1):25-9.

17. Rimm EB, Stampfer MJ, Ascherio A, et al, "Vitamin E Consumption and the Risk of Coronary Heart Disease in Men," *N Engl J Med*, 1993, 328(20):1450-6.

18. Stampfer MJ, Hennekens CH, Manson JE, et al, "Vitamin E Consumption and the Risk of Coronary Disease in Women," *N Engl J Med*, 1993, 328(20):1444-9.

19. Gomez Vida JM, Bayes Garcia R, and Molina Font JA, "Materno-Fetal Nutritional Status Related to Vitamin E," *An Esp Pediatr*, 1992, 36(3):197-200.

References

Anderson R, "Assessment of the Roles of Vitamin C, Vitamin E, and Beta-Carotene in the Modulation of Oxidant Stress Mediated by Cigarette Smoke-Activated Phagocytes," *Am J Clin Nutr*, 1991, 53(1 Suppl):358S-61S.

Burtis CA and Ashwood ER, *Tietz Textbook of Clinical Chemistry*, 2nd ed, Philadelphia, PA: WB Saunders Co, 1994, 1285-8.

Havel RJ and Kane JP, "Abetalipoproteinemia - Introduction: Structure and Metabolism of Plasma Lipoproteins," *The Metabolic Basis of Inherited Disease*, 6th ed, Chapter 44A, Scriver CR, Beaudet AL, Sly WS, et al, eds, New York, NY: McGraw-Hill Inc, 1989, 1145-51.

Kelleher J, Miller MG, Littlewood JM, et al, "The Clinical Effect of Correction of Vitamin E Depletion in Cystic Fibrosis," *Int J Vitam Nutr Res*, 1987, 57(3):253-9.

Munoz SJ, Heubi JE, Balistreri WF, et al, "Vitamin E Deficiency in Primary Biliary Cirrhosis: Gastrointestinal Malabsorption, Frequency and Relationship to Other Lipid-Soluble Vitamins," *Hepatology*, 1989, 9(4):525-31.

Seddon JM, Ajani UA, Sperduto RD, et al, "Dietary Carotenoids, Vitamins A, C, and E, and Advanced Age-Related Macular Degeneration. Eye Disease Case-Control Study Group," *JAMA*, 1994, 272(18):1413-20.

VLDL *see* Triglycerides *on page 209*

VMA *see* Vanillylmandelic Acid, Urine *on page 216*

Watson-Schwartz Test *see* Porphobilinogen, Qualitative, Urine *on page 185*

Weisberg Formula *see* Osmolality, Calculated *on page 172*

Wellness Programs *see* Chemistry Profile *on page 107*

Xylose Absorption Test *see* d-Xylose Absorption Test *on page 122*

Xylose Tolerance Test *see* d-Xylose Absorption Test *on page 122*

Zinc Protoporphyrin *see* Protoporphyrin, Zinc, Blood *on page 196*

ZPP *see* Protoporphyrin, Zinc, Blood *on page 196*

International Unit (SI Unit) Conversion Tables

Analyte	Conventional Units	Conventional to SI (multiply by)	SI Units	SI to Conventional (multiply by)
Acetaminophen (Datril®, Tylenol®)	µg/mL	6.62	µmol/L	0.151
Acid phosphatase	units/L	NA	units/L	NA
Adrenocorticotropic hormone (ACTH)	pg/mL	1	ng/L	1
Albumin, serum	g/dL	10	g/L	0.10
Aldolase, serum	units/L	NA	units/L	NA
Aldosterone				
blood	ng/dL	0.0277	nmol/L	36.10
urine	µg/24 h	2.77	nmol/d	0.361
Alkaline phosphatase	units/L	NA	units/L	NA
Alpha$_1$-antitrypsin	mg/dL	0.01	g/L	100
Alpha$_1$-fetoprotein				
amniotic fluid	µg/mL	1	mg/L	1
serum	ng/mL	1	µg/L	1
Alanine aminotransferase (ALT)	units/L	NA	units/L	NA
Aluminum, serum	ng/mL	0.0371	µmol/L	26.95
Amikacin	µg/mL	1.71	µmol/L	0.585
Ammonia, blood	µg/dL	0.714	µmol/L	1.4
Amylase, serum	units/L	NA	units/L	NA
Androstenedione	ng/dL	0.0349	nmol/L	28.7
Angiotensin	ng/dL	10	ng/L	0.1
Angiotensin converting enzyme (ACE)	nmol/min/mL	1	units/L	1
Anion gap	mEq/L	1	mmol/L	1
Antidiuretic hormone (ADH) (vasopressin)	pg/mL	1	ng/L	1
Arsenic				
serum	µg/dL	0.133	µmol/L	7.52
urine	µg/L	0.0133	µmol/d	75.2
Ascorbic acid, blood	mg/dL	56.78	µmol/L	0.018
Aspartate aminotransferase (AST)	units/L	NA	units/L	NA
Base excess	mEq/L	1	mmol/L	1
Bicarbonate (HCO_3^-)	mEq/L	1	mmol/L	1
Bilirubin, serum				
direct	mg/dL	17.1	µmol/L	0.584
total	mg/dL	17.1	µmol/L	0.584
Bromide	mg/dL	0.125	mmol/L	79.9
CA 15-3	units/mL	1	kU/L	1
CA 125	units/mL	1	kU/L	1
Cadmium	µg/L	8.897	nmol/L	0.112
Caffeine	µg/mL	5.15	µmol/L	0.194
Calcitonin	pg/mL	1	ng/L	1
Calcium				
ionized	mg/dL	0.25	mmol/L	4
serum	mg/dL	0.25	mmol/L	4
urine	mg/24 h	0.025	mmol/d	40
Carbamazepine (Tegretol®)	µg/mL	4.23	µmol/L	0.236
Carbon dioxide	mEq/L	1	mmol/L	1
Carboxyhemoglobin	%	NA	%	NA
Carcinoembryonic antigen (CEA)	ng/mL	1	µg/L	1
Carotene, serum	µg/dL	0.0186	µmol/L	53.7
Catecholamines, fractionation, urine	µg/24 h	5.91	nmol/d	0.169
Ceruloplasmin	mg/dL	10	µmol/L	0.10
Chloramphenicol	µg/mL	3.09	µmol/L	0.323
Chlordiazepoxide (Librium®)	µg/mL	3.33	µmol/L	0.30
Chloride				
serum	mEq/L	1	mmol/L	1
sweat	mEq/L	1	nmol/L	1
urine	mmol/24 h	1	mmol/d	1
Cholesterol	mg/dL	0.0259	mmol/L	38.61
HDL	mg/dL	0.0259	mmol/L	38.61
LDL	mg/dL	0.0259	mmol/L	38.61
Cholinesterase, serum	units/mL	1	kU/L	1
Chromium, serum	ng/mL	19.2	nmol/L	0.052
Clonazepam (Klonopin™)	ng/mL	3.17	nmol/L	0.316
Codeine	ng/mL	3.34	nmol/L	0.299
Compound S (11-deoxycortisol)	µg/dL	0.029	µmol/L	34.5

(continued)

Analyte	Conventional Units	Conventional to SI (multiply by)	SI Units	SI to Conventional (multiply by)
Copper				
serum	µg/dL	0.157	µmol/L	6.37
urine	µg/24 h	0.0157	µmol/d	63.69
Coproporphyrins (I and III)				
blood	µg/dL	15	nmol/L	0.067
fluid	µg/g	1.5	nmol/g	0.67
urine	µg/24 h	1.5	nmol/d	0.67
Cortisol				
blood	µg/dL	27.6	nmol/L	0.036
urine	µg/24 h	2.76	nmol/d	0.362
C-Peptide	ng/mL	0.33	nmol/L	3.03
Creatine kinase (CK)	units/L	NA	units/L	NA
Creatinine				
serum	mg/dL	88.4	µmol/L	0.0113
urine	mg/kg/24 h	8.84	µmol/kg/d	0.113
Creatinine Clearance	mL/minute/1.73 m^2	0.0166	mL/second/1.73 m^2	60
Cyanide, blood	mg/24 h	0.0088	µmol/d	113.1
	mg/L	38.4	µmol/L	0.026
Cyclic AMP				
plasma	ng/mL	3.04	nmol/L	0.329
urine	µg/L	3.04	µmol/L	0.329
Cystine, urine	mg/24 h	8.32	µmol/24 h	0.120
Delta aminolevulinic acid, urine	mg/24 h	7.626	µmol/d	0.131
DHEA	ng/mL	3.47	nmol/L	0.288
DHEA sulfate	µg/mL	2.6	µmol/L	0.38
Diazepam (Valium®)	ng/mL	0.0035	µmol/L	0.286
Digitoxin	ng/mL	1.31	nmol/L	0.765
Digoxin (Lanoxin®)	ng/mL	1.28	nmol/L	0.781
Diphenhydramine (Benadryl®)	µg/mL	3.92	µmol/L	0.255
Diphenylhydantoin (Dilantin®)	µg/mL	3.96	µmol/L	0.253
Disopyramide (Norpace®)	µg/mL	2.95	µmol/L	0.339
Doxepin (Sinequan®)	ng/mL	3.58	nmol/L	0.279
d-Xylose	mg/dL	0.066	mmol/L	15.01
Erythropoietin, serum	mIU/mL	1	IU/L	1
Estradiol (E$_2$), serum	pg/mL	3.67	pmol/L	0.272
Estriol (E$_3$), serum	µg/L	3.47	nmol/L	0.288
Estrone (E$_1$), serum	ng/dL	37	pmol/L	0.027
Ethanol	mg/dL	0.217	mmol/L	4.61
Ethchlorvynol (Placidyl®)	µg/mL	6.92	µmol/L	0.145
Ethosuximide (Zarontin®)	µg/mL	7.08	µmol/L	0.141
Ethylene glycol	mg/L	16.1	µmol/L	0.0621
Factor B (properdin)	mg/dL	10	mg/L	0.10
Fatty acids, free, serum	mg/dL	0.0354	mmol/L	28.25
Fecal fat	g/24 h	1	g/d	1
Ferritin, serum	ng/mL	1	µg/L	1
Fluoride	µg/mL	52.6	µmol/L	0.019
Folate				
red cell	ng/mL	2.265	nmol/L	0.442
serum	ng/mL	2.265	nmol/L	0.442
Follicle stimulating hormone (FSH)	mIU/mL	1	IU/L	1
Gamma glutamyl transferase (GGT)	units/L	NA	units/L	NA
Gastrin, serum	pg/mL	1	ng/L	1
Gentamicin	µg/mL	2.09	µmol/L	0.478
Glucagon, plasma	pg/mL	1	ng/L	1
Glucose				
blood	mg/dL	0.0555	mmol/L	18.02
CSF	mg/dL	0.0555	mmol/L	18.02
urine	mg/dL	0.0555	mmol/L	18.02
Glutamine, CSF	mg/dL	68.5	µmol/L	0.0146
Glutethimide (Doriden®)	µg/mL	4.60	µmol/L	0.217
Glycated hemoglobin	% of total Hb	0.01	Fraction of total Hb	100
Gold	µg/dL	0.0508	µmol/L	19.68
Growth hormone (GH)	ng/mL	1	µg/L	1
Haloperidol (Haldol®)	ng/mL	2.66	nmol/L	0.376
Haptoglobin, serum	mg/dL	10	mg/L	0.10

(continued)

Analyte	Conventional Units	Conventional to SI (multiply by)	SI Units	SI to Conventional (multiply by)
Homovanillic acid (HVA), urine	mg/24 h	5.49	μmol/d	0.182
	μg/mg of creatinine	0.621	mmol/mol of creatinine	1.61
Human chorionic gonadotropin (hCG), serum	mIU/mL	1	IU/L	1
17-Hydroxycorticosteroids (17-OHCS), urine	mg/24 h	2.76	μmol/d	0.362
5-Hydroxyindoleacetic acid (5-HIAA), urine	mg/24 h	5.2	μmol/d	0.19
17-Hydroxyprogesterone	ng/dL	0.030	nmol/L	33.3
Imipramine (Tofranil®)	ng/mL	3.57	nmol/L	0.280
Insulin, blood	μIU/mL	1	mIU/L	1
Iron	μg/dL	0.179	μmol/L	5.587
Iron binding capacity, total (TIBC)	μg/dL	0.179	μmol/L	5.587
Isopropanol	mg/L	0.0166	mmol/L	60.1
17-Ketogenic steroids, urine	mg/24 h	3.467	μmol/d	0.288
17-Ketosteroids	mg/24 h	3.467	μmol/d	0.288
Lactate dehydrogenase (LDH)	units/L	NA	units/L	NA
Lactic acid				
blood	mg/dL	0.111	mmol/L	9.01
CSF	mg/dL	0.111	mmol/L	9.01
Lead				
serum	μg/dL	0.0483	μmol/L	20.70
urine	μg/24 h	0.00483	μmol/d	207.04
Leucine aminopeptidase (LAP)	units/L	NA	units/L	NA
Lidocaine (Xylocaine®)	μg/mL	4.27	μmol/L	0.234
Lipase, serum	units/L	NA	units/L	NA
Lipids, total	mg/dL	0.01	g/L	100
Lithium	mEq/L	1	mmol/L	1
Lorazepam	ng/mL	3.11	nmol/L	0.321
Luteinizing hormone (LH)	mIU/mL	1	IU/L	1
Lysergic acid diethylamide (LSD)	μg/mL	3.09	μmol/L	0.323
Magnesium				
serum	mEq/L	0.50	mmol/L	2
urine	mEq/24 h	0.50	mmol/d	2
Manganese				
serum	μg/L	18.2	nmol/L	0.055
urine	μg/L	18.2	nmol/L	0.055
Mercury				
blood	μg/dL	0.0499	μmol/L	20.0
urine	μg/L	0.00499	μmol/d	200
Meperidine (Demerol®)	μg/mL	4.04	nmol/L	0.247
Meprobamate	μg/mL	4.58	μmol/L	0.218
Metanephrines, urine	mg/24 h	5.07	μmol/d	0.197
Methadone	ng/mL	0.00323	μmol/L	309
Methanol	mg/dL	0.312	mmol/L	3.2
Methsuximide (Celontin®)	μg/mL	5.29	μmol/L	0.189
Methyldopa (Aldomet®)	μg/mL	4.73	μmol/L	0.211
Methyprylon (Noludar®)	μg/mL	5.46	μmol/L	0.183
Myoglobin, blood	μg/L	NA	μg/L	NA
N-Acetylprocainamide (NAPA)	μg/mL	3.61	μmol/L	0.277
Nortriptyline (Aventyl®)	ng/mL	3.80	nmol/L	0.263
5' Nucleotidase	units/L	NA	units/L	NA
Osmolality				
serum	mOsm/kg	NA	mmol/kg	NA
urine	mOsm/kg	NA	mmol/kg	NA
Oxalate, urine	mg/24 h	11.4	μmol/d	0.088
Oxazepam (Serax®)	μg/mL	3.49	μmol/L	0.287
Pancreatic polypeptide, human	pg/mL	1	mmol/L	1
Parathyroid hormone	pg/mL	1	ng/L	1
Pentobarbital (Nembutal®)	μg/mL	4.42	μmol/L	0.266
Phencyclidine (PCP)	ng/mL	4.11	nmol/L	0.243
Phenobarbital	μg/mL	4.31	μmol/L	0.232
Phenylalanine, blood	mg/dL	60.5	μmol/L	0.016
Phenytoin (Dilantin®)				
free	μg/mL	3.96	μmol/L	0.253
total	μg/mL	3.96	μmol/L	0.253

(continued)

Analyte	Conventional Units	Conventional to SI (multiply by)	SI Units	SI to Conventional (multiply by)
Phosphorus				
serum	mg/dL	0.323	mmol/L	3.10
urine	g/24 h	32.3	mmol/d	0.031
Porphobilinogen (PBG), urine	mg/24 h	4.42	µmol/d	0.226
Potassium				
blood	mEq/L	1	mmol/L	1
urine	mEq/24 h	1	mmol/d	1
Pregnanediol, urine	mg/24 h	3.12	µmol/24 h	0.321
Pregnanetriol, urine	mg/24 h	2.97	µmol/24 h	0.337
Primidone (Mysoline®)	µg/mL	4.58	µmol/L	0.218
Procainamide (Pronestyl®)	µg/mL	4.23	µmol/L	0.236
Progesterone	ng/mL	3.18	nmol/L	0.314
Prolactin	ng/mL	1	µg/L	1
Propoxyphene (Darvon®)	µg/mL	2.95	µmol/L	0.339
Propranolol (Inderal®)	ng/mL	3.86	nmol/L	0.259
Protein				
CSF	mg/dL	10	mg/L	0.10
serum	g/dL	10	g/L	0.10
urine	mg/24 h	0.001	g/d	1000
Protoporphyrin, free erythrocyte	µg/dL	0.0178	µmol/L	56.18
Protoporphyrin, zinc (ZPP)	µg/dL	0.016	µmol/L	62.5
Quinidine	µg/mL	3.08	µmol/L	0.250
Renin, plasma	ng/mL/h	0.77	nmol/L/h	1.30
Salicylate	mg/dL	0.0724	mmol/L	13.81
Secobarbital (Seconal™)	µg/mL	4.20	µmol/L	0.238
Serotonin	ng/mL	0.00568	µmol/L	176
Sodium				
blood	mEq/L	1	mmol/L	1
urine	mEq/24 h	1	mmol/d	1
T_3 uptake (T_3U)	%	1	AU*	1
Testosterone	ng/dL	0.0347	nmol/L	28.8
Theophylline	µg/mL	5.55	µmol/L	0.18
Thiocyanate	µg/mL	0.0172	mmol/L	58.0
Thyroglobulin	ng/mL	1	µg/L	1
Thyroid stimulating hormone (TSH)	µIU/mL	1	mIU/L	1
Thyrotropin-releasing hormone (TRH)	pg/mL	1	ng/L	1
Thyroxine binding globulin (TBG)	mg/dL	10	mg/L	0.10
Thyroxine (T_4)	µg/dL	12.9	nmol/L	0.0075
Thyroxine, free (FT_4)	ng/dL	12.9	pmol/L	0.0075
Tobramycin	µg/mL	2.14	µmol/L	0.467
Transferrin	mg/dL	0.01	g/L	100
Triglycerides	mg/dL	0.0113	mmol/L	88.5
Triiodothyronine (T_3)	ng/dL	0.0154	nmol/L	65.1
Troponin	µg/L	NA	µg/L	NA
Urea nitrogen, blood (BUN)	mg/dL	0.357	mmol/L	2.80
Uric acid				
serum	mg/dL	0.059	mmol/L	16.9
urine	mg/24 h	0.0059	mmol/d	169
Valproic acid (Depakene®)	µg/mL	6.93	µmol/L	0.144
Vancomycin	µg/mL	0.690	µmol/L	1.45
Vanillylmandelic acid (VMA), urine	mg/24 h	5.05	µmol/d	0.198
Vasoactive intestinal polypeptide	pg/mL	1	ng/L	1
Vitamin				
A	µg/dL	0.0349	µmol/L	28.65
B_6	ng/mL	4.046	nmol/L	0.247
B_{12}	pg/mL	0.738	pmol/L	1.355
D_3 (calcitriol, 1,25-dihydroxy)	pg/mL	2.4	pmol/L	0.417
E	mg/dL	23.22	µmol/L	0.043
Warfarin (Coumadin®)	µg/mL	3.24	µmol/L	0.308
Zinc				
blood	µg/dL	0.153	µmol/L	6.54
urine	µg/24 h	0.0153	µmol/d	65.36

NA = not applicable.

AU = arbitrary unit.

COAGULATION

Wayne R. DeMott, MD

The prime functions of the coagulation mechanism are to protect the integrity of the blood vascular compartment, while reasonably maintaining its fluid state. Death may attend either the inability to stem the loss of blood or the conversion of blood to a solid. The illustrative comparable clinical problems are hemorrhage due to inability to form a normal clot on one hand versus intravascular thrombosis on the other. Thus, the modern medical environment focuses upon the results of panels of tests to assess hemorrhage (possibly due to consumptive coagulopathy) versus thrombosis (possibly the result of hypercoagulability). The exquisite and critically important equilibrium between these two states – irreversible sol vs irreversible gel – is inherent in the concept "disseminated intravascular coagulation" (consumptive coagulation). Excessive clotting occurs but mechanisms to maintain fluidity are activated resulting in coagulation failure-hemorrhage.

The following test listings describe clinical laboratory maneuvers that assist the clinician in the investigation and management of disorders of coagulation. Included importantly are the dichotomous states, intravascular coagulation, and hypercoagulation. Dichotomy of a different nature, a generation gap of sorts, must also be noted. Currently, the nature of many if not all coagulation abnormalities are biochemically highly defined. Earlier generations of tests, many of which persist (and are included amongst the entries which follow), suffer from lack of specificity. They are in reality crude screening procedures. On the other hand, they are not costly or difficult to perform and have some frequency of clinical applicability. Thus, they are readily maintained and are offered by many hospital clinical laboratories. Great strides in the understanding of diseases of coagulation at the molecular level have made possible analyses that are technically demanding and require a certain level of investment (in reagents, equipment, and personnel). Results of these more specific tests may have critical importance in defining a coagulation abnormality (eg, multimer analysis in von Willebrand disease). The conditions defined by these "modern generation" procedures are usually clinically uncommon. In the "modern generation" fiscal environment in which most hospital clinical laboratories function, a high cost/low volume procedure equates to "refer" (to a reference laboratory). Thus, a certain "functional generation gap" has evolved which may not always have favorable implications to the welfare of particular patients.

The following listings attempt to include some of the "old" and some of the "new." There are hopefully sufficient footnote and reference citations to allow the user satisfactory access to additional detail.

Ac-Globulin *see* Factor V *on page 239*

ACT *see* Activated Coagulation Time *on this page*

Activated Clotting Time *see* Activated Coagulation Time *on this page*

Activated Coagulation Time

CPT 85347

Related Information

Activated Partial Thromboplastin Time *on next page*

Antithrombin III Test *on page 230*

Heparin Assay Using Activated Factor X *on page 248*

Heparin Effect, Test for (Using Heparinase) *on page 249*

Lee-White Clotting Time *on page 254*

Synonyms ACT; Activated Clotting Time; Ground Glass Clotting Time

Applies to Protamine Sulfate

Abstract Screening test for coagulation deficiencies, with special application to the monitoring of heparin effect. The test is utilized, in particular, to monitor heparin effect during cardiopulmonary bypass surgical procedures.

Patient Preparation Tubes and syringes used to collect blood should be warmed to 37°C.

Specimen Whole blood

Container Blood sample is added or drawn into a tube containing an activator (silica, Celite, siliceous earth/diatomaceous earth or finely crushed ground glass). The Vacutainer® (Becton-Dickinson) line of evacuated glass tubes includes an appropriate tube reorder #6522. This gray stoppered tube contains 12 mg of purified siliceous earth.

Collection Test is done at bedside by the medical technologist. Whole blood is collected into syringes/tubes warmed to 37°C.

Causes for Rejection Tube not full; specimen hemolyzed; specimen clotted; specimen contaminated by anticoagulant, effect of which is not of interest

Turnaround Time Usually under 5 minutes

Special Instructions A two-syringe or two-tube collection method should be used. The initial 1 mL of blood collected into a plastic syringe or into a tube is discarded without removing needle from vein and the sample to be used for testing is then drawn into the tube containing siliceous earth.

Reference Range Varies between laboratories as it is procedure, activator, and lot number of activator dependent. Normal result is generally 70-120 seconds. Hattersley originally found a normal range of 107 seconds (2SD ±26 seconds[1]) (5000 routine presurgical studies). Becton-Dickinson cautions that use of Vacutainer® tube #6522 will result in shorter ACT normal range than that reported by Hattersley.

Critical Values A minimum ACT value for adequacy of heparinization has not yet been determined but there is evidence that it is under 400 seconds.[2] Gravlee et al suggest that during cardiopulmonary bypass the ACT range be kept within 300-500 seconds.

Use Screen for coagulation deficiencies using whole blood; establish baseline before heparin administration; monitor postheparin injection. ACT has been used to monitor the anticoagulant effect of heparin during percutaneous transluminal coronary angioplasty and coronary artery bypass surgery where heparin concentrations in the range of 1-5 units/mL may cause the APTT to become prolonged beyond measurable levels. Use of an arterial blood sample may avoid a falsely low ACT level.[3]

Limitations Test is insensitive to factor VII deficiency and to some platelet abnormalities. Different activators and methods respond variably to heparinized blood so that heparin dose/response experience in one laboratory setting is not necessarily transferable to a different laboratory. Some authorities feel that the normal range is not sufficiently removed (different from) the heparin anticoagulated therapeutic desirable range.[4] Response to heparin anticoagulation may need to be considered with knowledge of other drugs being taken by the patient (see following information). Lysed platelets shortened the ACT of heparinized whole blood from 248 seconds (controls) to 127 seconds indicating the ACT can be artifactually low in the presence of heparin. There is evidence that platelet membrane fragments (rather than cytosol particles which contain platelet factor 4) are responsible for this effect.[5] This could present a problem in the use of the ACT for monitoring of heparin neutralization as platelet membrane fragmentation occurs during bypass open heart surgery.[6] See Additional Information for recommendation that baseline ACTs be determined after surgical incision.

Methodology Tubes of freshly drawn blood (usually 1 mL) are incubated at 37°C and tilted at 30-second intervals until flow of blood stops. The tilting, detection, and recording of clotting is performed manually or by relatively low cost and compact automated devices. **Manual and even machine results are dependent upon differences in test volume,** intermachine variability, agitation speed and direction, and variation in individual technique.[7] Quality control/assurance procedures must be in place and in practice.

Additional Information While this test could readily replace the Lee and White and other older clotting time tests (which are considered obsolete by many and have not been offered in some laboratories for several years), it has found its greatest application in monitoring the results of heparin anticoagulation.

At least 12 different (some closely related) tests have been proposed to measure heparin's anticoagulant effect.[4] These include clotting time, plasma recalcification time, partial thromboplastin time, thrombin time, polybrene titration, and synthetic substrate assay tests. That such diverse tests can be applied to this task reflects heparin's multisite inhibition of the coagulation mechanism. The APTT is most commonly used. This is in part because the APTT fits into laboratory routine of performance (it is fast, semiautomated, and, therefore, lends itself to batching and performance in the laboratory). The ACT, however, is justifiably preferred by some, including in particular, the cardiovascular surgeons.[8]

The following protocol of Hattersley et al was used in a study of 134 patients with thromboembolic disorders and resulted in no heparin failures and only two cases of dangerous bleeding.[9] Heparin used: porcine gut (Liquaemin®) made up 100 units/mL in 250 mL bag; I.V. bolus 50 units/kg body weight; subsequent infusion 15-25 units/kg/hour; modification of infusion rate to maintain ACT of 150-190 seconds; ACT obtained 4 hours after start of pump infusion, 4 hours after each change of rate, and at least once/24 hours. After 2-3 days of target range ACT, oral warfarin is given 5-10 mg/day according to body weight. After 3-5 days warfarin therapy and with PT at 2 to 2.5 times control, heparin is discontinued (warfarin continued).

The importance of laboratory monitoring of heparin anticoagulation is underscored by the known considerable individual variation in response. **Dose required for adequate anticoagulation is dependent on a variety of factors including severity of thrombotic process, potential risk for bleeding, variations in the heparin preparation (polymer length, degree of sulfonation), and medications that inactivate or inhibit heparin (antihistamines, digitalis, nicotine, penicillin, tetracyclines, streptomycin, erythromycin, gentamicin, ascorbic acid, chlorpromazine, and protamine).** The ACT, while favored by cardiovascular surgeons and recently considered operationally superior to the APTT for bedside monitoring of postpercutaneous transluminal coronary angioplasty patients,[10] suffers a potential drawback. It assays overall coagulation activity. Prolonged values may not be exclusively the result of heparin. There is risk in giving protamine sulfate (heparin antagonist). When the protamine exceeds the amount of heparin, it begins to act as an anticoagulant; the ACT will lack specificity in this situation. It is likely that ACT is decreased as a result of a thromboplastic response induced with the surgical incision. Thus, in order to avoid false diagnosis of adequate protamine neutralization after cardiopulmonary bypass, baseline ACT should be determined after surgical incision.[11]

Footnotes

1. Hattersley PG, "Activated Coagulation of Whole Blood," *JAMA*, 1966, 196:436-40.
2. Metz S and Keats AS, "Low Activated Coagulation Time During Cardiopulmonary Bypass Does Not Increase Postoperative Bleeding," *Ann Thorac Surg*, 1990, 49(3):440-4.
3. Rath B and Bennett DH, "Monitoring the Effect of Heparin by Measurement of Activated Clotting Time During and After Percutaneous Transluminal Coronary Angioplasty," *Br Heart J*, 1990, 63(1):18-21.
4. Triplett DA, "Heparin: Clinical Use and Laboratory Monitoring," *Laboratory Evaluation of Coagulation*, Chicago, IL: American Society of Clinical Pathologists, 1982, 291-2.
5. Bode AP and Eick L, "Lysed Platelets Shorten the Activated Coagulation Time (ACT) of Heparinized Blood," *Am J Clin Pathol*, 1989, 91(4):430-4.
6. George JN, Pickett EB, Saucerman S, et al, "Platelet Surface Glycoproteins. Studies on Resting and Activated Platelets and Platelet Membrane Microparticles in Normal Subjects, and Observations in Patients During Adult Respiratory Distress Syndrome and Cardiac Surgery," *J Clin Invest*, 1986, 78(2):340-8.
7. Uden DL, Payne NR, Kriesmer P, et al, "Procedural Variables Which Affect Activated Clotting Time Test Results During Extracorporeal Membrane Oxygenation Therapy," *Crit Care Med*, 1989, 17(10):1048-51.
8. Dauchot PJ, Berzina-Moettus L, Rabinovitch A, et al, "Activated Coagulation and Activated Partial Thromboplastin Times in Assessment and Reversal of Heparin-Induced Anticoagulation for Cardiopulmonary Bypass," *Anesth Analg*, 1983, 62:710-9.
9. Hattersley PG, Mitsuoka JC, and King JH, "Heparin Therapy for Thromboembolic Disorders. A Prospective Evaluation of 134 Cases Monitored by the Activated Coagulation Time," *JAMA*, 1983, 250:1413-6.
10. Varah N, Smith J, and Baugh RF, "Heparin Monitoring in the Coronary Care Unit After Percutaneous Transluminal Coronary Angioplasty," *Heart-Lung*, 1990, 19(3):265-70.
11. Gravlee GP, Whitaker CL, Mark LJ, et al, "Baseline Activated Coagulation Time Should Be Measured After Surgical Incision," *Anesth Analg*, 1990, 71(5):549-53.

References

Gravlee GP, Haddon WS, Rothberger HK, et al, "Heparin Dosing and Monitoring for Cardiopulmonary Bypass," *J Thorac Cardiovasc Surg*, 1990, 99(3):518-27.

Activated Partial Thromboplastin Substitution Test

CPT 85732

Related Information

Activated Partial Thromboplastin Time *on this page*

Synonyms APTT Correction Studies; Differential APTT Test; PTT Substitution

Test Commonly Includes Correction of patient's abnormal plasma with normal aged serum, normal absorbed plasma and normal plasma

Abstract Modification of the APTT to screen for specific coagulation factor deficiencies

Specimen Plasma

Container Blue top (sodium citrate) tube

Collection Routine venipuncture. If multiple tests are being drawn, draw coagulation studies last. If only coagulation tests are being drawn, use two-syringe/tube technique, draw 1-2 mL into first syringe or Vacutainer®, discard, and then collect coagulation tests. This collection procedure avoids contamination of the specimen with tissue thromboplastins.

Storage Instructions Keep refrigerated

Causes for Rejection Tube not full, specimen hemolyzed, specimen clotted, specimen received more than 2 hours after collection

Special Instructions These substitution correction studies are not offered routinely by all clinical laboratories. Schedule and arrange with laboratory before ordering.

Activated Partial Thromboplastin Substitution Test

Plasma Deficient in:	APTT Corrected by:			
	Normal Plasma	Aged Normal Serum	BaSO₄ Plasma	Celite Plasma
V	+		+	+
VIII	+		+	+
IX	+	+		+
X	+	+		+
XI	+	+	+	
XII	+	+	+	+

Reference Range The deficient factor is indicated by the results of APTT performed on mixtures of the patient's plasma and prepared correcting reagents (aged serum or absorbed normal plasma). Normal plasma contains factors VIII, IX, X, XI, and XII. The prepared reagents are deficient as indicated in the table. A factor V deficient plasma can be prepared by adsorption with a monoclonal antibody to factor V.[1] Tabulation and analysis will indicate the presumptive deficiency causing prolongation of patient's plasma APTT.

Use Presumptive identification of single coagulation factor deficiencies. Confirmation of the deficient factor requires specific factor assays/comparison with plasmas with known deficiencies.

Limitations Only useful with single coagulation factor deficiencies. Correction reactions may be difficult to interpret if patient's APTT is only modestly prolonged.

Contraindications Current anticoagulant therapy

Footnotes

1. Katzmann JA, Nesheim ME, Hibbard LS, et al, "Isolation of Functional Human Coagulation Factor V by Using a Hybridoma Antibody," *Proc Natl Acad Sci U S A*, 1981, 78:162-6.

References

Bowie EJ and Owen CA Jr, "Clinical and Laboratory Diagnosis of Hemorrhagic Disorders," *Disorders of Hemostasis*, Chapter 3, Ratnoff OD and Forbes CD, eds, Philadelphia, PA: WB Saunders Co, 1991, 55.

Activated Partial Thromboplastin Time

CPT 85730

Related Information

Synonyms APTT; Partial Thromboplastin Time, Activated; PTT

Applies to Antiaggregating Agents; Heparin Inhibitors; Low Molecular Weight; Protamine Sulfate; Thrombin Clotting Time Heparin Assay

Test Commonly Includes Patient time and control time

Abstract The activated partial thromboplastin time (APTT) is a readily available low cost screening test. The test procedure is usually automated, batch processing is efficient, and the turnaround time is reasonably rapid in the individual or stat mode. The test finds application in screening for intrinsic factor deficiencies and for monitoring of heparin anticoagulation.

Patient Preparation Draw specimen 1 hour before next dose of heparin if heparin is being given by intermittent injection; not applicable to patients on continuous heparin infusion therapy. Do not draw from an arm with a heparin lock or heparinized catheter.

Specimen Plasma

Container Blue top (sodium citrate) tube

Collection Routine venipuncture. If multiple tests are being drawn, draw coagulation studies last. If only a PTT is being drawn, draw 1-2 mL into another Vacutainer®, discard, and then collect the PTT (two-tube or two-syringe technique). This collection procedure avoids contamination of the specimen with tissue thromboplastins. Transport the specimen to the Hematology Laboratory as soon as possible.

Storage Instructions Keep refrigerated. If specimen cannot be tested within 4 hours after collection, centrifuge and freeze resultant platelet poor plasma and freeze as soon as possible. If transporting specimen, keep frozen and test after thawing at 37°C (NCCLS published guidelines H21-A2).

Causes for Rejection Tube not full, specimen hemolyzed, specimen clotted, specimen received more than 2 hours after collection, specimen improperly labeled, specimen contaminated by anticoagulant effect of which is not being measured

Reference Range 25-39 seconds, usually stated to be within 10 seconds of control. The APTT ratio (observed APTT/mean of the laboratory control APTT) is often applied to the monitoring of heparin therapy. In the normal anticoagulant-free individual, this ratio would fluctuate modestly about unity. Healthy premature newborns have prolonged coagulation test screening results (eg, PT, PTT, TT) which return to normal adult values at about 6 months of age. Healthy prematures, however, do not develop spontaneous hemorrhage or thrombotic complications because of a balance between procoagulants and inhibitors. The normal range in childhood (ages 1-16) is similar to that in adults. (See references by Andrew et al).

Possible Panic Range Over 70 seconds

Use Evaluate intrinsic coagulation system. Useful in monitoring heparin therapy. Aid in screening for presence of classical hemophilia A and B; congenital deficiencies of factors II, V, VIII, IX, X, XI, and XII; dysfibrinogenemia; disseminated intravascular coagulation; liver failure; congenital hypofibrinogenemia; vitamin K deficiency; congenital deficiency of Fitzgerald factor; congenital deficiency of prekallikrein (Fletcher factor).

Limitations Use of the APTT to monitor heparin anticoagulation is complicated by variation in response between individuals due to difference in plasma levels of heparin neutralizing proteins and variations in response between individuals due to difference in plasma levels of heparin neutralizing proteins and variations in levels of factor VIII (as occur with the acute-phase inflammatory reaction). There is resultant reduction in APTT response in relation to heparin levels. Because of variation in reagent thromboplastins supplied by different manufacturers, a single APTT ratio (observed APTT/mean of control APTT) cannot be used to determine therapeutic effect (the same APTT ratio cannot be used for all reagents). The therapeutic range for each reagent should be calibrated to be equivalent to an antifactor Xa level of about 0.3-0.7 units/mL. The APTT should not be used to monitor heparin dosage resulting in heparin concentrations >1 unit/mL (eg, as used in high-risk angioplasty patients and in cardiac bypass patients). Heparin levels >5 units/mL may be required to prevent the bypass circuit from clotting. The activated clotting time can be used in these situations (provides graded response to heparin in the range of 1-5 units/mL).

Contraindications Specimen obtained less than 3 hours after dose of heparin.

Methodology Methods involve addition of a contact activator (eg, Celite, kaolin, microsilicate, elagic acid). Plasma sample is added to activator and incubated at 37°C, usually for 5 minutes. Thromboplastin preparation is added, mixed, and with addition of CaCl₂, a timer is started. A variety of automated instruments have been designed to perform this test, often with the capability of also performing the prothrombin time test. A variety of instruments and reagents are used in the field resulting in many combinations, most monitored by the College of American (Continued)

Activated Partial Thromboplastin Time

(Continued)

Pathologists survey process. A handheld portable instrument that determines the APTT using a fingerstick sample of capillary whole blood has recently been developed.[1]

Additional Information Hemolysis significantly shortens the activated partial thromboplastin time in normal but not in abnormal persons.[2] The APTT may be normal in persons with mild hereditary bleeding disorders. About 30% of normal concentration of factors V, VIII, IX, X, XI, and XII will maintain a rate of thrombin formation sufficient to produce a normal APTT. Prolongation of the APTT clotting time occurs if the concentration of any of the above single clotting factors falls below this level. Fibrinogen level, if <80 mg/dL, may result in an abnormal APTT. If Fletcher or Fitzgerald factors are <5% of normal the APTT may be abnormal. A prolonged APTT can be caused by inherited factor deficiency (I, II, V, VIII-XII), Fletcher or Fitzgerald factor, Coumadin® type therapy, liver disease, circulating anticoagulant (heparin, lupus anticoagulant, fibrin breakdown products), specific factor inhibitor (rheumatoid arthritis, penicillin reaction, occasional hemophiliacs), or intravascular coagulation.

The results of the College of American Pathologists surveys indicate that the source and type of heparinized specimen is important to consider when interpreting APTT test results.[3] Different reagent/instrument combinations effect the APTT response to heparin. Sensitivity is most influenced by the APTT reagent used while precision is most effected by the instrument utilized.

Control of heparin therapy: The control of heparin anticoagulant therapy is complex, controversial, and problematic. Recommendations for dosage and laboratory monitoring will be followed by a consideration of factors that may be responsible for "failures" (failure to achieve anticoagulated state, and/or excessive anticoagulation).

Heparin: Heparin is an acidic mucopolysaccharide found in mast cells and basophils, has a strong negative charge, a circulating half-life of only a few hours, and inhibits all of the active serine proteases (IIa, Xa, IXa, XIa, and XIIa). It is stable for 24 hours in a 5% dextrose solution. Low dose heparin activity relates to inactivation of Xa and possibly to cell surface repulsion effects. On the basis of minimum dose of heparin effective in producing comparable prolongations of clotting time, the whole blood PTT, APTT, whole blood clotting time, and PTT are about equivalent in measuring response to heparin. While some inactivation of heparin may occur in the liver (through action of heparinase), elimination is largely by the kidney so that heparin must be used cautiously in patients with impaired glomerular filtration.

Administration, dosage: Heparin is best administered intravenously, intermittently, or better as continuous infusion in a dosage of 400-500 units/kg body weight/day divided into every 6-hour dosage (so that 100-125 units/kg body weight is given each 6 hours). Laboratory monitoring can be accomplished using the Lee-White clotting time, APTT, or activated clotting time (ACT). Dosage is adjusted to maintain the coagulation test result at about two times the control or "normal" level (APTT target range 60-85 seconds or APTT ratio which is equivalent to a heparin level by antifactor Xa assay of 0.3-0.7 units/mL).

There are three levels of heparin therapy: low dose, moderate dose, and large dose. Low dose refers to small amounts of heparin (10,000-20,000 units/day) given subcutaneously and useful in the prophylaxis against venous thrombosis (selected patients). Measurable change in APTT does not usually occur. See review by Hirsh and Levine listed in references. Moderate dose implies full anticoagulation, requires 20,000-60,000 units/day, the APTT is adjusted to 1.5 to 2 times the control, and the regimen is applied to patients without active thromboembolic disease. Large dose heparin therapy utilizes dosage levels of 60,000-100,000 units/day during the first 24-48 hours and then reverting to 30,000-45,000 units/day. Large dose therapy is for patients with active thromboembolic disease.

Heparin should not be given intramuscularly. There is a trend to favor subcutaneous administration in the initial treatment of deep vein thrombosis. In support of this trend are studies claiming efficacy and safety, procedural simplification allowing outpatient or home therapy (see reference by Hommes et al).

Drugs which antagonize the action of heparin include streptomycin, erythromycin, gentamicin, chlorpromazine, ascorbic acid, antihistamines, and digitalis.

Complications: Not all individuals respond ideally or predictably to heparin. A voluminous literature deals with these exceptions and one must conclude that there is no shortcut to adequate and safe heparin anticoagulation. Investigation of the cause and management of aberrant cases must be undertaken. Anaphylaxis and erythematous reactions may occur with the use of heparin in some individuals.

Untoward effects of heparin include development of osteoporosis with fractures (doses of 20,000 units/day over 6 months) for which a calcium intake of 1 g or more per day may be protective, anti-inflammatory effect, and inhibition of antidiuretic effect resulting in diuresis. Unusual reactions to heparin include anaphylaxis and erythematous reactions (species specific), alopecia, urticaria, headache, and bronchospasm.

An especially important complication of high dose heparin therapy is the development of thrombocytopenia which relates to heparin-induced aggregation. Because of the dangers attendant to a minority of heparin anticoagulated individuals, pretherapeutic laboratory evaluation has been recommended.[4] Abnormalities in platelet count, whole blood clotting time, activated PTT, or antithrombin III may indicate that the patient has a predisposition to an unusual heparin response. Hussey et al have emphasized the significant morbidity (including amputation of extremities) and mortality associated with heparin induced platelet aggregation resulting in new thrombosis and thrombocytopenia.[5] This phenomenon appears to have immune etiology and occurs in the presence of either an IgG or IgM heparin dependent platelet aggregating antibody.

The **progressive thromboembolic syndrome** appears to be always associated with thrombocytopenia. Monitoring of the heparinized patient has been recommended and includes daily physical examination for evidence of further thrombosis and periodic platelet counts, the need for which is determined clinically. Evidence of new thrombosis or decrease in platelet count to <100,000/mm³ should be further investigated with aggregation studies to see if an abnormal response to platelet aggregation is present.

The platelet abnormality quickly reverses when heparin is discontinued. Added beneficial therapy includes antiaggregating agents such as dextran (Rheomacrodex®) I.V., 25 mL/hour; acetylsalicylic acid; dipyridamole; and Coumadin®. Iloprost® has been utilized to prevent heparin-induced thrombocytopenia during open heart surgery.[6,7]

The table summarizes the relation of three coagulation tests that have been and can be utilized to adjust the heparin anticoagulant effect.

Early studies[8,9] suggested that thrombi do not propagate when the heparin level is such as to prolong the Lee and White (L&W) clotting time to twice that of a normal control. The level of heparin required or desirable, however, varies on an individual basis depending on the severity of the thrombotic process, the potential bleeding risk, variations in the heparin preparation - varying polymer length, sulfonation of polymers, medications that inactivate or inhibit heparin (antihistamines, digitalis, nicotine, penicillin, tetracyclines, phenothiazines and protamine), poor coordination in timing the dose and collection of specimens, antithrombin III level, platelet factor IV level, and fibrinogen level. If the latter factors are in normal range, heparin level of 0.3 units/mL of plasma is required to result in a Lee-White clotting time of twice the normal control.

Monitoring: A number of coagulation tests and protocols have been recommended for monitoring heparin effect. The Lee and White clotting time, activated clotting time (ACT), and the activated plasma thromboplastin time (APTT) are used, the latter most commonly (see table).

Heparin Anticoagulant Effect

Test	Usual Normal Control Results	Anticoagulant Range (Heparin Level 0.2-0.4 units/mL)
Lee-White clotting time	8-15 min	20-30 min
Activated clotting time	70-120 sec	180-240 sec
Activated PTT	25-39 sec	60-80 sec

(About twice the normal control value)

The **ACT** has been favored during cardiovascular operations to monitor heparin dosage and neutralization. The ACT, however, assays overall coagulation activity such that prolonged values may not be exclusively the result of heparin.

A significantly larger amount of heparin is required for effective anticoagulation in the presence of active thromboembolic disease. The heparin dosage required to maintain a target APTT of 1.5-2.5 times the control may have diagnostic importance and contribute to an understanding of whether or not thromboembolic disease is present.

Simultaneous monitoring of APTT, WBCT, and the thrombin clotting time appears to have identified a population of patients in which a significant increase (more than double) in the level of factor VIII activity occurs.[10] This results in a misleading shortening of the APTT. To detect this situation, a combination of APTT and a thrombin clotting time heparin assay (TCT) has been recommended.[10] Discrepancy between a normal APTT and a prolonged TCT may indicate presence of antithrombin III deficiency. With dysfibrinogenemia, the TCT would be especially prolonged.

The APTT may be excessively sensitive, and while many studies show correlation with the whole blood clotting time, the series usually lack cases with prolonged APTT or the data show poor correlation with high levels of anticoagulation.

The Lee-White clotting time (WBCT) provides useable results but may require 30-40 minutes to achieve endpoint (clot formation) at high heparin levels. The microsilicate activated clotting time (ACT) obviates some of the difficulties with the WBCT, providing shorter clotting times.

Low molecular weight heparin (LMWH): Standard heparin is composed of sulfated mucopolysaccharides, heterogeneous fragments of different molecular weights. LMWH is less heterogeneous, consists of fragments with high and low affinity for AT III but LMWH use is associated with decreased antithrombin activity while anti-Xa activity is largely preserved. There is evidence that LMWH is able to protect against thromboembolic events while the risk of hemorrhage is reduced.[11] Conventional tests used in monitoring of standard heparin treatment (eg, APTT, TT, ACT) are not affected by LMWH at the doses usually employed. Laboratory control of the use of LMWH is, therefore, not applicable. Heparin-induced thrombocytopenia is usually seen, however, some 7-12 days after LMWH therapy begins so that periodic platelet counts are recommended.[11]

In recent years, increased emphasis has been placed on prevention of bleeding as a complication of anticoagulation, one of the goals of laboratory monitoring. To this end, use of a bleeding risk index for prospective evaluation has been developed and found to provide a valid estimate of the probability of major bleeding during anticoagulation.[12]

Lupus anticoagulant: Patients with a prolonged APTT not corrected by mixing with normal plasma but with no family or clinical/surgical history of bleeding are (in screening situations) most commonly due to a phospholipid (lupus type) anticoagulant. College of American Pathologists surveys have found significant difference in the sensitivity of different APTT reagents to the presence of lupus anticoagulants. The difference in reagent responsiveness can affect the apparent factor activity and also the dilutional effect on mixing patient with normal plasma samples, thus impairing the ability to differentiate a lupus anticoagulant from a specific factor inhibitor.[13]

Appropriateness of prothrombin and partial thromboplastin time testing on the medical service of a teaching hospital (ordering patterns in relation to clinical indications) concludes that these tests are overutilized (at least 70% were not clinically indicated).[14,15]

Specially designed devices have been developed (eg, paramagnetic iron oxide technology based thrombolytic assessment system) for use in point-of-care testing.[16] In some clinical situations, the reliability of point-of-care APTT assays has been found similar to that of conventional assays,[17,18] perhaps with some caveats.

Over 50% of cases of Noonan's syndrome (congenital heart disease, short stature, and dysmorphic facies) also have abnormal bleeding. Prolonged APTT was found in 40% of patients with the syndrome. A variety of specific individual and combined deficiencies were identified.[19]

Footnotes

1. Ansell J, Tiarks C, Hirsh J, et al, "Measurement of the Activated Partial Thromboplastin Time From a Capillary (Fingerstick) Sample of Whole Blood. A New Method for Monitoring Heparin Therapy," *Am J Clin Pathol*, 1991, 95(2):222-7.
2. Garton S and Larsen AE, "Effect of Hemolysis on the Partial Thromboplastin Time," *Am J Med Technol*, 1972, 38:408-10.
3. Gawoski JM, Arkin CF, Bovill T, et al, "The Effects of Heparin on the Activated Partial Thromboplastin Time of the College of American Pathologists Survey Specimens: Responsiveness, Precision, and Sample Effects," *Arch Pathol Lab Med*, 1987, 111(9):785-90.
4. Forman WB, "The Risks of Heparin Therapy," *Hosp Formulary*, 1978, 779-84.
5. Hussey CU, Bernhard VM, McLean MR, et al, "Heparin Induced Platelet Aggregation: In Vitro Confirmation of Thrombotic Complications," *Ann Clin Lab Sci*, 1979, 9:487-93.
6. Addonizio VP Jr, Fisher CA, Kappa JR, et al, "Prevention of Heparin-Induced Thrombocytopenia During Open Heart Surgery With Iloprost® (ZK36374)," *Surgery*, 1987, 102(5):796-807.
7. Sobel M, Adelman B, Sezntpetery S, et al, "Surgical Management of Heparin-Associated Thrombocytopenia. Strategies in the Treatment of Venous and Arterial Thromboembolism," *J Vasc Surg*, 1988, 8(4):395-401.
8. Wessler S and Morris CE, "Studies in Intravascular Coagulation: IV. The Effect of Heparin and Dicumarol on Serum Induced Venous Thrombosis," *Circulation*, 1955, 12:553-6.
9. Carey LC and Williams RD, "Comparative Effects of Dicumarol, Tromexan, and Heparin on Thrombus Propagation," *Ann Surg*, 1960, 152:919-22.
10. Glynn MF, "Heparin Monitoring and Thrombosis," *Am J Clin Pathol*, 1979, 71:397-400.
11. Samama M, "Low Molecular Weight Heparin," *ASCP Check Sample®*, Chicago, IL: American Society of Clinical Pathologists, 1987.
12. Landefeld CS, McGuire E 3d, and Rosenblatt MW, "A Bleeding Risk Index for Estimating the Probability of Major Bleeding in Hospitalized Patients Starting Anticoagulant Therapy," *Am J Med*, 1990, 89(5):569-78.
13. Brandt JT, Triplett DA, Rock WA, et al, "Effect of Lupus Anticoagulants on the Activated Partial Thromboplastin Time. Results of the College of American Pathologists Survey Program," *Arch Pathol Lab Med*, 1991, 115(2):109-14.
14. Erban SB, Kinman SL, and Schwartz JS, "Routine Use of the Prothrombin and Partial Thromboplastin Times," *JAMA*, 1989, 262(17):2428-32.
15. Janvier G, Winnock S, and Freyburger G, "Value of the Activated Partial Thromboplastin Time for Preoperative Detection of Coagulation Disorders Not Revealed by a Specific Questionnaire," *Anesthesiology*, 1991, 75(5):920-1.
16. Oberhardt BJ, "Thrombosis and Hemostasis Testing at the Point of Care," *Am J Clin Pathol*, 1995, 104(Suppl 1):S72-8.
17. Werner M, Gallagher JV, Ballo MS, et al, "Effect of Analytic Uncertainty of Conventional and Point-of-Care Assays of Activated Partial Thromboplastin Time on Clinical Decisions in Heparin Therapy," *Am J Clin Pathol*, 1994, 102(2):237-41.
18. Arkin CF, "Coagulation Screening Tests," *Am J Clin Pathol*, 1994, 102(2):150-1.
19. Sharland M, Patton MA, Talbot S, et al, "Coagulation-Factor Deficiencies and Abnormal Bleeding in Noonan's Syndrome," *Lancet*, 1992, 339(8784):19-21.

References

Andrew M, "Developmental Hemostasis: Relevance to Hemostatic Problems During Childhood," *Semin Thromb Hemost*, 1995, 21(4):341-56.

Andrew M, Paes B, Milner R, et al, "Development of the Human Coagulation System in the Healthy Premature Infant," *Blood*, 1988, 72(5):1651-7.

Andrew M, Vegh P, Johnston M, et al, "Maturation of the Hemostatic System During Childhood," *Blood*, 1992, 80(8):1998-2005.

Brill-Edwards P, Ginsberg JS, Johnston M, et al, "Establishing a Therapeutic Range for Heparin Therapy," *Ann Intern Med*, 1993, 119(2):104-9.

Colvin BT and Barrowcliffe TW, "The British Society for Haematology Guidelines on the Use and Monitoring of Heparin 1992: Second Revision," *J Clin Pathol*, 1993, 46(2):97-103.

D'Angelo A, Seveso MP, D'Angelo SV, et al, "Effect of Clot-Detection Methods and Reagents on Activated Partial Thromboplastin Time (APTT). Implications in Heparin Monitoring by APTT," *Am J Clin Pathol*, 1990, 94(3):297-306.

Dhami MS and Bona RD, "Using Anticoagulants Safely. Guidelines for Therapeutic and Prophylactic Regimens," *Postgrad Med*, 1991, 90(1):121-2, 127-32.

Hirsh J and Fuster V, "Guide to Anticoagulant Therapy. Part 1: Heparin. American Heart Association," *Circulation*, 1994, 89(3):1449-68.

Hirsh J and Levine MN, "Low Molecular Weight Heparin," *Blood*, 1992, 79(1):1-17.

Hirsh J, Raschke R, Warkentin TE, et al, "Heparin: Mechanism of Action, Pharmacokinetics, Dosing Considerations, Monitoring, Efficacy, and Safety," *Chest*, 1995, 108(4 Suppl):258S-75S.

Hommes DW, Bura A, Mazzolai L, et al, "Subcutaneous Heparin Compared With Continuous Intravenous Heparin Administration in the Initial Treatment of Deep Vein Thrombosis. A Meta-Analysis," *Ann Intern Med*, 1992, 116(4):279-84.

Joch LE, Lutomski DM, Williams DJ, et al, "Accuracy of a First-Order Model for Estimating Initial Heparin Dosage," *Clin Pharm*, 1993, 12(8):597-601.

Turpie AG, Robinson JG, and Doyle DJ, "Comparison of High-Dose With Low-Dose Subcutaneous Heparin to Prevent Left Ventricular Mural Thrombosis in Patients With Acute Transmural Anterior Myocardial Infarction," *N Engl J Med*, 1989, 320(6):352-7.

Weinmann EE and Salzman EW, "Deep-Vein Thrombosis," *N Engl J Med*, 1994, 331(24):1630-41.

Yedinak KC and Sproat TT, "Heparin and Warfarin Therapy After Acute Myocardial Infarction," *Clin Pharm*, 1993, 12(3):197-215.

Acute Phase Reactants *see* Fibrinogen *on page 246*

Aggregometer Test *see* Platelet Aggregation *on page 257*

AHF *see* Factor VIII *on page 240*

Antiaggregating Agents *see* Activated Partial Thromboplastin Time *on page 227*

Anticoagulant, Circulating

CPT 85732

Related Information

Activated Partial Thromboplastin Time *on page 227*
Anticardiolipin Antibody *on page 364*
Antinuclear Antibody *on page 368*
Cryoprecipitate *on page 606*
Factor VIII *on page 240*
Factor VIII Concentrate *on page 608*
Factor IX Complex (Human) *on page 609*
Inhibitor, Lupus, Phospholipid Type *on page 251*
VDRL, Serum *on page 438*

Synonyms CAC; Lupus Anticoagulant

Abstract Circulating anticoagulants include antibodies (immunoglobulins) to coagulation factors that develop in cases of inherited deficiency, in cases of autoimmune/malignant neoplastic conditions, as a result of the use of some medications and include the lupus (phospholipid type) anticoagulant.

Patient Preparation Coumadin® therapy should be discontinued for 2 weeks prior to test; heparin therapy should be discontinued 2 days prior to collection of the specimen.

Specimen Plasma

Container Blue top (3.2% or 3.8% sodium citrate) tube

Collection Routine clean venipuncture. If multiple tests are being drawn, draw coagulation studies last. If only circulating anticoagulant is being drawn, use two-syringe (or Vacutainer® tube) technique. Avoid contamination of specimen with tissue thromboplastin. Draw first 1-2 mL in one syringe (or tube), discard, and (without moving needle) draw specimen into second tube (or with second syringe). Use only plastic syringes.

Storage Instructions Place specimen tube on ice and transport immediately to the laboratory.

Causes for Rejection Patient receiving Coumadin® or heparin therapy; specimen hemolyzed, clotted, diluted or contaminated; specimen not on ice or received over 1 hour after collection

Reference Range No circulating anticoagulant identified. Previous prothrombin and activated partial thromboplastin times are useful in interpretation of results.

Use Detection of circulating anticoagulants as may occur in multiple-transfused, factor-deficient patients, as associated with dysproteinemias (multiple myeloma), lupus erythematosus, rheumatoid arthritis, ulcerative colitis, postpartum complication and other conditions
(Continued)

Anticoagulant, Circulating *(Continued)*

Limitations Accurate quantitation of inhibitor may not be possible if patient is or has been receiving replacement or anticoagulant therapy or if test is done more than 2 hours after collection. Determination of presence of inhibitor may, however, be possible in some of these situations.

Methodology Serial dilutions of patient's plasma with fresh normal plasma incubated at room temperature and at 37°C for 2 hours followed by APTT. Factor specificity can be determined by measuring the specific factor activity remaining after incubation of normal plasma and dilutions of patient plasma. (For example, incubate equal parts of normal and test plasma for 30 minutes and compare factor levels before and after incubation).

Additional Information Acquired circulating anticoagulants are of different types (usually immunoglobulins) and occur in a variety of disorders. In classic hemophilia, factor VIII antibody (usually of IgG class) can act as a circulating anticoagulant, negating the effect of exogenously administered factor VIII. These are the most common and important of the stage I inhibitors (against factors VIII, IX, XI, or XII) occurring in 5% to 20% of factor VIII deficient patients. They are more common in severe than mild cases of hemophilia A. They apparently arise as an immune response to that part of the factor VIII molecule (VIII:C or VIII:CAg) that is decreased or absent in these patients.[1] Less commonly, they may occur spontaneously (in patients without hemophilia) in some chronic inflammatory states, collagen diseases, postpartum, and in association with some drugs and some malignancies.[2] More common are the "lupus-like" or lupus anticoagulants, one of the most common causes of prolonged APTT (in absence of liver disease) and most often found during preoperative screening. These do not appear to be directed against a specific clotting factor. Rather, they are heterogeneous, including autoantibodies directed against phospholipid-binding plasma proteins.[3] At least some lupus anticoagulants are directed against phospholipid-bound prothrombin or against β_2-glycoprotein I (one of the complement control proteins). They may interfere with hemostatic reactions that have an *in vivo* requirement for anionic phospholipid membrane surfaces such as the platelet phospholipid platform. The clinical effect may be thrombosis rather than "anticoagulant." Clinically, significant bleeding is not usually associated with presence of a "lupus anticoagulant."

Detection of a circulating anticoagulant depends upon finding a prolonged clotting test result which is not corrected by adding normal plasma. Such inhibitors occur in some 5% to 10% of cases of systemic lupus erythematosus but are more often found in patients with other autoimmune processes or without demonstrable associated disease. A 32% incidence of this inhibitor has been reported in patients on long-term phenothiazine therapy.[4] Patients with lupus anticoagulant have a high incidence of positive ANA tests and may have a false-positive serology for syphilis. Lupus anticoagulant may appear as part of the procainamide-induced lupus syndrome. Patients with lupus anticoagulant often have prolonged prothrombin time, occasionally severe, due to associated deficiency of prothrombin activity.

Of most importance clinically is that many patients (25% to 30%) with lupus "anticoagulant" have thromboembolism.[5] Cerebral ischemic episodes may be the result of cardioembolism occurring in patients who have a circulating lupus anticoagulant.[6] There is evidence that immunoadsorption (using extracorporeal staphylococcal protein A columns in hemophiliac patients) removes coagulation factor inhibitors and may allow successful factor replacement therapy.[7] Incubation with protein A bound to Sepharose (which removes IgG) has been used to show that a patient with acquired deficiency of both factor VII activity and antigen was likely the result of an IgG able to bind factor VII without neutralizing its activity. The bound immunoglobulin is hypothesized to have induced rapid plasma clearance of the factor VII molecule or to have modified its synthesis.[8]

Clinically significant inhibitors of factor XIII (eg, inhibitor New Haven) have been described.[9] Perioperative hemostasis has been achieved in patients with hemophilia who have developed inhibitors by use of recombinant activated factor VII, thus bypassing factor VIII.[10]

Footnotes

1. White GC II, McMillan CW, Blatt PM, et al, "Factor VIII Inhibitors: A Clinical Overview," *Am J Hematol*, 1982, 13:335-42.
2. Kessler CM, "An Introduction to Factor VIII Inhibitors: The Detection and Quantitation," *Am J Med*, 1991, 91(5A):1S-5S.
3. Roubey RA, "Autoantibodies to Phospholipid-Binding Plasma Proteins: A New View of Lupus Anticoagulants and Other "Antiphospholipid" Autoantibodies," *Blood*, 1994, 84(9):2854-67.
4. Canoso RT, Hutton RA, and Deykin D, "A Chlorpromazine-Induced Inhibitor of Blood Coagulation," *Am J Hematol*, 1977, 2:183-91.
5. Carreras LO, Defreyn G, Machin SJ, et al, "Arterial Thrombosis, Intrauterine Death, and "Lupus" Anticoagulant: Detection of Immunoglobulin Interfering With Prostacyclin Formation," *Lancet*, 1981, 1:244-6.
6. Young SM, Fisher M, Sigsbee A, et al, "Cardiogenic Brain Embolism and Lupus Anticoagulant," *Ann Neurol*, 1989, 26(3):390-2.
7. Uehlinger J, Button GR, McCarthy J, et al, "Immunoadsorption for Coagulation Factor Inhibitors," *Transfusion*, 1991, 31(3):265-9.

8. Weisdorf D, Hasegawa D, and Fair DS, "Acquired Factor VII Deficiency Associated With Aplastic Anemia: Correction with Bone Marrow Transplantation," *Br J Haematol*, 1989, 71(3):409-13.
9. Fukue H, Anderson K, McPhedran P, et al, "A Unique Factor XIII Inhibitor to a Fibrin-Binding Site on Factor XIIIA," *Blood*, 1992, 79(1):65-74.
10. O'Marcaigh AS, Schmalz BJ, Shaughnessy WJ, et al, "Successful Hemostasis During a Major Orthopedic Operation By Using Recombinant Activated Factor VII in a Patient With Severe Hemophilia A and a Potent Inhibitor," *Mayo Clin Proc*, 1994, 69(7):641-4.

References
Aledort L, "Inhibitors in Hemophilia Patients: Current Status and Management," *Am J Hematol*, 1994, 47(3):208-17.

Kaczor DA, Bickford NN, and Triplett DA, "Evaluation of Different Mixing Study Reagents and Dilution Effect in Lupus Anticoagulant Testing," *Am J Clin Pathol*, 1991, 95(3):408-11.

Kasper CK, "Treatment of Factor VIII Inhibitors," *Prog Hemost Thromb*, 1989, 9:57-86.

Peacock NW and Levine SP, "Case Report: The Lupus Anticoagulant-Hypoprothrombinemia Syndrome," *Am J Med Sci*, 1994, 307(5):346-9.

Triplett DA, "Coagulation Assays for the Lupus Anticoagulant: Review and Critique of Current Methodology," *Stroke*, 1992, 23(2 Suppl):111-4.

Antifactor Xa *see* Heparin Assay Using Activated Factor X *on page 248*

Antihemophilic Factor *see* Factor VIII *on page 240*

Antiphospholipid Antibody *see* Inhibitor, Lupus, Phospholipid Type *on page 251*

Antiphospholipid Antibody (APA) *see* Inhibitor, Lupus, Phospholipid Type *on page 251*

α_2-Antiplasmin *see* Plasminogen Assay *on page 256*

Antithrombin III Assay, Functional AT III *see* Antithrombin III Test *on this page*

Antithrombin III Test

CPT 85300 (activity); 85301 (antigen assay)

Related Information

Activated Coagulation Time *on page 226*
Activated Partial Thromboplastin Time *on page 227*
Hypercoagulable State Coagulation Screen *on page 250*
Platelet Aggregation, Hypercoagulable State *on page 258*
Prothrombin Fragment 1.2 *on page 261*

Synonyms Antithrombin III Assay, Functional AT III; Heparin Cofactor Activity; Immunologic Antithrombin III; Serine Protease Inhibitor

Abstract Test for antithrombin III level with applicability to testing for thromboembolic disease states.

Specimen Plasma

Container Two blue top (sodium citrate) tubes

Collection Routine venipuncture. If multiple tests are being drawn, draw AT III with coagulation studies, last. If only antithrombin III is being drawn, draw 1-2 mL in another Vacutainer®, discard, and draw specimen into second tube (with citrate anticoagulant) avoiding contamination with tissue thromboplastin. Immediately invert gently at least five times, mixing thoroughly. Avoid excessively vigorous mixing. Tubes must be sufficiently full (eg, 4.5 mL blood added to 0.5 mL of liquid citrate anticoagulant). Place tubes on ice and deliver immediately to the laboratory.

Storage Instructions Separate plasma and keep refrigerated; deliver refrigerated specimen for testing within 2 hours.

Causes for Rejection Specimen received more than 2 hours after collection, specimen not refrigerated, citrate tubes insufficiently filled, tubes not labeled, clotted specimens, specimen contaminated with heparin (as with heparin flush procedures)

Turnaround Time 2-4 hours

Reference Range 17-30 mg/dL (SI: 170-300 mg/L); 80% to 120% of normal activity, considerable method dependent variation. AT III is lower in serum than in plasma when using the thrombin neutralization test (some antithrombin is consumed when blood clots). Healthy premature infants at birth have decreased AT III, heparin cofactor II, protein C and protein S inhibitor levels, approximately 50% below normal adult values. With the exception of protein C and protein S, values have risen to those of normal adults by 6 months of age. Spontaneous hemorrhage or thromboses do not develop in healthy prematures, however, because of a balance that is maintained between procoagulants and inhibitors (see following references by Andrew et al). Potentially fatal hemorrhagic and thrombotic complications occur in sick (eg, respiratory distress, necrotizing enterocolitis, sepsis) prematures. There may be DIC, severe AT III deficiency, and/or dysfunctional AT III (see following references by Andrew et al and by Manco-Johnson).

Use Evaluate hypercoagulable state, fibrinogenolytic state, and response to heparin. Test for the hereditary deficiency of antithrombin III (autosomal dominant) which is characterized by predisposition to thrombosis. Acquired deficiency associated with severe cirrhosis, chronic liver failure, DIC, thrombolytic therapy, pulmonary embolism, nephrotic syndrome, or postsurgical state (especially liver transplant or partial hepatectomy). Also used to evaluate decreased synthesis or increased loss/consumption. Changes induced by drugs must be considered. Antithrombin III levels might also be of use in cases of suspected heparin failure, suspected DIC, or personal or familial history of thromboembolic disease. The test is indicated in the latter cases especially prior to heparinization, general or orthopedic surgery, prolonged bedrest, pregnancy, postpartum, or postoperative state or oral contraceptive use. AT III deficiency has been found **not** to be an inherent feature of SLE.[1] See table.

Antithrombin III Levels

Increased With	Decreased With
Elevated ESR	Use of oral contraceptives
Elevated CRP	Pulmonary embolism
Hyperglobulinemia	Acute myocardial infarction
Coumarin-type anticoagulation	Intravascular coagulation
	Thrombophlebitis
	Neoplastic disease of the liver

Limitations Test may measure functional or immunologic levels only. The functional anticoagulant effect may be variable. Presence of additional "antithrombins" (distinct from AT III, in particular heparin cofactor II) may contribute to functional "AT III" activity as determined variously by different clinical assays complicating their interpretation and comparability.[2] Antithrombin III activity may be decreased due to oral contraceptive use in women, in the third trimester of pregnancy, and in blood type O women taking high estrogen dose contraceptive preparations.[3] If specimen contains heparin (as with specimen drawn after heparin flush or patient receiving heparin), results may be erroneous. Patients receiving coumarin type anticoagulants may have increased AT III levels.

Methodology The numerous available methods (see references) fall into either functional (ie, thrombin neutralization, von Kaulla chromogenic/fluorogenic synthetic substrate) or immunologic based (ie, radial immunodiffusion (RID), electroimmunoassay, radioimmunoassay (RIA), enzyme-linked immunosorbent assay (ELISA)) groups. While RIA and ELISA methods are sensitive, they may give unreliable, misleading results in cases of inherited deficiency due to a functionally abnormal but antigenically nearly normal molecule. Increased heparin cofactor II in patients with type I diabetes and possibly in other clinical situations may lead to overestimation of functionally active AT III by the thrombin inhibition assay. Use of a factor Xa inhibition assay for functionally active AT III has been shown to give results similar to an immunoreactive method.[4] Synthetic chromogenic substrate-based methodology may now be considered the method of choice for determination of AT III activity.[5]

Additional Information Antithrombin III has been shown to inhibit the activity of activated factors XII, XI, IX and X, as well as, II (thrombin). Antithrombin III is the main physiologic inhibitor of serine proteases generated during coagulation, in particular factor Xa, where it appears to exert its most critical effect. AT III is a "heparin cofactor." Heparin interacts with AT III and thrombin, increasing the rate of thrombin neutralization (inhibition) but decreasing the total quantity (of thrombin) inhibited. The understanding of "antithrombins" began in the early 1900s, is colorful as well as complex, and is still incomplete.[2] Two protein fractions were separated in 1974 and designated heparin cofactors A and B.[6] Heparin cofactor A (HC A) has an absolute requirement for heparin and did not inhibit activated factor X. AT III (heparin cofactor B) which neutralizes both thrombin and factor Xa was characterized and studied to the exclusion of HC A. An inhibitor (of thrombin) distinct from AT III has been purified,[7,8] partially sequenced, and designated heparin cofactor II (HC II). HC II has, essentially, the properties of HC A, is structurally similar to but different from AT III.[9] AT III and heparin, each alone or together, inhibit both the classical and alternative pathways of complement. AT III may act as a serine protease inhibitor of enzymatic stages of the complement system.[10]

Patients with low AT III levels usually exhibit some degree of resistance to heparin anticoagulation. AT III deficiency affects 1/2000 of the general population; 40% to 70% of these become symptomatic (experience thrombosis). Only some 2% to 3% of hospitalized patients with recurrent or extensive thrombosis have AT III deficiency.[5] In the more common forms of AT III deficiency, genetic molecular heterogeneity has been shown by the application of recombinant DNA techniques for molecular analysis.[11] Decrease in AT III may be associated with tendency to thrombosis with seemingly minor trauma in early adult years.

Thrombotic symptoms in cases of hereditary deficiency of antithrombin III have been reported with levels ranging from 40% to 60% of normal. Clinical picture of AT III deficiency may be similar to that of protein C deficiency.[12] Individuals with antithrombin III deficiency will show resistance to anticoagulation with heparin but can be anticoagulated with

coumarin derivatives, in which case antithrombin III levels have been shown to rise. Antithrombin III levels may be decreased in women during hormonal contraceptive therapy. A significant number of patients with mesenteric venous thrombosis may have AT III deficiency. It has been recommended that patients with such thrombotic disease be screened for AT III levels to identify those patients that may benefit from coumarin anticoagulant prophylaxis.[13]

Synthetic nucleotides have been developed and applied to the analysis of AT III variants, AT III Northwick Park and AT III Glasgow. Inheritance of these variants is associated with thrombosis. Oligonucleotides, used as specific hybridization probes, have shown that these AT III variants result from a single base substitution that causes an amino acid substitution at Arg 393. Such nucleotide probe procedures could provide for early detection of AT III variants.[14]

Footnotes

1. Jarrett MP, Green D, and Ts'ao CH, "Relation Between Antithrombin III and Clinical and Serologic Parameters in Systemic Lupus Erythematosus," *J Clin Pathol*, 1983, 36:357-60.
2. Brandt JT, "The Role of Natural Coagulation Inhibitors in Hemostasis," *Clin Lab Med*, 1984, 4(2):245-84.
3. Burkman RT, Bell WR, Zacur HA, et al, "Oral Contraceptives and Antithrombin III: Variations by Dosage and ABO Blood Group," *Am J Obstet Gynecol*, 1991, 164(6 Pt 1):1453-8.
4. Gram J and Jespersen J, "Increased Concentrations of Heparin Cofactor II in Diabetic Patients, and Possible Effects on Thrombin Inhibition Assay of Antithrombin III," *Clin Chem*, 1989, 35(1):52-5.
5. Bick RL, *Disorders of Thrombosis and Hemostasis: Clinical and Laboratory Practice*, Chicago, IL, American Society of Clinical Pathologists, 1992, 270.
6. Briginshaw GF and Shanberge JN, "Identification of Two Distinct Heparin Cofactors in Human Plasma: II. Inhibition of Thrombin and Activated Factor X," *Thromb Res*, 1974, 4:463-77.
7. Tollefsen DM and Blank MK, "Detection of a New Heparin-Dependent Inhibitor of Thrombin in Human Plasma," *J Clin Invest*, 1981, 68:589-96.
8. Tollefsen DM, Majerus DW, and Blank MK, "Heparin Cofactor II: Purification and Properties of a Heparin-Dependent Inhibitor of Thrombin in Human Plasma," *J Biol Chem*, 1982, 257:2162-9.
9. Griffith MJ, Noyes CM, and Church FC, "Reactive Site Peptide Structural Similarity Between Heparin Cofactor II and Antithrombin III," *J Biol Chem*, 1985, 260(4):2218-25.
10. Weiler JM and Linhardt RJ, "Antithrombin III Regulates Complement Activity In Vitro," *J Immunol*, 1991, 146(11):3889-94.
11. Prochownik EV, Antonarakis SE, Bauer KA, et al, "Molecular Heterogeneity of Inherited Antithrombin III Deficiency," *N Engl J Med*, 1983, 308:1549-52.
12. Broekmans AW, Veltkamp MD, and Bertina RM, "Congenital Protein C Deficiency and Venous Thromboembolism. A Study of Three Dutch Families," *N Engl J Med*, 1983, 309:340-4.
13. Wilson C, Walker ID, Davidson JF, et al, "Mesenteric Venous Thrombosis and Antithrombin III Deficiency," *J Clin Pathol*, 1987, 40(8):906-8.
14. Thein SL and Lane DA, "Use of Synthetic Oligonucleotides in the Characterization of Antithrombin III Northwick Park (393 CGT-TGT), and Antithrombin III Glasgow (393 CGT-CAT)," *Blood*, 1988, 72(5):1817-21.

References

Andrew M, "Developmental Hemostasis: Relevance to Hemostatic Problems During Childhood," *Semin Thromb Hemost*, 1995, 21(4):341-56.

Andrew M, Massicotte-Nolan P, Mitchell L, et al, "Dysfunctional Antithrombin III in Sick Premature Infants," *Pediatr Res*, 1985, 19(2):237-9.

Andrew M, Vegh P, Johnston M, et al, "Maturation of the Hemostatic System During Childhood," *Blood*, 1992, 80(8):1998-2005.

Bauer KA and Rosenberg RD, "Role of Antithrombin III as a Regulator of In Vivo Coagulation," *Semin Hematol*, 1991, 28(1):10-8.

Blajchman MA, Austin RC, Fernandez-Rachubinski F, et al, "Molecular Basis of Inherited Human Antithrombin III Deficiency," *Blood*, 1992, 80(9):2159-71.

Brandt JT and Ezenagu L, "Heparin Cofactor II, Thrombosis and Hemostasis," *ASCP Check Sample®*, Chicago, IL: American Society of Clinical Pathologists, 1987.

Buller HR and ten Cate JW, "Acquired Antithrombin III Deficiency: Laboratory Diagnosis, Incidence, Clinical Implications, and Treatment With Antithrombin III Concentrate," *Am J Med*, 1989, 87(3B):44S-48S.

Chuansumrit A, Manco-Johnson MJ, and Hathaway WE, "Heparin Cofactor II in Adults and Infants With Thrombosis and DIC," *Am J Hematol*, 1989, 31(2):109-13.

Demers C, Ginsberg JS, Hirsh J, et al, "Thrombosis in Antithrombin-III-Deficient Persons: Report of a Large Kindred and Literature Review," *Ann Intern Med*, 1992, 116(9):754-61.

De Stefano V, Finazzi G, and Mannucci PM, "Inherited Thrombophilia: Pathogenesis, Clinical Syndromes, and Management," *Blood*, 1996, 87(9):3531-44.

Edgar P, Jennings I, and Harper P, "Enzyme Linked Immunosorbent Assay for Measuring Antithrombin III," *J Clin Pathol*, 1989, 42(9):985-7.

Manco-Johnson MJ, "Neonatal Antithrombin III Deficiency," *Am J Med*, 1989, 87(3B):49S-52S.

Menache D, "Antithrombin III: Introduction," *Semin Hematol*, 1991, 28(1):1-2.

Olds RJ, Lane DA, Mille B, et al, "Antithrombin: The Principal Inhibitor of Thrombin," *Semin Thromb Hemost*, 1994, 20(4):353-72.

Owen MC, Borg JY, and Carrell RW, "Antithrombin III Rouen-I (47 Arg to his) and (47 ser). Two New Variants With Decreased Heparin Affinity," *N Z Med J*, 1987, 100:566-7.

van Boven HH, Olds RJ, Thein SL, et al, "Hereditary Antithrombin Deficiency: Heterogeneity of the Molecular Basis and Mortality in Dutch Families," *Blood*, 1994, 84(12):4209-13.

Vinazzer H, "Therapeutic Use of Antithrombin III in Shock and Disseminated Intravascular Coagulation," *Semin Thromb Hemost*, 1989, 15(3):347-52.

APC-R *see* Resistance to Activated Protein C *on page 265*

APC Resistance *see* Resistance to Activated Protein C *on page 265*

APTT *see* Activated Partial Thromboplastin Time *on page 227*

aPTT/APC Screening Test *see* Resistance to Activated Protein C *on page 265*

APTT Correction Studies *see* Activated Partial Thromboplastin Substitution Test *on page 226*

ASA Tolerance Test *see* Aspirin Tolerance Test *on this page*

Aspirin Tolerance Test

CPT 85002 (x 2)

Related Information

Bleeding Time, Duke *on next page*

Bleeding Time, Ivy *on next page*

Clot Retraction *on page 235*

Platelet Force Development by Clot Retractometry *on page 259*

von Willebrand Factor Antigen *on page 267*

Synonyms ASA Tolerance Test; Bleeding Time Aspirin Tolerance Test; Tolerance Test for Aspirin

Test Commonly Includes Bleeding time measurement before and after ingestion of aspirin

Patient Preparation Patient must not have consumed aspirin (acetylsalicylic acid) or aspirin-containing preparations for the 10 days prior to testing. In adults, 10 grains (600 mg) of acetylsalicylic acid are given after the initial bleeding time has been performed. In children weighing less than 70 pounds, the dose of aspirin is 5 grains.

Specimen Blood; an *in vivo* test performed directly on the patient

Collection Test is performed at patient's bedside by medical technologist.

Causes for Rejection History of aspirin intake, presence of known abnormal bleeding time possibly due to abnormality of capillary vasculature

Reference Range Test is to assess the degree of change that can be detected (using the bleeding time procedure) as a result of aspirin ingestion. The bleeding time will usually be prolonged by 2-3 minutes. If a vascular or platelet function defect is present or if the subject is a hyper-responder, there may be greater prolongation of the bleeding time after aspirin ingestion.

Use Assess the magnitude of aspirin effect on the bleeding time as an indirect reflection of the effect on platelet function; identify aspirin hyper-responders; may serve as a provocative test for von Willebrand disease

Limitations Invalid if previous aspirin ingestion has occurred

Contraindications Previous aspirin ingestion; markedly prolonged bleeding time before aspirin ingestion

Methodology A bleeding time test (preferably Mielke, template bleeding time) is performed before the patient ingests 600 mg of aspirin; 2 hours later the bleeding time is repeated using the opposite arm.[1]

Additional Information There is evidence that some 15% of individuals may be aspirin "hyper-responders". These subjects are characterized by prolongation of over 5.9 minutes above normal baseline when the template bleeding time is determined 7 hours after a single 325 mg dose of aspirin is given.[2]

An *in vitro* bleeding time test device and procedure have been described and applied to the detection of aspirin effect.[1] The device consists of a conical tube with a coated membrane covered window in which a slit has been placed. The nylon membrane is coated with collagen types I and III, factor VIII - von Willebrand factor and fibronectin and then dried. A second square of nylon membrane is applied, dried, $CaCl_2$-$MgCl_2$ solution added and dried. This is the "subendothelial membrane." The conical-shaped tube is prepared from polyethylene tubing, a bulge produced, and a window cut into the tube. The membrane is then glued, coated side on the inside over the window. Within run precision had a coefficient of variation of 17%. Normal bleeding time by this method was less than 1 minute, postaspirin bleeding times were more than 7 minutes. The study group consisted, however, of only eight individuals.[3] See footnote by Mammen et al and discussion in test entry Bleeding Time, Ivy *on page 233* for additional information about *in vitro* bleeding time tests.

Aspirin, by suppressing thromboxane A_2 (through inhibition of cyclo-oxygenase pathway) is used to decrease the risk of thrombosis in coronary artery disease (CAD). Presence of noncyclo-oxygenase dependent mechanisms of platelet activity contributing to coronary thrombosis have led to interest in more reliable measures of clot retraction and stability. A "clot retractometer" has been used to monitor platelet function by measuring platelet force and clot elastic modulus during clot retraction. Despite aspirin therapy, there is evidence that at least some patients with severe CAD have persistent platelet activation and rigid clot structure.[4]

Footnotes

1. Bick RL, Adams T, and Schmalhorst WR, "Bleeding Times, Platelet Adhesion, and Aspirin," *Am J Clin Pathol*, 1976, 65:69-72.

2. Fiore LD, Brophy MT, Lopez A, et al, "The Bleeding Time Response to Aspirin. Identifying the Hyperresponder," *Am J Clin Pathol*, 1990, 94(3):292-6.

3. Brubaker DB, "An *In Vitro* Bleeding Time Test," *Am J Clin Pathol*, 1989, 91(4):422-9.

4. Greilich PE, Carr ME, Zekert SL, et al, "Quantitative Assessment of Platelet Function and Clot Structure in Patients With Severe Coronary Artery Disease," *Am J Med Sci*, 1994, 307(1):15-20.

References

Mielke CH Jr, "Aspirin Prolongation of the Template Bleeding Time: Influence of Venostasis and Direction of Incision," *Blood*, 1982, 60:1134-42.

Patrono C, "Aspirin as an Antiplatelet Drug," *N Engl J Med*, 1994, 330(18):1287-94.

Pappas JM, Westengard JC, and Bull BS, "Population Variability in the Effect of Aspirin on Platelet Function: Implications for Clinical Trials and Therapy," *Arch Pathol Lab Med*, 1994, 118(8):801-4.

Autoprothrombin I *see* Factor VII *on page 240*

Autoprothrombin II *see* Factor IX *on page 241*

Beta-Thromboglobulin

CPT 85999

Related Information

Fibrinopeptide A *on page 247*

Hypercoagulable State Coagulation Screen *on page 250*

Intravascular Coagulation Screen *on page 253*

Synonyms βTG; β-TG; β-Thromboglobulin

Abstract Beta-thromboglobulin (βTG) is a platelet α granule polypeptide protein formed of 81 amino acids. It is a marker of platelet activation applicable to the study of both prothrombotic states (hypercoagulability) and disseminated intravascular coagulation (DIC).

Specimen Blood or urine

Container Special siliconized tube containing EDTA, prostaglandin E_1, and theophylline must be used in order to stabilize platelets so that βTG will not be released during preparation of platelet-poor plasma.[1]

Collection Blood should be harvested from a carefully performed clean venipuncture using a "two-tube" (or two-syringe) technique. The first 2-5 mL of blood (first tube) is discarded. The following 2.5 mL of blood is collected in special βTG assay tubes (see Container), usually supplied by the manufacturer. Specimen must be transported on ice.

Storage Instructions Whole blood may be stored at 0°C to 4°C for up to 72 hours before processing. Platelet-poor plasma should be prepared from whole blood using a refrigerated centrifuge.

Causes for Rejection Specimen improperly collected, specimen clotted, specimen not submitted in special βTG assay tubes or not submitted on ice

Special Instructions This test will most commonly be performed by a referral or research laboratory. Platelet-poor plasma should be prepared from whole blood using a refrigerated centrifuge (0°C to 4°C), centrifugation at 1900 g for 60 minutes. This will reduce the amount of βTG released from platelets during preparation to a minimum so that the plasma concentration will more closely reflect the true circulating level *in vivo*.[1]

Reference Range 10-50 ng/mL

Use Differentiate DIC from primary lysis (βTG is elevated in the former); assess platelet hyperreactivity as in hypercoagulable states; studies of the prothrombotic state and of the effects of thrombolytic regimens in vascular occlusive disease,[2] heart failure,[3] coronary atherosclerosis,[4] inflammatory bowel disease,[5] and chronic uremia,[6] including diabetic nephropathy.[7] Urine, as well as plasma, levels of βTG may be increased in patients with diabetic nephropathy. It was considered that the study of urine levels were less subject to methodological error.[7]

Limitations Dependent upon method of analysis, in particular specimen handling/processing, plasma levels of βTG may be artifactually increased due to platelet activation *in vitro*. Study of the ratio of plasma beta-thromboglobulin to plasma platelet factor 4 may allow distinction between *in vivo* and artifactual *in vitro* release.[8]

Methodology Radioimmunoassay (RIA), enzyme-linked immunosorbent assay (ELISA), procedure and reagents are commercially available

Additional Information Beta-thromboglobulin (βTG) is a platelet-secreted protein, with a molecular weight of 8800 daltons. It is present exclusively in megakaryocytes and in the α granules of platelets. βTG has a primary structure similar to platelet factor 4 (PF4). Platelet basic protein, another resident of α granules, is the apparent precursor for both βTG and PT4. βTG is a fibroblast chemoattractant and as such is involved in inflammatory reactions. Plasma βTG levels provide a specific marker of the *in vivo* platelet release reaction and are thus indicative of platelet activation.[2] Such activation may occur upon interaction of platelets with subendothelial collagen, or by the action of thrombin, ADP, or catecholamines. There is evidence that platelets from elderly individuals have increased levels of βTG.[9] Presence of a circadian rhythm of plasma βTG has been reported.[10]

Footnotes

1. Ludlam CA and Cash JD, "Studies on the Liberation of β-Thromboglobulin From Human Platelets In Vitro," *Br J Haematol*, 1976, 33:239-47.

2. Lonsdale RJ, Heptinstall S, Westby JC, et al, "A Study of the Use of the Thromboxane A_2 Antagonist, Sulotroban, in Combination With Streptokinase for Local Thrombolysis

in Patients With Recent Peripheral Arterial Occlusions: Clinical Effects, Platelet Function, and Fibrinolytic Parameters," *Thromb Haemost*, 1993, 69(2):103-11.

3. Jafri SM, Ozawa T, Mammen E, et al, "Platelet Function, Thrombin and Fibrinolytic Activity in Patients With Heart Failure," *Eur Heart J*, 1993, 14(2):205-12.
4. Nilsson J, Volk-Jovinge S, Svensson J, et al, "Association Between High Levels of Growth Factors in Plasma and Progression of Coronary Atherosclerosis," *J Intern Med*, 1992, 232(5):397-404.
5. Webberley MJ, Hart MT, and Melikian V, "Thromboembolism in Inflammatory Bowel Disease: Role of Platelets," *Gut*, 1993, 34(2):247-51.
6. Sagripanti A, Cupisti A, Baicchi U, et al, "Plasma Parameters of the Prothrombotic State in Chronic Uremia," *Nephron*, 1993, 63(3):273-8.
7. Tóth L, Szénási P, Varsányi MN, et al, "Elevated Levels of Plasma and Urine Beta-Thromboglobulin or Thromboxane-B_2 as Markers of Real Platelet Hyperactivation in Diabetic Nephropathy," *Haemostasis*, 1992, 22(6):334-9.
8. Kaplan KL and Owen J, "Plasma Levels of β-Thromboglobulin and Platelet Factor 4 as Indices of Platelet Activation *In Vivo*," *Blood*, 1981, 57(2):199-202.
9. Abbate R, Prisco D, Rostagno C, et al, "Age-Related Changes in the Hemostatic System," *Int J Clin Lab Res*, 1993, 23(1):1-3.
10. Stubbs F, "Circadian Rhythm of Plasma Beta-Thromboglobulin in Healthy Human Subjects," *Blood Coagul Fibrinolysis*, 1992, 3(4):497.

References

Brozović M and Mackie I, "Investigation of Thrombotic Tendency," *Practical Haematology*, 7th ed, Chapter 20, Dacie JV and Lewis SM, eds, New York, NY: Churchill Livingstone, 1991, 328-9.

Kerry PJ and Curtis AD, "Standardization of β-Thromboglobulin (β-TG) and Platelet Factor 4 (PF4): A Collaborative Study to Establish International Standards for β-TG and PF4," *Thromb Haemost*, 1985, 53(1):51-5.

Miller MD and Krangel MS, "Biology and Biochemistry of the Chemokines: A Family of Chemotactic and Inflammatory Cytokines," *Crit Rev Immunol*, 1992, 12(1-2):17-46.

Bleeding Time *see* Bleeding Time, Duke *on this page*

Bleeding Time Aspirin Tolerance Test *see* Aspirin Tolerance Test *on previous page*

Bleeding Time, Duke
CPT 85002

Related Information
Aspirin Tolerance Test *on previous page*
Bleeding Time, Ivy *on this page*
Bleeding Time, Mielke *on next page*

Synonyms Bleeding Time

Abstract An *in vivo* screening test, largely of historic interest, for platelet and capillary function.

Specimen Blood; an *in vivo* test performed directly on the patient

Container Filter paper

Causes for Rejection Low platelet count

Turnaround Time Same day, usually within minutes or hours

Reference Range 5 minutes; there is marked variation between laboratories in reported bleeding times performed on normal subjects.[1] As a corollary, each laboratory should have established its own normal range.

Use Evaluate platelet function

Limitations Not as sensitive as bleeding time, Ivy template

Methodology Ear lobe (after cleansing with 70% alcohol and allowing to dry) is punctured with a sterile lancet. Duration of flow of blood is timed (beginning with time of puncture and ending when flow stops). Filter paper is used to blot the drops of blood (must be done without touching skin or disturbing clot) at 15- to 30-second intervals. An *in vitro* bleeding time test device and procedure has been described. See Aspirin Tolerance Test *on page 232*.

Additional Information Use is recommended only under special circumstances. Most laboratories no longer perform this test. The Ivy template bleeding time is a more standardized measure of the bleeding time. It is recommended in place of the Duke bleeding time except under unusual circumstances, such as bilateral arm casts. Test should be performed no sooner than 1 week after last dose of aspirin-containing medication.

Footnotes
1. Poller L, Thomson JM, and Tomenson JA, "The Bleeding Time: Current Practice in the UK," *Clin Lab Haematol*, 1984, 6(4):369-73.

References

Duke WW, "The Relation of Blood Platelets to Hemorrhagic Disease: Description of a Method for Determining the Bleeding Time and Coagulation Time and Report of Three Cases of Hemorrhagic Disease Relieved by Transfusion," *JAMA*, 1910, 55:1185-92.

"Guidelines on Platelet Function Testing. The British Society for Haematology BCSH Haemostasis and Thrombosis Task Force," *J Clin Pathol*, 1988, 41(12):1322-30.

Bleeding Time, Ivy
CPT 85002

Related Information
Aspirin Tolerance Test *on previous page*
Bleeding Time, Duke *on this page*
Bleeding Time, Mielke *on next page*
Clot Retraction *on page 235*
Platelet Adhesion Test *on page 256*
Platelet Aggregation *on page 257*
von Willebrand Factor Antigen *on page 267*

Synonyms Ivy Bleeding Time

Abstract An *in vivo* functional test for platelet and capillary function

Patient Preparation The skin of the volar surface of patient's forearm is prepared with alcohol wash and allowed to dry.

Aftercare If brisk bleeding has occurred (as with puncturing a vein) or if bleeding is prolonged, a pressure bandage should be placed over the puncture site.

Specimen Blood; an *in vivo* test performed directly on patient

Container Filter paper

Collection Performed at bedside by a medical technologist.

Causes for Rejection If the patient needs to be restrained, has excessively cold or edematous arms, or cannot have blood pressure cuff placed on either arm (as with casts, dressings, infection, or extensive rash). History of keloid formation. Some laboratories may require that patient or guardian signs informed consent.

Turnaround Time Same day, usually within minutes or hours

Reference Range 2-7 minutes, shorter in men than women, shorter in those older than 50 years of age

Possible Panic Range Greater than 12-15 minutes

Use A screening test used to assess capillary function, platelet number and function, and ability of platelets to adhere to vessel wall and form a plug. See reference by Burns and Lawrence for a comprehensive assessment of clinical utility. Useful in evaluation of ecchymosis, spontaneous bruising and bleeding, bleeding tendency. Prolonged in some patients after aspirin ingestion, in qualitative platelet disorders (eg, von Willebrand disease, Bernard-Soulier syndrome, Glanzmann's thrombasthenia, and the "gray platelet syndrome"), with fibrinogen disorders, macroglobulinemia, some cases of myeloproliferative disease, renal failure, and with abnormalities of blood vessels. There is inconclusive evidence that the bleeding time is a good predictor of operative hemorrhage in patients with a negative history of bleeding diathesis.

Limitations Scarring of skin may occur. Patients with low platelet count ($<100,000/mm^3$) and some patients on aspirin therapy may have prolongation of the bleeding time.

Contraindications Low platelet count ($<50,000/mm^3$); patient receiving medication containing aspirin; patient with established severe bleeding diathesis; patient with infectious disease of skin or taking any drug with acetyl groups; senile skin changes; prior history of keloid formation

Methodology A blood pressure cuff, placed on the arm above the elbow, is inflated and adjusted to 40 mm Hg. After the alcohol-cleansed puncture site has dried, the skin is held taut and two approximately 3 mm deep puncture wounds (test is performed in duplicate) are made in the volar skin of patient's forearm, immediately after which a stopwatch is started. Superficial veins should be avoided. At 30-second intervals the drops of blood are blotted using filter paper. When the flow of blood ceases, the stop watch is triggered off. The classical Ivy bleeding time suffers from poor reproducibility. The test depends importantly on the ability to produce a uniform precise incision (freehand in the Ivy method). Characteristics of the incision may vary with the technologist, as well as, the site chosen for the test and the direction of the puncture wound. The use of template methods may not increase sensitivity or reproducibility (precision).[1] See listing Bleeding Time, Mielke *on page 234*. Commercial versions with disposable equipment are available. A comparison of two such commercial adaptations have shown that the devices are fairly comparable, with some evidence that the horizontal incision may be more sensitive in detection of primary hemostasis.[2] There are compelling operational and practical reasons for preferring the Mielke (template) bleeding time over the nonstandardized Ivy bleeding time and for producing vertical (cephalocaudal, elbow to wrist) rather than horizontal cuts.[3] An *in vitro* bleeding time device and procedure has been described. See Aspirin Tolerance Test *on page 232*.

Additional Information Test should be performed no sooner than 1 week after last dose of medication containing aspirin. Low platelet count or aspirin therapy will prolong the bleeding time. It may be prolonged in patients with senile skin changes in the presence of normal platelet function. Bleeding time is prolonged in both constitutional and acquired forms of von Willebrand syndrome. The latter may relate to presence of dysproteinemia associated with lymphoproliferative disease.[4] There may be prolonged bleeding time in some patients with advanced renal failure who, however, have largely intact measurable parameters of platelet function.[5]

Either intravenous or subcutaneous administration of 1-deamino-8-D-arginine vasopressin (DDAVP®) has been shown to shorten the bleeding time in patients with uremia.[6]

The bleeding time may find application as a marker of thrombolytic activity in patients treated with streptokinase for deep vein thrombosis.[7] Oral administration of conjugated estrogens may decrease the bleeding time and improve clinical bleeding in patients with renal failure.[8]

(Continued)

Bleeding Time, Ivy *(Continued)*

Gray platelet syndrome is a rare autosomal recessive inherited isolated deficiency of platelet alpha granule content. It is associated with modest prolongation of the bleeding time, large degranulated (pale gray) platelets on the peripheral blood smear, increased plasma beta-thromboglobulin, decreased platelet factor 4, and decreased platelet aggregation with epinephrine, ADP, thrombin and collagen. Aggregation with ristocetin is normal.[9] Alpha granule depletion has also been reported with cardiopulmonary bypass[10] and as an *in vitro* artifact caused by EDTA-dependent platelet agglutinin.[11]

A current study found prolonged Ivy bleeding time in 33% of women with severe pre-eclampsia. Most of these subjects had an adequate number of platelets (>100,000/mm³).Correlation of bleeding time with platelet count occurred only with platelet counts <100,000/mm³.[12]

There is evidence that platelet storage pool deficiency may present with a prolonged bleeding time but without platelet aggregation abnormalities. Thus, storage pool deficiency enters into the differential consideration in all patients with unexplained prolongation of the bleeding time.[13]

An improved model of an *in vitro* bleeding time device is recently commercially available (initially in Europe). The system (PFA-100™ for Platelet Function Analyzer) measures primary, platelet dependent hemostasis in citrated whole blood. It has been found that the system identifies normals and abnormals with greater sensitivity and specificity than the manual *in vivo* bleeding time test.[14]

Footnotes
1. Koster T, Caekebeke-Peerlinck KM, and Briet E, "A Randomized and Blinded Comparison of the Sensitivity and the Reproducibility of the Ivy and Simplate® II Bleeding Time Techniques," *Am J Clin Pathol*, 1989, 92(3):315-20.
2. Buchanan GR and Holtkamp CA, "A Comparative Study of Variables Affecting the Bleeding Time Using Two Disposable Devices," *Am J Clin Pathol*, 1989, 91(1):45-51.
3. Bick RL, *Disorders of Thrombosis and Hemostasis: Clinical and Laboratory Practice*, Chicago, IL: American Society of Clinical Pathologists, 1992, 44.
4. Gan TE, Sawers RJ, and Koutts J, "Pathogenesis of Antibody-Induced Acquired von Willebrand Syndrome," *Am J Hematol*, 1980, 9:363-71.
5. Gordge MP, Faint RW, Rylance PB, et al, "Platelet Function and the Bleeding Time in Progressive Renal Failure," *Thromb Haemost*, 1988, 60(1):83-7.
6. Vigano GL, Mannucci M, Lattuada A, et al, "Subcutaneous Desmopressin (DDAVP®) Shortens the Bleeding Time in Uremia," *Am J Hematol*, 1989, 31(1):32-5.
7. Hirsch DR, Reis SE, Polak JF, et al, "Prolonged Bleeding Time as a Marker of Venous Clot Lysis During Streptokinase Therapy," *Am Heart J*, 1991, 122(4 Pt 1):965-71.
8. Shemin D, Elnour M, Amarantes B, et al, "Oral Estrogens Decrease Bleeding Time and Improve Clinical Bleeding in Patients With Renal Failure," *Am J Med*, 1990, 89(4):436-40.
9. Peerschke EI, "The Gray Platelet Syndrome," *ASCP Check Sample®*, Chicago, IL: American Society of Clinical Pathologists, 1988.
10. Pumphrey CW and Dawes J, "Platelet Alpha Granule Depletion: Findings in Patients With Prosthetic Heart Valves and Following Cardiopulmonary Bypass Surgery," *Thromb Res*, 1983, 30:257-64.
11. Pegels JG, Bruynes ECE, Engelfriet CP, et al, "Pseudothrombocytopenia: An Immunologic Study on Platelet Antibodies Dependent on Ethylene Diamine Tetra-Acetate," *Blood*, 1982, 59:157-61.
12. Ramanathan J, Sibai BM, Vu T, et al, "Correlation Between Bleeding Times and Platelet Counts in Women With Pre-Eclampsia Undergoing Caesarean Section," *Anesthesiology*, 1989, 71(2):188-91.
13. Israels SJ, McNicole A, Robertson C, et al, "Platelet Storage Pool Deficiency: Diagnosis in Patients With Prolonged Bleeding Times and Normal Platelet Aggregation," *Br J Haematol*, 1990, 75(1):118-21.
14. Mammen EF, Alshameeri RS, and Comp PC, "Preliminary Data From a Field Trial of the PFA-100™ System," *Semin Thromb Hemost*, 1995, 21(Suppl 2):113-21.

References
Burns ER and Lawrence C, "Bleeding Time: A Guide to Its Diagnostic and Clinical Utility," *Arch Pathol Lab Med*, 1989, 113(11):1219-24.

Davis JM and Schwartz KA, "Bleeding Time," *Lab Med*, 1989, 20:759-62.

Ellinger P and Peterson P, "Demonstrating Proficiency for the Bleeding-Time Test," *Lab Med*, 1995, 26(12):776-7.

Lind SE, "The Bleeding Time Does Not Predict Surgical Bleeding," *Blood*, 1991, 77(12):2547-52.

Sirridge MS and Shannon R, *Laboratory Evaluation of Hemostasis and Thrombosis*, 3rd ed, Philadelphia, PA: Lea & Febiger, 1983, 72.

Bleeding Time, Mielke

CPT 85002

Related Information
Bleeding Time, Duke *on previous page*

Bleeding Time, Ivy *on previous page*

Clot Retraction *on next page*

Platelet Concentrate, Donation and Transfusion *on page 616*

Synonyms Bleeding Time, Simplate®; Bleeding Time, Template; Surgicutt®

Abstract An *in vivo* test for platelet function and capillary integrity

Patient Preparation The advisability of informing patient as to the possibility of scar/keloid formation should be considered.

Aftercare Butterfly closure of puncture for 24 hours

Specimen Blood; an *in vivo* test performed directly on the patient

Container Filter paper

Collection Performed at bedside by a laboratory technologist.

Causes for Rejection Patient needs to be restrained, has excessively cold or edematous arms, or cannot have blood pressure cuff placed on either arm (as with casts, dressings, infection, or extensive rash). History of keloid formation. Some laboratories may require that patient or guardian sign informed consent.

Turnaround Time Same day, usually within minutes or hours

Reference Range 2.5-10 minutes; using the Surgicutt® pediatric device the normal range in children 1-10 years of age is reported as 2.5-13 minutes; 11-16 years of age, 3-8 minutes; compared to an adult range of 1-7 minutes (using a Surgicutt® adult automated device). The children studied had no history of bleeding and did not have pathologic bleeding during their surgery. The difference between pediatric and adult bleeding time may relate to the length of the cut with the pediatric device.[1]

Use Screening for coagulation abnormality, in particular to assess capillary and platelet function. Useful in evaluation of ecchymosis, spontaneous bruising and bleeding, bleeding tendency. May be prolonged after aspirin ingestion, in cases of von Willebrand disease, Bernard-Soulier syndrome, and Glanzmann's thrombasthenia (qualitative platelet disorders), macroglobulinemia, some case of myeloproliferative disease, fibrinogen disorders, and in renal failure.[2]

Limitations Low platelet count (<100,000/mm³) or aspirin therapy may prolong the bleeding time. Scarring of skin may occur. If disease, injury, or I.V. therapy precludes access to the skin of the arm, test may be performed using medial aspect of the thigh. Results using normal controls and sensitivity to aspirin-induced prolongation are comparable at these two sites (arm compared to thigh).[3]

Contraindications Low platelet count; patient receiving medication containing aspirin

Methodology This test is a modification of the Ivy bleeding time (see Bleeding Time, Ivy *on page 233*) and has replaced the classical Ivy bleeding time in most laboratories. The patient preparation (including use of a blood pressure cuff) is the same. Sensitivity and reproducibility of the test theoretically is increased by standardizing the method of production and length of the incision. This is achieved by use of a template or by use of the commercially available Simplate® or Surgicutt® devices, the latter two giving fairly comparable results. A study comparing Ivy method and Simplate® II, however, did not find that the Simplate® II method was superior in sensitivity or reproducibility (precision) to the Ivy method.[5] There are significant practical reasons for producing vertical (elbow to wrist oriented) rather than horizontal cuts.[6] An *in vitro* bleeding time device and procedure have been described (see Aspirin Tolerance Test *on page 232*).

Additional Information Test should be performed no sooner than 10 days after the last dose of medication containing aspirin. There is no significant effect of therapeutic propranolol on template bleeding time.[7] In newborns, use of an automated bleeding time device resulted in bleeding times similar to or shorter than those of adults.[8]

An *in vitro* bleeding time device (the PFA-100™) is recently commercially available (initially in Europe). See footnote by Mammen et al in listing Bleeding Time, Ivy *on page 233*.

Footnotes
1. Andrew M, Vegh P, Johnston M, et al, "Maturation of the Hemostatic System During Childhood," *Blood*, 1992, 80(8):1998-2005.
2. Gordge MP, Faint RW, Rylance PB, et al, "Platelet Function and the Bleeding Time in Progressive Renal Failure," *Thromb Haemost*, 1988, 60(1):83-7.
3. Hertzendorf LR, Stehling L, Kurec AS, et al, "Comparison of Bleeding Times Performed on the Arm and the Leg," *Am J Clin Pathol*, 1987, 87(3):393-6.
4. Buchanan GR and Holtkamp CA, "A Comparative Study of Variables Affecting the Bleeding Time Using Two Disposable Devices," *Am J Clin Pathol*, 1989, 91(1):45-51.
5. Koster T, Caekebeke-Peerlinck KM, and Briet E, "A Randomized and Blinded Comparison of the Sensitivity and the Reproducibility of the Ivy and Simplate® II Bleeding Time Techniques," *Am J Clin Pathol*, 1989, 92(3):315-20.
6. Bick RL, *Disorders of Thrombosis and Hemostasis: Clinical and Laboratory Practice*, Chicago, IL: American Society of Clinical Pathologists, 1992, 44.
7. Pamphilon DH, Boon RJ, Prentice AG, et al, "Lack of Significant Effect of Therapeutic Propranolol on Measurable Platelet Function in Healthy Subjects," *J Clin Pathol*, 1989, 42(8):793-6.
8. Andrew M, Paes B, Bowker J, et al, "Evaluation of an Automated Bleeding Time Device in the Newborn," *Am J Hematol*, 1990, 35(4):275-7.

References
Braman AM and Schwartz KA, "Platelet Disorders," *Lab Med*, 1989, 20:831-5.

BSCH Haemostasis and Thrombosis Task Force of the British Society for Haematology, "Guidelines on Platelet Function Testing," *J Clin Pathol*, 1988, 41(12):1322-30.

Montgomery RR and Scott JP, "Hemostasis: Diseases of the Fluid Phase," *Hematology of Infancy and Childhood*, 4th ed, Chapter 44, Nathan DG and Oski FA, eds, Philadelphia, PA: WB Saunders Co, 1993, 1609-10.

Sirridge MS and Shannon R, *Laboratory Evaluation of Hemostasis and Thrombosis*, 3rd ed, Philadelphia, PA: Lea & Febiger, 1983, 73-4.

Bleeding Time, Simplate® *see Bleeding Time, Mielke on this page*

Bleeding Time, Template *see Bleeding Time, Mielke on this page*

CAC *see Anticoagulant, Circulating on page 229*

Capillary Fragility Test

CPT 85999

Synonyms Negative Pressure Suction Cup Capillary Fragility; Rumpel-Leede Test; Rumpel-Leede Tourniquet Test; Tourniquet Test

Abstract Test for evaluation of capillary integrity

Collection Performed at bedside by medical technologist

Causes for Rejection Presence of petechiae, ecchymoses, extensive infection, vesicle or bullae formation involving skin of patient's arms, casts on arms, or extensive intravenous attachments or wrappings impeding access to patient's upper extremities

Reference Range Presence of 5 or less petechiae in men and 10 or less petechiae in women and children in an area of 2.5 cm radius. Normal range varies, dependent on technical differences in method.

Use Evaluate capillary endothelial integrity, ecchymosis, easy bruising, easy bleeding, spontaneous bruising, spontaneous bleeding

Limitations Results may be difficult to interpret if petechiae or other forms of hemorrhage in the skin are present before the test begins. Some normal individuals may show capillary fragility. Test may be normal in some patients with thrombocytopenia.

Methodology Negative- and/or positive-pressure methods may be employed.[1] Negative-pressure method uses a suction cup which is applied to the skin. Capillary resistance is the least negative pressure required for 1 minute to produce one or more petechiae. In the positive-pressure method, blood pressure cuff is maintained on the arm with pressure halfway between diastolic and systolic (maximum of 100 mm Hg) for 5 minutes. Cuff pressure is released and arm is observed for petechiae. The number of petechiae appearing in a given area is reported.

Additional Information This test provides a relatively crude measure of capillary integrity. Positive reactions may occur with thrombocytopenia (platelet count <10,000/mm^3), toxic vascular reactions, and hereditary vascular abnormalities. Generally, large petechiae relate to thrombocytopenia while tiny pinpoint examples are more often associated with increase in vascular permeability. The results may vary with age and menstrual cycle. Positive results may occur prior to and immediately after menstruation and in the postmenopausal state. Hormones of the estrogen and cortisone type often improve capillary resistance. The prolonged use of steroids, however, eventually results in increased capillary fragility, possibly due to loss of subcutaneous tissue.

The tourniquet test lacks specificity and has been referred to as "abandoned by most laboratories." For use in children and the elderly, a standard petechiometer is commercially available.[2]

Footnotes

1. Bennington JL, *Saunders Dictionary & Encyclopedia of Laboratory Medicine and Technology*, Philadelphia, PA: WB Saunders Co, 1984, 251.
2. Bick RL, *Disorders of Thrombosis and Hemostasis: Clinical and Laboratory Practice*, Chicago, IL: American Society of Clinical Pathologists, 1992, 44, 51.

CBA see von Willebrand Factor Collagen Binding Assay *on page 269*

Christmas Disease Factor see Factor IX *on page 241*

Clot Lysis Time see Diluted Whole Blood Clot Lysis *on page 237*

Clot Retraction

CPT 85170

Related Information

Aspirin Tolerance Test *on page 232*
Bleeding Time, Ivy *on page 233*
Bleeding Time, Mielke *on previous page*
Factor XIII *on page 243*
Fibrinogen *on page 246*
Platelet Aggregation *on page 257*
Platelet Force Development by Clot Retractometry *on page 259*

Test Commonly Includes Description of clot retraction, size, firmness and RBC fallout. May include serum "drip-out" and serum and RBC escaping from clot.

Abstract Evaluation of clot formation, providing a window for possible platelet function (and/or number) abnormalities and/or fibrinogen level/function

Specimen Blood

Container Red top tube

Collection Transport specimen to the laboratory within 1 hour of collection. May require special collection.

Causes for Rejection Hemolyzed specimen, specimen received more than 1 hour after collection, tubes inadequately filled

Special Instructions Method may require collection directly into graduated centrifuge tube by laboratory technologist.

Reference Range Amount of serum and RBC escaping from clot: ≥40%; RBC fallout: <5%; serum retained in clot: <20%; serum "drip-out": two drops or less in 2 minutes. Normally clot retraction starts in 1 hour and is complete within 24 hours.

Use Assess platelet function and fibrin structure in inducing clot retraction; a coagulation parameter used to investigate possibility of Glanzmann's disease

Limitations Concentration and functional ability of fibrinogen and hematocrit level should be within normal limits for valid interpretation and conclusions about platelet function. With low platelet count, aspirin therapy, increased fibrinolysis, altered fibrinogen/fibrin structure, or hypofibrinogenemia, abnormal clot retraction may occur and limit the ability to assess platelet function. In disseminated intravascular coagulation, afibrinogenemia, and severe hemophilic states, clot formation may not occur.

Contraindications Patients with low platelet counts, hypofibrinogenemia, or those taking aspirin-containing medications

Methodology Whole blood without anticoagulant is placed in a clean, glass, graduated centrifuge tube. After 1 hour at 37°C a number of parameters can be measured (eg, amount of fluid remaining, RBC fallout, serum "dripout," others). The older literature describes a variety of quantitative methods using platelet-rich plasma.[1]

Additional Information Clot retraction depends upon normal platelet function, a contractile protein present in the platelet membrane (thrombosthenin), and magnesium, ATP, and pyruvate kinase.[2] It is also influenced by the hematocrit level and fibrinogen structure and concentration. Thrombocytopenia and thrombasthenia are characterized by a soft friable clot with increased serum "drip-out" and decreased amount of serum expressed. With hypofibrinogenemia, the clot should be small, firm, and show increase in RBC fallout. With increased fibrinolysis, the clot should be soft and shaggy with increased RBC fallout. With disseminated intravascular coagulation, the clot is small and ragged with increased RBC fallout.[3] With congenital dysfibrinogenemia the clot should be of normal size but with increased RBC fallout. Coating of platelets with paraproteins (as in macroglobulinemia) may result in poor clot retraction. Thrombasthenia (Glanzmann's disease) is an inherited hemorrhagic condition with normal platelet count but with prolonged bleeding time, markedly decreased clot retraction, and abnormal platelet aggregation and adhesion. The defective clot retraction may reflect a failure of ADP activation of actin in the platelet membrane. A decrease in the amount of membrane glycoproteins II$_b$ and III$_a$ is accepted as the characteristic membrane abnormality in Glanzmann's thrombasthenia.[4] Clot retraction procedures have been largely replaced by platelet aggregation, platelet adhesion, and platelet release studies. An instrument has been developed, however, that measures force development during clot retraction. Force generated is transduced to a voltage change that is recorded. In this manner, the effect on clot retraction of change in platelet function and fibrin structure can be quantified. This device may extend the life of clot retraction studies by allowing quantification of retraction parameters in a more specific and reproducible manner. Qualitative platelet dysfunction may thus be characterized in part by measured functional abnormality of clot retraction. Practical clinical application must await results of patient studies. It has been shown that clot retraction parameters are temperature dependent with total inhibition at 15°C.[5]

Footnotes

1. Bang NU, Beller FK, Deutsch E, et al, *Thrombosis and Bleeding Disorders: Theory and Methods*, New York, NY: Academic Press, 1971, 441-5.
2. Corriveau DM and Fritsma GA, *Hemostasis and Thrombosis in the Clinical Laboratory*, Philadelphia, PA: JB Lippincott Co, 1988, 302.
3. Harmening DM, *Clinical Hematology and Fundamentals of Hemostasis*, Philadelphia, PA: FA Davis Co, 1992, 588.
4. Forbes CD and Cuschieri A, *Management of Bleeding Disorders in Surgical Practice*, Oxford, UK: Blackwell Scientific Publications, 1993, 43.
5. Carr ME and Zekert SL, "Measurement of Platelet-Mediated Force During Plasma Clot Formation," *Am J Med Sci*, 1991, 302(1):13-8.

References

Coller BS, "Inherited Disorders of Platelet Function," *Haemostasis and Thrombosis*, 3rd ed, Vol 1, Chapter 32, Bloom AL, Forbes CD, Thomas DP, et al, eds, New York, NY: Churchill Livingstone, 1994, 721-66.

Owen CA Jr, "Historical Account of Tests of Hemostasis," *Am J Clin Pathol*, 1990, 93(4 Suppl 1):S3-8.

Sirridge MS and Shannon R, *Laboratory Evaluation of Hemostasis and Thrombosis*, 3rd ed, Philadelphia, PA: Lea & Febiger, 1983, 66, 83-5.

Clot Time see Lee-White Clotting Time *on page 254*

Coagulation Factor Assay

CPT 85611 (PT substitution); 85732 (PTT substitution)

Related Information

Activated Partial Thromboplastin Time *on page 227*
Factor II *on page 238*
Factor V *on page 239*
(Continued)

Coagulation Factor Assay *(Continued)*

Synonyms Factor Assay

Applies to Coagulation Factor(s) II, V, VII, VIII, IX, X, XI, XII, and XIII (Screen)

Abstract Tests for specific clotting factors

Patient Preparation Avoid Coumadin® therapy for 2 weeks and heparin therapy for 2 days prior to test

Specimen Plasma

Container Two blue top (sodium citrate) tubes

Collection Routine venipuncture. If multiple tests are being drawn, draw coagulation studies last. If only factor assay is being drawn, draw 1-2 mL into another Vacutainer®, discard, and then collect the factor assay. This collection procedure avoids contamination of the specimen with tissue thromboplastins. Transport specimen to the laboratory immediately.

Storage Instructions Keep refrigerated.

Causes for Rejection Tubes not full, tubes clotted, specimen hemolyzed, specimen received more than 2 hours after collection, specimen improperly labeled, specimen not refrigerated

Turnaround Time Commonly sent to reference laboratories.

Special Instructions These assays are not usually routinely available. They may require referral to a specialized coagulation laboratory. Make arrangements with your local laboratory facility before drawing and submitting specimen.

Reference Range Normal range varies with each factor and between laboratories but is generally broad, approximately 50% to 150% of normal activity. Factor XIII is usually estimated as present or absent on the basis of a urea solubility screening test. The normal finding is for the clot to be insoluble in 5M urea at 24 hours. Healthy premature infants have levels of vitamin K dependent factors (II, VII, IX, and X) and contact factors (XI, XII, PK, and HMWK) that are <50% of the level of normal adults (with the exception of VII which is somewhat higher). Healthy prematures, however, do not develop spontaneous hemorrhage because of a balance between procoagulant and inhibitors.[1]

Use Detect specific coagulation factor deficiency which may be present on a congenital basis or may be acquired secondary to a number of organ specific or generalized disease processes. Triplett[2] has provided a broad discussion of abnormalities that have been seen in association with liver, renal, immune, lymphoproliferative, and other disease processes.

Use of Differential APTT in the Identification of Hemophilia

Hemophilia	PT	PTT	Adsorbed Plasma	Aged Normal Serum
A (VIII def)	Normal	↑	Corrects	No change
B (IX def)	Normal	↑	No change	Corrects
C (XI def)	Normal	↑	Corrects (partial)	Corrects (partial)
XII def	Normal	↑	Corrects	Corrects

Limitations Factors II, VII, IX, X may be increased in patients taking oral contraceptives. Interpretations of results may be limited if patient is receiving anticoagulant therapy or if test is done more than 2 hours after collection.

Contraindications Patient on anticoagulant therapy

Methodology Results of mixing patient's plasma with naturally or treated deficient plasma and serum preparations are determined by using prothrombin time and activated partial thromboplastin time tests. Absorbed plasma and aged serum can be prepared and maintained locally. Storage and maintenance of a full set of known deficient plasmas, while commercially available (George King Biomedical, Olathe, Kansas), is usually only attempted by the specialized coagulation laboratory.

Additional Information Stage II, intrinsic pathway coagulation deficiency states include the hemophilias, A (factor VIII deficiency), B (factor IX deficiency), and C (factor XI deficiency). Results of differential APTT testing using specially treated normal plasma and serum can be used to support these diagnoses. The reagents are commercially available or may be prepared in the laboratory. Consult the references for additional information. After absorption with $BaSO_4$ or $Al(OH)_3$ factors I, V, VIII, XI, and XII remain in the plasma (II, VII, IX, and X, the vitamin K dependent factors are removed). Adsorbed serum contains only factors XI and XII. Aged serum contains factor VII, IX, X, XI, and XII (lacks factors I, V, and VIII). Specific factor assay using known deficient plasma should be used to confirm results of differential (crossmixing) studies.

Footnotes

1. Andrew M, Paes B, Milner R, et al, "Development of the Human Coagulation System in the Healthy Premature Infant," *Blood*, 1988, 72(5):1651-7.
2. Triplett DA, "Acquired Abnormalities of Hemostasis," *Laboratory Evaluation of Coagulation*, Chicago, IL: American Society of Clinical Pathologists, 1982, 209-44.

References

Bloom AL, Forbes CD, Thomas DP, et al, eds, "Blood Coagulation," *Haemostasis and Thrombosis*, 3rd ed, Vol 1, Section 4, New York, NY: Churchill Livingstone, 1994, 289-546.
Sirridge MS and Shannon R, *Laboratory Evaluation of Hemostasis and Thrombosis*, 3rd ed, Philadelphia, PA: Lea & Febiger, 1983, 115-33, 204-19.

Coagulation Factor(s) II, V, VII, VIII, IX, X, XI, XII, and XIII (Screen) *see Coagulation Factor Assay on previous page*

Coagulation Screen, Intravascular *see Intravascular Coagulation Screen on page 253*

Coagulation Time *see Lee-White Clotting Time on page 254*

Collagen Binding Assay for vWF *see von Willebrand Factor Collagen Binding Assay on page 269*

Consumptive Coagulopathy Screen *see Intravascular Coagulation Screen on page 253*

Coumarins *see Prothrombin Time on page 262*

Cryocrit *see Cryofibrinogen on this page*

Cryofibrinogen

CPT 82585

Related Information

Cryoglobulin, Qualitative, Serum *on page 388*

Applies to Cryocrit

Abstract A test for one of the cold-precipitable plasma proteins in patients with cold intolerance.

Specimen Plasma

Container Blue top (sodium citrate) tube

Causes for Rejection Improper tube, specimen more than 2 hours in transit to the laboratory

Turnaround Time 24 hours

Special Instructions Transport to the laboratory immediately following collection. Must be allowed to clot at 37°C.

Reference Range Negative: no cryofibrinogen detected

Use Detect cold precipitable fibrinogen. Cryofibrinogen has been reported in association with coagulation disorders, malignancies, phlebitis of pregnancy, inflammatory processes including neonatal infections, the use of oral contraceptives, and with scleroderma.[1]

Contraindications Patients anticoagulated with heparin

Methodology Tube of plasma refrigerated overnight is compared to a control tube of patient's plasma kept covered at room temperature. Cryofibrinogen (precipitate from **plasma** on cooling) must be differentiated from cryoglobulin (precipitates or gels from **serum or plasma** when cooled at 4°C for 24 hours). Either of these may disappear on warming to 32°C. A "cold-precipitable protein study" to identify these cryoproteins is desirable. This involves keeping a sample of both patient's serum and plasma refrigerated for 24-72 hours. If samples are studied in Wintrobe tubes, any precipitating material can be measured by centrifuging (using a refrigerated centrifuge) and quantitated using the sedimentation scale (each mm of precipitate equates to 1% of "cryocrit").

Additional Information Cryofibrinogenemia can produce a clinical picture similar to that of cryoglobulinemia (cold sensitivity with purpura, vascular damage with bleeding, bullae, chronic ulcerations, and cold urticaria). Cryoprecipitable complexes between fibrinogen, globulins, and fibrinogen degradation products occur, such as fragments X and Y, forming complexes with fibrinogen and fibrin monomer and precipitating in the cold and in heparinized plasma.

Footnotes

1. Beightler E, Diven DG, Sanchez RL, et al, "Thrombotic Vasculopathy Associated With Cryofibrinogenemia," *J Am Acad Dermatol*, 1991, 24(2 Pt 2):342-5.

References

Klein AD and Kerdel FA, "Purpura and Recurrent Ulcers on the Lower Extremities. Essential Cryofibrinogenemia," *Arch Dermatol*, 1991, 127(1):113-8.
Schneiderman P, "The Vascular Purpuras," *Williams Hematology*, 5th ed, Chapter 134, Part X, Beutler E, Lichtman MA, Coller BS, et al, eds, New York, NY: McGraw-Hill Inc, 1995, 1409.

D-Dimer

CPT 85378 (semiquantitative); 85379 (quantitative)

Related Information

Fibrin Breakdown Products *on page 245*
Fibrinogen *on page 246*
Fibrin Split Products, Protamine Sulfate *on page 248*
Intravascular Coagulation Screen *on page 253*

Abstract Test for the D-dimer fragment of fibrin in plasma. D-dimer appears in plasma of patients with disseminated intravascular coagulation, deep vein thrombosis, and acute myocardial infarction.

Specimen Plasma

Container Collect whole blood in plastic tube that contains 0.11 mol/L sodium citrate and aprotinin (100 TIU/L (trypsin inhibiting units))

Storage Instructions Test plasma may be stored at -80°C. The clinical situation in which these tests are employed, however, usually requires that samples be tested immediately.

Turnaround Time Latex particle immunoassay, 30 minutes (applicable to clinical emergency situations); enzyme immunoassay (Dimertest EIA), 4-5 hours

Use Screening test for the detection of deep vein thrombosis (DVT); evaluation of acute myocardial infarction, unstable angina, and disseminated intravascular coagulation (DIC)[1]

Limitations Elevated D-dimer levels are not specific for the presence of DIC or of deep vein thrombosis. False-positive or false-negative results may occur when attempting to confirm a diagnosis of DIC.[2]

Methodology Enzyme-linked immunosorbent assay (ELISA), latex particle assay, immunoblotting[3]

Additional Information The D-dimer is a fragment of fibrin that contains one intermolecular cross-link between the gamma chains of two fibrin monomers. This cross-linkage occurs in fibrin but not fibrinogen. It is thus specific for fibrin. Increased levels of D-dimer (cross-linked fibrin fragments) have been found in patients with deep vein thrombosis,[4] acute myocardial infarction,[5] acute pulmonary embolism,[6] unstable angina,[7] and disseminated intravascular coagulation.[1] D-dimer level <500 µg/L has been considered to exclude the diagnosis of acute pulmonary embolism.[6] In one study,[7] plasma from nearly 40% of pregnant women with pre-eclampsia was positive for D-dimer. Patients with D-dimer had more severe disease. Some latex clumping tests have been found to have a low sensitivity, rendering them unsuitable for emergency screening.[8,9] Some assays may not be able to consistently detect D-dimer levels as claimed by the manufacturer (as in package insert).[10] While detection limits of 200 µg/L for one test and 500 µg/L for the other latex test are claimed, a low level of specificity (47%) does not allow a positive diagnosis of DVT when the level of D-dimer is >200 µg/L. On the other hand, a level of D-dimer by ELISA <200 µg/L appears reliably to exclude presence of DVT. Results of D-dimer test by ELISA are 100% predictive for the absence of DVT (level <200 µg/L).[7,9] In an emergency room setting, sensitivity of D-dimer ELISA and a latex method with cut-off limit of 200 µg/L was found to be 94% with negative predictive value of 92% and 93% for distal DVT. Both tests had negative predictive value of 100% for proximal DVT.[11] Results of D-dimer by ELISA may be considered to screen for those patients needing further evaluation to establish the presence of DVT.[9] Presence of increase in D-dimer supports the interpretation of presence of FDP, X, Y, D, and E fragments as indicative of acute DIC (eg, fibrin rather than fibrinogen fragments).[12] A lack of correlation has been found between thrombolysis (with resultant reperfusion) and increase in D-dimer levels (eg, D-dimer measurement does not distinguish between thrombolysis and fibrinolysis).[13,14] D-dimer values may be dissociated from (lower than expected) elevated FDP levels in cases of accelerated fibrinogenolysis.[15]

On the other hand, presence of D-dimer confirms that both thrombin generation and plasmin generation have occurred. The in tandem use of fibrin degradation products (FDP) test and D-dimer measurement in the evaluation of DIC has been recommended. Sensitivity and specificity are thereby maximized. The FDP measurement, highly sensitive, is confirmed with the D-dimer test, relatively specific. Elevated FDP confirmed by D-dimer test result >0.5 mg/L is highly predictive of DIC in patients at risk.[1]

The use of plasma D-dimer levels in conjunction with other tests to follow clot lysis during thrombolytic therapy has been studied.[16,17] It is uncertain whether or not D-dimer originating from the degradation of soluble plasma fibrin should be subtracted from the total post-treatment level to obtain D-dimer resulting from lysis of thrombi.[18] D-dimer fragment in the plasma can then be considered a marker of solid-phase fibrin dissolution.[19] D-dimer analysis of cerebrospinal fluid has been found to accurately and rapidly differentiate cases of subarachnoid hemorrhage from traumatic lumbar puncture. D-dimer was superior to the use of xanthochromia or declining RBC count in sequential tubes for this distinction.[20]

Footnotes

1. Carr JM, McKinney M, and McDonagh J, "Diagnosis of Disseminated Intravascular Coagulation: Role of D-Dimer," *Am J Clin Pathol*, 1989, 91(3):280-7.
2. Bleyer AJ and Bell WR, "Disseminated Intravascular Coagulation," *Current Therapy in Hematology-Oncology*, 4th ed, Brain MC and Carbone PP, eds, Philadelphia, PA: BC Decker, 1992, 119-21.
3. Francis CW, Connaghan DG, Scott WL, et al, "Increased Plasma Concentration of Cross-Linked Fibrin Polymers in Acute Myocardial Infarction," *Circulation*, 1987, 75(6):1170-7.
4. Kruskal JB, Commerford PJ, Franks JJ, et al, "Fibrin and Fibrinogen-Related Antigens in Patients With Stable and Unstable Coronary Artery Disease," *N Engl J Med*, 1987, 317(22):1361-5.
5. Bounameaux H, Cirafici P, de-Moerloose P, et al, "Measurement of D-dimer in Plasma as Diagnostic Aid in Suspected Pulmonary Embolism," *Lancet*, 1991, 337(8735):196-200.
6. Trofatter KF Jr, Howell ML, Greenberg CS, et al, "Use of the Fibrin D-Dimer in Screening for Coagulation Abnormalities in Pre-eclampsia," *Obstet Gynecol*, 1989, 73(3 Pt 1):435-40.
7. Rowbotham BJ, Carroll P, Whitaker AN, et al, "Measurement of Cross Linked Fibrin Derivatives - Use in the Diagnosis of Venous Thrombosis," *Thromb Haemost*, 1987, 57(1):59-61.
8. Heaton DC, Billings JD, and Hickton CM, "Assessment of D Dimer Assays for the Diagnosis of Deep Vein Thrombosis," *J Lab Clin Med*, 1987, 110(5):588-91.
9. Bounameaux H, Schneider P-A, Reber G, et al, "Measurement of Plasma D-Dimer for Diagnosis of Deep Venous Thrombosis," *Am J Clin Pathol*, 1989, 91(1):82-5.
10. Charles LA, Edwards T, and Macik BG, "Evaluation of Sensitivity and Specificity of Six D-Dimer Latex Assays," *Arch Pathol Lab Med*, 1994, 118(11):1102-5.
11. Hansson PO, Eriksson H, Eriksson E, et al, "Can Laboratory Testing Improve Screening Strategies for Deep Vein Thrombosis at an Emergency Unit?" *J Intern Med*, 1994, 235(2):143-51.
12. Bick RL, "Disseminated Intravascular Coagulation and Related Syndromes: A Clinical Review," *Semin Thromb Hemost*, 1988, 14(4):299-338.
13. Brenner B, Francis CW, and Marder VJ, "The Role of Soluble Cross-Linked Fibrin in D-Dimer Immunoreactivity of Plasmic Digests," *J Lab Clin Med*, 1989, 113(6):682-8.
14. Mosesson MW, "D-Dimer, An Ambiguous Marker of Thrombolysis," *J Lab Clin Med*, 1989, 113(6):662.
15. Sato N, Takahashi H, and Shibata A, "Fibrinogen/Fibrin Degradation Products and D-Dimer in Clinical Practice: Interpretation of Discrepant Results," *Am J Hematol*, 1995, 48(3):168-74.
16. Lawler CM, Bovill EG, Stump DC, et al, "Fibrin Fragment D-Dimer and Fibrinogen Bβ Peptides in Plasma as Markers of Clot Lysis During Thrombolytic Therapy in Acute Myocardial Infarction," *Blood*, 1990, 76(7):1341-8.
17. Boisclair MD, Lane DA, Wilde JT, et al, "A Comparative Evaluation of Assays for Markers of Activated Coagulation and/or Fibrinolysis: Thrombin-Antithrobmin Complex, D-Dimer and Fibrinogen/Fibrin Fragment E Antigen," *Br J Haematol*, 1990, 74(4):471-9.
18. Brenner B, Francis CW, Totterman S, et al, "Quantitation of Venous Clot Lysis With the D-Dimer Immunoassay During Fibrinolytic Therapy Requires Correction for Soluble Fibrin Degradation," *Circulation*, 1990, 81(6):1818-25.
19. Eisenberg PR, Jaffe AS, Stump DC, et al, "Validity of Enzyme-Linked Immunosorbent Assays of Cross-Linked Fibrin Degradation Products as a Measure of Clot Lysis," *Circulation*, 1990, 82(4):1159-68.
20. Lang DT, Berberian LB, Lee S, et al, "Rapid Differentiation of Subarachnoid Hemorrhage From Traumatic Lumbar Puncture Using the D-Dimer Assay," *Am J Clin Pathol*, 1990, 93(3):403-5.

DIC Screen *see Intravascular Coagulation Screen on page 253*

Differential APTT Test *see Activated Partial Thromboplastin Substitution Test on page 226*

Diluted Whole Blood Clot Lysis

CPT 85175

Related Information

Euglobulin Clot Lysis *on next page*
Plasminogen Activator Inhibitor *on page 255*
Plasminogen Assay *on page 256*

Synonyms Clot Lysis Time; Fibrinolysis Time

Specimen Laboratory personnel will usually collect specimen and initiate this test at the patient's bedside.

Reference Range Rapid lysis implies excessive fibrinolytic activity. Clot still intact after 2 hours is "normal." Clot which lyses in less than 2 hours reflects lytic activity, time of dissolution is reported. A "control" tube with clot is kept in the refrigerator; lysis does not occur at that temperature. (Fibrinolytic activity of plasmin is inhibited.)

Possible Panic Range 100% lysis in 1 hour or less

Use Monitor urokinase and streptokinase therapy, fibrinolytic activity; evaluate abnormal fibrinolysis; aids in differentiating primary pathologic fibrinolysis from secondary (physiologic) fibrinolysis with low levels of circulating plasmins

Limitations Testing must begin immediately upon drawing blood unless citrate-anticoagulated, chilled, platelet-poor plasma is tested.[1] Aspirin may influence fibrinolytic activity in addition to its antiplatelet activity. An inverse relationship has been shown between the degree of acetylation of fibrinogen and the clot lysis time.[2]

Methodology Whole blood is obtained and a 1:10 dilution in iced buffer solution is prepared. Test is started with the addition of 0.1 mL thrombin and is set up in triplicate. After 30 minutes refrigerator incubation (inactivates inhibitors), two of the tubes are heated at 37°C and the time to lysis noted. A clot in the refrigerated control tube assures that sufficient functional fibrinogen was present.
(Continued)

Diluted Whole Blood Clot Lysis *(Continued)*

Additional Information A tabular comparison of clot lysis tests is included in the listing Euglobulin Clot Lysis *on page 238*.

Footnotes

1. Graeff H and Beller FK, "Fibrinolytic Activity in Whole Blood, Dilute Blood, and Euglobulin Clot Lysis Time Tests," *Thrombosis and Bleeding Disorders: Theory and Methods*, Bang NU, Beller FK, Deutsch E, et al, eds, New York, NY: Academic Press, 1971, 328-31.
2. Bjornsson TD, Schneider DE, and Berger H Jr, "Aspirin Acetylates Fibrinogen and Enhances Fibrinolysis. Fibrinolytic Effect Is Independent of Changes in Plasminogen Activator Levels," *J Pharmacol Exp Ther*, 1989, 250(1):154-61.

References

Sirridge MS and Shannon R, *Laboratory Evaluation of Hemostasis and Thrombosis*, 3rd ed, Philadelphia, PA: Lea & Febiger, 1983, 11-6, 169-74.

Disseminated Intravascular Coagulation Screen *see* Intravascular Coagulation Screen *on page 253*

Endothelial Cofactor *see* Thrombomodulin *on page 266*

Euglobulin Clot Lysis

CPT 85360

Related Information

Diluted Whole Blood Clot Lysis *on previous page*
Fibrin Breakdown Products *on page 245*
Fibrinogen *on page 246*
Intravascular Coagulation Screen *on page 253*
Plasminogen Assay *on page 256*

Synonyms Euglobulin Clot Lysis Time; Euglobulin Lysis Time; Fibrinolysis Time

Abstract A measure of fibrinolytic activity, an older generation procedure

Patient Preparation Prohibit exercise prior to drawing sample.

Specimen Plasma. Use of platelet-poor plasma is desirable, as platelets have antiplasmin activity and may prolong the lysis time.

Container Blue top (sodium citrate) tube

Collection Use two-syringe or two-tube collection technique to avoid contamination by tissue proteins. A clean venipuncture is a necessity. To avoid release of plasminogen activator (which shortens the lysis time), do not massage vein vigorously, pump fist excessively, or leave tourniquet in place for a prolonged period.

Storage Instructions Deliver specimen immediately to the laboratory on ice. After centrifugation, the separated plasma should be kept on ice and tested within 90 minutes of blood withdrawal. Alternatively, the test may be performed on platelet-poor plasma stored at -80°C or on euglobulin precipitates undissolved and stored at -20°C for 24 hours.[1]

Causes for Rejection Specimen not delivered promptly (within 15-20 minutes), hemolysis, clotted blood, dilution by I.V. fluids, specimen not iced, tubes not filled with correct amount of sample

Special Instructions It may be necessary to schedule this test with the laboratory.

Reference Range Lysis time greater than 90 minutes. Shortened time to lysis indicates excessive fibrinolytic activity. Bleeding danger may exist if there is 100% lysis in 1 hour or less.

Use Detect and evaluate pathologic fibrinolytic activity; monitor urokinase or streptokinase fibrinolytic therapy. May be normal in cases of DIC. Useful in evaluation of lytic states during cardiovascular surgery, as the harvest of euglobulin fraction separates out inhibitors including heparin.

Limitations Decreased fibrinogen (<80 mg/dL) causes shortened (rapid) lysis time. Increased fibrinogen prolongs lysis time. Dysfibrinogen may be responsible for abnormal lysis time. If plasminogen is depleted (by *in vivo* fibrinolysis as in long-term cases of disseminated intravascular coagulation), a false normal lysis time may result. Clot dissolution will not occur because of the lack of plasminogen. See Methodology for use of control to detect this possibility. The euglobulin clot lysis test is nonspecific and is considered obsolete by some.

Methodology Plasma is acidified to form a "euglobulin clot" (antiplasmins are removed during treatment). Time required for lysis to occur is measured and reported. The lower the pH of plasma/acid, the longer the lysis time. (Maximal lysis results from precipitating euglobulins at pH 6.2.) With precipitation at pH 5.3, lysis may require 10-24 hours. Positive and negative plasma controls, as well as patient activated control (PAC), should be run concurrently with the test plasma. PAC consists of patient euglobulin fraction with streptokinase added. This should cause rapid clot dissolution. If plasminogen is depleted, the PAC will show no dissolution of clot, and the euglobulin lysis time will appear normal. A normal result in the PAC indicates that the actual test is unreliable.[2]

Additional Information Lysis time of less than 60 minutes may be associated with presence of fibrin degradation products. Increased fibrinolysis may be associated with shock/circulatory collapse, epinephrine injection, pyrogen reactions, obstetric complication, and sudden death. See table. There is evidence that some (apparently most) patients with vascular ulcers have a prolonged euglobulin lysis time and an increased plasma fibrinogen level.[3] The exact role (primary or secondary) of the change in fibrinolytic activity has not been established.

Comparison of Clot Lysis Tests

Test	Measures	Sensitivity	Time Required (hours)
Whole blood clot lysis	Activator Plasminogen (plasmin) Fibrinogen Inhibitors	+/–	24
Diluted whole blood clot lysis	Activator Plasminogen (plasmin) Fibrinogen Inhibitors (decreased)	++	2-12
Euglobulin clot lysis	Activator Plasminogen (plasmin) Fibrinogen (decreased) Inhibitors (eliminated)	++ or +++	2

From Sirridge MS and Shannon R, *Laboratory Evaluation of Hemostasis and Thrombosis*, 3rd ed, Philadelphia, PA: Lea and Febiger, 1983, 171.

Footnotes

1. Prisco D, Paniccia R, Bandinelli B, et al, "Euglobulin Lysis Time in Fresh and Stored Samples," *Am J Clin Pathol*, 1994, 102(6):794-6.
2. Fritsma GA, "Clot Based Assays of Coagulation," *Hemostasis and Thrombosis in the Clinical Laboratory*, eds, Corriveau DM and Fritsma GA, Philadelphia, PA: JB Lippincott Co, 1988, 124-5.
3. Falanga V, Moosa HH, Nemeth AJ, et al, "Dermal Pericapillary Fibrin in Venous Disease and Venous Ulceration," *Arch Dermatol*, 1987, 123(5):620-3.

References

Graeff H and Beller FK, "Fibrinolytic Activity in Whole Blood, Dilute Blood, and Euglobulin Clot Lysis Time Tests," Bang NU, Beller FK, Deutsch E, et al, eds, *Thrombosis and Bleeding Disorders: Theory and Methods*, New York, NY: Academic Press, 1971, 328-31.

Laffan MA and Bradshaw AE, "Investigation of a Thrombotic Tendency," *Practical Hematology*, 8th ed, Chapter 18, Dacie JV and Lewis SM, eds, New York, NY: Churchill Livingstone, 1995, 357-8.

Sirridge MS and Shannon R, *Laboratory Evaluation of Hemostasis and Thrombosis*, 3rd ed, Philadelphia, PA: Lea & Febiger, 1983, 69, 173-4.

Euglobulin Clot Lysis Time *see* Euglobulin Clot Lysis *on this page*

Euglobulin Lysis Time *see* Euglobulin Clot Lysis *on this page*

F 1.2 *see* Prothrombin Fragment 1.2 *on page 261*

F1+2 *see* Prothrombin Fragment 1.2 *on page 261*

Factor II

CPT 85210

Related Information

Coagulation Factor Assay *on page 235*
Prothrombin Time *on page 262*

Synonyms Prothrombin

Abstract Factor II (prothrombin) is measured by functional or immunologic assays, results of which assist in identifying the presence of qualitative or quantitative deficiency. Such autosomal recessive defects are rare. If homozygous, they may be responsible for severe clinical bleeding and will be characterized by prolonged prothrombin time and partial thromboplastin time with normal thrombin time.

Patient Preparation Avoid Coumadin® therapy for 2 weeks and heparin therapy for 2 days prior to test.

Specimen Plasma

Container Blue top (sodium citrate) tube

Collection Routine venipuncture. If multiple tests are being drawn, draw coagulation studies last. If only coagulation tests are being drawn, draw 1-2 mL into another Vacutainer®, discard, and then collect coagulation tests. This collection procedure avoids contamination of the specimen with tissue thromboplastins.

Storage Instructions Keep refrigerated.

Causes for Rejection Tube not full, specimen hemolyzed, specimen clotted, specimen received more than 2 hours after collection

Special Instructions Schedule or arrange for referral testing with laboratory, as prothrombin assay is not commonly available and is not the same test as a "prothrombin time" determination.

Reference Range 83% to 117% of normal

Use Document specific factor deficiency

Limitations Interpretation of results may be limited if patient is receiving anticoagulant therapy or if test is done more than 2 hours after collection.

Contraindications Patient on anticoagulant therapy

Methodology Test (patient's) plasma is diluted, mixed with factor II deficient substrate, clotting (prothrombin) time determined, and result obtained by comparison with dilution curve prepared by testing mixtures of factor II deficient plasma and dilutions of normal serum. Two-stage prothrombin assay may be used (does not require a factor II deficient preparation).[1] These are "functional" assays. Confirmation of prothrombin deficiency should include tests for both biologic (functional) and immunologically (amidolytic-chromogenic substrate assay or native prothrombin radioimmunoassay) defined prothrombin protein. Normal level determined by an immunologic- or chromogenic substrate-based method but decrease in function by biologic assay (eg, two-stage assay) indicates presence of dysprothrombinemia. One-stage assays for prothrombin using trypsin, tiger snake, taipan snake, and *Echis carinatus* snake venoms have been applied to the analysis of molecular defects of prothrombin.

Additional Information Prothrombin, a vitamin K dependent, single polypeptide chain coagulation protein is synthesized in the liver. It achieves a plasma concentration of about 10 mg/dL and has a half-life of about 3 days.[2] It is formed of 581 amino acid residues organized into three domains and has a molecular weight of some 70,000. The enzyme factor Xa activates prothrombin (a zymogen) with the resultant formation of the enzyme thrombin. The prothrombin molecule is unique in that carboxylation of glutamic acid residues (by a vitamin K dependent carboxylase) occurs and is necessary for the binding of the protein to phospholipid surfaces and subsequent conversion to thrombin. Factor V, phospholipids, and calcium ions accelerate the rate of this conversion.

Two classes of autosomal recessive inherited abnormalities manifest, clinically; both are uncommon. Quantitative and qualitative (dysfunctional) defects occur. The latter are termed "dysprothrombinemias". The term "CRM-" (cross reacting material negative) is applied if factor II protein is absent while "CRM+" (cross reacting material positive) indicates presence of dysfunctional prothrombin. Inherited prothrombin deficiency is a rare coagulopathy. True hypoprothrombinemia is the most common form of congenital prothrombin deficiency.[3] Hypoprothrombinemia may be homozygous (prothrombin levels of 1% to 25%) or heterozygous (levels of 50% to 60%). Severe bleeding occurs in homozygous individuals with epistaxis, easy bruising, hematoma formation, menorrhagia, and post-trauma/postsurgical hemorrhage. Heterozygotes may have bleeding but usually very mild. Homozygotes have prolonged whole blood clotting times, APTT, and PT tests (prothrombin is required in the final common pathway of coagulation). A variety of genetic mechanisms underlie the dysprothrombinemias. Bick, in his recent text (see reference), lists 19 examples of dysprothrombinemias described over the past two decades.

Transient acquired factor II deficiency has been briefly described, associated with *Mycoplasma pneumoniae* infection.[4]

Use of a native prothrombin antigen assay to monitor warfarin-anticoagulated patients may result in a significantly lower incidence of bleeding and thrombotic complications as compared to use of the prothrombin time test for monitoring.[5] Such assay, however, is not yet readily available at reasonable cost.

Footnotes

1. Dacie JV and Lewis SM, *Practical Haematology*, 8th ed, New York, NY: Churchill Livingstone, 1995, 304-5, 325-8.
2. Seegers WH, "Purification of Prothrombin and Thrombin," *Semin Thromb Hemost*, 1981, 7:199-212.
3. Bithell TC, "Hereditary Coagulation Disorders," *Wintrobe's Clinical Hematology*, 9th ed, Vol 2, Chapter 56, Lee GR, Bithell TC, Foerster J, et al, eds, Philadelphia, PA: Lea and Febiger, 1993, 1442-3.
4. Collazos J, Egurbide MV, Atucha K, et al, "Transient Acquired Factor II Deficiency With *Mycoplasma pneumoniae* Infection," *J Infect Dis*, 1991, 164(2):434-5.
5. Furie B, Diuguid CF, Jacobs M, et al, "Randomized Prospective Trial Comparing the Native Prothrombin Antigen With the Prothrombin Time for Monitoring Oral Anticoagulant Therapy," *Blood*, 1990, 75(2):344-9.

References

Bick RL, "Hereditary Coagulation Protein Defects," *Disorders of Thrombosis and Hemostasis: Clinical and Laboratory Practice*, Chapter 6, Chicago, IL: American Society of Clinical Pathologists, 1992, 112-4.

Mammen EF, "Nature of Inherited Disorders," *Prothrombin and Other Vitamin K Proteins*, Vol 1, Seegers WA and Walz DA, eds, Boca Raton, FL: CRC Press, 1986, 115.

Factor V

CPT 85220

Related Information

Coagulation Factor Assay *on page 235*
Hypercoagulable State Coagulation Screen *on page 250*
Plasma, Fresh Frozen *on page 615*
Protein C *on page 260*
Resistance to Activated Protein C *on page 265*
Thrombomodulin *on page 266*

Synonyms Ac-Globulin; Labile Factor; Proaccelerin

Patient Preparation Avoid Coumadin® therapy for 2 weeks and heparin therapy for 2 days prior to test.

Specimen Plasma

Container Blue top (sodium citrate) tube

Collection Routine venipuncture. If multiple tests are being drawn, draw coagulation studies last. If only coagulation tests are being drawn, draw 1-2 mL into another Vacutainer®, discard, and then collect coagulation tests. This collection procedure avoids contamination of the specimen with tissue thromboplastins.

Storage Instructions Deliver specimen immediately to the laboratory on ice. Centrifuge (in refrigerated centrifuge at 4°C) and separate plasma. Keep refrigerated and test immediately, preferably within 1-2 hours.

Causes for Rejection Tube not full, specimen hemolyzed, specimen clotted, specimen received more than 2 hours after collection

Special Instructions Not available in most general clinical laboratories. Communicate with laboratory for scheduling and referral as required.

Reference Range 50% to 150% of normal. Homozygous factor V deficient patients have <10% (often <5%) activity.

Use Document specific factor deficiency

Limitations Interpretation of results may be limited if patient is receiving anticoagulant therapy or if test is done more than 2 hours after collection.

Methodology Modified one-stage prothrombin time using commercially available factor V deficient preparation, known factor V deficient patient plasma or artificially prepared factor V deficient plasma. Chromogenic substrate assay.

Additional Information Factor V, a glycoprotein with molecular weight of 300,000, is synthesized in the liver. It is converted in the plasma from a single chain to a two chain molecule under the influence of thrombin activation. Activated V (Va) is a part of the prothrombin converting complex. Va is inactivated by protein Ca.[1] The molecular characterization of Va, in particular identification of the structural determinants responsible for acceleration of prothrombin activation and those that bind to phospholipid surfaces, have been described.[2] Factor V deficiency is inherited as an autosomal recessive, males and females are equally affected. Only homozygotes have bleeding symptoms; heterozygotes are largely asymptomatic. Symptoms include ecchymoses, epistaxis, menorrhagia, and bleeding following trauma and tooth extraction. GI hemorrhage and hemarthrosis may occur. Severity of bleeding does not correlate directly with factor V level, and symptoms are often mild, even in homozygotes. Homozygous V deficient individuals usually have prolonged whole blood clotting time, prothrombin time, and APTT. Platelet factor V is present in α-granules of platelets and is necessary to the binding of Xa to the platelet surface. Factor V deficient patients have varying levels of platelet factor V (may not be fully deficient). Platelet transfusion may have a role in the treatment of factor V deficient patients.[3] It has been shown that commercial preparations of bovine thrombin may contain bovine factor V and patients exposed to topical thrombin (bovine) may develop antibodies to factor V.[4] Antithrombin antibodies may also develop and mask the factor V inhibitor (antibody) of activity that is responsible in part for clinical bleeding.

Protein C (a vitamin K-dependent serine protease zymogen), when activated (by thrombin, plasmin, or trypsin), destroys activated factors V and VIII, thus exerting a braking effect on the coagulation mechanism, and acting as an anticoagulant. Recently, patients with a factor V gene mutation (factor V Leiden) have been identified. An Agr 506 to G1n mutation results in resistance to activated protein C (APC). Such patients, as would be expected, have a hypercoagulable state.[5] Resistance to APC is apparently the most common cause of unexplained thrombosis, accounting for some 20% to 60% of such patients.[6] At least some patients with recurrent deep vein and/or other thrombotic conditions previously attributed to a variety of mechanisms (eg, oral contraceptive therapy)[7] may prove in reality to be the result of resistance to activated protein C. Factor V Leiden may have a similar distribution worldwide.[8]

Footnotes

1. Heeb MJ, España, and Griffin JH, "Inhibition and Complexation of Activated Protein C by Two Major Inhibitors in Plasma," *Blood*, 1989, 73(2):446-54.
2. White GC 2nd, "Coagulation Factors V and VIII: Normal Function and Clinical Disorders," *Blood: Principles and Practice of Hematology*, Chapter 39, Handin RI, Lux SE, and Stossel TP, eds, Philadelphia, PA: JB Lippincott, 1995, 1151-79.
3. Triplett DA, *Laboratory Evaluation of Coagulation*, Chicago, IL: American Society of Clinical Pathologists, 1982, 78.
4. Zehnder JL and Leung LL, "Development of Antibodies to Thrombin and Factor V With Recurrent Bleeding in a Patient Exposed to Topical Bovine Thrombin," *Blood*, 1990, 76(10):2011-6.
5. Dahlbäck B, "Molecular Genetics of Thrombophilia: Factor V Gene Mutation Causing Resistance to Activated Protein C as a Basis of the Hypercoagulable State," *J Lab Clin Med*, 1995, 125(5):566-71.
6. Griffin JH, Evatt B, Wideman C, et al, "Anticoagulant Protein C Pathway Defective in Majority of Thrombophilic Patients," *Blood*, 1993, 82(7):1989-93.
7. Aslam S, Standen GR, Morse C, et al, "DVT Following Oral Contraceptive Therapy in Association With Homozygous Factor V Leiden," *Clin Lab Haematol*, 1995, 17(1):99-100.
8. Arruda VR, Annichino-Bizzacchi JM, Costa FF, et al, "Factor V Leiden (FVQ 506) Is Common in a Brazilian Population," *Am J Hematol*, 1995, 49(3):242-3.

(Continued)

Factor V *(Continued)*

References
Janeway CM, Rivard GE, Tracy PB, et al, "Factor V Quebec Revisited," *Blood*, 1996, 87(9):3571-8.

Mammen EF, "Factor V Deficiency; Congenital Coagulation Disorders," *Semin Thromb Hemost*, 1983, 9:17-8.

Svensson PJ and Dahlbäck B, "Resistance to Activated Protein C as a Basis for Venous Thrombosis," *N Engl J Med*, 1994, 330(8):517-22.

Factor VII

CPT 85230

Related Information
Coagulation Factor Assay *on page 235*
Hypercoagulable State Coagulation Screen *on page 250*
Plasma, Fresh Frozen *on page 615*
Prothrombin Time *on page 262*

Synonyms Autoprothrombin I; Proconvertin; Stable Factor

Patient Preparation Avoid coumarin-type anticoagulants for 2 weeks and heparin therapy for 2 days prior to test.

Specimen Plasma

Container Blue top (sodium citrate) tube

Collection Routine venipuncture. If multiple tests are being drawn, draw coagulation studies last. If only coagulation tests are being drawn, draw 1-2 mL into another Vacutainer®, discard, and then collect coagulation tests. This collection procedure avoids contamination of the specimen with tissue thromboplastins.

Storage Instructions Keep refrigerated.

Causes for Rejection Tube not full, specimen hemolyzed, specimen clotted, specimen received more than 2 hours after collection

Special Instructions Schedule with laboratory in advance as this test is not routinely available and usually requires transport to a specialized coagulation laboratory.

Reference Range 50% to 150% of normal. Homozygous VII deficient patients have a <10% level of this factor.

Use Document specific factor deficiency

Limitations Interpretation of result may be limited if patient is receiving anticoagulant therapy or if test is done more than 2 hours after collection.

Methodology Modified one-stage prothrombin time utilizing commercially available factor VII deficient substrates or known factor VII deficient patient plasma (as condition is rare this is uncommonly available). A coupled amidolytic assay, tritiated peptide release assay, and an enzyme immunoassay (EIA) have been developed.[1] Use of a factor VII antigen assay (EIA) may be superior as it is not affected by the level of extrinsic pathway inhibitor.

Additional Information Factor VII, a vitamin K dependent coagulation glycoprotein is synthesized in the liver. It is a single peptide chain of molecular weight 45,000-53,000 and is formed of 408 amino acids. Acute deficiencies may occur with severe hepatocellular disease. Glutamic acid residues are carboxylated (vitamin K dependent) as with prothrombin. At these γ-carboxyglutamic acid residues calcium binds factor VII to phospholipid surfaces. Factor VII is activated to VIIa by thrombin, IXa, Xa, or XIIa fragments. The activated enzymic form of factor VII is a two chain molecule with the serine active site present on the heavy chain. Factor VII is unique in that it is the only factor in the extrinsic pathway of factor X activation. It is recently claimed, however, that under basal conditions (absence of thrombosis) IXa is the protease primarily responsible for generation of free factor VIIa *in vivo*.[2] Deficiency of factor VII should be considered in patients with a prolonged prothrombin time but a normal APTT. Over 150 cases of hereditary deficiency have been described in the literature. About 20% of patients with functional hereditary factor VII defect are due to factor VII molecular variants (phenotypically abnormal proteins). While deficiency is rare, two forms exist. Both are autosomal recessive and affect both sexes. In one form the VII molecules are decreased while in the second group an abnormally formed molecule is produced. Bleeding symptoms may be severe in homozygotes and include epistaxis, ecchymoses, GI bleeding, hemarthroses, menorrhagia, and umbilical cord hemorrhage. Fatal cerebral hemorrhage may occur. Heterozygotes are usually asymptomatic. Homozygotes have prolonged prothrombin time (corrected by adding normal plasma) but normal APTT, cephalin activated clotting time, and thrombin time.

Phenotype expression in the form of hemorrhagic symptoms is quite variable; symptomatology does not always correlate with the degree of factor VII deficiency. There are some patients reported to have thrombotic episodes.[3] It is not clear if some of the clinical variation relates to molecular structural variants.

Homozygous homocystinuria is associated with thromboembolism. Factor VII, AT III, and protein C levels have been reported as decreased in two sisters with this disease.[4] Decreased synthesis of liver produced coagulation factors may occur in homocystinuria.

A growing body of evidence indicates greater risk of coronary artery disease with both higher plasma fibrinogen and factor VII coagulant activity (VIIc) relating to apparently associated lipid parameters.[5,6,7,8,9] Increase in dietary fat intake has been associated with increases in factor VII coagulant activity, serum lipids, and coronary heart disease.[10] Specifically, plasma VII level has been found higher in women than men and, in both sexes, increased relative to body size, triglyceride, LDL cholesterol, and HDL cholesterol.[11] Factor VII levels have been found inversely proportional to ethanol intake.[11] Postprandial triglyceridemia has been associated with an acute effect (increase) in VII activity.[12]

Footnotes
1. Hultin MB, "Fibrinogen and Factor VII as Risk Factors in Vascular Disease," *Prog Hemost Thromb*, 1991, 10:215-41.
2. Eichinger S, Mannucci PM, Tradati F, et al, "Determinants of Plasma Factor VIIa Levels in Humans," *Blood*, 1995, 86(8):3021-5.
3. Ogston D, *Venous Thrombosis: Causation and Prediction*, New York, NY: John Wiley and Sons, 1987.
4. Palareti G, Salardi S, Legnani C, et al, "Reduced Levels of Antithrombin III, Protein C and Factor VII in Homocystinuria. Long-Term Changes in Relation to Treatment," *Thromb Haemost*, 1985, 54:35.
5. Meade TW, Mellows S, Brozovic M, et al, "Haemostatic Function and Ischaemic Heart Disease: Principal Results of the Northwick Park Heart Study," *Lancet*, 1986, 2(8506):533-7.
6. Broadhurst P, Kelleher C, Hughes L, et al, "Fibrogen, Factor VII Clotting Activity and Coronary Artery Disease Severity," *Atherosclerosis*, 1990, 85(2-3):169-73.
7. Hubbard AR and Parr LJ, "The Effect of Phospholipase C on Plasma Factor VII," *Br J Haematol*, 1989, 73(3):360-4.
8. Hoffman CJ, Miller RH, Lawson WE, et al, "Elevation of Factor VII Activity and Mass in Young Adults at Risk of Ischemic Heart Disease," *J Am Coll Cardiol*, 1989, 14(4):941-6.
9. Mitropoulos KA, Miller GJ, Reeves BE, et al, "Factor VII Coagulant Activity Is Strongly Associated With the Plasma Concentration of Large Lipoprotein Particles in Middle-Aged Men," *Atherosclerosis*, 1989, 76(2-3):203-8.
10. Miller GJ, Cruickshank JK, Ellis LJ, et al, "Fat Consumption and Factor VII Coagulant Activity in Middle-Aged Men - An Association Between a Dietary and Thrombogenic Coronary Risk Factor," *Atherosclerosis*, 1989, 78(1):19-24.
11. Folsom AR, Wu KK, Davis CE, et al, "Population Correlates of Plasma Fibrinogen and Factor VII, Putative Cardiovascular Risk Factors," *Atherosclerosis*, 1991, 91(3):191-205.
12. Miller GJ, Martin JC, Mitropoulos KA, et al, "Plasma Factor VII Is Activated by Postprandial Triglyceridaemia, Irrespective of Dietary Fat Composition," *Atherosclerosis*, 1991, 86(2-3):163-71.

References
Fadel HE and Krauss JS, "Factor VII Deficiency and Pregnancy," *Obstet Gynecol*, 1989, 73(3 Pt 2):453-4.

Giddings JC, *Molecular Genetics and Immunoanalysis in Blood Coagulation*, Chichester, England: Ellis Horwood Ltd, 1988, 42-7.

Hayes TE, Pike J, and Tracy RP, "Factor VII Assays," *Arch Pathol Lab Med*, 1993, 117(1):52-7.

Rao LV and Rapaport SI, "Factor VIIa-Catalyzed Activation of Factor X Independent of Tissue Factor: Its Possible Significance for Control of Hemophilic Bleeding by Infused Factor VIIa," *Blood*, 1990, 75(5):1069-73.

Factor VIII

CPT 85240

Related Information
Activated Partial Thromboplastin Time *on page 227*
Anticoagulant, Circulating *on page 229*
Coagulation Factor Assay *on page 235*
Cryoprecipitate *on page 606*
Factor VIII Concentrate *on page 608*
Factor IX *on next page*
Factor IX Complex (Human) *on page 609*
Plasma, Fresh Frozen *on page 615*
von Willebrand Factor Antigen *on page 267*
von Willebrand Factor Multimer Assay *on page 269*

Synonyms AHF; Antihemophilic Factor; F VIII; VIIIC:Ag

Applies to von Willebrand Protein; vWF

Specimen Plasma

Container Blue top (sodium citrate) tube

Collection Routine venipuncture. If multiple tests are being drawn, draw coagulation studies last. If only coagulation tests are being drawn, draw 1-2 mL into another Vacutainer®, discard, and then collect coagulation tests. This collection procedure avoids contamination of the specimen with tissue thromboplastins.

Storage Instructions Deliver immediately on ice to the laboratory. Separate off platelet poor plasma. May store up to 2 hours at 2°C to 8°C or up to 2 weeks at -35°C.

Causes for Rejection Clotted, hemolyzed or I.V. fluid diluted specimens, heparin contamination, improperly filled specimen tube, tube not iced, specimen received more than 1 hour after collection

Special Instructions Is not a routinely performed assay. May require scheduling or referral to a specialized or reference laboratory.

Reference Range 50% to 150% of normal, plasma concentration is about 100 µg/L. See table in von Willebrand Factor Antigen *on page 267*.

Use Detect coagulant factor VIII deficiency

Limitations Increased in patients taking oral contraceptives. Does not measure antigenic reactivity. See listing von Willebrand Factor Antigen *on page 267.*

Methodology Clotting times (one-stage or two-stage APTT) are performed on dilutions of patient plasma which have been mixed with APTT reagent and specific factor deficient plasma. The level of activity is determined by graphing results and comparing with those from pooled normal plasma similarly treated. Electroimmunoassay (Laurell rocket assay), two-dimensional crossed immunoelectrophoresis, immunoautoradiography, immunoblotting, radioimmunoassay (RIA), enzyme immunoassay (EIA) using monoclonal antibody.

Additional Information Factor VIII deficiency (**hemophilia A**) is one of the most common of the hereditary bleeding disorders with an incidence of about 1 in 5000 to 10,000 males. Clinical features are the same as for factor IX deficiency. See listing Factor IX *on page 241.* Deficiencies of factor VIII or IX are inherited as sex-linked recessive disorders.

Factor VIII is a molecular complex consisting of VIII:C, which corrects the abnormal clotting time, and VIII:R the "related protein" (the von Willebrand protein) which corrects the defect in von Willebrand disease. VIII:C portion of the complex is a glycoprotein with molecular weight of about 285,000. There are both VIII:C deficient patients (cross reacting material negative (CRM⁻) type also named hemophilia A⁻, the common form) and VIII:C nonfunctional molecular variant patients (CRM⁺ type also named hemophilia A⁺).

Factor VIII circulates as a heterodimer bound to vWF through a C-terminal light chain.[1] The latter is metal ion-bridged to a N-terminal heavy chain. Proteolytic processing by thrombin produces expression of cofactor activity which correlates with cleavages at amino acid positions 372, 740, and 1689. Cleavages at positions 1689 and 372 are essential for cofactor activity in recombinant F VIII.[2] The factor VIII gene is large (186 kilobases). There is a high frequency of *de novo* mutations but in only about 50% of patients with severe hemophilia A are mutations in the gene itself detected.[3,4] It is hypothesized that mutations occur in locus-controlling regions or other sequences outside the gene that are important for its expression or in other genes necessary for factor VIII expression.[4] Use of factor VIII gene probes have confirmed the thesis that multiple different molecular abnormalities may result in clinical hemophilia A.[5] A case of severe hemophilia A, factor VIII 1689-Cys, a point mutation of a C to T transition in codon 1689 converting Arg to Cys at the light chain thrombin cleavage site has been shown to result in a failure to release the acidic peptide from the light chain on thrombin activation.[6]

Desmopressin (1-deamino-8-D-arginine vasopressin, DDAVP®), a synthetic analogue of ADH L-arginine vasopressin, can raise circulating levels of F VIII and vWF. As such, it has become established as a nontransfusional form for the therapy of mild and moderate forms of hemophilia A and von Willebrand disease. In addition, there is evidence that DDAVP® reduces blood loss and transfusion requirements in cardiopulmonary bypass patients (who have defective hemostasis) and also in hemostatically normal individuals (eg, spinal fusion patients). DDAVP® may cause increase in factor VIII and vWF by increasing their release from storage sites. Mannucci has reviewed this important subject (see following reference).

Factor VIII concentrates, produced using recombinant technology, have been undergoing human clinical trials[7,8] and are available for clinical use (eg, Kogenate®, antihemophilic factor, recombinant). The manufacture of recombinant factor VIII, however, suffers from inefficiencies of production relating to the large size of this heterogeneous glycoprotein. To circumvent these difficulties, a B-domain-deleted form of FVIII has been developed. Residues 760-1639 are absent in this form (LA-VIII) of the molecule. It has been shown that the biochemical, immunologic, and *in vivo* functional characteristics are those of wild type rFVIII.[9] Potentially this source of factor VIII will allow large supply, low cost, and freedom from the threat of human virus infection. Molecular biologic techniques such as cloning of the VIII and IX genes and recombinant genetic technology may allow therapy to be directed at the underlying cause of the disease. On the near horizon is cure of factor VIII deficiency by "gene therapy."[10,11] See listing Anticoagulant, Circulating *on page 229* for information about inhibitors of (antibody to) factor VIII.

Family studies, combined with DNA (restriction fragment length polymorphism) and discriminant analyses, can determine if at-risk women are carriers for hemophilia A in most cases.[12]

Footnotes

1. Eaton DL and Vehar GA, "Factor VIII Structure and Proteolytic Processing," *Prog Hemost Thromb*, 1986, 8:47-70.
2. Pittman DD and Kaufman RJ, "Proteolytic Requirements for Thrombin Activation of Anti-Hemophilic Factor (Factor VIII)," *Proc Natl Acad Sci U S A*, 1988, 85(8):2429-33.
3. Randall T, "Gene Scene: Factor VIII Gene Explains Just Half of Severe Cases of Hemophilia A," *JAMA* 1991, 226(12):1612-3.
4. Higuchi M, Kazazian HH Jr, Kasch L, et al, "Molecular Characterization of Severe Hemophilia A Suggests That About Half the Mutations Are Not Within the Coding Regions and Splice Junctions of the Factor VIII Gene," *Proc Natl Acad Sci U S A*, 1991, 88(16):7405-9.

5. Higuchi M, Kochhan L, Schwaab R, et al, "Molecular Defects in Hemophilia A: Identification and Characterization of Mutations in the Factor VIII Gene and Family Analysis," *Blood*, 1989, 74(3):1045-51.
6. O'Brien DP and Tuddenham EG, "Purification and Characterization of Factor VIII 1,689-Cys: A Nonfunctional Cofactor Occurring in a Patient With Severe Hemophilia A," *Blood*, 1989, 73(8):2117-22.
7. Aronson DL, "The Current Status of Recombinant Human Factor VIII," *Semin Hematol*, 1991, 28(2 Suppl 1):55-6.
8. Schwartz RS and Rousell RH, "A Summary of the World-Wide Clinical Investigations of Recombinant Factor VIII," *Semin Hematol*, 1991, 28(2 Suppl 1):53-4.
9. Pittman DD, Alderman EM, Tomkinson KN, et al, "Biochemical, Immunological, and *In Vivo* Functional Characterization of B-Domain-Deleted Factor VIII," *Blood*, 1993, 81(11):2925-35.
10. Roberts HR, High VA, White GL, et al, "Ultra-Pure Factor VIII Products: The Impact for the Future of Hemophilia Care," Presented at the XVIII International Congress of the World Federation of Hemophilia, Madrid, May 26-31, 1988.
11. Israel DI and Kaufman RJ, "Retroviral-Mediated Transfer and Amplification of a Functional Human Factor VIII Gene," *Blood*, 1990, 75(5):1074-80.
12. Poon M-C, Hoar DI, Low S, et al, "Hemophilia A Carrier Detection by Restriction Fragment Length Polymorphism Analysis and Discriminant Analysis Based on ELISA of Factor VIII and vWF," *J Lab Clin Med*, 1992, 119(6):751-62.

References

Aledort L, "Inhibitors in Hemophilia Patients: Current Status and Management," *Am J Hematol*, 1994, 47(3):208-17.

Antonarakis SE, Rossiter JP, Young M, et al, "Factor VIII Gene Inversions in Severe Hemophilia A: Results of an International Consortium Study," *Blood*, 1995, 86(6):2206-12.

Arkin CF, Bovill EG, Brandt JT, et al, "Factors Affecting the Performance of Factor VIII Coagulant Activity Assays," *Arch Pathol Lab Med*, 1992, 116(9):908-15.

Brandt JT, "Measurement of Factor VIII: A Potential Risk Factor for Vascular Disease," *Arch Pathol Lab Med*, 1993, 117(1):48-51.

Brettler DB and Levine PH, "Factor Concentrates for Treatment of Hemophilia: Which One to Choose?" *Blood*, 1989, 73(8):2067-73.

Cohen AJ and Kessler CM, "Treatment of Inherited Coagulation Disorders," *Am J Med*, 1995, 99(6):675-82.

Mannucci PM, "Desmopressin: A Nontransfusional Form of Treatment for Congenital and Acquired Bleeding Disorders," *Blood*, 1988, 72(5):1449-55.

O'Brien DP and Tuddenham EG, "The Structure and Function of Factor VIII," *Haemostasis and Thrombosis*, 3rd ed, Vol 1, Bloom AL, Forbes CD, Thomas DP, et al, eds, New York, NY: Churchill Livingstone, 1994, 333-48.

Rao LV and Rapaport SI, "Factor VIIa-Catalyzed Activation of Factor X Independent of Tissue Factor: Its Possible Significance for Control of Hemophilic Bleeding by Infused Factor VIIa," *Blood*, 1990, 75(5):1069-73.

Schwaab R, Oldenburg J, Tuddenham EG, et al, "Mutations in Haemophilia A," *Br J Haematol*, 1993, 83(3):450-8.

Thompson AR, "Molecular Biology of the Hemophilias," *Prog Hemost Thromb*, 1991, 10:175-214.

White GC 2d and Shoemaker CB, "Factor VIII Gene and Hemophilia A," *Blood*, 1989, 73(1):1-12.

Factor IX

CPT 85250

Related Information

Activated Partial Thromboplastin Time *on page 227*
Coagulation Factor Assay *on page 235*
Factor VIII *on previous page*
Factor IX Complex (Human) *on page 609*
Plasma, Fresh Frozen *on page 615*

Synonyms Autoprothrombin II; Christmas Disease Factor; Hemophilia B; Plasma Thromboplastin Component

Patient Preparation Avoid Coumadin® therapy for 2 weeks and heparin therapy for 2 days prior to test

Specimen Plasma

Container Blue top (sodium citrate) tube

Collection Routine venipuncture. If multiple tests are being drawn, draw coagulation studies second. If only coagulation studies are being drawn, draw 1-2 mL into another Vacutainer®, discard, and then collect coagulation tests. This avoids contamination of the specimen with tissue thromboplastins.

Storage Instructions Keep refrigerated.

Causes for Rejection Tube not full, specimen hemolyzed, specimen clotted, specimen received more than 2 hours after collection

Special Instructions Contact testing facility to schedule and possibly arrange for referral as this is an uncommonly available procedure unless you have access to a special coagulation laboratory.

Reference Range 50% to 150% of normal. Patients with severe hemophilia will have levels <1%, often undetectable. Moderate forms of the disease have levels of 1% to 10% while some mild cases may have 11% to 49% of normal factor IX. Plasma concentration is about 4 mg/L, biological half-life is 18-24 hours. Caution has been recommended in the interpretation of factor IX levels in prepubertal children and in particular, FIX functional to FIX antigen determined ratios, as there is evidence that values are lower in normal children than in adults.[1]

Use Document specific factor deficiency

Limitations Interpretation of results may be limited if patient is receiving anticoagulant therapy or if test is done more than 2 hours after collection.

Contraindications Patient on anticoagulant therapy

Methodology One-stage and two-stage assays have been described. One-stage assay based on APTT involves testing mixtures of factor IX (Continued)

Factor IX (Continued)

deficient plasma and dilutions of normal and test plasma. APTT results are obtained, and corrective effect of test plasma, as compared to normal plasma, is expressed as a percentage.[2] A 1988 College of American Pathologists Survey Program found that factor IX assay performance by participating laboratories showed improved assay precision as compared with performance in a 1980 survey.[3] There was significant difference, however, in the sensitivity of APTT reagents to factor IX deficiency. In addition, the least sensitive reagents included some that are in common use.[3]

Additional Information Factor IX is a vitamin K dependent liver produced coagulation protein (a zymogen). It is a single chain glycoprotein with molecular weight of about 55,000 and plasma concentration of 4 µg/mL. It is about 18% carbohydrate; the complete amino acid sequence has been determined. As with factor II, glutamic acid residues are converted by a carboxylase (vitamin K dependent process) to γ-carboxyglutamic acid. Factor IX is activated to the enzyme IXa by XIa and calcium or, and perhaps predominantly by, VIIa, a tissue factor substance, and calcium.[4]

Factor IX deficiency (PTC, plasma thromboplastin component or **Christmas disease**) is commonly referred to as **hemophilia B**. It has a recessive sex-linked mode of inheritance, males are affected, females are carriers. It occurs in 1 of 25,000 males. There is genetic heterogeneity, not all cases are clinically severe; mild forms are more prevalent than severe, some may not be associated with spontaneous bleeding episodes. Carriers are asymptomatic, but some variants may have moderately prolonged prothrombin time (see following information). In some cases, the functional abnormality relates to production of an abnormal factor IX molecule. Over 20 variants have been described. Factor IX deficiency can be characterized and phenotypically classified on the basis of functional activity, level of antigenic-reacting material and reaction with bovine thromboplastin in relation to the presence of CRM (cross reacting material).[5] Clinical symptoms of hemophilia B include hematuria; GI hemorrhage; muscle and mucous membrane hemorrhage; intracranial, post-traumatic, and postsurgical bleeding; and joint hematomas (not significantly different from the features of hemophilia A - factor VIII deficiency). Low levels of factor IX may be present in patients with liver disease. Severity of the symptoms correlate directly with the degree of prolongation of APTT test (level of factor IX deficiency). Mildly affected patients may show excessive bleeding only with major trauma or surgery. The APTT may not be prolonged if the factor IX level is >25%. In most cases of hemophilia B, the prothrombin time and thrombin times are normal. A subgroup of cross reacting material positive hemophilia B patients, however, is defined by its markedly prolonged ox-brain prothrombin time. The molecular defect of this "hemophilia B$_m$" (factor IX$Hilo$) has recently been described.[6]

A considerable body of knowledge concerning the molecular diversity of factor IX deficiency and the responsible genetic mechanisms has accumulated and is expanding. Application of oligonucleotide probes and endonuclease restriction enzymes has been applied to the study of factor IX polymorphisms. Recently a procedure based on DNA amplification using the polymerase chain reaction has been described.[7] It is described as rapid, avoids the use of radioisotopes, can be performed on small samples (under 1 mL) of whole blood, and has shown a high level of sensitivity. It is said to be applicable to any genetic polymorphism that overlaps a restriction enzyme recognition site.

A novel possibly curative therapy for factor IX deficiency has been described and could have application to other coagulation deficient states or abnormalities.[8] A retroviral vector encoding human clotting factor IX was introduced into normal human skin fibroblasts. More than 3 µg of factor IX per 1 million cultured cells was secreted over 24 hours. More than 70% of this protein was structurally and functionally indistinguishable from normal human factor IX. While this work was performed in rats and mice, it suggests that infected autologous fibroblasts might be capable of providing therapeutic levels of factor IX if transplanted into some hemophilia B patients.

Footnotes

1. Sweeney JD and Hoernig LA, "Age-Dependent Effect on the Level of Factor IX," *Am J Clin Pathol*, 1993, 99(6):687-8.
2. Dacie JV and Lewis SM, *Practical Haematology*, 7th ed, New York, NY: Churchill Livingstone, 1991, 275-6.
3. Brandt JT, Arkin CF, Bovill EG, et al, "Evaluation of APTT Reagent Sensitivity to Factor IX and Factor IX Assay Performance," *Arch Pathol Lab Med*, 1990, 114(2):135-41.
4. Bauer KA, Kass BL, ten Cate H, et al, "Factor IX Is Activated *In Vivo* by the Tissue Factor Mechanism," *Blood*, 1990, 76(4):731-6.
5. Giddings JC, *Molecular Genetics and Immunoanalysis in Blood Coagulation*, Chichester, England: Ellis Horwood Ltd, 1988, 51-71.
6. Huang M-N, Kasper CK, Roberts HR, et al, "Molecular Defect in Factor IX$_{Hilo}$, a Hemophilia B$_m$ Variant: Arg → Gln at the Carboxyterminal Cleavage Site of the Activation Peptide," *Blood*, 1989, 73(3):718-21.
7. Graham JB, Kunkel GR, Tennyson GS, et al, "The Malmö Polymorphism of Factor IX: Establishing the Genotypes by Rapid Analysis of DNA," *Blood*, 1989, 73(8):2104-7.

8. Palmer TD, Thompson AR, and Miller AD, "Production of Human Factor IX in Animals by Genetically Modified Skin Fibroblasts: Potential Therapy for Hemophilia B," *Blood*, 1989, 73(2):438-45.

References

Goldsmith JC, Kasper CK, Blatt PM, et al, "Coagulation Factor IX: Successful Surgical Experience With a Purified Factor IX Concentrate," *Am J Hematol*, 1992, 40(3):210-5.

Mammen EF, "Congenital Coagulation Disorders," *Semin Thromb Hemost*, 1983, 9:28-33.

Thompson AR, "Molecular Biology of the Hemophilias," *Prog Hemost Thromb*, 1991, 10:175-214.

Wilbers LL and Triplett DA, "Acquired Factor IX Inhibitors," *ASCP Check Sample®*, Chicago, IL: American Society of Clinical Pathologists, 1987.

Factor X

CPT 85260

Related Information

Coagulation Factor Assay *on page 235*

Plasma, Fresh Frozen *on page 615*

Synonyms Stuart Factor; Stuart-Prower Factor

Patient Preparation Avoid Coumadin® therapy for 2 weeks and heparin therapy for 2 days prior to test.

Specimen Plasma

Container Blue top (sodium citrate) tube

Collection Routine venipuncture. If multiple tests are being drawn, draw coagulation studies last. If only coagulation tests are being drawn, draw 1-2 mL into another Vacutainer®, discard, and then collect coagulation tests. This collection procedure avoids contamination of the specimen with tissue thromboplastins.

Storage Instructions Keep refrigerated.

Causes for Rejection Tube not full, specimen hemolyzed, specimen clotted, specimen received more than 2 hours after collection

Special Instructions Test is not commonly available. Communicate with laboratory for scheduling and referral to a specialized coagulation laboratory.

Reference Range 50% to 150%. Homozygotes have <2% activity, heterozygotes, 40% to 60%.[1] Plasma concentration is about 12 mg/L.

Use Document specific factor deficiency

Limitations Interpretation of result may be limited if patient is receiving anticoagulant therapy or if test is done more than 2 hours after collection.

Methodology Modified one-stage prothrombin time utilizing commercially available factor X deficient substrate with test result read from normal plasma dilution curve; enzyme-linked immunosorbent assay (ELISA): chromogenic assay

Additional Information Factor X is a vitamin K dependent glycoprotein coagulation factor (molecular weight of 59,000) produced by the liver. It circulates in plasma as a two chain molecule with a serine active center in the heavy chain. A 43,000 dalton heavy chain and a 16,000 dalton light chain are held together by a disulfide bond; the protein contains some 15% carbohydrate. Glutamic acid residues on the light chain are converted to γ-carboxyglutamic acid by carboxylase (vitamin K required). This process allows for binding (calcium dependent) to phospholipid surfaces during coagulation. Factor X activation occurs by the extrinsic path (thromboplastin) and by the intrinsic path (IXa, VIIa, Ca^{++}, and phospholipids). A protease in Russell's viper venom produces nonphysiological activation. All activation pathways cleave the same arginyl-isoleucyl heavy chain bond. Activated X (Xa) converts prothrombin to thrombin. The rare clinical condition (X deficiency) is inherited as autosomal, incompletely recessive, consanguinity present in <50% of affected families. About 50 families with hereditary factor X deficiency have been reported. Symptoms (homozygotes) include hematoma formation, hemorrhage, menorrhagia, hematuria, and umbilical cord hemorrhage. Hemarthrosis, petechiae, and cerebral hemorrhage occur only rarely. Acquired deficiencies occur with significant hepatic dysfunction and with oral anticoagulant (coumarin) therapy. Whole blood clotting time, prothrombin time (corrected by giving aged plasma), and APTT are prolonged while thrombin time, bleeding time, platelet count, platelet function, and other coagulation factor levels are normal. Factor X deficiency may be associated with primary systemic amyloidosis.[2] Successful treatment has been reported with the use of Autoplex® T (activated prothrombin complex).[3]

Coagulation profiles of known factor X variants indicate a number of molecular aberrations of factor X/Xa function. There are cases without detectable factor X antigen or function, cases with selective abnormalities involving one of the pathways of activation and a population (Friuli region of Italy) with moderate bleeding tendency, functional decrease in factor X (as defined by PT and APTT testing) but normal clotting times with Russell's viper venom and normal levels of factor X antigen. A structural defect in the heavy chain of factor X Friuli has been identified. The defect is probably produced by a point mutation affecting the activated heavy chain within the 195-424 segment of the amino acid sequences. The functional result is an approximately 33% decrease in the rate of activation of prothrombin to thrombin by activated factor X

Friuli as compared to normal factor X.[4] Factor X Santo Domingo, a cause of severe bleeding, is caused by a homozygous transition in exon I which causes a substitution in the carboxy-terminus of the signal peptide, preventing cleavage by the signal peptidase resulting in impaired factor X secretion.[5] Major abnormalities of chromosome 13 and partial deletion of the factor X gene (resulting in severe deficiency of factor X activity and antigen) have also been reported.[6]

Footnotes

1. Mori K, Sakai H, Nakano N, et al, "Congenital Factor X Deficiency in Japan," *Tohoku J Exp Med*, 1981, 133:1-19.
2. McPherson RA, Onstad JW, Ugoretz RJ, et al, "Coagulopathy in Amyloidosis: Combined Deficiency of Factors IX and X," *Am J Hematol*, 1977, 3:225-35.
3. Henson K, Files JC, and Morrison FS, "Transient Acquired Factor X Deficiency: Report of the Use of Activated Clotting Concentrate to Control a Life-Threatening Hemorrhage," *Am J Med*, 1989, 87(5):583-5.
4. Fair DS, Revak DJ, Hubbard JG, et al, "Isolation and Characterization of the Factor X Friuli Variant," *Blood*, 1989, 73(8):2108-16.
5. Watzke HH, Wallmark A, Hamaguchi H, et al, "Factor X Santo Domingo. Evidence That the Severe Clinical Phenotype Arises From a Mutation Blocking Secretion," *J Clin Invest*, 1991, 88(5):1685-9.
6. Bernardi F, Marchetti G, Patracchini P, et al, "Partial Gene Deletion in a Family With Factor X Deficiency," *Blood*, 1989, 73(8):2123-7.

References

Jackson CM, "Factor X," *Prog Hemost Thromb*, 1984, 7:55-109.
Mammen EF, "Factor X Abnormalities," *Semin Thromb Hemost*, 1983, 9:31-3.

Factor XI

CPT 85270

Related Information

Coagulation Factor Assay *on page 235*
Plasma, Fresh Frozen *on page 615*

Synonyms Plasma Thromboplastin Antecedent; PTA

Patient Preparation Avoid Coumadin® therapy for 2 weeks and heparin therapy for 2 days prior to test.

Specimen Plasma

Container Blue top (sodium citrate) tube

Collection Routine venipuncture. If multiple tests are being drawn, draw coagulation studies last. If only coagulation tests are being drawn, draw 1-2 mL into another Vacutainer®, discard, and then collect coagulation tests. This collection procedure avoids contamination of the specimen with tissue thromboplastins.

Storage Instructions Keep refrigerated.

Causes for Rejection Tube not full, specimen hemolyzed, specimen clotted, specimen received more than 2 hours after collection

Special Instructions Schedule with laboratory in advance. Test is not routinely available, done by specialized coagulation laboratory.

Reference Range 50% to 150% of normal. Homozygotes usually have levels of 1% to 10% while heterozygotes have about 50%.

Use Document specific factor deficiency

Limitations Interpretation of result may be limited if patient is receiving anticoagulant therapy or if test is done more than 2 hours after collection.

Methodology Modified APTT using commercially available factor XI deficient substrate with test result read from normal plasma dilution curve

Additional Information Factor XI, a coagulation glycoprotein produced in the liver, circulates in the plasma as a dimer, the two chains held by disulfide bonds. Factor XI is activated (to XIa) by factor XIIa, and the dimer is broken into two chains. The serine active center is resident on the light chain. Activation of XI requires surfaces (usually phospholipid) and presence of prekallikrein and HMWK (high molecular weight kininogen). Structural organization of the complete factor XI gene has been described.[1] Inherited factor XI deficiency, while uncommon, is one of the more frequently encountered inherited defects of the coagulation mechanism. This condition is transmitted as an incomplete autosomal recessive, affecting males and females, and is seen especially in Ashkenazi Jews. Only homozygous patients have bleeding symptoms. They suffer post-trauma/postsurgical hemorrhage, epistaxis, hematuria, and menorrhagia. Excessive postpartum hemorrhage is especially common. Severity of bleeding does not always correlate with the plasma level of factor XI.[1] This may relate in part to the mechanism of activation of factor XI[2] and/or to use of aspirin. Heterozygotes are asymptomatic. Homozygotes have prolonged whole blood clotting time and APTT. Prothrombin time, thrombin time, bleeding time, platelet count, and platelet function tests are normal.

Footnotes

1. Fujikawa K and Chung DW, "Factor XI," *Molecular Basis of Thrombosis and Hemostasis*, Chapter 12, High KA and Roberts HR, eds, New York, NY: Marcel Dekker Inc, 1995, 257-68.
2. Gailani D and Broze GJ Jr, "Factor XI Activation in a Revised Model of Blood Coagulation," *Science*, 1991, 253(5022):909-12.

References

Kitchens CS, "Factor XI: A Review of Its Biochemistry and Deficiency," *Semin Thromb Hemost*, 1991, 17(1):55-72.
Mammen EF, "Factor XI Deficiency," *Semin Thromb Hemost*, 1983, 9:34-5.

Factor XII

CPT 85280

Related Information

Coagulation Factor Assay *on page 235*
Hypercoagulable State Coagulation Screen *on page 250*
Plasma, Fresh Frozen *on page 615*

Synonyms Hageman Factor; XIIa

Patient Preparation Avoid Coumadin® therapy for 2 weeks and heparin therapy for 2 days prior to test.

Specimen Plasma

Container Blue top (sodium citrate) tube

Collection Routine venipuncture. If multiple tests are being drawn, draw coagulation studies last. If only coagulation tests are being drawn, draw 1-2 mL into another Vacutainer®, discard, and then collect coagulation tests. This collection procedure avoids contamination of the specimen with tissue thromboplastins.

Storage Instructions Keep refrigerated.

Causes for Rejection Tube not full, specimen hemolyzed, specimen clotted, specimen received more than 2 hours after collection

Special Instructions Schedule with laboratory in advance as this is an uncommonly available test and is usually done only by specialized coagulation laboratories.

Reference Range 50% to 150% of normal; homozygotes have levels <1%; heterozygotes have levels of 15% to 80%.

Use Document specific coagulation deficiency

Limitations Interpretation of results may be limited if patient is receiving anticoagulant therapy or if test is done more than 2 hours after collection.

Methodology Modified APTT using a known factor XII deficient substrate, test result read from normal plasma dilution curve

Additional Information Hageman factor (factor XII) is one of three proteins, XII, prekallikrein, and high molecular weight kininogen (HMWK), involved in the contact activation system. Factor XII is the first protein adsorbed onto negatively-charged surfaces (collagen fibers, platelet membranes, and other tissue surfaces) exposed after endothelial damage. With activation to XIIa, there is interaction with prekallikrein, HMWK, and XIIa fragments in a complex circular reinforcement loop in which activation of the fibrinolytic system (plasminogen), complement system (C1), and vasoactive system (HMWK to bradykinin) also occur. Factor XII is a single chain glycoprotein molecule synthesized and secreted by hepatocytes.[1] Upon activation by kallikrein, it is transformed to an enzyme with a light and heavy chain. The light chain contains the active enzymatic (serine) site, while the heavy chain is concerned with surface binding. Factor XII deficiency is usually inherited as an autosomal recessive condition, but a rare example appears to have autosomal dominant mode of inheritance. The condition affects both males and females. Patients, however, do not have bleeding symptoms as the clotting system can be activated by alternate paths that bypass the contact system. Occasionally, patients suffer thromboembolic episodes which can be fatal and apparently relate to impaired fibrinolytic activity (one of the functions of XIIa is to activate plasminogen to plasmin). Homozygous XII deficient patients have prolonged whole blood clotting times and APTT results. Euglobulin clot lysis time is usually significantly prolonged. Prothrombin time, thrombin time, and bleeding time are normal in the XII deficient patient.

A structurally abnormal F XII (F XII Bern) has been shown to have a defect in the light chain region (wherein the enzymatic active site is situated).[2]

While there are some apparent clinical associations between eosinophilia (marked) and thrombosis, a recent study indicates that eosinophils in suspension or eosinophil peroxidase, eosinophil major basic protein or eosinophil cationic protein, inhibit activation of Hageman factor.[3]

Footnotes

1. Gordon EM, Gallagher CA, Johnson TR, et al, "Hepatocytes Express Blood Coagulation Factor XII (Hageman Factor)," *J Lab Clin Med*, 1990, 115(4):463-9.
2. Wuillemin WA, Huber I, Furlan M, et al, "Functional Characterization of an Abnormal Factor XII Molecule (F XII Bern)," *Blood*, 1991, 78(4):997-1004.
3. Ratnoff OD, Gleich GJ, Shurin SB, et al, "Inhibition of the Activation of Hageman Factor (Factor XII) by Eosinophils and Eosinophilic Constituents," *Am J Hematol*, 1993, 42(1):138-45.

References

Braulke I, Pruggmayer M, Melloh P, et al, "Factor XII (Hageman) Deficiency in Women With Habitual Abortion: New Subpopulation of Recurrent Aborters?" *Fertil Steril*, 1993, 59(1):98-101.
Mammen EF, "Contact Factor Abnormalities," *Semin Thromb Hemost*, 1983, 9:36-41.
McDonough RJ and Nelson CL, "Clinical Implications of Factor XII Deficiency," *Oral Surg Oral Med Oral Pathol*, 1989, 68(3):264-6.

Factor XIII

CPT 85290; 85291 (screen)

Related Information

Clot Retraction *on page 235*
(Continued)

Factor XIII (Continued)

Coagulation Factor Assay *on page 235*
Plasma, Fresh Frozen *on page 615*

Synonyms Fibrin Stabilizing Factor; Fibrinoligase; Laki-Lorand Factor

Specimen Plasma

Container Blue top (sodium citrate) tube

Collection Routine venipuncture

Storage Instructions Keep refrigerated.

Causes for Rejection Tubes not full, blood clotted, hemolyzed specimen, specimen received more than 2 hours after collection, specimen not refrigerated

Reference Range Clot stable in 5M urea for at least 24 hours. If factor XIII deficiency is present, clot will usually dissolve in 1-2 hours.

Use Evaluate bleeding disorders due to homozygous deficiency of factor XIII

Methodology Citrated plasma is recalcified, clotted at 37°C, and after 30 minutes placed in 5M urea at 37°C (screening test). A quantitative assay is based on the incorporation of monodansylcadaverine into casein (transaminase activity).[1]

Additional Information Factor XIII converts loose hydrogen bonded monomers into covalently bonded fibrin polymer. The resultant end product of fibrin formation has increased tensile strength and is resistant to fibrinolysis. Inactive factor XIII is present in plasma at a concentration of about 1 mg/dL. It is converted into its active transglutaminase enzymic form by thrombin. Then, in the presence of calcium, it causes covalent cross-linkage of fibrin molecules. Clinical symptoms and abnormal result in the factor XIII screening test do not occur unless only 1% to 2% or less of factor XIII activity remains (patients have near total deficiency) - there are no mild to moderate forms. The deficiency is inherited as an autosomal recessive condition, heterozygotes (with 50% of levels of XIII) are asymptomatic. Homozygotes have slow progressive bleeding, often hematomas-hemorrhagic cysts, bleeding after cuts, and poor wound healing. Death may be due to intracranial hemorrhage. An important early sign is persistent umbilical stump hemorrhage. Cases of liver disease, pregnancy, sickle cell disease, and Henoch-Schönlein purpura may have moderately decreased factor XIII levels (without resultant bleeding).

Activated factor XIII levels and cross-linked fibrin polymers are increased in patients with acute myocardial infarction.[2]

Intracranial hemorrhage, reported in infants with XIII deficiency, has lead to a recommendation that prophylactic life-long factor XIII concentrate (eg, Fibrogammin®) replacement therapy be considered in patients with severe deficiency.[3]

Hemorrhagic diarrhea in some patients with active Crohn's disease may be due (at least in part) to acquired factor XIII deficiency.[4,5] Clinically significant inhibitors of factor XIII have been described but are encountered only rarely, some 12 cases having been reported.[6]

Footnotes
1. Lorand L, Urayama T, de Kiewiet JW, et al, "Diagnostic and Genetic Studies on Fibrin-Stabilizing Factor With a New Assay Based on Amine Incorporation," *J Clin Invest*, 1969, 48:1054-64.
2. Francis CW, Connaghan DG, Scott WL, et al, "Increased Plasma Concentration of Cross-Linked Fibrin Polymers in Acute Myocardial Infarction," *Circulation*, 1987, 75(6):1170-7.
3. Abbondanzo SL, Gootenberg JE, Lofts RS, et al, "Intracranial Hemorrhage in Congenital Deficiency of Factor XIII," *Am J Pediatr Hematol Oncol*, 1988, 10(1):65-8.
4. Wisen O and Gardlund B, "Hemostasis in Crohn's Disease: Low Factor XIII Levels in Active Disease," *Scand J Gastroenterol*, 1988, 23(8):961-6.
5. Mamel JJ, "Gastrointestinal Bleeding in Crohn's Disease: The Role of Acquired Factor Deficiency," *Am J Gastroenterol*, 1990, 85(3):321-2.
6. Fukue H, Anderson K, McPhedran P, et al, "A Unique Factor XIII Inhibitor to a Fibrin-Binding Site on Factor XIIIA," *Blood*, 1992, 79(1):65-74.

References
Duckert F, Jung E, Shmerling DH, et al, "A Hitherto Undescribed Congenital Hemorrhagic Diathesis Probably Due to Fibrin Stabilizing Factor Deficiency," *Thromb Diath Hemorrh*, 1960, 5:179.
McDonagh J, Kaczmarek E, and Lee MH, "Fibrinogen and Factor XIII: Biology and Disorders of Fibrin Formation and Cross-Linking," *Blood: Principles and Practice of Hematology*, Chapter 41, Handin RI, Lux SE, and Stossel TP, eds, Philadelphia, PA: JB Lippincott, 1995, 1219-59.

Factor Assay *see* Coagulation Factor Assay *on page 235*

Factor, Fitzgerald

CPT 85293

Related Information

Coagulation Factor Assay *on page 235*
Factor, Fletcher *on this page*

Synonyms Fitzgerald Factor Assay; High Molecular Weight Kininogen; HMW Kininogen; Williams-Fitzgerald-Flaujeac Factor

Patient Preparation Avoid Coumadin® therapy for 2 weeks and heparin therapy for 2 days prior to test.

Specimen Plasma

Container Blue top (sodium citrate) tube

Collection Routine venipuncture. If multiple tests are being drawn, draw coagulation studies last. If only coagulation tests are being drawn, draw 1-2 mL into another Vacutainer®, discard, and then collect coagulation tests. This collection procedure avoids contamination of the specimen with tissue thromboplastins. Place specimen in ice and transport immediately to the laboratory.

Storage Instructions Keep refrigerated (2°C to 8°C for up to 2 hours). May store frozen (at -35°C) for up to 2 weeks.

Causes for Rejection Specimen hemolyzed, clotted, diluted, or contaminated with heparin; tubes not full, not iced, or received more than 1 hour after collection

Special Instructions Not a routine test. Contact laboratory to learn of availability and need for special arrangements.

Reference Range Patient's plasma is normal if upon mixing with known deficient plasma the combination has normal APTT, 90 mg/L (bioassay)

Use Investigate cause of prolonged APTT; confirmation of Fitzgerald factor deficiency

Limitations Interpretation of results may be limited if patient is receiving anticoagulant therapy

Contraindications Patient on anticoagulant therapy

Methodology Measurement of functional coagulant activity of a mixture of test (patient's) plasma with Fitzgerald factor deficient plasma, bioassay based on kinin formation, radioimmunoassay (RIA), enzyme-linked immunosorbent assay (ELISA), particle concentration fluorescence immunoassay[1]

Additional Information Previous prothrombin time and activated partial thromboplastin time are useful for interpretation. Patients with deficiency of Fitzgerald factor deficiency do not have clinical bleeding disease. Some patients have been reported to have thromboembolic episodes. This rare condition is considered when an abnormal APTT is not explained by other significant factor deficiency. The prolonged APTT clotting time may be shortened or even normalized after incubation with contact activators. HMWK (high molecular weight kininogen), Hageman factor (factor XII), and prekallikrein are functionally and structurally closely related. The gene for human kininogen has been isolated and characterized.[2] HMWK augments the formation of activated Hageman factor. A functional domain for the binding of HMWK is present within the heavy chain region of factor XI.[3] HMWK has a binding site for prekallikrein (Fletcher factor).[4] These proteins are involved in the contact phase of coagulation and immune system mechanisms. As deficient states of these proteins lack bleeding manifestations, it could be considered that they are not true coagulation factors. The intrinsic pathway of coagulation is initiated when the four plasma proteins (Hageman factor, prekallikrein, HMWK, and factor XI) interact with particular negatively charged surfaces. Plasminogen activation, immune pathway activation (release of kinins and complement activation) may also be involved. HMWK is one of the proteins required for the generation of bradykinin (a vasoactive peptide).

Footnotes
1. Scott CF and Colman RW, "Sensitive Antigenic Determinations of High Molecular Weight Kininogen Performed by Covalent Coupling of Capture Antibody," *J Lab Clin Med*, 1992, 119(1):77-86.
2. Kitamura N, Kitagawa H, Fukushima D, et al, "Structural Organization of the Human Kininogen Gene and a Model for Its Evolution," *J Biol Chem*, 1985, 260(14):8610-7.
3. Baglia FA, Sinha D, and Walsh PN, "Functional Domains in the Heavy-Chain Region of Factor XI: A High Molecular Weight Kininogen-Binding Site and a Substrate-Binding Site for Factor IX," *Blood*, 1989, 74(1):244-51.
4. Reddigari SR and Kaplan AP, "Monoclonal Antibody to Human High-Molecular-Weight Kininogen Recognizes Its Prekallikrein Binding Site and Inhibits Its Coagulant Activity," *Blood*, 1989, 74(2):695-702.

References
Giddings JC, *Molecular Genetics and Immunoanalysis in Blood Coagulation*, Chichester, England: Ellis Horwood Ltd, 1988, 30-2.

Factor, Fletcher

CPT 85292

Related Information

Coagulation Factor Assay *on page 235*
Factor, Fitzgerald *on this page*

Synonyms Fletcher Factor Assay; Prekallikrein Assay

Patient Preparation Avoid Coumadin® therapy for 2 weeks and heparin therapy for 2 days prior to test.

Specimen Plasma

Container Blue top (sodium citrate) tube

Collection Routine venipuncture. If multiple tests are being drawn, draw coagulation studies last. If only coagulation tests are being drawn, draw 1-2 mL into another Vacutainer®, discard, and then collect coagulation tests. This collection procedure avoids contamination of the specimen with tissue thromboplastins.

Storage Instructions Keep refrigerated. Centrifuge at 2500 g for 15 minutes at 4°C and remove platelet-poor plasma with plastic pipette. Test immediately or freeze and store at -70°C.

Causes for Rejection Tube not full, specimen hemolyzed, specimen clotted, specimen received more than 2 hours after collection

Special Instructions Not a routine test. Contact laboratory for special arrangements and scheduling.

Reference Range Patient's plasma is normal if upon addition to known deficient plasma the mixture has normal APTT. A level of only 2% of prekallikrein provides complete correction. 50 mg/L (RIA), 100 mg/L (RID).

Use Investigate cause of prolonged APTT; identify prekallikrein deficiency (Fletcher factor deficit)[1]

Limitations Interpretation of results may be limited if patient is receiving anticoagulant therapy. Use of an ellagic acid-activated thromboplastin will usually not detect Fletcher factor deficiency.

Contraindications Patient on anticoagulant therapy

Methodology Measurement of coagulant activity of a mixture of test (patient's) plasma with Fletcher factor deficient plasma; radioimmuno-assay (RIA), radial immunodiffusion (RID)

Additional Information Previous prothrombin time and activated partial thromboplastin time are useful for interpretation. Prekallikrein is one of the coagulation proteins involved in the generation of bradykinin (a vaso-active peptide), and one of the major factors required for contact activation (others are Hageman factor and high molecular weight kininogen (HMWK)). Prekallikrein is a single-chain glycoprotein with molecular weight of about 88,000. In plasma, complexes form between prekalli-krein and HMWK (up to 70% of prekallikrein may be so bound); immune-based assays, therefore, may overestimate the actual value. Deficiency of any of the contact factors is associated with prolongation of APTT test. Prolonged APTT times may be shortened or even normal after incubation with contact activators. Deficiency is thought to be inherited as an autosomal recessive trait and does not result in bleeding tendency. Some patients may have thromboembolic episodes. Prekallikrein may be decreased in some newborns. Levels may be decreased in some patients with liver disease and in patients with uremia.[2]

Footnotes
1. LaDuca FM and Tourbaf KD, "Fletcher Factor Deficiency, Source of Variations of the Activated Partial Thromboplastin Time Test," *Am J Clin Pathol*, 1981, 75:626-8.
2. Saito H and Ratnoff OD, "Alteration of Factor VII Activity by Activated Fletcher Factor (A Plasma Kallikrein): A Potential Link Between the Intrinsic and Extrinsic Blood-Clotting Systems," *J Lab Clin Med*, 1975, 85:405-15.

References
DeLa Cadena RA, "Fletcher Factor Deficiency in a 9-Year-Old Girl: Mechanisms of the Contact Pathway of Blood Coagulation," *Am J Hematol*, 1995, 48(4):273-7.
Giddings JC, *Molecular Genetics and Immunoanalysis in Blood Coagulation*, Chichester, England: Ellis Horwood Ltd, 1988, 27-30.
Triplett DA, "Congenital Coagulation Factor Deficiencies (Excluding Abnormalities of Factor VIII)," *Laboratory Evaluation of Coagulation*, Chicago, IL: American Society of Clinical Pathologists, 1982, 96-7.

Factor I *see Fibrinogen on next page*

Factor VIIIR:Ag *see von Willebrand Factor Antigen on page 267*

Factor VIII-Related Antigen *see von Willebrand Factor Antigen on page 267*

FBP *see Fibrin Breakdown Products on this page*

FDP *see Fibrin Breakdown Products on this page*

Fibrin Breakdown Products

CPT 85362 (semiquantitative); 85370 (quantitative)

Related Information
Activated Partial Thromboplastin Time *on page 227*
D-Dimer *on page 237*
Euglobulin Clot Lysis *on page 238*
Fibrinogen *on next page*
Fibrinopeptide A *on page 247*
Fibrin Split Products, Protamine Sulfate *on page 248*
Intravascular Coagulation Screen *on page 253*

Synonyms FBP; FDP; Fibrin Degradation Products; Fibrin Split Products; Staphylococcal Clumping Test; Thrombo-Wellcotest® for Fibrin Split Products

Abstract Test for disseminated intravascular coagulation (DIC). Test results, if positive, are indicative of clot formation and subsequent lysis or partial lysis by fibrinolytic activity.

Patient Preparation Draw sample for fibrin breakdown products before instituting heparin therapy

Specimen Plasma

Container Special tube for fibrin split products, containing thrombin and an antifibrinolytic agent (protease inhibitor)

Collection Routine venipuncture. Blood placed in special tube obtained from Coagulation Laboratory. Mix gently. The specimen will clot.

Storage Instructions Separate and refrigerate serum as soon as possible if test is not run immediately.

Causes for Rejection Nonclotted blood, improper collection tube, tube overfilled, inadequate labeling, improper storage of serum

Reference Range <10 µg/mL

Possible Panic Range >40 µg/mL

Use Detect fibrin breakdown products (FBP) in serum. Helpful in establishing the diagnosis of disseminated intravascular coagulation. The presence of fibrin breakdown products at the higher titer level (>40 µg/mL - Thrombo-Wellcotest®) indicates that a fibrinolytic process has high likelihood of being associated with DIC. FBP are also elevated in primary fibrinolysis. May be of use in monitoring fibrinolytic therapy. Of use in study of pulmonary embolism, myocardial infarct, inflammation, and some liver diseases (in which clot formation and lysis occur or increased fibrinolytic activity is present).[1]

Limitations May be normal in fibrinolytic states if fragments have been degraded into portions too small to detect (method dependent). The presence of rheumatoid factor may rarely interfere and cause falsely high results. If rheumatoid arthritis (RA) is clinically suspect, it is advisable to perform RA testing. If the patient's RA is negative, the test is valid. However, if the RA is positive, the FBP should be interpreted with caution. The presence of fibrinogen in the test serum will cause a false-positive result. The collection tube must be fully clotted.

Contraindications Patient on heparin therapy

Methodology Latex agglutination (LA) /clumping (Thrombo-Wellcotest®), tanned RBC hemagglutination inhibition, staphylococcal clumping test, radioimmunoassay (RIA), others, a variety of immunologic-based methods incorporating antisera to one or more of the fragments of fibrinogen (X, Y, D, and E). A comparative study of three different methods has found significant variation in sensitivity when dealing with normal and "suspicious" range samples but comparable results in the detection of abnormal levels of fibrin split products.[2]

Additional Information Breakdown products of fibrinogen and fibrin (X, Y, D, and E) are released during the process of fibrinolysis. Fragment X (large) can polymerize slowly with thrombin but usually forms aggregates with fibrinogen, fibrin monomer, or other X and Y fragments. Fragment Y does not polymerize but interferes with the action of thrombin (acts as an antithrombin). Fragments D and E are small, D inhibits fibrin polymerization, while E is relatively inert. In addition, it has been shown (using B β-1-24 determinations) that FBP provide a surface for tissue plasminogen activator and plasminogen binding potentiating fibrinogen proteolysis by promoting plasmin generation.[3] Previous and recent red cell morphology, thrombin time, prothrombin time, activated partial thromboplastin time, fibrinogen, and platelet count are useful for interpretation.

Increased levels of fibrin degradation products may occur with a variety of pathologic processes in which clot formation and lysis are involved. In particular, application to the differentiation of pulmonary embolic lung disease from nonthromboembolic processes has been suggested. FBP and soluble fibrin complexes (measured using the serial dilution protamine sulfate test of Gurewich and Hutchinson) are positive in 55% of patients with pulmonary embolism but in only 4% of patients with nonthromboembolic disease. Eighty-three percent of 29 patients with pulmonary emboli were positive for FBP, but 50% of 80 patients with nonthromboembolic pulmonary disease were positive (indicative of poor specificity). Carcinoma was especially associated with presence of FBP. Use of the two tests together provides greater specificity, but this approach, generally, is not specific for the diagnosis of pulmonary embolism.[4,5] Reference must be made to the patient's clinical status (eg, results of lung scan studies) to establish presence of pulmonary embolus. Use of plasma FBP levels to exclude diagnosis of pulmonary embolism may be of value but is not firmly established.[4]

Presence of FBP in the urine does not correlate with serum FBP level. Over 2 mg/day of urinary FBP may indicate fibrin deposition and lysis in the kidney (if marked proteinuria is not present).[6]

Footnotes
1. Triplett DA, "Acquired Abnormalities of Hemostasis," *Laboratory Evaluation of Coagulation*, Chicago, IL: American Society of Clinical Pathologists, 1982, 215-7.
2. Drewinko B, Surgeon J, Cobb P, et al, "Comparative Sensitivity of Different Methods to Detect and Quantify Circulating Fibrinogen/Fibrin Split Products," *Am J Clin Pathol*, 1985, 84(1):58-66.
3. Weitz JI, Leslie B, and Ginsberg J, "Soluble Fibrin Degradation Products Potentiate Tissue Plasminogen Activator-Induced Fibrinogen Proteolysis," *J Clin Invest*, 1991, 87(3):1082-90.
4. Bynum LJ, Crotty C, and Wilson JE 3d, "Use of Fibrinogen/Fibrin Degradation Products and Soluble Fibrin Complexes for Differentiating Pulmonary Embolism From Nonthromboembolic Lung Disease," *Am Rev Respir Dis*, 1976, 114:285-9.
5. Rowbotham BJ, Egerton-Vernon J, Whitaker AN, et al, "Plasma Cross Linked Fibrin Degradation Products in Pulmonary Embolism," *Thorax*, 1990, 45(9):684-7.
6. Stiehm ER, Kuplic LS, and Uehling DT, "Urinary Fibrin Split Products in Human Renal Disease," *J Lab Clin Med*, 1971, 77:843-52.

References
Bick RL, "Disseminated Intravascular Coagulation," *Disorders of Thrombosis and Hemostasis*, Chapter 7, Chicago, IL: American Society of Clinical Pathologists, 1992, 137-73.

(Continued)

Fibrin Breakdown Products (Continued)

Graeff H and Hafter R, "Detection and Relevance of Cross-linked Fibrin Derivatives in Blood," *Semin Thromb Hemost*, 1982, 8:57-68.

Triplett DA, *Laboratory Evaluation of Coagulation*, Chicago, IL: American Society of Clinical Pathologists, 1982, 42-5, 175-8, 185-8.

Fibrin Degradation Products *see* Fibrin Breakdown Products *on previous page*

Fibrindex™ *see* Thrombin Time *on page 266*

Fibrinogen

CPT 85384 (activity); 85385 (antigen)

Related Information
Albumin and Plasma Protein Fraction for Infusion *on page 601*
Clot Retraction *on page 235*
Cryoprecipitate *on page 606*
D-Dimer *on page 237*
Euglobulin Clot Lysis *on page 238*
Fibrin Breakdown Products *on previous page*
Fibrinopeptide A *on next page*
Fibrin Split Products, Protamine Sulfate *on page 248*
Intravascular Coagulation Screen *on page 253*
Plasma, Fresh Frozen *on page 615*
Sedimentation Rate, Erythrocyte *on page 347*
Thrombin Time *on page 266*
Zeta Sedimentation Ratio *on page 354*

Synonyms Factor I; Fibrinogen Level; Quantitative Fibrinogen

Applies to Acute Phase Reactants; Sedimentation Rate

Abstract Precursor of fibrin, major contributor to the meshwork of blood clots. Meaningful assay of fibrinogen is uniquely challenging. Fibrinogen is an acute phase reactant as well as the focal point in the coagulation process. Consumption of fibrinogen is a major and clinically threatening aspect of disseminated intravascular coagulation.

Specimen Plasma

Container Blue top (sodium citrate) tube

Collection If multiple tests are being drawn, draw coagulation studies last. If only a fibrinogen is being drawn, draw 1-2 mL into another Vacutainer® or syringe (two-syringe technique), discard, and then collect the fibrinogen tube. This collection procedure avoids contamination of the specimen with tissue thromboplastin.

Storage Instructions Separate and freeze plasma as soon as possible if test is not run immediately.

Causes for Rejection Tube not full, tube clotted, specimen improperly labeled, specimen hemolyzed, specimen more than 1 hour old, stored specimen not frozen

Reference Range Quantitative: 200-400 mg/dL. The normal range in childhood (ages 1-16) is similar to that in adults (see reference by Andrew et al).

Possible Panic Range <100 mg/dL

Use Identify congenital afibrinogenemia, disseminated intravascular coagulation, and fibrinolytic activity

Limitations Increased in patients on oral contraceptives. Interpretations of results may be limited if patient is receiving anticoagulant therapy depending upon method of analysis. In cases of dysfibrinogenemia, results of fibrinogen determination will vary widely (method dependent). Individual methods may very widely (see following information) and suffer specific, occasionally significant, limitation.

Contraindications Patient receiving heparin less than 1 hour prior to specimen collection (depending upon method of analysis)

Methodology The many tests for fibrinogen proposed and in use over the past generation are a reflection of difficulties encountered in their clinical application. Generally, the most useful clinical information is obtained from "functional" based methods (ie, those that determine clottable plasma protein). These, however, are dependent upon fibrinogen activation with subsequent assessment of fibrin (which may or may not be contaminated with other protein). Functional methods are "blind" to the presence of nonclottable fibrinogen (molecular aberrant forms - dysfibrinogens). Most immunologic-based methods give misleading high results (from the vantage point of availability in the patient of useable-clottable fibrinogen). They will usually detect altered molecular forms but may include breakdown products (largely fragment X). Consideration should be given to employing two different methodologies depending on the clinical situation. Functional methods with different modes of activation and/or end point detection or one "functional" and one immunologic-based method, as available in the individual laboratory situation.

Earlier literature describes many methods based on harvesting the fibrin clot from plasma, washing, and determining the protein in the clot (by weight or chemically). These methods are generally time consuming, technically difficult, and suffer from inaccuracy due to inclusion of nonfibrinogen proteins in the clot, loss of clot fragments, and inaccuracies in measuring the clot protein. They will not measure the nonclottable fibrinogen derived protein.

Modified thrombin time method, the Clauss assay (in which a high concentration of thrombin is added to diluted plasma, resultant clotting time then proportional to the fibrinogen concentration) has the advantage that the endpoint is measured as a rate reaction. It is a rapid and simple procedure. The Clauss assay, however, depends upon the reliable maintenance of an accurate reference dilution curve and may give falsely low results in patients with circulating FBPs or paraproteins.[1]

A method (Ellis and Stransky[2]) similar to the Clauss assay is growing in use due to its adaptation to several automated instruments. Thrombin and calcium are added to citrated plasma, and the change in resultant turbidity is measured. The extent of fibrin polymerization rather than the rate of fibrinogen conversion is the parameter utilized. A similar automated method, but based on the kinetic reaction of the developing fibrin clot rather than measurement of total turbidity is said to be reliable and accurate.[3]

A variety of immunologic-based tests have been and continue to be developed. The FI™ test was a screening procedure utilizing antibody coated latex particles. When modified, it was used as a screen for FBP, a forerunner of the Thrombo-Wellcotest®. Radioimmunoassays have been developed for fibrinogen fragments, monomers, and fibrinopeptides A and B. Interest exists in RIA for released fibrinopeptide A as an indication of presence of thromboembolic process.[4] See also test listing Fibrinopeptide A *on page 247*.

A number of less well established (and uncommonly available) approaches to the determination of fibrinogen have been proposed. As an example, the method of Frigola et al[5] combines electrophoresis and thrombin clotting of fibrinogen. Following protein electrophoresis of plasma, thrombin is applied to "fix" fibrinogen (it is converted to fibrin on the cellulose acetate electrophoretic membrane) and nonclotted proteins are washed away with saline. The membrane is then stained and quantitated by densitometry.

Additional Information Fibrinogen is a complex polypeptide which upon enzyme action (physiologically by thrombin but pathologically by other substances such as occur in snake venom, eg, Reptilase®-R) is converted to fibrin that forms along with platelets the meshwork of the common blood clot. Fibrinogen is formed of three different pairs of polypeptide chains (α, β, γ) linked by disulfide bonds and forming a dimer. With conversion to fibrin, two pairs of peptides are released from the N-terminals of the α- and β-chains (fibrinopeptides A are released from the α-chains, fibrinopeptides B from the β-chains). The detailed and intricate molecular biochemistry has been explored, and the primary structure completely established.[6] Fibrinogen levels are decreased with hereditary afibrinogenemia, intravascular coagulation, primary and secondary fibrinolysis, and liver disease. Increased levels may be seen with inflammation, pregnancy, and in women taking oral contraceptives. Very high levels of heparin or fibrin breakdown products may affect results of some assays. See Methodology for a discussion of clinical implications of assay method. Some clinical problems may benefit from application of more than one test method (eg, in the assessment of cardiovascular risk).[7]

Fibrinogen, while of primary importance as a coagulation protein, is also an acute-phase protein reactant. As such, it is increased in disease processes involving tissue damage/inflammation. It is not often employed clinically as a measure of acute phase response as concurrent hemorrhage (fibrinogen concentration rises initially) and DIC (rise or fall in fibrinogen depending on method) renders interpretation problematic. Fibrinogen is one of the major determinants of the ESR/ZSR (sedimentation rate) phenomenon. Changes in fibrinogen may impair the reliability of erythrocyte sedimentation measurements.[8] There is evidence that increase in dietary fish oils results in decreased fibrinogen levels.[9]

Congenital hypofibrinogenemia may be responsible for mild hemorrhagic symptoms, fibrinogen levels are usually <100 mg/dL, and screening tests (eg, PT, APTT) may be normal or only slightly prolonged. There are a growing number of patients with fibrinogen variants. About 150 varieties of such dysfibrinogenemia have been recorded. These individuals are usually detected when prolonged clotting times are discovered as a result of routine laboratory testing. Over 50% of the cases are asymptomatic; only in about 33% of the cases has a mild bleeding tendency been noted. Some 20 cases have been associated with thrombocytopenia, recurrent thrombosis, or spontaneous abortion. Most cases show a pattern of autosomal dominant inheritance. Most are heterozygous, but in some there is a negative family history. Most cases of dysfibrinogenemia show discrepancy between the results of fibrinogen assays based on the thrombin clotting time (functional) and immune or chemical based methods.[10]

Plasma fibrinogen levels correlate with response to therapy in small cell carcinoma of lung. Higher pretreatment levels at diagnosis are associated with reduced overall survival and with decreased likelihood of tumor regression with combined chemotherapy.[11]

Footnotes

1. Timmis GC, Mammen EF, Ramos RG, et al, "Hemorrhage vs Rethrombosis After Thrombolysis for Acute Myocardial Infarction," *Arch Intern Med*, 1986, 146(4):667-72.
2. Ellis BC and Stransky A, "A Quick and Accurate Method for the Determination of Fibrinogen in Plasma," *J Lab Clin Med*, 1961, 58:477-88.
3. Tan V, Doyle CJ, and Budzynski AZ, "Comparison of the Kinetic Fibrinogen Assay With the von Clauss Method and the Clot Recovery Method in Plasma of Patients With Conditions Affecting Fibrinogen Coagulability," *Am J Clin Pathol*, 1995, 104(4):455-62.
4. Joist JH, "Fibrinopeptide A in the Diagnosis and Treatment of Deep Venous Thrombosis and Pulmonary Embolism," *Clin Lab Med*, 1984, 4(2):363-80.
5. Frigola A, Angeloni S, and Cerqueti AR, "New Method for Determining Thrombin-Clottable Fibrinogen," *Clin Chem*, 1977, 23:2103-6.
6. Mosesson MW and Finlayson JS, "The Search for the Structure of Fibrinogen," *Prog Hemost Thromb*, 1976, 3:61-107.
7. Knapp ML, Feher MD, Carey H, et al, "Comparison of an Immunochemical Assay for Plasma Fibrinogen and a Turbidimetric Thrombin Clotting Technique to Discriminate Hyperlipidaemic Patients From Healthy Controls," *J Clin Pathol*, 1990, 43(6):508-10.
8. Fischer CL and Gill CW, "Acute Phase Proteins," *Serum Protein Abnormalities: Diagnostic and Clinical Aspects*, Ritzmann SE and Daniels JC, eds, New York, NY: Alan R Liss Inc, 1982, 336-7.
9. Radack K, Deck C, and Huster G, "Dietary Supplementation With Low-Dose Fish Oils Lowers Fibrinogen Levels: A Double-Blind Controlled Study," *Ann Intern Med*, 1989, 111(10):757-8.
10. Giddings JC, *Molecular Genetics and Immunoanalysis in Blood Coagulation*, Chichester, England: Ellis Horwood Ltd, 1988, 120-36.
11. Meehan KR, Zacharski LR, Moritz TE, et al, "Pretreatment Fibrinogen Levels Are Associated With Response to Chemotherapy in Patients With Small Cell Carcinoma of the Lung: Department of Veterans Affairs Cooperative Study 188," *Am J Hematol*, 1995, 49(2):143-8.

References

Andrew M, Vegh P, Johnston M, et al, "Maturation of the Hemostatic System During Childhood," *Blood*, 1992, 80(8):1998-2005.
Bovill EG, McDonagh J, Triplett DA, et al, "Performance Characteristics of Fibrinogen Assays - Results of the College of American Pathologists Proficiency Testing Program 1988-1991," *Arch Pathol Lab Med*, 1993, 117(1):58-66.
Galanakis DK, "Dysfibrinogenemia: A Current Perspective," *Clin Lab Med*, 1984, 4(2):395-418.
Geffken DF, Keating FG, Kennedy MH, et al, "The Measurement of Fibrinogen in Population-Based Research. Studies on Instrumentation and Methodology," *Arch Pathol Lab Med*, 1994, 118(11):1106-9.
Hermans J and McDonagh J, "Fibrin: Structure and Interactions," *Semin Thromb Hemost*, 1982, 8:11-24.
Hollensead SC and Triplett DA, "Review of Fibrinogen Methods: Clinical Considerations," *ASCP Check Sample*®, Chicago, IL: American Society of Clinical Pathologists, 1988.
Lord ST, "Fibrinogen," *Molecular Basis of Thrombosis and Hemostasis*, Chapter 3, High KA and Roberts HR, eds, New York, NY: Marcel Dekker Inc, 1995, 51-75.
Palareti G, Maccaferri M, Manotti C, et al, "Fibrinogen Assays: A Collaborative Study of Six Different Methods," *Clin Chem*, 1991, 37(5):714-9.
Schorer AE, Singh J, and Basara ML, "Dysfibrinogenemia: A Case With Thrombosis (Fibrinogen Richfield) and an Overview of the Clinical and Laboratory Spectrum," *Am J Hematol*, 1995, 50(3):200-8.

Fibrinogen Level *see* Fibrinogen *on previous page*

Fibrinogen Screen *see* Thrombin Time *on page 266*

Fibrinoligase *see* Factor XIII *on page 243*

Fibrinolysis Time *see* Diluted Whole Blood Clot Lysis *on page 237*

Fibrinolysis Time *see* Euglobulin Clot Lysis *on page 238*

Fibrinopeptide A

CPT 85999

Related Information

Beta-Thromboglobulin *on page 232*
Fibrin Breakdown Products *on page 245*
Fibrinogen *on previous page*
Hypercoagulable State Coagulation Screen *on page 250*
Inhibitor, Lupus, Phospholipid Type *on page 251*
Intravascular Coagulation Screen *on page 253*

Synonyms FpA; FPA

Abstract Fibrinopeptides A and B are removed proteolytically from fibrinogen by thrombin. Fibrinogen is a dimer formed of three polypeptide chains, alpha, beta, and gamma. Presence of FPA indicates that the enzyme thrombin is present and has acted on fibrinogen. FPA is elevated in patients with disseminated intravascular coagulation and is also increased in hypercoagulable states.[1]

Specimen Plasma, urine, cerebrospinal fluid, ascitic fluid

Collection Specimen drawn into special anticoagulant (supplied by manufacturer) which contains EDTA, aprotinin, and a thrombin inhibitor. Special precautions are required during sample collection and handling to avoid exogenous conversion of fibrinogen. Clean venipuncture and gentle handling of the specimen is required. Double syringe technique should be used with the first 2-3 mL of blood being discarded. Draw sample into a prechilled collection tube and place immediately on ice.

Storage Instructions Centrifuge specimen at 4°C within 30 minutes of collection. Perform analysis immediately or freeze plasma specimen at -70°C.

Causes for Rejection Specimen not collected in special anticoagulant, specimen not iced, specimen clotted, specimen improperly labeled

Special Instructions Special anticoagulant, handling, and processing as indicated above.

Reference Range Male: 1.5±1.1 ng/mL, female: 1.9±1.2 ng/mL[2]

Use Results of FPA determinations are applicable to the study of hypercoagulable states, procoagulant conditions, and disseminated intravascular coagulation (DIC) in which FPA levels are increased. Levels are also elevated in a range of conditions in which there is activation of coagulation (eg, numerous malignancies, postoperative states, and disorders of fibrinolysis). FPA levels are decreased during therapeutic heparinization.

Limitations Careful attention must be given to proper specimen collection and handling to avoid artifactual elevation of FPA levels as the result of coagulation activation with exogenous conversion of fibrinogen.

Methodology Radioimmunoassay (RIA),[2] enzyme immunoassay (EIA),[3] established procedures are commercially available from a number of manufacturers

Additional Information Fibrinopeptide A is a small peptide formed of 16 amino acids with a molecular weight of 1535 daltons. It is released from the N-terminus of the alpha chain of fibrinogen. Fibrinogen serves as a substrate for the enzymatic activity of thrombin which cleaves FPA from the amino terminal end of the Aα chain. FPA is a specific marker of the *in vivo* generation of thrombin and, as such, provides a measure of endogenous activation of coagulation. Assays of such peptides and of platelet-specific proteins (see also test listing Beta-Thromboglobulin *on page 232*) been applied to the study of a variety of clinical problems involving the prethrombotic state and its control. A limited sampling of recent reports include applications of FPA levels in the fields of cardiology, hematology/oncology, nephrology, gastroenterology, and neurology. The threat of thromboembolism in patients with heart failure has been studied. Increased platelet and thrombin activation and fibrinolytic activity correlate with the severity of the cardiac failure.[4] FPA levels are elevated in cases of acute coronary thrombosis with transmural infarction within the first 10 hours after onset of symptoms.[5] While FPA levels are considered a sensitive marker for coronary artery thrombosis in acute ischemic coronary artery syndromes, results of single determinations did not provide prognostic information additional to that available on the basis of history, physical examination, or electrocardiogram.[6] FPA levels have been used to monitor fibrin formation in patients with acute myocardial infarction who have been heparinized. Findings suggested that higher than standard doses of heparin may be required to fully inhibit fibrin formation.[7] On the basis of FPA levels, there is evidence that the process of DIC does not contribute to the coagulopathy of chronic liver disease (cirrhosis).[8] In the field of dermatology, the condition livedo vasculitis is considered to represent a thrombogenic vasculopathy (rather than a small vessel vasculitis) on the basis of elevated FPA levels.[9] Hemostatic activation in patients with carcinoma of prostate has been studied using measurements of FPA and D-dimer. In 40% of such patients, FPA levels were elevated. Higher levels were found in those patients with bone scan positive disease. Neither FPA nor D-dimer levels correlated with prostate specific antigen levels. These studies were interpreted as suggesting that changes of subclinical DIC occur in many patients on first presentation with prostate cancer.[10]

Footnotes

1. Bick RL, "Physiology of Hemostasis," *Disorders of Thrombosis and Hemostasis: Clinical and Laboratory Practice*, Chapter 1, Chicago, IL: American Society of Clinical Pathologists, 1992, 12, 15.
2. Walenga JM, Hoppensteadt D, Emanuele RM, et al, "Performance Characteristics of a Simple Radioimmunoassay for Fibrinopeptide A," *Semin Thromb Hemost*, 1984, 10(4):219-27.
3. Amiral J, Walenga JM, and Fareed J, "Development and Performance Characteristics of a Competitive Enzyme Immunoassay for Fibrinopeptide A," *Semin Thromb Hemost*, 1984, 10(4):228-42.
4. Jafri SM, Ozawa T, Mammen E, et al, "Platelet Function, Thrombin and Fibrinolytic Activity in Patients With Heart Failure," *Eur Heart J*, 1993, 14(2):205-12.
5. Eisenberg PR, Sherman LA, Schectman K, et al, "Fibrinopeptide A: A Marker of Acute Coronary Thrombosis," *Circulation*, 1985, 71(5):912-8.
6. Alemán-Gómez JA, López-Candalez A, Freytes CO, et al, "Usefulness of Single Fibrinopeptide a Determination in Patients With Acute Ischemic Coronary Artery Syndromes," *Bol Asoc Med P R*, 1992, 84(4-5):134-8.
7. Mombelli G, Im Hof V, Haerberli A, et al, "Effect of Heparin on Plasma Fibrinopeptide A in Patients With Acute Myocardial Infarction," *Circulation*, 1984, 69(4):684-9.
8. Mombelli G, Fiori G, Monotti R, et al, "Fibrinopeptide A in Liver Cirrhosis: Evidence Against a Major Contribution of Disseminated Intravascular Coagulation to Coagulopathy of Chronic Liver Disease," *J Lab Clin Med*, 1993, 121(1):83-90.
9. McCalmont CS, McCalmont TH, Jorizzo JL, et al, "Livedo Vasculitis: Vasculitis or Thrombotic Vasculopathy," *Clin Exp Dermatol*, 1992, 17(1):4-8.
10. Adamson AS, Francis JL, Witherow RO, et al, "Coagulopathy in the Prostate Cancer Patient: Prevalence and Clinical Relevance," *Ann R Coll Surg Engl*, 1993, 75(2):100-4.

(Continued)

Fibrinopeptide A *(Continued)*

References

Bick RL, "Disseminated Intravascular Coagulation," Chapter 7, and "Hypercoagulability and Thrombosis," Chapter 13, *Disorders of Thrombosis and Hemostasis: Clinical and Laboratory Practice*, Chicago, IL: American Society of Clinical Pathologists, 1992, 137-73, 261-89.

Fibrin Split Products *see* Fibrin Breakdown Products *on page 245*

Fibrin Split Products *see* Fibrin Split Products, Protamine Sulfate *on this page*

Fibrin Split Products, Protamine Sulfate

CPT 85366 (paracoagulation); 85370 (quantitative)

Related Information

Cryoprecipitate *on page 606*
D-Dimer *on page 237*
Fibrin Breakdown Products *on page 245*
Fibrinogen *on page 246*
Intravascular Coagulation Screen *on page 253*

Synonyms Fibrin Split Products; Plasma Protamine Paracoagulation; Protamine Sulfate Test for Fibrin Split Products; 3P Test; Triple P Test

Patient Preparation Perform test prior to instituting heparin therapy for DIC.

Specimen Plasma

Container Blue top (sodium citrate) tube

Collection Routine nontraumatic venipuncture. If multiple tests being drawn, draw coagulation studies last. If only a protamine sulfate test is being drawn, draw 1-2 mL into another Vacutainer® tube, discard, and then collect the blue top tube. This collection procedure avoids contamination of the specimen with tissue thromboplastin.

Causes for Rejection Sample received more than 2 hours after collection, sample clotted, improperly labeled sample

Reference Range Negative

Use Detection of fibrin monomers and early stage fibrin split products in plasma; useful in the diagnosis of disseminated intravascular coagulation, DIC

Limitations Latex particle test for fibrin breakdown products (eg, Thrombo-Wellcotest®) is more specific.

Additional Information Previous activated partial thromboplastin time, latex particle test for fibrin breakdown products, prothrombin time, and platelet count are often useful in interpretation of results. Protamine sulfate dissociates soluble fibrin monomer complexes, allowing fibrin monomers or early degradation products (fragment X) to polymerize, forming clot-like strands (precipitates) - the "paracoagulation" reaction. A positive test result reflects the presence of fibrin monomers, which is indicative of thrombin activity and is consistent with a diagnosis of intravascular coagulation (IVC). A negative result does not mean that IVC is not present. A positive result may also be seen in some cases of severe liver disease and inflammatory disorders due to accumulation of products of coagulation in the circulation. See table Findings Indicative of DIC in the listing Intravascular Coagulation Screen *on page 253*.

References

Baglini RL, "Laboratory Evaluation of Fibrinolysis," *Clinical Hematology: Principles, Procedures, Correlations*, Lotspeich-Steininger CA, Stiene-Martin EA, and Koepke JA, eds, Philadelphia, PA: JB Lippincott Co, 1992, 622-3.

Fibrin Stabilizing Factor *see* Factor XIII *on page 243*

Fibrin Time *see* Thrombin Time *on page 266*

Fitzgerald Factor Assay *see* Factor, Fitzgerald *on page 244*

Fletcher Factor Assay *see* Factor, Fletcher *on page 244*

FpA *see* Fibrinopeptide A *on previous page*

FPA *see* Fibrinopeptide A *on previous page*

F VIII *see* Factor VIII *on page 240*

Glass Bead Platelet Retention Test *see* Platelet Adhesion Test *on page 256*

Ground Glass Clotting Time *see* Activated Coagulation Time *on page 226*

Hageman Factor *see* Factor XII *on page 243*

Hemophilia B *see* Factor IX *on page 241*

Heparinase Test for Heparin *see* Heparin Effect, Test for (Using Heparinase) *on next page*

Heparin Assay Using Activated Factor X

Related Information

Activated Coagulation Time *on page 226*
Activated Partial Thromboplastin Time *on page 227*

Heparin Effect, Test for (Using Heparinase) *on next page*

Synonyms Antifactor Xa

Abstract This test, a two stage assay, determines concentration of heparin in plasma and can be used to monitor heparin anticoagulation. Concentration of heparin is derived from heparin's neutralization of fixed amounts of factor Xa added to plasma.

Specimen Plasma

Container Blue top (sodium citrate) siliconized tube. Collection in a polystyrene tube containing one volume of 0.1 M sodium citrate solution, one volume to nine volumes of blood is preferred.

Collection See under test listing Activated Partial Thromboplastin Time *on page 227*.

Storage Instructions Centrifuge 1600 g for 15 minutes at room temperature, transfer plasma to polystyrene tube, centrifuge again at 1000 g, transfer to clean tube, cap, and keep on ice until assayed or freeze at -70°C if assay cannot be performed within 1-2 hours.

Reference Range Therapeutic range for treatment of venous thromboembolism is 0.3-0.75 units/mL. See table.

Recommendations for Monitoring Heparin Therapy

Intravenous heparin therapy
Prolong the APTT* to ≥1.5 x initial (preheparin) APTT
Treatment with dose-adjusted subcutaneous unfractionated heparin (options)
Prolong the APTT to ≥1.5 x initial (preheparin) APTT
Adjust heparin level (antifactor Xa activity) to 0.3> ≤0.75 units/mL
Treatment with fixed-dose subcutaneous unfractionated heparin (options)
No monitoring generally needed
Adjust heparin level (antifactor Xa activity) to 0.3> ≤0.75 units/mL
Treatment with subcutaneous low-molecular-weight heparin (options)
No monitoring generally needed
Adjust heparin level (antifactor Xa activity) to 0.3> ≤0.75 units/mL
Prophylaxis with subcutaneous unfractionated heparin (options)
No monitoring generally needed
Adjust heparin level (antifactor Xa activity) to 0.05> ≤0.40 units/mL
Prophylaxis with subcutaneous low-molecular-weight heparin (options)
No monitoring generally needed
Adjust heparin level (antifactor Xa activity) to 0.05> ≤0.40 units/mL

*APTT indicates activated partial thromboplastin time

From Bick RL, "Monitoring Heparin Therapy to Manage Thrombotic Disease," *Lab Med*, 1995, 26(4):261-5, with permission.

Use Laboratory control of heparin therapy. Heparin monitoring in patients with antiphospholipid syndrome (lupus anticoagulant or anticardiolipin antibody) in which use of APTT is especially likely to be unreliable. Monitoring of low molecular weight heparin.[1]

Contraindications Test is costly as compared to the APTT and may not be routinely available. Unless the method of Teien is used (in which AT III is added), it is important to obtain pretherapeutic AT III level to establish that patient does not have AT III deficiency.

Methodology Test plasma is mixed with pooled plasma to add antithrombin III (AT III) to compensate for varying AT III level in test plasmas. Activated factor X (Xa) is incubated with test plasma diluted in buffer (stage I). In stage II, remaining Xa activity is determined by amidolysis of the chromogenic substrate B_3-Ile-Glu-Gly-Arg-pNA (method of Teien AN, et al).[2]

Additional Information Use of I.V. heparin (for management of acute-phase thromboembolic disease) is most commonly monitored with the APTT test. Heparin dosage is adjusted to at least maintain some prolongation of the APTT ideally to a level 1.5 times or greater than patient's initial value or the laboratory's control range. APTT is utilized in large part because of its ready availability which in turn derives from its low cost and ease of performance. Bick, however, has emphasized that prolongation of the APTT has not been shown to correlate with bleeding complications of heparin therapy or with rethrombosis (see references below). The effect of heparin on prolongation of the APTT may be quite variable dependent upon the type of heparin and the type of APTT reagent. In addition, with increase in level of factor VIII and/or fibrinogen (and competition with AT III by heparin binding proteins) as occurs with the acute phase reaction associated with acute thrombosis, responsiveness of the APTT test system is decreased.

Ideally, the appropriate therapeutic range should be determined by each laboratory using its reagent/instrument combination and heparin preparation(s) being utilized rather than depending upon a generic range of 1.5-2.5 times normal as the therapeutic range. Perhaps most reliable is the determination of both heparin concentration and APTT on plasma from patients receiving heparin. Assay (using Xa) may be used to assess effect of subcutaneously administered unfractionated heparin or fractionated (LMW) heparin in which APTT may be insensitive (APTT may not be significantly prolonged). Heparin assay also has value in patients with acute thromboembolism whose APTT is persistently subtherapeutic (because of variable levels of coagulation factors) even in the face of large daily doses of heparin. (See reference by Levine et al.)

Footnotes
1. Colvin BT and Barrowcliffe TW, "The British Society of Haematology Guidelines on the Use and Monitoring of Heparin 1992: Second Revision. BCSH Haemostasis and Thrombosis Task Force," *J Clin Pathol*, 1993, 46(2):97-103.
2. Teien AN, Lie M, and Abildgaard U, "Assay of Heparin in Plasma Using a Chromogenic Substrate for Activated Factor X," *Thromb Res*, 1976, 8(3):413-6.

References
Bick RL, "Antithrombotic Therapy," *Disorders of Thrombosis and Hemostasis: Clinical and Laboratory Practice*, Chapter 14, Chicago, IL: ASCP Press, American Society of Clinical Pathologists, 1992, 304-5.
Bick RL, "Monitoring Heparin Therapy to Manage Thrombotic Disease," *Lab Med*, 1995, 26(4):261-5.
Friberger P, Urig E, Eriksson-Skoog L, et al, "Coacute Heparin: A New Simple Monotest for Monitoring Heparin Treatment," *Semin Thromb Hemost*, 1994, 20(4):328-32.
Levine MN, Hirsh J, Gent M, et al, "A Randomized Trial Comparing Activated Thromboplastin Time With Heparin Assay in Patients With Acute Venous Thromboembolism Requiring Large Daily Doses of Heparin," *Arch Intern Med*, 1994, 154(1):49-56.

Heparin Cofactor Activity see Antithrombin III Test on page 230

Heparin Effect, Test for (Using Heparinase)

Related Information
Activated Coagulation Time *on page 226*
Activated Partial Thromboplastin Time *on page 227*
Heparin Assay Using Activated Factor X *on previous page*

Synonyms Heparinase Test for Heparin

Abstract Test utilizes heparinase for evaluation of prolonged APTT test result possibly due to unsuspected heparin in patient plasma sample.

Specimen Plasma

Container Blue top (3.8% sodium citrate anticoagulant) tube

Collection Routine venipuncture. If multiple tests are being drawn, draw coagulation studies last. If only coagulation tests are being drawn, use two-syringe/tube technique, draw 1-2 mL into first syringe or Vacutainer®, discard, and then collect coagulation tests. This collection procedure avoids contamination of the specimen with tissue thromboplastins.

Storage Instructions Test should be performed within 2-3 hours of sample collection.

Causes for Rejection Tube not full, specimen hemolyzed, specimen clotted

Turnaround Time 1 hour

Special Instructions Centrifuge samples at 4000 RPM for 10 minutes to obtain platelet poor plasma. Keep refrigerated.

Reference Range A "positive" test results when addition of heparinase to plasma causes normalization of previously prolonged test result.

Use Identify heparin contamination of plasma samples. Determine actual heparin free prothrombin time (PT), activated partial thromboplastin time (APTT), and/or activated coagulation time (ACT) in heparin-containing plasma. Study patients with clinical disseminated intravascular coagulation who are receiving heparin therapy. Study patients with venous thromboembolic disease or myocardial infarction who are being changed from heparin to coumadin-type therapy.

Methodology Test in question is performed on initial sample (eg, preoperative) and is repeated after addition of heparinase (1 mL of platelet poor plasma added to test vial, mixture inverted, and left at room temperature for 15 minutes).

Additional Information A number of clinical situations arise in which plasma submitted for coagulation testing has been unknowingly and inadvertently contaminated by heparin. Resultant abnormal ACT, APTT, and/or PT test values may lead to inappropriate diagnosis and/or therapeutic error when screening for coagulation deficiency, with preoperative coagulation screening, evaluation of disseminated intravascular coagulation (DIC), and evaluation of nonheparin-related changes in coagulation during cardiopulmonary bypass surgery. Inappropriate transfusion with fresh frozen plasma may result from heparin contamination with prolongation of the APTT. Newman and Fagin found that 39% of APTT results over 45 seconds (patients taking neither heparin nor Coumadin®) underwent complete correction when samples were treated with heparinase.

Heparinase cleaves heparin (a sulfated polymer of uronic acid and glucosamine) to produce oligosaccharides that have no anticoagulant activity. Prolonged APTT corrected only in part by treatment of the sample with heparinase bears implication of a coagulation abnormality in addition to heparin effect (eg, factor deficiency or inhibitory activity including that seen with DIC).

A test cartridge containing heparinase has been developed for use with the ACT assay.[1] Heparin is removed at the initiation of ACT testing with production of heparin-independent test results. The heparinase/ACT assay was useful in monitoring baseline drift and protamine reversal.

An additional indication of the presence of heparin in a plasma sample is presence of anodal slurring of alpha and beta lipoprotein bands on high resolution serum protein electrophoresis using lipoprotein staining. This effect relates to heparin activation of lipoprotein lipase.[2]

Footnotes
1. Baugh RF, Deemar KA, and Zimmermann JJ, "Heparinase in the Activated Clotting Time Assay: Monitoring Heparin-Independent Alterations in Coagulation Function," *Anesth Analg*, 1992, 74(2):201-5.
2. Pearson JP and Keren DF, "The Effects of Heparin on Lipoproteins in High-Resolution Electrophoresis of Serum," *Am J Clin Pathol*, 1995, 104:(4)468-71.

References
Hutt ED and Kingdon HS, "Use of Heparinase to Eliminate Heparin Inhibition in Routine Coagulation Assays," *J Lab Clin Med*, 1972, 79(6):1027-34.
Newman RS and Fagin AR, "Heparin Contamination in Coagulation Testing and a Protocol to Avoid It and the Risk of Inappropriate FFP Transfusion," *Am J Clin Pathol*, 1995, 104(4):447-9.

Heparin Inhibitors see Activated Partial Thromboplastin Time on page 227

High Molecular Weight Kininogen see Factor, Fitzgerald on page 244

Hirudin Determination

CPT 85999

Related Information
Thrombin Time *on page 266*

Abstract Hirudin, an anticoagulant from medicinal leeches, was used in the late 1800s and is currently being produced by recombinant DNA techniques. Members of the hirudin family are potent inhibitors of thrombin. Clinical effects of this anticoagulant are preferentially monitored by results of the thrombin time in routine use.

Specimen Method dependent; citrate anticoagulated plasma (thrombin time assay); for chromogenic assay using plasma, heat-defibrinogenated, acid treated plasma must be used; ELISA method can measure hirudin in buffer or urine

Use Largely of use in nonclinical (in-laboratory) applications. Such uses include quantitation of thrombin or prothrombin, screening for abnormal plasma prothrombin activation, verification of the therapeutic range of oral anticoagulation, studies on fibrinopeptide release, studies on structure of fibrin and fibrinogen fragment/fibrin monomer interaction, research studies on thrombin binding to membrane receptors and applications in which removal of unwanted thrombin is of benefit.

Limitations The limits of sensitivity (ELISA) method are 8-7700 ng/mL.

Methodology Clotting methods (eg, thrombin titration[1]) based on the selective reaction between 1 mol of hirudin and 1 mol of thrombin (prolongation of thrombin time correlates linearly with the plasma concentration of hirudin); enzyme-linked immunosorbent assay (ELISA);[2] chromogenic substrate based procedures are the recommended method.[3] In the latter, patient's sample (containing hirudin) is mixed with standardized thrombin solution, chromogenic peptide substrate is added, and the residual thrombin activity determined by spectrophotometry. The residual thrombin activity is related to the amount of hirudin.[4]

Additional Information Hirudin consists of a family of closely related small proteins, proteinase inhibitors with potent antithrombin effects. John Haycraft, in 1884, found that medicinal leeches (*Hirudo medicinalis*) contained a substance with anticoagulant properties. Markwardt et al isolated hirudin from leeches in the late 1950s.[5] It was characterized as a highly specific, very high affinity thrombin inhibitor, a polypeptide with 65 amino acids with a molecular weight of about 7000. The primary structures of members of the hirudin family are similar (eg, hirudins HV1 and PA, for which molecular sequences have been established and isoforms). In hirudins HV1 and PA, part of the active site of the inhibitor, a Lys residue flanked by two Pro residues, is thought to occupy the specificity pocket of thrombin.[6]

Methods for determining hirudin concentration are, in general, for in-laboratory/research applications. The most practical test for monitoring the clinical effects of hirudin anticoagulation is the thrombin time although in some clinical situations (eg, monitoring therapy of severe venous thromboembolism) it may be excessively sensitive.[7] The multiple nonclinical applications of hirudin have been reviewed by Stocker.[8] He considers three applications to be of special interest. These include use of hirudin as an inhibitor of meizothrombin, for discrimination between thrombin and other plasma proteinases, and use of hirudin as an anticoagulant to allow testing of blood and blood cell characteristics. The potential clinical applications of recombinant hirudin (r-hirudin) have been discussed.[9] These include postoperative prophylaxis against deep vein thrombosis and pulmonary embolus, prevention of reocclusion after

(Continued)

Hirudin Determination *(Continued)*

percutaneous transluminal coronary angioplasty, anticoagulation during cardiovascular bypass surgery, and treatment of disseminated intravascular coagulation. Recombinant hirudin has been administered (on compassionate grounds and with benefit) to a patient with heparin-associated thrombocytopenia and deep vein thrombosis.[10] A specific antagonist for neutralization of hirudin is not available. This is seen as a significant current impediment to the clinical development and application of hirudin.[9]

Footnotes

1. Markwardt F, Nowak G, Stürzebecher J, et al, "Pharmacokinetics and Anticoagulant Effect of Hirudin in Man," *Thromb Haemost*, 1984, 52(2):160-3.
2. Spinner S, Stöffler G, and Fink E, "Quantitative Enzyme-Linked Immunosorbent Assay (ELISA) for Hirudin," *J Immunol Methods*, 1986, 87(1):79-83.
3. Stürzebecher J, "Methods for Determination of Hirudin," *Semin Thromb Hemost*, 1991, 17(2):99-112.
4. Griessbach U, Stürzebecher J, and Markwardt F, "Assay of Hirudin in Plasma Using a Chromogenic Thrombin Substrate," *Thromb Res*, 1985, 37(2):347-50.
5. Markwardt F, "The Comeback of Hirudin as an Antithrombotic Agent," *Semin Thromb Hemost*, 1991, 17(2):79-82.
6. Stürzebecher J and Walsmann P, "Structure-Activity Relationships of Recombinant Hirudins," *Semin Thromb Hemost*, 1991, 17(2):94-8
7. Bridey F, Dreyfus M, Parent F, et al, "Recombinant Hirudin (HBW 023): Biological Data of Ten Patients With Severe Venous Thrombo-Embolism," *Am J Hematol*, 1995, 49(1):67-72.
8. Stocker K, "Laboratory Use of Hirudin," *Semin Thromb Hemost*, 1991, 17(2):113-21.
9. Walenga JM, Markwardt F, Breddin K, et al, "Report on a Discussion Forum: Medical and Surgical Application of Recombinant Hirudin," *Semin Thromb Hemost*, 1991, 17(2):150-6.
10. Nand S, "Hirudin Therapy for Heparin-Associated Thrombocytopenia and Deep Venous Thrombosis," *Am J Hematol*, 1993, 43(4):310-1.

References

Dodt J, Müller H-P, Seemüller U, et al, "The Complete Amino Acid Sequence of Hirudin, a Thrombin Specific Inhibitor," *FEBS Lett*, 1983, 165(2):180-3.

HMW Kininogen *see* Factor, Fitzgerald *on page 244*

Hypercoagulable State Coagulation Screen

CPT 85230 (factor VII); 85280 (factor XII); 85300 (antithrombin III); 85303 (protein C); 85305 (protein S); 85575 (platelet aggregation)

Related Information

Anticardiolipin Antibody *on page 364*
Antithrombin III Test *on page 230*
Beta-Thromboglobulin *on page 232*
Factor V *on page 239*
Factor VII *on page 240*
Factor XII *on page 243*
Fibrinopeptide A *on page 247*
Inhibitor, Lupus, Phospholipid Type *on next page*
Plasminogen Activator Inhibitor *on page 255*
Platelet Aggregation, Hypercoagulable State *on page 258*
Protein C *on page 260*
Protein S *on page 261*
Prothrombin Fragment 1.2 *on page 261*
Resistance to Activated Protein C *on page 265*
Thrombomodulin *on page 266*

Synonyms Screen for Hypercoagulation; Thrombotic Disease Screen

Test Commonly Includes Availability and composition of screen may vary between laboratories. Commonly included are antithrombin III, protein C, protein S, resistance to activated protein C, factor VII, factor XII, platelet aggregation (spontaneous, second wave of aggregation with weak ADP, and response to dilutions of epinephrine). See the following listings: Platelet Aggregation, Hypercoagulable State *on page 258*; Plasminogen Activator Inhibitor *on page 255*; Plasminogen Assay *on page 256*; Euglobulin Clot Lysis *on page 238*; Diluted Whole Blood Clot Lysis *on page 237*; Fibrinogen *on page 246*; Platelet Count *on page 340*; Thrombin Time *on page 266*; and also tests for fibrin monomer and/or fibrin degradation products. Also applicable but less commonly available are plasma beta-thromboglobulin, fibrinopeptide A and B, tissue plasminogen activator, tissue plasminogen activator inhibitor, test for D-dimer fragment of fibrin, heparin cofactor II, and studies for dysfibrinogenemia/dysplasminogenemia.

Specimen Requires multiple specimens, approximately 30-50 mL of blood, dependent on the needs of constituent tests and whether some or all tests are performed "in-house" or by a reference laboratory

Collection As for individual constituent tests. Sample for dilute clot lysis must be placed immediately into diluent after collection.

Causes for Rejection Presence of anticoagulants (eg, heparin) may significantly alter the results of many tests in the screen, in particular, thrombin time, antithrombin III, and platelet aggregation studies

Turnaround Time Dependent upon composition of screen and need to utilize reference laboratories. As some hypercoagulable clinical situations are of emergent nature an abbreviated screen ideally should have same day or even 2-4 hour turnaround time.

Special Instructions Initiate a dialogue with the Coagulation Laboratory concerning availability of, composition of, and special requirements for hypercoagulable screen.

Reference Range See individual constituent tests. See table. Note that some tests employed in the study of the hypercoagulable state (eg, AT III, protein C, and protein S) may measure "functional" or "antigenic" (immunologic based) levels. Results may be incomplete or even misleading if both functional and antigenic based tests are not employed.

Findings Indicative of Hypercoagulable State

Test Parameter	Finding
Antithrombin III	
antigenic	↓ or N
functional	↓
APTT	↓ or N
Beta-thromboglobulin	↑
Clot lysis tests	↓
Fibrinogen	↓
Fibrinopeptide A	↑
Inhibitor, lupus, phospholipid type	present
Plasminogen	↓
Platelet aggregation	
spontaneous	↑
weak dilutions of epinephrine	↑
Platelet count	±
Protein C/S	
antigenic	↓ or N
functional	↓↓
Prothrombin fragment 1.2	↑
Resistance to protein C	present
Thrombin time	↓ or N

Use Screen for imbalance between procoagulants (factors that effect the conversion of prothrombin to thrombin) and anticoagulants (regulators of the formation of thrombin). Identify presence of hypercoagulable state. Dependent on the structure of the screen may be able to determine if the predisposition to clotting is due to a primary or secondary disorder. If primary, the screen may indicate or disclose the underlying etiology.

Limitations Test results must be considered in relation to the clinical situation. Test results may be misleading if obtained in close temporal proximity to an acute thrombotic disorder. Some apparent abnormalities may reflect physiologic as opposed to pathophysiologic thrombosis.

Methodology As per the individual test, many of the more specific tests may not be routinely available in most healthcare facilities.

Additional Information Venous thromboembolic episodes result in approximately 600,000 hospitalizations annually.[1] Screening tests for hypercoagulable states have as their goal the detection of abnormalities of the coagulation mechanism that predispose to thrombosis and thromboembolic disease.

Primary hypercoagulable states usually have their basis in an inherited quantitative or qualitative deficiency in one of the components of the coagulation system. Increased clotting occurs when there are significant deficiencies in the regulators AT III, heparin cofactor II, protein S or protein C, conditions usually inherited as autosomal dominant. The recently discovered condition "resistance to activated protein C" due in some or all cases to a factor V mutation (factor V Leiden) appears to be the most common cause of inherited thrombotic disease being responsible for some 20% to 60% of cases of unexplained thrombosis (see also listings Factor V *on page 239*, Protein C *on page 260*, and Resistance to Activated Protein C *on page 265*.)[2,3] See accompanying table for estimates of incidence. Note also that resistance to activated protein C (presence of factor V Leiden) may cause a false-positive test result for protein S deficiency when a functional protein S assay is used.[4] Increased risk of thromboembolism may also occur with decrease in fibrinolysis, seen in patients with dysplasminogenemia, decreased plasminogen activator, or increased tissue plasminogen activator inhibitor plasma levels.

Acquired (secondary) hypercoagulable states are associated with clinical conditions that manifest wholly or in part by increased thromboembolism. Changes in platelet number and/or function, vessel wall and/or blood flow parameters may also predispose to thromboembolic episodes.

The primary thrombotic disorders include antithrombin III deficiency (present in 1 of 2000 individuals), protein C or S deficiency,[5,6] dysfibrinogenemia,[7] and dysplasminogenemia. A wide variety of disease processes are associated with secondary thrombotic states. See table. Any condition in which there is disruption of the endothelium of vessel wall or in which significant venous stasis occurs will increase the risk of

Estimated Prevalence of Inherited Thrombotic Disorders (as causes of unexplained thrombosis)

Disorder	Prevalence (%)
Antithrombin III deficiency	1-4
Protein C deficiency	5-6
Protein S deficiency	5-6
APC resistance	20-60

From Rodgers GM, "Activated Protein C Resistance and Inherited Thrombosis," *Am J Clin Pathol*, 1995, 103(3):261, with permission.

thrombosis. Hereditary deficiency of heparin cofactor II (HC II) (see also Antithrombin III Test *on page 230*) is apparently very rare. The level of HC II in acquired disorders parallels activity of AT III and may not contribute to clinical evaluation of the hypercoagulable state. Measurement of HC II (in conjunction with AT III) may assist in differentiating acquired from hereditary changes in these inhibitors.[8]

Clinical Associations of Secondary Thrombotic States

Advanced age	Kawasaki disease
Collagen/vascular disorders	Neoplastic disease
Diabetes mellitus	Nephrotic syndrome
Hormone therapy	Myeloproliferative disease
estrogen	PNH
pregnancy	Severe serum protein abnormalities
birth control regimens	Postoperative status
Hyperlipidemia	Previous episode of thromboembolism
Hyperviscosity	Sepsis
Immobilization	Thrombotic thrombocytopenic purpura
Inflammatory bowel disease	

Women with cerebrovascular accidents during oral contraceptive use were found to have persistent platelet coagulant hyperactivity (decreased plasma AT III, increased plasma β-thromboglobulin, normal platelet aggregation) even though use of contraceptives had been discontinued from 4 weeks to 14 years before the study.[9]

In patients younger than 51 years of age with lower limb ischemia, a high incidence of hypercoagulable states was found.[10] Presence of platelet aggregation showing increased activity, protein S or C deficiency, plasminogen deficiency, or lupus-like anticoagulant were common, only 24% of patients were normal. Arterial or graft thrombosis was common (20% incidence) in the early postoperative period.[11]

End-stage renal disease, while usually characterized by propensity to bleed, may also be predisposed to thromboembolic complications. Measures of fibrinolytic activity (euglobulin lysis activity, t-PA, urokinase), initially decreased, normalized after renal transplantation.[12] Thromboembolism (including renal vein thrombosis) is a serious complication of nephrotic syndrome, in particular with membranous nephropathy. Renal vein thrombosis complicating nephrotic syndrome has an overall incidence of some 35%. Thrombotic complications other than renal vein thrombosis occur in some 20% of nephrotic patients (pulmonary emboli account for 8%).[13] A variety of mechanisms, many involving impaired fibrinolysis, may be involved.[14,15,16,17,18]

Homocystinuria has been associated with thromboembolism and decreased AT III and protein C levels.[19]

Patients who have thrombotic disease on the basis of an inherited abnormality of the coagulation mechanism should be considered for lifetime anticoagulation.[20] The apparent frequency (9.5%) of hypercoagulable states in some vascular surgery populations has been considered to support the practice of routine preoperative screening in such populations.[21]

Footnotes
1. Schafer, AI, "The Hypercoagulable States," *Ann Intern Med*, 1985, 102(6):814-28.
2. Dahlbäck B, "Molecular Genetics of Thrombophilia: Factor V Gene Mutation Causing Resistance to Activated Protein C as a Basis of the Hypercoagulable State," *J Lab Clin Med*, 1995, 125(5):566-71.
3. Griffin JH, Evatt B, Wideman C, et al, "Anticoagulant Protein C Pathway Defective in Majority of Thrombophilic Patients," *Blood*, 1993, 82(7):1989-93.
4. Faioni EM, Franchi F, Asti D, et al, "Resistance to Activated Protein C in Nine Thrombophilic Families: Interference in a Protein S Functional Assay," *Thromb Haemost*, 1993, 70(6):1067-71.
5. Hill RJ and Ens GE, "The Protein C Pathway," *Clin Hemost Rev*, 1987, 1:1-6.
6. Comp PC and Esmon CT, "Recurrent Venous Thromboembolism in Patients With a Partial Deficiency of Protein S," *N Engl J Med*, 1984, 311(24):1525-8.
7. Carrell N, Gabriel DA, Blatt PM, et al, "Hereditary Dysfibrinogenemia in a Patient With Thrombotic Disease," *Blood*, 1983, 62:439-47.
8. Brandt JT and Ezenagu L, "Heparin Cofactor II, Thrombosis and Hemostasis," *ASCP Check Sample®*, Chicago, IL: American Society of Clinical Pathologists, 1987.

9. Elam MB, Viar MJ, Ratts TE, et al, "Mitral Valve Prolapse in Women With Oral Contraceptive-Related Cerebrovascular Insufficiency Associated Persistent Hypercoagulable State," *Arch Intern Med*, 1986, 146(1):73-7.
10. Eldrup-Jorgensen J, Flanigan DP, Brace L, et al, "Hypercoagulable States and Lower Limb Ischemia in Young Adults," *J Vasc Surg*, 1989, 9(2):334-41.
11. Gomez MJ, Carroll RC, Hansard MR, et al, "Regulation or Fibrinolysis in Aortic Surgery," *J Vasc Surg*, 1988, 8(4):384-8.
12. Hong SY and Yang DH, "Fibrinolytic Activity in End-Stage Renal Disease," *Nephron*, 1993, 63(2):188-92.
13. Llach F, "Hypercoagulability, Renal Vein Thrombosis, and Other Thrombotic Complications of Nephrotic Syndrome," *Kidney Int*, 1985, 28(3):429-39.
14. Kanfer A, "Coagulation Factors in Nephrotic Syndrome," *Am J Nephrol*, 1990, 10(S1):63-8.
15. Ono T, Kanatsu K, Doi T, et al, "Relationship of Intraglomerular Coagulation and Platelet Aggregation to Glomerular Sclerosis," *Nephron*, 1991, 58(4):429-36.
16. Nakamura Y, Tomura S, Tachibana K, et al, "Enhanced Fibrinolytic Activity During the Course of Hemodialysis," *Clin Nephrol*, 1992, 38(2):90-6.
17. Du XH, Glas-Greenwalt P, Kant KS, et al, "Nephrotic Syndrome With Renal Vein Thrombosis: Pathogenetic Importance of a Plasmin Inhibitor (α₂-Antiplasmin)," *Clin Nephrol*, 1985, 24(4):186-91.
18. Vaziri ND, Gonzales EC, Shayestehfar B, et al, "Plasma Levels and Urinary Excretion of Fibrinolytic and Protease Inhibitory Proteins in Nephrotic Syndrome," *J Lab Clin Med*, 1994, 124(1):118-24.
19. Palareti G, Salardi S, Legnani C, et al, "Reduced Levels of Antithrombin III, Protein C and Factor VII in Homocystinuria. Long-Term Changes in Relation to Treatment," *Thromb Haemost*, 1985, 54:35.
20. Bowen KJ and Vukelja SJ, "Hypercoagulable States. Their Causes and Management," *Postgrad Med*, 1992, 91(3):117-8, 123-5, 128.
21. Donaldson MC, Weinberg DS, Belkin M, et al, "Screening for Hypercoagulable States in Vascular Surgical Practice: A Preliminary Study," *J Vasc Surg*, 1990, 11(6):825-31.

References
Bick RL and Tse N, "Hemostasis Abnormalities Associated With Prosthetic Devices and Organ Transplantation," *Lab Med*, 1992, 23(7):462-8.

Bick RL and Ucar K, "Hypercoagulability and Thrombosis," *Hematol Oncol Clin North Am*, 1992, 6(6):1421-31.

Bolan CD and Alving BM, "Recurrent Venous Thrombosis and Hypercoagulable States," *Am Fam Physician*, 1991, 44(5):1741-51.

Büller HR and ten Cate JW, "Acquired Antithrombin III Deficiency: Laboratory Diagnosis, Incidence, Clinical Implications, and Treatment With Antithrombin III Concentrate," *Am J Med*, 1989, 87(3B):44S-48S.

De Stefano V, Finazzi G, and Mannucci PM, "Inherited Thrombophilia: Pathogenesis, Clinical Syndromes, and Management," *Blood*, 1996, 87(9):3531-44.

Freed JA, "Hypercoagulability - Should Every Patient With Venous Thrombosis Be Tested?" *Postgrad Med*, 1991, 90(6):157-60, 165-6, 168.

Janssen HF, Schachner J, Hubbard J, et al, "The Risk of Deep Venous Thrombosis: A Computerized Epidemiologic Approach," *Surgery*, 1987, 101(2):205-12.

Lottenberg R, Dolly FR, and Kitchens CS, "Recurring Thromboembolic Disease and Pulmonary Hypertension Associated With Severe Hypoplasminogenemia," *Am J Hematol*, 1985, 19(2):181-93.

Moake JL, "Hypercoagulable States: New Knowledge About Old Problems," *Hosp Pract (Off Ed)*, 1991, 26(3A):31-42.

Nachman RL and Silverstein R, "Hypercoagulable States," *Ann Intern Med*, 1993, 119(8):819-27.

Whitlock JA, Janco RL, and Phillips JA III, "Inherited Hypercoagulable States in Children," *Am J Pediatr Hematol Oncol*, 1989, 11(2):170-3.

Hypercoagulable State, Platelet Aggregation *see* Platelet Aggregation, Hypercoagulable State *on page 258*

Immunologic Antithrombin III *see* Antithrombin III Test *on page 230*

Inhibitor, Lupus, Phospholipid Type
CPT 85705

Related Information
Activated Partial Thromboplastin Time *on page 227*
Anticardiolipin Antibody *on page 364*
Anticoagulant, Circulating *on page 229*
Antinuclear Antibody *on page 368*
Fibrinopeptide A *on page 247*
HIV-1/HIV-2 Serology *on page 403*
Hypercoagulable State Coagulation Screen *on previous page*
Plasminogen Activator Inhibitor *on page 255*
Protein S *on page 261*

Synonyms Antiphospholipid Antibody (APA); Lupus Anticoagulant (LA); Phospholipid Type Anticoagulant

Applies to Antiphospholipid Antibody

Patient Preparation Discontinue heparin therapy for 2 days and coumarin therapy for 2 weeks prior to collection of the specimen.

Specimen Plasma

Container Blue top (sodium citrate) tube

Collection Obtain blood, using plastic syringe, from clean venipuncture without contamination by tissue thromboplastins. If blood is being drawn only for this test, use two-syringe technique. First draw 1-2 mL in one syringe (or tube if using Vacutainer® equipment), discard, and (without moving needle) draw specimen into second syringe (or tube).

Storage Instructions Centrifuge at 4°C for 20 minutes at 1500 g. Transfer plasma specimen using plastic pipettes.

Reference Range Prolongation of APTT may result from presence of lupus anticoagulant[1]

Use Evaluate prolonged APTT, thrombotic states, fetal death
(Continued)

Inhibitor, Lupus, Phospholipid Type *(Continued)*

Methodology Dilute tissue thromboplastin time, platelet neutralization procedure,[2] APTT, enzyme immunoassay (EIA), enzyme-linked immunosorbent assay (ELISA) for anticardiolipin antibody. The more specific assays may not be routinely available. The dilute tissue thromboplastin inhibition test lacks specificity for lupus anticoagulant. Modifications have been described that assist in distinguishing lupus anticoagulant from other causes of a prolonged APTT.[3] Results of survey programs of the College of American Pathologists (1986 and 1987) have found significant variation in the sensitivity of APTT reagents to the presence of lupus-type anticoagulants. Use of the less responsive reagents could impair detection of such anticoagulants and in other cases the differentiation of a lupus anticoagulant from a specific factor inhibitor.[4]

Additional Information Lupus anticoagulants (and also anticardiolipin antibodies) are immunoglobulins that cross react with phospholipids and interfere with phospholipid-dependent coagulation tests.[5] They are associated, therefore, with prolongation of the APTT, snake venom assays, plasma recalcification times and to a lesser extent, the prothrombin time. Presence of anticardiolipin antibody (by ELISA) may occur independent of demonstrable lupus anticoagulant activity. When the two occur together, adverse clinical events, thrombosis, or thrombocytopenia are of more common occurrence than if only anticardiolipin antibody is present.[6] The "lupus anticoagulant" while present in up to 10% of patients with systemic lupus erythematosus (SLE) is usually present in patients who do not have SLE. Patients with lupus anticoagulant are usually detected as the result of a prolonged APTT. While they usually do not manifest with abnormal bleeding, about 30% may have development of thromboses. Increased plasma levels of tissue plasminogen activator inhibitor, fibrinopeptide A, fibrinopeptide B beta 15-42 and thromboxane B_2 may have predictive value for occurrence of thrombotic events in cases of SLE who have lupus anticoagulant.[7,8] The lupus inhibitor may be present in otherwise normal individuals. It may occur as a complication of drug therapy, in particular, it is seen in association with the use of chlorpromazine. In some cases of valvular disease, the thrombotic tendency associated with lupus anticoagulant/phospholipid antibodies may be responsible for rheumatic-type deformities and severe **valvular heart disease**[9] (distortion of valve by layers of thrombus as in some patients with SLE, patients without a history of rheumatic fever).

There is evidence that lipoprotein-associated coagulation inhibitor contains three tandemly repeated serine protease inhibitory domains. When the inhibitory complex is generated, one domain binds to active site of Xa, two domains are required for the inhibition of VIIa/tissue factor (TF), and a third domain has no effect on the function of Xa or TF.[10] Some antiphospholipid antibodies decrease endothelial cell prostacyclin production apparently due to inhibition of phospholipase A_2 and thus predisposing to vascular thrombi.[11] See also additional discussion of the mechanism of phospholipid type inhibitors under test entry Anticoagulant, Circulating *on page 229.*

At least some examples of anticardiolipin antibody appear to be directed against a cardiolipin cofactor, notably with activity against B_2-glycoprotein 1 (GP1). Factor Va degradation by activated protein C/protein S may be inhibited by anti-GP1, thus, predisposing patients with such antiphospholipid antibody to thrombosis.[12]

Pregnant women with high antiphospholipid antibody titers have an increased incidence of **midterm fetal death**. Steroid therapy does not improve (and may worsen) fetal outcome in asymptomatic pregnant women with antiphospholipid antibody and previous episode of fetal death.[13]

A limited literature deals with lupus anticoagulants occurring in children. Nonhemophiliac examples of this condition have occurred in children 3-14 years of age, largely not associated with lupus erythematosus. Some have been associated with the use of antibiotics or antecedent viral infections. Presence of the inhibitor may be transient and not associated with bleeding or thrombotic episodes.[14] However, a recent study of 78 consecutive children with thromboses from a university pediatric service over the 7-year period 1987-1993, found 19 cases with LA, 5/19 with SLE. Of these, 2/5 children had thrombosis as the presenting sign of SLE. APA syndrome was diagnosed in 14/78 of the children with thromboses, most of whom had speckled antinuclear antibody pattern.[15]

There is a high incidence (20% to 50%) of lupus anticoagulant in patients with **AIDS**. Rarely, associated inhibition of a specific coagulation factor has also been found.[16,17,18]

It has been recommended that patients undergoing evaluation for hypercoagulability be tested for the antiphospholipid syndrome even in the absence of a prolonged PTT.[19] This recommendation (made in 1989) follows upon the results of a study of young patients with unusual thrombotic events (eg, cerebral thrombosis and coumarin associated skin necrosis), presence of "lupus anticoagulant," and binding of protein S by C4b-binding protein. Presumably, the decrease in free protein S is related to the hypercoagulable state in these patients, however, possibility of resistance to activated protein C due to factor V Leiden with interference in the protein S assay could not have been considered (in 1989).[20] See also listing Resistance to Activated Protein C *on page 265.*

Potentially fatal complications of the antiphospholipid antibody syndrome include hemorrhagic necrosis of the adrenal gland due to thrombosis of the adrenal vein.[21]

Footnotes

1. Shapiro SS and Thiagarajan P, "Lupus Anticoagulants," *Prog Hemost Thromb*, 1982, 6:263-85.
2. Triplett DA, Brandt JT, Kaczor D, et al, "Laboratory Diagnosis of Lupus Inhibitor. A Comparison of the Tissue Thromboplastin Inhibition Procedure With a New Platelet Neutralization Procedure," *Am J Clin Pathol*, 1983, 79:678-82.
3. Liu HW, Wong KL, Lin CK, et al, "The Reappraisal of Dilute Tissue Thromboplastin Inhibition Test in the Diagnosis of Lupus Anticoagulant," *Br J Haematol*, 1989, 72(2):229-34.
4. Brandt JT, Triplett DA, Rock WA, et al, "Effect of Lupus Anticoagulants on the Activated Partial Thromboplastin Time. Results of the College of American Pathologists Survey Program," *Arch Pathol Lab Med*, 1991, 115(2):109-14.
5. Kushner M and Simonian N, "Lupus Anticoagulants, Anticardiolipin Antibodies, and Cerebral Ischemia," *Stroke*, 1989, 20(2):225-9.
6. McHugh NJ, Moye DA, James IE, et al, "Lupus Anticoagulant: Clinical Significance in Anticardiolipin Positive Patients With Systemic Lupus Erythematosus," *Ann Rheum Dis*, 1991, 50(8):548-52.
7. Violi F, Ferro D, Valesini G, et al, "Tissue Plasminogen Activator Inhibitor in Patients With Systemic Lupus Erythematosus and Thrombosis," *Br Med J*, 1990, 300(6732):1099-102.
8. Mayumi T, Nagasawa K, Inoguchi T, et al, "Haemostatic Factors Associated With Vascular Thrombosis in Patients With Systemic Lupus Erythematosus and the Lupus Anticoagulant," *Ann Rheum Dis*, 1991, 50(8):543-7.
9. Ford SE, Lillicrap D, Brunet D, et al, "Thrombotic Endocarditis and Lupus Anticoagulant. A Pathogenetic Possibility for Idiopathic Type Valvular Heart Disease," *Arch Pathol Lab Med*, 1989, 113(4):350-3.
10. Girard TJ, Warren LA, Novotny WF, et al, "Functional Significance of the Kunitz-Type Inhibitory Domains of Lipoprotein-Associated Coagulation Inhibitor," *Nature*, 1989, 338(6215):518-20.
11. Schorer AE, Duane PG, Woods VL, et al, "Some Antiphospholipid Antibodies Inhibit Phospholipase A_2 Activity," *J Lab Clin Med*, 1992, 120(20):67-77.
12. Matsuda J, Gohchi K, Kawasugi K, et al, "Inhibitory Activity of Anti-B_2-Glycoprotein I Antibody on Factor Va Degradation by Activated Protein C and Its Cofactor Protein S," *Am J Hematol*, 1995, 49(1):89-91.
13. Lockshin MD, Druzin ML, and Qamar T, "Prednisone Does Not Prevent Recurrent Fetal Death in Women With Antiphospholipid Antibody," *Am J Obstet Gynecol*, 1989, 160(2):439-43.
14. Singh AK, Rao KP, Kizer J, et al, "Lupus Anticoagulants in Children," *Ann Clin Lab Sci*, 1988, 18(5):384-7.
15. Manco-Johnson MJ and Nuss R, "Lupus Anticoagulant in Children With Thrombosis," *Am J Hematol*, 1995, 48(4):240-3.
16. Ndimbie OK, Raman BKS, and Saeed SM, "Lupus Anticoagulant Associated With Specific Inhibition of Factor VII in a Patient With AIDS," *Am J Clin Pathol*, 1989, 91(4):491-3.
17. Taillan B, Roul C, Fuzibet JG, et al, "Circulating Anticoagulant in Patients Seropositive for Human Immunodeficiency Virus," *Am J Med*, 1989, 87(2):238.
18. Gotoh M and Matsuda J, "Human Immunodeficiency Virus Rather Than Hepatitis C Virus Infection Is Relevant to the Development of an Anti-Cardiolipin Antibody," *Am J Hematol*, 1995, 50(3):220-2.
19. Moreb J and Kitchens CS, "Acquired Functional Protein S Deficiency, Cerebral Venous Thrombosis, and Coumarin Skin Necrosis in Association With Antiphospholipid Syndrome: Report of Two Cases," *Am J Med*, 1989, 87(2):207-10.
20. Faioni EM, Franchi F, Asti D, et al, "Resistance to Activated Protein C in Nine Thrombophilic Families: Interference in a Protein S Functional Assay," *Thromb Haemost*, 1993, 70(6):1067-71.
21. Arnason JA and Graziano FM, "Adrenal Insufficiency in the Antiphospholipid Antibody Syndrome," *Semin Arthritis Rheum*, 1995, 25(2):109-16.

References

Abu-Shakra M, Gladman DD, Urowitz MB, et al, "Anticardiolipin Antibodies in Systemic Lupus Erythematosus: Clinical and Laboratory Correlations," *Am J Med*, 1995, 99(6):624-8.
Branch DW, "Antiphospholipid Antibodies and Pregnancy: Maternal Implications," *Semin Perinatol*, 1990, 14(2):139-46.
Branch DW, "Antiphospholipid Syndrome: Laboratory Concerns, Fetal Loss, and Pregnancy Management," *Semin Perinatol*, 1991, 15(3):230-7.
Cervera R, Asherson RA, and Lie JT, "Clinicopathologic Correlations of the Antiphospholipid Syndrome," *Semin Arthritis Rheum*, 1995, 24(4):262-72.
Eisenberg GM, "Antiphospholipid Syndrome: The Reality and Implications," *Hosp Pract*, 1992, 27(6):119-22, 127-31.
Farrugia E, Torres VE, Gastineau D, et al, "Lupus Anticoagulant in Systemic Lupus Erythematosus: A Clinical and Renal Pathological Study," *Am J Kidney Dis*, 1992, 20(5): 463-71.
Feinstein DI, "Lupus Anticoagulant, Anticardiolipin Antibodies, Fetal Loss, and Systemic Lupus Erythematosus," *Blood*, 1992, 80(4):859-62.
Feldman E and Levine SR, "Cerebrovascular Disease With Antiphospholipid Antibodies: Immune Mechanisms, Significance, and Therapeutic Options," *Ann Neurol*, 1995, 37(S1):S114-30.
Ferro D, Saliola M, Quintarelli C, et al, "Methods for Detecting Lupus Anticoagulants and Their Relation to Thrombosis and Miscarriage in Patients With Systemic Lupus Erythematosus," *J Clin Pathol*, 1992, 45(4):332-8.
"Guidelines on Testing for the Lupus Anticoagulant. Lupus Anticoagulant Working Party on Behalf of the BCSH Haemostasis and Thrombosis Task Force," *J Clin Pathol*, 1991, 44(11):885-9.
Harris EN, "Syndrome of the Black Swan," *Br J Rheumatol*, 1987, 26(5):324-6.
Harris EN, Pierangeli S, and Birch D, "Anticardiolipin Wet Workshop Report. Fifth International Symposium on Antiphospholipid Antibodies," *Am J Clin Pathol*, 1994, 101(5):616-24.
Kaczor DA, Bickford NN, and Triplett DA, "Evaluation of Different Mixing Study Reagents and Dilution Effect in Lupus Anticoagulant Testing," *Am J Clin Pathol*, 1991, 95(3):408-11.

Mackie IJ, Colaco CB, and Machin SJ, "Familial Lupus Anticoagulants," *Br J Haematol*, 1987, 67(3):359-63.

Mammen EF and Fujii Y, "Hypercoagulable States," *Lab Med*, 1989, 20:611-6.

Peacock NW and Levine SP, "Case Report: The Lupus Anticoagulant-Hypoprothrombinemia Syndrome," *Am J Med Sci*, 1994, 307(5):346-9.

Petri M "Diagnosis of Antiphospholipid Antibodies," *Rheum Dis Clin North Am*, 1994, 20(2):443-69.

Pope JM, Canny CL, and Bell DA, "Cerebral Ischemic Events Associated With Endocarditis, Retinal Vascular Disease, and Lupus Anticoagulant," *Am J Med*, 1991, 90(3):299-309.

Raz E, Michaeli J, Rosenmann E, et al, "Antinuclear Antibody-Negative Systemic Lupus Erythematosus (SLE) and Severe Renal Involvement: Close Correlation Between Disease Activity and Appearance of Circulating Anticoagulant," *Isr J Med Sci*, 1988, 24(2):105-8.

Rosner E, Pauzner R, Lusky A, et al, "Detection and Quantitative Evaluation of Lupus Circulating Anticoagulant Activity," *Thromb Haemost*, 1987, 57(2):144-7.

Saxena R, Saraya AK, Kotte VK, et al, "Inosithin Neutralization Test to Measure Lupus Anticoagulants," *Am J Clin Pathol*, 1993, 99(1):61-4.

Seaman DE, Londino AV Jr, Kwoh CK, et al, "Antiphospholipid Antibodies in Pediatric Systemic Lupus Erythematosus," *Pediatrics*, 1995, 96(6):1040-5.

Triplett DA, "Antiphospholipid Antibodies and Thrombosis: A Consequence, Coincidence, or Cause?" *Arch Pathol Lab Med*, 1993, 117(1):78-88.

INR *see* Prothrombin Time *on page 262*

International Normalized Ratio *see* Prothrombin Time *on page 262*

Intravascular Coagulation Screen

CPT 85023 (CBC, platelet count, manual differential); 85362 (fibrin degradation products); 85384 (fibrinogen quantitative); 85610 (prothrombin time); 85730 (PTT)

Related Information

Activated Partial Thromboplastin Time *on page 227*
Beta-Thromboglobulin *on page 232*
D-Dimer *on page 237*
Euglobulin Clot Lysis *on page 238*
Fibrin Breakdown Products *on page 245*
Fibrinogen *on page 246*
Fibrinopeptide A *on page 247*
Fibrin Split Products, Protamine Sulfate *on page 248*
Plasminogen Assay *on page 256*
Platelet Count *on page 340*
Risks of Transfusion *on page 623*
Thrombin Time *on page 266*

Synonyms Coagulation Screen, Intravascular; Consumptive Coagulopathy Screen; DIC Screen; Disseminated Intravascular Coagulation Screen; Screen for Disseminated Intravascular Coagulation

Test Commonly Includes Availability and composition of screen varies between laboratories. Commonly included are platelet estimate or platelet count, PTT, dilute clot lysis or euglobulin clot lysis, fibrinogen, thrombin time, fibrin breakdown products (FBPs) (fibrin degradation-FDPs- or "split" products), and review of peripheral blood smear for microangiopathic changes in red blood cells. Prothrombin time and APTT have limited use in evaluation of DIC, each may be normal or shortened in up to 50% to 60% of such patients and cannot be used to exclude the diagnosis. Tests for D-dimer, antithrombin III, heparin cofactor II, beta-thromboglobulin, and fibrinopeptide A may also be included. A comparison of the value of screen components concluded that increased levels of both FDPs and D-dimer (in a patient clinically at risk) were the most helpful in establishing a diagnosis of DIC.[1] Sensitivity and specificity were maximized by screening with FDP (highly sensitive) and confirming with D-dimer (highly specific). One approach to screening for DIC suggests a panel consisting of PT, PTT, TT, and platelet count as the initial screen with use of plasma fibrinogen, plasma D-dimer, and serum FDP titer as confirmatory tests.[2]

Abstract Screens for DIC generally incorporate multiple tests which are individually sensitive but not specific. Individual test protocols must result in rapid turnaround time with limited expenditure of technologist resources. Correlation of the multiple test results usually allows specific conclusion as to the existence of a consumptive coagulopathy.

Specimen Approximately 15 mL of blood, see individual test listings for specific requirements.

Collection As for individual constituent tests. Sample for dilute clot lysis must be collected at patient's side and placed directly into diluent.

Turnaround Time It is possible and desirable that the DIC screen include largely tests that can be rapidly performed, so that a single experienced technologist can complete the tests in 60-90 minutes.

Special Instructions Initiate a dialogue with the Coagulation Laboratory concerning availability of, composition of, and special requirements for the DIC screen.

Reference Range See individual constituent tests and additional information. See table.

Findings Indicative of DIC

Test Parameter	Acute DIC	Chronic DIC
Antithrombin III	↓	
APTT (activated partial thromboplastin time)	↑ to ↑↑ or N	N
β-thromboglobulin	↑	
Clotting factor assays	Unreliable	N or ↑
D-dimer, monoclonal antibody	↑	Usually ↑
Fibrin(ogen) breakdown products present	++	+
Fibrinogen (clottable)	↓↓ or ↓↓↓	N or ↑
Fibrinolytic activity	N rarely ↑	N rarely ↑
Plasminogen	↓	N or ↓
Platelet count	↓↓ to ↓↓↓	N to ↑
Platelet factor IV	↑	
PT (prothrombin time)	↑ or N	N
RBC microangiopathy	++	+
Reptilase time	↑	
Soluble fibrin/monomer complexes (protamine sulfate or ethanol gelation)	++	+
Thrombin time	↑↑	↑

Use Identify the presence of or to follow course of the process of disseminated intravascular coagulation (DIC) including abnormalities in platelet count, fibrinogen, fibrin split products, fibrinolytic activity

Limitations One cannot distinguish physiologic from pathophysiologic clot formation and lysis in all cases. Results should be reviewed in relation to the clinical situation.

Additional Information Platelet adhesion and aggregation with subsequent intravascular coagulation occur physiologically as early states in the reparative response to vascular injury, in which the nonthrombogenic endothelium has been torn or rubbed away. Naturally occurring inhibitors, including prostacyclin, antithrombin III, and protein C/factor V, normally control the intravascular clotting process. With severe injury and/or entrance of thromboplastins into the circulation, the process may become pathologic and result in morbidity and/or mortality. The amount and rate of entry of thromboplastins into the circulation determine the severity and rapidity of the process. A corollary of primary importance in therapy is removal of the source of thromboplastic agents if possible.

The process of intravascular coagulation results in the partial to nearly complete conversion of plasma to serum. Clotting factors are variously converted with factors V and VIII completely utilized, with small amounts of VII, IX, and X activated and lost due to the action of antithrombin. Platelets undergo changes in configuration and release reactions. Later and concurrently, fibrinogen is cleared and fibrin lysed to give rise to fibrin monomer aggregates and fibrin degradation products. Marked decrease in levels of heparin cofactor II have been reported in infants with DIC.[3]

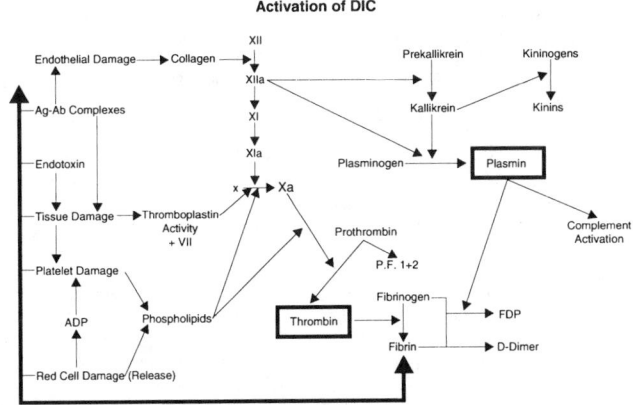

Activation of DIC

From Bick RL, "Disseminated Intravascular Coagulation, Objective Laboratory Diagnostic Criteria and Guidelines for Management," *Clin Lab Med*, 1994, 14(4):729-68, with permission.

Varying levels of complexity in interpretation are introduced by the multitest nature of the DIC screen and the need for clinical correlation. If all test results are normal, it is very unlikely that any significant degree of intravascular coagulation and lysis is in progress. With levels of fibrin breakdown products (FBP) <10 µg/mL, any significant level of DIC is unlikely. This is also a finding against physiologic clot formation and lysis of any significant degree. Intermediate levels of FBP (10-40 µg/mL) may
(Continued)

Intravascular Coagulation Screen *(Continued)*

Trigger Factors That Can Alter Hemostatic Balance and Initiate DIC

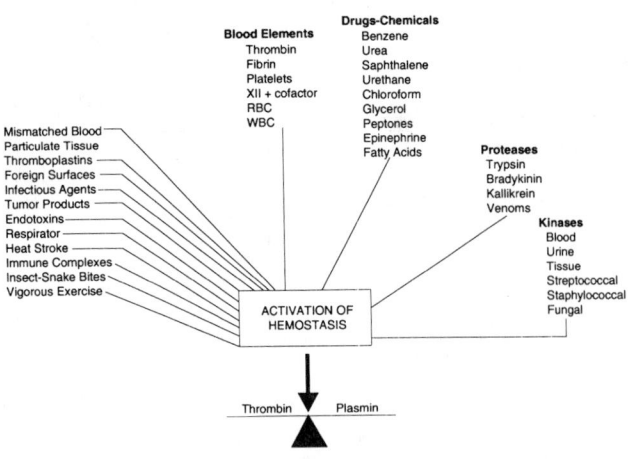

From Bell WR, "The Pathophysiology of Disseminated Intravascular Coagulation," *Sem Hematol*, 1994, 31(2 suppl 1):19-24, with permission.

be associated with mild or early DIC or with physiologic clot formation and lysis. Levels of FBP >40 µg/mL may still reflect only a physiologic process, but if associated with decreased (or decreasing) fibrinogen and/or platelet levels, possibility of DIC is likely. Process of DIC is frequently dynamic with changes occurring rapidly (acute DIC). Close monitoring of fibrinogen level and platelet count will reflect the rapidly changing picture and provide prognostic insight. With well developed, advanced DIC, PT and PTT become prolonged. Clot lysis may be active and shortened along with significantly decreased levels of fibrinogen and platelets and increased levels of FBP. The protamine sulfate paracoagulation test may be a useful adjunct for indication of increased levels of fibrin monomers.

Clinical states associated with intravascular coagulation (IVC) include gram-negative sepsis (endotoxin effect); gram-positive sepsis (some bacterial strains with a peptidoglycan that aggregates platelets in the presence of staphylococcal A protein);[4] pneumonia, severe (tissue destruction with thromboplastin generation); malaria (release of lipids from RBCs); malignancies involving pancreas, prostate, lung (necrosis and thromboplastin generation); Hodgkin's disease (necrosis and thromboplastin generation); some acute leukemias[5]; shock and trauma (stasis and thromboplastin); end state disease with tissue necrosis; placenta praevia and abruptio; toxemia of pregnancy; amniotic fluid embolus; dead fetus syndrome; ruptured uterus. Resulting from the observation that plasma D-dimer and serum FBP levels follow one another closely in cases of DIC, it has been considered that FBPs arise predominantly from plasmin's action on cross-linked fibrin rather than on fibrinogen.[6]

The rare association of severe thrombocytopenia and chronic consumptive coagulopathy with the Klippel-Trenaunay syndrome has been successfully treated with epsilon-aminocaproic acid (EACA).[7] The therapy was associated with a rise in platelet count to normal levels and technetium-99m-labeled autologous RBC imaging demonstration of regression of abnormal vascular channels. The Klippel-Trenaunay syndrome is an inherited abnormality which includes vascular malformations and varicose veins.

Therapy is based on removal of the inciting cause, replacement of deficient factors, and in some cases, heparin anticoagulant therapy. Replacement includes especially platelet infusion, whole blood, and fibrinogen rich cryoprecipitates. The risk of aggravation of bleeding must be carefully weighed in considering heparin therapy. In cases with evidence or threat of shock, renovascular thrombosis and necrosis, heparin (in the form of a constant I.V. infusion to maintain the APTT or activated coagulation time at 2.5 to 3 times control value) may be of protective value. Heparin should not be used until bleeding is controlled with replacement therapy and should never be used in patients with head injury or evidence of CNS bleeding. Use of antithrombin III concentrates may be of value in therapy of at least some forms of DIC (see references by Bell and by Bick, 1994, given below).

Subgroups that may be helped by AT-III therapy:

- septic shock
- shock
- acute fatty liver pregnancy
- eclampsia?
- pre-eclampsia?
- postoperative total joint replacement
- tamoxifen?
- pancreatitis?

Footnotes

1. Carr JM, McKinney M, and McDonagh J, "Diagnosis of Disseminated Intravascular Coagulation. Role of D-Dimer," *Am J Clin Pathol*, 1989, 91(3):280-7.
2. Bovill EG, "Laboratory Diagnosis of Disseminated Intravascular Coagulation," *Semin Hematol*, 1994, 31(2 Suppl 1):35-9.
3. Chuansumrit A, Manco-Johnson MJ, and Hathaway WE, "Heparin Cofactor II in Adults and Infants With Thrombosis and DIC," *Am J Hematol*, 1989, 31(2):109-13.
4. Kessler CM, Nussbaum E, and Tuazon CU, "Disseminated Intravascular Coagulation Associated With *Staphylococcus aureus* Septicemia Is Mediated by Peptidoglycan-Induced Platelet Aggregation," *J Infect Dis*, 1991, 164(1):101-7.
5. Lisiewicz J, "Disseminated Intravascular Coagulation in Acute Leukemia," *Semin Thromb Hemost*, 1988, 14(4):339-50.
6. Wilde JT, Kitchen S, Kinsey S, et al, "Plasma D-Dimer Levels and Their Relationship to Serum Fibrinogen/Fibrin Degradation Products in Hypercoagulable States," *Br J Haematol*, 1989, 71(1):65-70.
7. Poon M-C, Kloiber R, and Birdsell DC, "Epsilon-Aminocaproic Acid in the Reversal of Consumption Coagulopathy With Platelet Sequestration in a Vascular Malformation of Klippel-Trenaunay Syndrome," *Am J Med*, 1989, 87(2):211-13.

References

Baker WF Jr, "Clinical Aspects of Disseminated Intravascular Coagulation: A Clinician's Point of View," *Semin Thromb Hemost*, 1989, 15(1):1-57.

Bell WR, "The Pathophysiology of Disseminated Intravascular Coagulation," *Semin Hematol*, 1994, 31(2 Suppl 1):19-24.

Bick RL, "Disseminated Intravascular Coagulation: Objective Laboratory Diagnostic Criteria and Guidelines for Management," *Clin Lab Med*, 1994, 14(4):729-68.

Bick RL, "Disseminated Intravascular Coagulation," *Hematol Oncol Clin North Am*, 1992, 6(6):1259-85.

Bick RL and Tse N, "Hemostasis Abnormalities Associated With Prosthetic Devices and Organ Transplantation," *Lab Med*, 1992, 23(7):462-8.

Büller HR and ten Cate JW, "Acquired Antithrombin III Deficiency: Laboratory Diagnosis, Incidence, Clinical Implications, and Treatment With Antithrombin III Concentrate," *Am J Med*, 1989, 87(3B):44S-48S.

Colman RW and Rubin RN, "Disseminated Intravascular Coagulation Due to Malignancy," *Semin Oncol*, 1990, 17(2):172-86.

Fareed J, Bick RL, Hoppensteadt DA, et al, "Molecular Markers of Hemostatic Activation: Implications in the Diagnosis of Thrombosis, Vascular, and Cardiovascular Disorders," Thrombosis and Hemostasis for the Clinical Laboratory: Part II, *Clin Lab Med*, 1995, 15(1):39-61.

Marder VJ, Feinstein DI, Francis CW, et al, "Consumptive Thrombohemorrhagic Disorders," *Hemostasis and Thrombosis: Basic Principles and Clinical Practice*, 3rd ed, Chapter 52, Colman RW, Hirsh J, Marder VJ, et al, eds, Philadelphia, PA: JB Lippincott Co, 1994, 1023-63.

Muller-Berghaus G, "Pathophysiologic and Biochemical Events in Disseminated Intravascular Coagulation: Dysregulation of Procoagulant and Anticoagulant Pathways," *Semin Thromb Hemost*, 1989, 15(1):58-87.

Okajima K, Fujise R, Motosato Y, et al, "Plasma Levels of Granulocyte Elastase-Alpha$_1$-Proteinase Inhibitor Complex in Patients With Disseminated Intravascular Coagulation: Pathophysiologic Implications," *Am J Hematol*, 1994, 47(2):82-8.

Ivy Bleeding Time *see* Bleeding Time, Ivy *on page 233*

Labile Factor *see* Factor V *on page 239*

Laki-Lorand Factor *see* Factor XIII *on page 243*

Lee-White *see* Lee-White Clotting Time *on this page*

Lee-White Clotting Time

CPT 85345

Related Information
Activated Coagulation Time *on page 226*
Activated Partial Thromboplastin Time *on page 227*

Synonyms Clot Time; Coagulation Time; Lee-White; Lee-White Coagulation Time; L-W

Patient Preparation No heparin therapy for a minimum of 3 hours prior to specimen collection.

Specimen Blood

Container Three 12 x 75 mm glass test tubes and syringe

Collection Use two-syringe technique, draw blood into a plastic syringe. 1 mL of blood is placed into each of three tubes. Kept at 37°C. Start stopwatch upon filling of third tube. The test is complete when the last tube has clotted.

Causes for Rejection Traumatic venipuncture, patient receiving heparin therapy within 3 hours of collection

Reference Range 8-15 minutes

Use Evaluate whole blood clotting system; monitor therapy with heparin

Limitations Specimen obtained less than 3 hours after a dose of heparin will have markedly prolonged clotting time. The standard Lee-White clotting time lacks precision, as it is difficult to perform the test under truly standard conditions between individual technologists and individual laboratories. Prolonged CTs (as encountered when monitoring heparin use) are especially subject to inaccuracy. **A number of laboratories no longer offer this test.**

Methodology Time required for visual detection of clotting is determined after freshly drawn blood is subjected to standardized activation stimulus (timed periodic tube tilting)

Additional Information Clotting time may be used to monitor effect of heparin therapy, but with occasional patients, no single test will allow unambiguous monitoring of such therapy. The addition of accelerators of coagulation (such as phospholipids or excessive contact activation as with some APTT reagents) will tend to overcome or mask the anticoagulant action of heparin. Heparin action is through the activation of antithrombin III. If AT III is greatly decreased, heparin will have little anticoagulant effect without the addition of plasma infusion. This may especially pertain to patients with disseminated intravascular coagulation. With severe lipemia, there will be a competitive attraction by lipase for heparin.

A table in the listing Activated Partial Thromboplastin Time *on page 227*, provides relationships of three coagulation tests which can be utilized to adjust heparin.

References

Sirridge MS and Shannon R, *Laboratory Evaluation of Hemostasis and Thrombosis*, 3rd ed, Philadelphia, PA: Lea & Febiger, 1983, 68, 112-5.

Lee-White Coagulation Time see Lee-White Clotting Time *on previous page*

Low Molecular Weight see Activated Partial Thromboplastin Time *on page 227*

Lumi-Aggregometry see Platelet Aggregation *on page 257*

Lupus Anticoagulant see Anticoagulant, Circulating *on page 229*

Lupus Anticoagulant (LA) see Inhibitor, Lupus, Phospholipid Type *on page 251*

L-W see Lee-White Clotting Time *on previous page*

Negative Pressure Suction Cup Capillary Fragility see Capillary Fragility Test *on page 235*

P62 see Platelet Aggregation *on page 257*

PAI see Plasminogen Activator Inhibitor *on this page*

PAI Chromogenic Assay see Plasminogen Activator Inhibitor *on this page*

Partial Thromboplastin Time, Activated see Activated Partial Thromboplastin Time *on page 227*

PC see Protein C *on page 260*

Phospholipid Type Anticoagulant see Inhibitor, Lupus, Phospholipid Type *on page 251*

Plasma Plasminogen Activator Inhibitor see Plasminogen Activator Inhibitor *on this page*

Plasma Protamine Paracoagulation see Fibrin Split Products, Protamine Sulfate *on page 248*

Plasma Thromboplastin Antecedent see Factor XI *on page 243*

Plasma Thromboplastin Component see Factor IX *on page 241*

Plasminogen Activator Inhibitor

CPT 85415

Related Information

Diluted Whole Blood Clot Lysis *on page 237*
Hypercoagulable State Coagulation Screen *on page 250*
Inhibitor, Lupus, Phospholipid Type *on page 251*
Plasminogen Assay *on next page*
Protein C *on page 260*
Protein S *on page 261*

Synonyms PAI; PAI Chromogenic Assay; Plasma Plasminogen Activator Inhibitor; Spectrolyse™/pL Procedure

Specimen Plasma

Container Blue top (sodium citrate) tube

Sampling Time PAI-1 has a circadian rhythm, high in the early morning but falling in the afternoon and evening. This change should be considered when planning PAI-1 plasma studies.

Collection Obtain **free flowing** venous blood sample using a two-syringe technique. If indwelling catheter is in place or Vacutainer® technique is utilized, use sample from second or third tube. Discard the first 3-5 mL of free flowing blood. Place gently mixed tube on ice and process (centrifuge) within 60 minutes.

Storage Instructions Plasma may be stored at -70°C (until analyzed).

Causes for Rejection Correction procedure may be necessary if plasma sample is hemolyzed or has increase in bilirubin levels

Special Instructions Plasma must be absolutely platelet-free. Centrifugal force of at least 30,000 g/min used during centrifugation.[1]

Reference Range 0-15 units/mL (average 4.5 units/mL).[2] Men generally have higher values than women.

Use Evaluate deep vein thrombosis, myocardial infarction (MI), and risk of postoperative thrombosis. Use in evaluation of familial thrombosis is uncertain.[3]

Limitations Results may be affected by abnormally high levels of hemoglobin, bilirubin, or lipid levels present concurrently in the plasma test sample. There is evidence of significant intra-individual variation for 30 days following surgery or onset of deep vein thrombosis. Due to this acute phase reaction, it has been recommended that study of the fibrinolytic system should be postponed for at least 1 month after an acute episode.[4]

Methodology Two-stage indirect enzymatic assay (principle first developed by Chmielewska et al[5]), available commercially as Spectrolyse™/pL. In the first step a fixed amount of t-PA reacts with PAI in the test plasma, and sample is acidified to destroy other plasmin inhibitors. In the second step residual t-PA activity is measured by determining the color developed after any residual t-PA has generated plasmin that effects hydrolysis of the chromogen substrate.

Additional Information There are two distinct plasminogen activator inhibitors, PAI-1 (present in normal plasma and platelet releasates) and PAI-2 (present in pregnancy plasma and leukocytes).[6] PAI-1 is a single chain glycoprotein, molecular weight of about 50,000. It is a serine protease inhibitor, a member of the "serpin" gene family. PAI-1 exists in latent (inactive), active, and complex (t-PA/PAI-1) forms in the blood. Increase in plasma PAI may be a cause of decreased fibrinolytic activity and may relate to clinical thrombotic disease. Patients postmyocardial infarct and those with recurrent myocardial infarction, coronary artery disease, and deep vein thrombosis may have increased plasma PAI levels.[7] There is increase in risk of recurrent MI in survivors of a first infarctive episode.[8] If plasma PAI is elevated prior to surgery, there is increase in risk of postoperative thrombosis. As PAI is an acute phase reactant of the inflammatory process, levels increase after surgery. Plasma PAI levels are increased with endotoxemia and with pregnancy. Perioperative (aortic surgery patients) increase in PAI may be due in part to release of inhibitor from platelets.[9]

There is evidence that human recombinant lymphotoxin, α and β interleukin-1, and recombinant tumor necrosis factor increase the production of plasminogen activator inhibitor. Increase in PAI activity might decrease fibrinolysis.[10]

Utilizing a radioimmunoassay to measure PAI-1 antigen levels before and after platelet aggregation, 85% of PAI-1 (in platelet-rich plasma) was found to be associated with platelets, about 4000 molecules per platelet.[5]

Plasminogen activation may play an important role in atherogenesis. Lipoprotein (a) (Lp(a)), a variant of low density lipoprotein, is a physiological inhibitor of plasminogen activation. Lp(a) competes with plasminogen for plasminogen binding sites, decreases binding of plasminogen by endothelial cells, thus suppressing fibrinolysis and contributing to a procoagulant state.[11]

Impaired fibrinolysis with elevated plasma plasminogen activator inhibitor levels was noted in a group of patients with malignant disease.[12] This finding may relate to the development of deep-vein thrombosis in some patients with malignant conditions.

Footnotes

1. Macy EM, Meilahn EN, Declerck PJ, et al, "Sample Preparation for Plasma Measurement of Plasminogen Activator Inhibitor-1 Antigen in Large Population Studies," *Arch Pathol Lab Med*, 1993, 117(1):67-70.
2. Wiman B, "The Role of the Fibrinolytic System in Thrombotic Disease," *Acta Med Scand Suppl*, 1987, 715:169-71.
3. Bolan CD, Krishnamurti C, Tang DB, et al, "Association of Protein S Deficiency With Thrombosis in a Kindred With Increased Levels of Plasminogen Activator Inhibitor-1," *Ann Intern Med*, 1993, 119(8):779-85.
4. Jansson J-H, Norberg B, and Nilsson TK, "Impact of Acute Phase on Concentrations of Tissue Plasminogen Activator and Plasminogen Activator Inhibitor in Plasma After Deep Vein Thrombosis or Open Heart Surgery," *Clin Chem*, 1989, 35(7):1544-5.
5. Chmielewska J and Wiman B, "Determination of Tissue Plasminogen Activator and Its "Fast" Inhibitor in Plasma," *Clin Chem*, 1986, 32(3):482-5.
6. Kruithof EK, Nicolasa G, and Bachmann F, "Plasminogen Activator Inhibitor 1: Development of a Radioimmunoassay and Observations on Its Plasma Concentration During Venous Occlusion and After Platelet Aggregation," *Blood*, 1987, 70(5):1645-53.
7. Chandler WL and Stratton JR, "Laboratory Evaluation of Fibrinolysis in Patients With a History of Myocardial Infarction," *Am J Clin Pathol*, 1994, 102(2):248-52.
8. Hamsten A, de Faire U, Walldius G, et al, "Plasminogen Activator Inhibitor in Plasma: Risk Factor for Recurrent Myocardial Infarction," *Lancet*, 1987, 2(8549):3-9.
9. Gomez MJ, Carroll RC, Hansard MR, et al, "Regulation of Fibrinolysis in Aortic Surgery," *J Vasc Surg*, 1988, 8(4):384-8.
10. van Hinsbergh VW, Kooistra T, van den Berg EA, et al, "Tumor Necrosis Factor Increases the Production of Plasminogen Activator Inhibitor in Human Endothelial Cells *In Vitro* and Rats *In Vivo*," *Blood*, 1988, 72(5):1467-73.
11. Scott J, "Lipoprotein(a) Thrombogenesis Linked to Atherogenesis at Last?" *Nature*, 1989, 341(6237):22-3.
12. Newland JR and Haire WD, "Elevated Plasminogen Activator Inhibitor Levels Found in Patients With Malignant Conditions," *Am J Clin Pathol*, 1991, 96(5):602-4.

References

Chandler WL, Loo SC, Nguyen SV, et al, "Standardization of Methods for Measuring Plasminogen Activator Inhibitor Activity in Human Plasma," *Clin Chem*, 1989, 35(5):787-93.

(Continued)

Plasminogen Activator Inhibitor *(Continued)*

Duncan A and Hunter RL, "Plasminogen Activator (PAI) in Plasma Samples," *Manual of Procedures for the Seminar on Diagnostic Hematology*, Sunderman FW, ed, Philadelphia, PA: Institute for Clinical Science, 1988, 29-37.

Krishnamurti C, Tang DB, Barr CF, et al, "Plasminogen Activator and Plasminogen Activator Inhibitor Activities in a Reference Population," *Am J Clin Pathol*, 1988, 89(6):747-52.

Lawrence DA and Ginsburg D, "Plasminogen Activator Inhibitors," *Molecular Basis of Thrombosis and Hemostasis*, Chapter 25, High KA and Roberts HR, eds, New York, NY: Marcel Dekker, Inc, 1995, 517-43.

Loskutoff DJ, Sawdey M, and Mimuro J, "Type 1 Plasminogen Activator Inhibitor," *Prog Hemost Thromb*, 1989, 9:87-115.

Ranby M, Bergsdorf N, Nilsson T, et al, "Age Dependence of Tissue Plasminogen Activator Concentrations in Plasma, as Studied by an Improved Enzyme-Linked Immunosorbent Assay," *Clin Chem*, 1986, 32(12):2160-5.

Plasminogen Assay

CPT 85420

Related Information

Diluted Whole Blood Clot Lysis *on page 237*
Euglobulin Clot Lysis *on page 238*
Intravascular Coagulation Screen *on page 253*
Plasminogen Activator Inhibitor *on previous page*

Synonyms Plasminogen, Quantitative

Applies to α_2-Antiplasmin

Specimen Plasma

Container Blue top (sodium citrate) tube

Collection Routine venipuncture. If multiple tests are being drawn, draw coagulation studies last. If only coagulation tests are being drawn, draw 1-2 mL into another Vacutainer® tube, discard, and then collect coagulation tests (double syringe/tube technique). This collection procedure avoids contamination of the specimen with tissue thromboplastins.

Storage Instructions Keep refrigerated.

Causes for Rejection Tube not full, specimen hemolyzed, specimen clotted, specimen received more than 2 hours after collection

Special Instructions Schedule with laboratory.

Reference Range 3.8-8.4 CTA (Council on Thrombolytic Agents) units/mL (α-Caseinolytic method), may also be reported as percentage of normal for human plasma or in absolute concentration (immunologic assays). Levels are reduced in the newborn (in comparison with the mother).[1,2]

Use Determine plasminogen and plasmin activity in plasma, study dysplasminogens, monitor thrombolytic therapy, evaluate DIC

Methodology Caseinolytic method[3] and synthetic substrate based (amidolytic, chromogenic, fluorogenic)[4,5]

Additional Information Plasminogen is a glycoprotein (molecular weight about 90,000 daltons) and is present in plasma as an inactive protein (zymogen) at a concentration of about 200 µg/mL and has an *in vivo* half-life of 2.2 days. Molecular structure/function relationships are known and are nicely summarized in the following references. A series of five triple-loop structures (kringles) form a major part of the N-terminal region of the molecule and are binding sites for fibrin as well as for antifibrinolytic agents (eg, EACA). Activation of plasminogen (a single-chain protein) to the two-chain serine protease-plasmin, a potent enzyme, is accomplished by either an intrinsic pathway (factor XIIa is involved) or an extrinsic mechanism (serine proteases including urokinase are involved). Decreased plasminogen activity may be on an acquired or familial basis. Acquired decrease is seen in some cases of DIC, liver disease, L-asparaginase therapy (of acute leukemia), neonatal hyaline membrane disease, and following surgery.[6] Plasminogen assay has application to the monitoring of antifibrinolytic therapy.[7] After streptokinase therapy for acute myocardial infarction, the radial immunodiffusion assay did not show as great a decrease in plasma plasminogen as did a fluorogenic synthetic substrate assay.[8] This was shown to be the apparent result of a lack of specificity of the RID assay antibody to plasminogen. Decrease in plasminogen activity may be associated with tendency to thrombosis; altered molecular forms have been described.[9] Inhibitors of plasmin (eg, α_2-antiplasmin) are important in the regulation of fibrinolysis. There is evidence that regular vigorous physical exercise (participation in sporting activities) increases fibrinolytic activity of blood by decreasing plasminogen activator inhibitor capacity.[10]

Plasminogen polymorphism has been applied in the field of forensic hemogenetics.[11]

Footnotes

1. Biland L and Duckert F, "Coagulation Factors of the Newborn and His Mother," *Thromb Diath Haemorrh*, 1973, 29:644-51.
2. Corrigan JJ, Sleeth JJ, Jeter M, et al, "Newborn's Fibrinolytic Mechanism: Components and Plasmin Generation," *Am J Hematol*, 1989, 32(4):273-8.
3. Triplett DA and Harms CS, "Plasminogen Assay by α-Caseinolytic Method," *Procedures for the Coagulation Laboratory*, Chicago, IL: American Society of Clinical Pathologists, 1981, 144-6.

4. Fareed J, Messmore HL, Walenga JM, et al, "Diagnostic Efficacy of Newer Synthetic-Substrates Methods for Assessing Coagulation Variables: A Critical Overview," *Clin Chem*, 1983, 29:225-36.
5. Friberger P, "Chromogenic Peptide Substrates. Their Use for the Assay of Factors in the Fibrinolytic and the Plasma Kallikrein-Kinin Systems," *Scand J Clin Lab Invest Suppl*, 1982, 162:1-298.
6. Pierson-Perry JF, Wehrly JA, and Siefring GE Jr, "Coagulation Testing With the Du Pont aca® Discrete Clinical Analyzer," *Semin Thromb Hemost*, 1983, 9:321-33.
7. Marder VJ and Bell WR, "Fibrinolytic Therapy," *Hemostasis and Thrombosis*, Colman RW, Hirsch J, Marder VJ, et al, eds, Philadelphia, PA: JB Lippincott Co, 1982, 1037-57.
8. Hysell DC, Smith MR, Brewster PS, et al, "Discrepant Changes in Plasminogen by Two Different Assays in Patients Receiving Streptokinase," *Am J Clin Pathol*, 1988, 90(2):200-5.
9. Giddings JC, "Components of the Fibrinolytic Mechanism," *Molecular Genetics and Immunoanalysis in Blood Coagulation*, Chapter 7, Chichester, England: Ellis Horwood Ltd, 1988, 161-6.
10. Speiser W, Langer W, Pschaick A, et al, "Increased Blood Fibrinolytic Activity After Physical Exercise: Comparative Study in Individuals With Different Sporting Activities and in Patients After Myocardial Infarction Taking Part in a Rehabilitation Sports Program," *Thromb Res*, 1988, 51(5):543-55.
11. Skoda U, Klein A, Lübcke I, et al, "Application of Plasminogen Polymorphism to Forensic Hemogenetics," *Electrophoresis*, 1989, 9(8):422-6.

References

Benedict CR, Mueller S, Anderson HV, et al, "Thrombolytic Therapy: A State of the Art Review," *Hosp Pract*, 1992, 27(6):61-72.

Castellino FJ, "Plasminogen," *Molecular Basis of Thrombosis and Hemostasis*, Chapter 24, High KA and Roberts HR, eds, New York, NY: Marcel Dekker, Inc, 1995, 495-515.

Collen D and Lijnen HR, "Basic and Clinical Aspects of Fibrinolysis and Thrombolysis," *Blood*, 1991, 78(12):3114-24.

Laffan MA and Bradshaw AE, "Investigation of Fibrinolytic System," *Practical Haematology*, 8th ed, Dacie JV and Lewis SM, eds, New York, NY: Churchill Livingstone, 1995, 356-60.

Soff GA and Rosenberg RD, "Physiology of Hemostasis: The Fluid Phase," *Hematology of Infancy and Childhood*, 4th ed, Nathan DG and Oski FA, eds, Philadelphia, PA: WB Saunders Co, 1993, 1534-60.

Plasminogen, Quantitative *see* Plasminogen Assay *on this page*

Platelet Adhesion Test

CPT 85999

Related Information

Bleeding Time, Ivy *on page 233*
Platelet Aggregation *on next page*
Platelet Count *on page 340*

Synonyms Glass Bead Platelet Retention Test; Platelet Adhesiveness; Platelet Retention; Salzman Column Test

Patient Preparation Avoid aspirin, phenylbutazone, antihistamines, phenothiazines for 10 days prior to test

Specimen Whole blood

Collection Specimen will usually be collected by Hematology technologist.

Causes for Rejection Specimen clotted

Special Instructions Schedule with laboratory in advance.

Reference Range Method dependent. Normals usually have at least 75% platelet retention by glass bead column, commonly 90% to 95%; 35% to 75% may be considered borderline.

Use Evaluate platelet function; aid in the diagnosis of von Willebrand disease, thrombasthenia (Glanzmann's disease), storage pool disease, and the Bernard-Soulier syndrome

Limitations This test is offered by very few laboratories because of difficulty in obtaining glass beads and columns of glass beads, in standardizing the technique and keeping glass beads (in the column) from settling. Procedure given in the reference by Zacharski and McIntyre provides for a low cost, reliable standardized test. Settling of beads is avoided by agitation with a vibrating hair management device just before use. A current authoritative reference indicates that *in vitro* platelet adhesion testing is **"unreliable"** and "has no clinical relevance" - thus, "should not be used".[1]

Contraindications Thrombocytopenia or therapy with drugs listed above under patient preparation

Methodology Glass bead column. The relationship between the platelet count done on a presample (not exposed to glass beads) compared to a postsample (glass bead filtered) will give an indication of the adhesiveness of the platelets.

Additional Information Useful in the evaluation of some thrombopathies. A defect in adhesion is present in **von Willebrand disease**, **thrombasthenia**, **storage pool disease**, and the **Bernard-Soulier syndrome**. The Bernard-Soulier syndrome is a severe congenital hemorrhagic disorder characterized by large platelets, deficiency of platelet membrane glycoprotein I, and the inability of platelets to bind von Willebrand factor. Glass bead retention is decreased in vWD, the percent retention returns to normal, however, in columns that have been pretreated with normal plasma.[2] Platelet adhesion is defective in cases of complete afibrinogenemia. In a study designed to standardize platelet function tests there was wide variation between glass bead columns.[3]

Some columns showed wide variation in normal subjects. It was felt columns would not detect abnormal platelet retention. These studies however, may not have controlled for glass bead settling in the column.

In normal individuals ingesting 200 IU of alpha-tocopherol (vitamin E) per day, platelet adhesion was decreased on average by 75%. A dose of 400 IU/day resulted in reduction of platelet adhesion by 82%. Scanning EM study showed decrease in pseudopodium formation in the alpha-tocopherol enriched platelets.[4]

There is evidence that some cases of mild bleeding disorders of von Willebrand disease type may be detected only by use of the McPherson and Zucker two-stage platelet retention assay.[5] In such cases platelets were defective in the second stage (platelet-platelet interaction) of the assay. The platelet retention defects normalized after treatment with desmopressin (d-DAVP). Thus, platelet adhesion studies may identify mild bleeding disorder patients who may improve after treatment with d-DAVP.[6]

Dietary supplementation with vitamin E (alpha-tocopherol) may result in significant decrease in platelet adhesion.[4]

Footnotes

1. Bick RL, "Qualitative (Functional) Platelet Disorders," *Disorders of Thrombosis and Hemostasis: Clinical and Laboratory Practice*, Chapter 4, Chicago, IL: American Society of Clinical Pathologists, 1992, 49.
2. Davis GL and Fritsma GA, "Platelet Disorders," *Hemostasis and Thrombosis in the Clinical Laboratory*, Corriveau DM and Fritsma GA, eds, Philadelphia, PA: JB Lippincott Co, 1988, 334.
3. Roper-Drewinko PR, Drewinko B, Corrigan G, et al, "Standardization of Platelet Function Tests," *Am J Hematol*, 1981, 11:182-203.
4. Jandak J, Steiner M, and Richardson PD, "α-Tocopherol, an Effective Inhibitor of Platelet Adhesion," *Blood*, 1989, 73(1):141-9.
5. McPherson J and Zucker MB, "Platelet Retention in Glass Bead Columns: Adhesion to Glass and Subsequent Platelet-Platelet Interactions," *Blood*, 1976, 47:55-67.
6. Zeigler ZR, "Platelet Glass Bead Retention Is Useful in Monitoring Response to 1-Deamino-8-D-Arginine-Vasopressin (d-DAVP)," *Am J Hematol*, 1989, 31(4):248-52.

References

Giddings JC and Yamamoto J, "Changing Concepts in Investigations of Haemostasis," *Clin Lab Haematol*, 1995, 17(1):85-91.

de Groot PG and Sixma JJ, "Platelet Adhesion," *Br J Haematol*, 1990, 75(3):308-12.

Packham MA and Mustard JF, "Platelet Adhesion," *Prog Hemost Thromb*, 1984, 7:211-88.

Zacharski LR and McIntyre OR, "A Standardized Test of Platelet Adhesiveness," *Am J Clin Pathol*, 1972, 58:422-7.

Platelet Adhesiveness *see* Platelet Adhesion Test *on previous page*

Platelet Aggregation

CPT 85576 (each agent)

Related Information

Bleeding Time, Ivy *on page 233*
Clot Retraction *on page 235*
Platelet Adhesion Test *on previous page*
Platelet Aggregation, Hypercoagulable State *on next page*
Platelet Count *on page 340*
von Willebrand Factor Assay *on page 268*

Synonyms Aggregometer Test; Platelet Function Studies

Applies to Lumi-Aggregometry; P62; Platelet Impedance Aggregation in Whole Blood

Test Commonly Includes Response to ADP, epinephrine, collagen, ristocetin, optionally arachidonic acid, thrombin

Patient Preparation For 10 days prior to testing, drugs that inhibit platelet aggregation are contraindicated. See accompanying list. Any caffeine-containing products must not be consumed the day of test. Aspirin, ubiquitous in our society, will impair platelet aggregation.

Drugs That Inhibit Platelet Aggregation

Acetylsalicylic acid (ASA, Aspirin)	Indomethacin (Indocin)
Antihistamines	Marijuana
Chlordiazepoxide (Librium)	Phenothiazines
Clofibrate (Atromid)	Phenylbutazone (Butazolidin)
Cocaine	Propranolol (Inderal)
Corticosteroids	Pyrimidine compounds
Diazepam (Valium)	Sulfinpyrazone (Anturane)
Dipyridamole (Persantine)	Theophylline
Furosemide (Lasix)	Tricyclic antidepressants
Gentamicin	Others
Ibuprofen (Motrin)	

Specimen Plasma

Container Plastic or siliconized glass syringe

Collection Specimen may need to be specially drawn by laboratory. Keep at room temperature and transport to the laboratory immediately.

Storage Instructions Test should be run within 2 hours of obtaining the sample. Do not chill specimen, platelets are activated at low temperatures. Blood should be processed at 20°C to 25°C and stored at 20°C to 37°C until tested.

Causes for Rejection Platelet count <100,000/mm^3, clotted specimen, hemolysis, patient receiving therapy with drugs, particularly aspirin, antihistamines, anti-inflammatory drugs, psychotropic drugs, some antibiotics and others (unless one wishes to study effect of such medication upon platelet function)

Special Instructions Must usually be scheduled with laboratory.

Reference Range ADP: 60% to 100%; epinephrine: 60% to 100%; collagen: 60% to 100%; ristocetin: 60% to 100%. Diagnostic information is present in the graphical representation of results. Response of normal platelets may vary with concentration of aggregating agent.

Use Evaluate platelet function; aid in diagnosis of von Willebrand disease, Glanzmann's disease, storage pool disease (including Hermansky-Pudlak and Chédiak-Higashi syndromes), Bernard-Soulier syndrome, "gray platelet syndrome," and Raynaud's phenomenon

Limitations If drugs (as indicated above) are exerting an inhibitory effect, evaluation of pre-existing disease of platelet function may be impaired. Presence of lipemia or cryoglobulins may cause difficulty in interpretation.

Methodology Aggregating agent is added to platelet-rich plasma. Resultant change in optical density (if any) that occurs as the dispersed platelets form clumps is measured and recorded. Whole blood platelet aggregation methods have been developed and utilized (impedance aggregation).[1] Some aggregometers are fitted with a luminescence detector which monitors ATP release simultaneously with platelet aggregation (Lumi-aggregometers). Luciferase (firefly extract) acts on ATP as a substrate to emit light.

Additional Information Ristocetin stimulated aggregation is of special value in study of von Willebrand disease. Latter is characterized by decreased aggregation with ristocetin. It is suggested that about 50% of patients with chronic ITP have abnormal (decreased or absent) aggregation with ADP, collagen and epinephrine (using albumin density gradient concentrated platelets). These patients (with thrombopathy) also have demonstrable antiplatelet antibodies.[2] Abnormal platelet aggregation has been found in nearly one-half (44%) of beta-thalassemia major patients.[3] Enhanced platelet aggregation has been noted in insulin stress test induced by hypoglycemia, coinciding with the lowest blood glucose levels and with clinical signs of adrenaline release but without correlation with changes in cortisol, growth hormone, prolactin, or levodopa administration.[4] Platelets from diabetics are more sensitive to aggregating agents.[5] Aggregation responses with platelet concentration <100,000/mm^3, samples processed 90 minutes or longer at room temperature and ADP-induced responses in males as compared to females result in significantly lower values.[6]

Platelet aggregation and/or release is absent in a variety of conditions with qualitative platelet defects, generally termed thrombocytopathy. There are familial forms such as **Bernard-Soulier syndrome, Wiskott-Aldrich syndrome**, **storage pool disease, Hermansky-Pudlak syndrome**, and others.

Acquired disorders that affect platelet function are **uremia, macroglobulinemia, drug ingestion**, and others. Patients with **thrombasthenia** show no aggregation with ADP, epinephrine, or collagen.

Patients with **von Willebrand disease** and **Bernard-Soulier syndrome** show defective aggregation with ristocetin. Whole blood platelet aggregation (along with RIA for platelet glycoprotein expression and monoclonal antibody immunochemical staining of whole blood smears) has been applied to establishing the diagnosis of Bernard-Soulier syndrome. Such patients have large platelets with decreased glycoprotein Ib expression. Platelet aggregation with ristocetin is absent.[7]

Patients with the **"gray platelet syndrome"** have large alpha granule content-depleted, pale staining platelets that aggregate with ristocetin but not with ADP, epinephrine, thrombin, or collagens[8]. See listing Bleeding Time, Ivy *on page 233*.

Patients with primary and secondary **Raynaud's phenomenon** have increased aggregation to the agonists serotonin and ADP but normal responses to adrenalin and collagen.[9] Aspirin effect is characterized by inhibition of collagen aggregation and absence of the secondary waves (release reaction) of ADP, epinephrine, and ristocetin. Aspirin and aspirin-containing drugs will inhibit platelet aggregation for about 7-10 days after ingestion.

Therapeutic propranolol levels have no significant influence on platelet function as determined by platelet aggregation studies with the possible exception of the agonists collagen and noradrenaline in which minor changes without likely biological import were noted.[10] On the other hand, a reversible effect of nitroglycerine (at therapeutic doses) has been (Continued)

Platelet Aggregation *(Continued)*

shown on platelet function (platelet aggregation with ADP using an impedance aggregometer at bedside).[11]

A critical retrospective review of 188 patients with bleeding abnormalities resulted in the conclusion that results of aggregation and bleeding times were not highly correlated and that only rarely were previously undiagnosed platelet function diseases identified.[12] The authors find that 75% of patients with an abnormal bleeding time had normal aggregation while 26% of those with normal bleeding times had abnormal aggregation.

Four types of granules are present in human platelets (alpha granules, dense granules, lysosomes, and peroxisomes). Alpha granules contain adhesive proteins and growth factors. Dense granules contain serotonin, calcium, ADP, ATP, and pyrophosphate. Alpha and dense granule content contribute to platelet aggregation. Storage pool deficiencies (SPD) are characterized by decrease in number and content of dense granules. It has been shown that features of platelet storage pool deficiency may be present in some patients with prolonged bleeding times but no demonstrable abnormalities in platelet aggregation or von Willebrand factor.[13] More commonly, however, platelets of SPD do not aggregate with collagen and do not show secondary stage response to ADP or epinephrine. SPD (including Hermansky-Pudlak and Chédiak-Higashi syndromes) may have decreased serotonin, calcium, and serotonin uptake and high ATP:ADP ratios. Some patients with dense granule storage pool deficiency have decreased levels of granulophysin (CD63),[14] a protein constituent of the platelet dense granule membrane.[15] Hermansky-Pudlak syndrome patients have marked decrease in both dense granules and the membrane protein granulophysin. An apparently rare condition, the "empty sack syndrome" has been identified in which membrane dense granules are present but lack granulophysin (are "empty").[16] These patients have history of bleeding tendency since birth, abnormal platelet aggregation to epinephrine and collagen, marked decrease in serotonin and ATP secretion and decreased platelet content of serotonin, ADP, and ATP.

A patient with deficiency of P62 (a putative collagen receptor found in at least some patients with idiopathic thrombocytopenic purpura) has been shown to have defective collagen-induced platelet aggregation.[17] Hemostatic complications occurring with cardiopulmonary bypass (CPB) surgery have a complex pathogenesis. Decrease in platelet and neutrophil number and function play major roles. Platelet count falls due in part to adhesion of platelets to membrane oxygenators. In addition to this partially reversible platelet adhesion, changes in platelet membrane receptors (including measurable decrease in fibrinogen and α_2-adrenergic receptors) result in decreased aggregation to ADP, epinephrine, collagen, and thrombin.[18] Use of aprotinin decreases blood loss due to CPB from an average of 400-600 mL. Mechanism of action of aprotinin involves inhibition of kallikrein C1-inhibitor complexes with resultant decrease in neutrophil degranulation and thus decreased secretion of the potent platelet agonists cathepsin G and platelet-activating factor.

Footnotes
1. Mackie IJ, Jones R, and Machin SJ, "Platelet Impedance Aggregation in Whole Blood and Its Inhibition by Antiplatelet Drugs," *J Clin Pathol*, 1984, 37(8):874-8.
2. Heyns AD, Fraser J, and Retief FP, "Platelet Aggregation in Chronic Idiopathic Thrombocytopenia Purpura," *J Clin Pathol*, 1978, 31:1239-43.
3. Hussain MA, Hutton RA, Pavlidou O, et al, "Platelet Function in Beta-Thalassemia Major," *J Clin Pathol*, 1979, 32:429-33.
4. Hutton RA, Mikhailidis D, Dormandy KM, et al, "Platelet Aggregation Studies During Transient Hypoglycemia: A Potential Method for Evaluating Platelet Function," *J Clin Pathol*, 1979, 32:434-8.
5. DiMinno G, Silver MJ, Cerbone AM, et al, "Increased Binding of Fibrinogen to Platelets in Diabetes: The Role of Prostaglandins and Thromboxane," *Blood*, 1985, 65(1):156-62.
6. Roper P, Drewinko B, Hasler D, et al, "Effects of Time, Platelet Concentrations, and Sex on the Human Platelet Aggregation Response," *Am J Clin Pathol*, 1979, 71:263-8.
7. Nichols WL, Kaese SE, Gastineau DA, et al, "Bernard-Soulier Syndrome: Whole Blood Diagnostic Assays of Platelets," *Mayo Clin Proc*, 1989, 64(5):522-30.
8. Peerschke EI, "The Gray Platelet Syndrome," *ASCP Check Sample®*, Chicago, IL: American Society of Clinical Pathologists, 1988.
9. Biondi ML and Marasini B, "Abnormal Platelet Aggregation in Patients With Raynaud's Phenomenon," *J Clin Pathol*, 1989, 42(7):716-8.
10. Pomphilon DH, Boon RJ, Prentice AG, et al, "Lack of Significant Effect of Therapeutic Propranolol on Measurable Platelet Function in Healthy Subjects," *J Clin Pathol*, 1989, 42(9):793-6.
11. Diodati J, Théroux P, Latour J-G, et al, "Effects of Nitroglycerin at Therapeutic Doses on Platelet Aggregation in Unstable Angina Pectoris and Acute Myocardial Infarction," *Am J Cardiol*, 1990, 66(7):683-8.
12. Remaley AT, Kennedy JM, and Laposata M, "Evaluation of the Clinical Utility of Platelet Aggregation Studies," *Am J Hematol*, 1989, 31(3):188-93.
13. Israels SJ, McNicole A, Robertson C, et al, "Platelet Storage Pool Deficiency: Diagnosis in Patients With Prolonged Bleeding Times and Normal Platelet Aggregation," *Br J Haematol*, 1990, 75(1):118-21.
14. Nishibori M, Cham B, McNicol A, et al, "The Protein CD63 Is in Platelet Dense Granules, Is Deficient in a Patient With Hermansky-Pudlak Syndrome, and Appears Identical to Granulophysin," *J Clin Invest*, 1993, 91(4):1775-82.
15. Shalev A, Michaud G, Israels SJ, et al, "Quantification of a Novel Dense Granule Protein (Granulophysin) in Platelets of Patients With Dense Granule Storage Pool Deficiency," *Blood*, 1992, 80(5):1231-7.
16. McNicol A, Israels SJ, Robertson C, et al, "The Empty Sack Syndrome: A Platelet Storage Pool Deficiency Associated With Empty Dense Granules," *Br J Haematol*, 1994, 86(3):574-82.

17. Ryo R, Yoshida A, Sugano W, et al, "Deficiency of P62, a Putative Collagen Receptor, in Platelets From a Patient With Defective Collagen-Induced Platelet Aggregation," *Am J Hematol*, 1992, 39(1):25-31.
18. Colman RW, "Hemostatic Complications of Cardiopulmonary Bypass," *Am J Hematol*, 1995, 48(4):267-72.

References
Bick RL, "Acquired Platelet Function Defects," *Hematol Oncol Clin North Am*, 1992, 6(6):1203-28.
Braman AM and Schwartz KA, "Platelet Disorders," *Lab Med*, 1989, 20:831-5.
BSCH Haemostasis and Thrombosis Task Force of the British Society for Haematology, "Guidelines on Platelet Function Testing," *J Clin Pathol*, 1988, 41(12):1322-30.
Fratantoni JC and Poindexter BJ, "Measuring Platelet Aggregation With Microplate Reader. A New Technical Approach to Platelet Aggregation Studies," *Am J Clin Pathol*, 1990, 94(5):613-7.
Hutton RA and Ludlam CA, "ACP Broadsheet #122 Platelet Function Testing," *J Clin Pathol*, 1989, 42(8):858-64.

Platelet Aggregation, Hypercoagulable State
CPT 85575

Related Information
Antithrombin III Test *on page 230*
Hypercoagulable State Coagulation Screen *on page 250*
Platelet Aggregation *on previous page*
Protein C *on page 260*
Protein S *on page 261*
Resistance to Activated Protein C *on page 265*

Synonyms Hypercoagulable State, Platelet Aggregation; Platelet Autoaggregation

Test Commonly Includes Evaluation of spontaneous aggregation, second wave of aggregation with weak ADP, and platelet response to dilutions of epinephrine

Patient Preparation The patient should not receive aspirin, phenylbutazone, phenothiazines, antihistamines, or other drugs (see Platelet Aggregation *on page 257*) for 7-10 days prior to testing.

Specimen Plasma

Container Plastic tube or syringe with sodium citrate

Collection Specimen is usually specially collected by Hematology technologist.

Special Instructions Consult laboratory as to availability of and need for scheduling this analysis. While a simple modification of standard platelet aggregation studies, in most laboratories such hypercoagulable aggregation tests are not routinely available.

Reference Range Rapid spontaneous aggregation or aggregation with very dilute concentrations of epinephrine (as compared to control) may correlate with presence of hypercoagulable state.

Use Coagulation parameter used for evaluation of hypercoagulable states

Limitations Miale has noted that platelet autoaggregation should be a part of platelet aggregation studies but has not found hyperaggregability studies with dilute ADP or epinephrine reagents helpful.[1]

Contraindications Thrombocytopenia, therapy with drugs as indicated under patient preparation

Methodology Platelet aggregation study techniques are used to evaluate platelet function for spontaneous aggregation and enhanced platelet response to standard aggregating agents, using platelet-rich plasma or whole blood (impedance method study of aggregation).

Additional Information Spontaneous aggregation, second wave of aggregation with weak ADP, and enhanced platelet response with dilutions of epinephrine may be indications of platelet hyperactivity and may reflect presence of a hypercoagulable state. The results of whole blood aggregometry have been found significantly more sensitive than those of platelet-rich plasma optical aggregometry in the investigation of platelet hyperaggregability in patients with thromboembolic disease.[2] Hyperaggregation to ADP and to collagen, as well as, spontaneous aggregation has been reported in some but not all cases of myeloproliferative disease whose clinical characteristics included recurrent arterial and venous thromboses.[3]

Footnotes
1. Miale JB, *Laboratory Medicine: Hematology*, 6th ed, St Louis, MO: Mosby-Year Book Inc, 1982, 853-4.
2. Abbate R, Boddi M, Prisco D, et al, "Ability of Whole Blood Aggregometer to Detect Platelet Hyperaggregability," *Am J Clin Pathol*, 1989, 91(2):159-64.
3. Raman BKS, Van Slyck EJ, Riddle J, et al, "Platelet Function and Structure in Myeloproliferative Disease, Myelodysplastic Syndrome, and Secondary Thrombocytosis," *Am J Clin Pathol*, 1989, 91(6):647-55.

Platelet Antibody
CPT 86022

Related Information
Platelet Antibody, Immunohematologic *on page 616*
Platelet Count *on page 340*
Platelets, Apheresis, Donation *on page 617*

Synonyms Serotonin Release

Specimen Plasma

Container Two blue top (sodium citrate) tubes

Collection Routine venipuncture. If multiple tests are being drawn, draw coagulation test last.

Storage Instructions Separate plasma from red cells, transfer to plastic tube (12 x 75 mm) and freeze at -25°C. If the specimen is to be referred to a central laboratory (with resultant delay) for a test measuring platelet associated IgG, optimal collection is of whole blood into acid citrate dextrose, samples kept at 4°C.[1] This results in maximal yield of platelets without change in level of platelet associated IgG. A simplified test using preserved platelets has been described.[2]

Causes for Rejection Specimen clotted, stored plasma not frozen, specimen hemolyzed

Special Instructions Communicate with laboratory before ordering. Platelet antibody tests are not commonly available.

Reference Range Within control range that is determined with each test run

Use Detect the presence of an antibody that destroys platelets; diagnose and follow instances of immune thrombocytopenia

Limitations The serotonin release test may not reliably detect platelet antibodies in patients with idiopathic thrombocytopenia purpura[1] (ITP)

Methodology Serotonin release: Plasma from patient is mixed with a suspension of normal platelets labeled with ^{14}C-serotonin, and the amount of radioactivity (serotonin) released is measured.[2] More recently developed methods include direct and indirect antiplatelet antibody procedures utilizing fluorescein-conjugated antisera with immunofluorescence quantitated by flow cytometry;[3,4,5] direct and indirect immunoprecipitation utilizing polyacrylamide gel electrophoresis;[6] enzyme-linked immunosorbent assay (ELISA);[5] radiolabeled protein staph A assay;[7] direct chemiluminescence assay;[8] and immunoblot analysis.[9] Flow cytometry-based methods using platelets and lymphocytes can distinguish anti-HLA from platelet-specific antibodies.[10]

Additional Information Determination of and significance of platelet antibodies presents an array of intriguing and complex issues. IgG is present on platelets of apparently normal nonthrombocytopenic individuals (about 4000 molecules per platelet).[1] Platelet-bound IgG is not necessarily pathogenic and might reflect immune complex binding or nonspecifically bound IgG, as well as, true antiplatelet antibody of probable more potential significance to immune platelet destruction. The many problems involved in developing an ideal test for platelet-associated IgG is reflected by the over 20 different tests available for platelet antibodies or complexes. The current status of this difficult area and its relation to the diagnosis of ITP has been the subject of informative reviews (see references). Platelet-associated autoantibodies against glycoprotein IIb/IIIa, as well as, against unidentified proteins have been reported in cases of ITP.[6] Radiolabeled allogeneic platelet kinetic (survival) studies indicate that platelet crossmatch tests, using radiolabeled protein staph A assay combined with the IgA ELISA test, provide the best indication of post-transfusion donor platelet survival.[7]

For additional information from the perspective of platelet transfusion see the listing Platelet Antibody, Immunohematologic on page 616.

Footnotes

1. Kelton JG and Gibbons S, "Autoimmune Platelet Destruction: Idiopathic Thrombocytopenic Purpura," Semin Thromb Hemost, 1982, 8:88-91.
2. Marmer DJ, Bowman RP, and Kennedy PS, "A Simplified (^{3}H) Serotonin Release Assay for the Detection of Platelet Antibodies," Am J Hematol, 1979, 6:45-50.
3. Lazarchick J and Jones T, "Antiplatelet Antibody Assay (Indirect Method)," Manual of Procedures for the Seminar on Diagnostic Hematology, Sunderman FW, Institute for Clinical Science, 1988, 101-8.
4. Tazzari PL, Ricci F, Vianelli N, et al, "Detection of Platelet-Associated Antibodies By Flow Cytometry in Hematological Autoimmune Disorders," Ann Hematol, 1995, 70(5):267-72.
5. Lin RY, Levin M, Nygren EN, et al, "Assessment of Platelet Antibody by Flow Cytometric and ELISA Techniques: A Comparison Study," J Lab Clin Med, 1990, 116:(4)479-86.
6. Tomiyama Y, Take H, Honda S, et al, "Demonstration of Platelet Antigens That Bind Platelet-Associated Autoantibodies in Chronic ITP by Direct Immunoprecipitation Procedure," Br J Haematol, 1990, 75(1):92-8.
7. Bensinger WI, Hadlock D, and Slichter SJ, "Identification of Alloimmunized Patients: Use of Radiolabeled Allogeneic Platelet Kinetic Measurements and Platelet Antibody Tests," Blood, 1991, 77(11):2372-8.
8. Kazemi A, Singh AK, and Slater NGP, "An In Vitro Direct Chemiluminescence Assay for Assessment of Platelet-Bound Antibody in Thrombocytopenic Patients," Br J Haematol, 1991, 79(4):624-7.
9. Lazarchick J, Russell R, and Horn B, "Maternal Platelet Antibody Levels in Neonatal Isoimmune Thrombocytopenia," Ann Clin Lab Sci, 1990, 20(3):200-4.
10. Freedman J and Hornstein A, "Simple Method for Differentiating Between HLA and Platelet-Specific Antibodies by Flow Cytometry," Am J Hematol, 1991, 38(4):314-20.

References

Andersen JC, "Response of Resistant Idiopathic Thrombocytopenic Purpura to Pulsed High-Dose Dexamethasone Therapy," N Engl J Med, 1994, 330(22):1560-4.
Deckmyn H and DeReys S, "Functional Effects of Human Antiplatelet Antibodies," Semin Thromb Hemost, 1995, 21(1):46-59.
George JN, "Platelet IgG: Measurement, Interpretation, and Clinical Significance," Prog Hemost Thromb, 1991, 10:97-126.
Karpatkin S, "Autoimmune Thrombocytopenic Purpura," Semin Hematol, 1985, 22(4):260-88.

McMillan R, "Clinical Role of Antiplatelet Antibody Assays," Semin Thromb Hemost, 1995, 21(1):37-45.
Schwartz KA, "Platelet Antibody: Review of Detection Methods," Am J Hematol, 1988, 29(2):106-14.
Waters AH, "Platelet and Neutrophil Antigens and Antibodies," Practical Haematology, 8th ed, Chapter 25, Dacie JV and Lewis SM, eds, New York, NY: Churchill Livingstone, 1995, 465-78.

Platelet Autoaggregation see Platelet Aggregation, Hypercoagulable State on previous page

Platelet Force Development by Clot Retractometry

Related Information

Aspirin Tolerance Test on page 232
Clot Retraction on page 235

Test Commonly Includes Lag phase prior to force development, maximum rate of force development (MRFD), maximum force generated (MFG)

Abstract This test provides quantitation of components of force developed during clot retraction. It is a research procedure that has been applied to the study of platelet function in patients with coronary artery disease (CAD), some of whom received aspirin therapy.

Specimen Whole blood for preparation of platelet rich plasma (PRP)

Container Blue top (sodium citrate, 3.8%) siliconized tube

Collection Blood obtained by venipuncture or from pre-existing arterial line

Storage Instructions Test is performed as soon as blood is obtained.

Special Instructions Either whole blood or platelet rich plasma may serve as the test sample. PRP is prepared by centrifugation at 500 g for 5 minutes at room temperature.

Reference Range At 37°C and platelet count 7.5×10^4:
- Lag phase: 160 seconds
- MRFD: 1.06 $dyne/cm^2$ seconds
- MFG: 4400 dynes
- Elastic modulus: 11.4 ±0.9 x 10^3 $dynes/cm^2$

Use Quantify some elements of clot retraction and thereby provide a marker of platelet function. May aid in delineating contributions of thromboxane and noncyclo-oygenase-mediated platelet activation in antiplatelet therapy.

Limitations Procedure is recently developed at Medical College of Virginia (Coagulation Special Studies Laboratory) and McGuire VA Medical Center. As such it currently has research status.

Methodology Clots are formed in a thermostated aluminum cup with an upper plate lowered into the clotting solution. Force is measured using a force displacement transducer, the transducer arm generating a voltage proportional to the force applied by platelets pulling the fibrin strands inward. A compression elastic modulus can be determined at the same time by monitoring the amount of downward deflection of the upper plate after application of a known force. The applied force (stress) and the amount of deflection (induced strain) when ratioed (stress/strain) results in the elastic modulus. Standard clotting conditions must be maintained as the procedure is ionic strength, calcium, fibrinogen, and temperature dependent.

Additional Information Application of this test procedure to platelet rich plasma of patients with CAD and either taking aspirin or aspirin free has indicated that significant noncyclo-oxygenase-dependent platelet activation persists despite more than 95% suppression of thromboxane B_2. Despite aspirin therapy, patients with severe CAD had apparent persistent platelet activation with rigid clot structure.[1]

Footnotes

1. Greilich PE, Carr ME, Zekert SL, et al, "Quantitative Assessment of Platelet Function and Clot Structure in Patients With Severe Coronary Artery Disease," Am J Med Sci, 1994, 307(1):15-20.

References

Carr ME Jr and Zekert SL, "Measurement of Platelet-Mediated Force Development During Plasma Clot Formation," Am J Med Sci, 1991, 302(1):13-8.

Platelet Function Studies see Platelet Aggregation on page 257

Platelet Impedance Aggregation in Whole Blood see Platelet Aggregation on page 257

Platelet Retention see Platelet Adhesion Test on page 256

Prekallikrein Assay see Factor, Fletcher on page 244

Proaccelerin see Factor V on page 239

Proconvertin see Factor VII on page 240

Protamine Sulfate see Activated Coagulation Time on page 226

Protamine Sulfate see Activated Partial Thromboplastin Time on page 227

Protamine Sulfate Test for Fibrin Split Products *see* Fibrin Split Products, Protamine Sulfate *on page 248*

Protein C

CPT 85302 (antigen); 85303 (activity)

Related Information

Factor V *on page 239*
Hypercoagulable State Coagulation Screen *on page 250*
Plasminogen Activator Inhibitor *on page 255*
Platelet Aggregation, Hypercoagulable State *on page 258*
Protein S *on next page*
Resistance to Activated Protein C *on page 265*
Thrombomodulin *on page 266*

Synonyms PC; Protein C Antigen; Protein C, Functional

Applies to Protein Ca; Tissue Plasminogen Activator (t-PA)

Specimen Plasma

Container Blue top (sodium citrate) tube

Collection Routine venipuncture. If multiple tests are being drawn, draw coagulation studies last. If only coagulation tests are being drawn, draw 1-2 mL into another Vacutainer® tube, discard, and then collect coagulation tests (double syringe/tube technique). This collection procedure avoids contamination of the specimen with tissue thromboplastins.

Storage Instructions May be stable for 1 month at -70°C.

Causes for Rejection Patient receiving heparin (exception: chromogenic substrate based methods)[1]

Turnaround Time 1 hour (automated synthetic substrate methods)

Special Instructions Determine if patient is on oral anticoagulants. Protein C (vitamin K dependent) levels may be decreased as a result of anticoagulation (as with coumarin derivatives). Snake venom activated chromogenic substrate based methods are not importantly affected by therapeutic levels of heparin.

Reference Range 70% to 150% of normal pooled plasma, 0.60-1.13 units/mL (chromogenic assay and ELISA).[2] Quantitative antigen and activity are decreased (one-third adult normal) at birth, gradually increase but remain low during the first month of life.[3] Values are significantly decreased in children (ages 1-16 years) as compared to adults; 1-5 years of age: 0.40-0.92 units/mL; 6-10 years of age: 0.45-0.93 units/mL; 11-16 years of age: 0.55-1.11 units/mL.[2]

Use Investigate patients with thromboses, especially venous thromboses in young adults; study of patients with hypercoagulable state

Limitations Caution must be used in interpreting decreased protein C levels obtained from coumarin-anticoagulated patient samples (protein C level is decreased in patients taking Coumadin®).

Methodology Enzyme-linked immunosorbent assay (ELISA), radioimmunoassay (RIA), rocket immunoelectrophoresis (Laurell), particle concentration fluorescent immunoassay.[4] Functional assays include determination of activated protein C by chromogenic substrate after harvesting with immobilized antiprotein C antibody or determination of the effect of Ca on prolonging the APTT of normal plasma. Recently, automated chromogenic synthetic substrate methods suited to batch testing and screening have been developed utilizing a snake venom protein C activator derived from the Southern copperhead snake (*Agkistrodon contortix*).[1,5] The generation of *p*-nitroaniline measured at 405 nm is proportional to the level of protein Ca.

Additional Information Protein C, a vitamin K dependent zymogen of a serine protease (activated protein C or Ca), has a molecular weight of 62,000 and neutralizes an inhibitor of tissue plasminogen activator (t-PA). It inactivates factors Va and VIIIa with prolongation of the conversion of prothrombin to thrombin by factor Xa. It thus has both profibrinolytic and anticoagulant properties. Protein C is synthesized in the liver and is activated to Ca rapidly by thrombin that has been bound by its endothelial cell receptor thrombomodulin. Protein Ca in the presence of protein S inhibits factor Va. By increasing the activity of t-PA, protein Ca enhances fibrinolysis. The protein C mechanism thus functions to prevent extension of intravascular thrombi.

Deficiency or functionally deficient forms of protein Ca are clinically, as would be expected, associated with thrombotic episodes. Griffin et al in 1981 described familial recurrent thrombophlebitis-associated with hereditary protein C deficiency.[6] Patients with partial protein C or with partial protein S deficiency (heterozygotes) may suffer venous thrombotic episodes, usually in early adult years. There may be deep vein thromboses, episodes of thrombophlebitis and/or pulmonary emboli, manifestations of a hypercoagulable state. Heterozygous protein C deficiency is an independent risk factor for the development of thrombotic episodes in some pedigrees.[7]

Homozygous protein C deficient patients have absent or near absent levels of C antigen and usually succumb in infancy with the picture of purpura fulminans neonatalis including lower extremity skin ecchymoses, anemia, fever, and shock. Heterozygous protein C deficient

patients are of type I in which there is decreased C antigen or type II with normal C antigen levels but decreased functional activity. Some 40% of type I protein C deficiencies may be caused by missense mutations resulting (by various mechanisms) in abnormal polypeptide chain structure and stability and responsible (at least in part) for the known phenotypic heterogeneity.[8] Protein C deficiency may be involved in some cases of Coumadin®-induced skin necrosis. Acquired deficiency may occur as with decreased protein C synthesis associated with liver disease. Patients may have combined deficiencies of protein C, antithrombin III, or protein S.[9]

The possible association of changes in protein C and/or protein S in patients having glomerular pathology with or without nephrosis has been studied (nephrotic patients are at risk for the development of thromboses). The mean levels of protein C, total protein S, and free protein S did not differ between patients with nephrosis and those without nephrosis. While mean free protein S levels were in the normal range for the four types of glomerular pathology studied, patients with diabetic glomerulopathy had significantly lower levels than those with membranous glomerulopathy. Hypercoagulability, however, is uncommon in patients with diabetic glomerulopathy but occurs with membranous glomerulonephritis. The presence of nephrosis, degree of proteinuria, or level of serum albumin did not correlate with changes in protein C or S.[10]

Resistance to protein Ca caused by an inherited defect in the factor V gene (factor V Leiden) with an Arg 506 to Gln replacement has recently been recognized.[11] It is inherited as autosomal dominant, causes significantly increased risk of thrombosis and is apparently the underlying defect in 20% to 60% of patients with unexplained thrombosis.[12] Resistance to protein Ca is perhaps the most common cause of pathologic thrombosis.

Decreased levels of protein C have been found during vaso-occlusive crises in children with sickle cell disease. With clinical improvement, protein C returned to preattack levels. In such cases, decreased levels of protein C may be due to increased consumption, as well as decreased production relating to changes in liver function.[13]

See tables, including Findings Indicative of Hypercoagulable State, in the listing Hypercoagulable State Coagulation Screen *on page 250*.

Footnotes

1. Walker PA, Bauer KA, and McDonagh J, "A Simple, Automated Functional Assay for Protein C," *Am J Clin Pathol*, 1989, 92(2):210-3.
2. Andrew M, Vegh P, Johnston M, et al, "Maturation of the Hemostatic System During Childhood," *Blood*, 1992, 80(8):1998-2005.
3. Takamiya O, Kinoshita S, Niinomi K, et al, "Protein C in the Neonatal Period," *Haemostasis*, 1989, 19(1):45-50.
4. Miletech JP and Broze GJ, "Plasma Protein C Antigen in the Normal Population: What Is a Deficiency?" *Circulation*, 1986, 74(2):92.
5. Hales SC, "Measurement of Protein C Activity on the Multistat III Plus," *Lab Med*, 1989, 20:484-6.
6. Griffin JH, Evatt B, Zimmerman TS, et al, "Deficiency of Protein C in Congenital Thrombotic Disease," *J Clin Invest*, 1981, 68:1370-3.
7. Bovill EG, Bauer KA, Dickerman JD, et al, "The Clinical Spectrum of Heterozygous Protein C Deficiency in a Large New England Kindred," *Blood*, 1989, 73(3):712-7.
8. Gandrille S and Aiach M, "Identification of Mutations in 90 of 121 Consecutive Symptomatic French Patients With a Type I Protein C Deficiency. The French INSERM Network on Molecular Abnormalities Responsible for Protein C and Protein S Deficiencies," *Blood*, 1995, 86(7):2598-605.
9. Bauer KA, Broekmans AW, Bertina RM, et al, "Hemostatic Enzyme Generation in the Blood of Patients With Hereditary Protein C Deficiency," *Blood*, 1988, 71(5):1418-26.
10. Allon M, Soffer O, Evatt BL, et al, "Protein S and C Antigen Levels in Proteinuric Patients: Dependence on Type of Glomerular Pathology," *Am J Hematol*, 1989, 31(2):96-101.
11. Dahlbäck B, "Molecular Genetics of Thrombophilia: Factor V Gene Mutation Causing Resistance to Activated Protein C as a Basis of the Hypercoagulable State," *J Lab Clin Med*, 1995, 125(5):566-711.
12. Griffin JH, Evatt B, Wideman C, et al, "Anticoagulant Protein C Pathway Defective in Majority of Thrombophilic Patients," *Blood*, 1993, 82(7):1989-93.
13. Karayalcin G and Lanzkowsky P, "Plasma Protein C Levels in Children With Sickle Cell Disease," *Am J Pediatr Hematol Oncol*, 1989, 11(3):320-3.

References

Berdeaux DH, Abshire TC, and Marlar RA, "Dysfunctional Protein C Deficiency (Type II) - A Report of 11 Cases in 3 American Families and Review of the Literature," *Am J Clin Pathol*, 1993, 99(6):677-86.

Brenner B, Shapira A, Bahari C, et al, "Hereditary Protein C Deficiency During Pregnancy," *Am J Obstet Gynecol*, 1987, 157(5):1160-1.

De Stefano V, Finazzi G, and Mannucci PM, "Inherited Thrombophilia: Pathogenesis, Clinical Syndromes, and Management," *Blood*, 1996, 87(9):3531-44.

Esmon NL, "Thrombomodulin," *Prog Hemost Thromb*, 1989, 9:29-55.

Harrison RL and Alperin JB, "Concurrent Protein C Deficiency and Lupus Anticoagulants," *Am J Hematol*, 1992, 40(1):33-7.

Manco-Johnson M and Nuss R, "Protein C Concentrate Prevents Peripartum Thrombosis," *Am J Hematol*, 1992, 40(1):69-70.

Marchetti G, Patracchini P, Gemmati D, et al, "Symptomatic Type II Protein C Deficiency Caused by a Missense Mutation (Gly 381 → Ser) in the Substrate-Binding Pocket," *Br J Haematol*, 1993, 84(2):285-9.

Melissari E and Kakkar VV, "Congenital Severe Protein C Deficiency in Adults," *Br J Haematol*, 1989, 72(2):222-8.

Rosenberg RD and Bauer KA, "New Insights Into Hypercoagulable States," *Hosp Pract (Off Ed)*, 1986, 21(3):131-8, 143, 147.

Schofield KP, Thomson JM, and Poller L, "Protein C Response to Induction and Withdrawal of Oral Anticoagulant Treatment," *Clin Lab Haematol*, 1987, 9(3):255-62.

Tollefson DF, Friedman KD, Marlar RA, et al, "Protein C Deficiency: A Cause of Unusual or Unexplained Thrombosis," *Arch Surg*, 1988, 123(7):881-4.

Protein Ca *see* Protein C *on previous page*

Protein C Antigen *see* Protein C *on previous page*

Protein C, Functional *see* Protein C *on previous page*

Protein S

CPT 85305 (total); 85306 (free)

Related Information

Hypercoagulable State Coagulation Screen *on page 250*

Inhibitor, Lupus, Phospholipid Type *on page 251*

Plasminogen Activator Inhibitor *on page 255*

Platelet Aggregation, Hypercoagulable State *on page 258*

Protein C *on previous page*

Resistance to Activated Protein C *on page 265*

Specimen Plasma

Container Blue top (sodium citrate) tube

Storage Instructions Sample may be stored up to 30 days at -20°C (preferably -70°C) prior to assay.

Turnaround Time 48 hours

Reference Range Total protein S, males: 78% to 103%; females: 70% to 122%; free protein S, males: 69% to 149%, females: 50% to 130%[1]; 0.60-1.13 units/mL using ELISA method, low end of ranges lower in children ages 1-16 (see reference by Andrew, et al).

Use Investigate the possibility of protein S deficiency. Of use in the evaluation of hypercoagulable states.

Limitations There is evidence that functional deficiency of protein S may occur in patients who have demonstrable protein S antigen.[2] Spurious low results may be obtained with plasma-based functional protein S assay in patients who have activated protein C resistance.[3]

Methodology Electroimmunodiffusion (Laurell rocket), enzyme immunoassay (EIA)[4] commercially available in kit form (both involve measurement of antigen by immunologic means after precipitation of S complexed C4b-binding protein). Functional screening procedure has been developed. This test measures the contribution of patient's plasma to a mixture of purified protein C activated by a venom activator, protein S deficient plasma, cephalin, and CaCl$_2$. The clotting time is compared to results obtained with assayed standards using a standard curve.[5]

Additional Information The activity of protein C is dependent upon a cofactor, protein S. Both protein C and protein S are vitamin K dependent coagulation proteins. Slightly over one-half of protein S is complexed with C 4b-binding protein and is inactive. The unbound fraction circulates in the plasma as the active form. Since protein S is required for the action of protein C, tendency to thrombosis would be expected (on a theoretic basis) in individuals with low levels of protein S. Recurrent thrombosis has been reported associated with congenital protein S deficiency.[6] Decrease in plasma protein S level has also been noted with use of oral contraceptives.[1] Before protein S deficiency can be excluded, both functional and antigenic levels should be studied.

Nonfamilial protein S deficiency has been reported in a 28-year old patient with inflammatory bowel disease and multiple episodes of deep vein thrombosis.[7] A possible role of congenital protein S deficiency in the development of intestinal arteriovenous malformations has been suggested.[8]

Presence of hypercoagulable state associated with decrease in free protein S levels has been reported with diabetic nephropathy, chronic renal failure due to hypertension, and antiphospholipid syndrome with cerebral venous thrombosis and coumarin-induced skin necrosis.[9,10]

Endothelial cells (which produce protein S) are the target of some anticardiolipin antibodies. Such antibodies have been found in association with deep vein thrombosis and decreased protein S activity with normal protein S antigen levels.[11]

See tables, including Findings Indicative of Hypercoagulable State, in listing Hypercoagulable State Coagulation Screen *on page 250*.

Footnotes

1. Boerger LM, Morris PC, Thurnau GR, et al, "Oral Contraceptives and Gender Affect Protein S Status," *Blood*, 1987, 69(2):692-4.
2. Comp PC, Doray D, Patton D, et al, "An Abnormal Plasma Distribution of Protein S Occurs in Functional Protein S Deficiency," *Blood*, 1986, 67(2):504-8.
3. Faioni EM, Franchi F, Asti D, et al, "Resistance to Activated Protein C in Nine Thrombophilic Families: Interference in a Protein S Functional Assay," *Thromb Haemost*, 1993, 70(6):1067-71.
4. Deutz-Terlouw P, Ballering L, van Wijngaarden A, et al, "Two ELISA's for Measurement of Protein S, and Their Use in the Laboratory Diagnosis of Protein S Deficiency," *Clin Chim Acta*, 1990, 186(3):321-34.
5. Kobayashi I, Amemiya N, Endo T, et al, "Functional Activity of Protein S Determined With Use of Protein C Activated by Venom Activator," *Clin Chem*, 1989, 35(8):1644-8.
6. Comp PC, Nixon RR, Cooper MR, et al, "Familial Protein S Deficiency Is Associated With Recurrent Thrombosis," *J Clin Invest*, 1984, 74(6):2082-8.
7. Wyshock E, Caldwell M, and Crowley JP, "Deep Venous Thrombosis, Inflammatory Bowel Disease, and Protein S Deficiency," *Am J Clin Pathol*, 1989, 90(5):633-5.
8. Guarner J, Grossman B, Judd R, et al, "Multiple Arteriovenous Malformations of the Small Intestine in a Patient With Protein S Deficiency," *Am J Clin Pathol*, 1989, 92(3):374-8.

9. Allon M, Soffer O, Evatt BL, et al, "Protein S and C Antigen Levels in Proteinuric Patients: Dependence on Type of Glomerular Pathology," *Am J Hematol*, 1989, 31(2):96-101.
10. Moreb J and Kitchens CS, "Acquired Functional Protein S Deficiency, Cerebral Venous Thrombosis, and Coumarin Skin Necrosis in Association With Antiphospholipid Syndrome: Report of Two Cases," *Am J Med*, 1989, 87(2):207-10.
11. Malnick SD and Sthoeger ZM, "Autoimmune Protein S Deficiency," *N Engl J Med*, 1993, 329(25):1898.

References

Andrew M, Vegh P, Johnston M, et al, "Maturation of the Hemostatic System During Childhood," *Blood*, 1992, 80(8):1998-2005.

Formstone CJ, Wacey AI, Berg LP, et al, "Detection and Characterization of Seven Novel Protein S (PROS) Gene Lesions: Evaluation of Reverse Transcript-Polymerase Chain Reaction as a Mutation Screening Strategy," *Blood*, 1995, 86(7):2632-41.

Graves-Hoagland RL and Walker FJ, "Laboratory Determination of Protein S," *Manual of Procedures for the Seminar on Diagnostic Hematology*, compiled by FW Sunderman, Institute for Clinical Science, Philadelphia, 1988.

Schwarz HP, Heeb MJ, Lottenberg R, et al, "Familial Protein S Deficiency With a Variant Protein S Molecule in Plasma and Platelets," *Blood*, 1989, 74(1):213-21.

Stahl CP, Wideman CS, Spira TJ, et al, "Protein S Deficiency in Men With Long-Term Human Immunodeficiency Virus Infection," *Blood*, 1993, 81(7):1801-7.

Prothrombin *see* Factor II *on page 238*

Prothrombin Fragment 1.2

CPT 85999

Related Information

Antithrombin III Test *on page 230*

Hypercoagulable State Coagulation Screen *on page 250*

Prothrombin Time *on next page*

Synonyms F 1.2; F1+2; Prothrombin Fragment F1+2

Abstract Prothrombin fragment 1.2 is released from prothrombin during thrombin formation. Thus it is a prothrombin activation fragment. This test has clinical application as a marker of thrombin formation. F 1.2 levels may assist in study of the hypercoagulable state, assessment of thrombotic risk, and in monitoring anticoagulant therapy.

Specimen Plasma, lithium heparin anticoagulant. Some ELISA methods use plasma from 3.8% sodium citrate anticoagulated blood

Storage Instructions Dilute plasma 9:1 (by volume) with an EDTA-containing anticoagulant for use with heparinized plasma, assay immediately or store at -20°C (stable for at least 3 months).[1]

Turnaround Time Currently, this test is not commonly available in most clinical environments and will be performed by a referral or reference laboratory. Some applications, however, would benefit from a rapid turnaround time.

Reference Range 0.21-2.78 nmol/L in healthy individuals up to 44 years of age. F 1.2 levels rise slightly with age older than 44 years (ELISA, monoclonal antibody based)

Use Assessment of prethrombotic (hypercoagulable) state, risk of thrombosis, efficacy of anticoagulant therapy[1]

Methodology Enzyme-linked immunosorbent assay (ELISA), monoclonal antibody based,[1,2] polyclonal

Additional Information With activation of prothrombin, factor Xa cleaves the bond Arg 273-Thr 274 resulting in liberation of prothrombin fragment F 1.2 and prethrombin 2. With cleavage of prethrombin, α-thrombin is formed. The latter enzyme converts fibrinogen to fibrin. Plasma F 1.2 is increased in clinical conditions in which there is increased risk of thrombosis. Such conditions have included patients with leukemia, severe liver disease, and postmyocardial infarction.[3] F 1.2 is decreased with oral anticoagulant therapy and in patients treated with antithrombin III.[1,4] Sample collection site, sex, and smoking status do not correlate significantly with the plasma concentration of F 1.2.[5] Venous occlusion for 2 minutes during sampling has not been noted to significantly alter plasma levels of F 1.2.[3]

Footnotes

1. Hursting MJ, Butman BT, Steiner JP, et al, "Monoclonal Antibodies Specific for Prothrombin Fragment 1.2 and Their Use in a Quantitative Enzyme-Linked Immunosorbent Assay," *Clin Chem*, 1993, 39(4):583-91.
2. Greenberg CS, Hursting MJ, Macik BG, et al, "Evaluation of Preanalytical Variables Associated With Measurement of Prothrombin Fragment 1.2," *Clin Chem*, 1994, 40(10):1962-9.
3. Bruhn HD, Conard J, Mannucci M, et al, "Multicentric Evaluation of a New Assay for Prothrombin Fragment F 1+2 Determination," *Thromb Haemost*, 1992, 68(4):413-7.
4. Rodeghiero F, Castaman G, Gugliotta L, et al, "Supranormal Antithrombin III Levels Induced by Concentrate Administration Are Ineffective in Quenching Thrombin Generation in Acute Promyelocytic Leukemia," *Thromb Res*, 1993, 69(4):377-85.
5. Hursting MJ, Stead AG, Crout FV, et al, "Effects of Age, Race, Sex, and Smoking on Prothrombin Fragment 1.2 in a Healthy Population," *Clin Chem*, 1993, 39(4):683-6.

References

Bauer KA and Rosenberg RD, "Congenital Antithrombin III Deficiency: Insights into the Pathogenesis of the Hypercoagulable State and Its Management Using Markers of Hemostatic System Activation," *Am J Med*, 1989, 87(3B):39S-43S.

Bauer KA and Rosenberg RD, "The Pathophysiology of the Prethrombotic State in Humans: Insights Gained From Studies Using Markers of Hemostatic System Activation," *Blood*, 1987, 70(2):343-50.

Millenson MM, Bauer KA, Kistler JP, et al, "Monitoring ©Mini-Intensity' Anticoagulation With Warfarin: Comparison of the Prothrombin Time Using a Sensitive Thromboplastin With Prothrombin Fragment F 1+2 Levels," *Blood*, 1992, 79(8):2034-8.

(Continued)

Prothrombin Fragment 1.2 *(Continued)*

Solymoss S and Bovill EG, "Markers of *In Vivo* Activation of Anticoagulation. Interrelationships Change With Intensity of Oral Anticoagulation," *Am J Clin Pathol*, 1996, 105(3):293-7.

Prothrombin Fragment F1+2 *see* Prothrombin Fragment 1.2 *on previous page*

Prothrombin Time

CPT 85610

Related Information

Albumin and Plasma Protein Fraction for Infusion *on page 601*
Blood, Urine *on page 631*
Coagulation Factor Assay *on page 235*
Cryoprecipitate *on page 606*
Factor II *on page 238*
Factor VII *on page 240*
Liver Profile *on page 161*
Plasma, Fresh Frozen *on page 615*
Prothrombin Fragment 1.2 *on previous page*
Warfarin *on page 579*

Synonyms Protime; PT

Applies to Coumarins; INR; International Normalized Ratio; PT Ratio

Test Commonly Includes Patient time and control time

Abstract A simple, low cost test useful for the evaluation of the extrinsic system of coagulation as it is sensitive to reduced levels of factors II, VII, and X. It is the time, in seconds, required for clot formation after addition of calcium and thromboplastin. A common application is monitoring the effect of warfarin type anticoagulation.

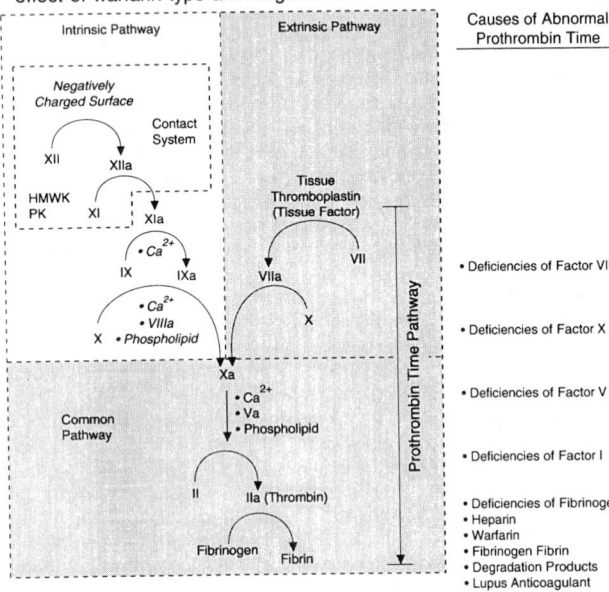

The prothrombin time (PT) of plasma was developed by Quick in 1935. Clotting is initiated by the addition of calcium and tissue thromboplastin, an extract containing both phospholipid and the glycoprotein now known as tissue factor. Because acquired fibrinogen deficiency was thought to be uncommon, and factors V, VII and X had not been discovered, Quick concluded that a prolongation of PT was due to prothrombin deficiency. It is now recognized that this test depends on the functional integrity of the entire extrinsic pathway.

From Lind SE, "The Hemostatic System," *Blood: Principles and Practice of Hematology*, Chapter 33, Handin RI, Lux SE, and Stossel EP, eds, Philadelphia, PA: JB Lippincott Co, 1995, 961, with permission.

Specimen Plasma

Container Blue top (sodium citrate) tube

Collection Routine venipuncture. If multiple tests are being drawn, draw coagulation studies last. If only a prothrombin time is being drawn, two-syringe collection technique is recommended to avoid contamination of the specimen with tissue thromboplastins.

Storage Instructions Plasma should be separated from cells as soon as possible and refrigerated if testing cannot be immediately performed. Testing should be performed within 4 hours.

Causes for Rejection Tube not full; specimen clotted; specimen hemolyzed, lipemic, or icteric (possible interference with photo-optical clot detection); specimen received more than 3-4 hours after collection;

specimen contaminated by anticoagulant, effect of which is not the primary reason for performing the test (eg, heparin)

Special Instructions Transport specimen to the Hematology Laboratory as soon as possible.

Reference Range 10-13 seconds. Healthy premature newborns have prolonged coagulation test screening results (eg, PT, APTT, TT) which return to normal adult values at about 6 months of age. Healthy prematures, however, do not develop spontaneous hemorrhage or thrombotic complications because of a balance between procoagulants and inhibitors (see references by Andrew et al). See table. The normal range in childhood (ages 1-16) is similar to that in adults.[1]

Effect of Drugs on Anticoagulation and Monitoring Using the Prothrombin Time

Drug	PT	Increase in Coumarin*
Amiodarone	↑	S
Anabolic steroids	↑	S
Ancrod	↑	S
Antacids	↓	R
Barbiturates	↓	R
Carbamazepine	↓	R
Cephalosporins, 2nd, 3rd generation	↑	S
Cefamandole, 2nd, 3rd generation	↑	S
Chloral hydrate		None
Chloramphenicol		S
Cholestyramine	↓	R
Cimetidine (rarely)	↑	S
Clofibrate	↑	S
Corticosteroids		R
Disulfiram	↑	S
Erythromycin	↑	S
Estrogen	↑	S
Ethchlorvynol	↓	R
Fluconazole	↑	S
Glucagon		S
Glutethimide	↓	R
Griseofulvin	↓	R
Ibuprofen	↑	S
Ketoconazole	↑	
Meprobamate		R
Metronidazole	↑	S
Miconazole		S
Nafcillin	↓	R
Nonsteroidal AID, many		S
Oral contraceptives	↓	R
Oral hypoglycemic agents		S
Phenylbutazone	↑	S
Phenytoin sodium	↑	S
Piroxicam	↑	S
Primidone	↓	R
Propafenone	↑	S
Quinidine	↑	S
Rifampin	↓	R
Salicylates (aspirin)		
Sucralfate	↓	R
Sulfamethoxazole trimethoprim	↑	S
Sulfinpyrazone	↑	S
Tamoxifen	↑	
Tolbutamide		S
Tolmetin	↑	S
Vitamin E (large amount)	↑	S

*R = resistance, S = sensitivity.

Possible Panic Range Nonanticoagulated: >20 seconds; anticoagulated: more than three times control

Use Evaluate extrinsic coagulation system; aid in screening for congenital deficiencies of factors II, V, VII, X; screen for deficiency of prothrombin; evaluate dysfibrinogenemia, afibrinogenemia (complete); evaluate heparin effect, coumarin or warfarin effect; liver failure; disseminated intravascular coagulation (DIC); screen for vitamin K deficiency

Limitations Prothrombin times drawn less than 2 hours after heparin administration will be prolonged (sensitivity to heparin effect is reagent thromboplastin dependent). The number of drugs which modify the hypo-prothrombinemic action of the coumarins is remarkable.[2] Included are barbiturates, chloral hydrate, chloramphenicol, clofibrate, ethchlorvynol, glutethimide, phenylbutazone, phenyramidol, quinidine, allopurinol, anabolic steroids, MAO-inhibitors, nortriptyline, phenytoin, propylthiour-acil, antacids, sulfonamides, salicylates, carbamazepine, estrogenic contraceptives, and griseofulvin.[2] Drugs lowering the PT include ethchlorvynol, glutethimide, anabolic steroids, antacids, estrogenic contraceptives, and griseofulvin. Nafcillin has been associated with warfarin resistance.[3]

The prothrombin time determination is sensitive to the ratio of plasma to citrate anticoagulant. That is, if enough blood is not added to the liquid citrate-containing tube when the specimen is drawn (tube usually contains 0.5 mL of 3.2% or 3.8% sodium citrate), a falsely elevated prothrombin time may result. The minimum amount of blood in the tube necessary to a reliable PT is therefore not readily predictable. **The citrate tube for PT/PTT must be completely filled.** An excellent discussion of important technical considerations in performance of the prothrombin time is given in the text by Sirridge and Shannon (reference following).

Antibiotic therapy and prolonged prothrombin time: Broad-spectrum antibiotics, in particular second- and third-generation cephalosporins exert a hypoprothrombinemic effect. Destruction of menaquinone-producing GI bacteria and/or interference with prothrombin synthesis by N-methyl-thio-tetrazole side chains has resulted in recommendations that prophylactic vitamin K administration be considered.[4,5] A study controlled for condition and treatment variables by univariate and multi-variate statistical analyses revealed, after multiple logistic regression analyses, increased risk of bleeding with the β-lactam antibiotics, moxa-lactam and possibly cefoxitin.[6]

Methodology The clotting time of citrate anticoagulated plasma is deter-mined after the addition of an optimum concentration of calcium and an excess of thromboplastin. Clot detection is by manual (tilt tube visual) or, more commonly by an automated device for fibrin clot detection, elec-trode, electro-optical or other method. The result is always reported with that obtained on a commercial normal control plasma run at the same time. Coumatrak Protime Monitor® is a capillary whole blood (25 μL) method suitable for bedside testing.[7] A laser photometer detects cessa-tion of flow by sensing change in light scatter from red blood cells. Time elapsed is converted to a plasma equivalent PT. Attempts to standardize prothrombin time results has led to growing interest in reporting of the "international normalized ratio" (INR).[8,9] See comments under Additional Information concerning INR and International Sensitivity Index (ISI). Chromogenic assays for determination of prothrombin have been devel-oped. If the PT is prolonged repeat testing using half patient and half normal control plasma will identify presence of a circulating anticoagu-lant (prolonged PT will not correct). Further testing with aged serum (source of VII and X) and adsorbed plasma (source of V) may define the nature of the abnormality (see reference by Sirridge).

Additional Information Control of coumarin derivative (warfarin) therapy: The warfarin type anticoagulants act by inhibiting enzymes (vitamin K epoxide reductase and vitamin K quinone reductase) respon-sible for the conversion of vitamin K epoxide to vitamin KH_2. The latter has an obligatory role in the activation (through carboxylation) of the proenzyme forms of factors II, VII, IX, and X. Long-term anticoagulant therapy usually involves the use of a coumarin derivative (eg, Coumadin®). The prothrombin time (PT) provides for "control" of the dosage. The attempt is to impede thrombus formation without the threat of morbidity or mortality from hemorrhage. In the past this goal has been approached by administering a Coumadin® dosage that prolongs the PT to twice that of a normal control plasma. More recently it is considered that lower dosage of warfarin derivatives (Coumadin®, dicumarol, Tromexan®) provide effective prophylaxis against thrombosis without excessive risk of hemorrhage. Warfarin anticoagulant effect occurs gradually. Without a loading dose, 7.5 mg/day of warfarin anticoagulant will produce desired therapeutic effect in 5-7 days. With a loading dose of 10-15 mg the anticoagulant effect can be achieved in some 3 days but with greater risk of bleeding. When warfarin compounds are discon-tinued the PT will require 2-4 days to return to normal. If oral vitamin K is given PT returns to normal within about 24 hours. The overanticoagu-lated state can be quickly reversed by giving intramuscular vitamin K.

As a result of a series of conferences on antithrombotic therapy held in 1985, 1989, 1992, and most recently in 1995 (Fourth American College of Chest Physicians (ACCP) Consensus Conference on Antithrombotic Therapy), the earlier recommendation that the intensity of warfarin therapy be reduced (for most indications) has found support in the results of subsequent clinical trials. The ACCP recommends use of the INR for monitoring oral (warfarin-coumarin derivative) therapy. INR of 2.0-3.0 is recommended for all conditions with the exception of patients anticoagulated for thrombotic complications of mechanical heart valves for which an INR of 2.5-3.5 is recommended.[10] Use of a thromboplastin with high sensitivity is recommended.

Warfarin therapy can be started soon after the onset of heparin therapy in patients with venous thromboembolic disease with resultant savings in hospitalization costs.[11] A 1-year course of warfarin therapy may be needed for patients with prior deep vein thrombosis and indefinite treat-ment if there have been over two previous episodes.[12]

The characteristics of thromboplastins including results of human brain vs rabbit brain thromboplastin and the ISI (International Sensitivity Index) have been studied.[13] Consistency in the practice of warfarin (coumarin) anticoagulation relating to its control by use of prothrombin time results has been elusive. This is due to variability in the sensitivity of thrombo-plastins. Historically, thromboplastins prepared locally by hospital labora-tories and the human brain thromboplastin Manchester Comparative Reagent, used as a reference plasma in the United Kingdom (UK), were more sensitive than rabbit brain or mixed commercial thromboplastin reagents introduced subsequently in North America.[14] Continued adher-ence to a 1948 American Heart Association recommendation that the therapeutic ranges for oral anticoagulation be kept at 2.0-2.5 that of a control PT (prothrombin time ratio of 2.0-2.5) led to a higher degree of anticoagulation. There was resultant increase in morbidity/mortality from bleeding. Nonhuman (largely rabbit) thromboplastins have also come into routine use throughout the UK (with advice to use the International Normalized Ratio) since withdrawal of Manchester Comparative Reagent in 1986.[15]

The variability in sensitivity of thromboplastins with resultant lack of between laboratory comparability of PT test results provided stimulus for standardization. In 1983, the International Normalized Ratio (INR) system was adopted by the International Committee for Standardization in Haematology, International Committee on Thrombosis and Haemos-tasis (ISCH/ICTH).[16] This system is based on the first World Health Organization (WHO) primary international reference preparation of thromboplastin. It has been considered to be an accepted international standard for clinical use.[14] The system is centered about the concept of an International Sensitivity Index (ISI). The ISI represents the respon-siveness of a thromboplastin to reduction in vitamin K-dependent factors. The ISI is derived by calibrating a thromboplastin reagent with a refer-ence preparation. Use is made of a linear relation between the logarithm of the prothrombin time ratio of the reference material and that of the test thromboplastin. The goal of standardized reporting of the prothrombin time would be met with a reliable ISI in hand (provided by the manufac-turer of the reagent thromboplastin) allowing conversion of the prothrombin time ratio measured with that reagent thromboplastin into an INR according to the formula: INR = (PT ratio)^{ISI} = (patient PT/mean normal PT)^{ISI} where ISI is the International Sensitivity Index. The "mean normal PT" should be the geometric as opposed to the arithmetic mean PT. It is important to avoid large biases in determining the reference mean.[17] Recent generation coagulation instruments, when provided with the ISI value, will calculate and report the INR value. Theoretically, the INR is the PT ratio that would result if the WHO reference thromboplastin had been used in performing the test.

Acceptance (use) of the INR system by the North American medical community has been slow, leading to criticism and impassioned pleas for education and compliance.[14,18,19,20] Reliability of the INR system, however, which depends upon a valid ISI has recently come into ques-tion.[21,22,23,24,25,26,27] Ng et al could not obtain consistent reagent-inde-pendent INR values within three related laboratories and note reports that some automated coagulation analyzers produce inconsistent INR values.[21] Swaim emphasizes the importance of ensuring that "ISI assign-ments permit accurate "normalization" of PT ratios." He has provided nine general recommendations to improve the INR system.[22] These include use of a single master International Reference Plasma, instru-ment-specific ISIs, commercial ISI assignments appropriate to specific instrument-thromboplastin combinations, ISI assignments based on three or more ISI determinations, and use of reagents with low ISI values (high sensitivity thromboplastins).

A growing number of recent reports appear to reflect continuing uncer-tainty and controversy about both the INR and the appropriate level (intensity) of warfarin anticoagulation. The following represents only a sampling of concerns and recommendations.

- Need for use of a reliable plasma calibrant and local ISI determina-tion.[28,29,30]

- Use of thromboplastins insensitive to heparin (eg, recombinant tissue factor) to avoid heparin-induced increase in the INR.[31]

- Dutch Thrombosis Centers find risk of hemorrhage acceptable and urge more intensive anticoagulation than current British/American "moderate intensity" warfarin regimens (eg, recommend levels of 3.0-4.0 INR dependent upon clinical condition).[32] Others find that even with reduced intensity of treatment, bleeding remains the most

(Continued)

Prothrombin Time *(Continued)*

common side effect.[33] Attention to drug interactions and careful monitoring can minimize risk.[32,33]

- Delta method (use of product of ISI and coefficient of variance for the PT assay) has been proposed to assess random error.[34]
- Avoidance of overshooting and resultant "ping-pong" effect in dosage adjustment as the result of random fluctuation in serial INR determinations.[35]

Recombinant human tissue factor, with very low ISI of 1.0 ±0.1, has been developed and is commercially available. rTF reagents are more sensitive to lower levels of factors II, VII, IX, and X. Thromboplastin reagents are not equivalent. Results from use of rTF reagents are not comparable to those obtained with mammalian thromboplastins when testing oral anticoagulated patients.[36] Use of such a thromboplastin reagent may allow for accurate and uniform reporting of PT results as an INR.

Use of a native prothrombin assay to monitor warfarin anticoagulation is reported to result in a lower incidence of bleeding and thrombotic complications as compared to use of the prothrombin time.[37] This radioimmunoassay utilizes an antibody specific for native prothrombin and as such is not yet available for routine coagulation testing.

The prothrombin time has been shown to lack sensitivity (in its current form) as a monitor for the anticoagulant effect of recombinant hirudin (originally an anticoagulant from the medicinal leech *Hirudo medicinalis*).[38] See listing Hirudin Determination *on page 249*.

A study involving warfarin-derivative anticoagulated outpatients (562) found a 2% incidence of fatal bleeding, a 10% incidence of nonfatal major bleeding and a 12% incidence of minor bleeding. Important remedial lesions were present in 38% of cases with major bleeding. These lesions were unknown prior to bleeding, however, and represent a diagnostic yield from investigation of patients who bleed.[39,40]

Specially designed devices have been developed (eg, paramagnetic iron-oxide technology based Thrombolytic Assessment System) for use in point-of-care testing.[42]

Footnotes

1. Andrew M, Vegh P, Johnston M, et al, "Maturation of the Hemostatic System During Childhood," *Blood*, 1992, 80(8):1998-2005.
2. Bick RL, *Disorders of Thrombosis and Hemostasis: Clinical and Laboratory Practice*, Chicago, IL: American Society of Clinical Pathologists, 1992, 297.
3. Fraser GL, Miller M, and Kane K, "Warfarin Resistance Associated With Nafcillin Therapy," *Am J Med*, 1989, 87(2):237-8.
4. Lipsky JJ, "N-methyl-thio-tetrazole Inhibition of the Gamma Carboxylation of Glutamic Acid: Possible Mechanism for Antibiotic-Associated Hypoprothrombinemia," *Lancet*, 1983, 2:192-3.
5. Bechtold H, Andrassy K, Jahnchen E, et al, "Evidence for Impaired Hepatic Vitamin K$_1$ Metabolism in Patients Treated With N-methyl-thiotetrazole Cephalosporins," *Thromb Haemost*, 1984, 51(3):358-61.
6. Brown RB, Klar J, Lemeshow S, et al, "Enhanced Bleeding With Cefoxitin or Moxalactam. Statistical Analysis Within a Defined Population of 1493 Patients," *Arch Intern Med*, 1986, 146(11):2159-64.
7. Ansell JE, Hamke AK, Holden A, et al, "Cost-Effectiveness of Monitoring Warfarin Therapy Using Standard Versus Capillary Prothrombin Times," *Am J Clin Pathol*, 1989, 91(5):587-9.
8. Hirsh J, "Is the Dose of Warfarin Prescribed by American Physicians Unnecessarily High?" *Arch Intern Med*, 1987, 147(4):769-71.
9. Poller L, "A Simple Nomogram for the Derivation of International Normalized Ratios for the Standardization of Prothrombin Times," *Thromb Haemost*, 1988, 60(1):18-20.
10. Hirsh J, Dalen JE, Deykin D, et al, "Oral Anticoagulants: Mechanism of Action, Clinical Effectiveness, and Optimal Therapeutic Ranges," *Chest*, 1995, 108(Suppl 4):231S-46S.
11. Rosiello RA, Chan CK, Tencza F, et al, "Timing of Oral Anticoagulation Therapy in the Treatment of Angiographically Proven Acute Pulmonary Embolism," *Arch Intern Med*, 1987, 147(8):1469-73.
12. Hirsh J and Hull RD, "Treatment of Venous Thromboembolism," *Chest*, 1986, 89(5 Suppl):426S-33S.
13. Denson KW, "Thromboplastin - Sensitivity, Precision, and Other Characteristics," *Clin Lab Haematol*, 1988, 10(3):315-28.
14. Hirsh J, "Oral Anticoagulant Drugs," *N Engl J Med*, 1991, 324(26):1865-75.
15. Poller L, Taberner DA, Thomson JM, et al, "Survey of Prothrombin Time in National External Quality Assessment Scheme Exercises (1980-87)," *J Clin Pathol*, 1988, 41(4):361-4.
16. "International Committee for Standardization in Haematology, International Committee on Thrombosis and Haemostasis: ICSH/ICTH Recommendations for Reporting Prothrombin Time in Oral Anticoagulant Control," *Thromb Haemost*, 1985, 53(1):155-6.
17. Critchfield GC and Bennett ST, "The Influence of the Reference Mean Prothrombin Time on the International Normalized Ratio," *Am J Clin Pathol*, 1994, 102(6):806-11.
18. Bussey HI, Force RW, Bianco TM, et al, "Reliance on Prothrombin Time Ratios Causes Significant Errors in Anticoagulation Therapy," *Arch Intern Med*, 1992, 152(2):278-82.
19. Hirsh J, "Substandard Monitoring of Warfarin in North America: Time for Change," *Arch Intern Med*, 1992, 152(2):257-8.
20. Ansell JE, "Imprecision of Prothrombin Time Monitoring of Oral Anticoagulation: A Survey of Hospital Laboratories," *Am J Clin Pathol*, 1992, 98(2):237-9.
21. Ng VL, Levin J, Corash L, et al, "Failure of the International Normalized Ratio to Generate Consistent Results Within a Local Medical Community," *Am J Clin Pathol*, 1993, 99(6):689-94.
22. Swaim WR, "Prothrombin Time Reporting and the International Normalized Ratio System: Improvements Are Needed," *Am J Clin Pathol*, 1993, 99(6):653-5.
23. Poller L, Thomson JM, and Taberner DA, "Effect of Automation on Prothrombin Time Test in NEQAS Surveys," *J Clin Pathol*, 1989, 42(10):97-100.
24. Taberner DA, Poller L, Thomson JM, et al, "Effect of International Sensitivity Index (ISI) of Thromboplastins on Precision of International Normalised Ratios (INR)," *J Clin Pathol*, 1989, 42(10):92-6.
25. Poller L, Taberner DA, Thomson JM, et al, "Effect of the Choice of WHO International Reference Preparation for Thromboplastin on International Normalised Ratios," *J Clin Pathol*, 1993, 46(1):64-6.
26. Hirsh J, "Inadequate Monitoring of Warfarin Dosage," *Blood*, 1992, 80(2):562-3.
27. Le DT, Weibert RT, Sevilla BK, et al, "The International Normalized Ratio (INR) for Monitoring Warfarin Therapy: Reliability and Relation to Other Monitoring Methods," *Ann Intern Med*, 1994, 120(7):552-8.
28. Ford K, McArdle B, and Kesteven PJ, "A Comparison of Five Commercial Thromboplastins: ISI Re-Evaluation on an Automated Coagulometer," *Clin Lab Haematol*, 1995, 17(1):41-5.
29. Poller L, Triplett DA, Hirsh J, et al, "A Comparison of Lyophilized Artificially Depleted Plasmas and Lyophilized Plasmas From Patients Receiving Warfarin in Correcting for Coagulometer Effects on International Normalized Ratios," *Am J Clin Pathol*, 1995, 103(3):366-71.
30. Poller L, Triplett DA, Hirsh J, et al, "The Value of Plasma Calibrants in Correcting Coagulometer Effects on International Normalized Ratios: An International Multicenter Study," *Am J Clin Pathol*, 1995, 103(3):358-65.
31. Solomon HM, Randall JR, and Simmons VL, "Heparin-Induced Increase in the International Normalized Ratio - Responses of 10 Commercial Thromboplastin Reagents," *Am J Clin Pathol*, 1995, 103(6):735-9.
32. Loeliger EA, "Therapeutic Target Values in Oral Anticoagulation - Justification of Dutch Policy and a Warning Against the So-Called Moderate-Intensity Regimens," *Ann Hematol*, 1992, 64(2):60-5.
33. Raj G, Kumar R, and McKinney WP, "Long-Term Oral Anticoagulant Therapy: Update on Indications, Therapeutic Ranges, and Monitoring," *Am J Med Sci*, 1994, 307(2):128-32.
34. Inciardi JF, "Assessing Random Error in the International Normalized Ratio," *Ther Drug Monit*, 1994, 16(4):425-6.
35. Lassen JF, Kjeldsen J, Antonsen S, et al, "Interpretation of Serial Measurements of International Normalized Ratio for Prothrombin Times in Monitoring Oral Anticoagulant Therapy," *Clin Chem*, 1995, 41(8 Pt 1):1171-6.
36. Hoppensteadt DA, Walena JM, Fareed J, et al, "Comparing r-Tissue Factor and Mammalian Tissue Reagents for Prothrombin Time," *Lab Med*, 1995, 26(3):198-203.
37. Furie B, Diguid CF, Jacobs M, et al, "Randomized Prospective Trial Comparing the Native Prothrombin Antigen With the Prothrombin Time for Monitoring Oral Anticoagulant Therapy," *Blood*, 1990, 75(2):344-9.
38. Walenga JM, Pifarre R, Hoppensteadt DA, et al, "Development of Recombinant Hirudin as a Therapeutic Anticoagulant and Antithrombotic Agent: Some Objective Considerations," *Semin Thromb Hemost*, 1989, 15(3):316-33.
39. Landefeld CS and Goldman L, "Major Bleeding in Outpatients Treated With Warfarin: Incidence and Prediction by Factors Known at the Start of Outpatient Therapy," *Am J Med*, 1989, 87(2):144-52.
40. Landefeld CS, Rosenblatt MW, and Goldman L, "Bleeding in Outpatients Treated With Warfarin: Relation to the Prothrombin Time and Important Remedial Lesions," *Am J Med*, 1989, 87(2):153-9.
42. Oberhardt BJ, "Thrombosis and Hemostasis Testing at the Point of Care," *Am J Clin Pathol*, 1995, 104(Suppl 1):S72-8.

References

Andrew M, "Developmental Hemostasis: Relevance to Hemostatic Problems During Childhood," *Semin Thromb Hemost*, 1995, 21(4):341-56.

Andrew M, Paes B, Milner R, et al, "Development of the Human Coagulation System in the Healthy Premature Infant," *Blood*, 1988, 72(5):1651-7.

Cunningham MT and Olson JD, "Lower Interinstrument Variability of the International Normalized Ratio With the Coagamate X2/Simplastin Excel System," *Am J Clin Pathol*, 1996, 105(3):301-4.

D'Angelo A, Seveso MP, D'Angelo SV, et al, "Comparison of Two Automated Coagulometers and the Manual Tilt Tube Method for the Determination of Prothrombin Time," *Am J Clin Pathol*, 1989, 92(3):321-8.

James AH, Britt RP, Raskino CL, et al, "Factors Affecting the Maintenance Dose of Warfarin," *J Clin Pathol*, 1992, 45(8):704-6.

Litin SC and Gastineau DA, "Current Concepts in Anticoagulant Therapy," *Mayo Clin Proc*, 1995, 70(3):266-72.

Millenson MM, Bauer KA, Kistler JP, et al, "Monitoring ©Mini-Intensity' Anticoagulation With Warfarin: Comparison of the Prothrombin Time Using a Sensitive Thromboplastin With Prothrombin Fragment F 1+2 Levels," *Blood*, 1992, 79(8):2034-8.

Poller L and Hirsh J, "Special Report: A Simple System for the Derivation of International Normalized Ratios for the Reporting of Prothrombin Time Results With North American Thromboplastin Reagents," *Am J Clin Pathol*, 1989, 92(1):124-6.

Weinmann EE and Salzman EW, "Deep-Vein Thrombosis," *N Engl J Med*, 1994, 331(24):1630-41 (review).

Protime see Prothrombin Time *on page 262*

PT see Prothrombin Time *on page 262*

PTA see Factor XI *on page 243*

3P Test see Fibrin Split Products, Protamine Sulfate *on page 248*

PT Ratio see Prothrombin Time *on page 262*

PTT see Activated Partial Thromboplastin Time *on page 227*

PTT Substitution see Activated Partial Thromboplastin Substitution Test *on page 226*

Quantitative Fibrinogen see Fibrinogen *on page 246*

RAPC see Resistance to Activated Protein C *on next page*

Reptilase®-R Time

CPT 85635

Related Information

Thrombin Time *on page 266*

Abstract A clotting time procedure similar to the thrombin time but clotting is produced by action of the snake venom enzyme, Reptilase®.

Specimen Plasma

Container Plastic (preferred) coagulation tube with sodium citrate liquid anticoagulant. Invert tube gently 5-10 times to mix and prevent clotting.

Collection By venipuncture only. Avoid contamination of specimen with tissue thromboplastin. Deliver immediately to the laboratory.

Causes for Rejection Specimen clotted, hemolyzed, received in laboratory more than 2 hours after collection

Turnaround Time Approximately 45 minutes

Reference Range 18-22 seconds

Use Aids in distinguishing hypofibrinogenemias from heparin contamination and from effects of fibrin degradation products

Methodology A plasma clotting time is determined using Reptilase®-R reagent to activate and transform fibrinogen

Additional Information Reptilase®-R has an action similar to that of thrombin, it clots fibrinogen. It is isolated from *Bothrops atrox* snake venom. It differs from thrombin's action on fibrinogen by releasing only fibrinopeptide A (thrombin hydrolyzes both fibrinopeptide A and B from fibrinogen). Reptilase®-R time is not inhibited by heparin and can be substituted for the thrombin time in fibrinogen evaluation in heparinized patients. In cases of afibrinogenemia and some cases of dysfibrinogenemia both the thrombin time and the Reptilase®-R time will be prolonged. In evaluation of a patient with hypercoagulability normal thrombin time or Reptilase® time essentially excludes presence of an abnormal fibrinogen.[1] Reptilase® time is infinitely prolonged in cases of congenital afibrinogenemia and cases of dysfibrinogenemias with the exception of fibrinogen Oklahoma and fibrinogen Oslow. If heparin effect is the only cause of a prolonged prothrombin time, the Reptilase®-R time will be normal.

Footnotes

1. Mammen EF and Fujii Y, "Hypercoagulable States," *Lab Med*, 1989, 20:611-2.

References

Wyrick-Glatzel J and Gwaltney-Krause S, "Laboratory Methods in Hematology and Hemostasis," *Clinical Hematology and Fundamentals of Hemostasis*, Chapter 31, Harmening DM, ed, Philadelphia, PA: FA Davis Co, 1992.

Resistance to Activated Protein C

Related Information

Activated Partial Thromboplastin Time *on page 227*
Factor V *on page 239*
Hypercoagulable State Coagulation Screen *on page 250*
Platelet Aggregation, Hypercoagulable State *on page 258*
Protein C *on page 260*
Protein S *on page 261*
Thrombomodulin *on next page*

Synonyms APC-R; APC Resistance; aPTT/APC Screening Test; RAPC

Abstract The effect of activated protein C (APC) on patient's activated partial thromboplastin time (APTT) is used to detect presence of resistance to APC (as occurs in individuals with the gene mutation factor V Leiden).

Specimen Plasma

Container Blue top (sodium citrate) tube

Collection Routine venipuncture. If multiple tests are being drawn, draw sample for this test and any other coagulation tests last. If only this modified APTT test is being drawn, draw 1-2 mL into another Vacutainer®, discard, and then collect specimen (two-tube or two-syringe technique).

Causes for Rejection Tube not full, specimen hemolyzed, specimen clotted, specimen received more than 2 hours after collection, specimen improperly labeled, patient on anticoagulation therapy

Reference Range Affected individuals will show APC-dependent prolongation of the clotting time below the 5th percentile of controls.

Contraindications Concurrent warfarin type anticoagulation or heparin/heparin analogue therapy

Methodology APTT-based determination of the anticoagulant response in patient plasma to added purified APC.[1] Commercial versions of this "APC-APTT" test are available. (Coatest APC resistance kit from Chromogenix). Test provides a measure of the APC-dependent prolongation of the clotting time (APTT), in essence, of the ability of APC to act as an anticoagulant. PCR (polymerase chain reaction) method has been developed and is not affected by anticoagulants.[2,3]

Additional Information Resistance to APC is a major cause of unexplained recurrent thrombosis.[4] Initially recognized as a poor anticoagulant response to activated protein C, a cofactor to activated protein C was suspected. It now appears that the "cofactor" in the great majority, if not all cases, is a mutant factor V molecule.[3] The anticoagulant function of protein C is initiated after the binding of thrombin to thrombomodulin on the endothelial cell membrane. Protein C is then converted to its active enzyme form and as such inactivates factor V (active) and factor VIII (active). Most patients with APC resistance have an abnormal factor

V molecule (factor V Leiden) which in its active form is resistant to the proteolytic effect of APC. Thus, the anticoagulant effect of activated protein C is diminished, and the patient has increased tendency to thrombosis. Factor V Leidin is characterized by a single point mutation in the factor V gene (at nucleotide position 1,691 G → A substitution) which results in the synthesis of a factor V protein with an Agr 506 → Gln replacement.[3] This mutant factor V cannot be properly cleaved (inactivated) by APC. It appears that resistance to APC is the most common cause of unexplained thrombosis, accounting for some 13% to 60% of such patients dependent in part upon study group selection criteria.[4,5,6] A population-based case-control study found a 5% incidence of resistance to APC among 301 healthy control subjects.[5] Factor V Leiden, with a gene frequency of some 2%,[3] has been considered to be the most common hereditary coagulation disorder yet described.[2] At least some patients with recurrent deep vein and/or other thrombotic conditions previously attributed to a variety of mechanisms (eg, oral contraceptive therapy) are in reality the result of resistance to activated protein C.[2]

Protein C activator reagent (PCA) is more stable than APC. Use of PCA forms the basis of a recently proposed screening test for resistance to APC as well as for protein C and/or protein S deficiency.[7]

Footnotes

1. Dahlbäck B, Carlsson M, and Svensson PJ, "Familial Thrombophilia Due to a Previously Unrecognized Mechanism Characterized by Poor Anticoagulant Response to Activated Protein C: Prediction of a Cofactor to Activated Protein C," *Proc Natl Acad Sci USA*, 1993, 90(3):1004-8.
2. Aslam S, Standen GR, Morse C, et al, "DVT Following Oral Contraceptive Therapy in Association With Homozygous Factor V Leiden," *Clin Lab Haematol*, 1995, 17(1):99-100.
3. Bertina RM, Koeleman BP, Koster T, et al, "Mutation in Blood Coagulation Factor V Associated With Resistance to Activated Protein C," *Nature*, 1994, 369(6475):64-7.
4. Griffin JH, Evatt B, Wideman C, et al, "Anticoagulant Protein C Pathway Defective in Majority of Thrombophilic Patients," *Blood*, 1993, 82(7):1989-93.
5. Koster T, Rosendaal FR, de Ronde H, et al, "Venous Thrombosis Due to Poor Anticoagulant Response to Activated Protein C: Leiden Thrombophilia Study," *Lancet*, 1993, 342(8886-7):1503-6.
6. Samaha M, Trossaert M, Conard J, et al, "Prevalence and Patient Profile in Activated Protein C Resistance," *Am J Clin Pathol*, 1995, 104(4):450-4.
7. Denson KW, Haddon ME, Reed SV, et al, "A More Discriminating Test for APC Resistance and a Possible Screening Test to Include Protein C and Protein S," *Thromb Res*, 1996, 81(1):151-6.

References

Dahlbäck B, "Molecular Genetics of Thrombophilia: Factor V Gene Mutation Causing Resistance to Activated Protein C as a Basis of the Hypercoagulable State," *J Lab Clin Med*, 1995, 125(5):566-71.

De Stefano V, Finazzi G, and Mannucci PM, "Inherited Thrombophilia: Pathogenesis, Clinical Syndromes, and Management," *Blood*, 1996, 87(9):3531-44.

Hillarp A, Dahlbäck B, and Zöller B, "Activated Protein C Resistance: From Phenotype to Genotype and Clinical Practice," *Blood Reviews*, 1995, 9(4):201-12.

Svensson PJ and Dahlbäck B, "Resistance to Activated Protein C as a Basis for Venous Thrombosis," *N Engl J Med*, 1994, 330(8):517-22.

Ristocetin Cofactor *see* von Willebrand Factor Assay *on page 268*

Rumpel-Leede Test *see* Capillary Fragility Test *on page 235*

Rumpel-Leede Tourniquet Test *see* Capillary Fragility Test *on page 235*

Salzman Column Test *see* Platelet Adhesion Test *on page 256*

Screen for Disseminated Intravascular Coagulation *see* Intravascular Coagulation Screen *on page 253*

Screen for Hypercoagulation *see* Hypercoagulable State Coagulation Screen *on page 250*

Sedimentation Rate *see* Fibrinogen *on page 246*

Serine Protease Inhibitor *see* Antithrombin III Test *on page 230*

Serotonin Release *see* Platelet Antibody *on page 258*

Spectrolyse™/pL Procedure *see* Plasminogen Activator Inhibitor *on page 255*

Stable Factor *see* Factor VII *on page 240*

Staphylococcal Clumping Test *see* Fibrin Breakdown Products *on page 245*

Stuart Factor *see* Factor X *on page 242*

Stuart-Prower Factor *see* Factor X *on page 242*

Surgicutt® *see* Bleeding Time, Mielke *on page 234*

βTG *see* Beta-Thromboglobulin *on page 232*

β-TG *see* Beta-Thromboglobulin *on page 232*

Thrombin Clotting Time Heparin Assay *see* Activated Partial Thromboplastin Time *on page 227*

Thrombin-Fibrindex *see* Thrombin Time *on next page*

Thrombin Time

CPT 85670; 85675 (titer)

Related Information

Activated Partial Thromboplastin Time *on page 227*
Cryoprecipitate *on page 606*
Fibrinogen *on page 246*
Hirudin Determination *on page 249*
Intravascular Coagulation Screen *on page 253*
Reptilase®-R Time *on page 264*

Synonyms Fibrin Time; Fibrindex™; Fibrinogen Screen; Thrombin-Fibrindex

Test Commonly Includes Patient time and control time

Specimen Plasma

Container Blue top (sodium citrate) tube

Collection Routine venipuncture as for coagulation studies. If multiple tests are being drawn, draw coagulation studies last. If only a thrombin time is being drawn, draw 1-2 mL into another Vacutainer® or syringe (two-syringe technique), discard, and then collect the thrombin time. This collection procedure avoids contamination of the specimen with tissue thromboplastins.

Storage Instructions Keep refrigerated. Freeze plasma if test is not to be performed promptly.

Causes for Rejection Tube not full, specimen clotted, hemolyzed specimen, specimen received more than 2 hours after collection

Special Instructions Transport the specimen to the hematology laboratory as soon as possible.

Reference Range Less than $1\frac{1}{2}$ times control value

Use Determination of severe hypofibrinogenemia, dysfibrinogenemia, and presence of heparin-like anticoagulants; useful in diagnosis and monitoring of disseminated intravascular coagulation (DIC) and fibrinolysis; useful in monitoring fibrinolytic therapy.[1] The thrombin time test can be used to monitor therapy with heparin. See Limitations.

Limitations Affected by concentration and reactivity of fibrinogen, increased amounts of fibrin degradation products (FDP), and the presence of inhibitory substances, such as heparin and large amounts of fibrin degradation products. Use of this test to monitor heparin will be unreliable if hypofibrinogenemia is present or if fibrin breakdown products (FBP) have been generated by a process of DIC. See also test listing Reptilase®-R Time *on page 264*.

Contraindications Patient on heparin therapy

Methodology Clotting time is measured after exogenous thrombin is added. Reliable results and use depends upon the addition of a standard concentration of thrombin to test and control plasmas. Concentration of thrombin in commercial preparations varies. The amount of calcium chloride added in the test environment should be adjusted to give a "normal" plasma clotting time of 8-9 seconds. Loss of sensitivity (with resultant inability to detect some clinical abnormalities) will occur if the thrombin time control has risen into the 11-14 second range.

Additional Information Thrombin time is a screening test for presence of sufficient amount of functional (clottable) fibrinogen. The thrombin time is often included as part of a panel of tests for detection and evaluation of DIC. Fibrinogen/FBP act as powerful antithrombins, prolong the thrombin time, and thereby indicate presence of DIC. If the thrombin time is prolonged, additional information can be obtained by repeating the analysis on a 1:1 mixture of patient's plasma and normal (control) plasma. If the clotting time of such a 1:1 mix approximates that of the control plasma, hypofibrinogenemia or a defective molecular form of fibrinogen (dysfibrinogenemia) may be present. If the clotting time after mixing does not correct (is closer to the patient's originally prolonged thrombin time) presence of a thrombin inhibitor in the patient's plasma is likely (eg, heparin, FBP). The thrombin time is nearly always prolonged with dysfibrinogenemia.[2]

See tables, including Findings Indicative of Hypercoagulable State, in the listing Hypercoagulable State Coagulation Screen *on page 250* and the table, Findings Indicative of DIC, in the listing Intravascular Coagulation Screen *on page 253*.

Footnotes

1. Bick RL and Strauss J, "Thrombolytic Therapy and Its Uses," *Lab Med*, 1995, 26(5):330-7.
2. Mammen EF and Fujii Y, "Hypercoagulable States," *Lab Med*, 1989, 20:611-2.

References

Brozović M, "Investigation of Acute Haemostatic Failure," *Practical Haematology*, Chapter 18, Dacie JV and Lewis SM, eds, New York, NY: Churchill Livingstone, 1991, 284.

Sirridge MS and Shannon R, *Laboratory Evaluation of Hemostasis and Thrombosis*, 3rd ed, Philadelphia, PA: Lea & Febiger, 1983, 161-3.

β-Thromboglobulin *see Beta-Thromboglobulin on page 232*

Thrombomodulin

CPT 85337

Related Information

Factor V *on page 239*
Hypercoagulable State Coagulation Screen *on page 250*
Protein C *on page 260*
Resistance to Activated Protein C *on previous page*

Synonyms Endothelial Cofactor; TM

Abstract Thrombomodulin (TM) is the endothelial cell thrombin receptor. The thrombin-thrombomodulin complex activates protein C. TM is thus an anticoagulant protein cofactor modulating the specificity of thrombin for its receptor and activating the central enzyme (protein C) of a major anticoagulant pathway resulting in the inactivation of factors Va and VIIIa. Soluble TM is increased in the sera of patients with systemic lupus erythematosus (SLE), disseminating cancer, and a variety of conditions in which there is endothelial cell injury.

Specimen Plasma

Container Citrated blood drawn into siliconized tubes

Storage Instructions Centrifuge at 2000 g at 4°C for 20 minutes. May store plasma at -70°C.

Special Instructions This test will likely be available only from reference or research laboratories.

Reference Range 44 ± 10.5 ng/mL[1]

Use TM fragments measured in plasma likely reflect endothelial cell injury occurring in diverse conditions including systemic lupus erythematosus,[2] cancer, in particular, disseminated forms,[1] disseminated intravascular coagulation (DIC),[3,4] pulmonary thromboembolism, adult respiratory distress syndrome, renal failure including diabetic nephropathy, acute hepatic failure,[4] liver transplantation,[5] and thrombotic thrombocytopenic purpura (TTP).[6] Plasma TM levels may have value in assessing prognosis in DIC and TTP.[6]

Limitations Results using tests based on different monoclonal antibodies may vary, dependent upon sensitivity of reagent antibody to fragments of TM.[6]

Methodology Enzyme-linked immunosorbent assay (ELISA), procedure and reagents available commercially

Additional Information Thrombomodulin (TM) is an endothelial cell receptor with high affinity for thrombin. It exerts anticoagulant influence acting as a cofactor for thrombin-catalyzed activation of protein C. The latter is an important anticoagulant protease zymogen. Thrombin binding to endothelial cell thrombomodulin activates protein C which then inactivates factors V and VIII (their active forms) in the presence of protein S. In 1994 a mutant factor V (factor V Leiden) was described which resists proteolysis by activated protein C and which appears to be the most common cause of unexplained thrombosis (present in some 20% to 60% of such patients).[7]

TM is a single chain glycoprotein. It has six consecutive epidermal growth factor-like structural domains in an extracellular position. Monoclonal ELISA analytic systems have recently been developed.[1,2,4] Plasma thrombomodulin fragments reflect endothelial cell injury. They are reportedly increased in a variety of conditions with microvascular injury including SLE, DIC, acute hepatic failure, acute respiratory distress syndrome, and renal dysfunction.[1] A study of plasma TM levels in cancer patients found significant increase with the development of disseminated disease.[1] Marked variation in individual plasma TM levels were noted. Patients with colorectal cancer had normal levels at the time of diagnosis while some patients with pancreatic cancer had initial elevation of plasma TM.

Footnotes

1. Lindahl AK, Boffa MC, and Abildgaard U, "Increased Plasma Thrombomodulin in Cancer Patients," *Thromb Haemost*, 1993, 69(2):112-4.
2. Kodama S, Uchijima E, Nagai M, et al, "One-Step Sandwich Enzyme Immunoassay for Soluble Human Thrombomodulin Using Monoclonal Antibodies," *Clin Chim Acta*, 1990, 192(3):191-9.
3. Asakura H, Jokaji H, Saito M, et al, "Plasma Levels of Soluble Thrombomodulin Increase in Cases of Disseminated Intravascular Coagulation With Organ Failure," *Am J Hematol*, 1991, 38(4):281-7.
4. Takano S, Kimura S, Ohdama S, et al, "Plasma Thrombomodulin in Health and Diseases," *Blood*, 1990, 76(10):2024-9.
5. Himmelreich G, Riewald M, Rosch R, et al, "Thrombomodulin: A Marker for Endothelial Damage During Orthotopic Liver Transplantation," *Am J Hematol*, 1994, 47(1):1-5.
6. Wada H, Ohiwa M, Kaneko T, et al, "Plasma Thrombomodulin as a Marker of Vascular Disorders in Thrombotic Thrombocytopenic Purpura and Disseminated Intravascular Coagulation," *Am J Hematol*, 1992, 39(1):20-4.
7. Rodgers GM, "Activated Protein C Resistance and Inherited Thrombosis," *Am J Clin Pathol*, 1995, 103(3):261-2.

References

Dittman WA and Majerus PW, "Structure and Function of Thrombomodulin: A Natural Anticoagulant," *Blood*, 1990, 75(2):329-36.

Esmon NL, "Thrombomodulin," *Prog Hemost Thromb*, 1989, 9:29-55.

Sadler JE, Lentz SR, Sheehan JP, et al, "Structure-Function Relationships of the Thrombin-Thrombomodulin Interaction," *Haemostasis*, 1993, 23(Suppl 1):183-93.

Thrombotic Disease Screen *see* Hypercoagulable State Coagulation Screen *on page 250*

Thrombo-Wellcotest® for Fibrin Split Products *see* Fibrin Breakdown Products *on page 245*

Tissue Plasminogen Activator (t-PA) *see* Protein C *on page 260*

TM *see* Thrombomodulin *on previous page*

Tolerance Test for Aspirin *see* Aspirin Tolerance Test *on page 232*

Tourniquet Test *see* Capillary Fragility Test *on page 235*

Triple P Test *see* Fibrin Split Products, Protamine Sulfate *on page 248*

VIIIC:Ag *see* Factor VIII *on page 240*

VIIIR Antigen *see* von Willebrand Factor Antigen *on this page*

von Willebrand Factor Antigen

CPT 85246

Related Information

Aspirin Tolerance Test *on page 232*
Bleeding Time, Ivy *on page 233*
Cryoprecipitate *on page 606*
Factor VIII *on page 240*
von Willebrand Factor Assay *on next page*
von Willebrand Factor Collagen Binding Assay *on page 269*
von Willebrand Factor Multimer Assay *on page 269*

Synonyms Factor VIIIR:Ag; Factor VIII-Related Antigen; VIIIR Antigen; vWF Ag

Abstract This test measures the quantity of von Willebrand factor protein but may not reflect functional activity.

Specimen Plasma

Container Two blue top (sodium citrate) tubes

Collection Routine venipuncture. If multiple tests are being drawn, draw coagulation studies last. If only a factor VIIIR antigen is being drawn, draw 1-2 mL into another Vacutainer®, discard, and then collect the factor VIIIR antigen. This collection procedure avoids contamination of the specimen with tissue thromboplastins.

Storage Instructions Keep refrigerated

Causes for Rejection Specimen hemolyzed, specimen received more than 2 hours after collection, stored specimen not refrigerated

Special Instructions Transport the specimen to the laboratory as soon as possible. May not be available as a routine test.

Factor VIII/von Willebrand Factor Terminology

vWD	von Willebrand disease
VIII:C	Factor VIII procoagulant activity, the AHF factor (protein which corrects abnormality in hemophilia A)
	Factor VIII-related protein
VIIIC:Ag	The immunologic determinant of VIIIC
VIIIR	von Willebrand factor, factor VIII carrier protein (corrects bleeding time abnormality in von Willebrand disease)
VIIIR:Ag	Antigenic expression of von Willebrand factor
VIIIR:RCo VIIIR:RCF VIIIR:WF	Ristocetin cofactor (property of VIIIR which in presence of ristocetin, strongly aggregates platelets)

Factor VIII/von Willebrand Disease Terminologic Equivalents

Current (Intl Committee Thrombosis/ Hemostasis)	Previous Terminology or Equivalents
Factor VIII (FVIII)	AHF; VIIIC
Factor VIII antigen (FVIII Ag)	VIIIC Ag
von Willebrand factor (vWF)	RiCoF; VIIIR:RCo; VIIIR:RCF
von Willebrand factor antigen (vWF Ag)	VIIIR Ag; FVIIIR Ag

Reference Range Results of patient's diluted plasma are referenced to a standard curve constructed from results of dilutions of normal pooled plasma. Results of electroimmunoassay may be falsely elevated in patients who have disproportionate increase in small vWF multimers. In normal individuals, vWF Ag and ristocetin cofactor are within 5% to 15% of each other.[1] Factor VIII assay results aid in interpretation of antigen level. Plasma level of vWF Ag is about 10 μg/mL.[2] A number of factors influence the antigen level including ABO blood type (vWF levels are lower with type O and may vary with Lewis blood type).[3,4] Levels vary with adrenergic stimulation (eg, as occurs with exercise, trauma,

surgery, etc) and are increased with some chimic conditions (eg, pregnancy, oral estrogen therapy, liver disease, hyperthyroidism, renal disease, cancer, inflammation, diabetes, and atherosclerosis).[2]

Use A coagulation parameter useful in establishing the presence of von Willebrand disease (vWD), usually in conjunction with one or more other tests for vWD (see Related Information)

Limitations Interpretation of results may be limited if specimen is received more than 2 hours after collection or if specimen is stored unrefrigerated. Does not measure functional activity. Improper handling of specimen may result in degradation of the larger vWF multimers.

Methodology Crossed immunoelectrophoresis, Laurell one-dimensional electroimmunoassay, radioimmunoassay (RIA), enzyme-linked immunosorbent assay (ELISA), or radiocrossed immunoelectrophoresis

Additional Information

Molecular Structure/Function

The test for vWF antigen determines the quantitative amount of a unique polypeptide coagulation protein circulating in the peripheral blood. The result reflects the physical presence of protein but does not determine its functional ability. The vWF consists of a family of proteins that vary in size and functional capability, a series of multimers, molecular weight from 800,000 to 20,000,000. They are formed from a single subunit with molecular weight (M_r) of about 250,000. Minor circulating units (M_r about 120,000-189,000) represent proteolytic fragments of the base 250,000 M_r unit. In the circulation, vWF exists as multimers of a basic repeating dimer of the M_r 250,000 subunit. The larger multimers (formed of more than 4 or 5 dimers) appear to have the greatest binding activity (greatest functional activity). Synthesis occurs in endothelial cells and megakaryocytes. Initially, a precursor protein of 2813 amino acid residues with M_r of about 360,000 is produced which includes the mature subunit with M_r of about 250,000. vWF is cysteine-rich with multimers formed by interchain disulfide binding.[5] Glycoprotein constitutes nearly 20% of vWF. After formation in the endoplasmic reticulum, glycosylation occurs in the Golgi apparatus and mature vWF is stored in Weibel-Palade bodies, intracellular organelles, unique to the endothelial cell.[6]

vWF acts as a carrier protein for factor VIII (ratio of the mass of factor VIII to the VIII vWF complex is about 1:100) and as a bridge between collagen and platelets, appropriate binding sites forming a part of its molecular structure. Subendothelial collagen type VI is a likely *in vivo* receptor. There are also binding sites for activated platelet membrane GP IIb-IIIa and for factor VIII. The integrin, $\alpha v \beta_3$, serves as an endothelial cell receptor for vWF.[7] The test, vWF assay, (see von Willebrand Factor Assay *on page 268*) as distinct from the test for vWF antigen, reflects vWF activity, the antibiotic ristocetin causing platelet aggregation in normal individuals but not in those with vWD. Characteristics of vWF multimers can be established using electrophoretic techniques.

Classification

With the understanding that vWF is a spectrum of multimers, each with as yet incompletely understood function (eg, binding activity) and with a number of reciprocal receptor structures, it is not surprising that vWD shows considerable clinical variation both on an acquired basis and as the result of genetic diversity. Classification of the different forms of vWD has undergone evolution in keeping with the detection and description of new varieties of the disease. Common to most classifications is the recognition of three groups: type I - residual vWF **qualitatively** normal; type II - vWF qualitatively abnormal; and type III - vWF protein essentially undetectable. Each of these categories, however, is heterogeneous, eg, while type I is characterized by quantitative reduction in qualitatively normal multimers, variants are recognized which include a qualitative component (functionally abnormal protein). In 1994, a simplified phenotypic classification was proposed by the Subcommittee on von Willebrand Factor of the Scientific and Standardization Committee of the International Society on Thrombosis and Haemostasis.[8] (See also the table of comparison of von Willebrand disease classifications from Ewenstein and Hardin.) The new classification defines major categories of vWD in terms of quantitative or qualitative defects with further division of qualitative defects by specific pathophysiologic mechanism. It is an extension of Ruggeri and Zimmerman's pathophysiology based system of 1987.[9]

The new classification embodies the following quantitative defects:
- Type 1: Partial quantitative deficiency of vWF
- Type 3: Essentially complete deficiency of vWF

The new classification embodies the following qualitative defects (type 2):
- Type 2A: Variants with decreased platelet-dependent function with loss of high molecular weight (HMW) vWF multimers
- Type 2B: Variants with increased affinity for platelet glycoprotein Ib
- Type 2M: Variants with decreased platelet-dependent function not caused by absence of HMW vWF multimers
- Type 2N: Variants with decreased affinity for factor VIII

The accompanying table compares vWD classifications
(Continued)

von Willebrand Factor Antigen (Continued)

Correspondence Between vWD Classifications

New/Revised	Previous Type
1	I platelet normal
	I platelet low
	IA
	I-1, I-2, I-3
2A	IIA
	IB
	I platelet discordant
	IIC
	IID
	IIE
	IIF
	IIG
	IIH
	II-I
	IIA-1, IIA-2, IIA-3
2B	IIB
	I New York
	Malmo
2M	B
	Vicenza
	IC
	ID
2N	Defective binding to factor VIII
	Normandy
3	III

From Ewenstein BM and Handin RI, "von Willebrand's Disease," *Blood, Principles and Practice of Hematology*, Chapter 36, Handin RI, Lux SE, and Stossel TP, eds, Philadelphia, PA: JB Lippincott Co, 1995, 1069-94, with permission.

A platelet type vWD (pseudo-vWD) is caused by an abnormal platelet receptor for vWF.

Clinical Features

von Willebrand disease, the most common inherited bleeding disorder, clinically and biochemically diverse, has a spectrum of clinical presentation that relates to underlying inherited or acquired abnormality in vW multimer structure/function. Familiarity with variation (over time) in test results when dealing with some cases of mild vWD or when attempting to exclude the diagnosis is necessary.

von Willebrand syndrome is characterized clinically by easy/spontaneous bruising, petechiae/purpura, mucosal (GI, GU, nasal, gingival) membrane bleeding and hemorrhage, occasionally severe, with surgery/trauma. Bilateral epistaxis and easy bruising may begin in early childhood. There is broad variation in clinical severity, some forms of vWD being essentially asymptomatic with negligible or mild bleeding defect. Bleeding time is prolonged. Platelet count, clot retraction, and coagulation time are normal. With type III vWD, there is severe hemorrhage, high incidence of consanguinity, and very long bleeding time with

Terminology: Factor VIII and von Willebrand Factor*

FVIII (FVIIIC)	Factor VIII	Procoagulant activity (deficient in hemophilia A)
FVIII Ag	Factor VIII antigen	Factor VIII, immunologic definition
vWD		von Willebrand disease
vWF (VIIIR)	von Willebrand factor	Activity of protein deficient in von Willebrand disease measured using ristocetin cofactor assays (RiCoF)
vWF Ag	von Willebrand factor antigen	Immunologic determinants of von Willebrand factor previously termed factor VIII related antigen (VIIIR Ag)

*Recommendations of the International Committee for Thrombosis and Hemostasis, 1985

absence/near absence of vWF multimer proteins. Laboratory diagnosis may require the use of two or more tests for vWF.

Acquired von Willebrand syndrome with evidence of proteolysis of or antibodies against the factor VIII complex occur with a variety of lymphoproliferative and myeloproliferative disorders, in particular, multiple myeloma, chronic lymphocytic leukemia, and monoclonal gammopathy of undetermined significance. Lupus erythematosus, nephroblastoma, GI telangiectasia, hypothyroidism, and hemoglobin E-beta thalassemia have also been reported with acquired von Willebrand disease. Acquired disease may occur occasionally with use of the drugs valproic acid and ciprofloxacin.[10]

The increased platelet agglutinating activity occurring with thrombotic thrombocytopenic purpura (TTP) appears to result from release of platelet-agglutinating factor and unusually large vWF multimers.[11] Platelet agglutination in patients with TTP can be inhibited by large dose infusion of human immunoglobulin G with resultant remission (in a majority of cases) of this once usually fatal disease.[12]

Familiarity with the possible considerable variation (over time) in test results when dealing with mild vWD or when attempting to exclude the diagnosis has been re-emphasized.[13]

Footnotes

1. Rick ME, "Laboratory Diagnosis of von Willebrand's Disease," *Clin Lab Med*, 1994, 14(4):781-94.
2. Sadler JE and Davie EW, "von Willebrand Factor and von Willebrand Disease," *The Molecular Basis of Blood Diseases*, Stamatoyannopoulos G, Neinhuis AW, Majerus PW, et al, eds, 2nd ed, Chapter 19, Philadelphia, PA: WB Saunders Co, 1994, 675-700.
3. Gill JC, Endres-Brooks J, Bauer PJ, et al, "The Effect of ABO Blood Group on the Diagnosis of von Willebrand Disease," *Blood*, 1987, 69(6):1691-5.
4. Orstavik KH, Kornstad L, Reisner H, et al, "Possible Effect of Secretor Locus on Plasma Concentration of Factor VIII and von Willebrand Factor," *Blood*, 1989, 73(4):990-3.
5. Wagner DD and Bonfanti R, "von Willebrand Factor and Endothelium," *Mayo Clin Proc*, 1991, 66(6):621-7.
6. Wagner DD, Urban-Pickering M, and Marder VJ, "von Willebrand Protein Binds to Extracellular Matrices Independently of Collagen," *Proc Natl Acad Sci U S A*, 1984, 81(2):471-5.
7. Cheresh DA, "Human Endothelial Cells Synthesize and Express an Arg-Gly-Asp-Directed Adhesion Receptor Involved in Attachment to Fibrinogen and von Willebrand Factor," *Proc Natl Acad Sci U S A*, 1987, 84(18):6471-5.
8. Sadler JE and Gralnick HR, "Commentary: A New Classification for von Willebrand Disease," *Blood*, 1994, 84(3):676-9.
9. Ruggeri ZM and Zimmerman TS, "von Willebrand Factor and von Willebrand Disease," *Blood*, 1987, 70(4):895-904.
10. Jakway JL, "Acquired von Willebrand's Disease," *Hematol Oncol Clin North Am*, 1992, 6(6):1409-19.
11. Schmidt JL, "Thrombotic Thrombocytopenic Purpura: Successful Treatment Unlocks Etiologic Secrets," *Mayo Clin Proc*, 1989, 64(8):956-61.
12. Lian EC, Mui PT, Siddiqui FA, et al, "Inhibition of Platelet-Aggregating Activity in Thrombotic Thrombocytopenic Purpura Plasma by Normal Adult Immunoglobulin G," *J Clin Invest*, 1984, 73(2):548-55.
13. Blombäck M, Eneroth P, Andersson O, et al, "On Laboratory Problems in Diagnosing Mild von Willebrand's Disease," *Am J Hematol*, 1992, 40(2):117-20.

References

Bick RL, "Hereditary Coagulation Protein Defects - von Willebrand's Disease," *Disorders of Thrombosis and Hemostasis: Clinical and Laboratory Practice*, Chapter 6, Chicago, IL: American Society of Clinical Pathologists, 1992, 123-6.

Bona RD, "von Willebrand Factor and von Willebrand's Disease: A Complex Protein and a Complex Disease," *Ann Clin Lab Sci*, 1989, 19(3):184-9.

Fujimura Y and Titani K, "Structure and Function of von Willebrand Factor," *Hemostasis and Thrombosis*, Chapter 16, Bloom AL, Forbes CD, Thomas DP, et al, eds, New York, NY: Churchill Livingstone, 1994, 379-95.

Giddings JC and Yamamoto J, "Changing Concepts in Investigations of Haemostasis," *Clin Lab Haematol*, 1995, 17(1):85-91.

Ginsburg D, "The von Willebrand Factor Gene and Genetics of von Willebrand's Disease," *Mayo Clin Proc*, 1991, 66(5):506-15.

Hill RJ and Ens GE, "Thrombotic Thrombocytopenic Purpura," *Clin Hemost Rev*, 1989, 3:1-4.

Meyer D, Piétu G, Fressinaud E, et al, "von Willebrand Factor: Structure and Function," *Mayo Clin Proc*, 1991, 66(5):516-23.

Miller JL, "von Willebrand Disease," *Hematology/Oncology Clinics of North America: Platelets in Health and Disease*, Vol 4, Colman RW and Rao AK, eds, Philadelphia, PA: WB Saunders Co, 1990, 107-28.

Sadler JE, "von Willebrand Disease," *The Metabolic and Molecular Basis of Inherited Disease*, 7th ed, Vol 3, Scriver CR, Beaudet AL, Sly WS, et al, eds, New York, NY: McGraw-Hill Inc, 1995, 3269-87.

Sadler JE, "von Willebrand Disease," *Hemostasis and Thrombosis*, Chapter 35, Bloom AL, Forbes CD, Thomas DP, et al, eds, New York, NY: Churchill Livingstone, 1994, 843-57.

Triplett DA, "Laboratory Diagnosis of von Willebrand's Disease," *Mayo Clin Proc*, 1991, 66(8):832-40.

von Willebrand Factor Assay

CPT 85245

Related Information

Platelet Aggregation *on page 257*
von Willebrand Factor Antigen *on previous page*
von Willebrand Factor Multimer Assay *on next page*

Synonyms Ristocetin Cofactor; vW Factor Assay

Aftercare A functional assay for vWF activity based on platelet aggregation with ristocetin. vWD patient's platelets do not aggregate with ristocetin as do those from normal individuals.

Specimen Plasma

Container Blue top (sodium citrate) tube

Collection Specimen may be drawn by clinic or laboratory technologist.

Storage Instructions Separate into plastic vial, freeze immediately and send frozen.

Causes for Rejection Tube not full, specimen hemolyzed, specimen clotted, specimen received more than 2 hours after collection

Special Instructions Must schedule with laboratory in advance.

Reference Range Interpretation of platelet aggregation patterns, normal plasma/platelets aggregate when exposed to ristocetin

Use Aid with the differential diagnosis of hemophilia and von Willebrand disease

Methodology Modified platelet aggregation (aggregation as stimulated by ristocetin - a measure of vWF binding to platelet glycoprotein Ib); measurement of agglutination of fresh washed or formalin-fixed platelets by patient's plasma as compared to agglutination produced by a "standard plasma" (donor pool or reference plasma) used to prepare a standard curve;[1] botrocetin snake venom based platelet agglutinating test[2]

Additional Information Plasma from von Willebrand disease patients lacks the ability to cause platelet aggregation in response to ristocetin. See Additional Information under the entry von Willebrand Factor Antigen *on page 267* for additional discussion.

Footnotes

1. Laffan MA and Bradshaw AE, "Investigation of a Bleeding Tendency," *Practical Haematology*, 8th ed, Chapter 17, Dacie JV and Lewis SM, eds, New York, NY: Churchill Livingstone, 1995, 336-8.
2. Brinkhous KM and Read MS, "Use of Venom Coagglutinin and Lyophilized Platelets in Testing for Platelet-Aggregating von Willebrand Factor," *Blood*, 1980, 55(3):517-20.

References

Bloom AL, "von Willebrand Factor: Clinical Features of Inherited and Acquired Disorders," *Mayo Clin Proc*, 1991, 66(7):743-51.

Cheresh DA, "Structural and Biologic Properties of Integrin-Mediated Cell Adhesion," *Clin Lab Med*, 1992, 12(2):217-36.

Triplett DA, "Laboratory Diagnosis of von Willebrand's Disease," *Mayo Clin Proc*, 1991, 66(8):832-40.

von Willebrand Factor Collagen Binding Assay

Related Information

von Willebrand Factor Antigen *on page 267*

Synonyms CBA; Collagen Binding Assay for vWF; vWF:CBA

Test Commonly Includes von Willebrand factor antigen (vWF:Ag), von Willebrand factor collagen binding (vWF:CBA), and vWF Ag/vWF CBA ratio

Abstract This test measures the ability of von Willebrand factor (vWF) to bind to collagen with sensitivity for the large (more functionally active) vWF multimers. It has been proposed as a screening functional test for von Willebrand disease (vWD) which can replace the technically more difficult platelet aggregation based ristocetin cofactor assay.

Specimen Plasma

Container Blue top tube, 0.105 M buffered sodium citrate

Storage Instructions May be transported for assay after plasma is separated from cells and snap frozen at -70°C. Otherwise, assay should be performed just after plasma is harvested.

Causes for Rejection Filtered plasma and serum are inappropriate specimens.

Turnaround Time 4 hours, 52 hours if collagen-coated plates must be prepared prior to testing.

Reference Range 50% to 250% of pooled normal plasma[1]

Use Test for vWF functional activity incorporated as one of a panel of screening tests for vWD

Limitations Ability of this test to respond to large vWF multimers critically depends upon characteristics of the collagen reagent.

Methodology Enzyme-linked immunosorbent assay (ELISA) utilizing collagen-coated microtiter plates and horseradish peroxidase/tetramethyl benzidine detection system

Additional Information This assay, originally proposed in 1986,[2] is capable of identifying type 2 (subtypes 2A and 2B) vWD and discriminating such cases from type 1 vWD patients and normal individuals. The test has application as one of a panel of screening tests including also ELISA assay for vWF antigen. The vWF:CBA assay appears to selectively detect depletion of the higher molecular weight forms of vWF multimers.[3] High vWF:Ag to vWF:CBA ratios >2.5 suggest the presence of type 2A or type 2B vWD. Low ratios (<2.5) occur in normal individuals or those persons with type I vWD. The CBA has been proposed as a measure of functional responsiveness to (laboratory monitoring of) desmopressin (DDAVP) therapy.[4] The CBA to vWF:Ag ratio is increased (as compared to baseline pre-DDAVP levels) in patients receiving desmopressin.

Footnotes

1. Favaloro EJ, Grispo L, Dinale A, et al, "von Willebrand's Disease: Laboratory Investigation Using an Improved Functional Assay for von Willebrand Factor," *Pathology*, 1993, 25(2):152-8.

2. Brown JE and Bosak JO, "An ELISA Test for the Binding of von Willebrand Antigen to Collagen," *Thromb Res*, 1986, 43(3):303-11.
3. Favaloro EJ, Facey D, and Grispo L, "Laboratory Assessment of von Willebrand Factor. Use of Different Assays Can Influence the Diagnosis of von Willebrand's Disease, Dependent on Differing Sensitivity to Sample Preparation and Differential Recognition of High Molecular Weight VWF Forms," *Am J Clin Pathol*, 1995, 104(3):264-71.
4. Favaloro EJ, Dean M, Grispo L, et al, "von Willebrand's Disease: Use of Collagen Binding Assay Provides Potential Improvement to Laboratory Monitoring of Desmopressin (DDAVP) Therapy," *Am J Hematol*, 1994, 45(3):205-11.

von Willebrand Factor Multimer Assay

CPT 85247

Related Information

Factor VIII *on page 240*

von Willebrand Factor Antigen *on page 267*

von Willebrand Factor Assay *on previous page*

Synonyms vWF Multimer Assays

Specimen Plasma

Container Blue top (sodium citrate) tube

Collection Routine venipuncture. If multiple tests are being drawn, draw coagulation studies last. If only a sample for this test is being drawn, two-syringe collection technique is recommended.

Turnaround Time This is not a routine clinical laboratory procedure and will usually be performed at a reference laboratory. As such 5-7 days may be required before analytic results are available.

Use Classification of von Willebrand disease variants

Methodology Immunoelectrophoresis using agarose gel and ^{125}I labeled anti-vWF followed by autoradiography for detection of vWF multimers. A Western blot nonradioactive chemiluminescence assay has been developed.[1]

Additional Information The von Willebrand factor (vWF) is a family of protein multimers varying in molecular weight from 1-20 million daltons. There is evidence that a large, fully polymerized vWF multimer is released from vascular endothelial cells. vWF is found in plasma, α granules of platelets and subendothelial connective tissue. Plasma and basement membrane vWF are largely of endothelial cell origin. Extensive intracellular processing occurs before active vWF multimers are formed. A large precursor pro-vWF protein dimerizes, is transported to the Golgi apparatus after N-linked glycosylation and in subsequent acidic environment pro vWF dimers multimerize by formation of interchain disulfide bonds.[2] The protein accumulates in Weibel-Palade bodies of endothelial cells and is released from these compartments basolaterally.[3] The integrin $\alpha v \beta_3$ serves as an endothelial cell receptor for von Willebrand factor.[4] Plasma multimers are generated from the polymer after it is released into the circulation.[5] See table.

Subtypes of von Willebrand Disease

Subtype	Multimer Composition	Multimer Level	Platelet Aggregation
I	Complete	↓	
II	Highest MW multimers absent		
III (clinically severe)	All multimers involved	Absent	
IIb	Highest MW multimers absent		↓ with ristocetin
Platelet type	Highest MW multimers absent		↓ with ristocetin

Terminology: Factor VIII and von Willebrand Factor*

FVIII (FVIIIC)	Factor VIII	Procoagulant activity (deficient in hemophilia A)
FVIII Ag	Factor VIII antigen	Factor VIII, immunologic definition
vWD		von Willebrand disease
vWF (VIIIR)	von Willebrand factor	Activity of protein deficient in von Willebrand disease measured using ristocetin cofactor assays (RiCoF)
vWF Ag	von Willebrand factor antigen	Immunologic determinants of von Willebrand factor previously termed factor VIII related antigen (VIIIR Ag)

*Recommendations of the International Committee for Thrombosis and Hemostasis, 1985

(Continued)

von Willebrand Factor Multimer Assay
(Continued)

The spectrum of von Willebrand disease may involve qualitative and/or quantitative abnormalities of plasma and/or platelet vWF.[6] Multimer analysis has formed the basis of subtype classification of vWD. See table. A platelet-type vWD (pseudo-vWD) is caused by an abnormal platelet receptor for vWF.[7,8]

There is evidence that some, probably rare, cases of type I vWD are acquired and result from accelerated clearance of vWF from the circulation with or without involvement of inactivating antibodies against vWF:Ag.[9]

See Additional Information under von Willebrand Factor Antigen *on page 267* for additional discussion.

Footnotes

1. Wen LT, McPherson RA, and Smolec JM, "A Chemiluminographic Detection of von Willebrand's (Factor VIII-Related Antigen) Multimeric Composition," *Am J Clin Pathol*, 1993, 99(3):343.
2. Wagner DD and Bonfanti R, "Von Willebrand Factor and the Endothelium," *Mayo Clin Proc*, 1991, 66(6):621-7.
3. Wagner DD, Urban-Pickering M, and Marder VJ, "von Willebrand Protein Binds to Extracellular Matrices Independently of Collagen," *Proc Natl Acad Sci U S A*, 1984, 81(2):471-5.
4. Cheresh DA, "Human Endothelial Cells Synthesize and Express an Arg-Gly-Asp-Directed Adhesion Receptor Involved in Attachment to Fibrinogen and von Willebrand Factor," *Proc Natl Acad Sci U S A*, 1987, 84(18):6471-5.
5. Tsai H-M, Nagel RL, Hatcher VB, et al, "Multimeric Composition of Endothelial Cell-Derived von Willebrand Factor," *Blood*, 1989, 73(8):2074-6.
6. Ruggeri ZM and Zimmerman TS, "von Willebrand Factor and von Willebrand Disease," *Blood*, 1987, 70(4):895-904.
7. Bloom AL, "Von Willebrand Factor: Clinical Features of Inherited and Acquired Disorders," *Mayo Clin Proc*, 1991, 66(7):743-51.
8. Scott JP and Montogmery RR, "The Rapid Differentiation of Type IIb von Willebrand's Disease From Platelet-Type (Pseudo-) von Willebrand's Disease by the ©Neutral' Monoclonal Antibody Binding Assay," *Am J Clin Pathol*, 1991, 96(6):723-8.
9. Igarashi N, Miura M, Kato E, et al, "Acquired von Willebrand's Syndrome With Lupus-Like Serology," *Am J Ped Hemat/Oncol*, 1989, 11(1):32-5.

References

Bona RD and Carta CA, "von Willebrand Factor Multimer Assay," *Manual of Procedures for the Seminar on Diagnostic Hematology*, FW Sunderman, Philadelphia, PA: Institute for Clinical Science Inc, 1988, 193-8.

Gralnick HR, Williams SB, McKeown LP, et al, "Platelet von Willebrand Factor," *Mayo Clin Proc*, 1991, 66(6):634-40.

Lian EC, "Pathogenesis of Thrombotic Thrombocytopenic Purpura," *Semin Hematol*, 1987, 24(2):82-100.

Ruggeri ZM, "Structure and Function of von Willebrand Factor: Relationship to von Willebrand's Disease," *Mayo Clin Proc*, 1991, 66(8):847-61.

Triplett DA, "Laboratory Diagnosis of von Willebrand's Disease," *Mayo Clin Proc*, 1991, 66(8):832-40.

von Willebrand Protein *see* Factor VIII *on page 240*

vWF *see* Factor VIII *on page 240*

vW Factor Assay *see* von Willebrand Factor Assay *on page 268*

vWF Ag *see* von Willebrand Factor Antigen *on page 267*

vWF:CBA *see* von Willebrand Factor Collagen Binding Assay *on previous page*

vWF Multimer Assays *see* von Willebrand Factor Multimer Assay *on previous page*

Williams-Fitzgerald-Flaujeac Factor *see* Factor, Fitzgerald *on page 244*

XIIa *see* Factor XII *on page 243*

CYTOGENETICS

Julia Bridge, MD

Diane Persons, MD

Chromosomes, as they appear in a metaphase spread, consist of tightly coiled DNA and protein. A karyotype is the somatic chromosomal complement of an individual or species. For the human, a normal karyotype consists of 46 chromosomes including 22 pairs of autosomes, identical in males and females, and one pair of sex chromosomes, XX in the female and XY in the male. The primary constriction of a chromosome, the centromere, divides the chromosome into an upper (short) arm and lower (long) arm designated "p" (petite) and "q", respectively. The chromosomes are aligned in a standard sequence on the basis of size, centromere location, and banding pattern. The karyotype is one of the basic tools of the cytogeneticist.

Chromosomal abnormalities are defined according to a uniform system, The International System for Cytogenetic Nomenclature. An example of the abbreviations provided in this system include the use of a plus sign to signify gain of a chromosome: +21 is interpreted as gain of one copy of chromosome 21. A translocation is designated by "t" and is defined as the exchange of chromosomal material between two or more nonhomologous chromosomes. A list of some of the most commonly utilized terms is provided in the following table.

Partial Listing of Cytogenetic Symbols and Abbreviated Terms

del	Deletion
der	Derivative chromosome
dmin	Double minute
hsr	Homogeneously staining region
i	Isochromosome
ins	Insertion
inv	Inversion
mar	Marker chromosome
mat	Maternal origin
minus (-)	Loss of
p	Short arm
pat	Paternal origin
plus (+)	Gain of
q	Long arm
r	Ring chromosome
t	Translocation

From Mitelman F, *An International System of Human Cytogenetic Nomenclature*, 1995.

The greatest advancement in the field of cytogenetics over the last decade has been the development of molecular cytogenetic techniques. Traditionally, cytogenetic data have been obtained through the direct microscopic analysis of chromosomes displaying characteristic bands with Giemsa, quinacrine, or other staining methods from cells arrested in metaphase. Progress in the study of the organization and function of nucleic acid sequences has made it possible to gain information about the chromosomes in an interphase or terminally differentiated cell by means of specially developed chromosome-specific probes and *in situ* hybridization (ISH). Most commonly, these probes are labeled with fluorescent dyes, either directly or indirectly (fluorescence *in situ* hybridization, FISH). Different combinations of haptenated probes (eg, labeled with biotin, digoxigenin, or dinitrophenol) and different fluorophores [green (fluorescein), red (rhodamine or Texas Red), and blue (AMCA or Cascade Blue)] allows visualization of three or more separate chromosomal DNA sequences concurrently. Specific DNA or RNA target sequences in individual cells in tissue sections, single-cell, or chromosome preparations can be detected with *in situ* hybridization.

Interactive efforts between clinicians and cytogeneticists armed with these new technologies have been highly productive. As a result, new diagnostic tests have emerged. With this approach, DNA sequences can be mapped on specific chromosomes; repositioning of sequences between chromosomes or within a particular chromosome, as a result of a chromosomal rearrangement, can be determined; small rearrangements, not detectable with standard karyotypic analysis, can be uncovered; breakpoints using probes for defined DNA sequences can be detected and characterized; and numerical chromosomal abnormalities can be ascertained in interphase and/or metaphase cells. With respect to the latter, cell culture can be omitted resulting in an expedited diagnosis. Prenatal evaluation for Down syndrome performed on amniotic fluid or chorionic villi interphase cells with a probe specific for 21q22 (this region on chromosome 21 must be present in three copies for the Down syndrome phenotype) is one illustration of this diagnostic improvement.

Another central area of diagnostic testing that has profited from advances in cytogenetic technology is cancer genetics. Cancer is a genetic disease resulting from loss of normal regulation of cell growth. This loss is manifested in a number of different ways, including alteration of the normal chromosomal complement. Cytogenetic analysis of both benign and malignant neoplasms has resulted in the definition of characteristic chromosomal anomalies which serve as important, if not essential, diagnostic aids. Identification of the aberrant chromosomal bands has provided a basis for molecular approaches in establishing the definitive genes affected and the associated consequences of these gene alterations. Moreover, many of these abnormalities are important prognostically.

More recently, a new molecular cytogenetic technique has been developed which is not dependent on the availability of probes homologous to the nucleic acid sequence carrying the genetic aberration of interest. This approach, termed "comparative genomic hybridization"(CGH) can provide an overview of DNA sequence copy number changes (including losses or deletions and gains or amplifications) in a tumor specimen and maps these changes on normal chromosomes in a single hybridization. With this assay, dual-color fluorescence *in situ* hybridization is performed to normal metaphase spread using DNA from a test population (eg, a tumor) and from a comparison DNA sample (eg, normal DNA). DNA labeling and hybridization are performed so that the test DNA is detected at one wavelength and the comparison DNA is detected at a different wavelength. Analysis with fluorescence microscopy reveals the chromosomal locations of copy number changes in DNA sequences between the two complements by measuring the tumor/normal fluorescence intensity ratio for each locus in the target metaphase chromosomes. CGH is particularly useful for analysis of DNA sequence copy number changes in tumors where high quality metaphase preparations are often difficult to make, and karyotypes are complex. CGH can be performed using total genomic DNA from fresh, frozen, or paraffin-embedded tissue.

Amniotic Fluid, Chromosome and Genetic Abnormality Analysis

CPT 88235 (culture); 88267 (chromosome analysis); 88283 (specialized banding technique)

Related Information

Synonyms Chromosome Studies, Amniotic Fluid; Karyotype, Amniotic Fluid

Test Commonly Includes Chromosomal complement of fetal cells in amniotic fluid are examined for determination of abnormalities.

Abstract A karyotype is the somatic chromosomal complement of an individual or species. For the human, a normal karyotype consists of 46 chromosomes aligned in a standard sequence on the basis of size, centromere location, and banding pattern. Amniocentesis is performed to obtain cells of fetal origin in the amniotic fluid for culturing and chromosomal analysis. Examination of the chromosomes by banding techniques can reveal numerical and/or structural abnormalities. Additionally, fetal sex is determined.

Patient Preparation The patient should be placed on her abdomen for approximately 20 minutes prior to the amniocentesis. The pregnancy should be at least 16 weeks gestation. Ultrasound studies (to verify fetal life, detect multiple gestation, confirm fetal age, localize placenta, and detect fetal/uterine/adnexal abnormality) are usually carried out.

Specimen Amniotic fluid

Container Sterile container

Sampling Time At or after 16 weeks gestation

Collection An optimum quantity of 20 mL should be obtained by amniocentesis using strict aseptic technique. Pertinent medical findings should accompany the request, including maternal age, gestational age by sonography, reason for study, relevant history, medication history, transfusion history, note of any viral infection, number of pregnancies and miscarriages, and suspected diagnosis. In the case of twins or triplets, amniotic fluid must be collected separately from each amniotic sac.

Storage Instructions Maintain specimen at room temperature. Specimen should be transported to the laboratory, however, as quickly as possible for successful culture.

Causes for Rejection Specimen frozen or clotted (due to excess contamination with blood)

Turnaround Time 2-3 weeks may be needed.

Reference Range Forty-six chromosomes to include 22 sets of normal autosomal chromosomes and one set of normal sex chromosomes (XX for female; XY for male). Interpretative information is usually included.

Use Prenatal detection of chromosomal abnormalities, especially Down syndrome, in groups of pregnant women at risk. Such groups include women age 35 years or older, previous child with a chromosomal abnormality or multiple congenital abnormalities, three or more previous spontaneous abortions, familial history of a chromosomal abnormality, or known carrier of an X-linked disorder. At the same time that amniotic fluid is collected for chromosomal analysis, additional sample can be obtained for testing of inherited metabolic disorders (enzyme deficiency analyses on cultured cells) or neural tube defects (alpha₁-fetoprotein).

Limitations Failure of cells to grow in culture and/or contamination precludes complete analysis (molecular cytogenetic techniques (chromosome *in situ* hybridization) may be of use if this occurs). Overall culture success rate has been reported as 97% with a fetal loss (within 4 weeks of the amniocentesis) of 1.2%.

Contraindications Environment lacking capability in ultrasonography, genetic counseling, amniocentesis, amniotic fluid culturing, and chromosomal analysis techniques

Methodology Cell culturing of fetal cells, subsequent harvesting and chromosome analysis with Giemsa or quinacrine banding techniques

Additional Information At least 0.5% of newborns are born with a chromosomal abnormality. Among these, the most common is trisomy 21 or Down syndrome. It affects approximately 1 in 800 newborns and is a major cause of mental retardation. The incidence is higher in children born to mothers 35 years of age and older. For example, the incidence is 1 in 25 liveborn children of mothers older than 45 years of age. The risk of obstetric complications for amniocentesis is <0.5%. Because the risk of having a child with a chromosomal abnormality for a mother older than 35 years of age is greater than the risk of the procedure for amniocentesis or chorionic villus sampling, maternal age is an indication for prenatal testing.

Birth defects and genetic disorders are encountered in approximately 3% of liveborn infants (less than $1/3$ of which are the result of a chromosomal abnormality). Prenatal diagnosis is possible for more than 1000 inherited diseases, including inborn errors of metabolism. See table for some of the most common disorders. Most follow Mendelian inheritance (autosomal recessive, autosomal dominant, and sex-linked). Many disorders can be detected with metabolic/biochemical tests. Prenatal diagnosis using **gene probes** is available for cystic fibrosis, muscular dystrophy, sickle cell anemia, hemophilia, fragile X syndrome, and many other genetic abnormalities. This can be done by either using cultured amni-

Methods for Prenatal Diagnosis of Genetic Disorders

Biochemical Analysis

Adenosine deaminase deficiency	Lesch-Nyhan disease
Argininosuccinic aciduria	Mannosidosis
Batten disease	Maple syrup urine disease
Citrullinemia	Menkes' disease
Cystinosis	Methylmalonic aciduria
Fabry's disease	Mucopolysaccharidosis (I, II, III, VI, VII)
Farber's disease	Niemann-Pick
Fucosidosis	Orotic aciduria
Galactosemia	Pyruvate decarboxylate deficiency
Gaucher's disease	Refsum's disease
Generalized gangliosidosis	Sandhoff's disease
Glycogen storage disease (II, III, IV)	Steroid sulfatase deficiency
Homocystinuria	Tay-Sachs disease
I-cell disease	Wolman's disease
Krabbe's disease	

Cytogenetic Analysis

Cri Du Chat syndrome (deletion 5)	**Chromosome Instability**
Down syndrome (trisomy 21)	Ataxia telangiectasia
Edwards' syndrome (trisomy 18)	Bloom's syndrome
Klinefelter syndrome (XXY)	Fanconi's anemia
Miller-Dieker syndrome (deletion 17)	
Patau syndrome (trisomy 13)	
Prader-Willi syndrome (deletion 15)	
Retinoblastoma (deletion 13)	
Wiedemann-Beckwith syndrome (deletion 11)	
Wilms' tumor (deletion 11)	
XXX syndrome (XXX)	

Genetic Analysis

Adult polycystic kidney disease	Lesch-Nyhan syndrome
Alpha₁-antitrypsin deficiency	Multiple endocrine neoplasia (types 1 and 2a)
Alpha-thalassemia	Myotonic muscular dystrophy
Beta-thalassemia	Neurofibromatosis I
Carbamyl phosphate synthetase I deficiency	Norrie's disease
Congenital adrenal hyperplasia	Ornithine transcarbamylase deficiency
Cystic fibrosis	Osteogenesis imperfecta
Duchenne/Becker muscular dystrophy	Phenylketonuria
Ehlers-Danlos syndrome	Retinoblastoma
Familial amyloidosis	Sickle cell disease
Fragile X syndrome	Tay-Sachs disease
Friedrich ataxia	Wiskott-Aldrich syndrome
Hemophilias A and B	X-linked lymphoproliferative disease
Huntington disease	

(Continued)

Amniotic Fluid, Chromosome and Genetic Abnormality Analysis *(Continued)*

otic fluid cells or direct chorionic villus sampling. The techniques require isolation of DNA with subsequent digestion of DNA using certain restriction endonucleases. The DNA is electrophoresed, transferred to nitrocellulose and hybridized with specific DNA probes which bind to or very near (restriction fragment length polymorphisms) the genes of interest. The patterns obtained after development of the blot can determine with a high degree of certainty, the presence or absence of disease in the fetus.

References

Beaudet AL, Scriver CR, Sty WS, et al, "Genetics and Biochemistry of Variant Human Phenotypes," *The Metabolic Basis of Inherited Disease*, 6th ed, Chapter 1, New York, NY: McGraw-Hill Inc, 1989, 3-163.

Bridge JA and Sandberg AA, "Cytogenetics," *Anderson's Textbook of Pathology*, 10th ed, Damjanov I and Linder J, eds, 1996, 223-57.

DiLiberti JH, Greenstein MA, and Rosengren SS, "Prenatal Diagnosis," *Pediatr Rev*, 1992, 13(9):334-42.

Kiechle FL and Quattrociocchi-Longe TM, "The Role of the Molecular Probe Laboratory in the 21st Century," *Lab Med*, 1992, 23:758-63.

Shapiro LJ, Gross I, and Hill HR, "Advances in Human Genetics: Current Applications and Prospects for the Future," *Semin Perinatol*, 1991, 15(Suppl 1):1-56.

Aneuploidy *see* Chromosome Analysis, Bone Marrow *on page 277*

Aneusomy *see* Chromosome Analysis, Bone Marrow *on page 277*

Ataxia-Telangiectasia, Chromosome Breakage Study

CPT 88230 (tissue culture for chromosome analysis, lymphocyte); 88248 (chromosome analysis for breakage syndromes, score 100 cells)

Related Information

Bloom's Syndrome, Chromosome Breakage Study *on this page*
Breast Biopsy *on page 35*
Breast Cancer, Hereditary (BRCA1) *on page 504*
Fanconi's Anemia, Chromosome Breakage Study *on page 282*
Follicle Stimulating Hormone *on page 129*
Glucose Tolerance Test *on page 139*
Immunoglobulin A *on page 408*
Immunoglobulin E *on page 409*
Immunoglobulin G *on page 409*
Immunoglobulin G Subclasses *on page 410*
Immunoglobulin M *on page 410*
Leukocyte Immunophenotyping *on page 414*
Luteinizing Hormone, Blood or Urine *on page 163*
Lymphocyte Transformation Test *on page 416*
Xeroderma Pigmentosum, Chromosome Breakage Study *on page 283*

Synonyms Bleomycin Stress Test; Chromosome Breakage Study, Ataxia-Telangiectasia; Chromosome Breakage Syndrome Test; Chromosome Instability Test; Chromosome Stress Test; X-Irradiation Stress Test

Test Commonly Includes Detection of increased spontaneous and chemically-induced chromosome breakage in the patient's lymphocytes compared to control lymphocytes.

Abstract Ataxia-telangiectasia (A-T), a chromosome breakage syndrome, is estimated to affect 1 in 40,000 individuals. The clinical findings of this rare autosomal recessive disorder include progressive cerebellar ataxia, ocular apraxia, telangiectasia, humoral and cellular immune deficiency, susceptibility to T-cell leukemia, muscular weakness, endocrine malfunction, and intellectual decline. A-T is a lethal disorder, and death, due to either recurrent infections or a neoplastic disease, usually occurs by the third decade of life. Carriers (heterozygotes) constitute approximately 1% of the U.S. Caucasian population.[1] Studies have indicated that female relatives of A-T patients have an increased risk (relative risk of 3.9) of breast cancer.[2] Cytogenetic diagnostic abnormalities of homozygotes include both spontaneous chromosome breakage and rearrangements and hypersensitivity to ionizing radiation and radiomimetic agents (chemicals in which the mode of action mimics that of radiation). IgA and IgE deficiencies are commonplace, as are IgG_2 and IgG_4 deficiencies. B- and T-lymphocyte deficiencies are variable.

Specimen Whole blood

Container Green top (sodium heparin) tube; EDTA, citrate, or lithium heparin anticoagulants should not be used

Storage Instructions Specimen should be delivered to the laboratory immediately.

Causes for Rejection Clotted or hemolyzed specimen, specimen more than 24 hours old, use of improper anticoagulant

Reference Range An increased frequency of chromosomal damage is observed compared to control specimens for both spontaneous breakage and chemically- or radiologically-induced chromosome breakage. The induced aberrations may be 10- to 20-fold higher than those observed in controls. Interpretation should be provided with report.

Use Increased levels of chromosome instability provide an important aid to clinical diagnosis of A-T.

Limitations Spontaneous chromosome damage is usually observed but may be absent in any given single specimen from a patient. Spontaneous breakage may need to be measured repeatedly over a period of time. In approximately 10% of families, the level of x-ray induced damage may not be significantly higher than in controls. However, within this group, spontaneous breakage is usually higher than controls.

Methodology Peripheral T cells from PHA-stimulated white blood cell cultures of the patient and a control are exposed to either X-irradiation or a radiomimetic agent such as bleomycin (a chemotherapeutic antibiotic leading to chromosome breakage effects which have been demonstrated in lymphocytes and fibroblasts of A-T patients). In addition, spontaneous breakage is evaluated from untreated specimens from both the patient and control. Cells are harvested in a routine fashion and either banded or unbanded chromosomes are evaluated for chromosome breakage and rearrangements.

Additional Information A gene, ATM (A-T, mutated), has recently been identified and is located on chromosome 11q22-q23.[3,4] Although previous studies identified complementation groups (different genetic defects with the ability to correct for one another), suggesting the possibility of involvement of multiple genes,[5] the ATM gene was found to be mutated in A-T patients from all complementation groups, indicating the ATM may be the sole gene involved in A-T.[4] In cytogenetic analysis of homozygotes, in addition to chromosomal breakage, nonrandom translocations and inversions of chromosomes 7 and 14 occur.[6] Molecular characterizations of these rearrangements suggest that a DNA repair/processing defect may be responsible for the different chromosomal abnormalities observed in A-T cells.[7] Because of the increased risk for breast cancer, identification of carriers (heterozygotes) of the A-T gene would be valuable. Cultured cells from heterozygotes may show some increased sensitivity to ionizing radiation, however, carriers generally cannot be readily identified by cellular or cytogenetic methods. The discovery of the ATM gene should now make it possible to identify heterozygotes. Unfortunately, the size of the gene and abundant mutational sites will complicate the development of a simple DNA screening test for identification of abnormalities of the ATM gene. See also the listing Bloom's Syndrome, Chromosome Breakage Study *on page 274*.

Footnotes

1. Swift M, Morrell D, Massey RB, et al, "Incidence of Cancer in 161 Families Affected by Ataxia-Telangietasia," *N Engl J Med*, 1991, 325(6):1831-6.
2. Easton DF, "Cancer Risks in A-T Heterozygotes," *Int J Radiat Biol*, 1994, 66(6 Suppl):S177-82.
3. McConville CM, Byrd PJ, Ambrose HJ, et al, "Genetic and Physical Mapping of the Ataxia-Telangiectasia Locus on Chromosome 11q22-11q23," *Int J Radiat Biol*, 1994, 66(6 Suppl):S45-56.
4. Savitsky K, Bar-Shira A, Gilad S, et al, "A Single Ataxia-Telangiectasia Gene With a Product Similar to PI-3 Kinase," *Science*, 1995, 268(5218):1749-53.
5. Jaspers NG, Gatti RA, Baan C, et al, "Genetic Complementation Analysis of Ataxia-Telangiectasia and Nijmegen Breakage Syndrome: A Survey of 50 Patients," *Cytogenet Cell Genet*, 1988, 49(4):259-63.
6. Aurias A, Dutrillaux B, Buriot D, et al, "High Frequencies of Inversions and Translocations of Chromosome 7 and 14 in Ataxia-Telangiectasia," *Mutat Res*, 1980, 69:369-74.
7. Kojis TL, Gatti RA, and Sparkes RS, "The Cytogenetics of Ataxia-Telangiectasia," *Cancer Genet Cytogenet*, 1991, 56(2):143-56.

References

Cohn MM, "Chromosome Breakage Syndromes," *Clinical Laboratory Medicine*, Chapter 28, McClatchey KD, ed, Baltimore, MD: Williams and Wilkins, 1994, 685-701.

Howell RT and Taylor MR, "Chromosome Instability Syndromes," *Human Cytogenetics: A Practical Approach*, Rooney DE and Czepulkowski BH, 2nd, ed, New York, NY: Oxford University Press, 1992.

McKusick VA, *Mendelian Inheritance in Man: A Catalog of Human Genes and Genetic Disorders*, 11th ed, Vol 2, Baltimore, MD: Johns Hopkins University Press, 1994, 1649-56.

Barr Bodies *see* Buccal Smear for Sex Chromatin Evaluation *on next page*

Bleomycin Stress Test *see* Ataxia-Telangiectasia, Chromosome Breakage Study *on this page*

Bloom's Syndrome, Chromosome Breakage Study

CPT 88230 (tissue culture for chromosome analysis, lymphocyte); 88245 (chromosome analysis for breakage syndromes, score 25 cells)

Related Information

Ataxia-Telangiectasia, Chromosome Breakage Study *on this page*
Bone Marrow *on page 307*
Fanconi's Anemia, Chromosome Breakage Study *on page 282*
Lymph Node Biopsy *on page 50*

Skin Biopsy *on page 54*

Xeroderma Pigmentosum, Chromosome Breakage Study *on page 283*

Synonyms Chromosome Breakage Syndrome, Bloom's Syndrome; Chromosome Instability Test; Sister Chromatid Exchange

Test Commonly Includes Evaluation for increased spontaneous sister chromatid exchange

Abstract Bloom's syndrome (BS) is a rare autosomal recessive disease characterized by a high incidence of cancer at a young age. Phenotypically, patients present with marked short stature, growth retardation, typical facies, and sun sensitivity in infancy and childhood characterized by erythema and telangiectasia over the facial butterfly area and dorsa of the hands. Immune deficiency occurs. Approximately one in four patients develops malignancy. The types and sites of the neoplasms, including leukemia, lymphoma, and solid tumors, are similar to the general population, however, develop early in life. Cytogenetically, BS is considered a chromosome breakage syndrome because of the increased spontaneous interchanges between homologous chromosomes. These exchanges, referred to as "sister chromatid exchange (SCE)", represent a cytologic marker useful for diagnosis of BS.

Specimen Whole blood

Container Green top (sodium heparin) tube. **Note:** Specimens in lavender top (EDTA) tubes, blue top (sodium citrate) tubes, or green top (lithium heparin) tubes are not acceptable.

Storage Instructions Specimen should be delivered to the laboratory immediately.

Causes for Rejection Clotted or hemolyzed specimen, specimen more than 24 hours old, use of improper anticoagulant

Special Instructions Call laboratory so that the test can be arranged and scheduled.

Reference Range An increased frequency of spontaneous sister chromatid exchange (SCE) is observed compared to control specimens. Interpretation should be provided with report.

Use Increased levels of spontaneous SCE are almost pathognomonic for the diagnosis of BS.[1]

Limitations The coexistence of a minor population of cells with a normal SCE frequency has been noted in some BS patients.[2]

Methodology Peripheral T cells from PHA-stimulated blood cultures of the patient and a control are exposed to 5-bromo-2'-deoxyuridine (BrdU). The majority of SCE occur during the second cell cycle in culture where DNA containing BrdU is used as the template for replication. Following photodegradation, the asymmetric incorporation of the BrdU is visualized as different degrees of fluorescence within the unifiliarly BrdU-incorporated chromatid and the bifiliarly BrdU-incorporated chromatid. Such differential staining allows for the detection of rearrangements between the sister chromatids.

Additional Information Abnormalities of DNA ligase I have been demonstrated in BS.[3,4] However, it has been shown that the DNA ligase I was unchanged in at least two cases with aberrant DNA ligase I molecular phenotypes.[5] This suggests a factor other than mutation in the ligase I gene must be involved as the basic defect. Spontaneous mutations in somatic cells occur more frequently in patients with BS. The major clinical features are thought to be due to the excessive mutation rate in somatic cells.[6] SCE is not increased in heterozygotes, and heterozygotes do not appear to have an increased risk for malignancy.

See also the listing Ataxia-Telangiectasia, Chromosome Breakage Study *on page 274.*

Footnotes

1. Cohn MM, "Chromosome Breakage Syndromes," *Clinical Laboratory Medicine*, Chapter 28, McClatchey KD, ed, Baltimore, MD: Williams and Wilkins, 1994, 685-701.
2. Weksberg R, Smith C, Anson-Cartwright L, et al, "Bloom Syndrome: A Single Complementation Group Defines Patients of Diverse Ethnic Origin," *Am J Hum Genet*, 1988, 42(6):816-24.
3. Willis AE and Lindahl T, "DNA Ligase I Deficiency in Bloom's Syndrome," *Nature*, 1987, 325(6102):355-7.
4. Chan JY, Becker FF, German J, et al, "Altered DNA Ligase I Activity in Bloom's Syndrome Cells," *Nature*, 1987, 325(6102):357-9.
5. Petrini JH, Huwiler KG, and Weaver DT, "A Wild-Type DNA Ligase I Gene Is Expressed in Bloom's Syndrome Cells," *Proc Natl Acad Sci USA*, 1991, 88(17):7615-9.
6. German J, "Bloom Syndrome: A Mendelian Prototype of Somatic Mutational Disease," *Medicine*, 1993, 72(6):393-406.

References

Howell RT and Taylor MR, "Chromosome Instability Syndromes," *Human Cytogenetics: A Practical Approach*, Rooney DE and Czepulkowski BH, 2nd ed, New York, NY: Oxford University Press, 1992.
McKusick VA, *Mendelian Inheritance in Man: A Catalog of Human Genes and Genetic Disorders*, 10th ed, Vol 2, Baltimore, MD: Johns Hopkins University Press, 1994, 1667-70.

Bone Marrow Chromosome Analysis *see* Chromosome Analysis, Bone Marrow *on page 277*

Buccal Smear for Sex Chromatin Evaluation

CPT 88130

Related Information

Amniotic Fluid, Chromosome and Genetic Abnormality Analysis *on page 273*

Chromosome Analysis, Blood *on next page*

Chromosome Analysis, Bone Marrow *on page 277*

Chromosome *In Situ* Hybridization *on page 281*

Oral Cavity Cytology *on page 298*

Synonyms Barr Bodies; Sex Chromatin

Test Commonly Includes Cell count of Barr bodies under oil immersion; fluorescent Y chromosome examination

Patient Preparation Rinse mouth prior to obtaining specimens for adults. In infants, collection should be performed between feedings.

Aftercare Usually not needed but saline rinses may be used.

Specimen Scrape of buccal mucosa (right and left sides submitted separately)

Collection Scrape buccal mucosa with tongue depressor and **discard.** Then firmly scrape again with **clean** tongue depressor and spread evenly on frosted side of glass slides; fix immediately in 95% ethanol. Label frosted slide with patient's name. Label bottle.

Causes for Rejection Improper fixation, air drying

Special Instructions Provide age, phenotype, sex, and pertinent clinical information including tentative diagnosis to the laboratory.

Reference Range For practical purposes, the presence of ≥4% cells in which clear sex chromatin bodies are found is diagnostic of XX chromosomal constitution.[1]

Use Confirm the presence or absence of sex chromatin and the presence or absence of fluorescent portion of the "Y" chromosome

Limitations Chromatin testing of newborn infants should be deferred for 1 week. The incidence of chromatin-positive cells may fall in both the mother and in a normal female infant; thus, the buccal smear of an infant female may be erroneously interpreted as chromatin negative in the first few days of life. The incidence of chromatin-positive nuclei rises slowly to reach normal ranges within 3-4 days. **This is a screening test only.** It is subject to marked technical variability in interpretation. It is also unable to detect chimeric states reliably. For complete sex chromatin evaluation, a formal karyotype is needed.

This is not a contemporary procedure.

Contraindications Mouth lesions, bleeding abnormalities

Additional Information In a phenotypic mature female, vaginal wall scrapings are suitable and possibly more accurate than buccal scrapings.

Footnotes

1. Koss LG, ed, *Diagnostic Cytology and Its Histopathologic Bases*, 4th ed, Philadelphia, PA: JB Lippincott Co, 1992, 867.

Chorionic Villus Sampling (CVS), Chromosome and Genetic Abnormality Analysis

CPT 88173-26 (interpretation and report); 88235 (culture); 88267 (chromosome analysis); 88280 (additional karyotypes)

Related Information

Amniotic Fluid, Chromosome and Genetic Abnormality Analysis *on page 273*

Bone Marrow *on page 307*

Chromosome Analysis, Blood *on next page*

Chromosome Analysis, Bone Marrow *on page 277*

Chromosome Analysis, Lymph Node and Solid Tumor *on page 279*

Chromosome Analysis, Products of Conception *on page 280*

Chromosome *In Situ* Hybridization *on page 281*

Cystic Fibrosis DNA Detection *on page 507*

Duchenne/Becker Muscular Dystrophy DNA Detection *on page 509*

Fragile X DNA Detection *on page 511*

Inherited Diseases of Metabolism and Cell Structure Tests *on page 327*

Polymerase Chain Reaction *on page 523*

Synonyms Chromosome Karyotype, Chorionic Villus Sampling; Chromosome Studies, Chorionic Villus Sampling

Test Commonly Includes Chromosomal complement of fetal trophoblast cells are examined for determination of abnormalities

Specimen Chorionic villi

Container Sterile container

Sampling Time 8-12 weeks gestation

Collection Fetal trophoblast tissue is aspirated from placental chorionic villi transcervically or transabdominally with ultrasound guidance as early as the 8th week of gestation, usually performed at 9-12 weeks of gestation.

(Continued)

Chorionic Villus Sampling (CVS), Chromosome and Genetic Abnormality Analysis *(Continued)*

Vascularized and budding villi of the chorion frondosum are collected transcervically or transabdominally by aseptic technique with ultrasound guidance between the 8th and 12th weeks of gestation. Maternally derived tissue such as maternal blood, decidua, and cervical mucus is carefully separated from other tissues under a dissecting microscope to prevent maternal cell contamination.

Pertinent medical findings should accompany the request including maternal age, gestational age by sonography, reason for study, relevant history, medication history, transfusion history, note of viral infection, number of pregnancies and miscarriages, and suspected diagnosis.

Storage Instructions Specimen should be transported to the laboratory at room temperature and under sterile conditions as quickly as possible.

Causes for Rejection Specimen frozen or lacking in viable chorionic villi

Turnaround Time 1-2.5 weeks may be needed to process material for final results.

Reference Range Forty-six chromosomes to include 22 sets of normal autosomal chromosomes and one set of normal sex chromosomes (XX for female; XY for male). Interpretative information is usually included.

Use Prenatal detection of chromosomal abnormalities, especially Down syndrome, in groups of pregnant women at risk. Such groups include women age 35 years or older, previous child with a chromosomal abnormality or multiple congenital abnormalities, three or more previous spontaneous abortions, familial history of a chromosomal abnormality, or known carrier of an X-linked disorder. At the same time that chorionic villi are collected for chromosomal analysis, additional sample can be obtained for testing of inherited metabolic disorders.

Limitations Failure of cells to grow in culture and/or contamination precludes complete analysis (molecular cytogenetic techniques (chromosome *in situ* hybridization) may be of use if this occurs). The overall success rate of chromosome analysis is slightly lower than with amniocentesis. The rate of fetal loss due to CVS, when the fetus is viable at 8-12 weeks gestation, is approximately 1% to 3%.

Contraindications Environment lacking capability in ultrasonography, genetic counseling, CVS, chorionic villi culturing, and chromosomal analysis techniques

Methodology Cell culturing of fetal trophoblast, subsequent harvesting and chromosome analysis with Giemsa or quinacrine banding techniques

Additional Information CVS is still a limited service in many centers. A distinct advantage of CVS is the earlier gestational age in which the specimen may be collected, thus reducing the period of uncertainty and allowing termination, if elected, to be performed on an outpatient basis, in the first trimester. Additionally, there is a rapid technique to visualize spontaneous metaphases in the cytotrophoblast layer yielding results in 1-3 days if desired. A disadvantage is that amniotic fluid alpha-fetoprotein (AFAFP) measurement cannot be performed at this stage; it must be done later.

References
Goldberg JD and Golbus MS, "Chorionic Villus Sampling," *Adv Hum Genet*, 1988, 17:1-25.

Thompson MW, McInnes RR, and Willard HF, "Prenatal Diagnosis," *Genetics in Medicine*, 5th ed, Chapter 19, Philadelphia, PA: WB Saunders Co, 1991, 411-25.

Chromosome Analysis, Blood

CPT 88230 (culture, lymphocytes); 88262 (chromosome analysis, count 15-20 cells)

Related Information

Synonyms Chromosome Karyotype, Blood; Chromosome Studies, Blood; Cytogenetics, Blood; Karyotype, Blood

Abstract The constitutional karyotype (chromosome complement) of each individual is determined during fertilization or during the first few cell divisions. If the karyotype is abnormal, development may be altered.

In general, chromosome abnormalities with gains or losses of large amounts of chromatin will manifest early in development and often result in spontaneous abortion. Examples of such abnormalities include trisomies, monosomy X, triploids, and large unbalanced structural rearrangements. Approximately 1 in 156 live births have a major chromosome abnormality. Congenital anomalies and/or mental retardation or phenotypic abnormalities which appear later on in life are observed in about half of these cases. Some chromosome abnormalities go undetected during prenatal and perinatal periods. Physical and mental developmental delays first noted during childhood may be associated with small unbalanced rearrangements, small interstitial deletions (microdeletions), and mosaic trisomies. Sex chromosome abnormalities may not be clinically evident until puberty when inappropriate secondary sexual development occurs or when infertility is recognized later in life. Finally, normal individuals who are carriers of balanced rearrangements may remain unrecognized until adulthood, at which time they can present with multiple miscarriages or abnormal offspring.

Specimen Whole blood

Container Green top (sodium heparin) tube. **Note:** Specimens in lavender top (EDTA) tubes, blue top (sodium citrate) tubes, or green top (lithium heparin) tubes are not acceptable.

Storage Instructions Specimen should be delivered to the laboratory immediately; do not freeze.

Causes for Rejection Clotted or hemolyzed specimen, use of improper anticoagulant, improper storage

Reference Range Forty-six chromosomes including 22 sets of normal autosomal chromosomes and one set of normal sex chromosomes (XX for female, XY for male). Interpretive information should be included.

Use Evaluate congenital anomaly (birth defect), developmental delay, ambiguous genitalia, mental retardation, cryptorchidism, hypogonadism, primary amenorrhea, infertility, multiple miscarriages, or the carrier status in relatives of patients with known chromosome abnormalities.

Limitations Failure to obtain metaphases occurs infrequently and may be due to collection in inappropriate anticoagulant or improper specimen storage (eg, frozen specimen).

Methodology Accessibility of peripheral blood along with the success of mitogen stimulation has made lymphocyte culture the test of choice in studying constitutional chromosomes. At times, other tissues, such as skin biopsy, may be used for studying the mosaic status of an abnormality or for detection of tissue-specific abnormalities. The method for lymphocyte analysis involves phytohemagglutinin stimulation during lymphocyte culture, colchicine arrest of cells in metaphase, methanol:acetic acid fixation, spread preparation using hypotonic solution, banding of chromosomes, microscopic chromosome analysis, and preparation of karyotypes by photography or computerized image analysis. Conventional banding techniques employ trypsin treatment of chromosomes followed by staining with Giemsa (or a similar stain). Alternative banding techniques and special stains for identification of specific chromosome regions include quinacrine banding, reverse banding, C-banding (constitutive heterochromatin banding), DAPI technique, Ag-Nor technique (silver stain), and fluorescence *in situ* hybridization.

Additional Information The highest proportion of chromosome abnormalities occurs in early spontaneous abortions (50%) (see Chromosome Analysis, Products of Conception *on page 280*). Approximately 7% of stillbirths and perinatal deaths are chromosomally abnormal, and 0.65% of newborns have a major chromosome abnormality. Trisomy 21 (Down syndrome) is the most frequent chromosome anomaly, with an incidence of 1 in 700-850 births. Sex chromosome aneusomies are the next most common. One XXY and one XYY is present in every 1000 male births, and one XXX is seen in every 1000 female births. Structural balanced rearrangements have a frequency of about 1 in 500 live births. Carriers of such balanced rearrangements are phenotypically normal but have an increased risk for having abnormal offspring and multiple miscarriages.

Chromosome abnormalities are present in about 10% of mentally retarded children. When mentally retarded children are examined who also have multiple birth defects or low birthweights, the incidence of chromosome abnormalities increases to 23%, half of which are Down syndrome. In addition, 3% to 6% of males and 3% to 4% of females with mental retardation will have the fragile X syndrome. (See listing Fragile X DNA Detection *on page 511*.)

No single phenotype is exclusive to any chromosome syndrome. The combination of phenotypic abnormalities, however, allows certain syndromes to be recognized (see table). In general, complex organ systems are often adversely affected by a great variety of chromosomal abnormalities. The heart, brain (mental retardation), head, eyes, genitourinary system, hands, and feet frequently are abnormal when an autosomal chromosome anomaly is present. In contrast, sex chromosome anomalies usually have less severe phenotypic abnormalities, with the reproductive organs most commonly involved, and mental retardation being only rarely observed. In addition to the classic chromosome syndromes listed in the table, syndromes associated with minute deletions (microdeletion syndromes) are detected using special high-resolution chromosome analysis (see Chromosome Analysis, High-Resolution *on page 278*).

Common Chromosomal Syndromes

Autosome Syndromes		
Syndrome	Chromosome Abnormality	Features
Down syndrome	Trisomy 21	Epicanthal folds, simian crease of palm, flat nasal bridge, congenital heart disease, mental retardation
Patau syndrome	Trisomy 13	Microcephaly, cleft lip/palate, congenital heart disease, polydactaly, mental retardation
Edward syndrome	Trisomy 18	Micrognathia, congenital heart disease, mental retardation, clenched 3rd/4th fingers/overlapped fifth, rocker-bottom feet
Wolf-Hirschhorn syndrome	Deletion 4p	Microcephaly, growth retardation, mental retardation, carp mouth
Cri-du-chat syndrome	Deletion 5p	Cat-like cry, microcephaly, hypertelorism, retrognathia, mental retardation
Warkam syndrome	Mosaic trisomy 8	Malformed ears, bulbous nose, deep palmer creases, absent or hypoplastic patellae
Beckwith-Weidemann syndrome	Duplication 11p15	Macroglossia, omphalocele, ear lobe creases
Pallister-Killian syndrome	Trisomy 12p	Psychomotor delay, sparse anterior scalp hair, micrognathia, hypotonia
Cat's eye syndrome	Trisomy 22q11-pter	Anal atresia, coloboma
Sex Chromosome Syndromes		
Syndrome	Chromosome Abnormality	Features
Klinefelter syndrome	47,XXY	Hypogonadism, infertility, underdeveloped secondary sexual characteristics, learning disabilities
XYY syndrome	47,XYY	Tall stature, increased risk of behavior problems
Triple X syndrome	47,XXX	Increased risk of infertility and learning disabilities
Turner-Ullrich syndrome	45,X (and other structural abnormalities of X)	Short stature, gonadal dysgenesis, webbed neck, broad chest, low posterior hairline, renal and cardiovascular anomalies

References

Gosden CM, Davidson C, and Robertson M, "Lymphocyte Culture," *Human Cytogenetics: A Practical Approach*, 2nd ed, Rooney DE and Czepulkowski BH, eds, New York, NY: Oxford University Press, 1992.

McKusick VA, *Mendelian Inheritance in Man: A Catalog of Human Genes and Genetic Disorders*, 11th ed, Baltimore, MD: Johns Hopkins University Press, 1995.

Mulinsky A, *Genetic Disorders and the Fetus*, 3rd ed, Baltimore, MD: Johns Hopkins University Press, 1992.

Robinson A and Linden M, *Clinical Genetics Handbook*, 2nd ed, Boston, MA: Blackwell Scientific Publications, 1993.

Thompson MW, McInnes RR, and Willard HF, *Genetics in Medicine*, 5th ed, Philadelphia, PA: WB Saunders Co, 1991.

Thurman E and Susman M, *Human Chromosomes*, 3rd ed, New York, NY: Springer-Verlag, 1992.

Van Dyke DL and Wiktor A, "Clinical Cytogenetics," *Clinical Laboratory Medicine*, McClatchey KD, ed, Baltimore, MD: Williams and Wilkins, 1994.

Chromosome Analysis, Bone Marrow

CPT 88237 (tissue culture for chromosome analysis, bone marrow); 88262 (chromosome analysis, count 15-20 cells)

Related Information

Amniotic Fluid, Chromosome and Genetic Abnormality Analysis *on page 273*
Bone Marrow *on page 307*
Breakpoint Cluster Region Rearrangement in CML *on page 503*
Buccal Smear for Sex Chromatin Evaluation *on page 275*
Chorionic Villus Sampling (CVS), Chromosome and Genetic Abnormality Analysis *on page 275*
Chromosome Analysis, Lymph Node and Solid Tumor *on page 279*
Chromosome Analysis, Products of Conception *on page 280*
Chromosome *In Situ* Hybridization *on page 281*
Lymph Node Biopsy *on page 50*
Oral Cavity Cytology *on page 298*
White Blood Count *on page 353*

Synonyms Bone Marrow Chromosome Analysis; Cytogenetics, Bone Marrow; Karyotype, Bone Marrow

Applies to Aneuploidy; Aneusomy; Fluorescence *In Situ* Hybridization (FISH); Monosomy; Philadelphia Chromosome; Retinoic Acid Receptor Alpha; Translocation; Trisomy

Abstract Cytogenetic analysis is often routinely used in the diagnostic study of patients with or suspected of having, a hematologic disorder. Numerous consistently occurring primary chromosome abnormalities have been well established in both acute and chronic hematologic diseases. Select abnormalities have specific associations with morphologic subtypes of disorders, and are therefore useful in establishing specific diagnoses. Cytogenetic findings at diagnosis have also been shown to be an independent prognostic factor associated with complete remission, duration of remission, and ultimate survival in many hematologic disorders. Chromosome analysis is also used for monitoring patients following standard treatment or bone marrow transplantation.

Specimen Bone marrow aspirate

Container 1-3 mL bone marrow should be transported in a sterile container containing preservative-free sodium heparin; specimens in EDTA, citrate, or heparin anticoagulants are not acceptable.

Storage Instructions Maintain the specimen at room temperature and transport **immediately** to the Cytogenetics laboratory.

Causes for Rejection Clotted or hemolyzed specimen

Use Chromosome analysis of bone marrow aids in diagnosis of hematologic disorders, supplies prognostic information, and is used to monitor patients following therapy or bone marrow transplantation.

Limitations Neoplastic cells may fail to grow in culture. Since normal bone marrow stem cells can divide *in vitro*, a normal cytogenetic result may reflect either a diploid neoplastic population or the analysis of normal cells. Sensitivity may be limited in detecting minimal residual disease since only 20-30 metaphases are routinely analyzed.

Methodology Bone marrow aspirates are the specimen of choice for cytogenetic analysis of hematologic disorders. In cases of lymphoma, lymph node biopsies or aspirates are more appropriate. At times, unstimulated peripheral blood cultures may be useful, for example, in chronic lymphocytic leukemia, or following a dry bone marrow tap. A combination of two to three methods for obtaining metaphases is normally employed for bone marrow specimens. A "direct harvest" technique is used to analyze cells undergoing spontaneous division. One or more short-term cultures (24- and/or 48-hour) are also performed. Short-term cultures, in contrast to the direct technique, may be necessary for consistent detection of certain abnormalities including t(8;21) and t(15;17). Culturing of cells in chronic lymphocytic diseases may be enhanced with the use of B- or T-cell mitogens. Colchicine arrest of cells in metaphase, followed by routine harvesting of metaphases is performed prior to banding and microscopic analysis of chromosomes.

Additional Information Acute myelogenous leukemia: More than 30 different structural chromosome abnormalities have been implicated as primary rearrangements in AML (see table 1). Several abnormalities are specifically associated with FAB (French-American-British) subclasses. For example, t(8;21) typically occurs in FAB group M2, t(15;17) in M3, inv(16)/del(16) in M4 with eosinophilia, and t(9;11) in M5. High complete remission rates have been noted in patients with t(8;21), while patients with hyperdiploid karyotypes or combined abnormalities of chromosome 5 and 7 have low remission rates. Although a significant loss of patients with M3 may occur early in the disease because of hemorrhagic complications, the t(15;17) subgroup of AML patients go into remission readily. The duration of complete remission has been shown to be long for patients with t(8;21), t(15;17), and inv(16). However, a subset of patients with t(8;21) has a high incidence of relapse. Short durations of complete remission have been associated with abnormalities of chromosomes 5 or 7. Abnormalities of chromosomes 5 and 7, +8, and 11q23 rearrangements generally are associated with a short mean disease-free survival. In adult patients, inv(16) has been associated with relatively long survival, while in children, a more intermediate survival has been observed. In general, patients with abnormalities of chromosome 5 have a poor prognosis, while those with inv(16), t(8;21), or t(15;17) have a good prognosis. Secondary AML (therapy-related or environmental mutagen-related) usually has a larger number of chromosome abnormalities than *de novo* AML. Hypodiploidy, -7, del(5q), der(11q), del(7q), and der(1;7) are among the characteristic chromosome abnormalities observed in secondary AML.

Chronic myeloproliferative disorders: The first chromosome abnormality found to be consistently associated with a neoplastic process, was a small marker chromosome, referred to as the Philadelphia chromosome (Ph). Greater than 90% of patients with chronic myelogenous leukemia (CML) were found to be Ph-positive. It was later shown that the Ph originated from a balanced translocation, t(9;22)(q34;q11.2). Complex-variant translocations are found in 5% to 10% of CML patients and have the same molecular rearrangement as the classic t(9;22). (Continued)

Chromosome Analysis, Bone Marrow *(Continued)*

Table 1. Common Chromosome Abnormalities in Acute Myeloid Leukemia

FAB Correlation	Karyotypic Abnormality	Comments
M1	t(9;22)(q34;q11)	Also seen in M2
	inv(3)(q21q26), ins(3;3)(q26;q21q26), t(3;3)9q21;q26)	Platelet and megakaryocytic abnormalities, also seen in M7 and MDS
M2	t(8;21)(q22;q22)	Auer rod positive
	t(6;9)(p23;q34)	Basophilia, also seen in M1, M4, and MDS
M3	t(15;17)(q22;q12)	
M4	trans 11q23 with 1q21, 2p21, 6q27, 10p11-15, 17q25, 19p13	
	del(11)(q23)	
	inv(16)(p13q22) del(16)(q22)	M4Eo, with eosinophilia
	+4	Also seen in M2
M5	t(9;11)(p22;q23)	Mostly M5a
ALL classes	+8	Also seen in MDS, MPD
Therapy-related AML	-5/del(5q)	Also seen in MDS
	-7/del(7q)	Also seen in MDS
	t(1;7)(p10;q10)	Also seen in MDS

FAB = French-American-British

Actual Ph-negative CML may be quite rare. Many of the cases thought to be Ph-negative in the past have been reclassified into disorders other than CML or have been shown, by molecular methods, to have a submicroscopic *bcr/abl* rearrangement. Since the Ph-positive clone persists following most modes of standard chemotherapy, the use of cytogenetics in monitoring such patients is of limited value. However, the detection of additional cytogenetic abnormalities (most commonly +Ph, +8, iso(17q), +19) can be very helpful in diagnosing the accelerated phase or impending blast crisis. Secondary cytogenetic abnormalities often precede clinical blast crisis by several months. Although no karyotypic abnormality is specific for the other myeloproliferative disorders (polycythemia vera, idiopathic myelofibrosis, and essential thrombocythemia), the most frequently observed chromosome changes include rearrangements of the long arm of chromosome 1, -7, del(7q), del(5q), +8, +9, del(13q), and del(20q).

Myelodysplastic syndrome: Chromosome abnormalities are detected in approximately one-third to one-half of all *de novo* myelodysplastic syndromes (MDS), varying in frequency among the FAB subgroups. Among the most common recurring, nonrandom chromosome aberrations are del(5q), -7, +8, del(20q), del(7q), and del(13q). Although these abnormalities do not aid in subclassification of the FAB subgroups and can also be seen in other disorders, the detection of an acquired clonal abnormality within bone marrow cells establishes the diagnosis of a neoplastic disorder. This is especially helpful in cases of refractory anemia in which morphological changes may be subtle. Deletion of 5q is the most common chromosome abnormality in MDS (approximately 30% of abnormal cases). 5q can be observed in any subgroup of MDS and in some other hematologic disorders. A subgroup of patients with del(5q) as the sole abnormality have specific clinicohematologic characteristics referred to as the "5q- syndrome". These patients characteristically are elderly women with refractory macrocytic anemia, elevated or normal platelet counts, and hypolobulated megakaryocytes. The clinical course is generally mild with only rare transformation to AML. A poorer prognosis is associated with del(5q) when accompanied by additional chromosome abnormalities. In addition to the prognostic significance associated with del(5q), the presence of monosomy 7 or complex karyotypes has been associated with a poor prognosis of MDS. The frequency of chromosome abnormalities is generally higher in secondary MDS. Deletions or monosomy of chromosomes 5 and/or chromosome 7 are often observed especially following exposure to alkylating agents. Likewise, rearrangements involving 11q23 have been associated with exposure to drugs targeted against topoisomerase II.

Acute lymphocytic leukemia: Approximately two-thirds of all acute lymphocytic leukemias (ALL) have abnormal karyotypes. Table 2 illustrates some of the most common abnormalities and the FAB subgroups and cell types with which they are associated. Loci involved in normal development of lymphocytes are often part of a chromosome rearrangement observed in both acute and chronic lymphocytic disorders. These loci include immunoglobulin genes; the heavy-chain locus (IGH) at 14q32, the kappa light-chain locus (IGK) at 2p12, the lambda light-chain

locus (IGL) at 22q11, and T-cell receptor molecules; the α-chain locus (TCRA) at 14q11, the β-chain locus (TCRB) at 7q34-36, and the γ-chain locus (TCRG) at 7p13. The karyotype has been shown to be an important independent prognostic factor in ALL. Patients with a modal chromosome number >50 (hyperdiploid) have the most favorable cytogenetic prognosis. When, however, structural abnormalities co-exist within the hyperdiploid karyotype, the prognosis is no longer favorable. Hypodiploidy is associated with a poor prognosis, as are specific translocations such as t(1;19), t(4;11), t(9;22) and t(8;14). A normal karyotype appears to have an intermediate prognosis.

Table 2. Common Chromosome Abnormalities in Acute Lymphocytic Leukemia

Karyotypic Abnormality	FAB Type	Cell Type
t(8;14)(q24;q32)	L3	B
t(8;22)(q24;q11)	L3	B
t(2;8)(p12q24)	L3	B
t(1;19)(q23;p13)	L1, L2	Pre-B
t(8;14)(q24;q11)	L1, L2	T
t(11;14)(p13;q11)	L1, L2	T
del(9p)	L1, L2	T
del(6)(q21q25)	L1, L2	CALLA and early pre-B
t(9;22)(q34;q11)	L1, L2	Pre-B
t(4;11)(q21;q23)	L1, L2	Mixed lineage

FAB = French-American British

Chronic lymphoproliferative disorders: As in acute lymphocytic leukemias, immunoglobulin gene and T-cell receptor gene loci are often involved in clonal chromosome rearrangements. Other characteristic cytogenetic findings include trisomy 12 and del(13q) in chronic lymphocytic leukemia, del(6q) in numerous B- and T-cell derived chronic disorders, and 2p rearrangements in Sezary's syndrome.

Fluorescence *in situ* hybridization (FISH): FISH is becoming an important adjunct to conventional cytogenetic methods for detection of numerous classic abnormalities, including t(9;22), t(15;17), +8, +12, in both metaphase and interphase nuclei[1] (see Chromosome *In Situ* Hybridization on page 281).

Footnotes

1. Wolman SR, "Fluorescence *In Situ* Hybridization: A New Tool for the Pathologist," *Hum Pathol,* 1994, 25(6):586-90.

References

Dewald GW, Morris MA, and Lilla VC, "Chromosome Studies in Neoplastic Hematologic Disorders," *Clinical Laboratory Medicine,* McClatchey KD, ed, Baltimore, MD: Williams and Wilkins, 1994.

Heim S and Metelman F, *Cancer Cytogenetics: Chromosomal and Molecular Genetic Aberrations of Tumor Cells,* 2nd ed, New York, NY: Wiley-Liss, 1995.

Rooney DE and Czepulkowski BH, *Human Cytogenetics: Malignancy and Acquired Abnormalities,* 2nd ed, Vol II, New York, NY: Oxford University Press, 1992.

Sandberg AA, *The Chromosomes in Human Cancer and Leukemia,* 2nd ed, New York, NY: Elsevier, 1990.

Chromosome Analysis, High-Resolution

CPT 88230 (culture, lymphocytes); 88262 (chromosome analysis, count 15-20 cells); 88289 (chromosome analysis, additional high resolution study)

Related Information

Chromosome Analysis, Blood *on page 276*
Chromosome *In Situ* Hybridization *on page 281*

Synonyms Microdeletion Study; Prometaphase Study; Prophase Study

Applies to Fluorescence *In Situ* Hybridization (FISH)

Abstract Standard blood culture and chromosome-staining techniques result in metaphase chromosomes with 400 to 500 total bands per haploid set of chromosomes. The recognition of various chromosome abnormalities resulting from subtle gains or losses of genetic material consisting of single bands or even smaller portions of chromosomes, has resulted in the development of techniques for detection of these minute abnormalities. High-resolution techniques arrest cells in prophase or prometaphase resulting in elongated chromosomes with identifiable bands in the 550 to 1200 band stage. Such techniques are used when microdeletions or other subtle chromosome abnormalities are suspected.

Specimen Whole blood

Container Green top (sodium heparin) tube. **Note:** Specimens in lavender top (EDTA) tubes, blue top (sodium citrate) tubes, or green top (lithium heparin) tubes are not acceptable.

Storage Instructions Specimen should be delivered to the laboratory immediately; do not freeze.

Causes for Rejection Clotted or hemolyzed specimen, use of improper anticoagulant, improper storage (frozen specimen)

Reference Range Forty-six chromosomes including 22 sets of normal autosomal chromosomes and one set of normal sex chromosomes (XX for female, XY for male). Interpretive information is usually included.

Use Detect small chromosomal deletions, duplications, or rearrangements

Limitations Failure to obtain metaphases occurs infrequently and may be due to collection in inappropriate anticoagulant or improper specimen storage (eg, frozen specimen). The detection limit is a function of the resolution of the microscopic; therefore, submicroscopic abnormalities (deletions, duplications, or rearrangements) may remain undetected by these methods. Fluorescence *in situ* hybridization is a useful adjunct in detecting microdeletions (see listing Chromosome Analysis, Bone Marrow *on page 277*).

Methodology High-resolution chromosomes can be obtained by synchronizing cells in particular stages of prophase or prometaphase. Antimetabolites, such as methotrexate, can be used to arrest cells in S-phase, followed by release with thymidine resulting in synchronization. Alternatively, addition of substances such as actinomycin D or ethidium bromide will interfere with condensation, resulting in elongated chromosomes.

Additional Information High-resolution chromosome analysis is useful in situations in which a small chromosome deletion, duplication, or rearrangement may be clinically suspected. A number of disorders have been shown to be associated with minute deletions or duplications of chromatin. Examples of the major microdeletion/duplication syndromes and their clinical characteristics are shown in the table. These disorders are often referred to as "contiguous gene syndromes". It is thought that each of several contiguous genes involved in the abnormality is responsible for a portion of the clinical manifestations associated with the disorder. Therefore, clinical manifestations can be variable depending on the extent of material deleted or duplicated. Some individuals with these syndromes have no chromosome abnormality, and others may have abnormalities too small (submicroscopic) to be detected even by high-resolution cytogenetic methods. DNA probes for select microdeletion syndromes are now commercially available. They are used in conjunction with high-resolution chromosome analysis for confirmation of microdeletions within metaphases using fluorescence *in situ* hybridization (FISH). In some cases, FISH may confirm the presence of a submicroscopic deletion that is beyond the resolution of high-resolution cytogenetic analysis.

Major Microdeletion Syndromes

Syndrome	Deletion	Features
Langer-Giedion	8q24.11-q24.13	Multiple exostoses, mental retardation, sparse hair, bulbous nose
Anirida/Wilms' tumor (WAGR)	11p13	Wilms' tumor with aniridia, gonodoblastoma, and retardation
Retinoblastoma	13q14	Retinoblastoma, osteosarcoma, bossed head
Angelman	15q11-q13	Hypotonia, ataxia, seizures, mental retardation, excessive laughter
Prader-Willi	15q11-q13	Neonatal hypotonia, hypogonadism, obesity, small hands and feet, mental retardation
Smith-Magenis	17p11.2	Hyperactive, self-destructive behavior, facial dysmorphism, mental retardation
Miller-Dieker	17p13.3	Lissencephaly, facial dysmorphism, mental retardation
DiGeorge/ Velocardiofacial	22q11.2	Hypoplasia of parathyroid and thymus, facial anomalies, congenital heart disease

References
Gosden CM, Davidson C, and Robertson M, "Lymphocyte Culture," *Human Cytogenetics: A Practical Approach*, 2nd ed, Rooney DE and Czepulkowski BH, eds, New York, NY: Oxford University Press, 1992.
McKusick VA, *Mendelian Inheritance in Man: A Catalog of Human Genes and Genetic Disorders*, 11th ed, Baltimore, MD: Johns Hopkins University Press, 1995.
Thompson MW, McInnes RR, and Willard HF, *Genetics in Medicine*, 5th ed, Philadelphia, PA: WB Saunders Co, 1991.
Van Dyke DL and Wiktor A, "Clinical Cytogenetics," *Clinical Laboratory Medicine*, McClatchey KD, ed, Baltimore, MD: Williams and Wilkins, 1994.

Chromosome Analysis, Lymph Node and Solid Tumor

CPT 88173-26 (interpretation and report); 88233 (solid tissue culture); 88239 (lymph node culture); 88262 (chromosome analysis); 88280 (additional karyotypes)

Related Information
Amniotic Fluid, Chromosome and Genetic Abnormality Analysis *on page 273*
Breast Cancer, Hereditary (BRCA1) *on page 504*
Chorionic Villus Sampling (CVS), Chromosome and Genetic Abnormality Analysis *on page 275*
Chromosome Analysis, Blood *on page 276*
Chromosome Analysis, Bone Marrow *on page 277*
Chromosome Analysis, Products of Conception *on next page*
Chromosome *In Situ* Hybridization *on page 281*
Colon Cancer, Hereditary Nonpolyposis Type *on page 506*
Gene Rearrangement for Leukemia and Lymphoma *on page 512*
Histopathology *on page 42*
Immunophenotypic Analysis of Tissues by Flow Cytometry *on page 45*
Lymph Node Biopsy *on page 50*
MIC2 *on page 52*
Muscle Biopsy *on page 53*
N-*myc* Amplification *on page 522*
Tumor Aneuploidy by Flow Cytometry *on page 57*

Synonyms Chromosome Studies, Lymph Node and Solid Tumor; Karyotype, Lymph Node and Solid Tumor

Test Commonly Includes Lymph nodal or solid tumor tissue is examined cytogenetically for clonal chromosomal abnormalities

Abstract Cytogenetic analyses of both benign and malignant solid tumors and lymphoma have revealed abnormalities in the number and/or structure of chromosomes. Many such changes are specific for a particular tumor type and thus, play a direct, potentially decisive role in examination and therapy of these lesions. In addition to adding a new dimension to the formulation of diagnosis, the cytogenetic findings provide prognostic information and resolution of cellular origin. Identification of aberrant chromosomal bands has served as a basis of molecular approaches to establish the definitive genes affected and the associated consequences of these gene alterations. In some instances, recognition of the cytogenetic abnormality is the first clue that a mutated gene resides at a particular locus.

Specimen Lymph node or solid tumor

Container Sterile container

Collection A portion of lymph node or tumor specimen surgically removed for histopathologic diagnosis is submitted fresh and aseptically for cytogenetic analysis. The sample should represent the neoplastic process and adjacent normal tissue should be discarded.

A 1-2 cm^3 sample (approximately 0.5-1 g) should be provided for analysis, preferably as part of the specimen submitted for surgical pathology. Pertinent medical findings such as age and sex of the patient, location of the lesion, indication, relevant history, note of any viral infection, and suspected diagnosis should be submitted.

Storage Instructions Specimen should be submitted to the laboratory as soon as possible. If overnight storage is necessary, the sample can be refrigerated in sterile isotonic saline or culture media containing serum.

Causes for Rejection Specimen frozen

Turnaround Time 2-14 days

Reference Range Normal lymph node and solid tissue cells contain 46 chromosomes with 22 pairs of autosomal chromosomes and one set of sex chromosomes (XX for female; XY for male). Clonal numerical and/or structural chromosomal abnormalities are detected in neoplastic tissue. An abnormal clone is defined as two or more cells exhibiting a gain of the same chromosome or structural alteration, or three or more cells exhibiting loss of the same chromosome. Many of the characteristic or tumor-specific chromosomal abnormalities are listed (see tables).

Use Cytogenetic analysis of lymphoma and solid tumors (in particular sarcomas), is a useful and sometimes, essential diagnostic adjunct. Cytogenetic analysis also provides prognostic information for some malignancies, see table.

Limitations Failure of cells to grow in culture, overgrowth of normal supporting stromal cells (fibroblasts) and/or contamination precludes complete analysis (molecular cytogenetic techniques (chromosome *in situ* hybridization) may be of use if this occurs).

Methodology Cell culturing of neoplastic cells, subsequent harvesting, and chromosome analysis with Giemsa or quinacrine banding techniques

Additional Information In some cases, molecular methods are subsequently used to further define chromosomal abnormalities.

References
Bridge JA, "Cytogenetic and Molecular Cytogenetic Techniques in Orthopaedic Surgery," *J Bone Joint Surg*, 1993, 75(4):606-14.
Sandberg AA, *The Chromosomes in Human Cancer and Leukemia*, 2nd ed, New York, NY: Elsevier, 1990.
Sandberg AA and Bridge JA, "Techniques in Cancer Cytogenetics. An Overview and Update," *Cancer Invest*, 1992, 10(2):163-72.

(Continued)

Chromosome Analysis, Lymph Node and Solid Tumor (Continued)

Chromosomal Abnormalities in Lymphoma and Solid Tumors

Diagnosis	Chromosomal Abnormality
B-cell non-Hodgkin's lymphoma	
(Burkitt) small non-cleaved cell	t(8;14) (q24;q32)
(Burkitt) small non-cleaved cell	t(2;8) (p12;q24)
(Burkitt) small non-cleaved cell	t(8;22); (q24;q11)
Small lymphocytic or diffuse large cell	+12
Diffuse large cell	t(3;14) (q27;q32)
Diffuse large cell	t(3;22) (q27;q11)
Centrocytic (variable zone) with CD5-positive cells	t(11;14) (q13;q32)
Mixed, small cleaved and large cell follicular	t(14;18) (q32;q21)
T-cell lymphoma	t(11;14) (p13;q11)
	inv(14) (q11;?)
	t(14;?) (q11;?)
Anaplastic large cell (Ki-1)	t(2;5) (p23;q35)
Solid Tumors	
Transitional cell bladder carcinoma	+7
	del(8p)
	-9/del(9q)
Breast cancer	t or del(1) (p35)
	del (3p)
	t or del(16q)
	del(17q)
Clear cell sarcoma	t(12;22) (q13;q12)
Colon cancer	Abnormalities involving 1, 17, and 18
	+7
	+12
	del(5q)
	del(10q)
Desmoplastic small round cell tumor	t(11;22) (p13;q12)
Ewing's sarcoma	t(11;22) (q24;q12)
Glioma	double minutes
	+7
	-10
Germ-cell tumors	i(12) (p10)
Leiomyoma	t(12;14) (q14;q23)
Lipoma	t(12;?) (q14;?)
Medulloblastoma	i(17) (q10)
Melanoma	t or del(1) (p12-22)
	t(1;19) (q12;p13)
	t or del(6q) or i(6) (p10)
	+7
Meningioma	-22/del(22q)
Myxoid liposarcoma	t(12;16) (q13;p11)
Neuroblastoma	double minutes
	homogeneously staining regions
	del(1) (p31-32)
Pleomorphic adenoma	t(3;8) (p21;q12)
Prostate cancer	del(7) (q22)
	del(10) (q24)
Renal cell carcinoma	del(3p)
Retinoblastoma	del(13) (q14)
Rhabdomyosarcoma (alveolar)	t(2;13) (q37;q14)
Small cell lung carcinoma	del(3) (p14;p23)
Synovial sarcoma	t(X;18) (p11;q11)
Wilms' tumor	del(11p)

Sandberg AA and Bridge JA, *The Cytogenetics of Bone and Soft Tissue Tumors*, Austin, TX: RG Landes Co, 1994.

Secondary Chromosomal Abnormalities of Possible Prognostic Relevance in Lymphoma

Chromosomal Anomaly	Clinical Relevance
1q21-22	Poor survival in intermediate/high grade lymphoma
2p	Skin infiltration
+3	High grade lymphoma
+5, +6, +18	Short survival
rea(5) or rea(14q11)	Short survival
rea(6q13-16)	B-cell disease and short survival
10q22-24	Short survival
13q21-24	Bulky disease
+17 or i(7) (q10)	Diffuse histology and short survival
+der(18) t(14;18)	Disease progression
Many abnormalities and no normal cells	Rapid progression and short survival
Normal cells present with abnormal clone	Better prognosis than those cases without normal cells

From Sanger W, University of Nebraska Medical Center, Omaha, NE, with permission.

Chromosome Analysis, Products of Conception

CPT 88173-26 (interpretation and report); 88239 (culture); 88262 (chromosome analysis); 88280 (additional karyotypes)

Related Information

Amniotic Fluid, Chromosome and Genetic Abnormality Analysis *on page 273*

Chorionic Villus Sampling (CVS), Chromosome and Genetic Abnormality Analysis *on page 275*

Chromosome Analysis, Blood *on page 276*

Chromosome Analysis, Bone Marrow *on page 277*

Chromosome Analysis, Lymph Node and Solid Tumor *on previous page*

Chromosome *In Situ* Hybridization *on next page*

Endometrial Cytology *on page 293*

Synonyms Chromosome Karyotype, Products of Conception, Spontaneous Miscarriage or Abortion; Chromosome Studies, Products of Conception, Spontaneous Miscarriage or Abortion

Test Commonly Includes Chromosomal complement of products of conception are examined for determination of abnormalities

Abstract The overall incidence of chromosomal abnormalities in spontaneous abortions is at least 50%. More is known about the occurrence and effects of chromosomal abnormalities in the human population than any other group of animals. This is not necessarily because it occurs more frequently in humans, but because of its readily recognized clinical effects, which are always severe except in the case of mosaicism. Trisomy has been identified for all the human autosomes except chromosome 1. Generally, trisomies result in spontaneous abortions. Appreciable numbers of live births occur only for trisomies 13, 18, and 21, and these children are always abnormal. Chromosomal abnormalities most commonly seen in spontaneous abortions include the following in order of frequency: 45, -X (Turner syndrome), +16, and triploidy.

Specimen Products of conception

Container Sterile container

Collection Products of conception are the evacuated contents of the uterus after termination of an early pregnancy or the spontaneously aborted material collected after early miscarriage. The latter specimen generally consists of variably recognizable fetal parts and remnants of the sac and placenta. Although some fetal specimens may be severely autolyzed (depending on the time elapsed between death and specimen collection), it is important not to be dissuaded from attempting culture because the placenta will have recently been attached to the maternal circulation and may still contain viable cells.

Causes for Rejection Specimen frozen or lacking in viable fetal cells

Turnaround Time 1-3 weeks

Reference Range Forty-six chromosomes to include 22 sets of normal autosomal chromosomes and one set of normal sex chromosomes (XX for female; XY for male). Interpretative information is usually included.

Use Detect chromosomal abnormality in a spontaneously aborted fetus is important for genetic counseling and assessing risks for future abnormal pregnancies. For example, young women (younger than 35 years of age) who have previously given birth to a trisomic infant or who have had a trisomic fetus detected prenatally are at high risk for having a second trisomic abortion.

Limitations Failure of cells to grow in culture and/or contamination precludes complete analysis (molecular cytogenetic techniques (chromosome *in situ* hybridization) may be of use if this occurs).

Contraindications Environment lacking capability in genetic counseling, products of conception culture, and chromosomal analysis techniques

Methodology Cell culture most commonly of fetal fibroblasts, subsequent harvesting and chromosome analysis with Giemsa or quinacrine banding techniques

References
Bridge JA and Sandberg AA, "Cytogenetics," *Anderson's Textbook of Pathology*, 10th ed, Damjanov I and Linder J, eds, 1996, 223-57.
Warburton D, Kline J, Stein Z, et al, "Does the Karyotype of a Spontaneous Abortion Predict the Karyotype of a Subsequent Abortion? Evidence From 273 Women With Two Karyotyped Spontaneous Abortions?" *Am J Hum Genet*, 1987, 41(3):465-83.

Chromosome Breakage Study, Ataxia-Telangiectasia *see*
Ataxia-Telangiectasia, Chromosome Breakage Study *on page 274*

Chromosome Breakage Syndrome, Bloom's Syndrome *see*
Bloom's Syndrome, Chromosome Breakage Study *on page 274*

Chromosome Breakage Syndrome, Fanconi's Anemia *see*
Fanconi's Anemia, Chromosome Breakage Study *on next page*

Chromosome Breakage Syndrome Test *see* Ataxia-Telangiectasia, Chromosome Breakage Study *on page 274*

Chromosome Breakage Syndrome Test *see* Xeroderma Pigmentosum, Chromosome Breakage Study *on page 283*

Chromosome *In Situ* Hybridization
CPT 88283
Related Information
Alpha$_1$-Fetoprotein, Amniotic Fluid *on page 71*
Amniotic Fluid, Chromosome and Genetic Abnormality Analysis *on page 273*
Bone Marrow *on page 307*
Buccal Smear for Sex Chromatin Evaluation *on page 275*
Chorionic Villus Sampling (CVS), Chromosome and Genetic Abnormality Analysis *on page 275*
Chromosome Analysis, Blood *on page 276*
Chromosome Analysis, Bone Marrow *on page 277*
Chromosome Analysis, High-Resolution *on page 278*
Chromosome Analysis, Lymph Node and Solid Tumor *on page 279*
Chromosome Analysis, Products of Conception *on previous page*
Histopathology *on page 42*
Lymph Node Biopsy *on page 50*

Synonyms Fluorescent *In Situ* Hybridization (FISH); *In Situ* Chromosome Hybridization; Molecular Cytogenetics

Abstract Chromosome *in situ* hybridization is a technique in which specific nucleic acid sequences can be visualized utilizing fluorescent-labeled probes in individual metaphase or interphase cells from fresh or aged samples such as blood smears, touch and cytospin preparations, or paraffin-embedded tissue. Chromosome *in situ* hybridization, a powerful technique which has revolutionized the field of cytogenetics, has numerous applications. Importantly, analysis with *in situ* hybridization is not contingent on dividing or mitosing cells and is the only form of analysis which provides cellular localization of DNA and RNA sequences in a heterogeneous cell population.

Several different types of chromosomal probes are commercially available. Those most commonly used include probes to chromosome-specific repeated sequences (such as alpha satellite and satellite III DNA, regions around the chromosomal centromere); sequence or loci-specific probes such as those which are unique for the different chromosomal regions of deletion in the microdeletion syndromes (see table in the listing Chromosome Analysis, High-Resolution *on page 279*) or translocation breakpoint flanking or spanning probes (eg, the Philadelphia chromosome or t(9;22) in CML); and whole chromosome "painting" probes. The latter are composed of a mixture of sequences that will bind to the entire length of a particular chromosome and are useful for resolving structural rearrangements.

Specimen The specimen required will depend on the reason the test is requested; may include blood, bone marrow, amniotic fluid, chorionic villus sample, products of conception, lymph nodes, or solid tumors. All specimens should be sent fresh if standard cytogenetic studies will also be performed. Frozen, fixed, or paraffin-embedded samples are acceptable for detection of numerical abnormalities and some translocations and deletions but are not suitable for all types of structural rearrangements.

Container Blood should be collected in a green top (sodium heparin) tube, 5 mL minimum; bone marrow should be collected in a heparinized syringe (20-25 units heparin), 1-2 mL minimum; amniotic fluid, chorionic villi, products of conception, lymph node and solid tumor tissue should be submitted in a sterile container. See listings Amniotic Fluid, Chromosome and Genetic Abnormality Analysis *on page 273*; Chorionic Villus Sampling (CVS), Chromosome and Genetic Abnormality Analysis *on page 275*; Chromosome Analysis, Blood *on page 276*; Chromosome Analysis, Bone Marrow *on page 277*; Chromosome Analysis, Lymph Node and Solid Tumor *on page 279*; Chromosome Analysis, Products of Conception *on page 280* for further collection instructions.

Storage Instructions All fresh specimens must be sent to the laboratory immediately after collection. Maintain at room temperature.

Causes for Rejection Specimen more than 48 hours old, specimen clotted or hemolyzed due to the use of improper anticoagulant will yield suboptimal results, specimens that are unlabeled or mislabeled are not acceptable

Turnaround Time 24-72 hours

Reference Range Normal chromosome number and structure. Interpretation is usually provided with the report.

Use Numerous applications of chromosome *in situ* hybridization exist. Chromosome *in situ* hybridization is useful for prenatal diagnosis in the detection of aneusomy (loss or gain of one or more chromosomes) such as Turner syndrome (45,X), trisomy 21 (Down syndrome), or other autosomal or sex chromosomal disorders such as Klinefelter syndrome, trisomy 13, and trisomy 18. An advantage of chromosome *in situ* hybridization is that mitosing cells are not required and results for a suspected disorder can be obtained with 24 hours if necessary. Chromosome *in situ* hybridization can uncover small rearrangements that are not detectable with standard karyotypic analysis (eg, the presence of a microdeletion (see table in Chromosome Analysis, High-Resolution *on page 279*) can be detected by the absence of signal on one of a homologous chromosome pair).

Chromosome *in situ* hybridization is also useful in the evaluation of neoplasia. For example, the 9;22 translocation characteristic of CML can be detected quickly in interphase cells with high sensitivity (useful for determination of residual disease) and may be seen in the absence of the translocation visible cytogenetically (cryptic rearrangement). Chromosome *in situ* hybridization is used to determine bone marrow transplant engraftment in sex-mismatched donors and recipients. Chromosome *in situ* hybridization is often used to characterize chromosomal abnormalities that are difficult to define with traditional cytogenetic analysis such as marker and supernumerary chromosomes.

Limitations Chromosome *in situ* hybridization can only provide information with respect to the specific probe being utilized. For example, using an X chromosome-specific probe to rule out Turner syndrome will not disclose chromosomal abnormalities involving other chromosomes such as trisomy 21, 18, or 13. Therefore, unless there is a high suspicion for a particular diagnosis, it is recommended that chromosome *in situ* hybridization studies are performed in conjunction with standard cytogenetic analysis.

Methodology Cells from the specimen are first immobilized on a microscope slide and fixed with a methanol:acetic acid fixative. Chromosome *in situ* hybridization is performed using probes selected for specific chromosomes or chromosomal regions. DNA sequences in the target and probe (which are complementary) are denatured and then mixed together so that the probe binds to the chromosomal regions in which it has high homology. The bound probe is detected using a series of fluorescent-labeled reagents and a fluorescent microscope.

Additional Information Chromosome *in situ* hybridization is utilized for detection of aneusomy (loss or gain of one or more chromosomes) or structural rearrangements (most commonly deletions and translocations) in metaphase or interphase cells in amniotic fluid, peripheral blood lymphocytes, bone marrow, chorionic villi, products of conception, and tumor cells.

References
Bridge JA and Sandberg AA, "Cytogenetics," *Anderson's Textbook of Pathology*, 10th ed, Damjanov I and Linder J, eds, 1996, 223-57.
De Lellis RA, "*In Situ* Hybridization Techniques for the Analysis of Gene Expression: Applications in Tumor Pathology," *Hum Pathol*, 1994, 25(6):580-5.
Jenkins RB, Le Beau MM, Kraker WJ, et al, "Fluorescence *In Situ* Hybridization: A Sensitive Method for Trisomy 8 Detection in Bone Marrow Specimens," *Blood*, 1992, 79(12):3307-15.
Tkachuk DC, Westbrook CA, Andreeff M, et al, "Detection of *bcr-abl* Fusion in Chronic Myelogenous Leukemia by *In Situ* Hybridization," *Science*, 1990, 250(4980):559-62.
Trask BJ, "Fluorescence *In Situ* Hybridization: Applications in Cytogenetics and Gene Mapping," *Trends Genet*, 1991, 7:149-54.
Wolman SR, "Fluorescence *In Situ* Hybridization: A New Tool for the Pathologist," *Hum Pathol*, 1994, 25(6):586-90.

Chromosome Instability Test *see* Ataxia-Telangiectasia, Chromosome Breakage Study *on page 274*

Chromosome Instability Test *see* Bloom's Syndrome, Chromosome Breakage Study *on page 274*

Chromosome Instability Test *see* Fanconi's Anemia, Chromosome Breakage Study *on next page*

Chromosome Instability Test see Xeroderma Pigmentosum, Chromosome Breakage Study on next page

Chromosome Karyotype, Blood see Chromosome Analysis, Blood on page 276

Chromosome Karyotype, Chorionic Villus Sampling see Chorionic Villus Sampling (CVS), Chromosome and Genetic Abnormality Analysis on page 275

Chromosome Karyotype, Products of Conception, Spontaneous Miscarriage or Abortion see Chromosome Analysis, Products of Conception on page 280

Chromosome Stress Test see Ataxia-Telangiectasia, Chromosome Breakage Study on page 274

Chromosome Stress Test see Fanconi's Anemia, Chromosome Breakage Study on this page

Chromosome Stress Test see Xeroderma Pigmentosum, Chromosome Breakage Study on next page

Chromosome Studies, Amniotic Fluid see Amniotic Fluid, Chromosome and Genetic Abnormality Analysis on page 273

Chromosome Studies, Blood see Chromosome Analysis, Blood on page 276

Chromosome Studies, Chorionic Villus Sampling see Chorionic Villus Sampling (CVS), Chromosome and Genetic Abnormality Analysis on page 275

Chromosome Studies, Lymph Node and Solid Tumor see Chromosome Analysis, Lymph Node and Solid Tumor on page 279

Chromosome Studies, Products of Conception, Spontaneous Miscarriage or Abortion see Chromosome Analysis, Products of Conception on page 280

Cytogenetics, Blood see Chromosome Analysis, Blood on page 276

Cytogenetics, Bone Marrow see Chromosome Analysis, Bone Marrow on page 277

Diepoxybutane Stress Test see Fanconi's Anemia, Chromosome Breakage Study on this page

Fanconi's Anemia, Chromosome Breakage Study

CPT 88230 (tissue culture for chromosome analysis, lymphocyte); 88248 (chromosome analysis for breakage syndromes, score 100 cells)

Related Information
Ataxia-Telangiectasia, Chromosome Breakage Study on page 274
Bloom's Syndrome, Chromosome Breakage Study on page 274
Bone Marrow on page 307
Complete Blood Count on page 312
Lymphocyte Transformation Test on page 416
Platelet Count on page 340
Xeroderma Pigmentosum, Chromosome Breakage Study on next page

Synonyms Chromosome Breakage Syndrome, Fanconi's Anemia; Chromosome Instability Test; Chromosome Stress Test; Diepoxybutane Stress Test; Mitomycin C Stress Test

Test Commonly Includes Detection of increased spontaneous and chemically-induced chromosome breakage in the patient's lymphocytes compared to control lymphocytes

Abstract Fanconi's anemia (FA) is an autosomal recessive disorder affecting approximately 1 in 360,000 people. The molecular nature of the defect in this chromosome breakage syndrome is unknown. However, the cytogenetic hypersensitivity to bifunctional alkylating agents is suggestive of a defect in the repair of DNA interstrand crosslinks. Clinical features include involvement of all marrow elements resulting in anemia, leukopenia, and thrombocytopenia. Frequent congenital malformations include radial ray defects, microcephaly, renal malformations, and mental retardation. FA is associated with increased risk of malignancy, especially acute myeloid leukemia which occurs in approximately 9% of patients. FA cells manifest spontaneous chromosome breakage and display enhanced chromosome breakage upon exposure to bifunctional DNA cross-linking agents including mitomycin C, diepoxybutane (DEB), and nitrogen mustard.

Specimen Whole blood

Container Green top (sodium heparin) tube; EDTA, citrate, or lithium heparin anticoagulants should not be used

Storage Instructions Specimen should be delivered to the laboratory immediately.

Causes for Rejection Clotted or hemolyzed specimen, specimen more than 24 hours old, use of improper anticoagulant

Special Instructions Call laboratory so that test can be arranged and scheduled.

Reference Range An increased frequency of chromosomal damage is observed compared to control specimens for both spontaneous breakage and chemically-induced chromosome breakage following exposure to DEB or mitomycin C. Interpretation is usually provided with report.

Use Increased levels of chromosome instability provide an important aid to clinical diagnosis of Fanconi's anemia (FA)

Limitations Discrepancies exist between the clinical classification of some patients and the diagnosis suggested by in vitro cytogenetic findings. Therefore, the definitive diagnosis should not be based solely on cytogenetic results.

Methodology Peripheral T cells from PHA-stimulated blood cultures of the patient and a control are exposed to a bifunctional DNA cross-linking agent such as mitomycin C or diepoxybutane (DEB). In addition, spontaneous breakage is evaluated from untreated specimens from both the patient and control. Cells are harvested in a routine fashion and either banded or unbanded chromosomes are evaluated for chromosome breakage and rearrangements. The chromosomal instability in FA is primarily characterized by breaks and gaps and nonhomologous multiradials.

Additional Information At least four complementation groups (different genetic defects with the ability to correct for one another) have been identified in FA suggesting the presence of at least four different genes involved in the disease.[1] Genes located on chromosome 20q13.2-q13.3 and 9q22.3 have been associated with complementation groups FA(A) and FA(C), respectively.[1,2] Carriers (heterozygotes) have an increased risk of cancer, although no excess of any specific cancer type has been noted. The study of chromosome breakage by use of DEB and mitomycin C is usually a reliable technique for identification of homozygotes. However, cytogenetic analysis is not dependable for identification of FA heterozygotes.[3] Successful prenatal diagnosis using amniotic cells in at risk pregnancies has been demonstrated.[4,5]

See also listings Ataxia-Telangiectasia, Chromosome Breakage Study on page 274 and Bloom's Syndrome, Chromosome Breakage Study on page 274.

Footnotes
1. Strathdee CA, Duncan AM, and Buchwald M, "Evidence for at Least Four Fanconi Anaemia Genes Including FACC on Chromosome 9," Nature Genet, 1992, 1(3):196-8.
2. Mann WR, Venkatraj VS, Allen RG, et al, "Fanconi's Anemia: Evidence for Linkage Heterogeneity on Chromosome 20q," Genomics, 1991, 9(2):329-37.
3. Rosendorff J, and Bernstein R, "Fanconi's Anemia: Chromosome Breakage Studies in Homozygotes and Heterozygotes," Cancer Genet Cytogenet, 1988, 33(2):175-83.
4. Auerbach AD, Sagi M, and Adler B, "Fanconi Anemia: Prenatal Diagnosis of 30 Fetuses at Risk," Pediatrics, 1985, 76(5):794-800.
5. Auerbach AD, Min Z, Ghosh R, et al, "Clastogen-Induced Chromosomal Breakage as a Marker for First Trimester Prenatal Diagnosis of Fanconi's Anemia," Hum Genet, 1986, 73(1):86-8.

References
Auerbach AD, Rogatko A, and Schroeder-Kurth TM, "International Fanconi's Anemia Registry: Relation of Clinical Symptoms to Diepoxybutane Sensitivity," Blood, 1989, 73(2):391-6.
Cohn MM, "Chromosome Breakage Syndromes," Clinical Laboratory Medicine, Chapter 28, McClatchey KD, ed, Baltimore, MD: Williams and Wilkins, 1994, 693.
Gordon-Smith EC and Rutherford TR, "Fanconi's Anemia: Constitutional Aplastic Anemia," Semin Hematol, 1991, 28(2):104-12.
Howell RT and Taylor MR, "Chromosome Instability Syndromes," Human Cytogenetics: A Practical Approach, Rooney DE and Czepulkowski BH, 2nd ed, New York, NY: Oxford University Press, 1992.
McKusick VA, Mendelian Inheritance in Man: A Catalog of Human Genes and Genetic Disorders, 11th ed, Vol 2, Baltimore, MD: Johns Hopkins University Press, 1994, 1805-11.

Fluorescence In Situ Hybridization (FISH) see Chromosome Analysis, Bone Marrow on page 277

Fluorescence In Situ Hybridization (FISH) see Chromosome Analysis, High-Resolution on page 278

Fluorescent In Situ Hybridization (FISH) see Chromosome In Situ Hybridization on previous page

In Situ Chromosome Hybridization see Chromosome In Situ Hybridization on previous page

Karyotype, Amniotic Fluid see Amniotic Fluid, Chromosome and Genetic Abnormality Analysis on page 273

Karyotype, Blood see Chromosome Analysis, Blood on page 276

Karyotype, Bone Marrow see Chromosome Analysis, Bone Marrow on page 277

Karyotype, Lymph Node and Solid Tumor see Chromosome Analysis, Lymph Node and Solid Tumor on page 279

Microdeletion Study *see* Chromosome Analysis, High-Resolution *on page 278*

Mitomycin C Stress Test *see* Fanconi's Anemia, Chromosome Breakage Study *on previous page*

Molecular Cytogenetics *see* Chromosome *In Situ* Hybridization *on page 281*

Monosomy *see* Chromosome Analysis, Bone Marrow *on page 277*

Philadelphia Chromosome *see* Chromosome Analysis, Bone Marrow *on page 277*

Prometaphase Study *see* Chromosome Analysis, High-Resolution *on page 278*

Prophase Study *see* Chromosome Analysis, High-Resolution *on page 278*

Retinoic Acid Receptor Alpha *see* Chromosome Analysis, Bone Marrow *on page 277*

Sex Chromatin *see* Buccal Smear for Sex Chromatin Evaluation *on page 275*

Sister Chromatid Exchange *see* Bloom's Syndrome, Chromosome Breakage Study *on page 274*

Translocation *see* Chromosome Analysis, Bone Marrow *on page 277*

Trisomy *see* Chromosome Analysis, Bone Marrow *on page 277*

UV Stress Test *see* Xeroderma Pigmentosum, Chromosome Breakage Study *on this page*

Xeroderma Pigmentosum, Chromosome Breakage Study

CPT 88230 (tissue culture for chromosome analysis, lymphocyte); 88248 (chromosome analysis for breakage syndromes, score 100 cells)

Related Information

Ataxia-Telangiectasia, Chromosome Breakage Study *on page 274*
Bloom's Syndrome, Chromosome Breakage Study *on page 274*
Fanconi's Anemia, Chromosome Breakage Study *on previous page*
Skin Biopsy *on page 54*

Synonyms Chromosome Breakage Syndrome Test; Chromosome Instability Test; Chromosome Stress Test; UV Stress Test

Test Commonly Includes Detection of increased chromosome breakage in the patient's lymphocytes after UV (ultraviolet radiation)-exposure or exposure to UV-mimetic drugs.

Abstract Xeroderma pigmentosum (XP) is an autosomal recessive disorder with a worldwide estimated frequency of 1 in 250,000. Clinical manifestations include sensitivity to UV radiation resulting in cutaneous (numerous freckles, hypopigmentation, hyperpigmentation, cutaneous atrophy) and ocular (photophobia, corneal ulcerations, atrophy of eyelids) abnormalities.[1] Patients have an increased risk for development of skin tumors early in life in sun-exposed areas. Basal cell carcinoma and squamous cell carcinoma represent the most common skin tumors; however, malignant melanoma also commonly occurs and may result in the patient's death. In most cases of XP, a defect of excision repair of UV-induced damage is present.

Specimen Whole blood

Container Green top (sodium heparin) tube; EDTA, citrate, or lithium heparin anticoagulants should not be used

Storage Instructions Specimen should be delivered to the laboratory immediately.

Causes for Rejection Clotted or hemolyzed specimen, specimen more than 24 hours old, use of improper anticoagulant

Special Instructions Call laboratory so that test can be arranged and scheduled.

Reference Range An increased frequency of chromosomal damage following UV-exposure is observed in XP patient lymphocytes compared to control lymphocytes. Interpretation is usually provided with report.

Use Increased levels of chromosome instability provide an aid to clinical diagnosis of xeroderma pigmentosum (XP)

Limitations The level of repair synthesis can vary depending on complementation groups. It is important, therefore, to determine the extent of abnormal synthesis in a proband before attempting prenatal diagnosis.

Methodology Peripheral T cells from PHA-stimulated blood cultures of the patient and a control are exposed to UV radiation. Cells are harvested in a routine fashion and either banded or unbanded chromosomes are evaluated for chromosome breakage and rearrangements. XP cells display a higher level of induced sister chromatid exchange and other chromatid breakage anomalies.

Additional Information At least seven complementation groups (different genetic defects with the ability to correct for one another) have been described in XP, and in the majority of groups, the incision step of UV damage repair is defective.[2] Central nervous system symptoms occur in approximately 18% of cases. A clinical subtype of XP, De Sanctis-Cacchione syndrome is characterized by severe neurologic involvement.[3] Cancers, other than skin-related cancers, are rare in XP patients, although the risk for developing other malignancies is increased approximately 12% over the general population.

See also listings Bloom's Syndrome, Chromosome Breakage Study *on page 274*, Ataxia-Telangiectasia, Chromosome Breakage Study *on page 274*, and Fanconi's Anemia, Chromosome Breakage Study *on page 282*.

Footnotes

1. Kraemer KH, Lee MM, and Scotto J, "Xeroderma Pigmentosum: Cutaneous, Ocular, and Neurologic Abnormalities in 830 Published Cases," *Arch Dermatol*, 1987, 123(2):241-50.

2. Bootsma D and Hoeijmakers JH, "The Genetic Basis of Xeroderma Pigmentosum," *Ann Genet*, 1991, 34(3-4):143-50.

3. Kanda T, Oda M, Yonezawa M, et al, "Peripheral Neuropathy in Xeroderma Pigmentosum," *Brain*, 1990, 113(Pt 4):1025-44.

References

Cohn MM, "Chromosome Breakage Syndromes," *Clinical Laboratory Medicine*, Chapter 28, McClatchey KD, ed, Baltimore, MD: Williams and Wilkins, 1994, 693.

Howell RT and Taylor MR, "Chromosome Instability Syndromes," *Human Cytogenetics: A Practical Approach*, Rooney DE and Czepulkowski BH, 2nd ed, New York, NY: Oxford University Press, 1992.

McKusick VA, *Mendelian Inheritance in Man: A Catalog of Human Genes and Genetic Disorders*, 11th ed, Vol 2, Baltimore, MD: Johns Hopkins University Press, 1994, 2275-80.

Sandberg AA, *The Chromosomes in Human Cancer and Leukemia*, 2nd ed, New York, NY: Elsevier, 1990.

X-Irradiation Stress Test *see* Ataxia-Telangiectasia, Chromosome Breakage Study *on page 274*

CYTOPATHOLOGY

Melanie J. Castelli, MD

Russell M. Fiorella, MD

Patricia G. Tweeddale, EdD, CT (ASCP)

David S. Jacobs, MD

Paolo Gattuso, MD

Yeh Peng, MD

Susan B. Yokota Dubey, CT (ASCP), CMIAC

Cytopathology is the study of pathologic alterations in individual cells that reflect changes in their environment and also in the spectrum from premalignant to neoplastic conditions. The accurate interpretation of cytologic changes cannot be separated from the clinical presentation. All pertinent clinical and radiologic information is of inestimable value to a good cytomorphologist. Other factors are of importance also, and these include an adequate specimen: good cellularity, correct site sampled, and proper fixation.

The most commonly performed cytologic examination is the familiar "Pap" smear, a cervicovaginal specimen, introduced in 1943[1] by Dr George Papanicolaou. This screening procedure has played a role in reducing morbidity and mortality in women from cervical carcinoma.

Cytologic screening of many body sites is now routine. Exfoliated cells in urine, spinal fluid, effusion fluids (ascites, pleural, pericardial, joint), and fiberoptic endoscopically obtained brushings of the oropharyngeal, gastrointestinal, and upper genitourinary tract are all obtained without difficulty and frequently will yield a diagnosis for the clinician.

In addition, the development of fine needle aspiration cytology of palpable masses as well as deep seated lesions (available with radiographic assistance) has greatly enlarged the scope of cytopathologic practice. The place for fine needle aspiration diagnosis is at the forefront of cytopathology; however, the decision as to indications for use must be made jointly by clinician and pathologist.

In addition, cytologic material can be studied at present with numerous special modalities, including flow cytometry, electron microscopy, immunoperoxidase staining, immunofluorescence, and standard tissue special stains. The studies may elucidate specific etiologies of neoplasms; however, the diagnosis of a neoplastic versus a non-neoplastic process remains a morphologic one.

In order for the Cytopathology Laboratory to maintain high standards of diagnostic accuracy, close communication with the clinical staff must be regarded as essential. In addition, the patients' welfare is of the utmost importance, and in no case in which a question exists, either on the part of clinician or cytopathologist, should the suggestion for tissue confirmation be withheld. A well trained, experienced cytopathology staff is an invaluable asset to clinicians and patients alike.

Footnotes

1. Papanicolaou GN and Traut HF, *Diagnosis of Uterine Cancer by the Vaginal Smear*, New York, NY: The Commonwealth Fund, 1943.

Abdominal Mass Aspiration *see* Fine Needle Aspiration, Deep Seated Lesions *on page 294*

Amniotic Fluid Cytology

CPT 88313

Related Information

Amniotic Fluid, Chromosome and Genetic Abnormality Analysis *on page 273*

Amniotic Fluid Lecithin/Sphingomyelin Ratio and Phosphatidylglycerol *on page 77*

Cytomegalic Inclusion Disease Cytology *on page 293*

Nile Blue Fat Stain *on page 297*

Synonyms Premature Rupture of Bag of Waters (BOW); Premature Rupture of Fetal Membranes

Test Commonly Includes Simple smear from external os in patients suspected of having prematurely ruptured the amniotic sac (bag of waters)

Abstract Amniotic fluid is used for fetal evaluation using a variety of methods including biochemical, biophysical, and immunological techniques. Fluid obtained from the external os is a useful indicator for rupture of fetal membranes.

Specimen Amniotic fluid

Sampling Time Less than 15 minutes

Collection Obtain fluid with simple spatula or even wooden tongue depressor from the external os, fresh, smeared onto either a plain glass or frosted glass slide, and fixed in 95% ethyl alcohol.

Reference Range In nonrupture, the fluid will show a smooth, even pattern when examined under the microscope.

Use Assess leakage of amniotic fluid from the cervical os in cases of rupture of the fetal membranes

Contraindications Extensive bleeding precludes use of this method

Methodology Alcohol-fixed, Papanicolaou-stained smear, examined for "ferning" of the fluid obtained. The smear will show branching in the pattern of fern leaves induced by the presence of sodium in high concentration leaking from the amniotic fluid secondary to the high estrogen content of the fluid.

Additional Information One may sometimes be called upon to distinguish between maternal urine and amniotic fluid. Typically amniotic fluid contains more protein than urine and has concentrations of urea and creatinine similar to serum concentrations. Maternal urine typically contains higher urea and creatinine concentrations than amniotic fluid. Protein, urea, and creatinine concentrations may vary with the age of pregnancy.[1]

Footnotes

1. Schumann GB and Schweitzer SC, "Examination of Urine," *Todd-Sanford-Davidsohn Clinical Diagnosis and Management by Laboratory Methods*, 18th ed, Henry JB, ed, Philadelphia, PA: WB Saunders Co, 1991, 388-9.

References

Cunningham FG, MacDonald PC, Leveno KJ, et al, *Williams Obstetrics*, 19th ed, Norwalk, CT: Appleton and Lange, 1993, 373.

Romero R, Quintero R, Nores J, et al, "Amniotic Fluid White Blood Cell Count: A Rapid and Simple Test to Diagnose Microbial Invasion of the Amniotic Cavity and Predict Preterm Delivery," *Am J Obstet Gynecol*, 1991, 165(4 Pt 1):821-30.

Ascitic Fluid Cytology *see* Body Fluid Cytology *on this page*

BAL Cytology *see* Bronchoalveolar Lavage Cytology *on page 288*

Bladder, Ureteral, and Pelvicocalyceal Barbotage Specimens *see* Urine Cytology *on page 301*

Bladder Washings Cytology *see* Urine Cytology *on page 301*

Body Cavity Fluid Cytology *see* Body Fluid Cytology *on this page*

Body Fluid Cytology

CPT 88108

Related Information

Bacterial Culture, Biopsy or Body Fluid *on page 456*

Body Fluid *on page 89*

Body Fluid Amylase *on page 91*

Body Fluid Analysis, Cell Count *on page 306*

Body Fluid Glucose *on page 91*

Body Fluid Lactate Dehydrogenase *on page 92*

Body Fluid pH *on page 92*

CA 125 *on page 94*

Carcinoembryonic Antigen *on page 100*

Cyst Fluid Cytology *on page 292*

Fungal Culture, Biopsy or Body Fluid *on page 476*

Gene Rearrangement for Leukemia and Lymphoma *on page 512*

Gram's Stain *on page 481*

Immunoperoxidase Procedures *on page 43*

Immunophenotypic Analysis of Tissues by Flow Cytometry *on page 45*

Mycobacterial Culture, Biopsy or Body Fluid *on page 487*

Polymerase Chain Reaction *on page 523*

Synovial Fluid Analysis *on page 656*

Tumor Aneuploidy by Flow Cytometry *on page 57*

Viral Culture *on page 675*

Viral Culture, Body Fluid *on page 677*

Washing Cytology *on page 302*

Synonyms Body Cavity Fluid Cytology; Effusion Cytology; Fluids Cytology; Serous Effusion Cytology; Serous Fluid Cytology

Applies to Ascitic Fluid Cytology; Culdocentesis; Paracentesis Fluid Cytology; Pericardial Fluid Cytology; Peritoneal Fluid Cytology; Pleural Fluid Cytology; Synovial Fluid Cytology; Thoracentesis Fluid Cytology

Test Commonly Includes Cytologic evaluation of smears, cytocentrifuge preparations, filter preparations, and cell block preparations when indicated

Abstract Cytologic evaluation of body fluids, in conjunction with chemical analysis and clinical profile, can render and/or enhance diagnosis of a variety of benign and malignant conditions. Fluid may be obtained during staging surgical procedures (see listing Washing Cytology *on page 302*) or by puncture.

Patient Preparation Patient should sign informed consent prior to procedure. Puncture site should be carefully cleaned and prepared as for any tap. In cases of suspected malignancy, the smallest gauge needle (22 g) should be used, as tract seeding has been reported postthoracentesis with large bore needles.

Specimen Fresh body fluid

Container Use clear container to which anticoagulant can be added prior to collection. The optimal amount of fluid for cytology is 200-500 mL. The practice of salvaging large amounts (in excess of 500 mL) of fluid for cytologic examination is not recommended. The best diagnostic aliquot is the last portion that is drawn off, not the first. See Special Instructions.

Collection Gently agitate the container as fluid is collected in order to mix the heparin with the fluid; fluid may also be collected fresh without anticoagulant and sent to the laboratory in the fresh state immediately. Other tests are usually needed as well; see Related Information above. **Venous blood** drawn at the same time may be helpful; comparisons between serum and body fluid protein, LD, glucose, and other tests are often useful. See listing Body Fluid *on page 89*. When pleural fluid is sampled, a **pleural biopsy** may provide diagnosis, especially of granulomatous diseases as well as carcinoma.

Storage Instructions Fluid with or without anticoagulant may be stored at 4°C; cells in the fluid can be preserved at this temperature for up to 1 week, without appreciable deterioration of cellular detail. With special techniques, specimens may be kept frozen at -70°C for 1 year without serious loss of cellular details.[1]

Causes for Rejection Added fixation of any type, unless previously discussed with Cytology Laboratory personnel; prolonged period (over 2 hours) at room temperature; improper container (thoracentesis and paracentesis drainage bags and large syringes are not acceptable containers)

Special Instructions Add 1 mL of heparin per 100 mL of fluid anticipated (each mL of heparin contains 1000 units). The common anticoagulants that can be used are heparin, 5-10 units per mL of fluid to be placed in the collecting vessel; or 3.8% sodium citrate, 1 mL per 10 mL of fluid; or EDTA, 1 mg per 1 mL of fluid. The cells in these fluids do not deteriorate rapidly if refrigerated, and no fixative need be added if the **fluid is refrigerated** within 30 minutes of collection. Fixation precludes the use of certain stains which may be useful for particular diagnoses. Include pertinent clinical information on requisition including previous malignancy, drugs, radiation therapy, or history of alcohol abuse.

Use Establish the presence of primary or metastatic neoplasms. Aid in the diagnosis of rheumatoid pleuritis; systemic lupus erythematosus; myeloproliferative and lymphoproliferative disorders; viral, fungal, and parasitic infestation of serous cavities, and fistulas involving serous cavities. Examination of effusion is more sensitive and specific than blind pleural biopsy in the diagnosis of malignant pleural disease. The presence of malignant neoplastic cells in the fluid usually indicates that the patient has widespread metastases, with the exception of patients with primary pulmonary lesions. Effusion fluid may be submitted for flow cytometric analysis in those cases suspected of myeloproliferative or lymphoproliferative disorder.

Examination of **synovial fluid** from a joint effusion may aid in the diagnosis of metabolic arthritis (gout or pseudogout), rheumatoid arthritis, or traumatic arthritis as well as septic arthritis (gonococcal arthritis). Useful in staging of neoplasms.

Limitations Allowing fluid to stand for prolonged period before processing may cause deterioration and artifacts. In such fluids a second tap may be required after the reaccumulation of fluid for optimal cytologic interpretation. Clots may contain diagnostic cells which are available for recovery by preparation of a cell block; routine smears may fail to reveal such cells. Malignant cells cannot be recovered from all fluids from all subjects with malignant disease. Very well differentiated carcinomas may be difficult to distinguish from reactive states.

The most common cause of pleural transudate is congestive heart failure.

Contraindications Relative contraindications include documented bleeding diathesis and full anticoagulated state.

Additional Information Fluids should be submitted **fresh, unfixed**, and **heparinized** with anticoagulant added before collection to provide well-preserved, representative, diagnostic material. Exfoliated cells deteriorate rapidly in effusions, both in and out of the body. The amount of anticoagulant recommended is minimal but adequate to prevent clotting of body cavity fluids and to act as a preservative; excess amounts will not alter cytologic detail. Cytologic evaluation may classify the type of neoplasm and suggest its site of origin. Fixatives, such as formalin and alcohol, or other types of fixatives must not be used since they prevent adherence of the cells to the slides, do not allow cells to flatten out for optimal presentation of cellular details, and hinder quality staining by the Papanicolaou method. Alcohol also causes precipitation of protein which may interfere with cell analysis. If feasible, cell blocks can be prepared from the fluid sediment. Immunocytochemical studies can be performed on the cytology slides and cell blocks as additional diagnostic methods.[2,3,4,5,6,7]

Tumor markers support discrimination between benign and malignant effusions. **Carcinoembryonic antigen** (CEA) is used both as an immunocytochemical marker and as a test available for serum and other body fluids. As a fluid marker, it is significantly increased with many carcinomas of lung, especially adenocarcinomas,[8] while mesotheliomas do not cause significant elevations of fluid CEA. Other primary sites likely to cause CEA elevations include breast and gastrointestinal tract.

CA 125 elevation with negative CEA assay occurs with serous and endometrioid carcinomas of ovary and adenocarcinoma of endometrium and fallopian tube.[9,10] By contrast, increased fluid CEA with negative CA 125 results are found with mucinous adenocarcinomas of ovary, lungs, gastrointestinal tract (including pancreas), or breast.[10] Both antigens are within normal range with lymphoma, melanoma, and benign effusions. See listing CA 125 *on page 94.*

Lymphoblastic lymphoma classically presents as a mediastinal mass, with which pleural effusion is often found.[11]

Ascitic fluid from patients with cirrhosis may contain markedly atypical cells which may be derived from mesothelial cells.[12]

When fluids are examined in the clinical microscopy laboratory, detection of neoplastic cells cannot be expected to compare with the capabilities of the cytopathology laboratory.[13]

See also the listing Washing Cytology *on page 302.*

Footnotes
1. McCorriston J, "New Method for Preserving Cytology Specimens," *J Clin Pathol,* 1989, 42(10):1101-3.
2. Bedrossian CW, Bonsib S, and Moran C, "Differential Diagnosis Between Mesothelioma and Adenocarcinoma: A Multimodal Approach Based on Ultrastructure and Immunocytochemistry," *Semin Diagn Pathol,* 1992, 9(2):124-40.
3. Nance KV and Silverman JF, "Immunocytochemical Panel for the Identification of Malignant Cells in Serous Effusions," *Am J Clin Pathol,* 1991, 95(6):887-94.
4. Kuhlmann L, Berghauser KH, and Schaffer R, "Distinction of Mesothelioma From Carcinoma in Pleural Effusions. An Immunocytochemical Study on Routinely Processed Cytoblock Preparations," *Pathol Res Pract,* 1991, 187(4):467-71.
5. Wirth PR, Legier J, and Wright GL Jr, "Immunohistochemical Evaluation of Seven Monoclonal Antibodies for Differentiation of Pleural Mesothelioma From Lung Adenocarcinoma," *Cancer,* 1991, 67(3):655-62.
6. Tickman RJ, Cohen C, Varma VA, et al, "Distinction Between Carcinoma Cells and Mesothelial Cells in Serous Effusions. Usefulness of Immunohistochemistry," *Acta Cytol,* 1990, 34(4):491-6.
7. Flens MJ, van der Valk P, Tadema TM, et al, "The Contribution of Immunocytochemistry in Diagnostic Cytology. Comparison and Evaluation With Immunohistology," *Cancer,* 1990, 65(12):2704-11.
8. Kjeldsberg CR and Knight JA, *Body Fluids - Laboratory Examination of Amniotic, Cerebrospinal, Seminal, Serous, and Synovial Fluids,* 3rd ed, Chicago, IL: American Society of Clinical Pathologists, 1993, 159-254.
9. Pinto MM, Bernstein LH, Brogan DA, et al, "Immunoradiometric Assay of CA 125 in Effusions. Comparison With Carcinoembryonic Antigen," *Cancer,* 1987, 59(2):218-22.
10. Rudolph RA, Pinto MM, and Bernstein LH, "Measuring Decision Values for CEA and CA 125 in Effusions," *Lab Med,* 1990, 21(9):574-8.
11. Sandlund JT, Downing JR, and Crist WM, "Non-Hodgkin's Lymphoma in Childhood," *N Engl J Med,* 1996, 334(19):1238-48.
12. Guzman J, Bross KJ, Schölmerich J, et al, "Immunocytochemical Analysis of Ascitic Fluid Due to Cirrhosis - A Contribution to Understanding the Origin of Markedly Atypical Cells," *Acta Cytol,* 1992, 36(2):236-40
13. Ben-Ezra J, Stastny JF, Harris AC, et al, "Comparison of the Clinical Microscopy Laboratory With the Cytopathology Laboratory in the Detection of Malignant Cells in Body Fluids," *Am J Clin Pathol,* 1994, 102(4):439-42.

References
Bedrossian CW, Mason MR, and Gupta PK, "Rapid Cytologic Diagnosis of *Pneumocystis:* A Comparison of Effective Techniques," *Semin Diagn Pathol,* 1989, 6(3):245-61.

Bottles K, Reznicek MJ, Holly EA, et al, "Cytologic Criteria Used to Diagnose Adenocarcinoma in Pleural Effusions," *Mod Pathol,* 1991, 4(6):677-81.

Brandstetter RD, Velazquez V, Viejo C, et al, "Postural Changes in Pleural Fluid Constituents," *Chest,* 1994, 105(5):1458-61.

Covell JL, Lowry EH, and Feldman PS, "Cytologic Diagnosis of Blastomycosis in Pleural Fluid," *Acta Cytol,* 1982, 26:833-6.

Drew PA and Krauss JS, "Identification of *Giardia lamblia* in Peritoneal Fluid of Trauma Patients," *Acta Cytol,* 1989, 33(2):283-4.

Ehya H, "The Cytologic Diagnosis of Mesothelioma," *Semin Diagn Pathol,* 1986, 3(3):196-203.

Fam AG, Voorneveld C, Robinson JB, et al, "Synovial Fluid Immunocytology in the Diagnosis of Leukemic Synovitis," *J Rheumatol,* 1991, 18(2):293-6.

Gerbes AL, Jüngst D, Xie Y, et al, "Ascitic Fluid Analysis for the Differentiation of Malignancy-Related and Nonmalignant Ascites: Proposal of a Diagnostic Sequence," *Cancer,* 1991, 68(8):1808-14.

Goodman ZD, Gupta PK, Frost JK, et al, "Cytodiagnosis of Viral Infections in Body Cavity Fluids," *Acta Cytol,* 1979, 23:204-8.

Hallman JR and Geisinger KR, "Cytology of Fluids From Pleural, Peritoneal and Pericardial Cavities in Children. A Comprehensive Survey," *Acta Cytol,* 1994, 38(2):209-17.

Hira PR, Lindberg LG, Ryd W, et al, "Cytologic Diagnosis of Bancroftian Filariasis in a Nonendemic Area," *Acta Cytol,* 1988, 32(2):267-9.

Koss, LG, *Diagnostic Cytology and Its Histopathologic Bases,* 4th ed, Philadelphia, PA: Lippincott Co, 1992.

Lidang Jensen M and Johansen P, "Immunocytochemical Staining of Serous Effusions: An Additional Method in the Routine Cytology Practice?" *Cytopathology,* 1994, 5(2):93-103.

Mezger J, Stötzer O, Schilli G, et al, "Identification of Carcinoma Cells in Ascitic and Pleural Fluid - Comparison of Four Panepithelial Antigens With Carcinoembryonic Antigen," *Acta Cytol,* 1992, 36(1):75-81.

Naylor B, "Cytological Aspects of Pleural, Peritoneal, and Pericardial Fluids From in Patients With Systemic Lupus Erythematosus," *Cytopathology,* 1992, 3(1):1-8.

Naylor B, "The Pathognomonic Cytologic Picture of Rheumatoid Pleuritis," *Acta Cytol,* 1990, 34(4):465-73.

O'Hara MF, Cousar JB, Glick AD, et al, "Multiparameter Approach to the Diagnosis of Hematopoietic-Lymphoid Neoplasms in Body Fluids," *Diagn Cytopathol,* 1985, 1(1):33-8.

Okuyama T, Imai S, and Tsuburu Y, "Egg of *Schistosoma japonicum* in Ascitic Fluid," *Acta Cytol,* 1985, 29(4):651-2.

Reda MG and Baigelman W, "Pleural Effusion in Systemic Lupus Erythematosus," *Acta Cytol,* 1980, 24:553-7.

Sherman ME, "Cytopathology," *Blaustein's Pathology of the Female Genital Tract,* 4th ed, Chapter 25, Kurman RJ, ed, New York, NY: Springer-Verlag, 1994, 1097-130.

Stanley MW and Henry MJ, "The Significance of Leukemia and Lymphoma Cells in Cerebrospinal Fluid Contaminated by Blood Containing Malignant Cells: A Probabilistic Approach Based on the Poisson Frequency Distribution," *Diagn Cytopathol,* 1988, 4(3):193-5.

Stephenson RW, Britt DA, and Schumann GB, "Primary Cytodiagnosis of Peritoneal Extramedullary Hematopoiesis," *Diagn Cytopathol,* 1986, 2(3):241-3.

Wahl RW, "Curschmann's Spirals in Pleural and Peritoneal Fluids," *Acta Cytol,* 1986, 30(2):147-51.

Weaver KM, Novak PM, and Naylor B, "Vegetable Cell Contaminants in Cytologic Specimens. Their Resemblance to Cells Associated With Various Normal and Pathologic States," *Acta Cytol,* 1981, 25:210-4.

Wojno KJ, Olson JL, and Sherman ME, "Cytopathology of Pleural Effusions After Radiotherapy," *Acta Cytol,* 1994, 38(1):1-8.

Bronchial Washings Cytology

CPT 88104 (smears with interpretation); 88106 (filter method with interpretation); 88107 (smears and filter preparation with interpretation); 88108 (concentration technique, smears and interpretation)

Related Information
(Continued)

Bronchial Washings Cytology *(Continued)*

Pneumocystis carinii Preparation *on page 299*
Pneumocystis Immunofluorescence *on page 423*
Sputum Cytology *on page 300*
Viral Culture, Respiratory Symptoms *on page 680*
Virus, Direct Detection by Fluorescent Antibody *on page 682*

Synonyms Bronchial Aspirate Cytology; Bronchial Wash Cytology

Applies to Tracheal and Bronchial Washings; Tracheal Aspiration Cytology

Test Commonly Includes Cytologic evaluation of smears and cell block routinely; cytocentrifuge (cytospin) and filter preparations may be included. After the washings or aspirates have been centrifuged, direct smears and cell blocks can be prepared from the sediment or the fluid samples may be prepared using a membrane filtration technique. Use of both cytocentrifugation and membrane filtration techniques may be appropriate in some cases.[1,2]

Abstract Provides evaluation and diagnosis of diseases of the bronchial mucosa, particularly for patients with suspected primary or secondary lung cancer.

Patient Preparation Informed consent for bronchoscopy

Aftercare Postbronchoscopy sputum for cytology is advisable, as it may yield a more diagnostic specimen than that obtained during bronchoscopy.

Specimen Bronchial washings, unfixed

Container Clean container (eg, centrifuge tube, bronchoscopy trap, etc)

Collection Washings or aspirates are collected during endoscopic examination by instilling 3-5 mL of physiologic saline solution through the bronchoscope and reaspirating the fluid; the samples should be delivered to the laboratory immediately.

Storage Instructions After hours place in refrigerator.

Causes for Rejection Prolonged period (more than 1 hour) at room temperature

Special Instructions Include type of specimen and pertinent clinical information on requisition (ie, age, clinical impression, past diagnoses, radiographic findings, and history of radiation or chemotherapy). Infectious diseases suspected and immunocompromised status of patient (ie, status postorgan or marrow transplant or AIDS) should be specified. Special handling of all cytologic specimens regarding infectious etiology is routine (universal precautions).

Use Establish the presence of primary or metastatic neoplasms; aid in the diagnosis of respiratory infections with herpesvirus, cytomegalovirus, measles virus, fungal diseases, *Strongyloides*, *Echinococcus*, and *Paragonimus*; may be helpful in the diagnosis of lipoid pneumonitis, hemosiderosis (Goodpasture's syndrome), asbestosis, alveolar proteinosis, and allergic processes; diagnose some opportunistic infections in immunocompromised patients

Limitations Specimen is considered unsatisfactory if respiratory epithelium is not present.

Additional Information Special stains may be necessary for identification of organisms. The most commonly used are silver methenamine (Grocott), Diff-Quik™, or Giemsa for fungus and *Pneumocystis* and Ziehl-Neelsen for acid-fast bacteria. Immunoperoxidase staining for further diagnostic information can also be performed.[3] In addition, smears for immunofluorescence may be of use.

Footnotes

1. Taskinen E, Tukiainen P, and Renkonen R, "Bronchoalveolar Lavage - Influence of Cytologic Methods on the Cellular Picture," *Acta Cytol*, 1992, 36(5):680-6.

2. Thompson AB, Robbins RA, Ghafouri MA, et al, "Bronchoalveolar Lavage Fluid - Effect of Membrane Filtration Preparation on Neutrophil Recovery," *Acta Cytol*, 1989, 33(4):544-9.

3. Lyubsky S and Thorn R, "Application of Immunoperoxidase Staining to the Cell Blocks From Sputa and Bronchial Washings," *Arch Pathol Lab Med*, 1989, 113(1):94-5.

References

Broaddus C, Dake MD, Stulbarg MS, et al, "Bronchoalveolar Lavage and Transbronchial Biopsy for the Diagnosis of Pulmonary Infections in the Acquired Immunodeficiency Syndrome," *Ann Intern Med*, 1985, 102(6):747-52.

Chandra P, Delaney MD, and Tuazon CU, "Role of Special Stains in the Diagnosis of *Pneumocystis carinii* Infection From Bronchial Washing Specimens in Patients With the Acquired Immune Deficiency Syndrome," *Acta Cytol*, 1988, 32(1):105-8.

Chaudhuri B, Nanos S, Soco JN, et al, "Disseminated *Strongyloides stercoralis* Infestation Detected by Sputum Cytology," *Acta Cytol*, 1980, 24:360-2.

Corwin RW and Irwin RS, "The Lipid-Laden Alveolar Macrophage as a Marker of Aspiration in Parenchymal Lung Disease," *Am Rev Respir Dis*, 1985, 132(3):576-81.

Riazmontazer N and Bedayat G, "Cytology of Plasma Cell Myeloma in Bronchial Washings," *Acta Cytol*, 1989, 33(4):519-22.

Strigle SM and Gal AA, "A Review of Pulmonary Cytopathology in the Acquired Immunodeficiency Syndrome," *Diagn Cytopathol*, 1989, 5(1):44-54.

Wheeler TM, Johnson EH, Coughlin D, et al, "The Sensitivity of Detection of Asbestos Bodies in Sputa and Bronchial Washings," *Acta Cytol*, 1988, 32(5):647-50.

Bronchoalveolar Lavage Cytology

CPT 88104

Related Information

Bacterial Culture, Bronchoscopy Specimen *on page 459*
Bacterial Culture, Sputum *on page 465*
Brushings Cytology *on next page*
Cytomegalic Inclusion Disease Cytology *on page 293*
Cytomegalovirus Antibody *on page 389*
Cytomegalovirus Culture *on page 664*
Fungal Culture, Sputum *on page 479*
Histoplasmosis Antibody *on page 402*
Mycobacterial Culture, Sputum *on page 490*
Pneumocystis carinii Preparation *on page 299*
Pneumocystis Immunofluorescence *on page 423*
Sputum Cytology *on page 300*
Transbronchial Fine Needle Aspiration *on page 300*
Viral Culture, Respiratory Symptoms *on page 680*
Virus, Direct Detection by Fluorescent Antibody *on page 682*

Synonyms BAL Cytology

Test Commonly Includes Cytologic evaluation of smears after processing. Special stains for microorganisms and/or cell count with differential; identification of hemosiderin-laden macrophages. Combined use of cytocentrifugation and membrane filtration techniques may be desirable in some circumstances.[1]

Abstract Useful in diagnosis, clinical staging, and therapy, of a variety of pulmonary diseases including airway disease, interstitial lung disease, opportunistic pulmonary infections, and malignancy

Patient Preparation Informed consent for procedure. Premedication is often given. Topical anesthesia of the pharynx and upper respiratory tree is necessary. Sedation is useful but often precluded by patient's clinical status.

Aftercare Transient fever, chills, and myalgias have been reported to occur in up to 50% of cases. Antipyretic analgesics may be indicated.

Specimen Lavage fluid

Container Centrifuge tubes or other sterile, leakproof disposable containers

Collection More than 80% of pulmonologists use the right middle lobe as the sampling site. Both volume recovered and total cell count are higher from this area. The bronchoscope is wedged in a distal bronchial segment. 100-300 mL of warm, pyrogen-free, isotonic, sterile solution is infused with recovery of 40% to 60%. Fixative should not be used. Collection into nonsiliconized glass containers placed on ice.[2]

Storage Instructions Specimen should be forwarded to the Cytology Laboratory immediately. Cold storage is less than optimal but essential if processing is delayed. Detection of *Pneumocystis* is not compromised by delayed processing; however, it is more difficult to identify in patients who are already receiving treatment for this organism.

Special Instructions Specify need for special stains for microorganisms or cell count. Routine processing in many cytology laboratories includes only Papanicolaou stained smears.

Reference Range 10-15 x 10^6 cells/100 mL, 80% to 90% macrophages, 10% lymphocytes

Use Useful in the diagnosis of infection of the lungs, bronchoalveolar lavage (BAL) is now commonly used as the preliminary diagnostic procedure in severe diffuse lung infections in both normal and immunocompromised hosts, particularly opportunistic infectious organisms (CMV, *Pneumocystis*, herpes, atypical mycobacteria, and fungi).[3,4,5] BAL is also useful in the diagnosis and management of sarcoid, fibrosing alveolitis, eosinophilic pneumonia, pneumoconioses including silica particles, asbestosis, alveolar proteinosis, idiopathic pulmonary hemosiderosis, and interstitial lung disease.[6,7,8] Neoplastic cells are identified by this method[9,10] including bronchoalveolar adenocarcinoma, metastatic tumors, leukemias, and lymphomas.[2] Atypical type II pneumocytes in the lavage fluid due to toxic injury may indicate progression of damage. BAL is useful in evaluation of response to therapy and follow up (eg, allergic alveolitis).[2]

Limitations Wide variability in cell type and numbers recovered, particularly in smokers. Standardized volumes and concentrations not yet established.

Contraindications Severe hypoxemia with impending respiratory failure

Methodology Fractionated analysis, millipore and cytocentrifuge techniques; Papanicolaou, May-Gruenwald-Giemsa staining, immunofluorescence, immunoperoxidase, Cyto-Tek techniques, PAS, PAS diastase, alcian blue PAS, iron stains, silver methenamine; flow cytometry

Additional Information Interstitial lung disease can be divided into BAL lymphocyte predominant groups (sarcoid, hypersensitivity pneumonitis) and neutrophil predominant (smoking, idiopathic pulmonary fibrosis, and histiocytosis-X). A Diff-Quik™ stained cytospin preparation of BAL is an excellent rapid screening procedure for pathogens, particularly in the immunocompromised patient. It can detect *Pneumocystis*, CMV, herpes, *Cryptococcus*, *Candida*, blastomycosis, and aspergillosis as well as *Nocardia* and *Actinomyces*. Detection of fat-laden macrophages in increased numbers (>40% of cells) correlates well with chronic aspiration pneumonia.

Footnotes

1. Thompson AB, Robbins RA, Ghafouri MA, et al, "Bronchoalveolar Lavage Fluid Processing - Effect of Membrane Filtration Preparation on Neutrophil Recovery," *Acta Cytol*, 1989, 33(4):544-9.
2. Taskinen EI, Tukizinen PS, Alitalo RL, et al, "Bronchoalveolar Lavage Cytological Techniques and Interpretation of the Cellular Profiles," *Pathology Annual*, Vol 29, Part 2, Rosen PP and Fechner RE, eds, Norwalk, CT: Appleton & Lange, 1994, 121-54.
3. DeFine LA, Saleba KP, Gibson BB, et al, "Cytologic Evaluation of Bronchoalveolar Lavage Specimens in Immunosuppressed Patients With Suspected Opportunistic Infections," *Acta Cytol*, 1987, 31(3):235-42.
4. Ognibene FP, Shelhamer J, Gill V, et al, "The Diagnosis of *Pneumocystis carinii* Pneumonia in Patients With the Acquired Immunodeficiency Syndrome Using Subsegmental Bronchoalveolar Lavage," *Am Rev Respir Dis*, 1984, 129(6):929-32.
5. Strigle SM and Gal AA, "A Review of Pulmonary Cytopathology in the Acquired Immunodeficiency Syndrome," *Diagn Cytopathol*, 1989, 5(1):44-54.
6. Corwin RW and Irwin RS, "The Lipid-Laden Alveolar Macrophage as a Marker of Aspiration in Parenchymal Lung Disease," *Am Rev Respir Dis*, 1985, 132(3):576-81.
7. Daniele RP, Elias JA, Epstein PE, et al, "Bronchoalveolar Lavage: Role in the Pathogenesis, Diagnosis and Management of Interstitial Lung Disease," *Ann Intern Med*, 1985, 102(1):93-108.
8. Martin WJ, Williams DE, Dines DE, et al, "Interstitial Lung Disease Assessment by Bronchoalveolar Lavage," *Mayo Clin Proc*, 1983, 58:751-7.
9. Linder J, Radio SJ, Robbins RA, et al, "Bronchoalveolar Lavage in the Cytologic Diagnosis of Carcinoma of the Lung," *Acta Cytol*, 1987, 31(6):796-801.
10. Wisecarver J, Ness MJ, Rennard SI, et al, "Bronchoalveolar Lavage in the Assessment of Pulmonary Hodgkin's Disease," *Acta Cytol*, 1989, 33(4):527-32.

References

Allen JN, Davis WB, and Pacht ER, "Diagnostic Significance of Increased Bronchoalveolar Lavage Fluid Eosinophils," *Am Rev Respir Dis*, 1990, 142(3):642-7.

Baughman R, Strohofer S, and Kim CK, "Variation of Differential Cell Counts of Bronchoalveolar Lavage Fluid," *Arch Pathol Lab Med*, 1986, 110(4):341-3.

Baughman RP, Dohn MN, Loudon RG, et al, "Bronchoscopy With Bronchoalveolar Lavage in Tuberculosis and Fungal Infections," *Chest*, 1991, 99(1):92-7.

Buhl R, Stahl E, and Meier-Sydow J, "*In Vivo* Assessment of Pulmonary Oxidant Damage: The Role of Bronchoalveolar Lavage," *Monaldi Arch Chest Dis*, 1994, 49(3 Suppl 1):1-8.

Chamberlain DW, Braude AC, and Rebuck AS, "A Critical Evaluation of Bronchoalveolar Lavage; Criteria for Identifying Unsatisfactory Specimens," *Acta Cytol*, 1987, 31(5):599-605.

Fleury-Feith J, Escudier E, Pocholle MJ, et al, "The Effects of Cytocentrifugation on Differential Cell Counts in Samples Obtained by Bronchoalveolar Lavage," *Acta Cytol*, 1987, 31(5):606-10.

Konstan MW, Hilliard KA, Norvell TM, et al, "Bronchoalveolar Lavage Findings in Cystic Fibrosis Patients With Stable, Clinically Mild Lung Disease Suggest Ongoing Infection and Inflammation," *Am J Respir Crit Care Med*, 1994, 150(2):448-54.

Martin WJ 2d, "Diagnostic Bronchoalveolar Lavage in Immunosuppressed Patients With New Pulmonary Infiltrates," *Mayo Clin Proc*, 1992, 67(3):296-8.

Meduri GU, Stover DE, Greeno RA, et al, "Bilateral Bronchoalveolar Lavage in the Diagnosis of Opportunistic Pulmonary Infections," *Chest*, 1991, 100(5):1272-6.

Moumouni H, Garaud P, Diot P, et al, "Quantification of Cell Loss During Bronchoalveolar Lavage Fluid Processing. Effects of Fixation and Staining Methods," *Am J Respir Crit Care Med*, 1994, 149(3 Pt 1):636-40.

Mylius EA and Gullvag B, "Alveolar Macrophage Count as an Indicator of Lung Reaction to Industrial Air Pollution," *Acta Cytol*, 1986, 30(2):157-62.

Pisani RJ, Witzig TE, Li CY, et al, "Confirmation of Lymphomatous Pulmonary Involvement by Immunophenotypic and Gene Rearrangement Analysis of Bronchoalveolar Lavage Fluid," *Mayo Clin Proc*, 1990, 65(5):651-6.

Popp W, Ritschka L, Scherak O, et al, "Bronchoalveolar Lavage in Rheumatoid Arthritis and Secondary Sjögren's Syndrome," *Lung*, 1990, 168(4):221-31.

Radio SJ, Rennard SI, Kessinger A, et al, "Breast Carcinoma in Bronchoalveolar Lavage. A Cytologic and Immunocytochemical Study," *Arch Pathol Lab Med*, 1989, 113(4):333-6.

Rennard SI, "Bronchoalveolar Lavage in the Diagnosis of Cancer," *Lung*, 1990, 168(Suppl):1035-40.

Rennard SI, "Future Directions for Bronchoalveolar Lavage," *Lung*, 1990, 168(Suppl):1050-6.

Roggli VL, Piantadosi CA, and Bell DY, "Asbestos Bodies in Bronchoalveolar Lavage Fluid: A Study of 20 Asbestos-Exposed Individuals and Comparison to Patients With Other Chronic Interstitial Lung Disease," *Acta Cytol*, 1986, 30(5):470-6.

Schumann GB and Swensen JJ, "Comparison of Papanicolaou's Stain With the Gomori Methenamine Silver (GMS) Stain for the Cytodiagnosis of *Pneumocystis carinii* in Bronchoalveolar Lavage (BAL) Fluid," *Am J Clin Pathol*, 1991, 95(4):583-6.

Silverman JF, Turner RC, West RL, et al, "Bronchoalveolar Lavage in the Diagnosis of Lipoid Pneumonia," *Diagn Cytopathol*, 1989, 5(1):3-8.

Stanley MW, Henry-Stanley MJ, and Iber C, "Bronchoalveolar Lavage," *Cytology and Clinical Application*, New York, NY: Igaku-Shoin, 1991.

Woods GL, Thompson AB, Rennard SL, et al, "Detection of Cytomegalovirus in Bronchoalveolar Lavage Specimens. Spin Amplification and Staining With a Monoclonal Antibody to the Early Nuclear Antigen for Diagnosis of Cytomegalovirus Pneumonia," *Chest*, 1990, 98(3):568-75.

Bronchopulmonary Lavage for *Pneumocystis* see *Pneumocystis carinii* Preparation on page 299

Brushings Cytology

CPT 88104

Related Information

Bronchoalveolar Lavage Cytology *on previous page*
Cytomegalic Inclusion Disease Cytology *on page 293*

Applies to Bronchial Brushings Cytology; Colonic Brushings Cytology; Esophageal Brushings Cytology; Gastric Brushings Cytology; Oropharyngeal Brushings Cytology; Small Bowel Brushings Cytology; Tracheal Brushings Cytology; Ureteral Brushings Cytology

Test Commonly Includes Examination of prepared smears; cytocentrifuge preparations may be prepared if the brush is submitted to the laboratory in physiologic saline solution.

Abstract Bronchial brushings are usually done in conjunction with bronchial washings during bronchoscopy, primarily for the diagnosis of bronchogenic lung cancer. Visualization of tumor results in excellent diagnostic yield.

Patient Preparation Informed consent for procedure

Specimen Brush suspected lesions via a flexible fiberoptic bronchoscope or other endoscopic devices to examine and brush suspected lesions[1,2,3,4]

Container Coplin jar containing 95% ethanol

Collection Roll brush gently over fully frosted or plain glass slide and fix immediately in 95% ethanol or Saccomanno® fixative. Label one end of glass slide as well as Coplin jar with patient's identification. The exact site brushed should be indicated on the jar label and the requisition. For assistance in the diagnosis of infectious disease, a special double-sheathed brush should be sent sterile, separately, to the Microbiology Laboratory for cultures.

Special Instructions Specify the site brushed; indicate requests for special stains to identify unusual organisms (eg, ameba, fungus).

Use Most bronchogenic carcinomas are detectable by exfoliative respiratory cytology, which is used to establish the presence of primary or metastatic neoplasms; aid in the diagnosis of certain infections with herpesvirus, cytomegalovirus, measles virus, fungal diseases, *Pneumocystis carinii*, *Strongyloides*, *Echinococcus*, *Giardia lamblia*, *Entamoeba*, *Paragonimus*; aid in the diagnosis of Legionnaires' disease; aid in the diagnosis of anaerobic pulmonary infections; aid in the diagnosis of lipoid pneumonia, hemosiderosis (Goodpasture's syndrome), asbestosis, allergic processes, metaplastic glandular epithelium of esophagus (Barrett's esophagus). Brushing smears are suitable for immunocytochemical staining for bacterial or tumor antigens.

Limitations Technically adequate specimens are needed for diagnosis. Allowing smears and brushes to dry before they are well fixed will introduce many artifacts and distortions hampering reliable interpretation. Such dried slides are reported as **unsatisfactory** for cytologic evaluation. If smears have not been air dried for longer than 30 minutes, a 30 second rehydration in normal saline prior to fixing in 95% alcohol may rehydrate cells sufficiently for smear to be interpretable.[5] Detailed clinical history is necessary as exemplified by a case report of marked post-tracheostomy atypia simulating squamous cell carcinoma.[6] False-positive bronchial washing and brushing interpretations have been reported from highly respected sources. An incidence >0.02% false-positives is published.[7] Conditions which may give rise to false-positive reports of **adenocarcinoma** include lung infarct, bronchiectasis, oxygen toxicity, radiation pneumonitis, reactive pneumonitis caused by chemotherapy, viral pneumonitis, thermal lung damage, toxin inhalation, vasculitis, interstitial pneumonitis, and adult respiratory distress syndrome. Entities which may cause atypical **squamous** metaplasias include granulomatous diseases, lung infarcts, asthma, chronic bronchitis, bronchiectasis, and pneumonia. Problems exist too regarding **small cell/neuroendocrine carcinomas**. In some instances transthoracic or transbronchial fine needle aspiration may help to avoid misinterpretation.[7]

Additional Information Special stains and culture may be indicated, especially in the diagnosis of infectious processes or inflammatory conditions.

Footnotes

1. Chen YL, "The Diagnosis of Colorectal Cancer With Cytologic Brushings Under Direct Vision at Fiberoptic Colonoscopy," *Dis Colon Rectum*, 1987, 30(5):342-4.
2. Dowlwatshahi K, Skinner DB, DeMeester TR, et al, "Evaluation of Brush Cytology as an Independent Technique for Detection of Esophageal Cancer," *J Thorac Cardiovasc Surg*, 1988, 89:849-51.
3. Festa VI, Hajdu SI, and Winawar SJ, "Colorectal Cytology in Chronic Ulcerative Colitis," *Acta Cytol*, 1985, 29(3):262-8.
4. Ryan ME, "Cytologic Brushing of Ductal Lesions During ERCP," *Gastrointest Endosc*, 1991, 37(2):139-42.
5. Chan JK and Kung IT, "Rehydration of Air-Dried Smears With Normal Saline - Application in Fine-Needle Aspiration Cytologic Examination," *Am J Clin Pathol*, 1988, 89(1):30-4.
6. Berman JJ, Murray RJ, and Lopez-Plaza IM, "Widespread Post-tracheostomy Atypia Simulating Squamous Cell Carcinoma - A Case Report," *Acta Cytol*, 1991, 35(6):713.
7. Ritter JH, Wick MR, Reyes A, et al, "False-Positive Interpretations of Carcinoma in Exfoliative Respiratory Cytology. Report of Two Cases and a Review of Underlying Disorders," *Am J Clin Pathol*, 1995, 104(2):133-40.

References

Chambers LA and Clark WE 2d, "The Endoscopic Diagnosis of Gastroesophageal Malignancy: A Cytologic Review," *Acta Cytol*, 1986, 30(2):110-4.

Cook IJ, de Carle DJ, and Haneman B, "The Role of Brush Cytology in the Diagnosis of Gastric Malignancy," *Acta Cytol*, 1988, 32(4):461-4.

(Continued)

Brushings Cytology *(Continued)*

Geisinger KR, Teot LA, and Richter JE, "A Comparative Cytopathologic and Histologic Study of Atypia, Dysplasia, and Adenocarcinoma in Barrett's Esophagus," *Cancer*, 1992, 69(1):8-16.

Jeevanandaur V, Treat MR, and Forde KA, "A Comparison of Direct Brush Cytology and Biopsy in the Diagnosis of Colorectal Cancer," *Gastrointest Endosc*, 1987, 33(5):370-1.

Melville DM, Richman PI, Shepherd NA, et al, "Brush Cytology of the Colon and Rectum in Ulcerative Colitis: An Aid to Cancer Diagnosis," *J Clin Pathol*, 1988, 41(11):1180-6.

Stanley MW, "False-Positive Diagnoses in Exfoliative Cytology," *Am J Clin Pathol*, 1995, 104(2):117-9.

Catheterized Urine Cytology *see* Urine Cytology *on page 301*

Cerebrospinal Fluid Cytology

CPT 88107 (smears and filter preparation); 88108 (concentration technique, smears)

Related Information
Bacterial Culture, Cerebrospinal Fluid *on page 460*
Beta$_2$-Microglobulin *on page 371*
Bone Marrow *on page 307*
Cerebrospinal Fluid Analysis *on page 309*
Cerebrospinal Fluid LD *on page 106*
Fungal Culture, Cerebrospinal Fluid *on page 477*
Immunoperoxidase Procedures *on page 43*
Immunophenotypic Analysis of Tissues by Flow Cytometry *on page 45*
Mycobacterial Culture, Cerebrospinal Fluid *on page 489*
Polymerase Chain Reaction *on page 523*
Tumor Aneuploidy by Flow Cytometry *on page 57*
Viral Culture, Central Nervous System Symptoms *on page 677*

Synonyms CSF Cytology; Spinal Fluid Cytology

Applies to Cisternal Tap Cytology; Lumbar Tap Cytology; Ventricular Tap Cytology

Test Commonly Includes Smears, filter preparations, cytocentrifuge preparations, and immunocytochemistry when indicated[1]

Patient Preparation Signed informed consent should be obtained. The patient is then prepped establishing a sterile field; 1% lidocaine is used for local anesthesia.

Aftercare A "fibrin patch" using the patient's own plasma may be necessary if severe headache and/or vertigo develops and persists.

Specimen Fresh cerebrospinal fluid

Container Use sterile tube from lumbar puncture tray or sterile, leakproof screw-top container

Collection A 23-gauge spinal needle with stylet is inserted through the L1-L2 interspinous space, and dura mater into the cerebrospinal fluid space. In a three part collection, the third tube should be submitted in its entirety to the Cytology Laboratory immediately. Specimen must be labeled with patient's identification.

Storage Instructions Spinal taps for cytology should be done when the specimen can be processed immediately. If it is not possible to process the cellular sample immediately, it must be refrigerated. It is imperative to note that **without immediate processing, degeneration of cells within the spinal fluid begins within 20 minutes at room temperature.**

Causes for Rejection Prolonged period (more than 3 hours) at room temperature

Special Instructions Include pertinent clinical data on requisition. It is of utmost importance to alert the Cytology Laboratory if the fluid has been recovered from any type of ventricular shunt.

Reference Range Adults and children: acellular, or up to 3-5 mononuclear cells/µL; infants: 20-30 mononuclear cells/µL

Use Establish the presence of **primary or metastatic neoplasm**; aid in the diagnosis of fungal (particularly cryptococcal), bacterial, viral, and aseptic meningitis; may be of assistance in patients with demyelinating disease (ie, multiple sclerosis). Of patients with untreated acute lymphoblastic leukemia (ALL), approximately 80% will have leukemic cells in CSF at some time. Of patients with acute myeloblastic leukemia, about 60% will be shown to have such cells in the CSF. Other malignant neoplasms metastatic to the CNS include primaries of the lung, breast, kidney, gastrointestinal tract, melanomas, and choriocarcinomas. Of the primary tumors from the lung, small cell undifferentiated carcinoma is the most common source of CNS metastases.[2] Cytologic studies may provide evidence of **cytomegalovirus infection** of the CNS (eg, in subjects with AIDS). Examination of CSF in AIDS patients is also helpful in detection of **cryptococcal meningitis** and lymphoma but less helpful in diagnosis of *Toxoplasma*.[3]

Limitations Malignant cells are shed into cerebrospinal fluid only from tumors which extend the subarachnoid space or into the ventricles. Metastatic tumors and leukemias have better detection rates than primary CNS tumors. Meningeal carcinomatosis or lymphoma may be

diagnosed in this fluid, however they shed fewer cells at intermittent periods. Herpes meningitis **cannot** be diagnosed by CSF cytology: brain biopsy is required.

Contraindications Elevated intracranial pressure; abnormal coagulation profile

Additional Information Myelography, radiation, and especially intrathecal therapy can all produce striking cytologic changes.

The outcome of **chronic idiopathic meningitis** is usually benign. Extensive studies are recommended including cultures for viruses, mycobacteria, fungi, bacteria, CSF syphilis serology, other CSF and serum studies, and CSF cytology. Of 49 patients, **neoplastic meningitis** was found in 8 of 10 in whom diagnosis was established.[4]

Footnotes
1. Vick WW, Wikstrand CJ, Bullard DE, et al, "The Use of a Panel of Monoclonal Antibodies in the Evaluation of Cytologic Specimens From the Central Nervous System," *Acta Cytol*, 1987, 31(6):815-24.
2. Kjeldsberg CR and Knight JA, "Cerebrospinal Fluid," *Body Fluids - Laboratory Examination of Amniotic, Cerebrospinal, Seminal, Serous, and Synovial Fluids*, 3rd ed, Chapter 2, Chicago, IL: American Society of Clinical Pathologists, 1993, 65-157.
3. Katz RL, Alappattu C, Glass JP, et al, "Cerebrospinal Fluid Manifestations of the Neurologic Complications of Human Immunodeficiency Virus Infection," *Acta Cytol*, 1989, 33(2):233-44.
4. Smith JE and Aksamit AJ Jr, "Outcome of Chronic Idiopathic Meningitis," *Mayo Clin Proc*, 1994, 69(6):548-56.

References
Bigner SH, "Cerebrospinal Fluid (CSF) Cytology: Current Status and Diagnostic Applications," *J Neuropathol Exp Neurol*, 1992, 51(3):235-45.
Bigner SH and Johnston WW, *Cytopathology of the Central Nervous System*, Chicago, IL: ASCP Press, 1994.
Craver RD and Carson TH, "Hematopoietic Elements in Cerebrospinal Fluid in Children," *Am J Clin Pathol*, 1991, 95(4):532-5.
Travlos A, Anton HA, and Wing PC, "Cerebrospinal Fluid Cell Count Following Spinal Cord Injury," *Arch Phys Med Rehabil*, 1994, 75(3):293-6.
Yurdakok M and Kocabas CN, "CSF Erythrocyte Volume Analysis: A Simple Method for the Diagnosis of Traumatic Tap in Newborn Infants," *Pediatr Neurosurg*, 1991-92, 17(4):199.

Cervical Smear *see* Cervical/Vaginal Cytology *on this page*

Cervical/Vaginal Cytology

CPT 88150; 88156 (Bethesda system)

Related Information
Chlamydia trachomatis Culture *on page 662*
Chlamydia trachomatis Direct FA Test *on page 663*
Cytomegalovirus Culture *on page 664*
Endometrial Cytology *on page 293*
Hormonal Evaluation, Cytologic *on page 296*
Human Papillomavirus DNA Probe Test *on page 516*
Neisseria gonorrhoeae Culture and Smear *on page 492*
Trichomonas Preparation *on page 498*
Viral Culture *on page 675*
Viral Culture, Urogenital *on page 681*

Synonyms Cervical Smear; Pap Smear; Vaginal Cytology

Applies to Herpes Smear; Human Papilloma Viruses (HPV); The Bethesda System; Vira Pap®; Vira Type®; Vulvar Cytology

Test Commonly Includes Fast smear, cervical scraping smear, vaginal pool smear, lateral vaginal wall smear, direct scraping smear

Abstract The spectrum of abnormality of cervical epithelium includes inflammatory processes (bacterial, fungal, parasitic, viral, and helminthic), low grade squamous intraepithelial lesions (**LSIL**, mild dysplasia, **CIN 1**), high grade squamous intraepithelial lesions (**HSIL**, moderate and severe dysplasia, **CIS, CIN 2-3**), and squamous carcinoma. About 80% of carcinomas of the uterine cervix are squamous. Most of the remainder are adenocarcinomas and mixed adenosquamous carcinomas. Other entities which may be detected include adenocarcinoma of endometrium, sarcomas, carcinoids, endocrine carcinomas, and other rare epithelial tumors and metastatic cancers.

A reduction in mortality from cervical cancer followed implementation of cytologic screening, but problems in sampling, specimen adequacy, screening, and interpretation remain. Even in very good laboratories, false-negatives occur.

Patient Preparation Patients are advised to avoid douches 48-72 hours prior to examination; however, this should not preclude taking of the smear. Provide relevant information including age and last menstrual period (LMP).

Specimen Cervical scrape and endocervical brush samples are recommended in all cases. The optimal sample for hormonal evaluation is a lateral vaginal wall scrape, but aspiration of posterior vaginal fornix fluid (vaginal pool) may be used. Endometrial aspirations are not advised for routine use. For lesions of the vagina or vulva, scrapings made directly from the lesion are most diagnostic.

Container Glass slides with frosted ends; spray fixative containing 95% ethanol and water or liquid fixative such as PRO-FIXX™ (Lerner Laboratories, Stanford, CT), also containing ethanol and water. **Hair spray**

should never be used to fix Pap smear slides. The slides may be sent to the laboratory in cardboard or plastic slide containers; if the smears are wet-fixed in 95% alcohol in a Coplin jar, this may be sent to the laboratory.

Collection Preferred fixatives: Spray or liquid fixatives as mentioned above or 95% ethanol. Patient identification of specimen: Each slide must be labeled with patient's name, medical record number or date of birth, and site sampled, written with graphite pencil on the frosted end of the slide. It is possible to label nonfrosted slides only with a diamond point pen. The speculum must be introduced **without** lubricant; in certain cases, running the speculum through warm saline will prove helpful prior to insertion into atrophic, stenotic, or small introitus.

Sampling:

Endocervix: Gentle scrape or brush of endocervical canal
- Scrape - Rotate narrow end of spatula in the cervical os and gently smear onto labeled glass slide and fix immediately.
- Brush - Use a tapered synthetic fiber brush to sample endocervical cells; remove mucous plug if present, before sampling the endocervical canal. Do not rub onto the slide; rather, lightly roll brush over the slide.

Ectocervical scrape: With spatula thoroughly scrape the entire ectocervix with emphasis on the squamocolumnar junction (transformation zone). Spread material evenly onto labeled glass slide and fix immediately. Immediate fixation is imperative.

Lateral vaginal wall smear: Scraping from upper lateral one-third of vaginal mucosa. Used for cytohormonal evaluations.

Direct scraping smear: Direct scrape of grossly visible lesion, smeared and fixed as previously described.

Special Instructions Include pertinent clinical history such as age, LMP, parity, postmenopausal status, surgery, exogenous hormones, history of carcinoma, radiation, chemotherapy, abnormal vaginal bleeding, and history of previous abnormal Pap smears.

Possible Panic Range Any smear with definitely malignant cells should ideally be verbally relayed directly to the clinician if possible, in addition to forwarding the formal report.

Use Diagnose primary or metastatic neoplasms; diagnose cervical dysplasia (cervical intraepithelial neoplasia (CIN)); diagnose genital infections with herpes, *Candida* sp, *Trichomonas vaginalis*, cytomegalovirus and *Actinomyces*; aid in the diagnosis of vaginal adenosis, cervicovaginal endometriosis, condyloma, human papillomavirus infection, lymphogranuloma venereum; aid in evaluation of hormonal function (formerly referred to as maturation index); useful in suggesting chlamydial infection.

Limitations Statement of adequacy:

"Satisfactory for evaluation" indicates that the specimen has all of the following:
- appropriate labeling and identifying information
- relevant clinical information
- adequate numbers of well-preserved and well-visualized squamous epithelial cells
- an adequate endocervical/transformation zone component (from those patients who have a cervix)[1]

A specimen is **"satisfactory for evaluation but limited by..."** if:
- lack of pertinent clinical patient information (age, date of last menstrual period as a minimum; additional information as appropriate)
- partially obscuring blood, inflammation, thick areas, poor fixation, air-drying artifact, contaminant, etc, that precludes interpretation of approximately 50% to 70% of the epithelial cells.
- absence of an endocervical/transformation zone component as defined above

The above implies that a diagnosis can be made, however interpretation might be compromised due to the above.[1]

A specimen is **"unsatisfactory for evaluation..."** if any of the following apply:
- lack of patient identification on the specimen and/or requisition form
- a slide that is broken and cannot be repaired
- scant squamous epithelial component (well preserved and well visualized squamous epithelial cells covering <10% of the slide surface)
- obscuring blood, inflammation, thick areas, poor fixation, air-drying artifact, contaminant, etc, that precludes interpretation of approximately 75% or more of the epithelial cells.[1]

The "unsatisfactory" designation indicates that the specimen is unreliable for the detection of cervical epithelial abnormalities. A diagnosis should not be made.

Contraindications Air drying of smears prior to fixation must not be permitted.

Additional Information The earliest identified event in the etiology of carcinogenesis of the uterine cervix is infection with types of human papillomavirus (HPV). HPV infections may lead to low grade squamous intraepithelial lesion (LGSIL) (mild dysplasia) (CIN 1 on biopsy), which can be expressed as koilocytotic condylomatous atypia. Such infections are common, and ultimately tend to resolve even at the molecular level. Less commonly, such infections persist and may progress to higher grade lesions. Infrequently, biopsy of patients with smear results of LGSIL reveal CIN 2 or 3. Risk factors include HPV type but other steps, factors, or cofactors exist as well.[2] Important pitfalls exist with analysis for human papillomavirus (HPV) infection in cervix and its correlation with smears and biopsies.[3] Detection of genital human papillomavirus (HPV) can be done by polymerase chain reaction,[4] Southern blot hybridization, dot blot hybridization, and Hybrid capture liquid hybridization kit. Although most of the ±440,000 global cases of cervical cancer are attributed to HPV infection, carcinoma of cervix is uncommon when compared to lifetime cumulative incidence of HPV infection of the cervix. Cytologic diagnosis of low grade SIL represents only up to about 30% of HPV infection which can be detected by DNA technology.[2] See listing Human Papillomavirus DNA Probe Test *on page 516.*

Traditional Class	Bethesda System
	ADEQUACY OF THE SPECIMEN
	Satisfactory for evaluation
	Satisfactory for evaluation but limited by...(specify reason)
	Unsatisfactory for evaluation...(specify reason)
	GENERAL CATEGORIZATION (optional)
1	Within normal limits
2	Benign cellular changes: see Descriptive Diagnoses.
3, 4, 5	Epithelial cell abnormality: see Descriptive Diagnoses.
	DESCRIPTIVE DIAGNOSES
	Benign Cellular Changes
2	Infection
	Trichomonas vaginalis
	Fungal organisms morphologically consistent with *Candida* sp
	Predominance of coccobacilli consistent with shift in vaginal flora
	Bacteria morphologically consistent with *Actinomyces* sp
	Cellular changes associated with herpes simplex virus
	Other*
2	Reactive Changes
	Reactive cellular changes associated with:
	Inflammation (includes typical repair)
	Atrophy with inflammation ("atrophic vaginitis")
	Radiation
	Intrauterine contraceptive device (IUD)
	Other
3, 4, 5	**Epithelial Cell Abnormalities**
	Squamous Cell
2 or 3†	Atypical squamous cells of undetermined significance (**ASCUS**): qualify†
3	Low grade squamous intraepithelial lesion (**LSIL**) encompassing:
	HPV* mild dysplasia/**CIN 1**
3 or 4	High grade squamous intraepithelial lesion (**HSIL**) encompassing:
	moderate and severe dysplasia, **CIS/CIN 2**, and **CIN 3**
5	Squamous cell carcinoma (**SCC**)
	Glandular Cell
2	Endometrial cells, cytologically benign in a postmenopausal woman
2 or 3†	Atypical glandular cells of undetermined significance (**AGUS**): qualify†
5	Endocervical adenocarcinoma
5	Endometrial adenocarcinoma
5	Extrauterine adenocarcinoma
5	Adenocarcinoma, NOS
5	**Other Malignant Neoplasms:** Specify
	Hormonal Evaluation (applies to vaginal smears only)
	Hormonal pattern compatible with age and history
	Hormonal pattern incompatible with age and history: specify
	Hormonal evaluation not possible due to: specify

*Cellular changes of human papillomavirus (**HPV**) — previously termed **koilocytosis, koilocytotic atypia,** and **condylomatous atypia** — are included in the category of **LSIL.**

†Atypical squamous or glandular cells of undetermined significance should be further qualified, if possible, as to whether a reactive or premalignant/malignant process is favored.

(Continued)

Cervical/Vaginal Cytology *(Continued)*

Discrepancies occur between cervicovaginal smears even when done by quality laboratories, and subsequent biopsies. The most common cause for such discrepancy at the University of Kentucky was colposcopic biopsy sampling. Other causes included errors in cytologic interpretation, cytologic sampling, histotechnical processing, and cytologic screening.[5] Sampling problems making smears inadequate are reported in 12.3% of cases. SIL may be underestimated in 17.5% of cases. About 15% to 25% of individuals with SIL are reported to have normal cervical/vaginal cytology.[6]

The practitioner and patients should insist on smear review by licensed cytotechnologists and board certified pathologists and should be cautious about simply seeking the lowest price.

Conferences of leading cytopathologists and gynecologists, held at Bethesda in 1988 and 1991, formulated recommendations for uniform diagnostic terminology for cervical/vaginal cytology. Such recommendations eliminated reporting by classes. These conferences, sponsored by the National Cancer Institute, led to a new classification, the Bethesda System (TBS). See table.

Footnotes

1. Solomon D and Kurman RJ, *The Bethesda System for Reporting Cervical/Vaginal Cytologic Diagnoses*, New York, NY: Springer-Verlag, 1994, 6-8.
2. Schiffman MH and Brinton LA, "The Epidemiology of Cervical Carcinogenesis," *Cancer*, 1995, 76(10 Suppl):1888-901.
3. Herrington CS, Evans MF, Gray W, et al, "Morphological Correlation of Human Papillomavirus Infection of Matched Cervical Smears and Biopsies From Patients With Persistent Mild Cervical Cytological Abnormalities," *Hum Pathol*, 1995, 26(9):951-5.
4. Mayelo V, Garaud P, Renjard L, et al, "Cell Abnormalities Associated With Human Papillomavirus-Induced Squamous Intraepithelial Cervical Lesions. Multivariate Data Analysis," *Am J Clin Pathol*, 1994, 101(1):13-8.
5. Tritz DM, Weeks JA, Spires SE, et al, "Etiologies for Non-Correlating Cervical Cytologies and Biopsies," *Am J Clin Pathol*, 1995, 103(5):594-7.
6. Cannistra SA and Niloff JM, "Cancer of the Uterine Cervix," *N Engl J Med*, 1996, 334(16):1030-8.

References

Allen KA, Zaleski S, and Cohen MB, "Review of Negative Papanicolaou Tests. Is the Retrospective 5-Year Review Necessary?" *Am J Clin Pathol*, 1994, 101(1):19-21.

Atkinson B, *Atlas of Diagnostic Cytopathology*, Philadelphia, PA: WB Saunders Co, 1992.

Betsill WL Jr and Clark AH, "Early Endocervical Glandular Neoplasia," *Acta Cytol*, 1986, 30(2):115-26.

Bibbo M and Wied GL, "Inflammation Reaction and Microbiology of the Female Productive Tract," *Compendium on Diagnostic Cytology*, Wied GL, Keebler Da CM, Koss LG, et al, eds, Chicago, IL: Tutorials of Cytology, 1992, 63-8.

Buntinx F, Knottnerus JA, Andre J, et al, "The Effect of Different Sampling Devices on the Presence of Endocervical Cells in Cervical Smears. A Systematic Literature Review," *Eur J Cancer Prev*, 1994, 3(1):23-30.

Chakrabarti S, Guijon FB, and Paraskevas M, "Brush vs Spatula for Cervical Smears. Histologic Correlation With Concurrent Biopsies," *Acta Cytol*, 1994, 38(3):315-8.

Chua KL and Hjerpe A, "Persistance of Human Papillomavirus (HPV) Infections Preceding Cervical Carcinoma," *Cancer*, 1996, 77(1):121-7.

Crum CP, "Papillomavirus-Related Changes and Premalignant and Malignant Squamous Lesions of the Uterine Cervix," *Tumors and Tumor-Like Lesions of the Uterine Corpus and Cervix*, Vol 19, Clement PB and Young RH, eds, New York, NY: Churchill Livingstone, 1993, 51-83.

Davey DD, Nielsen MI, Rosenstock W, et al, "Terminology and Specimen Adequacy in Cervicovaginal Cytology: The College of American Pathologists' Interlaboratory Comparison Experience," *Arch Pathol Lab Med*, 1992, 116(9):903-7.

Davila RM, "Cervicovaginal Smear, True or False?" *Am J Clin Pathol*, 1994, 101(1):1-2.

Gay JD, Donaldson LD, and Goellner JR, "False-Negative Results in Cervical Cytologic Studies," *Acta Cytol*, 1985, 29(6):1043-6.

Genest DR, Stein L, Cibas E, et al, "A Binary (Bethesda) System for Classifying Cervical Cancer Precursors: Criteria, Reproducibility, and Viral Correlates," *Hum Pathol*, 1993, 24(7):730-6.

Gupta PK, "Microbiology, Inflammation, and Viral Infection," *Comprehensive Cytopathology*, Bibbo M, ed, Philadelphia, PA: WB Saunders Co, 1991, 115-52.

Jones BA, "Rescreening in Gynecologic Cytology, Rescreening of 3762 Previous Cases for Current High-Grade Squamous Intraepithelial Lesions and Carcinoma - A College of American Pathologists Q-Probes Study of 312 Institutions," *Arch Pathol Lab Med*, 1995, 119(12):1097-103.

Jones HW 3d, "Impact of the Bethesda System," *Cancer*, 1995, 76(10):1914-8.

Levine AJ, Harper J, Hilborne L, et al, "HPV DNA and the Risk of Squamous Intraepithelial Lesions of the Uterine Cervix in Young Women," *Am J Clin Pathol*, 1993, 100(1):6-11.

Luff RD, "The Bethesda System for Reporting Cervical/Vaginal Cytologic Diagnoses. Report of 1991 Bethesda Workshop," *JAMA*, 1992, 98(2): 152-4.

Meyer MP, Carbonell RI, Mauser NA, et al, "Detection of Human Papillomavirus in Cervical Swab Samples by ViraPap® and in Cervical Biopsy Specimens by *In Situ* Hybridization," *Am J Clin Pathol*, 1993, 100(1):12-7.

National Cancer Institute Workshop, "The 1988 Bethesda System for Reporting Cervical/Vaginal Cytologic Diagnoses," *JAMA*, 1989, 262(7):931-4.

Nielsen ML, Davey DD, and Kline TS, "Specimen Adequacy Evaluation in Gynecologic Cytopathology: Current Laboratory Practice in the College of American Pathologists Interlaboratory Comparison Program and Tentative Guidelines for Future Practice," *Diagn Cytopathol*, 1993, 9(4):394-403.

Schumann JL, O'Connor DM, Covell JL, et al, "Pap Smear Collection Devices: Technical, Clinical, Diagnostic, and Legal Considerations Associated With Their Use," *Diagn Cytopathol*, 1992, 8(5):492-503.

Shroyer KR, Brookes CG, Markham NE, et al, "Detection of Human Papillomavirus in Anorectal Squamous Cell Carcinoma: Correlation With Basaloid Pattern of Differentiation," *Am J Clin Pathol*, 1995, 104(3):299-305.

***Chlamydia* Smears Cytology** *see* Ocular Cytology *on page 298*

Cisternal Tap Cytology *see* Cerebrospinal Fluid Cytology *on page 290*

CMV Smear *see* Cytomegalic Inclusion Disease Cytology *on next page*

Colonic Brushings Cytology *see* Brushings Cytology *on page 289*

Colon Washings Cytology *see* Washing Cytology *on page 302*

Conjunctival Smear Cytology *see* Ocular Cytology *on page 298*

Corneal Cytology *see* Ocular Cytology *on page 298*

Cornification Count *replaced by* Hormonal Evaluation, Cytologic *on page 296*

CSF Cytology *see* Cerebrospinal Fluid Cytology *on page 290*

CT-Guided FNA *see* Fine Needle Aspiration, Deep Seated Lesions *on page 294*

Cul-de-sac Fluid Cytology *see* Cyst Fluid Cytology *on this page*

Culdocentesis *see* Body Fluid Cytology *on page 286*

Cyst Fluid Cytology

CPT 88104 (smears); 88107 (smears and filter preparation); 88108 (concentration techniques, smears)

Related Information

Alpha$_1$-Fetoprotein, Serum *on page 72*
Body Fluid Cytology *on page 286*
Breast Biopsy *on page 35*
CA 125 *on page 94*
Carcinoembryonic Antigen *on page 100*
Fine Needle Aspiration, Deep Seated Lesions *on page 294*
Fine Needle Aspiration, Superficial Palpable Masses *on page 294*
Nipple Discharge Cytology *on page 297*

Applies to Brain Cyst Fluid Cytology; Breast Cyst Fluid Cytology; Cul-de-sac Fluid Cytology; Hydrocele Fluid Cytology; Ovarian Cyst Fluid Cytology; Pancreatic Cyst Fluid Cytology; Renal Cyst Fluid Cytology

Test Commonly Includes Filter preparation, smears, cytocentrifuge preparations

Abstract Palpable masses not associated with any specific organ, as well as cysts within organs, readily lend themselves to aspiration and subsequent cytologic examination. A variety of benign lesions and occasional malignant tumors can be diagnosed by cytologic examination of cyst fluid.

Specimen Freshly aspirated fluid

Container Sterile, leakproof, screw-top tube

Collection Label with identification and anatomic site.

Storage Instructions Specimen should be processed as soon as possible; specimens must be kept refrigerated, but not frozen, if processing is delayed.

Use Establish nature of cystic process (ie, malignancy, inflammatory, retention, infection). The most frequently aspirated ovarian entity is follicular cyst, a benign physiologic structure.

Limitations Diagnosis of ovarian tumors of low malignant potential usually requires histopathologic assessment of infiltration.

Additional Information After aspiration of a palpable cyst, the area should be re-examined for evidence of a residual mass. If the lesion has not entirely disappeared after fluid aspiration, aspiration biopsy of the residual mass is required in order to exclude cystic malignant lesion.

Breast cyst fluid is usually sparsely cellular and may contain a few apocrine and/or foam cells. Bloody, cellular fluids may indicate papilloma or intracystic papillary carcinoma (older age groups).

Benign **thyroid cysts** often reveal dark green to brown fluid containing numerous hemosiderin-laden macrophages, a result of intracystic hemorrhage. However, cystic variants of papillary thyroid carcinoma do exist, and a remaining mass should also be aspirated to exclude this possibility.

During laparoscopy, **ovarian cysts** are encountered for which aspiration may be indicated.[1,2] Tumor-associated antigens CEA, CA 125, and alpha-fetoprotein (AFP) are low in follicular and lutein cysts. Both benign and malignant serous cystadenomas contain fluid low in CEA and AFP but marked by high CA 125. High CEA with normal CA 125 is described in adenocarcinoma of colon metastatic to ovary,[3] an entity easily mistaken in histopathology for primary ovarian carcinoma. Elevated AFP was reported with a malignant teratoma and is increased with yolk sac tumor. Granulosa cells usually are not decorated with antikeratin antibodies AE-1/AE-3, while mesothelial cells are immunoreactive. The diagnosis of follicular cyst is supported by increased estrogen-17β levels.

Footnotes

1. Patel KR and Boon AP, "Metastatic Breast Cancer Presenting as an Ovarian Cyst: Diagnosis by Fine Needle Aspiration Cytology," *Cytopathology*, 1992, 3(3):191-5.
2. Stanley MW, Horwitz CA, and Frable WJ, "Cellular Follicular Cyst of the Ovary: Fluid Cytology Mimicking Malignancy," *Diagn Cytopathol*, 1991, 7(1):48-52.
3. Pinto MM, Bernstein LH, Brogan DA, et al, "Measurement of CA 125, Carcinoembryonic Antigen, and Alpha-Fetoprotein in Ovarian Cyst Fluid: Diagnostic Adjunct to Cytology," *Diagn Cytopathol*, 1990, 6(3):160-3.

References

Gaetje R and Popp LW, "Is Differentiation of Benign and Malignant Cystic Adnexal Masses Possible by Evaluation of Cysts Fluids With Respect to Color, Cytology, Steroid Hormones, and Tumor Markers?" *Acta Obstet Gynecol Scand*, 1994, 73(6):502-7.

Ingram EA and Helikson MA, "Echinococcosis (Hydatid Disease) in Missouri: Diagnosis by Fine Needle Aspiration of a Lung Cyst," *Diagn Cytopathol*, 1991, 7(5):527-31.

Katz LB and Ehya H, "Aspiration Cytology of Papillary Cystic Neoplasm of the Pancreas," *Am J Clin Pathol*, 1990, 94(3):328-33.

Lewandrowski KB, Southern JF, Pins MR, et al, "Cyst Fluid Analysis in the Differential Diagnosis of Pancreatic Cysts. A Comparison of Pseudocysts, Serous Cystadenoma, Mucinous Cystic Neoplasm, and Mucinous Cystadenocarcinoma," *Ann Surg*, 1993, 217(1):41-7.

Orell SR, Sterrett GF, Walters MN, et al, *Manual and Atlas of Fine Needle Aspiration Cytology*, New York, NY: Churchill Livingstone, 1992.

Rogers LR and Barnett G, "Percutaneous Aspiration of Brain Tumor Cysts Via the Ommaya Reservoir System," *Neurology*, 1991, 41(2 Pt 1):279-82.

Sherman ME, "Cytopathology," *Blaustein's Pathology of the Female Genital Tract*, 4th ed, Chapter 25, Kurman RJ, ed, New York, NY: Springer-Verlag, 1994, 1097-130.

Cytology, Sputum see Sputum Cytology on page 300

Cytomegalic Inclusion Bodies see Cytomegalic Inclusion Disease Cytology on this page

Cytomegalic Inclusion Disease Cytology

CPT 87207; 88108

Related Information

Amniotic Fluid Cytology on page 286

Bacterial Culture, Bronchoscopy Specimen on page 459

Bronchial Washings Cytology on page 287

Bronchoalveolar Lavage Cytology on page 288

Brushings Cytology on page 289

Cytomegalovirus Antibody on page 389

Cytomegalovirus Antigen Detection on page 664

Cytomegalovirus Culture on page 664

Cytomegalovirus DNA Detection on page 508

Urine Cytology on page 301

Viral Culture, Urine on page 681

Synonyms CMV Smear; Cytomegalic Inclusion Bodies; Cytomegalovirus Cytology; Viral Study

Test Commonly Includes Filter or cytocentrifuge preparations for identification of nuclear and/or cytoplasmic viral inclusion bodies

Abstract Although definitive viral diagnosis is not usually made only on the basis of cytology, cytology can provide a rapid, preliminary diagnosis which is most useful. CMV viral inclusions can be identified in specimens from the urinary, respiratory, and genital tracts, and in serous effusions and cerebrospinal fluid. Bronchoalveolar lavage is a superb means for detection of CMV infection of the lower respiratory tract.[1]

Specimen Fresh urine, lavage fluid, washing fluid, or alcohol-fixed brushing specimen

Causes for Rejection Nonfixed specimen not processed within 1 hour

Special Instructions History of immunosuppression, radiation, and/or chemotherapy especially is needed.

Use Establish the presence of cytomegalovirus infection, especially in immunosuppressed patients, including those with bone marrow and other transplantation procedures and AIDS.

Limitations Viral culture is often described as the method of choice for definitive diagnosis of CMV, but cytology can provide more rapid information. Although cytology is often described as less sensitive than culture for CMV even when immunohistochemical staining is employed, Solans et al have reported biopsy is more helpful in lung transplant recipients who are clinically symptomatic. A negative cytologic examination for CMV does not exclude the possibility of this etiology, and culture results are usually needed. Separation between CMV as a cause of clinical disease versus its presence as an incidental finding in a given patient remains a problem.[2]

Methodology Conventional cytologic methods, immunofluorescence microscopy

Additional Information Immunohistochemistry, applying monoclonal antibodies to immediate-early and early CMV nuclear antigens, is reported to provide evidence of evolution of CMV pneumonitis prior to development of cytopathic biopsy changes.[1]

Footnotes

1. Solans EP, Garrity ER Jr, McCabe M, et al, "Early Diagnosis of Cytomegalovirus Pneumonitis in Lung Transplant Patients," *Arch Pathol Lab Med*, 1995, 119(1):33-5.

2. Martin WJ II, "Diagnostic Bronchoalveolar Lavage in Immunosuppressed Patients With New Pulmonary Infiltrates," *Mayo Clin Proc*, 1992, 67(3):296-8.

References

Bibbo M, *Comprehensive Cytopathology*, Philadelphia, PA: WB Saunders Co, 1991, 340-1.

Crawford SW, Bowden RA, Hackman RC, et al, "Rapid Detection of Cytomegalovirus Pulmonary Infection by Bronchoalveolar Lavage and Centrifugation Culture," *Ann Intern Med*, 1988, 108(2):180-5.

Emanuel D, Peppard J, Stover D, et al, "Rapid Immunodiagnosis of Cytomegalovirus Pneumonia in Bone Marrow Transplant Recipients by Bronchoalveolar Lavage Using Human and Murine Monoclonal Antibodies," *Ann Intern Med*, 1986, 104(4):476-81.

Linder J and Rennard SI, *Bronchoalveolar Lavage*, Chicago, IL: American Society of Clinical Pathologists, 1988, 89-90.

Traystman MD, Gupta PK, Shah KV, et al, "Identification of Viruses in the Urine of Renal Transplant Recipients by Cytomorphology," *Acta Cytol*, 1980, 24:501-10.

Cytomegalovirus Cytology see Cytomegalic Inclusion Disease Cytology on this page

Effusion Cytology see Body Fluid Cytology on page 286

Endometrial Cytology

CPT 88305

Related Information

Cervical/Vaginal Cytology on page 290

Chromosome Analysis, Products of Conception on page 280

Synonyms Endo-Pap®; Gravlee Jet® Wash; Isaac's Aspirator®; Medhosa Cannula®; Mi-Mark® Procedure; Vakutage®

Test Commonly Includes Smears, filter, cytocentrifuge, and cell block preparations

Abstract The frequency of endometrial carcinoma has increased during the last several decades. The Pap smear, proven so very successful as a screening test for cervical cancer, is not a reliable source for the diagnosis of endometrial neoplasia, although the diagnosis is rendered from time to time. Nonetheless, cytology can provide a means of diagnosis of endometrial cancer, if a direct and optimal sample is obtained. Widespread use of the office endometrial biopsy has diminished the need for endometrial cytology.

Specimen Endometrial scrape, wash, or aspiration

Collection Smear cellular material from collecting instrument thinly and evenly on a clean glass slide. Immediately spray or wet fix. Any remaining cellular material is deposited in a formalin bottle for cell block preparation. Slides and specimen bottle are labeled with patient's name and identification number. Aspirated fluid must be brought to the laboratory at once. Fluid specimens may be processed either by cytocentrifuge or cell block method.

Special Instructions Include all relevant clinical data on requisition including LMP, age, prior diagnoses, history of bleeding, hypertension, diabetes, parity, as well as hormone use.

Use Evaluate possible endometrial carcinoma or hyperplasia

Limitations Hypocellular specimen, poorly fixed specimen limits interpretation

Contraindications Cervical or vaginal infections, cervical stenosis

Methodology Smears and cytocentrifuged specimens are examined microscopically; cell blocks and tissue fragments are processed as surgical tissue specimens for histopathologic examination.

Additional Information This procedure may be useful in women who are at high risk of developing endometrial carcinoma or in women on whose routine cervical Pap smear endometrial cells were identified. Evidence supporting screening for endometrial carcinoma is scanty. Moreover, patients may be screened with a well performed combined Fast smear. The presence of noncyclic endometrial cells in a routine PAP smear may be abnormal depending upon clinical history and cellular appearance.[1]

Footnotes

1. Means M, "The Significance of Noncyclic Endometrial Cells," *Cytopathology II*, The American Society of Clinical Pathologists Continuing Education Program, 1991, 2.

References

Bibbo M, *Comprehensive Cytopathology*, Philadelphia, PA: WB Saunders Co, 1991.

Byrne AJ, "Endocyte Endometrial Smears in the Cytodiagnosis of Endometrial Carcinoma," *Acta Cytol*, 1990, 34(3):373-81.

Coscia-Porrazzi LO, Maiello FM, and de Falco ML, "The Cytology of the Normal Cyclic Endometrium," *Diagn Cytopathol*, 1986, 2(3):198-203.

Koss LG, Schreiber K, Oberlander SG, et al, "Detection of Endometrial Carcinoma and Hyperplasia in Asymptomatic Women," *Obstet Gynecol*, 1984, 64(1):1-11.

Meisels A and Jolicoeur C, "Criteria for the Cytologic Assessment of Hyperplasias in Endometrial Samples Obtained by the Endopap Endometrial Sampler," *Acta Cytol*, 1985, 29(3):297-302.

Mencaglia L, "Endometrial Cytology: Six Years of Experience," *Diagn Cytopathol*, 1987, 3(3):185-90.

Osmers RG and Kuhn W, "Endometrial Cancer Screening," *Curr Opin Obstet Gynecol*, 1994, 6(1):75-9.

Pritchard KI, "Screening for Endometrial Cancer: Is It Effective?" *Ann Intern Med*, 1989, 110(3):177-9.

Tao, L-C, *Cytopathology of the Endometrium*, Chicago, IL: ASCP Press, 1993.

Endo-Pap® see Endometrial Cytology on this page

Esophageal Brushings Cytology *see* Brushings Cytology *on page 289*

Esophageal Washings Cytology *see* Washing Cytology *on page 302*

Estrogen Effect, Cytologic *see* Hormonal Evaluation, Cytologic *on page 296*

Eye Smear for Cytology *see* Ocular Cytology *on page 298*

Fat Cells *see* Nile Blue Fat Stain *on page 297*

Fetal Maturity Determination *see* Nile Blue Fat Stain *on page 297*

Fine Needle Aspiration Biopsy Cytology *see* Fine Needle Aspiration, Superficial Palpable Masses *on this page*

Fine Needle Aspiration, Deep Seated Lesions

CPT 88162 (for pathology interpretation); 88171

Related Information

Bacterial Culture, Abscess *on page 454*
Bacterial Culture, Biopsy or Body Fluid *on page 456*
Cyst Fluid Cytology *on page 292*
Electron Microscopy *on page 37*
Fine Needle Aspiration, Superficial Palpable Masses *on this page*
Fungal Culture, Biopsy or Body Fluid *on page 476*
Immunoperoxidase Procedures *on page 43*
Immunophenotypic Analysis of Tissues by Flow Cytometry *on page 45*
Mycobacterial Culture, Biopsy or Body Fluid *on page 487*
Transbronchial Fine Needle Aspiration *on page 300*

Synonyms CT-Guided FNA; FNA; FNAB; Ultrasound Guided FNA

Applies to Abdominal Mass Aspiration; Bone Needle Aspiration Cytology; Brain Needle Aspiration; Liver Needle Aspiration Cytology; Lung Needle Aspiration Cytology; Lymph Node Aspiration Cytology; Mediastinal Mass Aspiration; Neck Mass Aspiration; Needle Biopsy Cytology; Pancreas Needle Aspiration Cytology; Retroperitoneal Mass Aspiration; Thyroid Needle Aspiration Cytology

Test Commonly Includes Examination of air-dried, Diff-Quik™ stained, and/or ethanol-fixed, Papanicolaou stained direct smears, cytospin or cell block preparations. Useful adjuncts include microbiological cultures, special stains, flow cytometry, and immunohistochemistry. Rinses can be processed for electron microscopy if indicated.

Abstract Radiological techniques for imaging deep organs and lesions has led to a reliable means of sampling, using fine needle aspiration biopsy technique. Successful cytologic diagnosis is dependent upon adequate sampling and correct preparation.

Patient Preparation Signed informed consent from the patient is required. The patient is prepped surgically to produce a sterile field. One percent lidocaine is used for local anesthesia of skin and overlying subcutaneous tissue. Sedation and/or analgesics may be needed. The suite in which the biopsies are done should be equipped for the handling of complications, such as pneumothorax (chest tube trays, etc).

Aftercare Patient should be advised of possible discomfort, local pain, and bleeding. A postpulmonary biopsy routine chest x-ray is obtained, as are routine cuts of liver, etc; post-CT biopsy to exclude hematoma. Occasionally, antibiotics may be required, dependent upon clinical circumstances.[1]

Specimen Needle aspirated material, needle rinse

Container Plain glass slides with frosted end for labeling with patient information; Coplin jar containing 95% ethanol; container with 25 mL RPMI culture medium and/or container with 10-20 mL normal saline

Collection Aspiration equipment needed includes a 15 cm graduated 22-gauge sterile Chiba needle with stylet and attached 10-20 mL plastic syringe. The aspiration is usually performed by the radiologist, surgeon, or pathologist in the CT or ultrasound suites. Most important is the localization of the needle tip within the mass. Smears and needle rinse are usually prepared by a cytotechnologist or cytopathologist present at the procedure. Immediate evaluation of air-dried Diff-Quik™ stained smears is possible, and rapidly determines the adequacy of the specimen, and need for more material or ending of the procedure. Appropriate material for culture may be obtained by this method (eg, bacterial, fungal, and mycobacterial species, for *Legionella* if thoracic, and so forth).

Storage Instructions All material should be immediately brought to the Cytology Laboratory. All slides must be labeled with the patient's name. The needle rinse, if immediate delivery to the laboratory is not possible, should be refrigerated at 4°C.

Causes for Rejection Insufficient material can result in an "unsatisfactory" reading.

Turnaround Time Immediate evaluation can usually be given within 30 minutes.

Use Diagnosis of deep-seated lesions not accessible to superficial aspiration but visible and approachable with radiologic assistance. Most of the lesions examined so are clinically perceived as neoplasms, but infectious diseases are recognized as well. These include anaerobic pulmonary infection,[2] tuberculosis and other mycobacteria, syphilis, trypanosomiasis, actinomycosis, nocardiosis, blastomycosis, *Aspergillus*, *Candida*, *Cryptococcus*, *Histoplasma*, *Coccidioides*, phaeohyphomycosis, zygomycetes, *Echinococcus*, *Entamoeba*, *Legionella*, *Pneumocystis*, and filaria among others. Viral entities which may be recognized include adenovirus, herpesviruses, CMV, respiratory syncytial virus, and others for which monoclonal antibodies may be pivotal.

Limitations Sampling error, particularly with small (1 cm or less) pulmonary nodules; lesions completely surrounded by bone; or when the procedure must be terminated due to complications or patient discomfort

Contraindications Severe chronic obstructive pulmonary disease is a contraindication to pulmonary aspiration, which has a 15% to 30% risk of pneumothorax; abnormal coagulation profile; adrenal or extra-adrenal mass in which the diagnosis of pheochromocytoma is being considered.

Methodology Papanicolaou, Wright staining

Additional Information The smallest gauge needle should be used, routinely a 22-gauge needle is used. Needle tracking of malignancy has been reported in the literature but occurs only rarely. Although the majority of these cases were 18-gauge or greater needles, incidents of tracking with 22- and 23-gauge needles, especially of high-grade pancreatic carcinoma, have been reported. Other significant complications include pneumothorax, empyema, hemorrhage, nerve damage, and sudden death due to aspiration or to pheochromocytoma. Most deep-seated FNA biopsies proceed uneventfully. Good communication among radiologist, cytopathologist, and clinician maximizes the usefulness of this procedure.

Footnotes

1. Ulich TR and Layfield LJ, "Fatal Septic Shock After Fine Needle Aspiration of a Pancreatic Pseudocyst," *Acta Cytol*, 1985, 29(5):879-81.
2. Yungbluth M, "The Laboratory Diagnosis of Pneumonia. The Role of the Community Hospital Pathologist," *Clin Lab Med*, 1995, 15(2):209-34.

References

Koss LG, Wayke S, and Olsewski W, *Aspiration Biopsy: Cytologic Interpretation and Histologic Bases*, 2nd ed, New York, NY: Igaku-Shoin, 1992.

Orell SR, Sterrett GF, Walters MN, et al, *Manual and Atlas of Fine Needle Aspiration Cytology*, New York, NY: Churchill Livingstone, 1992.

Salzman AJ, "Imaging Techniques in Aspiration Biopsy," *Clinical Aspiration Cytology*, 2nd ed, Linsk JA and Franzen S, eds, 1989.

Silverman JF and Gay RM, "Fine-Needle Aspiration and Surgical Pathology of Infectious Lesions: Morphologic Features and the Role of the Clinical Microbiology Laboratory for Rapid Diagnosis," *Clin Lab Med*, 1995, 15(2):251-78.

Stanley MW and Löwhagen T, *Fine Needle Aspiration of Palpable Masses*, Stoneham, MA: Butterworth-Heinemann, 1993.

Tao L, *Guides to Clinical Aspiration Biopsy: Pleura and Mediastinum*, New York, NY: Igaku-Shoin, 1988.

Tao L, *Transabdominal Fine Needle Aspiration Biopsy*, New York, NY: Igaku-Shoin, 1990.

Fine Needle Aspiration of Lung *see* Transbronchial Fine Needle Aspiration *on page 300*

Fine Needle Aspiration, Superficial Palpable Masses

CPT 88162 (for pathology interpretation); 88170

Related Information

Bacterial Culture, Abscess *on page 454*
Bacterial Culture, Biopsy or Body Fluid *on page 456*
Breast Biopsy *on page 35*
Cyst Fluid Cytology *on page 292*
Electron Microscopy *on page 37*
Fine Needle Aspiration, Deep Seated Lesions *on this page*
Fungal Culture, Biopsy or Body Fluid *on page 476*
Histopathology *on page 42*
Image Analysis *on page 43*
Immunoperoxidase Procedures *on page 43*
Immunophenotypic Analysis of Tissues by Flow Cytometry *on page 45*
Mycobacterial Culture, Biopsy or Body Fluid *on page 487*
Transbronchial Fine Needle Aspiration *on page 300*
Tumor Aneuploidy by Flow Cytometry *on page 57*

Synonyms Fine Needle Aspiration Biopsy Cytology; FNA; FNAB; "Skinny" or "Thin" Needle Aspiration

Applies to Breast Cyst Aspiration Cytology; Intraoral Needle Aspiration; Lymph Node Needle Aspiration; Neck Mass Needle Aspiration; Needle Biopsy Cytology; Prostate Needle Aspiration; Subcutaneous Fat Pad Aspiration; Subcutaneous Mass Needle Aspiration; Thyroid Needle Aspiration

Test Commonly Includes Examination of both air-dried Diff-Quik™ and 95% ethanol-fixed Papanicolaou stained smears, with needle rinsed material submitted for cytospins or cell block preparation. Useful adjuncts include microbiological cultures, special stains for organisms (ethanol-fixed smears); direct fluorescent antibody (DFA) staining (air-dried smears): flow cytometric immunophenotyping for cell surface markers (RPMI media used for needle rinse); DNA ploidy analysis (Hank's balanced salt solution used in needle rinse); estrogen receptor immunohistochemical analysis (ethanol-fixed smears); and special stains for amyloid, copper, or iron (ethanol-fixed smears)

Abstract Superficial palpable masses readily lend themselves to fine needle aspiration. The procedure is relatively easy, safe, painless and economical. Successful cytologic diagnosis is dependent upon adequate sampling and correct preparation.

Patient Preparation A signed informed consent should be obtained. The patient should be comfortably seated or supine in a position which maximizes exposure of and access to the area to be biopsied. The overlying skin should be cleansed with an alcohol or Betadine® wipe and allowed to dry. Local anesthesia with 1% lidocaine is used only in rare cases (ie, possible traumatic neuroma). Intraoral lesions should be sprayed with topical anesthetic spray. Assistance of an otolaryngologist is recommended for biopsies of the posterior mouth and pharynx.

Aftercare Adequate pressure of at least 5 minutes is essential to prevent significant deep hematoma, especially in hyperplastic lymph nodes, thyroid gland, and salivary gland aspirates. If the patient regularly takes aspirin, longer pressure with ice pack may be required, as in patients on Coumadin®. Mild analgesics may be needed by the patients for 24-48 hours postbiopsy if the area is painful.

Specimen Aspirated cellular material from nodule with needle rinse material saved in a balanced salt solution and/or RPMI culture medium

Container Plain glass slides with frosted end for labeling with patient information; Coplin jar containing 95% ethanol; plastic container with 25 mL of a balanced salt solution and/or RPMI culture medium

Collection Aspiration equipment needed includes a 1" to 1.5" long 22- to 25-gauge sterile needle with a **clear hub** and an attached 10 or 20 mL syringe. The clear-hubbed needle allows the aspirated material to be seen easily. Commercially available syringe holders ("guns") are available. Fine needle aspiration technique requires extensive familiarization and experience. (See figures.) The table outlines the aspiration steps.

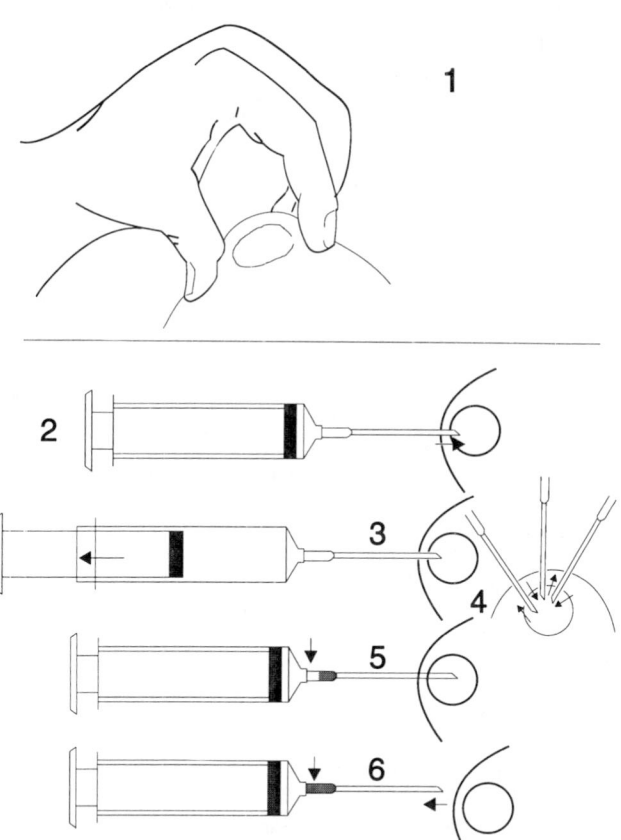

Aspiration Procedure Steps		Suction Applied
1.	Locate, palpate, and stabilize the target lesion (figure 1)	No
2.	Pass the needle through the skin and into the lesion (figure 2)	No
3.	Apply suction by pulling back on the syringe plunger (figure 3)	Yes
4.	Move the tip of the needle with quick tiny movements through the mass, in multiple directions (figure 4)	Yes
5.	Release suction by releasing the plunger, **do not pull back or push forward - simply release it** (figure 5)	No
6.	Remove the needle from the mass (figure 6)	No
7.	Give the syringe and needle to the cytotechnologist for immediate preparation of slides	No
Slides are prepared as follows:		
1.	Detach the needle from the syringe and fill the syringe with air	
2.	Replace the needle onto the syringe	
3.	Touch the needle to a glass slide and express a drop of specimen	
4.	Gently spread drop using care to avoid mechanical distortion	
5.	Alternate slides are air-dried and alcohol-fixed	
6.	Rinse needle and syringe with saline and collect for processing	

As noted in Cyst Fluid Cytology, if a cystic lesion is drained, the area should be re-examined for residual mass, and if present this mass should be aspirated. If an infectious process is suspected, appropriate cultures should be inoculated and immediately sent to the Microbiology Laboratory.

Storage Instructions All materials should be forwarded immediately to the Cytology Laboratory. If the needle rinse cannot be immediately brought to the laboratory, it should be kept refrigerated at 4°C.

Special Instructions The clinician should consider discussing the case and biopsy with the cytopathologist before it is performed, as this sometimes improves handling of the specimen especially when special studies are needed. All pertinent clinical history is needed.

Use Screen and diagnose superficial palpable masses including both primary benign and malignant lesions as well as metastatic lesions; particularly useful in situations where a rapid diagnosis is important to the clinician and patient. FNA can assist in the diagnosis of bacterial and fungal infections, and amyloidosis (abdominal fat pad aspiration). Aspirated material may be used for immunophenotyping, DNA ploidy analysis, estrogen receptor immunohistochemistry, and electron microscopy.

Limitations Needle aspiration is subject to sampling error (1% to 10%). Intraepidermal lesions, small, mobile subcutaneous lesions, extensively necrotic lesions, and diffuse plaque-like lesions may cause the most difficulty. Thyroid aspirations of neoplasm cannot usually reliably indicate if the lesion is an adenoma or carcinoma; histopathologic examination is needed. When an aspiration primary diagnosis of lymphoma is made, an excisional biopsy is sometimes preferable and usually definitive for classification of the lymphoma. In addition, a primary diagnosis of soft tissue sarcoma requires histopathologic evaluation for definitive classification.

Contraindications Significantly abnormal coagulation profile. Patients on Coumadin® may be biopsied, however, extensive and lengthy postbiopsy pressure and application of ice are advised. Such a case should be discussed with the cytopathologist beforehand.

Additional Information Routinely, FNA of palpable masses is a procedure causing only minor discomfort with local bruising and 24-58 hours of tenderness in the area biopsied. However, some situations **must** be considered if doing FNA, including the following. A neck mass in an elderly patient may represent a calcified atherosclerotic carotid; ultrasound prior to biopsy may be needed to exclude this possibility, as FNA may induce embolization of atheromatous plaque. Thyroid laceration with extensive bleeding may occur if the patient moves during thyroid aspiration. Rarely, tracheal laceration can complicate aspiration if the needle enters the trachea during aspiration and the patient coughs. Pneumothorax can be induced by aspiration of a mass in the supraclavicular fossa, most frequently in a markedly cachectic patient. Infarction of nodule due to FNA and, rarely, infection of aspiration site or nerve damage may occur.

Good communication between clinician and cytopathologist maximizes the usefulness of this procedure. FNA has a high degree of accuracy when in the hands of experienced physicians and cytopathologists. Its
(Continued)

Fine Needle Aspiration, Superficial Palpable Masses (Continued)

use has been steadily increasing in the United States as a consequence of its low morbidity, rapid turnaround time, and high accuracy. FNA of the prostate gland has essentially been replaced by use of the "biopty" gun method.

References

Abele JS and Miller TR, "Implementation of an Outpatient Needle Aspiration Biopsy Service and Clinic," *Personal Perspective Cytopathology Annual 1993*, Baltimore, MD: Williams & Wilkins, 1993, 113-7.

Abele JS, Miller TR, King EB, et al, "Smearing Techniques for the Concentration of Particles From Fine Needle Aspiration Biopsy," *Diagn Cytopathol*, 1985, 1(1):59-65.

Austin JH and Cohen MB, "Value of Having a Cytopathologist Present During Percutaneous Fine-Needle Aspiration Biopsy of Lung: Report of 55 Cancer Patients and Metaanalysis of the Literature," *AJR Am J Roentgenol*, 1993, 160(1):175-7.

Frable WJ, *Thin Needle Aspiration Biopsy*, Philadelphia, PA: WB Saunders Co, 1983.

Koss LG, Wayke S, and Olsewski W, *Aspiration Biopsy: Cytologic Interpretation and Histologic Bases*, 2nd ed, New York, NY: Igaku-Shoin, 1992.

Linsk JA and Franzen S, *Clinical Aspiration Cytology*, 2nd ed, New York, NY: JB Lippincott Co, 1989, 1-15.

Orell SR, Sterrett GF, Walters MN, et al, *Manual and Atlas of Fine Needle Aspiration Cytology*, New York, NY: Churchill Livingstone, 1992.

Qizilbash A and Young JE, *Guides to Clinical Aspiration Biopsy: Head and Neck*, New York, NY: Iguku-Shorn, 1988.

Silverman JF and Gay RM, "Fine-Needle Aspiration and Surgical Pathology of Infectious Lesions - Morphologic Features and the Role of the Clinical Microbiology Laboratory for Rapid Diagnosis," *Clin Lab Med*, 1995, 15(2):251-78.

Stanley MW and Löwhagen T, *Fine Needle Aspiration of Palpable Masses*, Boston, MA: Butterworth-Heinemann, 1993.

Fluids Cytology *see* Body Fluid Cytology *on page 286*

FNA *see* Fine Needle Aspiration, Deep Seated Lesions *on page 294*

FNA *see* Fine Needle Aspiration, Superficial Palpable Masses *on page 294*

FNAB *see* Fine Needle Aspiration, Deep Seated Lesions *on page 294*

FNAB *see* Fine Needle Aspiration, Superficial Palpable Masses *on page 294*

Gastric Brushings Cytology *see* Brushings Cytology *on page 289*

Gastric Washings Cytology *see* Washing Cytology *on page 302*

Gravlee Jet® Wash *see* Endometrial Cytology *on page 293*

Herpes Cytology

CPT 87207

Related Information

Herpes Simplex Antibody *on page 401*
Herpes Simplex Virus Antigen Detection *on page 667*
Herpes Simplex Virus Culture *on page 668*
Herpes Simplex Virus DNA Detection *on page 514*
Skin Biopsy *on page 54*
Varicella-Zoster Virus Serology *on page 437*
Viral Culture *on page 675*
Viral Culture, Dermatological Symptoms *on page 679*

Synonyms Herpetic Inclusion Bodies; Inclusion Body Cytology; Tzanck Smear

Applies to Polymerase Chain Reaction Detection of HSV, VZV

Test Commonly Includes Preparation of cytological smears, both air-dried and Diff-Quik™ stained, as well as alcohol-fixed Papanicolaou stained, with microscopic examination for cellular features of herpes virus infection.

Abstract Tzanck smears may be difficult to interpret. They are positive in approximately 50% of herpes simplex virus (HSV) infections and 80% of varicella-zoster virus (VZV) infections. Herpes may cause aseptic meningitis. Genital herpes simplex virus may be transmitted to neonates; such transmission may be catastrophic.

Specimen Scrape of lesion. If a blister is present, the smear should be taken at the edge of the lesion after the blister has been "deroofed". A direct scrape of the area under the blister will be useless, and will reveal only neutrophils.

Collection Firmly scrape the edge of the lesion, preferably a bullous lesion after removal of the bulla. The edge of normal skin and ulcer is to be scraped. In sites other than skin, a direct scrape is done. The scrape may be done with a wooden spatula or tongue blade. Use of cotton swab or Culturette® will recover fewer cells. If a nonblistering lesion is to be scraped, it may be moistened first with sterile saline before scraping. Label slides with patient's name.

Causes for Rejection Hypocellular smears or smears composed only of neutrophilic exudate

Use Establish the presence of herpes virus infection

Limitations Tzanck smears cannot provide distinction between HSV 1 and HSV 2, and treatment is not the same for each. Herpes inclusions may not be seen in 50% of active lesions, however, peripheral margination of nuclear chromatin, multinucleated giant cells, and other cellular changes suggestive of herpes infection may point to the correct diagnosis. Interpretation can be difficult. **Viral culture is the definitive diagnostic method.** Polymerase chain reaction has been utilized successfully in detection of HSV and VZV DNA sequences and has been reported as equivalent or superior to viral culture. Biopsy is also useful.

Methodology Air-dried, Diff-Quik™ stained or alcohol-fixed, Pap-stained smear. Both types of smears may be submitted for immunoperoxidase stain for herpes viral antigen. Giemsa or Wright's stain may also be used.

Additional Information Diagnostic yield is increased by immunoperoxidase or immunofluorescent procedures, which become positive before characteristic viral cytopathic changes develop. Smears with a heavy inflammatory exudate may be especially difficult to interpret because of nonspecific staining. Smears must be done with and without the primary antibody, and positive and negative controls must be run concurrently.

References

Arvin AM and Prober CG, "Herpes Simplex Virus," *Manual of Clinical Microbiology*, 6th ed, Murray PR, Baron EJ, Pfaller MA, et al, eds, Washington, DC: American Society of Microbiology, 1995, 876-83.

Koelle DM, Benedetti J, Langenberg A, et al, "Asymptomatic Reactivation of Herpes Simplex Virus in Women After the First Episode of Genital Herpes," *Ann Intern Med*, 1992, 116(6):433-7.

Mertz GJ, Benedetti J, Ashley R, et al, "Risk Factors for the Sexual Transmission of Genital Herpes," *Ann Intern Med*, 1992, 116(3):197-202.

Nahass GT, Goldstein BA, Zhu WY, et al, "Comparison of Tzanck Smear, Viral Culture, and DNA Diagnostic Methods in Detection of Herpes Simplex and Varicella-Zoster Infection," *JAMA*, 1992, 268(18):2541-4.

Herpes Smear *see* Cervical/Vaginal Cytology *on page 290*

Herpetic Inclusion Bodies *see* Herpes Cytology *on this page*

Hormonal Evaluation, Cytologic

CPT 88155

Related Information

Cervical/Vaginal Cytology *on page 290*

Synonyms Estrogen Effect, Cytologic; Maturation Index

Replaces Cornification Count

Test Commonly Includes Count of at least 200 squamous cells, with assessment of maturation as to parabasal, intermediate, or superficial (mature)

Abstract Cytology provides a simple, efficient, inexpensive method for a general evaluation of hormonal status. While vaginal epithelium is responsive to multihormonal substances, generally hormonal cytology is used to assist in determination of need for hormonal treatment, to monitor hormonal treatments, time of ovulation estimation, and to play a role in evaluation of ovarian dysfunction.

Patient Preparation Douches should be avoided for 24 hours prior to obtaining the smear.

Specimen Scrape of lateral vaginal wall; distal third is preferred

Container Smear on plain glass slide

Collection Prelabel frosted end of plain glass slide with graphite pencil with patient's name and LVW (lateral vaginal wall). The scrape, with a wooden spatula or tongue blade, is smeared across a glass slide and immediately fixed in 95% ethanol.

Causes for Rejection Air drying, specimen taken from site other than lateral vaginal wall, presence of inflammatory changes due to trichomonads, *Candida* sp, severe bacterial cytolysis

Special Instructions Slide should be labeled LVW (lateral vaginal wall). Include age, last menstrual period (LMP), pertinent history (ie, drugs, history of radiation therapy hormone use, previous gynecological surgery).

Reference Range Hormonal evaluation is reported in general terms, such as "normal for age and menstrual status", or "hormonal pattern incompatible with patient's age and menstrual status". When specifically requested, a count or maturation index can be given and is reported in in percentages of cell types, parabasal:intermediate:superficial (ie, 10/60/20 indicating 10% parabasal, 60% intermediate, and 20% superficial). Interpretation of this test is dependent upon the clinical situation.

Use Evaluate the maturation status of the vaginal squamous epithelium, which reflects the balance of estrogen and progesterone effects upon this target tissue; also useful in the diagnosis of conditions producing abnormal cytohormonal balance (ie, pituitary dysfunction, ovarian dysfunction, feminizing tumor, and virilizing tumor). **Note:** Any dysplastic or malignant changes noted are treated as they would be on a routine smear, and must be reported to the clinician.

Limitations This test cannot be performed in the presence of inflammation of the vaginal or cervical mucosa. Maturation index is of extremely limited value when applied to a given individual as an isolated procedure because of the great overlap of normal indices and because of great interobserver variability in counts. A series of smears for MI is more useful, but seldom warranted now that sensitive hormonal assays are available.

Contraindications Cervicitis, vaginitis

Additional Information A few agents affecting cytohormonal pattern are estrogen, cortisone, digitalis, and tetracycline suppositories (causing misleading massive desquamation).

References
Bibbo M, *Comprehensive Cytopathology*, Philadelphia, PA: WB Saunders Co, 1991.
Erozan Y, *Manual for the Thirty-Third Postgraduate Institute for Pathologists in Cytopathology*, Baltimore, MD: John Hopkins University School of Medicine and John Hopkins Hospital, 1992.
Wied GL and Bibbo M, "Hormonal Cytology," *Comprehensive Cytopathology*, Bibbo M, ed, Philadelphia, PA: WB Saunders Co, 1991, 85-114.

Human Papilloma Viruses (HPV) *see* Cervical/Vaginal Cytology *on page 290*

Hydrocele Fluid Cytology *see* Cyst Fluid Cytology *on page 292*

Inclusion Body Cytology *see* Herpes Cytology *on previous page*

Inclusion Conjunctivitis *see* Ocular Cytology *on next page*

Induced Sputum Technique *see Pneumocystis carinii* Preparation *on page 299*

Intraoral Needle Aspiration *see* Fine Needle Aspiration, Superficial Palpable Masses *on page 294*

Isaac's Aspirator® *see* Endometrial Cytology *on page 293*

Lavage Cytology *see* Washing Cytology *on page 302*

Lipid, Cytology *see* Nile Blue Fat Stain *on this page*

Liver Needle Aspiration Cytology *see* Fine Needle Aspiration, Deep Seated Lesions *on page 294*

Lumbar Tap Cytology *see* Cerebrospinal Fluid Cytology *on page 290*

Lung Needle Aspiration Cytology *see* Fine Needle Aspiration, Deep Seated Lesions *on page 294*

Lymph Node Aspiration Cytology *see* Fine Needle Aspiration, Deep Seated Lesions *on page 294*

Lymph Node Needle Aspiration *see* Fine Needle Aspiration, Superficial Palpable Masses *on page 294*

Maturation Index *see* Hormonal Evaluation, Cytologic *on previous page*

Medhosa Cannula® *see* Endometrial Cytology *on page 293*

Mediastinal Mass Aspiration *see* Fine Needle Aspiration, Deep Seated Lesions *on page 294*

Mi-Mark® Procedure *see* Endometrial Cytology *on page 293*

Neck Mass Aspiration *see* Fine Needle Aspiration, Deep Seated Lesions *on page 294*

Neck Mass Needle Aspiration *see* Fine Needle Aspiration, Superficial Palpable Masses *on page 294*

Needle Biopsy Cytology *see* Fine Needle Aspiration, Deep Seated Lesions *on page 294*

Needle Biopsy Cytology *see* Fine Needle Aspiration, Superficial Palpable Masses *on page 294*

Nile Blue Fat Stain

CPT 88313

Related Information
Amniotic Fluid Cytology *on page 286*
Amniotic Fluid Lecithin/Sphingomyelin Ratio and Phosphatidylglycerol *on page 77*

Applies to Fat Cells; Fetal Maturity Determination; Lipid, Cytology

Test Commonly Includes Special stain and count of cells positive for intracellular fat

Abstract This test was an early study to try to assess fetal maturity. This is essentially an obsolescent test.

Specimen Amniotic fluid

Container Sealed test tube

Storage Instructions If immediate processing is not possible, place in refrigerator.

Reference Range Negative for fat to positive for fat. Amniotic fluid: less than 34 weeks maturity: <1% of cells positive for intracellular fat; 34-38 weeks maturity: 1% to 10% of cells positive; 38-40 weeks maturity: 10% to 50% or more of cells positive; more than 40 weeks maturity: >50% of cells positive.

Use Determine the presence of intracellular fat; amniotic fluid test for fetal maturity

Limitations Not as specific as more recent tests including the lecithin/sphingomyelin ratio measured on amniotic fluid; additional spectrophotometric determinations on amniotic fluid are more precise than the Nile Blue fat stain.

Methodology Test based on the staining of neutral lipid in fetal cells obtained by amniocentesis. The neutral lipid is stained by oxazone present in commercial Nile blue sulfate. A smear of the amniotic fluid is made on a clean slide. No fixative is required. The stain solution is a 0.1% aqueous solution of Nile Blue sulfate, which is a differential stain for neutral fat. The preparation is examined under low power (10x) for the presence of fetal cells. Notation is made between the anucleate fetal cells with the orange lipid droplets and the blue nucleated, lipid-free cells. The test is based on staining characteristics and detailed knowledge of cellular morphology is not required by the examiner.

References
Kjeldsberg CR and Knight JA, "Amniotic Fluid," *Body Fluids - Laboratory Examination of Amniotic, Cerebrospinal, Seminal, Serous, and Synovial Fluids*, 3rd ed, Chapter 1, Chicago, IL: American Society of Clinical Pathologists, 1993, 1-63.

Nipple Discharge Cytology

CPT 88104

Related Information
Breast Biopsy *on page 35*
Cyst Fluid Cytology *on page 292*

Synonyms Breast Discharge Cytology

Test Commonly Includes Examination of smeared stained slides

Abstract Examination of nipple discharge may aid in the evaluation of inflammatory or neoplastic lesions of the breast.

Specimen Nipple discharge

Collection Clean nipple and areola with warm saline; then gently grip subareolar area and nipple with thumb and forefinger. Using a milking action, when liquid appears, allow a pea sized drop to accumulate on the nipple apex. Place a plain glass slide (with one frosted end for labeling) upon the nipple and slide across quickly. Place slide immediately in 95% ethanol. See diagram. Prepare four to six smears, as the amount of specimen allows. If clinician has difficulty expressing liquid, allow the patient to do it herself. If an eczematous areolar lesion exists, a separate scraping should be made with a wooden spatula or tongue blade for examination for Paget's disease of breast.

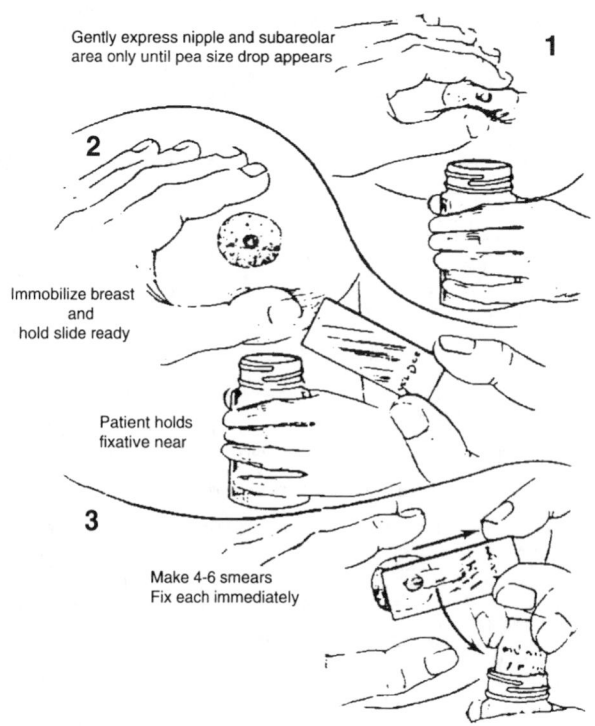

Gently express nipple and subareolar area only until pea size drop appears **1**

2

Immobilize breast and hold slide ready

Patient holds fixative near

3

Make 4-6 smears Fix each immediately

(Continued)

Nipple Discharge Cytology *(Continued)*

Special Instructions Specify nipple discharge. Provide pertinent clinical data, specifically indicating presence of subareolar mass, other dominant breast masses, or fibrocystic disease.

Use Assist in the diagnosis of neoplastic and inflammatory disease

Limitations Drying of smear before fixation will render it unsatisfactory for evaluation. Hypocellular smears with poor cytologic detail are unlikely to support accurate diagnosis.

Additional Information If material obtained is scanty and quickly air dries, submit the air-dried smear for Diff-Quik™ or Giemsa stains.

References

Fung A, Rayter Z, Fisher C, et al, "Preoperative Cytology and Mammography in Patients With Single-Duct Nipple Discharge Treated by Surgery," *Br J Surg*, 1990, 77(11):1211-2.

Johnson TL and Kini SR, "Cytologic and Clinicopathologic Features of Abnormal Nipple Secretions: 225 Cases," *Diagn Cytopathol*, 1991, 7(1):17-22.

Lee MM, Petrakis NL, Wrensch MR, et al, "Association of Abnormal Nipple Aspirate Cytology and Mammographic Pattern and Density," *Cancer Epidemiol Biomarkers Prev*, 1994, 3(1):33-6.

Takeda T, Matsui A, Sato Y, et al, "Nipple Discharge Cytology in Mass Screening for Breast Cancer," *Acta Cytol*, 1990, 34(2):161-4.

Ocular Cytology

CPT 88104 (smears); 88312 (special stains)

Related Information

Bacterial Culture, Conjunctiva *on page 461*
Chlamydia trachomatis Direct FA Test *on page 663*
Viral Culture, Eye or Ocular Symptoms *on page 679*

Synonyms *Chlamydia* Smears Cytology; Conjunctival Smear Cytology; Corneal Cytology; Eye Smear for Cytology

Applies to Inclusion Conjunctivitis

Test Commonly Includes Smears fixed in 95% ethanol and stained with Papanicolaou stain; or air-dried smears stained with Giemsa or Diff-Quik™ stain

Abstract Useful for diagnosis of infections, inflammatory conditions, and primary as well as metastatic malignancies

Specimen Direct smear (scraping, washing) of ocular lesion or fine needle aspiration specimen[1,2,3]

Collection Swab lesion with cotton-tipped applicator or scrape with sterile ophthalmic spatula and smear on two clean, glass slides, **immediately** spray-fix one slide, let other air dry. Label frosted end of slide with patient's identification. FNA is performed in standard manner. (See Fine Needle Aspiration, Superficial Palpable Masses *on page 294*.)

Use Diagnose trachoma-inclusion conjunctivitis and evaluate possible dysplastic or malignant conjunctival lesions; diagnose intraocular and/or orbital tumors

Additional Information Diagnosis of viral and chlamydial infections is considerably improved by immunofluorescent and immunoperoxidase stains for organisms. A study of 292 palpable orbital and eyelid tumors reported a false-positive rate for malignancy of 1.6% and a false-negative rate of 1.8%.[4] Experience with intraocular fine needle aspirations is limited, but published reports exist.[3]

Footnotes

1. Scroggs MW, Johnston WW, and Klintworth GK, "Intraocular Tumors: A Cytopathologic Study," *Acta Cytol*, 1990, 34(3):401-8.
2. Arora R, Rewari R, and Betharia SM, "Fine Needle Aspiration Cytology of Orbital and Adnexal Masses," *Acta Cytol*, 1992, 36(4):483-91.
3. O'Hara BJ, Ehya H, Shields JA, et al, "Fine Needle Aspiration Biopsy in Pediatric Ophthalmic Tumors and Pseudotumors," *Acta Cytol*, 1993, 37(2):125-30.
4. Zajdela A, Vielh P, Schlienger P, et al, "Fine Needle Cytology of 292 Palpable Orbital and Eyelid Tumors," *Am J Clin Pathol*, 1990, 93(1):100-4.

References

Arora R, Rewari R, and Betharia SM, "Fine Needle Aspiration Cytology of Eyelid Tumors," *Acta Cytol*, 1990, 34(2):227-32.

Carlier C, Coste J, Etchepare M, et al, "Conjunctival Impression Cytology With Transfer as a Field-Applicable Indicator of vitamin A Status for Mass Screening," *Int J Epidemiol*, 1992, 21(2):373-80.

Char DH and Miller T, "Orbital Pseudotumor. Fine-Needle Aspiration Biopsy and Response to Therapy," *Ophthalmology*, 1993, 100(11):1702-10.

Char DH, Kroll SM, Stoloff A, et al, "Cytomorphometry of Uveal Melanoma. Comparison of Fine Needle Aspiration Biopsy Samples With Histologic Sections," *Anal Quant Cytol Histol*, 1991, 13(4):293-9.

Connor CG, Campbell JB, Tirey WW, et al, "Modification of Impression Cytology for In-Office Use," *J Am Optom Assoc*, 1991, 62(12):898-901.

Cristallini EG, Bolis GB, and Ottaviano P, "Fine Needle Aspiration Biopsy of Orbital Meningioma - Report of a Case," *Acta Cytol*, 1990, 34(2):236-8.

de Rojas MV, Rodriguez MT, Ces Blanco JA, et al, "Impression Cytology in Patients With Keratoconjunctivitis Sicca," *Cytopathology*, 1993, 4(6):347-55.

Dewan S, Mittal S, D'Souza A, et al, "Cytological Evaluation of Conjunctival Scrape Smears in Cases of Conjunctivitis," *Indian J Pathol Microbiol*, 1992, 35(2):118-24.

Fuchs GJ, Ausayakhun S, Ruckphaopunt S, et al, "Relationship Between Vitamin A Deficiency, Malnutrition, and Conjunctival Impression Cytology," *Am J Clin Nutr*, 1994, 60(2):293-8.

Fuller DG, "Cytology in Anterior Segment Disease," *Optom Clin*, 1992, 2(1):27-40.

Gadkari SS, Adrianwala SD, Prayag AS, et al, "Conjunctival Impression Cytology - A Study of Normal Conjunctiva," *J Postgrad Med*, 1992, 38(1):21-3.

Glasgow BJ and Foos RY, *Ocular Cytopathology*, Boston, MA: Butterworth Heinemen, 1993.

Knop E and Brewitt H, "Conjunctival Cytology in Asymptomatic Wearers of Soft Contact Lenses," *Graefes Arch Clin Exp Ophthalmol*, 1992, 230(4):340-7.

Kobayashi TK, Tsubota K, Ugajin Y, et al, "Presence of Bar-Shaped Nuclear Chromatin in Cell Samples From the Conjunctiva," *Acta Cytol*, 1992, 36(2):163-6.

Paridaens AD, McCartney AC, Curling OM, et al, "Impression Cytology of Conjunctival Melanosis and Melanoma," *Br J Ophthalmol*, 1992, 76(4):198-201.

Resnikoff S, Luzeau R, Filliard G, et al, "Impression Cytology With Transfer in Xerophthalmia and Conjunctival Diseases," *Int Ophthalmol*, 1992, 16(6):445-51.

Rivas L, Oroza MA, Perez-Esteban A, et al, "Morphological Changes in Ocular Surface in Dry Eyes and Other Disorders by Impression Cytology," *Graefes Arch Clin Exp Ophthalmol*, 1992, 230(4):329-34.

Rivas L, Rodriguez JJ, Alvarez MI, et al, "Correlation Between Impression Cytology and Tear Function Parameters in Sjögren's Syndrome," *Acta Ophthalmol*, 1993, 71(3):353-9.

Schwartz D, Sobottka I, Leitch GJ, et al, "Pathology of Microsporidiosis: Emerging Parasitic Infections in Patients With Acquired Immunodeficiency Syndrome," *Arch Pathol Lab Med*, 1996, 120:173-88.

Tsubota K, Kajiwara K, Ugajin S, et al, "Conjunctival Brush Cytology," *Acta Cytol*, 1990, 34(2):233-5.

Tsubota K, Takamura E, Hasegawa T, et al, "Detection by Brush Cytology of Mast Cells and Eosinophils in Allergic and Vernal Conjunctivitis," *Cornea*, 1991, 10(6):525-31.

Tsubota K, Yamada M, Kajiwara K, et al, "Cytologic Evaluation of Conjunctival Epithelium After Cataract Surgery," *Cornea*, 1992, 11(5):418-26.

Vadrevu VL and Fullard RJ, "Enhancements to the Conjunctival Impression Cytology Technique and Examples of Applications in a Clinico-Biochemical Study of Dry Eye," *CLAO J*, 1994, 20(1):59-63.

Oral Cavity Cytology

CPT 88104

Related Information

Buccal Smear for Sex Chromatin Evaluation *on page 275*
Chromosome Analysis, Blood *on page 276*
Chromosome Analysis, Bone Marrow *on page 277*
Herpes Simplex Virus Antigen Detection *on page 667*
Herpes Simplex Virus Culture *on page 668*
Morphine, Urine *on page 564*
Skin Biopsy *on page 54*
Skin Biopsy, Immunofluorescence *on page 56*

Synonyms Oral Scraping Cytology; Pemphigus Smear

Test Commonly Includes Evaluation of 95% ethanol-fixed, Papanicolaou-stained smears or 95% ethanol-fixed, Aceto-Orcein-stained smears; smears may also be used for immunofluorescent studies screening for monosomies or trisomies.

Abstract Used to diagnose various conditions of the oral cavity including, but not limited to, dysplastic and neoplastic lesions.

Patient Preparation Patient should rinse mouth vigorously several times before scrape is done.

Specimen For grossly visible lesion, a direct scrape of the area with a tongue blade or wooden spatula is done.

Container Glass slides, with one frosted end; Coplin jar filled with 95% ethanol

Sampling Time 10-15 minutes

Collection Scrape grossly visible lesion with spatula or tongue blade. Smear gently on labeled glass slide and fix **immediately** in 95% ethanol or with spray or liquid fixative (described in Cervical/Vaginal Cytology). For genetic assessments, a scraping is taken from the lateral buccal mucosa just above the dentate line along the anterior two-thirds of the buccal mucosa. All materials should be submitted to the laboratory with a completed requisition containing full history.

Special Instructions Requisition should include age, physical findings, history of smoking, presence of dentures, skin lesions, reverse smoking, radiation or chemotherapy, and clinical findings suggestive of chromosomal abnormality. If pemphigus is suspected, the lesion should be scraped at the edge, where normal mucosa and affected mucosa are identified.

Use Diagnose dysplastic and malignant disease of the oral cavity, oral pemphigus, oral herpes or *Candida* sp, and rarely, neoplasm of minor palatal salivary glands; screen for Turner syndrome, Klinefelter syndrome, multiple X syndrome, and trisomy 21, 13, and 18.

In AIDS, oral ulcers can be caused by tuberculosis, bacillary angiomatosis, *Enterobacteriaceae*, *Candida*, *Histoplasma*, *Cryptococcus*, cytomegalovirus, herpes simplex virus, lymphoma, Kaposi's sarcoma, squamous cell carcinoma as well as autoimmune and idiopathic ulcers and stomatitis not otherwise defined.[1]

Limitations Poorly fixed or hypocellular specimens

Methodology Tissue biopsy may be more rewarding in cases of neoplasm, as many oral cancers show extensive overlying hyperkeratosis (leukoplakia) which reveals only anucleate squames on smear. Buccal smears for Barr body analysis have been almost replaced by karyotyping studies. With the advent of monoclonal anticentromeric antibodies for specific chromosomes, rapid screening for Turner syndrome, trisomy 21, 13, and 18 is becoming increasingly efficacious.

Footnotes

1. "Case Records of the Massachusetts General Hospital. Weekly Clinicopathological Exercises. Case 3-1995. A 29-Year-Old Man With AIDS and Multiple Splenic Abscesses," *N Engl J Med*, 1995, 332(4):249-57.

References

Bibbo M, *Comprehensive Cytopathology*, Philadelphia, PA: WB Saunders Co, 1991, 399.

Das DK, Gulati A, Bhatt NC, et al, "Fine Needle Aspiration Cytology of Oral and Pharyngeal Lesions - A Study of 45 Cases," *Acta Cytol*, 1993, 37(3):333-42.

Günhan O, Doğan N, Celasun B, et al, "Fine Needle Aspiration Cytology of Oral Cavity and Jaw Bone Lesions - A Report of 102 Cases," *Acta Cytol*, 1993, 37(2):135-41.

Medak H and Burlakow P, "Cytology of Pemphigus Vulgaris," *ASCP Check Sample®*, Chicago, IL: American Society of Clinical Pathologists, 1981.

Oral Scraping Cytology *see* Oral Cavity Cytology *on previous page*

Oropharyngeal Brushings Cytology *see* Brushings Cytology *on page 289*

Ovarian Cyst Fluid Cytology *see* Cyst Fluid Cytology *on page 292*

Pancreas Needle Aspiration Cytology *see* Fine Needle Aspiration, Deep Seated Lesions *on page 294*

Pancreatic Cyst Fluid Cytology *see* Cyst Fluid Cytology *on page 292*

Pap Smear *see* Cervical/Vaginal Cytology *on page 290*

Paracentesis Fluid Cytology *see* Body Fluid Cytology *on page 286*

Pemphigus Smear *see* Oral Cavity Cytology *on previous page*

Pericardial Fluid Cytology *see* Body Fluid Cytology *on page 286*

Peritoneal Fluid Cytology *see* Body Fluid Cytology *on page 286*

Peritoneal Washings Cytology *see* Washing Cytology *on page 302*

Pleural Fluid Cytology *see* Body Fluid Cytology *on page 286*

Pneumocystis carinii Preparation

CPT 88108; 88312 (special stains, microorganisms)

Related Information

Bacterial Culture, Bronchoscopy Specimen *on page 459*
Bronchial Washings Cytology *on page 287*
Bronchoalveolar Lavage Cytology *on page 288*
Pneumocystis Immunofluorescence *on page 423*
Sputum Cytology *on next page*
Viral Culture, Respiratory Symptoms *on page 680*

Applies to Bronchial Aspiration for *Pneumocystis*; Bronchopulmonary Lavage for *Pneumocystis*; Induced Sputum Technique; Transbronchial Aspiration Biopsy for *Pneumocystis*; Transthoracic Needle Aspiration for *Pneumocystis*

Test Commonly Includes Papanicolaou, Diff-Quik™, Giemsa, methenamine silver stains, or monoclonal antibodies to *Pneumocystis*

Abstract Diagnosis of *Pneumocystis* pneumonia in any immunocompromised subject, including individuals with AIDS, postorgan transplant patients, those with hematologic malignant diseases, inflammatory disorders, and those receiving chemotherapeutic regimens. Corticosteroids had been given to most of the patients without AIDS in the month prior to onset.[1]

Patient Preparation Induced sputum technique: A common method used consists of using a heated (37°C) solution of 15% NaCl and 20% propylene glycol, the vapors of which the patient inhales for 15-20 minutes. Subsequent to this inhalation, the patient usually will produce a large amount of satisfactory sputum.

Specimen Lung biopsy, transthoracic needle aspirate, bronchoalveolar lavage fluid, or induced sputum. **Routine sputum is not acceptable** for identification of *Pneumocystis*.

Container Sterile jar, clean glass slides

Collection For bronchoalveolar lavage, see Bronchoalveolar Lavage Cytology *on page 288*. For tissue lung biopsy, touch preparations made from the fresh surgical specimen are made by lightly touching the fresh tissue in rapid succession along the length of three to four slides. Induced sputum is sent to the laboratory fresh, and prepared in the laboratory.

Use Identify *Pneumocystis carinii* organisms, predominantly in immunocompromised patients

Limitations *Pneumocystis* preparations applied to spontaneously expectorated sputum have an extremely low yield. In about 40% of individuals with AIDS and symptomatic pneumonia caused by other agents, one may anticipate *P. carinii* in bronchoalveolar lavage fluid, unless the patient is receiving treatment for this organism prophylactically. *P. carinii* was correctly identified in 94% of adequate transbronchial biopsies, 95%

of bronchoalveolar lavage cell block specimens, 88% of bronchoalveolar smears, and 79% of brushings in a series of 36 autopsy-proven cases.[2] Although a paper from the city of New York indicates that *Pneumocystis* can be reliably identified in smears of bronchial washes,[3] others recommend lavage cytologic procedures.[4,5] Martin explains that although sputum analysis remains useful for the diagnosis of *P. carinii* pneumonia in subjects who have AIDS, its utility for diagnosis of *P. carinii* in immunosuppressed patients who do not have AIDS is limited.[5] An NIH paper recommends the induced sputum technique and provides details of methods.[6] PCR detection of *P. carinii* is more sensitive than cytology or immunofluorescence.[7]

Methodology In the hands of an experienced cytopathologist, *P. carinii* can be identified with Pap, Giemsa, Diff-Quik™, and methenamine silver stains.

Additional Information Impaired cellular immunity is the major predisposing background for *Pneumocystis carinii* infection: AIDS, malnutrition, prematurity, immunodeficiency disease entities, and use of immunosuppressive drugs and/or corticosteroids. In subjects with AIDS, the risk of *P. carinii* correlates with the number of CD4 lymphocytes.[8]

This entity is found in patients with clinical diffuse interstitial pneumonitis. Immunocompromised patients have a high incidence of *Pneumocystis carinii* infection (as high as 44% in some series). *Pneumocystis carinii* pneumonia may be, but is not always, rapidly progressive. It may be life-threatening, so that rapid diagnosis is important to allow prompt institution of therapy. *Pneumocystis carinii* is the most frequent cause of death in children with ALL in remission, such that some institutions routinely give prophylactic trimethoprim-sulfamethoxazole to their leukemic children undergoing antineoplastic therapy. *P. carinii* is also the most common infection and most common cause of death in patients with AIDS. If a patient has been receiving prophylactic therapy for *P. carinii* and presents with pneumonitis, the cytopathologist must be notified, because if organisms are present, they will have destroyed or partially destroyed cyst walls, and examination must be extremely meticulous to identify the organisms. Under circumstances of prophylactic therapy for *Pneumocystis*, such organisms are best identified through use of an immunohistochemical or immunofluorescent method.

P. carinii causes extrapulmonary infections in patients with or without AIDS. It involves liver and spleen, eyes, ears, lymph nodes, thymus, skin, ascitic fluid, portions of the gastrointestinal tract, kidneys, bone marrow, pancreas, adrenals and other tissues. Some of the sites can be diagnosed by aspiration.[9]

Serum carcinoembryonic antigen has been proposed but not proven prognostic in HIV-related *P. carinii* pneumonia.[10]

Footnotes

1. Yale SH and Limper AH, "*Pneumocystis carinii* Pneumonia in Patients Without Acquired Immunodeficiency Syndrome: Associated Illness and Prior Corticosteroid Therapy," *Mayo Clin Proc*, 1996, 71(1):5-13.

2. Gal AA, Klatt EC, Koss MN, et al, "The Effectiveness of Bronchoscopy in the Diagnosis of *Pneumocystis carinii* and Cytomegalovirus Pulmonary Infections in Acquired Immunodeficiency Syndrome," *Arch Pathol Lab Med*, 1987, 111(3):238-41.

3. Rorat E, Garcia RL, and Skolom J, "Diagnosis of *Pneumocystis carinii* Pneumonia by Cytologic Examination of Bronchial Washings," *JAMA*, 1985, 254(14):1950-1.

4. DeFine LA, Saleba KP, Gibson BB, et al, "Cytologic Evaluation of Bronchoalveolar Lavage Specimens in Immunosuppressed Patients With Suspected Opportunistic Infections," *Acta Cytol*, 1987, 31(3):235-42.

5. Martin WJ 2nd, "Diagnostic Bronchoalveolar Lavage in Immunosuppressed Patients With New Pulmonary Infiltrates," *Mayo Clin Proc*, 1992, 67(3):296-8.

6. Masur H, Gill VJ, Ognibene FP, et al, "Diagnosis of *Pneumocystis* Pneumonia by Induced Sputum Technique in Patients Without the Acquired Immunodeficiency Syndrome," *Ann Intern Med*, 1988, 109(9):755-6.

7. Leibovitz E, Pollack H, Moore T, et al, "Comparison of PCR and Standard Cytological Staining for Detection of *Pneumocystis carinii* From Respiratory Specimens From Patients With or at High Risk for Infection by Human Immunodeficiency Virus," *J Clin Microbiol*, 1995, 33(11):3004-7.

8. Walzer PD, "*Pneumocystis carinii* - New Clinical Spectrum?" *N Engl J Med*, 1991, 324(4):263-5.

9. "Case Records of the Massachusetts General Hospital. Weekly Clinicopathological Exercises. Case 3-1995. A 29-Year-Old Man With AIDS and Multiple Splenic Abscesses," *N Engl J Med*, 1995, 332(4):249-57.

10. Bedos JP, Hignette C, Lucet JC, et al, "Serum Carcinoembryonic Antigen: A Prognostic Marker in HIV-Related *Pneumocystis carinii* Pneumonia," *Scand J Infect Dis*, 1992, 24(3):309-15.

References

Bibbo M, *Comprehensive Cytopathology*, Philadelphia, PA: WB Saunders Co, 1991.

"Case Records of the Massachusetts General Hospital. Weekly Clinicopathological Exercises. Case 8-1987. A 44 Month-Old Girl With Fever of Unknown Origin After Repair of Tetralogy of Fallot," *N Engl J Med*, 1987, 316(8):466-75.

Koss LG, *Diagnostic Cytology and Its Histopathologic Bases*, 4th ed, Philadelphia, PA: JB Lippincott Co, 1992, 741-2.

Polymerase Chain Reaction Detection of HSV, VZV *see* Herpes Cytology *on page 296*

Premature Rupture of Bag of Waters (BOW) *see* Amniotic Fluid Cytology *on page 286*

Premature Rupture of Fetal Membranes *see* Amniotic Fluid Cytology *on page 286*

Prostate Needle Aspiration see Fine Needle Aspiration, Superficial Palpable Masses on page 294

Pulmonary Cytology Series see Sputum Cytology on this page

Renal Cyst Fluid Cytology see Cyst Fluid Cytology on page 292

Renal Pelvic Washings Cytology see Urine Cytology on next page

Retroperitoneal Mass Aspiration see Fine Needle Aspiration, Deep Seated Lesions on page 294

Serous Effusion Cytology see Body Fluid Cytology on page 286

Serous Fluid Cytology see Body Fluid Cytology on page 286

"Skinny" or "Thin" Needle Aspiration see Fine Needle Aspiration, Superficial Palpable Masses on page 294

Small Bowel Brushings Cytology see Brushings Cytology on page 289

Spinal Fluid Cytology see Cerebrospinal Fluid Cytology on page 290

Sputum Cytology

CPT 88104; 88108 (concentration technique, smears and interpretation)

Related Information

Bacterial Culture, Sputum on page 465
Bronchial Washings Cytology on page 287
Bronchoalveolar Lavage Cytology on page 288
Coccidioidomycosis Antibodies on page 384
Cytomegalovirus Antibody on page 389
Cytomegalovirus Culture on page 664
Fungal Culture, Sputum on page 479
Mycobacterial Culture, Sputum on page 490
Pneumocystis carinii Preparation on previous page
Pneumocystis Immunofluorescence on page 423
Uric Acid, Serum on page 213
Viral Culture, Respiratory Symptoms on page 680
Virus, Direct Detection by Fluorescent Antibody on page 682

Synonyms Cytology, Sputum; Pulmonary Cytology Series

Test Commonly Includes Three to five consecutive first morning deep cough specimens

Abstract Cytopathological examination of sputum may aid in the evaluation of respiratory infections or neoplasms.

Patient Preparation It should be explained to the patient that the contents of the collection container (fixative material) should not be consumed by the patient.

Specimen Expectorated sputum, **not saliva or nasal aspirates**

Container 50 mL screw-top plastic container; for sputum series it will contain cytologic fixative (ie, Saccomanno® fixative, Carbowax®). Antibiotic to prevent bacterial overgrowth is sometimes used.

Collection Upon arising the patient rinses his mouth with water and expectorates a deep cough into the container. The **first** cough specimen is the most rewarding.

Storage Instructions Specimens not delivered during laboratory hours should be placed in a refrigerator (but not allowed to freeze) and delivered as soon as possible. If it is not possible to bring unfixed material to the laboratory, a prefixed specimen (using Carbowax® or 70% ethanol) may be substituted. The best preparations are from **fresh** sputum.

Causes for Rejection Specimen consists of saliva or nasal secretions

Special Instructions Include admitting diagnosis and pertinent clinical history on requisition (ie, age, clinical diagnosis, exposure to carcinogens, radiographic findings, and history of radiation or chemotherapy).

Use Establish the presence of neoplasm; aid in the diagnosis of respiratory infections with herpesvirus, cytomegalovirus,[1] fungal diseases, Strongyloides, Echinococcus, and Paragonimus; aid in the diagnosis of lipoid pneumonitis, allergic processes, hemosiderosis, Goodpasture's syndrome, asbestosis, and alveolar proteinosis

Limitations If no carbon bearing histiocytes are identified in the specimen, it is considered to be an unsatisfactory specimen (not a deep cough specimen).

Methodology Sputa may be collected fresh, without fixative; make direct smears from white flecks and blood-tinged areas;[2,3] fix smears immediately in 95% ethanol. Sputa may be collected in Carbowax® if Saccomanno's technique is used.[4] Saccomanno's technique involves the collection of sputum material in a mixture of 50% ethanol and 2% polyethylene glycol. If the patient cannot produce sputum spontaneously by deep coughing, it should be induced as described in the listing Pneumocystis carinii Preparation on page 299.

Additional Information Special stains are sometimes needed. When a pulmonary lesion is suspected, a complete sputum series should be examined. The complete sputum series consists of a fresh, early morning, deep cough specimen each day for 3-5 days. A postbronchoscopy sputum should be included in the series. The complete sputum series increases the detection of primary bronchogenic carcinoma from 45% (one specimen) to 86% (three specimens). A 12- to 24-hour specimen is collected in Carbowax® in patients with scanty sputum, when previous single sputum contains rare malignant cells, or cells highly suspicious for malignancy are present. Sputum cytology can distinguish between undifferentiated carcinoma, small cell type and other (nonsmall cell) bronchogenic carcinomas In cases where infectious agents are identified by cytology, culture confirmation is advised. Although some institutions report high accuracy of diagnosis of P. carinii with induced sputa, our laboratory has not been able to duplicate these results.

Footnotes

1. Lyubski S and Thorn R, "Application of Immunoperoxidase Staining to the Cell Blocks From Sputa and Bronchial Washings," Arch Pathol Lab Med, 1989, 113(1):94-5.
2. Risse EK, Van't Hof MA, and Vooijs GP, "Relationship Between Patient Characteristics and the Sputum Cytologic Diagnosis of Lung Cancer," Acta Cytol, 1987, 31(2):159-65.
3. Risse EK, Vooijs GP, and Van't Hof MA, "Relationship Between the Cellular Composition of Sputum and the Cytologic Diagnosis of Lung Cancer," Acta Cytol, 1987, 31(2):170-6.
4. Saccomanno G, Saunders RP, Ellis H, et al, "Concentration of Carcinoma or Atypical Cells in Sputum," Acta Cytol, 1963, 7:305-10.

References

Bibbo M, Comprehensive Cytopathology, Philadelphia, PA: WB Saunders Co, 1991, 320-98.
Blumenfeld W and Griffiss JM, "Pneumocystis carinii in Sputum," Arch Pathol Lab Med, 1988, 112(8):816-20.
Dao AH, "Entamoeba gingivalis in Sputum Smears," Acta Cytol, 1985, 29(4):632-3.
Fontana RS, Sanderson DR, Woolner LB, et al, "Screening for Lung Cancer. A Critique of the Mayo Lung Project," Cancer, 1991, 67(4 Suppl):1155-64.
Gupta RK, "Diagnosis of Unsuspected Pulmonary Cryptococcosis With Sputum Cytology," Acta Cytol, 1985, 29(2):154-6.
Koss LG, Diagnostic Cytology and Its Histopathologic Bases, 4th ed, Philadelphia, PA: JB Lippincott Co, 1992, 687-768.
Midgley J, Parsons PA, Shanson DC, et al, "Monoclonal Immunofluorescence Compared With Silver Stain for Investigating Pneumocystis carinii Pneumonia," J Clin Pathol, 1991, 44(1):75-6.
O'Brien RF, Quinn JL, Miyahara BT, et al, "Diagnosis of Pneumocystis carinii Pneumonia by Induced Sputum in a City With Moderate Incidence of AIDS," Chest, 1989, 95(1):136-8.
Schwartz D, Sobottka I, Leitch GJ, et al, "Pathology of Microsporidiosis: Emerging Parasitic Infections in Patients With Acquired Immunodeficiency Syndrome," Arch Pathol Lab Med, 1996, 120:173-88.

Subcutaneous Fat Pad Aspiration see Fine Needle Aspiration, Superficial Palpable Masses on page 294

Subcutaneous Mass Needle Aspiration see Fine Needle Aspiration, Superficial Palpable Masses on page 294

Synovial Fluid Cytology see Body Fluid Cytology on page 286

The Bethesda System see Cervical/Vaginal Cytology on page 290

Thoracentesis Fluid Cytology see Body Fluid Cytology on page 286

Thyroid Needle Aspiration see Fine Needle Aspiration, Superficial Palpable Masses on page 294

Thyroid Needle Aspiration Cytology see Fine Needle Aspiration, Deep Seated Lesions on page 294

Tracheal and Bronchial Washings see Bronchial Washings Cytology on page 287

Tracheal Aspiration Cytology see Bronchial Washings Cytology on page 287

Tracheal Brushings Cytology see Brushings Cytology on page 289

Transbronchial Aspiration Biopsy for *Pneumocystis* see Pneumocystis carinii Preparation on previous page

Transbronchial Fine Needle Aspiration

CPT 88162 (cytopathology, smears, extended study); 88170 (fine needle aspiration, superficial tissue)

Related Information

Bronchoalveolar Lavage Cytology on page 288
Fine Needle Aspiration, Deep Seated Lesions on page 294
Fine Needle Aspiration, Superficial Palpable Masses on page 294
Washing Cytology on page 302

Synonyms Fine Needle Aspiration of Lung; Wang Needle Biopsy of Lung

Test Commonly Includes Examination of direct air-dried, Diff-Quik™ stained or 95% ethanol-fixed, Papanicolaou stained smears; cytospin or cell block preparations may be included.

Abstract Cytopathological examination of transbronchial aspirates may aid in the evaluation of infections or neoplastic central pulmonary lesions.

Patient Preparation Radiographic studies (ie, CT scan) for exact location of lesion. Informed consent from patient. Topical anesthesia of the pharynx and upper respiratory tree is necessary. Sedation may be used.

Specimen Needle aspirate smears; needle rinse in balanced salt solution or RPMI culture medium

Container Plain glass slides with frosted end for labeling; Coplin jar containing 95% ethanol; 50 mL plastic tube

Collection Fiberoptic bronchoscopic placement of a long flexible tube with attached fine needle and subsequent placement of needle into mass through the bronchial wall;[1,2] subsequent aspiration with preparation of aspirated material as described under Fine Needle Aspiration, Superficial Palpable Masses.

Storage Instructions All material should be forwarded to the Cytology Laboratory as soon as possible. The needle rinse material should be refrigerated if immediate delivery to the laboratory is not possible. This technique may also be applied to submucosal gastrointestinal lesions with an endoscope.[3]

Special Instructions The diagnoses of this type of biopsy depends greatly on the skill of the pulmonologist who is obtaining the specimen. Bloody specimens should be smeared as soon as possible to avoid clotting. If the specimen appears to consist almost entirely of blood, it may be entirely placed in the salt solution or RPMI for cell block preparation. Requisition should contain all pertinent clinical information, particularly if infection is suspected, and culture to exclude tuberculosis and histoplasmosis may be indicated in selected cases.

Use Diagnose neoplastic or infectious central pulmonary lesions

Limitations Sampling error may be as high as 10% to 25%. Lack of lymphocytes in transbronchial aspirates should be regarded as tantamount to an inadequate specimen.[4]

Contraindications Abnormal coagulation profile; severe hypoxemia with impending respiratory failure

Additional Information Bronchoalveolar lavage and/or bronchial brushings are usually performed in association with the FNA. At times, a simultaneous transbronchial biopsy may also be obtained. Lesions which ulcerate the bronchial mucosa may be more accessible to direct forceps tissue biopsy or bronchial brushing. An alternative approach to deep seated thoracic lesions is a percutaneous CT-guided fine needle aspiration. Although transbronchial FNA specimens tend to be scanty, specimens provided by experienced pulmonologists often include sufficient and adequate material to permit cytologic diagnosis. Transbronchial fine needle aspiration is likely to be of benefit when a submucosal mass is present, extrinsic compression of bronchi is present, or when an extrabronchial mass is found radiographically.[5]

Footnotes
1. Horsley JR, Miller RE, Amy RW, et al, "Bronchial Submucosal Needle Aspiration Performed Through the Fiberoptic Bronchoscope," *Acta Cytol*, 1984, 28(3):211-7.
2. Rosenthal DL and Wallace JM, "Fine Needle Aspiration of Pulmonary Lesions via Fiberoptic Bronchoscopy," *Acta Cytol*, 1984, 28(3):203-10.
3. Ingoldby CJ, Mason MK, and Hall RI, "Endoscopic Needle Aspiration Cytology: A New Method for the Diagnosis of Upper Gastrointestinal Cancer," *Gut*, 1987, 28(9):1142-4.
4. Baker JJ, Solanki PH, Schenk DA, et al, "Transbronchial Fine Needle Aspiration of the Mediastinum - Importance of Lymphocytes as an Indicator of Specimen Adequacy," *Acta Cytol*, 1990, 34(4):517-23.
5. Gay PC and Brutinel WM, "Transbronchial Needle Aspiration in the Practice of Bronchoscopy," *Mayo Clin Proc*, 1989, 64(2):158-62.

References
Wagner ED, Ramzy I, Greenberg SD, et al, "Transbronchial Fine Needle Aspiration, Reliability and Limitations" *Am J Clin Pathol*, 1989, 92(1):36-50.

Transthoracic Needle Aspiration for *Pneumocystis* see *Pneumocystis carinii* Preparation *on page 299*

Tzanck Smear see Herpes Cytology *on page 296*

Ultrasound Guided FNA see Fine Needle Aspiration, Deep Seated Lesions *on page 294*

Ureteral Brushings Cytology see Brushings Cytology *on page 289*

Ureteral Washings Cytology see Urine Cytology *on this page*

Urine Cytology

CPT 88104 (smears); 88107 (smears and filter preparation); 88108 (concentration technique, smears)

Related Information
Blood, Urine *on page 631*
Cytomegalic Inclusion Disease Cytology *on page 293*
Cytomegalovirus Culture *on page 664*
Fungal Culture, Urine *on page 480*
Herpes Simplex Virus Antigen Detection *on page 667*
Ova and Parasites, Urine *on page 495*

Tumor Aneuploidy by Flow Cytometry *on page 57*
Viral Culture *on page 675*
Viral Culture, Urine *on page 681*

Applies to Bladder, Ureteral, and Pelvicocalyceal Barbotage Specimens; Bladder Washings Cytology; Catheterized Urine Cytology; Renal Pelvic Washings Cytology; Ureteral Washings Cytology; Voided Urine Cytology

Test Commonly Includes Smears, cytocentrifuge preparations, millipore filter preparations, flow cytometry, immunocytochemistry

Abstract Urine cytology may be useful in the evaluation of inflammatory and neoplastic conditions in the urinary system.

Patient Preparation Hydrate patient (give several glasses of water) 30 minutes to 1 hour prior to collection. Patient should **not** have had mineral oil cathartics. Inform patient to discard first early morning voided urine. Taking 1 g vitamin C at bedtime the night before the examination can help to improve cell preservation.

Specimen Voided or catheterized urine; intraoperative washings of urinary bladder, ureters, or renal pelvis; ileal conduit urine

Container 100 mL plastic, leakproof, screw-top container; specimen should be submitted in the fresh state as soon as possible to the Cytology Laboratory. If a delay of more than 1 hour is anticipated, addition of Saccomanno or other suitable fixative (1:1 specimen to fixative) is recommended.

Sampling Time Ideally, the specimen should be as fresh as possible. Urine which has been in the bladder for prolonged periods shows extensive cellular degeneration. Specimens sitting fresh at room temperature demonstrate cellular degeneration within 1 hour.

Collection For detection of upper urinary tract lesions: Catheterize ureters to pelvis for suspected renal or pelvic lesions. Repeat procedure using either ureter for control. For ureteral lesion, catheterize ureter to a point just below the level of the suspected lesion. Catheterize other ureter for control. Collect urine for 30 minutes. Label appropriately, right and left ureteral or right and left pelvic specimen. Bring specimen immediately to the Cytology Laboratory.

Storage Instructions If the specimen cannot be brought immediately to the Cytology Laboratory, it must be refrigerated at 4°C and fixed with a suitable fixative.

Causes for Rejection 24-hour collection, prolonged period at room temperature with extensive degeneration of cellular detail

Special Instructions First morning voided specimen is unsatisfactory, due to cellular degeneration. Bladder washings should not be collected in a hypotonic solution. Voided urine is the specimen of choice for male patients, and catheterized urine is the specimen of choice for female patients (to avoid vaginal-vulvar squamous contamination). If cytomegalovirus infection is suspected, this concern should be noted. The type of collection must be made known to the cytology service, as the cellular presentation varies with the collection method. Failure to do so, could possibly result in a false-positive diagnosis.

Use Recognition of primary benign or malignant as well as metastatic disease; routine surveillance for recurrent transitional cell carcinoma; follow-up patients receiving intravesicular therapy for transitional cell carcinoma; aid in diagnoses of infections with herpesvirus, polymovirus, cytomegalovirus, fungal diseases, and *Schistosoma*; detect malacoplakia, renal hemosiderosis, hemolytic anemia, cerebral metachromatic leukodystrophy, and endometriosis of the urinary tract

Limitations Low grade (grade 1) papillary transitional cell carcinoma cannot be diagnosed reliably by cytology alone. Polyoma virus infections may sometimes be confused with high grade transitional cell carcinoma.[1] Recent instrumentation and calculi may produce atypical changes in urothelial cells simulating malignancy. History of instrumentation of the bladder must be provided. Numerous chemotherapeutic agents (Cytoxan®, thiotepa, BCG) may produce cell changes almost indistinguishable from true dysplasia or neoplasia. For these reasons, complete clinical history is of utmost importance. Urine cytology has a very low sensitivity for detection of primary renal and prostate neoplasms. Diagnostic accuracy of urine cytology appears closely related to the grade of bladder tumors, pretreatment and post-treatment status, and minimally to the type of therapy (radiation, chemotherapy, surgery).[2]

Methodology Two preparatory methods to evaluate urine cytology have been compared.[3]

Additional Information Voided urine is much preferred over a catheterized sample due to atypical cell changes induced by trauma of the catheter itself. Barbotage (instilled saline insufflated with air in tiny bubbles to gently exfoliate the urothelium) cytology has the highest sensitivity for the detection of transitional cell carcinoma. Although poorly-differentiated carcinomas are diagnosed with relative ease, well-differentiated (low grade) carcinomas may not be diagnosed by usual cytologic methods. DNA flow cytometry (DNA analysis) may detect the presence of an aneuploid population of cells with or without an increased S phase. It is a sensitive indicator for recurrent transitional neoplasia but (Continued)

Urine Cytology *(Continued)*

is of no use in cases in which the primary transitional cell carcinoma is diploid. Maximum sensitivity is obtained using both cell morphology and DNA analysis. Renal tubular cells may be found in the urine secondary to acute tubular injury.[4] Lymphomas may rarely be diagnosed in urine cytology.[5]

Footnotes

1. Boon ME, van Keep J-P, and Kok LP, "Polyomavirus Infection Versus High-Grade Bladder Carcinoma - The Importance of Cytologic and Comparative Morphometric Studies of Plastic-Embedded Voided Urine Sediments," *Acta Cytol*, 1989, 33(6):887-93.

2. Wiener HG, Vooijs GP, Van't Hof-Grootenboer B, "Accuracy of Urinary Cytology in the Diagnosis of Primary and Recurrent Bladder Cancer," *Acta Cytol*, 1993, 37(2):163-9.

3. Dhundee J and Rigby HS, "Comparison of Two Preparatory Techniques for Urine Cytology," *J Clin Pathol*, 1990, 43(12):1034-5.

4. Tanaka T, Yoshimi N, Sawada K, et al, "Ki-1-Positive Large Cell Anaplastic Lymphoma Diagnosed by Urinary Cytology - A Case Report," *Acta Cytol*, 1993, 37(4):520-4.

5. Racusen LC and Solez K, "Ideas in Pathology. Exfoliation of Renal Tubular Cells," *Mod Pathol*, 1991, 4(3):368-70.

References

Betz SA, See WA, and Cohen MB, "Granulomatous Inflammation in Bladder Wash Specimens After Intravesical Bacillus Calmette-Guérin Therapy for Transitional Cell Carcinoma of the Bladder," *Am J Clin Pathol*, 1993, 99(3):244-8.

Crosby JH, Allsbrook WC Jr, Koss LG, et al, "Cytologic Detection of Urothelial Cancer and Other Abnormalities in a Cohort of Workers Exposed to Aromatic Amines," *Acta Cytol*, 1991, 35(3):263.

Koss LG, Czerniak B, Herz F, et al, "Flow Cytometric Measurements of DNA and Other Cell Components in Human Tumors: A Critical Appraisal," *Hum Pathol*, 1989, 20(6):528-48.

Matzkin H, Moinuddin SM, and Soloway MS, "Value of Urine Cytology Versus Bladder Washing in Bladder Cancer," *Urology*, 1992, 39(3):201-3.

Murphy WM, "Current Status of Urinary Cytology in the Evaluation of Bladder Neoplasms," *Hum Pathol*, 1990, 21(9):886-96.

Radio SJ, Stratta RJ, Linder J, et al, "Histologic Confirmation of Acute Rejection Detected by Urine Cytology in Pancreas Transplant Recipients," *Transplant Proc*, 1994, 26(2):529-30.

Schwartz D, Sobottka I, Leitch GJ, et al, "Pathology of Microsporidiosis: Emerging Parasitic Infections in Patients With Acquired Immunodeficiency Syndrome," *Arch Pathol Lab Med*, 1996, 120:173-88.

Vaginal Cytology *see* Cervical/Vaginal Cytology *on page 290*

Vakutage® *see* Endometrial Cytology *on page 293*

Ventricular Tap Cytology *see* Cerebrospinal Fluid Cytology *on page 290*

Viral Study *see* Cytomegalic Inclusion Disease Cytology *on page 293*

Vira Pap® *see* Cervical/Vaginal Cytology *on page 290*

Vira Type® *see* Cervical/Vaginal Cytology *on page 290*

Voided Urine Cytology *see* Urine Cytology *on previous page*

Vulvar Cytology *see* Cervical/Vaginal Cytology *on page 290*

Wang Needle Biopsy of Lung *see* Transbronchial Fine Needle Aspiration *on page 300*

Washing Cytology

CPT 88104 (smears); 88107 (smears and filter preparation); 88108 (concentration technique, smears)

Related Information

Body Fluid *on page 89*
Body Fluid Cytology *on page 286*
Transbronchial Fine Needle Aspiration *on page 300*

Synonyms Lavage Cytology

Applies to Colon Washings Cytology; Esophageal Washings Cytology; Gastric Washings Cytology; Peritoneal Washings Cytology

Test Commonly Includes Smears, cytocentrifuge preparations, filter preparations, cell block

Abstract Used to establish the presence of inflammatory or neoplastic lesions in various body sites.

Patient Preparation For gastric or esophageal washings, patient must be fasting at least 12 hours prior to procedure. Soft supper the night before, water ad lib 1 hour before. For intubation patient should be sitting upright. Dentures, if worn, should be removed. Colon washings specimens should be collected prior to barium examination. If this is not possible, wait at least 24 hours after the barium exam before attempting a cytologic study.

Specimen Gastric washings, colon washings, esophageal washings, peritoneal washings in a fresh unfixed state

Container Plastic, screw-top container, 50 mL; may contain 50% ethanol; **packed in ice**

Collection Gastric washing: Evaluation for neoplasm: Collect resting gastric contents and discard. Then instill 300 mL of a balanced salt solution through the gastric tube. Have patient then sit, lie on back, lie on stomach, lie on right side, and lie on left side. Aspirate as much of injected saline as possible and place in container packed in ice. Label with patient name, identification number, and date. Deliver immediately on ice to the Cytology Laboratory.

Peritoneal washings: Wash peritoneal site vigorously with several hundred mL of a balanced salt solution. Retrieve as much as possible and submit as above, labeled by anatomic site (ie, "subdiaphragm", "cul-de-sac", "left gutter wash", "right gutter wash").

Storage Instructions Due to rapid degeneration of cellular material, storage, even at 4°C for any extended length of time, is not recommended.

Special Instructions Provide pertinent clinical history (eg, suspicion for neoplasm, history of peptic ulcer, endoscopic findings).

Use Establish the presence of primary or metastatic neoplasms, recognition of reactive processes and infectious disease. Aids especially in staging of gynecologic and gastrointestinal neoplasms. Cytopathology may provide the only evidence of extraovarian spread of primary ovarian tumors in approximately 3% to 10% of patients.

Limitations Nondiagnostic if epithelium is not present or poorly preserved; if specimen is grossly contaminated with food or barium sulfate; if no mesothelial cells are identified in peritoneal washings, the specimen is unsatisfactory; may be of limited value in intestinal cases where the lesion is submucosal; a Wang transmucosal needle aspirate may be helpful (see Transbronchial Fine Needle Aspirate *on page 300*).

Contraindications Collection of specimen at a time when it cannot be immediately processed.

Additional Information Lavage is not as sensitive or specific as endoscopically directed brushings or biopsy (aspiration biopsy or tissue forceps biopsy). However, a complete set of peritoneal, pelvic, and diaphragmatic washings are an essential part of the staging of gynecologic, particularly ovarian carcinomas.

References

Drake M, "Esophageal and Gastric Cytology," *Compendium on Diagnostic Cytology*, 6th ed, Wied GL, Keebler CM, Koss LG, et al, eds, Chicago, IL: Tutorials of Cytology, 1988, 364-78.

Gupta RK and Rogers KE, "Endoscopic Cytology and Biopsy in the Diagnosis of Gastroesophageal Malignancy," *Acta Cytol*, 1983, 27:17-22.

Ingoldby CJ, Mason MK, and Hall RI, "Endoscopic Needle Aspiration Cytology: A New Method for the Diagnosis of Upper Gastrointestinal Cancer," *Gut*, 1987, 28(9):1142-4.

Layfield LJ, Reichman A, and Weinstein WM, "Endoscopically Directed Fine Needle Aspiration Biopsy of Gastric and Esophageal Lesions," *Acta Cytol*, 1992, 36(1):69-74.

Ravinsky E, "Cytology of Peritoneal Washings in Gynecologic Patients. Diagnostic Criteria and Pitfalls," *Acta Cytol*, 1986, 30(1):8-16.

Sherman ME, "Cytopathology," *Blaustein's Pathology of the Female Genital Tract*, 4th ed, Chapter 25, Kurman RJ, ed, New York, NY: Springer-Verlag, 1994, 1097-130.

Shida S and Ishioka K, "Gastric Cytology: Its Evaluation for the Diagnosis of Early Gastric Cancer," *Compendium on Diagnostic Cytology*, 6th ed, Wied GL, Keebler CM, Koss LG, et al, eds, Chicago, IL: Tutorials of Cytology, 1988, 382-7.

Wang HH, Jonasson JG, and Ducatman BS, "Brushing Cytology of the Upper Gastrointestinal Tract: Obsolete or Not?" *Acta Cytol*, 1991, 35(2):195-8.

HEMATOLOGY

Wayne R. DeMott, MD

Hematology involves the study of blood, bone marrow, and components of the reticuloendothelial system as found in a number of discreet and diffuse organs and systems including liver, spleen, gastrointestinal tract, and lymph nodes. Physiologic and biochemical processes that affect the quantity, quality, and function of the cellular components of blood (erythrocytes, leukocytes, and platelets) are an integral part of this discipline of medicine.

While hematology has deep roots in morphology, there has been significant progress in unraveling and establishing the genetic and molecular biologic bases of hematologic disorders. Our knowledge of hemoglobinopathies (including the thalassemias), red cell enzyme deficiencies, and red cell membrane/structural protein abnormalities, to mention but a few, is undergoing exponential expansion. A new generation of analytic techniques are being applied to the analysis of molecular biologic and cell-based mechanisms of the hematologic diseases. These new methods complement and, in many cases, supplant the earlier generation of morphologic-based observations and concepts. Dissection of lymphocyte function and pathology at the molecular level is of particular importance to a variety of human afflictions that have abnormalities of cell structure, immunology, and/or neoplasia as their basis. Analytic techniques such as electrophoresis of nucleic acid fragments with Southern (DNA) or Northern (RNA) hybridization, cell *in situ* hybridization, fluorescence *in situ* hybridization (FISH), polymerase chain reaction (PCR),[1,2] restriction fragment length polymorphism (RFLP) analyses, and applications involving use of flow cytometry[3,4,5] are moving from research laboratory status increasingly to practical and often critical (albeit expensive) patient applications. In spite of budgetary restraints, this migration from research to patient benefit appears destined to continue.

Table of Unit Equivalency

Procedure	Conventional Unit	SI Equivalent
Red blood cell count	$10^6/\mu L$ ($10^6/mm^3$)	$10^{12}/L$
White blood cell count	$10^3/\mu L$ ($10^3/mm^3$)	$10^9/L$
Platelet count	$10^3/\mu L$ ($10^3/mm^3$)	$10^9/L$
Reticulocyte count	% (or .../mm³)	% (or ... x $10^9/L$)
Hemoglobin	g/dL	g/L
Mean cell volume	fL	fL
Mean cell hemoglobin	pg	pg
Mean cell hemoglobin concentration	g/dL	g/L
Mean cell diameter	μm	μm
Plasma hemoglobin	mg/dL	mg/L
Vitamin B_{12}, Serum	pg/mL	pmol/L
Folate, serum	ng/mL	nmol/L

Footnotes

1. McPherson RA, "Evolution of Polymerase Chain Reaction to a Quantitative Laboratory Tool," *Clin Chem*, 1995, 41(8):1065-7.
2. Abdel-Reheim FA, Edwards E, and Arber DA, "Utility of a Rapid Polymerase Chain Reaction Panel for the Detection of Molecular Changes in B-Cell Lymphomas," *Arch Pathol Lab Med*, 1996, 120(4):357-63.
3. McCoy JP Jr, Johnson E, Catalano E, et al, Detection and Monitoring of a Concomitant Atypical Myeloproliferative Disorder and Chronic Lymphocytic Leukemia by Flow-Cytometric Immunophenotyping, Arch Pathol Lab Med, 1995, 119(1):1038-43.
4. Kilo MN and Dorfman DM, "The Utility of Flow Cytometric Immunophenotypic Analysis in the Distinction of Small Lymphocytic Lymphoma/Chronic Lymphocytic Leukemia From Mantle Cell Lymphoma," *Am J Clin Pathol*, 1996, 105(4):451-7.
5. Johnson RL, "Flow Cytometry: From Research to Clinical Laboratory Applications," *Clin Lab Med*, 1993, 13(4):831-52.

Absence of Phosphorylatin-induced Gelation of Red Cell Membrane Skeletons see Gelation Assay on page 318

Absolute Eosinophil Count see Eosinophil Count on page 315

Acid β-Galactosidase see Inherited Diseases of Metabolism and Cell Structure Tests on page 327

Acid Elution for Fetal Hemoglobin see Kleihauer-Betke on page 329

Acid-Fast, Ziehl-Neelsen, Stain for Intracellular Pigment see Leukocyte Cytochemistry on page 331

Acidified Glycerol Lysis Test see Glycerol Lysis Test, Acidified, Modified on page 320

Acidified Serum Test see Ham Test on page 320

Acid Phosphatase Stain With and Without Tartrate see Leukocyte Cytochemistry on page 331

Acid Phosphatase, Tartrate Resistant, Leukocytes see Tartrate Resistant Leukocyte Acid Phosphatase on page 349

Acid Serum Test see Ham Test on page 320

Acid Serum Test for PNH see Ham Test on page 320

Adrenal Function Eosinophil Count see Thorn Test on page 350

AGLT see Glycerol Lysis Test, Acidified, Modified on page 320

Alpha-Naphthyl Esterase Stain With and Without Fluoride see Leukocyte Cytochemistry on page 331

Amyloid see Leukocyte Cytochemistry on page 331

Antipernicious Anemia Factor see Vitamin B_{12} on page 351

APT Test

CPT 83033

Synonyms Apt Test for Swallowed Blood Syndrome; Fetal Hemoglobin Test in Newborn

Abstract This test uses alkali denaturation of fetal hemoglobin to determine if blood present in the stool of a newborn is the result of swallowing maternal blood or is due to perinatal/neonatal GI hemorrhage.

Specimen Blood stained diaper, grossly bloody (red) stool, or bloody vomitus or mucus

Container Use clean uncontaminated glass or plastic container for specimen or send blood stained diaper.

Causes for Rejection Specimen is not grossly bloody or there is evidence of melena/coffee ground aspirate.

Reference Range Report will provide indication if blood is of maternal or infant origin (adult or fetal hemoglobin).

Use Diagnose swallowed blood syndrome and differentiate this condition from gastrointestinal hemorrhage in the newborn. The test is performed infrequently.

Limitations The specimen must be grossly bloody, red, not tarry. Test performed in cases of melena or with coffee ground material (denatured blood) may produce a false-positive result as oxyhemoglobin has been converted to hematin.[1] Visual judgment of color produced by test procedure may lead to error if only a small amount of blood is present. Bilirubin containing meconium and possibly other substances may cause stool color interference. Use of a spectrophotometric-based procedure may avoid these problems.[2]

Methodology Dissolved blood (one volume of bloody stool or vomitus mixed with five volumes of water) is treated with 1% NaOH, 1-4 mL of hemolysate (alkali denaturation test). The mixture is then centrifuged at 2000 rpm for 1-2 minutes. Fetal hemoglobin is alkali resistant, and the solution will remain pink. Maternal blood will be converted to alkaline hematin in 1-2 minutes, and the solution becomes yellow brown. Thus, if the supernatant remains pink (indicative of fetal blood), additional clinical investigation must be pursued.[3] The newborn's blood should be tested concurrently as a control to exclude the possibility of adult Hgb in the test infant.

Additional Information In the swallowed blood syndrome, blood or bloody stools are passed usually on the second or third day of life. The blood may be swallowed during delivery or may be from a fissure of the mother's nipple. This condition must be differentiated from gastrointestinal hemorrhage of the newborn. The test is based on the fact that the infant's blood contains >60% fetal hemoglobin that is alkali resistant. Swallowed blood of maternal origin contains adult hemoglobin which is converted to brownish alkaline hematin on the addition of alkali. In a study of 94 infants younger than 30 days of age with gastrointestinal bleeding, 49 had no obvious source of bleeding, in 19 definite evidence of a bleeding diathesis was found, and in 12 hematemesis or melena resulted from previously swallowed maternal blood as demonstrated by the Apt Test.[4] A sensitive and accurate spectrophotometric-based procedure has been developed.[2] It should be of special value when the sample is small and/or only a small amount of blood is present in the sample. The ratio of absorbance of oxyhemoglobin before and after the addition of sodium hydroxide is determined spectrophotometrically at 576 nm. This ratio has been found to be linearly proportional to the percentage of HbF in the specimen.[2]

Footnotes
1. Apt L and Downey WS, "Melena Neonatorum: The Swallowed Blood Syndrome. A Simple Test for the Differentiation of Adult and Fetal Hemoglobin in Bloody Stools," *J Pediatr*, 1955, 47:6-12.
2. Liu N, Wu AH, and Wong SS, "Improved Quantitative Apt Test for Detecting Fetal Hemoglobin in Bloody Stools of Newborns," *Clin Chem*, 1993, 39(11 Pt 1):2326-9.
3. Glader BE, "Recognition of Anemia and Red Blood Cell Disorders During Infancy," *Perinatal Hematology*, Vol 21, Chapter 6, Alter BD, ed, New York, NY: Churchill Livingstone, 1989, 158-9.
4. Sherman NJ and Clatworthy HW Jr, "Gastrointestinal Bleeding in Neonates: A Study of 94 Cases," *Surgery*, 1967, 62:614-9.

References
Apt L, "Melena Neonatorum: An Experimental Study of the Effect of the Oral Administration of Blood on the Stools," *J Pediatr*, 1955, 47:1-5.
Berry R and Perrault J, "Gastrointestinal Bleeding," *Pediatric Gastrointestinal Disease: Pathophysiology-Diagnosis-Management*, Vol 1, Chapter 10, Walker WA, Durie PR, Hamilton JR, et al, eds, Philadelphia, PA: BC Decker Inc, 1991, 111-31.
Mougenot JF, "Gastrointestinal Haemorrhage," *Paediatric Gastroenterology*, Chapter 38, New York, NY: Oxford University Press, 1992, 446-57.
Silber G, "Lower Gastrointestinal Bleeding," *Pediatr Rev*, 1990, 12(3):85-93.

Apt Test for Swallowed Blood Syndrome see APT Test on this page

Ascitic Fluid Analysis see Body Fluid Analysis, Cell Count on page 306

ASD Chloroacetate Esterase Stain see Leukocyte Cytochemistry on page 331

Autohemolysis Test

CPT 86940 (screen); 86941 (incubated)

Related Information
Glucose-6-Phosphate Dehydrogenase, Quantitative, Blood on page 319
Glucose-6-Phosphate Dehydrogenase Screen, Blood on page 319
Osmotic Fragility on page 334
Osmotic Fragility, Incubated on page 335
Peripheral Blood: Red Blood Cell Morphology on page 339
Pyruvate Kinase Assay, Erythrocytes on page 342
Red Blood Cell Enzyme Deficiency, Quantitative on page 342

Abstract Autohemolysis test measures the degree to which patient's red cells lyse without additives, with glucose, and with ATP. Sterile conditions are required. Test has some application to diagnosis of hereditary spherocytosis and RBC enzyme deficiencies but is tedious to perform and is of limited value.

Specimen Defibrinated sterile blood

Container Sterile syringe

Collection Using sterile technique, 25 mL of blood is drawn and immediately defibrinated by swirling in a bottle which contains glass beads.

Storage Instructions Specimen is immediately taken to the laboratory, blood defibrinated, and tubes prepared for incubation.

Causes for Rejection Specimen hemolyzed, specimen clotted, specimen more than 5 minutes in transit, specimen with bacteria (as from a patient with septicemia)

Special Instructions Defibrinated blood must usually be obtained by laboratory personnel.

Reference Range Percent of red cell lysis at 48 hours: blood alone: 0.2-2.0; blood and 10% glucose: 0-0.9; blood and 0.4M ATP: 0.5-2.5

Use Diagnose hereditary spherocytosis; detect conditions producing spontaneous hemolysis, particularly hereditary spherocytosis; categorize RBC enzyme deficiencies; work up hemolytic anemia

Limitations Large sample of blood required and must be obtained by a trauma-free venipuncture. Test lacks sensitivity and specificity. While this test finds application in the diagnosis of hereditary spherocytosis, it has largely been supplanted by specific enzyme spot assays for the diagnosis of nonspherocytic congenital hemolytic anemia.[1,2]

Contraindications Bacteremic patients

Methodology Defibrinated blood from patient and from a control are incubated without additives, with glucose, and with ATP. Subsequently absorbance determinations are used to calculate the percent hemolysis. Procedure is technically laborious. Sterile glassware must be used.

Additional Information The test must always be run with and compared to a control. Test should be run in duplicate. This may allow detection of reagent inactivity or bacterial contamination of specimen or reagent. It is difficult to maintain sterility but also full activity of ATP. Normal red cells hemolyze minimally when incubated. G-6-PD deficient RBCs (Dacie type I hemolytic anemia) have increased autohemolysis which corrects significantly with glucose or ATP. Pyruvate kinase deficiency (Dacie type II hemolytic anemia) has increased autohemolysis which does not correct and may be aggravated with glucose but does correct toward normal with ATP. Triosephosphate isomerase deficiency corrects completely with glucose or ATP. Hereditary spherocytosis is a type I hemolytic anemia; the addition of glucose usually, but not always, decreases the rate of autohemolysis to about the same proportion as normal blood.

Glucose by itself can induce hemolysis in the autohemolysis test in patients with hereditary spherocytosis.[3] Streichman et al suggest this was the result of a direct effect of glucose on already swollen red cells. They found that the problem could be ameliorated by adding NaCl to isotonic conditions. With autoimmune hemolytic anemia, autohemolysis may be increased, but the effect of adding glucose is unpredictable. Autohemolysis is usually normal in cases of paroxysmal nocturnal hemoglobinuria. Hemolytic anemia due to oxidant drugs is usually associated with increased autohemolysis. Generally, failure of glucose to decrease autohemolysis indicates presence of a glycolytic block. Schröter et al have found the autohemolysis test, along with the fresh osmotic fragility test, to be highly diagnostic for hereditary spherocytosis in the newborn.[4] This is especially important since the MCHC may not be elevated in hereditary spherocytosis in the newborn and because spherocytes are not uncommon in newborns without hereditary spherocytosis. See table.

Autohemolysis Test

Condition	Incubation at 37°C for 48 Hours	Incubation + 10% Glucose	Incubation + ATP
Normal	0.2%-2.0%	0.0%-0.9%	0.5%-2.5%
G-6-PD deficiency	3.0%-5.0%	Normal	Normal
Pyruvate kinase deficiency	12%-16%	12%-16%	Normal
Hereditary spherocytosis	12.0%-15.0%	3.0%-5.0%	3.0%-5.0%

The acidified glycerol lysis test, a modification called the "pink test," and the onalain autohemolysis test have also been applied to the diagnosis of HS. Histogram of MCHC provided by some automated hematology analyses (eg, Technicon-Miles H Series) may also be useful in the diagnosis of HS.[5]

Footnotes

1. Beutler E, "Why Has the Autohemolysis Test Not Gone the Way of the Cephalin Flocculation Test?" *Blood*, 1978, 51:109-10.
2. Fukagawa N, Friedman S, Gill FM, et al, "Hereditary Spherocytosis With Normal Osmotic Fragility After Incubation: Is the Autohemolysis Test Really Obsolete?" *JAMA*, 1979, 242:63-4.
3. Streichman S, Cohen S, and Tatarsky J, "Glucose-Induced Hemolysis of Spheric Red Blood Cells in Hereditary Spherocytosis: New Aspects of the Autohemolysis Test," *Am J Clin Pathol*, 1984, 81(1):122-7.
4. Schröter W and Kahsnitz E, "Diagnosis of Hereditary Spherocytosis in Newborn Infants," *J Pediatr*, 1983, 103:460-3.
5. Becker PS and Lux SE, "Disorders of the Red Cell Membrane," *Hematology of Infancy and Childhood*, 4th ed, Chapter 17, Nathan DG and Oski FA, eds, Philadelphia, PA: WB Saunders Co, 1993, 958-9.

References

Dacie J, "Haemolytic Anaemia in Man: Clinical Findings, Blood Picture and Other Pathological Changes, Methods of Investigation, Diagnosis and Treatment," *The Haemolytic Anaemias: The Hereditary Haemolytic Anaemias*, Vol 1, Part 1, Chapter 3, New York, NY: Churchill Livingstone, 1985, 101-5.

Dacie JV and Lewis SM, *Practical Haematology*, 8th ed, New York, NY: Churchill Livingstone, 1995, 222-5.

Grimes AJ, Leets I, and Dacie JV, "The Autohemolysis Test: Appraisal of the Method for the Diagnosis of Pyruvate Kinase Deficiency and the Effect of pH and Additives," *Br J Haematol*, 1968, 14:309-22.

Lee GR, "The Hemolytic Disorders: General Considerations," *Wintrobe's Clinical Hematology*, 9th ed, Chapter 32, Lee RG, Bithell TC, Foerster J, et al, eds, Philadelphia, PA: Lea & Febiger, 1993, 958-9.

Selwyn J and Dacie J, "Autohemolysis and Other Changes Resulting From the Incubation *In Vitro* of Red Cells From Patients With Congenital Hemolytic Anemia," *Blood*, 1954, 9:414.

Automated Differential see Peripheral Blood: Differential Leukocyte Count *on page 336*

B₁₂ see Vitamin B₁₂ *on page 351*

Bacteremia Detection, Buffy Coat Micromethod

CPT 85060

Related Information

Bacterial Antigens, Rapid Detection Methods *on page 454*
Bacterial Culture, Blood *on page 457*
Buffy Coat Smear Study of Peripheral Blood *on page 309*
Microfilariae, Peripheral Blood Preparation *on page 333*
Peripheral Blood: Differential Leukocyte Count *on page 336*

Synonyms Buffy Coat Method for Detection of Bacteremia; Microbuffy Coat Method for Detection of Bacteremia; Septicemia Detection, Buffy Coat Micromethod

Abstract Glass slide smears of buffy coat of blood (relatively concentrated white cells) are stained for pathogenic microorganisms. The procedure is a simple, quick, cost efficient method that can assist in establishing the presence of bacteremia but lacks sensitivity and to some extent, specificity.

Specimen Blood

Container Heparinized capillary tubes

Collection Transport immediately to the laboratory for processing. Blood should be cultured concurrently.

Turnaround Time 1-2 hours

Reference Range Negative

Possible Panic Range Positive

Use Aid in the diagnosis of acute bacterial blood infection, bacteremia

Limitations There have been conflicting reports on the usefulness of this technique. A high incidence of false-positives and negatives has been reported.[1]

Methodology Gram's stain is applied to smear of buffy coat; Wright stain of buffy coat can show histoplasmosis; Ziehl-Neelsen stain can show mycobacteria

Additional Information A variety of unusual organisms, sites of infection and clinical circumstances may produce septicemia. Attempts to stain buffy coat of blood samples obtained from children with suspected bacteremia using acridine orange (a DNA-intercalating agent) has proven to be of low diagnostic efficiency.[2] The QBC® tube (quantitative buffy coat, utilizing tubes precoated with acridine orange) has been considered to have value in the rapid detection of *Wuchereria bancrofti* microfilarial organisms[3] but had low sensitivity and was frequently (40% of specimens) unable to provide species identification when utilized for malaria case identification in the field.[4] The ability to detect and diagnose *Mycobacterium avium-intracellulare* and *Cryptococcus neoformans* using both a stain of the buffy coat and culture of the buffy coat from AIDS patients has been studied. The results showed that culture of buffy coat was much more effective in early diagnosis of those organisms than examining the stained buffy coat smear microscopically.[5] Another group found that use of the buffy coat smear was rapid and specific for detection of *Mycobacterium avium* complex infection in AIDS patients although lacking in sensitivity (positive predictive value of 100%, negative predictive value of 22%).[6] Buffy coat smears have been employed in the diagnosis of histoplasmosis in AIDS patients[7] and in the detection of *Malassezia* sp deep-line catheter-associated sepsis.[8]

Footnotes

1. Coppen MJ, Noble CJ, and Aubrey C, "Evaluation of Buffy Coat Microscopy for the Early Diagnosis of Bacteremia," *J Clin Pathol*, 1981, 34:1375-7.
2. Henrickson KJ, Powell KR, and Ryan DH, "Evaluation of Acridine Orange Stained Buffy Coat Smears for Identification of Bacteremia in Children," *J Pediatr*, 1988, 112(1):65-6.
3. Freedman DO and Berry RS, "Rapid Diagnosis of Bancroftian Filariasis by Acridine Orange Staining of Centrifuged Parasites," *Am J Trop Med Hyg*, 1992, 47(6):787-93.
4. Mak JW, Normaznah Y, and Chiang GL, "Comparison of the Quantitative Buffy Coat Technique With the Conventional Thick Blood Film Technique for Malaria Case Detection in the Field," *Singapore Med J*, 1992, 33(5):452-4.
5. Damsker B and Bottone EJ, "Mycobacteria and Cryptococci Cultured From the Buffy Coat of AIDS Patients Prior to Symptomatology: A Rationale for Early Therapy," *AIDS Res*, 1986, 2(4):343-8.
6. Nussbaum JM, Dealist C, Lewis W, et al, "Rapid Diagnosis by Buffy Coat Smear of Disseminated *Mycobacterium avium* Complex Infection in Patients With Acquired Immunodeficiency Syndrome," *J Clin Microbiol*, 1990, 28(3):631-2.
7. Kurtin PJ, McKinsey DS, Gupta MR, et al, "Histoplasmosis in Patients With Acquired Immunodeficiency Syndrome," *Am J Clin Pathol*, 1990, 93(3):367-72.
8. Marcon MJ and Powell DA, "Human Infections Due to *Malassezia* spp," *Clin Microbiol Rev*, 1992, 5(2):101-19.

References

Kleiman MB, Reynolds JK, Schreiner RL, et al, "Rapid Diagnosis of Neonatal Bacteremia With Acridine Orange-Stained Buffy Coat Smears," *J Pediatr*, 1984, 105(3):419-21.

Kostiala AA, Jormalainen S, and Kosunen TU, "Detection of Experimental Bacteremia and Fungemia by Examination of Buffy Coat Prepared by a Micromethod," *Am J Clin Pathol*, 1979, 72:437-43.

Studer JP, Glauser MP, and Schapira M, "Value of Examining Buffy Coats for Intragranulocytic Microorganisms in Patients With Fever," *Br Med J*, 1979, 1:85-6.

Band 4.2, Red Cell Membrane

Related Information

Osmotic Fragility *on page 334*

Synonyms Pallidin

Abstract Complete or partial deficiency of band 4.2, a red cell membrane protein, may be responsible for uncompensated hemolysis and in some cases modest anemia.

Specimen Whole blood (to obtain red blood cells)

Container Lavender top (EDTA) tube

Special Instructions This test is likely to be available only on a research/referral basis. Consult your clinical laboratory for availability and additional details.

Use Evaluate hemolytic states; assist in determining cause of red cell stomatocytosis
(Continued)

Band 4.2, Red Cell Membrane *(Continued)*

Methodology 1% sodium dodecylsulfate (SDS) polyacrylamide gel electrophoresis (PAGE) with Coomassie blue staining; immunoblotting with antiband 4.2 antibody

Additional Information Band 4.2 is one of a number of red cell membrane proteins. It has a molecular weight of 72 kDa (on SDS-PAGE) and accounts for about 5% of total membrane protein. The cDNA of band 4.2 is 2.35 kb long, encoding 619 amino acids. Chromosome location is at 15q15.[1] Isoforms are largely P4.2L (721 amino acids) and P4.2S (691 amino acids). In healthy Japanese, P4.2S has an incidence of about 97%. Congenital band 4.2 abnormalities are of three types: complete deficiency, partial deficiency, and band 4.2 variants (doublet cases). "Complete" deficiency of band 4.2 is responsible for uncompensated hemolysis and in some cases normochromic anemia. Osmotic fragility is increased into the range seen with hereditary spherocytosis but peripheral blood smear shows ovalostomatocytosis with few or absent spherocytes. Band 4.2 variant cases are associated with stomatocytosis. The red cell morphologic abnormalities persist after splenectomy.

This condition is uncommon clinically and apparently largely isolated to the Japanese (estimated incidences of 1% of all red cell membrane disorders in Japan). Acquired band 4.2 deficiency has been reported with biliary obstruction.[2]

Footnotes
1. Najfeld V, Ballard SG, Menninger J, et al, "The Gene for Human Erythrocyte Protein 4.2 Maps to Chromosome 15q15," *Am J Hum Genet*, 1992, 50(1):71-5.
2. Iida H, Hasegawa I, and Nozawa Y, "Biochemical Studies on Abnormal Erythrocyte Membranes Protein Abnormality of Erythrocyte Membrane in Biliary Obstruction," *Biochim Biophys Acta*, 1976, 443:394-401.

References
Cohen CM, Dotimas E, and Korsgren C, "Human Erythrocyte Membrane Protein Band 4.2 (Pallidin)," *Semin Hematol*, 1993, 30(2):119-37.

Rybicki AC, Qiu JJ, Mustro S, et al, "Human Erythrocyte Protein 4.2 Deficiency Associated With Hemolytic Anemia and a Homozygous [40]Glutamic Acid - Lysine Substitution in the Cytoplasmic Domain of Band 3 (Band 3[Montefiore])," *Blood*, 1993, 81(8):2155-65.

Yawata Y, "Band 4.2 Abnormalities in Human Red Cells," *Am J Med Sci*, 1994, 307(3):190-203.

Beta-Glucuronidase Stain *see* Leukocyte Cytochemistry *on page 331*

Blood Cell Profile *see* Complete Blood Count *on page 312*

Blood Count *see* Complete Blood Count *on page 312*

Blood Smear for Malarial Parasites *see* Malaria Smear *on page 332*

Blood Smear for Trypanosomal/Filarial Parasites *see* Microfilariae, Peripheral Blood Preparation *on page 333*

Blood Smear Morphology *see* Peripheral Blood: Red Blood Cell Morphology *on page 339*

Blood Viscosity *see* Viscosity, Blood *on page 350*

Blood Volume

CPT 78120 (red cell volume single sample); 78121 (multiple samples)

Related Information
Erythropoietin, Serum *on page 124*
Hematocrit *on page 322*
Peripheral Blood: Red Blood Cell Morphology *on page 339*
Phlebotomy, Therapeutic *on page 614*
Red Blood Cell Indices *on page 343*
Red Cell Mass *on page 345*

Synonyms Plasma/Blood Volume; Total Blood Volume

Applies to Plasma Volume Measurement; Red Cell Volume

Test Commonly Includes Total blood volume, red cell mass, and plasma volume, measured and predicted

Abstract This procedure measures the patient's total circulating volume of blood and/or fractions (eg, red cell mass) of the blood volume. A component of the blood (eg, albumin) is labeled, usually with a radioisotope. The dilution of the label is inversely proportional to the size (volume) of the compartment in which it has been diluted. Blood volume study may be an invaluable contribution to some clinical situations (eg, polycythemia, acute blood loss) in which determination of Hgb, a concentration, or Hct, a fraction, could be misleading.

Patient Preparation Patient should have all RIA blood work performed, at least drawn, prior to injection of any radioactive material. Technologist will administer injected dose to patient and withdraw blood samples after the appropriate interval (usually 10 minutes). Patient must be available since timing is important.

Specimen Whole blood

Container Method dependent. For ^{51}Cr-labeled red cell methods, ACD-NIH or Strumia's ACD solution, ratio of one part ACD to five parts blood.

EDTA anticoagulated blood may be used, but excess EDTA must be avoided. EDTA causes shrinkage of red cells, the resultant red cell volume is too low unless used in a concentration of 1.5 ± 0.25 mg/mL of blood. Samples of blood for [125]I- or ^{131}I-labeled albumin plasma volume methods may be collected in heparinized syringe.

Reference Range Normal values are method dependent. Blood volume varies with body habitus, age, sex, weight, and height. There is special correlation with body surface area. As the amount of blood in fat is about 2/35 that of lean tissue, the normal value for an obese individual is less than that for a lean person of same weight. Careful clinical assessment as to degree of obesity, edema, etc, must be a part of the determination of normal. See table.

Blood Volume Parameters Normal Adult Males and Females ^{51}Cr RBC Label Method

Measurement	Male (mL/kg)	Female (mL/kg)
Blood volume	61.54 ± 8.59	58.95 ± 4.94
Erythrocyte volume	28.27 ± 4.11	24.24 ± 2.59
Plasma volume	33.45 ± 5.18	34.77 ± 3.24

Use Differentiate relative from absolute polycythemia. Polycythemia may be defined as increased red cells and, in a sense, is the opposite of anemia. Polycythemia is usually considered when hemoglobin is 18 g/dL, hematocrit is 52%, and RBC count is 6 million/mm[3]. These values do not tell whether the red cell mass is increased or the plasma volume is decreased. Relative polycythemias are caused by decreased plasma volumes such as in burns, severe sweating, shock, dehydration, or any other cause of hemoconcentration. Absolute polycythemia occurs when red cell mass is increased. This can be because of increased erythropoietin in secondary polycythemia (appropriate or inappropriate[1]) or occurs spontaneously as in the myeloproliferative syndrome, polycythemia vera (splenomegaly usually present).

Limitations Any *in vivo* isotope test may affect radioisotope determined blood volume (eg, bone scans, liver scans, brain scans). Check with the laboratory to see if blood volume determination will be valid. Cost of radioisotope label has increased substantially in recent years. A decline in orders for blood volume determination has occurred over the past two decades relating to technical variations, accuracy concerns, and in part to FDA related-withdrawal of some partially automated analytic systems. A dependable, accurate, "double tag" method (simultaneous use of ^{125}I albumin and ^{51}Cr-labeled RBCs) is technically rigorous and time consuming compared to other clinical laboratory procedures.

Contraindications Patient actively bleeding, edema

Methodology General concept of dilution technique using ^{125}I-tagged albumin and/or ^{51}Cr-tagged red blood cells. Technetium (Tc-99m) or indium ([113m]In or ^{111}In) labeled red cells have also been used for red cell volume measurements.

Additional Information Hgb, Hct, or RBC count determinations are concentration expressed parameters and may be misleading when the clinical situation requires assessment of the absolute volume of blood or one of its components. Acute shift in body fluids between the intravascular and extravascular spaces as may occur with heart failure, shock, and third space pooling are examples of such misleading circumstances. There is increase in plasma volume in the last trimester of pregnancy, toxemia of pregnancy, and in uremia. Blood volume may be as much as 16% higher in the evening than in the morning.[2] See references for further information and comprehensive table of predicted normal blood volumes.

Footnotes
1. Shouval D, Anton M, Galun E, et al, "Erythropoietin-Induced Polycythemia in Athymic Mice Following Transplantation of Human Renal Carcinoma Cell Line," *Cancer Res*, 1988, 48(12):3430-4.
2. Finlayson DC, "Diurnal Variation in Blood Volume of Man," *J Surg Res*, 1964, 4:286.

References
Dacie JV and Lewis SM, "Blood Volume," *Practical Haematology*, 8th ed, Chapter 21, New York, NY: Churchill Livingstone, 1995, 391-7.

Erslev AJ and Beutler E, "Production and Destruction of Erythrocytes," *Williams Hematology*, 5th ed, Chapter 39, Beutler E, Lichtman MA, Coller BS, et al, eds, New York, NY: McGraw-Hill Inc, 1995, 425-7.

Langan JK, Scheffel U, and McIntyre PA, "The Hematopoietic System," *Nuclear Medicine Technology and Techniques*, Chapter 18, Bernier DR, Christian PE, Langan JK, et al, eds, St Louis, MO: Mosby-Year Book Inc, 1989, 485.

Pollycove M and Tono M, "Blood Volume," *Diagnostic Nuclear Medicine*, 2nd ed, Vol 2, Chapter 42, Gottschalk A, Hoffer PB, Potchen EJ, et al, eds, Baltimore, MD: Williams & Wilkins, 1988, 690-7.

"Recommended Methods for Measurement of Red-Cell and Plasma Volume: International Committee for Standardization in Haematology," *J Nucl Med*, 1980, 21:793-800.

Body Fluid Analysis, Cell Count

CPT 89050 (cell count); 89051 (with differential)

Related Information
Bacterial Culture, Biopsy or Body Fluid *on page 456*
Body Fluid *on page 89*

Body Fluid Amylase *on page 91*
Body Fluid Cytology *on page 286*
Body Fluid Glucose *on page 91*
Body Fluid Lactate Dehydrogenase *on page 92*
Body Fluid pH *on page 92*
CA 125 *on page 94*
Carcinoembryonic Antigen *on page 100*
Cerebrospinal Fluid Analysis *on page 309*
Fungal Culture, Biopsy or Body Fluid *on page 476*
Mycobacterial Culture, Biopsy or Body Fluid *on page 487*
Synovial Fluid Analysis *on page 656*
Viral Culture, Body Fluid *on page 677*

Applies to Ascitic Fluid Analysis; Cyst Fluid Analysis; Joint Fluid Analysis; Paracentesis Fluid Analysis; Pericardial Fluid Analysis; Peritoneal Fluid Analysis; Pleural Fluid Analysis; Thoracentesis Fluid Analysis

Test Commonly Includes Total WBC count and differential, total RBC count (protein, sugar, LD (LDH), amylase, and multiple additional tests are commonly done on body fluids)

Patient Preparation Aseptic preparation for aspiration

Specimen Body fluid (ie, pleural fluid, synovial fluid, cyst fluid, paracentesis fluid, pericardial fluid, etc)

Container Glass test tube or large glass container

Collection Add heparin to specimen.

Storage Instructions Specimen should be brought directly to the laboratory after collection. Do **not** store.

Causes for Rejection Clotted specimen, inadequate volume of specimen for the procedures requested

Special Instructions Requisition must state site of origin. Commonly cytologic, microbiologic and chemical examinations are also helpful.

Reference Range See table. Glucose and amylase levels in fluids approximate whole blood levels. A pleural fluid LD to serum LD ratio >0.6 suggests exudate. In pleural fluids, total protein >3.0 g/dL indicates exudate, protein <3.0 g/dL indicates transudate. For peritoneal fluid, the cutoff point is lower, 2.0-2.5. Pericardial fluids have no established cutoff point in differentiating transudates from exudates.

Expected Normal Findings – Body Fluids

Type of Fluid	Appearance	Amount (mL)	Cells	Glucose	Total Protein
Pleural	Clear, colorless to pale yellow	1-10	<1000/mm^3 <25% polys 0 RBC	Approximates WB glucose	
Peritoneal	Clear, colorless to pale yellow	<100	<500/mm^3 <25% polys <100,000 RBC/mm^3		
Pericardial	Clear, colorless to pale yellow	20-25	<500 WBC/mm^3 <25% polys 0 RBC		
Synovial	No crystals	<4	<200 WBC/mm^3 <25% polys	Blood/synovial difference <10 mg/dL	1.0-3.0 g/dL

Use Evaluate body fluids; differential diagnosis of exudate, transudate

Additional Information Cultures, cytology, and chemical studies usually must be requested separately and should have a separate specimen if possible. See listings Body Fluid *on page 89*; Body Fluid Glucose *on page 91*; Body Fluid Amylase *on page 91*; Body Fluid pH *on page 92*; and Body Fluid Cytology *on page 286*. Elevated lymphocytes can be associated with congestive heart failure (pleural fluid), tuberculosis, tumors, lymphomas, lymphatic leukemia, rheumatoid arthritis, and postpneumonic effusions. Elevated polymorphonuclear leukocytes are associated with acute infectious processes (ie, bacterial inflammation, eg, bacterial peritonitis). The difference between uninfected ascitic fluid and that of bacterial peritonitis is reported as WBC count of 122/mm^3 vs 2686/mm^3. PMN count provides the highest sensitivity; its reliability is enhanced with pH (low with peritonitis, <7.35).[1] Elevated eosinophils are associated with tumors, infarcts, SLE, rheumatoid arthritis, rheumatic fever, parasites, postpneumonic effusions, pneumothorax, or may have no clinical significance. Elevated plasma cells can be associated with lymphoma, especially Hodgkin's disease or with chronic inflammation. Sometimes atypical plasma cells are seen in the presence of multiple myeloma. A low glucose level supports diagnosis of rheumatoid effusion. Creatinine level distinguishes ascitic collection from tap of an overdistended bladder.

A cost efficient management of body fluid clinical laboratory testing is recommended by Albright et al with the description of "transport and rapid accessioning for additional procedures," a two-tiered analytic

system.[2] Physician understanding and logistic considerations for standardized handling are involved. Storage of and access to body fluid samples for subsequent testing after limited initial study are the cornerstone of this concept. Cell count, however, must be performed as soon as possible to avoid distortions produced by storage. Microbiologic study and cytology must also receive timely consideration.

Footnotes
1. Garcia-Tsao G, Conn HO, and Lerner E, "The Diagnosis of Bacterial Peritonitis: Comparison of pH, Lactate Concentration and Leukocyte Count," *Hepatology*, 1985, 5(1):91-6.
2. Albright RE Jr, Christenson RH, Habig RL, et al, "Cerebrospinal Fluid (CSF) TRAP: A Method to Improve CSF Laboratory Efficiency," *Am J Clin Pathol*, 1988, 90(6):707-10.

References
Albright RE Jr, "Management of Cerebrospinal Fluid and Other Body Fluids," *Practical Laboratory Hematology*, Chapter 13, Koepke JA, ed, New York, NY: Churchill Livingstone, 1991, 295-310.
Kjeldsberg CR and Knight JA, *Body Fluids - Laboratory Examination of Amniotic, Cerebrospinal, Seminal, Serous, and Synovial Fluids*, 3rd ed, Chicago, IL: American Society of Clinical Pathologists, 1993, 159-253, 265-301.
Strasinger SK, *Urinalysis and Body Fluids: A Self-Instructional Test*, Philadelphia, PA: FA Davis Co, 1985, 169-74.

Bone Marrow

CPT 85095 (aspiration); 85097 (smear interpretation)

Related Information

Bacterial Culture, Biopsy or Body Fluid *on page 456*
Bloom's Syndrome, Chromosome Breakage Study *on page 274*
Breakpoint Cluster Region Rearrangement in CML *on page 503*
Buffy Coat Smear Study of Peripheral Blood *on page 309*
Cerebrospinal Fluid Cytology *on page 290*
Chorionic Villus Sampling (CVS), Chromosome and Genetic Abnormality Analysis *on page 275*
Chromosome Analysis, Blood *on page 276*
Chromosome Analysis, Bone Marrow *on page 277*
Chromosome *In Situ* Hybridization *on page 281*
Complete Blood Count *on page 312*
Fanconi's Anemia, Chromosome Breakage Study *on page 282*
Fungal Culture, Biopsy or Body Fluid *on page 476*
Gene Rearrangement for Leukemia and Lymphoma *on page 512*
Immunofixation Electrophoresis *on page 408*
Iron Stain, Bone Marrow *on page 328*
Leishmaniasis Serological Test *on page 413*
Leukocyte Alkaline Phosphatase *on page 330*
Leukocyte Cytochemistry *on page 331*
Lymph Node Biopsy *on page 50*
Mycobacterial Culture, Biopsy or Body Fluid *on page 487*
Peripheral Blood: Differential Leukocyte Count *on page 336*
Schilling Test *on page 346*
Terminal Deoxynucleotidyl Transferase *on page 349*
Viral Culture *on page 675*
Viral Culture, Body Fluid *on page 677*
Vitamin B$_{12}$ *on page 351*
White Blood Count *on page 353*

Synonyms Bone Marrow Aspirate; Bone Marrow Biopsy

Test Commonly Includes H & E stain, Wright or Wright/Giemsa type stain, and iron stain; special histochemistry in certain indicated circumstances. Study of peripheral blood and marrow smears, sections of marrow clot, and sections of decalcified bone biopsy.

Abstract A glass or plastic syringe is used to suck marrow (the "aspirate") from cancellous bone and/or a "core" biopsy is obtained by using special needles (eg, Jamshidi needle). The specimens can be studied microscopically using a variety of routine and special stains, tested for the presence of microorganisms, and/or studied using molecular biologic techniques. Marrow study has broad application to disease processes.

Patient Preparation Physician explains procedure to patient. Hopefully, patient apprehension is allayed. Aseptic aspiration under local anesthetic is performed.

Aftercare Keep site dry for 24 hours.

Specimen Bone marrow aspirate and/or biopsy

Container Coverslips are prepared at bedside, and biopsy and clot are placed in fixative (formalin or Zenker's solution).

Special Instructions Marrow procedures must generally be planned in advance with coordination and scheduling allowing for indicated cultures, biopsy, or other special studies (eg, electron microscopy, flow cytometry, gene rearrangement, or chromosome analysis).

Reference Range Results interpreted by pathologist/hematologist/oncologist. Values for marrow cell populations have been determined in a group of 88 normal American infants of diverse racial origin from birth to 18 months of age.[1]

Use Evaluate bone marrow morphology, erythropoiesis, myelopoiesis, myeloid/erythroid ratio, megakaryocytes, cellularity, and marrow iron stores; evaluate platelet dependent clotting dysfunction; evaluate (Continued)

Bone Marrow *(Continued)*

anemia; marrow culture can make a valuable contribution to the study of fever of undetermined origin and possible systemic infection, in particular, histoplasmosis and tuberculosis; establish the presence of, classify, or follow up neoplasia (myeloma, macroglobulinemia of Waldenström, carcinomatosis, lymphoproliferative diseases, myeloproliferative diseases, ie, myelofibrosis, leukemias). In general, serum ferritin level with the CBC, serum iron, TIBC, and peripheral smear evaluation can supplant bone marrow exam when the **only** indication for marrow exam is evaluation of iron stores.

Limitations Presence of normal or nondiagnostic marrow at one site may not exclude the possibility of disease elsewhere in the marrow. Aspiration prior to biopsy does not disturb the estimation of cellularity of the biopsy at that same site (provided an adequate sized biopsy is obtained).[2]

Contraindications Sternal site - aneurysm of thoracic aorta; very severe bleeding diathesis

Methodology A variety of sites and needles are available. Jamshidi needle for marrow biopsy is effective and currently enjoys widespread use. Sternum or posterosuperior iliac spine are common sites for marrow aspirate. Posterosuperior iliac spine is the most common site for biopsy and is usually favored over the anterior iliac crest.[3] Anterior iliac crest and vertebral spinous process may also be used in adults; anterior tibia is the desirable site in infants and young children.

Additional Information A bone marrow biopsy may not be part of the routine marrow study but is desirable in most cases. Biopsy may be necessary in cases of "packed marrow" as with some forms of malignancy, myeloproliferative disease, and with granulomatous entities. Information obtained from the study of different types of marrow specimens is complementary. An unusual cause of depleted iron stores may be iron storage preferentially by tumor cells.[4] The marrow is said to be always involved in cases of hairy cell leukemia. Marrow study is important in the classification of a number of diseases involving the reticuloendothelial system. The French, American, British (FAB) classifications have achieved increasing acceptance.[5,6]

FAB Classifications

Acute Lymphoblastic

L1: Small lymphoblasts, scant cytoplasm, inconspicuous nucleoli

L2: Larger and variable cell size, more cytoplasm and nucleolar prominence than L1

L3: Large Burkitt's lymphoma-like blast cells with large single nucleolus

Acute Myelogenous

M1: Myeloblastic leukemia without maturation:
Type I blast: primitive cell without granules and one or more nucleoli
Type II blast: larger than type I, lower N/C ratio, 1-6 granules
Few blasts are myeloperoxidase and/or Sudan black positive and/or with Auer rods, over 90% of nonerythroid cells are blasts.

M2: Myeloblastic leukemia with maturation:
Type I and II blasts are 30% to 84% of the nonerythroid cells
Maturation to promyelocyte stage or beyond
Monocytic cells <20%
Myeloblasts with nucleoli and/or azurophilic granules and/or Auer rods are common

M3: Hypergranular promyelocytic leukemia:
Promyelocytes with prominent granules
Reniform nuclei, coalescent cytoplasmic granules in some cells
Numerous cells with Auer rods, some with bundles of Auer rods

M3 Variant: Microgranular promyelocytic leukemia:
Promyelocytes with many tiny granules may appear agranular
Strongly myeloperoxidase-positive cytoplasm, many Auer rods
t(15:17) translocation on cytogenetic analysis

M4: Myelomonocytic leukemia:
>30% of nonerythroid cells must be blasts
>20% but <80% of nonerythroid cells must be monocytes
Absolute peripheral blood monocyte level >5000/mm^3 promonocytes or serum/urine lysozyme level greater than 3 times normal

M5: Monocytic leukemia:
M5a: >80% marrow nonerythroid cells are monoblasts
M5b: <80% nonerythroid cells are monoblasts but >80% are monoblasts, promonocytes, or monocytes

M6: Erythroleukemia:
>30% of nonerythroid cells are type I or II blasts
>50% of marrow cells are erythroblasts
If <30% of nonerythroid cells are myeloblasts, classify as myelodysplastic syndrome - refractory anemia with excess blasts in transition

M7: Megakaryoblastic leukemia:
Blasts are polymorphic with round nuclei
May have cytoplasmic blebs and/or nuclei with platelets
Peripheral blood may have megakaryocyte fragments
Blasts are peroxidase and Sudan black negative

Blasts are often PAS and/or acid phosphatase positive
Bone marrow fibrosis often present
Platelet peroxidase, platelet membrane glycoprotein, immunophenotype studies may be helpful to confirm diagnosis

Myelodysplastic Syndromes

Refractory anemia (RA)
Patient's age usually older than 50 years
Reticulocytopenia (peripheral blood)
Absent to 1% or less blasts (peripheral blood)
Normo- or hypercellular marrow
Marrow erythroid series shows hyperplasia and/or dyserythropoiesis
Marrow granulocytic/megakaryocytic series usually normal, <5% blasts

Refractory anemia with ring sideroblasts
Features of RA but ringed sideroblasts are >15% of all nucleated marrow cells
Dimorphic erythrocyte population (peripheral blood)

Refractory anemia with excess of blasts (RAEB)
Patient's age usually older than 50 years
Dysgranulopoiesis (peripheral blood), with <5% blasts
Marrow hyperplasia with dysgranulopoiesis, dyserythropoiesis and/or dysmegakaryocytopoiesis; ringed sideroblasts may be present
Marrow blasts (type I and II) are from 5% to 20%

Chronic myelomonocytic leukemia (CMML)
Absolute monocytosis (>1000/mm^3) (peripheral blood)
<5% blasts (peripheral blood)
Dysgranulopoiesis (hypogranularity and/or Pelger-type cells) may be present (peripheral blood)
Marrow similar to RAEB but with increase in promonocytes, may be <5% blasts but with increasing monocyte precursor blasts, may rise to >5% up to 20%

RAEB in transformation (RAEBT)
Patients any age
Includes cases of cytopenia
Symptoms often of brief duration
Cellular features of RAEB but may have >5% blasts in peripheral blood and/or >20% up to 30% marrow blasts (type I and II) and/or Auer rods in granulocyte precursors

The concept of myeloproliferative disease includes a spectrum of developmental/maturational defects involving the hematopoietic system. Occasionally, patients have characteristics that may not fit readily into one of the FAB categories and are then considered (by some) as a "new" myeloproliferative process.[7]

FAB Criteria for Classification of Myelodysplastic Syndromes (Quantitative Abnormalities)

FAB Type	Peripheral Blood	Bone Marrow
Refractory Anemia (RA)	Blasts <1%	Blasts <5%
RA with ringed sideroblasts (RARS)	Blasts <1%	Blasts <5% with ringed sideroblasts >15%
RA with excess of blasts (RAEB)	Blasts <5%	Blasts 5%-20%
RAEB in transformation (RAEBt)	Blasts ≥5%	Blasts 20%-29% and/or Auer rods
Chronic myelomonocytic leukemia (CMML)	Blasts <5% with >1 x 10^9/L of monocytes	Blasts <20%
Acute myeloid leukemia (AML)		Blasts >30%

Bone marrow culture is sometimes helpful, for instance, in diagnosis of miliary tuberculosis and of histoplasmosis. Orders for appropriate cultures must accompany such samples, which require sterile containers.

Serial bone marrow biopsy samples have been utilized to follow the course of *in vivo* differentiation of myeloid cells in cases of acute leukemia that are receiving chemotherapy. The method uses monoclonal antibody to a purine analogue with subsequent identification by immunofluorescence. *In vivo* differentiation as detected in this manner has been found to indicate favorable long-term prognosis and may assist in the choice of effective therapeutic regimens.[8]

Application of current immunologic/molecular biologic analytic techniques (eg, flow cytometry and tissue-based cluster of differentiation (CD) antigen studies, restriction fragment-linked polymorphisms (RFLP), polymerase chain reaction (PCR), cytogenetic analyses utilizing appropriate fresh or fixed samples) can assist in the solution of difficult marrow interpretive problems. Bone marrow transplantation, performed on selected patients, may utilize some of these techniques for the detection of minimal resistant disease.[9]

Footnotes

1. Rosse C, Kraemer MJ, Dillon TL, et al, "Bone Marrow Cell Populations of Normal Infants: The Predominance of Lymphocytes," *J Lab Clin Med*, 1977, 89(6):1225-40.
2. Wolff SN, Katzenstein AL, Phillips GL, et al, "Aspiration Does Not Influence Interpretation of Bone Marrow Biopsy Cellularity," *Am J Clin Pathol*, 1983, 80:60-2.
3. Hernández-García MT, Hernández-Nieto L, Pérez-González E, et al, "Bone Marrow Trephine Biopsy: Anterior Superior Iliac Spine *Versus* Posterior Superior Iliac Spine," *Clin Lab Haematol*, 1993, 15(1):15-9.
4. Udoji WC and Husain I, "Microcytic Normochromic Anemia Associated With Iron Storage by Hypernephroma," *Am J Clin Pathol*, 1978, 70:944-6. 51:189-99.
5. Bennett JM, Catovsky D, Daniel MT, et al, "Proposed Revised Criteria for the Classification of Acute Myeloid Leukemia. A Report of the French-American-British Cooperative Group," *Ann Intern Med*, 1985, 103(4):620-5.
6. Bennett JM, Catovsky D, Daniel MT, et al, "Criteria for the Diagnosis of Acute Leukemia of Megakaryocyte Lineage (M7). A Report of the French-American-British Cooperative Group," *Ann Intern Med*, 1985, 103(3):460-2.
7. Schofield JR and Robinson WA, "A New Myeloproliferative Syndrome," *Am J Hematol*, 1995, 48(3):186-91.
8. Raza A, Preisler H, Lampkin B, et al, "Clinical and Prognostic Significance of *In Vivo* Differentiation in Acute Myeloid Leukemia," *Am J Hematol*, 1993, 42(2):147-57.
9. Negrin RS and Cleary ML, "Laboratory Evaluation of Minimal Residual Disease," *Bone Marrow Transplantation*, Chapter 15, Forman SJ, Blume KG, and Thomas ED, eds, Boston, MA: Blackwell Scientific Publications, 1994, 179.

References

Armitage JO, "Bone Marrow Transplantation," *N Engl J Med*, 1994, 330(12):827-38.
Bain BJ, Clark DM, and Lampert IA, *Bone Marrow Pathology*, Boston, MA: Blackwell Scientific Publications, 1992.
Bartl R, Frisch B, and Wilmanns W, "Potential of Bone Marrow Biopsy in Chronic Myeloproliferative Disorders (MPD)," *Eur J Haematol*, 1993, 50(1):41-52.
Bennett JM, Catovsky D, Daniel MT, et al, "Proposals for the Classification of the Myelodysplastic Syndromes," *Br J Haematol*, 1982, 51(2):189-99.
Bloomfield CD and Brunning RD, "The Revised French-American-British Classification of Acute Myeloid Leukemia: Is New Better?" *Ann Intern Med*, 1985, 103(4):614-5.
Brunning RD and McKenna RW, *Tumors of the Bone Marrow*, Washington, DC: Armed Forces Institute of Pathology, 1994.
Cline MJ, "Histiocytes and Histiocytosis," *Blood*, 1994, 84(9):2840-53.
Dunbar CE and Nienhuis AW, "Myelodysplastic Syndromes," Chapter 12, *Blood: Principles and Practice of Hematology*, Handin RI, Lux SE, and Stossel TP, eds, Philadelphia, PA: JB Lippincott, 1995, 377-414.
Foucar K, *Bone Marrow Pathology*, Chicago, IL: ASCP Press, 1994.
Haase D, Fonatsch C, Freund M, et al, "Cytogenetic Findings in 179 Patients With Myelodysplastic Syndromes," *Ann Hematol*, 1995, 70(4):171-87.
Hyun BH, Gulati GL, and Ashton JK, *Color Atlas of Clinical Hematology*, New York, NY: Igaku-Shoin, 1986.
Hyun BH, Stevenson AJ, and Hanau CA, "Fundamentals of Bone Marrow Examination," *Hematol/Oncol Clin North Am*, 1994, 8(4):651-63.
Karcher DS and Frost AR, "The Bone Marrow in Human Immunodeficiency Virus (HIV)-Related Disease: Morphology and Clinical Correlation," *Am J Clin Pathol*, 1991, 95(1):63-71.
Li C-Y, Yam LT, and Sun T, *Modern Modalities for the Diagnosis of Hematologic Neoplasms: Color Atlas/Test*, New York, NY: Igaku-Shoin, 1996.
Paulman PM, "Bone Marrow Sampling," *Am Fam Physician*, 1989, 40(6):85-9.
Rothstein G, "Origin and Development of the Blood and Blood Forming Tissues," *Wintrobe's Clinical Hematology*, 9th ed, Chapter 3, Lee GR, Bithell TC, Foerster J, et al, eds, Philadelphia, PA: Lea and Febiger, 1993, 41-78.
Verhoef GE, Pittaluga S, DeWolf-Peeters C, et al, "FAB Classification of Myelodysplastic Syndromes: Merits and Controversies," *Ann Hematol*, 1995, 71(1):3-11.
Weinstein HJ and Griffin JD, "Acute Myelogenous Leukemia," Chapter 18, *Blood: Principles and Practice of Hematology*, Handin RI, Lux SE, and Stossel TP, eds, Philadelphia, PA: JB Lippincott, 1995, 543-74.

Bone Marrow Aspirate see Bone Marrow *on page 307*

Bone Marrow Biopsy see Bone Marrow *on page 307*

Bone Marrow Iron Stain see Iron Stain, Bone Marrow *on page 328*

Buffy Coat Method for Detection of Bacteremia see Bacteremia Detection, Buffy Coat Micromethod *on page 305*

Buffy Coat Smear Study of Peripheral Blood

CPT 85009

Related Information
Bacteremia Detection, Buffy Coat Micromethod *on page 305*
Bacterial Culture, Blood *on page 457*
Bone Marrow *on page 307*
Lymph Node Biopsy *on page 50*

Abstract The detection of some pathologic elements potentially present in peripheral blood can be enhanced by preparing and staining the concentrated white cell fraction ("buffy coat") of blood

Specimen Blood

Container Lavender top (EDTA) tube

Use Low cost maneuver to detect uncommon cells or organisms in blood, largely for detection of abnormal, immature, blast, or malignant white blood cell or other nucleated cell forms; usually used to detect leukemic cells, circulating malignant cells, or immature blood cells in cases of myelofibrosis or other marrow myelophthisic processes; may be used in histochemical evaluation of leukemias when a "dry tap" of the marrow occurs

Limitations Preparation of buffy coat smears may distort cells; artifact affects especially fragile cells

Methodology Wright's stained smear of buffy coat developing in centrifuged tube or capillary of anticoagulated whole blood

Additional Information Utility of buffy coat study has been questioned. In a series of 96 children with ALL, buffy coat study found no cases of relapse not detected by WBC count or usual peripheral blood smear.[1] On the other hand, it has been suggested that erroneous results from buffy coat study are the result of an uneven distribution of WBCs in the buffy coat layer. Removal and mixing of the entire buffy coat layer prior to making smears prevents uneven distribution of the leukocytes and avoids artifactual distortion of WBC morphology.[2] Unusual microorganisms, tumor cells, and cells with inclusions (eg, *Strongyloides stercoralis* hyperinfection in an immune-suppressed individual,[3] microfilaria[4], AIDS, Howell-Jolly body-like inclusions,[5] RBC-associated bacillus *Tropheryma whippelii* [proposed causative agent of Whipple's disease],[6] *Ehrlichia* neutrophil inclusions in human ehrlichiosis,[7] myeloma[8], and other circulating malignant cells) may be more readily detected by buffy coat study.

Footnotes

1. Franklin IM, "A Comparison of Peripheral Blood and Buffy Coat Smear Examination for the Prediction of Bone Marrow Relapse of Acute Lymphoblastic Leukemia in Childhood," *J Clin Pathol*, 1983, 36:192-4.
2. Pereira TT, Hargrove GH, and Combleet PJ, "Preparation of Buffy Coat Smears in Leukopenic Patients," *Lab Med*, 1981, 12:2, 96-8.
3. Gambino R, "Examination of the Buffy Coat in Patients With FUO," *Lab Report for Physicians*, 1983, 5:43-4.
4. Freedman DO and Berry RS, "Rapid Diagnosis of Bancroftian Filariasis by Acridine Orange Staining of Centrifuged Parasites," *Am J Trop Med Hyg*, 1992, 47(6):787-93.
5. Slagel DD, Lager DJ, and Dick FR, "Howell-Jolly Body-Like Inclusions in the Neutrophils of Patients With Acquired Immunodeficiency Syndrome," *Am J Clin Pathol*, 1994, 101(4):429-31.
6. Lowsky R, Archer GL, Fyles G, et al, "Brief Report: Diagnosis of Whipple's Disease by Molecular Analysis of Peripheral Blood," *N Engl J Med*, 1994, 331(20):1343-6.
7. Rynkiewicz DL and Liu LX, "Human Ehrlichiosis in New England," *N Engl J Med*, 1994, 330(4):292-3.
8. Witzig TE, "Detection of Malignant Gels in the Peripheral Blood of Patients With Multiple Myeloma: Clinical Implications and Research Applications," *Mayo Clin Proc*, 1994, 69(9):903-7.

References

Brown BA, "Routine Hematology Procedures," *Hematology: Principles and Procedures*, 6th ed, Philadelphia, PA: Lea & Febiger, 1993, 99.
Goodman JL, Nelson C, Vitale B, et al, "Direct Cultivation of the Causative Agent of Human Granulocytic Ehrlichiosis," *N Engl J Med*, 1996, 334(4):209-15.

CBC see Complete Blood Count *on page 312*

Cell Count, CSF see Cerebrospinal Fluid Analysis *on this page*

Ceramidase see Inherited Diseases of Metabolism and Cell Structure Tests *on page 327*

Ceramidetrihexoside α-Galactosidase see Inherited Diseases of Metabolism and Cell Structure Tests *on page 327*

Cerebrospinal Fluid Analysis

CPT 82947 (glucose); 84155 (protein quantitative); 89050 (cell count); 89051 (with differential count)

Related Information
Bacterial Antigens, Rapid Detection Methods *on page 454*
Bacterial Culture, Cerebrospinal Fluid *on page 460*
Body Fluid Analysis, Cell Count *on page 306*
Cerebrospinal Fluid Cytology *on page 290*
Cerebrospinal Fluid Glucose *on page 105*
Cerebrospinal Fluid IgG Ratios and IgG Index *on page 377*
Cerebrospinal Fluid Lactic Acid *on page 106*
Cerebrospinal Fluid LD *on page 106*
Cerebrospinal Fluid Protein *on page 380*
Enterovirus Genome Detection *on page 510*
FTA-ABS, Cerebrospinal Fluid *on page 394*
Fungal Culture, Cerebrospinal Fluid *on page 477*
Gram's Stain *on page 481*
Mycobacterial Culture, Cerebrospinal Fluid *on page 489*
Viral Culture, Central Nervous System Symptoms *on page 677*

Synonyms Cell Count, CSF; CSF Analysis; Spinal Fluid Analysis

Test Commonly Includes Color of supernatant, volume, turbidity, WBC/mm^3, polys/mm^3, lymphs/mm^3, RBC/mm^3, percent of crenated RBC, protein, sugar, sometimes VDRL, sometimes FTA-ABS, and protein electrophoresis may be helpful in selected cases.

Abstract Cerebrospinal fluid (CSF) exists in the cerebral ventricles and subarachnoid spaces. Examination of CSF contributes to diagnosis and sometimes management of various disease entities of the central nervous system including meningitis, encephalitis, instances of vasculitis, demyelinating diseases, tumors, paraneoplastic entities, polyneuritis, instances of cerebrovascular disease, cases of seizure disorders and confusional states.[1] For diagnosis of meningitis, culture, and then Gram's stain study have priority over all other testing, when only a small quantity of cerebrospinal fluid (CSF) is available. Cell count with differential deserves the next priority, followed by glucose and protein.

Patient Preparation Aseptic preparation for aspiration

Specimen Cerebrospinal fluid. A sample of peripheral blood for serum should be obtained concurrently if CSF is being studied for presence of
(Continued)

Cerebrospinal Fluid Analysis *(Continued)*

oligoclonal bands (eg, as in demyelinating diseases, in particular multiple sclerosis) or when glucose and protein levels are needed as in cases of possible infection (eg, meningitis or encephalitis). Blood culture and plasma glucose should be drawn in cases of possible meningitis as well as CBC and differential.

Container Sterile test tubes from lumbar puncture tray

Collection Specimens of spinal fluid and blood for culture should be obtained prior to initiation of antibiotic treatment of meningitis. Tubes must be labeled with patient's name, date, and labeled with number indicating sequence in which tubes were obtained. Specimen should be delivered to the laboratory **promptly**.

Storage Instructions Do **not** store; place in the hands of a laboratory technologist.

Causes for Rejection Unlabeled tubes, insufficient or clotted specimen

Special Instructions When a diagnosis of meningitis is considered, culture of other materials as well as culture of CSF may be helpful. Most children with bacterial meningitis are initially bacteremic, and blood cultures are of value. In neonates and small children, urine culture may be positive. Culture and Gram's stain of petechiae may provide immediate diagnosis.

Reference Range Adults: 0-5 cells/mm^3, all lymphocytes and monocytes; 0 red blood cells; protein: lumbar 15-50 mg/dL, cisternal 15-25 mg/dL, ventricular 6-15 mg/dL; glucose 50-80 mg/dL. Younger than 1 month: <32 cells/mm^3, 1 month to 1 year: <10 cells/mm^3, 1-4 years: <8 cells/mm^3, 5 years to puberty: <5 cells/mm^3; in the premature neonate: <29 cells/mm^3

Possible Panic Range Increased number of cells

Use Evaluate bacterial or viral encephalitis, meningitis, meningoencephalitis, mycobacterial or fungal infection, parasitic infestations, primary or secondary malignancy, leukemia/malignant lymphoma of CNS, trauma, vascular occlusive disease, vasculitis, heredofamilial and/or degenerative processes. The table outlines findings, including those with subdural empyema, brain abscess, ventricular empyema, cerebral epidural abscess, spinal epidural abscess, tuberculosis, syphilis, sarcoidosis, and other entities.[1]

The nucleated blood cell count in the cerebrospinal fluid is described as superior to any combination of the other CSF tests for bacterial meningitis. In patients who have not received antimicrobial agents the ultimate diagnosis of bacterial meningitis is based on results of culture.[2] The cell count and differential count are mandatory, and a Gram's stain must be examined promptly in work-up of possible meningitis. Glucose and protein are necessary, as well, in the work-up for possible meningitis.[3] In a study of aseptic versus bacterial meningitis, the mean CSF cell counts in aseptic and bacterial meningitis were respectively 228 cells/mm^3 (range 6-2650) and 4035 cells/mm^3 (range 16-17,650).[4] **Early viral infection** as well as **bacterial meningitis** can elicit neutrophil leukocytosis in blood and CSF. In viral meningitis, a shift to mononuclear predominance often occurs subsequently.[5,6,7] In 205 cases of acute **viral** meningitis, the 25th percentile, median, and 75th percentile leukocyte counts (10^6/L) were 37/100/250, with 3%, 33%, and 75%, respectively PMNs. In 217 cases of acute **bacterial** meningitis, leukocyte counts (10^6/L) were 330/1195/4400 with 70%, 86%, and 97% PMNs, respectively.[8] Seasonal curves for viral and bacterial infection go in opposite directions; viral meningitis is a disease of midsummer, while bacterial meningitis is relatively more common in the winter.[8]

Signals of possible meningeal infection in the newborn: Leukocyte count >30 cells/mm^3 with more than 60% PMNs, CSF protein >100 mg/dL, CSF glucose lower than 40% of the level in blood are findings in bacterial meningitis.[9] CSF WBC >10 cells/mm^3 in very young infants, and 5 cells/mm^3 in older infants and children with >1 PMN/mm^3 is abnormal.

Limitations A traumatic (bloody) tap may make interpretation difficult. Normal CSF may be found early in meningitis.

Methodology Manual cell count using hemacytometer. Electronic cell counters lack precision and validity when used to analyze most CSF specimens (background is high relative to total white cell count). Differential cell study using manually prepared smears or cytocentrifuge methods. Bovine albumin, 22%, mixed with spinal fluid specimen is helpful in maintaining the morphologic integrity of smeared cells. For chemical, microbiologic, and other analyses, see appropriate entries.

Additional Information More extensive testing: Cytology, conventional cultures and cultures for mycobacteria, fungi, and viruses, additional chemistry and serologic determinations must usually be ordered separately.

Correction for traumatic tap: If cell counts and protein determinations are performed on CSF and blood obtained at the same time, correction

for "bloody tap" can be calculated. All CSF measurements should be made from the same tube. The ratio of RBC count CSF to RBC count blood provides a factor which when multiplied by the blood WBC count or blood protein level indicates the expected level of contribution of these parameters from the blood to the spinal fluid. These contributed WBC or protein values can then be subtracted from the respective values measured in the spinal fluid. For example:

1. RBCs (CSF)/RBCs (blood) x WBCs (blood) or x protein (blood).
2. WBCs (CSF) or protein (CSF) - product calculated in 1 = true CSF WBC or true CSF protein.

If the peripheral blood is normal and traumatic tap occurs, about 1 WBC is added to the CSF for each 700 RBCs that have been transferred into the CSF.[10] RBC contamination from a traumatic tap does not adversely affect the laboratory diagnosis of bacterial meningitis.

When only a small amount of CSF can be obtained, Gram's stain and culture must always have priority over antigen detection testing.[11] Antigen detection methods cannot replace culture and Gram's stain. A bacterial culture is the first test to be performed on cerebrospinal fluid for meningitis. It is the "gold standard" for diagnosis.[12] A requirement for 50 or more leukocytes per µL of CSF has been proposed as justification for bacterial antigen testing.[11] Another group found a CSF nucleated blood cell count <6/mm^3 provided a criterion for an abbreviated CSF evaluation.[2] Correlation exists between bacterial concentration in CSF and the numbers of PMNs found.[13]

There is substantial mortality and morbidity in subjects with bacterial meningitis. Neurologic sequelae are found in as many as 33% of all survivors in one study.[14] Sequelae occur especially in newborns and children.[11] Particularly when bacterial meningitis follows an insidious pattern, diagnostic delay may be unavoidable.[15] Eight of 21 survivors of neonatal meningitis were normal, eight had mild sequelae, and five had moderate to severe sequelae in a culture-proven series.[16] Despite early diagnosis and the use of appropriate therapy, both complications of meningitis and death may occur. As many as 50% of survivors of meningitis have some sequelae, as summarized by the Task Force on Diagnosis and Management of Meningitis.[17]

White cell pleocytosis is found in only 33% of patients with multiple sclerosis (MS). The white count rarely exceeds 20 cells/mm^3. Most patients with MS (66%) have normal total protein. In contrast, patients with Guillain-Barré syndrome usually have no excess white cells but show elevated CSF protein of 100-500 mg/dL.[18]

Footnotes

1. Felgin RD and Cherry JD, *Textbook of Pediatric Infectious Diseases*, Philadelphia, PA: WB Saunders Co, 1987, 488.
2. Rodewald LE, Woodin KA, Szilagyi PG, et al, "Relevance of Common Tests of Cerebrospinal Fluid in Screening for Bacterial Meningitis," *J Pediatr*, 1991, 119(3):363-9.
3. Fishman RA, *Cerebrospinal Fluid in Diseases of the Nervous System*, 2nd ed, Philadelphia, PA: WB Saunders Co, 1992, 157-351.
4. Walsh-Kelly C, Nelson DB, Smith DS, et al, "Clinical Predictors of Bacterial Versus Aseptic Meningitis in Childhood," *Ann Emerg Med*, 1992, 21(8):910-4.
5. Connolly KJ and Hammer SM, "The Acute Aseptic Meningitis Syndrome," *Infect Dis Clin North Am*, 1990, 4(4):599-622.
6. Hammer SM and Connolly KJ, "Viral Aseptic Meningitis in the United States: Clinical Features, Viral Etiologies, and Differential Diagnosis," *Curr Clin Top Infect Dis*, 1992, 12:1-25.
7. Amir J, Harel L, Frydman M, et al, "Shift of Cerebrospinal Polymorphonuclear Cell Percentage in the Early Stage of Aseptic Meningitis," *J Pediatr*, 1991, 119(6):938-41.
8. Spanos A, Harrell FE Jr, and Durack DT, "Differential Diagnosis of Acute Meningitis: An Analysis of the Predictive Value of Initial Observations," *JAMA*, 1989, 262(19):2700-7.
9. McCracken GH Jr, "Current Management of Bacterial Meningitis in Infants and Children," *Pediatr Infect Dis J*, 1992, 11(2):169-74.
10. Bauer JD, *Clinical Laboratory Methods*, 9th ed, St Louis, MO: Mosby-Year Book Inc, 1982, 759.
11. Gray LD and Fedorko DP, "Laboratory Diagnosis of Bacterial Meningitis," *Clin Microbiol Rev*, 1992, 5(2):130-45.
12. Smith AL, "Bacterial Meningitis," *Pediatr Rev*, 1993, 14(1):11-8.
13. La Scolea LJ Jr and Dryja D, "Quantitation of Bacteria in Cerebrospinal Fluid and Blood of Children With Meningitis and Its Diagnostic Significance," *J Clin Microbiol*, 1984, 19(2):187-90.
14. Sáez-Llorens X, Ramilo O, Mustafa MM, et al, "Molecular Pathophysiology of Bacterial Meningitis: Current Concepts and Therapeutic Implications," *J Pediatr*, 1990, 116(5):671-84.
15. Kilpi T, Anttila M, Kallio MJ, et al, "Severity of Childhood Bacterial Meningitis and Duration of Illness Before Diagnosis," *Lancet*, 1991, 338(8764):406-9.
16. Franco SM, Cornelius VE, and Andrews BF, "Long-Term Outcome of Neonatal Meningitis," *Am J Dis Child*, 1992, 146(6):567-71.
17. Klein JO, Feigin RD, and McCracken GH Jr, "Report of the Task Force on Diagnosis and Management of Meningitis," *Pediatrics*, 1986, 78(5):959-82.
18. Harrington MG and Kennedy PG, "The Clinical Use of Cerebrospinal Fluid Studies in Demyelinating Neurological Diseases," *Postgrad Med J*, 1987, 63(743):735-40.

References

Bonadio WA, Smith DS, Goddard S, et al, "Distinguishing Cerebrospinal Fluid Abnormalities in Children With Bacterial Meningitis and Traumatic Lumbar Puncture," *J Infect Dis*, 1990, 162(1):251-4.

Feigin RD, McCracken GH Jr, and Klein JO, "Diagnosis and Management of Meningitis," *Pediatr Infect Dis J*, 1992, 11:785-814.

Levy M, Wong E, and Fried D, "Diseases That Mimic Meningitis. Analysis of 650 Lumbar Punctures," *Clin Pediatr (Phila)*, 1990, 29(5):258-61.

Initial Cerebrospinal Fluid Findings in Suppurative Diseases of the Central Nervous System and Meninges

Condition	Pressure (mm H$_2$O)	Leukocytes/mm^3	Protein (mg/dL)	Sugar (mg/dL)	Specific Findings
Acute bacterial meningitis	Usually elevated; average, 300	Several hundred to more than 60,000; usually a few thousand; occasionally fewer than 100 (especially meningococcal or early in disease); PMNs* predominate	Usually 100-500, occasionally >1000	<40 in >50% of cases	Organism usually seen on smear or culture in >90% of cases
Subdural empyema	Usually elevated; average, 300	Fewer than 100 to a few thousand; PMNs predominate	Usually 100-500	Normal	No organisms seen on smear or culture unless concurrent meningitis
Brain abscess	Usually elevated	Usually 10-200; fluid is rarely acellular; lymphocytes predominate	Usually 75-400	Normal	No organisms seen on smear or culture
Ventricular empyema (rupture of brain abscess)	Considerably elevated	Several thousand to 100,000; usually >90% PMNs	Usually several hundred	Usually <40	Organism may be seen on smear or culture
Cerebral epidural abscess	Slightly to modestly elevated	Few to several hundred or more cells; lymphocytes predominate	Usually 50-200	Normal	No organisms seen on smear or culture
Spinal epidural abscess	Usually reduced with spinal block	Usually 10-100; lymphocytes predominate	Usually several hundred	Normal	No organisms seen on smear or culture
Thrombophlebitis (often associated with subdural empyema)	Often elevated	Few to several hundred; PMNs and lymphocytes	Slightly to moderately elevated	Normal	No organisms seen on smear or culture
Bacterial endocarditis (with embolism)	Normal or slightly elevated	Few to fewer than 100; lymphocytes and PMNs	Slightly elevated	Normal	No organisms seen on smear or culture
Acute hemorrhagic encephalitis	Usually elevated	Few to more than 1000; PMNs predominate	Moderately elevated	Normal	No organisms seen on smear or culture
Tuberculous infection	Usually elevated; may be low with dynamic block in advanced stages	Usually 25-100, rarely more than 500; lymphocytes predominate, except in early stages when PMNs may account for 80% of the cells	Nearly always elevated, usually 100-200; may be much higher if dynamic block	Usually reduced; <50 in 75% of cases	Acid-fast organisms may be seen on smear of protein coagulum (pellicle) or recovered from inoculated guinea pig or by culture
Cryptococcal infection	Usually elevated; average, 225	Average, 50 (0-800); lymphocytes predominate	Average, 100; usually 20-500	Reduced in >50% the cases; average 30; often higher in patients with concomitant diabetes mellitus	Organisms may be seen in India ink preparation and on culture (Sabouraud's medium); will usually grow on blood agar; may produce alcohol in cerebrospinal fluid from fermentation of glucose
Syphilis (acute)	Usually elevated	Average, 500; usually lymphocytes; rare PMNs	Average, 100; - globulin often high, with abnormal colloidal gold curve	Normal (rarely reduced)	Positive results of reagin test for syphilis; spirochetes not demonstrable by usual techniques of smear or culture
Sarcoidosis	Normal to considerably elevated	0 to <100 mononuclear cells	Slight to moderate elevation	Normal	No specific findings

*Polymorphonuclear leukocytes

From Feigin RD and Cherry JD, eds, *Textbook of Pediatric Infectious Diseases*, Vol 1, Philadelphia, PA: WB Saunders, 1992, 410, with permission.

Travlos A, Anton HA, and Wing PC, "Cerebrospinal Fluid Cell Count Following Spinal Cord Injury," *Arch Phys Med Rehabil*, 1994, 75(3):293-6.

Yurdakok M and Kocabas CN, "CSF Erythrocyte Volume Analysis: A Simple Method for the Diagnosis of Traumatic Tap in Newborn Infants," *Pediatr Neurosurg*, 1991-92, 17(4):199.

CHBHA *see* Heinz Body Stain *on page 321*

Chromium-51 Tagged RBC Survival Test *see* ^{51}Cr Red Cell Survival *on page 314*

Cold Hemolysin Test

CPT 86941

Related Information

Cold Agglutinin Screen *on page 605*

Synonyms Donath-Landsteiner Test; PCH Test; Test for D-L Antibody; Test for Paroxysmal Cold Hemoglobinuria

Abstract Test for paroxysmal cold hemoglobinuria (PCH), a condition caused by sensitization of red blood cells (at temperatures less than 30°C) by a complement binding IgG biphasic hemolysin. Warming to 37°C causes hemolysis of patient's RBCs.

Specimen Blood

Container Red top tube

Collection Obtain 7 mL of blood by routine venipuncture from patient in previously warmed (37°C) red top tube and another 7 mL of blood in previously cooled (3°C to 4°C) red top tube in an ice water bath. Collect similar samples from a normal individual for a negative control. Deliver to hematology laboratory immediately.

Special Instructions Consult laboratory as test may need to be arranged in advance.

Reference Range Negative

Use Diagnosis of the uncommon disorder, paroxysmal cold hemoglobinuria. PCH may occur with syphilis, infectious mononucleosis, influenza, measles, mumps, chickenpox, and other viral illnesses.

Methodology Observation of red cell lysis by patient's cold activated serum

Additional Information There are two types of cold autoantibodies, the cold autoagglutinins/hemolysins (as found in cold-antibody autoimmune hemolytic anemia) and the biphasic hemolysins. These antibodies are characterized by optimal reaction at temperatures less than 30°C. The cold autoagglutinins are usually monoclonal or polyclonal IgM antibodies with anti-H, anti-IH, or anti-i immunospecificity. Anti-Pr is the second most commonly associated antibody. Classic paroxysmal cold hemoglobinuria is caused by an IgG complement binding biphasic hemolysin,[1] an autoantibody that attaches to the RBC membrane at 4°C to 20°C. The antibody causes only weak agglutination of red cells in saline. When the temperature rises to 37°C, hemolysis occurs. The immunohematologic specificity of the Donath-Landsteiner type PCH antibody is usually anti-P.[2] While PCH was the first hemolytic anemia to be recognized, it has become the least common type of autoimmune hemolytic anemia. Previously associated with syphilis, it is now more commonly seen in viral-like illness, largely in children.[3] The re-emergence of syphilis associated with AIDS may cause a comeback of PCH.

Footnotes

1. Engelfriet CP, Overbeeke MA, and von dem Borne AE, "Autoimmune Hemolytic Anemia," *Semin Hematol*, 1992, 29(1):3-12.

2. Judd WJ, Wilkinson SL, Issitt PD, et al, "Donath-Landsteiner Hemolytic Anemia Due to an Anti-Pr-Like Biphasic Hemolysin," *Transfusion*, 1986, 26(5):423-5.

3. Nordhagen R, Stensvold A, Winses A, et al, "Paroxysmal Cold Hemoglobinuria. The Most Frequent Acute Autoimmune Haemolytic Anaemia in Children?" *Acta Paediatr Scand*, 1984, 73(2):258-62.

(Continued)

Cold Hemolysin Test *(Continued)*

References

Dacie JV and Lewis SM, *Practical Haematology*, 8th ed, New York, NY: Churchill Livingstone, 1995, 520-4.

Mollison PL, Engelfriet CP, and Contreras M, *Blood Transfusion in Clinical Medicine*, 9th ed, Oxford, UK: Blackwell Scientific Publications, 1993, 293-5.

Packman CH and Leddy JP, "Cryopathic Hemolytic Syndromes," *Williams Hematology*, 5th ed, Chapter 65, Beutler E, Lichtman MA, Coller BS, et al, eds, New York, NY: McGraw-Hill Inc, 1995, 688-90.

Sherry C Sr, "Acquired Immune Anemia of Increased Destruction," *Clinical Hematology: Principles, Procedures, Correlations*, Chapter 19, Lotspeich-Steininger CA, Stiene-Martin EA, and Koepke JA, eds, Philadelphia, PA: JB Lippincott Co, 1992, 274.

Complete Blood Count

CPT 85021 (hemogram, automated [RBC, WBC, Hgb, Hct, and indices only]); 85022 (hemogram, automated and manual differential WBC count [CBC]); 85023 (hemogram and platelet count, automated and manual differential WBC count [CBC]); 85024 (hemogram and platelet count, automated and automated partial differential WBC count [CBC]); 85025 (hemogram and platelet count, automated and automated complete, differential WBC count [CBC])

Related Information

Ammonia, Blood *on page 75*
Bone Marrow *on page 307*
CD4/CD8 Enumeration *on page 375*
Cold Agglutinin Screen *on page 605*
Eosinophil Count *on page 315*
Fanconi's Anemia, Chromosome Breakage Study *on page 282*
Ferritin, Serum *on page 127*
Folic Acid, RBC *on page 317*
Folic Acid, Serum *on page 317*
Hematocrit *on page 322*
Hemoglobin *on page 323*
Iron and Total Iron Binding Capacity/Transferrin *on page 150*
Kidney Profile *on page 153*
Lymph Node Biopsy *on page 50*
Peripheral Blood: Differential Leukocyte Count *on page 336*
Peripheral Blood: Red Blood Cell Morphology *on page 339*
Platelet Count *on page 340*
Platelet Sizing *on page 341*
Red Blood Cell Indices *on page 343*
Red Cell Count *on page 344*
Uric Acid, Serum *on page 213*
Vitamin B$_{12}$ *on page 351*
White Blood Count *on page 353*

Synonyms Blood Cell Profile; Blood Count; CBC; Hematology Profile; Hemogram

Test Commonly Includes WBC, Hct, Hgb, differential count, RBC, WBC and RBC morphology, RBC indices, platelet estimate, platelet count, RDW, and histograms. Although RBC, hemoglobin concentration (of individual RBCs), WBC, and platelet histograms are not usually available on patient charts, they are helpful to the technologist in detecting problems with patients and quality control. Even though the histograms are not on the chart, they can be viewed in the laboratory along with the blood smear. New analyzers also provide automated 5-part white cell differentials: granulocytes, monocytes, lymphocytes, eosinophils, basophils, and additional RBC and platelet indices.

Abstract The CBC is a profile of tests rather than a single test. It is the standard, broadly inclusive, usually automated test for evaluation of RBC, WBC, and platelets. The majority of CBC results are generated by highly automated electronic and pneumatic multichannel analyzers based on aperture-impedance and/or laser beam cell sizing and counting (see reference by Koepke).

Specimen Whole blood

Container Lavender top (EDTA) tube. International Council for Standardization in Hematology recommendation is for use of K$_2$-EDTA, 1.5-2.2 mg/mL of blood as anticoagulant for blood cell counting and sizing.[1]

Collection Mix specimen 10 times by gentle inversion. If specimen is not brought to the laboratory immediately refrigeration is required. If the anticipated delay in arrival is more than 4 hours, two blood smears should be prepared immediately after the venipuncture and submitted with the blood specimen.

Storage Instructions EDTA-anticoagulated sample should be analyzed within 6 hours at room temperature and within 24 hours when stored at 4°C.

Causes for Rejection Improper tube, clotted specimen, hemolyzed specimen, dilution of blood with I.V. fluid

Special Instructions Blood specimen and diluent may require prewarming to obtain meaningful results if cold agglutinins are present.

Reference Range Accompanying tables summarize differences in red cell parameter normal ranges, note especially important age and sex variances. Refer to tables.

Red Cell Values on First Postnatal Day*

Gestational Age (wk)	24-25	26-27	28-29	30-31	32-33	34-35	36-37	Term
RBC (x 10^6/mm^3)	4.65 ±0.43	4.73 ±0.45	4.62 ±0.75	4.79 ±0.74	5.0 ±0.76	5.09 ±0.5	5.27 ±0.68	5.14 ±0.7
Hgb (g/dL)	19.4 ±1.5	19.0 ±2.5	19.3 ±1.8	19.1 ±2.2	18.5 ±2.0	19.6 ±2.1	19.2 ±1.7	19.3 ±2.2
Hct (%)	63 ±4	62 ±8	60 ±7	60 ±8	60 ±8	61 ±7	64 ±7	61 ±7.4
MCV (fL)	135 ±0.2	132 ±14.4	131 ±13.5	127 ±12.7	123 ±15.7	122 ±10.0	121 ±12.5	119 ±9.4
Retic (%)	6.0 ±0.5	9.6 ±3.2	7.5 ±2.5	5.8 ±2.0	5.0 ±1.9	3.9 ±1.6	4.2 ±1.8	3.2 ±1.4

From Zaizov R and Matoth Y,[1] "Red Cell Values on the First Postnatal Day During the Last 16 Weeks of Gestation," *Amer J Hematol*, 1976, 1:2, 275-8, with permission.
*Mean values ±1 SD.

Mean Hematologic Values for Full-Term Infants, Children, and Adults*

Age	Hgb (g/dL)	Hct (%)	RBC (x 10^6/mm^3)	MCV (fL)	MCH (pg)	MCHC (g/dL)
Birth (cord blood)	17.1±1.8	52.0±5	4.64±0.5	113±6	37±2	33±1
1 d	19.4±2.1	58.0±7	5.30±0.5	110±6	37±2	33±1
2-6 d	19.8±2.4	66.0±8	5.40±0.7	122±14	37±4	30±3
14-23 d	15.7±1.5	52.0±5	4.92±0.6	106±11	32±3	30±2
24-37 d	14.1±1.9	45.0±7	4.35±0.6	104±11	32±3	31±3
40-50 d	12.8±1.9	42.0±6	4.10±0.5	103±11	31±3	30±2
2-2.5 mo	11.4±1.1	38.0±4	3.75±0.5	101±10	30±3	30±2
3-3.5 mo	11.2±0.8	37.0±3	3.88±0.4	95±9	29±3	30±2
5-7 mo	11.5±0.7	38.0±3	4.21±0.5	91±9	27±3	30±2
8-10 mo	11.7±0.6	39.0±2	4.35±0.4	90±8	27±3	30±1
11-13.5 mo	11.9±0.6	39.0±2	4.44±0.4	88±7	27±2	30±1
1.5-3 y	11.8±0.5	39.0±2	4.45±0.4	87±7	27±2	30±2
5 y	12.7±1.0	37.0±3	4.65±0.5	80±4	27±2	34±1
10 y	13.2±1.2	39.0±3	4.80±0.5	81±6	28±3	34±1
Male	15.5±1.1	46.0±3.1	5.11±0.38	—	—	—
Female	13.7±1.0	40.9±3	4.51±0.36	—	—	—
Male and female	—	—	—	90.1±4.8	30.2±1.8	33.7±1.1

From Johnson TR, 'How Growing Up Can Alter Lab Values in Pediatric Laboratory Medicine,' *Diag Med* (special issue), 1982, 5:13-8, with permission.
*Mean ±1 SD.

Critical Values Critical values: Hematocrit: <18% or >54%; hemoglobin: <6.0 g/dL or >18.0 g/dL; WBC on admission: <2500/mm^3 or >30,000/mm^3; platelets: <20,000/mm^3 or >1,000,000/mm^3

Use Evaluate anemia, leukemia, reaction to inflammation and infections, peripheral blood cellular characteristics, state of hydration and dehydration, polycythemia, hemolytic disease of the newborn; manage chemotherapy decisions

Limitations Hemoglobin (and thus the derived MCH and MCHC) may be falsely high if the plasma is lipemic or if the white count is >50,000 cells/mm^3. "Spun" (manual centrifuged) microhematocrits are approximately 3% higher (due to plasma trapping) compared to automated hematocrit levels. The increase is especially pronounced in cases of polycythemia (increased Hct levels) and when the cells are hypochromic and microcytic. The spun Hct level (as compared to automated instruments' calculated level) may be 12% higher at Hct levels of 70% and MCV of 48 fL with decrease in change to 3% higher at Hct levels of 70% with MCV of 100 fL.[2] Cold agglutinins (high titer) may cause spurious macrocytosis and low RBC count. This results when RBC couplets are "seen" and processed as single cells by the detection circuitry. Keeping the blood warm and warming the diluent prior to and during counting can correct this problem. See also discussion under listing Hematocrit *on page 322*. Cryoproteinemia may cause pseudoleukocytosis or pseudothrombocytosis.

Methodology Varies considerably between institutions. Most laboratories have high capacity multichannel instruments in place (available

Proposed Classification of Anemic Disorders Based on Red Cell Mean (MCV) and Heterogeneity (RDW)

MCV Low RDW Normal (microcytic homogeneous)	MCV Low RDW High (microcytic heterogeneous)	MCV Normal RDW Normal (normocytic homogeneous)	MCV Normal RDW High (normocytic heterogeneous)	MCV High RDW Normal (macrocytic homogeneous)	MCV High RDW High (macrocytic heterogeneous)
Heterozygous thalassemia*	Iron deficiency*	Normal	Mixed deficiency*	Aplastic anemia	Folate deficiency*
Chronic disease*	S/β -thalassemia	Chronic disease* chronic liver disease*†	Early iron or folate deficiency*	Preleukemia†	Vitamin B$_{12}$ deficiency
	Hemoglobin H	Nonanemic hemoglobinopathy (eg, AS, AC)	Anemic hemoglobinopathy (eg, SS, SC)*		Immune hemolytic anemia
	Red cell fragmentation	Transfusion†	Myelofibrosis		Cold agglutinins
		Chemotherapy	Sideroblastic*		Chronic lymphocytic leukemia, high count
		Chronic lymphocytic leukemia			
		Chronic myelocytic leukemia†			
		Hemorrhage			
		Hereditary spherocytosis			

From Bessman JD Jr, Gilmer PR, and Gardner FH, "Improved Classification of Anemias by MCV and RDW," *Am J Clin Pathol*, 1983, 80:324, with permission. The data for sensitivity of RDW and MCV in each disease category can be obtained from the authors.

*MCV alone <90% sensitive.

†RDW alone <90% sensitive.

Mean Hematologic Values for Low-Birth-Weight Infants*

Weight and Gestational Age at Birth	Age at Testing	Hemoglobin (g/dL)	Hematocrit (%)	Reticulocytes (%)
<1500 g, 28-32 wk	3 d	17.5±1.5	54±5	8.0±3.5
	1 wk	15.5±1.5	48±5	3.0±1.0
	2 wk	13.5±1.1	42±4	3.0±1.0
	3 wk	11.5±1.0	35±4	—
	4 wk	10.0±0.9	30±3	6.0±2.0
	6 wk	8.5±0.5	25±2	11.0±3.5
	8 wk	8.5±0.5	25±2	8.5±3.5
	10 wk	9.0±0.5	28±3	7.0±3.0
1500-2000 g, 32-36 wk	3 d	19.0±2.0	59±6	6.0±2.0
	1 wk	16.5±1.5	51±5	3.0±1.0
	2 wk	14.5±1.1	44±5	2.5±1.0
	3 wk	13.0±1.1	39±4	—
	4 wk	12.0±1.0	36±4	3.0±1.0
	6 wk	9.5±0.8	28±3	6.0±2.0
	8 wk	9.5±0.5	28±3	5.0±1.5
	10 wk	9.5±0.5	29±3	4.5±1.5
2000-2500 g, 36-40 wk	3 d	19.0±2.0	59±6	4.0±1.0
	1 wk	16.5±1.5	51±5	3.0±1.0
	2 wk	15.0±1.5	45±5	2.5±1.0
	3 wk	14.0±1.1	43±4	—
	4 wk	12.5±1.0	37±4	2.0±1.0
	6 wk	10.5±0.9	31±3	3.0±1.0
	8 wk	10.5±0.9	31±3	3.0±1.0
	10 wk	11.0±1.0	33±3	3.0±1.0

From Johnson TR, "How Growing Up Can Alter Lab Values in Pediatric Laboratory Medicine," *Diag Med* (special issue), 1982, 5:13-8, with permission.

*Mean ±1 SD.

from multiple commercial sources). The majority measure RBC and WBC parameters on the basis of changes in electrical impedance as cells and platelets are pulled through a tiny aperture. These are highly automated devices with extensive computer processing of the electrical signals after analog/digital conversion. Accuracy (with proper standardization) and precision (usually in the 0.5% to 2% range) is significantly improved over older manual and semiautomated methods. Some instruments count light impulses that are generated as cells flow across a laser beam. Proper calibration is a prime requisite (see references by Koepke, Lewis et al, and Rowan et al).

Additional Information Presence of one or more of the following may be indications for further investigation: hemoglobin <10 g/dL, hemoglobin >18 g/dL, MCV >100 fL, MCV <80 fL, MCHC >37%, WBC >20,000/mm^3, WBC <2000/mm^3, presence of sickle cells, significant spherocytosis, basophilic stippling, stomatocytes, significant schistocytosis, oval macrocytes, tear drop red blood cells, eosinophilia (>10%) monocytosis

(>15%), nucleated red blood cells in other than the newborn, malarial organisms or the possibility of malarial organisms, hypersegmented (five or more nuclear segments) PMNs, agranular PMNs, Pelger-Huët anomaly, Auer rods, Döhle bodies, marked toxic granulation, mononuclears in which apparent nucleoli are prominent (blast type cells), presence of metamyelocytes, myelocytes, promyelocytes, neutropenia, presence of plasma cells, peculiar atypical lymphocytes, significant increase or decrease in platelets. Some quantitative elements of the CBC are related to each other, normally, such that examination of the results of any individual analysis allow for the application of a simple but effective case individualized quality control maneuver. The RBC count, hemoglobin, and hematocrit may be analyzed by applying a "rule of three." If red cells are normochromic/normocytic, the RBC count times three should approximately equal the hemoglobin and the hemoglobin multiplied by three should approximate the hematocrit.[3] If there is significant deviation from this relation, one should check for supporting abnormalities in RBC indices and peripheral smear. The indices themselves offer a quick quality control check of the CBC. If patient transfusion can be excluded, then RBC indices should vary little consecutively from day to day.

Histograms of red cell, white cell, platelet, and hemoglobin distributions have important application to quality assurance, analyzer trouble shooting, and patient diagnosis. Such histograms are usually not charted in patients' medical records but are available for review in the clinical laboratory. See reference by Gulati and Hyun, below, for review of the "Value of Histograms."

Anemias have been classified on the basis of their MCV and RDW (RBC heterogeneity). This classification has been especially helpful in the separation of iron deficiency from thalassemia. Heterozygous thalassemia (thalassemia minor) when associated with normal hemoglobin has a normal RDW (13.4 ±1.2%) while RDW is high with iron deficiency (16.3 ±1.8%).[4] RDW will be increased slightly in cases of thalassemia with slight anemia.[4] Some studies have found that the RDW does not reliably separate iron deficiency from thalassemia minor unless, possibly, a higher cutoff value of 17.0% is utilized.[5] See also the listing Ferritin, Serum *on page 127* and references by Jiménez and by Erler BS, et al, concerning, respectively, discriminant analysis and neural networks using elements of the CBC in differentiating thalassemia trait from iron deficiency.

In patients who do not have disorders known to result in anisocytosis (eg, liver disease, alcoholism, combined nutritional deficiency) and who have not received a recent blood transfusion, it has been claimed RDW may be helpful in separating the anemia of chronic disease (RDW in normal range) from iron deficiency (RDW increased) thereby reducing the need for marrow study to determine iron stores.[6] It has also been reported, however, on the basis of serum ferritin levels in relatively undefined patient populations that RDW is not clinically useful in distinguishing the anemia of chronic disease from iron deficiency.[7] In some 30% to 50% of patients with anemia of chronic disease, red cells are hypochromic and microcytic, often with decreased serum iron, iron (Continued)

Complete Blood Count *(Continued)*

binding capacity and transferrin saturation even with demonstrably adequate iron stores.[8]

Bessman claims that the RDW is increased before the MCV decreases in iron deficiency.[9] Although this is somewhat controversial,[10] perhaps even a simple marketing tool copied by all hematology instrument manufacturers, it serves as an inexpensive screen for the common iron deficiency anemia. See tables. The histogram of MCHCs as provided by Technicon® H series of instruments is of value in the diagnosis of hereditary spherocytosis[11] and the differentiation of α- from β-thalassemic red cells.[12]

As might be anticipated, the RDW is an insensitive parameter for the diagnosis of vitamin B_{12} deficiency, as well as for the diagnosis of folate deficiency, and the RDW has no value in separating alcohol-related macrocytosis from B_{12}/folate deficiency.[13] It has been found that in a hospitalized urban patient population, zidovudine treatment of AIDS is the most common cause of macrocytosis (44%) and B_{12}/folate deficiency are relatively decreased (3% and 4%, respectively).[14]

For consideration of the differential leukocyte count see listing Peripheral Blood: Differential Leukocyte Count *on page 336* and also reference by Krause JR.

Footnotes

1. "Recommendations of the International Council for Standardization in Haematology for Ethylenediaminetetraacetic Acid Anticoagulation of Blood for Blood Cell Counting and Sizing," *Am J Clin Pathol*, 1993, 100(4):371-2.
2. Dosik H and Prasad B, "Coulter S Hematocrit and Microhematocrit in Polycythemic Patients," *Am J Hematol*, 1978, 5:51-4.
3. Lofsness KG, "Correlation of Hematologic Data From the Individual Patient as a Quality Control Tool," *Am J Med Technol*, 1983, 49:655-9.
4. Bessman JD Jr, Gilmer PR, and Gardner FH, "Improved Classification of Anemias by MCV and RDW," *Am J Clin Pathol*, 1983, 80:322-6.
5. van Zeben D, Bieger R, van Wermeskerken RK, et al, "Evaluation of Microcytosis Using Serum Ferritin and Red Blood Cell Distribution Width," *Eur J Haematol*, 1990, 44(2):106-9.
6. Kaye FJ and Alter BP, "Red-Cell Size Distribution Analysis: An Evaluation of Microcytic Anemia in Chronically Ill Patients," *Mt Sinai J Med*, 1985, 52(5):319-23.
7. Rice LE, Saleem A, Dunn K, et al, "RDW Fails to Distinguish Iron-Deficiency From Anemia of Chronic Disease," *Blood*, 1987, 70:55a.
8. Krantz SB, "Pathogenesis and Treatment of the Anemia of Chronic Disease," *Am J Med Sci*, 1994, 307(5):353-9.
9. McClure S, Custer E, and Bessman JD, "Improved Detection of Early Iron Deficiency in Nonanemic Subjects," *JAMA*, 1985, 253(7):1021-3.
10. Flynn MM, Reppun TS, and Bhagavan NV, "Limitations of Red Cell Distribution Width (RDW) in Evaluation of Microcytosis," *Am J Clin Pathol*, 1986, 85(4):445-9.
11. Lux SE and Palek J, "Disorders of the Red Cell Membrane," *Blood: Principles and Practice of Hematology*, Chapter 54, Handin RI, Lux SE, and Stossel TP, eds, Philadelphia, PA: JB Lippincott Co, 1995, 1701.
12. Bunyaratvej A, Fucharoen S, Greenbaum A, et al, "Hydration of Red Cells in Alpha and Beta Thalassemias Differs. A Useful Approach to Distinguish Between These Red Cell Phenotypes," *Am J Clin Pathol*, 1994, 102(2):217-22.
13. Zuiable A and Wickramasinghe SN, "RDW in Vitamin B_{12} and Folate Deficiency and in Patients With Alcohol-Related Macrocytosis," *Clin Lab Haematol*, 1992, 14(2):164-6.
14. Snower DP and Weil SC, "Changing Etiology of Macrocytosis: Zidovudine as a Frequent Causative Factor," *Am J Clin Pathol*, 1993, 99(1):57-60.

References

Al-Ismail SA, Bond K, Carter AB, et al, "Two-Centre Evaluation of the Abbott CD3500 Blood Counter," *Clin Lab Haematol*, 1995, 17(1):11-21.

Bentley SA, Johnson A, and Bishop CA, "A Parallel Evaluation of Four Automated Hematology Analyzers," *Am J Clin Pathol*, 1993, 100(6):626-32.

Burgess PR, Kershaw GW, "A Computerized Expert System for Handling the Output of the Technicon H-1 Haematology Analyser," *Clin Lab Haematol*, 1993, 15(1):21-32.

Cornbleet PJ, Myrick D, and Levy R, "Evaluation of the Coulter STKS Five-Part Differential," *Am J Clin Pathol*, 1993, 99(1):72-81.

Dot D, Miró J, and Fuentes-Arderiu X, "Within-Subject Biological Variation of Hematological Quantities and Analytical Goals," *Arch Pathol Lab Med*, 1992, 116(8):825-6.

Erler BS, Vitagliano P, and Lee S, "Superiority of Neural Networks Over Discriminant Functions for Thalassemia Minor Screening of Red Blood Cell Microcytosis," *Arch Pathol Lab Med*, 1995, 119(4):350-4.

Fraser CG, Wilkinson SP, Neville RG, et al, "Biologic Variation of Common Hematologic Laboratory Quantities in the Elderly," *Am J Clin Pathol*, 1989, 92(4):465-70.

Gulati GL and Hyun BH, "An Unusual WBC Scattergram and Its Possible Causes," *Lab Med*, 1996, 27(6):398-9.

Gulati GL and Hyun BH, "The Automated CBC: A Current Perspective," *Hematol Oncol Clin North Am*, 8(4):593-603.

Hoyer JD, "Leukocyte Differential," *Mayo Clin Proc*, 1993, 68(10):1027-8.

Hübl W, Hauptlorenz S, Tlustos L, et al, "Precision and Accuracy of Monocyte Counting: Comparison of Two Hematology Analyzers, the Manual Differential and Flow Cytometry," *Am J Clin Pathol*, 1995, 103(2):167-70.

Jiménez CV, "Iron-Deficiency Anemia and Thalassemia Trait Differentiated by Simple Hematological Tests and Serum Iron Concentrations," *Clin Chem*, 1993, 39(11):2271-5.

Johnson CL, Gerson B, Nunez M, et al, "Field Evaluation of the NOVA Celltrak 12 Hematology Analyzer," *Am J Clin Pathol*, 1994, 100:36-9.

Jones RG, Faust AM, and Matthews RA, "Quality Team Approach in Evaluating Three Automated Hematology Analyzers With Five-Part Differential Capability," *Am J Clin Pathol*, 1995, 103(2):159-66.

Koepke J, "Quantitative Blood Cell Counting," *Practical Laboratory Hematology*, Chapter 3, Koepke JA, ed, New York, NY: Churchill Livingstone, 1991, 43-60.

Krause JR, "The Automated White Blood Cell Differential: A Current Perspective," *Hematol Oncol Clin North Am*, 1994, 8(4):605-16.

Lee GR, "Microcytosis and the Anemias Associated With Impaired Hemoglobin Synthesis," *Wintrobe's Clinical Hematology*, 9th ed, Vol 1, Chapter 25, Lee GR, Bithell TC, Foerster J, et al, eds, Philadelphia, PA: Lea & Febiger, 1993, 791-807.

Lewis SM, England JM, and Rowan RM, "Current Concerns in Haematology 3: Blood Count Calibration," *J Clin Pathol*, 1991, 44(11):881-4.

Rowan RM and England JM, "Special Aspects in Haematology," *Evaluation Methods in Laboratory Medicine*, Chapter 7, Haeckel R, ed, New York, NY: VCH Publishers, 1993, 141-51.

Second National Health and Nutrition Examination Survey, "Hematological and Nutritional Biochemistry Reference Data for Persons 6 Months-74 Years of Age: United States, 1976-80," *Vital and Health Statistics*, DHHS Publication No (PHS) 83-1682, 1982.

Sheridan BL, Lollo M, Howe S, et al, "Evaluation of the Roche Cobas Argos 5Diff Automated Haematology Analyser With Comparison to a Coulter STKS," *Clin Lab Haematol*, 1994, 16(2):117-30.

van Duijnhoven HL and Treskes M, "Marked Interference of Hyperglycemia in Measurements of Mean (Red) Cell Volume by Technicon H Analyzers," *Clin Chem*, 1996, 42(1):76-80.

Viteri FE, deTuna V, and Guzmán MA, "Normal Haematological Values in the Central American Population," *Br J Haematol*, 1972, 23(2):189-213.

^{51}Cr-Labeled Red Cell Volume *see* Red Cell Mass *on page 345*

^{51}Cr Red Cell Survival

CPT 78130; 78135 (with splenic and/or hepatic sequestration)

Related Information

Occult Blood, Stool *on page 645*

Reticulocyte Count *on page 345*

Synonyms Chromium-51 Tagged RBC Survival Test; Erythrocyte Survival; Red Cell Survival; Survival of Red Blood Cells

Patient Preparation Obtain signed procedure permit for "^{51}Cr red cell survival." Patient's own ^{51}Cr-labeled red cells are infused. Patient should be provided a schedule for serial blood samples to be drawn.

Specimen Whole blood is drawn, processed (tagged with ^{51}Cr), and reinfused into the patient.

Container Lavender top (EDTA) tube

Collection Scheduled periodic blood samples are drawn for determination of residual radioactivity.

Causes for Rejection Previous isotope procedure with significant radioactivity remaining in patient's blood, significant transfused blood, intermittent bleeding episodes

Turnaround Time Time required for procedure depends on half-time of disappearance of labeled cells and averages 3 weeks.

Special Instructions At least 21 days should be allowed for this study. When selective splenic sequestration as cause of hemolysis is suspected, liver and spleen readings may be performed in conjunction with ^{51}Cr RBC Survival Test.

Reference Range Presence of half of ^{51}Cr label remaining at 25-35 days (red cell survival half-life of 25-35 days).[1] Given an isotope label that would act as a "perfect" tracer (no loss through elution), one would expect half of the label to disappear at about 55-60 days, half of the average red cell life span of 110-120 days (see discussion that follows). The ratio of spleen to liver counts is usually 1:1 in normal individuals.

Use Provide proof of hemolytic process (ie, determine if patient's RBCs have decreased survival); determine red cell survival in cases of increased red cell destruction (ie, immunohemolytic anemia;[2] spherocytosis, red cell enzyme deficiency, and hemoglobinopathies); evaluate occult blood loss, especially subdural hematomas,[3] and splenic sequestration. In the spleen/liver (S/L) ratio, the average patient with splenomegaly ratio is 1:1; hemolytic anemias show 3:1 or 4:1.

Limitations This test cannot discriminate between red cell loss due to intravascular hemolysis and red cell loss due to bleeding that results in blood loss from the intravascular compartment. Test is expensive.

Methodology Patient's own RBCs incubated with ^{51}Cr under sterile conditions are injected back into the patient's vascular system and periodic blood samples are obtained for measurement of residual radioactivity over a 2- to 3-week period. Activity (counts/minute/mL of RBCs) obtained at 24 hours is usually taken as the starting point (is given a value of 100%). A plot is constructed (should include hematocrit correction)[4] and the ^{51}Cr half-life is determined.

Additional Information The ^{51}Cr red cell survival does not equate numerically with one-half of the physiologic RBC lifespan (110-120 days). This is due to elution of the ^{51}Cr label from red cells during the procedure. As a result, the ^{51}Cr survival time does not relate in a simple or direct manner to the red cell lifespan and is best viewed as a semiquantitative index of survival. Given a "perfect" label, half of the activity would be lost at 55-60 days. Di-isopropylfluorophosphate (DFP) ^{14}C, ^{32}P, or tritium labels act, essentially, as a perfect label but are not in common routine clinical use as, lacking gamma emission, imaging or organ uptake studies cannot be performed. In patients with hemolysis, the RBC survival curve results from the rate of elution of the label combined with the rate of random hemolysis. In addition to DFP, red cells may be labeled for survival studies with ^{14}C cyanate, ^{75}Se selenomethionine, ^{14}C or ^{15}N glycine or ^{55}Fe or ^{59}Fe iron. Because of the penetrance capability of gamma emitting ^{51}Cr, patients with ^{51}Cr-labeled RBCs can undergo *in* *vivo* count rate measurements over the spleen and liver during red cell survival study. See reference by Landaw for clinical significance of spleen/liver ratio, RBC sequestration index, and RBC survival.

Footnotes

1. International Committee for Standardization in Haematology, "Recommended Method for Radioisotope Red-Cell Survival Studies," *Br J Haematol*, 1980, 45:659-66.
2. Levy GJ, Selset G, McQuiston D, et al, "Clinical Significance of Anti-Yt^b. Report of a Case Using ^51Chromium Red Cell Survival Study," *Transfusion*, 1988, 28(3):265-7.
3. Ito H, Yamamoto S, Saito K, et al, "Quantitative Estimation of Hemorrhage in Chronic Subdural Hematoma Using the ^51Cr Erythrocyte Labeling Method," *J Neurosurg*, 1987, 66(6):862-4.
4. Milam JD, Samuels MS, Hidalgo JU, et al, "Use of Hematocrit Values in Evaluation of Red Cell Survival With Chromium-51," *Am J Clin Pathol*, 1966, 45:56-60.

References

Brucer M, "How Long Will Red Cells Last?" "Development of the Red Cell Survival Test," *Vignettes in Nuclear Medicine*, St Louis, MO: Mallinckrodt Chemical Works, 1973, 55.
Henry JB, Nelson DA, Tomar RH, et al, *Todd-Sanford-Davidsohn Clinical Diagnosis and Management by Laboratory Methods*, 18th ed, Philadelphia, PA: WB Saunders Co, 1991, 642-3.
Landaw SA, "Hemostasis, Survival, and Red Cell Kinetics: Measurement and Imaging of Red Cell Production," *Hematology Basic Principles and Practice*, 2nd ed, Chapter 34, Hoffman R, Benz EJ Jr, Shattil SJ, et al, eds, New York, NY: Churchill Livingstone, 1995, 448-58.
Langan JK, Scheffel U, and McIntyre PA, "The Hematopoietic System," *Nuclear Medicine Technology and Techniques*, Chapter 18, Bernier DR, Christian PE, Langan JK, et al, eds, St Louis, MO: Mosby-Year Book Inc, 1989, 493-5.

CSF Analysis *see* Cerebrospinal Fluid Analysis *on page 309*

Cyanocobalamin, True *see* Vitamin B$_{12}$ *on page 351*

Cyst Fluid Analysis *see* Body Fluid Analysis, Cell Count *on page 306*

Cytochemistry, Leukocyte *see* Leukocyte Cytochemistry *on page 331*

Cytokines *see* Eosinophil Count *on this page*

Differential *see* Peripheral Blood: Differential Leukocyte Count *on page 336*

Differential Smear *see* Peripheral Blood: Differential Leukocyte Count *on page 336*

Dithionite Test *see* Sickle Cell Tests *on page 347*

Donath-Landsteiner Test *see* Cold Hemolysin Test *on page 311*

Eos Count *see* Eosinophil Count *on this page*

Eosinophil Count

CPT 85999

Related Information

Complete Blood Count *on page 312*
Eosinophil Smear *on next page*
Muramidase, Blood and Urine *on page 333*
Ova and Parasites, Stool *on page 494*
Ova and Parasites, Urine *on page 495*
Parasite Antibodies *on page 421*
Peripheral Blood: Differential Leukocyte Count *on page 336*
Thorn Test *on page 350*

Synonyms Absolute Eosinophil Count; Eos Count; Total Eosinophil Count

Applies to Cytokines; Granulocyte/Macrophage Colony Stimulating Factor; Interleukin-3; Interleukin-5

Abstract Manual (using phloxine stain) or automated absolute eosinophil count is requested in certain clinical situations because of expected greater precision/accuracy than is usually obtained using the relative number of eosinophils from the manual differential count. Eosinophil count is increased in a wide variety of conditions including especially, allergy, drug reaction, parasitism, collagen vascular disease, and some malignant states. Eosinophils are decreased with hyperadrenalism.

Specimen Whole blood

Container Lavender top (EDTA) tube

Causes for Rejection Clotted specimen, specimen more than 4 hours old

Reference Range 50-350/mm³

Use Aid in the diagnosis of allergy, drug reaction, parasitic infestations, collagen disease, Hodgkin's disease, and myeloproliferative diseases. Increased also in a broad range of less common conditions including the acute hypereosinophilic syndrome, angioneurotic edema, acute renal allograft rejection, eosinophilic nonallergic rhinitis, anisakiasis,[1] eosinophilic gastroenteritis,[2] eosinophilia myalgia syndrome,[3] and others. Decrease in eosinophils occurs in Cushing's disease (hyperadrenalism).

Limitations Manual method is subject to an inherent error of 20% to 30%.[4]

Methodology Manual, using Fuchs-Rosenthal or Speirs-Levy special large volume hemocytometer and eosinophil stain diluent (eg, Pilot's

solution or phloxine B solution as used in the Unopette™ Brand System, Becton Dickinson, Rutherford, NJ). Automated method (eg, Technicon®, Coulter, Sysmex) should provide greater precision/accuracy and is recommended for obtaining an absolute eosinophil count.[4]

Additional Information Toxocaral disease (visceral larva migrans) is a typical parasitic disease in which eosinophil counts (eosinophils >30% on differential) are usually elevated. Taylor et al[5] point out, however, that up to 27% of children with toxocariasis have normal eosinophil counts. Thus, normal eosinophil counts do not rule out toxocaral disease or other parasitic infestations. The T-cell produced cytokines interleukin-3, granulocyte/macrophage colony stimulating factor, and interleukin-5 (IL-5) stimulate eosinophil production *in vitro*. Murine eosinophil differentiation factor (IL-5) has its most specific effect on eosinophil growth in culture with no significant effect on growth/development of other myeloid cell lines.[6] IL-5 appears to be the prime mediator of eosinophilia in patients with certain parasitic diseases.[7,8] Type 2 helper T cells (CD4+,CD3-), which can produce interleukin-4 (stimulates IgE antibody production) and interleukin-5 (promotes the differentiation and activation of eosinophils) may be involved in causing the hypereosinophilic syndrome.[9]

An important although rare cause of increased eosinophils in the peripheral blood is the acute hypereosinophilic syndrome (HES). Reported mortalities range from 81% to 95% in 1-3 years. The HES syndrome includes high peripheral WBC count, circulating early eosinophil forms without blast cells, mental confusion, delusions, near coma, and severe cardiac symptoms. Consistently associated with a poor prognosis are WBC count ≥90,000/mm³, blast forms in blood, heart failure, and severe CNS symptoms (confusion, organic psychosis and coma). This condition may not be a true leukemic myeloproliferative disease, although concepts of HES are controversial.

Infiltrative lung diseases, in which peripheral blood eosinophils may be increased, include eosinophilic pneumonia, Löffler's syndrome (often related to *Ascaris* infestation), and tropical eosinophilia (usually related to filariasis).[10]

Eosinophilic gastroenteritis may occur with blood eosinophilia.[2]

Eosinophilia myalgia syndrome (EMS) characterized by an eosinophil count of 1000 cells/mm³ or more and severe often incapacitating myalgia is possibly associated with the use of L-tryptophan-containing products (LTCPs). Further definition of this syndrome, causal association between LTCPs and EMS, and modifying etiologic factors/cofactors has been recommended and is being pursued by CDC.[3,11] An EMS-like syndrome has been considered to result from several factors including ingestion of tryptophan, inactivation of indoleamine-2,3-dioxygenase, and possible impairment of the hypothalamic-pituitary-adrenal axis.[12] The differential diagnosis of EMS (causes other than L-tryptophan) is discussed by Dicker et al (see References). Sarcoidosis, granulomatous myositis, collagen vascular diseases, neoplastic myositis, and other entities should be considered. EMS is potentially fatal (Guillain-Barré like ascending polyneuropathy) with a clinical course resembling the toxic oil syndrome that was epidemic in Spain in 1981.[13]

Footnotes

1. Valdiserri, RO, "Intestinal Anisakiasis. Report of a Case and Recovery of Larvae From Market Fish," *Am J Clin Pathol*, 1981, 76:329-33.
2. Pavli P and Doe WF, "The Alimentary Tract in Disorders of the Immune System," *Gastrointestinal and Oesophageal Pathology*, Whitehead R, ed, Edinburgh, England: Churchill Livingstone, 1989, 187.
3. Centers for Disease Control, "Eosinophilia-Myalgia Syndrome - New Mexico," *MMWR Morb Mortal Wkly Rep*, 1989, 38(45):765-7.
4. McNeely JC and Brown D, "Laboratory Evaluation of Leukocytes: Absolute Eosinophil Counting Procedure," *Clinical Hematology: Principles, Procedures, Correlations*, Chapter 25, Lotspeich-Steininger CA, Stiene-Martin EA, and Koepke JA, eds, Philadelphia, PA: JB Lippincott Co, 1992, 329-31.
5. Taylor MR, Keane CT, O'Connor P, et al, "The Expanded Spectrum of Toxocaral Disease," *Lancet*, 1988, 1(8587):692-5.
6. Clutterbuck EJ, Hirst EM, and Sanderson CJ, "Human Interleukin-5 (IL-5) Regulates the Production of Eosinophils in Human Bone Marrow Cultures: Comparison and Interaction With IL-1, IL-3, IL-6, and GMCSF," *Blood*, 1989, 73(6):1504-12.
7. Limaye AP, Abrams JS, Silver JE, et al, "Regulation of Parasitic Induced Eosinophilia: Selectively Increased Interleukin-5 Production in Helminth-Infected Patients," *J Exp Med*, 1990, 172(1):399-402.
8. Limaye AP, Abrams JS, Silver JE, et al, "Interleukin-5 and the Post-treatment Eosinophilia in Patients With Onchocerciasis," *J Clin Invest*, 1991, 88(4):1418-21.
9. Cogan E, Schandené L, Crusiaux A, et al, "Brief Report: Clonal Proliferation of Type 2 Helper T Cells in a Man With the Hypereosinophilic Syndrome," *N Engl J Med*, 1994, 330(8):535-8.
10. Colby TV and Carrington CB, "Infiltrative Lung Disease," Chapter 20, *Pathology of the Lung*, Thurlbeck WM, ed, New York, NY: Thieme Medical Publishers Inc, 1988, 425-517.
11. Centers for Disease Control, "Eosinophilia-Myalgia Syndrome and L-Tryptophan-Containing Products - New Mexico, Minnesota, Oregon and New York," *MMWR Morb Mortal Wkly Rep*, 1989, 38(46):785-8.
12. Silver RM, Heyes MP, Maize JC, et al, "Scleroderma, Fasciitis, and Eosinophilia Associated With the Ingestion of Tryptophan," *N Engl J Med*, 1990, 322(13):874-81.
13. Kilbourne EM, Rigau-Perez JG, Heath CW Jr, et al, "Clinical Epidemiology of Toxic-Oil Syndrome: Manifestations of a New Illness," *N Engl J Med*, 1983, 309:1408-14.

References

Dicker RM, James N, and Cunha BA, "The Eosinophilia-Myalgia Syndrome With Neuritis Associated With L-Tryptophan Use," *Ann Intern Med*, 1990, 112(12):957-8.
Duffy J, "Eosinophilia-Myalgia Syndrome," *Mayo Clin Proc*, 1992, 67(12):1201-2.

(Continued)

Eosinophil Count *(Continued)*

Galli SJ and Goetzl EJ, "Eosinophils, Basophils, and Mast Cells," *Blood: Principles and Practice of Hematology*, Chapter 20, Handin RI, Lux E, and Stossel TP, eds, Philadelphia, PA: JB Lippincott Co, 1995, 621-40.

Martin RW, Duffy J, Engel AG, et al, "The Clinical Spectrum of the Eosinophilia-Myalgia Syndrome Associated With L-Tryptophan Ingestion. Clinical Features in 20 Patients and Aspects of Pathophysiology," *Ann Intern Med*, 1990, 113(9):124-34.

Mayeno AN, Belongia EA, Lin F, et al, "3-(Phenylamino)alanine, a Novel Aniline-Derived Amino Acid Associated With the Eosinophilia-Myalgia Syndrome: A Link to the Toxic Oil Syndrome?" *Mayo Clin Proc*, 1992, 67(12):1134-9.

Randolph TG, "Differentiation and Enumeration of Eosinophils in the Counting Chamber With a Glycol Stain; A Valuable Technique in Appraising ACTH Dosage," *J Lab Clin Med*, 1949, 34:1696-1701.

Van Slyck EJ and Adamson TC III, "Acute Hypereosinophilic Syndrome. Successful Treatment With Vincristine, Cytarabine, and Prednisone," *JAMA*, 1979, 242:175-6.

Smith H and Cook RM, *Immunopharmacology of Eosinophils, The Handbook of Immunopharmacology*, San Diego, CA: Academic Press, 1993, 1-250.

Eosinophil Smear

CPT 89190

Related Information

Eosinophil Count *on previous page*

Synonyms Fecal Smear for Eosinophils; Nasal Smear for Eosinophils; Sputum Smear for Eosinophils

Specimen Two slides of nasal secretion, smear or swab of feces or sputum. No fixation is required for slides. Nasal secretions may be submitted on wax paper or plastic wrap.

Container Slides or nasal secretions on wax paper

Causes for Rejection Slides received in cytology fixative, no specimen on slide, smear, or swab

Special Instructions Requisition must state site of specimen.

Reference Range No eosinophils identified

Use Investigate allergy, asthmatic disorders, and parasitic infestations

Methodology Wright's stain and microscopic examination of smear

Additional Information Eosinophils are often increased in the blood and sputum of patients with asthma, usually in relation to the severity of the process.[1] There is no percentage of eosinophils in sputum diagnostic of asthma, but levels >80% (related to proportion of neutrophils) are very suggestive of asthma or of chronic bronchitis with wheezing. There is evidence of an inverse correlation between the numbers of eosinophils in the circulation and/or sputum and pulmonary function (eg, airway flow rates).[2,3,4] Gram's stained smears of microbiology specimens will not stain eosinophils.

Footnotes

1. Busse WW and Sedgwick JB, "Eosinophils in Asthma," *Ann Allergy*, 1992, 68(3):286-90.
2. Griffin E, Håkansson L, Formgren H, et al, "Blood Eosinophil Number and Activity in Relation to Lung Function in Patients With Asthma and With Eosinophilia," *J Allergy Clin Immunol*, 1991, 87(2):548-57.
3. O'Connor GT, Sparrow D, and Weiss ST, "The Role of Allergy and Nonspecific Airway Hyperresponsiveness in the Pathogenesis of Chronic Obstructive Pulmonary Disease," *Am Rev Respir Dis*, 1989, 140(1):225-52.
4. Alfaro C, Sharma OP, Navarro L, et al, "Inverse Correlation of Expiratory Lung Flows and Sputum Eosinophils in Status Asthmaticus," *Ann Allergy*, 1989, 63(3):251-4.

References

Middleton E Jr, "Chronic Rhinitis in Adults," *J Allergy Clin Immunol*, 1988, 81(5 Pt 2):971-5.

Viera VG and Prolla JC, "Clinical Evaluation of Eosinophils in the Sputum," *J Clin Pathol*, 1979, 32:1054-7.

Erythrocyte Count *see* Red Cell Count *on page 344*

Erythrocyte Enzyme Deficiency, Quantitative *see* Red Blood Cell Enzyme Deficiency, Quantitative *on page 342*

Erythrocyte Enzyme Deficiency Screen *see* Red Blood Cell Enzyme Deficiency Screen *on page 343*

Erythrocyte Indices *see* Red Blood Cell Indices *on page 343*

Erythrocyte Membrane Skeleton Gelation Assay *see* Gelation Assay *on page 318*

Erythrocyte Sedimentation Rate *see* Zeta Sedimentation Ratio *on page 354*

Erythrocyte Survival *see* ^{51}Cr Red Cell Survival *on page 314*

Extrinsic Factor of Castle *see* Vitamin B_{12} *on page 351*

Fecal Smear for Eosinophils *see* Eosinophil Smear *on this page*

Fetal Hemoglobin

CPT 83030

Related Information

Hemoglobin Electrophoresis *on page 324*
Kleihauer-Betke *on page 329*
Sickle Cell Tests *on page 347*

Synonyms Hb F; Hemoglobin, Fetal

Specimen Whole blood

Container Lavender top (EDTA) tube for venipuncture specimen; lavender top Microtainer™ tube for capillary specimen

Reference Range 6 months to adult: up to 2% of the total hemoglobin; 0-6 months: up to 75%

Use Evaluate hemoglobinopathies, hemolytic anemia; diagnose hereditary persistence of fetal hemoglobin, thalassemia; evaluate sickling hemoglobins

Limitations Carboxyhemoglobin A is also resistant to alkali denaturation. Assay for Hb F should initially convert carboxyhemoglobin to cyanmethemoglobin or false-positive elevations of Hb F may be obtained.[1]

Methodology Alkali denaturation, high resolution hemoglobin electrophoresis (some methods), acid elution (Kleihauer-Betke), radial immunodiffusion (RID), isoelectric focusing, high performance liquid chromatography (HPLC), enzyme immunoassay (EIA)[2]

Additional Information Fetal hemoglobin is formed of two α-chains and two γ-chains. It is the major hemoglobin during fetal life. Hb F levels decrease after birth by about 3% to 4% per week. In 2-3 weeks fetal hemoglobin is about 65%. By 6 months of age fetal hemoglobin is <2% of the total hemoglobin. See graph. The oxygen dissociation curve of Hb F is shifted to the left as compared with normal Hb A. This may be due to decreased binding of 2,3-DPG by Hb F (γ-chains). This facilitates placental oxygen transfer. With erythroblastosis fetalis and anoxic states of the newborn, however, Hb F is proportionally lower than in a normal newborn. Over 15 inherited abnormalities of γ-chain structure have been described[3], but most are without clinical significance (fetal Hgb normally forms <2% of total hemoglobin). An exception is Hb F Poole which has been reported as a cause of hemolytic disease of the newborn.[4]

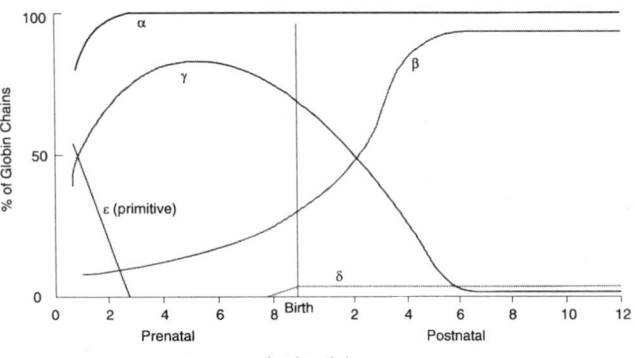

Relative amounts of the several globin chains (ε, α, γ, β, and δ) present during fetal development and the first year of life.

In the adult, hereditary persistence of fetal hemoglobin (HPFH) of multiple varieties, is associated with varying elevations of Hb F. The homozygous form of HPFH is found only in African-Americans. In the heterozygous state, the Hb F level is 15% to 35% in the black type, and 5% to 20% in the Greek type. Homozygous β-thalassemia is associated with Hb F levels >10% to <90%. About 50% of heterozygotes for β-thalassemia have elevated levels around 2%, rarely >5%. The remainder have normal Hb F. Using elements of the CBC, discriminant analysis[5] and use of neural networks have been applied to the differentiation of heterozygous thalassemia from iron deficiency anemia.[6] Heterozygous S/β thalassemia may have Hb F in the 5% to 20% range. With homozygous Hb S disease the level of Hb F varies from 0% to 20%.[7] Hgb F inhibits the polymerization of sickle hemoglobin exerting an ameliorating effect on the sickle disease process. Other conditions associated with elevated Hb F include various anemias, spherocytosis, Fanconi's, acquired aplastic, hemolytic, hypoplastic, megaloblastic, myelophthisic, and untreated pernicious anemia; all types of leukemia (especially erythroleukemia and juvenile chronic myelogenous leukemia), multiple myeloma and lymphomas, metastatic disease of the bone marrow; pregnancy; miscellaneous disorders reported include infants small for gestational age, infants with chronic intrauterine anoxia with developmental anomalies; during anticonvulsant drug therapy; diabetes; hyper and hypothyroidism; and macroglobulin. Elevation of Hb F should, then, raise the question of possible underlying disease.

The oxyhemoglobin dissociation curve for Hb F compared to Hb A shows a "left shift" (greater affinity of Hb F c.f. Hb A). Mutant Hb F with decreased oxygen affinity is in the differential diagnosis of newborns presenting with cyanosis of unknown cause.[10] Hb F also causes interference with the laboratory measurement of percent saturation with O_2 and with measurement of fraction of oxygenated hemoglobin. There are a variety of approaches to correction for the effect of Hb F.[8] Modern Co-oximeter instruments nearly eliminate interference by Hb F through appropriate selection of light wavelengths. Neither Hb F nor bilirubin in

Nonmalignant Conditions Associated With Increased Proportions of Hb F

Condition	Hb F Value (%)
Anemias	
Aplastic anemia (both congenital and acquired)	5-25
Pernicious anemia	2-6
Hereditary spherocytosis	2-5
Hereditary elliptocytosis	2-5
Congenital nonspherocytic hemolytic anemia	3-4
Anemia of chronic infection	2-3
Anemia of blood loss	2-8
Erythropoietic porphyria	2-10
Paroxysmal nocturnal hemoglobinuria	2-25
Hemoglobinopathies	
Unstable hemoglobins	<10
Homozygous Hb S disease	<20
Hb Lepore trait	<5
Hb Kenya trait	6-13
Thalassemias	
β-thalassemia minor	<5
δβ-thalassemia minor	5-20
β-thalassemia major	30-95
α-thalassemia minor	~ 1
Hb H disease	5-15
Hemoglobinopathy-thalassemia interactions	
S/β-thalassemia	10-30
E/β-thalassemia	10-50
C/β-thalassemia	10-30
Hereditary persistence of fetal hemoglobin (HPFH)	
African-type	
heterozygous	15-40
homozygous	100
Greek-type	
heterozygous	10-20
Swiss-type	
heterozygous	1-3

blood causes clinically significant interference with COHb measurement such that COHb could be used to assist in the diagnosis of hemolysis in the newborn.[9]

Footnotes

1. Hoagland HC, "Interpretation of Increased Concentration of Hemoglobin F," *Hemoglobinopathies and Thalassemias: Laboratory Methods and Case Studies*, Fairbanks VF, ed, New York, NY: Thieme-Stratton Inc, 1980, 69.
2. Moscoso H, Shyamala M, Kiefer CR, et al, "Monoclonal Antibody to the γ-Chain of Human Fetal Hemoglobin Used to Develop an Enzyme Immunoassay," *Clin Chem*, 1989, 35(10):2066-9.
3. Weatherall DJ, Clegg JB, Higgs DR, et al, "The Hemoglobinopathies," *The Metabolic and Molecular Basis of Inherited Disease*, 7th ed, vol 111, Scriver CR, Beaudet AL, Sly WS, et al, eds, New York, NY: McGraw-Hill Inc, 1995, 3417-84.
4. Lee-Potter JP, Deacon-Smith RA, Simpkiss MJ, et al, "A New Cause of Hemolytic Anemia in the Newborn. A Description of an Unstable Fetal Hemoglobin: F. Poole, $\alpha_2\gamma_2$ 130 Tryptophan Yields Glycine," *J Clin Pathol*, 1975, 28:317-20.
5. Jiménez CV, "Iron-Deficiency Anemia and Thalassemia Trait Differentiated by Simple Hematological Tests and Serum Iron Concentrations," *Clin Chem*, 1993, 39(11 Pt 1):2271-5.
6. Erler BS, Vitagliano P, and Lee S, "Superiority of Neural Networks Over Discriminant Functions for Thalassemia Minor Screening of Red Blood Cell Microcytosis," *Arch Pathol Lab Med*, 1995, 119(4):350-4.
7. Warth JA and Rucknagal DL, "The Increasing Complexity of Sickle Cell Anemia," *Prog Hematol*, 1983, 13:25-47.
8. Moran RF, "Hemoglobin F and Measurement of Oxygen Saturation and Fractional Oxyhemoglobin," *Clin Lab Sci*, 1994, 7(3):162-4.
9. Vreman HJ and Stevenson DK, "Carboxyhemoglobin Determined in Neonatal Blood with a CO-Oximeter Unaffected by Fetal Oxyhemoglobin," *Clin Chem*, 1994, 40(8):1522-7.
10. Kohli-Kumar M, Zwerdling T, and Rucknagel DL, "Hemoglobin F-Cincinnati, $\alpha_2{}^G\gamma_2$ 41 (C7) Phe → Ser in a Newborn With Cyanosis," *Am J Hematol*, 1995, 49(1):43-7.

References

Bunn HF and Forget BG, *Hemoglobin: Molecular, Genetic and Clinical Aspects*, Philadelphia, PA: WB Saunders Co, 1986, 68-75.

Castro O, Winter WP, Lee TC, et al, "Prevalence of α-Chain Variants at Birth," *Am J Clin Pathol*, 1981, 75:56-9.

Embury SH and Mentzer WC, "The Thalassemia Syndromes," *The Hereditary Hemolytic Anemias*, Chapter 3, Mentzer WC and Wagner GM, New York, NY: Churchill Livingstone, 1989, 93-144.

Fucharoen S, Rowley PT, Paul NW, et al, *Thalassemia: Pathophysiology and Management*, March of Dimes Birth Defects Foundation Original Article Series, Vol 23, No 5A, New York, NY: Alan R Liss Inc, 1987.

Kaufman RE, "Analysis of Abnormal Hemoglobins," *Practical Laboratory Hematology*, Koepke JA, ed, New York, NY: Churchill Livingstone, 1991, 251-94.

Papadea C and Cate JC 4th, "Identification and Quantification of Hemoglobins A, F, S, and C by Automated Chromatography," *Clin Chem*, 1996, 42(1):57-63.

Steinberg MH, "Sickle Cell Anemia and Fetal Hemoglobin," *Am J Med Sci*, 1994, 308(5):259-65.

Fetal Hemoglobin Test in Newborn *see* APT Test *on page 304*

Filarial Infestation *see* Microfilariae, Peripheral Blood Preparation *on page 333*

Filariasis Peripheral Blood Preparation *see* Microfilariae, Peripheral Blood Preparation *on page 333*

Folate Level *see* Folic Acid, Serum *on this page*

Folic Acid, RBC

CPT 82747

Related Information

Complete Blood Count *on page 312*
d-Xylose Absorption Test *on page 122*
Folic Acid, Serum *on this page*
Hemoglobin *on page 323*
Parietal Cell Antibody *on page 421*
Schilling Test *on page 346*
Vitamin B$_{12}$ *on page 351*
Vitamin B$_{12}$ Unsaturated Binding Capacity *on page 352*

Synonyms RBC Folate; Red Cell Folate

Patient Preparation Avoid radioisotope scan prior to collection of specimen if RIA is used for assay.

Specimen Erythrocytes

Container Lavender top (EDTA) tube. Green top (heparin) tube may also be used for folate assay, but heparin interferes with vitamin B$_{12}$ determinations, which are often performed simultaneously.

Sampling Time Fasting specimen is preferred.

Storage Instructions Red cells (or hemolysate) can be stored at 4°C or frozen until assay.

Reference Range 125-600 ng/mL (SI: 283-1360 nmol/L). The megaloblastic anemia of folate deficiency is usually associated with red cell folate levels <100 ng/mL (SI: <227 nmol/L) RBCs.[1,2]

Use Detect folate deficiency

Methodology Radioimmunoassay (RIA), competitive protein binding

Additional Information Since serum folate values fluctuate significantly with diet, measurement of red cell folate is a better measure of tissue folate stores. It is widespread practice to measure serum and red cell folate with vitamin B$_{12}$ levels. A study of patients in an inner city area geriatric unit disclosed 50 cases with decreased vitamin B$_{12}$ and/or folate (serum and RBC levels) but without hematologic signs of megaloblastosis (all had MCV <100 fL).[3] Attention to clinical setting is important since a normal red cell folate level can be found in a rapidly developing folic acid deficiency such as the stress of pregnancy.[4] There is evidence that when RBC folate and D-xylose absorption tests, used as a noninvasive screen, are both normal, the predictive accuracy for absence of celiac disease is 100%. When used together, these tests were found ideal for selecting patients for jejunal biopsy from an otherwise unmanageable number with symptoms suggestive of celiac disease.[5]

Footnotes

1. McNeely MD, "Folic Acid," *Clinical Chemistry: Theory, Analysis, and Correlation*, 2nd ed, Kaplan LA and Pesce AJP, St Louis, MO: Mosby-Year Book Inc, 1989, 1131-2.
2. Bauer JD, *Clinical Laboratory Methods*, 9th ed, St Louis, MO: Mosby-Year Book Inc, 1982, 95-6.
3. Craig GM, Elliot C, and Hughes KR, "Masked Vitamin B$_{12}$ and Folate Deficiency in the Elderly," *Br J Nutr*, 1985, 54(3):613-9.
4. Williams WJ, Beutler E, Erslev AJ, et al, *Hematology*, 4th ed, New York, NY: McGraw-Hill Inc, 1990, 456-9.
5. Labib M, Gama R, and Marks V, "Predictive Value of D-Xylose Absorption Test and Erythrocyte Folate in Adult Coeliac Disease: A Parallel Approach," *Ann Clin Biochem*, 1990, 27(Pt 1):75-7.

References

Chanarin I, "Megaloblastic Anaemia, Cobalamin, and Folate," *J Clin Pathol*, 1987, 40(9):978-84.

Davis RE and Nicol DJ, "Folic Acid," *Int J Biochem*, 1988, 20(2):133-9.

Miller SM, "Old and New Rationales for Serum B$_{12}$ and Folate Determinations," *Clin Lab Sci*, 1993, 6(5):272-4.

Folic Acid, Serum

CPT 82746

Related Information

Complete Blood Count *on page 312*
Folic Acid, RBC *on this page*
Hemoglobin *on page 323*
Intrinsic Factor Antibody *on page 411*
Parietal Cell Antibody *on page 421*
Schilling Test *on page 346*

(Continued)

Folic Acid, Serum *(Continued)*

Vitamin B$_{12}$ *on page 351*
Vitamin B$_{12}$ Unsaturated Binding Capacity *on page 352*

Synonyms Folate Level; Serum Folate

Patient Preparation Patient should be fasting overnight. Collect prior to transfusion or initiation of folate therapy.

Specimen Serum

Container Red top tube

Collection Avoid hemolysis. Transport specimen to the laboratory promptly after collection. Avoid exposure to light. Significant (12% to 19%) loss of folate occurs over 24 hours in specimens kept at room temperature and exposed to light. Specimens exposed to light for more than 8 hours should be redrawn.[1]

Storage Instructions Stable 24 hours at 4°C or store frozen early in hospital stay (feeding malnourished patient may rapidly elevate folate level to normal). Protect from light.

Causes for Rejection Hemolyzed specimen, stored specimen not frozen or protected from light, patient having had isotope scan or Schilling's test prior to collection of specimen

Reference Range >2 ng/mL (SI: >5 nmol/L). See table for pediatric reference ranges.

Pediatric Serum Folate Reference Chart

Age	Male (nmol/L)		Female (nmol/L)	
	Low	High	Low	High
0-1 y	16.3	50.8	14.3	51.5
2-3 y	5.7	34.0	3.9	35.6
4-6 y	1.1	29.4	6.1	31.9
7-9 y	5.2	27.0	5.4	30.4
10-12 y	3.4	24.5	2.3	23.1
13-18 y	2.7	19.9	2.7	16.3

From Hicks JM, Cook J, Godwin ID, et al, "Vitamin B$_{12}$ and Folate – Pediatric Reference Ranges," *Arch Pathol Lab Med*, 1993, 117:705, with permission.

Use Detect folate deficiency; monitor therapy with folate; evaluate megaloblastic and macrocytic anemia; evaluate alcoholic patients and those with prior jejunoileal bypass for morbid obesity or those with intestinal blind-loop syndrome

Limitations May be decreased in patients on oral contraceptives. Folate will deteriorate on exposure to light. Usually measured with red cell folate and vitamin B$_{12}$ levels.

Methodology Competitive protein binding radioimmunoassay. Patient's endogenous unlabeled serum folate competes with radiolabeled folate for specific sites on a binding protein (eg, as derived from milk) and is compared to a standard curve. A chemiluminescence receptor assay has been developed. It employs an acridinium-ester-coupled folate molecule as tracer and folate binding protein on magnetic particles as the solid phase.[2]

Additional Information Naturally occurring folates are present widely in plant and animal foods taken in the diet and absorbed in the small intestine. Folic acid (pteroylglutamic acid) has a number of biologically active forms (largely conjugates of glutamic acid, eg, N-5-methyltetrahydrofolic acid and N-5-formyltetrahydrofolic acid - folinic acid) that function as coenzymes. Lack of folic acid inhibits DNA synthesis in rapidly dividing cells, thus producing megaloblastic anemia. While a specific folate-binding protein is present in the serum, some 90% of folate is unbound. The binding protein increases with folate deficiency and returns to normal with treatment.

Serum levels are affected by present dietary intake. Drugs that are folate antagonists, such as methotrexate and pentamidine, may induce a deficiency state. Some drugs, such as oral contraceptives, phenytoin, and ethanol impair absorption of folate. In the pH range of physiologic significance, folate binds to aluminum hydroxide. Chronic use of antacids or H$_2$-receptor antagonists by patients with diets marginal in folate has been considered as a cause of folic acid deficiency.[3] Levels are commonly high in patients with B$_{12}$ deficiency since this vitamin is needed to allow incorporation of folate into tissue cells. Folate (folic acid) deficiency is present in some 33% of pregnant women, many alcoholics, patients with a wide variety of malabsorption syndromes including celiac disease, sprue, Crohn's disease, and jejunal/ileal bypass procedure.

Measurement of both serum and red cell folate levels constitutes a reliable means of determining the existence of folate deficiency. These tests are recommended for all patients who have megaloblastic anemia, as well as for patients who have anemia, hypersegmentation of the granulocytic nuclei, and coincident evidence of iron deficiency. The finding of a low serum folate means that the patient's recent diet has been subnormal in folate content and/or that recent absorption of folate has been subnormal, but does not prove that the patient either has or will develop tissue folate depletion requiring folate therapy. Therefore, serum folate assays have a very poor predictive value in diagnosis and should be interpreted with caution. A low red cell folate can mean either that there is tissue folate depletion due to folate deficiency requiring folate therapy, or alternatively, that the patient has primary vitamin B$_{12}$ deficiency blocking the ability of cells to take up folate. In the latter case, the proper therapy would be with vitamin B$_{12}$ rather than with folic acid. It is for these reasons that it is advisable to determine red cell folate in addition to serum folate, and thereby definitively determine that the diagnosis is folate deficiency for which the proper treatment is folic acid. For thoroughness, the serum vitamin B$_{12}$ level should also be determined. In some geographic areas (hospitalized urban patient populations), zidovudine, used in the treatment of acquired immune deficiency syndrome, has been the most common condition associated with macrocytosis.[4]

Folate deficient diets have been proposed for methotrexate responsive malignancy. It has also been suggested that plasma folate concentrations in patients who do and do not respond to folate deprivation/antagonism be compared and ratioed to methotrexate levels as part of tumor therapy regimes.[5] The levels of serum and RBC folate may be significantly increased in hyperthyroidism.[6] The biochemical events underlying the phenomenon of megaloblastosis and the pathways of thymidylate synthesis has recently been reviewed.[7]

Footnotes

1. Mastropaolo W and Wilson MA, "Effect of Light on Serum B$_{12}$ and Folate Stability," *Clin Chem*, 1993, 39(5):913.
2. Klukas C, Comerci C, Campbell J, et al, "A Chemiluminescence Receptor Assay for Folate," *Clin Chem*, 1989, 35:1194.
3. Russell RM, Golner BB, Krasinski SD, et al, "Effect of Antacid and H$_2$ Receptor Antagonists on the Intestinal Absorption of Folic Acid," *J Lab Clin Med*, 1988, 112(4):458-63.
4. Snower DP and Weil SC, "Changing Etiology of Macrocytosis: Zidovudine as a Frequent Causative Factor," *Am J Clin Pathol*, 1993, 99(1):57-60.
5. Cohen P and Dix D, "On the Role of Folate Deficiency in Cancer Therapy," *Clin Chem*, 1988, 34(9):1945-6.
6. Ford HC, Carter JM, and Rendle MA, "Serum and Red Cell Folate and Serum Vitamin B$_{12}$ Levels in Hyperthyroidism," *Am J Hematol*, 1989, 31(4):233-6.
7. Das KC and Herbert V, "*In Vitro* DNA Synthesis by Megaloblastic Bone Marrow: Effect of Folates and Cobalamins on Thymidine Incorporation and De Novo Thymidylate Synthesis," *Am J Hematol*, 1989, 31(1):11-20.

References

Chanarin I, "Megaloblastic Anaemia, Cobalamin, and Folate," *J Clin Pathol*, 1987, 40(9):978-84.
Craig GM, Elliot C, and Hughes KR, "Masked Vitamin B$_{12}$ and Folate Deficiency in the Elderly," *Br J Nutr*, 1985, 54(3):613-9.
Davis RE and Nicol DJ, "Folic Acid," *Int J Biochem*, 1988, 20(2):133-9.
Hicks JM, Cook J, Godwin ID, et al, "Vitamin B$_{12}$ and Folate: Pediatric Reference Ranges," *Arch Pathol Lab Med*, 1993, 117(7):704-6.

Free Hemoglobin *see* Hemoglobin, Plasma *on page 325*

α-Fucosidase *see* Inherited Diseases of Metabolism and Cell Structure Tests *on page 327*

G-6-PD, Qualitative *see* Glucose-6-Phosphate Dehydrogenase Screen, Blood *on next page*

G-6-PD, Quantitative, Blood *see* Glucose-6-Phosphate Dehydrogenase, Quantitative, Blood *on next page*

G-6-PD Screen, Blood *see* Glucose-6-Phosphate Dehydrogenase Screen, Blood *on next page*

Galactocerebroside *see* Inherited Diseases of Metabolism and Cell Structure Tests *on page 327*

β-Galactosidase *see* Inherited Diseases of Metabolism and Cell Structure Tests *on page 327*

Gelation Assay

Related Information

Glycerol Lysis Test, Acidified, Modified *on page 320*
Osmotic Fragility *on page 334*
Osmotic Fragility, Incubated *on page 335*

Synonyms Absence of Phosphorylatin-induced Gelation of Red Cell Membrane Skeletons; Erythrocyte Membrane Skeleton Gelation Assay; Gelation Failing Test

Applies to Hemolytic Anemia; Hereditary Spherocytosis

Abstract A recently developed test, initially reported to be specific for the diagnosis of hereditary spherocytosis (HS).

Specimen Whole blood

Container Green top (heparin) tube

Storage Instructions Blood is collected and processed within the same day. cAMP-independent protein kinase may be stored at -20°C.

Reference Range Normal individuals and patients with a variety of hemolytic anemias show gelation after 30-50 minutes. Patients with hereditary spherocytosis show absence of gelation of erythrocyte membranes including after incubation for 12 hours (positive test is absence of gelation).

Use Diagnosis of hereditary spherocytosis

Limitations Assay is currently available on a research basis only. Preparation requires considerable laboratory manual processing. Documentation of sensitivity and specificity is based on small patient samples.

Methodology Red cell membrane (ghosts) and partially purified cAMP-independent kinase are prepared, mixed under standardized conditions in a pipette, and observation for gelation is conducted by visual inspection.

Additional Information This test, based on a visually detectable change in the behavior of erythrocyte membrane ghosts, was developed and investigated as a possibly specific test for hereditary spherocytosis. HS appears in many patients to be the result of an abnormally functioning or deficient spectrin component of the red cell membrane skeleton. The gelation assay is based on the observation of Pinder et al that upon phosphorylation with cAMP-independent protein kinase, normal red cell membrane ("ghost") preparations set to a gelatinous mass (negative reaction) while those from spherocytosis red cells do not gel (positive reaction). There is evidence that this failure of gelation is specific for HS. Negative reactions have been observed in cases of hereditary elliptocytosis, hereditary stomatocytosis, β-thalassemia, pyruvate kinase deficiency, glucose phosphate isomerase deficiency, and glucose-6-phosphate dehydrogenase deficiency as well as in normal individuals (reference by Armbrust et al). The gelation test is technically more involved and time consuming than the modified acidified glycerol lysis or osmotic fragility screening tests.

References

Agre P, Asimos A, Casella JF, et al, "Inheritance Pattern and Clinical Response to Splenectomy as a Reflection of Erythrocyte Spectrin Deficiency in Hereditary Spherocytosis," *N Engl J Med*, 1986, 315(25):1579-83.

Armbrust R, Eber SW, and Schröter W, "Absence of Phosphorylation-Induced Gelation of Erythrocyte Membrane Skeletons: A Diagnostic Tool for Hereditary Spherocytosis," *Ann Hematol*, 1992, 64(2):93-6.

Pinder JC, Dhermy D, Baines AJ, et al, "A Phenomenological Difference Between Membrane Skeletal Protein Complexes Isolated From Normal and Hereditary Spherocytosis Erythrocytes," *Br J Haematol*, 1983, 55(3):455-63.

Gelation Failing Test *see* Gelation Assay *on previous page*

Glucocerebroside *see* Inherited Diseases of Metabolism and Cell Structure Tests *on page 327*

Glucose-6-Phosphate Dehydrogenase, Quantitative, Blood

CPT 82955

Related Information

Autohemolysis Test *on page 304*

Glucose-6-Phosphate Dehydrogenase Screen, Blood *on this page*

Heinz Body Stain *on page 321*

Red Blood Cell Enzyme Deficiency, Quantitative *on page 342*

Red Blood Cell Enzyme Deficiency Screen *on page 343*

Synonyms G-6-PD, Quantitative, Blood

Applies to Heinz Bodies

Specimen Erythrocytes

Container Lavender top (EDTA) tube, green top (heparin) tube, or acid-citrate-dextrose (ACD) solution

Storage Instructions In above anticoagulants, RBC enzymes stable at 4°C for at least 6 days and stable at 25°C for at least 24 hours. If sample must be sent to a referral laboratory, ship on wet ice, do not freeze.[1]

Reference Range 8.34±1.59 IU/g hemoglobin

Use Evaluate G-6-PD deficiency; determine the cause of drug-induced hemolysis or hemolysis secondary to acute bacterial or viral infection or metabolic disorder such as acidosis

Limitations False normal results after hemolysis may occur; *vide infra*.

Contraindications Normal G-6-PD screen, marked reticulocytosis

Methodology Using hemolysate, measurement of formation of NADPH by following change in absorbance at 340 nm at 37°C

Additional Information The active G-6-PD enzyme exists as a dimer, each monomer consisting of 515 amino acids. Aggregation of monomers into active forms (largely dimers) is NADP dependent. G-6-PD catalyzes the first step in the hexose monophosphate pathway which acts to remove peroxide, thus protecting the red cell from oxidative damage. The enzyme provides reducing power in the form of NADPH which with glutathione is requisite for detoxification of H_2O_2. Over 440 G-6-PD mutations have been described of which some 60 mutations or combinations of mutations have been documented in G-6-PD deficiency. Total deficiency is thought to be incompatible with life.

A G-6-PD screen is recommended before G-6-PD quantitative is requested (see Glucose-6-Phosphate Dehydrogenase Screen, Blood *on page 319*). G-6-PD hemolysis is associated with formation of Heinz bodies in peripheral red blood cells. It is the older erythrocytes which are most G-6-PD deficient in affected individuals. These cells are first eliminated in a hemolytic crisis. The younger cells and reticulocytes contain more G-6-PD. For these reasons after a hemolytic crisis, when only younger erythrocytes and reticulocytes are present, the G-6-PD values may be spuriously normal. Quantitative assay of G-6-PD may be helpful in establishing the diagnosis in female patients (who have two RBC populations) or in males with mild G-6-PD deficiency who have had recent hemolysis. In such cases, assay of the reticulocyte-poor bottom fraction of a centrifuged blood sample may be useful.[2] Mutations responsible for the G-6-PD deficient state have been identified by use of molecular biologic techniques.[3]

Footnotes

1. Beutler E, Blume KG, Kaplan JC, et al, "International Committee for Standardization in Haematology: Recommended Methods for Red-Cell Enzyme Analysis," *Br J Haematol*, 1977, 35:331-40.
2. Beutler E, "Glucose-6-Phosphate Dehydrogenase Deficiency," *N Engl J Med*, 1991, 324(3):169-74.
3. Huang CS, Tang CJ, Huang MJ, et al, "Diagnosis of Glucose-6-Phosphate Dehydrogenase (G6PD) Mutations by DNA Amplification and Allele-Specific Oligonucleotide Probes," *Acta Haematol*, 1992, 88(2-3):92-5.

References

Beutler E, "G6PD Deficiency," *Blood*, 1994, 84(11):3613-36.

Beutler E, "Study of Glucose-6-Phosphate Dehydrogenase: History and Molecular Biology," *Am J Hematol*, 1993, 42(1):53-8.

Mentzer WC and Wagner GM, *The Hereditary Haemolytic Anaemias*, Chapter 6, New York, NY: Churchill Livingstone, 1989, 289-92.

Glucose-6-Phosphate Dehydrogenase Screen, Blood

CPT 82960

Related Information

Autohemolysis Test *on page 304*

Glucose-6-Phosphate Dehydrogenase, Quantitative, Blood *on this page*

Red Blood Cell Enzyme Deficiency, Quantitative *on page 342*

Red Blood Cell Enzyme Deficiency Screen *on page 343*

Synonyms G-6-PD, Qualitative; G-6-PD Screen, Blood

Abstract G-6-PD is a red cell enzyme with an X-linked mode of inheritance that is important in maintaining RBC proteins in the reduced state. There are over 440 different mutations recorded,[1] of which 60 by themselves or in combination with other mutations result in premature hemolysis of red cells when the mutant enzyme is stressed.

Specimen Erythrocytes

Container Lavender top (EDTA) tube

Reference Range G-6-PD enzyme activity detected

Use Detect drug sensitive populations of red cells due to G-6-PD deficiency; determine the cause of hemolysis. G-6-PD deficient hemolysis may also be secondary to acute bacterial or viral infection and metabolic disorder such as acidosis.

Limitations A blood enzyme screen, performed after a hemolytic episode often will not detect G-6-PD deficiency even if present because the most deficient cells have been destroyed. This procedure can only differentiate between normal and grossly deficient samples. **Test may need to be repeated (if initial result is normal) after the patient recovers from an undiagnosed episode of anemia.**

Contraindications Marked reticulocytosis

Methodology Fluorescent NADPH spot test

Additional Information G-6-PD quantitation may be useful if a deficiency is detected in the screening test. In a large group of American black males the incidence of G-6-PD deficiency was found to be 11% (methemoglobin reduction test and fluorescent spot test). Approximately 20% of female are heterozygous. G-6-PD deficiency had no adverse effect on the course and fatality rates of a spectrum of diseases (including those with thrombotic associations).[2] While usually mild in black children G-6-PD deficiency may be severe and life-threatening with oxidative stress, especially that relating to infection (viral in particular), fava bean ingestion, and less often relating to naphthalene exposure. A number of commonly used drugs/chemicals can induce hemolysis in individuals with G-6-PD deficiency (see table), while evidence has accumulated that some occasionally suspect drugs can be given in therapeutic doses without inducing hemolysis.[3] Distinctive abnormal RBC "eccentrocytes" may occur. While G-6-PD screens may be normal after hemolytic episodes significant reticulocytosis (usually >7%) will reflect presence of the deficiency.[4] Infection rather than use of ASA appears to precipitate hemolytic episodes in cases of G-6-PD deficiency. If deficiency is severe, impaired granulocyte function occurs with increased susceptibility to infection.[5] Occasionally, a few of this group can be symptomatic. There are many genetic variants of G-6-PD, some causing marked clinical manifestations, others none. The nonblack variant found in high frequency in such areas as India, Japan, Southeast Asia, and certain Mediterranean countries tends to present as a more severe form of the disease. Rare sporadic cases occurring anywhere in the world (Continued)

Glucose-6-Phosphate Dehydrogenase Screen,
Blood (Continued)

may present as chronic nonspherocytic hemolytic anemia.[6] Molecular heterogeneity, as reflected by the numerous mutant isoenzymes, is accompanied by biochemical functional diversity including decreased catalytic effectiveness, impaired substrate and cofactor kinetics, variable reactivity with substrate analogues, and variations in electrophoretic migration rates and pH optima. Cloning of the G-6-PD gene has been accomplished, and there is ongoing activity in cDNA sequencing of G-6-PD variants.[3,7,8,9]

Drugs and Chemicals That Should Be Avoided by Persons With G-6-PD Deficiency

Acetanilid	Primaquine
Furazolidone (Furoxone®)	Sulfacetamide
Isobutyl nitrite	Sulfamethoxazole (Gantanol®)
Methylene blue	Sulfanilamide
Nalidixic acid (NegGram®)	Sulfapyridine
Naphthalene	Thiazolesulfone
Niridazole (Ambilhar®)	Toluidine blue
Nitrofurantoin (Furadantin®)	Trinitrotoluene (TNT)
Phenazopyridine (Pyridium®)	Urate oxidase
Phenylhydrazine	

From Beutler E, "G6PD Deficiency," Blood, 1994, 84(11):3614.

Footnotes

1. Beutler E, "G6PD Deficiency," Blood, 1994, 84(11):3613-36.
2. Heller P, Best WR, Nelson RB, et al, "Clinical Implications of Sickle Cell Trait and Glucose-6-Phosphate Dehydrogenase Deficiency in Hospitalized Black Male Patients," N Engl J Med, 1979, 300:1001-5.
3. Beutler E, "Glucose-6-Phosphate Dehydrogenase Deficiency," N Engl J Med, 1991, 324(3):169-74.
4. Shannon K and Buchanan GR, "Severe Hemolytic Anemia in Black Children With Glucose-6-Phosphate Dehydrogenase Deficiency," Pediatrics, 1982, 70(3):364-9.
5. Vives Corrons JL, Feliu E, Pujades MA, et al, "Severe Glucose-6-Phosphate Dehydrogenase Deficiency (G-6-PD) Associated With Chronic Hemolytic Anemia, Granulocyte Dysfunction and Increased Susceptibility to Infections: Description of a New Molecular Variant (G-6-PD Barcelona)," Blood, 1982, 59:428-34.
6. Mason PJ, Sonati MF, MacDonald D, et al, "New Glucose-6-Phosphate Dehydrogenase Mutations Associated With Chronic Anemia," Blood, 1995, 85(5):1377-80.
7. Martini G, Toniolo D, Vulliamy T, et al, "Structural Analysis of the X-Linked Gene Encoding Human Glucose-6-Phosphate Dehydrogenase," EMBO J, 1986, 5(8):1849-55.
8. Chiu DT, Zuo L, Chao L, et al, "Molecular Characterization of Glucose-6-Phosphate Dehydrogenase (G6PD) Deficiency in Patients of Chinese Descent and Identification of New Base Substitutions in the Human G6PD Gene," Blood, 1993, 81(8):2150-4.
9. Saha S, Saha N, Tay JS, et al, "Molecular Characterisation of Red Cell Glucose-6-Phosphate Dehydrogenase Deficiency in Singapore Chinese," Am J Hematol, 1994, 47(4):273-7.

References

Beutler E, "Study of Glucose-6-Phosphate Dehydrogenase: History and Molecular Biology," Am J Hematol, 1993, 42(1):53-8.

Luzzatto L, "Glucose-6-Phosphate Dehydrogenase Deficiency and the Pentose Phosphate Pathway," Blood: Principles and Practice of Hematology, Chapter 58, Handin RI, Lux SE, and Stossel TP, eds, Philadelphia, PA: JB Lippincott Co, 1995, 1897-923.

Naylor CE, Rowland P, Basak AK, et al, "Glucose-6 Phosphate Dehydrogenase Mutations Causing Enzyme Deficiency in a Model of the Tertiary Structure of the Human Enzyme," Blood, 1996, 87(7):2974-82.

β-Glucosidase see Inherited Diseases of Metabolism and Cell Structure Tests on page 327

Glutathione Reductase Deficiency, RBC see Red Blood Cell Enzyme Deficiency, Quantitative on page 342

Glycerol Lysis Test see Glycerol Lysis Test, Acidified, Modified on this page

Glycerol Lysis Test, Acidified, Modified

Related Information

Gelation Assay on page 318
Osmotic Fragility on page 334
Osmotic Fragility, Incubated on page 335

Synonyms Acidified Glycerol Lysis Test; AGLT; Glycerol Lysis Test; Pink Test

Applies to Hemolytic Anemia; Hereditary Spherocytosis

Abstract A sensitive, specific, simple, inexpensive test applicable to population screening and provisional diagnosis of hereditary spherocytosis (HS). The test is a measure of glycerol's ability to retard osmotic swelling of red blood cells.

Specimen EDTA anticoagulated whole blood; test is performed on less than 100 µL of blood, amenable to finger puncture collection

Container Lavender top (EDTA) tube, microsample container, or buffer containing tube

Collection Whole blood collected by venipuncture or by finger puncture

Storage Instructions Test is usually started by placing skin puncture obtained whole blood into appropriate buffer solution immediately upon collection, but whole blood collected within 24 hours and kept at room temperature can be used.

Turnaround Time 1-2 hours

Reference Range Half-time for AGLT lysis: normal is over 30 minutes; result is less than 5 minutes in cases of hereditary spherocytosis (major portion of HS cases have half-time between 1 and 2 minutes).[1]

Use Screening test for diagnosis of hereditary spherocytosis

Limitations While 100% specificity is claimed, some 7% of apparent normals may give results of between 5 and 30 minutes ("possibly pathologic"). In the series of 1464 healthy blood donors of Eber, et al, these individuals were hematologically normal and did not have increased osmotic fragility.

Methodology Sample (20 µL) of EDTA anticoagulated whole blood is diluted in buffered saline (0.0093 M sodium phosphate, pH 6.90) and 1 part added to 2 parts of a buffered 0.3 M glycerol solution. Temperature must be controlled at 25°C. Fall in absorbance (625 nm) is measured as the solution's turbidity decreases due to hemolysis of red cells. Results are given as the half time for AGLT lysis.

Additional Information Development of a screening test for HS might be considered unfeasible due to the heterogeneous nature of the disease process. Clinically, the hemolytic anemia of HS ranges from mild, asymptomatic fully compensated forms to those with severe hemolysis requiring transfusion. There is not a single underlying molecular red cell structural defect (dependent upon one's definition of "hereditary spherocytosis"). HS or HS-like clinical picture occurs with primary structural defects of spectrin, ankyrin, band 3, and band 4.2 (pallidin) red cell proteins. It is thus somewhat surprising that after a series of modifications over the past 20 years (see reference) following Gottfried and Robertson's original procedure[2] that the current AGLT has been found to be 100% sensitive and nearly 100% specific!

Footnotes

1. Eber SW, Pekrun A, Neufeldt A, et al, "Prevalence of Increased Osmotic Fragility of Erythrocytes in German Blood Donors: Screening Using a Modified Glycerol Lysis Test," Ann Hematol, 1992, 64(2):88-92.
2. Gottfried EL and Robertson NA, "Glycerol Lysis Time as a Screening Test for Erythrocyte Disorders," J Lab Clin Med, 1974, 83(2):323-33.

References

Bucx MJ, Breed WP, and Hoffmann JJ, "Comparison of Acidified Glycerol Lysis Test, Pink Test and Osmotic Fragility Test in Hereditary Spherocytosis: Effect of Incubation," Eur J Haematol, 1988, 40(3):227-31.

Lux SE and Palek J, "Disorders of the Red Cell Membrane," Blood: Principles and Practice of Hematology, Chapter 54, Handin RI, Lux SE, and Stossel TP, eds, Philadelphia, PA: JB Lippincott Co, 1995, 1759.

Glycogen Storage Diseases see Inherited Diseases of Metabolism and Cell Structure Tests on page 327

Granulocyte/Macrophage Colony Stimulating Factor see Eosinophil Count on page 315

Hairy Cell Leukemia Test see Tartrate Resistant Leukocyte Acid Phosphatase on page 349

Ham Test

CPT 85475

Related Information

Hemosiderin Stain, Urine on page 637
Peripheral Blood: Red Blood Cell Morphology on page 339
Red Blood Cells, Washed on page 622
Sugar Water Test Screen on page 348

Synonyms Acid Serum Test; Acid Serum Test for PNH; Acidified Serum Test; Paroxysmal Nocturnal Hemoglobinuria Test; PNH Test; Serum Lysis

Abstract A positive Ham test (lysis of patient red cells in acidified serum) is used as a test for paroxysmal nocturnal hemoglobinuria (PNH) and indicates unusual sensitivity of such red cells to the action of complement. PNH is characterized clinically by nocturnal hemoglobinuria, chronic hemolytic anemia, hypoplastic or aplastic hematopoiesis, and tendency to thrombosis. It is the result of an acquired defect of hematopoietic stem cells. At least some cases of PNH result from defective synthesis of glycosyl-phosphatidylinositol. The latter acts to anchor proteins (CD55 and CD59) which protect red blood cells from the action of complement.

Specimen Erythrocytes

Container Lavender top (EDTA) tube

Causes for Rejection Improper tube, specimen clotted, specimen hemolyzed

Reference Range A positive result shows lysis of red cells in acidified serum samples with patient's cells (not with normal cells).

Use Evaluate patients with suspected PNH (paroxysmal nocturnal hemoglobinuria) or suspected congenital dyserythropoietic anemia, type II (HEMPAS); evaluate hemolytic anemia, especially with hemosiderinuria, pancytopenia, decreased RBC acetylcholinesterase, decreased leukocyte alkaline phosphatase, negative direct Coombs' test, and/or apparent marrow failure. Positive in PNH: 10% to 50% lysis in acidified noninactivated serum. Can be as low as 5% or as much as 80%. Low or negative after transfusion. Diagnosis of PNH rests upon showing that the suspected patient's red cells have a high sensitivity to complement mediated hemolysis.[1]

Limitations False-positive results may occur in other hematologic diseases: hereditary and acquired spherocytosis, hereditary dyserythropoietic anemia (CDA type II, HEMPAS, vide infra), aged red cells (as with old transfused blood), aplastic anemia, leukemia, and myeloproliferative syndromes. In these conditions hemolysis will also occur in the acidified inactivated serum. The latter is negative in PNH since hemolysis is complement dependent.

Contraindications Transfusion

Methodology Acidified serum test of Ham. PNH suspect RBCs will lyse in acidified normal and acidified patient's serum. The normal serum used must be fresh and ABO blood group compatible with test RBCs. Sensitivity is maximized by optimizing pH and serum concentration (see reference by Rosse). Alternatives to acidification of the testing serum are the addition of bovine thrombin, cobra venom factor, insulin, heating, or use of specific antibodies to activate complement. Probably these tests do not offer advantages over the Ham test. False-negative results may occur with any of these tests in which the PNH patient's serum (which may have low serum complement activity) is used.[1]

Additional Information PNH red cells are unusually susceptible to lysis by complement. The Ham (acidified serum) and sucrose hemolysis test can demonstrate this lysis in vitro. A positive acidified-serum test (performed with careful attention to proper controls) defines the PNH condition. A positive test is necessary for the diagnosis. In PNH, 10% to 50% of lysis (measured as liberated hemoglobin) is usually obtained but lysis may be as great as 80% or as little as 5%.

In some cases, three populations of cells exist in patients with PNH. One is markedly hypersensitive to complement (type III cells), one has a midlevel of sensitivity (type II cells), and the third population has normal sensitivity (type I cells). Type III cells are variably present, are the population which undergoes lysis in the Ham test and relate to the severity of illness.[2] The young PNH cells (reticulocyte-rich) are more susceptible to lysis than the older red cells. PNH RBCs will undergo lysis in acidified normal serum and in the patient's acidified serum.[2]

The membrane defect is complex, involving importantly, a protein, the membrane inhibitor of reactive lysis (MIRL, "protectin", also called CD59). This protein regulates the assembly of polymerized C9 in the membrane attack complex, the effector and final stage of the complement activation sequence. MIRL (protectin or CD59) is an 18,000-20,000 MW complement lysis restricting factor that inhibits C5b-8 catalyzed insertion of C9 into lipid bilayers. The protein is also expressed in granulocytes, monocytes, and on platelets; its absence plays a role in the hypercoagulable state present in PNH. The underlying gene defect (in the gene, "pig A") is located on the short arm of the X chromosome and is acquired (present only in somatic hematopoietic cells). As of 1995, 84 pig A mutations in 72 patients had been reported; 53 of the 84 were deletion or insertion mutations.[3,4]

The only other disorder which may give a positive Ham test is one of the congenital dyserythropoietic anemias. In CDA type II (HEMPAS - hereditary erythroblastic multinuclearity with positive acidified serum test) the red cells undergo lysis in only a proportion (about 30%) of normal sera, and these RBCs do not undergo lysis in the patient's own acidified serum. The sucrose lysis test is negative in cases of HEMPAS. Heating at 56°C, which destroys the complement in serum, inactivates the lytic system so that if lysis occurs with inactivated serum this cannot be considered positive.

Another type of cell that may lyse in inactivated serum is the spherocyte. Spherocytes may lyse in acidified serum possibly due to the lowered pH.[2]

PNH has been considered a "candidate" myeloproliferative disease, a myelodysplastic syndrome.[5] A 55% to 65% incidence of PNH occurs in primary myelofibrosis and myeloid metaplasia.

PNH is a disease not only of increased complement sensitivity of red cell membranes, but also granulocytes and platelet membranes, the latter predisposing to venous thrombosis at unusual sites including abdomen and liver. A new diagnostic test using flow cytometry and monoclonal antibodies has been developed.[6] This technique reveals and detects missing proteins from granulocytes in patients with PNH. The method correlates well with the Ham test for abnormal red cells.

Footnotes

1. Harruff RC and Rohn RJ, "Potential Errors in the Laboratory Diagnosis of Paroxysmal Nocturnal Hemoglobinuria," *Am J Clin Pathol*, 1983, 80:152-8.
2. Luzzato L and Hillmen P, "Laboratory Methods Used in the Investigation of Paroxysmal Nocturnal Hemoglobinuria (PNH)," *Practical Haematology*, Dacie JV and Lewis SM, eds, 8th ed, Chapter 15, New York, NY: Churchill Livingstone, 1995, 287-96.

3. Rosse WF and Ware RE, "The Molecular Basis of Paroxysmal Nocturnal Hemoglobinuria," *Blood*, 1995, 86(9):3277-86.
4. Miyata T, Yamada N, Iida Y, et al, "Abnormalities of PIG-A Transcripts in Granulocytes From Patients With Paroxysmal Nocturnal Hemoglobinuria," *N Engl J Med*, 1994, 330(4):249-55.
5. Dameshek W, "Foreword and a Proposal for Considering Paroxysmal Nocturnal Hemoglobinuria (PNH) as a "Candidate" Myeloproliferative Disorder," *Blood*, 1969, 33:263-4.
6. van der Schoot CE, Huizinga TW, van't Veer Korthof ET, et al, "Deficiency of Glycosyl-Phosphatidylinositol-Linked Membrane Glycoproteins of Leukocytes in Paroxysmal Nocturnal Hemoglobinuria, Description of a New Diagnostic Cytofluorometric Assay," *Blood*, 1990, 76(7):1853-9.

References

Beutler E, "Paroxysmal Nocturnal Hemoglobinuria," *Williams Hematology*, 5th ed, Chapter 25, Beutler E, Lichtman MA, Coller BS, et al, eds, New York, NY: McGraw-Hill Inc, 1995, 252-6.

Grenier KA, "Hemolytic Anemias: Intracorpuscular Defects: V. Paroxysmal Nocturnal Hemoglobinuria," *Clinical Hematology and Fundamentals of Hemostasis*, 2nd ed, Chapter 13, Harmening DM, ed, Philadelphia, PA: FA Davis Co, 1992, 183-92.

Marks PW and Mitus AJ, "Congenital Dyserythropoietic Anemias," *Am J Clin Hematol*, 1996, 51(1):55-63.

Rosse WF, "Paroxysmal Nocturnal Hemoglobinuria," *Blood: Principles and Practice of Hematology*, Chapter 11, Handin RI, Lux SE, and Stossel TP, eds, Philadelphia, PA: JB Lippincott Co, 1995, 367-76.

H and H see Hematocrit *on next page*

H and H see Hemoglobin *on page 323*

Hb see Hemoglobin *on page 323*

Hb A₂ see Hemoglobin A₂ *on page 323*

Hb F see Fetal Hemoglobin *on page 316*

Hct see Hematocrit *on next page*

Heat Denaturation see Hemoglobin, Unstable, Heat Labile Test *on page 326*

Heinz Bodies see Glucose-6-Phosphate Dehydrogenase, Quantitative, Blood *on page 319*

Heinz Bodies see Hemoglobin, Unstable, Heat Labile Test *on page 326*

Heinz Bodies see Hemoglobin, Unstable - Isopropanol Precipitation Test *on page 326*

Heinz Bodies see Red Blood Cell Enzyme Deficiency, Quantitative *on page 342*

Heinz Bodies see Red Blood Cell Enzyme Deficiency Screen *on page 343*

Heinz Body Stain

CPT 85441

Related Information

Glucose-6-Phosphate Dehydrogenase, Quantitative, Blood *on page 319*
Hemoglobin, Unstable, Heat Labile Test *on page 326*
Hemoglobin, Unstable - Isopropanol Precipitation Test *on page 326*
Peripheral Blood: Red Blood Cell Morphology *on page 339*
Red Blood Cell Enzyme Deficiency, Quantitative *on page 342*
Red Blood Cell Enzyme Deficiency Screen *on page 343*
Reticulocyte Count *on page 345*

Synonyms Methyl Violet Stain for Heinz Bodies

Applies to CHBHA

Abstract Heinz bodies are intraerythrocyte insoluble inclusions of oxidatively denatured hemoglobin. They reflect the presence of a metabolic derangement of or abnormality in the secondary structure of hemoglobin.

Specimen Whole blood

Container Lavender top (EDTA) tube, green top (heparin) tube

Collection Obtain a tube of normal control blood at the time patient sample is drawn.

Storage Instructions Refrigerate

Causes for Rejection Clotted specimen, hemolyzed specimen

Reference Range No Heinz bodies identified. Using blood incubated with acetylphenylhydrazine, normal control may have one to a few (under five) Heinz bodies in about one-third of the RBCs. A positive result (indicative of a defective reducing system) will find five or more Heinz bodies in about one-third or more of the RBCs. The definition of "abnormal" may vary somewhat between different laboratories.

Use Test for hemolytic disorders associated with Heinz body formation (eg, G-6-PD deficiency, thalassemia, unstable hemoglobin)

Methodology Supravital stain (methyl violet, new methylene blue, crystal violet, or brilliant cresyl blue) using blood incubated (60 minutes or more) at room temperature with acetylphenylhydrazine or sterile blood incubated 24 and 48 hours at 37°C. Heinz bodies are intraerythrocytic, purple, vary in shape (round, oval, serrated), 1-3 μm across, single or multiple, and close to the cell membrane.

(Continued)

Heinz Body Stain (Continued)

Additional Information Heinz bodies are uncommon except with G-6-PD deficiency immediately following hemolysis and in patients with unstable hemoglobin variants. They are present characteristically in the congenital Heinz body hemolytic anemias (CHBHA). There are over 30 different molecular variants of hemoglobin underlying CHBHA. The three major causes for Heinz body formation and increased hemolysis are exposure to certain chemicals and drugs, deficiency of one of the reducing systems of blood, and presence of an unstable hemoglobin. Oxidative denaturation of the hemoglobin molecule leads to Heinz body formation with the first two situations and is probably the mechanism for the precipitation of unstable hemoglobin. A variety of detailed molecular mechanisms have been proposed and defined to underlie the actual production of the Heinz body phenomenon.[1] Heinz bodies are usually removed by the spleen; postsplenectomy they increase in the peripheral blood. It has also been proposed that they may be actively extruded in cases of drug-induced hemolytic anemia.[2] While absent in the blood of normal individuals presplenectomy, they occur in sulfonamide-induced hemolytic crisis in cases of Hb Zurich and in cases of Hb Shepherd's Bush, Hb Gun Hill, and Hb Philly. Postsplenectomy, Heinz bodies occur in >50% of cells in blood stained supravitally, especially with methyl violet. They can be generated in red cells of unsplenectomized patients by 60 minutes or more incubation with acetylphenylhydrazine or by incubation of sterile blood for 24-48 hours at 37°C. Ability to demonstrate the bodies relates to the degree of instability of the hemoglobin. Cells of Hb Koln require up to 48 hours incubation and the Heinz bodies are small. With Hb Seattle and Hb Shepherd's Bush the bodies are seen readily after 24 hours incubation.[3] Heinz bodies may be found after the administration of sulfonamides, nitrofurans, Dilantin®, streptomycin, fava beans, chlorates, phenylhydrazine, primaquine (in sensitive individuals), and likely, other compounds.

Footnotes

1. Dacie J, "The Haemolytic Anaemias," *The Hereditary Haemolytic Anaemias*, 3rd ed, Vol 1, Part 1, Chapter 3, New York, NY: Churchill Livingstone, 1985, 84-6.
2. Amare M, Lawson B, and Larsen WE, "Active Extrusion of Heinz Bodies in Drug-Induced Hemolytic Anemia," *Br J Haematol*, 1972, 23:215-9.
3. White JM and Dacie JV, "The Unstable Hemoglobins - Molecular and Clinical Features," *Prog Hematol*, 1971, 7:85-9.

References

Beutler E, "Heinz Body Staining," *Williams Hematology*, 5th ed, Chapter 5, Beutler E, Lichtman MA, Coller BS, et al, eds, New York, NY: McGraw-Hill Inc, 1995, 356 and L26.

Brown BA, *Hematology: Principles and Procedures*, 6th ed, Philadelphia, PA: Lea & Febiger, 1993, 143-5.

Jaffe ER, "Oxidative Hemolysis or What Made the Red Cell Break?" *N Engl J Med*, 1972, 286:156-7.

Jandl JH, "Heinz Body Hemolytic Anemia," *Blood*, 1st ed, Boston, MA: Little, Brown and Co, 1987, 335-9.

Wyrick-Glatzel J and Gwaltney-Krause S, *Laboratory Methods in Hematology and Hemostasis, Clinical Hematology and Fundamentals of Hemostasis*, 2nd ed, Chapter 30, Section 1, Harmening DM, ed, Philadelphia, PA: FA Davis Co, 1992, 540.

Helminths, Blood *see* Microfilariae, Peripheral Blood Preparation *on page 333*

Hematocrit

CPT 85013 (spun hematocrit); 85014 (other than spun hematocrit)

Related Information

Blood Volume *on page 306*
Complete Blood Count *on page 312*
Hemoglobin *on next page*
Peripheral Blood: Red Blood Cell Morphology *on page 339*
Red Blood Cell Indices *on page 343*
Red Blood Cells *on page 621*
Red Cell Count *on page 344*
Red Cell Mass *on page 345*
Reticulocyte Count *on page 345*

Synonyms Hct; Microhematocrit; Packed Cell Volume; PCV

Applies to H and H

Abstract Percent of whole blood that is red blood cells. A determination that is of importance in the detection and follow-up of anemia and polycythemia. The hematocrit value is used in the calculation of the MCV and MCHC.

Specimen Whole blood

Container Lavender top (EDTA) tube

Collection Routine venipuncture. Invert tube gently to mix. For capillary puncture, establish free flow of blood to minimize dilution with tissue fluid.

Storage Instructions If specimen is not brought to the laboratory within 4 hours, refrigeration should be provided.

Causes for Rejection Clotted or hemolyzed specimen

Reference Range Males: 2 years of age: 35% to 44%, 6 years of age: 31% to 43%, adult: 42% to 52%; females: 2 years of age: 35% to 44%, 6

years of age: 31% to 43%, adult: 35% to 47%. In general, spun hematocrits are 2% to 3% higher than automated hematocrits, due to plasma trapping. See tables.

Hematocrit Values – First Postnatal Day[5]

Gestational Age (wk)	Hct (%)
24-25	63
26-27	62
28-29	60
30-31	60
32-33	60
34-35	61
36-37	64
Term	61

Normal Hematocrit Values – Newborn

Age	Hct (%)
Birth - 2 d	54-68
2-3 d	54-66
3-4 d	52-71
4-5 d	39-55
5-6 d	50-64
6-7 d	47-61
7-8 d	47-64
1-2 wk	50-62
2-3 wk	39-53
3-4 wk	37-49

Use Evaluate anemia, blood loss, hemolytic anemia, polycythemia, and other conditions

Limitations When dealing with results of automated instruments falsely high results may occur with cryoproteins, significant leukocytosis, giant platelets; false low results may be seen with microcytosis, *in vitro* hemolysis or in presence of autoagglutinins.

Methodology Manual microhematocrit centrifugation; automated - electronic cell counters such as Coulter S, Coulter S Plus, subsequent Coulter S models including STKR® and JT series, H-1, Sysmex, others; derived by electronic calculation considering that Hct = RBC x MCV / 10 (latter two are directly measured). Data ReCap, a summary compilation of data of College of American Pathologists indicates that for the year 1980, hematocrit had a SD of 2.2 and CV of 5.3%.[1] Reference to the results of current CAP surveys indicate a trend toward a further decrease in SD and CV of the hematocrit.

Additional Information The degree of plasma trapping is increased in disease with less deformable RBCs (eg, sickle cell disease, hereditary spherocytosis, and iron deficiency). A study[2] using ^{125}I labeled human serum albumin found trapped plasma volume to be 1.53% (25 normals), somewhat less than earlier work[3] which found a level of 3% and the work of Miale, who reported the calculated hematocrit (Coulter S and Coulter S Plus derived) to be 2% lower than the microhematocrit at the 40% level.[4]

A large study (17,274 children in apparent good health and residing in the Washington, DC, metropolitan area) found that the lower mean Hct and Hgb value in African-American children (as compared to white children) was the result not only of α- and β-thalassemia but also of the presence of Hb AS and Hb AC. The mean Hct of children with Hb AC and Hb AS was 1.5 and 1.0 point lower, respectively, than that of subjects with Hb AA.[5]

Hct levels in the highest quintile have been associated with increased morbidity and mortality from cardiovascular disease.[6] Elevated Hct (51 or higher) has been noted to increase the risk of stroke.[7]

The red cell indices, MCV and MCHC, depend on the Hct for their derivation and are of use in the evaluation of anemia. See also discussion under the listing Complete Blood Count *on page 312*.

A six parameter (includes Hct) point-of-care handheld portable analyzer that requires just 2 minutes for analyses is currently available.[8]

Footnotes

1. Elevitch FR and Noce PS, eds, *Data ReCap: 1970-1980. A Compilation of Data From the College of American Pathologists Clinical Laboratory Improvement Programs*, Skokie, IL: College of American Pathologists, 1981, 208-10.
2. Pearson TC and Guthrie DL, "Trapped Plasma in the Microhematocrit," *Am J Clin Pathol*, 1982, 78:770-2.
3. England JM, Walford DM, Waters DA, et al, "Reassessment of the Reliability of the Hematocrit," *Br J Haematol*, 1972, 23:247-56.

4. Miale JB, *Laboratory Medicine: Hematology*, 6th ed, St Louis, MO: Mosby-Year Book Inc, 1982, 360.
5. Rana SR, Sekhsaria S, and Castro OL, "Hemoglobin S and C Traits: Contributing Causes for Decreased Mean Hematocrit in African-American Children," *Pediatrics*, 1993, 91(4):800-2.
6. Gagnon DR, Zhang TJ, Brand FN, et al, "Hematocrit and the Risk of Cardiovascular Disease - The Framingham Study: A 34-Year Follow-Up," *Am Heart J*, 1994, 127(3):674-82.
7. Wannamethee G, Perry IJ, and Shaper AG, "Haematocrit, Hypertension and Risk of Stroke," *J Intern Med*, 1994, 235(2):163-8.
8. Woo J, McCabe JB, Chauncey D, et al, "The Evaluation of a Portable Clinical Analyzer in the Emergency Department," *Am J Clin Pathol*, 1993, 100(6):599-605.

References

Brown BA, *Hematology: Principles and Procedures*, 6th ed, Philadelphia, PA: Lea & Febiger, 1993, 85-7, 345-79.

Henry JB, Nelson DA, Tomar RH, et al, *Todd-Sanford-Davidsohn Clinical Diagnosis and Management by Laboratory Methods*, 18th ed, Philadelphia, PA: WB Saunders Co, 1991, 560-1, 582, 597-8.

Second National Health and Nutrition Examination Survey, "Hematological and Nutritional Biochemistry Reference Data for Persons 6 Months-74 Years of Age: United States, 1976-80," *Vital and Health Statistics*, DHHS Publication No (PHS), 83-1682, 1982.

Wyrick-Glatzel J and Gwaltney-Krause S, *Laboratory Methods in Hematology and Hemostasis, Clinical Hematology and Fundamentals of Hemostasis*, 2nd ed, Chapter 30, Section 1, Harmening DM, ed, Philadelphia, PA: FA Davis Co, 1992, 523-53.

Zaizov R and Matoth Y, "Red Cell Values on the First Postnatal Day During the Last 16 Weeks of Gestation," *Am J Hematol*, 1976, 1:275-8.

Hematology Profile *see* Complete Blood Count *on page 312*

Hemoflagellates *see* Microfilariae, Peripheral Blood Preparation *on page 333*

Hemoglobin

CPT 85018

Related Information

Complete Blood Count *on page 312*
Cyanide, Blood *on page 544*
Erythropoietin, Serum *on page 124*
Ferritin, Serum *on page 127*
Folic Acid, RBC *on page 317*
Folic Acid, Serum *on page 317*
Hematocrit *on previous page*
Iron and Total Iron Binding Capacity/Transferrin *on page 150*
Oxygen Saturation, Blood *on page 175*
P-50 Blood Gas *on page 176*
Protoporphyrin, Free Erythrocyte *on page 195*
Red Blood Cell Indices *on page 343*
Red Blood Cells *on page 621*
Red Cell Count *on page 344*
Red Cell Mass *on page 345*
Reticulocyte Count *on page 345*
Sickle Cell Tests *on page 347*
Vitamin B_{12} *on page 351*

Synonyms Hb; Hgb

Applies to H and H

Abstract This procedure determines the concentration of hemoglobin (Hgb) in whole blood. Hemoglobin is the major component of the red cell and functions to transport oxygen. It also acts to buffer carbon dioxide formed during metabolic activity. The Hgb level is important in the detection and follow up of anemia and polycythemia. The Hgb value is used in the calculation of the MCH and MCHC.

Specimen Whole blood

Container Lavender top (EDTA) tube

Collection Routine venipuncture. Invert tube gently to mix.

Causes for Rejection Clotted or hemolyzed specimen

Reference Range See tables in the listing Complete Blood Count *on page 312*.

Use Evaluate anemia, blood loss, hemolysis, polycythemia, and other conditions

Limitations Hyperlipemic plasma (especially Fredrickson and Lees type I and V in which chylomicronemia is present) or white count >50,000/mm³ may falsely elevate the hemoglobin result with corresponding increase in the MCH and MCHC. A method correcting for lipemia has been suggested.[1] Increased turbidity (with resultant interference in sample absorbance) may also be due to presence of a paraprotein or of an abnormal hemoglobin (S or C). A variety of corrective procedures are available,[2] (see also reference by Brown).

Methodology While oxyhemoglobin and other chemical approaches to hemoglobinometry exist, nearly all current procedures involve a one or two step procedure in which RBC lysis/dilution occurs with the formation of a cyanmethemoglobin compound. Dilutions are read by spectrophotometer at 540 nm. The majority of routine hematology laboratories obtain the hemoglobin level as one of a number of parameters from an automated multichannel instrument.

Additional Information The hemoglobin determination is one of the best standardized and accurate of available clinical laboratory analyses. Data ReCap, a summary compilation of data of College of American Pathologists, indicates that for the year 1980, the hemoglobin determination had a SD of 0.3 and a CV of 2.2%.[3] The results of current CAP surveys continue to show good interlaboratory performance for the Hgb procedure with low SD and CV values. The clinical utility of subject-specific reference values has been delineated and emphasized.[4]

In cyanide poisoned individuals treated with methemoglobin-forming agents (to protect cytochrome oxidase) oxygen carrying capacity is decreased in direct proportion to the amount of methemoglobin (nonoxygen carrying) that is formed. A multiwavelength spectrophotometric method has been developed which allows monitoring of hemoglobin derivatives present in the blood of treated cyanide poisoned patients.[5]

The red cell indices, MCH and MCHC, depend on the Hgb for their derivation and are of use in the evaluation of anemia. See also the discussion under Complete Blood Count *on page 312*.

Footnotes

1. Williams GJ, (letters to the editor), *Coulter Currents*, 1980, 3:2.
2. Linz LJ, "Elevation of Hemoglobin, MCH, and MCHC by Paraprotein: How to Recognize and Correct the Interference," *Clin Lab Sci*, 1994, 7(4):211-2.
3. Elevitch FR and Noce PS, eds, *Data ReCap: 1970-1980. A Complication of Data From the College of American Pathologists Clinical Laboratory Improvement Programs*, Skokie, IL: College of American Pathologists, 1981, 211-3.
4. Fraser CG, Wilkinson SP, Neville RG, et al, "Biologic Variation of Common Hematologic Laboratory Quantities in the Elderly," *Am J Clin Pathol*, 1989, 92(4):465-70.
5. Zijlstra WG and Buursma A, "Rapid Multicomponent Analysis of Hemoglobin Derivatives for Controlled Antidotal Use of Methemoglobin-Forming Agents in Cyanide Poisoning," *Clin Chem*, 1993, 39(8):1685-9.

References

Brown BA, *Hematology: Principles and Procedures*, 6th ed, Philadelphia, PA: Lea & Febiger, 1993, 83-5, 345-79.

Henry JB, Nelson DA, Tomar RH, et al, *Todd-Sanford-Davidsohn Clinical Diagnosis and Management by Laboratory Methods*, 18th ed, Philadelphia, PA: WB Saunders Co, 1991, 555-60, 608-13, 627-76.

Second National Health and Nutrition Examination Survey, "Hematological and Nutritional Biochemistry Reference Data for Persons 6 Months-74 Years of Age: United States, 1976-80," *Vital and Health Statistics*, DHHS Publication No (PHS) 83-1682, 1982.

Wyrick-Glatzel J and Gwaltney-Krause S, *Laboratory Methods in Hematology and Hemostasis, Clinical Hematology and Fundamentals of Hemostasis*, 2nd ed, Chapter 30, Section 1, Harmening DM, ed, Philadelphia, PA: FA Davis Co, 1992, 523-53.

Zwart A, "Spectrophotometry of Hemoglobin: Various Perspectives," *Clin Chem*, 1993, 39(8):1570-2.

Hemoglobin A_2

CPT 83020 (electrophoresis)

Related Information

Hemoglobin Electrophoresis *on next page*
Peripheral Blood: Red Blood Cell Morphology *on page 339*
Red Blood Cell Indices *on page 343*

Synonyms Hb A_2

Abstract Hemoglobin A_2 (Hb A_2) is a tetramer of α- and δ-globulin chains (α_2 δ_2). Concentration fluctuates in the thalassemia syndromes and some acquired diseases.

Specimen Whole blood

Container Lavender top (EDTA) tube

Causes for Rejection Specimen clotted

Reference Range The stable adult Hb A_2 level is 2.5% to 3.5% of total hemoglobin. See table.

Alterations in Hb A_2 in Various Disorders

	Elevated	Reduced
Congenital	β-thalassemia trait	α-thalassemia
	Unstable hemoglobin variants	δβ-thalassemia
	Sickle trait (AS)	δ-thalassemia
	SS with α-thalassemia	HPFH
Acquired	Megaloblastic anemias	Iron deficiency
	Hyperthyroidism	Sideroblastic anemias

From Bunn HF and Forget BG, *Hemoglobin: Molecular, Genetic, and Clinical Aspects*, Philadelphia, PA: WB Saunders Co, 1986, 61-7, with permission.

Use Investigate microcytic anemia, for hemoglobinopathies, especially thalassemia, particularly beta-thalassemia trait

Limitations Blood transfusion prior to hemoglobin electrophoresis may make interpretation inconsistent. High levels of hemoglobin F usually are accompanied by lower levels of A_2. Sickle cell trait range is from 1.7% to 4.5% hemoglobin A_2. Presence of Hb S or Hb C will interfere with column chromatographic method. Presence of Hb C interferes with routine electrophoretic method. Quantitation of Hb A_2 by densitometric scanning of electrophoretic pattern may result in misleading (high) results as this method is not uniformly reliable.

Contraindications Recent blood transfusion

(Continued)

Hemoglobin A₂ (Continued)

Methodology Electrophoresis, DEAE cellulose chromatography is preferred; radial immunodiffusion (RID) has also been used.

Additional Information This test is done in many laboratories as part of the hemoglobin electrophoresis. Hemoglobin A₂ levels have special application to the diagnosis of beta-thalassemia trait, which may be present even though peripheral blood smear is normal. (This reflects the underlying genetic spectrum of beta-thalassemia which in reality is a complex of 20-30 distinct conditions and over 50 different mutations.) The microcytosis and other morphologic changes of beta-thalassemia trait must be differentiated from iron deficiency. Low MCV may include the majority of beta-thalassemia trait patients but does not differentiate iron deficient individuals. Low Hb A₂ levels occur in untreated iron deficiency. If the beta-thalassemia is associated with iron deficiency, the Hb A₂ level falls, making the differentiation even more difficult (corrected after iron therapy).[1]

The most definitive evidence for presence of beta-thalassemia trait is genetic (family study). A well documented report, however, indicates the occurrence of beta-thalassemia minor as a result of a spontaneous initiation codon mutation.[2] Offspring of a person with thalassemia major will have beta-thalassemia trait. Apart from such genetic studies (which are subject to practical difficulties) gene probes are the most definitive method for identifying beta-thalassemia trait. This method identifies "silent" carriers but is a research level procedure. Elevated percent Hb A₂ is the next best evidence for the diagnosis of beta-thalassemia trait. Sufficient criteria for the diagnosis of thalassemia trait are an elevated Hb A₂ percentage by a reliable method (Hgb electrophoresis with elution and quantitation by spectrophotometry) or column chromatography (assuming Hb S, C, or an unstable hemoglobin are not present).

Hb A₂ may be increased in megaloblastic anemia and may be decreased in sideroblastic anemia, Hb H disease, and erythroleukemia. Approximately one-third of zidovudine (AZT) treated human immunodeficiency virus-1 positive individuals have elevated Hb A₂ levels.[3]

Footnotes

1. Wasi P, Disthasongchan P, and Na-Nakorn S, "The Effect of Iron Deficiency on the Levels of Hemoglobins A₂ and E," *J Lab Clin Med*, 1968, 71:85-91.
2. Beris P, Darbellay R, Speiser D, et al, "De Novo Initiation Codon Mutation (ATG → ACG) of the β-Globin Gene Causing β-Thalassemia in a Swiss Family," *Am J Hematol*, 1993, 42(3):248-53.
3. Routy JP, Monte M, Beaulieu R, et al, "Increase of Hemoglobin A₂ in Human Immunodeficiency Virus-1-Infected Patients Treated With Zidovudine," *Am J Hematol*, 1993, 43(2):86-90.

References

Adams JG 3d and Coleman MB, "Structural Hemoglobin Variants That Produce the Phenotype of Thalassemia," *Semin Hematol*, 1990, 27(3):229-38.

Bunn HF and Forget BG, *Hemoglobin: Molecular, Genetic, and Clinical Aspects*, Philadelphia, PA: WB Saunders Co, 1986, 61-7.

Kazazian HH Jr, "The Thalassemia Syndromes: Molecular Basis and Prenatal Diagnosis in 1990," *Semin Hematol*, 1990, 27(3):209-28.

Lukens JN, "The Thalassemias and Related Disorders: Quantitative Disorders of Hemoglobin Synthesis," *Wintrobe's Clinical Hematology*, 9th ed, Vol 1, Chapter 39, Lee GR, Bithell TC, Foerster J, et al, eds, Philadelphia, PA: Lea & Febiger, 1993, 1102-45.

Steinberg MH and Adams JG 3d, "Hemoglobin A₂: Origin, Evolution, and Aftermath," *Blood*, 1991, 78(9):2165-77.

Thonglairoam V, Winichagoon P, Fucharoen S, et al, "Hemoglobin Constant Spring in Bangkok: Molecular Screening by Selective Enzymatic Amplification of the α₂-Globin Gene," *Am J Hematol*, 1991, 38(4):277-80.

Hemoglobin Electrophoresis

CPT 83020

Related Information

Fetal Hemoglobin *on page 316*
Hemoglobin A₂ *on previous page*
Methemoglobin *on page 166*
P-50 Blood Gas *on page 176*
Peripheral Blood: Red Blood Cell Morphology *on page 339*
Reticulocyte Count *on page 345*
Sickle Cell Tests *on page 347*

Test Commonly Includes Electrophoresis for separation and distribution of hemoglobins

Abstract In this procedure, hemoglobins are caused to separate and migrate. A variety of techniques are utilized. Most commonly bands are developed on a substrate in a buffer solution across an electric field with subsequent visualization after fixation and staining. Clinical applications include detection and identification of hemoglobin variants and the investigation of some hemolytic anemias resulting from red cell intracorpuscular defects.

Specimen Whole blood

Container Lavender top (EDTA) tube for venipuncture specimen; lavender top Microtainer™ tube for capillary specimen

Causes for Rejection Specimen clotted

Turnaround Time Method dependent, usually 1-2 days

Reference Range Hemoglobin A: 95% to 98%; hemoglobin A₂: 1.5% to 3.5%; hemoglobin F: 0% to 2%; hemoglobin C: absent; hemoglobin S: absent

Use Diagnose hemoglobinopathies; evaluate hemolytic anemia; diagnose thalassemia; evaluate sickling hemoglobins, hemoglobin C; with other and specialized techniques, evaluate unstable, low and high oxygen affinity hemoglobinopathies (eg, one cause of polycythemia)

Limitations Blood transfusion prior to hemoglobin electrophoresis may make interpretations inconsistent. Many abnormal hemoglobins will not separate from normal adult Hb A during application of routine electrophoretic techniques. Rarely, there may be lack of specificity for Hgb (eg, monoclonal immunoglobulin).[1]

Methodology Electrophoresis using cellulose acetate, agarose gel, citrate agar gel, or starch gel substrates; isoelectric focusing using polyacrylamide or agarose gel substrates; alkali denaturation for fetal hemoglobin; anion exchange resin chromatography for hemoglobin A₂ quantitation; globin chain electrophoresis

	CELLULOSE ACETATE PATTERN							AGAR (CITRATE) GEL PATTERN					
	ORIGIN	CA	A₂,C,E	D,S G,F	A	H,	Bart's	C	ORIGIN S	D,E,A	F		
Normal (A₁A₂)			■		■				■				Normal
Sickle Trait (A₁SA₂)			■	■	■				■	■			Sickle Trait
S-C Disease (SC)			■	■					■	■			S-C Disease
Sickle Disease (S)			■	■				■		■			Sickle Disease
C Disease (C)			■					■		■			C Disease
Cord Blood (A, F)				■	■			■		■	■		Cord Blood
S Thal (A₁ FSA₂)			■	■	■				■				
Control (A₁ FSC)		■	■	■	■			■		■			Control

Additional Information In this procedure, hemoglobin (Hgb), released from lysed red blood cells, is caused to migrate through a substrate in a buffer by application of an electric current. Different types of hemoglobin are separated into specific bands that are subsequently visualized by application of one of a variety of staining procedures. Migration of hemoglobin is defined by interaction of a specific hemoglobin molecule with substrate structure, buffer pH, ionic strength, and other characteristics. The test is of central importance in establishing the presence of common hemoglobinopathies (Hb S, C, D, and E) and in the evaluation of some cases of hemolytic anemia. Study of peripheral blood smear RBC morphology can assist in the decision to order hemoglobin electrophoresis. Hemoglobin electrophoresis (including determination of Hb F) is indicated if a positive sickle screening test has been obtained. Hb F and Hb A₂ quantitation (often included as part of an "Hb electrophoresis" package) are important in establishing the presence of thalassemia. In some cases additional study will be needed. Depending upon the abnormality encountered this might include reticulocyte count, haptoglobin level, citrate agar gel electrophoresis at acidic pH, globin chain electrophoresis, and family studies.

Complete characterization of abnormal hemoglobin states may require sophisticated laboratory studies usually available only in a research setting (eg, some of the thalassemia syndromes).[2] Amino acid globin chain sequencing may be used to establish the presence of a hemoglobinopathy.

Hemoglobin electrophoresis of umbilical cord blood can detect α-chain variants Hb F/G and Hb G as well as S and C gene products. Results have been reported as consistent with the predicted frequency (1 in 625) of sickle anemia at birth.[3] Newer techniques of analysis, globin chain electrophoresis,[4,5] isoelectric focusing,[6,7] restriction endonuclease studies,[8] and polymerase chain reaction[9] are powerful additions to the laboratory's ability to detect and identify hemoglobin variants. A multiplex polymerase chain reaction for the detection of α-thalassemia (caused by α-globin gene deletion - the most common genetic abnormality in the world) is said to be applicable to routine performance by clinical laboratories.[10]

Some alkaline gel electrophoretic systems may offer advantages in glycohemoglobin quantitation because of their ability to discriminate Hb F and to simultaneously detect common hemoglobinopathies.[11] Cation exchange HPLC has delineated over 10 minor hemoglobins including HbA₁c and HbA₁d₃ with evidence that the latter is useful for assessment of the uremic state.[12] It has been shown that capillary electrophoresis can separate hemoglobin variants within 10 minutes.[13]

Screening of the general population for sickle cell and other hemoglobinopathies had vocal proponents in the late 1960s and early 1970s. Interest waned, largely the result of possible socioeconomic implications of case detection. During the past decade, however, there has been growing activity in (and state support of) newborn screening for sickle

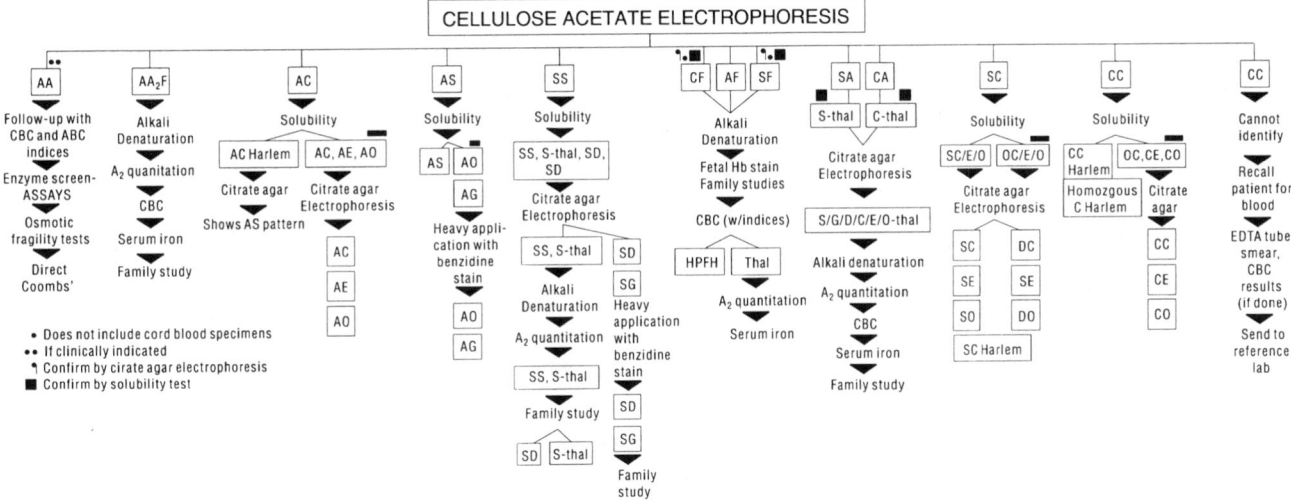

cell and other hemoglobinopathies. Problem areas include false-negative results (associated with the use of dried blood filter paper samples) and the detection of maternal contamination of cord blood.[14,15,16]

Footnotes

1. Sughayer MA and Arkin CF, "Unusual Band on Hemoglobin Electrophoresis Produced by a Monoclonal Immunoglobulin in Serum," *Clin Chem*, 1989, 35(8):1794.
2. Huisman TH, "Sickle Cell Anemia as a Syndrome: A Review of Diagnostic Features," *Am J Hematol*, 1979, 6:173-84.
3. Castro O, Winter WP, Lee TC, et al, "Prevalence of α-Chain Variants at Birth," *Am J Clin Pathol*, 1981, 75:56-9.
4. Alter BP, "Gel Electrophoretic Separation of Globin Chains," *Prog Clin Biol Res*, 1981, 60:157-75.
5. Alter BP, Coupal E, and Forget BG, "Globin Chain Electrophoresis for Prenatal Diagnosis of Beta Thalassemia," *Hemoglobin*, 1981, 5:357-70.
6. Basset P, Beuzard Y, Garel MC, et al, "Isoelectric Focusing of Human Hemoglobin: Its Application to Screening, to the Characterization of 70 Variants, and to the Study of Modified Fractions of Normal Hemoglobins," *Blood*, 1978, 51:971-82.
7. Cossu G, Manca M, Pirastu G, et al, "Neonatal Screening of β-Thalassemias by Thin Layer Isoelectric Focusing," *Am J Hematol*, 1982, 13:149-57.
8. Gutmann DH, "The Use of Restriction Endonucleases in the Prenatal Diagnosis of Hemoglobinopathies," *Am J Med Technol*, 1982, 48:361-6.
9. Skogerboe KJ, West SF, Murillo MD, et al, "Genetic Screening of Newborns for Sickle Cell Disease: Correlation of DNA Analysis With Hemoglobin Electrophoresis," *Clin Chem*, 1991, 37(3):454-8.
10. Bowie LJ, Reddy PL, and Nagabhushan M, et al, "Detection of α-Thalassemias by Multiplex Polymerase Chain Reaction," *Clin Chem*, 1994, 40(12):2260-6.
11. Bayliss KM, Kopinski WS, and Kueck BD, "Glycohemoglobin Quantitation by Alkaline Gel Electrophoresis. A Reliable Technique with Practical Clinical Advantages," *Am J Clin Pathol*, 1989, 91(5):570-4.
12. Bissé E, Huaman-Guillen P, and Wieland H, "Chromatographic Evaluation of Minor Hemoglobins: Clinical Significance of Hemoglobin A_{1d}, Comparison With Hemoglobin, A_{1c}, and Possible Interferences," *Clin Chem*, 1995, 41(5):658-63.
13. Chen FT, Liu CM, Hsieh YZ, et al, "Capillary Electrophoresis - A New Clinical Tool," *Clin Chem*, 1991, 37(1):14-9.
14. Kutlar A, Ozcan O, Brisco JT, et al, "The Detection of Hemoglobin Variants by Isoelectrofocusing Using EDTA-Collected and Filter Paper-Dried Cord Blood Specimens," *Am J Clin Pathol*, 1990, 94(2):199-202.
15. Githens JH, Lane PA, McCurdy RS, et al, "Newborn Screening for Hemoglobinopathies in Colorado. The First 10 Years," *Am J Dis Child*, 1990, 144(4):466-70.
16. Scott RB, "Newborn Screening for Sickle Cell Disease and Other Hemoglobinopathies," *Pediatrics* , 1989, 83(5 Pt 2):908-9.

References

Alter BP, "Prenatal Diagnosis of Hemoglobinopathies and Other Hematologic Diseases," *J Pediatr*, 1979, 95:501-3.
Bunn HF and Forget BG, *Hemoglobin: Molecular, Genetic and Clinical Aspects*, Philadelphia, PA: WB Saunders Co, 1986.
Dickerson RE and Geis I, *Hemoglobin: Structure, Function, Evolution and Pathology*, Menlo Park, CA: The Benjamin/Cummings Publishing Co Inc, 1983.
Fairbanks VF, *Hemoglobinopathies and Thalassemias: Laboratory Methods and Case Studies*, Chapter 6, New York, NY: Thieme-Stratton Inc, 1980.
Harrison CR, "Hemolytic Anemias: Intracorpuscular Defects, IV. Thalassemia," *Clinical Hematology and Fundamentals of Hemostasis* 2nd ed, Chapter 12, Harmening DM, ed, Philadelphia, PA: FA Davis Co, 1992.
Papadea C and Cate JC 4th, "Identification and Quantification of Hemoglobins A, F, S, and C by Automated Chromatography," *Clin Chem*, 1996, 42(1):57-63.
Sandhaus LM and Harvey FG, "Laboratory Methods for the Detection of Hemoglobinopathies in the Community Hospital," *Clin Lab Med*, 1993, 13(4):801-16.
Stamatoyannopoulos G, Nienhuis AW, Majerus PW, et al, eds, *The Molecular Basis of Blood Diseases*, 2nd ed, Chapters 4-6, Philadelphia, PA: WB Saunders Co, 1994, 107-256.

Thonglairoam V, Winichagoon P, Fucharoen S, et al, "Hemoglobin Constant Spring in Bangkok: Molecular Screening by Selective Enzymatic Amplification of the $α_2$-Globin Gene," *Am J Hematol*, 1991, 38(4):277-80.
Zeringer H and Harmening DM, "Hemolytic Anemias: Intracorpuscular Defects, III. The Hemoglobinopathies," *Clinical Hematology and Fundamentals of Hemostasis* 2nd ed, Chapters 11, Harmening DM, ed, Philadelphia, PA: FA Davis Co, 1992.

Hemoglobin, Fetal *see* Fetal Hemoglobin *on page 316*

Hemoglobin, Free *see* Hemoglobin, Plasma *on this page*

Hemoglobin, Plasma

CPT 83051

Related Information

Haptoglobin, Serum *on page 141*
Hemoglobin, Qualitative, Urine *on page 637*

Synonyms Free Hemoglobin; Hemoglobin, Free; Plasma Free Hemoglobin

Abstract Test used to detect intravascular hemolysis

Patient Preparation Special precautions and patient preparation are usually required to draw the specimen. Laboratory should be contacted directly.

Aftercare A pressure bandage should be applied to the site of 18-gauge needle puncture (following the puncture) to stop residual bleeding.

Specimen Plasma

Container Lavender top (EDTA) tube

Collection Recommended procedure for collecting sample without inducing hemolysis: Use 18-gauge needle with attached infusion tubing. Observing HIV precautions, place tourniquet lightly around the upper arm. Puncture antecubital vein with as little trauma as possible. Release tourniquet and clamp tubing off as soon as blood return is seen. Collect 3 mL of blood first in a red top tube with the rubber stopper off. Follow by a 5 mL collection in a green top (heparin) tube with the stopper off. Clamp tubing, withdraw needle, and apply pressure to the site until residual bleeding is stopped. Cap green top tube and gently mix three to five times. Use this specimen for the plasma hemoglobin determination.

Storage Instructions Separate and freeze plasma as soon as possible if test is not run immediately.

Causes for Rejection Traumatic venipuncture causing hemolysis

Reference Range <10 mg/dL,[1] optimally (with absence of artifactual hemolysis during collection of blood) <1 mg/dL

Use Evaluate hemolytic anemia, especially intravascular hemolysis

Limitations Plasma hemoglobin is increased with intravascular hemolysis, ABO incompatible transfusion, traumatic hemolysis, falciparum malaria, burns, and march hemoglobinuria. Increase may occur in some cases of extravascular hemolysis, delayed transfusion reaction, slight increase in sickle cell anemia, and β-thalassemia. High bilirubin, turbidity, methemalbuminemia, lipemic plasma, and hemolysis during or after venipuncture may cause falsely elevated values in the plasma hemoglobin test (method based on peroxide oxidation of benzidine). Method based on the fractional absorbance of oxyhemoglobin at 578 nm

(Continued)

Hemoglobin, Plasma *(Continued)*

is proportional even in the presence of those interfering substances. Use of benzidine has been restricted because of reports that it is carcinogenic.

Methodology An established method utilizes fractional absorbance of oxyhemoglobin at 578 nm. A method utilizing first-derivative spectroscopy (procedure of Soloni et al) has undergone evaluation. It is rapid and not affected by bilirubin, myoglobin, lipemia, or turbidity. It is sensitive down to a level of 1 mg/dL.[2]

Additional Information High bilirubin (up to 36 mg/dL), turbidity of the specimen, or a fair amount of methemalbumin will not affect the method based on fractional absorbance of oxyhemoglobin at 578 nm or the method of Soloni et al.[3] Hemoglobinemia can be easily detected by gross examination of centrifuged blood when plasma hemoglobin is >50 mg/dL.

Footnotes

1. Copeland BE, Dyer PJ, and Pesce AJ, "Hemoglobin by First Derivative Spectrophotometry: Extent of Hemolysis in Plasma and Serum Collected in Vacuum Container Devices," *Ann Clin Lab Sci*, 1989, 19(5):383-8.
2. Soloni FG, Cunningham MT, and Amazon K, "Plasma Hemoglobin Determination by Recording Derivative Spectrophotometry," *Am J Clin Pathol*, 1986, 85(3):342-7.
3. Copeland BE, Dyer PJ, and Pesce AJ, "Hemoglobin Determination in Plasma or Serum by First-Derivative Recording Spectrophotometry," *Am J Clin Pathol*, 1989, 92(5):619-24.

References

Fairbanks VF, Ziesmer SC, and O'Brien PC, "Methods for Measuring Plasma Hemoglobin in Micromolar Concentration Compared," *Clin Chem*, 1992, 38(1):132-40.

Lee GR, "The Hemolytic Disorders: General Considerations," *Wintrobe's Clinical Hematology*, 9th ed, Vol 1, Chapter 32, Lee GR, Bithell TC, Foerster J, et al, eds, Philadelphia, PA: Lea & Febiger, 1993, 944-64.

Hemoglobin, Unstable, Heat Labile Test

CPT 83065

Related Information

Heinz Body Stain *on page 321*

Hemoglobin, Unstable - Isopropanol Precipitation Test *on this page*

Synonyms Heat Denaturation; Test for Congenital Heinz Body Hemolytic Anemia; Unstable Hemoglobins

Applies to Heinz Bodies

Abstract A simple, low cost test for the detection of unstable hemoglobin. Most of such variant hemoglobins will not separate from Hb A on routine electrophoresis.

Specimen Whole blood

Container Lavender top (EDTA) tube

Causes for Rejection Specimen more than 4 hours old

Reference Range Less than 1% unstable hemoglobin (quantitation by hemoglobinometry of centrifuged lysate). Normally, test should result in little or no precipitate. A positive result (denatured hemoglobin present) is the presence of turbidity and/or fine flocculation, a readily visible precipitate.

Use Determine the presence of unstable hemoglobins, most of which will not be identified by routine hemoglobin electrophoresis

Limitations The visual end point in this test may be difficult to interpret. Test should be run along with a normal control. Some degree of slight precipitation may occur in an erratic manner in normals. Quantitation of % unstable hemoglobin (by hemoglobinometry) is desirable. Result can be compared to the isopropanol precipitation test for unstable hemoglobin (see Hemoglobin, Unstable - Isopropanol Precipitation Test *on page 326*).

Methodology Washed cells lysed, acidified, lysate heated at 50°C for 1 hour and examined for turbidity/flocculation (compared to control). Percent unstable hemoglobin may be reported.

Additional Information Another approach to detection of unstable hemoglobins is to search for Heinz bodies. Heinz body test is less specific than heat instability study. Hemolysates containing unstable hemoglobin may precipitate spontaneously on standing a few days in the refrigerator. Some unstable hemoglobins are associated with hemolytic anemia and an appropriate clinical picture including intermittent jaundice and usually splenomegaly. If hypersplenism is present there may be thrombocytopenia. There have been many different unstable hemoglobins reported after the early study of Hb Köln.[1] Lukens and Lee in the 9th edition (1993) of *Wintrobe's Clinical Hematology* indicate that over 125 unstable hemoglobins have been identified. On the basis of clinical severity, these authors have divided the unstable hemoglobin variants into five groups. Eleven are classified as "severe hemolytic disease, no response to splenectomy"; 15 are associated with "moderately severe hemolytic disease improved by splenectomy"; 52 are classified as "moderate to mild hemolytic disease with hemolytic crises"; 33 have "no clinical or hematologic abnormality"; and 28 are considered to have "insufficient data to classify". The most common unstable Hb variant is

Hb Köln which has wide geographic distribution. Most unstable hemoglobins have been demonstrated only in single individuals or families. Most unstable hemoglobin diseases have an autosomal dominant mode of inheritance, however, in over 40 some cases the disease has occurred as a result of a spontaneous mutation.[2] Some of these unstable hemoglobins also have abnormal affinity for oxygen.

Footnotes

1. White JM and Dacie JV, "The Unstable Hemoglobins - Molecular and Clinical Features," *Prog Hematol*, 1971, 7:69-109.
2. Lukens JN and Lee GR, "Unstable Hemoglobin Disease," *Wintrobe's Clinical Hematology*, 9th ed, Vol 1, Chapter 37, Lee GR, Bithell TC, Foerster J, et al, eds, Philadelphia, PA: Lea & Febiger, 1993, 1054-60.

References

Beutler E, Lichtman MA, and Coller BS, *Williams Hematology*, 5th ed, Chapters 57 and L9, New York, NY: McGraw-Hill Inc, 1995, 650-4 and L33.

Bunn HF and Forget BG, *Hemoglobin: Molecular, Genetic and Clinical Aspects*, Philadelphia, PA: WB Saunders Co, 1986, 565-94.

Nagel RL, "Disorders of Hemoglobin Function and Stability," Chapter 52, Handin RI, Lux SE, and Stossel TP, eds, Philadelphia, PA: JB Lippincott Co, 1995, 1591-644.

Zinkham WH and Winslow RM, "Unstable Hemoglobins: Influence of Environment on Phenotypic Expression of a Genetic Disorder," *Medicine (Baltimore)*, 1989, 68(5):309-20.

Hemoglobin, Unstable - Isopropanol Precipitation Test

CPT 83068

Related Information

Heinz Body Stain *on page 321*

Hemoglobin, Unstable, Heat Labile Test *on this page*

Synonyms Unstable Hemoglobins

Applies to Heinz Bodies

Abstract A simple, low cost test for unstable hemoglobins. Most of such variant hemoglobins will not be detected by routine hemoglobin electrophoresis as they migrate with Hb A.

Specimen Whole blood

Container Lavender top (EDTA) tube

Reference Range Absence of a precipitate in buffered isopropanol. Solution should remain clear for 30-40 minutes.

Use Differential diagnosis of hemolytic anemias; detect unstable hemoglobins many of which will not be identified (separated from Hb A) by standard electrophoretic techniques

Limitations Hemoglobin F begins to precipitate about halfway through the incubation period - about the time that one expects unstable Hgb to appear. If the patient's Hb F is increased, a false-positive result for unstable Hgb may result.[1]

Methodology Mix 2 mL of 17% (unit/unit) isopropanol with 0.2 mL of hemolysate. Incubate at 37°C; check for precipitate at 20 minutes.

Additional Information Heat lability and Heinz body tests are also applicable to the detection and study of unstable hemoglobins. While simple to perform, interpretation may be difficult. A multitest approach has been suggested.[2]

Footnotes

1. Dacie JV and Lewis SM, *Practical Haematology*, 7th ed, New York, NY: Churchill Livingstone, 1991, 252.
2. Carrell RW, "Hemoglobin Stability Tests," *The Detection of Hemoglobinopathies*, Schmidt RM, et al, eds, Cleveland, OH: CRC Press, 1974.

References

Beutler E, Lichtman MA, Coller BS, et al, *Williams Hematology*, 5th ed, Chapters 57 and L34, New York, NY: McGraw-Hill Inc, 1995, 650-4 and L34.

Bunn HF and Forget BG, *Hemoglobin: Molecular, Genetic and Clinical Aspects*, Philadelphia, PA: WB Saunders Co, 1986, 565-94.

Carrell RW and Kay R, "A Simple Method for the Detection of Unstable Hemoglobins," *Br J Haematol*, 1972, 23:615-9.

Zinkham WH and Winslow RM, "Unstable Hemoglobins: Influence of Environment on Phenotypic Expression of a Genetic Disorder," *Medicine (Baltimore)*, 1989, 68(5):309-20.

Hemogram *see* Complete Blood Count *on page 312*

Hemolytic Anemia *see* Gelation Assay *on page 318*

Hemolytic Anemia *see* Glycerol Lysis Test, Acidified, Modified *on page 320*

Hemosiderin Stain *see* Iron Stain, Bone Marrow *on page 328*

Hemosiderin Stain *see* Siderocyte Stain *on page 348*

Hereditary Spherocytosis *see* Gelation Assay *on page 318*

Hereditary Spherocytosis *see* Glycerol Lysis Test, Acidified, Modified *on page 320*

Hexosaminidase A *see* Inherited Diseases of Metabolism and Cell Structure Tests *on next page*

Hexosaminidase A and B *see* Inherited Diseases of Metabolism and Cell Structure Tests *on next page*

Hgb *see* Hemoglobin *on page 323*

Inborn Errors of Metabolism *see* Inherited Diseases of Metabolism and Cell Structure Tests *on this page*

Incubated Osmotic Fragility *see* Osmotic Fragility *on page 334*

Indices *see* Red Blood Cell Indices *on page 343*

Inherited Diseases of Metabolism and Cell Structure Tests

CPT 85999

Related Information

Amniotic Fluid, Chromosome and Genetic Abnormality Analysis *on page 273*

Chorionic Villus Sampling (CVS), Chromosome and Genetic Abnormality Analysis *on page 275*

Muscle Biopsy *on page 53*

Urinalysis *on page 658*

Synonyms Glycogen Storage Diseases; Inborn Errors of Metabolism; Large Molecule Diseases; Lysosomal Storage Diseases; Mucopolysaccharidoses; Small Molecule Diseases; Sphingolipidoses; Test for Uncommon Inherited Diseases of Metabolism and Cell Structure

Applies to Acid β-Galactosidase; Ceramidase; Ceramidetrihexoside α-Galactosidase; α-Fucosidase; Galactocerebroside; β-Galactosidase; Glucocerebroside; β-Glucosidase; Hexosaminidase A; Hexosaminidase A and B; Neutral β-Galactosidase; Sphingomyelinase; Sulfatidase

Test Commonly Includes Under this heading recognition is given to an ever growing number of genetically determined disorders having a biochemical/metabolic defect (usually an enzyme deficiency or abnormality). The limitations of space allow only brief mention. Most of these disorders can be categorized as to biochemical type (eg, sphingolipidoses, mucopolysaccharidoses, lysosomal storage diseases) with overlap between these concepts and with some independent entities.

Of some 500 diseases with a defined biochemical basis, a majority involve abnormalities in enzymes, receptors, and/or structural proteins. The 7th (1995) edition of the monumental text, *The Metabolic and Molecular Bases of Inherited Disease* (with 302 authors) has descriptions of inborn errors of metabolism that include some 900 entities tabulated over 4605 pages. They are grouped by biochemical type (eg, carbohydrate, amino acid, lipoprotein/lipid, purine/pyrimidine, acid lipase), tissue/function type (eg, blood and blood forming organs, transport, peroxisome, immune, etc) and include some 70 **disorders of lysosomal enzymes**, with which this listing will be largely concerned. Clinical features (eg, age at onset, severity, signs and symptoms) may show considerable variation within diagnostic groups. Over 54 specific mutations responsible for the G_{m2} gangliosidoses (includes Tay-Sachs disease and Sandhoff disease) have been characterized. The 11th edition of McKusick's *Mendelian Inheritance in Man* lists 6678 human genes and their disorders as of early March 1994 with 51,879 journal reference citations and including 933 clinical disorders that have been mapped to specific chromosomal sites. This synopsis of the Kown map of the human genome is updated nearly daily in a computer accessible on line database (catalog) available from the William H Welch Medical Library (Johns Hopkins University School of Medicine).

Abstract Inherited diseases of metabolism/cell structure include a very large array of clinical disorders with a variety of underlying genetic bases. Many represent a specific enzyme deficiency with resultant excessive accumulation of substances (substrates) usually present in only small amounts. The disorders range from acute life-threatening crises to episodic conditions with prolonged asymptomatic periods or with developmental delay. Presentation in the pediatric age group is common and as indicated in the reference by Linder and Karnes, rapid diagnosis and institution of therapy may be lifesaving or may be important to optimizing long-term outcome.

Patient Preparation Appropriate preliminary studies may be critically important to allow narrowing the range of diagnostic testing possibilities. Such investigation might include eye examination (cherry red macula occurs in some gangliosidoses; corneal opacities in Fabry disease; optic atrophy in metachromatic leukodystrophy and Krabbe disease), blood/urine screening tests (Berry spot test positive in G_{M1} gangliosidosis, cetylpyridinium chloride citrate, or thin-layer chromatography for mucopolysaccharidoses (see reference by Pennock); anemia; vacuolated lymphocytes in fucosidosis), x-ray studies (for developmental changes in bone as with mucopolysaccharidoses, EEG, nerve conduction time, and bone marrow in search of inclusion bearing or foamy histocytes, eg, as with Gaucher cells).

Specimen The majority of tests in this area involve lysosomal enzymes, present in body tissues and fluids. Blood (serum, plasma, or white cells), urine, and tears are the most easily obtained samples for analysis. Solid tissue may be biopsied (eg, skin, liver, muscle). Most commonly used are serum, leukocytes, and culture fibroblasts (from tissue biopsy). Heparin anticoagulated whole blood, usually at least 5 mL is needed,

along with the serum. Specimen preference may be disease dependent (eg, the α-glucosidase deficiency of Pompe disease is best detected by using cultured skin fibroblasts or skeletal muscle).[1] Leukocytes provide a favorable substrate for sphingolipidosis testing but for detection of heterozygotes of Niemann-Pick or Krabbe disease cultured fibroblasts are preferred.[1] Referral of a leukocyte pellet or biopsy in culture media or even a growing culture of fibroblasts may be required. Molecular analysis for identification of a specific gene defect may be applicable usually with more readily obtained specimen (eg, whole blood).

Special Instructions For a number of reasons (a sampling follows), the reference laboratory should be contacted before specimens are sent. Details of the preliminary findings can be reviewed, appropriate tests recommended, the preferred samples obtained, need for a clinical photograph established, mode of transport decided, and any other special requirement arranged.

Use Assist in the diagnosis of sphingolipid and mucopolysaccharide lysosomal storage diseases by demonstrating presence of a partial or complete enzyme deficiency. Major symptoms, lipids accumulating, and enzymes involved in the sphingolipidoses are given in the table.

Sphingolipid Storage Diseases (Sphingolipidoses)

Disease	Signs and Symptoms	Enzyme Defect
Fabry's disease	Reddish-purple skin rash, kidney failure, pain in lower extremities	Ceramidetrihexoside-α-galactosidase
Farber's disease	Hoarseness, dermatitis, skeletal deformation, mental retardation	Ceramidase
Fucosidosis	Cerebral degeneration, muscle spasticity, thick skin	α-fucosidase
Gaucher disease	Spleen and liver enlargement, erosion of long bones and pelvis, mental retardation only in infantile form	Glucocerebroside-β-glucosidase
Generalized gangliosidosis	Mental retardation, liver enlargement, skeletal deformities, about 50% with red spot in retina	β-galactosidase
Krabbe's disease (globoid leukodystrophy)	Mental retardation, almost total absence of myelin, globoid bodies in white matter of brain	Galactocerebroside-β-galactosidase
Niemann-Pick disease type I, II and subtypes	Liver and spleen enlargement, mental retardation, about 30% with red spot in retina	Sphingomyelinase
Metachromatic leukodystrophy	Mental retardation, psychological disturbances in adult form, nerves stain yellow-brown with cresyl violet dye	Sulfatidase
Sandhoff's disease	Same as Tay-Sachs disease but progressing more rapidly	Hexosaminidase A and B
Shindler disease	Neurodegeneration, psychomotor retardation, cortical blindness, myoclonic seizures	α-N-acetyl-galactosaminidase
Tay-Sachs disease	Mental retardation, red spot in retina, blindness, muscular weakness	Hexosaminidase A

From Brady RO and Kolodny EH, "The Sphingolipid Storage Disorders: Diagnosis and Detection," *Lab Management*, 1982, 20:28, with permission.

Methodology Tests for enzyme deficiency utilizing synthetic substrates (eg, monosaccharide derivatives of 4-methylumbelliferone) have found growing application in this group of diseases.[2] In addition to serum or plasma assays, tests utilizing pelleted leukocytes and fibroblast cultures are used. Molecular analyses for identification of a specific gene defect with use of specific restriction fragment length polymorphism S, synthetic oligonucleotide probes, DNA sequencing, and/or study of linked chromosomal anonymous DNA sequences may be used, in particular for identification of heterozygosity.

Additional Information One group of lysosomal storage diseases, the mucopolysaccharidoses are due to genetic defects in enzymes that degrade connective tissue glycosaminoglycan. The table relates the type of mucopolysaccharidosis to the enzyme defect. Urine screening tests are available for initial diagnosis of these diseases.

A table of glycogen storage diseases follows. Most of these disorders of carbohydrate metabolism are not lysosomal storage diseases. They are all autosomal recessive except one form of liver phosphorylase kinase deficiency in which only males are affected and the inheritance is X-linked.[3]

Disease severity and symptoms vary widely with type and organ site of the defective enzyme activity.

The recognized spectrum of inherited abnormalities of metabolism and structure is continually enlarging. The majority are uncommon to rare, so (Continued)

327

Inherited Diseases of Metabolism and Cell Structure Tests *(Continued)*

Mucopolysaccharidoses

Type	Eponymic Designation	Lysosomal Enzyme Defect
I	Three allelic disorders Hurler-Scheie	α-L-iduronidase
II	Hunter severe, mild	Iduronate sulfatase
III (A-D)	Four nonallelic disorders Sanfilippo syndromes A-D	IIIA Heparan N-sulfatase
		IIIB N-acetyl-α-D-glucosaminidase
		IIIC Acetyl-CoA: α-glucosaminide N-acetyl transferase
		IIID N-acetyl-α-D-glucosaminide 6-sulfate sulfatase
IV (A,B)	Two nonallelic disorders Morquio syndromes A,B	IVA Galactosamine 6-sulfate sulfatase
		IVB β-galactosidase
VI	Several allelic types Maroteaux-Lamy syndrome	Arylsulfatase B
VII	Sly syndrome	β-glucuronidase

Glycogen Storage Diseases

I	von Gierke's Ia, Ib	Glucose-6-phosphatase
II	Pompe's infantile, adult form	Lysosomal α-1,4-glucosidase
III	Cori's Forbe's	Amylo-1,6-glucosidase (debrancher enzyme)
IV	Andersen's	Amylo-(1,4:1,6)-transglucosidase (brancher enzyme)
V	McArdle's	Muscle phosphorylase
VI	Hers', glycogenoses	Hepatic phosphorylase X-linked phosphorylase-β-kinase Autosomal phosphorylase-β-kinase
VII	Tarui's	Muscle phosphofructokinase

that resources of equipment and experienced personnel for testing are justifiably limited to the specialized laboratory. Even so there are a sufficient number of laboratories performing these assays so as to raise the question if any one can develop necessary case experience. Dialogue between the referring physician and the specialty laboratory is essential (discussed above in relation to technical considerations) in particular because of the biochemical heterogeneity frequently seen with these conditions. Clinical expression may be variable and unpredictable.

Each of the sphingolipidoses represents not one but several diseases differing in clinical signs and/or enzyme activity. They are characterized by differing age of onset, site of pathology, and amount of residual enzyme activity (total or partial deficiency). As in Tay-Sachs disease more than one form of the involved enzyme may be present. Two lysosomal glycoproteins (hexosaminidase A and G_{M2} activator protein) account for the enzymatic hydrolysis of glycolipids (largely ganglioside G_{M2}). With defective lysosomal degradation, glycolipid accumulates in neurones. Hexosaminidase A is formed of subunits α and β, each under different chromosome control. Hexosaminidase, the enzyme involved exists as two isoenzymes, A and B. In Tay-Sachs disease, hexosaminidase A is decreased or absent while hexosaminidase B is increased. In Sandhoff's disease, a variant form of Tay-Sachs, there is deficiency of both hexosaminidase A and B due to hexosaminidase β-subunit defect (encoded on chromosome 5).[4] In addition, the usual sources of variance may affect enzyme deficiency testing. The activity of β-N-acetyl hexosaminidases in Tay-Sachs is affected by pregnancy, chronic diseases of liver, heart, joints, endocrine system, skin and medications including oral contraceptives, some steroids, thyroid, and Butazolidin®. These factors do not affect the result of hexosaminidase assays performed on leukocytes, fibroblasts, or tears.

Sphingolipid storage diseases involve most cells of the body and thus are expressed as multisystem diseases. Gaucher disease is the most common and may show hepatosplenomegaly, thrombocytopenia, erosion of bone with tendency to pathologic fracture and in a few cases, CNS involvement. All of the lipid storage diseases show autosomal

recessive inheritance with the exception of Fabry's disease (which is transmitted as X-linked).

The advent of treatment strategies (eg, enzyme infusion,[5,6,7] use of recombinant enzymes, and gene therapy) may add further impetus to establishing the diagnosis, detection of carriers, and monitoring of pregnancies at risk (through amniocentesis and culturing of epithelial cells in the amniotic fluid).[8] Macrophage-targeted natural and recombinant glucocerebrosidase is now available for the treatment of Gaucher disease.[7]

Steroid sulfatase deficiency, characterized clinically by low maternal estrogen excretion with normal fetal growth/development, is important to recognize by antenatal diagnosis so that it can be differentiated from more serious fetal defects that are associated with low estrogen levels.[9]

Peroxisomes, cellular organelles involved in oxidative functions are deficient in cases of Zellweger syndrome. There is accumulation of long chain fatty acids, phytanic acid, pipecolic acid, bile acid intermediates, and lack of plasmalogen biosynthesis. Other diseases in this group include adrenoleukodystrophy and a form of chondrodysplasia punctata.[10]

See the references by Applegarth et al and the text by Scriver et al for investigation of small molecule diseases; organic acid, urea cycle, and peroxisomal disorders.

The rapidly expanding field of molecular genetics as it applies to the diagnosis of inherited disease has been succinctly discussed with emphasis on the nature of available tests in a review by Ostrer and Hejtmancik (see references).

Footnotes

1. Kolodny EH, "General Principles and Techniques of Case Identification, Carrier Testing, and Prenatal Diagnosis," *Practical Enzymology of the Sphingolipidoses, Laboratory and Research Methods in Biology and Medicine*, Glew RH and Peters SP, eds, New York, NY: Alan R Liss Inc, 1977, 1:35-7, 17.
2. Brady RO and Kolodny EH, "The Sphingolipid Storage Disorders: Diagnosis and Detection," *Lab Management*, 1982, 20:7, 30-2.
3. Hers H-G, Van Hoof F, and de Barsy T, "Glycogen Storage Diseases," *The Metabolic Basis of Inherited Disease*, 6th ed, Chapter 12, Scriver CR, Beaudet AL, Sly WS, et al, eds, New York, NY: McGraw-Hill Inc, 1989, 425-52.
4. Sandhoff K, Conzelmann E, Neufeld EF, et al, "The G_{M2} Gangliosidoses," *The Metabolic Basis of Inherited Disease*, 6th ed, Scriver CR, Beaudet AL, Sly WS, et al, eds, New York, NY: McGraw-Hill Inc, 1989, 1807.
5. Brady RO, Barranger JA, Gal AE, et al, "Treatment of Lipidoses by Enzyme Infusion," *Lysosomes and Lysosomal Storage Diseases*, Callahan JW and Lowden JA, eds, New York, NY: Raven Press, 1981, 373-9.
6. Neuwelt EA, Barranger JA, Brady RO, et al, "Delivery of Hexosaminidase A to the Cerebrum After Osmotic Modification of the Blood-Brain Barrier," *Proc Natl Acad Sci USA*, 1981, 78:5838-41.
7. Duursma SA, guest ed, "Gaucher Disease, Hematologic, Skeletal, Visceral, and Biochemical Effects: Current Understanding, Recent Advances, and Future Directions," *Semin Hematol*, 1995, 32(3 Suppl 1):1-52.
8. Kudoh T, Kikuchi K, Nakamura F, et al, "Prenatal Diagnosis of G_{M1}-gangliosidosis: Biochemical Manifestations in Fetal Tissues," *Hum Genet*, 1978, 44:287-93.
9. Sherwood RA and Rocks BF, "Antenatal Diagnosis of Steroid Sulfatase Deficiency: Case Report and Literature Survey," *J Clin Pathol*, 1982, 35:1236-9.
10. Moser HW, "Peroxisomal Disorders," *Clin Biochem*, 1991, 24(4):343-51.

References

Applegarth DA, Dimmick JE, and Toone JR, "Laboratory Detection of Metabolic Disease," *Pediatr Clin North Am*, 1989, 36(1):49-65.

Borgaonkar DS, *Chromosomal Variation in Man: A Catalog of Chromosomal Variants and Anomalies*, 7th ed, New York, NY: Wiley-Liss, 1994.

Beutler E, Demina A, Laubscher K, et al, "The Clinical Course of Treated and Untreated Gaucher Disease. A Study of 45 Patients," *Blood Cells Mol Dis*, 1995, 21(2):73-85.

Dowton SB and Slaugh RA, "Diagnosis of Human Heritable Diseases - Laboratory Approaches and Outcomes," *Clin Chem*, 1995, 41(5):785-94.

Lindor NM and Karnes PS, "Initial Assessment of Infants and Children With Suspected Inborn Errors of Metabolism," *Mayo Clin Proc*, 1995, 70(10):987-8.

McKusick VA, *Mendelian Inheritance in Man: A Catalog of Human Genes and Genes Disorders*, 11th ed, Baltimore, MD: John Hopkins University Press, 1994.

Ostrer H and Hejtmancik JF, "Prenatal Diagnosis and Carrier Detection of Genetic Diseases by Analysis of Deoxyribonucleic Acid," *J Pediatr*, 1988, 112(5):679-87.

Pennock CA, "A Review and Selection of Simple Laboratory Methods Used for the Study of Glycosaminoglycan Excretion and the Diagnosis of the Mucopolysaccharidoses," *J Clin Pathol*, 1976, 29:111-23.

Rhead WJ, "Inborn Errors of Fatty Acid Oxidation in Man," *Clin Biochem*, 1991, 24(4):319-29.

Roth KS, "Inborn Errors of Metabolism: The Essentials of Clinical Diagnosis," *Clin Pediatr (Phila)*, 1991, 30(3):183-90.

Scriver CR, Beaudet Al, Sly WS, et al, eds, Part 12, "Lysosomal Enzymes," Vol II, *The Metabolic and Molecular Bases of Inherited Disease*, 7th ed, New York, NY: McGraw-Hill Inc, 1995, 2427-879.

Shih VE, "Detection of Hereditary Metabolic Disorders Involving Amino Acids and Organic Acids," *Clin Biochem*, 1991, 24(4):301-9.

Interleukin-3 *see* Eosinophil Count *on page 315*

Interleukin-5 *see* Eosinophil Count *on page 315*

Iron Stain *see* Siderocyte Stain *on page 348*

Iron Stain, Bone Marrow

CPT 85535

Related Information

Bone Marrow *on page 307*

Ferritin, Serum *on page 127*

Iron and Total Iron Binding Capacity/Transferrin *on page 150*
Siderocyte Stain *on page 348*

Synonyms Bone Marrow Iron Stain; Hemosiderin Stain; Marrow Iron Stores; Perls' Test; Prussian Blue Stain; Sideroblast Stain

Test Commonly Includes Iron stain on sections of marrow aspirate clot and/or bone marrow biopsy and iron stain marrow cover slip smears

Specimen Bone marrow glass coverslip or slide smears, marrow aspirate, or biopsy

Container Coverslips or glass microslides are prepared at the bedside. Biopsy and clot fixed in formalin or other fixative (eg, B5 or Zenker's solution).

Collection Physician obtains bone marrow aspirate specimen by aseptic aspiration technique. Phlebotomist simultaneously obtains blood specimen for the preparation of peripheral blood smears.

Causes for Rejection No marrow obtained ("dry tap") or no bone marrow particles on smears

Special Instructions Requisition should include a brief clinical history.

Reference Range Results should be interpreted in light of clinical background. Peripheral blood: no stainable iron is usually present (ie, no siderocytes are normally found). Bone marrow: stainable iron present as extracellular granules/globules and/or intracellular in cytoplasm of histiocytes - cells of the RE system. About one-third of the rubricytes in the marrow may be iron-positive sideroblasts (but not "ringed sideroblasts").

Use Semiquantitation of bone marrow iron stores; sensitive test for the evaluation of iron reserve; aid in the diagnosis of iron deficiency; aid in the diagnosis of hemosiderosis/hemochromatosis; aid in the diagnosis of sideroblastic anemia (including refractory anemia with ringed sideroblasts) and in the detection of hemophagocytosis

Limitations Specimen should include sufficiently large spicules of marrow.

Methodology Ferrocyanide ion reacts in acid with ferric ion to form a dark blue precipitate called Prussian blue. A silver stain has been proposed as a sensitive alternative for the demonstration of ringed sideroblasts.[1]

Additional Information It would appear that when a bone biopsy specimen is decalcified for over 2 hours, "leaching" of iron may occur so that a bone biopsy may be negative for iron while aspirate smear is positive. Krause et al, however, found that in only 35% of 270 cases with iron negative aspirate smears were there also iron negative biopsies (65% iron positive biopsies with iron negative smears).[2] Therefore, without evaluation of both types of specimens a significant overdiagnosis of iron deficiency may occur. Hemochromatosis, hemolytic anemias, and those with ineffective erythropoiesis (eg, thalassemia, megaloblastic and sideroblastic anemias) and anemias of chronic disease (especially inflammation) are characterized by increase in iron stores. The usual sideroblast has small iron positive granules without pattern in the cytoplasm. Ringed sideroblasts are rubricytes with tiny particles of iron located in mitochondria forming a ring around at least two-thirds of the nucleus. These pathologic sideroblasts occur in cases of normoblastic refractory anemia, B_6 responsive anemia including inherited (X-linked) pyridoxine-responsive sideroblastic anemia due to mutant erythroid 5-aminolevulinate synthase,[3] thalassemia, a variety of sideroblastic anemias, in some cases of B_{12}/folic acid deficiency, and in chloramphenicol toxicity.

Siderocytes in Peripheral Blood Normal vs Hemolytic States

	Average (%)	Range (%)
Normal	0	0
Normal, postsplenectomy	4	0-14
Hereditary spherocytosis	0-2	0-2
Hereditary spherocytosis, postsplenectomy	10	2-45
Acquired hemolytic anemia	2.3	0-21
Acquired hemolytic anemia, postsplenectomy	20	1-67
Thalassemia	0	0
Sickle cell anemia	0.2	0.2
Hemolytic disease newborn	3.7	0-35

From Miale JB, *Laboratory Medicine: Hematology*, 6th ed, St Louis, MO: Mosby-Year Book Inc, 1982, 582, with permission.

Review of iron-stained marrow preparations also finds application in the identification of hemophagocytic histiocytosis (evidence of erythrophagocytosis and/or leukophagocytosis).[4]

A proposed silver stain for ringed sideroblasts may have as its chemical basis the demonstration of insoluble phosphates and/or carbonates of iron or other metals. Thus, when marrow iron is decreased (eg, sideroblastic anemia with iron deficiency due to GI bleeding), silver staining

may be used to demonstrate ringed sideroblasts that would not be seen with Perls' reaction. Decalcified bone biopsy specimens, however, cannot be used to demonstrate sideroblasts (reaction is negative) by this method.[1] Silver staining is not considered to substitute for the Prussian blue reaction in identification of ringed sideroblasts.[1]

A cost efficient and noninvasive alternative to bone marrow iron study is the proposed combined determination of zinc protoporphyrin/heme ratio and serum ferritin.[5,6] In a study of the anemia of chronic disease (rheumatoid arthritis) it was concluded that a combination of peripheral blood parameters (MCV, ferritin, and transferrin) could detect iron deficiency without resorting to marrow aspiration.[7]

Footnotes

1. Tham KT, Cousar JB, and Macon WR, "Silver Stain for Ringed Sideroblasts. A Sensitive Method That Differs From Perls' Reaction in Mechanism and Clinical Application," *Am J Clin Pathol*, 1990, 94(1):73-6.
2. Krause JR, Brubaker D, and Kaplan S, "Comparison of Stainable Iron in Aspirated and Needle Biopsy Specimens of Bone Marrow," *Am J Clin Pathol*, 1979, 72:68-70.
3. Cox TC, Bottomley SS, Wiley JS, et al, "X-Linked Pyridoxine-Responsive Sideroblastic Anemia Due to a Thr[388]-to-Ser Substitution in Erythroid 5-Aminolevulinate Synthase," *N Engl J Med*, 1994, 330(10):675-9.
4. Koduri PR, "Prussian Blue Reaction and Hemophagocytosis: A New Use for an Old Test," *Am J Hematol*, 1995, 49(2):167.
5. Labbe RF, "Zinc Protoporphyrin/Heme Ratio as an Indicator of Marrow Iron Stores," *Am J Clin Pathol*, 1991, 95(5):758.
6. Labbe RF and Rettmer RL, "Zinc Protoporphyrin: A Product of Iron-Deficient Erythropoiesis," *Semin Hematol*, 1989, 26(1):40-6.
7. Vreugdenhil G, Baltus CA, Van Eijk HG, et al, "Anaemia of Chronic Disease: Diagnostic Significance of Erythrocyte and Serological Parameters in Iron Deficient Rheumatoid Arthritis Patients," *Br J Rheumatol*, 1990, 29(2):105-10.

References

Krantz SB, "Pathogenesis and Treatment of the Anemia of Chronic Disease," *Am J Med Sci*, 1994, 307(5):353-9.

Itano Solubility Test *see* Sickle Cell Tests *on page 347*

Joint Fluid Analysis *see* Body Fluid Analysis, Cell Count *on page 306*

K-B *see* Kleihauer-Betke *on this page*

Kleihauer-Betke

CPT 85460

Related Information

D^u *on page 608*
Fetal Hemoglobin *on page 316*
Prenatal Screen, Immunohematology *on page 618*
Rh_o(D) Immune Globulin (Human) *on page 623*
Rosette Test for Fetomaternal Hemorrhage *on page 625*

Synonyms Acid Elution for Fetal Hemoglobin; K-B

Abstract Staining of a postpartum maternal blood specimen for identification of percentage of fetal cells present

Specimen Whole blood

Container Lavender top (EDTA) tube

Storage Instructions Blood must be less than 6 hours old. Smears must be fixed within 1 hour after preparation.

Causes for Rejection Clotted specimen, improper labeling, inadequate specimen, gross hemolysis

Special Instructions A cord blood specimen should also be sent as a source of fetal blood (for use as a positive control).

Reference Range Full-term newborns: Hb F cells are >90%; normal adults: Hb F cells are <0.01%

Use Determine possible fetal-maternal hemorrhage in the newborn; aid in diagnosis of certain types of anemia in adults; assess the magnitude of fetal-maternal hemorrhage; calculate dosage of Rh immune globulin (eg, RhoGAM™) to be given. A study by Emery concludes (on the basis of 523 tests performed in 1993) that the Kleihauer-Betke test should be performed on all screening test positive Rh-negative mothers of Rh-positive infants and in cases of maternal trauma, unexplained increased maternal alpha-fetoprotein levels, fetal distress with abnormal cardiac tracings, intrauterine fetal death, and in cases of unexplained neonatal anemia.[1]

Limitations Possibility of presence of a hemoglobinopathy with increase in Hb F must be considered when this test is used to assess fetal-maternal hemorrhage. Specimens must be obtained prior to transfusion.

Contraindications Known pre-existing elevation of maternal Hb F (eg, mothers with hereditary persistence of fetal hemoglobin)[2,3]

Methodology Acid elution. After fixation with alcohol Hb F remains as a precipitate within the cell while Hb A is soluble in citric acid phosphate buffer. The adult RBCs containing little or no Hb F appear as ghosts under microscope.

Additional Information The Kleihauer-Betke test is helpful in distinguishing some forms of thalassemia from hereditary persistence of fetal hemoglobin (HPFH). The hereditary persistence of fetal hemoglobin reveals a uniform distribution of fetal hemoglobin in each red cell. $\Delta\beta$-
(Continued)

Kleihauer-Betke *(Continued)*

thalassemia, in contrast, demonstrates a heterogeneous distribution of fetal hemoglobin (ie, some cells are stained and others are ghost RBCs).

Some RhoGAM™ failures are due to a failure to suspect and diagnose fetal-maternal hemorrhage that may require more than one dose of RhoGAM™. Ultimate purpose is to prevent generation of anti-D antibodies in the postpartum woman and subsequent evolution hemolytic disease of the newborn (erythroblastosis fetalis). The amount of fetal blood contamination can be calculated. Each vial of Rh immune globulin contains 300 μg of anti-D. This is enough to prevent maternal immunization when the fetal bleed is up to 30 mL of whole blood (15 mL packed cells). One vial of Rh immune globulin is given to the Rh-negative mother for every 30 mL of fetal blood contamination from an Rh-positive fetus.

In cases of maternal hereditary persistence of fetal hemoglobin, an alternative method for detection and quantification of fetal Rh(D)-positive hemorrhage has been developed.[2] In this method, a flow cytometer is used to quantitate an indirect immunofluorescent reaction in which IgG anti-D is used as the primary antibody.

A study designed to determine the incidence of fetomaternal hemorrhage following cesarean section utilizing Kleihauer-Betke testing found some degree of hemorrhage in 18.5% of the study patients. In 2.5%, there was evidence of more than 30 mL of fetal blood lost into the maternal circulation. This finding led to the recommendation that all Rh-negative patients having a C-section be screened (Kleihauer-Betke test) for fetomaternal hemorrhage.[4]

Footnotes
1. Emery CL, Morway CF, Chung-Park M, et al, "The Kleihauer-Betke Test. Clinical Utility, Indication, and Correlation in Patients With Placental Abruption and Cocaine Use," *Arch Pathol Lab Med*, 1995, 119(11):1032-7.
2. Patton WN, Nicholson GS, Sawers AH, et al, "Assessment of Fetal-Maternal Haemorrhage in Mothers With Hereditary Persistence of Fetal Haemoglobin," *J Clin Pathol*, 1990, 43(9):728-31.
3. Holcomb WL, Gunderson E, and Petrie RH, "Clinical Use of the Kleihauer-Betke Test," *J Perinat Med*, 1990, 18(5):331-7.
4. Feldman N, Skoll A, and Sibai B, "The Incidence of Significant Fetomaternal Hemorrhage in Patients Undergoing Cesarean Section," *Am J Obstet Gynecol*, 1990, 163(3):855-8.

References
Henry JB, Nelson DA, Tomar RH, et al, *Todd-Sanford-Davidsohn Clinical Diagnosis and Management by Laboratory Methods*, 18th ed, Philadelphia, PA: WB Saunders Co, 1991, 493-4.
Kleihauer E, "Determination of Fetal Hemoglobin: Elution Technique," *The Detection of Hemoglobinopathies*, Schmidt RM, et al, eds, Cleveland, OH: CRC Press, 1974.
Von Stein GA, Munsick RA, Stiver K, et al, "Fetomaternal Hemorrhage in Threatened Abortion," *Obstet Gynecol*, 1992, 79(3):383-6.

LAP *see* Leukocyte Alkaline Phosphatase *on this page*

LAP Score *see* Leukocyte Alkaline Phosphatase *on this page*

LAP Smear *see* Leukocyte Alkaline Phosphatase *on this page*

Large Molecule Diseases *see* Inherited Diseases of Metabolism and Cell Structure Tests *on page 327*

LE Cell Test
CPT 87205

Related Information
Anti-DNA *on page 365*
Antinuclear Antibody *on page 368*
Scleroderma Antibody *on page 430*
Sjögren's Antibodies *on page 430*
Smooth Muscle Antibody *on page 431*

Synonyms LE Prep; LE Preparation; LE Slide Cell Test; Lupus Test

Abstract Historically, an important test for systemic lupus erythematosus (SLE), it is currently outmoded.

Patient Preparation Avoid heparin therapy for 2 days prior to collection. Large doses of heparin may increase the incidence of false-negative results.

Specimen Whole blood

Container Green top (heparin) tube; EDTA anticoagulated blood may cause false-negative results

Collection Routine venipuncture. Invert gently to mix. Transport to the laboratory within 30 minutes.

Causes for Rejection Insufficient volume, clotted specimen, patient on heparin

Reference Range Negative

Use Evaluate autoimmune diseases, specifically SLE (systemic lupus erythematosus); aid in the diagnosis of "lupoid" hepatitis (chronic active hepatitis). The discovery of the LE cell more than 40 years ago has been important in understanding autoimmune disease. As stated by Tan and associates, however, "It has been superseded by modern ANA tests with greater sensitivity and rapidity, but its fundamental contribution to understanding of ANAs cannot be overlooked."[1] A few authors[2,3] still advocate the use of this test.

Limitations This test is an indirect method for detecting one of the antinuclear antibodies. It is less sensitive than fluorescent antibody techniques for ANA and not specific for lupus erythematosus. Positive tests have been reported in a variety of drug induced lupus syndromes, in rheumatoid arthritis, chronic and active hepatitis, drug hypersensitivity, and other collagen diseases. One negative result should not be considered to rule out the possibility of LE. EDTA anticoagulated blood may cause a false-negative reaction.

Contraindications Patients receiving large doses of heparin or with severe leukopenia/neutropenia

Methodology Blood cells are ruptured by a variety of methods - glass beads are commonly used. Nuclear material is thereby released to interact with any antibody that may be present. One hour incubation at 37°C allows time for interaction of nuclear material and antibody and for the altered nuclear material to be phagocytosed (a complement dependent process). Buffy coat smears are prepared, stained, and studied for presence of phagocytosed homogenous lavender staining material. Presence of extracellular LE material or formation of rosettes does not add specific diagnostic information.

Additional Information SLE is a disease of protean clinical manifestations commonly with rash, arthralgia, fever, anemia, leukopenia, thrombocytopenia, and hypocomplementemia, occurring especially in women. The LE slide cell test is relatively insensitive. It is positive in only 60% to 80% of acutely ill cases of LE. A negative LE slide cell test does not exclude the diagnosis of lupus erythematosus. The patient's serum should be studied for antinuclear antibody (ANA). The antibody may be of IgG, A, or M specificity but is most commonly of IgG class. A negative ANA test nearly excludes the diagnosis of LE (>95% sensitivity) if the patient is not being treated with corticosteroid or immunosuppressive drugs. Some drugs (in particular Dilantin®) may relate to lupus erythematosus and cause positive LE slide cell tests. Up to 25% of individuals taking Dilantin® (diphenylhydantoin) develop antinuclear antibodies. See table.

Drugs Capable of Inducing Lupus Syndromes Positive LE Slide Tests

Dilantin	Phenelzine sulfate
Ethosuximide	Phenylbutazone
Griseofulvin	Primidone
Hydralazine	Procainamide
Isoniazid	Propylthiouracil
Mesantoin	Reserpine
Methyldopa	Streptomycin
Methylthiouracil	Sulfonamides
Oral contraceptives	Tetracycline
Penicillin	Tridione

Footnotes
1. Tan EM, Robinson CA, and Nakamura RM, "ANAs in Systemic Rheumatic Disease. Diagnostic Significance," *Postgrad Med*, 1985, 78(3):141-2, 145-8.
2. Hidalgo C and Vladutiu AO, "Lupus Erythematosus Cells in Serum and Pleural Fluid of a Patient With Negative Fluorescent Antinuclear Antibody Test," *Am J Clin Pathol*, 1987, 87(5):660-2.
3. Wallace DJ, "Lupus Erythematosus Cell Test," *Am J Clin Pathol*, 1995, 104(1):110-1.

References
Dacie JV and Lewis SM, "Demonstration of LE Cells," *Practical Haematology*, 8th ed, New York, NY: Churchill Livingstone, 1995, 569-71.
Hargraves MM, "Discovery of the LE Cell and Its Morphology," *Mayo Clin Proc*, 1969, 44:579.
Hargraves MM, Richmond H, and Morton R, "Presentation of Two Bone Marrow Elements: The "Tart" Cell and the "LE" Cell," *Proc Staff Meet Mayo Clin*, 1948, 23:25.
Nakamura RM, Peebles CL, Rubin RL, et al, *Autoantibodies to Nuclear Antigens (ANA): Advances in Laboratory Tests and Significance in Systemic Rheumatic Disease*, 1st ed, Chicago, IL: American Society of Clinical Pathologists, 1985, 7-33.
Steinberg AD, Gourley MF, Klinman DM, et al, "NIH Conference. Systemic Lupus Erythematosus," *Ann Intern Med*, 1991, 115(7):548-59.

LE Prep *see* LE Cell Test *on this page*

LE Preparation *see* LE Cell Test *on this page*

LE Slide Cell Test *see* LE Cell Test *on this page*

Leukemic Reticuloendotheliosis Test *see* Tartrate Resistant Leukocyte Acid Phosphatase *on page 349*

Leukocyte Acid Phosphatase *see* Tartrate Resistant Leukocyte Acid Phosphatase *on page 349*

Leukocyte Alkaline Phosphatase
CPT 85540

Related Information
Bone Marrow *on page 307*
Breakpoint Cluster Region Rearrangement in CML *on page 503*
Leukocyte Cytochemistry *on next page*

White Blood Count *on page 353*

Synonyms LAP; LAP Score; LAP Smear

Abstract A cytochemical reaction useful in differential diagnosis of myelo-proliferative diseases, in particular, distinguishing leukemoid reaction from leukemia.

Specimen Whole blood

Container Slides with smears of blood

Collection Make six smears on long slides from fingerstick blood. Air dry the slides. Transport to Hematology immediately (ie, within 30 minutes).

Storage Instructions Slides must be fixed with cold 10% formalin methanol or citrated buffered acetone, rinsed, air dried, and frozen within 8 hours (preferably within 30 minutes) after obtaining the blood. After fixation, smears can be stored for up to 8 weeks before staining.

Causes for Rejection Blood collected in EDTA anticoagulant, transit time to the laboratory in excess of 30 minutes, neutrophil count <1000/mm^3 in peripheral blood

Reference Range 11-95

Use Aid in the differential diagnosis of chronic granulocytic leukemia versus leukemoid reaction; aid in the evaluation of polycythemia and myelofibrosis

Limitations Pregnancy, increased number of immature forms of neutrophils, and postoperative or "stressful" states are associated with increased scores. The differential must have adequate numbers of mature neutrophilic granulocytes to perform the LAP.

Methodology Enzyme reaction with leukocyte alkaline phosphatase liberating naphthol or a substituted naphthol compound which then couples with fast blue RR or other chromogen to form an insoluble precipitate. Color of the precipitate relates to the type of substituted naphthol substrate and diazonium dye used (color is reagent dependent). Cells are scored as to the degree of phosphatase activity present, 0 to 4+. One hundred cells are counted and the score totaled.

Additional Information Low scores have been associated with CML, PNH, thrombocytopenic purpura, and hereditary hypophosphatasia. In CML regardless of the total white count, the score remains low. Occasionally, an apparent new myeloproliferative disorder is described. One such is characterized by low LAP score and also by leukocytosis, polycythemia, thrombocytopenia, splenomegaly, and generalized lymphoadenopathy but without Philadelphia chromosome, *bcr* gene rearrangement, or other karyotypic abnormalities.[1] In CML, it has been demonstrated that the mRNA for leukocyte alkaline phosphatase by Northern blotting is undetectable.[2] This suggests either rapid degradation of the message or no transcription of the LAP gene. In nonleukemic neutrophilia, the LAP rises as the WBC rises. High scores have been seen in polycythemia vera, myelofibrosis, aplastic anemia, mongolism, hairy cell leukemia, leukemoid reactions, and neutrophilia either physiological or secondary to infection. LAP is also increased in Hodgkin's disease. Serial activity can be a useful adjunct in evaluating the activity of Hodgkin's disease as well as its response to therapy. Increase in LAP does not occur in cases of sickle cell crisis, possibly due to zinc deficiency (leukocyte alkaline phosphatase is a zinc metalloenzyme) but more likely relating to a mild defect in the hypothalamic-pituitary-adrenal axis with decreased plasma cortisol response in patients with sickle cell crisis.[3]

Footnotes

1. Schofield JR and Robinson WA, "A New Myeloproliferative Syndrome," *Am J Hematol*, 1995, 48(3):186-91.
2. Rambaldi A, Terao M, Bettoni S, et al, "Differences in the Expression of Alkaline Phosphatase mRNA in Chronic Myelogenous Leukemia and Paroxysmal Nocturnal Hemoglobinuria Polymorphonuclear Leukocytes," *Blood*, 1989, 73(5):1113-5.
3. Rosenbloom BE, Odell WD, and Tanaka KR, "Pituitary-Adrenal Axis Function in Sickle Cell Anemia and Its Relationship to Leukocyte Alkaline Phosphatase," *Am J Hematol*, 1980, 9:373-9.

References

Catovsky D, "Leukocyte Cytochemical and Immunological Techniques," *Practical Haematology*, 8th ed, Chapter 9, Dacie JV and Lewis SM, eds, New York, NY: Churchill Livingstone, 1995, 143-74.
Cline MJ, "Laboratory Evaluation of Benign Quantitative Granulocyte and Monocyte Disorders," *Hematology: Clinical and Laboratory Practice*, Vol 2, Chapter 75, Bick RL, ed, St Louis, MO: Mosby-Year Book Inc, 1993, 1155-60.
Kaplow LS, "Cytochemistry of Leukocyte Alkaline Phosphatase: Use of Complex Naphthol AS Phosphates in Azo Dye-Coupling Technics," *Am J Clin Pathol*, 1963, 39:439-49.

Leukocyte Count *see* White Blood Count *on page 353*

Leukocyte Cytochemistry

CPT 88313 (each stain)

Related Information

Bone Marrow *on page 307*
Breakpoint Cluster Region Rearrangement in CML *on page 503*
Leukocyte Alkaline Phosphatase *on previous page*
Muramidase, Blood and Urine *on page 333*
Peripheral Blood: Differential Leukocyte Count *on page 336*
Tartrate Resistant Leukocyte Acid Phosphatase *on page 349*

White Blood Count *on page 353*

Synonyms Cytochemistry, Leukocyte

Applies to Acid-Fast, Ziehl-Neelsen, Stain for Intracellular Pigment; Acid Phosphatase Stain With and Without Tartrate; Alpha-Naphthyl Esterase Stain With and Without Fluoride; Amyloid; ASD Chloroacetate Esterase Stain; Beta-Glucuronidase Stain; Methenamine Silver; Methyl Green-Pyronine; Nonspecific Esterase; Oil Red O Stain; PAS Stain; Peroxidase Stain; Sudan Black Stain

Test Commonly Includes Any of the above stains indicated by examination of routinely stained preparations or specific request

Abstract Cytochemical reactions are useful in differential diagnosis, in particular, in the study and characterization of acute leukemia.

Specimen Blood or bone marrow smears, imprints or smears of cell suspensions

Container Green top (heparin) tube

Collection Smears are prepared at the patient's bedside.

Storage Instructions Transport specimen to the laboratory immediately.

Reference Range Interpretation and significance usually requires correlation with other cytologic and cytochemical aspects of the specific case.

Use Cytochemically evaluate neoplasms and abnormal cells in bone marrow, peripheral blood, or other specimens such as imprints; detect amyloidosis; classify leukemias and plasma cell dyscrasias; evaluate myeloproliferative/lymphoproliferative disorders

Additional Information See also test listing Tartrate Resistant Leukocyte Acid Phosphatase *on page 349*, for hairy cell leukemia. In the technique of Yam et al for esterase reactions, a single slide preparation is consecutively stained for two different enzyme activities.[1] The nonspecific esterase (α-naphthyl acetate substrate - black granulation) is monocyte specific, while the chloroacetate esterase (naphthol ASD chloroacetate - red granulation) is granulocyte specific.[1] These reactions should be helpful in some cases in distinguishing acute granulocytic from acute monocytic leukemia and are of value in distinguishing acute myelomonocytic leukemia from acute granulocytic leukemia and acute monocytic leukemia (Schilling type). In acute myelomonocytic leukemia, both granulocytic and monocytic markers are present simultaneously in the leukemic cells. Nonspecific esterase activity inhibited by fluoride has been described in red cell precursors - including megaloblasts in cases of untreated pernicious anemia, megaloblastoid rubricytes in cases of DiGuglielmo syndrome, and rubricytes in cases of severe untreated iron deficiency. Rubricytes from normal marrow lack nonspecific esterase activity.[2] By use of high resolution isoelectric focusing in polyacrylamide gel, isoenzymes of nonspecific esterases extracted from leukemic blasts can be visualized. For each type of leukemic blast (ie, lymphoblast, myeloblast, and monoblast), a consistent and distinctive pattern of nonspecific esterase activity has been reported.[3] Isoenzyme fractions of acid phosphatases and nonspecific esterases appear to be unique for lymphoblasts, myeloblasts, and immature or leukemic monocytes. The fluoride inhibited nonspecific esterase reaction indicates monocytic origin and is unusual in T- lymphocyte cell malignancy. The laboratory may be unable to perform the peroxidase reaction as this test utilizes a chemical, benzidine, which has been shown to be carcinogenic. Alternate methods are available.[4] The table lists cytochemical reactions for leukemias. A current study was designed to assess the value of PAS (periodic acid-Schiff) stain in delineating lymphoblastic and myeloblastic leukemia. It was concluded that a positive PAS reaction combined with negative myeloperoxidase, Sudan black B, and alpha-naphthyl butyrate esterase results continues to have a diagnostic role in differentiating lymphoblastic and myeloblastic leukemia.[5] Another study showed that PAS and iron stain together or PAS and double esterase together was helpful in excluding a diagnosis of myelodysplastic syndrome.[6] Flow cytochemistry study has been applied to the differentiation of acute leukemias.[7] Immunocytochemical marker, enzyme and cytokine studies can be applied to the differentiation of macrophages, Langerhans cells, and dendritic cells and their disease processes (see reference by Cline).

Footnotes

1. Yam LT, Li CY, Crosby WH, et al, "Cytochemical Identification of Monocytes and Granulocytes," *Am J Clin Pathol*, 1971, 55:283-90.
2. Kass L and Peters CL, "Nonspecific Esterase Activity in Pernicious Anemia and Chronic Erythremic Myelosis: A Cytochemical and Electrophoretic Study," *Am J Clin Pathol*, 1977, 68:273-5.
3. Tavassoli M, Shaklai M, and Crosby WH, "Cytochemical Diagnosis of Acute Myelomonocytic Leukemia," *Am J Clin Pathol*, 1979, 72:59-62.
4. Hanker JS, Yates PE, Metz CB, et al, "A New Specific, Sensitive and Noncarcinogenic Reagent for the Demonstration of Horseradish Peroxidase," *Histochem J*, 1977, 9:789-92.
5. Snower DP, Smith BR, Munz UJ, et al, "Re-Evaluation of the Periodic Acid-Schiff Stain in Acute Leukemia With Immunophenotypic Analyses," *Arch Pathol Lab Med*, 1991, 115(4):346-50.
6. Seo IS, Li CY, and Yam LT, "Myelodysplastic Syndrome: Diagnostic Implications of Cytochemical and Immunocytochemical Studies," *Mayo Clin Proc*, 1993, 68(1):47-53
7. Tsakona CP, Kinsey SE, and Goldstone AH, "Use of Flow Cytometry Via the H*1 in FAB Identification of Acute Leukaemias," *Acta Haematol*, 1992, 88(2-3):72-7.

(Continued)

Leukocyte Cytochemistry (Continued)

Cytochemical Reactions in Normal Blood Cells and Blast Cells of Acute Leukemias

	Peroxidase Sudan Black B	α-Naphthyl Acetate	α-Naphthyl Butyrate	Naphthol-AS-D Chloroacetate	PAS	Acid Phosphatase
Promyelocyte	+/++	–/±	–	+/++	± /+	+/++
Neutrophil	++	–/±	–	+/++	+++	+
Monocyte	–/±	+++	++/+++	–/±	±	++
Lymphocyte	–	–/±[a]	–/±[a]	–	–/+	–/++
Erythroblast	–	–/±[b]	–	–	–	±/–
Megakaryocyte	–	+++	±	–	++	++
ALL	–	–/+[c]	–	–	+/++[d]	–/+[c]
AML(M1)	+	–	–	+	+	–
AML(M2)	++	–/+	–/+	++	+	+
APL(M3)	+++	–/++	–	+++	± /++	++
AMML(M4)	++	++/+++	++	++	–/++	++
AMoL(M5)	–/±	+++	+++	–/±	++	+
EL(M6)	–	++	+	–	++	–
MegL(M7)	–	+	–/±	–	++	+
AUL	–	–	–	–	–	–

From Williams WJ, Beutler E, Erslev AJ, et al, eds, *Hematology*, 4th ed, New York, NY: McGraw-Hill Inc, 1990, 1745-53, with permission.

– = negative

± = weak or few positive cells

+ = moderate

++ = moderately strong

+++ = strongly positive (most cells)

ALL = acute lymphocytic leukemia

AML(M1) = acute myeloblastic leukemia

AML(M2) = acute myeloblastic leukemia with maturation

APL(M3) = acute promyelocytic leukemia

AMML(M4) = acute myelomonocytic leukemia

AMoL(M5) = acute monocytic leukemia

EL(M6) = acute erythroleukemia

MegL(M7) = acute megakaryocytic leukemia

AUL = acute undifferentiated leukemia

[a] Positivity is focal, not diffuse.

[b] In erythroleukemia and in some erythroid maturation defects, positivity is strong.

[c] Focal cytoplasmic positivity in a small proportion of ALL.

[d] Coarse blocks are typical.

Note: In M1 through M5, the cytochemical reactions for the esterases apply to all the mononuclear nonerythroid, nonlymphocytic cells. In M6, the cytochemical reactions in the table apply to the erythroblasts. Myeloblasts are also present and are likely to be Sudan black B- or peroxidase-positive.

References
Cline MJ, "Histiocytes and Histiocytosis," *Blood*, 1994, 84(9):2840-53.

Goasguen J and Bennett JM, "The Acute Myeloid Leukemias: Morphology and Cytochemistry," *Hematology: Clinical and Laboratory Practice*, Vol 2, Chapter 77, Bick RL, ed, St Louis, MO: Mosby-Year Book Inc, 1993, 1195-216.

Kass L and Elias JM, "Cytochemistry and Immunocytochemistry in Bone Marrow Examination: Contemporary Techniques for the Diagnosis of Acute Leukemia and Myelodysplastic Syndrome," *Hematol Oncol Clin North Am*, 1988, 2(4):537-55.

Li CY, Yam LT, and Sun T, *Modern Modalities for the Diagnosis of Hematologic Neoplasms: Color Atlas/Text*, New York, NY: Igaku-Shoin, 1996, 7-19 and 112-40.

Li CY and Yam LT, "Cytochemistry and Immunochemistry in Hematologic Diagnoses," *Hematol Oncol Clin North Am*, 1994, 8(4):665-81.

Nelson DA and Davey FR, "Leukocyte Peroxidase," *Williams Hematology*, 5th ed, Chapter L23, Beutler E, Lichtman MA, Coller BS, et al, eds, New York, NY: McGraw-Hill Inc, 1995, L65-72.

Lupus Test *see* LE Cell Test *on page 330*

Lysosomal Storage Diseases *see* Inherited Diseases of Metabolism and Cell Structure Tests *on page 327*

Lysozyme, Blood *see* Muramidase, Blood and Urine *on next page*

Lysozyme, Urine *see* Muramidase, Blood and Urine *on next page*

Malarial Parasites *see* Malaria Smear *on this page*

Malaria Smear
CPT 87207
Related Information
Babesiosis Serological Test *on page 370*

Chagas' Disease Serological Test *on page 383*

Myoglobin, Qualitative, Urine *on page 644*

Parasite Antibodies *on page 421*

Peripheral Blood: Red Blood Cell Morphology *on page 339*

Synonyms Blood Smear for Malarial Parasites; Malarial Parasites

Test Commonly Includes Examination of thick and thin smears

Abstract Malaria is still the most common infectious disease in the world. Its rapid diagnosis in the laboratory is extremely important. Although there are not many cases in the United States, with more world travel, it can be expected to increase.

Specimen Fresh blood - fresh fingerstick smears (two or three of each thick and thin film type) made at bedside preferred, EDTA anticoagulated blood for saponin lysis.[1] To make a thick film smear, spread a drop of blood centrally placed on a slide into a square about four times area of original drop. Spreading is conveniently achieved with the corner of another slide. Ideally, blood should be thinned until small newsprint is just visible.[2]

Malaria Species Infecting Human Red Cells

Plasmodium Species	Malaria	Length of Cycle (hours)
P. vivax	Tertian	45
P. falciparum	Malignant tertian	48
P. ovale	Ovale	48
P. malariae	Quartan	72

Container Slides and lavender top (EDTA) tube

Collection Specimen should be drawn immediately before a fever spike is anticipated.

Causes for Rejection Specimen clotted

Special Instructions If the patient has traveled to a malaria endemic area the date and area traveled should be specified on the requisition. Most cases of malaria seen in the U.S. are found in foreign nationals traveling in the United States.[3]

Reference Range No organisms identified

Use Diagnose malaria, parasitic infestation of blood; evaluate febrile disease of unknown origin

Limitations One negative result does not rule out the possibility of parasitic infestation. If protozoal, filarial, or trypanosomal infection is strongly suspected, test should be performed at least three times with samples obtained at different times in the fever cycle.

Changes in Infected RBCs Useful in Identification of Malaria Species

Plasmodium Species	Infected RBC Enlarged	Presence of Schüffner Dots	Presence of Maurer Dots	Multiple Parasites per RBC	Parasite With Double Chromatin Dots	Parasite With Sausage-Shaped Gametocytes
P. vivax	+	+	—	Rare	Rare	—
P. falciparum	—	—	+	+	+	+
P. ovale	±	+	—	—	—	—
P. malariae	—	—	+	—	—	—

Methodology Microscopic examination of thick and thin peripheral blood Romanovsky dye (in particular Giemsa) stained smears. Thick films are more difficult to interpret but greatly increase sensitivity (by concentrating cells and organisms). Thick smears require considerable experience with malaria. They increase the number of cells examined in a given time period by a factor of about 12.[2] Screening for malaria can also be accomplished by fluorescent microscopy using acridine orange or benzothiocarboxypurine.[3,4,5,6,7] These methods are sensitive and can provide consistent results without the need for highly experienced observers. DNA hybridization probes for detection of malaria have been described,[8,9] but in one study, sensitivity was not comparable to that obtained with use of thick films.[9] Thin smears, although not as sensitive, are far superior for determining the species of *Plasmodium* on morphological grounds.[10] A "magnet test" has recently been developed, is not yet commercially available, but is expected to be sensitive, rapid, and inexpensive.[11]

Additional Information Proper therapy depends upon identification of the specific variety of malaria parasite. Release of trophozoites and RBC debris results in a febrile response. Periodicity of fever correlates with type of malaria (see table). Organisms are most likely to be detected just before onset of fever which is predictable in many cases. Sampling immediately upon onset of fever is the most desirable time to obtain blood. Alternatively in cases negative by these means but with a strong clinical history, multiple sampling at different times in the fever cycle may prove successful. Hemozoin, a component of malarial pigment, is present in mature trophozoites and gametocytes of all human malarial species. It is a polymer of ferriprotoporphyrin and has paramagnetic and birefringent properties. It allows parasitized red cells to separate in a magnetic field forming the basis of the "magnet test" (see above).[11] Malarial parasites are destroyed in AS and SS patients. The cause of parasite death in AS cells is potassium loss, in SS cells Hb S aggregates destroy the parasites by physical penetration.[12]

Footnotes

1. Keffer JH, "Malarial Parasites. Concentration by Saponin Hemolysis," *Tech Bull Regist Med Technol*, 1966, 36:153-5.
2. Dacie JV and Lewis SM, *Practical Haematology*, 7th ed, New York, NY: Churchill Livingstone, 1991, 80-1.
3. Gordon S, Brennessel DJ, Goldstein JA, et al, "Malaria: A City Hospital Experience," *Arch Intern Med*, 1988, 148(7):1569-71.
4. Jahanmehr SA, Hyde K, Geary CG, et al, "Simple Technique for Fluorescence Staining of Blood Cells With Acridine Orange," *J Clin Pathol*, 1987, 40(8):926-9.
5. Rickman LS, Long GW, Oberst R, et al, "Rapid Diagnosis of Malaria by Acridine Orange Staining of Centrifuged Parasites," *Lancet*, 1989, 1(8629):68-71.
6. Long GW, Jones TR, Rickman LS, et al, "Acridine Orange Detection of *Plasmodium falciparum* Malaria: Relationship Between Sensitivity and Optical Configuration," *Am J Trop Med Hyg*, 1991, 44(4):402-5.
7. Makler MT, Ries LK, Ries J, et al, "Detection of *Plasmodium falciparum* Infection With the Fluorescent Dye, Benzothiocarboxypurine," *Am J Trop Med Hyg*, 1991, 44(1):11-6.
8. Barker RH Jr, Suebsaeng L, Rooney W, et al, "Detection of *Plasmodium falciparum* Infection in Human Patients: A Comparison of the DNA Probe Method to Microscopic Diagnosis," *Am J Trop Med Hyg*, 1989, 41(3):266-72.
9. Lanar DE, McLaughlin GL, Wirth DF, et al, "Comparison of Thick Films, *In Vitro* Culture and DNA Hybridization Probes for Detecting *Plasmodium falciparum* Malaria," *Am J Trop Med Hyg*, 1989, 40(1):3-6.
10. Pammenter MD, "Techniques for the Diagnosis of Malaria," *S Afr Med J*, 1988, 74(2):55-7.
11. Nalbandian RM, Sammons DW, Manley M, et al, "A Molecular-Based Magnet Test for Malaria," *Am J Clin Pathol*, 1995, 103(1):57-64.
12. Friedman MJ and Trager W, "The Biochemistry of Resistance to Malaria," *Sci Am*, 1981, 244(2):154-5, 158-64.

References

Henry JB, Nelson DA, Tomar RH, et al, *Todd-Sanford-Davidsohn Clinical Diagnosis and Management by Laboratory Methods*, 18th ed, Philadelphia, PA: WB Saunders Co, 1991, 1168-72.

Makler MT and Gibbins B, "Laboratory Diagnosis of Malaria," *Clin Lab Med*, 1991, 11(4):941-56.

Marrow Iron Stores *see* Iron Stain, Bone Marrow *on page 328*

MCHC (Mean Corpuscular Hemoglobin Concentration) MCH (Mean Corpuscular Hemoglobin) *see* Red Blood Cell Indices *on page 343*

MCV (Mean Corpuscular Volume) *see* Red Blood Cell Indices *on page 343*

Methenamine Silver *see* Leukocyte Cytochemistry *on page 331*

Methyl Green-Pyronine *see* Leukocyte Cytochemistry *on page 331*

Methylmalonic Acid *see* Vitamin B$_{12}$ *on page 351*

Methyl Violet Stain for Heinz Bodies *see* Heinz Body Stain *on page 321*

Microbuffy Coat Method for Detection of Bacteremia *see* Bacteremia Detection, Buffy Coat Micromethod *on page 305*

Microfilariae, Peripheral Blood Preparation

CPT 87207

Related Information

Bacteremia Detection, Buffy Coat Micromethod *on page 305*
Filariasis Serological Test *on page 393*
Peripheral Blood: Red Blood Cell Morphology *on page 339*

Synonyms Blood Smear for Trypanosomal/Filarial Parasites; Filariasis Peripheral Blood Preparation; Helminths, Blood; Trypanosomiasis, Peripheral Blood Preparation

Applies to Filarial Infestation; Hemoflagellates

Test Commonly Includes Examination of both thick and thin smears, wet preparation

Specimen Fresh blood from fingerstick

Container Slides

Collection Recommended procedure is for specimen to be obtained when patient spikes a fever. Optimal yield results from examination of a daytime specimen (ie, noon), and a night time specimen (ie, midnight). Timing of sampling relates to geographic place of exposure.

Causes for Rejection Specimen clotted

Special Instructions If patient has traveled to an endemic area, the date of travel, the area, and the parasite suspected should be specified.

Reference Range No parasites identified

Use Diagnose trypanosomiasis or microfilariasis; work up of elephantiasis, parasitic infestation of blood

Limitations One negative result does not rule out the possibility of parasitic infestation. Since some species of blood parasites can be found during the day and others are nocturnal, both day and night specimens enhance identification. Most filariae generate microfilariae which can be found in peripheral blood, but *Onchocerca volvulus* and *Dipetalonema streptocerca* give rise to microfilariae which do not circulate.

Methodology Fresh wet blood film, with a coverslip, in which motile microfilariae cause agitation of adjacent red cells. Stained films are used as well.

Additional Information Biopsy of skin and subcutaneous mass is used in diagnosis of *D. streptocerca* and *O. volvulus*. Differential diagnosis of species of circulating microfilariae requires distinction between the presence or absence of a sheath, the pattern of nuclei in the tail and sometimes the history of geographic exposure and time of sampling.

References

Garcia LS, "Laboratory Methods for Diagnosis of Parasitic Infections," *Bailey and Scott's Diagnostic Microbiology*, Chapter 44, Finegold SM and Baron EJ, eds, St Louis, MO: Mosby-Year Book Inc, 1986, 838-42, 854-6.

Microhematocrit *see* Hematocrit *on page 322*

Morphology *see* Peripheral Blood: Red Blood Cell Morphology *on page 339*

MPV *see* Platelet Sizing *on page 341*

Mucopolysaccharidoses *see* Inherited Diseases of Metabolism and Cell Structure Tests *on page 327*

Muramidase, Blood and Urine

CPT 85549

Related Information

Eosinophil Count *on page 315*
Leukocyte Cytochemistry *on page 331*
Lymph Node Biopsy *on page 50*
Urine Collection, 24-Hour *on page 30*

Synonyms Lysozyme, Blood; Lysozyme, Urine

Specimen Serum, 24-hour urine

Container Red top tube; EDTA plasma (lavender top tube) may also be used; 24-hour urine container

Collection Collect urine for 24-hour period on ice, no preservative. (Continued)

Muramidase, Blood and Urine *(Continued)*

Storage Instructions Separate serum and freeze **immediately** in plastic vial on dry ice. Upon receipt of urine specimen, freeze on dry ice **immediately** in plastic vial.

Reference Range Serum: 4.0-15.6 µg/mL (0.28-1.10 µmol/L); urine: 0-1.4 µg/mL (0-0.097 µmol/L)[1]

Use Differential diagnosis of leukemia; present in association with some cases of myelogenous and most cases of monocytic leukemia

Methodology Turbidimetric, immunochemical (nephelometry), enzymatic - colorimetric, radioimmunoassay (RIA), agarose gel diffusion (recommended method)[1]

Additional Information Lysozyme when present in large amounts, may appear as a far cathodal migrating ("cationic") band occasionally on serum or urine protein electrophoresis. It is elevated in some cases of myelogenous, and most cases of myelomonocytic and monocytic leukemia. Lysozyme has been found within the granules of normal and leukemic eosinophils by immunoelectron microscopic study. Elevated serum lysozyme may not establish presence of monocytic differentiation in cases of acute myelogenous leukemia with eosinophilia.[3] The level of serum lysozyme has been used as a predictor of CNS involvement in these leukemias.[2] Serum lysozyme has been shown to be elevated in a number of conditions, including tuberculosis and sarcoidosis as well as leukemia, and it is markedly elevated in sarcoid lymph nodes.[4]

Footnotes
1. Schultz AL, "Lysozyme," *Methods in Clinical Chemistry*, Chapter 95, Pesce AJ and Kaplan LA, eds, St Louis, MO: Mosby-Year Book Inc, 1987, 742-6.
2. Peterson BA, Brunning RD, Bloomfield CD, et al, "Central Nervous System Involvement in Acute Nonlymphocytic Leukemia. A Prospective Study of Adults in Remission," *Am J Med*, 1987, 83(3):464-70.
3. Moscinski LC, Kasnic G Jr, and Saker A Jr, "The Significance of an Elevated Serum Lysozyme Value in Acute Myelogenous Leukemia With Eosinophilia," *Am J Clin Pathol*, 1992, 97(2):195-201.
4. Silverstein E, Friedland J, and Ackerman T, "Elevation of Granulomatous Lymph-Node and Serum Lysozyme in Sarcoidosis and Correlation With Angiotensin-Converting Enzyme," *Am J Clin Pathol*, 1977, 68:219-24.

References
Zucker S, Hanes DJ, Vogler WR, et al, "Plasma Muramidase: A Study of Methods and Clinical Applications," *J Lab Clin Med*, 1970, 75:83-92.

Murayama Test *see* Sickle Cell Tests *on page 347*

Nasal Smear for Eosinophils *see* Eosinophil Smear *on page 316*

NBT Test *see* Nitroblue Tetrazolium Test *on this page*

Neutral β-Galactosidase *see* Inherited Diseases of Metabolism and Cell Structure Tests *on page 327*

Nitroblue Tetrazolium Test

CPT 86384

Synonyms NBT Test; Tetrazolium Reduction Test

Abstract NBT test is used mainly for the diagnosis of chronic granulomatous disease (CGD), an X-linked inherited disease, characterized by disabled phagocyte NADPH oxidase with inability to efficiently kill phagocytized bacteria.

Specimen Whole blood

Container Green top (heparin) tube

Storage Instructions Specimen cannot be stored (test utilizes live granulocytes).

Causes for Rejection Transit to the laboratory of more than 1 hour, specimen clotted

Special Instructions Advance scheduling with the laboratory may be required as the specimen must be tested while the neutrophils are still viable. Transport to the laboratory **immediately** following collection.

Reference Range 2% to 8% segmented neutrophils reduce dye

Use Diagnose chronic granulomatous disease (CGD) of childhood

Limitations Requires fresh blood for live white blood cells.

Methodology Assessment of reduction of a tetrazolium dye by stimulated and unstimulated neutrophils. Neutrophils reduce the dye to a dark blue-black formazan pigment upon phagocytosis.

Additional Information Usually a reliable aid in the diagnosis of CGD in which neutrophils are unable to reduce the dye (which correlates with their inability to kill bacteria). In patients with CGD, the NADPH oxidase system fails to generate superoxide and related oxygen intermediates with resultant susceptibility to recurrent bacterial and fungal infections. The NBT test is unreliable in the differentiation of bacterial from viral and other infections, producing unacceptable false-negative and false-positive results. Forty-three nonbacterial infections and other clinical states have been associated with false-positive NBT tests.[1] There are also reports of bacterial infections accompanied by false-negative results. One study suggests that peripheral segmented neutrophils from patients with solid cancer (nonlymphomatous tumors) have decreased capacity

to reduce NBT dye to formazan when maximally stimulated with endotoxin.[2] NBT reduction in lymphoma patients was comparable to that of controls. It was also found that stimulated NBT reduction apparently declines with age.[2] Chronic granulomatous disease can now be diagnosed using restriction fragment length polymorphism with labeled gene probes.[3] The abnormal gene located on the short arm of the X chromosome codes for cytochrome b558.[4] The CGD may result from genetic defects in at least four different components of the multicomponent NADPH oxidase system.[5]

Treatment of CGD patients with recombinant interferon-γ has been shown to result in a near-normal level of superoxide production and return of granulocyte bactericidal capacity to normal control levels. Interferon-γ (rIFN-γ) stimulates progenitor cells and their mature progeny. Colonies of such cells regain the ability to generate superoxide.[5] Therapy with rIFN-γ is considered safe and effective with decrease in the number and severity of infections.[6]

Footnotes
1. Lace JV, Tan JS, and Watanakunakorn C, "An Appraisal of the Nitroblue Tetrazolium Reduction Test," *Am J Med*, 1975, 58:685-94.
2. Haim N, Obedeanu N, Meshulam T, et al, "Comparative Study of the Endotoxin-Stimulated Nitroblue Tetrazolium Test in Disease and Health," *J Clin Pathol*, 1978, 31:1249-52.
3. Antonarakis SE, "Diagnosis of Genetic Disorders at the DNA Level," *N Engl J Med*, 1989, 320(3):153-63.
4. Francke U, Ochs HD, Darras BT, et al, "Origin of Mutations in Two Families With X-Linked Chronic Granulomatous Disease," *Blood*, 1990, 76(3):602-6.
5. Ezekowitz RAB, "Chronic Granulomatous Disease: An Update and a Paradigm for the Use of Interferon-γ as Adjunct Immunotherapy in Infectious Diseases," *Curr Top Microbiol Immunol*, 1992, 181:283-92.
6. Bemiller LS, Roberts DH, Starko KM, et al, "Safety and Effectiveness of Long-Term Interferon Gamma Therapy in Patients With Chronic Granulomatous Disease," *Blood Cells Mol Dis*, 1995, 21(3):239-47.

References
Babior BM and Woodman RC, "Chronic Granulomatous Disease," *Semin Hematol*, 1990, 27(3):247-59.
Forrest CB, Forehand JR, Axtell RA, et al, "Clinical Features and Current Management of Chronic Granulomatous Disease," *Hematol/Oncol Clin North Am*, 1988, 2(2):253-66.
Quie PG, "Chronic Granulomatous Disease of Childhood: A Saga of Discovery and Understanding," *Pediatr Infect Dis J*, 1993, 12(5):395-8.
Smith RM and Curnutte JT, "Molecular Basis of Chronic Granulomatous Disease," *Blood*, 1991, 77(4):673-86.
Van der Valk P and Herman CJ, "Leukocyte Functions," *Lab Invest*, 1987, 56(2):127-37.

Nonspecific Esterase *see* Leukocyte Cytochemistry *on page 331*

Oil Red O Stain *see* Leukocyte Cytochemistry *on page 331*

Osmotic Fragility

CPT 85555

Related Information
Autohemolysis Test *on page 304*
Band 4.2, Red Cell Membrane *on page 305*
Gelation Assay *on page 318*
Glycerol Lysis Test, Acidified, Modified *on page 320*
Osmotic Fragility, Incubated *on next page*
Peripheral Blood: Red Blood Cell Morphology *on page 339*
Red Blood Cell Indices *on page 343*
Reticulocyte Count *on page 345*

Synonyms Incubated Osmotic Fragility; RBC Fragility; Red Cell Fragility

Specimen Whole blood

Container Lavender top (EDTA) tube or green top (heparin) tube

Storage Instructions Store refrigerated (4°C) if test performance must be delayed.

Causes for Rejection Hemolysis, clotted specimen, blood more than 6 hours old, oxalate or citrate anticoagulated blood collected

Special Instructions May need to schedule this test in advance.

Reference Range Hemolysis begins 0.45%, hemolysis complete 0.35%

Use Evaluate hemolytic anemia, especially hereditary spherocytosis; evaluate immune hemolytic states

Limitations Any severe anemia including iron deficiency will yield an abnormal curve. Test measures presence of spherocytes and "spheroidal" cells. Test is **not** specific for hereditary spherocytosis. Trauma-free venipuncture is needed.

Methodology Erythrocytes are placed in graded dilutions of sodium chloride solution; swelling and hemolysis in the lower dilutions provide an index of the resistance of the cells to hypotonic saline. Percent hemolysis is determined using optical density measurements. A modification of osmotic fragility using glycerol and Bis-Tris, is purportedly more sensitive for the diagnosis of hereditary spherocytosis.[1]

Additional Information Hereditary spherocytosis may be the result of an autosomal dominant transmitted defect in red cell structural proteins.[2] It is associated with a compensated or uncompensated hemolytic state which is relieved by splenectomy. Uncompensated forms of the disease (ie, with anemia) may be associated with reticulocytosis (usually mild to moderate) and mild elevation of serum indirect bilirubin. Patients are susceptible to pigment stones of the gallbladder and to aplastic marrow crises. Spherocytes are more susceptible than are normal red cells to hemolysis in dilute (hypotonic) saline. They show increased osmotic fragility. Spherocytes of any origin (including conditions other than hereditary spherocytosis, eg, autoimmune hemolytic anemia) will cause increased osmotic fragility. Generally, fully expanded cells (eg, spheroidal cells or spherocytes) have increased osmotic fragility while cells with higher surface area to volume ratios (eg, thin cells, hypochromic, target) have decreased osmotic fragility, including some cases of stomatocytosis.[3] The molecular pathology of spherocytosis and other red cell membrane structural protein defects has been partially established and described (see references). Most hereditary hemolytic anemias (including spherocytosis and elliptocytosis) involve mutations of membrane structural proteins, the majority code for abnormal spectrin molecules. Red cell protein 4.2 deficiency has been described. It has been reported recently in Japanese individuals who have related anemia and whose red cells show osmotic fragility.[4] (See also test listing Band 4.2, Red Cell Membrane on page 305.)

Osmotic fragility is increased in cases of malaria infestation. Both infected and uninfected cells show the increased osmotic fragility. Both osmotic and mechanical fragility of RBCs in patients with multiple sclerosis has been reported as increased.[6] See table.

Decreased osmotic fragility (resistance to lysis) may be seen with iron deficiency (hypochromic cell population), other hemoglobinopathies (especially hemoglobin C disease)[5] likely due to the target cell population, and is characteristic of thalassemia.

See test listing Red Blood Cell Indices on page 343 for value of histogram of MCHC in detection of hereditary spherocytosis.

Footnotes
1. Vettore L, Zanella A, Molaro GL, et al, "A New Test for the Laboratory Diagnosis of Spherocytosis," Acta Haematol, 1984, 72(4):258-63.
2. Boivin P and Galand C, "Isoelectric Focusing of Spectrin Components in Hereditary Spherocytosis," Clin Chim Acta, 1976, 71:165-71.
3. McGrath KM, Collecutt MF, Gordon A, et al, "Dehydrated Hereditary Stomatocytosis - A Report of Two Families and A Review of the Literature," Pathology, 1984, 16(2):146-50.
4. Rybicki AC, Qiu JJ, Musto S, et al, "Human Erythrocyte Protein 4.2 Deficiency Associated With Hemolytic Anemia and a Homozygous 40Glutamic Acid → Lysine Substitution in the Cytoplasmic Domain of Band 3 (Band 3Montefiore)," Blood, 1993, 81(8):2155-65.
5. Booth F and Mead SV, "Resistance to Lysis of Erythrocytes Containing Hemoglobin C - Detected in a Differential White Cell Counting System," J Clin Pathol, 1983, 36:816-8.
6. Schauf CL, Frischer H, and Davis FA, "Mechanical Fragility of Erythrocytes in Multiple Sclerosis," Neurology, 1980, 30:323-5.

References
DiPaolo BR, Speicher KD, and Speicher DW, "Identification of the Amino Acid Mutations Associated With Human Erythrocyte Spectrin αII Domain Polymorphisms," Blood, 1993, 82(1):284-91.
Henry JB, Nelson DA, Tomar RH, et al, Todd-Sanford-Davidsohn Clinical Diagnosis and Management by Laboratory Methods, 18th ed, Henry JB, ed, Philadelphia, PA: WB Saunders Co, 1991, 644-5.
Luzzato L and Roper D, "Osmotic Fragility as Measured by Lysis in Hypotonic Saline," Practical Haematology, 8th ed, Chapter 13, Dacie JV and Lewis SM, eds, New York, NY: Churchill Livingstone, 1995, 216-20.
Palek J, "Introduction: Red Blood Cell Membrane Proteins, Their Genes and Mutations," Semin Hematol, 1993, 30(1):1-3.
Palek J and Jarolim P, "Clinical Expression and Laboratory Detection of Red Blood Cell Membrane Protein Mutations," Semin Hematol, 1993, 30(4):249-83.
Peters LL and Lux SE, "Ankyrins: Structure and Function in Normal Cells and Hereditary Spherocytes," Semin Hematol, 1993, 30(2):85-118.
Winkelmann JC and Forget BG, "Erythroid and Nonerythroid Spectrins," Blood, 1993, 81(12):3173-85.
Yawata Y, "Band 4.2 Abnormalities in Human Red Cells," Am J Med Sci, 1994, 307(3):190-203.

Osmotic Fragility, Incubated
CPT 85557
Related Information
Autohemolysis Test on page 304
Gelation Assay on page 318
Glycerol Lysis Test, Acidified, Modified on page 320
Osmotic Fragility on previous page
Synonyms RBC Fragility; Red Cell Fragility
Abstract The same as the previous test (osmotic fragility) except blood is incubated at 37°C for 24 hours. The test is mainly for diagnosis of hereditary spherocytosis.
Specimen Whole blood
Container Lavender top (EDTA) tube or green top (heparin) tube
Collection Sterile technique must be used.
Causes for Rejection Specimen hemolyzed, specimen clotted,

Osmotic Fragility of Erythrocytes in Various Diseases

Disease	Initial Hemolysis (% saline ±1 SD)	Complete Hemolysis (% saline ±1 SD)	Remarks
Normal	0.44±0.02	0.32±0.02	
Hereditary spherocytosis	0.68±0.14	0.46±0.10	Abnormal in all cases; initial hemolysis may occur in 0.85% saline solution
Acquired hemolytic anemia	0.52±0.04	0.42±0.04	Abnormal in most cases; degree varies with severity
Hemolytic disease caused by ABO incompatibility	0.50±0.02	0.40±0.02	Abnormal in many cases; degree varies with severity
Hemolytic disease caused by Rh incompatibility	0.60±0.06	0.40±0.04	Abnormal in many cases; degree varies with severity
Hemolytic anemia caused by drugs	0.50±0.04	0.40±0.04	Abnormal in most cases during onset; may be normal in later stages
Hemolytic anemia caused by burns	0.50±0.04	0.40±0.04	Abnormal in about 50% of cases during first few days; usually normal after a few days
Pernicious anemia	0.48±0.04	0.36±0.02	Occasionally very abnormal; normal in most cases
Congenital nonspherocytic hemolytic anemia	0.44±0.02	0.32±0.02	Fragility may be increased after blood is incubated
Elliptocytosis, asymptomatic	0.44	0.32	
Elliptocytosis with hemolytic anemia	0.50	0.32	
Thalassemia	0.38±0.04	0.20±0.06	Complete hemolysis may not be achieved until salt concentration of 0.1% is reached
Sickle cell anemia	0.36±0.02	0.20±0.04	Abnormal in all cases
Sickle cell trait (S/A)	0.44±0.04	0.32±0.04	Always normal
Hb C disease	0.34	0.22	Abnormal in almost all cases
Erythremia	0.40±0.02	0.28±0.02	Not a constant finding
Iron deficiency anemia	0.38±0.02	0.28±0.02	Typical in severe anemia; not common otherwise
Obstructive jaundice (severe)	0.36±0.02	0.28±0.04	Decreased fragility usually noted in severely jaundiced patients

From Miale JB, Laboratory Medicine: Hematology, 6th ed, St Louis, MO: Mosby-Year Book Inc, 1982, 584, with permission.

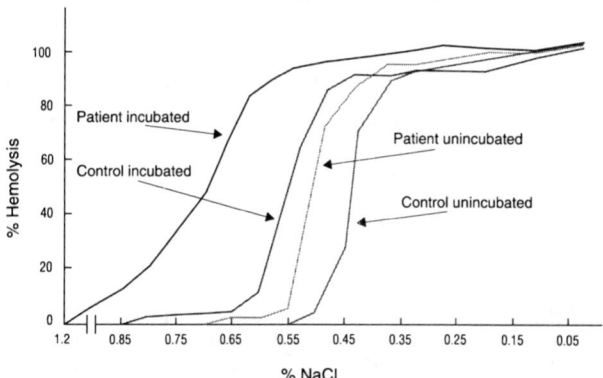

Osmotic fragility of unincubated and incubated RBCs from a normal individual and from a patient with hereditary spherocytosis. Note the increase in fragility produced by incubation of hereditary spherocytosis RBCs.

From Rapaport SI, Introduction to Hematology, 2nd ed, Philadelphia, PA: J.B. Lippincott Co., 1987, with permission.

improper anticoagulant (oxalate or citrate), improper venipuncture technique

Use Evaluate hemolytic anemia, particularly hereditary spherocytosis, congenital nonspherocytic hemolytic anemia, thalassemia

Additional Information Incubation accentuates increased osmotic fragility. In cases of nonspherocytic hemolytic anemia, fragility may be normal in the unincubated osmotic fragility test but increased after incubation. See graph.

References

Luzzatto L and Roper D, "Osmotic Fragility as Measured by Lysis in Hypotonic Saline," *Practical Haematology*, 8th ed, Chapter 13, Dacie JV and Lewis SM, eds, New York, NY: Churchill Livingstone, 1995, 216-20.

Ovalocytes Smear *see* Peripheral Blood: Red Blood Cell Morphology *on page 339*

Packed Cell Volume *see* Hematocrit *on page 322*

Pallidin *see* Band 4.2, Red Cell Membrane *on page 305*

Pappenheimer Body Stain *see* Siderocyte Stain *on page 348*

Paracentesis Fluid Analysis *see* Body Fluid Analysis, Cell Count *on page 306*

Paroxysmal Nocturnal Hemoglobinuria Test *see* Ham Test *on page 320*

PAS Stain *see* Leukocyte Cytochemistry *on page 331*

PCH Test *see* Cold Hemolysin Test *on page 311*

PCV *see* Hematocrit *on page 322*

PDW *see* Platelet Sizing *on page 341*

Pericardial Fluid Analysis *see* Body Fluid Analysis, Cell Count *on page 306*

Peripheral Blood: Differential Leukocyte Count

CPT 85007

Related Information

Bacteremia Detection, Buffy Coat Micromethod *on page 305*
Bone Marrow *on page 307*
CD4/CD8 Enumeration *on page 375*
Complete Blood Count *on page 312*
Eosinophil Count *on page 315*
Infectious Mononucleosis Screening Test *on page 410*
Leukocyte Cytochemistry *on page 331*
Lymph Node Biopsy *on page 50*
Peripheral Blood: Red Blood Cell Morphology *on page 339*
Platelet Count *on page 340*
Platelet Sizing *on page 341*
White Blood Count *on page 353*

Synonyms Automated Differential; Differential; Differential Smear; Peripheral Differential; White Blood Cell Morphology

Test Commonly Includes Relative frequency (%) of and also (in some laboratories) the absolute number of the different types of white blood cells in the peripheral blood, RBC morphology, platelet evaluation

Abstract This procedure, usually a part of the complete blood count, determines the relative and/or absolute number of different types of leukocytes circulating in the peripheral blood. There are significant differences between pediatric and adult reference ranges.

Specimen Whole blood, fresh, anticoagulated (EDTA preferred)

Differential Leukocyte Count

Age	Segs (%)	Bands (%)	Eos (%)	Basos (%)	Lymphs (%)	Monos (%)
Birth	47±15	14.1±4	2.2	0.6	31±5	5.8
12 h	53	15.2	2.0	0.4	24	5.3
24 h	47	14.2	2.4	0.5	31	5.8
1 wk	34	11.8	4.1	0.4	41	9.1
2 wk	29	10.5	3.1	0.4	48	8.8
2 mo	25	8.4	2.7	0.5	57	5.9
6 mo	23	8.8	2.5	0.4	61	4.8
10 mo	22	8.3	2.5	0.4	63	4.6
2 y	25	8.0	2.6	0.5	59	5.0
6 y	43	8.0	2.7	0.6	42	4.7
10 y	46±15	8.0±3	2.4	0.5	38±10	4.3
14 y	48	8.0	2.5	0.5	37	4.7
21 y	51±15	8.0±3	2.7	0.5	34±10	4.0

From Miale JB, *Laboratory Medicine: Hematology*, 6th ed, St Louis, MO: Mosby-Year Book Inc, 1982, with permission.

Container Lavender top (EDTA) tube or smears prepared directly from fingerstick or heelstick blood. Heparin or oxalate may produce artifactual distortion of morphology, especially of white blood cells. International Council for Standardization in Hematology recommendation is for use of K_2-EDTA, 1.5-2.2 mg/mL of blood as anticoagulant for blood cell counting and sizing.[1]

Reference Range See tables.

Use Determine qualitative and quantitative variations in white cell numbers and morphology, morphology of red cells and platelet evaluation; evaluate anemia, leukemia, infections, inflammatory states, and inherited disorders of red cells, white cells, and platelets; with automated instruments, generation of cell histograms

Limitations Because of sampling, large statistical variation exists, particularly with 100 cell count manual method and with low incidence cells. Day-to-day changes should be interpreted in relation to known method-related variation.

Methodology One or a combination of methods: manual enumeration of white cells on Wright-stained peripheral blood smear; automated WBC computer image analysis (such instruments are no longer being manufactured); continuous flow system (automated) using cytochemical/light scattering measurements; cell volume (impedance related/conductivity/light scattering) measurements, resultant electronic signals of combined methods are further manipulated with computer-assisted synthesis and derivations. See in particular the references by Shapiro MF and Banez EI below for details of how white blood cells (including eosinophils and basophils) are differentiated by different commercially available automated systems.

Additional Information Significantly abnormal findings (automated or manual method) should be the subject of further study and review. Changes in leukocyte fractions are a window to a spectrum of minor to serious physiologic and pathologic changes. Some of these are tabulated in the table and in tables in the Hematology Appendix *on page 355*.

The past decade has seen significant contributions to the definition of WBC differential reference values. The considerable increase in available data (as compared to that of the 1940-1970 period) cannot be summarized comprehensively in a simple manner. Variations, often not clinically significant, relate to differences in sex, race, physiologic state, and method of analysis. More significant variation is seen with age. A continuous flow cytochemical based automated analytic system (Miles Laboratory, Technicon®) determines immaturity of the neutrophilic granulocytic series on the basis of a peroxidase reaction. This is not directly comparable to identification of band (stab) population using morphologic criteria. It is possible to detect myeloperoxidase deficiency with this peroxidase reaction-based system. Enumeration of band population is definition dependent. Automated differential determinations may vary between instruments and manual techniques but clinical significance of such differences may be minimal. Black individuals have lower neutrophil values than whites.[2] The greatest variation, both in relative and absolute terms occurs as the result of age. High WBC levels are present in the newborn and lymphocytes are increased in childhood (as compared to adult values). Correlation of the manually performed vs automated differential is somewhat poorer in pediatric as compared to adult populations.[3] Both relative (%) and absolute (actual number of cells/mm³) values need to be considered in relation to the clinical situation.

The overuse of the manual differential has become an important issue in times of cost containment[4] and technologist shortages. Current hematology instruments can produce automated differentials by cytochemistry/light scattering or cell volume/conductivity/light scattering ("VCS") techniques. Conductivity measurements utilize a high frequency electromagnetic probe. Leukocytes are separated into granulocytes, lymphocytes, monocytes, eosinophils, and basophil categories and an immaturity index (not exactly bands) of the granulocytes. With modern hematology instruments, manual differentials are probably overordered. High white counts[5,6] and fever are better indicators of clinical infection than the percentage of bands. This is because of the high variability of manual differential band counts from technologist to technologist. In the words of Shapiro et al, "The leukocyte differential is overused, only occasionally useful, and amenable to real cost reduction."[4] On the other hand, any particular patient (albeit uncommonly encountered) may present with very few but very significantly abnormal peripheral red or white cells allowing timely diagnosis not possible by other initial methods of evaluation. Some morphologic abnormalities of peripheral blood neutrophils (degree of hypogranulation and of Pelger-Huet-like changes) reflect the degree of marrow dysplasia in myelodysplastic syndromes.[7] Detection of circulating myeloma cells is clinically important as they correlate with disease activity. The cells of multiple myeloma are most sensitively detected by the use of sensitive immunofluorescent, flow cytometric, or molecular genetic techniques.[8] See also comments under

Review of Peripheral Blood Smear

Red Cell Variant*†	Clinical Associations
Crenated cell (Echinocyte)	Variant form of normal RBC
Burr cell	DIC, I.V. fibrin deposition
Schizocyte	Microangiopathic hemolytic anemia
Helmet cell	Hypertension
(Schizocyte)	Cardiac valve disease
	Uremia, burns
	Metastatic malignancy
	Severe iron deficiency/bleeding lesion
	Normal newborn
Elliptocyte	Few seen normally
Ovalocyte	Many may mean primary elliptocytosis
	Iron deficiency
	Thalassemia
	Hb S or C
	Other hemolytic anemias
Target cell (Codocyte)	Hemoglobinopathies (S, C, D, thalassemia, esp)
	Iron deficiency
	Liver disease
	LCAT deficiency
Oval macrocyte (Megalocyte)	Megaloblastic anemia
	B_{12} /folate deficiency
	Myeloproliferative disease
	Chemotherapy patients
Spherocyte	Hereditary spherocytosis
	Immune and other hemolytic states
Tear drop cell (Dacryocyte)	Myeloproliferative diseases
	Myelophthisic processes
	Pernicious anemia
	Thalassemia
Sickle cell (Drepanocyte)	Sickle cell disease and variants (ie, sickle/thalassemia, SD disease, SC disease)
Acanthocyte	Abetalipoproteinemia
	Alcoholic cirrhosis with hemolysis
	Pyruvate kinase deficiency
	Postheparin in some individuals[1]
Stomatocyte	Hereditary stomatocytosis
	Alcoholism
	Rh null disease
Schistocyte	Microangiopathic hemolysis
Helmet cell	Cardiac valve disease
Spurr cell	DIC
(Schizocyte) (Keratocyte)	Severe burns
	Uremia
Triangulocytes[2]	Alcoholism
	Rarely, Hb C disease
	Thalassemia
	Nonalcohol liver disease
	TTP
	Antimitotic chemotherapy
Eccentrocytes[3] (Asymmetric distribution of Hgb)	G-6-PD deficiency
Bite cells[4,5]	Heinz body hemolytic anemia
(Degmacyte)	Oxidative hemolysis
	Methemoglobinemia due to phenazopyridine sulfanilamide
	Unstable hemoglobin (eg, Hb Köln)
	Thalassemia
Hemighosts[6]	Severe oxidative injury
	Heinz body hemolytic anemia
	Oxidative hemolysis
Polychromatophil	Increased erythropoiesis
Reticulocyte	Myelophthisic states
Nucleated RBC	Hemolytic states
	Postsplenectomy
Basophilic stippling	Lead poisoning
(Punctate basophilis)	Hemolytic states, other anemias
	Thalassemia
	Pyrimidine-5'-nucleotidase deficiency
Pappenheimer bodies	Some hemolytic anemias
(Siderocytes)	Postsplenectomy
	Some megaloblastic anemias
	Some sideroblastic states
Parasites	Plasmodium (malaria)
	Bartonella
	Microfilaria (not intracellular)
	Whipple's disease bacillus (Tropheryma whippelii)
	Babesia and Babesia-like organisms

Review of Peripheral Blood Smear

Red Cell Variant*†	Clinical Associations
Rouleaux of RBCs	Reflects increased protein concentration
	May be associated with multiple myeloma
	Waldenström's macroglobulinemia blue staining background
Howell-Jolly bodies	Hemolytic anemia
(Nuclear fragments)	Hyposplenism/asplenism (splenectomy)
	Megaloblastic anemia
Cabot Ring (Nuclear remnants)	Megaloblastic anemia
Heinz bodies	Some drug sensitive oxidative hemolytic anemias
(Denatured Hgb)	Unstable hemoglobinopathies
WBC Abnormalities	**Clinical Associations**
Leukocytosis	Acute reactive state metabolic basis infections (esp bacterial) basis
Increase in % bands (left shift)	
Toxic granulation	
Toxic vacuolation	
Döhle bodies	Acute infection, esp pneumonia
	Scarlet fever
	Measles,
	Septicemia
	May-Hegglin anomaly
Chediak-Higashi anomaly	Inherited, giant lysosomal granules
Pseudo-Chediak-Higashi anomaly	Few cases of acute myeloid leukemia
Hypersegmented neutrophils	Megaloblastic states as pernicious anemia
Hypogranular neutrophils	Some cases of chronic myelogenous leukemia
Intraleukocyte microorganisms	Bacteria
	Ehrlichia sennetsu (Sennetsu fever)
Intragranulocytic	Ehrlichia species
Intramonocytic and small lymphocytic	Ehrlichia chaffeensis (human ehrlichiosis)
Auer rods (present in blast cells)	Acute myelogenous leukemia
Chediak-Higashi inclusions	Congenital deficiency
	Lysosomal membrane
	Phospholipid
Alder-Rielly anomaly	Mucopolysaccharidosis
Pelger-Huët anomaly (mono and bilobed neutrophils with clumped nuclear chromatin)	Congenital form
	Acquired form - associated with myelogenous leukemia
Howell-Jolly body-like basophilic neutrophil inclusions	AIDS
Neutrophil cytoplasmic inclusion bodies	Human ehrlichiosis
Platelet Abnormalities	**Clinical Associations**
Platelet satellitosis	No definite causal clinical association
Platelet clumping	May cause spurious leukocytosis and thrombocytopenia[7]

From Bessis M, *Blood Smears Reinterpreted*, New York, NY: Springer International, 1977, with permission.

From Bessis M, Weed RI, and Leblond PF, Red Cell Shape: Physiology, Pathology, Ultrastructure, New York, NY: Springer Verlag, 1973, with permission.

[1] Silber R, 'Of Acanthocytes, Spurs, Burrs, and Membranes,' Blood, 1969, 34:111.

[2] Schumacher HR, Khanna S, and Moyer B, 'Letter: Triangulocytes in Alcoholism,' *JAMA*, 1976, 235:2285-6.

[3] Ham TH, Grauel JA, Dunn RF, et al, 'Physical Properties of Red Cells as Related to Effects In Vivo. IV. Oxidant Drugs Producing Abnormal Intracellular Concentration of Hemoglobin (Eccentrocytes) With a Rigid Red-Cell Hemolytic Syndrome,' J Lab Clin Med, 1973, 82:898-910.

[4] Ward PC, Schwartz BS, and White JG, 'Heinz Body Anemia: 'Bite Cell' Variant — A Light and Electron Microscopic Study,' *Am J Hematol*, 1983, 15:135-46.

[5] Greenberg MS, 'Heinz Body Hemolytic Anemia: 'Bite Cells' — A Clue to Diagnosis,' *Arch Intern Med*, 1976, 136:153-5.

[6] Chan TK, Chan WC, and Weed RI, 'Erythrocyte Hemighosts: A Hallmark of Severe Oxidative Injury In Vivo,' Br J Haematol, 1982, 50:575.

[7] Solanki DL and Blackburn BC, 'Spurious Leukocytosis and Thrombocytopenia. A Dual Phenomenon Caused by Clumping of Platelets In Vitro,' JAMA, 1983, 250:2514-5.

*Established terminology is followed (parentheses) by that of Bessis M, et al, introduced on the basis of ultrastructural analyses.

†Some abnormal red cell forms may represent artifact introduced during preparation of the blood smear (esp stomatocytes and elliptocytes, occasionally target like cells).

Peripheral Blood: Differential Leukocyte Count
(Continued)

Leukocyte Values From Birth to Maturity*

Age	Leukocyte count (x 10^3 /mm^3)	Neutrophils			Eosinophils	Basophils	Lymphocytes	Monocytes
		Total	Band	Segmented				
At birth	18.1 (0.0-30.0)	11.0 (6.0-26.0) 61%	1.65 9.1%	9.4 52%	0.40 (0.02-0.85) 2.2%	0.10 (0-0.64) 0.6%	5.5 (2.0-11.0) 31%	1.05 (0.40-3.1) 5.8%
12 h	22.8 (13.0-38.0)	15.5 (6.0-28.0) 68%	2.33 10.2%	13.2 58%	0.45 (0.02-0.95) 2.0%	0.10 (0-0.50) 0.4%	5.5 (2.0-11.0) 24%	1.20 (0.40-3.6) 5.3%
24 h	18.9 (9.4-34.0)	11.5 (5.0-21.0) 61%	1.75 9.2%	9.8 52%	0.45 (0.05-1.00) 2.4%	0.10 (0-0.30) 0.5%	5.8 (2.0-11.5) 31%	1.10 (0.20-3.1) 5.8%
1 wk	12.2 (5.0-21.0)	5.5 (1.5-10.0) 45%	0.83 6.8%	4.7 39%	0.50 (0.07-1.10) 4.1%	0.05 (0-0.25) 0.4%	5.0 (2.0-17.0) 41%	1.10 (0.30-2.7) 9.1%
2 wk	11.4 (5.0-20.0)	4.5 (1.0-9.5) 40%	0.63 5.5%	3.9 34%	0.35 (0.07-1.00) 3.1%	0.05 (0-0.23) 0.4%	5.5 (2.0-17.0) 48%	1.00 (0.20-2.4) 8.8%
4 wk	10.8 (5.0-19.5)	3.8 (1.0-9.0) 35%	0.49 4.5%	3.3 30%	0.30 (0.07-0.90) 2.8%	0.05 (0-0.20) 0.5%	6.0 (2.5-16.5) 56%	0.70 (0.15-2.0) 6.5%
2 mo	11.0 (5.5-18.0)	3.8 (1.0-9.0) 34%	0.49 4.4%	3.3 30%	0.30 (0.07-0.85) 2.7%	0.05 (0-0.20) 0.5%	6.3 (3.0-16.0) 57%	0.65 (0.13-1.8) 5.9%
4 mo	11.5 (6.0-17.5)	3.8 (1.0-9.0) 33%	0.45 3.9%	3.3 29%	0.30 (0.07-0.80) 2.6%	0.05 (0-0.20) 0.4%	6.8 (3.5-14.5) 59%	0.60 (0.10-1.5) 5.2%
6 mo	11.9 (6.0-17.5)	3.8 (1.0-8.5) 32%	0.45 3.8%	3.3 28%	0.30 (0.07-0.75) 2.5%	0.05 (0-0.20) 0.4%	7.3 (4.0-13.5) 61%	0.58 (0.10-1.3) 4.8%
8 mo	12.2 (6.0-17.5)	3.7 (1.0-8.5) 30%	0.41 3.3%	3.3 27%	0.30 (0.07-0.70) 2.5%	0.05 (0-0.20) 0.4%	7.6 (4.5-12.5) 62%	0.58 (0.08-1.2) 4.7%
10 mo	12.0 (6.0-17.5)	3.6 (1.0-8.5) 30%	0.40 3.3%	3.2 27%	0.30 (0.06-0.70) 2.5%	0.05 (0-0.20) 0.4%	7.5 (4.5-11.5) 63%	0.55 (0.05-1.2) 4.6%
12 mo	11.4 (6.0-17.5)	3.5 (1.5-8.5) 31%	0.35 3.1%	3.2 28%	0.30 (0.05-0.70) 2.6%	0.05 (0-0.20) 0.4%	7.0 (4.0-10.5) 61%	0.55 (0.05-1.1) 4.8%
2 y	10.6 (6.0-17.0)	3.5 (1.5-8.5) 33%	0.32 3.0%	3.2 30%	0.28 (0.04-0.65) 2.6%	0.05 (0-0.20) 0.5%	6.3 (3.0-9.5) 59%	0.53 (0.05-1.0) 5.0%
4 y	9.1 (5.5-15.5)	3.8 (1.5-8.5) 42%	0.27 (0-1.0) 3.0%	3.5 (1.5-7.5) 39%	0.25 (0.02-0.65) 2.8%	0.05 (0-0.20) 0.6%	4.5 (2.0-8.0) 50%	0.45 (0-0.8) 5.0%
6 y	8.5 (5.0-14.5)	4.3 (1.5-8.0) 51%	0.25 (0-1.0) 3.0%	4.0 (1.5-7.0) 48%	0.23 (0-0.65) 2.7%	0.05 (0-0.20) 0.6%	3.5 (1.5-7.0) 42%	0.40 (0-0.8) 4.7%
8 y	8.3 (4.5-13.5)	4.4 (1.5-8.0) 53%	0.25 (0-1.0) 3.0%	4.1 (1.5-7.0) 50%	0.20 (0-0.50) 2.4%	0.05 (0-0.20) 0.6%	3.3 (1.5-6.8) 39%	0.35 (0-0.8) 4.2%
10 y	8.1 (4.5-13.5)	4.4 (1.8-8.0) 54%	0.24 (0-1.0) 3.0%	4.2 (1.8-7.0) 51%	0.20 (0-0.60) 2.4%	0.04 (0-0.20) 0.5%	3.1 (1.5-6.5) 38%	0.35 (0-0.8) 4.3%
12 y	8.0 (4.5-13.5)	4.4 (1.8-8.0) 55%	0.25 (0-1.0) 3.0%	4.2 (1.8-7.0) 52%	0.20 (0-0.55) 2.5%	0.04 (0-0.20) 0.5%	3.0 (1.2-6.0) 38%	0.35 (0-0.8) 4.4%
14 y	7.9 (4.5-13.0)	4.4 (1.8-8.0) 56%	0.24 (0-1.0) 3.0%	4.2 (1.8-7.0) 53%	0.20 (0-0.50) 2.5%	0.04 (0-0.20) 0.5%	2.9 (1.2-5.8) 37%	0.38 (0-0.8) 4.7%
16 y	7.8 (4.5-13.0)	4.4 (1.8-8.0) 57%	0.23 3.0%	4.2 54%	0.20 (0-0.50) 2.6%	0.04 (0-0.20) 0.5%	2.8 (1.2-5.2) 35%	0.40 (0-0.8) 5.1%
18 y	7.7 (4.5-12.5)	4.4 (1.8-7.7) 57%	0.23 3.0%	4.2 54%	0.20 (0-0.45) 2.6%	0.04 (0-0.20) 0.5%	2.7 (1.0-5.0) 35%	0.40 (0-0.8) 5.2%
20 y	7.5 (4.5-11.5)	4.4 (1.8-7.7) 59%	0.23 (0-0.7) 3.0%	4.2 (1.8-7.0) 56%	0.20 (0-0.45) 2.7%	0.04 (0-0.20) 0.5%	2.5 (1.0-4.8) 33%	0.38 (0-0.8) 5.2%
21 y	7.4 (4.5-11.0)	4.4 (1.8-7.7) 59%	0.22 (0-0.7) 3.0%	4.2 (1.8-7.0) 56%	0.20 (0-0.45) 2.7%	0.04 (0-0.20) 0.5%	2.5 (1.0-4.8) 34%	0.30 (0-0.8) 4.0%

*From Altman PL and Dittmer DS, eds, *Blood and Other Body Fluids*, Bethesda, MD: Federation of American Societies for Experimental Biology, 1961, with permission.

Additional Information of Peripheral Blood: Red Blood Cell Morphology on page 339.

See also listings Platelet Count on page 340 and Platelet Sizing on page 341 for discussion of platelet morphology and abnormalities.

EDTA-induced leukoagglutination has been reported but is very uncommon. It has been seen with neutrophils and with both benign and malignant lymphocytes.[9]

Footnotes

1. "Recommendations of the International Council for Standardization in Haematology for Ethylenediaminetetraacetic Acid Anticoagulation of Blood for Blood Cell Counting and Sizing," *Am J Clin Pathol*, 1993, 100(4):371-2.
2. Karayalcin G, Rosner F, and Sawitsky A, "Pseudoneutropenia in Blacks: A Normal Phenomenon," *N Y State J Med*, 1972, 72:1815-7.
3. Goyzueta FG, Bailey CJ, and Billett HH, "Automated Differential White Blood Cell Counts in the Young Pediatric Population," *Lab Med*, 1996, 27(1):48-52.
4. Shapiro MF, Hatch RL, and Greenfield S, "Cost Containment and Labor-Intensive Tests. The Case of the Leukocyte Differential Count," *JAMA*, 1984, 252(2):231-4.
5. Banez EI and Bacaling JH, "An Evaluation of the Technicon® HI Automated Hematology Analyzer in Detecting Peripheral Blood Changes in Acute Inflammation," *Arch Pathol Lab Med*, 1988, 112(9):885-8.
6. Bentley SA, "Alternatives to the Neutrophil Band Count," *Arch Pathol Lab Med*, 1988, 112(9):883-4.
7. Widell S, Hellström-Lindberg E, Kock Y, et al, "Peripheral Blood Neutrophil Morphology Reflects Bone Marrow Dysplasia in Myelodysplastic Syndromes," *Am J Hematol*, 1995, 49(2):115-20.
8. Witzig TE, "Detection of Malignant Cells in the Peripheral Blood of Patients With Multiple Myeloma: Clinical Implications and Research Applications," *Mayo Clin Proc*, 1994, 69(9):903-7.
9. Deol I, Hernandez AM, and Pierre RV, "Ethylenediamine Tetraacetic Acid-Associated Leukoagglutination," *Am J Clin Pathol*, 1995, 103(3):338-40.

References

Ardron MJ, Westengard JC, and Dutcher TF, "Band Neutrophil Counts Are Unnecessary for the Diagnosis of Infection in Patients With Normal Total Leukocyte Counts," *Am J Clin Pathol*, 1994, 102(5):646-9.

Barenfanger J, Patel PG, Dumler JS, et al, "Identifying Human Ehrlichiosis," *Lab Med*, 1996, 27(6):372-3.

Brouqui P and Raoult D, "Human Ehrlichiosis," *N Engl J Med*, 1994, 330(24):1760-1.

Cornbleet J, "Spurious Results From Automated Hematology Cell Counters," *Lab Med*, 1983, 14:509-14.

Everett ED, Evans KA, Henry RB, et al, "Human Ehrlichiosis in Adults After Tick Exposure. Diagnosis Using Polymerase Chain Reaction," *Ann Intern Med*, 1994, 120(9):730-5.

Hope E and Peerschke EI, "Principles of Automated Differential Analysis," *Clinical Hematology and Fundamentals of Hemostasis*, 2nd ed, Chapter 30, Section II, Harmening DM, ed, Philadelphia, PA: FA Davis Co, 1992, 554-67.

Hoyer JD, "Leukocyte Differential," *Mayo Clin Proc*, 1993, 68(10):1027-8.

Krause JR, "The Automated White Blood Cell Differential: A Current Perspective," *Hematol Oncol Clin North Am*, 1994, 8(4):605-16.

Paddock CD, Suchard DP, Grumbach KL, et al, "Brief Report: Fatal Seronegative Ehrlichiosis in a Patient With HIV Infection," *N Engl J Med*, 1993, 329(16):1164-7.

Pierre RV, "Leukocyte Differential Counting," *Practical Laboratory Hematology*, Chapter 7, Koepke JA, ed, New York, NY: Churchill Livingstone, 1991, 131-56.

Reed KD, Mitchell PD, Persing DH, et al, "Transmission of Human Granulocytic Ehrlichiosis," *JAMA*, 1995, 273(1):23.

Rich EC, Crowson TW, and Connelly DP, "Effectiveness of Differential Leukocyte Count in Case Finding in the Ambulatory Care Setting," *JAMA*, 1983, 249:633-6.

Robertson EP, Lai HW, and Wei DC, "An Evaluation of Leukocyte Analysis on the Coulter STKS," *Clin Lab Haematol*, 1992, 14(1):53-68.

Swaim WR, "Laboratory and Clinical Evaluation of White Blood Cell Differential Counts: Comparison of the Coulter VCS, Technicon H-1, and 800-Cell Manual Method," *Am J Clin Pathol*, 1991, 95(3):381-8.

Wardlaw SC and Levine RA, "Quantitative Buffy Coat Analysis. A New Laboratory Tool Functioning as a Screening Complete Blood Cell Count," *JAMA*, 1983, 249:617-20.

Peripheral Blood: Red Blood Cell Morphology

CPT 85008

Related Information

Synonyms Blood Smear Morphology; Morphology; Peripheral Smear, Blood; RBC Morphology; RBC Smear; Red Blood Cell Morphology

Applies to Ovalocytes Smear; Schistocytes Smear; Sickle Cells Smear; Spherocytes Smear; Stippled RBCs Smear

Specimen Whole blood

Container Lavender top (EDTA) tube or smears prepared directly from fingerstick or heelstick blood. Heparin or oxalate may produce artifactual distortion especially of white blood cells.

Collection Routine venipuncture. Invert tube gently to mix.

Storage Instructions Refrigerate

Causes for Rejection Clotted or hemolyzed specimen

Reference Range Normal morphology. It may not be possible to correlate minor changes in RBC morphology (eg, 5% to 10% elliptocytosis) with identifiable disease.

Use Evaluate red cell disorders, white cell disorders, platelet disorders, and correlation of findings with CBC parameters as quality control function

Methodology Study of red blood cell morphology as it presents on Wright's stained peripheral blood. Red blood cell indices as determined by automated cell counters (eg, MCV, MCH, MCHC, RDW) also give insight into morphologic red cell abnormalities.

Additional Information Diverse trends at all levels of the medical care system have combined to focus attention on the utility/cost-effectiveness of manual review of the peripheral blood smear (PBS), in particular, as a routine incorporated in the CBC. The CBC has evolved from highly labor intensive to highly capital intensive, while the PBS has remained highly labor intensive. Automated devices continue to expand their repertoire, adding new parameters that digitize and in some cases improve upon information formerly gleaned from study of the PBS (eg, red cell distribution width which quantitates the morphologic observation anisocytosis). Radical changes in reimbursement, some in effect, others yet to occur, provide economic incentive to retain only laboratory procedures that have very strongly favorable cost/benefit ratios. Studies have suggested that physician criteria for ordering WBC differential on patients in the hospital are inconsistent (demand vs need is not clear)[1] and that differential leukocyte counting has no value in case finding in the "ambulatory care setting."[2] There appears to be a growing trend to perform WBC differential only in cases of abnormal WBC count or only upon specific order. That is, the trend is to delete the differential (blood smear review) from the "complete blood count" routine however the latter is defined. Differential counts have been found unproductive in a specialized clinical environment (healthy midshipmen being considered for nuclear submarine duty).[3] Patients requiring hospitalization, however, should present

with greater hematologic abnormality (variable with type of patient and institution). The review of PBS is a part of the quality control cross check system built into each CBC and available to the medical technologist performing the test and to physicians and others who may subsequently question the integrity of the results. Each CBC (when truly complete with review of PBS, WBC differential count, and RBC indices) is a self-contained case individualized quality control unit.[4] Spurious results from automated counters may arise from a surprisingly large number of different sources, many requiring review of the PBS for detection and/or analysis.[5]

Cost and utilization considerations briefly reviewed above seem to indicate that review of PBS and differential study of WBCs should be relegated to the occasional special situation (ie, on physician order or to assist with evaluation of an abnormal result from an automated cell counter). This role in itself would necessitate review of some 10% to 30% of CBC studies depending on the type of institution. Computer assisted automated differential analyzers flag and require some 10% to 20% of cases for manual review, also institution variable. While labor intensive, the study of PBS is nearly devoid of capital costs. On the other hand, automated counters are not free of labor costs and are highly capital intensive. These expensive units are not centralized, due in part to the perceived need for "stat" capability. They are, therefore, not efficiently utilized; they are idle for part of the day. In effect a costly instrument is used to screen (CBC without differential) for performance of a low cost but in some respects more definitive test. A "variable effort" approach to the WBC differential utilizing a computer and "linkage patterns" of linked abnormalities has been proposed.[6] Here, the number of cells examined per slide varies with the apparent abnormality of the slide. Another alternative, quantitative buffy coat analysis (QBCA), has been proposed and may find acceptance. It is based on lower cost technology in which WBCs are differentially stained with a fluorescent dye in a specialized hematocrit tube having a float that expands the buffy coat layer.[7] In a critique, QBCA has been challenged, somewhat unrealistically, as not cost-competitive with manual methods.[8] The clinician will likely find a variable and changing approach to these problems.

Efforts expended on technical and economic aspects of delivering a CBC for patient/physician use unfortunately may becloud the fact that a wealth of information may be hidden from the sensory mechanisms and microcomputers of automated counters (eg, presence of target, sickle, or tear drop cells, Howell-Jolly or Pappenheimer bodies, intracellular parasites, and other abnormalities). This data, beneficial to the patient, may be lost without the manual study of the PBS. Examples of blood cell morphologic abnormalities (not comprehensive) are given in tabular form in the listing Peripheral Blood: Differential Leukocyte Count *on page 336*. The possibility of confusing ring forms of *Babesia* (an intraerythrocytic protozoan which is also characterized by presence of red cell tetrad forms) with ring forms of the malarial organism *Plasmodium falciparum* is notable.[9,10]

Footnotes

1. Rock WA Jr and Grogan JE, "Demand vs Need vs Physician Prerogatives in the Use of the WBC Differential," *JAMA*, 1983, 249:613-6.
2. Rich EC, Crowson TW, and Connelly DP, "Effectiveness of Differential Leukocyte Count in Case Finding in the Ambulatory Care Setting," *JAMA*, 1983, 249:633-6.
3. Wesson SK, Mercado T, Austin M, et al, "Differential Counts and Overuse of the Laboratory," *Lancet*, 1980, 1:552.
4. Lafsness KG, "Correlation of Hematologic Data From the Individual Patient as a Quality Control Tool," *Am J Med Technol*, 1983, 49:655-9.
5. Cornbleet J, "Spurious Results From Automated Hematology Cell Counters," *Lab Med*, 1983, 14:509-14.
6. Korpman RA and Bull B, "Whither the WBC Differential? - Some Alternatives," *Blood Cells*, 1980, 6:421-9.
7. Wardlaw SC and Levine RA, "Quantitative Buffy Coat Analysis. A New Laboratory Tool Functioning as a Screening Complete Blood Cell Count," *JAMA*, 1983, 249:617-20.
8. Fischer P and Addison L, "Quantitative Buffy Coat Analysis," *JAMA*, 1983, 250:1272.
9. Quick RE, Herwaldt BL, Thomford JW, et al, "Babesiosis in Washington State: A New Species of *Babesia*?" *Ann Intern Med*, 1993, 119(4):284-90.
10. Persing DH, Herwaldt BL, Glaser C, et al, "Infection With a *Babesia*-Like Organism in Northern California," *N Engl J Med*, 1995, 332(5):298-303.

References

Beutler E, Lichtman MA, and Coller BS, *Williams Hematology*, 5th ed, New York, NY: McGraw-Hill Inc, 1995, 13-4.

Javidian P, Garshelis L, and Peterson P, "Pathologist Review of the Peripheral Smear: A Mandatory Quality Assurance Activity?" *Clin Lab Med*, 1993, 13(4):853-61.

Van Assendelft OW, "Interpretation of the Quantitative Blood Cell Count," *Practical Laboratory Hematology*, Chapter 4, Koepke JA, ed, New York, NY: Churchill Livingstone, 1991, 78-98.

Williams WJ, "Polychrome Staining," *Hematology*, 4th ed, Appendix, Chapter A2, Williams WJ, Beutler E, Ersler AJ, et al, eds, New York, NY: McGraw-Hill Publishing Co, 1990, 1699-700.

Peripheral Differential *see* Peripheral Blood: Differential Leukocyte Count *on page 336*

Peripheral Smear, Blood *see* Peripheral Blood: Red Blood Cell Morphology *on this page*

Peritoneal Fluid Analysis *see* Body Fluid Analysis, Cell Count *on page 306*

Perls' Test see Iron Stain, Bone Marrow on page 328

Peroxidase Stain see Leukocyte Cytochemistry on page 331

Pink Test see Glycerol Lysis Test, Acidified, Modified on page 320

PK Assay see Pyruvate Kinase Assay, Erythrocytes on page 342

Plasma/Blood Volume see Blood Volume on page 306

Plasma Free Hemoglobin see Hemoglobin, Plasma on page 325

Plasma Volume Measurement see Blood Volume on page 306

Platelet Count

CPT 85590 (manual); 85595 (automated)

Related Information

Activated Partial Thromboplastin Time on page 227
Blood, Urine on page 631
Complete Blood Count on page 312
Fanconi's Anemia, Chromosome Breakage Study on page 282
Intravascular Coagulation Screen on page 253
Kidney Profile on page 153
Peripheral Blood: Differential Leukocyte Count on page 336
Platelet Adhesion Test on page 256
Platelet Aggregation on page 257
Platelet Antibody on page 258
Platelet Antibody, Immunohematologic on page 616
Platelet Concentrate, Donation and Transfusion on page 616
Platelets, Apheresis, Donation on page 617
Platelet Sizing on next page

Synonyms Thrombocyte Count

Abstract Enumeration of platelets in the circulating peripheral blood. Platelet count is important in the assessment of bleeding, thrombotic, and malignant neoplastic processes, in evaluation of marrow function, and in study of effects of some diseases involving autoimmune mechanisms.

Specimen Whole blood

Container Lavender top (EDTA) tube

Causes for Rejection Clotted specimen, platelet clumping

Reference Range 150,000-450,000/mm^3 (150-450 x 10^9/L or 150,000-450,000/µL).[1] Considerable interlaboratory variation exists, manual vs electronic automated procedures. Count is method dependent; results of manual count have high coefficient of variation as compared to automated methods.[2] Occasionally, apparently normal children, in particular those under 24 months of age, may have platelet counts in the 500,000-750,000 range.[3]

Possible Panic Range <50,000/mm^3 or >1,000,000/mm^3

Use Evaluate, diagnose, and follow up bleeding disorders, purpura/petechiae, drug-induced thrombocytopenia, idiopathic thrombocytopenia purpura, disseminated intravascular coagulation, leukemia, hypercoagulable states, and chemotherapeutic management of malignant disease.

Limitations Clumping may cause false low count. Platelet satellitism around neutrophils may cause pseudothrombocytopenia. An IgG autoantibody is apparently involved with specificity against the platelet membrane glycoprotein IIb/IIIa complex and also against the neutrophil Fcγ receptor III (CD16).[4] RBC (eg, microspherocytes) or WBC fragments including fragmented fragile leukemic cells and neutrophil pseudoplatelets may cause falsely elevated counts. EDTA-induced platelet clumping is a frequent cause of spuriously low platelet counts[5] resulting from various platelet antigen/antibody reactions including antiplatelet with antiphospholipid antibodies[6] and occurring also in vitro (eg, IgM autoantibody against 78 kD platelet glycoprotein).[7]

Methodology Variety of automated/semiautomated devices are in use. Counts are performed on platelet-rich plasma or whole blood by optical or impedance matching counting techniques. Carefully controlled phase microscopy manual count is usually considered the reference method but suffers from a wide coefficient of variation (Brecher-Cronkite phase contrast method has CV of 7% to 17%). In a study documenting the reliability of automated platelet counts performed on one commercially available analyzer, the mean of low platelet counts (machine determined) had a CV of 10% while manual counts had a CV of 30%.[8]

Additional Information The platelet, of growing practical clinical importance in hemostatic considerations and a variety of medical/surgical processes, is also fundamental to etiologic considerations of arteriosclerotic and malignant disease.[9] Platelets are generally 2-3 microns in diameter but large forms (megathrombocytes) appear when production is increased. The production of platelets is controlled by thrombopoietin. Platelets survive for 8-10 days and are subject to circadian periodicity, highest platelet counts occurring during midday.[10] Some drugs may increase the platelet count by stimulating thrombopoietin production.

Deaths from cardiovascular disease may relate temporally to the circadian rhythm of platelet production.[10]

Careful estimate of platelet number from stained peripheral blood smear can provide useful information. A variety of factors affect the distribution of platelets on a peripheral blood smear, and thus platelet estimates lack precision. Capillary blood platelet counts (compared to venous blood counts) may be significantly underestimated. Platelets are often clumped on smears obtained from capillary blood, contributing to imprecision. A small whole blood clot or very small fibrin clots in the EDTA anticoagulated specimen will usually be associated with clumping of platelets on the slide and with a false low platelet count.

Quantitative platelet disorders have varied etiology. Thrombocytopenia may have an immunologic basis, the result of production deficiency due to the effect of drugs or physical agents, abnormal platelet pooling or increased destruction (eg, sequestration by large vascular tumor), or result from a variety of probably nonimmunologic mechanisms (eg, hypersplenism). Decreases may occur after severe bleeding, transfusion, infections, or relating to defective production of or regulation by thrombopoietin. Serum lactate dehydrogenase and platelet count may predict survival in thrombotic thrombocytopenic purpura.[11]

Drugs and chemicals associated with thrombocytopenia often on an immune mediated basis or as the result of marrow suppression include quinidine, quinine, heparin, gold salts, sulfas, rifampicin, ASA, digitoxin, apronal, chlorothiazides, chlorpropamide, meprobamate, antihistamines, chloramphenicol, penicillin, DDT, benzol, a variety of other industrial organic chemicals, diphenylhydantoin, PAS, hydrochlorothiazide, phenylbutazone, and a variety of antineoplastic chemotherapeutic agents. ASA acts by acetylating cyclo-oxygenase.

Thrombocytosis is less common, but likewise varied in etiology: physiologic (eg, postpartum or after exercise); myeloproliferative syndromes (eg, thrombocythemia, some cases of chronic myelogenous leukemia, myelofibrosis with myeloid metaplasia); rebound following thrombocytopenia, marrow regenerative activity after bleeding episode, hemophilia, iron deficiency; asplenism, infections, inflammatory or malignant disease, in particular, carcinomatosis but also in early (stage IB) cervical carcinoma.[10] Thrombocytosis in cases of malignancy may relate to the production of cytokines and/or growth factors (eg, interleukin-6, thrombopoietin). Interleukin-6 has been shown to be produced by some malig-

Inherited Abnormalities of Platelet Production (Characterized by Thrombocytopenia)

Condition	Inheritance	Abnormality	Therapy
May-Hegglin	Autosomal Dominant	Severe thrombocytopenia	Platelet replacement
Wiskott-Aldrich	Sex-linked	Severe thrombocytopenia with small platelets	Possibly splenectomy
Congenital thrombopoietin deficiency	? Autorecessive	Severe thrombocytopenia	Plasma transfusion
Thrombocytopenia with absent radius	Autorecessive	Moderate thrombocytopenia	Platelet replacement
Abnormalities of Platelet Function, Familial Transmission, Autorecessive			
Thrombasthenia		Absent clot retraction, absent aggregation, mild thrombocytopenia	Platelet replacement, steroids
Bernard-Soulier syndrome		Giant platelets, absent Ristocetin® aggregation	Platelet replacement
Platelet storage pool disease		Absent aggregation with collagen, mild thrombocytopenia, absent dense granules with decreased platelet serotonin	Splenectomy, platelet replacement
Hermansky-Pudlak syndrome		Aggregation abnormal with epinephrine and collagen, decreased dense granules and absent ADP stores	Platelet replacement
Release reaction abnormalities		Absent second wave aggregation with epinephrine and collagen, absent PF-3 release, varied inheritance	Platelet replacement

From Penner J, Blood Coagulation Laboratory Manual, University of Michigan Medical School, Sept, 1979, with permission.

nant cells, notably by a number of different cancer cell lines.[12] Oral contraceptives may cause slight increase in platelet count. Slight to moderate decrease in platelet count has been noted during pregnancy in most women who have essential thrombocythemia.[13]

Congenital causes of thrombocytopenia include Wiskott-Aldrich syndrome, May-Hegglin anomaly, thrombocytopenia with absent radius, Bernard-Soulier syndrome, and Paris-Trousseau syndrome.[14] See table. See listing Platelet Sizing *on page 341* for discussion of changes in platelet count and size in pre-eclampsia and the HELLP syndrome (hemolysis, elevated liver tests, and low platelet count).

Footnotes

1. Rowan RM, "Platelet Counting and the Assessment of Platelet Function," *Practical Laboratory Hematology*, Chapter 8, Koepke JA, ed, New York, NY: Churchill Livingstone, 1991, 164.
2. Lohmann RC, Crawford LN, and Wood DE, "Proficiency Testing of Platelet Counting in Ontario," *Am J Clin Pathol*, 1992, 98(2):231-6.
3. Novak RW, Tschantz JA, and Krill CE Jr, "Normal Platelet and Mean Platelet Volumes in Pediatric Patients," *Lab Med*, 1987, 18:613-4.
4. Bizzaro N, Goldschmeding R, and Von Dem Borne AE, "Platelet Satellitism Is FCγ RIII (CD16) Receptor-Mediated," *Am J Clin Pathol*, 1995, 103(6):740-4.
5. Payne BA and Pierre RV, "Pseudothrombocytopenia: A Laboratory Artifact With Potentially Serious Consequences," *Mayo Clin Proc*, 1984, 59(2):123-5.
6. Bizzaro N and Brandalise M, "EDTA-Dependent Pseudothrombocytopenia. Association With Antiplatelets and Antiphospholipid Antibodies," *Am J Clin Pathol*, 1995, 103(1):103-7.
7. De Caterina M, Fratellanza G, Grimaldi E, et al, "Evidence of a Cold Immunoglobulin M Autoantibody Against 78-kD Platelet Glycoprotein in a Case of EDTA-Dependent Pseudothrombocytopenia," *Am J Clin Pathol*, 1993, 99(2):163-7.
8. Lawrence JB, Yomtovian RA, Dillman C, et al, "Reliability of Automated Platelet Counts: Comparison With Manual Method and Utility for Prediction of Clinical Bleeding," *Am J Hematol*, 1995, 48:244-50.
9. Doolittle RF, Hunkapillar MW, Hood LE, et al, "Simian Sarcoma Virus onc Gene, v-sis, Is Derived From the Gene (or Genes) Encoding a Platelet-Derived Growth Factor," *Science*, 1983, 221:275-7.
10. de Nicola P and Casale G, "Platelets," *Blood Diseases in the Aged*, Stuttgart, West Germany: Schwer Verlag, 1988, 71-6.
11. Patton JF, Manning KR, Case D, et al, "Serum Lactate Dehydrogenase and Platelet Count Predict Survival in Thrombotic Thrombocytopenic Purpura," *Am J Hematol*, 1994, 47(2):94-9.
12. Rodriguez GC, Clarke-Pearson DL, Soper JT, et al, "The Negative Prognostic Implications of Thrombocytosis in Women With Stage IB Cervical Cancer," *Obstet Gynecol*, 1994, 83(3):445-8.
13. Chow EY, Haley LP, and Vickars LM, "Essential Thrombocythemia in Pregnancy: Platelet Count and Pregnancy Outcome," *Am J Hematol*, 1992, 41(4):249-51.
14. Breton-Gorius J, Favier R, Guichard J, et al, "A New Congenital Dysmegakaryocytic Thrombocytopenia (Paris-Trousseau) Associated With Giant Platelet α-Granules and Chromosome 11 Deletion at 11q23," *Blood*, 1995, 85(7):1805-14.

References

Bizzaro N, "EDTA-Dependent Pseudothrombocytopenia: A Clinical and Epidemiological Study of 112 Cases, With 10-Year Follow-Up," *Am J Hematol*, 1995, 50(2):103-9.

Cornbleet PJ and Kessinger S, "Accuracy of Low Platelet Counts on the Coulter S-Plus IV®," *Am J Clin Pathol*, 1985, 83(1):78-80.

Feusner JH, Behrens JA, Detter JC, et al, "Platelet Counts in Capillary Blood," *Am J Clin Pathol*, 1979, 72:410-4.

George JN, El-Harake MA, and Raskob GE, "Chronic Idiopathic Thrombocytopenic Purpura," *N Engl J Med*, 1994, 331(18):1207-11.

Kaushansky K, "Thrombopoietin: The Primary Regulator of Platelet Production," *Blood*, 1995, 86(2):419-31.

Rowan RM, "Platelet Counting and the Assessment of Platelet Function," *Practical Laboratory Hematology*, Chapter 8, Koepke JA, ed, New York, NY: Churchill Livingstone, 1991, 157-70.

Tefferi A and Hoagland HC, "Issues in the Diagnosis and Management of Essential Thrombocythemia," *Mayo Clin Proc*, 1994, 69(7):651-5.

Thompson CE, Damon LE, Ries CA, et al, "Thrombotic Microangiopathies in the 1980s: Clinical Features, Response to Treatment, and the Impact of the Human Immunodeficiency Virus Epidemic," *Blood*, 1992, 80(8):1890-5.

Vora AJ and Lilleyman JS, "Secondary Thrombocytosis," *Arch Dis Child*, 1993, 68(1):88-90.

Platelet Indices *see* Platelet Sizing *on this page*

Platelet Sizing

CPT 85029

Related Information

Complete Blood Count *on page 312*
Peripheral Blood: Differential Leukocyte Count *on page 336*
Peripheral Blood: Red Blood Cell Morphology *on page 339*
Platelet Count *on previous page*

Synonyms MPV; PDW; Platelet Indices

Test Commonly Includes MPV (mean platelet volume), platelet count, PDW (platelet distribution width)

Abstract Modern automated cell counters may generate platelet sizing parameters (eg, MPV and PDW) which may be abnormal in some clinical situations. Platelet indices are analogous to red blood cell indices (eg, MCV and RDW) but have only modest clinical application. MPV and PDW are increased in patients with idiopathic thrombocytopenic purpura (ITP).

Specimen Whole blood

Container Lavender top (EDTA) tube; green top (heparin) tube may cause platelet clumping

Storage Instructions Effects of EDTA anticoagulation on the reliability of MPV determination is uncertain.

Reference Range See tables for mean platelet volume and platelet "crit" reference values.

Platelet Parameters in Males (mean ±SD)*

Age	n	Platelet Count (x 10³/mm³) (x 10⁹/L)	MPV (fL)	PCT (%)
1-5 y	24	357±70	8.6±0.7	0.304±0.059
6-10 y	24	351±85	8.6±0.8	0.300±0.058
11-15 y	16	282±63	9.8±1.0	0.274±0.053
16-20 y	16	266±63	10.2±1.1	0.266±0.049
21-30 y	24	238±49	9.6±0.6	0.277±0.045
31-40 y	12	244±56	9.8±1.2	0.237±0.044
41-50 y	17	271±66	9.4±1.0	0.250±0.045
51-60 y	22	258±61	9.8±1.2	0.248±0.045
61-70 y	29	256±53	9.4±1.1	0.238±0.047
71-86 y	23	237±49	9.6±1.0	0.226±0.048

*SI conversion units for platelet count x 10³/mm³ is platelet count x 10⁹/L.

From Graham SS, Traub B, and Minic IB, 'Automated Platelet-Sizing Parameters on a Normal Population,' *Am J Clin Pathol*, 1987, 87:365-9, with permission.

Platelet Parameters in Females (mean ±SD)*

Age	n	Platelet Count (x 10³/mm³) (x 10⁹/L)	MPV (fL)	PCT (%)
1-5 y	25	381±76	8.9±0.8	0.337±0.069
6-10 y	18	336±76	9.7±1.1	0.326±0.080
11-15 y	31	298±72	9.8±1.2	0.288±0.058
16-20 y	22	270±58	9.7±0.7	0.262±0.058
21-30 y	43	270±58	9.8±1.0	0.261±0.046
31-40 y	30	282±56	9.8±1.2	0.271±0.046
41-50 y	26	279±65	9.8±0.9	0.274±0.072
51-60 y	21	285±54	9.7±0.7	0.276±0.045
61-70 y	30	274±61	9.6±0.9	0.262±0.052
71-83 y	24	279±65	9.5±1.0	0.261±0.054

*SI conversion units for platelet count x 10³/mm³ is platelet count x 10⁹/L.

From Graham SS, Traub B, and Minic IB, 'Automated Platelet-Sizing Parameters on a Normal Population,' *Am J Clin Pathol*, 1987, 87:365-9, with permission.

Use Differential diagnosis of hematologic disease, assess platelet function, and guide need for platelet transfusion in thrombocytopenic patients

Limitations May be unreliable if platelet count is <10,000/mm³

Methodology Flow cytometry (FC) with measurement of platelet volume and size parameters by changes in electrical impedance (resistance of an individual cell is proportional to its volume) and microprocessor assisted mathematical analysis. Electrical signals (proportional to particle size) are sorted according to magnitude. Upper and lower thresholds define the central platelet volume distribution (2-20 fL).[1]

Additional Information The clinical significance of variation in platelet size has only recently begun to be explored. Generally, large platelets are young platelets and have better hemostatic function than average age or old platelets.[2] MPV (in normal subjects) bears an inverse relation to platelet count. MPV rises with increased platelet turnover due to production of megathrombocytes. Platelet size parameters may be an example of a "test in search of a disease". Platelet sizing does find application in the evaluation of acute thrombocytopenia, in cases of suspected idiopathic thrombocytopenic purpura (ITP). MPV and PDW are increased with ITP. Use of increased platelet volume as an indicator of ITP versus acute leukemia will not likely replace bone marrow study for evaluation of megakaryocytes in cases of thrombocytopenia. Large platelets are present in the recovery stage of alcohol-induced thrombocytopenia.[3] Platelet size, while often a marker for platelet age, may in some cases reflect altered platelet production (eg, dyspoietic states such as the May-Hegglin anomaly in which increased platelet volume occurs).[1] Small platelets are seen in the Wiskott-Aldrich syndrome. Autoimmune thrombocytopenia and leukemia may be associated with presence of platelet fragments and decreased platelet volume. Hypersplenetic patients have smaller platelet size. Low MPV may be seen in patients with septic thrombocytopenia and in some cases of myeloproliferative disease after treatment with cytotoxic drugs. In the Bernard-Soulier syndrome, there is thrombocytopenia with large platelets.[4] Large platelets, occasionally with abnormal morphology, occur in the myeloproliferative syndromes. Increased MPV may also be seen in hyperthyroidism.[5] Mediterranean macrothrombocytopenia is characterized by low platelet count, large platelets, and a generally normal platelet
(Continued)

Platelet Sizing (Continued)

"crit".[6] There is evidence that mean platelet volume correlates with bleeding tendency in thrombocytopenic patients.[7] A significantly lower frequency of bleeding occurs with mean platelet volumes >6.4 fL. This measure, then, may be of use in assessing the need for platelet transfusion.

MPV and platelet count are normal and constant between the first trimester and the end of normal pregnancy, but MPV is increased in patients with pre-eclampsia. Platelet count is decreased in cases of pre-eclampsia but was also found to be decreased in 10% of normal pregnancies.[8] Platelet count is decreased in pre-eclamptic women with the HELLP syndrome (hemolysis, elevated liver tests, and low platelet count). Platelets have also been found to decrease in pre-eclamptic women with platelet count in the normal range.[9] Increase in MPV has been noted in neonates with coagulase-negative staphylococcal septicemia.[10] Platelet volume has been noted to decrease during cardiopulmonary bypass and to increase in atherosclerotic smokers.[11,12] Increase in MPV due to smoking has been proposed as a risk factor for atherosclerotic disease.[12]

The increase in platelet membrane fluidity with electron microscopic atypia (abundant internal system of smooth membrane) is apparently not associated with increase in MPV.[13]

Footnotes

1. Paulus JM, "Platelet Size in Man," *Blood*, 1975, 46:321-36.
2. Haver VM and Gear AR, "Functional Fractionation of Platelets," *J Lab Clin Med*, 1981, 97:187-204.
3. Sahud MA, "Platelet Size and Number in Alcoholic Thrombocytopenia," *N Engl J Med*, 1973, 286:355-6.
4. Howard MA, Hutton RA, and Hardisty RM, "Hereditary Giant Platelet Syndrome: A Disorder of a New Aspect of Platelet Function," *Br Med J (Clin Res Ed)*, 1983, 2:586-8.
5. Henry JB, Nelson DA, Tomar RH, et al, *Todd-Sanford-Davidsohn Clinical Diagnosis and Management by Laboratory Methods*, 18th ed, Henry JB, ed, Philadelphia, PA: WB Saunders Co, 1991, 567-8.
6. England JM, "Blood Cell Sizing," *Practical Laboratory Hematology*, Chapter 6, Koepke JA, ed, New York, NY: Churchill Livingstone, 1991, 127-8.
7. Eldor A, Avitzour M, Or R, et al, "Prediction of Hemorrhagic Diathesis in Thrombocytopenia by Mean Platelet Volume," *Br Med J (Clin Res Ed)*, 1982, 285:397-400.
8. Ahmed Y, van Iddekinge B, Paul C, et al, "Retrospective Analysis of Platelet Numbers and Volumes in Normal Pregnancy and in Pre-eclampsia," *Br J Obstet Gynaecol*, 1993, 100(3):216-20.
9. Neiger R, Contag SA, and Coustan DR, "Pre-eclampsia Effect on Platelet Count," *Am J Perinatol*, 1992, 9(5-6):378-80.
10. O'Connor TA, Ringer KM, and Gaddis ML, "Mean Platelet Volume During Coagulase-Negative Staphylococcal Sepsis in Neonates," *Am J Clin Pathol*, 1993, 99(1):69-71.
11. Boldt J, Zickmann B, Benson M, et al, "Does Platelet Size Correlate With Function in Patients Undergoing Cardiac Surgery?" *Intensive Care Med*, 1993, 19(1):44-7.
12. Kario K, Matsuo T, and Nakao K, "Cigarette Smoking Increases the Mean Platelet Volume in Elderly Patients With Risk Factors for Atherosclerosis," *Clin Lab Haematol*, 1992, 14(4):281-7.
13. Zubenko GS, Malinakova I, and Chojnacki B, "Proliferation of Internal Membranes in Platelets From Patients With Alzheimer's Disease," *J Neuropathol Exp Neurol*, 1987, 46(4):407-18.

References

Bithell TC, "Thrombocytopenia Caused by Immunologic Platelet Destruction," *Wintrobe's Clinical Hematology*, 9th ed, Vol 2, Chapter 50, Philadelphia, PA: Lea & Febiger, 1993, 1335.
Graham SS, Traub B, and Mink IB, "Automated Platelet-Sizing Parameters on a Normal Population," *Am J Clin Pathol*, 1987, 87(3):365-9.
Jackson SR and Carter JM, "Platelet Volume: Laboratory Measurement and Clinical Application," *Blood Rev*, 1993, 7(2):104-13.
Thompson CB, Diaz DD, Quinn PG, et al, "The Role of Anticoagulation in the Measurement of Platelet Volumes," *Am J Clin Pathol*, 1983, 80:327-32.
Threatte GA, "Usefulness of the Mean Platelet Volume," *Clin Lab Med*, 1993, 13(4):937-50.

Pleural Fluid Analysis see Body Fluid Analysis, Cell Count on page 306

PNH Test see Ham Test on page 320

PNH Test Screen see Sugar Water Test Screen on page 348

Prussian Blue Stain see Iron Stain, Bone Marrow on page 328

Pyruvate Kinase Assay see Pyruvate Kinase Assay, Erythrocytes on this page

Pyruvate Kinase Assay, Erythrocytes

CPT 84220

Related Information

Autohemolysis Test *on page 304*
Red Blood Cell Enzyme Deficiency, Quantitative *on this page*
Red Blood Cell Enzyme Deficiency Screen *on next page*

Synonyms PK Assay; Pyruvate Kinase Assay

Abstract A deficiency of this glycolytic enzyme is characterized by a decrease in RBC ATP level, consequent membrane defect, and resultant nonspherocytic chronic hemolytic anemia.

Specimen Erythrocytes (washed)

Container Yellow top (ACD) tube, green top (heparin) tube, or lavender top (EDTA) tube

Collection Mix tube three times by gentle inversion, place on ice.

Causes for Rejection Specimen not fresh

Special Instructions Notify laboratory before specimen collection. Deliver specimen on ice. Specimen **must** be received in the laboratory within 30 minutes of collection.

Reference Range Adults: 6-19 µmol NAD(H)₂/min/g Hgb (37°C)

Use Evaluate chronic hemolytic anemia

Limitations Some patients with PK-deficient variant hemolytic disease may not be identified if the enzyme is assayed only under conditions of substrate saturation.

Methodology Spectrophotometric kinetic assay

Additional Information Pyruvate kinase (PK) deficiency is the most common enzyme defect in anaerobic red cell glycolysis (Embden-Meyerhof glycolytic pathway) and the most common cause of congenital nonspherocytic hemolytic anemia.[1] PK is a glycolytic enzyme that converts phosphoenolpyruvate to pyruvate. The deficiency is inherited as an autosomal recessive trait. Current assay techniques preclude accurate distinction of all heterozygotes from normals. Specialized PK assays and the determination of red cell 2,3-DPG levels are often helpful in these cases. Most homozygous PK deficient children, younger than 2 years of age, have higher residual PK activities than those found in adult PK deficient homozygotes with comparable levels of reticulocytosis. Reductions of red cell pyruvate kinase activity to <20% of normal indicates hereditary PK deficiency. Application of molecular biologic techniques (polymerase chain reaction and restriction endonuclease analysis) may allow prenatal diagnosis (using amniotic fluid cells and/or cord blood).[2] Slight to moderate decrease of red cell PK activity can be seen in some patients with leukemia and in bone marrow aplasia. Further characterization may be necessary to diagnose hemolytic disease due to PK deficient variants, including doubly heterozygous individuals.

Footnotes

1. Miwa S and Fujii H, "Pyruvate Kinase Deficiency," *Clin Biochem*, 1990, 23(2):155-7.
2. Baronciani L and Beutler E, "Prenatal Diagnosis of Pyruvate Kinase Deficiency," *Blood*, 1994, 84(7):2354-6.

References

Baronciani L and Beutler E, "Molecular Study of Pyruvate Kinase Deficient Patients With Hereditary Nonspherocytic Hemolytic Anemia," *J Clin Invest*, 1995, 95(4):1702-9.
Baronciani L, Magalhães IQ, Mahoney DH Jr, "Study of the Molecular Defects in Pyruvate Kinase Deficient Patients Affected by Nonspherocytic Hemolytic Anemia," *Blood Cells Mol Dis*, 1995, 21(1):49-55.
Miwa S, Kanno H, and Fujii H, "Concise Review: Pyruvate Kinase Deficiency: Historical Perspective and Recent Progress of Molecular Genetics," *Am J Hematol*, 1993, 42(1):31-5.
Mosca A, Tagarelli A, Paleari R, et al, "Rapid Determination of Erythrocyte Pyruvate Kinase Activity," *Clin Chem*, 1993, 39(3):512-6.
Zachee P, Staal GE, Rijksen G, et al, "Pyruvate Kinase Deficiency and Delayed Clinical Response to Recombinant Human Erythropoietin Treatment," *Lancet*, 1989, 1(8650):1327-8.

Radioactive Vitamin B₁₂ Absorption Test With or Without Intrinsic Factor see Schilling Test on page 346

RBC see Red Cell Count on page 344

RBC Enzyme Screen see Red Blood Cell Enzyme Deficiency Screen on next page

RBC Enzymes, Quantitative see Red Blood Cell Enzyme Deficiency, Quantitative on this page

RBC Folate see Folic Acid, RBC on page 317

RBC Fragility see Osmotic Fragility on page 334

RBC Fragility see Osmotic Fragility, Incubated on page 335

RBC Indices see Red Blood Cell Indices on next page

RBC Morphology see Peripheral Blood: Red Blood Cell Morphology on page 339

RBC Smear see Peripheral Blood: Red Blood Cell Morphology on page 339

RDW (Red Cell Distribution Width) see Red Blood Cell Indices on next page

Red Blood Cell Count see Red Cell Count on page 344

Red Blood Cell Enzyme Deficiency, Quantitative

CPT 82955 (G-6-PD)

Related Information

Autohemolysis Test *on page 304*
Glucose-6-Phosphate Dehydrogenase, Quantitative, Blood *on page 319*
Glucose-6-Phosphate Dehydrogenase Screen, Blood *on page 319*
Heinz Body Stain *on page 321*
Pyruvate Kinase Assay, Erythrocytes *on this page*
Red Blood Cell Enzyme Deficiency Screen *on next page*

Synonyms Erythrocyte Enzyme Deficiency, Quantitative; RBC Enzymes, Quantitative

Applies to Glutathione Reductase Deficiency, RBC; Heinz Bodies

Test Commonly Includes Glucose-6-phosphate dehydrogenase, pyruvate kinase, and any of over 20 RBC enzymes included in the following reference by E. Beutler

Specimen Erythrocytes

Container Lavender top (EDTA) tube

Causes for Rejection Clotted or hemolyzed specimen

Reference Range G-6-PD: 8.6-18.6 IU/g hemoglobin; phosphohexoisomerase: 14.7-42.2 IU/g hemoglobin; pyruvate kinase: 2.0-8.8 IU/g hemoglobin

Use Investigation of hemolytic anemia

Limitations False normal results may occur if testing is performed on a sample obtained just after a hemolytic episode (deficiency may be obscured by the presence of a young, enzyme-rich population of RBCs, the older enzyme-deficient red cells having been destroyed).

Additional Information Individuals with low levels of RBC G-6-PD are susceptible to hemolytic episodes after exposure to certain chemicals, drugs, and fava beans. Drugs that may precipitate hemolysis in patients with G-6-PD deficiency include: analgesics/antipyretics: aspirin; sulfa drugs: sulfapyridine, sulfisoxazole; antimalarias: primaquine, pentaquine, quinine; nitrofurantoin; Chloromycetin®, quinidine, para-aminosalicylic acid; others. Deficient or absent RBC enzyme activity may relate to absence of or decreased level of the enzyme, presence of an inactive molecular form or of an isoenzyme with altered activity.[1] In some hematologic diseases (eg, PNH, aplastic anemia and acute leukemia), acquired red cell enzyme deficiency is not infrequently seen.[2] RBC glutathione reductase deficiency bears an association with a variety of chemotherapeutically treated malignant states (up to 43% in a study of hospitalized patients).[3] Glutathione reductase deficiency also occurred in some cases of malnutrition, liver disease, and sepsis.

Footnotes

1. Paglia DE, Valentine WN, Williams KD, et al, "An Isozyme of Erythrocyte Pyruvate Kinase (Pk-Los Angeles) With Impaired Kinetics Corrected by Fructose-1, 6-Diphosphate," *Am J Clin Pathol*, 1977, 68:229-34.
2. Miwa S, "Significance of the Determination of Red Cell Enzyme Activities," *Am J Hematol*, 1979, 6:163-72.
3. Frischer H, "Erythrocytic Glutathione Reductase Deficiency in a Hospital Population in the United States," *Am J Hematol*, 1977, 2:327-34.

References

Arya R, Layton DM, and Bellingham AJ, "Hereditary Red Cell Enzymopathies," *Blood Rev*, 1995, 9(3):167-75.

Beutler E, "Glucose-6-Phosphate Deficiency and Other Enzyme Abnormalities," *Williams Hematology*, 5th ed, Chapter 54, Beutler E, Lichtman MA, Coller BS, et al, eds, New York, NY: McGraw-Hill Inc, 1995, 564-81.

Beutler E, *Red Cell Metabolism: A Manual of Biochemical Methods*, 3rd ed, New York, NY: Grune and Stratton Inc, 1984.

Beutler E, "Study of Glucose-6-Phosphate Dehydrogenase: History and Molecular Biology," *Am J Hematol*, 1993, 42(1):53-8.

Brown KA, "Erythrocyte Metabolism and Enzyme Defects," *Lab Med*, 1996, 27(5):329-30.

Feng CS, Tsang SS, and Mak YT, "Prevalence of Pyruvate Kinase Deficiency Among the Chinese: Determination by the Quantitative Assay," *Am J Hematol*, 1993, 43(4):271-3.

Miwa S, Kanno H, and Fujii H, "Concise Review: Pyruvate Kinase Deficiency: Historical Perspective and Recent Progress of Molecular Genetics," *Am J Hematol*, 1993, 42(1):31-5.

Miwa S and Fujii H, "Molecular Basis of Erythroenzymopathies Associated With Hereditary Hemolytic Anemia: Tabulation of Mutant Enzymes," *Am J Hematol*, 1996, 51(2):122-32.

Red Blood Cell Enzyme Deficiency Screen

CPT 82960 (G-6-PD)

Related Information

Glucose-6-Phosphate Dehydrogenase, Quantitative, Blood *on page 319*

Glucose-6-Phosphate Dehydrogenase Screen, Blood *on page 319*

Heinz Body Stain *on page 321*

Pyruvate Kinase Assay, Erythrocytes *on previous page*

Red Blood Cell Enzyme Deficiency, Quantitative *on previous page*

Reticulocyte Count *on page 345*

Synonyms Erythrocyte Enzyme Deficiency Screen; RBC Enzyme Screen

Applies to Heinz Bodies

Test Commonly Includes G-6-PD qualitative, pyruvate kinase, triosephosphate isomerase, NADH diaphorase (NADH methemoglobin reductase), glutathione reductase. Completeness varies between laboratories.

Specimen Erythrocytes

Container Lavender top (EDTA) tube

Causes for Rejection Clotted or hemolyzed specimen

Reference Range Enzyme present, reported as normal

Use Detect etiology of hemolytic state

Limitations Does not detect heterozygotes. False normal results may occur if testing is performed on a sample obtained just after a hemolytic episode.

Additional Information Phenotyping of RBC enzymes has been applied to paternity testing.[1]

Footnotes

1. Lee CL and Ying RL, "Phenotyping of Eight Erythrocytic Enzymes in One Acrylamide Gel," *Am J Clin Pathol*, 1979, 71:672-6.

References

Luzzatto L and Mehta A, "Glucose 6-Phosphate Dehydrogenase Deficiency," *The Metabolic and Molecular Bases of Inherited Disease*, 7th ed, Chapter 111, Scriver CR, Beaudet AL, Sly WS, et al, eds, New York, NY: McGraw-Hill Inc, 1995, 3367-98.

Luzzatto L and Roper D, "Investigation of the Hereditary Haemolytic Anaemias: Membrane and Enzyme Abnormalities," *Practical Haematology*, 8th ed, Chapter 13, New York, NY: Churchill Livingstone, 1995, 215-47.

Meloon JR, "Introduction to Hemolytic Anemias: Intracorpuscular Defects, II. Hereditary Enzyme Deficiencies," *Clinical Hematology and Fundamentals of Hemostasis*, 2nd ed, Chapter 10, Harmening DM, ed, Philadelphia, PA: FA Davis Co, 1992, 134-41.

Tanaka KR and Paglia DE, "Pyruvate Kinase and Other Enzymopathies of the Erythrocyte," *The Metabolic and Molecular Bases of Inherited Disease*, 7th ed, Chapter 114, Scriver CR, Beaudet AL, Sly WS, et al, eds, New York, NY: McGraw-Hill Inc, 1995, 3485-3511.

Red Blood Cell Indices

CPT 85029 (1-3 indices); 85030 (4 or more indices)

Related Information

Aluminum, Serum *on page 586*

Blood Volume *on page 306*

Complete Blood Count *on page 312*

Hematocrit *on page 322*

Hemoglobin *on page 323*

Hemoglobin A_2 *on page 323*

Ketone Bodies, Blood *on page 152*

Osmotic Fragility *on page 334*

Peripheral Blood: Red Blood Cell Morphology *on page 339*

Red Cell Count *on next page*

Schilling Test *on page 346*

Vitamin B_{12} *on page 351*

Synonyms Erythrocyte Indices; Indices

Applies to MCHC (Mean Corpuscular Hemoglobin Concentration) MCH (Mean Corpuscular Hemoglobin); MCV (Mean Corpuscular Volume); RBC Indices; RDW (Red Cell Distribution Width)

Test Commonly Includes MCV, MCH, MCHC, RBC, RDW, Hct, Hgb

Abstract The RBC indices are measured or mathematically derived from Hgb, Hct, and red blood cell count. The values can be used for quick assessment of anemia.

Specimen Whole blood

Container Lavender top (EDTA) tube for venipuncture specimen; lavender top Microtainer™ tube for capillary specimen

Collection Routine venipuncture. Invert the tube 5 to 10 times gently to mix. There must be no clots.

Storage Instructions Specimen cannot be used if stored over 10 hours at room temperature or 18 hours at 4°C refrigerated temperature. Specimen must not be frozen.

Causes for Rejection Hemolyzed or clotted specimen

Reference Range Normal values: RBC indices, healthy white and black subjects data from Coulter S, Sysmex, or H-1 Counters as of Miale.[1] See table. Values represent the mean and 95% range.

Blood Indices

	MCV (fL)	MCH (pg)	MCHC (%)	RDW
Adult male	90 (80-100)	30 (25.4-34.6)	34 (31-37)	13.0 (11.5-14.5)
Adult female	88 (79-98)	30 (25.4-34.6)	33 (30-36)	13.0 (11.5-14.5)

Use Evaluate red cell parameters; differential diagnosis of anemia, iron deficiency, hereditary spherocytosis (about 50% of such individuals have MCHC >36%), immune spherocytosis, thalassemia, chronic lead poisoning, folate deficiency, vitamin B_{12} deficiency, vitamin B_6 deficiency, pernicious anemia, and anemia of pregnancy

Limitations Patients showing both macrocytosis and microcytosis of the red cells may have indices within the reference range because of the averaging method used in determining indices. Patients with autoagglutination will show spurious results. Although MCV is commonly elevated early in pernicious anemia, it may be normal, especially later when micropoikilocytosis develops.

Methodology The great majority of RBC indices are obtained by the use of microcomputerized, highly automated electronic and pneumatic multichannel analyzers based on aperture-impedance cell sizing and counting (see reference by Koepke).
(Continued)

Red Blood Cell Indices *(Continued)*

Additional Information The group of three red cell indices are a productive and economically efficient approach to screening for hematologic abnormality, in particular the compensated and uncompensated anemias. The MCV (mean corpuscular volume) is the size (volume) of the average red cell. The MCH (mean corpuscular hemoglobin) is the weight of hemoglobin in the average red cell. The MCHC (mean corpuscular hemoglobin concentration) is the amount of hemoglobin present in the average red cell as compared to its size. The RBC indices are a valuable guide to the choice of more specific measurements such as serum iron, ferritin, folic acid, and/or vitamin B_{12} levels. The MCV decreases before MCHC in evolving iron deficiency anemia[1] while the MCHC decreases before the MCV in evolving anemia of chronic disease.[2] In hemolytic anemias, particularly the hemoglobinopathies, the RBC indices are less helpful. Decreased MCV levels may be due to thalassemia minor although they are not specific for this condition; A_2 hemoglobin levels should be studied to follow-up low MCV levels in appropriate clinical settings. Screening for high A_2 hemoglobin levels will discriminate a population of beta-thalassemics with normal MCV levels. Hemoglobin A_2 levels are most useful using the column chromatography method. Technicon® (Miles Laboratory) series H analyzers provide a measure of heterogeneity in hemoglobin concentration of individual red cells (histogram of MCHCs). Decreased cell Hb concentration (increased cell hydration) have been noted to characterize α-thalassemia while both decreased and increased cell Hb concentration (cell hydration and dehydration) characterize β-thalassemia red cells.[3] Cell dehydration as reflected by histogram of MCHCs can also be used to identify most patients with hereditary spherocytosis.[4]

Changes in RBC Indices With Disease

Condition	MCV	MCH	MCHC	RDW
Iron deficiency anemia	↓	↓	↓	↑
Chronic inflammation	↓	N±	N±	N±
Pernicious anemia	↑	N or high N	high N	↑
B_{12}/folate deficiency	↑	N or high N	high N	↑
Hereditary spherocytosis	N or ↓	↑	↑	N±
Hemolytic/aplastic anemia	N±	N±	N±	N±
Anemia 2° acute blood loss	N±	N±	N±	N±
Polycythemia	N±	N±	N±	N±

A number of conditions (usually characterized by the generation of numerous RBC fragments) may show "relative microcytosis" as reflected by slightly decreased to low normal MCV. This has been described with sickle cell anemia. In children, low MCV for age suggests iron deficiency, lead poisoning, thalassemia syndrome, or very rarely, a pyridoxine-responsive anemia. Examination of the peripheral smear, family history, dietary history, and stool guaiac are helpful in this setting. MCV may be significantly increased in diabetic ketoacidosis[5] (this is due to plasma hyperosmolarity). The high molar concentration of glucose is the main contributing factor to the increased plasma osmolarity, producing a hypertonic intracellular state of RBCs. When such cells are put into a relatively hypotonic diluent (eg, Coulter cell counting), water enters the cell, it swells and may produce erroneously high MCV. Recognition of increase in MCV may alert the clinician to presence of the hyperosmolar state.[5]

Aluminum toxicity, occurring in uremic patients on chronic hemodialysis, is associated in some cases with decreased MCV, microcytic anemia.[6,7]

RDW is an electronic measurement of anisocytosis (red cell size variability). RDW is typically elevated in iron deficiency anemia while usually normal in beta thalassemia minor (heterozygous thalassemia). RDW is elevated in beta thalassemia major.

A recent study suggests that zidovudine (AZT) treatment of AIDS has become the most common cause of macrocytosis (increase in MCV) in the hospitalized urban patient population.[8]

Footnotes

1. Miale JB, *Laboratory Medicine: Hematology*, 6th ed, St Louis, MO: Mosby-Year Book Inc, 1982, 378.
2. England JM, Ward SM, and Down MC, "Microcytosis, Anisocytosis and the Red Cell Indices in Iron Deficiency," *Br J Haematol*, 1976, 34:589-97.
3. Bunyaratvej A, Fucharoen S, Greenbaum A, et al, "Hydration of Red Cells in Alpha and Beta Thalassemias Differs. A Useful Approach to Distinguish Between These Red Cell Phenotypes," *Am J Clin Pathol*, 1994, 102(2):217-22.
4. Lux SE and Palek J, "Disorders of the Red Cell Membrane," *Blood: Principles and Practice of Hematology*, Chapter 54, Handin RI, Lux SE, and Stossel TP, eds, Philadelphia, PA: JB Lippincott Co, 1995, 1758.

5. Evan-Wong LA and Davidson RJ, "Raised Coulter Mean Corpuscular Volume in Diabetic Ketoacidosis and Its Underlying Association With Marked Plasma Hyperosmolarity," *J Clin Pathol*, 1983, 36:334-6.
6. Touam M, Martinez F, Lacour B, et al, "Aluminum-Induced, Reversible Microcytic Anemia in Chronic Renal Failure: Clinical and Experimental Studies," *Clin Nephrol*, 1983, 19:295-8.
7. Mladenovic J, "Aluminum Inhibits Erythropoiesis *In Vitro*," *J Clin Invest*, 1988, 81(6):1661-5.
8. Snower DP and Weil SC, "Changing Etiology of Macrocytosis: Zidovudine as a Frequent Causative Factor," *Am J Clin Pathol*, 1993, 99(1):57-60.

References

Brown RG, "Normocytic and Macrocytic Anemias," *Postgrad Med*, 1991, 89(8):125-32, 135-6.

Fraser CG, Wilkinson SP, Neville RG, et al, "Biologic Variation of Common Hematologic Laboratory Quantities in the Elderly," *Am J Clin Pathol*, 1989, 92(4):465-70.

Kjeldsberg CR, "Principles of Hematologic Examination," *Wintrobe's Clinical Hematology*, 9th ed, Chapter 2, Lee GR, Bithell TC, Foerster J, et al, eds, Philadelphia, PA: Lea & Febiger, 1993, 7-37.

Koepke JA, "Quantitative Blood Cell Counting," *Practical Laboratory Hematology*, Chapter 3, Koepke JA, ed, New York, NY: Churchill Livingstone, 1991, 43-60.

Savage RA, "The Red Cell Indices: Yesterday, Today, and Tomorrow," *Clin Lab Med*, 1993, 13(4):773-85.

van Duijnhoven HL and Treskes M, "Marked Interference of Hyperglycemia in Measurements of Mean (Red) Cell Volume by Technicon H Analyzers," *Clin Chem*, 1996, 42(1):76-80.

van Assendelft OW, "Interpretation of the Quantitative Blood Cell Count," *Practical Laboratory Hematology*, Chapter 4, Koepke J, ed, New York, NY: Churchill Livingstone, 1991, 61-98.

Red Blood Cell Morphology *see* Peripheral Blood: Red Blood Cell Morphology *on page 339*

Red Cell Count

CPT 85041

Related Information

Complete Blood Count *on page 312*
Erythropoietin, Serum *on page 124*
Ferritin, Serum *on page 127*
Hematocrit *on page 322*
Hemoglobin *on page 323*
Peripheral Blood: Red Blood Cell Morphology *on page 339*
Red Blood Cell Indices *on previous page*
Vitamin B_{12} *on page 351*

Synonyms Erythrocyte Count; RBC; Red Blood Cell Count

Specimen Whole blood

Container Lavender top (EDTA) tube for venipuncture specimen; properly filled lavender top Microtainer™ tubes for capillary specimen

Causes for Rejection Hemolyzed or clotted specimen

Reference Range Male: $4.6-6.0 \times 10^6/mm^3$; female: $3.9-5.5 \times 10^6/mm^3$. See Complete Blood Count *on page 312* for age related normals.

Use Evaluate anemia, polycythemia

Limitations Presence of cold agglutinins may result in falsely low RBC counts. Modern electronic cell counters have a level of precision and accuracy greatly improved over manual counting techniques. With correct threshold setting, properly controlled and functioning instrumentation, reliability, and reproducibility of the RBC count is equivalent to or better than most laboratory tests. Surveys (College of American Pathologists) indicate a coefficient of variation (CV) of 1% to 2%. Some instruments commonly perform with CVs <1%. Between laboratory precision has been reported as 2.8%.[1]

Methodology Manual hemocytometer chamber count of diluted blood sample or electronic counting and sizing of red cells made to flow through a fine aperture or capillary, microcomputer control and analysis of data developed from changes in impedance or flow past a laser beam

Additional Information Decrease in RBC count may be the result of red cell loss by bleeding or hemolysis (intravascular or extravascular), failure of marrow production (due to a broad variety of causes), or may be secondary to dilutional factors (eg, intravenous fluids). Increase in RBC count may be the result of primary polycythemia (polycythemia vera) or secondary polycythemia (hypoxemia of lung or cardiovascular disease, increased erythropoietin production associated with renal cyst, renal cell carcinoma, cerebellar hemangioblastoma, or high O_2 affinity hemoglobinopathy) including stress polycythemia (hemoconcentration associated with exercise, exertion, fright, etc). RBC count is normally higher in individuals residing at high altitudes.

Footnotes

1. Elevitch FR and Noce PS, eds, *Data ReCap: 1970-1980. A Compilation of Data From College of American Pathologists Clinical Laboratory Improvement Programs*, Skokie, IL: College of American Pathologists, 1981, 216-7.

References

Henry JB, Nelson DA, Tomar RH, et al, *Todd-Sanford-Davidsohn Clinical Diagnosis and Management by Laboratory Methods*, 18th ed, Henry JB, ed, Philadelphia, PA: WB Saunders Co, 1991, 562-3.

Koepke JA, "Quantitative Blood Cell Counting," *Practical Laboratory Hematology*, Chapter 3, New York, NY: Churchill Livingstone, 1991, 43-60.

Red Cell Folate *see* Folic Acid, RBC *on page 317*

Red Cell Fragility *see* Osmotic Fragility *on page 334*

Red Cell Fragility *see* Osmotic Fragility, Incubated *on page 335*

Red Cell Mass

CPT 78120 (single sample); 78121 (multiple samples)

Related Information

Blood Volume *on page 306*

Erythropoietin, Serum *on page 124*

Hematocrit *on page 322*

Hemoglobin *on page 323*

Synonyms ^{51}Cr-Labeled Red Cell Volume; Red Cell Volume

Test Commonly Includes Red cell mass, plasma volume, and total blood volume

Specimen Laboratory will usually manage sampling and reinjecting.

Special Instructions May require scheduling with laboratory in order to procure radioisotope. Patient's weight and height must be made available to the laboratory.

Reference Range Male: 28.2±4 mL/kg; female: 24.2±2.6 mL/kg.[1] See table for reference values relating to body surface area.

Formulas for Calculating RBC Volume Reference Values From Body Surface Area (S)

Male	$RCV = (1100)(S)$
	$RCV = (1486)(S^2) - (4106)(S) + 4514$
	$RCV = (1550)(S) - 890$
Female	$RCV = (840)(S)$
	$RCV = (1167)(S) - 479$

From International Committee for Standardization in Hematology, "Recommended Methods for Measurement of Red Cell and Plasma Volume," *J Nucl Med*, 1980, 21:793-800, with permission.

Use Determine red cell mass; support the diagnosis of polycythemia vera; monitor therapy with antineoplastic drugs

Limitations Radiation from isotopes used in bone scans, liver scans, brain scans, and other isotope procedures may interfere with red cell mass determination. Application of "normal range" tables based on weight and height must be made cautiously. An individual patient may not be comparable to the normal (eg, severely edematous individuals). Dilutional relationship will be unrepresentative and RBC mass overestimated. Severe edema might also be associated with isotope loss but is especially problematic due to unrepresentative normal range comparisons. Test is expensive and time consuming.

Contraindications Severe active bleeding

Clinical Effect of Variable Relationship Between Red Cell Volume and Plasma Volume

Red Cell Volume	Plasma Volume	Cause	Effect
Normal	High	Pregnancy Cirrhosis Nephritis Congestive cardiac failure	Pseudoanemia
Normal	Low	Stress Peripheral circulatory failure Dehydration Edema Prolonged bedrest	Pseudopolycythemia
Low	Normal	Anemia	Accurate reflection of degree of anemia
Low	High	Anemia	Anemia less severe than indicated by blood count
Low	Low	Hemorrhage Severe anemia (when hematocrit <0.2)	Anemia more severe than indicated by blood count
High	Normal to low	Polycythemia	Accurate reflection of polycythemia or polycythemia less severe than apparent
High	High	Polycythemia (when hematocrit >0.5)	Polycythemia more severe than apparent
Normal or even high	High	Marked splenomegaly	Pseudoanemia

From Dacie JV and Lewis SM, *Practical Haematology*, 7th ed, New York, NY: Churchill Livingstone, 1991, 362, with permission.

Methodology Patient blood sample is drawn, red cells are labeled with ^{51}Cr and then reinjected into patient. Separate blood samples are obtained prior to injection and at a timed interval after injection. RBC mass is calculated on the basis of dilution principle. While other isotope labels are used, ^{51}Cr is the most convenient and widely used. Technetium-99m can be used for red cell mass determination after treatment of patient's red blood cells with stannous ion ($SnCl_2$) before incubation with pertechnetate. This results in the binding of nearly all of the added technetium to patient's red cells.

Additional Information The assessment of anemia and polycythemia (assessment of whether or not one of these conditions truly exists) depends foremost upon a reliable and direct determination of red cell volume. RBC count, Hgb level, and Hct provide only concentration parameters, the measured number or amount relative to the solution in which it exists. In a number of clinical situations (eg, acute blood loss) the RBC count, Hgb, and Hct will not indicate the actual decrease or increase in circulating red cell mass. Components (RBC count, etc) do correlate with RBC volume. Due to technical complexity (resulting in high cost and prolonged turnaround time) CBC is usually used, especially for follow-up or monitoring situations, even though RBC mass study would provide a more meaningful result. Nevertheless, some clinical situations (eg, polycythemia, complicated fluid and electrolyte management problems) will benefit from at least initial red cell volume determination.

Causes of decreased red cell volume include anemia, nutritional (iron, B_{12}, folate deficit, etc), hemolytic (intravascular or extravascular hemolysis), production deficit (marrow failure, drug or chemical related), acute and/or chronic blood loss; acute blood loss (decreased RBC volume may be present with normal or increased Hgb/Hct/RBC count); chronic disease (inflammation/infection); radiation, starvation, or severe edema.

Causes of increased red cell volume include: a) polycythemia vera ("primary" polycythemia); b) secondary polycythemia, hypoxia may be due to **lung disease** (eg, emphysema, Pickwickian syndrome), **CV disease** with right to left shunt or due to high altitude, **hemoglobin variants** (eg, high O_2 affinity hemoglobinopathies such as Hb M$_{Saskatoon}$ and Hb M$_{Hyde\ Park}$), methemoglobinemia, carboxyhemoglobinemia (increased CO due to smoking), **erythropoietin producing tumors/cysts**, rarely (eg, renal cyst, renal cell adenocarcinoma, hepatoma, large uterine myomas, cerebellar hemangioblastoma), or **hereditary overproduction of erythropoietin**;[2] and c) stress (relative, spurious, pseudo, benign) polycythemia due to decreased plasma volume, as in cases of severe dehydration, burns, and fluid and electrolyte abnormalities with Addison's or Cushing's diseases. Also relative polycythemia is seen in a population of "stressed" hypertensive middle aged males. The table shows relationship between increased and decreased red cell and plasma volum es.

Footnotes

1. Henry JB, *Todd-Sanford-Davidsohn Clinical Diagnosis and Management by Laboratory Methods*, 18th ed, Philadelphia, PA: WB Saunders Co, 1991, 1015-6.
2. Yonemitsu H, Yamaguchi K, Shigeta H, et al, "Two Cases of Familial Erythrocytosis With Increased Erythropoietin Activity in Plasma and Urine," *Blood*, 1973, 42:793-7.

References

Dacie JV and Lewis SM, *Practical Haematology*, 8th ed, New York, NY: Churchill Livingstone, 1995, 391-7.

"Recommended Methods for Measurement of Red Cell and Plasma Volume: International Committee for Standardization in Hematology," *J Nucl Med*, 1980, 21:793-800.

Red Cell Survival *see* [51]Cr Red Cell Survival *on page 314*

Red Cell Volume *see* Red Cell Mass *on this page*

Red Cell Volume *see* Blood Volume *on page 306*

Retic Count *see* Reticulocyte Count *on this page*

Reticulocyte Count

CPT 85044 (manual); 85045 (flow cytometry)

Related Information

[51]Cr Red Cell Survival *on page 314*

Heinz Body Stain *on page 321*

Hematocrit *on page 322*

Hemoglobin *on page 323*

Hemoglobin Electrophoresis *on page 324*

Osmotic Fragility *on page 334*

Red Blood Cell Enzyme Deficiency Screen *on page 343*

Sickle Cell Tests *on page 347*

Synonyms Retic Count

Specimen Whole blood

Container Lavender top (EDTA) tube or green top (heparin) tube for venipuncture specimen; heparinized capillary tube for capillary specimen

Storage Instructions Store EDTA anticoagulated blood at room temperature for up to 48 hours or up to 72 hours at 4°C.

Causes for Rejection Clotted or hemolyzed specimen

Reference Range Adults: 0.5% to 1.5%; newborns: ≤7%, expressed as a percentage of 1000 RBCs. Normal values at birth: 2.5% to 6.5%, falling
(Continued)

Reticulocyte Count *(Continued)*

to normal adult level by the end of the second week. The elderly (older than 70 years of age) have a slightly higher percent of reticulocytes than young individuals but still fall within the normal range.[1]

Use Evaluate erythropoietic activity. Increased in acute and chronic hemorrhage, hemolytic anemias. Evaluate erythropoietic response to therapy of various anemias. **The test is underutilized, especially when one considers it is at a pivotal decision-making juncture.** The reticulocyte production index will decide if one is working with a hyperproliferative or nonproliferative anemia, and thus, which tests should be subsequently ordered.

Limitations In recently transfused patients, reticulocytes may decrease on a dilutional basis due to transfusion. Automated flow cytometry methods using thiazole orange may give spuriously high counts in patients with chronic lymphocytic leukemia, Howell-Jolly bodies, intracellular parasites, large platelets, some drug therapies, erythropoietic protoporphyria, and in patients who have cold agglutinins (see NCCLS Document H44-P).

Contraindications Patients receiving a large number of blood transfusions

Methodology Vital stains, new methylene blue is commonly used; brilliant cresyl blue may be used. Flow cytometric and other methods using thioflavin T, thiazole orange auramine O, or Oxazine 750 have been developed that have the advantage of reproducibility.[2] Newer instruments allow derivation of the reticulocyte maturation index. The assay is a standard part of the repetoire of some multiparameter hematology instruments. Flow cytometry reticulocyte analysis using thiazole orange allows rapid analysis of 20,000-50,000 red cells per sample with resultant markedly improved reproducibility/precision as compared to manual methods.

Additional Information Demonstration of an increase in the number of circulating reticulocytes provides reliable and inexpensive evidence of increased red cell production. Care should be exercised during interpretation of results that an apparent increase in reticulocytes is not the result of decrease in the number of nonreticulated RBCs (ie, anemia with fewer mature red cells). A variety of corrections have been proposed and are in use. Absolute reticulocyte count = reticulocytes (%) x RBC count. This gives the number of reticulocytes per mm³ of blood. Reticulocyte index (RI) = reticulocytes (%) x patient Hct/normal Hct or patient RBC/normal RBC or patient Hgb/normal Hgb. This corrects the reticulocyte count for anemia. Reticulocyte production index (RPI) = RI x (1/maturation time), or RPI = patient's absolute reticulocyte count/normal absolute reticulocyte count x (1/maturation time). Maturation time is usually taken as 2. RPI corrects for the premature release of reticulocytes from the marrow as might occur in cases of brisk hemolysis or significant bleeding. RPI gives a reticulocyte percent value that reliably estimates RBC production. Current generation automated methods derive a reticulocyte maturity index (RMI) from semiquantitative study of reticulocyte RNA levels. Absolute reticulocyte count with RMI can be applied to classification and evaluation of anemia. Failure of marrow production results in anemia with absence of the expected increase in RPI. Reticulocyte count should be performed prior to transfusion. Image recognition and flow cytometry methods of reticulocyte determination provide greater precision and comparable accuracy compared to the manual method of reticulocyte counting.[3,4] An evaluation/comparison of three commercially available flow cytometers utilizing thiazole orange for reticulocyte enumeration found comparable performance with acceptable linearity, carryover (zero or near zero) and precision.[5] A multi-institutional study comparing different stains and instruments has also been reported.[6] In a comparison study the Miles (Technicon®) H3 analyzer reticulocyte count results were found acceptable with good precision and linearity.[7] The H3 also determines reticulocyte cellular indices. A rare case of myelodysplastic syndrome may have anemia with reticulocytosis, thus presenting some features of hemolytic disease.[8]

Footnotes

1. Kosower NS, "Altered Properties of Erythrocytes in the Aged," *Am J Hematol*, 1993, 42(3):241-7.

2. Metzger DK and Charache S, "Flow Cytometric Reticulocyte Counting With Thioflavin T in a Clinical Hematology Laboratory," *Arch Pathol Lab Med*, 1987, 111(6):540-4.

3. Pappas AA, Owens RB, and Flick JT, "Reticulocyte Counting by Flow Cytometry. A Comparison With Manual Methods," *Ann Clin Lab Sci*, 1992, 22(2):125-32.

4. Serke S and Huhn D, "Improved Specificity of Determination of Immature Erythrocytes (Reticulocytes) by Multiparameter Flow-Cytometry and Thiazole Orange Using Combined Staining With Monoclonal Antibody (anti-Glycophorin-A)," *Clin Lab Haematol*, 1993, 15(1):33-44.

5. Van Petegem M, Cartuyvels R, DeSchouwer P, et al, "Comparative Evaluation of Three Flow Cytometers for Reticulocyte Enumeration," *Clin Lab Haematol*, 1993, 15(2):103-11.

6. Davis BH, Bigelow NC, Koepke JA, et al, "Flow Cytometric Reticulocyte Analysis. Multi-Institutional Interlaboratory Correlation Study," *Am J Clin Pathol*, 1994, 102(4):468-77.

7. Brugnara C, Hipp MJ, Irving PJ, et al, "Automated Reticulocyte Counting and Measurement of Reticulocyte Cellular Indices. Evaluation of the Miles H*3 Blood Analyzer," *Am J Clin Pathol*, 1994, 102(5):623-32.

8. Sher GD, Pinkerton PH, Ali MA, et al, "Myelodysplastic Syndrome With Prolonged Reticulocyte Survival Mimicking Hemolytic Disease," *Am J Clin Pathol*, 1994, 101(2):149-53.

References

Brecher G, "New Methylene Blue as a Reticulocyte Stain," *Am J Pathol*, 1949, 19:895.

Brown BA, *Hematology: Principles and Procedures*, 6th ed, Philadelphia, PA: Lea & Febiger, 1993, 111-6, 279-80, 386-90.

Davis BH and Bigelow NC, "Automated Reticulocyte Analysis: Clinical Practice and Associated New Parameters," *Hematol Oncol Clin North Am*, 1994, 8(4):617-30.

Davis BH and Bigelow NC, "Flow Cytometric Reticulocyte Analysis and the Reticulocyte Maturity Index," *Ann N Y Acad Sci*, 1993, 677:281-92.

Houwen B, "Reticulocyte Maturation," *Blood Cells*, 1992, 18(2):167-86.

Koepke J, Broden P, Corash L, et al, "Reticulocyte Counting by Flow Cytometry; Proposed Guidelines," *NCCLS Document H44-P*, 1993, 13.

Lee GR, "The Hemolytic Disorders: General Considerations," *Wintrobe's Clinical Hematology*, 9th ed, Chapter 32, Lee GR, Bithell TC, Foerster J, et al, eds, Philadelphia, PA: Lea & Febiger, 1993, 944-64.

Schilling Test

CPT 78270 (without intrinsic factor); 78271 (with intrinsic factor)

Related Information

Bone Marrow *on page 307*
Folic Acid, RBC *on page 317*
Folic Acid, Serum *on page 317*
Gastrin, Serum *on page 135*
Intrinsic Factor Antibody *on page 411*
Iron and Total Iron Binding Capacity/Transferrin *on page 150*
Parietal Cell Antibody *on page 421*
Peripheral Blood: Red Blood Cell Morphology *on page 339*
Red Blood Cell Indices *on page 343*
Vitamin B_{12} *on page 351*
Vitamin B_{12} Unsaturated Binding Capacity *on page 352*

Synonyms Radioactive Vitamin B_{12} Absorption Test With or Without Intrinsic Factor; Vitamin B_{12} Absorption Test

Test Commonly Includes Measure of B_{12} absorption before and after administration of intrinsic factor (two stage procedure)

Abstract *In vivo* test for pernicious anemia, vitamin B_{12} malabsorption, and integrity of distal small intestine

Patient Preparation Patient must be fasting from midnight the day of the test. Patient should have received no B vitamins for a period of 3 days before the test.

Causes for Rejection Patient having radioisotope scan prior to test, patient receiving vitamin B_{12} prior to the test, patient not fasting, incomplete collection of urine, failure to administer the parenteral B_{12}, contamination of urine with stool (which will contain some unabsorbed B_{12})

Reference Range Normal values vary with the laboratory and procedure used. Generally, >10% excretion in the urine of radioactive B_{12} indicates intact intrinsic factor (IF) function. When only a few percent of B_{12} absorption occurs without IF, with improvement into normal range with exogenous IF, the presence of pernicious anemia is essentially established. Poor absorption (<6% or 7%) with, as well as without, IF suggests intestinal malabsorption.

Use Assess vitamin B_{12} absorption in the diagnosis of malabsorption due to the lack of intrinsic factor, [eg, Addisonian (pernicious) anemia], a diagnostic adjunct in other defects of small intestinal absorption; evaluate extent of Crohn's disease in terminal ileum. Part I of the Schilling test is ^{57}Co by itself. If abnormal, 5 days later it is repeated with intrinsic factor administered orally at the same time (Part II). If this part of the test is still abnormal, it suggests that the cause is not gastric in origin (PA) but lower in the GI tract. Dual tracer assays have been available to perform both assays at once but caution should be exercised, as described by Zuckler et al[1].

Limitations If other isotope tests are to be performed, Schilling test should be completed first. The presence of renal dysfunction, pancreatic insufficiency, bacterial overgrowth of intestinal content, antibodies against IF in gastric secretions, myxedema, liver disease, or any other condition resulting in the decreased absorption of B_{12} from the GI tract, its concentration in the liver, or its excretion in the urine may result in abnormal values. Incomplete urine collection may invalidate results.

Methodology Patient swallows radiolabeled B_{12} dose and receives a B_{12} intramuscular injection. The patient's urine is collected for 24 hours. The total activity from the B_{12} label is measured and calculated. The percent excretion of vitamin B_{12} is then determined.

Additional Information B_{12} tagged with ^{57}Co without (and on a repeat test, as indicated, with) intrinsic factor is given orally. A large parenteral dose of unlabeled B_{12} is given 1 hour later to load the cyanocobalamin serum binding sites. All orally absorbed (radioactively-tagged) B_{12} will be excreted in the urine. The 24-hour urine is analyzed, radioactive ^{57}Co is counted. This radiopharmaceutical should not be administered to patients who are pregnant or during lactation unless the information to be gained outweighs the potential hazards. The test should not be started within 2-3 days of a therapeutic dose (1000 μg) of B_{12} or previous Schilling test. Bone marrow examinations and B_{12} and folate levels must be obtained before the Schilling test is performed.

Fairbanks et al[2] have found that better separation of normal individuals from those with pernicious anemia occurs with oral B_{12} dose <1 μg (eg, 0.5 μg). They further confirmed earlier reports that some patients with pernicious anemia do not absorb B_{12} adequately, even when given with IF. Such malabsorption is reversible so that after B_{12} therapy, the vitamin then is normally absorbed with IF (reversible malabsorption). These findings complicate the diagnosis of pernicious anemia using the Schilling test. The importance of establishing the diagnosis and commencing life-long B_{12} maintenance therapy (so as to reverse the severe effects of the megaloblastic anemia and nervous system degenerative process - combined systems disease) dictates that a combination of clinical and laboratory findings be considered. The laboratory picture should include appropriate abnormalities of RBC indices (in particular high MCV), presence of anemia, peripheral blood smear findings of oval macrocytes, tear drop shaped RBCs, leukopenia, thrombocytopenia, hypersegmented PMNs, megaloblastic marrow picture, decreased serum B_{12} level, usually increased serum LD, all to be correlated with Schilling test result and the clinical presentation.

Footnotes
1. Zuckier LS and Chervu LR, "Schilling Evaluation of Pernicious Anemia: Current Status," *J Nucl Med*, 1984, 25(9):1032-9.
2. Fairbanks VF, Wahner HW, and Phyliky RL, "Tests for Pernicious Anemia: The Schilling Test," *Mayo Clin Proc*, 1983, 58:541-4.

References
Carethers M, "Diagnosing Vitamin B_{12} Deficiency, A Common Geriatric Disorder," *Geriatrics*, 1988, 43(3):89-94, 105-7, 111-2.

Lindenbaum J, "Status of Laboratory Testing in the Diagnosis of Megaloblastic Anemia," *Blood*, 1983, 61:624-7.

Pruthi RK and Tefferi A, "Pernicious Anemia Revisited," *Mayo Clin Proc*, 1994, 69(2):144-50.

Williams WJ, Beutler E, Erslev AJ, et al, *Hematology*, 4th ed, New York, NY: McGraw-Hill Inc, 1990, 462-4.

Schistocytes Smear *see* Peripheral Blood: Red Blood Cell Morphology *on page 339*

Sedimentation Rate *see* Sedimentation Rate, Erythrocyte *on this page*

Sedimentation Rate, Erythrocyte
CPT 85651 (nonautomated); 85652 (automated)

Related Information
C-Reactive Protein *on page 387*
Fibrinogen *on page 246*
Zeta Sedimentation Ratio *on page 354*

Synonyms Sedimentation Rate; Westergren Sed Rate

Abstract ESR is a generally nonspecific measure of inflammation and infection. It is used mainly to follow management of rheumatology patients.

Specimen Whole blood

Container Lavender top (EDTA) tube or citrated plasma in 4:1 dilution (9:1 dilution is **not** acceptable)

Collection Specimen must be received within 12 hours of collection.

Causes for Rejection Insufficient blood, clotted, hemolyzed specimen

Reference Range Male: younger than 50 year of age: 0-15 mm/hour, older than 50 years of age: 0-20 mm/hour; female: younger than 50 years of age: 0-25 mm/hour, older than 50 years of age: 0-30 mm/hour by Westergren method. See reference by Wolfe and Michaud for their extensive study of and application of the ESR in a number of different settings. Their study indicates that in a rheumatology clinic women younger than 60 years of age who have noninflammatory disorders have upper limit of normal for ESR of 38 mm/hour.

Use Evaluate the nonspecific activity of infections, inflammatory states, autoimmune disorders, and plasma cell dyscrasias; in particular to screen for, to assess severity of and follow clinical activity of rheumatic diseases, especially rheumatoid arthritis; important in clinical evaluation of temporal arteritis and polymyalgia rheumatica

Limitations Anemia and paraproteinemia invalidate results; some procedural methods may be associated with hazardous exposure of medical technologists to fresh whole blood.

Methodology Red cell sedimentation rate expressed in mm/hour, utilizing Westergren type sedimentation tubes. A validation procedure and method for the in laboratory production of a sedimentation rate reference material has been developed for and can be used for quality assurance programs.[1]

Additional Information Elevations in fibrinogen, alpha- and beta-globulins (acute phase reactants), and immunoglobulins increase the sedimentation rate of red cells through plasma. The test is important in the diagnosis and management of temporal arteritis and of polymyalgia

rheumatica.[2] Use of the ESR, ZSR, and/or CRP may aid in the differential diagnosis of the anemia of chronic disease from iron deficiency anemia.[3] ESR is elevated in about 50% of patients with newly diagnosed Hodgkin's disease, especially in advanced stage disease.

Footnotes
1. Thomas RD, Westengard JC, Hay KL, et al, "Calibration and Validation for Erythrocyte Sedimentation Tests: Role of the International Committee on Standardization in Hematology Reference Procedure," *Arch Pathol Lab Med*, 1993, 117(7):719-23.
2. Wong RL and Korn JH, "Temporal Arteritis Without an Elevated Erythrocyte Sedimentation Rate," *Am J Med*, 1986, 80(5):959-64.
3. Johnson MA, "Iron: Nutrition Monitoring and Nutrition Status Assessment," *J Nutr*, 1990, 120(Suppl 11):1486-91.

References
Gambino R, DiRe JJ, Monteleone M, et al, "The Westergren Sedimentation Rate, Using K_3 EDTA," *Am J Clin Pathol*, 1965, 43:173-80.

Lowe GD, "Should Plasma Viscosity Replace the ESR?" *Br J Haematol*, 1994, 86(1):6-11.

Salvarani C, Gabriel SE, O'Fallon WM, et al, "Epidemiology of Polymyalgia Rheumatica in Olmsted County, Minnesota, 1970-1991," *Arthritis Rheum*, 1995, 38(3):369-73.

Singer JI, Buchino JJ, and Chabali R, "Selected Laboratory in Pediatric Emergency Care," *Emerg Med Clin North Am*, 1986, 4(2):377-96.

Stuart J and Nash GB, "Technological Advances in Blood Rheology," *Crit Rev Clin Lab Sci*, 1990, 28(1):61-93.

Wolfe F and Michaud K, "The Clinical and Research Significance of the Erythrocyte Sedimentation Rate," *J Rheumatol*, 1994, 21(7):1227-37.

Zlonis M, "The Mystique of the Erythrocyte Sedimentation Rate: A Reappraisal of One of the Oldest Laboratory Tests Still in Use," *Clin Lab Med*, 1993, 13(4):787-800.

Sed Rate *see* Zeta Sedimentation Ratio *on page 354*

Septicemia Detection, Buffy Coat Micromethod *see* Bacteremia Detection, Buffy Coat Micromethod *on page 305*

Serum Folate *see* Folic Acid, Serum *on page 317*

Serum Lysis *see* Ham Test *on page 320*

Serum Viscosity *see* Viscosity, Serum/Plasma *on page 350*

Sickle Cell Preparation, Metabisulfite Test *see* Sickle Cell Tests *on this page*

Sickle Cell Solubility Test *see* Sickle Cell Tests *on this page*

Sickle Cells Smear *see* Peripheral Blood: Red Blood Cell Morphology *on page 339*

Sickle Cell Tests
CPT 83020 (electrophoresis); 85660 (reduction slide method)

Related Information
Cytapheresis, Therapeutic *on page 606*
Fetal Hemoglobin *on page 316*
Hemoglobin *on page 323*
Hemoglobin Electrophoresis *on page 324*
Reticulocyte Count *on page 345*

Synonyms Dithionite Test; Itano Solubility Test; Murayama Test; Sickle Cell Preparation, Metabisulfite Test; Sickle Cell Solubility Test; Sickledex™

Test Commonly Includes A variety of similar but usually slightly modified tests have been developed, described, and achieved varying degrees of acceptance. In some institutions a positive is confirmed by performing an alternate confirmatory sickle cell test and/or hemoglobin electrophoresis (the preferred procedure).

Abstract Screening tests for sickle cell anemia and related entities which include hemoglobin S.

Specimen Whole blood

Container Lavender top (EDTA) tube for venipuncture specimen; lavender top Microtainer™ for capillary specimen

Collection Routine venipuncture. Invert tube gently to mix.

Causes for Rejection Clotted specimen, hemolyzed specimen

Reference Range Negative

Use Detect sickling hemoglobins; evaluate hemolytic anemia, undiagnosed hereditary anemia with morphologic (sickle-like) abnormalities on peripheral blood smear

Limitations False-positive solubility test for sickling may be due to polycythemic blood; excess blood in relationship to the quantity of reagent; interference by some forms of hyperglobulinemia (if suspect, test should be repeated using patient's washed red cells); and a variety of abnormal hemoglobins including I, Bart's, $C_{Georgetown}$, Alexandra, C_{Harlem}, Porto Alegre, Memphis/S, $C_{Ziguinchor}$ and S_{Travis}. False-negative solubility test reaction may occur with inadequate quantities of blood from anemic patients (hemoglobin levels <8.0 g/dL); deterioration of reducing agents (detected by negative result on positive control); deterioration of the lytic agent (detected by negativity of positive control); improper illumination and visualization of the line-reader scale and high concentration of Hb F or of phenothiazines may inhibit the sickle reaction; quantities of hemoglobin S too small to detect, as at birth or with transfusions of nonhemoglobin S into patients with hemoglobin S. The appearance of
(Continued)

Sickle Cell Tests (Continued)

hemoglobin S is genetically delayed and is not usually present in sufficient quantity for a positive screening test result until after 3 months of age. Maximum levels are not reached until about 6 months of age. Solubility tests and sodium metabisulfite test are unlikely to be reliably positive until after 6 months of age.

Methodology Hgb high salt solubility - Sickledex™ and a number of other commercially available products; alternate: slide test with 2% sodium metabisulfite

Additional Information Hb S is the result of a single amino acid substitution (valine for the normally present glutamic acid) at the 6th position of the β-globin chain of the hemoglobin molecule. The homozygous state results in sickle cell disease, a condition with significant morbidity and mortality. The heterozygous state causes sickle trait, a condition ordinarily characterized by little or no morbidity. Sickle disease presents a spectrum of clinical severity. Amelioration results from coincidental occurrence of other hemoglobinopathies, notably those with increased levels of Hb F (eg, thalassemia and different types of hereditary persistence of fetal hemoglobin). Variation in clinical expression is also the result of DNA polymorphism in the β-globin gene cluster.[1,2]

The incidence of sickle cell trait amongst African Americans in the U.S. is 8.5%. Because of possible anterior segment ischemia (a significant complication of retinal detachment surgery) that may occur in otherwise asymptomatic sickle trait individuals, it has been recommended that African-Americans undergo preoperative sickle tests prior to such procedures.[3]

Distinction between Hb S beta-thalassemia and sickle cell anemia is not always possible on clinical, hematologic, or electrophoretic grounds. Thalassemia heterozygotes have hypochromia and microcytosis, but overlap values exist. Differentiation can best be made by family or molecular pathology methods. Regional prevalence in the midwest area of Hb S beta-thalassemia is estimated to be 1:23,000 of the black population. It is recommended that positive sickle cell screen patients be further evaluated with cellulose acetate or agarose gel hemoglobin electrophoresis at pH 8.6, citrate agar gel electrophoresis at pH 6.0, Hb F studies and family studies. Complete characterization may require sophisticated laboratory studies with DNA amplification.[4] Erythrocyte ecdysis (long free filamentous processes stripping away from the surface of red cells) has been described in sickle cell anemia associated with elevated cold agglutinin titer.[5]

Survey testing to determine the incidence and significance of hereditary anemias (including the sickle hemoglobinopathies) continues on a worldwide basis.[6,7,8] The application of molecular biologic (DNA) based techniques for population screening is currently cost prohibitive but in future years is likely to be the preferred method for detection of sickle hemoglobinopathies, in particular for detection of the heterozygous states.[9,10]

A survey of laboratory results, methods and problems in screening for sickle cell disease with emphasis on laboratory responsibilities has recently been published by the US Department of Health and Human Services.[11]

The rare condition, "hemoglobin Munchausen" has been reviewed.[12]

Footnotes

1. El-Hazmi MA, Bahakim HM, and Warsy AS, "DNA Polymorphism in the Beta-Globin Gene Cluster in Saudi Arabs: Relation to Severity of Sickle Cell Anaemia," *Acta Haematol*, 1992, 88(2-3):61-6.
2. El-Hazmi MA, "Heterogeneity and Variation of Clinical and Haematological Expression of Haemoglobin S in Saudi Arabs," *Acta Haematol*, 1992, 88(2-3):67-71.
3. Cartwright MJ, Blair CJ, Combs JL, et al, "Anterior Segment Ischemia: A Complication of Retinal Detachment Repair in a Patient With Sickle Cell Trait," *Ann Ophthalmol*, 1990, 22(9):333-4.
4. Chehab FF and Kan YW, "Detection of Sickle Cell Anaemia Mutation by Colour DNA Amplification," *Lancet*, 1990, 335(8680):15-7.
5. Ward PC, Smith CM, and White JG, "Erythrocytic Ecdysis: An Unusual Morphologic Finding in a Case of Sickle Cell Anemia With Intercurrent Cold Agglutinin Syndrome," *Am J Clin Pathol*, 1979, 72:479-85.
6. Aluoch JR and Aluoch LH, "Survey of Sickle Disease in Kenya," *Trop Geogr Med*, 1993, 45:18-21.
7. Ali M and Lafferty J, "The Clinical Significance of Hemoglobinopathies in the Hamilton Region: A Twenty Year Review," *Clin Invest Med*, 1992, 15(5):401-5.
8. Martins MC, Olim G, Melo J, et al, "Hereditary Anaemias in Portugal: Epidemiology, Public Health Significance, and Control," *J Med Genet*, 1993, 30(3):235-9.
9. Steinberg MH, "DNA Diagnosis for the Detection of Sickle Hemoglobinopathies," *Am J Hematol*, 1993, 43(2):110-5.
10. McCabe ER, "Genetic Screening for the Next Decade: Application of Present and New Technologies," *Yale J Biol Med*, 1991, 64(1):9-14.
11. Guideline: Laboratory Screening for Sickle Cell Disease, U.S. Department of Health and Human Services, *Lab Med*, 1993, 24(8):515-22.
12. Ballas SK, "Munchausen Sickle Cell Painful Crisis," *Ann Clin Lab Sci*, 1992, 22(4):226-8.

References

Koshy M, "Sickle Cell Disease and Pregnancy," *Blood Rev*, 1995, 9(3):157-64.
Platt OS, Brambilla DJ, Rosse WF, et al, "Mortality in Sickle Cell Disease: Life Expectancy and Risk Factors for Early Death," *N Engl J Med*, 1994, 330(23):1639-44.
Serjeant GR, *Sickle Cell Disease*, 2nd ed, Oxford, England: Oxford U Pr, 1992.
Steinberg MH, "Sickle Cell Anemia and Fetal Hemoglobin," *Am J Med Sci*, 1994, 308(5):259-65.

Sickledex™ see Sickle Cell Tests on previous page

Sideroblast Stain see Iron Stain, Bone Marrow on page 328

Siderocyte Stain

CPT 85535

Related Information

Iron Stain, Bone Marrow on page 328

Synonyms Hemosiderin Stain; Iron Stain; Pappenheimer Body Stain

Specimen Blood: coverslip or slide smears; bone marrow: coverslip smears preferred

Reference Range Peripheral blood: no siderocytes identified; bone marrow: stainable iron present

Use Detect sideroblastic anemias and hemolytic anemia; semiquantitation of marrow iron stores evaluation of iron reserve; assist in the diagnosis of iron deficiency and hemosiderosis/hemochromatosis

Limitations Siderocytes may be present in asplenic patients.

Methodology Prussian blue (potassium ferrocyanide) reaction

Additional Information Siderotic granules represent iron not yet incorporated into hemoglobin and occur primarily when there is impaired hemoglobin synthesis (eg, sideroblastic anemia, lead poisoning). Savage et al[1] have shown that 36% of alcoholic patients with bone marrow proven sideroblastic anemia have siderocytes in the peripheral blood. Otherwise, siderocytes are uncommon in the peripheral blood unless a splenectomy has been performed on the patient. Iron staining of bone marrow is more important in terms of deciding on questionable causes of anemia. Numerous siderocytes are noted postsplenectomy and in some hemoglobinopathies. They are absent with iron deficiency.

Footnotes

1. Savage D and Lindenbaum J, "Anemia in Alcoholics," *Medicine (Baltimore)*, 1986, 65(5):322-38.

References

Beutler E, "Blood, Marrow, and Urine Iron Stains," *Williams Hematology*, 5th ed, Chapter L6, Beutler E, Lichtman MA, Coller BS, et al, eds, New York, NY: McGraw-Hill Inc, 1995, L27.
Douglas AS and Dacie JV, "The Incidence and Significance of Iron Containing Granules in Human Erythrocytes and Their Precursors," *J Clin Pathol*, 1953, 6:307.

Small Molecule Diseases see Inherited Diseases of Metabolism and Cell Structure Tests on page 327

Spherocytes Smear see Peripheral Blood: Red Blood Cell Morphology on page 339

Sphingolipidoses see Inherited Diseases of Metabolism and Cell Structure Tests on page 327

Sphingomyelinase see Inherited Diseases of Metabolism and Cell Structure Tests on page 327

Spinal Fluid Analysis see Cerebrospinal Fluid Analysis on page 309

Sputum Smear for Eosinophils see Eosinophil Smear on page 316

Stippled RBCs Smear see Peripheral Blood: Red Blood Cell Morphology on page 339

Sucrose Hemolysis Test see Sugar Water Test Screen on this page

Sudan Black Stain see Leukocyte Cytochemistry on page 331

Sugar Water Test Screen

CPT 86941

Related Information

Ham Test on page 320
Hemosiderin Stain, Urine on page 637

Synonyms PNH Test Screen; Sucrose Hemolysis Test

Test Commonly Includes Sucrose hemolysis if hemolysis is found in the sugar water screen test

Abstract Screening test for suspected paroxysmal nocturnal hemoglobinuria (PNH). Confirm with the Ham test and/or membrane protein defect studies (see listing Ham Test on page 320).

Specimen Blood

Container Blue top (sodium citrate) tube

Causes for Rejection Specimen clotted, hemolyzed specimens

Reference Range Absence of hemolysis is the normal condition. If no hemolysis is present, the patient probably does not have PNH provided multiple recent transfusions have not reduced the proportion of abnormal cells. The screening test is not definitive.

Use Screen for PNH

Limitations False-positives may be seen in cases of megaloblastic anemias and autoimmune hemolytic anemias. False-negative results may occur if heparin or EDTA is used as an anticoagulant.

Methodology Erythrocytes exposed to a solution of low ionic strength (sucrose in water) will fix complement to the cell surface. PNH red cells have unusual susceptibility to complement and will hemolyze under these conditions.

Additional Information If the sugar water test is positive, a subsequent Ham test is strongly recommended. A negative sugar water test rules out PNH in most instances, provided the proportion of patient cells has not been reduced by previous transfusion. It has been demonstrated that the most complement sensitive cells in PNH are younger RBCs and reticulocytes. Increased sensitivity can be obtained for the assay by separating young RBCs from old by centrifugation.[1]

Footnotes
1. Shimoda M and Yawata Y, "An Increased Calcium Accumulation in ATP-Dependent Red Cells of the Patients With Paroxysmal Nocturnal Hemoglobinuria," *Am J Hematol*, 1985, 20(4):325-35.

References
Beutler E, "Paroxysmal Nocturnal Hemoglobinuria," *Williams Hematology*, 5th ed, Chapter 25, Beutler E, Lichtman MA, Coller BS, et al, eds, New York, NY: McGraw-Hill Inc, 1995, 252-6 and L48.
Hartmann RC and Jenkins DE, "The "Sugar Water" Test for Paroxysmal Nocturnal Hemoglobinuria," *N Engl J Med*, 1966, 275:155-7.

Sulfatidase *see* Inherited Diseases of Metabolism and Cell Structure Tests *on page 327*

Survival of Red Blood Cells *see* ^{51}Cr Red Cell Survival *on page 314*

Tartrate Resistant Leukocyte Acid Phosphatase

CPT 88313

Related Information
Leukocyte Cytochemistry *on page 331*
Lymph Node Biopsy *on page 50*

Synonyms Acid Phosphatase, Tartrate Resistant, Leukocytes; Hairy Cell Leukemia Test; Leukemic Reticuloendotheliosis Test; Leukocyte Acid Phosphatase; TRAP Test

Test Commonly Includes Leukocyte acid phosphatase reaction with and without tartrate inhibition

Specimen Glass microscope slide smears prepared from fresh capillary or heparinized whole blood, fixed immediately (glutaraldehyde-acetone) after preparation

Container Green top (heparin) tube

Storage Instructions Smeared glass slides may be stored at least 1 week prior to assay if fixed immediately after preparation.

Causes for Rejection Smears unfixed, blood not fresh

Reference Range Most white cells of peripheral blood as well as platelets are acid phosphatase positive. Most white cells of blood have the acid phosphatase reaction inhibited by L(+) tartrate.

Use Diagnose "hairy cell leukemia" ("leukemic reticuloendotheliosis")

Methodology Naphthol AS-BI, fast garnet GBC, with and without L(+) tartaric acid

Additional Information There are some six isoenzymes of leukocyte acid phosphatase. Of the six, isoenzyme V is not inhibited by L(+) tartrate acid. It has been found that the malignant mononuclear cells of leukemic reticuloendotheliosis ("hairy cell leukemia") contain isoenzyme V and are resistant to inhibition by L(+) tartaric acid. There is evidence the reaction is not entirely specific as tartrate resistant acid phosphatase reactions have been reported in cases of prolymphocytic leukemia and malignant lymphoma as well as some cases of infectious mononucleosis.[1] There have also been reports of rare false-negative results (patients with leukemic reticuloendotheliosis having negative tartrate resistant acid phosphatase reactions). Recently, a new assay based on antibody against band V acid phosphatase has been described. The immunoassay has greater specificity[2] than the standard cytochemical procedure.

Footnotes
1. Brown BA, *Hematology: Principles and Practice*, 6th ed, Philadelphia, PA: Lea & Febiger, 1993, 137-8.
2. Whitaker KB, Cox TM, and Moss DW, "An Immunoassay of Human Band-5 (Tartrate Resistant) Acid Phosphatase That Involves the Use of Antiporcine Uteroferrin Antibodies," *Clin Chem* 1989, 35(1):86-9.

References
Davey FR and Nelson DA, "Leukocyte Acid Phosphatase," *Williams Hematology*, 5th ed, Chapter L27, Beutler E, Lichtman MA, Coller BS, et al, eds, New York, NY: McGraw-Hill Inc, 1995, L69-70.
Yam LT, Phyliky RL, and Li CY, "Benign and Neoplastic Disorders Simulating Hairy Cell Leukemia," *Semin Oncol*, 1984, 11(4):353-61.

TdT *see* Terminal Deoxynucleotidyl Transferase *on this page*

Terminal Deoxynucleotidyl Transferase

CPT 85999

Related Information
Bone Marrow *on page 307*

Immunophenotypic Analysis of Tissues by Flow Cytometry *on page 45*
Lymph Node Biopsy *on page 50*

Synonyms TdT; Terminal Deoxyribonucleotidyl Transferase; Terminal Transferase

Specimen Blood or bone marrow (avoid heparin) for leukocyte separation, pelletization, and storage at -20°C. Glass slide smears, air dried, of blood or marrow.

Collection Store dried smears at room temperature for up to 5 days.

Reference Range Peripheral blood: negative for TdT-positive cells; bone marrow: <1.8% TdT-positive cells

Use Classify certain leukemias and lymphomas, normally used to distinguish lymphoblastic from nonlymphoblastic leukemia; diagnose acute lymphoblastic leukemia, lymphoid blast crisis of chronic myelogenous leukemia, and lymphoblastic lymphomas

Terminal Deoxynucleotidyl Transferase (TdT) in Hematologic Disease

Disease	Percent Positive
Acute lymphoblastic leukemia	80-90
Lymphoblastic lymphoma	90
Chronic granulocytic leukemia in blast crisis	30
Acute undifferentiated leukemia	60
Acute nonlymphocytic leukemia	2-5

From Rubin E, MD and Farber JL, MD, *Pathology*, Philadelphia, PA: JB Lippincott Co, 1077, with permission.

Methodology Enzyme-linked immunosorbent assay (ELISA), indirect fluorescent antibody (IFA), peroxidase-antiperoxidase, avidin-biotin, immunoperoxidase, and incorporation of radiolabeled thymidine. A variety of methods for the enzyme assay of Ficoll/Hypaque® separated cell extracts have been described.[1] The radiometric assays are technically difficult and are usually available only in a research setting. Avidin-biotin immunoperoxidase[2] and flow cytometric[3] methods have been developed.

Additional Information TdT acts to catalyze the polymerization of deoxynucleoside triphosphates (by addition to the 3' hydroxyl ends of oligodeoxynucleotides or polydeoxynucleotides without DNA template instructions). Thymus is the primary site of TdT-positive cells and TdT is found in the nucleus of the more primitive T cells. A thymus related population of TdT-positive cells resides in the bone marrow (normally a minor population - 1% to 2%). TdT is increased in more than 90% of the cases of ALL of childhood.[1] This is true for even pre-B cell as well as B-cell ALL.[4] A minor (5% to 10%) population of patients with acute nonlymphoblastic leukemia have TdT-positive blasts. TdT-positive blasts are prominent in some cases of chronic myelogenous leukemia relating to the development of an acute blast phase. TdT has been reported to assist in establishing the diagnosis of acute lymphoblastic leukemia.[5] TdT-positive cases of blast phase CML correlate with a positive response to chemotherapy (vincristine and prednisone).[6,7] Combined assessment of nuclear TdT and cell surface antigens may assist in the detection of minimal residual disease after therapy of acute leukemia.[8,9] A 1991 study found that frequency of response to chemotherapy, response duration, and overall survival did not correlate with TdT expression.[10]

Footnotes
1. Beutler E and Blume KG, "Terminal Deoxynucleotidyl Transferase: Biochemical Properties, Cellular Distribution, and Hematologic Significance," *Prog Hematol*, 1979, 11:47-63.
2. Miller RT and Groothuis CL, "Improved Avidin-Biotin Immunoperoxidase Method for Terminal Deoxyribonucleotidyl Transferase and Immunophenotypic Characterization of Blood Cells," *Am J Clin Pathol*, 1990, 93(5):670-4.
3. Almasri NM, Iturraspe JA, Benson NA, et al, "Flow Cytometric Analysis of Terminal Deoxynucleotidyl Transferase," *Am J Clin Pathol*, 1991, 95(3):376-80.
4. Michiels JJ, Adriaansen HJ, Hagemeijer A, et al, "TdT Positive B-Cell Acute Lymphoblastic Leukemia (B-ALL) Without Burkitt Characteristics," *Br J Haematol*, 1988, 68(4):423-6.
5. Braziel RM, Keneklis T, and Donlon JA, "Terminal Deoxynucleotidyl Transferase in Non-Hodgkin's Lymphoma," *Am J Clin Pathol*, 1983, 80:655-9.
6. Tanaka M, Kaneda T, Hirota Y, et al, "Terminal Deoxynucleotidyl Transferase in the Blastic Phase of Chronic Myelogenous Leukemia: An Indicator of Response to Vincristine and Prednisone Therapy," *Am J Hematol*, 1980, 9:287-93.
7. Paciucci PA, Keaveney C, Cuttner J, et al, "Mitoxantrone Vincristine, and Prednisone in Adults With Relapsed or Primarily Refractory Acute Lymphocytic Leukemia and Terminal Deoxynucleotidyl Transferase Positive Blastic Phase Chronic Myelocytic Leukemia," *Cancer Res*, 1987, 47(19):5234-7.
8. Drach J, Gattringer C, and Huber H, "Combined Flow Cytometric Assessment of Cell Surface Antigens and Nuclear TdT for the Detection of Minimal Residual Disease in Acute Leukaemia," *Br J Haematol*, 1991, 77(1):37-42.
9. Smith RG and Kitchens RL, "Phenotypic Heterogeneity of TdT$^+$ Cells in the Blood and Bone Marrow: Implications for Surveillance of Residual Leukemia," *Blood*, 1989, 74(1):312-9.
10. Gucalp R, Paietta E, Weinberg V, et al, "Terminal Transferase Expression in Acute Myeloid Leukaemia: Biology and Prognosis," *Br J Haematol*, 1991, 78(1):48-54.

Terminal Deoxyribonucleotidyl Transferase *see* Terminal Deoxynucleotidyl Transferase *on previous page*

Terminal Transferase *see* Terminal Deoxynucleotidyl Transferase *on previous page*

Test for Congenital Heinz Body Hemolytic Anemia *see* Hemoglobin, Unstable, Heat Labile Test *on page 326*

Test for D-L Antibody *see* Cold Hemolysin Test *on page 311*

Test for Paroxysmal Cold Hemoglobinuria *see* Cold Hemolysin Test *on page 311*

Test for Uncommon Inherited Diseases of Metabolism and Cell Structure *see* Inherited Diseases of Metabolism and Cell Structure Tests *on page 327*

Tetrazolium Reduction Test *see* Nitroblue Tetrazolium Test *on page 334*

Thoracentesis Fluid Analysis *see* Body Fluid Analysis, Cell Count *on page 306*

Thorn Test
CPT 85999
Related Information
Cortisol, Blood *on page 112*
Cortisol, Urine *on page 113*
Cosyntropin Test *on page 114*
Eosinophil Count *on page 315*
Synonyms Adrenal Function Eosinophil Count
Abstract Eosinophil count is performed before and 4 hours following an injection of ACTH as a test of adrenal cortical function.
Patient Preparation Hold breakfast. Draw blood for initial eosinophil count. Give 25 units ACTH intramuscularly. May eat breakfast. Hold lunch. Repeat eosinophil count 4 hours after ACTH is given. May have lunch after second count is taken.
Specimen Whole blood
Container Lavender top (EDTA) tube
Causes for Rejection Patient not fasting
Use This test is of largely historical interest.
Limitations The test is rather antiquated and nonspecific. Addison's disease is most appropriately diagnosed using modern ACTH and cortisol levels. Borderline values are further investigated by stimulation tests of the pituitary and adrenals.
Additional Information If adrenal cortical function is normal, the eosinophil count will act as follows: The eosinophil count before the injection will be about twice the value of the eosinophil count after the injection (eg, eosinophil count of 200 before injection vs 100 after injection). If the adrenal cortical function is decreased, eosinophil count before the injection will be approximately the same as the eosinophil count after the injection (eg, eosinophil count before the injection of 200, after the injection, 195). When adrenal cortical function is decreased, it indicates hypoadrenalism (Addison's disease).
References
McNeely JC and Brown D, "Laboratory Evaluation of Leukocytes," *Clinical Hematology: Principles, Procedures, Correlations,* Chapter 25, Lotspeich-Steininger CA, Stiene-Martin EA, and Koepke JA, eds, Philadelphia, PA: JB Lippincott Co, 1992, 331.

Thrombocyte Count *see* Platelet Count *on page 340*

Total Blood Volume *see* Blood Volume *on page 306*

Total Eosinophil Count *see* Eosinophil Count *on page 315*

Total WBC *see* White Blood Count *on page 353*

TRAP Test *see* Tartrate Resistant Leukocyte Acid Phosphatase *on previous page*

Trypanosomiasis, Peripheral Blood Preparation *see* Microfilariae, Peripheral Blood Preparation *on page 333*

UBBC *see* Vitamin B_{12} Unsaturated Binding Capacity *on page 352*

Unsaturated Vitamin B_{12} Binding Capacity *see* Vitamin B_{12} Unsaturated Binding Capacity *on page 352*

Unstable Hemoglobins *see* Hemoglobin, Unstable, Heat Labile Test *on page 326*

Unstable Hemoglobins *see* Hemoglobin, Unstable - Isopropanol Precipitation Test *on page 326*

Viscosity, Blood
CPT 85810
Related Information
Erythropoietin, Serum *on page 124*

Immunoglobulin M *on page 410*
Viscosity, Serum/Plasma *on this page*
Synonyms Blood Viscosity
Specimen Whole blood
Container Green top (heparin) tube
Causes for Rejection Specimen clotted or hemolyzed
Special Instructions While this is an infrequently performed test and may not be routinely available, there is evidence that neonatal hyperviscosity is common,[1] suggesting that the test should be more frequently utilized. Consult the laboratory to determine if the requisite microviscometer can be obtained.
Reference Range See references for normal range data. Viscosity normally rises with increase in hematocrit and is lower with lower shear rates. Study has shown that umbilical cord and venous hematocrits (not capillary) correlate with microviscometer readings in newborns.[2]
Use Detect hyperviscosity states including especially hyperviscosity in the neonatal period.
Methodology Wells-Brookfield microviscometer.[3] Viscosity is measured at low and high shear rates at 37°C.
Additional Information The relatively new fields of haemorheology and clinical haemorheology focus upon the characteristics and resultant clinical effects of the flow behavior of blood. Somer and Meiselman have classified the hematological hyperviscosity syndromes as of polycythemic, sclerocythemic, or plasma type.[4] The polycythemic category includes syndromes the result of erythrocytosis (primary or secondary) or of hyperleukocytic leukemia. Sclerocythemic cases are the result of decreased deformability of red cells (as occur with sickle hemoglobinopathies, other hemolytic anemias, some forms of malaria, and with rigid leukemic cells). In the plasma category are paraproteinemias (eg, multiple myeloma and Waldenström's macroglobulinemia) and reactive polyclonal dysproteinemias.

Neonatal hyperviscosity, usually but not always associated with polycythemia, may be accompanied by a fairly typical clinical picture. Plethora, hypoglycemia, lethargy, and jitteriness/seizures (CNS symptoms) occur. There may be symptoms and findings suggesting congenital heart disease (CHD) (ie, respiratory distress, cardiac enlargement, and cyanosis). False diagnoses of CHD have been made in such cases. About 50% of such infants have modest hyperbilirubinemia (bilirubin >12 mg/dL). Blood viscosity of small or large-for-gestational age infants does not differ from average-for-gestational age infants. About 50% of the cases have schistocytes and increased nucleated RBC on peripheral blood smear. The whole blood viscosity test can be used to follow the result of exchange transfusion therapy of neonatal hyperviscosity syndrome. Whole blood viscosity is increased after splenectomy (adults).[5]

Footnotes
1. Hathaway WE, "Neonatal Viscosity," *Pediatrics,* 1983, 72:567-9.
2. Ramamurthy RS and Berlanga M, "Postnatal Alteration in Hematocrit and Viscosity in Normal and Polycythemic Infants," *J Pediatr,* 1987, 110(6):929-34.
3. Wells RE, Denton R, and Merrill EW, "Measurement of Viscosity of Biologic Fluids by Cone Plate Viscometer," *J Lab Clin Med,* 1961, 57:646-56.
4. Somer T and Meiselman HJ, "Disorders of Blood Viscosity," *Ann Med,* 1993, 25(1):31-9.
5. Robertson DA, Simpson FG, and Losowsky MS, "Blood Viscosity After Splenectomy," *Br Med J (Clin Res Ed),* 1981, 283:573-5.

References
Black VD and Lubchenko LO, "Neonatal Polycythemia and Hyperviscosity," *Pediatr Clin North Am,* 1982, 29:1137-48.
Crowley JP, Metzger JB, Merrill EW, et al, "Whole Blood Viscosity in Beta Thalassemia Minor," *Ann Clin Lab Sci,* 1992, 22(4):229-35.
Williams WJ, Beutler E, Erslev AJ, et al, *Hematology,* 4th ed, New York, NY: McGraw-Hill Inc, 1990, 427-9.

Viscosity, Serum/Plasma
CPT 85810
Related Information
Immunofixation Electrophoresis *on page 408*
Protein Electrophoresis, Serum *on page 424*
Protein Electrophoresis, Urine *on page 425*
Viral Culture, Respiratory Symptoms *on page 680*
Viscosity, Blood *on this page*
Synonyms Serum Viscosity
Specimen Serum or plasma
Container Red top tube or lavender top (EDTA) tube
Reference Range 1.4-1.8 relative to water
Use Evaluate hyperviscosity syndromes associated with monoclonal gammopathy states (myeloma, macroglobulinemia of Waldenström and other dysproteinemias), including occasional cases of rheumatoid arthritis, systemic lupus erythematosus, hyperfibrinogenemia
Limitations Does not measure whole blood viscosity, which increases with high hemoglobin/hematocrit. Subjective endpoint, temperature dependent, large technical error, less than ideal correlation exists between measured viscosity levels and clinical symptoms.

Methodology Viscometer (Viscosimeter), Cannon-Feuske, Ostwald. Water and plasma "flow times" are determined with the use of a viscometer RBC or WBC pipette and stopwatch.[1] Test may be performed at room temperature or 37°C. The relative viscosity is expressed as a ratio of plasma "flow time" to water "flow time." A viscometer is commercially available which gives an automated measurement of plasma viscosity.[2]

Additional Information Hyperviscosity is most frequent (33% of cases)[3] with IgM monoclonal gammopathy (Waldenström's macroglobulinemia); next with IgA myeloma. When IgG myeloma leads to hyperviscosity IgG levels are usually very significantly elevated. Kappa light chain myeloma may (rarely) be responsible for hyperviscosity syndrome apparently as a result of true polymer formation.[4] A relative viscosity of 6-7 usually results in symptoms of the hyperviscosity syndrome, they have however been described with lower levels of relative viscosity (ie, 4). Results of plasma viscosity obtained with an automated capillary viscometer show good precision and close correlation with the Harkness manual method (standard method selected by the International Committee for Standardization in Hematology).[2]

Footnotes

1. Wright DJ and Jenkins DE Jr, "Simplified Method for Estimation of Serum and Plasma Viscosity in Multiple Myeloma and Related Disorders," *Blood*, 1970, 36:516-22.
2. Cooke BM and Stuart J, "Automated Measurement of Plasma Viscosity by Capillary Viscometer," *J Clin Pathol*, 1988, 41(11):1213-6.
3. Gandara DR and Mackenzie MR, "Differential Diagnosis of Monoclonal Gammopathy," *Med Clin North Am*, 1988, 72(5):1155-67.
4. Carter PW, Cohen HJ, and Crawford J, "Hyperviscosity Syndrome in Association With Kappa Light Chain Myeloma," *Am J Med*, 1989, 86(5):591-5.

References

Foerster J, "Plasma Cell Dyscrasias: General Considerations," *Wintrobe's Clinical Hematology*, 9th ed, Chapter 83, Section 4, Lee RG, Bithell TC, Foerster J, et al, eds, Philadelphia, PA: Lea & Febiger, 1993, 2202-10.

Henry JB, Nelson DA, Tomar RH, et al, *Todd-Sanford-Davidsohn Clinical Diagnosis and Management by Laboratory Methods*, 18th ed, Philadelphia, PA: WB Saunders Co, 1991, 709.

Lowe GD, "Should Plasma Viscosity Replace the ESR?" *Br J Haematol*, 1994, 86(1):6-11.

Murphy PT, Allen B, and Hutchinson RM, "Plasma Viscosity and Erythrocyte Sedimentation Rate in Suspected Cases of Temporal Arteritis," *Br J Haematol*, 1994, 87(3):671.

"Case Records of the Massachusetts General Hospital Clinicopathological Exercises. Case 13-1994. A 62-Year-Old Man With Epistaxis, Confusion, Renal Failure, and Bilateral Central Retinal-Vein Thrombosis," *N Engl J Med*, 1994, 330(13):920-7.

Somer T and Meiselman HJ, "Disorders of Blood Viscosity," *Ann Med*, 1993, 25(1):31-9.

Vitamin B₁₂

CPT 82607

Related Information

Bone Marrow *on page 307*
Complete Blood Count *on page 312*
Folic Acid, RBC *on page 317*
Folic Acid, Serum *on page 317*
Gastrin, Serum *on page 135*
Hemoglobin *on page 323*
Intrinsic Factor Antibody *on page 411*
Parietal Cell Antibody *on page 421*
Phlebotomy, Therapeutic *on page 614*
Red Blood Cell Indices *on page 343*
Red Cell Count *on page 344*
Schilling Test *on page 346*
Vitamin B₁₂ Unsaturated Binding Capacity *on next page*

Synonyms Antipernicious Anemia Factor; B₁₂; Cyanocobalamin, True; Extrinsic Factor of Castle

Applies to Methylmalonic Acid

Abstract Radioisotopic method replaces *Euglena* microbiological assay for detection of cobalamin deficiency. This assay has low (only slightly better than 20%) positive predictive value for clinical cobalamin deficiency. Additional evaluation is important in order to establish the presence of clinical B₁₂ deficiency.

Patient Preparation A fasting specimen is preferred; draw before transfusions or B₁₂ therapy is started.

Specimen Serum

Container Red top tube

Storage Instructions Separate serum and freeze; protect from light. Obtain hematocrit from EDTA tube before freezing the whole blood specimen.

Causes for Rejection Stored specimen not frozen

Reference Range The lower reference limit, which is critical to the diagnosis of B₁₂ deficiency/pernicious anemia, is not clearly established. It is likely in the range of 100-250 pg/mL (SI: 74-185 pmol/L).[1,2,3] Most commercial methods have in the past undergone modification, in particular after the report by Kolhouse et al.[1] Clinical correlation and multiple test documentation of the etiology of macrocytic anemia is advised. Occasionally, patients with significant neuropsychiatric abnormalities may have no hematologic abnormalities (absence of anemia or macrocytosis), but vitamin B₁₂ level >200 pg/mL (SI: >150 pmol/L), or

more commonly between 100 and 200 pg/mL (SI: 75-150 pmol/L).[4] See table for pediatric reference ranges.

Pediatric Serum B₁₂ Reference Ranges

Age	Male (pg/mL)		Female (pg/mL)	
	Low	High	Low	High
0-1 y	216	891	168	1117
2-3 y	195	897	307	892
4-6 y	181	795	231	1038
7-9 y	200	863	182	866
10-12 y	135	803	145	752
13-18 y	158	638	134	605

From Hicks JM, Cook J, Godwin ID, et al, "Vitamin B₁₂ and Folate — Pediatric Reference Ranges," *Arch Pathol Lab Med*, 1993, 117:705, with permission.

Use Detect B₁₂ deficiency as in pernicious anemia in those patients who have hematologic (weakness, anemia, oval macrocytosis, hypersegmented neutrophils, leukopenia/thrombocytopenia) or neurologic (numbness, tingling, loss of vibratory sensation in extremities) findings suggestive of such deficiency state. Because of problems associated with verifying the lower limits of "normal," this assay should not be employed as a screening test for functional cobalamin deficiency.[2,3,4] Diagnose folic acid deficiency[5]; evaluate hypersegmentation of granulocyte nuclei; investigate MCV >100 fL; diagnose macrocytic and megaloblastic anemia; work up alcoholism; prenatal care; evaluate malabsorption, including jejunoileal bypass patients operated for massive obesity; work up certain neurological disorders.

Limitations Drugs capable of interference with absorption of B₁₂ and/or folic acid include chemotherapeutic (methotrexate), antimalarial (pyrimethamine), diuretics (triamterene), protozoacides (pentamidine, isethionate), antibacterials (trimethoprim), anticonvulsants (phenytoin), sedatives (barbiturates), oral contraceptives, antituberculosis agents (cycloserine, para-aminosalicylic acid), antigout (colchicine), oral hypoglycemic, biguanide group (metformin, phenformin). See accompanying table concerning cautions in interpretation. Establishing functional cobalamin (B₁₂) sufficiency in any individual patient may require consideration of intra-individual variation, functional status of the gastric mucosa (in particular in elderly individuals) and transcobalamin II binding.[3,6] See following discussion of application of serum methylmalonic acid.

Contraindications B₁₂/folate levels should be drawn before performance of Schilling test and before administration of any other radioactivity.

Methodology Radioimmunoassay (RIA) based on competitive protein binding has largely replaced earlier microbiologic assays. Patient's unlabeled endogenous serum B₁₂ competes with radiolabeled B₁₂ for specific sites on a binding protein (intrinsic factor) and is compared to the behavior of a standard. Some commercially available procedures combine B₁₂ and folate testing in a single simultaneous method using two different isotopes (generally, with B₁₂, ⁵⁷Co and folate, ¹²⁵I labels). A chemiluminescence receptor assay utilizing intrinsic factor immobilized on magnetic particles (solid phase) has been developed.[7]

Additional Information Vitamin B₁₂ (cyanocobalamin) analogues form the base compound in coenzymes having important biologic functions. The vitamin has an intriguing ring structure, a planar tetrapyrrole corrin ring around an asymmetric cobalt atom. The structure is reminiscent of the relation of iron to heme. The corrin system, like porphyrin (heme), is synthesized from delta aminolevulinic acid. The basic compound is named cobalamin, the form with attached cyanide group (cyanocobalamin) is vitamin B₁₂. Two metabolically important cobamides (vitamin B₁₂ containing coenzymes) are adenosyl cobamide and methyl cobamide. Cobamides are required for DNA synthesis, methylation, and citric acid cycle reactions.[4]

Vitamin B₁₂ is not synthesized by humans. It is a requisite dietary component widely available in animal products (meat, fish, eggs, butter, milk, and cheese). The minimum daily requirement (MDR) is 1-5 µg/day, body stores are 2000-5000 µg, and daily loss is only about 0.1%. B₁₂ is absorbed by mucosal epithelial cells (microvilli) of the terminal ileum, a pH and divalent cation dependent process. The vitamin is ingested in food sources bound to protein. Its absorption is dependent upon a gastric glycoprotein, intrinsic factor (IF). Gastric acid splits the B₁₂ protein linkage. IF binding is by a benzimidazole nucleotide, which is independent of the analogue chemical form and which protects against digestive enzymes. After the B₁₂ intrinsic factor complex is absorbed by the ileal mucosa, the vitamin enters the portal circulation where it is bound by a system of carrier proteins, the transcobalamins I, II, and III. See the listing Vitamin B₁₂ Unsaturated Binding Capacity *on page 352*. Transcobalamins I and III are of leukocyte origin, transcobalamin II is synthesized by the liver.

(Continued)

Vitamin B$_{12}$ *(Continued)*

Competitive protein binding methods measure total or "true" cobalamin levels. Kolhouse et al[1] have shown that cobalamin analogues are present in some human plasmas and that these may have higher affinity for "R proteins" (B$_{12}$ binding proteins without intrinsic factor activity) than for intrinsic factor with resultant masking of cobalamin deficiency.[1] Defects in some assay procedures capable of producing falsely high levels of B$_{12}$ (eg, patients with true deficiency of cobalamin but with serum levels in the normal range) have been corrected. Currently, such assay procedures have been modified. Spurious high B$_{12}$ results have been reported in the past relating to anti-intrinsic factor-blocking antibodies and high or low results relating to endogenous B$_{12}$ binding proteins.

Conditions associated with decreased vitamin B$_{12}$ include hypochlorhydria; pernicious anemia (PA) in which cobalamin levels may vary from 0 to overlapping lower limits of patients without PA; dietary deficiency (uncommon); disorders of intestinal absorption; inflammatory bowel disease; bacterial overgrowth, small intestine; *Diphyllobothrium* fish tapeworm, small intestine; prior gastric surgery; intestinal surgery (diminished B$_{12}$ or folate or both are found in 88% of patients with jejunoileal bypass operated for morbid obesity;[8] resection of terminal ileum as for Crohn's disease which prevents absorption of B$_{12}$; oral contraceptives; abnormalities of cobalamin transport or metabolism;[6] Imerslund's syndrome.[9,10] **A significant rise in red blood cell mean corpuscular volume (MCV) may be an important early indicator of B$_{12}$ deficiency.** Conditions associated with increased vitamin B$_{12}$ include chronic granulocytic leukemia (and to a lesser degree leukemoid states); chronic renal failure; severe congestive heart failure; diabetes; obesity; COPD; and cases of liver cell damage (eg, acute hepatitis). Currently, macrocytosis in a hospitalized urban population is most commonly associated with AIDS patients undergoing zidovudine therapy. This may result from AIDS-associated malabsorption and/or a possible DNA-inhibiting effect of zidovudine.[11,12]

Elevated serum or urine methylmalonic acid (MMA) level is probably a more definitive indication of early cobalamin (B$_{12}$) deficiency than the serum cobalamin level. MMA serum level, when increased, reflects decreased tissue cobalamin and is an early indicator of B$_{12}$ deficiency. Cobalamin dependent neurologic disease with normal hematologic parameters and serum B$_{12}$ levels may be associated with significant elevations of serum methylmalonic acid.[4,13] GC/MS methodology for MMA determinations is preferred, is not currently in widespread use, but there have been important advances in sample preparation (simplification).[14] To avoid dietary influence serum MMA levels have preference over urine studies in nonfasting patients.[15]

Folate deficiency may be a cause of low levels of serum cobalamin. Low serum B$_{12}$ levels may be seen in some individuals deficient only in folate. It is important to note that a normal level of cobalamin in the serum does not always exclude cobalamin deficiency. Individuals with low serum B$_{12}$ require clinical confirmation of deficiency. In pregnancy low serum B$_{12}$ level does not usually indicate deficiency at the biochemicals level. Elevation of serum homocysteine concentrations (in the absence of folate deficiency) may be of value in establishing true B$_{12}$ deficiency. Serum MMA level may be independent of B$_{12}$ status in the pregnant patient.[16]

Footnotes

1. Kolhouse JF, Kondo H, Allen NC, et al, "Cobalamin Analogues Are Present in Human Plasma and Can Mask Cobalamin Deficiency Because Current Radioisotope Dilution Assays Are Not Specific for True Cobalamin," *N Engl J Med*, 1978, 299:785-92.
2. Schilling RF, Fairbanks VF, Miller R, et al, "Improved Vitamin B$_{12}$ Assays: A Report on Two Commercial Kits," *Clin Chem*, 1983, 29:582-3.
3. Lindstedt G, Lundberg P-A, Johansson P-M, et al, "High Prevalence of Atrophic Gastritis in the Elderly: Implications for Health-Associated Reference Limits for Cobalamin in Serum," *Clin Chem*, 1989, 35(7):1557-9.
4. Lindenbaum J, Healton EB, Savage DG, et al, "Neuropsychiatric Disorders Caused by Cobalamin Deficiency in the Absence of Anemia or Macrocytosis," *N Engl J Med*, 1988, 318(26):1720-8.
5. Tisman G and Herbert V, "B$_{12}$ Dependence of Cell Uptake of Serum Folate: An Explanation for High Serum Folate and Cell Folate Depletion in B$_{12}$ Deficiency," *Blood*, 1973, 41:465-9.
6. Herzlich B and Herbert V, "Depletion of Serum Holotranscobalamin II. An Early Sign of Negative Vitamin B$_{12}$ Balance," *Lab Invest*, 1988, 58(3):332-7.
7. Leonard H, Klukas C, Williams M, et al, "A Chemiluminescence Receptor Assay for Vitamin B$_{12}$," *Clin Chem*, 1989, 35:1194.
8. Hocking MP, Duerson MC, O'Leary JP, et al, "Jejunoileal Bypass for Morbid Obesity. Late Follow-up in 100 Cases," *N Engl J Med*, 1983, 308:995-9.
9. Abdelaal MA and Ahmed AF, "Imerslund-Gräsbeck Syndrome in a Saudi Family," *Acta Paediatr Scand*, 1991, 80(11):1109-12.
10. Russo CL, Hyman PE, and Oseas RS, "Megaloblastic Anemia Characterized by Microcytosis: Imerslund-Gräsbeck Syndrome With Coexistent Alpha-Thalassemia," *Pediatrics*, 1988, 81(6):875-6.
11. Snower DP and Weil SC, "Changing Etiology of Macrocytosis: Zidovudine as a Frequent Causative Factor," *Am J Clin Pathol*, 1993, 99(1):57-60.
12. Rule SA, Hooker M, Costello C, et al, "Serum Vitamin B$_{12}$ and Transcobalamin Levels in Early HIV Disease," *Am J Hematol*, 1994, 47(3):167-71.
13. Rasmussen K, Moelby L, and Jensen MK, "Studies on Methylmalonic Acid in Humans. II. Relationship Between Concentrations in Serum and Urinary Excretion, and the Correlation Between Serum Cobalamin and Accumulation of Methylmalonic Acid," *Clin Chem*, 1989, 35(12):2277-80.

14. Rasmussen K, "Solid Phase Sample Extraction for Rapid Determinations of Methylmalonic Acid in Serum and Urine by a Stable-Isotope-Dilution Method," *Clin Chem*, 1989, 35(2):260-4.
15. Rasmussen K, "Studies on Methylmalonic Acid in Humans. I. Concentrations in Serum and Urinary Excretion in Normal Subjects After Feeding and During Fasting and After Loading With Protein, Fat, Sugar, Isoleucine, and Valine," *Clin Chem*, 1989, 38(12):2271-6.
16. Metz J, McGrath K, Bennett M, et al, "Biochemical Indices of Vitamin B$_{12}$ Nutrition in Pregnant Patients With Subnormal Serum Vitamin B$_{12}$ Levels," *Am J Hematol*, 1995, 48:251-5.

References

Amos RJ, Dawson DW, Fish DI, et al, Working Party of the BCSH General Haematology Task Force, "Guidelines on the Investigation and Diagnosis of Cobalamin and Folate Deficiencies. A Publication of the British Committee for Standards in Haematology," *Clin Lab Haematol*, 1994, 16:101-15.

Carethers M, "Diagnosing Vitamin B$_{12}$ Deficiency, A Common Geriatric Disorder," *Geriatrics*, 1988, 43(3):89-94, 105-7, 111-2.

Chanarin I, "Megaloblastic Anaemia, Cobalamin, and Folate," *J Clin Pathol*, 1987, 40(9):978-84.

Cooper BA and Rosenblatt, "Disorders of Cobalamin and Folic Acid Metabolism," Chapter 47, Part 7 (Red Blood Cells), *Blood: Principles and Practice of Hematology*, Handin RI, Lux SE, and Stossel TP, eds, Philadelphia, PA: JB Lippincott Co, 1995, 1399-432.

Gimsing P and Nexo E, "Cobalamin-Binding Capacity of Haptocorrin and Transcobalamin: Age-Correlated Reference Intervals and Values From Patients," *Clin Chem*, 1989, 35(7):1447-51.

Herbert V, "Don't Ignore Low Serum Cobalamin (Vitamin B$_{12}$) Levels," *Arch Intern Med*, 1988, 148(8):1705-7.

Herbert V, "The 1986 Herman Award Lecture. Nutrition Science as a Continually Unfolding Story: The Folate and Vitamin B$_{12}$ Paradigm," *Am J Clin Nutr*, 1987, 46(3):387-402.

Hicks JM, Cook J, Godwin ID, et al, "Vitamin B$_{12}$ and Folate: Pediatric Reference Ranges," *Arch Pathol Lab Med*, 1993, 117(7):704-6.

Lee GR, "Megaloblastic and Nonmegaloblastic Macrocytic Anemias," *Wintrobe's Clinical Hematology*, 9th ed, Chapter 24, Lee GR, Bithell TC, Foerster J, et al, eds, Philadelphia, PA: Lea & Febiger, 1993, 745-90.

Matchar DB, McCrory DC, Millington DS, et al, "Performance of the Serum Cobalamin Assay for Diagnosis of Cobalamin Deficiency," *Am J Med Sci*, 1994, 308(5):276-83.

Pruthi RK and Tefferi A, "Pernicious Anemia Revisited," *Mayo Clin Proc*, 1994, 69(2):144-50.

Schilling RF and Williams WJ, "Vitamin B$_{12}$ Deficiency: Underdiagnosed, Overtreated?" *Hosp Pract*, 1995, 30(7):47-54.

Steiner I, Kidron D, Soffer D, et al, "Sensory Peripheral Neuropathy of Vitamin B$_{12}$ Deficiency: A Primary Demyelinating Disease?" *J Neurol*, 1988, 235(3):163-4.

Thompson WG, Babitz L, Cassino C, et al, "Evaluation of Current Criteria Used to Measure Vitamin B$_{12}$ Levels," *Am J Med*, 1987, 82(2):291-4.

Vitamin B$_{12}$ Absorption Test *see* Schilling Test *on page 346*

Vitamin B$_{12}$ UBC *see* Vitamin B$_{12}$ Unsaturated Binding Capacity *on this page*

Vitamin B$_{12}$ Unsaturated Binding Capacity

CPT 82608

Related Information

Erythropoietin, Serum *on page 124*
Folic Acid, RBC *on page 317*
Folic Acid, Serum *on page 317*
Intrinsic Factor Antibody *on page 411*
Parietal Cell Antibody *on page 421*
Schilling Test *on page 346*
Vitamin B$_{12}$ *on previous page*

Synonyms UBBC; Unsaturated Vitamin B$_{12}$ Binding Capacity; Vitamin B$_{12}$ UBC

Specimen Serum is most commonly used by most reference laboratories but use of EDTA plasma avoids increase in binding protein released from granulocytes (see following information).

Container Red top tube

Storage Instructions Refrigerate serum if not delivered to the laboratory immediately. Stable for days. Very stable when stored at -20°C.

Reference Range 1000-2000 pg/mL binding capacity

Use Differential diagnosis of polycythemia vera from secondary/relative polycythemias; evaluate macrocytic/megaloblastic anemia; diagnose congenital absence of transcobalamin II or cobalophilin (transcobalamin I and III)

Limitations Increased with pregnancy and use of contraceptive hormones. Unrepresentative increase may occur during clotting of blood samples by release of unsaturated binding protein (cobalophilin) from granulocytes.[1] May give low values in samples with low protein content. Usually available only at reference or research laboratories.

Methodology Binding proteins are determined by their B$_{12}$ binding capacity. Uptake of radiolabeled B$_{12}$ is quantitated after saturation of serum transport systems and removal of excess vitamin with albumin or hemoglobin-coated charcoal. DEAE cellulose ion-exchange chromatography and isoelectric focusing are also used (in research environments).

Additional Information Serum transport of vitamin B$_{12}$ is accomplished by normally occurring proteins termed transcobalamins including I (an α-globulin), II (a β-globulin), and III (a group of transport factors - "R-type" binders or binder III - found also in some tissues, saliva, milk, and tears).

The term "R-type" refers to binding protein with "rapid" mobility on electrophoresis. The term haptocorrin (TCO, I, II, R binder, cobalophyllin) refers to a family of immunologically similar proteins which are variably glycosylated and not all of which have rapid electrophoretic mobility. Transcobalamin I is the major B_{12} transport protein binding 80% to 90% of endogenous cobalamin which is delivered from peripheral tissues to the liver. It bears immunologic identity to granulocyte cobalophilin. Transcobalamin II binds only 10% to 25% of total plasma cobalamin but provides most of the total UBBC of plasma. Less than 2% of plasma TC II is saturated at any one point in time. The TC II bound B_{12} is decreased in untreated B_{12} deficiency. As the B_{12} deficient state develops, TC II UBBC increases.[1] See accompanying table for other clinical associations. Isoelectric focusing has shown that the cobalophilins (R-binders) are a microheterogenous group of plasma binding proteins. Stenman has reviewed this subject in detail.[2] Cobalophilin is increased in diseases characterized by excess granulocyte production, reactive leukocytosis, chronic myelogenous leukemia, and other myeloproliferative states, in particular polycythemia vera. UBBC levels are increased in >66% of the cases of polycythemia vera. Most cases of secondary/relative polycythemia patients have normal levels of UBBC. High levels occur in some patients with hepatoma.[3] The transcobalamins are normally about 25% saturated with vitamin B_{12}. UBBCs of transcobalamins I and II are increased in asymptomatic human immunodeficiency seropositive patients.[4]

Levels and Binding Capacity of Cobalamin-Binding Proteins in Disease

Binder	Disease
Increased TC I (R protein)	Myeloproliferative disorders
	Polycythemia vera
	Myelofibrosis
	Benign neutrophilia
	Chronic myelocytic leukemia
	Hepatoma (occasionally)
	Metastatic cancer
Increased TC II	Myeloproliferative disorders
	Liver disease
	Inflammatory disorders
	Gaucher disease
	Anti-TC II antibodies
Unsaturated cobalamin binders*	
Increased	Transient neutropenia
	Elevated TC I
Decreased	Liver disease
	Elevated serum cobalamin

*UBBC = unsaturated B_{12} binding capacity

From Babior BM, "Metabolic Aspects of Folic Acid and Cobalamin," *Williams Hematology*, 5th ed, Chapter 35, Beutler E, Lichtman MA, Coller BS, et al, eds, New York, NY: McGraw-Hill Inc, 1995, 390, with permission.

TC II deficiency (presents shortly after birth as failure to thrive) is an uncommon condition characterized by vomiting and weakness, megaloblastic anemia and later, neurologic disease. Serum cobalamin levels are normal or nearly normal (most serum cobalamin is carried by TC I, an R binder). Even more uncommon is R-binder deficiency (absent or deficient TC I) in which serum cobalamin level is decreased but there are no clinical signs of B_{12} deficiency. In such cases TC II cobalamin levels are normal.

Footnotes
1. Herzlich B and Herbert V, "Depletion of Serum Holotranscobalamin II. An Early Sign of Negative Vitamin B_{12} Balance," *Lab Invest*, 1988, 58(3):332-7.
2. Stenman U-H, "Intrinsic Factor and the Vitamin B_{12} Binding Proteins," *Megaloblastic Anemia, Clinics in Haematology*, Hoffbrand AV, ed, Philadelphia, PA: WB Saunders Co, 1976, 5:473-95.
3. Waxman S and Gilbert HS, "A Tumor-Related Vitamin B_{12} Binding Protein in Adolescent Hepatoma," *N Engl J Med*, 1973, 289:1053-6.
4. Rule SA, Hooker M, Costello C, et al, "Serum Vitamin B_{12} and Transcobalamin Levels in Early HIV Disease," *Am J Hematol*, 1994, 47(3):167-71.

References
Babior BM, "Metabolic Aspects of Folic Acid and Cobalamin," *Williams Hematology*, 5th ed, Chapter 35, Beutler E, Lichtman MA, Coller BS, et al, eds, New York, NY: McGraw-Hill Inc, 1995, 388-90.
Fenton WA and Rosenberg LE, "Inherited Disorders of Cobalamin Transport and Metabolism," *The Metabolic and Molecular Bases of Inherited Disease*, 7th ed, Chapter 102, McGraw-Hill Inc, 1995, 3129-49.
Hall CA, Horch C, and Begley JA, "The Forms and Transport of Plasma Cobalamins in Normal Man and in Myeloproliferative States," *J Lab Clin Med*, 1979, 94:772-83.
Zittoun J, Farcet JP, Marquet J, et al, "Cobalamin (Vitamin B_{12}) and B_{12} Binding Proteins in Hypereosinophilic Syndromes and Secondary Eosinophilia," *Blood*, 1984, 63(4):779-83.

WBC *see* White Blood Count *on this page*

Westergren Sed Rate *see* Sedimentation Rate, Erythrocyte *on page 347*

White Blood Cell Morphology *see* Peripheral Blood: Differential Leukocyte Count *on page 336*

White Blood Count

CPT 85048

Related Information
Antineutrophil Antibody *on page 366*
Bone Marrow *on page 307*
CD4/CD8 Enumeration *on page 375*
Chromosome Analysis, Blood *on page 276*
Chromosome Analysis, Bone Marrow *on page 277*
Complete Blood Count *on page 312*
HIV-1/HIV-2 Serology *on page 403*
Leukocyte Alkaline Phosphatase *on page 330*
Leukocyte Cytochemistry *on page 331*
Lymph Node Biopsy *on page 50*
Peripheral Blood: Differential Leukocyte Count *on page 336*

Synonyms Leukocyte Count; Total WBC; WBC; White Count

Abstract This procedure determines the white blood cell concentration in a body fluid, usually blood. The count is most commonly generated by an automated analyzer using aperture-impedance and/or laser beam technology. Different types of white blood cells (eg, granulocytes, monocytes, lymphocytes, etc) are included in the total count. The results have widespread application to the diagnosis and monitoring of a variety of clinical conditions including infectious, neoplastic, and immunologic disease states.

Specimen Whole blood or other body fluid

Container Lavender top (EDTA) tube

Causes for Rejection Clotted specimen, hemolyzed specimen

Reference Range Peripheral blood: 4500-11,000/mm³ (SI: 4.5-11.0 x 10^9/L)

Possible Panic Range On admission <2500/mm³ (SI: 2.5 x 10^9/L) or >30,000/mm³ (SI: >30.0 x 10^9/L)

Use White cell enumeration; evaluate myelopoiesis, bacterial and viral infections, toxic metabolic processes; diagnose/evaluate leukemic states

Limitations If nucleated RBCs are found in differential count, the white blood count should be corrected. Electronic counters are subject to spurious high WBC counts in cases where clumped platelet aggregates are "seen" as white cells.[1]

Methodology Manual - hemocytometer counting chambers. Most WBC count determinations are obtained from one channel of a highly automated multichannel electronic and pneumatic analyzer using aperture-impedance and/or aperture conductance and/or laser light scattering technologies. WBC differential determination is provided by recent generations of analyzers. Excellent performance (precision, linearity, and lack of carryover) has been found on field evaluation of a commonly utilized multichannel device.[2] A new automated hematology analyzer performs the differential leukocyte count (DLC) using flow-cytochemical technology. Evaluation has suggested that this method provides "the most reliable quantitative index of neutrophil left shift currently available in a commercial automated DLC analyzer."[3]

Additional Information In newborn infants WBC counts from different vascular sources (ie, capillary vs venous vs arterial blood) should not necessarily be considered equivalent. WBC counts from actively crying babies may show leukocytosis with left shift, possibly erroneously suggesting bacterial infections. Any stressful situation in newborns, children, or adults which leads to increase in endogenous epinephrine production may cause a rapid (15-30 minutes) increase in WBC count. In the evaluation of infection in newborns and young children, it is recommended that several counts be obtained from a consistent vascular source in resting individuals. A study of within subject and between subject variation has reaffirmed that hematologic parameters have significant individuality. Screening using conventional reference limits may be misleading. Subject specific reference values are likely to have greater clinical utility.[4,5] There is modest progressive leukocytosis (due to neutrophils) throughout pregnancy into the third trimester with subsequent decline in white count after about 34 weeks gestation.[6] Included in the broad differential consideration for the cause of neutropenia is collagen-vascular disease, notably lupus erythematosus and other autoimmune neutropenias (see References). Many drugs result in leukopenia including bezafibrate, an antihyperlipidemic fibric acid.[7]
(Continued)

White Blood Count *(Continued)*

Footnotes

1. Solanki DL and Blackburn BC, "Spurious Leukocytosis and Thrombocytopenia. A Dual Phenomenon Caused by Clumping of Platelets *In Vitro*," *JAMA*, 1983, 250:2514-5.

2. Warner BA and Reardon DM, "A Field Evaluation of the Coulter STKS®," *Am J Clin Pathol*, 1991, 95(2):207-17.

3. Bentley SA, Johnson TS, Sohier CH, et al, "Flow-Cytochemical Differential Leukocyte Analysis With Quantitation of Neutrophil Left Shift. An Evaluation of the Cobas-Helios Analyzer," *Am J Clin Pathol*, 1994, 102(2):223-30.

4. Fraser CG, Wilkinson SP, Neville RG, et al, "Biologic Variation of Common Hematologic Laboratory Quantities in the Elderly," *Am J Clin Pathol*, 1989, 92(4):465-70.

5. Dot D, Miró J, and Feuntes-Arderiu X, "Within-Subject Biological Variation of Hematological Quantities and Analytical Goals," *Arch Pathol Lab Med*, 1992, 116(8):825-6.

6. Balloch AJ and Cauchi MN, "Reference Ranges for Haematology Parameters in Pregnancy Derived From Patient Populations," *Clin Lab Haematol*, 1993, 15(1):7-14.

7. Ariad S and Hechtlinger V, "Bezafibrate-Induced Neutropenia," *Eur J Haematol*, 1993, 50(3):179.

References

Christensen RD and Rothstein G, "Pitfalls in the Interpretation of Leukocyte Counts of Newborn Infants," *Am J Clin Pathol*, 1979, 72:608-11.

Hartman KR, "Anti-Neutrophil Antibodies of the Immunoglobulin M Class in Autoimmune Neutropenia," *Am J Med Sci*, 1994, 308(2):102-5.

Hoyer JD, "Leukocyte Differential," *Mayo Clin Proc*, 1993, 68(10):1027-8.

Second National Health and Nutrition Examination Survey, "Hematological and Nutritional Biochemistry Reference Data for Persons 6 Months to 74 Years of Age: United States, 1976-80," *Vital and Health Statistics*, DHHS Publication No (PHS) 83-1682, 1982.

Shastri KA and Logue GL, "Autoimmune Neutropenia," *Blood*, 1993, 81(8):1984-95.

White Count *see* White Blood Count *on previous page*

Zeta Sedimentation Rate, ESR *see* Zeta Sedimentation Ratio *on this page*

Zeta Sedimentation Ratio

CPT 85651 (nonautomated); 85652 (automated)

Related Information

Bacterial Culture, Burn Sites *on page 460*
C-Reactive Protein *on page 387*
Fibrinogen *on page 246*
Sedimentation Rate, Erythrocyte *on page 347*

Synonyms Erythrocyte Sedimentation Rate; Sed Rate; Zeta Sedimentation Rate, ESR; ZSR

Test Commonly Includes Sedimentation rate expressed in percent

Abstract An automated sedimentation rate method, which however is not entirely analogous to other ESR methods. The ZSR requires a special centrifuge (which is no longer under manufacture) for its performance.

Aftercare If results are equivocal or inconsistent with clinical impression, the C-reactive protein (CRP) is a useful test which is comparable and which also is an acute phase reactant.

Specimen Whole blood

Container Lavender top (EDTA) tube

Collection Specimen must be received within 4 hours of collection.

Causes for Rejection Insufficient blood, clotted specimen, hemolyzed specimen

Reference Range Younger than 50 years: <55%; 50-80 years: 40% to 60%

Use Nonspecific indicator of infectious disease and inflammatory states, reflects acute phase reactant levels; screen for collagen diseases; screen for and follow activity of rheumatic diseases, especially rheumatoid arthritis

Limitations The ZSR centrifuge is no longer produced. There are, however, many instruments still in use in the country. The majority of laboratories use the manual Westergren sed rate method (see Sedimentation Rate, Erythrocyte *on page 347*).

Methodology Standardized stress is applied to a column of red cells and the extent of red cell packing is determined.

Additional Information The ZSR is rapidly performed, reproducible, and independent of the hematocrit, requiring no hematocrit correction. Sedimentation rate is increased, generally, in cases of infection/inflammation/tissue necrosis, especially where fibrinogen and inflammatory or macroglobulins are increased. May be increased with pregnancy, malignancy, and dysproteinemias (eg, especially macroglobulinemia and myeloma). Sedimentation rate may be decreased in sickle cell disease and spherocytosis. Poikilocytosis acts to inhibit red cell sedimentation. Use of the ESR, ZSR, and/or CRP may aid in the differentiation of the anemia of chronic disease from iron deficiency.[1] In a series of 981 measurements, Bucher et al found the ZSR a useful monitor of disease activity and found good correlation with the Wintrobe or Westergren ESR.[2] Comparison of ZSR with modified Westergren ESR and with clinical assessment of disease activity in rheumatoid arthritis has shown good correlation.[3] The erythrocyte sedimentation rate (including the ZSR) is usually markedly elevated in temporal (giant cell) arteritis.[4]

Footnotes

1. Johnson MA, "Iron: Nutrition Monitoring and Nutrition Status Assessment," *J Nutr*, 1990, 120(Suppl 11):1486-91.

2. Bucher WC, Gall EP, and Becker PT, "The Zeta Sedimentation Ratio (ZSR) as the Routine Monitor of Disease Activity in a General Hospital," *Am J Clin Pathol*, 1979, 72:65-7.

3. Morris MW, Pinals RS, and Nelson DA, "The Zeta Sedimentation Ratio (ZSR) and Activity of Disease in Rheumatoid Arthritis," *Am J Clin Pathol*, 1977, 68:760-2.

4. Molloy DW, Brooymans MA, and Borrie MJ, "Acute Chest Pain in An Elderly Woman," *Can J Cardiol*, 1988, 4(3):144-5.

References

Stuart J and Nash GB, "Technological Advances in Blood Rheology," *Crit Rev Clin Lab Sci*, 1990, 28(1):61-93.

ZSR *see* Zeta Sedimentation Ratio *on this page*

Anemia Flowchart

The flowchart that follows is intended as an aid in diagnosis of anemia and is a supplement to this chapter to demonstrate how the entries might be placed in a logical order. The flowchart is not meant to replace a standard history and physical for diagnosis. Instead, it is intended as a teaching tool to develop patterns for test ordering in the work-up of anemia. Cost-effectiveness is made a prime concern. Thus, the beginning is based on the initial screen by the CBC, including the RDW. (See Complete Blood Count *on page 312* and the tables in that listing.) The method of Bessman has been adapted for this beginning classification. In real life, some diagnoses may not fit the flowchart exactly, but the majority of cases do. The bulk of the flowchart centers around the reticulocyte count (section C) and the reticulocyte production index (RPI). See Reticulocyte Count *on page 345* entry for more information.

It will soon become apparent that the flowchart often ends with the diagnosis of iron deficiency anemia. This should not be surprising since iron deficiency anemia is the most common cause of decreased hemoglobin, especially in the outpatient setting. Normal values for many tests will vary between laboratories. Use reference ranges (normal values) from your own laboratory when appropriate. This flowchart is not intended to cover every hematologic possibility.

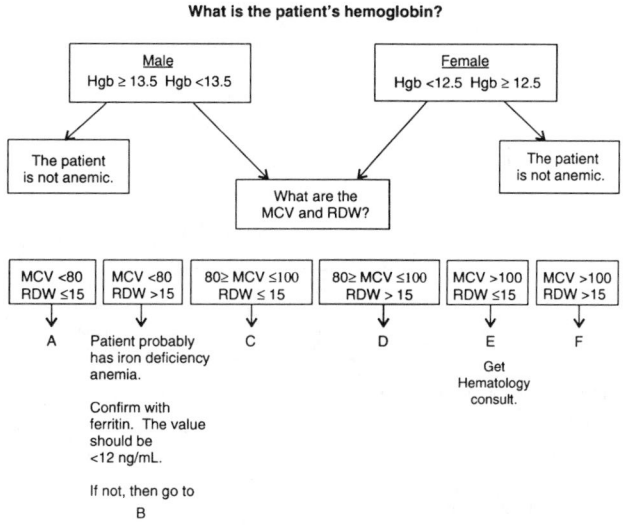

Footnotes
1. Bessman JD, "Improved Classification of Anemias by MCV and RDW," *Am J Clin Pathol,* 1983, 580:322-6.

A
What Is the RBC?

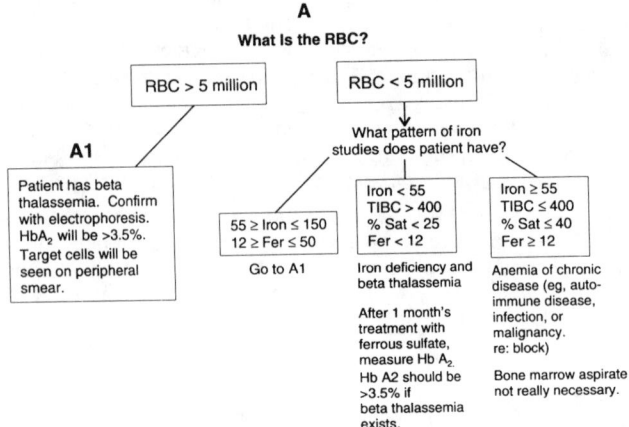

RBC > 5 million

RBC < 5 million

↓

What pattern of iron studies does patient have?

A1

Patient has beta thalassemia. Confirm with electrophoresis. HbA_2 will be >3.5%. Target cells will be seen on peripheral smear.

55 ≥ Iron ≤ 150
12 ≥ Fer ≤ 50

Go to A1

Iron < 55
TIBC > 400
% Sat < 25
Fer < 12

Iron deficiency and beta thalassemia

After 1 month's treatment with ferrous sulfate, measure Hb A_2. Hb A2 should be >3.5% if beta thalassemia exists.

Iron ≥ 55
TIBC ≤ 400
% Sat ≤ 40
Fer ≥ 12

Anemia of chronic disease (eg, auto-immune disease, infection, or malignancy. re: block)

Bone marrow aspirate not really necessary.

B

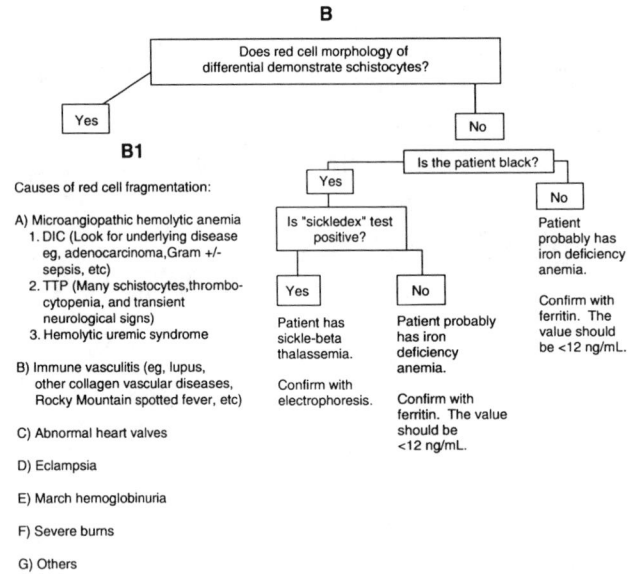

Does red cell morphology of differential demonstrate schistocytes?

Yes

No

B1

Causes of red cell fragmentation:

A) Microangiopathic hemolytic anemia
  1. DIC (Look for underlying disease eg, adenocarcinoma,Gram +/- sepsis, etc)
  2. TTP (Many schistocytes,thrombo-cytopenia, and transient neurological signs)
  3. Hemolytic uremic syndrome

B) Immune vasculitis (eg, lupus, other collagen vascular diseases, Rocky Mountain spotted fever, etc)

C) Abnormal heart valves

D) Eclampsia

E) March hemoglobinuria

F) Severe burns

G) Others

Is the patient black?

Yes

No

Is "sickledex" test positive?

No

Patient probably has iron deficiency anemia.

Confirm with ferritin. The value should be <12 ng/mL.

Yes

No

Patient has sickle-beta thalassemia.

Confirm with electrophoresis.

Patient probably has iron deficiency anemia.

Confirm with ferritin. The value should be <12 ng/mL.

C
What is the uncorrected reticulocyte count?

S = Single correction reticulocyte count

S = Ret Count x (.xx/.45), where .xx is patient's hematocrit

Double correction reticulocyte count or reticulocyte production index (RPI) is calculated by dividing the single correction reticulocyte count by the maturation index (T).

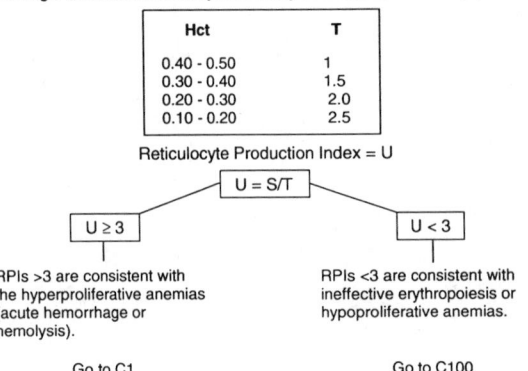

Hct	T
0.40 - 0.50	1
0.30 - 0.40	1.5
0.20 - 0.30	2.0
0.10 - 0.20	2.5

Reticulocyte Production Index = U

U = S/T

U ≥ 3

U < 3

RPIs >3 are consistent with the hyperproliferative anemias (acute hemorrhage or hemolysis).

Go to C1

RPIs <3 are consistent with ineffective erythropoiesis or hypoproliferative anemias.

Go to C100

C1

Tests to perform

Bilirubin
LDH
Urine Urobilinogen
Hemoglobinemia
Hemoglobinuria
Hemosiderinuria

and

Haptoglobin

Haptoglobin >25 mg/dL; Bleeding

Patient probably has an acute hemorrhage.

Of course, you are most likely aware of this because you are covered with the patient's blood.

However, patients can lose large volumes of blood internally and either have obvious sources (eg, esophogeal varices or duodenal ulcer) or not so obvious sources (eg, retroperitoneal blood or quadriceps bleed).

Haptoglobin <25 mg/dL; Hemolysis

The patient probably has a hemolytic anemia. Just a quick comment about the above tests. Bilirubin in hemolytic anemia is usually between 1.0 and 5.0 mg/dL. The majority (about 85%) should be indirect bilirubin. Urine urobilinogen may not be elevated unless the hemolysis is moderate to severe. The serum LDH isoezymes will show a flipped 1:2 pattern similar to that of an acute infarction of myocardium.

If the patient has intravascular hemolysis, hemoglobinemia, hemoglobinuria, and hemosiderinuria should be present. A bone marrow aspirate (usually not needed) will reveal erythroid hyperplasia with fairly normal maturation.

The next easiest and most cost-effective part of the work-up is to look at the differential.

C2

Does the patient have any of the following abnormal morphology?

C3) Sickle cells
C4) Hb C crystals
C5) Target cells
C6) Spherocytes
C7) Elliptocytes
C8) Acanthocytes
C9) Stomatocytes
C10) Schistocytes
C11) Malaria
C12) None of the above

C3

Do hemoglobin electrophoresis. The patient either has sickle cell disease (SS) or is doubly heterozygous (SC, SD, SO, S-thal, etc).

C4

The patient probably is homozygous Hb C. Confirm with electrophoresis.

C5

Three possibilities:

A) Liver disease...elevated enzymes, (AST, ALT, LDH, GGT, Alk Phos), decreased albumin, increased PT, etc.

B) Hemoglobin C trait or disease, confirm by electrophoresis.

C) Thalassemia, confirm with elevated A2 (>3.5%) by electrophoresis.

C6

Are the results of direct Coombs' test positive?

Yes

C13

Is IgG type positive?

Yes

1) Primary idiopathic warm reactive

2) Secondary warm reactive (eg, lymphoreticular malignancy, SLE, infectious mononucleosis)

3) Drug dependent warm reactive (eg, penicillin, quinidine, Aldomet®...take careful history)

No

Is complement only positive?

Yes

1) Idiopathic cold agglutinin disease

2) Secondary to *Mycoplasma*, infectious mononucleosis, lymphoma

3) PCH

No

Lab error IgG and/or complement are likely to be positive; repeat Coombs'.

Go to C2

No

What is MCHC?

Patient probably has hereditary spherocytosis.

The MCHC is usually >34 but can drop below during reticulocytosis, confirm diagnosis with osmotic fragility test.

The patient should have splenomegaly and a history of jaundice. The disease is inherited as an autosomal dominant.

C7

Have test repeated to assure that the result is not an artifact.

If results are repeatable then the diagnosis is hereditary elliptocytosis (very rarely of clinical significance).

C8

Due to:

1) Severe (end-stage) liver disease...do Liver Chem Profile.

2) Congenital abetalipoproteinemia Publish it!

C9

Patient has hereditary stomatocytosis, or smear may be an artifact.

C10

Causes of red cell fragmentation:

A) Microangiopathic hemolytic anemia.

   1) DIC (look for underlying disease eg, adenocarcinoma, Gram +/- sepsis, etc.)

   2) TTP (many schistocytes, thrombocytopenia, and transient neurological signs)

   3) Hemolytic uremic syndrome

B) Immune vasculitis (eg, lupus, other collagen vascular diseases, Rocky Mountain spotted fever, etc.)

C) Abnormal heart valves

D) Eclampsia

E) March hemoglobinuria

F) Severe burns

C12

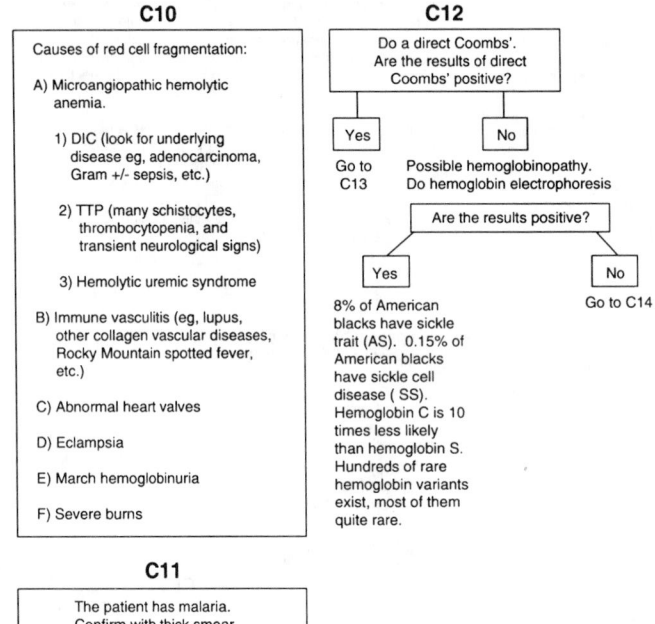

Do a direct Coombs'. Are the results of direct Coombs' positive?

Yes → Go to C13

No → Possible hemoglobinopathy. Do hemoglobin electrophoresis

Are the results positive?

Yes → 8% of American blacks have sickle trait (AS). 0.15% of American blacks have sickle cell disease (SS). Hemoglobin C is 10 times less likely than hemoglobin S. Hundreds of rare hemoglobin variants exist, most of them quite rare.

No → Go to C14

C11

The patient has malaria. Confirm with thick smear.

C14

Do PK and G-6-PD enzyme screens.

Is PK present?

Is G-6-PD present?

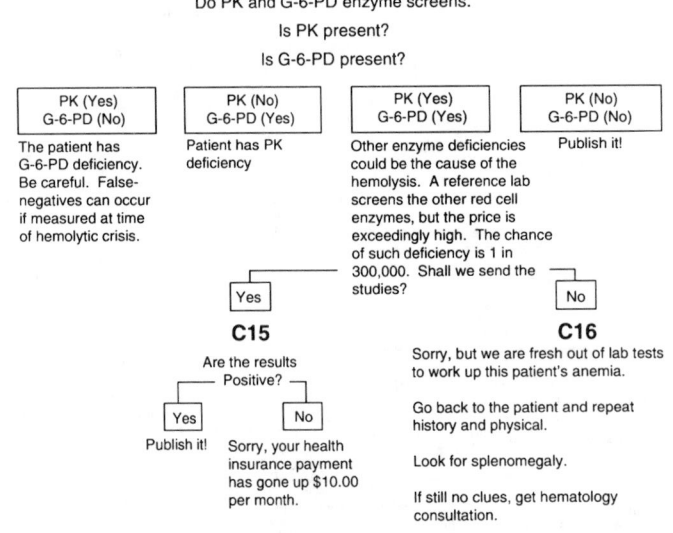

PK (Yes) G-6-PD (No)	PK (No) G-6-PD (Yes)	PK (Yes) G-6-PD (Yes)	PK (No) G-6-PD (No)
The patient has G-6-PD deficiency. Be careful. False-negatives can occur if measured at time of hemolytic crisis.	Patient has PK deficiency	Other enzyme deficiencies could be the cause of the hemolysis. A reference lab screens the other red cell enzymes, but the price is exceedingly high. The chance of such deficiency is 1 in 300,000. Shall we send the studies?	Publish it!

Yes

C15

Are the results Positive?

Yes → Publish it!

No → Sorry, your health insurance payment has gone up $10.00 per month.

No

C16

Sorry, but we are fresh out of lab tests to work up this patient's anemia.

Go back to the patient and repeat history and physical.

Look for splenomegaly.

If still no clues, get hematology consultation.

C25

What values does patient have?
B_{12} Folate and RBC Folate

300> B_{12} <1000 Folate <2 RBC Folate <200	B_{12} <300 Folate >2 RBC Folate >200	B_{12} <300 Folate <2 RBC Folate <200	Any other combination?
Patient has folate deficiency. The bone marrow aspirate will show hyperplastic, megaloblastic changes.	The patient has B_{12} deficiency. Do Schilling test, Parts 1 & 2, to distinguish gastric from ileal problem. The bone marrow aspirate will show hyperplastic, megaloblastic changes.	The patient has both B_{12} and folate deficiencies. The bone marrow aspirate will show hyperplastic, megaloblastic changes.	Do bone marrow aspirate and biopsy and evaluate microscopically. A) Myelophthisic state - this will show crowding out of the normal hematopoietic elements of the bone marrow by leukemia, metastic carcinoma, TB, etc. B) Hypoplasia/aplasia - bone marrow will show decrease in erythrocytic precursors only (pure red cell aplasia) or panhypoplasia of marrow elements. C) Endocrinopathy - slight hypoplasia due to Hashimoto's thyroiditis, Addison's disease, etc. Do appropriate endocrine tests. D) Normal marrow - get home consult.

C100

What pattern of iron studies does patient have?

Iron < 55 TIBC > 400 % Sat < 25 Fer < 12	Iron < 55 TIBC ≤ 400 % Sat ≤ 40 Fer > 12	Iron > 150 TIBC < 250 % Sat > 25 Fer > 50	55 ≥ Iron ≤ 150 12 ≥ Fer ≤ 50	Any other combination
The patient has iron deficiency. A bone marrow is not necessary, but would show absence of stainable iron.	Anemia of chronic disease, (autoimmune disease, infection, or malignancy... re: iron block)	The patient has sideroblastic anemia, either congenital, or acquired (lead poisoning, alcohol, isoniazid, etc).	**A1** Patient has beta thalassemia. Confirm with electrophoresis. Hb A will be >3.5%. Target cells will be seen on peripheral smear.	What is patient's BUN?

For "Any other combination":

What is patient's BUN?

BUN ≤ 50	BUN > 50
Go to C25	Chronic renal failure

Bone marrow will show hypoplasia due to lack of erythropoietin and toxicity of urea.

D

The patient has a normocytic, heterogeneous anemia.
Probable early iron, sideroblastic, or folate deficiency (or mixed deficiency)

What values does patient have for ferritin and RBC folate?

Fer <12 RBC Folate <200	Fer >12 RBC Folate <200	Fer >50 RBC Folate <200	Fer <12 RBC Folate >200	12< Fer <50 RBC Folate >200	Fer >50 RBC Folate >200
The patient has mixed iron and folate deficiency.	The patient has early folate deficiency.	The patient has a mixed sideroblastic anemia and folate deficiency... Publish It!	The patient has early iron deficiency anemia.	Is the patient black?	The patient has sideroblastic anemia, confirm with observation of ringed sideroblasts in the bone marrow.

For "Is the patient black?":

Yes	No
Do hemoglobin electrophoresis.	Go to D2

Results positive?

Yes	No
The patient has an "anemic" hemoglobinopathy, probably hemoglobin SS or SC.	

D2

The patient may have myelofibrosis. The differential should show a leukoerythroblastic reaction (nucleated RBCs and young WBC's).

Do bone marrow aspirate and biopsy to confirm.

If not myelofibrosis, repeat CBC and let's see what else might have caused the

F

Do Coombs' test
Are results of direct Coombs' test positive?

Yes

No
Go to F2

Is IgG type positive?

Yes

No

Is the complement only positive?

Yes

No

1) Primary idiopathic warm reactive

2) Secondary warm reactive (eg, lympho-reticular malignancy, SLE, infectious mono-nucleosis)

3) Drug dependent warm reactive (eg, penicillin, quinidine, Aldomet®... take careful history).

1) Idiopathic cold agglutinin disease

2) Secondary to *Mycoplasma,* infectious mononucleosis, lymphoma

3) PCH (actual IgG - do Donath-Landsteiner test).

Lab error; IgG and/or complement has to be positive: repeat Coombs'.

Go to F

F2

Macrocytic, heterogeneous anemia

What pattern of iron studies does patient have?

300> B_{12} <1000 Folate <2 RBC Folate <200	B_{12} <300 Folate >2 RBC Folate >200	B_{12} <300 RBC Folate <200	Any other combination?
The patient has folate deficiency.	The patient has B_{12} deficiency.	The patient has both B_{12} and folate deficiencies.	Do bone marrow aspirate and biopsy and evaluate microscopically.
Go to F3	Do Schilling test, Part 1 & 2 to distinguish gastric from ileal problems. Go to F3	Go to F3	If the diagnosis is not apparant then repeat CBC and begin work-up again.

F3

The bone marrow aspirate will show hyperplastic, megaloblastic changes.

IMMUNOLOGY AND SEROLOGY

David S. Jacobs, MD

Rebecca T. Horvat, PhD

Contributors:
Christopher J. Papasian, PhD
Wayne R. DeMott, MD
Phillip Munoz, MD
Fred V. Plapp, MD, PhD
Lowell Tilzer, MD, PhD
Christopher F. Bryan, PhD

The traditional approaches used to investigate serologic responses to disease were labor-intensive, as well as insensitive and nonspecific. Automation of serologic tests, broad availability of monoclonal antibody reagents, and dramatic improvements in flow cytometry instrumentation and software have combined to expand the readily available capabilities for immunologic evaluation of many clinical laboratories. Generally, diagnosis of disease by immunoassay involves either the detection of specific antibody or specific antigen.

The tests for antibodies may detect all classes of immunoglobulins or may be specific for IgG, IgM, or IgA. Often, detection of antibody requires paired sera, one drawn during the acute phase of disease and one during convalescence. Detection of autoimmune antibodies may require an interpretation of specific patterns. The Immunology and Serology tests in this book include useful assays that improve the diagnosis of specific diseases. However, the actual reading of some assays can be subjective. In addition, specifics of each test and potential problems and applications are included in each listing.

Many new assays and markers are available for subtyping lymphoproliferative disorders, following patients with immunodeficiency diseases, and detecting unusual infections. Whereas many of these provide diagnostically useful information, we must be cautious in our enthusiasm about new technologies to avoid unnecessary costs.

A table listing viruses that are nonculturable or that require animal inoculation or special technique is provided in a listing Viral Culture *on page 676*. Such entities bear serologic/immunologic considerations.

The authors express appreciation to Dr David F. Keren, who provided numerous additions and enhancements to the Immunology and Serology test listings in the 3rd edition of the *Laboratory Test Handbook*.

A₁AT *see* Alpha₁-Antitrypsin, Serum *on next page*

ACA *see* Anticardiolipin Antibody *on page 364*

Acetylcholine Modulating Antibody *see* Acetylcholine Receptor Antibody *on this page*

Acetylcholine Receptor Antibody

CPT 84238

Related Information

Antinuclear Antibody *on page 368*
Rheumatoid Factor *on page 427*
Striational Antibodies *on page 432*
Thyroid Antimicrosomal Antibody *on page 433*
Thyroid Antithyroglobulin Antibody *on page 434*

Synonyms Acetylcholine Modulating Antibody; Receptor Blocking Antibody; Receptor Modulating Antibody

Applies to Edrophonium Chloride Test; Prostigmin® Test; Rapid Nerve Stimulation Test; Single-Fiber Electromyographic Test

Abstract Myasthenia gravis (MG) represents autoimmune damage against postsynaptic acetylcholine receptors at the neuromuscular junction, causing muscular weakness and fatigability. Involvement of extraocular and general voluntary muscles is found. Ptosis and diplopia usually occur early. Swallowing is likely to be affected. MG is characterized by severe fatigue with exertion. There is some relief after rest.

Specimen Serum

Container Red top tube

Storage Instructions Separate serum and freeze in plastic vial

Causes for Rejection Recent radioactive scan

Reference Range Normal: <0.03 nmol/L; 1-20 nmol/L in 50% of patients; 20-400 nmol/L in 50% of patients

Critical Values A positive assay is specific.

Use Investigate myasthenia gravis

Limitations Poor concordance between antibody titer and clinical activity. Use of nonhuman substrates may produce false-negative results. Antibodies are not found in congenital (genetic) myasthenia. Uncommonly, false positives occur.

Contraindications Recent radioactive scan

Methodology Radioimmunoassay (RIA), enzyme-linked immunosorbent assay (ELISA). The target antigen is acetylcholine receptor.

Additional Information Antibodies to acetylcholine receptors are present in 90% of patients with generalized MG and in 75% to 80% of patients with ocular disease. Such antibodies bind to a site different from that which binds acetylcholine or α-bungarotoxin, and receptor injury may be mediated by complement. The specificity of the antibodies vary from patient to patient. Subjects with myasthenia gravis have heterogeneous types of acetylcholine receptor antibodies. Those patients with antibody that inhibits the binding of α-bungarotoxin (a snake toxin) pursue an aggressive course. Antibodies to the neurotransmitter binding site (receptor blocking antibodies) can be detected in 30% of patients with myasthenia. Receptor modulating antibodies are present in 90% of myasthenic patients, and may be useful in patients with recent onset of disease. MG is often associated with other autoantibodies (striational antibody 50%, thyroglobulin antibodies 40%) and with HLA-B8 and DR3. Sixty-six percent have thymic hyperplasia and up to 15% develop thymoma. Other autoimmune diseases associated with MG include thyroiditis, Graves' disease, rheumatoid arthritis, and lupus erythematosus.

Laboratory investigations recommended for myasthenia patients include antinuclear antibody, rheumatoid factor, antithyroid antibodies, thyroxine, and fasting glucose.

Genetically determined cases make up 5% to 10% of instances of MG and may be either presynaptic or postsynaptic.

Other tests for MG include the **edrophonium chloride test**, **Prostigmin® test**, and two electromyographic tests, **rapid nerve stimulation test** and **single-fiber electromyographic test**.

The diagnosis and differential diagnosis have recently been reviewed.[1,2] Treatment is with immunosuppression with or without therapeutic plasma exchange.

Footnotes

1. Drachman DB, "Myasthenia Gravis," *N Engl J Med*, 1994, 330(25):1797-810.
2. Faulkner WR, "Diagnosis and Misdiagnosis of Myasthenia Gravis," *Lab Rep* 1995, 17(2):9-14.

References

Bigazzi PE, Burek CL, and Rose NR, "Antibodies to Tissue-Specific Endocrine, Gastrointestinal, and Surface-Receptor Antigens," *Manual of Clinical Laboratory Immunology*, 4th ed, Vol 2, Rose NR, Conway de Macario E, Fahey JL, et al, eds, Washington, DC: American Society for Microbiology, 1992, 765-74.

Colvin RB, Bhan AK, and McCluskey RT, *Diagnostic Immunopathology*, New York, NY: Raven Press, 1988, 112.

Lennon VA and Howard FM, "Serological Diagnosis of Myasthenia Gravis" *Clinical Lab Molecular Analyses*, Nakamura RM and O'Sullivan MB, eds, New York, NY: Grune and Stratton Inc, 1985, 29-44.

Pachner AR, "Antiacetylcholine Receptor Antibodies Block Bungarotoxin Binding to Native Human Acetylcholine Receptor on the Surface of TE671 Cells," *Neurology*, 1989, 39(8):1057-61.

ACL *see* Anticardiolipin Antibody *on page 364*

Acquired Immune Deficiency Syndrome Serology *see* HIV-1/HIV-2 Serology *on page 403*

Acute Phase Reactant *see* Alpha₁-Antitrypsin, Serum *on next page*

Acute Phase Reactant *see* C-Reactive Protein *on page 387*

Adenovirus Antibody Titer

CPT 86603

Related Information

Adenovirus Culture *on page 662*
Bacterial Culture, Conjunctiva *on page 461*
Viral Culture *on page 675*
Viral Culture, Body Fluid *on page 677*
Viral Culture, Respiratory Symptoms *on page 680*
Virus, Direct Detection by Fluorescent Antibody *on page 682*

Synonyms Adenovirus Serology

Specimen Serum

Container Red top tube

Collection Acute and convalescent sera drawn 2-4 weeks apart

Special Instructions Acute and convalescent sera must be tested simultaneously. Tests should, therefore, not be performed unless both specimens are received.

Reference Range A fourfold or greater increase in titer in paired sera is indicative of a recent virus infection. Expected value single specimen: ≤1:2.

Use Establish adenovirus as the etiologic agent for respiratory ailments including pneumonia and tonsillitis, fever and chills, gastroenteritis, hemorrhagic cystitis and keratoconjunctivitis including swimming pool conjunctivitis.

Limitations Adenovirus infections are relatively common and circulating antibody may be long-lasting. Consequently, titers on unpaired sera are essentially uninterpretable.

Methodology Complement fixation (CF), hemagglutination inhibition (HAI), enzyme-linked immunosorbent assay (ELISA), serum neutralization

Additional Information There are 47 different types of adenovirus, and infections may vary from asymptomatic to persistent. Thus, serologic evidence of adenovirus, and even isolation of an adenovirus from a patient, may be coincidental rather than the cause of the patient's present complaints. Genus-reactive tests may be followed by serotype-specific tests, if epidemiologically warranted.

References

Abzug MJ and Levin MJ, "Neonatal Adenovirus Infection: Four Patients and Review of the Literature," *Pediatrics*, 1991, 87(6):890-6.

Hierholzer JC, "Adenoviruses," *Manual of Clinical Laboratory Immunology*, 4th ed, Vol 2, Rose NR, Conway de Macario E, Fahey JL, et al, eds, Washington, DC: American Society for Microbiology, 1992, 590-5.

Adenovirus Serology *see* Adenovirus Antibody Titer *on this page*

Adhesion Molecule CD31 *see* HLA Typing, Single Human Leukocyte Antigen *on page 405*

ADNase-B *see* Antideoxyribonuclease-B Titer, Serum *on page 365*

Agglutinins, Febrile *see* Febrile Agglutinins, Serum *on page 393*

AHT *see* Antihyaluronidase Titer *on page 365*

AIDS Screen *see* HIV-1/HIV-2 Serology *on page 403*

Alpha₁-Antitrypsin Phenotyping

CPT 82104

Related Information

Alpha₁-Antitrypsin, Serum *on next page*
Liver Biopsy *on page 48*
Liver Profile *on page 161*
Protein Electrophoresis, Serum *on page 424*

Synonyms α₁-AT Phenotype; Pi Phenotype

Applies to Protease Inhibitors

Test Commonly Includes Serum trypsin inhibitory capacity

Abstract Alpha₁-antitrypsin (α₁-AT) deficiency (alpha₁-protease inhibitor deficiency) is a genetic predisposition characterized by varying levels of severity. α_1-AT is a glycoprotein which is the largest fraction (65%) in the alpha$_1$ globulins. Patients are detected by lack or diminution of the alpha$_1$ band on serum protein electrophoresis, abnormal migration of the alpha$_1$ band or by decreased levels determined immunochemically.

Cases of emphysema which are caused by hereditary α_1-AT deficiency make up about 1% to 2% of the incidence of emphysema.

Patient Preparation Fasting preferred

Specimen Serum

Container Red top tube

Sampling Time Misleading results can follow sampling during acute illness; *vide infra*.

Storage Instructions Separate serum and refrigerate or freeze.

Reference Range Interpretation usually accompanies report; phenotypes are designated. Pi•MM phenotype is normal; Pi•MZ is heterozygous, intermediate deficient; and Pi•ZZ is homozygous, severely deficient. Over 75 alleles are described; over 30 deficient genetic variants are recognized.[1] Biosynthesis of α_1-AT is controlled at the Pi locus by a pair of genes. There is codominant expression. The phenotype is "Pi" for protease inhibitor. Z and S are mutant proteins. A null-null state occurs as well. In a dysfunctional type, α_1-AT is found in normal amounts but does not function normally.

Use Definitive analysis of hereditary α_1-AT deficiency, which is associated with chronic obstructive pulmonary disease (COPD) (panacinar or panlobular emphysema), hepatic cirrhosis, and hepatoma. α_1-AT deficiency is not an uncommon cause of neonatal cholestasis. Cholestasis with neonatal hepatitis is found in a minority of neonates with α_1-AT deficiency. Such neonatal hepatitis leads to cirrhosis. In addition to pulmonary and hepatic manifestations, evidence exists that α_1-AT deficiency may play a role in other entities in many of which inflammation and/or immune components exist. These diseases are thought to include severe erosive rheumatoid arthritis, panniculitis, membranoproliferative glomerulonephritis, uveitis, and vascular aneurysms, including aortic, large artery (eg, colic) and intracranial ones. Pi typing of patients with aneurysms is recommended.[2,3]

Methodology Crossed immunoelectrophoresis, isoelectric focusing in a narrow range pH gradient. Use of high-resolution electrophoresis which would detect the slower electrophoretic migration of the Z and S variants is preferred over quantification of α_1-AT by nephelometry as a screen for this deficiency. Further, a high-resolution electrophoretic system will detect heterozygotes which could lead to important family studies of potentially deficient first-degree relatives who may benefit from therapy.

Additional Information Most pathologic is homozygous ZZ. An M null genotype will have phenotype as MM but low serum level of α_1-AT. Alpha$_1$-antitrypsin deficiency may eventuate in or be associated with cholestatic hepatopathy in infants, a chronic hepatitis, familial infantile cirrhosis, or familial emphysema. The risks of cirrhosis and development of hepatoma are greater in males.

α_1-AT is a glycoprotein synthesized in the liver. It is the main component of the alpha$_1$ globulins. α_1-AT serves to counter the effects of several serine proteases including elastase and trypsin. α_1-AT represents about 90% of serum antiprotease capacity.[1] When α_1-AT is deficient, unopposed activity of these enzymes results in emphysema. Cigarette smoke is reported to inactivate α_1-AT.[1] The age of occurrence of emphysema varies with the type of deficiency, ZZ being most severe. Among children, severe ZZ α_1-AT deficiency most frequently presents as liver disease, cholestasis, and cirrhosis. Over 80% of individuals with ZZ ultimately develop chronic lung or liver disease.[1] ZS is less severe and SS least severe. SS is the second most common deficient category. Severity varies with the personal habits of the individual, especially regarding smoking.

In individuals with α_1-AT deficiency, PAS-positive diastase-resistant globules accumulate in periportal hepatocytes. The Z protein self-aggregates. An immunoperoxidase procedure for α_1-AT is available. Cirrhosis may develop.

It is especially important to detect α_1-AT deficiency early, as an experimental replacement therapy is now available.[1] Although the long-term effects of this therapy are still unknown, it does have great potential to decrease the severity of emphysema.

α_1-AT is a positive acute phase protein because it rises whenever there is tissue injury, necrosis, inflammation, or infection. Therefore, patients with α_1-AT deficiency who suffer from bronchitis, pneumonia, or similar respiratory inflammation may have falsely normal levels during acute illness. After the acute phase of illness has passed, repeat determinations often reveal the "true" or "resting" α_1-AT level which is indicative of the heterozygous phenotypic deficiency.

Serum α_1-AT may be increased in patients during normal pregnancy, chronic pulmonary diseases, hereditary angioneurotic edema, gastric diseases, liver diseases, pancreatitis, diabetes, carcinomas, renal

diseases, and rheumatic diseases and may be decreased in patients with severe protein loss or in improper storage of specimen.

More than 95% of subjects who are severely deficient are homozygous for the Z allele (Pi•ZZ). Pi•ZZ subjects who smoke have a shorter life expectancy than do nonsmoking Pi•ZZ persons. SS and SZ types bear association with decreased alpha$_1$-antitrypsin levels. Variation in severity of clinical manifestations is recognized; some subjects with deficiency do not have significant impairment, but development of airway disease is partly a function of age. Pulmonary disease develops in cigarette smokers about 15 years earlier.[1]

The significance of α_1-AT deficiency bears legal, insurance, and other implications which have recently been addressed.[1]

Footnotes

1. Wulfsberg EA, Hoffmann DE, and Cohen MM, "Alpha$_1$-Antitrypsin Deficiency. Impact of Genetic Discovery on Medicine and Society," *JAMA*, 1994, 271(3):217-22.
2. Cox DW, "Alpha$_1$-Antitrypsin: A Guardian of Vascular Tissue," *Mayo Clin Proc*, 1994, 69(11):1123-4 (editorial).
3. Schievink WI, Björnsson J, Parisi JE, et al, "Arterial Fibromuscular Dysplasia Associated With Severe Alpha$_1$-Antitrypsin Deficiency," *Mayo Clin Proc*, 1994, 69(11):1040-3.

References

Buist AS, "Alpha 1-Antitrypsin Deficiency - Diagnosing Treatment and Control: Identification of Patients," *Lung*, 1990, 168(Suppl):543-51.
Cohen AB, "Unraveling the Mysteries of Alpha$_1$-Antitrypsin Deficiency," *N Engl J Med*, 1986, 314(12):778-9.
Crystal RG, "Alpha-1-Antitrypsin Deficiency: Pathogenesis and Treatment," *Hosp Pract (Off Ed)*, 1991, 26(2):81-4, 88-9, 93-4.
Eriksson S, Carlson J, and Velez R, "Risk of Cirrhosis and Primary Liver Cancer in Alpha$_1$-Antitrypsin Deficiency," *N Engl J Med*, 1986, 314(12):736-9.
Garver RI Jr, Mornex JF, Nukiwa T, et al, "Alpha$_1$-Antitrypsin Deficiency and Emphysema Caused by Homozygous Inheritance of Nonexpressing Alpha$_1$-Antitrypsin Genes," *N Engl J Med*, 1986, 314(12):762-66.
Hutchison DC, "Natural History of Alpha-1-Protease Inhibitor Deficiency," *Am J Med*, 1988, 84(6A):3-12.
Keren DF, *High-Resolution Electrophoresis and Immunofixation: Techniques and Interpretation*, Boston, MA: Butterworth's Publishers, 1987, 31-5.
Schmidt EW, Rasche B, Ulmer WT, et al, "Replacement Therapy for Alpha-1-Protease Inhibitor Deficiency in PiZ Subjects With Chronic Obstructive Lung Disease," *Am J Med*, 1988, 84(6A):63-9.
Silverman EK, Pierce JA, Province MA, et al, "Variability of Pulmonary Function in Alpha$_1$-Antitrypsin Deficiency: Clinical Correlates," *Ann Intern Med*, 1989, 111(12):982-91.
Snider GL, "Pulmonary Disease in Alpha$_1$-Antitrypsin Deficiency," *Ann Intern Med*, 1989, 111(12):957-9.
Weinberger SE, "Recent Advances in Pulmonary Medicine," *N Engl J Med*, 1993, 328(19):1389-97.

Alpha$_1$-Antitrypsin, Serum

CPT 82103

Related Information

Alpha$_1$-Antitrypsin Phenotyping *on previous page*
C-Reactive Protein *on page 387*
Liver Profile *on page 161*
Protein Electrophoresis, Serum *on page 424*

Synonyms A$_1$AT; α_1-AT

Applies to Acute Phase Reactant; Protease Inhibitors

Abstract Deficiency of α_1-antitrypsin (α_1-AT) was described in 1963. It may present as emphysema, classically in smokers younger than 40 years of age. α_1-antitrypsin is the most abundant of proteinase inhibitors (Pi) in plasma.[1]

Specimen Serum. Prenatal diagnosis is possible.

Container Red top tube

Reference Range 126-226 mg/dL[1] (SI: 1.26-2.26 g/L), method dependent

Critical Values Levels <70 mg/dL (SI: <0.70 g/L) are likely to correlate with homozygous deficiency; subjects having levels <140 mg/dL (SI: <1.40 g/L) should be phenotyped.

Use Detect hereditary decreases in the production of alpha$_1$-antitrypsin (α_1-AT) (see listing Alpha$_1$-Antitrypsin Phenotyping *on page 362*). Decreased or nearly absent levels of α_1-AT is an important factor in chronic obstructive lung disease and liver disease. An increased prevalence of non-MM phenotypes is found with cryptogenic cirrhosis and with chronic liver disease. Cirrhosis in a child should raise consideration of α_1-AT deficiency or Wilson's disease.

Limitations α_1-AT may be elevated into normal range in heterozygous deficient patients during concurrent infection, pregnancy, estrogen therapy, steroid therapy, cancer, and during postoperative periods. Homozygous deficient patients will not show such elevation. Normal α_1-AT levels may occur in patients with liver disease who are heterozygotes. In normals, pregnancy and contraceptive medication may elevate levels. Levels are normally low at birth but rise soon thereafter. α_1-AT is often elevated in inflammatory states (eg, rheumatoid arthritis, bacterial infection, vasculitis, neoplasia).

Contraindications If CRP positive, retest α_1-AT in 10-14 days.

Methodology Radial immunodiffusion (RID), nephelometry

(Continued)

Alpha₁-Antitrypsin, Serum (Continued)

Additional Information This assay should be run when alpha₁ globulin in serum protein electrophoresis is low, when two bands are seen in the alpha₁ region, when the alpha₁ region is obscured by alpha₁ lipoprotein and especially on clinical indications. Heterozygous patients (Pi•MZ phenotype) exhibit α₁-AT levels which are commonly about 60% of normal. Homozygous (Pi•ZZ phenotype) patients exhibit activity levels of about 10% to 18% of normal. Phenotyping is desirable on patients with low values and on all patients being worked up for α₁-AT-deficient liver disease. Most pathologic is homozygous state ZZ. An M null genotype will have phenotype as MM but a low serum level. α₁-AT is one of the alpha globulins which together are called "acute phase reactants". These rise rapidly, but nonspecifically, in response to inflammatory insults.

Footnotes
1. Cox DW, "α₁-Antitrypsin: A Guardian of Vascular Tissue," *Mayo Clin Proc*, 1994, 69(11):1123-4 (editorial).

References
Brantly ML, Wittes JT, Vogelmeier CF, et al, "Use of a Highly Purified Alpha₁-Antitrypsin Standard to Establish Ranges for the Common Normal and Deficient Alpha₁-Antitrypsin Phenotypes," *Chest*, 1991, 100(3):703-8.
Hodges JR, Millward-Sadler GH, Barbatis C, et al, "Heterozygous MZ Alpha₁ Antitrypsin Deficiency in Adults With Chronic Active Hepatitis and Cryptogenic Cirrhosis," *N Engl J Med*, 1981, 304:557-68.

Alternate Complement Pathway *see* Factor B *on page 393*

AMA *see* Antimitochondrial Antibody *on page 366*

Amebiasis Serological Test *see* Entamoeba histolytica Serological Test *on page 391*

Amyloid A, Serum *see* C-Reactive Protein *on page 387*

Amyloid Beta Peptide *see* Cerebrospinal Fluid Amyloid Precursor Protein and Amyloid β-Protein *on page 376*

β-Amyloid Peptide *see* Cerebrospinal Fluid Tau Protein *on page 382*

Amyloid Precursor Protein (APP), CSF *see* Cerebrospinal Fluid Amyloid Precursor Protein and Amyloid β-Protein *on page 376*

ANA *see* Antinuclear Antibody *on page 368*

ANCA *see* Antineutrophil Cytoplasmic Antibody *on page 367*

ANF *see* Antinuclear Antibody *on page 368*

Antiactin Antibodies *see* Smooth Muscle Antibody *on page 431*

Anti-B19 IgG Antibodies *see* Parvovirus B19 Serology *on page 422*

Anti-B19 IgM Antibodies *see* Parvovirus B19 Serology *on page 422*

Antibody to Double-Stranded DNA *see* Anti-DNA *on next page*

Antibody to HAV, IgM *see* Hepatitis A Antibody, IgM *on page 396*

Antibody to Hepatitis B Core Antigen *see* Hepatitis B Core Antibody *on page 396*

Antibody to Hepatitis B Surface Antigen *see* Hepatitis B Surface Antibody *on page 398*

Antibody to Native DNA *see* Anti-DNA *on next page*

Anticardiolipin Antibody

CPT 86147

Related Information
Anticoagulant, Circulating *on page 229*
Antinuclear Antibody *on page 368*
Automated Reagin Test *on page 370*
Hypercoagulable State Coagulation Screen *on page 250*
Inhibitor, Lupus, Phospholipid Type *on page 251*
RPR *on page 428*
Sjögren's Antibodies *on page 430*
VDRL, Serum *on page 438*

Synonyms ACA; ACL

Applies to Antiphospholipid Antibody; Lupus Anticoagulant (LA)

Test Commonly Includes Detection of IgG, IgM, and IgA antibody to the phospholipid, cardiolipin

Abstract The **antiphospholipid antibody syndrome** is characterized by recurrent clinical events: noninflammatory thrombosis of small or large arteries and/or veins and fetal loss, with antiphospholipid antibodies, anticardiolipin antibody (ACA) or lupus anticoagulant. They are autoantibodies found in subjects with systemic lupus erythematosus and related entities[1], lupus-like diseases, infectious diseases, and drug reactions. The syndrome is primary if SLE is not present. When patients who have SLE and also have antiphospholipid antibodies with corresponding clinical features, cases are designated as the secondary antiphospholipid antibody syndrome.

Specimen Serum

Container Red top tube

Storage Instructions Repeated freeze-thaw cycles alters stability of anticardiolipin antibodies.[2]

Reference Range Negative

Critical Values Only moderately positive (16-80 G phospholipid [GPL] units) and highly positive (>80 GPL units) may be clinically relevant[3], but a question of adequacy of clinical data has been addressed.[4]

Use Differential diagnosis of recurrent thromboses, lupus-like syndromes, false-positive VDRL or RPR, recurrent fetal loss, and rarely, severe hemorrhage

Limitations Anticardiolipin levels by enzyme-linked immunosorbent assay (ELISA) are associated with poor reproducibility.

Methodology Enzyme-linked immunosorbent assay (ELISA)[5] for IgG or IgM anticardiolipin antibody

Additional Information Antibody to a cardiolipin, the diphosphatidyl glycerol component of many phospholipid membranes, is at least partially cross reactive with the reagin antibody of syphilis and the lupus anticoagulant. The commonality between these diseases is the antibody against phosphate groups (lupus-DNA; VDRL-phospholipid of cardiolipin; and ACA - the antibody against phospholipids of the coagulation system). ACA is associated with a host of clinical and laboratory abnormalities. Abnormal tests include thrombocytopenia, reactive VDRL or RPR, SS-A/Ro antibodies, and prolonged activated partial thromboplastin time (APTT) (lupus anticoagulant). Clinically, patients have lupus-like symptoms, often "ANA negative," recurrent venous and arterial thromboses, recurrent fetal loss (usually more than two episodes for a strong association), mitral valve endocarditis, chorea, and epilepsy. The entire constellation is sometimes called the antiphospholipid antibody syndrome. The association between thrombosis and recurrent fetal loss and ACA in patients with a prolonged APTT is especially strong in patients in whom ACA is not induced by infection or medication. IgG anticardiolipin is more influenced by disease activity than is IgM anticardiolipin. Plasmapheresis along with anticoagulant therapy is often used in symptomatic cases. Lupus anticoagulant and anticardiolipin antibodies are found together in about 70% of patients with antiphospholipid antibody syndrome. LA is found in about 34% and ACA is found in 44% of subjects with SLE.[6] An increased incidence of antiphospholipid antibodies has been found among patients with monoclonal gammopathy of undetermined significance.[7]

See listing Inhibitor, Lupus, Phospholipid Type *on page 251.*

Footnotes
1. Love PE and Santoro SA, "Antiphospholipid Antibodies: Anticardiolipin and the Lupus Anticoagulant in Systemic Lupus Erythematosus (SLE) and in Non-SLE Disorders," *Ann Intern Med*, 1990, 112(9):682-98.
2. Brey RL, Cote SA, McGlasson DL, et al, "Effects of Repeated Freeze-Thaw Cycles on Anticardiolipin Antibody Immunoreactivity," *Am J Clin Pathol*, 1994, 102(5):586-8.
3. Infante-Rivard C, David M, Gauthier R, et al, "Lupus Anticoagulants, Anticardiolipin Antibodies, and Fetal Loss," *N Engl J Med*, 1992, 326(14):953-4 (letter).
4. Lockshin MD and Sammaritano LR, "Antiphospholipid Antibodies and Fetal Loss," *N Engl J Med*, 1992, 326(14):951-4.
5. Harris EN, Pierangeli S, and Birch D, "Anticardiolipin Wet Workshop Report. Fifth International Symposium on Antiphospholipid Antibodies," *Am J Clin Pathol*, 1994, 101(5):616-24.
6. Arnold WJ and Ike RW, "Specialized Procedures in the Management of Patients With Rheumatic Diseases," *Cecil Textbook of Medicine*, Vol 2, Wyngaarden JB, Smith LH Jr, and Bennett JC, eds, Philadelphia, PA: WB Saunders Co, 1992, 1505.
7. Stern JJ, Ng RH, Triplett DA, et al, "Incidence of Antiphospholipid Antibodies in Patients With Monoclonal Gammopathy of Undetermined Significance," *Am J Clin Pathol*, 1994, 101(4):471-4.

References
Alving BM, Barr CF, and Tang DB, "Correlation Between Lupus Anticoagulants and Anticardiolipin Antibodies in Patients With Prolonged Activated Partial Thromboplastin Times," *Am J Med*, 1990, 88(2):112-6.
Boumpas DT, Fessler BJ, Austin HA 3rd, et al, "Systemic Lupus Erythematosus: Emerging Concepts. Part 2: Dermatologic and Joint Disease, the Antiphospholipid Antibody Syndrome, Pregnancy and Hormonal Therapy, Morbidity and Mortality, and Pathogenesis," *Ann Intern Med*, 1995, 123(1):42-53.
"Case Records of the Massachusetts General Hospital. Weekly Clinicopathological Exercises. Case 37-1988. A 35-Year-Old Woman With Recurrent Strokes, an Intracardiac Lesion, Anemia, and Thrombocytopenia," *N Engl J Med*, 1988, 319(11):699-712.
Creagh MD, Malia RG, Cooper SM, et al, "Screening for Lupus Anticoagulant and Anticardiolipin Antibodies in Women With Fetal Loss," *J Clin Pathol*, 1991, 44(1):45-7.
Deegan MJ, "Antiphospholipid Antibodies," *Am J Clin Pathol*, 1992, 98(4):390-1.
Greisman SG, Thayaparan RS, Godwin TA, et al, "Occlusive Vasculopathy in Systemic Lupus Erythematosus. Association With Anticardiolipin Antibody," *Arch Intern Med*, 1991, 151(2):389-92.
Khamashta MA, Cuadrado MJ, Mujic F, et al, "The Management of Thrombosis in the Antiphospholipid-Antibody Syndrome," *N Engl J Med*, 1995, 332(15):993-7.
Khamashta MA and Hughes GR, "Detection and Importance of Anticardiolipin Antibodies. ACP Broadsheet No 136," *J Clin Pathol*, 1993, 46(2):104-7.
Levine SR and Welch KM, "The Spectrum of Neurologic Disease Associated With Antiphospholipid Antibodies - Lupus Anticoagulants and Anticardiolipin Antibodies," *Arch Neurol*, 1987, 44(8):876-83.

Lockshin MD, "Answers to the Antiphospholipid-Antibody Syndrome?" *N Engl J Med*, 1995, 332(15):1025-7.

Lopez LR, Santos ME, Espinoza LR, et al, "Clinical Significance of Immunoglobulin A *Versus* Immunoglobulins G and M Anticardiolipin Antibodies in Patients With Systemic Lupus Erythematosus - Correlation with Thrombosis, Thrombocytopenia, and Recurrent Abortion," *Am J Clin Pathol*, 1992, 98(4):449-54.

Antideoxyribonuclease-B Titer, Serum

CPT 86215

Related Information

Antihyaluronidase Titer *on this page*

Antistreptolysin O Titer, Serum *on page 369*

Bacterial Culture, Throat *on page 468*

Group A *Streptococcus* Screen, Rapid *on page 483*

Streptozyme *on page 432*

Synonyms ADNase-B; Anti-DNase-B Titer; Antistreptococcal DNase-B Titer; Streptodornase

Specimen Serum

Container Red top tube

Reference Range Children: preschool: ≤60 units; school: ≤170 units; adults: ≤85 units; a rise in titer of two or more dilution increments between acute and convalescent sera is significant.

Use Document recent streptococcal infection

Limitations Normal ranges may vary in different populations; test must use a pure source of DNase-B to ensure specificity.

Contraindications Not valid in patients with hemorrhagic pancreatitis

Methodology Colorimetry based on hydrolysis of DNA

Additional Information DNase-B is antigenically the most consistent of four streptococcal DNases. Presence of antibodies to streptococcal DNase is an indicator of recent infection, especially if a rise in titer can be documented. This test has advantages over the ASO test: It is more sensitive to streptococcal pyoderma, it is not as subject to false-positives due to liver disease, reagents are not likely to oxidize, and it is not affected by the site of infection. It is positive, like ASO, in about 80% to 85% of patients with streptococcal infections. Application of both tests detects about 95%.[1] Used together, each is helpful.

Footnotes

1. Leavelle DE, *Mayo Medical Laboratories Interpretive Handbook*, Rochester, MN: Mayo Medical Laboratories, 1994, 404-5.

References

Pacifico L, Mancuso M, Properzi E, et al, "Comparison of Nephelometric and Hemolytic Techniques for Determination of Antistreptolysin O Antibodies," *Am J Clin Pathol*, 1995, 103(4):396-9.

Weinstein AJ and Farkas S, "Serologic Tests in Infectious Diseases: Clinical Utility and Interpretation," *Med Clin North Am*, 1978, 62:1099-1118.

Anti-DNA

CPT 86225 (double-stranded); 86226 (single-stranded)

Related Information

Antinuclear Antibody *on page 368*

C3 Complement, Serum *on page 373*

Complement, Total, Serum *on page 386*

Kidney Profile *on page 153*

LE Cell Test *on page 330*

Scleroderma Antibody *on page 430*

Sjögren's Antibodies *on page 430*

Urinalysis *on page 658*

Synonyms Antibody to Double-Stranded DNA; Antibody to Native DNA; Anti-Double-Stranded DNA; Anti-ds-DNA; DNA Antibody; n-DNA; ss-DNA

Applies to Anti-Sm

Test Commonly Includes Titers on positive specimens

Abstract IgG autoantibodies to ds-DNA are found characteristically in subjects with SLE and only rarely with other connective tissue diseases. The other autoantibody bearing relative specificity for SLE is anti-Sm, but its incidence is less. Anti-ss-DNA is less specific.

Specimen Serum

Container Red top tube

Storage Instructions Refrigerate immediately.

Reference Range Normal: low levels of antibody or none (units and reference range will depend on laboratory and methodology)

Use Confirmatory test for systemic lupus erythematosus (SLE); monitor clinical course and response to treatments

Limitations False-positive tests due to antibodies against histones have been reported with use of the *Crithidia luciliae* substrate assay but are rare using calf thymus DNA.[1]

Methodology Enzyme-linked immunosorbent assay (ELISA), indirect fluorescent antibody (IFA) using *Crithidia luciliae* substrate, radioimmunoassay (RIA), enzyme immunoassay (EIA)

Additional Information Antibodies to DNA, either single or double-stranded, are found primarily in systemic lupus erythematosus and are

important for diagnosis of that condition. IgG antibodies to ds-DNA are present in 60% of active SLE cases. They may be present in smaller fractions of patients with other rheumatic disorders and in chronic active hepatitis, infectious mononucleosis, and biliary cirrhosis. In part, sensitivity for the different diseases is methodology dependent, and correlation with local laboratory experience is necessary.

In the past it was a rule of thumb that it was unnecessary to test for anti-DNA in patients with a negative test for antinuclear antibodies. A group of "ANA-negative" lupus patients has been described with anti-ss-DNA and anti-SS-A/Ro and anti-SS-B/La. However, HEp-2 substrate is much more sensitive than frozen section substrates; and it is uncommon for anti-SS-A/Ro to be negative with such substrates.

Procainamide and hydralazine may induce anti-ss-DNA antibodies and antihistone antibodies.

Following titers of anti-DNA antibody may be of use in evaluating response to therapy, but should be regarded as a guide rather than a rigid dictator of treatment. Titers correlate with activity of lupus nephritis, but ANA and anti-DNA antibodies are less reliably related to active progressive lupus glomerulonephritis than are C3 and CH50 complement depression.[2]

Antibodies to ss-DNA are not as diagnostically useful as those against ds-DNA which are associated with renal disease and clinical activity. Patients at risk for severe nephritis are characterized by persistent abnormal urinalysis, high levels of anti-ds-DNA and/or diminished complement.[3]

Other tests relevant to SLE additional to the complements include CBC, ESR, urinalysis with urine sediment microscopy, urinary protein excretion, and creatinine. Creatinine and creatinine clearance, however, are relatively insensitive to deterioration of glomerular filtration rate in lupus nephritis.[2]

Footnotes

1. Leavelle DE, *Mayo Medical Laboratories Interpretive Handbook*, Rochester, MN: Mayo Medical Laboratories, 1994.
2. Boumpas DT, Austin HA 3d, Fessler BJ, et al, "Systemic Lupus Erythematosus: Emerging Concepts. Part 1: Renal, Neuropsychiatric, Cardiovascular, Pulmonary, and Hematologic Disease," *Ann Intern Med*, 1995, 122(12):940-50.
3. Hahn BH, "Systemic Lupus Erythematosus," *Harrison's Principles of Internal Medicine*, 13th ed, Isselbacher KJ, Braunwald E, Wilson JD, et al, eds, New York, NY: McGraw-Hill Inc, 1994.

References

Carson DA, "The Specificity of Anti-DNA Antibodies in Systemic Lupus Erythematosus," *J Immunol*, 1991, 146(1):1-2.

Homburger HA, "Cascade Testing for Autoantibodies in Connective Tissue Diseases," *Mayo Clin Proc*, 1995, 70(2):183-4.

James K and Meek G, "Evaluation of Commercial Enzyme Immunoassays Compared to Immunofluorescence and Double Diffusion for Autoantibodies Associated With Autoimmune Diseases," *Am J Clin Pathol*, 1992, 97(4):559-65.

Mills JA, "Systemic Lupus Erythematosus," *N Engl J Med*, 1994, 330(26):1871-9.

Anti-DNase-B Titer *see* Antideoxyribonuclease-B Titer, Serum *on this page*

Anti-Double-Stranded DNA *see* Anti-DNA *on this page*

Anti-ds-DNA *see* Anti-DNA *on this page*

Anti-ER Antibodies *see* Liver/Kidney Microsomal Type 1 Antibodies *on page 415*

Anti-F Actin *see* Smooth Muscle Antibody *on page 431*

Anti-GBM *see* Glomerular Basement Membrane Antibody *on page 395*

Antigliadin Antibody *see* Endomysial Antibodies *on page 391*

Antiglomerular Basement Membrane Antibody *see* Glomerular Basement Membrane Antibody *on page 395*

Anti-HAV, IgM *see* Hepatitis A Antibody, IgM *on page 396*

Anti-HB$_c$ *see* Hepatitis B Core Antibody *on page 396*

Anti-HB$_e$ *see* Hepatitis B$_e$ Antibody *on page 397*

Anti-HB$_s$ *see* Hepatitis B Surface Antibody *on page 398*

Anti-HCV (IgM) *see* Hepatitis C Serology *on page 399*

Antihistidyl-Transfer RNA (tRNA) Synthetase *see* Myositis-Specific Autoantibody *on page 420*

Antihistidyl Transfer tRNA Synthase *see* Jo-1 Antibody *on page 411*

Antihyaluronidase Titer

CPT 86060 (ASO titer); 86215 (antideoxyribonuclease-B titer)

Related Information

Antideoxyribonuclease-B Titer, Serum *on this page*

Antistreptolysin O Titer, Serum *on page 369*

Bacterial Culture, Throat *on page 468*

Kidney Biopsy *on page 47*

(Continued)

Antihyaluronidase Titer (Continued)

Streptozyme *on page 432*

Synonyms AHT; Antistreptococcal Hyaluronidase Titer

Test Commonly Includes Antideoxyribonuclease-B, antihyaluronidase titer, ASO titer

Patient Preparation A fasting specimen is preferred.

Specimen Serum

Container Red top tube

Reference Range A fourfold rise in titer between acute and convalescent specimens is significant, regardless of the magnitude of the titer. For a single specimen, titers ≤1:250 are considered normal.

Use Document recent streptococcal infection; investigation of glomerulonephritis

Limitations Test is less reproducible than ASO or anti-DNase-B.

Methodology Tube enzyme neutralization test

Additional Information In addition to ASO, antihyaluronidase is used to aid in the diagnosis of streptococcal infections. Combined with antideoxyribonuclease-B, it leads to nearly 100% proof of prior infection.[1] It is better than the ASO test for the detection of antibodies in acute glomerulonephritis which follows a streptococcal pyoderma.

Footnotes

1. Berry PH and Brewer ED, "Glomerular Nephritis and Nephrotic Syndrome," *Principles and Practice of Pediatrics*, 2nd ed, Oski FA, DeAngelis CD, Feigin RD, et al, eds, Philadelphia, PA: JB Lippincott Co, 1994, 1785-802.

Anti-immunoglobulin A *see* IgA Antibodies *on page 407*

Anti-Ku Autoantibodies *see* Myositis-Specific Autoantibody *on page 420*

Antiliver Cytosol 1 Antibodies *see* Liver/Kidney Microsomal Type 1 Antibodies *on page 415*

Antiliver/Kidney Microsomal Antibodies *see* Liver/Kidney Microsomal Type 1 Antibodies *on page 415*

Anti-LKM1 *see* Liver/Kidney Microsomal Type 1 Antibodies *on page 415*

Anti-Mi-2 Autoantibodies *see* Myositis-Specific Autoantibody *on page 420*

Antimitochondrial Antibody

CPT 86255 (IFA)

Related Information

Antineutrophil Antibody *on this page*
Antineutrophil Cytoplasmic Antibody *on next page*
Liver Biopsy *on page 48*
Liver/Kidney Microsomal Type 1 Antibodies *on page 415*
Liver Profile *on page 161*
Smooth Muscle Antibody *on page 431*

Synonyms AMA; Mitochondrial Antibody

Abstract Primary biliary cirrhosis (PBC) is a progressive cholestatic disease in which intrahepatic bile ducts undergo damage, leading ultimately to cirrhosis and hepatic failure. Mitochondrial antibodies are found in up to 90% of patients with primary biliary cirrhosis, but may be found in other circumstances as well.[1] They are usually absent in subjects with extrahepatic jaundice.

Specimen Serum

Container Red top tube

Reference Range ≤1:20 considered nondiagnostic

Use Tests for mitochondrial antibody are needed in differential diagnosis of chronic liver disease and to provide confirmatory evidence for diagnosis of PBC

Limitations Titers <1:16 seen in 10% of cases of primary biliary cirrhosis. Level of antibody does not correlate with severity or duration of disease. Low, transient titers are sometimes seen with chlorpromazine or halothane sensitivity. AMA negativity in sera of subjects with PBC may be induced by decreased immunoreactivity to M2 proteins,[2] *vide infra*.

Methodology Indirect fluorescent antibody (IFA), enzyme-linked immunosorbent assay (ELISA)

Additional Information AMA is also found in cryptogenic cirrhosis and in 25% to 30% of cases which have been classified as chronic active hepatitis. AMA is rarely found in patients with extrahepatic biliary obstruction, drug-induced hepatitis, viral hepatitis, alcoholic and other forms of cirrhosis, and hepatic malignancy. There is an incidence of 1% positives in a general hospital population, mostly people with autoimmune disease. PBC is a chronic intrahepatic cholestatic disease found most frequently in women with an incidence which is highest in the 35- to 60-year age group. The diagnosis of PBC is based upon clinical observations including pruritus and often fatigue, and malabsorption of fat soluble vitamins, histologic findings on liver biopsy, increased serum alkaline phosphatase activity and cholesterol, elevated IgM levels, and presence of mitochondrial antibodies. Increases of 5′-nucleotidase and gamma-glutamyl transferase parallel those of alkaline phosphatase. In >90% of patients, the key M2 antigen has been identified as the E_2 component of the pyruvate dehydrogenase complex. Enzyme-linked immunosorbent assays developed using pyruvate, branched-chain keto-acid, and alpha-ketoglutarate dehydrogenase promise to add objectivity to analysis of these antibodies.

An overlap syndrome is recognized in which histopathologic features of autoimmune hepatitis accompany antimitochondrial antibodies.[3]

A group of AMA-negative PBC patients all had ANA titers, often high.[4]

With pruritus and high serum alkaline phosphatase, autoimmune cholangiopathy resembles primary biliary cirrhosis or primary sclerosing cholangitis but lacks antimitochondrial antibodies.[3]

Antineutrophil cytoplasmic antibody may prove helpful in the differential diagnosis between PBC and primary sclerosing cholangitis.[5]

Footnotes

1. Kaplan MM, "Primary Biliary Cirrhosis," *N Engl J Med*, 1987, 316(9):521-8.
2. Kitami N, Ishii H, Shimizu H, et al, "Immunoreactivity to M2 Proteins in Antimitochondrial Antibody-Negative Patients With Primary Biliary Cirrhosis," *J Gastroenterol Hepatol*, 1994, 9(1):7-12.
3. Krawitt EL, "Autoimmune Hepatitis," *N Engl J Med*, 1996, 334(14):897-903.
4. Michieletti P, Wanless IR, Katz A, et al, "Antimitochondrial Antibody Negative Primary Biliary Cirrhosis: A Distinct Syndrome of Autoimmune Cholangitis," *Gut*, 1994, 35(2):260-5.
5. Hardarson S, Labrecque DR, Mitros FA, et al, "Antineutrophil Cytoplasmic Antibody in Inflammatory Bowel and Hepatobiliary Diseases. High Prevalence in Ulcerative Colitis, Primary Sclerosing Cholangitis, and Autoimmune Hepatitis," *Am J Clin Pathol*, 1993, 99(3):221-3.

References

Berg PA and Klein R, "Antimitochondrial Antibodies in Primary Biliary Cirrhosis and Other Disorders: Definition and Clinical Relevance," *Dig Dis*, 1992, 10(2):85-101.

Brenard R and Geubel AP, "Antimitochondrial and Antinuclear Antibodies in Primary Biliary Cirrhosis: An Update in Relation to Their Biochemical Characterization and Clinical Significance," *Acta Clin Belg*, 1991, 46(5):305-12.

Butler P, Valle F, and Burroughs AK, "Mitochondrial Antigens and Antibodies in Primary Biliary Cirrhosis," *Postgrad Med J*, 1991, 67(791):790-7.

Fussey SP, West SM, Lindsay JG, et al, "Clarification of the Identity of the Major M2 Autoantigen in Primary Biliary Cirrhosis," *Clin Sci*, 1991, 80(5):451-5.

Heseltine L, Turner IB, Fussey SP, et al, "Primary Biliary Cirrhosis. Quantitation of Autoantibodies to Purified Mitochondrial Enzymes and Correlation With Disease Progression," *Gastroenterology*, 1990, 99(6):1786-92.

Klein R, Huizenga JR, Gips CH, et al, "Antimitochondrial Antibody Profiles in Patients With Primary Biliary Cirrhosis Before Orthotopic Liver Transplantation and Titres of Antimitochondrial Antibody-Subtypes After Transplantation," *J Hepatol*, 1994, 20(2):181-9.

Klion FM, Fabry TL, Palmer M, et al, "Prediction of Survival of Patients With Primary Biliary Cirrhosis," *Gastroenterology*, 1992, 102(1):310-3.

Neuberger J, Lombard M, and Galbraith R, "Primary Biliary Cirrhosis," *Gut*, 1991, S73-8.

Perros P, Palmer JM, Yeaman SJ, et al, "Antimitochondrial Antibodies in Patients With Graves' Disease May Not Signify Primary Biliary Cirrhosis," *Postgrad Med J*, 1994, 70(819):17-8.

Provenzano G, Diquattro O, Craxi A, et al, "Immunoblotting as a Confirmatory Test for Antimitochondrial Antibodies in Primary Biliary Cirrhosis," *Gut*, 1993, 34(4):544-8.

Van de Water J, Cooper A, Surh CD, et al, "Detection of Autoantibodies to Recombinant Mitochondrial Proteins in Patients With Primary Biliary Cirrhosis," *N Engl J Med*, 1989, 320(21):1377-80.

Yeaman SJ, Fussey SP, Danner DJ, et al, "Primary Biliary Cirrhosis: Identification of Two Major M2 Mitochondrial Autoantigens," *Lancet*, 1988, 1(8594):1067-70.

Yoshida T, Bonkovsky H, Ansari A, et al, "Antibodies Against Mitochondrial Dehydrogenase Complexes in Primary Biliary Cirrhosis," *Gastroenterology*, 1990, 99(1):187-94.

Antineutrophil Antibody

CPT 86255 (screen); 86256 (titer)

Related Information

Antimitochondrial Antibody *on this page*
Transfusion Reaction Work-up *on page 625*
White Blood Count *on page 353*

Synonyms Granulocyte Antibody; Neutrophil Antibody

Abstract Neutrophil autoantibodies may be the result of prior transfusion or pregnancy and may cause transfusion-related acute lung injury (TRALI). It was felt in the past that antineutrophil antibodies were responsible for febrile reactions. It is now known that febrile reactions are caused by Interleukin-1, -6, and -8 as well as tumor necrosis factor (TNF). They may cause alloimmune neonatal neutropenia. The neutropenia of systemic lupus erythematosus, Felty's syndrome, and other autoimmune diseases may relate to neutrophil antigen-antibody complexes.

Specimen Serum

Container Red top tube

Collection Venipuncture

Storage Instructions Remove serum from clot as soon as possible. Freeze serum.

Reference Range Negative

Use Investigate for possible immune origin of neutropenia; detect antibodies against granulocyte-specific antigens to evaluate neonatal alloimmune neutropenia, autoimmune neutropenia, and transfusion reactions.

Limitations In cases of severe neutropenia, inability to obtain sufficient sample may preclude or impair testing. A positive result in autoimmune neutropenia does not distinguish between allo- and autoantibodies.

Methodology Antiglobulin assay (direct or indirect), immunofluorescence (direct or indirect) utilizing flow cytometry, agglutination, cytotoxicity, staphylococcal protein A binding

Additional Information Advances in antibody detection have made possible the detection of autoantibodies specific for neutrophils. Autoantibodies to the antigen sites NA-1, NA-2, NB-1, NC-1, and 9a may be detected providing compelling evidence for the existence of autoimmune neutropenia. In some patients with autoimmune neutropenia, autoantibodies have specificity to actin. This condition is associated with idiopathic thrombocytopenic purpura and responds to steroids. Resulting neutropenia may be moderate to severe.

References

Dale DC, "Neutropenia," *Williams Hematology*, 5th ed, Chapter 81, Beutler E, Lichtman MA, Coller BS, et al, eds, New York, NY: McGraw-Hill Inc, 1995, 815-24.

Ferrara JL, "The Febrile Platelet Transfusion Reaction: A Cytokine Shower," *Transfusion*, 1995, 35(2):89-90.

Hartman KR, Mallet MK, Nath J, et al, "Antibodies to Actin in Autoimmune Neutropenia," *Blood*, 1990, 75(3):736-43.

Logue GL, Shastri KA, Laughlin M, et al, "Idiopathic Neutropenia: Antineutrophil Antibodies and Clinical Correlations," *Am J Med*, 1991, 90(2):211-6.

Popovsky MA, Chaplin HC Jr, and Moore SB, "Transfusion-Related Acute Lung Injury: A Neglected, Serious Complication of Hemotherapy," *Transfusion*, 1992, 32(6):589-92.

Antineutrophil Cytoplasmic Antibody

CPT 86255 (screen); 86256 (titer)

Related Information

Antimitochondrial Antibody *on previous page*

Glomerular Basement Membrane Antibody *on page 395*

Kidney Biopsy *on page 47*

Kidney Profile *on page 153*

Synonyms ANCA

Applies to c-ANCA; p-ANCA; Proteinase 3 (PR3)

Abstract ANCAs are autoantibodies that are directed against neutrophil granules and lysosomes of monocytes.

Specimen Serum

Container Red top tube; do **not** use serum separator tube.

Reference Range Negative; titer falls with remission

Use The pathologic triad of Wegener's granulomatosis (WG) includes granulomatous inflammation of the upper and lower respiratory tract, vasculitis, and necrotizing-crescentic glomerulonephritis. **c-ANCA represents the most useful marker available for WG and its variants.**

Reactivity with **p-ANCA** includes subjects who have rheumatoid arthritis with or without vasculitis or Felty's syndrome, alveolar hemorrhage, angiitis/polyangiitis, vasculitis, leukocytoclastic skin vasculitis, necrotizing-crescentic glomerulonephritis, inflammatory bowel disease, autoimmune liver disease, and Churg-Strauss syndrome.[1] Differences in character of pulmonary disease respectively with c-ANCA and p-ANCA are described,[2] but relationships of each to pulmonary disease are established.[3,4]

ANCA determinations can be utilized to distinguish between vasculitic disease activity and effects of therapy.[5]

ANCA may be useful in the differential diagnosis of ulcerative colitis and to separate primary biliary cirrhosis from sclerosing cholangitis.[6,7]

Limitations Technically demanding; requires expert interpretation of fluorescent patterns. A negative result does not exclude the diagnosis of Wegener's granulomatosis.[8] Serum dilutions vary between laboratories. Titer readings between laboratories are not necessarily comparable.

Methodology Indirect immunofluorescence on ethanol-fixed neutrophil cytocentrifuge preparation, follow up with antimyeloperoxidase ELISA for p-ANCA

Additional Information Serum antibodies against components of neutrophil cytoplasm can be demonstrated in patients with Wegener's granulomatosis (WG) and other forms of vasculitis. Two major patterns of reactivity are seen when the indirect fluorescent antibody technique is used - diffuse (centrally accentuated) cytoplasmic staining (**c-ANCA**, formerly ACPA) and perinuclear staining (**p-ANCA**). The c-ANCA pattern is caused by antibodies to proteinase 3 (PR3) in neutrophil and monocyte granules[1], whereas the p-ANCA has several reactivities including myeloperoxidase, cathepsin G, and neutrophil elastase. c-ANCA is reported in 88% of patients with active WG and 43% of those in remission.[9] Unless the procedure is done with utmost critical evaluation of the patterns of immunofluorescence, there will be unacceptable nonspecificity.

Reactivity has been described in rare cases of SLE.

Footnotes

1. Specks U and Homburger HA, "Antineutrophil Cytoplasmic Antibodies," *Mayo Clin Proc*, 1994, 69(12):1197-8.

2. Jennette JC and Falk RJ, "The Coming of Age of Serologic Testing for Antineutrophil Cytoplasmic Autoantibodies," *Mayo Clin Proc*, 1994, 69(9):908-10.

3. Gal AA, Salinas FF, and Staton GW Jr, "The Clinical and Pathlogical Spectrum of Antineutrophil Cytoplasmic Autoantibody-Related Pulmonary Disease. A Comparison Between Perinuclear and Cytoplasmic Antineutrophil Cytoplasmic Autoantibodies," *Arch Pathol Lab Med*, 1994, 118(12):1209-14.

4. Gaudin PB, Askin FB, Falk RJ, et al, "The Pathologic Spectrum of Pulmonary Lesions in Patients With Anti-Neutrophil Cytoplasmic Autoantibodies Specific for Anti-Proteinase 3 and Anti-Myeloperoxidase," *Am J Clin Pathol*, 1995, 104(1):7-16.

5. Markey BA and Warren JS, "Use of Anti-Neutrophil Cytoplasmic Antibody Assay to Distinguish Between Vasculitic Disease Activity and Complications of Cytotoxic Therapy," *Am J Clin Pathol*, 1994, 102(5):589-94.

6. Hardarson S, LaBrecque DR, Mitros FA, et al, "Antineutrophil Cytoplasmic Antibody in Inflammatory Bowel and Hepatobiliary Diseases. High Prevalence in Ulcerative Colitis, Primary Sclerosing Cholangitis, and Autoimmune Hepatitis," *Am J Clin Pathol*, 1993, 99(3):277-81.

7. Sung JY, Chan KL, Hsu R, et al, "Ulcerative Colitis and Antineutrophil Cytoplasmic Antibodies in Hong Kong Chinese," *Am J Gastroenterol*, 1993, 88(6):864-9.

8. Colby TV, Tazelaar HD, Specks U, et al, "Nasal Biopsy in Wegener's Granulomatosis," *Hum Pathol*, 1991, 22(2):101-4.

9. Hoffman GS, Kerr GS, Leavitt RY, et al, "Wegener Granulomatosis: An Analysis of 158 Patients," *Ann Intern Med*, 1992, 116(6):488-98.

References

Bonsib SM, Goeken JA, Fandel T, et al, "Necrotizing Medullary Lesions in Patients With ANCA Associated Renal Disease," *Mod Pathol*, 1994, 7(2):181-5.

Bonsib SM, Goeken JA, Kemp JD, et al, "Coexistent Anti-Neutrophil Cytoplasmic Antibody and Antiglomerular Basement Membrane Antibody Associated Disease: Report of Six Cases," *Mod Pathol*, 1993, 6(5):526-30.

Braun MG, Csernok E, Gross WL, et al, "Proteinase 3, the Target Antigen of Anticytoplasmic Antibodies Circulating in Wegener's Granulomatosis. Immunolocalization in Normal and Pathologic Tissues," *Am J Pathol*, 1991, 139(4):831-8.

Broekroelofs J, Mulder AH, Nelis GF, et al, "Antineutrophil Cytoplasmic Antibodies (ANCA) in Sera From Patients With Inflammatory Bowel Disease (IBD). Relation to Disease Pattern and Disease Activity," *Dig Dis Sci*, 1994, 39(3):545-9.

Cats HA, Tervaert JW, van Wijk R, et al, "Anti-Neutrophil Cytoplasmic Antibodies in Giant Cell Arteritis and Polymyalgia Rheumatica," *Adv Exp Med Biol*, 1993, 336:363-6.

Cohen-Tervaert JW, van der Woude FJ, Fauci AS, et al, "Association Between Active Wegener's Granulomatosis and Anticytoplasmic Antibodies," *Arch Intern Med*, 1989, 149(11):2461-5.

Davenport A, Lock RJ, Wallington TB, et al, "Clinical Significance of Antineutrophil Cytoplasm Antibodies Detected by a Standardized Indirect Immunofluorescence Assay," *Q J Med*, 1994, 87(5):291-9.

De Remee RA, Homburger HA, and Specks U, "Lesions of the Respiratory Tract Associated With the Finding of Antineutrophil Cytoplasmic Autoantibodies With a Perinuclear Staining Pattern," *Mayo Clin Proc*, 1994, 69(9):819-24.

Fannin SW, Hagley MT, Seibert JD, et al, "Bronchocentric Granulomatosis, Acute Renal Failure, and High Titer Antineutrophil Cytoplasmic Antibodies: Possible Variants of Wegener's Granulomatosis," *J Rheumatol*, 1993, 20(3):507-9.

Fienberg R, Mark EJ, Goodman M, et al, "Correlation of Antineutrophil Cytoplasmic Antibodies With the Extrarenal Histopathology of Wegener's (Pathergic) Granulomatosis and Related Forms of Vasculitis," *Hum Pathol*, 1993, 24(2):160-8.

Gruber R, Brockmeyer C, Hoechtien-Vollmar W, et al, "Detection of Antineutrophil Cytoplasmic Antibodies (ANCA) and Their Association With Other Autoantibodies in Patients With Hepatobiliary Disorders," *Adv Exp Med Biol*, 1993, 336:539-44.

Guzman J, Fung M, and Petty RE, "Diagnostic Value of Anti-Neutrophil Cytoplasmic and Anti-Endothelial Cell Antibodies in Early Kawasaki Disease," *J Pediatr*, 1994, 124(6):917-20.

Jennette JC and Falk RJ, "Antineutrophil Cytoplasmic Autoantibodies in Inflammatory Bowel Disease," *Am J Clin Pathol*, 1993, 99(3):221-3.

Juby A, Johnston C, Davis P, et al, "Antinuclear and Antineutrophil Cytoplasmic Antibodies (ANCA) in the Sera of Patients With Felty's Syndrome," *Br J Rheumatol*, 1992, 31(3):185-8.

Kalina PH, Garrity JA, Herman DC, et al, "Role of Testing for Anticytoplasmic Autoantibodies in the Differential Diagnosis of Scleritis and Orbital Pseudotumor," *Mayo Clin Proc*, 1990, 65(8):1110-7.

Kerr GS, Fleisher TA, Hallahan CW, et al, "Limited Prognostic Value of Changes in Antineutrophil Cytoplasmic Antibody Titers in Patients With Wegener's Granulomatosis," *Adv Exp Med Biol*, 1993, 336:411-4.

Leaker B and Cambridge G, "Clinical Use of Antineutrophil Cytoplasmic Antibodies," *Br J Hosp Med*, 1993, 50(9):540-7.

Lesavre P, "Antineutrophil Cytoplasmic Autoantibodies Antigen Specificity," *Am J Kidney Dis*, 1991, 18(2):159-63.

Mulder AH, Broekroelofs J, Horst G, et al, "Antineutrophil Antibodies in Inflammatory Bowel Disease Recognize Different Antigens," *Adv Exp Med Biol*, 1993, 336:519-22.

Mulder AH, Horst G, van Leeuwen MA, et al, "Antineutrophil Cytoplasmic Antibodies in Rheumatoid Arthritis. Characterization and Clinical Correlations," *Arthritis Rheum*, 1993, 36(8):1054-60.

Nölle B, Specks U, Lüdemann J, et al, "Anticytoplasmic Autoantibodies: Their Immunodiagnostic Value in Wegener's Granulomatosis," *Ann Intern Med*, 1989, 111(1):28-40.

Proujansky R, Fawcett PT, Gibney KM, et al, "Examination of Anti-Neutrophil Cytoplasmic Antibodies in Childhood Inflammatory Bowel Disease," *J Pediatr Gastroenterol Nutr*, 1993, 17(2):193-7.

Specks U, Rohrbach MS, and De Remee RA, "Antineutrophil Cytoplasmic Autoantibodies," *N Engl J Med*, 1988, 319(21):1416-7.

Specks U, Wheatley CL, McDonald TJ, et al, "Anticytoplasmic Autoantibodies in the Diagnosis and Follow-Up of Wegener's Granulomatosis," *Mayo Clin Proc*, 1989, 64(1):28-36.

Sung JY, Chan FK, Lawton J, et al, "Anti-Neutrophil Cytoplasmic Antibodies (ANCA) and Inflammatory Bowel Diseases in Chinese," *Dig Dis Sci*, 1994, 39(4):886-92.

Ulmer M, Rautmann A, and Gross WL, "Immunodiagnostic Aspects of Autoantibodies Against Myeloperoxidase," *Clin Nephrol*, 1992, 37(4):161-8.

Velosa JA, Homburger HA, and Holley KE, "Prospective Study of Anti Neutrophil Cytoplasmic Autoantibody Tests in the Diagnosis of Idiopathic Necrotizing-Crescentic Glomerulonephritis and Renal Vasculitis," *Mayo Clin Proc*, 1993, 68(6):561-5.

Wieslander J, "How Are Antineutrophil Cytoplasmic Autoantibodies Detected?" *Am J Kidney Dis*, 1991, 18(2):154-8.

Antinuclear Antibody

CPT 86038; 86039 (titer); 86255 (fluorescent screen); 86256 (fluorescent titer)

Related Information

Synonyms ANA; ANF; FANA

Applies to Extractable Nuclear Antigens (ENA); MA Antibody; Nucleolar Antibody; RNP Antibody; Scl-70; Sm Antibody; SS-A/Ro; SS-B/La; U_1RNP

Test Commonly Includes Titers and pattern of nuclear fluorescence on positive samples

Abstract The antinuclear antibody (ANA) test detects autoantibodies which are directed against a variety of antigens which reside mainly in the nucleus. Such autoantibodies are found in a wide variety of connective tissue diseases; especially systemic lupus erythematosus (SLE), progressive systemic sclerosis (PSS), Sjögren's syndrome, and mixed connective tissue disease (MCTD). The specific autoantibody detected can be helpful in distinguishing between these and alternative diagnoses. ANA are found in more than 95% of SLE patients. Higher titers increase the positive predictive value of the test.[1] ANA is the best screening test for SLE but lacks specificity. A negative ANA makes SLE unlikely but does not rule out the possibility of the diagnosis.

Specimen Serum

Container Red top tube

Reference Range Negative. Reference ranges vary from one laboratory to another. A positive ANA test result may indicate need for additional investigation. For extractable nuclear antigen (ENA) antibodies, RNP and Smith (Sm) may be positive at about 40-80 units.

Use Screening test for systemic lupus erythematosus (SLE) and other rheumatic and autoimmune diseases, including autoimmune thyroid and liver diseases (eg, autoimmune hepatitis). ANA is a hallmark of SLE and related disorders. The most common clinical manifestations of SLE are polyarthritis and dermatitis.

Limitations This test is not specific for any one collagen vascular disease. For specific tests for SLE see listing Anti-DNA *on page 365*. Specimen is screened at a dilution which should be determined by each laboratory. Typically, dilutions of 1:20, 1:40, or 1:80 have been used. A small percent of SLE patients may have a titer of less than the screening dilution. Men and women older than 80 years of age have a 50% incidence of low titer ANA. Various medications can induce a "lupoid" condition and elevated ANA titers. Usually the titer decreases following removal of the drug. **Drugs** significantly associated with positive ANA tests include, among others: procainamide (Pronestyl®) causing a majority of such cases, para-aminosalicylic acid (PAS, Parasol®), carbamazepine (Tegretol®), chlorpromazine (Thorazine®), Dilantin®, ethosuximide (Zarontin®), griseofulvin (Fulvicin®, Grifulvin® V), hydralazine (Apresoline®), isoniazid (INH, Nydrazid®), mephenytoin (Mesantoin®), methyldopa (Aldomet®), penicillin, phenylbutazone (Butazolidin®, Azolid®), phenytoin (Dilantin®) - hydantoin group, primidone (Mysoline®), propylthiouracil, trimethadione (Tridione®). Subjects with drug-induced lupus may have antiphospholipid antibody with thromboembolic complications, as may 30% of patients with SLE.[1]

Viruses can transiently cause reactivity.

ANA-negative lupus patients are known; *vide infra*.

Methodology Indirect fluorescent antibody (IFA) on HEp-2 cell line (human epithelioid cells)

Additional Information Three elements to consider in results of the indirect fluorescent antibody test: 1. **Positive or negative fluorescence**. A negative test is strong evidence against a diagnosis of SLE but not conclusive. 2. The **titer** (dilution) to which fluorescence remains positive provides a reflection of the concentration or avidity of the antibody. Many individuals, particularly the elderly, may have low titer ANA without significant disease substantiated after work-up. 3. The **pattern** of nuclear fluorescence reflects specificity for various diseases. **Nuclear rim (peripheral) pattern** correlates with antibody to native DNA and deoxynucleoprotein and bears correlation with SLE, SLE activity, and lupus nephritis. **Homogenous (diffuse) pattern** suggests SLE or other connective tissue diseases. Using indirect immunofluorescence on HEp-2 cells, a homogeneous diffuse cytoplasmic staining pattern may indicate myositis;[2] see listing Myositis-Specific Autoantibody *on page 420*. **Speckled pattern** correlates with antibody to nuclear antigens extractable by saline; it is found in many disease states, including SLE and scleroderma. When antibodies to DNA and deoxyribonucleoprotein are present (rim and homogenous pattern), there may be interference with the detection of speckled pattern. **Nucleolar pattern** is seen in sera of patients with progressive systemic sclerosis and Sjögren's syndrome. **Centromere pattern** is seen in CREST syndrome. Maternal antibody to Ro is associated probably in <10% with risk of complete heart block in the newborn. The presence of antiphospholipid antibody bears risk of second trimester miscarriage.

Antinuclear Antibody

ANA Pattern	Corresponding Antibody	Found In
Rim and/or homogeneous	Double-stranded DNA	SLE
	Double and single-stranded DNA	SLE and other rheumatic diseases
	"LE cell antibody"	SLE, drug induced LE
Homogeneous	Histones	Drug induced LE
Speckled	Sm ('Smith')	SLE
	MA	SLE (severe)
	U1-RNP	Mixed connective tissue disease
Atypical speckled	Scl-70 (Scl-1)	Scleroderma
Speckled	SS-B/La, SS-A/Ro	Sjögren's syndrome
Nucleolar	Nucleolar	Progressive systemic sclerosis

The **extractable nuclear antigens** include U_1RNP, Sm, SS-A/Ro, and SS-B/La. Antibodies to U_1RNP and Sm are found in subjects who have SLE, and Sm reactivity is diagnostic. About 30% of patients with SLE have Sm. Antibody to U_1RNP is by definition found in mixed connective tissue disease; it is present in about 40% of patients with SLE, and occurs in Sjögren's syndrome. Anti-SS-A/Ro antibodies are found in about 25% of patients with SLE. Anti-SS-B/La antibodies are found in about 10% of subjects with SLE. See listing Sjögren's Antibodies *on page 430*.

Two percent of the apparently "normal population" demonstrate serum ANA, usually in low titer. Low titers of ANA reactivity may be seen in patients with rheumatoid arthritis (40% to 60% of patients), scleroderma (60% to 90%), discoid lupus, necrotizing vasculitis, Sjögren's syndrome (80%), autoimmune hepatitis, pulmonary interstitial fibrosis, pneumoconiosis, tuberculosis, malignancy, age older than 60 years (18%), as well as in SLE, especially if the disease is inactive or under treatment. Titers $\geq$1:160 usually indicate the presence of active SLE, although occasionally other autoimmune disease may induce such high titers. Using HEp-2 cell lines, some authorities do further testing if the ANA titer is 1:160 or more.[3] ANA cannot be regarded as a foolproof screening test for either SLE or other rheumatic disorders, since it detects some significant nuclear antibodies poorly or not at all. Some failures may be related to the substrate used (rat kidney, mouse kidney, liver, tissue culture), while others may be intrinsic failures of the test. Groups of "ANA-negative" lupus patients are known. About half have antibodies to SS-A/Ro antigen, which is not easily detected by the standard immunofluorescence assay. This disease is characterized by skin manifestations, photosensitivity, arthritis, and polyserositis.[1]

Ten percent of patients with SLE manifest biologic false-positive tests for syphilis; this may even be the initial manifestation. Other tests used in differentiation of autoimmune states include antibody to double-stranded DNA, rheumatoid factor, antibody to extractable nuclear antigens, total hemolytic complement (C3, C4, etc). Although ANA tests are occasionally ordered on cerebrospinal fluid or synovial fluid, current assays are not standardized for these fluids and such assays do not add to the diagnostic process.

Antiphospholipid antibody can be detected in 30% of patients with SLE, as well as in some subjects with drug-induced lupus. Patients with Libman-Sacks endocarditis often have antiphospholipid antibody.

Features of SLE include facial erythema, discoid lupus, Raynaud's phenomenon, alopecia, photosensitivity, oral or nasopharyngeal ulceration, arthritis without deformity, chronic false-positive syphilis serology, nephritis, profuse proteinuria >3.5 g/day, cellular casts, pleuritis and/or pericarditis, psychosis and/or convulsions, hemolytic anemia/leukopenia/thrombocytopenia, and antinuclear antibodies.

Footnotes

1. Mills JA, "Systemic Lupus Erythematosus," *N Engl J Med*, 1994, 330(26):1871-9.
2. Miller FW, "Myositis-Specific Autoantibodies. Touchstones for Understanding the Inflammatory Myopathies," *JAMA*, 1993, 270(15):1846-9.
3. Homburger HA, "Cascade Testing for Autoantibodies in Connective Tissue Diseases," *Mayo Clin Proc*, 1995, 70(2):183-4.

References

Aho K, Koskela P, Makitalo R, et al, "Antinuclear Antibodies Heralding the Onset of Systemic Lupus Erythematosus," *J Rheumatol*, 1992, 19(9):1377-9.
Astion ML, Orkand AR, Olsen GB, et al, "ANA-Tutor: A Computer Program That Teaches the Antinuclear Antibody Test," *Lab Med*, 1993, 24(6):341-4.
Bridges AJ, Anderson JD, McKay J et al, "Antinuclear Antibody Testing in a Referral Laboratory," *Lab Med*, 1993, 24(6):345-9.
Clegg DO, Williams HJ, Singer JZ, et al, "Early Undifferentiated Connective Tissue Disease. II. The Frequency of Circulating Antinuclear Antibodies in Patients With Early Rheumatic Diseases," *J Rheumatol*, 1991, 18(9):1340-3.
Moder KG, "Use and Interpretation of Rheumatologic Tests: A Guide for Clinicians," *Mayo Clin Proc*, 1996, 71(4):391-6.
Senecal JL and Raymond Y, "Autoantibodies to DNA, Lamins, and Pore Complex Proteins Produce Distinct Peripheral Fluorescent Antinuclear Antibody Patterns on the HEp-2 Substrate," *Arthritis Rheum*, 1991, 34(2):249-51.

Antiparietal Cell Antibody *see* Parietal Cell Antibody *on page 421*

Antiphospholipid Antibody *see* Anticardiolipin Antibody *on page 364*

Anti-PM-Scl Autoantibodies *see* Myositis-Specific Autoantibody *on page 420*

Antireticulin Antibody *see* Endomysial Antibodies *on page 391*

Antisignal Recognition (Anti-SRP) Autoantibodies *see* Myositis-Specific Autoantibody *on page 420*

Anti-Sm *see* Anti-DNA *on page 365*

Antismooth Muscle Antibody *see* Smooth Muscle Antibody *on page 431*

Anti-SRP Autoantibodies *see* Myositis-Specific Autoantibody *on page 420*

Antistreptococcal DNase-B Titer *see* Antideoxyribonuclease-B Titer, Serum *on page 365*

Antistreptococcal Hyaluronidase Titer *see* Antihyaluronidase Titer *on page 365*

Antistreptolysin O Titer, Serum

CPT 86060 (titer); 86063 (screen)

Related Information

Antideoxyribonuclease-B Titer, Serum *on page 365*
Antihyaluronidase Titer *on page 365*
Bacterial Culture, Throat *on page 468*
Group A *Streptococcus* Screen, Rapid *on page 483*
Streptozyme *on page 432*

Synonyms ASO

Abstract Detection of elevated ASO titer is useful to detect patients with acute rheumatic fever or nephritis evolving following streptococcal infection.

Specimen Serum

Container Red top tube

Reference Range Younger than 2 years of age: usually <50 Todd units; 2-5 years: <100 Todd units; 5-19 years: <166 Todd units; adults: <125 Todd units. A rise in titer of four or more dilution increments between acute and convalescent specimens is considered to be significant regardless of the magnitude of the titer. For a single specimen, ASO titers ≤166 Todd units are considered normal; but higher titers may be "normal" in demographic groups or may be associated with chronic pharyngeal carriage.

Use Used with antideoxyribonuclease-B and other investigations to document streptococcal infection including acute pharyngitis, tonsillitis, and scarlet fever. A marked rise in titer or a persistently elevated ASO titer indicates a recent or current infection with beta-hemolytic group A *Streptococcus* (*Streptococcus pyogenes*). Elevated titers are seen in 80% to 85% of patients with acute rheumatic fever and in 95% of patients with acute glomerulonephritis.

Limitations False-positive ASO titers can be caused by increased levels of serum beta-lipoprotein produced in liver disease and by contamination of the serum with *Bacillus cereus* and *Pseudomonas* sp. ASO is not

sensitive to sequelae of streptococcal pyoderma. Test is subject to technical false-positives due to a variety of technical and clinical circumstances.

Methodology Nephelometry (the nephelometric assay may provide optimal sensitivity[1]), hemolysis inhibition, latex agglutination (LA)

Additional Information Streptolysin is a hemolysin produced by group A streptococci. In an infected individual streptolysin O acts as a protein antigen, and the patient mounts an antibody response. A rise in titer begins about 1 week after infection and peaks 2-4 weeks later. In the absence of complications or reinfection, the ASO titer will usually fall to preinfection levels within 6-12 months. Both clinical and laboratory findings should be correlated in reaching a diagnosis.

Other relevant investigations include throat culture, streptozyme, WBC count, and ESR.

Footnotes

1. Pacifico L, Mancuso G, Properzi E, et al, "Comparison of Nephelometric and Hemolytic Techniques for Determination of Antistreptolysin O Antibodies," *Am J Clin Pathol*, 1995, 103(4):396-9.

References

Escobar MR, "Hemolytic Assays: Complement Fixation and Antistreptolysin O," *Manual of Clinical Microbiology*, 5th ed, Balows A, Hausler WJ Jr, Herrmann KL, et al, eds, Washington DC: American Society for Microbiology, 1991, 73-8.
Keren DF and Warren JS, *Diagnostic Immunology*, Baltimore, MD: Williams & Wilkins, 1992, 168-70.

Antisynthetases *see* Jo-1 Antibody *on page 411*

Antithyroglobulin Antibody *see* Thyroid Antithyroglobulin Antibody *on page 434*

Antithyroid Peroxidase Antibody *see* Thyroid Antimicrosomal Antibody *on page 433*

Anti-TPO *see* Thyroid Antimicrosomal Antibody *on page 433*

Anti-U1-Ribonucleoprotein Autoantibodies *see* Myositis-Specific Autoantibody *on page 420*

βA (or Aβ) Peptide *see* Cerebrospinal Fluid Amyloid Precursor Protein and Amyloid β-Protein *on page 376*

APP, CSF *see* Cerebrospinal Fluid Amyloid Precursor Protein and Amyloid β-Protein *on page 376*

Arbovirus Serology *see* Encephalitis Viral Serology *on page 391*

ART *see* Automated Reagin Test *on next page*

ART Test *replaced by* RPR *on page 428*

Asialoglycoprotein Receptor Antibodies *see* Smooth Muscle Antibody *on page 431*

ASO *see* Antistreptolysin O Titer, Serum *on this page*

Aspergillosis Complement Fixation Test *see* Aspergillus Serology *on this page*

Aspergillosis ID Test *see* Aspergillus Serology *on this page*

Aspergillus fumigatus Precipitating Antibodies *see* Hypersensitivity Pneumonitis Serology *on page 406*

Aspergillus niger Precipitating Antibodies *see* Hypersensitivity Pneumonitis Serology *on page 406*

Aspergillus Serology

CPT 86606

Related Information

Fungal Culture, Biopsy or Body Fluid *on page 476*
Fungal Culture, Blood *on page 477*
Fungal Culture, Sputum *on page 479*
Immunoglobulin E *on page 409*

Synonyms Aspergillosis Complement Fixation Test; Aspergillosis ID Test

Specimen Serum

Container Red top tube

Special Instructions Acute and convalescent serum specimens are desirable.

Reference Range Immunodiffusion: no precipitin bands detected; positive: at least one precipitin band detected. **Complement fixation:** titer <1:8 or less than fourfold increase.

Use Confirm the presence of serum precipitating antibodies to *Aspergillus* species

Limitations A negative test does not rule out aspergillosis. Nonspecific precipitin bands could be due to presence of C-reactive protein. Cross reactions may occur in cases of histoplasmosis, coccidioidomycosis and blastomycosis. Bands due to reaction with C-reactive protein can be removed by sodium citrate.

(Continued)

Aspergillus Serology *(Continued)*

The value of complement fixing antibodies in the diagnosis of pulmonary aspergillosis is not established.

Methodology Immunodiffusion (ID), complement fixation (CF), enzyme-linked immunosorbent assay (ELISA)

Additional Information Aspergillosis immunodiffusion: Sera can be tested against a polyvalent antigen mixture, or a series of species preparations. The greater the number of bands, the greater the likelihood of either a fungus ball or invasive aspergillosis. *Aspergillus* precipitins are seen in 90% of patients with **fungus balls**, 70% of patients with **allergic bronchopulmonary aspergillosis**, and less often in patients with **invasive aspergillosis**.

Primary criteria for the diagnosis of **allergic bronchopulmonary aspergillosis** include asthma, peripheral blood eosinophilia, immediate skin reactivity and precipitating antibody to *Aspergillus* antigen, elevated serum IgE, pulmonary infiltrates and central bronchiectasis. Secondary criteria include *Aspergillus fumigatus* in sputum, history of expectoration of brown plugs or flecks, and Arthus reaction (late skin reactivity) to *Aspergillus* antigen. Allergic bronchopulmonary aspergillosis is reported in 6% to 20% of patients with asthma and in 5.8% of patients with cystic fibrosis.[1] It is a hypersensitivity reaction which may progress to a fibrotic end stage.[2] Impacted mucin may contain large numbers of eosinophils and Charcot-Leyden crystals.[3] The demonstration of *Aspergillus* antigen in serum, urine, or other body fluids is extremely sensitive and specific for the diagnosis of aspergillosis. Many of these assays appear promising but are not yet widely available.[4,5]

Footnotes

1. "Case Records of the Massachusetts General Hospital. Weekly Clinicopathological Exercises. Case 45-1993. A 23-Year-Old Asthmatic Man With Pulmonary Infiltrates and Hilar Lymphadenopathy," *N Engl J Med*, 1993, 329(20):1484-91.
2. Hantsch CE and Tanus T, "Allergic Bronchopulmonary Aspergillosis With Adenopathy," *Ann Intern Med*, 1991, 115(7):546-7.
3. Bosken CH, Myers JL, Greenberger PA, et al, "Pathologic Features of Allergic Bronchopulmonary Aspergillosis," *Am J Surg Pathol*, 1988, 12(3):216-22.
4. Haynes KA, Latge JP, and Rogers TR, "Detection of *Aspergillus* Antigens Associated With Invasive Infection," *J Clin Microbiol*, 1990, 28(9):2040-4.
5. Warnock DW, Foot AB, Johnson EM, et al, "*Aspergillus* Antigen Latex Test for Diagnosis of Invasive Aspergillosis," *Lancet*, 1991, 338(8773):1023-4.

References

Brummund W, Resnick A, Fink JN, et al, "*Aspergillus fumigatus* Specific Antibodies in Allergic Bronchopulmonary Aspergillosis and Aspergilloma: Evidence for a Polyclonal Antibody Response," *J Clin Microbiol*, 1987, 25(1):5-9.

Kennedy MJ and Sigler L, "*Aspergillus, Fusarium*, and Other Opportunistic Moniliaceous Fungi," *Manual of Clinical Microbiology*, 6th ed, Washington, DC: American Society for Microbiology, 1995, 765-90.

Knutsen AP, Hutcheson PS, Mueller KR, et al, "Serum Immunoglobulins E and G Anti-*Aspergillus fumigatus* Antibody in Patients With Cystic Fibrosis Who Have Allergic Bronchopulmonary Aspergillosis," *J Lab Clin Med*, 1990, 116(5):724-7.

Kurup VP and Kumar A, "Immunodiagnosis of Aspergillosis," *Clin Microbiol Rev*, 1991, 4(4):439-56.

α$_1$-**AT** *see* Alpha$_1$-Antitrypsin, Serum *on page 363*

α$_1$-**AT Phenotype** *see* Alpha$_1$-Antitrypsin Phenotyping *on page 362*

Australian Antigen *replaced by* Hepatitis B Surface Antigen *on page 399*

Australian Antigen Antibody *replaced by* Hepatitis B Surface Antibody *on page 398*

Automated Reagin Test

CPT 86592

Related Information

Anticardiolipin Antibody *on page 364*
Darkfield Examination, Syphilis *on page 475*
FTA-ABS, Serum *on page 394*
MHA-TP *on page 418*
Risks of Transfusion *on page 623*
RPR *on page 428*
VDRL, Cerebrospinal Fluid *on page 438*
VDRL, Serum *on page 438*

Synonyms ART

Applies to Serologic Test for Syphilis; Syphilis Screening Test

Abstract A nontreponemal screening test. Positives should be retested by FTA-ABS or MHA-TP tests. The use of this test has essentially disappeared.

Specimen Serum

Container Red top tube

Reference Range Negative

Use Obsolescent screening test for syphilis

Limitations Biological false-positives have been reported in a large number of entities. The lack of sensitivity of the nontreponemal tests in late syphilis is noteworthy.

Methodology Autoanalyzer modification of reagin agglutination test

References

McGrew BE and Lantz MA, "Quantitative Automated Reagin Test for Syphilis," *Am J Med Technol*, 1970, 36.

Stevens RW and Stroebel E, "The Automated Reagin Test: Results Compared With VDRL and FTA-ABS Tests," *Am J Clin Pathol*, 1970, 53:32-4.

B27 *see* HLA-B27 *on page 404*

***Babesia* Species Serological Test** *see* Babesiosis Serological Test *on this page*

Babesiosis Serological Test

CPT 86317 (quantitative); 86318 (qualitative or semiqualitative)

Related Information

Arthropod Identification *on page 453*
Chagas' Disease Serological Test *on page 383*
Ehrlichiosis Serology *on page 390*
Lyme Disease Serology *on page 415*
Malaria Smear *on page 332*
Parasite Antibodies *on page 421*
Risks of Transfusion *on page 623*

Synonyms *Babesia* Species Serological Test; Nantucket Fever Serological Test

Applies to WA1-Antibody

Abstract This is an intraerythrocytic protozoan, *B. microti*, which can cause symptoms resembling those of *Plasmodium falciparum*. Like malaria, it causes hemolytic anemia. Asplenic, immunocompromised, and elderly subjects are especially at risk, but immunocompetent persons can develop the disease. These organisms are known to cause disease in cattle, including Texas fever.

Specimen Serum

Container Red top tube

Storage Instructions Refrigerate at 4°C.

Reference Range Negative

Critical Values Titers >1:64 are considered consistent with infection. A fourfold increase in titer establishes diagnosis.[1]

Use Diagnose babesiosis; prevent sequellae

Limitations False reactivity may be seen in patients with malaria.

Methodology Indirect immunofluorescent antibody (IFA). Intraerythrocytic ring forms and tetrads are found in the peripheral blood film. The former resemble those of *P. falciparum* malaria, but the rare tetrad forms are diagnostic. Organisms can resemble Pappenheimer bodies, which are found in asplenic persons. An acridine orange technique is available.[1] Finger puncture peripheral blood collected directly on glass slides for thick and thin films, Giemsa stained, are useful for detection of organisms, as with malaria and Chagas' disease. Polymerase chain reaction (PCR) is under development. It is more sensitive and as specific as hamster inoculation and direct smear.[2]

Additional Information *Babesia* is an intraerythrocytic parasite endemic in the northeastern U.S. *Babesia*-like piroplasms are described in the western U.S. with IFA reactivity for WA1.[3,4] *Babesia* can be transmitted by tick bite or blood transfusion. It is particularly severe in patients who have undergone splenectomy (and who lack the RBC "pitting" function of the spleen). It may be potentially life-threatening in immunosuppressed persons or those of advanced age. It also occurs in individuals with normal spleens and may be occult.[2] In a series of six patients with babesiosis, all had high titers of antibody while acutely ill. Titers declined with clinical improvement but remained elevated for 4-16 weeks. A tick, *Ixodes dammini*, which transmits one of the *Babesia* species (*B. microti*, a rodent parasite) also transmits Lyme disease. Subjects with either disease should be considered for the other. Another important vector is *I. racinus*. Diagnosis of babesiosis is established by examination of peripheral blood smears. A WA1-reactive case was originally misdiagnosed as an instance of *P. falciparum* malaria but intraerythrocytic tetrad forms were recognized.[3]

Footnotes

1. "Case Records of the Massachusetts General Hospital. Weekly Clinicopathological Exercises. Case 28-1993. A 63-Year-Old Man With Fever, Sweats, and Shaking Chills," *N Engl J Med*, 1993, 329(3):194-9.
2. Pruthi RK, Marshall WF, Wiltsie JC, et al, "Human Babesiosis," *Mayo Clin Proc*, 1995, 70(9):853-62.
3. Quick RE, Herwaldt BL, Thomford JW, "Babesiosis in Washington State: A New Species of *Babesia*?" *Ann Intern Med*, 1993, 119(4):284-90.
4. Persing DH, Herwaldt BL, Glaser C, et al, "Infection With a Babesia-Like Organism in Northern California," *N Engl J Med*, 1995, 332(5):298-303.

References

Ash LR and Orihel TC, *Atlas of Human Parasitology*, 3rd ed, Chicago, IL: American Society of Clinical Pathologists, 1990, 115-7.

Bove JR, "Transfusion-Transmitted Diseases Other Than AIDS and Hepatitis," *Yale J Biol Med*, 1990, 63(5):347-51.

Dammin GJ, Spielman A, Benach JL, et al, "The Rising Incidence of Clinical *Babesia microti* Infection," *Hum Pathol*, 1981, 12:398-400.

Bartonella **Antibodies** *see* Cat Scratch Disease Serology *on page 375*

Bence Jones Protein *replaced by* Protein Electrophoresis, Urine *on page 425*

Bence Jones Protein Test *replaced by* Immunoelectrophoresis, Serum or Urine *on page 408*

Bence Jones Protein Test *replaced by* Immunofixation Electrophoresis *on page 408*

Beta$_2$-Microglobulin

CPT 82232

Related Information

Aminoglycosides *on page 531*
Cadmium, Urine *on page 539*
CD4/CD8 Enumeration *on page 375*
Cerebrospinal Fluid Cytology *on page 290*
HIV-1/HIV-2 Serology *on page 403*
Urine Collection, 24-Hour *on page 30*
Zidovudine *on page 580*

Synonyms β_2-M; β_2-Microglobulin

Abstract β_2-Microglobulin is increased in entities in which cell turnover is increased, in B lymphocyte hematologic malignant diseases and other neoplastic states and in several non-neoplastic conditions.

Patient Preparation Avoid recent administration of radioisotopes if assay performed by RIA.

Specimen Serum or 24-hour urine

Container Red top tube, plastic urine container

Storage Instructions Urine β_2-M is unstable when pH is <5.5.

Reference Range Serum: <2 µg/mL (SI: <170 nmol/L); urine: <120 µg/ 24 hours (SI: <10 nmol/day)

Critical Values In myeloma, survival is shorter when β_2-microglobulin is >4 µg/mL.

Use Evaluate renal disease, prognosis of myeloma, activity of chronic lymphocytic leukemia, activity of AIDS; urinary β_2-microglobulin is increased with tubular damage (eg, in cadmium poisoning)

Limitations Increased synthesis of β_2-M in Crohn's disease, hepatitis, sarcoidosis, vasculitis, hyperthyroidism, viral infections, and some malignancies decreases the usefulness of serum levels.

Contraindications Recent radioactive scan

Methodology Radioimmunoassay (RIA), enzyme immunoassay (EIA)

Additional Information β_2-M is a cell membrane-associated 100 amino acid peptide, a component of the class I human leukocyte antigen (HLA) complex. It is increased nonspecifically in inflammatory reactions and in active chronic lymphocytic leukemia in which there is increased lymphocyte turnover. Serum β_2-M predicts response in subjects with low grade lymphoma: at 42 months no patient with a level ≥3.0 mg/L was projected to be in remission.[1] It is also a prognostic marker in multiple myeloma. It may be a useful differentiator of glomerular and tubular dysfunction: in glomerular disease β_2-M is increased in serum and decreased in urine, while in tubular disorders the opposite changes occur. Urinary retinol-binding protein and β_2-M levels may delineate those nephrotic subjects likelier to respond to steroids.[2] Urinary β_2-M becomes abnormal before serum creatinine in aminoglycoside nephrotoxicity. β_2-M is increased in AIDS patients with progressive disease, particularly those with opportunistic infection. Serum β_2-M has been a useful marker for *in vivo* antiretroviral drug activity. It decreases in response to therapy with AZT. Its use has been combined with CD4 lymphocyte counts to calculate the probability of an HIV-infected person developing AIDS within the next 3 years. β_2-M has been used with T-lymphocyte subsets to monitor factor VIII replacement therapy in hemophiliacs with HIV.[3]

Although some studies point to elevated β_2-M in the CSF of patients with neurologic involvement by HIV, this is unlikely to provide significant information to guide therapy.

It is reported to delineate a subset of subjects who have primary amyloidosis whose outcomes are unfavorable, but it is not useful in such patients as an index of response to therapy.[4]

Footnotes

1. Litam P, Swan F, Cabanillas F, et al, "Prognostic Value of Serum β-2 Microglobulin in Low-Grade Lymphoma," *Ann Intern Med*, 1991, 114(10):855-60.
2. Sesso R, Santos AP, Nishida SK, et al, "Prediction of Steroid Responsiveness in the Idiopathic Nephrotic Syndrome Using Urinary Retinol-Binding Protein and Beta-2-Microglobulin," *Ann Intern Med*, 1992, 116(11):905-9.
3. Mannucci PM, Brettler DB, Aledort LM, et al, "Immune Status of Human Immunodeficiency Virus Seropositive and Seronegative Hemophiliacs Infused for 3.5 Years With Recombinant Factor VIII. The Kogenate Study Group," *Blood*, 1994, 83(7):1958-62.
4. Gertz MA, Kyle RA, Greipp PR, et al, "Beta 2-Microglobulin Predicts Survival in Primary Amyloidosis," *Am J Med*, 1990, 89(5):609-14.

References

Leavelle DE, *Mayo Medical Laboratories Interpretive Handbook*, Rochester, MN: Mayo Medical Laboratories, 1994.

Lucey PR, McGuire SA, Clerici M, et al, "Comparison of Spinal Fluid β$_2$-Microglobulin Levels With CD4+ T-Cell Count, *In Vitro* T Helper Cell Function, and Spinal Fluid IgG Parameters in 163 Neurologically Normal Adults Infected With the Human Immunodeficiency Virus Type 1," *J Infect Dis*, 1991, 163(5):971-5.

Roiter I, Da Rin G, De Menis E, et al, "Increased Serum β$_2$-Microglobulin Concentrations in Hyperthyroid States," *J Clin Pathol*, 1991, 44(1):73-4.

Beta-Gamma Bridging *see* Protein Electrophoresis, Serum *on page 424*

Bilharziasis *see* Schistosomiasis Serological Test *on page 429*

Blastomycosis Serology

CPT 86612

Related Information

Fungal Culture, Biopsy or Body Fluid *on page 476*
Fungal Culture, Sputum *on page 479*
Fungal Culture, Urine *on page 480*
Fungus Smear, Stain *on page 481*

Abstract Blastomycosis is caused by the dimorphic fungus *Blastomyces dermatitidis*. This mold is a natural inhabitant of the soil, and most cases in the United States occur around the Great Lakes and Upper Mississippi River. The disease almost always begins as a pulmonary infection. It can become disseminated.

Specimen Serum

Container Red top tube

Reference Range Complement fixation: titers <1:8; immunodiffusion: no precipitin band; enzyme immunoassay: titers <1:32

Use Support the diagnosis of infection due to *Blastomyces dermatitidis*. Acute and convalescent titers are helpful. This diagnosis is established by demonstration of the organisms in smear and/or tissue section and optimally, culture.

Limitations Failure to demonstrate precipitin antibodies does not rule out blastomycosis. Cross reactions are seen in patients with histoplasmosis and coccidioidomycosis. Skin testing prior to the test may elevate the complement fixation titer. The complement fixation test lacks sensitivity and specificity and gives positive results in <50% of culture proven cases. Newer EIA tests for blastomycosis have shown greater sensitivity with no compromise in specificity compared to other tests. EIA for antibody to purified A antigen is 90% sensitive, with some cross reaction with cases of histoplasmosis.

Methodology Complement fixation (CF), immunodiffusion (ID), enzyme immunoassay (EIA)

Additional Information Blastomycosis immunodiffusion: A band of identity with the "A" reference antibody from an infected human indicates active infection or recent past infection. This detects about 80% of cases. A negative test has little value and in no way excludes the existence of blastomycosis. Cross reactions producing lines of partial identity are seen in patients with histoplasmosis and coccidioidomycosis. Repeated testing at 3-week intervals may be needed to secure a diagnosis. After diagnosis is established, falling titers are a good prognostic sign.

References

Kaufman L and Reiss E, "Serodiagnosis of Fungal Diseases," *Manual of Clinical Laboratory Immunology*, 4th ed, Vol 2, Chapter 78, Rose NR, Conway de Macario E, Fahey JL, et al, eds, Washington, DC: American Society for Microbiology, 1992, 506-28.

Lo CY and Notenboom RH, "A New Enzyme Immunoassay Specific for Blastomycosis," *Am Rev Respir Dis*, 1990, 141(1):84:8.

Turner S and Kaufman L, "Immunodiagnosis of Blastomycosis," *Semin Respir Infect*, 1986, 1(1):22-8.

Blood Mononuclear Cells *see* Mixed Lymphocyte Culture *on page 418*

Bordetella pertussis **Antibodies** *see Bordetella pertussis* Serology *on next page*

Bordetella pertussis Direct Fluorescent Antibody

CPT 87206

Related Information

Bordetella pertussis Culture *on page 471*
Bordetella pertussis Serology *on next page*

Synonyms *Bordetella pertussis* Smear; Nasopharyngeal Smear for *Bordetella pertussis*; Pertussis DFA

Replaces Cough Plate Culture for Pertussis

Patient Preparation Patient must not be on antimicrobial therapy.

Specimen Nasopharyngeal swab

Collection Swab is passed through nose gently and into nasopharynx. Stay near septum and floor of nose. Rotate and remove. Specimen must be hand transported to the laboratory immediately following collection.

Storage Instructions Do not refrigerate.

Causes for Rejection Specimen not received in appropriate sterile container or on appropriate isolation medium, specimen more than 2 hours old. Cough plates are unacceptable.

(Continued)

Bordetella pertussis Direct Fluorescent Antibody
(Continued)

Use Detect and identify *B. pertussis* and *B. parapertussis*, establish diagnosis of whooping cough

Limitations Direct detection assays are always limited by the adequacy of the sample. Bacteria may be difficult to detect if there are few bacteria present in the specimen or too much mucoid material. Direct assay should always be used in conjunction with culture. Negative direct detection assays do not rule out pertussis.

Contraindications Lack of clinical symptoms of pertussis; previous antibiotic therapy

Methodology Direct fluorescent antibody (DFA)

Additional Information The procedure enables early presumptive identification of *Bordetella pertussis*, the agent of whooping cough. An experienced laboratory will have a 60% sensitivity and a 90% specificity when compared with culture.[1,2] Definitive cultural identification should be completed. There is also available a test for serum agglutinating antibodies, which if present may be titered over time to indicate exposure.

Footnotes
1. Ewanowich CA, Chui LW, Paranchych MG, et al, "Major Outbreak of Pertussis in Northern Alberta, Canada: Analysis of Discrepant Direct Fluorescent-Antibody and Culture Results by Using Polymerase Chain Reaction Methodology," *J Clin Microbiol*, 1993, 31(7):1715-25.
2. Strebel PM, Cochi SL, Farizo KM, et al, "Pertussis in Missouri: Evaluation of Nasopharyngeal Culture, Direct Fluorescent Antibody Testing, and Clinical Case Definitions in the Diagnosis of Pertussis," *Clin Infect Dis*, 1993, 16(2):276-85.

References
Marcon MJ, "*Bordetella*," *Manual of Clinical Microbiology*, 6th ed, Murray PR, Baron EJ, Pfaller MA, et al, eds, Washington, DC: American Society for Microbiology, 1995, 566-73.

Bordetella pertussis Serology

CPT 86615

Related Information
Bacterial Culture, Sputum *on page 465*
Bordetella pertussis Culture *on page 471*
Bordetella pertussis Direct Fluorescent Antibody *on previous page*

Synonyms *Bordetella pertussis* Antibodies; *Bordetella pertussis* Titer; Pertussis Serology

Test Commonly Includes Enzyme-linked immunosorbent assay to detect antibodies to *Bordetella pertussis* and/or pertussis toxin

Specimen Serum

Container Red top tube

Storage Instructions Refrigerate serum at 4°C.

Reference Range Less than fourfold rise in titer in paired sera; IgM antibody: negative

Use Evaluate acute infection with or immunity following vaccination for *Bordetella pertussis*

Limitations Serologic diagnosis of acute pertussis is severely limited by the time required for seroconversion

Methodology Microhemagglutination, complement fixation (CF), toxin neutralization, enzyme-linked immunosorbent assay (ELISA)

Additional Information Patients with acute infection develop IgG, IgM, and IgA antibodies to febrile agglutinogens; and IgM and IgA antibodies are probably diagnostic. Following vaccination, IgG and IgM antibodies can be demonstrated, except in infants. IgA antibodies do not develop.

References
Cherry JD, Beer T, Chartrand SA, et al, "Comparison of Values of Antibody to *Bordetella pertussis* Antigens in Young German and American Men," *Clin Infect Dis*, 1995, 20(5):1271-4.
Mertsola J, Ruuskanen O, Kuronen T, et al, "Serologic Diagnosis of Pertussis: Evaluation of Pertussis Toxin and Other Antigens in Enzyme-Linked Immunosorbent Assay," *J Infect Dis*, 1990, 161(5):966-71.
Tomoda T, Ogura H, and Kurashige T, "Immune Responses to *Bordetella pertussis* Infection and Vaccination," *J Infect Dis*, 1991, 163(3):559-63.

Bordetella pertussis Smear *see Bordetella pertussis* Direct Fluorescent Antibody *on previous page*

Bordetella pertussis Titer *see Bordetella pertussis* Serology *on this page*

Borrelia burgdorferi Serology *see* Lyme Disease Serology *on page 415*

Breath Testing for *H. pylori* *see* Helicobacter pylori Serology *on page 395*

Brucella abortus *see* Brucellosis Agglutinins *on this page*

Brucella melitensis *see* Brucellosis Agglutinins *on this page*

Brucella suis *see* Brucellosis Agglutinins *on this page*

Brucellosis Agglutinins

CPT 86000

Related Information
Bacterial Culture, Blood *on page 457*
Brucella Culture *on page 472*
Febrile Agglutinins, Serum *on page 393*

Synonyms Undulant Fever

Applies to *Brucella abortus*; *Brucella melitensis*; *Brucella suis*

Abstract Brucellosis is a zoonotic infection caused by gram-negative intracellular coccobacilli, *Brucella melitensis*, *B. abortus*, *B. suis*, and *B. canis*. In the U.S., ingestion of unpasteurized goat's milk or cheese has led to an upsurge. Brucellosis can affect essentially any organ. Occupational exposure represents the predominant means of transmission (butchers, abattoir workers, farmers, veterinarians).

Specimen Serum

Container Red top tube

Special Instructions Paired specimens should be tested together in the same laboratory.

Reference Range Negative. A fourfold titer rise on paired (acute and convalescent) sera drawn 10-14 days apart is strongly indicative of the diagnosis. However, the insidious clinical presentation of brucellosis often precludes collection of acute specimens. Titers of 1:160 are suggestive of active past or present disease. Ninety percent of patients with titers ≥1:320 have bacteremia.

Use Diagnosis of *Brucella* infection by positive cultures is often difficult, consequently, serologic diagnosis is often the method of choice, by detection of antibody titers to *Brucella* antigens.

Limitations Previous vaccination may have an effect on the titer. Test must be done utilizing a standard antigen prepared from *B. abortus* strain 1119. This will not detect antibodies to *B. canis*. Blocking antibodies may interfere at low titers. There are cross reactions with *Proteus* OX-19, *Yersinia enterocolitica*, *Francisella tularensis*, and *Vibrio cholerae* including cholera vaccination, as well as with skin tests for *Brucella*.

Methodology Tube agglutination, complement fixation, enzyme linked immunosorbent assay (ELISA)

Additional Information Cultures of blood, bone marrow, and of specific sites are desirable. *Brucella* agglutinins appear during the second week in acute cases and peak in 3-6 weeks. The *B. abortus* antigen used in the *Brucella* agglutination test is group specific and not species specific. If infection with *B. canis* is possible, a specific test for those antibodies must be done. (*B. canis* rarely causes infection in humans.) Although cross reactions occur with several other organisms, usually homologous titers will be much higher than the cross reactants. With newer ELISA assays, IgG and IgM antibodies to *Brucella* are used both for initial diagnosis and for follow-up of the patient. Persistence of IgG antibody indicates active infection. **Diagnosis of brucellosis ideally requires isolation (blood and/or bone marrow cultures)** or cultures from infected sites, but only about 20% of cases are confirmed.

References
Ariza J, Pellicer T, Pallares R, et al, "Specific Antibody Profile in Human Brucellosis," *Clin Infect Dis*, 1992, 14(1):131-40.
Kaye D, "Brucellosis," *Harrison's Principles of Internal Medicine*, 13th ed, Isselbacher KJ, Braunwald E, Wilson J, et al, eds, New York, NY: McGraw-Hill Inc, 1994, 685-7.
Peiris V, Fraser S, Fairhurst M, et al, "Laboratory Diagnosis of *Brucella* Infection: Some Pitfalls," *Lancet*, 1992, 339(8806):1415-6.
Radolf JD, "Southwestern Internal Medicine Conference: Brucellosis: Don't Let It Get Your Goat," *Am J Med Sci*, 1994, 307(1):64-75.

Brugia malayi Serology *see* Filariasis Serological Test *on page 393*

Brugia timori Serology *see* Filariasis Serological Test *on page 393*

Bunya Virus Titer *see* California Encephalitis Virus Titer *on page 374*

C1 Esterase Inhibitor, Serum

CPT 85335

Related Information
Complement Components *on page 385*

Synonyms C1 Inactivator; C1 Inhibitor; Esterase Inhibitor; HANE Assay; Hereditary Angioneurotic Edema Test

Applies to Esterase, Subunit of C1

Test Commonly Includes Functional (activity) analysis by complement decay and total immunoreactive level by immunodiffusion and CH_{50}

Abstract C1 esterase inhibitor is decreased in both genetic and acquired angioedema.

Specimen Serum

Container Red top tube

Collection Collect sample on ice. Specimen must be chilled (in ice bath) during clotting. Separate from clot with minimum centrifugation. Freeze serum immediately.

Reference Range Total: 8-24 mg/dL; functional: "present"

Use C1 esterase inhibitor is decreased in hereditary angioneurotic edema; decrease may be functional or quantitative

Methodology Radial immunodiffusion (RID) or nephelometry for measurement of antigenic material; functional assay of C1 activity on acetyl-L-tyrosine ethyl ester or by antigenic masking

Additional Information The more common form (85% of patients) of hereditary angioneurotic edema is due to an absolute decrease in the amount of C1 esterase inhibitor. A less common form (15% of patients) is due to a functional defect. Both abnormalities must be tested for due to the potential life-threatening nature of the illness.

In addition to decreased C1 esterase inhibitor in the serum of patients with hereditary angioneurotic edema, a unique polypeptide kinin is increased in plasma from C1 esterase inhibitor deficient patient during attacks of swelling. Danazol, a synthetic androgenic inhibitor of gonadotropin release with little virilizing potential, decreases the number of clinical attacks in cases of hereditary angioneurotic edema. Patients with attacks of hereditary angioneurotic edema also have low total complement, C4 and C2. Consequently, measurement of serum C4 titer is an often used screening test. Hereditary angioneurotic edema is transmitted as an autosomal dominant trait. Heterozygotes also show decreased levels of C1 esterase inhibitor. During acute attacks of the disease, complement factors C4 and C2 can be markedly reduced, but C1 and C3 are normal. The initiating stimulus of clinical attacks is often unknown.

Angioedema may also be an acquired illness. The acquired form includes nonhereditary C1 esterase deficiency; drug-induced, allergic, and idiopathic forms; angioedema associated with autoimmune disease, especially with systemic lupus erythematosus and hypereosinophilia; angioedema occasionally associated with malignancy; and angioedema caused by physical stimuli. Angioedema has occasionally been known to precede development of lymphoproliferative disorders.

References

Alsenz J, Bork K, and Loos M, "Autoantibody-Mediated Acquired Deficiency of C1 Inhibitor," *N Engl J Med*, 1987, 316(22):1360-6.

Baldwin J, Pence HL, Karibo JM, et al, "C1-Esterase Inhibitor Deficiency: Three Presentations," *Ann Allergy*, 1991, 67(2 Pt 1):107-13.

Colten HR, "Hereditary Angioneurotic Edema, 1887-1987," *N Engl J Med*, 1987, 317(1):43-4.

Frank MM, "Hereditary Angio-Oedema," *Complement in Health and Disease*, 2nd ed, Vol 20, Chapter 8, Whaley K, Loos M and Weiler JM, eds, Boston, MA: Kluwer Academic Publishers, 1993, 229-43.

Greaves M and Lawlor F, "Angioedema: Manifestations and Management," *J Am Acad Dermatol*, 1991, 25(1 Pt 2):155-61.

C1 Inactivator *see C1 Esterase Inhibitor, Serum on previous page*

C1 Inhibitor *see C1 Esterase Inhibitor, Serum on previous page*

C1q Binding Test *see C1q Immune Complex Detection on this page*

C1q Immune Complex Detection

CPT 86332

Related Information

C3 Complement, Serum *on this page*
Complement Components *on page 385*
Complement, Total, Serum *on page 386*

Synonyms C1q Binding Test; Circulating Immune Complexes; Immune Complex Detection by C1q

Applies to Synovial Fluid C1q Immune Complexes Detection

Abstract An assay for immune complexes, different from complement component C1q. C1q is the recognition unit of the classical complement pathway.[1]

Specimen Serum

Container Red top tube

Reference Range None detected

Use Assays for circulating immune complexes have little practical use for following autoimmune diseases. Although they have been proposed to follow conditions such as systemic lupus erythematosus, glomerulonephritis, and even Lyme disease, they are not superior to tests such as CH_{50} or CH_{100}, which are better standardized between laboratories and less expensive. Further, assays such as C1q do not correlate well with other assays (eg, Raji cell or immune conglutinins). Therefore, these assays are considered to be of research use only. Elevated levels may contribute to support a diagnosis of chronic fatigue syndrome but are not specific for this condition.

Limitations Correlates poorly with other immune complex assays

Methodology Radioimmunoassay (RIA), protein precipitation, coagglutination

Additional Information C1q stimulates host defenses. The ability of monocytes to ingest pathogens is enhanced with C1q binding. It binds to other cell types as well.[1] The C1q assay is based on the binding of this component of complement to the Fc portion of immunoglobulins in antigen-antibody complexes. The entire complex can be precipitated with polyethylene glycol, and if the C1q is properly labeled, the complexes can be quantitated. Circulating immune complexes can be demonstrated in rheumatic, infectious, and neoplastic diseases, as well as most immunologically mediated illnesses (inflammatory bowel disease, thrombotic thrombocytopenic purpura. The 1981 WHO/IUIS survey of laboratory tests in clinical immunology concluded that the detection of circulating immune complexes is not essential to any specific diagnosis.

Footnotes

1. Tenner AJ, "Functional Aspects of the C1q Receptors," *Behring Inst Mitt*, 1993, 93:241-53.

References

Bates DW, Buchwald D, Lee J, et al, "Clinical Laboratory Test Findings in Patients With Chronic Fatigue Syndrome," *Arch Intern Med*, 1995, 155(1):97-103.

Endo L, Corman LC, and Panush RS, "Clinical Utility of Assays for Circulating Immune Complexes," *Med Clin North Am*, 1985, 69(4):623-36.

Keren DF, "Assays for Circulating Immune Complexes," *Clinical Laboratory Annual*, Batsakis JG and Homburger HA, eds, New York, NY: Appleton-Century-Crofts, 1985, 105-23.

Lanham RJ, "Chronic Fatigue Syndrome: A Diagnostic Challenge for the Laboratory," *Clin Lab Sci*, 1994, 7(5):279-82.

C3 Activator *see Factor B on page 393*

C3 Complement, Serum

CPT 86160 (antigen); 86161 (functional activity)

Related Information

Anti-DNA *on page 365*
C1q Immune Complex Detection *on this page*
C4 Complement, Serum *on next page*
Complement Components *on page 385*
Complement, Total, Serum *on page 386*
Factor B *on page 393*
Kidney Profile *on page 153*

Synonyms Complement C3

Abstract Complement levels can be a useful index for following autoimmune disease activity. Genetic deficiencies may be associated with pyogenic infections.

Specimen Serum

Container Red top tube

Storage Instructions Allow sample to clot 15-30 minutes at room temperature (cold activation of the complement system with loss of activity may occur at 0°C), then 30-60 minutes at 4°C. Centrifuge at 4°C. Freeze serum at -70°C if assay cannot be run at once.

Reference Range Fresh serum: 1200-1500 µg/mL (SI: 1.2-1.5 g/L)

Use Quantitation of C3 is used to detect individuals with congenital deficiency of this factor or those with immunologic disease in whom complement is consumed at an increased rate. These include chronic hepatitis, certain chronic infections, immune complex disease, poststreptococcal and membranoproliferative glomerulonephritis, and others. It is especially useful to assess disease activity in lupus erythematosus (SLE) and to investigate decreased total complement.

Limitations Detects both biologically active and inactive C3

Methodology Radial immunodiffusion (RID), rate nephelometry

Additional Information C3 is made in the liver and comprises about 70% of the total protein in the complement system. It is central to activation of both the classical and alternate pathways. Increased levels are found in numerous inflammatory states as an acute phase response. CH_{50} (total complement hemolytic activity), C3 and/or C4 may be decreased in cases of systemic lupus erythematosus, especially in cases with lupus nephritis, acute and chronic hypocomplementemic nephritis, infective endocarditis, DIC, and partial lipodystrophy (with associated nephritis-like activity in serum.) However, C3 level is a poor indicator of diagnosis or prognosis in many entities. The "nongamma" (C3) Coombs' test may detect C3 on red cell membranes in some cases of autoimmune hemolytic anemias, but C3 levels are seldom decreased. In cases of disseminated intravascular coagulation, plasmin attacks C3 directly, and C3 levels have been found low in the hemolytic uremic syndrome form of disseminated intravascular coagulation (DIC). Cases of hereditary C3 deficiency, while rare, have been reported and are characterized clinically by recurrent infections and by immune complex disease, in particular, membranoproliferative glomerulonephritis. The central role of C3 (classical and alternate pathways) place C3 deficient patients at risk for especially severe infections by the encapsulated organisms, *S. pneumoniae*, *H. influenzae*, and *N. meningitidis* (both gram-positive and gram-negative bacteria). Bacteremia, sinopulmonary infections, meningitis, paronychia, and impetigo may occur. C3 levels (Continued)

C3 Complement, Serum *(Continued)*

have also been found deficient in cases of uremia, chronic liver diseases, anorexia nervosa, and celiac disease. See table.

General Guide to Evaluation of C4 and C3 Protein Levels in Presence of Decreased Hemolytic Complement Activity

	Normal C4	Decreased C4
Normal C3	Alterations *in vitro* (eg, improper specimen handling) Coagulation-associated complement consumption Inborn errors (other than C4 or C3)	Immune complex disease Hypergammaglobulinemic states Cryoglobulinemia Hereditary angioedema Inborn C4 deficiency
Decreased C3	Acute glomerulonephritis Membranoproliferative glomerulonephritis Immune complex disease Active SLE Inborn C3 deficiency	Active SLE Serum sickness Autoimmune/chronic active hepatitis Infective endocarditis Immune complex disease

Modified from *Gradwohl's Clinical Laboratory Methods and Diagnosis*, 8th ed, Sonnenwirth AC and Jarett L, eds, St Louis, MO: Mosby-Year Book Inc, 1980, 1233.

References

Densen P, "Complement," *Principles and Practice of Infectious Diseases*, 4th ed, Vol 1, Chapter 6, Mandell GL, Bennett JE, and Dolin R, eds, New York, NY: Churchill Livingstone, 1995, 58-78.

Figueroa JE and Densen P, "Infectious Diseases Associated With Complement Deficiencies," *Clin Microbiol Rev*, 1991, 4(3):359-95.

Frank MM, "Complement in the Pathophysiology of Human Disease," *N Engl J Med*, 1987, 316(24):1525-30.

Nusinow SR, Zuraw BL, and Curd JG, "The Hereditary and Acquired Deficiencies of Complement," *Med Clin North Am*, 1985, 69(3):487-504.

C3 Proactivator *see* Factor B *on page 393*

C4 Complement, Serum

CPT 86160 (antigen); 86161 (functional activity)

Related Information

C3 Complement, Serum *on previous page*
Complement Components *on page 385*
Complement, Total, Serum *on page 386*
Factor B *on page 393*
Kidney Profile *on page 153*

Synonyms Complement C4

Specimen Serum

Container Red top tube

Storage Instructions Allow sample to clot 15-30 minutes at room temperature, then 30-60 minutes at 4°C. Freeze serum at -70°C if assay cannot be run at once.

Reference Range 350-600 μg/mL (SI: 0.35-0.60 g/L)

Use Quantitation of C4 is used to detect individuals with congenital deficiency of this factor or those with immunologic disease in whom hypercatabolism of complement causes reduced levels. These diseases include lupus erythematosus (SLE), rheumatoid arthritis, serum sickness, certain glomerulonephritides, chronic hepatitis, cryoglobulinemia, immune complex disease, and hereditary angioedema. C4 levels are sensitive indicators of lupus disease activity and C4 is a marker for activity as well with proliferative glomerulonephritis and other entities. It may be increased with autoimmune hemolytic anemia.

Limitations Complement proteins are acute phase reactants and have short half-lives. Serum level is a balance of synthesis and catabolism. Serial measurements are more useful than single values.

Methodology Radial immunodiffusion (RID), rate nephelometry

Additional Information C4 is utilized only by the classical pathway, so that it is decreased only when this arm is activated. In diseases activating the alternate pathway alone, C4 levels will be normal. Total hemolytic activity (CH$_{50}$), C3, and C4 are frequently decreased in a variety of conditions producing immune complexes. In hereditary angioedema, the lack of C1 esterase inhibitor allows unopposed lysis of C2 and C4 by C1 esterase, so C4 levels will be low. C4 deficiency has been described in association with a clinical SLE-like disease but with absence of LE cells, with variable immunoglobulin or C3 deposits in the skin biopsy, and with Henoch-Schönlein purpura or glomerulonephritis. The condition is inherited as an autosomal recessive trait with close HLA linkage. Nearly all patients with total absence of C4 have discoid or systemic lupus erythematosus often with associated glomerulonephritis. Hereditary C4 deficiency is associated with an increased incidence of pyogenic bacterial infections, in particular those caused by the encapsulated organism *S. pneumoniae*. See table in C3 Complement, Serum *on page 374*.

References

Bishof NA, Welch TR, and Beischel LS, "C4B Deficiency: A Risk Factor for Bacteremia With Encapsulated Organisms," *J Infect Dis*, 1990, 162(1):248-50.

Frank MM, "Complement in the Pathophysiology of Human Disease," *N Engl J Med*, 1987, 316(24):1525-30.

Ruddy S, "Complement," *Manual of Clinical Laboratory Immunology*, 4th ed, Chapter 18, Rose NR, Conway de Macario E, Fahey JL, et al, eds, Washington, DC: American Society for Microbiology, 1992, 114-23.

c100-3 *see* Hepatitis C Serology *on page 399*

CA2 *see* Thyroid Antithyroglobulin Antibody *on page 434*

California Encephalitis (LaCrosse) *see* Encephalitis Viral Serology *on page 391*

California Encephalitis Virus Titer

CPT 86651

Related Information

Eastern Equine Encephalitis Virus Serology *on page 389*
St Louis Encephalitis Virus Serology *on page 432*
Viral Culture, Central Nervous System Symptoms *on page 677*
Western Equine Encephalitis Virus Serology *on page 439*

Synonyms Bunya Virus Titer; Encephalitis Virus Titer, California; LaCrosse Virus Titer

Abstract The California encephalitis virus is a member of the Bunyaviridae family. It is often referred to as the LaCrosse virus. This virus commonly causes aseptic meningitis, especially during the summer. Other members of the California serogroup are the Jamestown Canyon virus and snowshoe hare virus.

Specimen Serum, cerebrospinal fluid

Container Red top tube, sterile container

Collection Acute and convalescent sera drawn 10-14 days apart are required.

Reference Range Less than a fourfold increase in titer in paired sera; IgM in CSF is considered diagnostic of CNS infection.

Use Support diagnosis of California encephalitis virus infection

Limitations Complement fixing antibodies appear slowly

Methodology Counterimmunoelectrophoresis (CIE), indirect fluorescent antibody (IFA), enzyme-linked immunosorbent assay (ELISA), complement fixation (CF), hemagglutination

Additional Information Despite its name, California virus is rare in western states. It is more commonly the cause of an encephalitis occurring in children (5-9 years of age) in the North Central states during the summer. The organism, a bunyavirus, is harbored in small field animals and rodents and is transmitted by mosquitoes.

References

Campbell GL, Eldridge BF, Reeves WC, et al, "Isolation of Jamestown Canyon Virus From Boreal *Aedes* Mosquitoes From the Sierra Nevada of California," *Am J Trop Med Hyg*, 1991, 44(3):244-9.

Tsai TF, "Arboviral Infections in the United States," *Infect Dis Clin North Am*, 1991, 5(1):73-102.

Tsai TF, "Arboviruses," *Manual of Clinical Laboratory Immunology*, 4th ed, Vol 2, Chapter 91, Rose NR, Conway de Macario E, Fahey JL, et al, eds, Washington, DC: American Society for Microbiology, 1992, 606-18.

***Campylobacter pylori* Serology** *see* Helicobacter pylori Serology *on page 395*

c-ANCA *see* Antineutrophil Cytoplasmic Antibody *on page 367*

Candida Antigen

CPT 86313 (immunoassay, multiple step); 86315 (immunoassay, single step)

Related Information

Candidiasis Serologic Test *on next page*
Fungal Culture, Biopsy or Body Fluid *on page 476*
Fungal Culture, Blood *on page 477*
Fungal Culture, Stool *on page 480*
Fungus Smear, Stain *on page 481*

Specimen Serum

Container Red top tube

Storage Instructions Separate and refrigerate serum at 4°C.

Reference Range Negative

Use Diagnosis of candidiasis in immunocompromised patients by detection of *Candida* antigens in serum specimen

Limitations *Candida* tests are relatively insensitive. Evaluation of these assays has been hampered by difficulty in establishing the diagnosis of disseminated candidiasis by other clinical and laboratory methods.

Methodology Latex agglutination (LA), enzyme-linked immunosorbent assay (ELISA)

Additional Information Detection of disseminated candidiasis is particularly important in immunocompromised patients due to the life-threatening nature of the illness. Unfortunately, the sensitivity of *Candida* antigen tests is too low to rule out candidiasis despite a negative test result. Consequently, a negative result does not preclude the use of empiric antifungal therapy. A positive test is usually reliable but many of these patients also have positive blood cultures.

References

Escuro RS, Jacobs M, Gerson SL, et al, "Prospective Evaluation of a *Candida* Antigen Detection for Invasive Candidiasis in Immunocompromised Adult Patients With Cancer," *Am J Med*, 1989, 87(6):621-7.

Gutierrez J, Maroto C, Peidrola G, et al, "Circulating *Candida* Antigens and Antibodies: Useful Markers of Candidemia," *J Clin Microbiol*, 1993, 31(9):2550-2.

Hayette MP, Strecker G, Faille C, et al, "Presence of Human Antibodies Reacting With *Candida albicans* O-Linked Oligomannosides Revealed by Using an Enzyme-Linked Immunosorbent Assay and Neoglycolipids," *J Clin Microbiol*, 1992, 30(2):411-7.

Morhart M, Rennie R, Ziola B, et al, "Evaluation of Enzyme Immunoassay for *Candida* Cytoplasmic Antigens in Neutropenic Cancer Patients," *J Clin Microbiol*, 1994, 32(3):766-76.

Reiss E and Morrison CJ, "Nonculture Methods for Diagnosis of Disseminated Candidiasis," *Clin Microbiol Rev*, 1993, 6(4):311-23.

Walsh TJ, Hathorn JW, Sobel JD, et al, "Detection of Circulating *Candida* Enolase by Immunoassay in Patients With Cancer and Invasive Candidiasis," *N Engl J Med*, 1991, 324(15):1026-31.

Candidiasis Serologic Test

CPT 86628

Related Information

Candida Antigen *on previous page*
Fungal Culture, Biopsy or Body Fluid *on page 476*
Fungal Culture, Blood *on page 477*
Fungal Culture, Sputum *on page 479*
Fungal Culture, Stool *on page 480*
Fungal Culture, Urine *on page 480*
Fungus Smear, Stain *on page 481*

Test Commonly Includes Precipitin test by agar gel diffusion

Specimen Serum

Container Red top tube

Storage Instructions Store serum at 4°C.

Reference Range Negative. A fourfold increase in titer in paired sera drawn 10-14 days apart is usually indicative of acute infection. Titer >1:8 in the latex agglutination test is presumptive for systemic disease.

Use In evaluation of suspected systemic candidiasis, rising titers of agglutinins are believed to be reliable indicators of the presence of visceral candidiasis. Quantitative tests on sera taken at biweekly intervals are of value in monitoring the progress of infection before and after therapy. Although limited data is available, the presence of IgM antibodies appears to provide a good indicator of disseminated candidiasis.

Limitations Cross reactions occur in cases of cryptococcosis and tuberculosis with the latex agglutination test. Negative results do not rule out candidiasis. This test is difficult to interpret because precipitins are found in 20% to 30% of the normal population. Very severe cases of vaginitis or mucocutaneous candidiasis can produce positive results. Clinical correlation must exist for the test to be useful.

Methodology Latex agglutination (LA), crossed electrophoresis, immunodiffusion (ID), enzyme-linked immunosorbent assay (ELISA)

References

Fujita S, Matsubara F, and Matsuda T, "Enzyme-Linked Immunosorbent Assay Measurement of Fluctuations in Antibody Titer and Antigenemia in Cancer Patients With and Without Candidiasis," *J Clin Microbiol*, 1986, 23(3):568-75.

Gutierrez J, Maroto C, Peidrola G, et al, "Circulating *Candida* Antigens and Antibodies: Useful Markers of Candidemia," *J Clin Microbiol*, 1993, 31(9):2550-2.

Hayette MP, Strecker G, Faille C, et al, "Presence of Human Antibodies Reacting With *Candida albicans* O-Linked Oligomannosides Revealed by Using an Enzyme-Linked Immunosorbent Assay and Neoglycolipids," *J Clin Microbiol*, 1992, 30(2):411-7.

Reiss E and Morrison CJ, "Nonculture Methods for Diagnosis of Disseminated Candidiasis," *Clin Microbiol Rev*, 1993, 6(4):311-23.

Cat Scratch Disease Serology

Related Information

Lymph Node Biopsy *on page 50*
Skin Biopsy *on page 54*

Synonyms *Bartonella* Antibodies; *Rochalimaea* Antibodies

Applies to PCR Assay for *Bartonella*; PCR Assay for *Rochalimaea*

Abstract *Bartonella*, small gram-negative rods, include *B. quintana* and *B. henselae*, both of which have been associated with bacillary angiomatosis, bacillary peliosis hepatis, and bacteremia. **Bacillary angiomatosis**, characterized by subcutaneous nodules and fever, occurs primarily in subjects with AIDS but has been found as well in immunocompetent patients and in recipients of organ transplants.

Cat scratch disease (CSD) is found in immunocompetent individuals, 80% of whom are younger than 21 years of age.[1] It is thought to be caused by *B. henselae*.[2]

Specimen Serum, separated quickly

Collection Paired serum samples are desirable, one drawn 2-4 weeks after the other. Blood cultures are indicated as well.

Causes for Rejection Plasma, severe lipemia, hemolysis

Reference Range IgG: <1:64; IgM: <1:16

Critical Values Fourfold increase in titer is meaningful. IgG: ≥1:256; IgM: ≥1:16; provide evidence of recent or present infection

Clinical Syndromes Associated With *Bartonella* Species

Cutaneous bacillary angiomatosis
Extracutaneous infection
Bacillary peliosis of the liver (bacillary peliosis hepatitis) and spleen
Fever and bacteremia (*Bartonella* bacteremic syndrome)
Cat scratch disease (associated only with *Bartonella henselae* to date)
Trench fever (associated only with *B. quintana*)

From Adal KA, Cockerell CJ, and Petri WA Jr, "Cat Scratch Disease, Bacillary Angiomatosis, and Other Infections Due to *Rochalimaea*," *N Engl J Med*, 1994, 330(21):1509, with permission.

Limitations Significance of these new serologic methods is not yet fully known. IgM titers without IgG increases must be interpreted with caution.

Methodology Indirect fluorescent antibody (IFA) testing to Centers for Disease Control and Prevention; enzyme immunoassay (EIA) detects IgG antibodies to *B. henselae* and is more sensitive than indirect fluorescent antibody testing.[1]

Additional Information Biopsies of skin and lymph node lesions include well described features. The pleomorphic bacilli may be recognized with the Warthin-Starry method in tissue sections and can be labeled by immunocytochemistry.[3] Detection of specific DNA sequences has enhanced epidemiologic investigations and polymerase chain reaction amplification in arthropods has provided understanding of such zoonotic infections.[4,5] Cat scratch disease is associated with kittens and cats.[5,6] Blood cultures should be obtained.[7,8]

Footnotes

1. Adal KA, Cockerell CJ, and Petri WA Jr, "Cat Scratch Disease, Bacillary Angiomatosis, and Other Infections Due to *Rochalimaea*," *N Engl J Med*, 1994, 330(21):1509-15.

2. Anderson B, Sims K, Regnery R, et al, "Detection of *Rochalimaea henselae* DNA in Specimens From Cat Scratch Disease Patients by PCR," *J Clin Microbiol*, 1994, 32(4):942-8.

3. Min KW, Reed JA, Welch DF, et al, "Morphologically Variable Bacilli of Cat Scratch Disease Are Identified by Immunocytochemical Labeling With Antibodies to *Rochalimaea henselae*," *Am J Clin Pathol*, 1994, 101(5):607-10.

4. Tompkins LS, "*Rochalimaea* Infections. Are They Zoonoses?" *JAMA*, 1994, 271(7):553-4.

5. Koehler JE, Glaser CA, and Tappero JW, "*Rochalimaea henselae* Infection. A New Zoonosis With the Domestic Cat as Reservoir," *JAMA*, 1994, 271(7):531-5.

6. Zangwill KM, Hamilton DH, Perkins BA, et al, "Cat Scratch Disease in Connecticut - Epidemiology, Risk Factors, and Evaluation of a New Diagnostic Test," *N Engl J Med*, 1993, 329(1):8-13.

7. Tierno PM Jr, Inglima K, and Parisi MT, "Detection of *Bartonella (Rochalimaea)* henselae Bacteremia Using BacT/Alert Blood Culture System," *Am J Clin Pathol*, 1995, 104(5):530-6.

8. Cockerell CJ and Bottone EJ, "*Bartonella* Infections. Evolution From the Esoteric," *Am J Clin Pathol*, 1995, 104(5):487-90.

References

"Case Records of the Massachusetts General Hospital. Weekly Clinicopathological Exercises. Case 22-1992. A 6½-Year-Old Girl With Status Epilepticus, Cervical Lymphadenopathy, Pleural Effusions, and Respiratory Distress," *N Engl J Med*, 1992, 326(22):1480-9.

Doyle MD, Eppes SC, and Klein JD, "Atypical Cat-Scratch Disease: Diagnosis by a Serologic test for *Rochalimaea* Species," *South Med J*, 1994, 87(4):485-7.

Reed JA, Brigati DJ, Flynn SD, et al, "Immunocytochemical Identification of *Rochalimaea henselae* in Bacillary (Epithelioid) Angiomatosis," *Am J Surg Pathol*, 1992, 16(7):650-7.

Yu X and Raoult D, "Monoclonal Antibodies to *Afipia felis* - A Putative Agent of Cat Scratch Disease," *Am J Clin Pathol*, 1994, 101(5):603-6.

CD4/CD8 Enumeration

CPT 88180

Related Information

Beta$_2$-Microglobulin *on page 371*
Complete Blood Count *on page 312*
HIV-1/HIV-2 Serology *on page 403*
Human Immunodeficiency Virus Culture *on page 669*
Leukocyte Immunophenotyping *on page 414*
Peripheral Blood: Differential Leukocyte Count *on page 336*
White Blood Count *on page 353*
Zidovudine *on page 580*

Synonyms Immunodeficiency Profile

Applies to Flow Cytometry; Lymphocyte CD4 Counts

Test Commonly Includes Lymphocyte subpopulation enumeration

Abstract Depletion of CD4$^+$ helper/inducer T lymphocytes is the single most significant surrogate marker to study progression of human immunodeficiency virus disease.[1]

Specimen Whole blood

Container Green top (heparin) tube
(Continued)

CD4/CD8 Enumeration *(Continued)*

Storage Instructions Blood ideally is delivered to the laboratory immediately, however whole blood may be held for 48 hours at room temperature prior to assay. Do not refrigerate or freeze sample.

Reference Range Total lymphocytes: 1500-4000/mm^3; CD20 cells: 64-475/mm^3; CD3 cells: 876-1900/mm^3; CD4 cells: 450-1400/mm^3; CD8 cells: 190-725/mm^3; CD4/CD8 ratio: 1.0-3.5

Use Follow patients with HIV infection (CD4 cells <200/mm^3 often indicate progression to clinical AIDS); evaluate thymus-dependent or cellular immunocompetence; enumerate T-helper:T-suppressor ratio; study lymphoproliferative disorders for clonality and lineage. CD4 counts are useful in prediction of the clinical course of *Cryptosporidium* infections[2] as well as prediction of prospects for survival.[3]

Limitations Values can be abnormal if patient is taking steroids or other immunosuppressives, has a severe intercurrent illness, or has had recent surgery requiring general anesthesia; patterns of maturation are disordered and inconsistent in lymphomas.

Methodology Flow cytometry (FC); enumeration of specific subpopulation with batteries of monoclonal antibodies to lymphocyte, myeloid, and precursor antigens (see table)

Antibodies Commonly Used in Lymphocyte Subset Enumeration

Use	Cluster Designation	Available Antibodies
Pan T	CD2	T11, Leu5
Pan T (T-cell antigen receptor)	CD3	T3, Leu4
T helper/inducer	CD4	T4, Leu3
T suppressor/cytotoxic	CD8	T8, Leu2
T-cell ALL/B-cell CLL	CD5	T1, Leu1
T-cell ALL	CD7	3A1, Leu9
CALLA, ALL	CD10	J5, BA-3
Pan B	CD19	B4, Leu12
B cell specific	CD20	B1, Leu16
Mature B (EBV receptor)	CD21	B2
Myeloid/monocytic	CD13	MY7
Myeloid/monocytic	CD33	MY9
Myeloid adhesion	CD11	Mo1, Mac1
Glycoprotein II b/Ma megakaryocytes	CDw41	J15

Additional Information With increased understanding of the functional and immunologic subpopulations of circulating and nodal lymphocytes, and with the commercial availability of monoclonal antibodies to the antigens that define those populations, enumeration of lymphocyte classes has become both possible and clinically important. In the diagnosis and classification of malignant lymphoproliferative disorders, the demonstration of a homogeneous B- or T-lymphocyte population often contributes to prognosis and therapeutic planning. The lineage and stages of development of the proliferating cells can be determined. The demonstration of a reversed T-helper:T-suppressor ratio (<1.0) is important in the diagnosis of acquired immune deficiency syndrome (AIDS) and also helps explain pathogenetically the multiple recurrent opportunistic infections which comprise that illness. The absolute number of T4 cells is crucial in instituting and following treatment with AZT.

Subjects whose CD4 count is <300-400/mm^3, with progressive decline in absolute CD4 count as well as CD4:CD8 ratio less than unity should be intensively worked up for HIV infection and other entities which cause immunodeficiency.

Idiopathic CD4$^+$ T lymphocytopenia is defined by the Centers for Disease Control and Prevention as CD4$^+$ T lymphocytopenia without serologic or virologic evidence of HIV-1 or HIV-2 infection. The diagnosis requires a CD4 count <300/mm^3 on two occasions.[1]

Footnotes

1. Laurence J, "T-Cell Subsets in Health, Infectious Disease, and Idiopathic CD4$^+$ T Lymphocytopenia," *Ann Intern Med*, 1993, 119(1):55-62.
2. Flanigan T, Whalen C, Turner J, et al, "*Cryptosporidium* Infection and CD4 Counts," *Ann Intern Med*, 1992, 116(10):840-2.
3. Phillips AN, Sabin CA, Elford J, et al, "Use of CD4 Lymphocyte Count to Predict Long-Term Survival Free of AIDS After HIV Infection," *BMJ*, 1994, 309(6950):309-13.

References

"Guidelines for the Performance of CD4$^+$ T-Cell Determinations in Persons With Human Immunodeficiency Virus Infection," *MMWR Morb Mortal Wkly Rep*, 1992, 41(RR-8):1-17.

Kagan J, Calvelli T, Denny TN, et al, "Guideline for Flow Cytometric Immunophenotypic, a Report From the National Institute of Allergy and Infectious Diseases, Division of AIDS," *Cytometry*, 1993, 14(7):702-15.

Keren DF, Hanson CA, and Hurtubise PE, *Flow Cytometry and Clinical Diagnosis*, Chicago, IL: American Society of Clinical Pathologists, 1994.

Landay A, Ohlsson-Wilhelm B, and Giorgi JV, "Application of Flow Cytometry to the Study of HIV INfection," *AIDS*, 1990, 4(6)479-9.

Nicholson JK, "Use of Flow Cytometry in the Evaluation and Diagnosis of Primary and Secondary Immunodeficiency Diseases," *Arch Pathol Lab Med*, 1989, 113(6):598-605.

Schmidt RE, "Monoclonal Antibodies for Diagnosis of Immunodeficiencies," *Blut*, 1989, 59(3):200-6.

Schroeder TJ, First MR, Hurtubise PE, et al, "Immunologic Monitoring With Orthoclone OKT3 Therapy," *J Heart Transplant*, 1989, 8(5):371-80.

Stein DS, Korvick JA, and Vermund SH, "CD4$^+$ Lymphocyte Cell Enumeration for Prediction of Clinical Course of Human Immmunodeficiency Virus Disease: A Review," *J Infect Dis*, 1992, 165(2):352-63.

Centromere/Kinetochore Antibody

CPT 86235

Related Information

Antinuclear Antibody *on page 368*
Scleroderma Antibody *on page 430*

Abstract Anticentromere antibodies are strongly associated with the CREST syndrome. They are a subset of antinuclear antibodies.

Specimen Serum

Container Red top tube

Reference Range Negative

Use Aid in diagnosis of CREST syndrome, for which the presence of such antibodies provides favorable prognostic information.[1]

Anticentromere pattern is found in up to a quarter of individuals with idiopathic Raynaud's phenomenon.[2]

Limitations May be absent in some patients with scleroderma or CREST syndrome

Methodology Indirect immunofluorescent antibody (IFA) detected on HEp-2 tissue culture cell substrate.

Additional Information The anticentromere pattern is seen in about 80% of patients with the CREST syndrome. CREST syndrome (calcinosis, Raynaud's phenomenon, esophageal dysfunction, sclerodactyly, telangiectasia) is a variant of progressive systemic sclerosis. Patients have changes largely confined to the skin and digits, without renal disease. Patients' sera demonstrate speckled fluorescent antinuclear antibody patterns. When indirect immunofluorescence is applied to substrates with mitotic cells, the serum antibody is associated with chromosome centromeres. Its presence in patients without scleroderma or CREST often indicates the presence of another sometimes serious underlying autoimmune disease.

Footnotes

1. Leavelle DE, *Mayo Medical Laboratories Interpretive Handbook*, Rochester, MN: Mayo Medical Laboratories, 1994.
2. Moder KG, "Use and Interpretation of Rheumatologic Tests: A Guide for Clinicians," *Mayo Clin Proc*, 1996, 71(4):391-6.

References

Gilliland BC, "Systemic Sclerosis (Scleroderma)," *Harrison's Principles of Internal Medicine*, 13th ed, Vol 2, Isselbacher KJ, Braunwald E, Wilson E, et al, eds, New York, NY: McGraw-Hill Inc, 1994, 1653-62.

Goldman JA, "Anticentromere Antibody in Patients Without CREST and Scleroderma: Association With Active Digital Vasculitis, Rheumatic and Connective Tissue Disease," *Ann Rheum Dis*, 1989, 48(9):771-5.

Cerebrospinal Fluid Amyloid Precursor Protein and Amyloid β-Protein

Related Information

Apolipoprotein E *on page 82*
Cerebrospinal Fluid Tau Protein *on page 382*

Synonyms Amyloid Beta Peptide; Amyloid Precursor Protein (APP), CSF; βA (or Aβ) Peptide; APP, CSF; CSF Amyloid Precursor Protein and Amyloid β-Protein

Applies to sAβ; Soluble Amyloid Beta

Abstract Alzheimer's disease appears to relate importantly to abnormalities in amyloid proteins and/or amyloid protein processing. The ε4 allele of apolipoprotein E might act as a "pathological chaperone" for β-amyloid precursor protein, while the ε2 allele may act as a "neuroprotective guardian"[1] (ie, ε4 is associated with faster deposition of β-amyloid protein deposition).[2]

Patient Preparation Patient should be informed, relaxed, and properly positioned for lumbar puncture. Signed consent form is required. Antiseptic agents must be carefully and properly applied to the proposed puncture site. Local anesthetic (to which patient is not allergic) is usually advised.

Aftercare Patient should be maintained supine for a few hours postpuncture in an attempt to avoid postpuncture headache.

Specimen Cerebrospinal fluid

Collection Lumbar (usual site) cerebrospinal fluid collection

Storage Instructions Freeze immediately on dry ice and store at -70°C.

Causes for Rejection Specimen contaminated with blood ("bloody tap"); specimen not frozen

Special Instructions Advance preparation (following the recommendations of research or referral laboratory) should be made prior to obtaining specimen.

Reference Range APP: 2.7 ±0.7 µg/mL. Alzheimer's disease patients have levels of APP about one-third of normal (0.8 ±0.4 µg/mL).[3] Absolute values will depend on antibody specificity.

Use Possible contribution to the diagnosis of Alzheimer's disease (AD). Aβ is present in CSF while APP is decreased in patients with AD.

Limitations Multiple forms of Aβ may occur in CSF from patients with meningitis and other neurologic disorders. Results are importantly dependent upon the sensitivity and specificity of the monoclonal antibody used in the test procedure and may vary among laboratories.

Methodology Immunoblotting, enzyme-linked immunosorbent assay (ELISA)

Additional Information Tests based on amyloid protein for diagnosis of Alzheimer's disease (AD) are in an early stage of evolution. AD is a central nervous system degenerative process characterized by the presence of senile plaques and congophilic vascular deposits. Aβ is the major component of fibrils forming the senile plaques and vascular deposits. Aβ is a 27-43 residue proteolytic degradation product of APP (amyloid precursor protein). Aβ deposits in Alzheimer plaques and vessels are largely of 39-42 residues. It has been established by a number of research teams that Aβ and APP are present in CSF. The CSF soluble form of amyloid beta (sAβ) has been shown to be complexed to SP-40,40 (apolipoprotein J) and that this interaction occurs in vivo.[4] sAβ occurs in CSF as a proteolytic product of APP but can also bind to CSF APP with high avidity. Abnormalities, some or possibly all, with a genetic basis in Aβ amyloid peptide binding, solubilization, transport and/or degradation may contribute importantly to the pathologic deposition of Aβ in brains of patients with AD. An accompanying finding may be a decrease in the CSF level of APP and/or its complexed forms.

Footnotes
1. Campion EW, "When a Mind Dies," *N Engl J Med*, 1996, 334(12):791-2.
2. Reiman EM, Caselli RJ, Yun LS, et al, "Preclinical Evidence of Alzheimer's Disease in Persons Homozygous for the ε4 Allele for Apolipoprotein E," *N Engl J Med*, 1996, 334(12):752-8.
3. Van Nostrand WE, Wagner SL, Shankle WR, et al, "Decreased Levels of Soluble Amyloid β-Protein Precursor in Cerebrospinal Fluid of Live Alzheimer Disease Patients," *Proc Natl Acad Sci USA*, 1992, 89(7):2551-5.
4. Ghiso J, Matsubara E, Koudinov A, et al, "The Cerebrospinal-Fluid Soluble Form of Alzheimer's Amyloid Beta Is Complexed to SP-40,40 (Apolipoprotein J), an Inhibitor of the Complement Membrane-Attack Complex," *Biochem J*, 1993, 293(Pt 1):27-30.

References
Henriksson T, Barbour RM, Braa S, et al, "Analysis and Quantitation of the Beta-Amyloid Precursor Protein in the Cerebrospinal Fluid of Alzheimer's Disease Patients With a Monoclonal Antibody-Based Immunoassay," *J Neurochem*, 1991, 56(3):1037-42.
Seubert P, Vigo-Pelfrey C, Esch F, et al, "Isolation and Quantification of Soluble Alzheimer's Beta-Peptide From Biological Fluids," *Nature*, 1992, 359(6393):325-7.
Shoyi M, Golde TE, Ghio J, et al, "Production of the Alzheimer Amyloid Beta Protein by Normal Proteolytic Processing," *Science*, 1992, 258(5079):126-9.
Strittmatter WJ, Huang DY, Bhasin R, et al, "Avid Binding of Beta A Amyloid Peptide to Its Own Precursor," *Exp Neurol*, 1993, 122(2):327-34.
Vigo-Pelfrey C, Lee D, Keim P, et al, "Characterization of Beta-Amyloid Peptide From Human Cerebrospinal Fluid," *J Neurochem*, 1993, 61(5):1965-8.
Wagner SL, Peskind ER, Nochlin D, et al, "Decreased Levels of Soluble Amyloid Beta-Protein Precursor Are Associated With Alzheimer's Disease in Concordant and Discordant Monozygous Twin Pairs," *Ann Neurol*, 1994, 36(2):215-20.

Cerebrospinal Fluid Cryptococcal Latex Agglutination see
Cryptococcal Antigen Titer on page 388

Cerebrospinal Fluid, FTA-ABS see FTA-ABS, Cerebrospinal Fluid
on page 394

Cerebrospinal Fluid IgG see Cerebrospinal Fluid Immunoglobulin
G on next page

Cerebrospinal Fluid IgG Ratios and IgG Index

CPT 82784 (IgG); 84165 (protein, electrophoretic quantitation)

Related Information
Cerebrospinal Fluid Analysis on page 309
Cerebrospinal Fluid Immunoglobulin G on next page
Cerebrospinal Fluid Myelin Basic Protein on page 379
Cerebrospinal Fluid Oligoclonal Bands on page 379
Cerebrospinal Fluid Protein on page 380

Synonyms CSF IgG/CSF α₂-Macroglobulin; CSF IgG/CSF Albumin Ratio; CSF IgG/CSF Total Protein Ratio; IgG Ratios and IgG Index, Cerebrospinal Fluid

Test Commonly Includes Protein measurements, frequently immunochemical, on CSF and/or serum with determination of ratio or ratios of one protein to another.

Abstract The IgG index can be calculated with use of serum and CSF albumin and IgG.

Patient Preparation Patient should be informed, relaxed, and properly positioned for lumbar puncture. Signed consent form is required. Antiseptic agents must be carefully and properly applied to the proposed puncture site. Local anesthetic (to which patient is not allergic) is usually advised.

Aftercare Patient should be maintained supine for a few hours postpuncture in an attempt to avoid postpuncture headache.

Specimen Cerebrospinal fluid and serum; usually at least 0.1-0.5 mL of CSF is required.

Container Clean, sterile CSF tube; red top tube

Collection Tube should be labeled with the number indicating the sequence in which tubes were obtained.

Storage Instructions Store CSF in refrigerator at 4°C.

Causes for Rejection CSF received without concurrently obtained serum, insufficient quantity of CSF, CSF contaminated with blood ("bloody tap")

Special Instructions Before performing lumbar puncture, communicate with laboratory to determine which measurements and ratios are offered or can be obtained on a referral basis. The third tube of routinely obtained three tube set of CSF should be used for these studies.

Reference Range CSF IgG index: 0.3-0.85.[1] Published information is relevant only to lumbar CSF. Ventricular, cisternal, or cervical CSF will have different reference ranges.

Use The level of IgG production by the central nervous system has been applied to support the diagnosis of multiple sclerosis (CSF IgG index, CSF immunoglobulin synthesis rate and CSF immunoglobulin "oligoclonal" bands).

Limitations Conditions in which lymphoreticular elements of the CNS produce immunoglobulins will result in false-positive (in relation to multiple sclerosis) elevations. Such conditions include but are not limited to aseptic meningitis, lymphoma, subacute sclerosing panencephalitis (SPE), sarcoid, neurosyphilis, Guillain-Barré syndrome, and cerebral lupus erythematosus. These conditions, however, are either uncommon or are not frequently associated with an increased IgG index. It has been asserted that without presence of CSF oligoclonal bands the IgG index has no diagnostic value for multiple sclerosis (MS). The index has been noted to have limitations even as a screening test. Even a small amount of bloody contamination elevates the IgG index and IgG synthesis rate.[1]

Methodology Wide variety of generally immunochemical based methods (eg, nephelometry). See also listing Cerebrospinal Fluid Immunoglobulin G on page 378.

Additional Information The finding that patients with multiple sclerosis frequently have increased CSF IgG has led to a quest for a test that would provide sensitive and specific support for the diagnosis. The three contenders, IgG index, synthesis rate, and oligoclonal bands, have shown sensitivity at the 80% to 90% level but are not uniformly specific. CSF IgG may be increased, generally with inflammatory disorders of the CNS (eg, idiopathic polyneuropathy, neurosyphilis). Rents in the interface between blood and CSF will allow increase in CSF IgG. The three contending methods attempt to differentiate between increased barrier permeability and increased CNS immunoglobulin synthesis, each in a different manner. The ratio technique relates CSF IgG level to another protein that hopefully reflects protein present on the basis of increased blood/CSF permeability. CSF IgG/CSF total protein is such a measure. CSF IgG/CSF albumin has been proposed by Tourtellotte et al as equally discriminative for MS as the CSF IgG/CSF total protein ratio. Both methods as originally described utilize electroimmunodiffusion described by Tourtellotte as "easy, rapid, sensitive, and reliable." The method requires only 5 µL of CSF (no concentration needed). This procedure, however, is being supplanted by less technically demanding automated immunochemical analyses. These ratios and a third, CSF IgG/CSF α₂-macroglobulin, are being supplanted by the IgG index, a ratio of ratios (CSF/serum IgG / CSF/serum albumin), which compares CSF with serum parameters. The index provides good separation of increased CNS IgG production from protein increases, the result of altered permeability of blood/CNS interface.

Results of IgG index testing appear to correlate with those of oligoclonal banding determinations, but the IgG index may have no specific value independent of the presence of oligoclonal bands.

Recommendations continue for careful clinical neurologic evaluation in cases of suspected multiple sclerosis as all of the laboratory testing procedures produce nonspecific results. Free kappa light chains in the CSF may represent a relatively specific laboratory abnormality to support a clinical diagnosis of multiple sclerosis.

In a population of 56 HIV-seropositive individuals in which five had AIDS, 30% showed an increase in the CSF:serum albumin/IgG ratio.[2]

Patients with sciatica caused by lumbar disk herniation may leak plasma proteins into the CSF resulting in increased CSF total protein. Disk patients with paresis may have significant increase in CSF total protein, CSF albumin and IgG, and in the CSF/serum albumin and IgG ratios but not in the IgG index (as compared to patients with lumbar disk herniation but without symptoms).[3] Because cigarette smoking may result in increased endoneural capillary permeability, plasma albumin may leak from the nerve root into the CSF. Regression analysis studies have (Continued)

Cerebrospinal Fluid IgG Ratios and IgG Index
(Continued)

shown an increase in CSF/serum albumin ratio, in particular, in men who are smokers and have paresis from lumbar disk herniation.[3]

Footnotes

1. Fishman RA, *Cerebrospinal Fluid in Diseases of the Nervous System*, 2nd ed, Philadelphia, PA: WB Saunders Co, 1992, 207-8.
2. Hall CD, Snyder CR, and Robertson KR, "Cerebrospinal Fluid Analysis in Human Immunodeficiency Virus Infection," *Ann Clin Lab Sci*, 1992, 22(3):139-43.
3. Skouen JS, Larsen JL, and Vollset SE, "Cerebrospinal Fluid Protein Concentrations Related to Clinical Findings in Patients With Sciatica Caused by Disk Herniation," *J Spinal Disord*, 1994, 7(1):12-8.

References

Barna BP, Valenzuela R, and Gupta MK, "Laboratory Analyses of Cerebrospinal Fluid," *Laboratory Handbook of Neuroimmunologic Disease*, Chapter 5, Barna BP, ed, Chicago, IL: American Society of Clinical Pathologists, 1987, 65-104.

Giles PD, Heath JP, and Wroe SJ, "Oligoclonal Bands and the IgG Index in Multiple Sclerosis: Uses and Limitations," *Ann Clin Biochem*, 1989, 26(Pt 4):317-23.

Keren DF, "Multiple Sclerosis and Oligoclonal Bands," *High-Resolution Electrophoresis: Techniques and Interpretation*, Chapter 3, Boston, MA: Butterworth's Publishers, 1987, 86-93.

Rudick RA, French CA, Breton D, et al, "Relative Diagnostic Value of Cerebrospinal Fluid Kappa Chains in MS: Comparison With Other Immunoglobulin Tests," *Neurology*, 1989, 39(7):964-8.

Tourtellotte WW, Tavolato B, Parker JA, et al, "Cerebrospinal Fluid Electroimmunodiffusion. An Easy, Rapid, Sensitive, Reliable, and Valid Method for the Simultaneous Determination of Immunoglobulin G and Albumin," *Arch Neurol*, 1971, 25:345-50.

Cerebrospinal Fluid IgG Synthesis Rate
CPT 82784

Related Information

Cerebrospinal Fluid Immunoglobulin G *on this page*
Cerebrospinal Fluid Oligoclonal Bands *on next page*
Cerebrospinal Fluid Protein Electrophoresis *on page 381*

Synonyms IgG Synthesis Rate, Cerebrospinal Fluid

Test Commonly Includes Serum and CSF IgG and albumin levels, calculation of IgG synthesis rate

Abstract Estimation of amount of IgG synthesized daily in the CNS, with the intention to correct for the amount of IgG entering from serum. Used to support the diagnosis of multiple sclerosis.

Patient Preparation Patient should be informed, relaxed, and properly positioned for lumbar puncture. Signed consent form is required. Antiseptic agents must be carefully and properly applied to the proposed puncture site. Local anesthetic (to which patient is not allergic) is usually advised.

Aftercare Patient should be maintained supine for a few hours postpuncture in an attempt to avoid postpuncture headache.

Specimen Cerebrospinal fluid and serum obtained concurrently. Usually at least 0.1-0.5 mL of CSF is required.

Container Clean, sterile CSF tube; red top tube

Storage Instructions Refrigerate CSF at 4°C.

Causes for Rejection CSF received without concurrently obtained serum, insufficient quantity of CSF, CSF contaminated with blood ("bloody tap")

Special Instructions Before performing lumbar puncture, communicate with laboratory to determine availability and specimen requirements. As a number of possibly helpful tests and ratios (applicable to the diagnosis of multiple sclerosis) based on protein immunochemical determinations have become available, individual laboratories may perform only a select few. Commercial (referral) laboratories may also be selective.

Reference Range 0.14 ±1.8 mg IgG synthesized/day, dependent upon the individual laboratory; normal values for CSF albumin and immunoglobulin G

Use Evaluate the *de novo* rate of synthesis of IgG in the CNS. Useful in diagnosis of inflammatory and autoimmune diseases involving the CNS, in particular, multiple sclerosis. Determination of IgG synthesis rate is based on the quotient of average normal serum IgG/average normal CSF IgG. As such it is dependent upon the validity of the IgG method and normal range of each individual laboratory. As indicated previously, there are a variety of different testing approaches in use. Good laboratory practice requires establishing one's own normal range, especially important in this area. A sufficiently large sample of "normal" CSF, however, is not easily obtained.

Limitations The formula involves a constant described as "a ratio constant that quantitatively determines the proportion of CSF IgG that normally passes by filtration from the serum into the CSF across an intact BBB" (blood-brain barrier). Even a small amount of bloody contamination elevates IgG index and IgG synthesis rate. Fishman notes a lack of unanimity of opinion regarding the virtues of the various calculations which have been advocated, and concludes that he prefers the IgG-albumin index.[1] Quantitative measurements of CNS IgG production are reported to be less sensitive than isoelectric focusing.[2]

Methodology A variety of usually immunochemical based methods are available. Nephelometry, rate immunonephelometry and electroimmunodiffusion have been used. See listing Cerebrospinal Fluid Immunoglobulin G *on page 378*.

Additional Information Tourtellotte's IgG synthesis rate is theoretically the most definitive approach to determining IgG production by the central nervous system. It is based upon an empirically derived formula, the validity of which, however, has been verified by radiolabeled IgG experiments. The formula is given as: *de novo* CNS $IgG_{syn} = ((IgG_{CSF} - IgG_s/369) - (Alb_{CSF} - Alb_s/230)(IgG_s/Alb_s) 0.43) \times 5$. The constants (eg, 369 and 230) are method dependent and may vary from laboratory to laboratory. Controversy concerning the accuracy of the IgG synthesis formula has been expressed. A study by Tourtellotte and associates has shown that about 90% of multiple sclerosis patients show evidence of enhanced IgG synthesis. A study from the Cleveland Clinic indicates a sensitivity and specificity comparable to that for the IgG index (see listing Cerebrospinal Fluid IgG Ratios and IgG Index *on page 377*) in predictive value for MS with sensitivity (96%) and specificity (98%) applied to a group considered as definite multiple sclerosis. A group of "possible multiple sclerosis" patients included a number of cases in which CNS IgG synthesis was normal - just 55% had an elevated rate. In the group with "neurologic diseases other than MS," 96% of patients had normal CNS IgG synthesis. The study suggests that determination of CSF IgG synthesis rate contributes importantly to the diagnosis of MS. The study also emphasizes that correlations between test results and diagnoses are dependent upon the validity of what must remain a clinical neurologic diagnosis.

Footnotes

1. Fishman RA, *Cerebrospinal Fluid in Diseases of the Nervous System*, 2nd ed, Philadelphia, PA: WB Saunders Co, 1992, 207-8.
2. Andersson M, Alvarez-Cermeno J, Bernardi G, et al, "Cerebrospinal Fluid in the Diagnosis of Multiple Sclerosis: A Consensus Report," *J Neurol Neurosurg Psychiatry*, 1994, 57(8):897-902.

References

Barna BP, Valenzuela R, and Gupta MK, "Laboratory Analyses of Cerebrospinal Fluid," *Laboratory Handbook of Neuroimmunologic Disease*, Chapter 5, Barna BP, ed, Chicago, IL: American Society of Clinical Pathologists, 1987, 65-104.

Thompson EJ and Keir G, "Laboratory Investigation of Cerebrospinal Fluid Proteins," *Ann Clin Biochem*, 1990, 27(Pt 5):425-35.

Tourtellotte WW, Potvin AR, Fleming JO, et al, "Multiple Sclerosis: Measurement and Validation of Central Nervous System IgG Synthesis Rate," *Neurology*, 1980, 30:240-4.

Tourtellotte WW, Staugaitis SM, Walsh MJ, et al, "The Basis of Intra-Blood-Brain-Barrier IgG Synthesis," *Ann Neurol*, 1985, 17(1):21-7.

Cerebrospinal Fluid Immunoglobulin G
CPT 82784

Related Information

Cerebrospinal Fluid IgG Ratios and IgG Index *on previous page*
Cerebrospinal Fluid IgG Synthesis Rate *on this page*
Cerebrospinal Fluid Oligoclonal Bands *on next page*
Cerebrospinal Fluid Protein *on page 380*

Synonyms Cerebrospinal Fluid IgG; CSF Gamma G; CSF IgG; CSF Immunoglobulin; Gamma G, CSF; IgG, CSF; Immunoglobulin G, Cerebrospinal Fluid; Spinal Fluid Globulin; Spinal Fluid Immunoglobulin

Replaces Colloidal Gold Curve

Patient Preparation Patient should be informed, relaxed, and properly positioned for lumbar puncture. Signed consent form is required. Antiseptic agents must be carefully and properly applied to the proposed puncture site. Local anesthetic (to which patient is not allergic) is usually advised.

Aftercare Patient should be maintained supine for a few hours postpuncture in an attempt to avoid postpuncture headache.

Specimen Cerebrospinal fluid; usually at least 0.1-0.5 mL of CSF is required.

Container Clean, sterile CSF tube

Collection Tube should be labeled with the sequence in which tubes were obtained.

Storage Instructions Store in refrigerator.

Causes for Rejection CSF received without concurrently obtained serum, insufficient quantity of CSF, CSF contaminated with blood ("bloody tap")

Special Instructions The third tube of a routinely obtained three tube set of CSF should be used for CSF IgG study.

Reference Range Normal CSF IgG: 5% to 12% of total CSF protein.[1] There is no evidence of diurnal variation.

Use Evaluate central nervous system involvement by infection, neoplasm, or primary neurologic disease (in particular, multiple sclerosis)

Limitations Normal levels do not exclude disease; clinical correlation is needed.

Methodology Radial immunodiffusion (RID), electroimmunodiffusion, immunofluorometry, immunoprecipitation, immunonephelometry, rate immunonephelometry. A comparison of immunochemical methods (RID, rate nephelometry, and nephelometric light scattering at quasi-equilibrium) showed that calibrator crossover studies agreed well although precipitating diameters were difficult to read below IgG levels <3 mg/dL (SI: <0.03 g/L).

Additional Information Cerebrospinal fluid protein is elevated in many conditions which affect the central nervous system primarily or secondarily. In inflammatory or destructive processes in which serum leaks into CSF, both IgG and albumin will be present in the CSF in increased amounts. Since albumin is not, but immunoglobulins are, synthesized in the central nervous system, a relative increase in CSF IgG indicates presence of a process involving the central nervous system primarily, in particular multiple sclerosis.

While MS patients are maintained on ACTH and/or steroid therapy or during remission, CSF IgG levels decrease but generally remain significantly elevated.

Electrophoresis of CSF may also be enlightening if oligoclonal gamma globulin bands are demonstrated, which also suggest multiple sclerosis. See also the test listing Cerebrospinal Fluid Oligoclonal Bands *on page 379.*

Footnotes
1. Fishman RA, *Cerebrospinal Fluid in Diseases of the Nervous System*, 2nd ed, Philadelphia, PA: WB Saunders Co, 1992, 206-14.

References

Barna BP, Valenzuela R, and Gupta MK, "Laboratory Analyses of Cerebrospinal Fluid," *Laboratory Handbook of Neuroimmunologic Disease*, Chapter 5, Barna BP, ed, Chicago, IL: American Society of Clinical Pathologists, 1987, 65-104.

Ben-Menachem E, Persson L, Schechter PJ, et al, "Cerebrospinal Fluid Parameters in Healthy Volunteers During Serial Lumbar Punctures," *J Neurochem*, 1989, 52(2):632-5.

Christenson RH, Russell ME, and Hassett BJ, "Cerebrospinal Fluid: Electrophoresis and Methods for Determining Immunoglobulin G Compared," *Clin Biochem*, 1989, 22(6):429-32.

Marshall DW, Brey RL, Cahill WT, et al, "Spectrum of Cerebrospinal Fluid Findings in Various Stages of Human Immunodeficiency Virus Infection," *Arch Neurol*, 1988, 45(9):954-8.

Cerebrospinal Fluid Myelin Basic Protein

CPT 83873

Related Information

Cerebrospinal Fluid IgG Ratios and IgG Index *on page 377*
Cerebrospinal Fluid Oligoclonal Bands *on this page*

Synonyms CSF Myelin Basic Protein; MBP Assay; Myelin Basic Protein, Cerebrospinal Fluid; Spinal Fluid Myelin Basic Protein

Abstract Myelin basic protein, a component of the myelin nerve sheath, is a product of oligodendroglia. Assay for MBP is more of an assessment of disease activity than a diagnostic test for any particular disease.

Patient Preparation Patient should be informed, relaxed, and properly positioned for lumbar puncture. Signed consent form is required. Antiseptic agents must be carefully and properly applied to the proposed puncture site. Local anesthetic (to which patient is not allergic) is usually advised.

Aftercare Patient should be maintained supine for a few hours postpuncture in an attempt to avoid postpuncture headache.

Specimen Cerebrospinal fluid

Container Clean, sterile CSF tube

Storage Instructions Freeze immediately after obtaining specimen.

Causes for Rejection CSF contaminated with blood ("bloody tap")

Special Instructions Communicate with laboratory to obtain details of specimen collection. Sample is usually referred to reference laboratory. CSF sample should preferably be obtained when patient is symptomatic (ie, not between acute episodes).

Reference Range (Immunoassay) no active demyelination: <4 ng/mL (or 4 μg/L);[1] weakly positive result: 5.1-6.0 μg/L; consistent with active demyelinating process: >6.0 μg/L

Use Estimate activity of demyelinating diseases of the central nervous system, in particular multiple sclerosis (MS)

Limitations Multiple sclerosis is often episodic. The MBP level may be low to undetectable between attacks. Patients in remission usually have no detectable MBP in their spinal fluid. MBP is optimally detected in CSF within 5-15 days of the onset of an acute exacerbation. The MBP molecule fragments readily undergo conformational changes in relation to solid surfaces versus liquid environment, and exhibit multiple immunologic determinants with different binding affinities. These and other considerations have led to disparate results of MBP RIA analyses from laboratory to laboratory. The variable expression of antigenic sites in relation to conformational changes occurring in the parent MBP molecule and its fragments also provide an explanation for the observation that MBP antigen and antibody to MBP antigen sometimes exist together in the same CSF or serum. Possibly, utilization of a radioligand of human MBP synthetic peptide 69-89 or human MBP peptide 43-88 as antigen

for radioimmunoassay may improve sensitivity, but the nature of specificity for MBP would remain to be established. The level is increased in a number of entities which cause breakdown of myelin, including stroke, hypoxia, trauma, neoplasms, leukodystrophies, Wernicke's disease, Guillain-Barré syndrome, and CNS LE.[2,3]

Methodology Radioimmunoassay (RIA), enzyme immunoassay (EIA)

Additional Information This test provides a measure of myelin fragments released into the spinal fluid as a result of the breakdown of myelin during acute phases in the course of demyelinating disease of the CNS (most common example of which is multiple sclerosis). MBP is a 169 amino acid peptide which comprises 30% of the protein of the myelin sheath. While MBP is a useful test in the diagnosis of active MS, some patients with this disorder will have normal levels, especially during remissions, and elevations may be seen in other disorders as well. Therefore, tests such as CSF oligoclonal bands and IgG index, which are positive in 90% of MS patients during active disease **or** revision, are preferred for laboratory support of the initial diagnosis. However, MBP is useful for providing objective evidence of disease activity.

CSF MBP levels were found to decrease to the level of controls in a group of 11 cases of chronic progressive multiple sclerosis receiving immunosuppressive therapy (cyclophosphamide and prednisone). These findings suggest that RIA for MBP might be used to monitor the hoped for beneficial effect of such therapy in some cases of MS.

It has been suggested that MBP levels in the CSF might be used in the assessment of radiation-induced myelopathy. MS patients in relapse have been shown to have increased interleukin 1 and interleukin 2 production as the result of MBP-stimulated peripheral blood mononuclear cells.

Initial evaluation of 130 HIV-infected patients for the presence of CSF myelin basic protein found none with MBP. Subsequent development of CNS symptoms with abnormal IgG parameters was not associated with abnormal MBP levels. MBP may play a role in the etiology of multiple sclerosis, acting as a target antigen in an autoimmune process. A study of Shanghai Chinese (genetically susceptible to MS), however, did not show correlation of polymorphisms (within the tetranucleotide repeat region of the MBP gene) with susceptibility to MS.[4]

Footnotes
1. Mukherjee A, Vogt RF, and Linthicum DS, "Measurement of Myelin Basic Protein by Radioimmunoassay in Closed Head Trauma, Multiple Sclerosis, and Other Neurological Diseases," *Clin Biochem*, 1985, 18(5):304-7.
2. Fishman RA, *Cerebrospinal Fluid in Diseases of the Nervous System*, 2nd ed, Philadelphia, PA: WB Saunders Co, 1992, 210.
3. Kjeldsberg CR and Knight JA, *Body Fluids - Laboratory Examination of Amniotic, Cerebrospinal, Seminal, Serous and Synovial Fluids*, 3rd ed, Chicago, IL: American Society of Clinical Pathologists, 1993, 93-4.
4. Kelly MA, Zhang Y, Mijovic CH, et al, "Genetic Susceptibility to Multiple Sclerosis in the Shanghai Chinese Is Not Linked to the Myelin Basic Protein Gene Microsatellite," *J Clin Pathol Mol Pathol*, 1995, 48(2):M111-2.

References

Lamers KJ, Uitdehaag BM, Hommes OR, et al, "The Short-Term Effect of an Immunosuppressive Treatment on CSF Myelin Basic Protein in Chronic Progressive Multiple Sclerosis," *J Neurol Neurosurg Psychiatry*, 1988, 51(10):1334-7.

Whitaker JN and Herman PK, "Human Myelin Basic Protein Peptide 69-89: Immunochemical Features and Use in Immunoassays of Cerebrospinal Fluid," *J Neuroimmunol*, 1988, 19(1-2):47-57.

Cerebrospinal Fluid Oligoclonal Bands

CPT 83916

Related Information

Apolipoprotein E *on page 82*
Cerebrospinal Fluid IgG Ratios and IgG Index *on page 377*
Cerebrospinal Fluid IgG Synthesis Rate *on previous page*
Cerebrospinal Fluid Immunoglobulin G *on previous page*
Cerebrospinal Fluid Myelin Basic Protein *on this page*
Cerebrospinal Fluid Protein Electrophoresis *on page 381*
Cerebrospinal Fluid Tau Protein *on page 382*

Synonyms Oligoclonal Bands, Cerebrospinal Fluid; Spinal Fluid Oligoclonal Bands

Test Commonly Includes High-resolution electrophoresis of cerebrospinal fluid and serum obtained concurrently

Abstract Oligoclonal bands on CSF electrophoresis are typical of but not pathognomonic for multiple sclerosis. Quantitative and qualitative tests for multiple sclerosis and other inflammatory and immunological disorders of the CNS are complementary.[1]

Patient Preparation Patient should be informed, relaxed, and properly positioned for lumbar puncture. Signed consent form is required. Antiseptic agents must be carefully and properly applied to the proposed puncture site. Local anesthetic (to which patient is not allergic) is usually advised.

Aftercare Patient should be maintained supine for a few hours postpuncture in an attempt to avoid postpuncture headache.

Specimen Cerebrospinal fluid and serum obtained concurrently

(Continued)

Cerebrospinal Fluid Oligoclonal Bands

(Continued)

Container Clean, sterile CSF tube; red top tube

Storage Instructions Refrigerate at 4°C.

Causes for Rejection CSF contaminated with blood ("bloody tap"), CSF submitted without accompanying serum specimen

Reference Range Normal CSF has no demonstrable oligoclonal bands.

Use Oligoclonal CSF bands contribute to the diagnosis of inflammatory and autoimmune disease of the CNS. In particular, they are found in 83% to 94% of subjects with clinically definite multiple sclerosis and in 100% of patients with subacute sclerosing panencephalitis,[1] and in other degenerative states as well (eg, presenile dementia).

CSF examination is useful in entities such as neuropsychiatric SLE to exclude infectious meningitis.[2]

Limitations Test has a satisfactorily high level of sensitivity (90%, approximately) for association with multiple sclerosis, but it is not specific. Serum protein electrophoresis must be run concurrently to assure that any CSF bands detected do not have origin in the serum.

Although oligoclonal bands have been seen in neuropsychiatric SLE, they lack specificity.[2]

Methodology Thin gel agarose high-resolution electrophoresis. Requires 80 times concentration of CSF. Cellulose acetate and agarose systems generally may detect "oligoclonal" bands but at a much lower level of sensitivity. Isoelectric focusing is preferred by some. Although it results in decreased specificity, it is reported to be the most sensitive method.[3]

Additional Information Important to the diagnosis of multiple sclerosis is the demonstration of "oligoclonal" bands either by high-resolution agarose electrophoresis or by isoelectric focusing. For practical technical/interpretive reasons, high-resolution agarose techniques are preferred over isoelectric focusing. See also listings Cerebrospinal Fluid IgG Synthesis Rate *on page 378* and Cerebrospinal Fluid IgG Ratios and IgG Index *on page 377*. The oligoclonal band test is a specialized CSF electrophoresis test using unique "high resolution" gels and particular equipment. It is not sufficient to order routine CSF electrophoresis and assume that oligoclonal banding will be detected. Many studies indicate a high frequency of oligoclonal bands occurring in CNS of patients with MS. Some have found isoelectric focusing to be more sensitive. IEF, however, is technically more demanding and is not routinely available in the majority of routine clinical laboratories. A combination of oligoclonal bands in CSF and an elevated CSF IgG index may provide the best biochemical indication of the presence of multiple sclerosis. It has also been considered, however, that in patients without oligoclonal bands the IgG index has no diagnostic value relative to multiple sclerosis. Oligoclonal bands are not specific for MS but have been described in many other disorders, including subacute sclerosing panencephalitis, Jakob-Creutzfeldt disease, encephalitis, Guillain-Barré syndrome, neurosyphilis, stroke, cerebral vasculitis, and neoplasms. However, in most of these diseases, oligoclonal bands are uncommon, whereas they are present in about 90% or more of patients with MS.

Evidence that multiple sclerosis is mediated by the immune system is persuasive but circumstantial. The initial target in multiple sclerosis may well be the oligodendrocyte, with degeneration of myelin processes secondary to damage to the myelin-forming function of those cells.[4,5] CNS antibody production may be directed in part against heat shock proteins (HSPs) of oligodendrocytes. CSF antibody titers to heat shock protein correlate with presence of oligoclonal bands.[6]

Oligoclonal banding was present in 26% of asymptomatic, HIV seropositive men.[7]

In a patient with acute myelitis, oligoclonal IgG bands in the CSF were shown to have immunospecificity for GFAP (glial fibrillary acidic protein).[8]

Footnotes

1. Fishman RA, *Cerebrospinal Fluid in Diseases of the Nervous System*, 2nd ed, Philadelphia, PA: WB Saunders Co, 1992, 208-10.
2. Boumpas DT, Austin HA 3d, Fessler BJ, et al, "Systemic Lupus Erythematosus: Emerging Concepts. Part 1: Renal, Neuropsychiatric, Cardiovascular, Pulmonary, and Hematologic Disease," *Ann Intern Med*, 1995, 122(12):940-50.
3. Andersson M, Alvarez-Cermeno J, Bernardi G, et al, "Cerebrospinal Fluid in the Diagnosis of Multiple Sclerosis: A Consensus Report," *J Neurol Neurosurg Psychiatry*, 1994, 57(8):897-902.
4. Ebers GC, "Multiple Sclerosis: New Insights From Old Tools," *Mayo Clin Proc*, 1993, 68(7):711-2.
5. Rodriguez M, Scheithauer BW, Forbes G, et al, "Oligodendrocyte Injury Is an Early Event in Lesions of Multiple Sclerosis," *Mayo Clin Proc*, 1993, 68(7):627-36.
6. Prabhakar S, Kurien E, Gupta RS, et al, "Heat Shock Protein Immunoreactivity in CSF: Correlation With Oligoclonal Banding and Demyelinating Disease," *Neurology*, 1994, 44(9):1644-8.
7. Chalmers AC, Aprill BS, and Shephard H, "Cerebrospinal Fluid and Human Immunodeficiency Virus - Findings in Healthy, Asymptomatic, Seropositive Men," *Arch Intern Med*, 1990, 150(7):1538-40.
8. Kaiser R and Lücking CH, "GFAP-Specific Oligoclonal Bands in the CSF of a Patient With Acute Myelitis," *Acta Neurol Scand*, 1993, 88(2):94-6.

References

Giles PD, Heath JP, and Wroe SJ, "Oligoclonal Bands and the IgG Index in Multiple Sclerosis: Uses and Limitations," *Ann Clin Biochem*, 1989, 26(Pt 4):317-23.

Hosein ZZ and Johnson KP, "Isoelectric Focusing of Cerebrospinal Fluid Proteins in the Diagnosis of Multiple Sclerosis," *Neurology*, 1981, 31:70-6.

Keren DF, "Multiple Sclerosis and Oligoclonal Bands," *High-Resolution Electrophoresis: Techniques and Interpretation*, Chapter 3, Boston, MA: Butterworth's Publishers, 1987, 86-93.

Wybo I, Van Blerk M, Malfoit R, et al, "Oligoclonal Bands in Cerebrospinal Fluid Detected by Phastsystem Isoelectric Focusing," *Clin Chem*, 1990, 36(1):123-5.

Cerebrospinal Fluid Protein

CPT 84155

Related Information

Bacterial Antigens, Rapid Detection Methods *on page 454*
Bacterial Culture, Cerebrospinal Fluid *on page 460*
Cerebrospinal Fluid Analysis *on page 309*
Cerebrospinal Fluid Glucose *on page 105*
Cerebrospinal Fluid IgG Ratios and IgG Index *on page 377*
Cerebrospinal Fluid Immunoglobulin G *on page 378*
Cerebrospinal Fluid Lactic Acid *on page 106*
Cerebrospinal Fluid LD *on page 106*
Cerebrospinal Fluid Protein Electrophoresis *on next page*
FTA-ABS, Cerebrospinal Fluid *on page 394*
Fungal Culture, Cerebrospinal Fluid *on page 477*
Gram's Stain *on page 481*
Mycobacterial Culture, Cerebrospinal Fluid *on page 489*
VDRL, Cerebrospinal Fluid *on page 438*
Viral Culture, Central Nervous System Symptoms *on page 677*

Synonyms CSF Protein; Protein, Cerebrospinal Fluid; Spinal Fluid Protein

Test Commonly Includes Culture, Gram's stain, glucose, and protein are usually ordered together.

Abstract Increased CSF protein may indicate presence of infections or hemorrhagic, malignant, or demyelinating disease of the CNS (central nervous system).

Patient Preparation Patient should be informed, relaxed, and properly positioned for lumbar puncture. Signed consent form is required. Antiseptic agents must be carefully and properly applied to the proposed puncture site. Local anesthetic (to which patient is not allergic) is usually advised. If increased intracranial pressure due to a mass lesion (eg, abscess) is suspected, lumbar puncture should be deferred until appropriate neuroimaging study is performed and the issue resolved.

Aftercare Patient should be maintained supine for a few hours postpuncture in an attempt to avoid postpuncture headache.

Specimen Cerebrospinal fluid, usually at least 0.1-0.5 mL of CSF is required.

Container Clean, sterile CSF tube

Collection Tubes should be labeled with patient's name, hospital number, and date and time of collection.

Storage Instructions Do not store. Must be delivered to clinical laboratory immediately.

Turnaround Time 1-2 hours

Special Instructions Usually three tubes of CSF are collected for count and culture in addition to protein and glucose with collection of 1 mL in each tube labeled #1, #2, #3 in order of collection. **For diagnosis of meningitis, culture and then Gram's staining have priority over all other testing**, when only a small quantity of cerebrospinal fluid (CSF) is available. **Cell count with differential deserves the next priority, followed by glucose and protein.**

Reference Range Lumbar CSF: 0-1 month: <150 mg/dL (SI: <1.5 g/L); 1-6 months: approximately 30-100 mg/dL (SI: 0.30-1.00 g/L); 6 months and up: approximately 15-50 mg/dL (SI: 0.15-0.50 g/L). Ventricular CSF protein is generally lower. A recent study found a reference interval (biuret method) of 14-62 mg/dL (SI: 0.14-0.62 g/L).[1]

Possible Panic Range Results above upper limits, especially with additional abnormalities (increased cells and/or decreased glucose)

Use Increased with bacterial meningitis, tuberculous meningitis, brain abscess, meningovascular syphilis, diabetes mellitus, CVA (including cases in which no hemorrhage has occurred), arachnoiditis, dehydration, some major depressive disorders, some patients with sciatica due to lumbar disk herniation, POEMS syndrome (polyneuropathy, organomegaly, endocrinopathy, M protein, and skin changes), drug effects, and subarachnoid hemorrhage. Protein is normal or **slightly** high in psychiatric disease. Used for differential diagnosis of multiple sclerosis; encephalomyelitis; other degenerative processes causing neurologic disease, some neoplastic diseases, some cases of myxedema and other instances of endocrine disorders, traumatic tap, and in CSF recovered from below the level of an obstruction of the spinal cord.

Decreased CSF protein may be seen in normal children 6-24 months of age, with dilution from water intoxication, CSF leak (CSF rhinorrhea or otorrhea, leaks following lumbar puncture, other fistulas), with removal of large volumes of CSF, in some patients with benign intracranial hypertension, in some leukemic subjects, and with hyperthyroidism. Low CSF protein is 10-20 mg/dL.[2]

Limitations Fresh blood in the specimen (traumatic tap) will invalidate the protein result; turbid samples may exhibit a positive interference; hemolyzed or xanthochromic specimens may falsely depress results; ampicillin, gentamicin, and vancomycin increase the apparent CSF protein in at least some cases when measured with Ektachem® slides.[1] Problems in the differential diagnosis of multiple sclerosis, meningitis, and other entities are discussed in following paragraphs.

Methodology Quantitative turbidimetric (sulfosalicylic acid, trichloroacetic acid, TCA); colorimetric (Biuret, Folin-Lowry phenol); dye binding (bromocresol green); Kjeldahl technique (reference method) and a number of other methods including UV spectrophotometry of diluted serum at wavelength 210-220 nm. Sulfosalicylic acid gives greater turbidity with albumin than with globulin. TCA method is less subject to inaccuracy from this source. Colorimetric methods may also suffer from the albumin/globulin specificity problem but in addition the reagents may react with nonprotein nitrogenous compounds. The use of gel filtration prior to direct UV spectrophotometry may eliminate chemical and drug interference. A micromethod utilizing benzethonium chloride and microtiter plates has been described.[3]

Additional Information Because of a less than sharply defined upper limit of normal,[2] a "borderline increased" range of 45-60 mg/dL (SI: 0.45-0.60 g/L) may be useful. The significance of elevated CSF protein should be carefully considered, in relation to the clinical findings, in particular if blood found its way into the CSF. This could occur at the time of needling the subarachnoid space ("bloody tap") and be clinically misleading, or reflect clinically significant CNS hemorrhage, trauma, vascular anomaly or tumor, and have prime clinical significance. The three tube collection procedure allows for helpful clinical differentiation; bloody CSF clearing between the first and third tubes usually indicates "traumatic tap." If such is the case, centrifuging the specimen should yield a supernatant fluid that is crystal clear. Pigmented (xanthochromic) supernatant indicates subarachnoid hemorrhage with lysis of RBCs as may occur if red cells reside more than a few hours in CSF. The fluid may be clear, however, up to 12 hours after subarachnoid hemorrhage in some cases while traumatic tap itself may be responsible for xanthochromia for as long as 2-5 days after lumbar puncture. If traumatic tap is reasonably certain clinically, the RBC count of patient's blood can be ratioed against the RBC count of CSF to obtain a factor that can be compared against total protein of blood vs CSF protein. This is not a particularly exacting or reliable procedure but may provide an indication that the CSF protein is higher than would be expected on the basis of contamination by peripheral blood. Patients with elevated CSF protein should have additional analyses (eg, IgG/albumin index, IgG synthetic rate, and high resolution agarose protein electrophoresis for demonstration of "oligoclonal" bands), in particular if there are clinical findings of multiple sclerosis. Total protein in CSF is within normal limits in 66% of subjects with MS. Protein levels >100 mg/dL are very atypical, and bring a diagnosis of MS or other neurologic disease into question.[2]

Protein may be normal or increased in viral meningitis but is usually slightly increased, 50-80 mg/dL. Protein in most cases of viral meningitis is <100 mg/dL.[4] It is usually 100-500 mg/dL in acute bacterial meningitis and is occasionally >1000 mg/dL. Protein was <45 mg/dL in fewer than 2% of a series of 157 patients with acute bacterial meningitis. It is almost always high in tuberculous meningitis.[2] Smith and Haas caution that for a premature or term newborn, CSF protein >100 mg/dL (among other criteria) places the baby at risk for bacterial meningitis.[5] **The gold standard for the diagnosis of bacterial meningitis is the culture, isolation of a bacterium from the CNS.**[6] For subjects who have not been given antimicrobial drugs, the ultimate diagnosis of bacterial meningitis is based on cultures.[7]

AIDS patients with primary CNS disease or secondary CNS infections may have elevated CSF protein. Studies of asymptomatic, HIV seropositive individuals, however, have shown that pleocytosis or elevated CSF protein occurs in some 50% of such patients, with 12% to 26% showing oligoclonal banding.[8,9] The percentage of protein abnormalities increases with inclusion of patients with AIDS and AIDS-related complex.[9]

CSF cellular and protein abnormalities occur with 10% to 20% of subjects who have primary syphilis and with 30% to 70% of those with secondary lues.[10]

Lumbar disk herniation with sciatica may be associated with increased CSF total protein (see comments in the listing Cerebrospinal Fluid IgG Ratios and IgG Index *on page 377*).[11]

There is evidence that mean CSF protein concentration is higher (high normal to slightly increased - mean ±SD of 40.9 ±15.8 mg/dL) in men with major depressive disorder (unipolar or bipolar depression) than in other subjects (in particular, women with similar diagnoses) and in controls.[12,13] The increase is polyclonal on protein electrophoretic study suggesting increased blood-brain capillary permeability.[12] There is also evidence that secretion of prealbumin into CSF may be increased in depression.[14]

Continuing investigation of two dimensional gel protein electrophoresis has led to development of a CSF protein database (see reference by Yun et al).

Footnotes

1. Lott JA and Warren P, "Estimation of Reference Intervals for Total Protein in Cerebrospinal Fluid," *Clin Chem*, 1989, 35(8):1766-70.
2. Fishman RA, *Cerebrospinal Fluid in Diseases of the Nervous System*, 2nd ed, Philadelphia, PA: WB Saunders Co, 1992, 197-214.
3. Luxton RW, Patel P, Keir G, et al, "A Micro-Method for Measuring Total Protein in Cerebrospinal Fluid by Using Benzethonium Chloride in Microtiter Plate Wells," *Clin Chem*, 1989, 35(8):1731-4.
4. Hammer SM and Connolly KJ, "Viral Aseptic Meningitis in the United States: Clinical Features, Viral Etiologies, and Differential Diagnosis," *Curr Clin Top Infect Dis*, 1992, 12:1-25.
5. Smith AL and Haas J, "Neonatal Bacterial Meningitis," *Infections of the Central Nervous System*, Scheld WM, Whitley RJ, and Durack DT, eds, New York, NY: Raven Press, 1991, 313-33.
6. Smith AL, "Bacterial Meningitis," *Pediatr Rev*, 1993, 14(1):11-8.
7. Rodewald LE, Woodin KA, Szilágyi PG, et al, "Relevance of Common Tests of Cerebrospinal Fluid in Screening for Bacterial Meningitis," *J Pediatr*, 1991, 119(3):363-9.
8. Chalmers AC, Aprill BS, and Shephard H, "Cerebrospinal Fluid and Human Immunodeficiency Virus - Findings in Healthy, Asymptomatic, Seropositive Men," *Arch Intern Med*, 1990, 150(7):1538-40.
9. Hall CD, Snyder CR, Robertson KR, et al, "Cerebrospinal Fluid Analysis in Human Immunodeficiency Virus Infection," *Ann Clin Lab Sci*, 1992, 22(3):139-43.
10. Hook EW 3d and Marra CM, "Acquired Syphilis in Adults," *N Engl J Med*, 1992, 326:1060-9.
11. Skouen JS, Larsen JL, and Vollset SE, "Cerebrospinal Fluid Protein Concentrations Related to Clinical Findings in Patients With Sciatica Caused by Disk Herniation," *J Spinal Disord*, 1994, 7(1):12-8.
12. Samuelson SD, Winokur G, and Pitts AF, "Elevated Cerebrospinal Fluid Protein in Men With Unipolar or Bipolar Depression," *Biol Psychiatry*, 1994, 35(8):539-44.
13. Pitts AF, Carroll BT, Gehris TL, et al, "Elevated CSF Protein in Male Patients With Depression," *Biol Psychiatry*, 1990, 28(7):629-37.
14. Jorgensen OS, "Neural Cell Adhesion Molecule and Prealbumin in Cerebrospinal Fluid From Depressed Patients," *Acta Psychiatr Scand*, 1988, 345:29-37.

References

Behrman RE, Kliegman RM, Nelson WE, et al, *Nelson Textbook of Pediatrics*, 14th ed, Philadelphia, PA: WB Saunders Co, 1992, 664-6, 683-91.
Kjeldsberg CR and Knight JA, *Body Fluids - Laboratory Examination of Amniotic, Cerebrospinal, Seminal, Serous and Synovial Fluids*, 3rd ed, Chicago, IL: American Society of Clinical Pathologists, 1993, 89-102.
Roos KL, Tunkel AR, and Scheld WM, "Acute Bacterial Meningitis in Children and Adults," *Infections of the Central Nervous System*, Scheld WM, Whitley RJ, and Durack DT, eds, New York, NY: Raven Press, 1991, 335-409.
Yun M, Wu W, Hood L, et al, "Human Cerebrospinal Fluid Protein Database: Edition 1992," *Electrophoresis*, 1992, 13(12):1002-13.

Cerebrospinal Fluid Protein Electrophoresis

CPT 84165

Related Information

Cerebrospinal Fluid IgG Synthesis Rate *on page 378*
Cerebrospinal Fluid Oligoclonal Bands *on page 379*
Cerebrospinal Fluid Protein *on previous page*
Protein Electrophoresis, Serum *on page 424*
Protein, Total, Serum *on page 194*

Synonyms CSF Electrophoresis; Protein Electrophoresis, Spinal Fluid; Spinal Fluid Electrophoresis

Applies to Tau Fraction; Transthyretin

Test Commonly Includes Total protein

Abstract On electrophoresis, CSF normally includes a prealbumin fraction and a tau fraction. Its gamma globulin proportionally is less in CSF than in serum.

Patient Preparation Patient should be informed, relaxed, and properly positioned for lumbar puncture. Signed consent form is required. Antiseptic agents must be carefully and properly applied to the proposed puncture site. Local anesthetic (to which patient is not allergic) is usually advised.

Aftercare Patient should be maintained supine for a few hours postpuncture in an attempt to avoid postpuncture headache.

Specimen Cerebrospinal fluid, serum obtained at the same time that lumbar puncture is performed

Container Clean, sterile CSF tube

Collection Tube should be labeled with the number indicating the sequence in which tubes were obtained.

Storage Instructions Store refrigerated.

Causes for Rejection Insufficient quantity of CSF, CSF contaminated with blood ("bloody tap")

Special Instructions The third tube of routinely obtained three tube set of CSF should be used for protein electrophoretic study.

Reference Range Depends on methodology. Gamma: 3% to 11%, beta: 7.3% to 17.9%, alpha$_2$: 3.0% to 12.6%, alpha$_1$: 1.1% to 6.6%, albumin: (Continued)

Cerebrospinal Fluid Protein Electrophoresis
(Continued)

56.8% to 76.9%, prealbumin: 2.2% to 7.1%, total protein: 15-50 mg/dL, CSF albumin: 13.4-23.7 mg/dL, beta-gamma ratio: 1.67-2.3, oligoclonal bands: absent. A recent study, using preconcentration of samples and agarose (high resolution) gels, found lower albumin and higher beta and gamma globulin fractions.

Use Quantitate CSF protein fractions, aid in diagnosis of inflammatory and demyelinating disease of CNS, although routine CSF protein electrophoresis is highly insensitive and nonspecific for presence of multiple sclerosis (MS). Routine CSF protein electrophoresis has no role in screening for demyelinating diseases (eg, MS). For this either high-resolution electrophoresis or isoelectric focusing is required. For tests with greater sensitivity/specificity for MS, see Cerebrospinal Fluid Oligoclonal Bands on page 379 and Cerebrospinal Fluid IgG Synthesis Rate on page 378.

Limitations Not specific; large volume of specimen needed (must be concentrated); insensitive and nonspecific for MS

Methodology Cellulose acetate, agarose electrophoresis, "high resolution" agarose gel systems

Additional Information Most CSF proteins reflect their counterparts in the serum (from which they are derived). CSF protein is only approximately 1/200 as concentrated as serum protein, necessitating concentration (usually 100 times) and therefore a minimal sample volume of 1 mL or greater is required. Serum protein electrophoresis should be performed simultaneously with CSF protein electrophoresis in order to determine if unique bands are of CNS origin or have been transferred in from the serum. Two protein populations usually not seen on serum protein electrophoretic studies (although possibly present in low concentration) are demonstrable routinely in CSF. These are **prealbumin**, now called **transthyretin** (just anodal to albumin) and the **tau fraction** (just cathodal to the β-fraction near the origin). The tau fraction is not present on serum protein electrophoretic patterns and represents asialated transferrin. Detection of asialated transferrin in samples obtained from nasal or auditory canals is strong evidence of CSF leakage due to skull fracture. CSF protein includes only small amounts of glycoproteins as compared to serum. As is the case with serum, they migrate as α_1-, α_2-, and β-globulins. Similarly there is very little lipoprotein (an α_1-globulin) in CSF as compared to serum. Severe craniocerebral trauma is characterized by a three- to fourfold increase in α_2 globulins over the first week post-trauma. Elevation of gamma globulin, increase in IgG to albumin ratio, IgG indices, increase in IgG synthetic rate and/or the presence of "oligoclonal" bands on thin gel agarose high resolution electrophoresis has special significance to the diagnosis of multiple sclerosis (see also discussion under these entries). Earlier studies indicated that a significant number (75%, even 89%) of patients with clinically documented multiple sclerosis had elevated gamma globulin (some studies using paper electrophoresis). Most of the increase in gamma globulin is due to an increase in IgG. IgA and IgM is present largely in cases with >80-100 mg/dL (SI: >0.8-1.0 g/L) total protein and appears to be without diagnostic significance. CSF protein from male patients with significant depressive illness is high normal to slightly increased as compared to controls and women with similar diagnoses. CSF protein electrophoresis has shown such CSF protein elevation to have polyclonal characteristics.[1]

Footnotes
1. Pitts AF, Carroll BT, Gehris TL, et al, "Elevated CSF Protein in Male Patients With Depression," Biol Psychiatry, 1990, 28(7):629-37.

References
Christenson RH, Russell ME, and Hassett BJ, "Cerebrospinal Fluid: Electrophoresis and Methods for Determining Immunoglobulin G Compared," Clin Biochem, 1989, 22(6):429-32.

Fishman RA, Cerebrospinal Fluid in Diseases of the Nervous System, 2nd ed, Philadelphia, PA: WB Saunders Co, 1992, 201-3.

Keren DF, "Interpretation of High-Resolution Electrophoresis Patterns in Serum, Urine, and Cerebrospinal Fluid," High Resolution Electrophoresis and Immunofixation: Techniques and Interpretation, Boston, MA: Butterworth's Publishers, 1987, 67-106.

Kjeldsberg CR and Knight JA, Body Fluids - Laboratory Examination of Amniotic, Cerebrospinal, Seminal, Serous and Synovial Fluids, 3rd ed, Chicago, IL: American Society of Clinical Pathologists, 1993, 89-102.

Zaret D, Morrison N, Gulbranson R, et al, "Immunofixation to Quantify β 2-Transferrin in Cerebrospinal Fluid to Detect Leakage of CSF From Skull Injury," Clin Chem, 1992, 38(9):1909-12.

Cerebrospinal Fluid Tau Protein
Related Information
Apolipoprotein E on page 82
Cerebrospinal Fluid Amyloid Precursor Protein and Amyloid β-Protein on page 376
Cerebrospinal Fluid Oligoclonal Bands on page 379

Synonyms CSF Tau Protein; Spinal Fluid Tau Protein

Applies to β-Amyloid Peptide; Ubiquitin

Abstract Cerebrospinal fluid (CSF) microtubule-associated protein tau concentration may reflect the progressive death of neurones in Alzheimer's disease (AD). Assay of CSF tau protein may serve as an early diagnostic test for AD.

Specimen Cerebrospinal fluid (CSF) from lumbar puncture

Collection CSF obtained using standard sterile technique

Storage Instructions May be stored after immediate freezing at -80°C until analysis.[1]

Turnaround Time Test is in early stages of commercial development and may be available currently only from research laboratories.

Special Instructions Maintain patient supine post-CSF removal in attempt to avoid postspinal headache.

Reference Range Method (monoclonal antibody) and standard dependent. Tau CSF concentration is in the low picogram range. AD patients have levels 2 to 10 times those of "control" groups.[1,2,3,4]

Use Support the diagnosis of AD; possibly provide for early detection of AD; monitor response to new pharmacologic AD interventions as they are developed

Limitations Test is in early stage of development and availability. Increased levels of CSF tau may also be seen with other disease processes in which neuronal degeneration occurs (eg, cerebrovascular disease, meningoencephalitis, AIDS), tau levels may be increased in some cases of Pick's, Creutzfeldt-Jacob, and other neurologic diseases. A subset of AD patients may have low CSF tau levels relating to insufficient number of neurofibrillary tangles characterizing their form of the disease.[5]

Methodology Enzyme-linked immunosorbent assay (ELISA) using monoclonal antibody AT 120, commercially available (Innogenetics, Belgium)

Additional Information Alzheimer's disease (AD) is the most common cause of dementia in the elderly. It is a central nervous system degenerative disorder characterized clinically by progressive and severe memory loss with cognitive decline occurring in the mid to late adult years and ultimately leading to death. Definitive therapy is not available. As elderly individuals are increasing in the population, AD is more commonly encountered. The pathologic findings are characterized, classically, by presence of cerebral atrophy with senile plaques and neurofibrillary tangles. The clinical diagnosis may require autopsy confirmation with some cases complicated by the finding of "mixed dementia" (eg, Alzheimer findings mixed with Lewy bodies that are more characteristic of Pick's disease).[6,7]

Rapidly evolving understanding of neurobiochemical and molecular genetic derangements indicates that the clinical diversity of AD relates to multifaceted underlying mechanism/mechanisms and/or coexisting non-AD dementing disease.

Early-onset AD is associated with mutations in the amyloid precursor protein gene (chromosome 21), an autosomal dominant condition.[8] Mutants of a gene on chromosome 14 may also lead to early onset autosomal dominant AD.[9] Apolipoprotein E (apo E) plays a major role in the regulation of lipid metabolism and the risk of developing coronary artery disease (see listing Apolipoprotein E on page 82), but is also involved in the genesis of at least some forms of AD. The three major isoforms of apo E (ε2, ε3, and ε4) are encoded by the alleles ε2, ε3, and ε4 of the apo E gene. APOε4 is a risk factor for both the sporadic and familial late-onset AD.[10] A Volga German kindred with high incidence of autosomal dominant early-onset AD relates to an abnormal locus on chromosome 1q31-42 but does not show linkage to loci on chromosomes 12 or 14.[11] Apo E isoforms are apparently important in the metabolism of amyloid B peptide.

The clinical phase of AD may follow after many years of gradual formation of senile plaques and neurofibrillary tangles. Development of effective therapy will likely involve preventive measures. As genetic studies can identify family members at risk, phenotypic analyses should find application in further defining risk, disease onset, and response to therapy.[3] Determination of CSF protein tau may represent such a phenotypic parameter. Abnormal highly phosphorylated forms of the microtubule-associated tau protein are major constituents of the paired helical filaments (PHF) that form neurofibrillary tangles in Alzheimer's disease. Four reports dealing with subjects of five different national origins have found statistically significant increase in CSF tau protein in AD patients as compared to members of "control" groups.[1,2,3,4] The variation about the mean, however, is considerable, generating overlap such that some cases of AD have low CSF tau levels while some non-AD neuronal degenerative diseases have increased levels. Some "overlap cases" can readily be separated on the basis of clinical features. While the level of tau elevation does not correlate with clinical stage, age at onset or apo E genotype,[1] there is evidence that tau levels may be a marker of clinical severity (reflect the number of neurofibrillary tangles).[3]

With the continuing rapid advances in delineating the pathogenesis of AD, a panel of diagnostic tests may evolve. Current candidates for such a panel might include CSF α_1-antichymotrypsin, ubiquitin, and/or β-amyloid peptide$_{42}$.[4,12]

Footnotes

1. Arai H, Terajima M, Miura M, et al, "Tau in Cerebrospinal Fluid: A Potential Diagnostic Marker in Alzheimer's Disease," *Ann Neurol*, 1995, 38(4):649-52.
2. Vigo-Pelfrey C, Seubert P, Barbour R, et al, "Elevation of Microtubule-Associated Protein Tau in the Cerebrospinal Fluid of Patients With Alzheimer's Disease," *Neurology*, 1995, 45(4):788-93.
3. Hock C, Golombowski S, Naser W, et al, "Increased Levels of Tau Protein in Cerebrospinal Fluid of Patients With Alzheimer's Disease - Correlation With Degree of Cognitive Impairment," *Ann Neurol*, 1995, 37(3):414-5.
4. Vandermeeren M, Mercken M, Vanmeehelen E, et al, "Detection of Tau Proteins in Normal and Alzheimer's Disease Cerebrospinal Fluid With a Sensitive Sandwich Enzyme-Linked Immunosorbent Assay," *J Neurochem*, 1993, 61(5):1828-34.
5. Terry RD, Hansen LA, De Teresa R, et al, "Senile Dementia of the Alzheimer Type Without Neocortical Neurofibrillary Tangles," *J Neuropathol Exp Neurol*, 1987, 46(3):262-8.
6. Hansen LA and Crain BJ, "Making the Diagnosis of Mixed and Non-Alzheimer's Dementias," *Arch Pathol Lab Med*, 1995, 119(11):1023-31.
7. Mirra SS, Hart MN, and Terry RD, "Making the Diagnosis of Alzheimer's Disease - A Primer for Practicing Pathologists," *Arch Pathol Lab Med*, 1993, 117(2):132-44.
8. Goate A, Chartier-Harlin MC, Mullan M, et al, "Segregation of a Missense Mutation in the Amyloid Precursor Protein Gene With Familial Alzheimer's Disease," *Nature*, 1991, 349(6311):704-6.
9. Sherrington R, Rogaev EI, Liang Y, et al, "Cloning of a Gene Bearing Missense Mutations in Early-Onset Familial Alzheimer's Disease," *Nature*, 1995, 375(6534):754-60.
10. Saunders AM, Strittmatter WJ, Schmechel D, et al, "Association of Apolipoprotein E Allele ε4 With Late-Onset Familial and Sporadic Alzheimer's Disease," *Neurology*, 1993, 43(8):1467-72.
11. Levy-Lahad E, Wijsman EM, Nemens E, et al, "A Familial Alzheimer's Disease Locus on Chromosome1," *Science*, 1995, 269(5226):970-3.
12. Motter R, Vigo-Pelfrey C, Kholodenko D, et al, "Reduction of β-Amyloid Peptide$_{42}$ in the Cerebrospinal Fluid of Patients With Alzheimer's Disease," *Ann Neurol*, 1995, 38(4):643-8.

References

Goedert M, "Tau Protein and the Neurofibrillary Pathology of Alzheimer's Disease," *Trends Neurosci*, 1993, 16(11):460-5.
Smith C and Anderson BH, "The Molecular Pathology of Alzheimer's Disease: Are We Any Closer to Understanding the Neurodegenerative Process?" *Neuropathol Appl Neurobiol*, 1994, 20(4):322-38.
Strittmatter WJ, Saunders AM, Goedert M, et al, "Isoform-Specific Interactions of Apolipoprotein E With Microtubule-Associated Protein Tau: Implications for Alzheimer Disease," *Proc Natl Acac Sci U S A*, 1994, 91(23):11183-6.

Cerebrospinal Fluid VDRL *see* VDRL, Cerebrospinal Fluid *on page 438*

CH$_{50}$ *see* Complement, Total, Serum *on page 386*

CH$_{100}$ *see* Complement, Total, Serum *on page 386*

Chagas' Disease Serological Test

CPT 86317 (quantitative); 86318 (qualitative or semiqualitative)

Related Information
Babesiosis Serological Test *on page 370*
Malaria Smear *on page 332*
Ova and Parasites, Stool *on page 494*
Parasite Antibodies *on page 421*
Risks of Transfusion *on page 623*

Applies to *Trypanosoma cruzi*

Abstract American trypanosomiasis (Chagas' disease) is caused by a protozoan, *Trypanosoma cruzi*. The chronic disease includes myocarditis, cardiomyopathy, and megadisease of esophagus and colon. It can cause placentitis, and maternal transmission to the fetus leads to congenital Chagas' disease or abortion. Laboratory workers may be accidentally infected. Found only in the Western hemisphere, Chagas' disease is thought to cause the deaths of 50,000 people annually. Severe recrudescence may occur with immunosuppression (eg, organ transplantation, AIDS). The correlation between infectivity and Chagas' antibodies is suboptimal.

Specimen Serum

Container Red top tube

Collection Thick and thin blood films may be collected as well for Giemsa staining

Reference Range Indirect hemagglutination titer: <1:128; complement fixation titer: <1:8; immunoelectrophoresis titer: <1:64

Use Support the clinical diagnosis of chronic Chagas' disease. In endemic areas, serologic testing is needed in blood banks, since transfusion from donors with chronic infection results in transmission of *T. cruzi* to the recipient in 13% to 23% of cases per contaminated unit.

Limitations False-positive serologic reactions occur in persons with leishmaniasis, malaria, toxoplasmosis, hepatitis, leprosy, syphilis, and collagen diseases. An individual can be serologically negative but still be infectious.

Methodology Indirect hemagglutination (IHA), complement fixation (CF), indirect fluorescent antibody (IFA), direct agglutination, enzyme-linked immunosorbent assay (ELISA), immunoelectrophoresis (IEP). Indirect immunofluorescence is more sensitive than CF. In patients with chronic infection, there may be diminution of CF titers. Radioimmunoprecipitation assay using purified glycoprotein antigens exists.[1]

Additional Information IHA is more sensitive but less specific than the CF. CF shows a high degree of sensitivity in the acute stages of the disease. Because of the chronicity of Chagas' disease, stable low to moderate titers by IHA or CF are difficult to interpret. Serum from patients with Chagas' heart disease contain antibodies which bind to endocardial, vascular, and interstitial elements of heart tissue. Such an "EVI" factor may be predictive of cardiac Chagas' disease. Serologic tests return to normal in a large majority of patients 12-24 months after treatment. A serum should test positive by at least two different assays before positivity is accepted.[2] Chagas' disease, usually transmitted as a zoonosis by reduviids (kissing bugs), is a life-long infection. Its highest incidence is found in Brazil, Argentina, Chile, Bolivia, and Venezuela.

Several cases of transfusion-transmitted Chagas' disease have been reported. Studies are being conducted to see if screening of the blood supply is necessary in certain areas of the country such as southern California.[3,4]

Footnotes

1. "Case Records of the Massachusetts General Hospital. Weekly Clinicopathological Exercises. Case 32-1993. A Native of El Salvador With Tachycardia and Syncope," *N Engl J Med*, 1993, 329(7):488-96.
2. Kirchhoff LV, "American Trypanosomiasis (Chagas' Disease) - A Tropical Disease Now in the United States," *N Engl J Med*, 1993, 329(9):639-44.
3. Brashear RJ, Winkler MA, Schur JD, et al, "Detection of Antibodies to *Trypanosoma cruzi* Among Blood Donors in the Southwestern and Western United States. I. Evaluation of the Sensitivity and Specificity of an Enzyme Immunoassay for Detecting Antibodies to *T. cruzi*," *Transfusion*, 1995, 35(3):213-8.
4. Winkler MA, Brashear RJ, Hall HJ, et al, "Detection of Antibodies to *Trypanosoma cruzi* Among Blood Donors in the Southwestern and Western United States. II. Evaluation of a Supplemental Enzyme Immunoassay and Radioimmunoprecipitation Assay for Confirmation of Seroreactivity," *Transfusion*, 1995, 35(3):219-25.

References

Araujo FG, "Serological Diagnosis - Perspectives for Confirmatory Tests," *Chagas' Disease (American Trypanosomiasis): Its Impact on Transfusion and Clinical Medicine*, Wendel S, Brener Z, Camargo ME, et al, eds, São Paulo, Brazil: Cartgraf Editoru Ltd, 1992, 219-23.
Kerndt PR, Waskin HA, Kirchhoff LV, et al, "Prevalence of Antibody to *Trypanosoma cruzi* Among Blood Donors in Los Angeles, California," *Transfusion*, 1991, 31(9):814-8.

Chickenpox Titer *see* Varicella-Zoster Virus Serology *on page 437*

Chlamydia Group Titer

CPT 86631; 86632 (IgM)

Related Information
Chlamydia trachomatis Culture *on page 662*
Chlamydia trachomatis Direct FA Test *on page 663*
Chlamydia trachomatis Genome Detection *on page 505*
Lymphogranuloma Venereum Titer *on page 417*
Psittacosis Titer *on page 425*

Test Commonly Includes Detection of antibody titer to *Chlamydia* species

Abstract Intracellular bacteria which multiply in living cells, *Chlamydia* are among the most successful pathogens.

Specimen Serum

Container Red top tube

Collection Collect acute phase blood as soon as possible after onset (no later than 1 week). Convalescent blood should be drawn 1-2 weeks after acute (no less than 2 weeks after onset).

Reference Range Negative. A fourfold increase in IgG titer in paired sera is usually indicative of chlamydial infection. Determination of IgM antibody indicates acute infection.

Use Evaluation of atypical pneumonias for possible chlamydial infection. *C. pneumoniae* is a common cause of community-acquired pneumonia, causing 5% to 10% of cases.[1] *Chlamydia* cause infantile pneumonia, blindness, ophthalmia neonatorum, lymphogranuloma venereum, pelvic inflammatory disease, ectopic pregnancy, urethritis, epididymitis, infertility, and reactive arthritis.

Limitations The antigen used in the test is group specific, not species specific. Conjunctivitis, urethritis, and pneumonia of the newborn do not usually induce an antibody response detectable by complement fixation. A very high "background" of immunity in the general population makes interpretation of levels difficult.

Methodology Complement fixation (CF), indirect fluorescence antibody (IFA), enzyme immunoassay (EIA)

Additional Information *Chlamydia* is the most common sexually transmitted bacterial pathogen in the United States. It is gaining increasing recognition as a respiratory pathogen. In a patient being evaluated for chlamydial disease, nonserologic methods (culture, PCR) are used. For genitourinary infections, serologic test for syphilis and culture for *Neisseria gonorrhoeae* are desirable as well. Chlamydial infection may lead to increased risk of ectopic gestation by damage to fallopian tubes. (Continued)

Chlamydia Group Titer *(Continued)*

Footnotes
1. Bartlett JG and Mundy LM, "Community-Acquired Pneumonia," *N Engl J Med*, 1995, 333(24):1618-24.

References
Blanchard TJ and Mabey DC, "Chlamydial Infections," *Br J Clin Pract*, 1994, 48(4):201-5.

Centers for Disease Control and Prevention, "Evaluation of Surveillance for *Chlamydia trachomatis* Infections in the United States, 1987 to 1991," *JAMA*, 1003, 270(14):1676-7.

Johnson DH and Cunha BA, "Atypical Pneumonias. Clinical and Extrapulmonary Features of *Chlamydia*, *Mycoplasma*, and *Legionella* Infections," *Postgrad Med*, 1993, 93(7):69-72, 75-6, 79-82.

Mahmoud E, Elshibly S, and Mardh PA, "Seroepidemiologic Study of *Chlamydia pneumoniae* and Other Chlamydial Species in a Hyperendemic Area for Trachoma in the Sudan," *Am J Trop Med Hyg*, 1994, 51(4):489-94.

Odland JO, Anestad G, Rasmussen S, et al, "Ectopic Pregnancy and Chlamydial Serology," *Int J Gynaecol Obstet*, 1993, 43(3):271-5.

Olliaro P, Regazzetti A, Marchetti AL, et al, "Prevalence of Chlamydial Antibody in Pregnancy. A Matched-Pair Study," *Eur J Epidemiol*, 1994, 10(1):47-50.

Rae R, Smith IW, Liston WA, et al, "Chlamydial Serologic Studies and Recurrent Spontaneous Abortion," *Am J Obstet Gynecol*, 1994, 170(3):782-5.

Weinstock H, Dean D, and Bolan G, "*Chlamydia trachomatis* Infections," *Infect Dis Clin North Am*, 1994, 8(4):797-819.

***Chlamydia psittaci* Antibodies** *see* Psittacosis Titer *on page 425*

***Chlamydia psittaci* Direct Immunofluorescent Antibody** *see* Psittacosis Titer *on page 425*

***Chlamydia psittaci* PCR** *see* Psittacosis Titer *on page 425*

***Chlamydia psittaci* Titer** *see* Psittacosis Titer *on page 425*

Circulating Immune Complexes *see* C1q Immune Complex Detection *on page 373*

Cluster Designations *see* Leukocyte Immunophenotyping *on page 414*

CMV-IFA *see* Cytomegalovirus Antibody *on page 389*

CMV-IFA, IgG *see* Cytomegalovirus Antibody *on page 389*

CMV-IFA, IgM *see* Cytomegalovirus Antibody *on page 389*

CMV Titer *see* Cytomegalovirus Antibody *on page 389*

***Coccidioides immitis* Antibody** *see* Coccidioidomycosis Antibodies *on this page*

Coccidioidomycosis Antibodies

CPT 86635

Related Information
Fungal Culture, Biopsy or Body Fluid *on page 476*
Fungal Culture, Blood *on page 477*
Fungal Culture, Sputum *on page 479*
Fungus Smear, Stain *on page 481*
Myoglobin, Qualitative, Urine *on page 644*
Sputum Cytology *on page 300*

Synonyms Desert Fever; Valley Fever

Applies to *Coccidioides immitis* Antibody; Spherulin®

Test Commonly Includes Complement fixing or precipitating antibodies

Abstract Coccidioidomycosis is an infection caused by the dimorphic fungus *Coccidioides immitis*. It is found in soil in portions of Arizona, California, Nevada, New Mexico, Texas, Utah, and Mexico. Diagnosis depends on identification of *C. immitis* by culture, cytologic, and/or histopathologic examination.

Specimen Serum, cerebrospinal fluid

Container Red top tube; clean, sterile CSF tube

Reference Range Negative

Possible Panic Range CF antibody titer ≥1:32 may indicate disseminated disease.[1]

Use Diagnose and evaluate the prognosis of coccidioidomycosis

Limitations A negative test does not exclude coccidioidomycosis. When low titers are obtained, a diagnosis of coccidioidomycosis must be based on subsequent serological tests and on clinical and mycological studies. Cross reactions may occur in sera from patients with active histoplasmosis. False-negative results often occur in patients with solitary pulmonary lesions. The sensitivity, specificity, and reproducibility of enzyme immunoassay and other new tests should be better defined.[2]

Methodology Complement fixation (CF), tube precipitin, enzyme-linked immunosorbent assay (ELISA), immunodiffusion (ID)

Additional Information Low titers are often associated with early, residual, or meningeal coccidioidomycosis with mild and localized disease. Patients with complement fixing (CF) titers ≥1:16 should be observed for evidence of pulmonary or extrapulmonary dissemination. The higher the CF titer, the poorer the prognosis in assessing the extent and severity of both acute and chronic coccidioidomycosis. Falling CF

titers indicate an improved clinical status. Specific IgM antibodies may be detected early in the course of the disease.

The tube precipitin test for IgM antibodies is effective in detection of early disease, 1-3 weeks after infection but becomes negative in 1-6 months. There are complement fixing antibodies to either coccidioidin (a culture filtrate) or Spherulin® (an extract of spherules). CF test for IgG antibodies becomes positive later and remains positive for years.[1] The agar gel test for precipitins is more specific than CF antibody testing and may be helpful when CF provides low titer reactivity.[1]

In immunodiffusion testing, a band of identity with coccidioidin indicates infection but may be negative early. Some individuals continue to produce detectable antibodies up to 1 year after clinical recovery from active disease. A negative test does not exclude coccidioidomycosis.

Finding CF antibody in CSF makes the diagnosis of coccidioidal meningitis (if fungal osteomyelitis of the base of the skull can be excluded).

Skin testing is not 100% sensitive nor 100% specific.[2]

Seroreactivity may take place before clinically recognized coccidioidomycosis in some HIV-positive individuals.[3]

Paracoccidioidomycosis (South American blastomycosis), endemic in Mexico, and Central and South America, is similar.

Footnotes
1. "Case Records of the Massachusetts General Hospital. Weekly Clinicopathological Exercises. Case 21-1994. A 20-Year-Old Mexican Immigrant With Recurrent Hemoptysis and a Pulmonary Cavitary Lesion," *N Engl J Med*, 1994, 330(21):1516-22.
2. Centers for Disease Control and Prevention, "Update: Coccidioidomycosis - California, 1991-1993," *JAMA*, 1994, 272(8):585.
3. Gambino R, "Coccidioidal Seropositivity Precedes Clinically Apparent Coccidioidomycosis," *Lab Rep*, 1995, 17(6):45.

References
Galgiani JN, Grace GM, and Lundergan LL, "New Serologic Tests for Early Detection of Coccidioidomycosis," *J Infect Dis*, 1991, 163(3):671-4.

Hedges E and Miller S, "Coccidioidomycosis: Office Diagnosis and Treatment," *Am Fam Physician*, 1990, 41(5):1499-506.

Kaufman L and Reiss E, "Serodiagnosis of Fungal Diseases," *Manual of Clinical Laboratory Immunology*, 4th ed, Vol 2, Chapter 78, Rose NR, Conway de Macario E, Fahey JL, et al, eds, Washington, DC: American Society for Microbiology, 1992, 506-28.

Cold Agglutinin Titer

CPT 86156 (screen); 86157 (titer)

Related Information
Cold Agglutinin Screen *on page 605*
Cold Autoabsorption *on page 605*
Mycoplasma pneumoniae Diagnostic Procedures *on page 671*
Mycoplasma pneumoniae DNA Probe Test *on page 520*
Mycoplasma Serology *on page 419*
Red Blood Cells *on page 621*
Risks of Transfusion *on page 623*
Warming, Blood *on page 627*

Applies to i Antigen; I Antigen of Red Cell Membranes

Specimen Serum

Container Red top tube

Storage Instructions After clotting at 37°C, separate serum from cells if specimen is to be stored overnight in refrigerator.

Causes for Rejection Refrigeration of the specimen before separating serum from cells, specimen not allowed to clot at 37°C

Special Instructions Transport blood immediately to the laboratory.

Reference Range Negative: less than a fourfold increase in titer or single titer <1:32

Critical Values Single titers ≥64 or a fourfold titer increase in specimens 5 or more days apart are relevant.

Use In primary atypical pneumonia (infection with *Mycoplasma pneumoniae*); IgM antibodies against I antigen of erythrocyte membranes are found in most subjects. Up to 80% of patients with *M. pneumoniae* infection have a positive test and 95% of subjects below 20 years of age. Investigate idiopathic cold agglutinin disease.

Limitations False-negatives may occur if serum is refrigerated on the clot. False-positive results are associated with rubeola, adenovirus pneumonia, infectious mononucleosis, some connective tissue diseases and tropical diseases. Antibiotic therapy may interfere with antibody formation.

Methodology Titer of patient's serum against type O blood cells at 2°C to 8°C

Additional Information *M. pneumoniae* has I-like antigen specificity. The i and I RBC antigens appear to be ceramide heptasaccharides and decasaccharides. The fetal i RBCs change after birth so that by 18 months red cells carry largely I. The i substance has been found in saliva, milk, amniotic fluid, ovarian cyst fluid, and serum.

Antibody to the I antigen is more specific for *Mycoplasma*, while i antigen is more commonly found in infectious mononucleosis. The most common cause of elevated cold agglutinin in high titers is an infection with *Mycoplasma pneumoniae*. Fifty-five percent of patients with disease have rising titers. In primary atypical *Mycoplasma pneumoniae*, cold agglutinins are demonstrated 1 week after onset; the titer increases in 8-10 days, peaks at 12-25 days, and rapidly falls after day 30.

Cold agglutinins are usually IgM autoantibodies directed against the Ii antigens of human RBCs. These antibodies may be found in patients with cold agglutinin disease or may occur transiently following a number of acute infectious illnesses. Cold agglutinins of cold agglutinin disease are usually monoclonal IgM kappa. Cold antibodies of IgG, IgA, or IgM type directed against Ii antigens may be found in infectious mononucleosis. Antibodies reacting near physiologic temperatures are more likely to be clinically important. Detection of cold agglutinins may be particularly important in patients in whom cold blood is to be used.

The differential diagnosis of atypical pneumonias, including features of *Chlamydia*, *Mycoplasma*, and *Legionella* infections, has been published.[1,2]

Footnotes

1. Johnson DH and Cunha BA, "Atypical Pneumonias. Clinical and Extrapulmonary Features of *Chlamydia*, *Mycoplasma*, and *Legionella* Infections," *Postgrad Med*, 1993, 93(7):69-72, 75-6, 79-82.
2. Clyde WA Jr, "*Mycoplasma* Infections," *Harrison's Principles of Internal Medicine*, 13th ed, Isselbacher KJ, Braunwald E, Wilson JD, et al, eds, New York, NY: McGraw-Hill Inc, 1994, 757-9.

References

Dake SB, Johnston MF, Brueggeman P, et al, "Detection of Cold Hemagglutination in a Blood Cardioplegia Unit Before Systemic Cooling of a Patient With Suspected Cold Agglutinin Disease," *Ann Thorac Surg*, 1989, 47(6):914-5.

Hadnagy C, "Agewise Distribution of Idiopathic Cold Agglutinin Disease," *Z Gerontol*, 1993, 26(3):199-201.

Silberstein LE, "B-Cell Origin of Cold Agglutinins," *Adv Exp Med Biol*, 1994, 347:193-205.

Colloidal Gold Curve *replaced by* Cerebrospinal Fluid Immunoglobulin G *on page 378*

Complement C3 *see* C3 Complement, Serum *on page 373*

Complement C4 *see* C4 Complement, Serum *on page 374*

Complement Components

CPT 86160 (antigen, each component); 86161 (activity, each component)

Related Information

C1 Esterase Inhibitor, Serum *on page 372*
C1q Immune Complex Detection *on page 373*
C3 Complement, Serum *on page 373*
C4 Complement, Serum *on page 374*
Complement, Total, Serum *on next page*
Factor B *on page 393*

Test Commonly Includes Quantitation of antigenic (immunologic) and/or functional complement components - C1, C1q, C1r, C1s, C2, C3, C4, C5, C6, C7, C8, C9; factor B; factor D

Abstract The complement system is a major participant in inflammatory reactions. It consists of cascading protein/enzymatic activities with associated receptors and inhibitors. During this process, potent low molecular weight peptide anaphylatoxins (C4a, C3a, and C5a) are generated. Complement components and their deficiency states relate importantly to pyogenic infection, neisserial infection (including, in particular, meningococcal meningitis), and connective tissue disease (eg, systemic lupus erythematosus (SLE)).

Specimen Serum

Container Red top tube

Collection Complement protein components are heat labile. Samples for complement analysis should be allowed to clot 15-30 minutes at room temperature (cold activation may occur at 0°C with loss of activity) and then 30-60 minutes at 4°C. If the assay cannot be run at once, serum should be stored at -70°C. Freezing at -20°C will result in significant loss of complement activity. If sample must be transported or there is delay in processing, a normal control specimen handled in the same manner should also be analyzed.

Reference Range The following reference values reflect the wide range of complement protein present in most "normal" populations. Null alleles (code for nonsynthesis of complement protein) may be common, as has been shown in the case of C4. Complement proteins are acute phase reactants. Increased levels may relate to a variety of recent clinical or subclinical infections and/or other illnesses. Levels may be elevated with pregnancy or with use of oral contraceptives. It is difficult to establish meaningful reference ranges. Vagaries in test reagent antisera, standardization, and intralaboratory technical variation make it difficult to interpret an isolated value. Interpretation should be made using reference ranges from a verified "normal" population, samples properly collected and handled by the same laboratory performing the patient's test.

Components of the classical complement system may be significantly decreased (on both an immunochemical and a functional basis) in neonates and during the first few weeks of life.

Complement Components

Component	Serum Concentrations (µg/mL)
Classical pathway	
C1q	70-300
C1r	34-100
C1s	30-80
C2	15-30
C4	350-600
Alternative pathway	
Factor B	140-240
Factor D	1-2
C3	1200-1500
Terminal pathway	
C5	70-85
C6	60-70
C7	55-70
C8	55-80
C9	50-160

Use Assess patients with hereditary deficiency of complement components or acquired decrease

Methodology Radial immunodiffusion (RID), nephelometry, functional analysis in hemolytic system. High voltage agarose gel electrophoresis and/or isoelectric focusing with subsequent visualization by functional overlay gel, immunofixation, or immunoblotting techniques for visualization of complement allotypes.

Additional Information The complement system is an array of over 30 proteins which can interact sequentially to produce a number of biologically active products which are implicated in the pathophysiology of numerous diseases with an immunologic basis. Complement is most often "activated" through either the "classical" pathway, beginning with antigen-antibody immune complexes (usually on some biologic surface) or the "alternate" pathway which is largely independent of antigen/antibody reaction and commonly relates to the action of bacterial products. Either mode of activation leads to formation of C3 convertase which then leads to production of the membrane attack complex (MAC). The classical pathway consists of the plasma proteins C1, C4, C2, and C3. C1 is a large complex formed of C1q (one molecule) and C1r and C1s (two molecules of each). C1 assembly requires calcium. C1q has six globular heads that bind immunoglobulin. Only IgG and IgM bind C1q and activate complement. The IgG$_3$ subset binds C1q efficiently; IgG$_4$ does not bind C1q. Activated C1 cleaves C4 to C4a and C4b. C4b then binds to the cell membrane beside C1. C2 binds to C4b and is cleaved by C1; C2a remains bound to C4b. C3 is then cleaved, C3b binding to the membrane after which C5 is bound and cleaved. The anaphylatoxin C5a is released. C6 is then bound, initiating the terminal path (formation of the membrane attack complex consisting of C5b-poly C9). Currently, it is considered that the MAC cylinder consists of up to 12 C9 molecules. See references by Morgan et al for review of considerable additional established detail concerning the process of complement activation and control. Complement proteins account for about 10% of the serum protein, C3 is present in the highest concentration (120-150 mg/dL). See figure.

In the course of activation several byproducts are produced which are active mediators of inflammation. C3a, C3b, C5a, and C5,6,7 are particularly important chemotactic factors and opsonins.

Measurement of total complement activity or components, particularly C3 and C4 which can reflect both complement pathways, may be useful in evaluating the activity of rheumatic disorders in which complement may be involved in pathogenesis. These include SLE, arteritis, and immune arthritis in particular.

There are congenital deficiencies of complement components associated with distinct clinical syndromes (see table).

The most common infections occurring in complement deficient individuals are those due to *Neisseria meningitidis* (some 75% of identified infections). Meningococcal disease may occur with any plasma protein complement deficiency but is most common in C5, C6, C7, C8, C9, or properdin deficiency.

Deficiency of C3 is associated with severe recurrent infections, usually with encapsulated microorganisms. Deficiencies of C1 components, C2 and C4 are associated with rheumatic diseases, including SLE, vasculitis, and dermatomyositis. Some individuals with deficiency may have no evidence of disease.

The most common complement deficiency is C2, which is a homozygous abnormality in 1 in 10,000 to 40,000 individuals, and is heterozygous in

(Continued)

Complement Components *(Continued)*

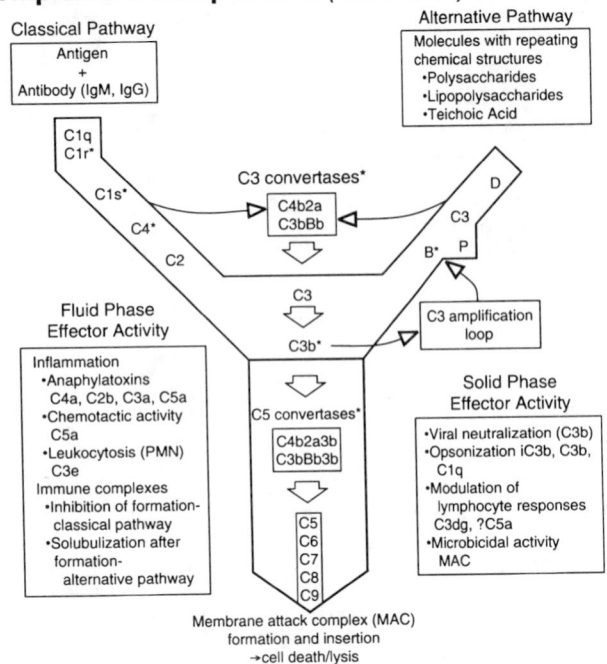

Asterisks indicate sites of downregulation of complement activity.

From Densen P, "Complement," *Principles and Practice of Infectious Diseases*, 4th ed, Chapter 6, Mandell GL, Bennett JE, and Dolin R, eds, New York, NY: Churchill Livingstone, 1995, 58-78.

Complement Deficiencies in Man

Component	Number of Cases*	Associated Diseases
C1q	13	
C1r/C1s	9	Pyogenic infections, SLE, GN
C4	13	
C2	77	About 50% healthy, remainder SLE, GN, infections
C3	14	Severe immune deficiency, SLE, GN
C5	13	Meningococcal meningitis, gonococcal sepsis, SLE
C6	33	
C7	22	Meningococcal meningitis, SLE (rare)
C8	31†	
C9	4‡	Healthy, meningococcal meningitis
Factor I	6	Severe pyogenic infections
Factor H	2	Hemolytic uremic syndrome
Properdin	4	Meningococcal meningitis, pneumonia

From Morgan BP, *Complement: Clinical Aspects and Relevance to Disease*, San Diego, CA: Academic Press, Inc, 1990, 82, with permission.

*Up to 1984, data in part from Ross and Densen, *Medicine*, 1984, 63:243-73.

†About 25% C8 A deficiency, 75% C8 B deficiency.

‡Non-Japanese patients only. In Japan, C9 deficiency is extremely common (about 1:1000) and is apparently asymptomatic.

1% to 2% of the general population. Patients with C2 deficiency and SLE often have negative or low titer ANA.

Complement components may drop in patients with active rheumatic diseases, particularly lupus nephritis, sometimes decreasing prior to the clinical attack.

Many complement proteins exhibit genetic polymorphism. Results of allotyping may be useful as major histocompatibility complex (MHC) markers for some diseases, in confirmation of inherited deficiency of a complement protein, and to assist with identification of donors for organ or tissue transplantation. Such allotyping has been referred to as "complotyping". (See reference by Marcus-Bagley.)

Complement research activity involves complement receptors and regulatory proteins including collectins, collectin receptors, and clusterin (complement lysis inhibitor). Collectins are collagen-containing mammalian multimeric lectins which resemble C1q in structure, bind to a C1q receptor, and function as opsonins. Clusterin upon binding to C5b-7

complexes blocks their membranolytic potential (complement lysis inhibition). Plasma clusterin is bound to high density lipoprotein and may be a regulatory apolipoprotein (apo-J) of HDLs.

References

Bearskeus F, Schornaged I, Krediet T, et al, "Functional Complement Deficiencies in Newborns," *Clin Exp Immunol*, 1994, 97(Suppl 2):17.

Densen P, "Complement," *Principles and Practice of Infectious Diseases*, 4th ed, Vol 1, Chapter 6, Mandell GL, Bennett JE, and Dolin R, eds, New York, NY: Churchill Livingstone, 1995, 58-78.

Frank MM, "Complement in the Pathophysiology of Human Disease," *N Engl J Med*, 1987, 316(24):1525-30.

Malhotra R, Lu J, Holmskov U, et al, "Collectins, Collectin Receptors and the Lectin Pathway of Complement Activation," *Clin Exp Immunol*, 1994, 97 (Suppl 2):4-9.

Marcus-Bagely D and Alper CA, "Methods for Allotyping Complement Proteins," *Manual of Clinical Laboratory Immmunology*, 4th ed, Chapter 19, Rose NR, Conway de Macario E, Fahey JL, et al, eds, Washington, DC: American Society for Microbiology, 1992, 124-41.

Morgan BP, *Complement: Clinical Aspects and Relevance to Disease*, San Diego, CA: Academic Press, Inc, 1990.

Ruddy S, "Complement," *Manual of Clinical Laboratory Immmunology*, 4th ed, Chapter 18, Rose NR, Conway de Macario E, Fahey JL, et al, eds, Washington, DC: American Society for Microbiology, 1992, 114-23.

Tschopp J and French LE, "Clusterin: Modulation of Complement Function," *Clin Exp Immunol*, 1994, 97 (Suppl 2):11-4.

Whaley K, Loos M, and Weiler JM, *Complement in Health and Disease*, 2nd ed, Vol 20, Boston, MA: Kluwer Academic Publishers, 1993.

Complement, Total, Serum

CPT 86162

Related Information

Anti-DNA *on page 365*

C1q Immune Complex Detection *on page 373*

C3 Complement, Serum *on page 373*

C4 Complement, Serum *on page 374*

Complement Components *on previous page*

Factor B *on page 393*

Kidney Profile *on page 153*

Synonyms CH_{50}; CH_{100}; Total Hemolytic Complement

Test Commonly Includes Quantitation of total functional serum complement

Abstract Complement is a system of over 30 cell membrane associated and plasma proteins, which when activated produce multiple inflammatory mediators, opsonins, lysins, and down-regulators vital to the normal function of the immune system. Complement components belong to a "classical" and "alternative" pathway in which activation steps differ.

Specimen Serum

Container Red top tube

Storage Instructions Allow sample to clot 15-30 minutes at room temperature, then 30-60 minutes at 4°C. Store serum at -70°C if assay cannot be run at once. Complement components may degrade if exposed to longer clotting times or higher temperatures.

Reference Range 40-100 CH_{50} units with some variation between laboratories. Synovial fluid levels are 33% to 50% of serum levels in patients with nonimmune processes.

Use Evaluate and follow-up response to therapy in SLE (systemic lupus erythematosus). Screen for complement component deficiency; evaluate complement activity in cases of immune complex disease, glomerulonephritis, rheumatoid arthritis, subacute bacterial endocarditis, cryoglobulinemia. The CH_{50} assay mainly evaluates the classical pathway.

Limitations Levels are affected by patient's age, stage and activity of disease, treatment, and genetic factors. A single normal result may be misleading; longitudinal studies are clinically more helpful.

Methodology Quantitative hemolysis (total complement hemolytic activity (CH_{50})), radial immunodiffusion (RID). CH_{50} unit reflects the reciprocal of the dilution of patient's serum required to hemolyze 50% of sheep red blood cells.

Additional Information Complement proteins can be increased as part of the acute phase response to inflammation or infection, and they can be decreased or absent due to hypercatabolism, expenditure in immune complexes, or hereditary deficiency. The end result of the CH_{50} assay is hemolysis of sheep RBCs. This assay, if normal, indicates that C1 through C9 are present in the test serum. Normal serum contains complement components in excess of that needed for a normal CH_{50} test result. Thus, absolute concentration of an individual C component may be lower than normal and undetected by CH_{50} result.

Patients with hereditary absence of a complement protein may have decreased total complement and recurrent bacterial infections or a rheumatic illness. Conversely, patients with rheumatic diseases, particularly with active illness and activation of complement and formation of immune complexes, may have low total complement. Falling complement levels may presage clinical flares, particularly of lupus nephritis.

References

Buyon JP, Tamerius J, Ordorica S, et al, "Activation of the Alternative Complement Pathway Accompanies Disease Flares in Systemic Lupus Erythematosus During Pregnancy," *Arthritis Rheum*, 1992, 35(1):55-61.

Frank MM, "Complement in the Pathophysiology of Human Disease," *N Engl J Med*, 1987, 316(24):1525-30.

McCavty-Farid GA, "Connective Tissue Diseases," *Laboratory Medicine: The Selection and Interpretation of Clinical Laboratory Studies*, Chapter 16, Noe DA and Rock RC, eds, Baltimore, MD: Williams and Wilkins, 1994, 280-1.

McPherson RA, "Serologic Evaluation of Renal Status," *Clin Lab Med*, 1993, 13(1):69-87.

Ruddy S, "Complement," *Manual of Clinical Laboratory Immunology*, 4th ed, Chapter 18, Rose NR, Conway de Macario E, Fahey JL, et al, eds, Washington, DC: American Society for Microbiology, 1992, 114-23.

Conglutinin Solid-Phase Assay *see* Immune Complex Assay *on page 407*

Cough Plate Culture for Pertussis *replaced by Bordetella pertussis* Direct Fluorescent Antibody *on page 371*

***Coxiella burnetii* Titer** *see* Q Fever Titer *on page 426*

Coxsackie A Virus Titer

CPT 86658

Related Information

Enterovirus Culture *on page 666*

Viral Culture, Blood *on page 677*

Viral Culture, Body Fluid *on page 677*

Viral Culture, Central Nervous System Symptoms *on page 677*

Viral Culture, Respiratory Symptoms *on page 680*

Test Commonly Includes Detection of antibody titer to Coxsackie A virus

Abstract The nonpolio enteroviruses include coxsackie viruses, echoviruses, and enteroviruses. Twenty-three coxsackie viruses group A are recognized.

Specimen Serum

Container Red top tube

Sampling Time Acute and convalescent sera drawn at least 14 days apart are required.

Reference Range Less than a fourfold increase in titer in paired sera

Use Coxsackie A virus produces a wide spectrum of disease including myositis, pericarditis, meningitis, respiratory illnesses, rash, and generalized systemic infection.

Limitations Documentation of infection by serology is difficult, and diagnosis may depend on culture and other methods. Neutralizing antibodies develop quickly and persist for many years after infection, making demonstration of a rise in titer difficult. Complement fixation test is not sensitive.

Methodology Viral neutralization, complement fixation (CF)

References

Melnick JL, "Enteroviruses," *Manual of Clinical Laboratory Immunology*, 4th ed, Vol 2, Chapter 93, Rose NR, Conway de Macario E, Fahey JL, et al, eds, Washington, DC: American Society for Microbiology, 1992, 631-3.

Coxsackie B Virus Titer

CPT 86658

Related Information

Enterovirus Culture *on page 666*

Viral Culture, Blood *on page 677*

Viral Culture, Body Fluid *on page 677*

Viral Culture, Central Nervous System Symptoms *on page 677*

Viral Culture, Respiratory Symptoms *on page 680*

Applies to Enteroviruses

Test Commonly Includes Coxsackie B_1, B_2, B_3, B_4, B_5, B_6 virus titers

Abstract Six coxsackie viruses group B are recognized

Specimen Serum

Container Red top tube

Sampling Time Acute and convalescent sera drawn 10-14 days apart are required.

Reference Range Less than a fourfold increase in titer in paired sera

Use Coxsackie B virus causes a wide variety of clinical illness, including pleurodynia (Bornholm's disease), meningitis, rash, pulmonary infection, myocarditis, pericarditis, and a generalized systemic infection. The coxsackie group B viruses are the viruses most commonly implicated in acute myocarditis.[1]

Limitations Neutralizing antibodies arise quickly and last for years and may make the demonstration of a rising titer difficult. Complement fixing antibodies are insensitive and nonspecific.

Methodology Complement fixation (CF), viral neutralization

Additional Information Since culture is frequently unrewarding, diagnosis may hinge on serologic studies. Recently there has been interest in various viral assays for postviral fatigue syndrome. Antibody to Coxsackie B virus is not helpful in this assessment.

Footnotes

1. "Case Records of the Massachusetts General Hospital. Weekly Clinicopathological Exercises. Case 47-1993. Presentation of Case. A 28-Year-Old Man With Recurrent

Ventricular Tachycardia and Dysfunction of Multiple Organs," *N Engl J Med*, 1993, 329(22):1639-47.

References

Miller NA, Carmichael HA, Calder BD, et al, "Antibody to Coxsackie B Virus in Diagnosing Postviral Fatigue Syndrome," *BMJ*, 1991, 302(6769):140-3.

See DM and Tilles JG, "Viral Myocarditis," *Rev Infect Dis*, 1991, 13(5):951-6.

C-Reactive Protein

CPT 86140

Related Information

Alpha$_1$-Antitrypsin, Serum *on page 363*

Insulin, Blood *on page 149*

Lipase, Serum *on page 158*

Sedimentation Rate, Erythrocyte *on page 347*

Zeta Sedimentation Ratio *on page 354*

Synonyms CRP

Applies to Acute Phase Reactant; Amyloid A, Serum

Abstract Produced by hepatocytes, C-reactive protein is a useful but nonspecific indicator of acute injury, bacterial infection, or inflammation, sensitive to activation of neutrophils. It is used to try to distinguish bacterial from viral infection, the former causing higher concentrations.

Specimen Serum

Container Red top tube

Storage Instructions Do not freeze.

Reference Range <8 µg/mL

Use Used similarly to erythrocyte sedimentation rate as a marker for inflammation, but each of the tests provides some information not available from the other.[1] CRP is nonspecific acute phase reactant used as an indicator of infectious disease and inflammatory states, including active rheumatic fever and rheumatoid arthritis. Progressive increases correlate with increases of inflammation/injury. CRP is a more sensitive, rapidly responding indicator than ESR. CRP may be used to detect early postoperative wound infection, support the differential diagnosis of appendicitis and acute pelvic inflammatory disease,[1] and to follow therapeutic response to anti-inflammatory agents. It may be a useful test to project severity of pancreatitis.[2] With serum amyloid A protein, it may predict outcome in subjects with unstable angina,[3] and it is reported as a screening test to distinguish pyonephrosis from uncomplicated hydronephrosis.[4]

Limitations Frozen specimens may give false-positive results; oral contraceptives may affect results.

Methodology Agglutination, nephelometry, radioimmunoassay (RIA)

Additional Information CRP is a pentameric globulin with mobility near the gamma zone. It rises rapidly, but nonspecifically in response to tissue injury and inflammation. It is particularly useful in detection of occult infections, acute appendicitis, particularly in leukemia and in postoperative patients. In uncomplicated postoperative recovery, CRP peaks on the 3rd postop day and returns to preop levels by day 7. It may also be helpful in evaluation of extension or reinfarction after myocardial infarction and in following response to therapy in rheumatic disorders. It may help to differentiate Crohn's disease (high CRP) from ulcerative colitis (low CRP) and rheumatoid arthritis (high CRP) from uncomplicated lupus (low CRP). When used to evaluate patients with arthritis, serum is the preferred specimen. There is no reason to examine synovial fluid for CRP.

Footnotes

1. Gambino R, "C-Reactive Protein (CRP) - How Much Proof Do We Need?" *Lab Rep*, 1994, 16(11):83-5.
2. Steinberg W and Tenner S, "Acute Pancreatitis," *N Engl J Med*, 1994, 330(17), 1198-210.
3. Liuzzo G, Biasucci LM, Gallimore JR, et al, "The Prognostic Value of C-Reactive Protein and Serum Amyloid A Protein in Severe Unstable Angina," *N Engl J Med*, 1994, 331(7):417-24.
4. Wu TT, Lee YH, Tzeng WS, et al, "The Role of C-Reactive Protein and Erythrocyte Sedimentation Rate in the Diagnosis of Infected Hydronephrosis and Pyonephrosis," *J Urol*, 1994, 152(1):26-8.

References

Delpuech P, Desch G, Magnan F, et al, "C-Reactive Protein in Inflammatory Articular Diseases: Comparison of Concentrations in Blood and Synovial Fluid," *Clin Biochem*, 1989, 22(4):305-8.

Dowton SR and Colten HR, "Acute Phase Reactants in Inflammation and Infection," *Semin Hematol*, 1988, 25(2):84-90.

Schofield KP, Voulgari F, Gozzard DI, et al, "C-Reactive Protein Concentration as a Guide to Antibiotic Therapy in Acute Leukemia," *J Clin Pathol*, 1982, 35:866-9.

Shaw AC, "Serum C-Reactive Protein and Neopterin Concentrations in Patients With Viral or Bacterial Infection," *J Clin Pathol*, 1991, 44(7):596-9.

Thimsen DA, Tong GK, and Gruenberg JC, "Prospective Evaluation of C-Reactive Protein in Patients Suspected to Have Acute Appendicitis," *Am J Surg*, 1989, 55(7):466-8.

Van Lente F, "The Diagnostic Utility of C-Reactive Protein," *Hum Pathol*, 1982, 13(12):1061-3.

Crossmatch, Lymphocyte *see* Tissue Typing *on page 434*

CRP *see* C-Reactive Protein *on this page*

Cryocrit *see* Cryoglobulin, Qualitative, Serum *on next page*

Cryoglobulin, Qualitative, Serum

CPT 82595

Related Information

Cryofibrinogen *on page 236*
Hepatitis C Serology *on page 399*
Kidney Profile *on page 153*
Rheumatoid Factor *on page 427*

Applies to Cryocrit

Patient Preparation Patient should be fasting.

Specimen Serum

Container Red top tube

Collection Specimen must be drawn in a prewarmed syringe and kept at 37°C while clotting.

Storage Instructions Separate serum from cells, recentrifuge serum if possible at 37°C and pour into clean test tube. Do not refrigerate or freeze.

Causes for Rejection Specimen not allowed to clot at 37°C.

Special Instructions Transport sample managed as above at ambient temperature.

Reference Range Negative

Use Cryoglobulins may be present in macroglobulinemia of Waldenström, myeloma, chronic lymphocytic leukemia, lupus, primary Sjögren's syndrome, liver diseases including chronic hepatitis, cirrhosis, and viral infections, in particular, hepatitis C virus (HCV).[1,2,3]

Methodology Precipitation of cryoglobulin at 4°C. After centrifugation, the "cryocrit" of precipitated cryoglobulin can be determined followed by immunochemical analysis of the precipitate.

Additional Information These are proteins which precipitate from blood at low temperatures. A precipitate from serum which forms overnight at 4°C and dissolves at 37°C is called a cryoglobulin. This qualitative test can be semiquantitated by spinning down the tube after incubation at 4°C and measuring the "cryocrit".

Cryoglobulins may be divided into three classes. **Type I** are monoclonal immunoglobulins and are usually associated with lymphoproliferative disorders. **Type II** are mixtures of a monoclonal IgM and polyclonal IgG, and are associated with macroglobulinemia and autoimmune/chronic active hepatitis. **Type III** are mixtures of polyclonal IgM and polyclonal IgG. These are found in a wide variety of disorders.

A high percentage of patients with cryoglobulinemia have clinical symptoms, and of these the most common are vascular (ie, purpura and digital necrosis). Raynaud's phenomenon is also common. Many idiopathic cases of cryoglobulinemia appear to be due to hepatitis C.

Patients with SLE who are rheumatoid factor negative but cryoglobulin positive are more likely to develop renal disease than those who are rheumatoid factor positive and cryoglobulin negative.

Footnotes

1. Lunel F, Musset L, Cacoub P, et al, "Cryoglobulinemia in Chronic Liver Diseases: Role of Hepatitis C Virus and Liver Damage," *Gastroenterology*, 1994, 106(5):1291-300.
2. Agnello V, "Mixed Cryoglobulinemia and Hepatitis C Virus," *Hosp Pract*, 1995, 30(3):35-42.
3. Cacoub P, Fabiani FL, Musset L, et al, "Mixed Cryoglobulinemia and Hepatitis C Virus," *Am J Med*, 1994, 96(2):124-32.

References

Howard TW, Iannini MJ, Burge JJ, et al, "Rheumatoid Factor, Cryoglobulinemia, Anti-DNA, and Renal Disease in Patients With Systemic Lupus Erythematous," *J Rheumatol*, 1991, 18(6):826-30.
Keren DF and Warren JS, *Diagnostic Immunology*, Baltimore, MD: Williams & Wilkins, 1992, 270-2.
Miescher PA, Huang YP, and Izui S, "Type II Cryoglobulinemia," *Semin Hematol*, 1995, 32(1):80-5.

Cryptococcal Antigen Titer

CPT 86313 (immunoassay, multiple step); 86315 (immunoassay, single step)

Related Information

Bacterial Antigens, Rapid Detection Methods *on page 454*
Fungal Culture, Cerebrospinal Fluid *on page 477*
Fungal Culture, Sputum *on page 479*
Fungus Smear, Stain *on page 481*
India Ink Preparation *on page 484*
Mycobacterial Culture, Cerebrospinal Fluid *on page 489*

Synonyms Cerebrospinal Fluid Cryptococcal Latex Agglutination

Test Commonly Includes Testing patient's serum or CSF for the presence of cryptococcal heteropolysaccharide capsular antigen

Abstract Cryptococcal antigen testing is the single most useful diagnostic test for cryptococcal meningitis.[1] Cryptococcosis is caused by *Cryptococcus neoformans*, a yeast-like fungal organism. Corticosteroids enhance development of this infection. Over half the cases in the U.S. presently are found in AIDS patients.

Specimen Serum or cerebrospinal fluid

Container Red top tube, sterile CSF tube

Reference Range Negative

Critical Values Positive results are phoned immediately to the physician.

Use Diagnose subacute or chronic meningitis, particularly in immunosuppressed patients; rapid diagnosis of cryptococcal meningitis; follow response of cryptococcal meningitis to therapy

Limitations False-positives and false-negatives occur. Lack of standardization between manufacturers exists; thus, titers from different kits are not comparable. False-positive results may be seen in patients with disseminated *Trichosporon beigelii* infections.

Methodology Latex agglutination (LA) with rheumatoid factor control and in some laboratories pronase pretreatment

Additional Information Serum and CSF are positive in at least 90% of patients with cryptococcal meningitis; these specimens are much less likely to provide positive results in cryptococcosis outside of the CNS.[1] Most commercially available kits employ controls for nonspecific agglutination by rheumatoid factor. Treatment of serum specimens with pronase may improve test results.

Footnotes

1. Greenlee JE, "Approach to Diagnosis of Meningitis - Cerebrospinal Fluid Evaluation," *Infect Dis Clin North Am*, 1990, 4(4):583-98.

References

Berlin L and Pincus JH, "Cryptococcal Meningitis: False-Negative Antigen Test Results and Cultures in Nonimmunosuppressed Patients," *Arch Neurol*, 1989, 46(12):1312-6.
Speed B and Dunt D, "Clinical and Host Differences Between Infections With the Two Varieties of *Cryptococcus neoformans*," *Clin Infect Dis*, 1995, 21(1):28-34.
Temstet A, Roux P, Poirot JL, et al, "Evaluation of a Monoclonal Antibody-Based Latex Agglutination Test for Diagnosis of Cryptococcosis: Comparison With Two Tests Using Polyclonal Antibodies," *J Clin Microbiol*, 1992, 30(10):2544-50.

CSF *see* VDRL, Cerebrospinal Fluid *on page 438*

CSF Amyloid Precursor Protein and Amyloid β-Protein *see* Cerebrospinal Fluid Amyloid Precursor Protein and Amyloid β-Protein *on page 376*

CSF Electrophoresis *see* Cerebrospinal Fluid Protein Electrophoresis *on page 381*

CSF FTA-ABS *see* FTA-ABS, Cerebrospinal Fluid *on page 394*

CSF Gamma G *see* Cerebrospinal Fluid Immunoglobulin G *on page 378*

CSF IgG *see* Cerebrospinal Fluid Immunoglobulin G *on page 378*

CSF IgG/CSF α₂-Macroglobulin *see* Cerebrospinal Fluid IgG Ratios and IgG Index *on page 377*

CSF IgG/CSF Albumin Ratio *see* Cerebrospinal Fluid IgG Ratios and IgG Index *on page 377*

CSF IgG/CSF Total Protein Ratio *see* Cerebrospinal Fluid IgG Ratios and IgG Index *on page 377*

CSF Immunoglobulin *see* Cerebrospinal Fluid Immunoglobulin G *on page 378*

CSF Myelin Basic Protein *see* Cerebrospinal Fluid Myelin Basic Protein *on page 379*

CSF Protein *see* Cerebrospinal Fluid Protein *on page 380*

CSF Tau Protein *see* Cerebrospinal Fluid Tau Protein *on page 382*

Cysticercosis Titer

CPT 86317 (immunoassay, quantitative); 86318 (immunoassay, qualitative or semiqualitative); 88347 (indirect immunofluorescence)

Related Information

Ova and Parasites, Stool *on page 494*
Parasite Antibodies *on page 421*

Applies to *Taenia solium*

Abstract Eggs of *Taenia solium*, the pork tapeworm acquired from contact with contaminated feces, lead to cysticercosis. Cysticercosis, larval forms in tissues, is endemic in Mexico, portions of South America, Africa, and Asia.

Specimen Serum, cerebrospinal fluid

Container Red top tube

Reference Range Negative

Use Cysticercosis is most commonly found in brain or muscle, in which a space-occupying mass presents with local inflammatory reaction. Diagnosis is usually established on the basis of imaging, clinical presentation and serology.

Limitations Cross reactions in patients with tapeworm or *Echinococcus* were found before immunoblotting techniques became available. Sensitivity remains limited when there is low parasite burden; ie, false-negatives occur.

Methodology Immunoblotting, enzyme-linked immunosorbent assay (ELISA)

Additional Information Ingestion of eggs of the pork tapeworm (*Taenia solium*) produces cysticercosis, an infection in which larval cysts are seen in various tissues. Water may also be contaminated with eggs, especially in areas with inadequate water purification systems. Serious infection occurs with CNS involvement. Recently, the number of cases of cysticercosis has increased in the U.S., likely due to increased levels of immigration from Latin America.[1]

In CNS involvement, CSF pleocytosis is found with increased CSF protein and decreased glucose.

Footnotes
1. Sorvillo FJ, Waterman SH, Richards FO, et al, "Cysticercosis Surveillance: Locally Acquired and Travel-Related Infections and Detection of Intestinal Tapeworm Carriers in Los Angeles County," *Am J Trop Med Hyg*, 1992, 47(3):365-71.

References
Ash LR and Orihel TC, *Atlas of Human Parasitology*, 3rd ed, Chicago, IL: American Society of Clinical Pathologists, 1990, 224-5.
Kagan IG and Maddison SE, "Serodiagnosis of Parasitic Diseases," *Manual of Clinical Laboratory Immunology*, 4th ed, Vol 2, Chapter 79, Rose NR, Conway de Macario E, Fahey JL, et al, eds, Washington, DC: American Society for Microbiology, 1992, 529-43.
Schantz PM, Moore AC, Munoz JL, et al, "Neurocysticercosis in an Orthodox Jewish Community in New York City," *N Engl J Med*, 1992, 327(10):692-5.
Sloan L, Schneider S, and Rosenblatt J, "Evaluation of Enzyme-Linked Immunoassay for Serological Diagnosis of Cysticercosis," *J Clin Microbiol*, 1995, 3124-8.
Wilson M, Bryan RT, Fried JA, et al, "Clinical Evaluation of the Cysticercosis Enzyme-Linked Immunoelectrotransfer Blot in Patients With Neurocysticeriosis," *J Infect Dis*, 1991, 164(5):1007-9.

Cytomegalic Inclusion Virus Titer *see* Cytomegalovirus Antibody *on this page*

Cytomegalovirus Antibody
CPT 86644; 86645 (IgM)
Related Information
Bacterial Culture, Bronchoscopy Specimen *on page 459*
Bronchial Washings Cytology *on page 287*
Bronchoalveolar Lavage Cytology *on page 288*
Cytomegalic Inclusion Disease Cytology *on page 293*
Cytomegalovirus Antigen Detection *on page 664*
Cytomegalovirus Culture *on page 664*
Cytomegalovirus DNA Detection *on page 508*
Risks of Transfusion *on page 623*
Sputum Cytology *on page 300*
TORCH *on page 435*
Synonyms CMV-IFA; CMV Titer; Cytomegalic Inclusion Virus Titer
Applies to CMV-IFA, IgG; CMV-IFA, IgM
Test Commonly Includes Both IgM and IgG antibodies can be tested.
Abstract The most common intrauterine infection is congenital cytomegalovirus infection. It is also an important problem in adult immunocompromised subjects including renal transplant recipients on immunosuppressive agents, patients with neoplastic diseases, and AIDS.
Specimen Serum
Container Red top tube
Sampling Time Sampling too early may miss acute infection. Acute and convalescent sera drawn 10-14 days apart are required for IgG CMV testing. A single specimen may be sufficient for IgM testing. For determination of prior exposure to CMV (for transplantation or transfusion), a single specimen may be satisfactory.
Storage Instructions 4°C
Special Instructions Neonatal specimens should be analyzed for specific IgM antibody only.
Reference Range IgM: <1:8 is considered nondiagnostic. Less than a fourfold increase in CMV-IgG titer in paired sera drawn 10-14 days apart.
Use Determine prior exposure to CMV for purposes of organ transplantation and provision of blood and blood fractions to selected recipients. Investigate patients with mononucleosis-like illness who are Monospot® negative. CMV serology is part of TORCH screen used to test pregnant women.
Limitations Heterophil antibodies and presence of rheumatoid factor may cause false-positive IgM results. Fetal IgM antibody to maternal IgG may also cause false-positive results. False-negatives occur. Because of high levels of "background" antibody in adult populations, a single antibody determination is not useful.
Methodology Indirect fluorescent antibody (IFA), enzyme immunoassay (EIA)
Additional Information Intrauterine transmission of CMV can occur whether or not prior maternal immunity exists. However, the presence of maternal antibody prior to conception does provide a significant degree of protection against neonatal damage of congenital CMV infection. Sequellae of congenital CMV infections are more severe in primary maternal infections occurring during pregnancy.[1]

A single titer is rarely significant if past history is unknown. A fourfold or greater rise in CMV titer between acute and convalescent specimens is evidence of infection. A single IgM specific titer >1:8 is also excellent evidence of acute infection. CMV causes an infectious mononucleosis syndrome clinically indistinguishable from heterophil positive mononucleosis. Significant CMV titers are found almost universally in patients with AIDS. CMV is a significant cause of postcardiotomy, post-transplant and postpump hepatitis syndromes.

Although serology is a useful method to detect CMV infections, the newer shell vial culture can more reliably identify symptomatic CMV infections in immunocompromised patients.

Several new EIA tests agree well with IFA serology and provide a more objective measure of infection status than the subjective IFA test.

See Related Information at the beginning of this listing for further tests relevant to CMV.

Footnotes
1. Fowler KB, Stagno S, Pass RF, et al, "The Outcome of Congenital Cytomegalovirus Infection in Relation to Maternal Antibody Status," *N Engl J Med*, 1992, 326(10):663-7.

References
Hughes JH, "Physical and Chemical Methods for Enhancing Rapid Detection of Viruses and Other Agents," *Clin Microbiol Rev*, 1993, 6(2):150-75.
Marsano L, Perrillo RP, Flye MW, et al, "Comparison of Culture and Serology for the Diagnosis of Cytomegalovirus Infection in Kidney and Liver Transplant Recipients," *J Infect Dis*, 1990, 161(3):454-61.
Paya CV, Smith TF, Ludwig J, et al, "Rapid Shell Vial Culture and Tissue Histology Compared With Serology for the Rapid Diagnosis of Cytomegalovirus Infection in Liver Transplantation," *Mayo Clin Proc*, 1989, 64(6):670-5.
Van Enk RA, James KK, and Thompson KD, "Evaluation of Three Commercial Enzyme Immunoassays for *Toxoplasma* and Cytomegalovirus Antibodies," *Am J Clin Pathol*, 1991, 95(3):428-34.

Davidsohn Differential *replaced by* Infectious Mononucleosis Screening Test *on page 410*

Davidsohn Slide Test *see* Infectious Mononucleosis Screening Test *on page 410*

Delta Agent Serology *see* Hepatitis D Serology *on page 400*

Delta Hepatitis Serology *see* Hepatitis D Serology *on page 400*

Desert Fever *see* Coccidioidomycosis Antibodies *on page 384*

DNA Antibody *see* Anti-DNA *on page 365*

DR-3 *see* Smooth Muscle Antibody *on page 431*

DR-4 *see* Smooth Muscle Antibody *on page 431*

DR52a *see* Smooth Muscle Antibody *on page 431*

Dysgammaglobulinemia *see* Immunoelectrophoresis, Serum or Urine *on page 408*

Dysgammaglobulinemia Evaluation *see* Immunofixation Electrophoresis *on page 408*

Eastern Equine Encephalitis *see* Encephalitis Viral Serology *on page 391*

Eastern Equine Encephalitis Virus Serology
CPT 86652
Related Information
California Encephalitis Virus Titer *on page 374*
St Louis Encephalitis Virus Serology *on page 432*
Viral Culture, Central Nervous System Symptoms *on page 677*
Western Equine Encephalitis Virus Serology *on page 439*
Synonyms Encephalitis Virus Titer, Eastern Equine
Abstract This is a low incidence disease. It occurs in late summer and early fall in the northeast United States. A 50% to 70% fatality rate is recognized.
Specimen Serum or cerebrospinal fluid
Container Red top tube
Sampling Time Acute and convalescent sera drawn 10-14 days apart
Reference Range Complement fixation: less than a fourfold increase in titer in paired sera
Use Support the diagnosis of Eastern equine encephalitis virus infection
Limitations Absence of IgM antibodies does not rule out the infection
Methodology Complement fixation (CF), hemagglutination inhibition (HAI), virus neutralization testing, enzyme-linked immunosorbent assay (ELISA) for IgM antibodies
Additional Information Eastern equine encephalitis virus is an alphavirus carried by a mosquito vector. It causes an acute illness which is either fatal or self-limited; chronic illness should suggest a different diagnosis. Syndromes include headache with fever, meningitis, and meningoencephalitis. The other alphavirus agents causing disease in the U.S. are Western equine encephalitis and Venezuelan equine encephalitis. These have been classified as group A arboviruses.
(Continued)

Eastern Equine Encephalitis Virus Serology
(Continued)

References

Centers for Disease Control, "Eastern Equine Encephalitis Virus - Florida," *JAMA*, 1992, 267(10):1324.

Monath TP, "Alphavirus (Eastern, Western, and Venezuelan Equine Encephalitis)," *Principles and Practice of Infectious Diseases*, 3rd ed, Mandell GL, Douglas RG Jr, and Bennett JE, eds, New York, NY: Churchill Livingstone, 1990, 1241-2.

Tsai TF, "Arboviruses," *Manual of Clinical Microbiology*, 6th ed, Washington, DC: American Society for Microbiology, 1995, 980-96.

Eaton Agent Titer *see Mycoplasma* Serology *on page 419*

EBNA *see* Epstein-Barr Virus Serology *on page 392*

EB Nuclear Antigen *see* Epstein-Barr Virus Serology *on page 392*

EB Virus Titer *see* Epstein-Barr Virus Serology *on page 392*

EBV Titer *see* Epstein-Barr Virus Serology *on page 392*

Echinococcosis Serological Test

CPT 86171 (complement fixation); 86403 (agglutination, screen); 86406 (agglutination, titer)

Related Information

Liver Profile *on page 161*
Ova and Parasites, Stool *on page 494*
Parasite Antibodies *on page 421*

Synonyms *Echinococcus granulosus* Serological Test; *Echinococcus multilocularis* Serological Test; Hydatid Disease Serological Test

Abstract Echinococcosis is a cestode parasitic disease important in livestock-raising areas in which dogs (the definitive hosts) are used. In humans, larval stages of *E. granulosus*, *E. multilocularis*, or *E. vogeli* cause the infection. *Echinococcus granulosus* causes unilocular cysts. The adult *E. granulosus* resides in the intestine of dogs. Sheep, caribou, deer, moose, pigs, or man are intermediate hosts. The cause of multilocular alveolar disease, a more invasive form, is a larval form of *E. multilocularis*. Polycystic hydatid disease is caused by *E. vogeli*.

Specimen Serum

Container Red top tube

Reference Range Indirect hemagglutination: 1:2-1:64

Use Support a diagnosis of echinococcosis. Cysts present in liver, lung, bone, or brain, in that order of frequency. Sensitivity and specificity of serologic assays is greater for hepatic than for pulmonary infections or those in other organs.

Limitations Serum from 50% of patients with cysticercosis cross react in this assay. False-positives are occasionally seen in patients with cirrhosis and lupus; false-negatives with some large cysts or dead cysts. Sensitivity of serological testing is no better than 60% to 90%, but serological testing is not definitive.

Methodology Complement fixation (CF), bentonite flocculation assay (BFA), indirect hemagglutination (IHA), latex agglutination (LA), enzyme-linked immunosorbent assay (ELISA); an immunoblot procedure is available at the CDC.

Additional Information Peripheral blood eosinophilia occurs, as in cyst rupture, but eosinophilia is not always found. After surgical removal of the cyst, there is generally a rapid decline in antibody within a year; failure to observe the decline indicates incomplete cyst removal. Cysts in the liver are more likely to elicit an immune response than cysts in the lungs. The newer ELISA tests are more sensitive than the more traditional hemagglutination and latex assays.

References

Ash LR and Orihel TC, *Atlas of Human Parasitology*, 3rd ed, Chicago, IL: American Society of Clinical Pathologists, 1990, 233-5.

Hira PR, Shweiki HM, and Francis I, "Cystic Hydatid Disease: Pitfalls in Diagnosis in the Middle East Endemic Area," *J Trop Med Hyg*, 1993, 96(6):363-9.

Kagan IG and Maddison SE, "Serodiagnosis of Parasitic Diseases," *Manual of Clinical Laboratory Immunology*, 4th ed, Vol 2, Chapter 79, Rose NR, Conway de Macario E, Fahey JL, et al, eds, Washington, DC: American Society for Microbiology, 1992, 529-43.

Maddison SE, "Serodiagnosis of Parasitic Diseases," *Clin Microbiol Rev*, 1991, 4(4):457-69.

Moir IL and Ho Yen DO, "The Use of Serology in Patients With Suspected Hydatid Diseases," *Scott Med J*, 1989, 34(3):466-8.

Verastegui M, Moro P, Guevara A, et al, "Enzyme-Linked Immunoelectrotransfer Blot Test for Diagnosis of Human Hydatid Disease," *J Clin Microbiol*, 1992, 30(6):1557-61.

Echinococcus granulosus Serological Test *see* Echinococcosis Serological Test *on this page*

Echinococcus multilocularis Serological Test *see* Echinococcosis Serological Test *on this page*

Edrophonium Chloride Test *see* Acetylcholine Receptor Antibody *on page 362*

Ehrlichia chaffeensis Antibodies *see* Ehrlichiosis Serology *on this page*

Ehrlichiosis Serology

Related Information

Arthropod Identification *on page 453*
Babesiosis Serological Test *on page 370*
Lyme Disease Serology *on page 415*
Rocky Mountain Spotted Fever Serology *on page 427*

Synonyms *Ehrlichia chaffeensis* Antibodies

Applies to Tickborne Diseases

Abstract Two distinct forms of ehrlichiosis have been recognized in the United States, **human monocytic ehrlichiosis (HME)** and **human granulocytic ehrlichiosis (HGE)**. Human granulocytic ehrlichiosis was first described in 1994 in Minnesota and Wisconsin. *Ehrlichia*, obligate intracellular bacteria, are transmitted to humans by ticks. They are rickettsia-like bacteria which localize in leukocytic phagosomes. Of the seven species of *Ehrlichia*, each infects leukocytoplasm or the cytoplasm of platelets. The disease is an acute febrile illness which resembles Rocky Mountain spotted fever. It can be mild but about a third of cases requires hospitalization.[1]

Specimen Serum

Container Red top tube

Collection Collect at time of illness, then 2-4 weeks after onset; ie, acute and convalescent samples.

Storage Instructions Refrigerate or freeze serum.

Reference Range Titer <1:80 with the source of antigen *E. chaffeensis*.

Critical Values Fourfold rise or fall in titer

Use Clinical features of ehrlichiosis may include rapid onset of fever with chills, myalgias, headache, and malaise. A rash may be seen, as may abdominal pain, vomiting, and diarrhea.

Limitations Positive cutoff titer for disease has not been standardized and varies between laboratories performing the test. Often, serologic results are initially negative.[2]

Methodology Indirect fluorescent antibody (IFA) for IgG and IgM antibodies. In a case of HME, *E. chaffeensis* were demonstrated in tissue by Brown and Brenn (tissue Gram's stain), and in Wright-stained peripheral blood smear and by immunocytochemistry.[3]

PCR provides early diagnosis, before antibodies are demonstrable.[4]

Additional Information Cases may be asymptomatic.

Relevant laboratory studies include thrombocytopenia, leukopenia, and increased AST and alkaline phosphatase. Inclusions (morulae) are found in neutrophils in HGE. A published photomicrograph is from a buffy coat smear, Wolbach Giemsa stain.[1] Wright's stain demonstrates *E. chaffeensis* in mononuclear cells and/or atypical lymphocytes.[3]

Nearly 400 cases have been confirmed in the U.S. with most of the cases occurring in western, south central, and south Atlantic states. The organism responsible for HME (*E. chaffeensis*) is most commonly found in the Lone Star tick (*Amblyomma americanum*) while the *E. equi*, responsible for HGE, has been found in the deer tick (*Ixodes scapularis*) and the dog tick (*Dermacentor variabilis*). HGE is found in the northern U.S., where Lyme disease and babesiosis are endemic. The latter two entities represent an important portion of the clinical differential diagnosis.[1] HME has mimicked thrombotic thrombocytopenic purpura.[3]

The agent of HGE has recently been cultivated in cell culture.[2]

Tickborne illnesses include ehrlichiosis, Lyme disease, babesiosis, relapsing fever, tularemia, Rocky Mountain spotted fever, and tick typhus.

Footnotes

1. Telford SR 3d, Lepore TJ, Snow P, et al, "Human Granulocytic Ehrlichiosis in Massachusetts," *Ann Intern Med*, 1995, 123(4):277-9.
2. Goodman JL, Nelson C, Vitale B, et al, "Direct Cultivation of the Causative Agent of Human Granulocytic Ehrlichiosis," *N Engl J Med*, 1996, 334(4):209-15.
3. Marty AM, Dumler JS, Imes G, et al, "Ehrlichiosis Mimicking Thrombotic Thrombocytopenic Purpura. Case Report and Pathological Correlation," *Hum Pathol*, 1995, 26(8):920-5.
4. Schaffner W and Standaert SM, "Ehrlichiosis - In Pursuit of an Emerging Infection," *N Engl J Med*, 1996, 334(4):262-3.

References

Dumler JS and Walker DH, "Diagnostic Tests for Rocky Mountain Spotted Fever and Other Rickettsial Diseases," *Dermatol Clin*, 1994, 12(1):25-36.

Feigin RD and Bloom ML, "Rickettsial Diseases," *Principles and Practice of Pediatrics*, 2nd ed, Oski FA, DeAngelis CD, Feigin RD, et al, eds, Philadelphia, PA: JB Lippincott Co, 1994, 1367-8.

Fishbein DB and Dennis DT, "Tick-Borne Diseases - A Growing Risk," *N Engl J Med*, 1995, 333(7):452-3 (editorial).

Spach DH, Liles WC, Campbell GL, et al, "Tick-Borne Diseases in the United States," *N Engl J Med*, 1993, 329(13):936-47.

EIA for Syphilis, IgG and IgM *see* MHA-TP *on page 418*

Electrophoresis, Protein, Urine *see* Protein Electrophoresis, Urine *on page 425*

Electrophoresis, Serum *see* Protein Electrophoresis, Serum *on page 424*

EMA *see* Endomysial Antibodies *on this page*

ENA *see* Sjögren's Antibodies *on page 430*

Encephalitis Viral Serology

Synonyms Arbovirus Serology

Applies to California Encephalitis (LaCrosse); Eastern Equine Encephalitis; St Louis Encephalitis Virus; Western Equine Encephalitis

Abstract Encephalitogenic arboviruses commonly seen in North America (ie, California encephalitis (LaCrosse), Western equine encephalitis, Eastern equine encephalitis, and St Louis encephalitis viruses). Arboviruses (arthropod-borne viruses) are a taxonomically heterogeneous group of viruses grouped together because they are all transmitted to humans via an arthropod vector.

Specimen Serum

Container Red top tube

Collection Acute and convalescent sera drawn 10-14 days apart

Reference Range Less than a fourfold titer increase in paired sera. CSF IgM: negative; hemagglutination inhibition: ≤1:80; complement fixation: ≤1:32; immunofluorescence: ≤1:128.

Use Support the diagnosis of infection with encephalitis viruses

Limitations Cross-reacting antibodies from previous infections or from immunization for yellow fever may produce false-positive results, particularly when assays are performed on unpaired sera.

Additional Information Central nervous system infection by California encephalitis (LaCrosse), Western equine encephalitis, Eastern equine encephalitis, or St Louis encephalitis viruses may manifest as aseptic meningitis, encephalitis, or meningoencephalitis. There is a seasonal distribution for these infections that reflects their mode of transmission to humans by mosquitos. In the United States, the incidence of arboviral infection is low as is the prevalence of antibodies to these agents in the general population. Consequently, a positive result in an unpaired specimen is **presumptive** evidence for a recent infection. A fourfold increase in titer or a positive CSF IgM test is confirmatory. Antibody detection is the diagnostic test of choice as these viruses are essentially nonculturable in routine diagnostic virology laboratories.

References
Bale JF Jr, "Viral Encephalitis," *Med Clin North Am*, 1993, 77(1):25-42.
Calisher CH, "Medically Important Arboviruses of the United States and Canada," *Clin Microbiol Rev*, 1994, 7(1):89-116.
Tsai TF, "Arboviruses," *Manual of Clinical Laboratory Immunology*, 4th ed, Chapter 91, Rose NR, Conway de Macario E, Fahey JL, et al, eds, Washington, DC: American Society for Microbiology, 1992, 606-18.

Encephalitis Virus Titer, California *see* California Encephalitis Virus Titer *on page 374*

Encephalitis Virus Titer, Eastern Equine *see* Eastern Equine Encephalitis Virus Serology *on page 389*

Encephalitis Virus Titer, Western Equine *see* Western Equine Encephalitis Virus Serology *on page 439*

Endomysial Antibodies

CPT 86255 (screen); 86256 (titer)

Related Information
Skin Biopsy, Immunofluorescence *on page 56*

Synonyms EMA

Applies to Antigliadin Antibody; Antireticulin Antibody

Test Commonly Includes Detection of antibodies to endomysin using immunofluorescence

Abstract The gold standard for diagnosis of celiac disease remains the jejunal biopsy.[1] Gliadin is the toxic moiety in wheat, and the alcohol-soluble fraction of wheat storage protein is gluten.[2]

Specimen Serum

Container Red top tube

Reference Range No antibody demonstrated

Use Diagnose dermatitis herpetiformis and gluten-sensitive enteropathy (nontropical sprue, celiac disease); follow response to gluten-free diet

Limitations Serum antigliadin antibodies, IgA and IgG, and IgA antiendomysial antibody lack specificity but may be helpful to measure patient compliance relevant to the gluten-free diet.[3] Gliadin antibody had 77% sensitivity.[4]

Methodology Diffusion in gel enzyme-linked immunosorbent assay;[3] indirect fluorescent antibody (IFA); immunofluorescence for endomysial and antireticulin antibody; enzyme-linked immunosorbent assay (ELISA) for gliadin antibodies. Immunofluorescent endomysial antibody is reported to have 100% sensitivity in one but not all series. Endomysial and IgA antireticulin antibody showed positive predictive value for disease detection in 91% of patients.[1]

Additional Information Dermatitis herpetiformis is a bullous skin disorder closely associated with gluten-sensitive enteropathy (celiac sprue, celiac disease). Strict observation of a gluten-free diet often induces remission of both the skin and bowel abnormalities. The presence of antibodies to endomysin (the basement membrane of smooth muscle fibers) has excellent sensitivity (80%) and specificity (96%) for dermatitis herpetiformis and sprue. There is no cross reaction with other bullous skin diseases. Further, these antibodies are not seen in control serum. Antibody titers and clinical findings respond to gluten-free diet. Antibodies reappear if the patient is challenged with a gluten-containing diet. See listings Skin Biopsy *on page 54* and Skin Biopsy, Immunofluorescence *on page 56*.

Footnotes
1. Ferreira M, Davies SL, Butler M, et al, "Endomysial Antibody: Is It the Best Screening Test for Coeliac Disease?" *Gut*, 1992, 33(12):1633-7.
2. "Case Records of the Massachusetts General Hospital. Weekly Clinicopathological Exercises. Case 30-1994. A 74 year-old Woman With Worsening Chronic Diarrhea, Weight Loss, and Abdominal Pain," *N Engl J Med*, 1994, 331(6):383-9.
3. Keating JP, "Gliadin Antibody Test Had Moderate Sensitivity for Celiac Disease in Adults," *ACP J Club*, September/October, 1994, 51 (commentary).
4. Bodé S and Gudmand-Hoyer E, "Evaluation of the Gliadin Antibody Test for Diagnosing Coeliac Disease," *Scand J Gastroenterol*, 1994, 29(2):148-52.

References
Beutner EH, Kumar V, and Chorzelski TP, "Screening for Celiac Disease," *N Engl J Med*, 1989, 320(16):1087-9.
Kapuscinska A, Zalewski T, and Chorzelski TP, "Disease Specificity and Dynamics of Changes in IgA Class Anti-Endomysial Antibodies in Celiac Disease," *J Pediatr Gastroenterol Nutr*, 1987, 6(4):529-34.
Kumar V, Hemedinger E, Chorzelski TP, et al, "Reticulin and Endomysial Antibodies in Bullous Diseases - Comparison of Specificity and Sensitivity," *Arch Dermatol*, 1987, 123(9):1179-82.
Ladinser B, Rossipal E, and Pittschieler K, "Endomysium Antibodies in Coeliac Disease: An Improved Method," *Gut*, 1994, 35(6):776-8.
Lindquist BL, Rogozinski T, Moi H, et al, "Endomysium and Gliadin IgA Antibodies in Children With Coeliac Disease," *Scand J Gastroenterol*, 1994, 29(5):452-6.
Patchett SE, Alstead EM, and Kumar PJ, "Case 30-1994: Antiendomysial Antibodies and Celiac Disease," *N Engl J Med*, 1994, 331(26):1776 (letter).
Volta U, Molinaro N, Fusconi M, et al, "IgA Antiendomysial Antibody Test. A Step Forward in Celiac Disease Screening," *Dig Dis Sci*, 1991, 36(6):752-6.

Entamoeba histolytica Serological Test

CPT 86171 (complement fixation); 86256 (immunofluorescence); 86329 (immunodiffusion)

Related Information
Bacterial Culture, Blood *on page 457*
Bacterial Culture, Stool *on page 466*
Methylene Blue Stain, Stool *on page 642*
Ova and Parasites, Stool *on page 494*
Parasite Antibodies *on page 421*
Viral Culture, Stool *on page 680*

Synonyms Amebiasis Serological Test

Test Commonly Includes Detection of antibodies to *Entamoeba histolytica* in serum

Patient Preparation Fasting blood sample required

Specimen Serum

Container Red top tube

Reference Range IHA titer: <1:128; CF titer: <1:8; immunodiffusion test: negative

Use Investigation of watery or bloody diarrhea, bearing varying numbers of leukocytes, to establish the diagnosis of systemic amebiasis. Serologic testing for amebiasis is the best single test to distinguish between the two major types of liver abscesses: amebic and pyogenic. The other major test in this differential diagnosis is blood culture. Since pyogenic liver abscesses usually require surgical drainage and prolonged intravenous antibiotic therapy, this differential diagnosis is a critical one. Overall mortality rates for pyogenic liver abscesses are about 40%, while the mortality rate for properly diagnosed and treated amebic liver abscess should approach 0%.[1] Extraintestinal amebiasis is frequently found without trophozoites or cysts in stool.

Limitations Sensitivity is highest in extraintestinal amebiasis, lower in amebic dysentery, and lowest in asymptomatic carriers. Some false-positives occur in patients with ulcerative colitis. A serine-rich recombinant *Entamoeba histolytica* protein has proven to be a useful antigen to assist in the serodiagnosis of *Entamoeba* which has disseminated.[2] The utility of the serologic marker is diminished in those parts of the world in which amebiasis is highly endemic with persistence of antibodies; *vide infra*.

Methodology Complement fixation (CF), indirect hemagglutination (IHA), immunodiffusion (ID), indirect immunofluorescent antibody (IFA), enzyme-linked immunosorbent assay (ELISA); rapid latex agglutination; cellulose acetate precipitin (CAP) test

Additional Information Indirect hemagglutination is positive in 87% to 100% of patients with amebic liver abscesses and >85% of patients with acute amebic dysentery. Fewer than 6% of uninfected individuals react in the test. Amebic serology when negative is strong evidence against (Continued)

Entamoeba histolytica Serological Test
(Continued)

amebic liver abscess. IHA titers ≥1:128 are considered to be clinically significant, and a fourfold rise in titer is firmer diagnostic evidence. It should be noted that although titers will decrease over time, serology may remain positive for as long as 2 years, even after curative therapy.

Footnotes
1. Pitt HA, "Surgical Management of Hepatic Abscesses," *World J Surg*, 1990, 14(4):498-504.
2. Stanley SL Jr, Jackson TF, Reed SL, et al, "Serodiagnosis of Invasive Amebiasis Using a Recombinant *Entamoeba histolytica* Protein," *JAMA*, 1991, 266(14):1984-6.

References
Cummins AJ, Moody AH, Lalloo K, et al, "Rapid Latex Agglutination Test for Extraluminal Amoebiasis," *J Clin Pathol*, 1994, 47(7):647-8.
Kagan IG, "Serodiagnosis of Parasitic Diseases," *Manual of Clinical Laboratory Immunology*, 4th ed, Vol 2, Rose NR, Conway de Macario E, Fahey JL, et al, eds, Washington, DC: American Society for Microbiology, 1992, 467-70.

Enteroviruses *see* Coxsackie B Virus Titer *on page 387*

Epstein-Barr Early Antigens *see* Epstein-Barr Virus Serology *on this page*

Epstein-Barr Viral Capsid Antigen *see* Epstein-Barr Virus Serology *on this page*

Epstein-Barr Virus Serology

CPT 86663 (early antigen); 86664 (nuclear antigen); 86665 (viral capsid antigen)

Related Information
Epstein-Barr Virus Culture *on page 666*
Heterophil Agglutinins *on page 401*
Infectious Mononucleosis Screening Test *on page 410*

Synonyms EB Virus Titer; EBV Titer

Applies to EBNA; EB Nuclear Antigen; Epstein-Barr Early Antigens; Epstein-Barr Viral Capsid Antigen; VCA; VCA Titer; Viral Capsid Antigen

Test Commonly Includes Titers on sera exhibiting a positive reaction at a 1:10 dilution

Abstract Since Epstein-Barr virus (EBV) was found in a Ugandan child with Burkitt's lymphoma three decades ago, a role for the virus has been shown or postulated for diseases additional to infectious mononucleosis. These include hairy leukoplakia (a disorder of the tongue), carcinoma of nasopharynx, lymphomas in patients following transplantation, other neoplastic entities, and with AIDS. Relationships to some T-cell lymphomas and to Hodgkin's disease have been recognized.[1]

Specimen Serum

Container Red top tube

Reference Range See table.

Epstein-Barr Virus Serology

	Uninfected	Previous Infection
IgG anti-VCA	<1:10	≥1:10
IgM anti-VCA*	<1:10	≤1:10
Anti-EBNA	<1:5	≥1:5

*IgM anti-VCA indicates a recent primary infection.

Use Diagnose Epstein-Barr virus infection, heterophil-negative mononucleosis, hereditary sex-linked lymphadenopathy

Limitations Despite much publicity, these tests are neither sensitive nor specific for chronic fatigue syndrome

Contraindications The Epstein-Barr viral test need not be done on patients who have heterophil antibodies with the symptoms, physical findings and lymphocyte morphology consistent with infectious mononucleosis.

Methodology Indirect fluorescent antibody (IFA), enzyme-linked immunosorbent assay (ELISA). EBV can be demonstrated in tissue with *in situ* hybridization, immunohistochemistry, and PCR. The EBV genome can be recognized by Southern blotting.[2]

Additional Information EBV is a ubiquitous human herpesvirus that infects epithelial cells and B lymphocytes. It causes classic infectious mononucleosis and is implicated in the pathogenesis of Burkitt's lymphoma, some nasopharyngeal carcinomas, a subset of gastric carcinomas, lymphoproliferative disorders in immunocompromised patients, hairy leukoplakia, non-Hodgkin's lymphomas in patients with AIDS, Hodgkin's disease, and smooth muscle tumors in immunosuppressed children.[3,4,5]

Although most cases of infectious mononucleosis can be diagnosed on the basis of clinical findings, blood count and morphology, with a positive test for heterophil antibody (infectious mononucleosis screening test), as many as 20% may be heterophil-negative, at least at presentation (heterophil may become positive when repeated in a few days). In some of these cases, a test for EBV antibodies may be useful, as well as investigation for other entities (eg, CMV).

The serologic response to EBV includes antibody to early antigen, which is usually short lived, IgM and IgG antibodies to viral capsid antigen (VCA), and antibodies to nuclear antigen (EBNA); of these, VCA are the most useful. A high presenting VCA titer is good evidence for EBV infection. Since titers are generally high by the time a patient is symptomatic, it may not be possible to demonstrate fourfold rise in titer. Even a very high titer may be due to past infection, so IgM titers should be measured to establish acute infection. Persistent absence of antibody to viral capsid is good evidence against EBV infection.

Antibody to EBV nuclear antigen (EBNA) usually develops 4-6 weeks after infection, so its presence early during an acute illness should lead one to consider diagnosis other than EBV infectious mononucleosis.

Patients with nonkeratinizing squamous carcinoma of nasopharynx may have elevated levels of IgG antibody to EB early antigen, but the rarity of this condition and the 10% to 20% false-positive rate vitiate its usefulness for screening. Such patients may also have IgA antibodies to VCA. The close relationship of EBV and nasopharyngeal carcinoma is established with EBV DNA, RNA and proteins in such tumor cells.[6]

The high levels of EBV antibodies in the general population, their long persistence, and the poor correlation of antibody titers with symptoms combine to make EBV serology useless in diagnosing, following, or ruling out chronic fatigue syndrome.

IgG antibody to early antigen occurs in patients with Hodgkin's disease in higher titer than expected. This observation suggests the possibility that EBV activation plays a pathogenetic role in Hodgkin's disease. EBV DNA has been detected in both Hodgkin's lymphoma and non-Hodgkin's lymphomas by *in situ* hybridization and DNA amplification. The EBV seems to be associated with non-Hodgkin's lymphomas in AIDS patients and transplant patients.[7,8] EBV-associated post-transplantation lymphoproliferative disease is found in 1% to 10% of transplant recipients.[9]

The pathogenesis of hemophagocytic syndrome remains uncertain. Detection of EBV RNA in some (but not all) cases is recently reported.[10]

See listings Epstein-Barr Virus Culture *on page 666* and Infectious Mononucleosis Screening Test *on page 410*.

Footnotes
1. Pagano JS, "Epstein-Barr Virus: Culprit or Consort?" *N Engl J Med*, 1992, 327(24):1750-2.
2. Pathmanathan R, Prasad U, Sadler R, et al, "Clonal Proliferations of Cells Infected With Epstein-Barr Virus in Preinvasive Lesions Related to Nasopharyngeal Carcinoma," *N Engl J Med*, 1995, 333(11):693-8.
3. McClain KL, Leach CT, Jenson HB, et al, "Association of Epstein-Barr Virus With Leiomyosarcomas in Children With AIDS," *N Engl J Med*, 1995, 332(1):12-8.
4. Lee ES, Locker J, Nalesnik M, et al, "The Association of Epstein-Barr Virus With Smooth-Muscle Tumors Occurring After Organ Transplantation," *N Engl J Med*, 1995, 332(1):19-25.
5. Liebowitz D, "Epstein-Barr Virus - An Old Dog With New Tricks," *N Engl J Med*, 1995, 332(1):55-7.
6. Kieff E, "Epstein-Barr Virus - Increasing Evidence of a Link to Carcinoma," *N Engl J Med*, 1995, 333(11):724-6 (editorial).
7. Borisch B, Finke J, Hennig I, et al, "Distribution and Localization of Epstein-Barr Virus Subtypes A and B in AIDS-Related Lymphomas and Lymphatic Tissue of HIV-Positive Patients," *J Pathol*, 1992, 168(2):229-36.
8. Telenti A, Marshall WF, and Smith TF, "Detection of Epstein-Barr Virus by Polymerase Chain Reaction," *J Clin Microbiol*, 1990, 28(10):2187-90.
9. Randhawa PS, Jaffe R, Demetris AJ, et al, "Expression of Epstein-Barr Virus-Encoded Small RNA (by the EBER-1 Gene) in Liver Specimens From Transplant Recipients With Post-Transplantation Lymphoproliferative Disease," *N Engl J Med*, 1992, 327(24):1710-4.
10. Gaffey MJ, Frierson HF Jr, Medeiros LJ, et al, "The Relationship of Epstein-Barr Virus to Infection-Related (Sporadic) and Familial Hemophagocytic Syndrome and Secondary (Lymphoma-Related) Hemophagocytosis: An *In Situ* Hybridization Study," *Hum Pathol*, 1993, 24(6):657-67.

References
Ambinder RF and Mann RB, "Detection and Characterization of Epstein-Barr Virus in Clinical Specimens," *Am J Pathol*, 1994, 145(2):239-52.
"Case Records of the Massachusetts General Hospital. Weekly Clinicopathological Exercises. Case 24-1994. A Two Year-Old Boy With Thrombocytopenia, Leukocytosis, and Hepatosplenomegaly," *N Engl J Med*, 1994, 330(24):1739-46.
Matheson BA, Chisholm SM, Ho-Yen DO, "Assessment of Rapid ELISA Test for Detection of Epstein-Barr Virus Infection," *J Clin Pathol*, 1990, 43(8):691-3.
Matthews DA, Lane TJ, and Manu P, "Antibodies to Epstein-Barr Virus in Patients With Chronic Fatigue," *South Med J*, 1991, 84(7):832-40.
Mueller N, Evans A, Harris NL, et al, "Hodgkin's Disease and Epstein-Barr Virus. Altered Antibody Pattern Before Diagnosis," *N Engl J Med*, 1989, 320(11):689-95.
Rowlands DC, Ito M, Mangham DC, et al, "Epstein-Barr Virus and Carcinomas: Rare Association of the Virus With Gastric Adenocarcinomas," *Br J Cancer*, 1993, 68(5):1014-9.
Sasajima Y, Yamabe H, Kobashi Y, et al, "High Expression of the Epstein-Barr Virus Latent Protein EB Nuclear Antigen-2 on Pyothorax-Associated Lymphomas," *Am J Pathol*, 1993, 143(5):1280-5.

Espundia Serological Test *see* Leishmaniasis Serological Test *on page 413*

Esterase Inhibitor *see* C1 Esterase Inhibitor, Serum *on page 372*

Esterase, Subunit of C1 *see* C1 Esterase Inhibitor, Serum *on page 372*

Extractable Nuclear Antibodies/Antigens *see* Sjögren's Antibodies *on page 430*

Extractable Nuclear Antigens (ENA) *see* Antinuclear Antibody *on page 368*

Extrinsic Allergic Alveolitis Serology *see* Hypersensitivity Pneumonitis Serology *on page 406*

Factor B

CPT 86160 (antigen); 86161 (functional activity)
Related Information
C3 Complement, Serum *on page 373*
C4 Complement, Serum *on page 374*
Complement Components *on page 385*
Complement, Total, Serum *on page 386*
Kidney Biopsy *on page 47*
Synonyms C3 Activator; C3 Proactivator; Properdin
Applies to Alternate Complement Pathway
Specimen Serum
Container Red top tube
Storage Instructions Allow sample to clot 15-30 minutes at room temperature, then 30-60 minutes at 4°C. Store serum at -70°C.
Reference Range 180-400 µg/mL
Use Decreased values are seen when the alternate pathway of complement is activated
Limitations Single values may be difficult or impossible to interpret.
Methodology Immunodiffusion (ID), isoelectric focusing/immunofixation
Additional Information The alternative pathway (AP) of the complement system consists of factors B, D, P (properdin) and C3b. A variety of externally derived substances may activate the AP (eg, cell walls of pathogenic microorganisms, cobra venom, virus infected cells, others). Initially, C3b or a C3b-like molecule is formed from C3 by one or more mechanisms. This C3b can find factor B to form a fluid phase C3 convertase. Factor B is a single chain glycoprotein formed of 739 amino acids. Factor D (adipsin), a 288 amino acid serine protease, cleaves factor B to Ba and Bb with release of Ba to the fluid phase and production of C3bBb which is stabilized by factor P (properdin) to C3bBbP. C3bBb (a C3 convertase) is Mg^{2+} dependent and cleaves C3, forming C3a and C3b.

Assay of factor B helps distinguish activation of the alternate from the classical complement pathway. Examples of conditions associated with alternate pathway activation are diffuse intravascular coagulation, systemic lupus erythematosus, infective endocarditis, bacteremia with shock, paroxysmal nocturnal hemoglobinuria, sickle cell disease, and hypocomplementemic chronic glomerulonephritis. Complement proteins are acute phase reactants and have very short half-lives. Their serum levels are a balance of synthesis and catabolism. Thus, serial measurements may be more informative than single values.

References
Kerr LD, Adelsberg BR, Schulman P, et al, "Factor B Activation Products in Patients With Systemic Lupus Erythematosus. A Marker of Severe Disease Activity," *Arthritis Rheum*, 1989, 32(11):1406-13.
Morgan BP, *Complement: Clinical Aspects and Relevance to Disease*, San Diego, CA: Academic Press, 1990, 18-20.
Ruddy S, "Complement," *Manual of Clinical Laboratory Immunology*, 4th ed, Chapter 18, Rose NR, Conway de Macario E, Fahey JL, et al, eds, Washington, DC: American Society for Microbiology, 1992, 114-23.
Weiler JM, *Complement in Health and Disease*, 2nd ed, Vol 20, Chapter 1, Whaley K, Loos M, and Weiler JM, eds, Boston MA: Kluwer Academic Publishers, 1993, 15-9.

FANA *see* Antinuclear Antibody *on page 368*

Farmer's Lung Disease Serology *see* Hypersensitivity Pneumonitis Serology *on page 406*

FA Smear for *Legionella pneumophila* *see* Legionnaires' Disease Direct Fluorescent Antibody Smear *on page 413*

Febrile Agglutinins, Serum

CPT 86000 (each antigen)
Related Information
Brucellosis Agglutinins *on page 372*
Rocky Mountain Spotted Fever Serology *on page 427*
Salmonella Titer *on page 429*
Tularemia Agglutinins *on page 436*
Weil-Felix Agglutinins *on page 439*
Synonyms Agglutinins, Febrile
Test Commonly Includes Detection of antibody titer to specific bacterial antigens such as *Salmonella* H antigens - *S. typhi* d, *S. paratyphi* a,

b, and c; testing patient's serum with *Salmonella* O antigens - *Salmonella* A, B, C, D and E; *Proteus* antigens - OX-19, OX-K, and OX-2; *Brucella* antigen; and *Francisella tularensis* antigen
Abstract Febrile agglutinins are scientifically obsolescent in most cases and are not cost effective.
Specimen Serum
Container Red top tube
Sampling Time Acute and convalescent sera drawn 10-14 days apart are recommended.
Reference Range Less than a fourfold increase in titer in paired sera. **Titers on a single sample are not diagnostically significant.**
Use Obsolescent screening tests to identify agglutinins in sera of patients suspected of having infectious bacterial diseases characterized by persistent fever
Limitations Many cross reactions; high background levels of antibody make interpretation difficult; requires two patient specimens obtained several weeks apart. Febrile antigen agglutination tests have no utility when performed on only one serum specimen. With the development of better culture methods and more specific serologic procedures, these rough screening tests are usually not recommended.
Methodology Agglutination

Filariasis Serological Test

CPT 86256 (immunofluorescence); 86403 (agglutination, screen); 86406 (agglutination, titer)
Related Information
Microfilariae, Peripheral Blood Preparation *on page 333*
Ova and Parasites, Stool *on page 494*
Ova and Parasites, Urine *on page 495*
Parasite Antibodies *on page 421*
Synonyms Microfilariae Serological Test
Applies to *Brugia malayi* Serology; *Brugia timori* Serology; *Loa loa* Serology; *Mansonella ozzardi* Serology; *Mansonella perstans* Serology; *Mansonella streptocerca* Serology; *Onchocerca volvulus* Serology; *Wuchereria bancrofti* Serology
Abstract Filariasis is a tropical disease. Filarial nematodes live in body cavities, subcutaneous tissue, or as adults, in the lymphatics of the host, leading to lymphatic inflammation and/or chronic lymphatic obstruction. Hydrocoele and elephantiasis develop secondarily in *Wuchereria* infestation. Microfilariae (embryos) are ingested by bloodsucking arthropods and develop to an infective phase. It is the microfilaria that are accessible for diagnosis. The term filariasis refers to invasion of lymphatics by the nematodes, *Wuchereria bancrofti*, *Brugia malayi*, or *Brugia timori*. **Although presently immunodiagnosis has little role**, means to detect filarial antigen should become available.[1]
Specimen Serum
Container Red top tube
Reference Range Varies with laboratory and methodology
Use Questionably useful, intended to support a diagnosis of filariasis, microfilariasis
Limitations Testing presently lacks sensitivity and specificity. Cross-reactivity between filarial antigens and antigens of other helminths complicates interpretation of serologic assays. False-positives occur in subjects residing in endemic areas.
Methodology Bentonite flocculation assay (BFA), complement fixation (CF), indirect fluorescent antibody (IFA), indirect hemagglutination (IHA), enzyme immunoassay (EIA)
Additional Information For screening, an antigen prepared from the dog heartworm, *Dirofilaria immitis*, detects antibody responses to several clinically significant microfilariae but sensitivity and specificity are poor. Testing with antigen prepared from homologous parasites is more specific but is essentially unavailable. **Morphologic examination of a blood film or hydrocoele fluid remains the bedrock of diagnosis.** Patients with other diseases or other types of parasites (helminths) may have antibodies, as may patients with eosinophilic infiltrates in the lungs, perhaps because of unrecognized dirofilariasis. Such cross reactions may be due to antibodies to phosphocholine, a molecule present in many organisms. IgG_4 antibodies are not developed to phosphocholine; antibodies of this class are specific for filaria. Eosinophilia and immunoglobulin E may be helpful additional tests.
Footnotes
1. Katz M, "The Nematodes," *Principles and Practice of Pediatrics*, 2nd ed, Oski FA, DeAngelis CD, Feigin RD, et al, eds, Philadelphia, PA: JB Lippincott Co, 1994, 1408-16.
References
Ash LR and Orihel TC, *Atlas of Human Parasitology*, 3rd ed, Chicago, IL: American Society of Clinical Pathologists, 1990, 22-5.
Kagan IG and Maddison SE, "Serodiagnosis of Parasitic Diseases," *Manual of Clinical Laboratory Immunology*, 4th ed, Vol 2, Chapter 79, Rose NR, Conway de Macario E, Fahey JL, et al, eds, Washington, DC: American Society for Microbiology, 1992, 529-43.

(Continued)

Filariasis Serological Test *(Continued)*

Lal RB and Ottesen EA, "Enhanced Diagnostic Specificity in Human Filariasis by IgG₄ Antibody Assessment," *J Infect Dis*, 1988, 158(5):1034-37.

Ro J, Tsakalakis PJ, White VA, et al, "Pulmonary Dirofilariasis: The Great Imitator of Primary or Metastatic Lung Tumor," *Hum Pathol*, 1989, 20(8):69-76.

Weil GJ, Ogunrinade AF, Chandrashekar R, et al, "IgG₄ Subclass Antibody Serology for Onchocerciasis," *J Infect Dis*, 1990, 161(3):549-54.

Flow Cytometry *see* CD4/CD8 Enumeration *on page 375*

Flow Cytometry *see* Leukocyte Immunophenotyping *on page 414*

Flukes *see* Schistosomiasis Serological Test *on page 429*

Fluorescent Treponemal Antibody-Absorption *see* FTA-ABS, Serum *on this page*

***Francisella tularensis* Antibodies** *see* Tularemia Agglutinins *on page 436*

***Francisella tularensis* Culture** *see* Tularemia Agglutinins *on page 436*

Frei Test *replaced by* Lymphogranuloma Venereum Titer *on page 417*

FTA-ABS, Cerebrospinal Fluid

CPT 86781

Related Information

Bacterial Culture, Cerebrospinal Fluid *on page 460*
Cerebrospinal Fluid Analysis *on page 309*
Cerebrospinal Fluid Protein *on page 380*
Darkfield Examination, Syphilis *on page 475*
FTA-ABS, Serum *on this page*
VDRL, Cerebrospinal Fluid *on page 438*

Synonyms Cerebrospinal Fluid, FTA-ABS; CSF FTA-ABS; *Treponema pallidum* Antibodies, CSF

Applies to Syphilis Serology

Test Commonly Includes CSF specimens are absorbed (FTA-ABS) and tested.

Abstract Syphilis has again become more common than it was between 1955-85. It is epidemiologically linked with HIV infection and the use of illegal drugs, especially crack cocaine. The FTA-ABS on CSF remains in investigational status.

Specimen Cerebrospinal fluid

Container Clean, sterile CSF tube

Causes for Rejection Bloody specimen

Reference Range Nonreactive

Critical Values Positive serology during pregnancy

Use Confirm the presence of *Treponema pallidum* antibodies; establish the diagnosis of neurosyphilis. Although the use of the FTA-ABS in analysis of CSF is not uniformly accepted, a negative CSF FTA-ABS eliminates the diagnostic possibility of neurosyphilis.[1,2] Many rely upon CSF-VDRL, but FTA testing on CSF is more sensitive.[2]

Limitations The interpretation of FTA results on CSF is not clearly defined. False-positive results may occur particularly if the specimen is not absorbed prior to testing. VDRL on cerebrospinal fluid is recommended by the Centers for Disease Control to help establish the diagnosis of neurosyphilis. However, while a positive CSF VDRL is strong evidence for active neurosyphilis, a negative does not rule it out. A FTA-ABS on CSF can be positive in cases of neurosyphilis when CSF VDRL is negative. Unfortunately, the CSF FTA-ABS test is less specific than CSF VDRL for distinguishing currently active neurosyphilis from past syphilis infection. Therefore, a correlation of the clinical facts with the serologic findings is essential for each case. One useful guide when screening for neurosyphilis is to first detect a serum FTA-ABS and/or a VDRL or RPR.

Methodology Indirect fluorescent antibody (IFA)

Additional Information Neurosyphilis encompasses a heterogeneous group of entities spanning all of the stages of lues. It includes syphilitic meningitis, gumma, general paresis, and tabes dorsalis.

Footnotes

1. Hook EW 3d and Marra CM, "Acquired Syphilis in Adults," *N Engl J Med*, 1992, 326(16):1060-9.
2. Larsen SA, Steiner BM, and Rudolph AH, "Laboratory Diagnosis and Interpretation of Tests for Syphilis," *Clin Microbiol Rev*, 1995, 8(1):1-21.

References

Davis LE and Schmitt JW, "Clinical Significance of Cerebrospinal Fluid Tests for Neurosyphilis," *Ann Neurol*, 1989, 25(1):50-5.

Young H, Moyes A, McMillan A, et al, "Enzyme Immunoassay for Antitreponemal IgG: Screening or Confirmatory Test?" *J Clin Pathol*, 1992, 45(1):37-41.

FTA-ABS, Serum

CPT 86781

Related Information

Automated Reagin Test *on page 370*
Darkfield Examination, Syphilis *on page 475*
FTA-ABS, Cerebrospinal Fluid *on this page*
MHA-TP *on page 418*
RPR *on page 428*
VDRL, Serum *on page 438*

Synonyms Fluorescent Treponemal Antibody-Absorption

Applies to Syphilis Serology

Test Commonly Includes Serum specimen is absorbed and then tested with immunofluorescence for antibody to *Treponema pallidum*

Abstract The FTA-ABS like the MHA-TP is a specific treponemal test. Although more sensitive than the reaginic tests, it is more expensive and more technically sophisticated. (Quantitative nontreponemal or reaginic tests include the VDRL and RPR.)[1] A reactive FTA-ABS in a patient also reactive to a nontreponemal test is highly specific.[2]

Patient Preparation Patient should be fasting if possible.

Specimen Serum

Container Red top tube

Reference Range Nonreactive. Results are reported as reactive, reactive minimal, equivocal, nonreactive, or atypical fluorescence observed; a titer is not determined.

Possible Panic Range Serodiagnosis of syphilis in pregnancy

Use Confirm the presence of antibodies to *Treponema pallidum* in patients who have tested positive for nontreponemal antibodies by VDRL or RPR screening test and to support a clinical impression of syphilis in patients in whom the nontreponemal test (eg, VDRL, RPR) is nonreactive.

Limitations FTA-ABS test for syphilis is reported positive in the treponemal diseases pinta, yaws and bejel, and falsely positive in patients with diseases associated with increased or abnormal globulins, antinuclear antibodies, lupus erythematosus (beaded pattern), pregnancy, and drug addiction (although drug addicts are likely to have true positives as well). Lyme disease, leprosy, malaria, infectious mononucleosis, relapsing fever, and leptospirosis are also listed as potential causes of false-positive FTA-ABS.[1] Fewer than 1% of healthy individuals will have a false-positive. Borderline results are inconclusive and cannot be interpreted; they may indicate a very low level of treponemal antibody or may be due to nonspecific factors. Further follow-up and serological confirmation with the treponemal immobilization test may be helpful. Potential causes of false-positive serologic tests for syphilis are tabulated in the listing VDRL, Serum *on page 438*.

Methodology Indirect fluorescent antibody (IFA) of killed *Treponema* after serum absorption

Additional Information FTA-ABS is a sensitive test in all stages of syphilis, and is the best standard confirmatory test for a serum reactive to a screening test such as RPR or VDRL. Occasionally, patients with ocular (uveitis) syphilis or otosyphilis will have a negative VDRL while their FTA-ABS is positive. FTA-ABS cannot be used to follow disease activity or response to treatment, since it will remain high for years or for life. A modification of the test can detect IgM specific antibodies, which may distinguish true congenital syphilis from placental transfer of maternal antibodies. When a positive serum FTA-ABS is required before performing CSF VDRL examination, the specificity of the CSF test is markedly improved. Although not officially recommended for testing cerebrospinal fluid, the FTA test, unabsorbed, can be performed on some spinal fluids with excellent specificity. At present this application of the test should be restricted to reference laboratories. See FTA-ABS, Cerebrospinal Fluid *on page 394*.

Treponema can be detected by direct immunofluorescence staining with polyclonal conjugates. PCR has been used to detect *T. pallidum* DNA in specimens including cerebrospinal fluid and amniotic fluid. This approach is described as highly sensitive and specific.[3]

Footnotes

1. Hook EW 3d and Marra CM, "Acquired Syphilis in Adults," *N Engl J Med*, 1992, 326(16):1060-9.
2. Larsen SA, Steiner BM, and Rudolph AH, "Laboratory Diagnosis and Interpretation of Tests for Syphilis," *Clin Microbiol Rev*, 1995, 8(1):1-21.
3. Horowitz HW, Valsamis MP, Wicher V, et al, "Brief Report: Cerebral Syphilitic Gumma Confirmed by the Polymerase Chain Reaction in Man With Human Immunodeficiency Virus Infection," *N Engl J Med*, 1994, 331(22):1488-91.

References

Albright RE Jr, Christenson RH, Emlet JL, et al, "Issues in Cerebrospinal Fluid Management. CSF Venereal Disease Research Laboratory Testing," *Am J Clin Pathol*, 1991, 95(3):397-401.

Birdsall HH, Baughn RE, and Jenkins HA, "The Diagnostic Dilemma of Otosyphilis. A New Western Blot Assay," *Arch Otolaryngol Head Neck Surg*, 1990, 116(5):617-21.

Davis LE and Schmitt JW, "Clinical Significance of Cerebrospinal Fluid Tests for Neurosyphilis," *Ann Neurol*, 1989, 25(1):50-5.

Farnes SW and Setness PA, "Serologic Tests for Syphilis," *Postgrad Med*, 1990, 87(3):37-41, 45-6.

Hart G, "Syphilis Tests in Diagnostic and Therapeutic Decision Making," *Ann Intern Med*, 1986, 104(3):368-76.

Musher DM and Baughn RE, "Neurosyphilis in HIV-Infected Persons," *N Engl J Med*, 1994, 331(22):1516-7.

Tamesis RR and Foster CS, "Ocular Syphilis," *Ophthalmology*, 1990, 97(10):1281-7.

Gag Gene of HIV *see* p24 Antigen *on page 420*

Gamma G, CSF *see* Cerebrospinal Fluid Immunoglobulin G *on page 378*

German Measles Serology *see* Rubella Serology *on page 428*

Globulin, Serum *see* Protein Electrophoresis, Serum *on page 424*

Globulins, Urine *see* Protein Electrophoresis, Urine *on page 425*

Glomerular Basement Membrane Antibody

CPT 88346

Related Information

Antineutrophil Cytoplasmic Antibody *on page 367*

Blood, Urine *on page 631*

Hemoglobin, Qualitative, Urine *on page 637*

Kidney Biopsy *on page 47*

Kidney Profile *on page 153*

Synonyms Anti-GBM; Antiglomerular Basement Membrane Antibody; Goodpasture's Antibody

Abstract Antibodies to the antigens of glomerular basement membranes may be detected in patients who have glomerulonephritis with or without pulmonary hemorrhage, idiopathic pulmonary hemosiderosis.

Specimen Serum or tissue (lung or kidney biopsy)

Container Red top tube

Special Instructions Tissue for immunofluorescence should be transported frozen in liquid nitrogen.

Reference Range Negative, <20 units

Use Detect presence of circulating glomerular basement membrane antibodies in Goodpasture's disease, which is defined as such; autoantibody with pulmonary hemorrhage and often glomerulonephritis. Quantitation may be useful in monitoring treatment. Investigate idiopathic pulmonary hemosiderosis. This test is often used in conjunction with the antineutrophil cytoplasmin antibody (ANCA) test for Wegener's granulomatosis and vasculitis.

Limitations 10% to 20% false-negatives; weak positives may be found in persons without disease mediated by anti-GBM.

Methodology Direct (DFA) or indirect fluorescent antibody (IFA), enzyme immunoassay (EIA), Western blot assay

Additional Information The two principal mechanisms of autoimmune renal disease are immune complex deposition with complement activation and specific antibody mediated damage to renal glomerular basement membrane. Antibody can be demonstrated by immunofluorescence in glomeruli, in renal tubular basement membranes, and in pulmonary capillary basement membranes. The 28 kD and 48-50 kD components of the GBM correspond to monomeric and dimeric NC1 fragments of type IV collagen in Western blot assay of serum for anti-GBM antibodies.[1]

Footnotes

1. "Case Records of the Massachusetts General Hospital. Weekly Clinicopathological Exercises. Case 16-1993. A 13 Year-Old Girl With Gross Hematuria Four Years After a Diagnosis of Idiopathic Pulmonary Hemosiderosis," *N Engl J Med*, 1993, 328(16):1183-90.

References

Savige JA, Dowling J, and Kincaid-Smith P, "Superimposed Glomerular Immune Complexes in Antiglomerular Basement Membrane Disease," *Am J Kidney Dis*, 1989, 14(2):145-53.

Goodpasture's Antibody *see* Glomerular Basement Membrane Antibody *on this page*

Granulocyte Antibody *see* Antineutrophil Antibody *on page 366*

HAA *see* Hepatitis B Surface Antigen *on page 399*

HANE Assay *see* C1 Esterase Inhibitor, Serum *on page 372*

Hantavirus Serology

Synonyms Muerto Canyon Strain Virus

Test Commonly Includes Detection of IgM and IgG antibody specific for the Muerto Canyon strain of hantavirus.

Abstract An outbreak of severe respiratory illness associated with respiratory failure, shock, and high mortality was recognized in May, 1993 in the southwestern part of the United States. The cause of the illness was identified as a unique hantavirus now known as the Muerto Canyon strain, and the disease is now called hantavirus pulmonary syndrome (HPS). Since the recognition of this disease, other cases have been recognized in 17 states, with most of the cases occurring west of the Mississippi. HPS begins with nonspecific symptoms such as fever and myalgia, which is followed in 3-6 days by progressive cough and shortness of breath. Common findings during this later stage include tachypnea, tachycardia, fever, and hypotension. Abnormalities on the chest radiograph are detected bilaterally, and pleural effusions are common. Hemoconcentration, thrombocytopenia, prolonged activated partial thromboplastin time, an increased proportion of immature granulocytes on the peripheral blood smear, leukocytosis, and elevated levels of serum lactate dehydrogenase and aspartate aminotransferase are found. Serum antibodies are detectable at the time of clinical presentation.

Specimen Serum from acute phase of illness

Container Red top tube

Storage Instructions Serum can be stored at 4°C up to 1 week; serum should be stored at -70°C after 1 week and during shipping.

Special Instructions Specimens should be sent to the CDC through state health departments.

Reference Range No detectable hantavirus IgM or less than a fourfold increase in IgG specific for the N and G1 proteins of the Muerto Canyon virus.

Use Confirm the diagnosis of hantavirus pulmonary syndrome

Limitations Assays for the detection of antibody to hantavirus are experimental and none have been approved by the Food and Drug Administration for use in the United States. All requests for testing must be sent to the CDC.

Methodology Western blot; enzyme-linked immunosorbent assay (ELISA)

Additional Information Hantaviruses are single-stranded RNA viruses of the family Bunyaviridae. Typically, rodents serve as the reservoir for hantaviruses, and infected rodents shed the virus in saliva, urine, and feces. Transmission to humans occurs most often by inhalation of infected rodent excreta. The Muerto Canyon strain of hantavirus has been found in a proportion of the deer mouse (*Peromyscus maniculatus*) population, which is prevalent in the western United States. Thus, this rodent species is thought to be the reservoir for the etiologic agent of HPS. Recommendations for prevention include avoidance of contact with the deer mouse and excreta from deer mice. Currently, no evidence exists for person-to-person transmission of HPS.

HPS can also be diagnosed by detection of hantavirus antigen in tissue by immunohistochemistry, with a monoclonal antibody reactive with conserved hantaviral nucleoproteins. In addition, hantaviral nucleotide sequences can be detected in tissue using a reverse transcriptase polymerase chain reaction.

References

Butler JC and Peters CJ, "Hantaviruses and Hantavirus Pulmonary Syndrome," *Clin Infect Dis*, 1994, 19(3):387-95.

Duchin JS, Koster FT, Peters CJ, et al, "Hantavirus Pulmonary Syndrome: A Clinical Description of 17 Patients With a Newly Recognized Disease. The Hantavirus Study Group," *N Engl J Med*, 1994, 330(14):949-55.

From the Centers for Disease Control and Prevention, "Progress in the Development of Hantavirus Diagnostic Assays - United States," *JAMA*, 1993, 270(16):1920-1.

Jenison S, Yamada T, Morris C, et al, "Characterization of Human Antibody Responses to Four Corners Hantavirus Infections Among Patients With Hantavirus Pulmonary Syndrome," *J Virol*, 1994, 68(5):3000-6.

HAVAB *see* Hepatitis A Antibody, IgM *on next page*

HB_cAb *see* Hepatitis B Core Antibody *on next page*

HB_eAb *see* Hepatitis B_e Antibody *on page 397*

HB_eAg *see* Hepatitis B_e Antigen *on page 397*

HB_sAb *see* Hepatitis B Surface Antibody *on page 398*

HB_sAg *see* Hepatitis B Surface Antigen *on page 399*

HB_sAg Ab *see* Hepatitis B Surface Antibody *on page 398*

HCV-PCR *see* Hepatitis C Serology *on page 399*

HCV Serology *see* Hepatitis C Serology *on page 399*

Helicobacter pylori Serology

CPT 86677

Related Information

Gastric Analysis *on page 133*

Helicobacter pylori Urease Test and Culture *on page 484*

Synonyms *Campylobacter pylori* Serology

Applies to Breath Testing for *H. pylori*

Test Commonly Includes Detection of IgG and IgA antibodies specific for *Helicobacter pylori*

Abstract Persons who have peptic ulcer disease either are users of nonsteroidal anti-inflammatory agents or have infection with *H. pylori*.[1] Patients with peptic ulcer disease associated with *H. pylori* have (Continued)

Helicobacter pylori Serology *(Continued)*

elevated levels of serum antibody against this bacterium. *H. pylori* is very strongly associated with duodenal and gastric ulcer and chronic active gastritis. Most instances of chronic gastritis are secondary to *H. pylori* infection. It is an independent risk factor for gastric cancer. However, antibodies persist up to a year after treatment.

Specimen Serum or plasma

Container Red top tube; some laboratories use lavender top (EDTA) tube or green top (heparin) tube

Collection Acute and convalescent samples may be useful.

Reference Range Undetectable or lower than cutoff limits in commercial assays

Use Increased antibody levels are associated with *H. pylori* infection, chronic active gastritis, and peptic ulcer. Negative serological results provide evidence against these diagnoses.

Limitations Serologic findings only provide evidence of past or present infection. A large number of people are infected with the organism but do not have apparent disease.[1] There is strain-to-strain antigenic variability in *H. pylori* which makes the test potentially insensitive. Sensitivities of commercially available assays range form 59% to 100% but specificities range from 29% to 65%.[2] In contrast, the sensitivity and specificity of histopathologic examination of gastric mucosal biopsy are well above 90%.[3] In some centers, application of *H. pylori* serology is limited to epidemiologic studies.

Methodology Enzyme-linked immunosorbent assay (ELISA)

Additional Information Large numbers of small, spiral-shaped bacteria, *Helicobacter pylori*, can be cultured from, or seen microscopically (especially with Dieterle or Giemsa stain) in gastric biopsies from most patients with chronic active gastritis and/or peptic ulcers. They can also be found in significant numbers of asymptomatic patients who have histologic gastritis, and from some individuals with no abnormality. Similarly, patients with chronic gastritis usually have elevated titers of IgG antibodies to *H. pylori*. The association of *H. pylori* infection in carcinogenesis of gastric cancer and primary malignant lymphoma of stomach is recognized. IgG antibody to *H. pylori* is increased in sera of patients with gastric cancer.[4] Culture is the gold standard for the presence of *H. pylori*, and biopsy with Giemsa or comparable staining to demonstrate disease with such organisms. Acridine orange staining and anti-*H. pylori* monoclonal antibody may be used as well.[4] Blecker et al have shown strong correlation between carbon-13 labeled urea breath tests and serologic testing for IgG antibodies, but in symptom-free subjects, such breath testing required use of a mass spectrometer.[5] Alternatives (ie, infrared spectrometry) will require FDA approval.[6]

Footnotes

1. Schieman J, "Serologic Test Kits for *Helicobacter pylori*," *ACP J Club*, 1993, 119(Suppl 2):49.
2. Taha AS, Reid J, Boothmann P, et al, "Serological Diagnosis of *Helicobacter pylori* - Evaluation of Four Tests in the Presence or Absence of Nonsteroidal Anti-inflammatory Drugs," *Gut*, 1993, 34(4):461-5.
3. Sipponen P, "*Helicobacter pylori*: A Cohort Phenomenon," *Am J Surg Pathol*, 1995, 19(Suppl 1):S30-6.
4. Endo S, Ohkusa T, Saito Y, et al, "Detection of *Helicobacter pylori* Infection in Early Stage Gastric Cancer: A Comparison Between Intestinal- and Diffuse-Type Gastric Adenocarcinomas," *Cancer*, 1995, 75(9):2203-8.
5. Blecker U, Lanciers S, Hauser B, et al, "Serology as a Valid Screening Test for *Helicobacter pylori* Infection in Asymptomatic Subjects," *Arch Pathol Lab Med*, 1995, 119(1):30-2.
6. Gambino R, "Is There a New Gold Standard for Detecting *Helicobacter pylori* Gastritis?" *Lab Rep*, 1995, 17(6):41-5.

References

Crabtree JE, Shallcross TM, Heatley RV, et al, "Evaluation of a Commercial ELISA for Serodiagnosis of *Helicobacter pylori*," *J Clin Pathol*, 1991, 44(4):326-8.

Graham DY, Malaty HM, Evans PG, et al, "Epidemiology of *Helicobacter pylori* in an Asymptomatic Population in the United States. Effect of Age, Race, and Socioeconomic Status," *Gastroenterology*, 1991, 100(6):1495-501.

Hentschel E, Brandstätter G, Dragosics B, et al, "Effect of Ranitidine and Amoxicillin Plus Metronidazole on the Eradication of *Helicobacter pylori* and the Recurrence of Duodenal Ulcer," *N Engl J Med*, 1993, 328(5):308-12.

Hirschl AM, Rathbone BJ, Wyatt JI, et al, "Comparison of ELISA Antigen Preparation Alone or in Combination for Serodiagnosing *Helicobacter pylori* Infections," *J Clin Pathol*, 1990, 43(6):511-3.

Isaacson PG, "Gastric Lymphoma and *Helicobacter pylori*," *N Engl J Med*, 1994, 330(18):1310-1.

Parsonnet J, Hansen S, Rodriguez L, et al, "*Helicobacter pylori* Infection and Gastric Lymphoma," *N Engl J Med*, 1994, 330(18):1267-71.

Rabeneck L and Ransohoff DF, "Is *Helicobacter pylori* a Cause of Duodenal Ulcer? A Methodologic Critique of Current Evidence," *Am J Med*, 1991, 91(6):566-72.

Roggero E, Zucca E, Pinotti G, et al, "Eradication of *Helicobacter pylori* Infection in Primary Low-Grade Gastric Lymphoma of Mucosa-Associated Lymphoid Tissue," *Ann Intern Med*, 1995, 122(10):767-9.

Sung JJ, Chung SC, Ling TK, et al, "Antibacterial Treatment of Gastric Ulcers Associated With *Helicobacter pylori*," *N Engl J Med*, 1995, 332(3):139-42.

Van Dam J and Graeme-Cook FM, "Case Records of the Massachusetts General Hospital. Weekly Clinicopathological Exercises. A 35-Year-Old Woman With Recurrent Bleeding From a Gastric Ulcer After Treatment for *Helicobacter pylori* Infection," *N Engl J Med*, 1995, 332(17):1153-9.

Hepatitis A Antibody, IgM

CPT 86296 (IgG and IgM); 86299 (IgM)

Related Information

Hepatitis B DNA Detection *on page 513*

Synonyms Antibody to HAV, IgM; Anti-HAV, IgM; HAVAB

Test Commonly Includes Detection of IgM antibody to hepatitis A virus

Abstract Hepatitis A virus (HAV) is a RNA-containing virus. The IgM antibody appears in acute hepatitis A by the clinical onset of symptoms and disappears 3-6 months later. While hepatitis A and E are transmitted by the fecal-oral route, hepatitis B, C, and D are bloodborne.

Patient Preparation Avoid recent administration of radioisotopes if assay performed by RIA.

Specimen Serum

Container Red top tube

Storage Instructions Remove serum and freeze.

Reference Range Negative

Use Differential diagnosis of hepatitis. Presence of IgM antibody to hepatitis A virus is good evidence for acute or subacute hepatitis A.

Methodology Radioimmunoassay (RIA), enzyme-linked immunosorbent assay (ELISA), microparticle enzyme immunoassay (MEIA)

Additional Information Hepatitis A is transmitted by the fecal-oral route, usually foodborne. Its incubation period is 2-7 weeks. Fecal excretion of HAV peaks before symptoms develop. If hepatitis A antibody is IgM, the hepatitis A infection is acute. IgM antibody develops within a week of symptom onset, peaks in 3 months, and is usually gone after 6 months. Hepatitis A antibody of IgG type is indicative of old infection, is found in almost half of adults, and is not usually clinically relevant. Many cases of hepatitis A are subclinical, particularly in children. Presence of IgG antibody to HAV does not exclude acute hepatitis B or hepatitis C.

Incubation	Early Acute	Acute	Recovery
Duration			
15-45 Days	0-14 Days	3-6 Months	Years

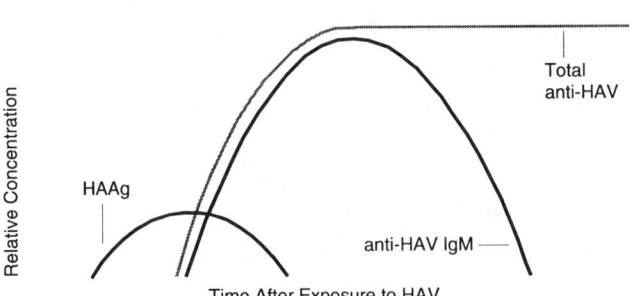

Reprinted from Abbott Diagnostics

References

Giacoia GP and Kasprisin DO, "Transfusion-Acquired Hepatitis A," *South Med J*, 1989, 82(11):1357-60.

Halliday ML, Kang LY, Zhou TK, et al, "An Epidemic of Hepatitis A Attributable to the Ingestion of Raw Clams in Shanghai, China," *J Infect Dis*, 1991, 164(5):852-9.

Kuhns MC, "Viral Hepatitis. Part 1: The Discovery, Diagnostic Tests, and New Viruses," *Lab Med*, 1995, 26(10):650.

Mahoney FJ, Farley TA, Kelso KY, et al, "An Outbreak of Hepatitis A Associated With Swimming in A Public Pool," *J Infect Dis*, 1992, 165(4):613-8.

Mbithi JN, Springthorpe VS, Boulet JR, et al, "Survival of Hepatitis A Virus on Human Hands and Its Transfer on Contact With Animate and Inanimate Surfaces," *J Clin Microbiol*, 1992, 30(4):757-63.

Mishu B, Hadler SC, Boaz VA, et al, "Foodborne Hepatitis A: Evidence That Microwaving Reduces Risk?" *J Infect Dis*, 1990, 162(3):655-8.

Shapiro CN, "Transmission of Hepatitis Viruses," *Ann Intern Med*, 1994, 120(1):82-4.

Summers PL, DuBois DR, Houston Cohen WH, et al, "Solid-Phase Antibody Capture Hemadsorption Assay for Detection of Hepatitis A Virus Immunoglobulin M Antibodies," *J Clin Microbiol*, 1993, 31(5):1299-302.

Hepatitis Associated Antigen *see* Hepatitis B Surface Antigen *on page 399*

Hepatitis B Core Antibody

CPT 86289 (IgG and IgM); 86290 (IgM)

Related Information

Donation, Blood *on page 607*
Hepatitis B DNA Detection *on page 513*
Hepatitis B$_e$ Antibody *on next page*
Hepatitis B$_e$ Antigen *on next page*

Synonyms Antibody to Hepatitis B Core Antigen; Anti-HB$_c$; HB$_c$Ab

Applies to Hepatitis B Core Antibody, IgM

Test Commonly Includes Detection of serologic response to hepatitis B infection; specifically, the antibody response to the core protein

Abstract For diagnosis of acute hepatitis, hepatitis B core antibody IgM and HB$_s$Ag are helpful. HB$_c$ antibody is found in resolved hepatitis and chronic hepatitis B. The antibody directed against HBV nucleocapsid or core protein, it may be the only serologic test that remains positive years after initial infection with hepatitis B.

Patient Preparation Avoid recent administration of radioisotopes if assay performed by RIA.

Specimen Serum

Container Red top tube

Reference Range Negative

Use Differential diagnosis of hepatitis syndromes. Is also used, in conjunction with other hepatitis B viral serologic markers, to assess the stage of hepatitis B infection. Utilized in screening volunteer blood donors for past hepatitis B infection, it can detect hepatitis in patients or donors in the window period after HB$_s$Ag has disappeared. Although the presence of Anti-HB$_c$ usually confers immunity, governmental regulations require such donors to be permanently deferred. Anti-HB$_c$ is used to look for past hepatitis B infections, since vaccination for hepatitis B produces antibodies to hepatitis B surface antigen. Thus, Anti-HB$_c$ was used as a surrogate marker for hepatitis non-A, non-B in the past, and now as a "lifestyle" marker since testing for hepatitis C began in 1990.

Limitations Weak positives without other positive markers or abnormalities in liver-related enzymes may represent false-positive reactions. Diagnostic use of this test is increased when it is part of a panel of hepatitis serologic markers.

Methodology Radioimmunoassay (RIA), enzyme-linked immunosorbent assay (ELISA). Both IgG and IgM antibodies can be differentiated.

Additional Information Anti-HB$_c$ appears 5-14 days after HB$_s$Ag and can be found shortly before HB$_s$Ag is no longer detectable. It may be negative in 9% of patients with acute hepatitis B in the first 2 weeks of illness, and should be repeated if clinically warranted. Anti-HB$_c$ and anti-HB$_e$ may be the only markers detectable in some patients at the time of presentation. The period between the disappearance of HB$_s$Ag and the appearance of HB$_s$Ab is often called the "core window." Anti-HB$_c$ persists for months to years after resolution of acute hepatitis B and persists in cases of chronic infection. However, **the demonstration of IgM-specific HB$_c$Ab is evidence that the patient has an acute infection.** Conversely, the absence of IgM core antibody in a patient with a chronic surface antigenemia and symptoms of acute hepatitis suggests acute

HEPATITIS B PROFILE

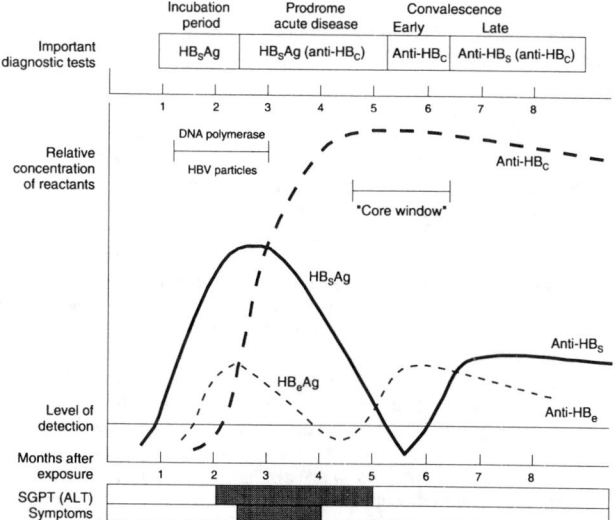

Serologic and clinical patterns observed during acute hepatitis B viral infection. From Hollinger FB and Dreesman GR, *Manual of Clinical Immunology*, 2nd ed, Rose NR and Friedman H, eds, Washington, DC: American Society for Microbiology, 1980, with permission.

non-A, non-B hepatitis or supervening delta hepatitis. The majority of patients with reactivation hepatitis will have detectable serum anti-HB$_c$ IgM. See figure.

References

Chambers LA and Popovsky MA, "Decrease in Reported Post-Transfusion Hepatitis. Contributions of Donor Screening for Alanine Aminotransferase and Antibodies to Hepatitis B Core Antigen and Changes in the General Population," *Arch Intern Med*, 1991, 151(12):2445-8.

Desforges JF, "Infectious Disease Testing for Blood Transfusions," *NIH Consensus Statement*, 1995, 13(1):1-27.

Gupta S, Govindarajan S, Fong TL, et al, "Spontaneous Reactivation in Chronic Hepatitis B: Patterns and Natural History," *J Clin Gastroenterol*, 1990, 12(5):562-8.

Herrera JL, "Serologic Diagnosis of Viral Hepatitis," *South Med J*, 1994, 87(7):677-84.

Klein HG, *Standards for Blood Banks and Transfusion Services*, 16th ed, Bethesda, MD: American Association of Blood Banks, 1994, 3-8.

Sjögren MH, "Serologic Diagnosis of Viral Hepatitis," *Gastroenterol Clin North Am*, 1994, 23(3):457-77.

Hepatitis B Core Antibody, IgM *see Hepatitis B Core Antibody on previous page*

Hepatitis B$_e$ Antibody

CPT 86295

Related Information

Synonyms Anti-HB$_e$; HB$_e$Ab

Test Commonly Includes Detection of antibody response to hepatitis e antigen

Abstract Anti-HB$_e$ appears in early convalescence in hepatitis B.

Patient Preparation Avoid recent administration of radioisotopes if assay performed by RIA.

Specimen Serum

Container Red top tube

Causes for Rejection Radioactive scan within 1 week if assay is RIA

Reference Range Negative

Use Differential diagnosis, staging, and prognosis of hepatitis B infection. Anti-HB$_e$ and anti-HB$_c$ together confirm the convalescent stage of hepatitis B after the disappearance of HB surface antigen (HB$_s$Ag).

Limitations Absence of anti-HB$_e$ does not rule out chronic hepatitis B carrier state or infectivity.

Methodology Radioimmunoassay (RIA), enzyme immunoassay (EIA)

Additional Information Hepatitis B$_e$ antigen is a proteolytic product of the HBV core protein.[1] The appearance of anti-HB$_e$ in patients who have previously been HB$_e$Ag positive indicates a reduced risk of infectivity. Failure of appearance implies disease activity and probable chronicity, but patients with HB$_e$Ab may have chronic hepatitis. Chronic HB$_s$Ag carriers can be positive for either HB$_e$Ag or anti-HB$_e$, but are less infectious when anti-HB$_e$ is present. Antibody to e antigen can persist for years, but usually disappears earlier than anti-HB$_s$ or anti-HB$_c$. HB$_e$Ab is not used as the sole serologic marker for hepatitis B infection. See figure in the listing Hepatitis B Core Antibody *on page 397*. Quantitation of HBV DNA, pre-S antigens, and IgM anti-HB$_c$ may prove helpful for monitoring antiviral therapy, particularly in anti-HB$_e$-positive HB$_s$Ag carriers.[2]

Footnotes

1. Jean-Jean O, Salhi S, Carlier D, et al, "Biosynthesis of Hepatitis B Virus e Antigen. Directed Mutagenesis of the Putative Aspartyl Protease Site," *J Virol*, 1989, 63(12):5497-500.
2. Zoulim F, Mimms L, Floreani M, et al, "New Assays for Quantitative Determination of Viral Markers in Management of Chronic Hepatitis B Virus Infection," *J Clin Microbiol*, 1992, 30(5):1111-9.

References

Bortolotti F, Calzia R, Cadrobbi P, et al, "Long-Term Evolution of Chronic Hepatitis B in Children With Antibody to Hepatitis B$_e$ Antigen," *J Pediatr*, 1990, 116(4):552-5.

Herrera JL, "Serologic Diagnosis of Viral Hepatitis," *South Med J*, 1994, 87(7):677-84.

Sjögren MH, "Serologic Diagnosis of Viral Hepatitis," *Gastroenterol Clin North Am*, 1994, 23(3):457-77.

Hepatitis B$_e$ Antigen

CPT 86293

Related Information

(Continued)

Hepatitis B$_e$ Antigen *(Continued)*

Hepatitis D Serology *on page 400*
Liver Biopsy *on page 48*
Liver Profile *on page 161*
Polymerase Chain Reaction *on page 523*

Synonyms HB$_e$Ag

Test Commonly Includes Detection of hepatitis B$_e$ antigen in patient's serum

Abstract HB$_e$Ag appears early in hepatitis B. Infectivity of a patient with hepatitis B virus (HBV) can be evaluated with HB$_e$Ag and HB$_s$Ag. Measurement of serum HBV DNA also provides evidence of infectivity.

Patient Preparation Avoid recent administration of radioisotopes if assay performed by RIA.

Specimen Serum

Container Red top tube

Storage Instructions Serum must be stored frozen or refrigerated, as HB$_e$Ag is thermolabile.

Causes for Rejection Radioactive scan within 1 week if assay is RIA

Reference Range Negative

Use Differential diagnosis, infectivity, and prognosis of hepatitis B infection. Hepatitis B$_e$ antigen is found during the most infectious period of hepatitis B. It is usually found for only 3-6 weeks. With appearance of anti-HB$_e$ and disappearance of HB$_e$Ag, resolution of hepatitis B can be recognized. Persistence beyond 10 weeks is evidence of development of the chronic carrier state and likely chronic hepatitis. Its presence bears correlation with infectivity, the number of Dane particles, detection of core antigen in hepatocyte nuclei, and with serum viral DNA polymerase.

Limitations Absence does not rule out infectivity or chronic hepatitis B carrier state.

Methodology Radioimmunoassay (RIA), enzyme immunoassay (EIA)

Additional Information HB$_e$Ag appears in acute B hepatitis with or shortly after HB$_s$Ag, when the patient is most infectious. HB$_e$Ag is a proteolytic product of HB$_c$Ag and is found only in HB$_s$Ag positive sera. During the HB$_e$Ag-positive state, usually 3-6 weeks, hepatitis B patients are at increased risk of transmitting the virus to their contacts, including babies born during this period. Exposure to serum or body fluid positive for HB$_e$Ag and HB$_s$Ag is associated with three to five times greater risk of infectivity than when HB$_s$Ag positivity occurs alone. This is probably related to increased amounts of circulating viral DNA. Persistence of HB$_e$Ag is associated with chronic liver disease. See figures and also the listing Hepatitis B Core Antibody *on page 396*. Modes of transmission of HBV include percutaneous (eg, drug use, blood or body fluid exposure in healthcare workers, transfusions); sexual (heterosexual or male homosexual); mother to infant (blood exposure at delivery). Other types of transmission occur as well.[1]

Hepatitis B Serological Profile

Core Window Identification

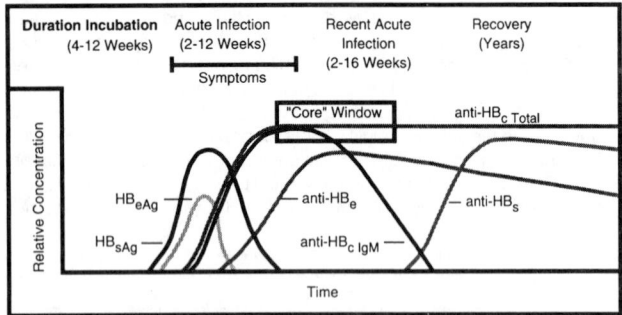

Hepatitis B Chronic Carrier

Late Seroconversion

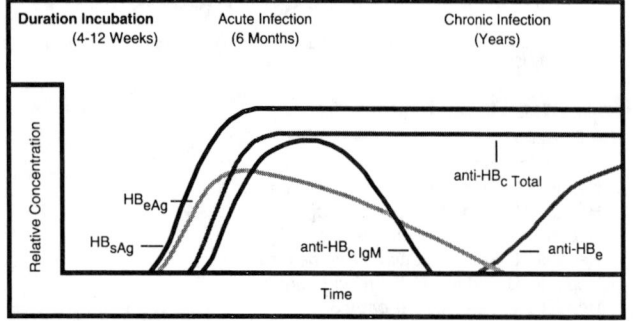

Hepatitis B Chronic Carrier

No Seroconversion

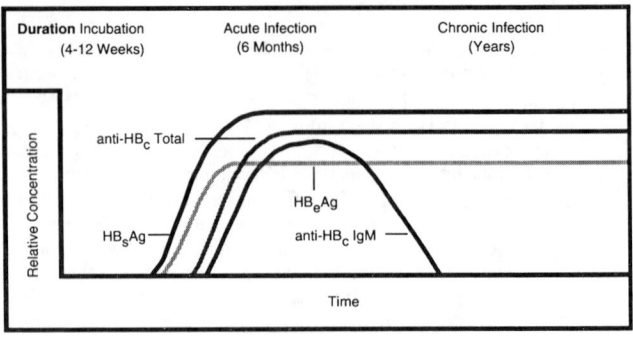

Footnotes

1. Shapiro CN, "Transmission of Hepatitis Viruses," *Ann Intern Med*, 1994, 120(1):82-4.

References

Edwards MS, "Hepatitis B Serology - Help in Interpretation," *Pediatr Clin North Am*, 1988, 35(3):503-15.
Lee HS and Vyas GN, "Diagnosis of Viral Hepatitis," *Clin Lab Med*, 1987, 7(4):741-57.

Hepatitis B$_s$ Antibody *see* Hepatitis B Surface Antibody *on this page*

Hepatitis B Surface Antibody

CPT 86291

Related Information

Hepatitis B Core Antibody *on page 396*
Hepatitis B DNA Detection *on page 513*
Hepatitis B$_e$ Antibody *on previous page*
Hepatitis B$_e$ Antigen *on previous page*
Hepatitis B Surface Antigen *on next page*
Hepatitis C Serology *on next page*
Hepatitis D Serology *on page 400*
Liver Biopsy *on page 48*
Liver Profile *on page 161*
Polymerase Chain Reaction *on page 523*

Synonyms Antibody to Hepatitis B Surface Antigen; Anti-HB$_s$; HB$_s$Ab; HB$_s$Ag Ab; Hepatitis B$_s$ Antibody

Applies to Hepatitis Vaccine

Replaces Australian Antigen Antibody

Test Commonly Includes Detection of serologic response to hepatitis B infection or hepatitis B vaccination; specifically, antibody response to surface protein

Abstract Anti-HB$_s$ develops following resolved hepatitis B. It is responsible for immunity.

Patient Preparation Avoid recent administration of radioisotopes if assay performed by RIA.

Specimen Serum

Container Red top tube

Causes for Rejection Recently administered radioisotopes if assay performed by RIA

Reference Range Varies with clinical circumstance

Use Presence of hepatitis B surface antibody indicates past infection with resolution of previous hepatitis B infection or vaccination against hepatitis B. Evaluate possible immunity in individuals who are at increased risks to further exposure to hepatitis B (ie, hemodialysis unit personnel, phlebotomists, etc). Evaluate need for hepatitis B immune globulin after needlestick injury. Evaluate need for hepatitis B vaccine. Evaluate efficacy of hepatitis B vaccine.

Limitations Presence of HB$_s$Ab is not an absolute indicator of resolved hepatitis infection, nor of protection from future infection. Since there are different serologic subtypes of hepatitis B virus, it is possible (and has been reported) for a patient to have antibody to one surface antigen type and to be acutely infected with virus of a different subtype. Thus, a patient may have coexisting HB$_s$Ag and HB$_s$Ab. Transfused individuals or hemophiliacs receiving plasma components may give false-positive tests for antibody to hepatitis B surface antigen, and passively acquired reactivity from transfusion or globulin therapy does not indicate immunity. Individuals vaccinated with HBV vaccine will have antibodies to the surface protein.

Methodology Radioimmunoassay (RIA), enzyme immunoassay (EIA)

Additional Information HB$_s$Ab usually can be detected several weeks to several years after HB$_s$Ag is no longer found, and it may persist for life after acute infection has been resolved. It may disappear in some patients with only antibody to hepatitis B core remaining. See figure in listing Hepatitis B Core Antibody *on page 397*. Patients with this antibody are not overtly infectious. Presence of the antibody without the presence of the antigen is evidence for immunity from reinfection, with virus of the same subtype (*vide supra*). HB$_s$Ab can be induced by vaccination with hepatitis vaccine, now genetically engineered preparations and free of any infective material. This vaccine so far has been safe and effective in protecting recipients from acute hepatitis B.

References
Centers for Disease Control, "Screening Donors of Blood, Plasma, Organs, Tissues, and Semen for Evidence of Hepatitis B and Hepatitis C," *Lab Med*, 1991, 22(8):555-63.

Devine P, Taswell HF, Moore SB, et al, "Passively Acquired Antibody to Hepatitis B Surface Antigen. Pitfall in Evaluating Immunity to Hepatitis B Viral Infections," *Arch Pathol Lab Med*, 1989, 113(5):529-31.

Edwards MS, "Hepatitis B Serology - Help in Interpretation," *Pediatr Clin North Am*, 1988, 35(3):503-15.

Hepatitis B Surface Antigen

CPT 86287

Related Information

Alanine Aminotransferase *on page 65*
Aspartate Aminotransferase *on page 84*
Blood and Fluid Precautions, Specimen Collection *on page 24*
Hepatitis B Core Antibody *on page 396*
Hepatitis B DNA Detection *on page 513*
Hepatitis B$_e$ Antibody *on page 397*
Hepatitis B$_e$ Antigen *on page 397*
Hepatitis B Surface Antibody *on previous page*
Hepatitis C Serology *on this page*
Hepatitis D Serology *on next page*
Liver Biopsy *on page 48*
Liver Profile *on page 161*
Polymerase Chain Reaction *on page 523*
Risks of Transfusion *on page 623*

Synonyms HAA; HB$_s$Ag; Hepatitis Associated Antigen

Replaces Australian Antigen; Serum Hepatitis Marker

Test Commonly Includes Detection of hepatitis B surface antigen in patient's serum

Abstract For evaluation of acute hepatitis, serologic testing is recommended for HB$_s$Ag, HB$_s$Ab, HB$_c$Ab (IgM), and HAV (IgM). HB$_s$Ag is the first marker to appear, detecting the HBV surface protein or envelope. Infectious mononucleosis screening test may be included, especially when the patient is youthful. Cytomegalovirus may cause a hepatitis-like clinical presentation. Persistence of HB$_s$Ag for periods in excess of 6 months indicates a chronic carrier state or chronic hepatitis. Hepatitis C and D also cause chronic hepatitis. Other useful tests include the transaminases; see listing Liver Profile *on page 161*.

Patient Preparation Avoid recent administration of radioisotopes if assay performed by RIA.

Specimen Serum

Container Red top tube

Causes for Rejection Recently administered radioisotopes if assay is by RIA

Reference Range Negative

Use Screen blood donors (HB$_s$Ag-positive individuals are rejected); differential diagnosis of hepatitis; evaluate risk in needlestick injuries in healthcare facilities, and guide use of hepatitis B immune globulin. Hepatitis B surface antigen is the earliest indicator of acute hepatitis B infection and is found, as well, in chronic carriers.

Limitations Patients who are negative for HB$_s$Ag may still have acute type B viral hepatitis. There is sometimes a "window" stage when HB$_s$Ag has become negative and the patient has not yet developed the antibody (anti-HB$_s$Ag). On such occasions the anti-HB$_c$Ag (IgM) is usually positive; and the patient should be treated as potentially infectious until anti-HB$_s$Ag is detected, at which time immunity is probable. In cases with strong clinical suspicion of viral hepatitis, serologic testing should not be limited to detecting HB$_s$Ag but should include a battery of tests to evaluate different stages of acute and convalescent hepatitis. These should include a test for hepatitis A antibody (IgM), and HB$_s$Ag, HB$_s$Ab, HB$_c$Ab (IgM), and hepatitis C virus (HCV).

Methodology Radioimmunoassay (RIA), enzyme immunoassay (EIA)

Additional Information Hepatitis B virus (HBV) is a DNA virus with a protein coat, surface antigen (HB$_s$Ag), and a core consisting of nucleoprotein (HB$_c$Ag is the core antigen). There are eight different serotypes. Early in infection, HB$_s$Ag, HBV DNA, and DNA polymerase can all be detected in serum.

Transmission is parenteral, sexual or perinatal. The incubation period of hepatitis B is 2-6 months. HB$_s$Ag can be detected 1-7 weeks **before** liver enzyme elevation or the appearance of clinical symptoms. Three weeks after the onset of acute hepatitis about 50% of the patients will still be positive for HB$_s$Ag, while at 17 weeks only 10% are positive. The best available markers for infectivity are HB$_s$Ag and HB$_e$Ag. The presence of HB$_s$Ab and HB$_e$Ab is associated with noninfectivity. The chronic carrier state is indicated by the persistence of HB$_s$Ag and/or HB$_e$Ag over long periods (6 months to years) without seroconversion to the corresponding antibodies. Such a condition has the potential to lead to serious liver damage, but may be an isolated asymptomatic serologic phenomenon. Persistence of HB$_s$Ag, without anti-HB$_s$, with combinations of positivity of anti-HB$_{core}$, HB$_e$Ag, or anti-HB$_e$ indicate infectivity and need for investigation for chronic persistent or chronic aggressive hepatitis. See figure in listing Hepatitis B Core Antibody *on page 397*. Chronic carrier states are found in up to 10% of cases. Some remain healthy, but evolution to chronic persistent hepatitis, chronic active hepatitis, cirrhosis, and hepatoma represent major problems of this disease. Prevention of hepatitis B for those at risk is available via vaccination,[1] as well as treatment for some chronic carriers.[2]

Footnotes
1. Mahoney FJ, Burkholder BT, and Matson CC, "Prevention of Hepatitis B Virus Infection," *Am Fam Physician*, 1993, 47(4):865-72.
2. Kaplan MM, "Twelve Questions Physicians Often Ask," *Consultant*, 1993, 33(3):145-52.

References
Jackson JB, "Polymerase Chain Reaction Assay for Detection of Hepatitis B Virus," *Am J Clin Pathol*, 1991, 95(4):442-4.

Repp R, Rhiel S, Heermann KH, et al, "Genotyping by Multiplex Polymerase Chain Reaction for Detection of Endemic Hepatitis B Virus Transmission," *J Clin Microbiol*, 1993, 31(5):1095-102.

Hepatitis C Serology

CPT 86302

Related Information

Cryoglobulin, Qualitative, Serum *on page 388*
Donation, Blood *on page 607*
Hepatitis B Core Antibody *on page 396*
Hepatitis B DNA Detection *on page 513*
Hepatitis B$_e$ Antibody *on page 397*
Hepatitis B$_e$ Antigen *on page 397*
Hepatitis B Surface Antibody *on previous page*
Hepatitis B Surface Antigen *on this page*
Hepatitis C RNA Detection *on page 513*
Liver Biopsy *on page 48*
Liver Profile *on page 161*
Polymerase Chain Reaction *on page 523*
Risks of Transfusion *on page 623*

Synonyms HCV Serology

Applies to Anti-HCV (IgM); c100-3; HCV-PCR; Non-A, non-B Hepatitis; Surrogate Tests

Test Commonly Includes Detection of antibody specific for hepatitis C in patient's serum

Abstract Most cases of post-transfusion non-A, non-B viral hepatitis are caused by HCV. Application of this test has virtually eliminated post-transfusion hepatitis. Six HCV genotypes are recognized, subdivided into 11 subtypes. Hepatitis C is characterized by a prolonged natural history. It is progressive, leading in some cases to chronic hepatitis, cirrhosis, hepatocellular carcinoma, and hepatic failure. Extrahepatic manifestations are recognized.

Specimen Serum

Container Red top tube

Reference Range Negative

Use Differential diagnosis of acute and chronic hepatitis; screen blood units for transfusion safety; evaluate patients with essential mixed cryoglobulinemia, membranoproliferative glomerulonephritis, and porphyria cutanea tarda.[1]

Limitations Since as many as 90% of commercial intravenous immunoglobulins test positive for hepatitis C antibody, a false-positive can result briefly after such transfusion. False-positive HCV immunoassays are found with hypergammaglobulinemia and connective tissue disorders.

Methodology Enzyme-linked immunosorbent assay (ELISA); enzyme immunoassay (EIA) is confirmed with recombinant strip immunoblot assay (RIBA). Second generation RIBA, RIBA-2, provides highly specific confirmation, but problems include false-negatives. RIBA-3 may resolve problems. HCV-PCR is more sensitive.

Additional Information Although first generation assays used only a single antigen, presently multiple HCV-specific antigen proteins provide better sensitivity.

There are approximately 170,000 new cases of hepatitis C in the U.S. each year. Between 1970 and 1990, hepatitis C, then called hepatitis (Continued)

Hepatitis C Serology *(Continued)*

non-A, non-B, caused more than 90% of transfusion-transmitted hepatitis. Before initiation of hepatitis B surface antigen testing in the 1970's, most significant post-transfusion hepatitis was due to hepatitis B. In 1989, a single-stranded RNA virus containing 3000 nucleotides was identified as the etiological agent we know as hepatitis C. The virus has 40% homology with the Flaviviridae family of RNA viruses. An ELISA assay was developed to detect antibody to hepatitis C for diagnostic purposes, as well as for screening blood donors. Non-A, non-B, and non-C hepatitis can still occur, probably due to CMV, hepatitis E, hepatitis G, and hepatitis GB.

For blood donors, hepatitis C serology correlates with surrogate tests for non-A, non-B hepatitis (ALT and anti-HB$_c$). Since hepatitis C serology identifies a broader group of infected individuals than surrogate testing, it reduces risk of HCV during transfusion. Studies in hemophiliacs indicate that antibody to HCV is a reliable marker of HCV; 70% to 90% of individuals with severe hemophilia are infected with HCV. Recently, IgM anti-HCV core has been shown to be a useful acute marker for HCV infection. Transmission is by intravenous drug abuse, dialysis, and other needlesticks. Although sexual transmission is much less common than that with hepatitis B, risk relates to exposure. In 50% of cases, no cause can be found for the infection. Before screening for hepatitis C antibody was in place, non-A, non-B hepatitis was said to occur in as many as 10% of transfusions. With the introduction of first generation hepatitis C screening tests, the number has fallen to 1 in 3300 units.[2,3,4,5] With a more sensitive second generation hepatitis C test being introduced in 1992, safety has increased even more. Michael Busch (personal communication, LT) puts the number of units of blood contaminated with hepatitis C to be less than 1 in 60,000. Chronic carrier states develop in more than 80% of patients, and chronic liver disease is a major problem. Substantial risk of chronic active hepatitis and cirrhosis exists in those who develop chronic non-A, non-B hepatitis, of whom about 90% develop anti-HCV. Of these, a risk of hepatocellular carcinoma exists. A series of patients who developed post-transfusion non-A, non-B hepatitis in the 1970s were followed for up to 15 years after initial diagnosis. Twenty percent of these patients developed liver failure.[6] The disease progression is slow. The time to detection by liver biopsy of chronic active hepatitis, cirrhosis, and hepatocellular carcinoma is 15, 20, and 25 years, respectively.[7] Some success has occurred in the treatment of hepatitis C using interferon alfa-2b.[8] Studies are currently being done on the detection of HCV in patient's specimens using reverse transcriptase and PCR.[9] Quantitative PCR is desirable but is a complex assay.[10,11]

Use of ALT remains important in evaluation of patients with HCV infection, but histopathologic abnormalities are found in HCV-infected patients whose serum enzyme levels are normal. Liver biopsy remains useful for patients with chronic hepatitis.[11,12]

HCV infection is linked with essential mixed cryoglobulinemia,[1,13] membranoproliferative glomerulonephritis, and porphyria cutanea tarda.[1]

Chronic hepatitis C often is a progressive disease, leading not infrequently to chronic active hepatitis and cirrhosis. Some develop hepatic failure or hepatocellular carcinoma.[14]

Footnotes

1. Gumber SC and Chopra S, "Hepatitis C: A Multifaceted Disease. Review of Extrahepatic Manifestations," *Ann Intern Med*, 1995, 123(8):615-20.
2. McCullough J, "The Nation's Changing Blood Supply System," *JAMA*, 1993, 269(17):2239-45.
3. Donahue JG, Muñoz A, Ness PM, et al, "The Declining Risk of Post-Transfusion Hepatitis C Virus Infection," *N Engl J Med*, 1992, 327(6):369-73.
4. Dodd RY, "The Risk of Transfusion-Transmitted Infection," *N Engl J Med*, 1992, 327(6):419-21.
5. Chaudhary RK and Maclean C, "Detection of Antibody to Hepatitis C Virus by Second-Generation Enzyme Immunoassay," *Am J Clin Pathol*, 1993, 99(6):702-4.
6. Koretz RL, Abbey H, Coleman E, et al, "Non-A, Non-B Post-Transfusion Hepatitis: Looking Back in the Second Decade," *Ann Intern Med* , 1993, 119(2):110-5.
7. Alter HJ, "To C or Not to C: These Are the Questions," *Blood*, 1995, 85(7):1681-95.
8. Poynard T, Bedossa P, Chevallier M, et al, "A Comparison of Three Interferon Alfa-2b Regimens for the Long-Term Treatment of Chronic Non-A, Non-B Hepatitis," *N Engl J Med*, 1995, 332(22):1457-62.
9. François M, Dubois F, Brand D, et al, "Prevalence and Significance of Hepatitis C Virus (HCV) Viremia in HCV Antibody-Positive Subjects from Various Populations," *J Clin Microbiol*, 1993, 31(5):1189-93.
10. Gretch DR, dela Rosa C, Carithers RL Jr, et al, "Assessment of Hepatitis C Viremia Using Molecular Amplification Technologies: Correlations and Clinical Implications," *Ann Intern Med*, 1995, 123(5):321-9.
11. Tedeschi V and Seeff LB, "Diagnostic Tests for Hepatitis C: Where Are We Now?" *Ann Intern Med*, 1995, 123(5):383-5 (editorial).
12. Serfaty L, Nousbaum JB, Elghouzzi MH, et al, "Prevalence, Severity, and Risk Factors of Liver Disease in Blood Donors Positive in a Second-Generation and Antihepatitis C Virus Screening Test," *Hepatology*, 1995, 21(3):725-9.
13. Lunel F, Musset L, Cacoub P, et al, "Cryoglobulinemia in Chronic Liver Diseases: Role of Hepatitis C Virus and Liver Damage," *Gastroenterology*, 1994, 106(5):1291-300.
14. Tong MJ, el-Farra NS, Reikes AR, et al, "Clinical Outcomes After Transfusion-Associated Hepatitis C," *N Engl J Med*, 1995, 332(22):1463-6.

References

Allain JP, Dailey SH, Laurian Y, et al, "Evidence for Persistent Hepatitis C Virus (HCV) Infection in Hemophiliacs," *J Clin Invest*, 1991, 88(5):1672-9.

Alter HJ, "Review of Serologic Testing for Hepatitis C Virus Infection and Risk of Post-Transfusion Hepatitis C," *Arch Pathol Lab Med*, 1994, 118(4):342-5.

Clemens JM, Taskar S, Chau K, et al, "IgM Antibody Response in Acute Hepatitis C Viral Infection," *Blood*, 1992, 79(1):169-72.

Desforges JF, "Infectious Disease Testing for Blood Transfusions," *NIH Consensus Statement*, 1995, 13(1):1-27.

Dodd LG, McBride JH, Gitnick GL, et al, "Prevalence of Non-A, Non-B Hepatitis/Hepatitis C Virus Antibody in Human Immunoglobulins," *Am J Clin Pathol*, 1992, 97(1):108-13.

Dodd RY, "Hepatitis C Virus, Antibodies and Infectivity - Paradox, Pragmatism, and Policy," *Am J Clin Pathol*, 1992, 97(1):4-6.

Hsieh TT, Yao DS, Sheen IS, et al, "Hepatitis C Virus in Peripheral Blood Mononuclear Cells," *Am J Clin Pathol*, 1992, 98(4):392-6.

Klein HG, *Standards for Blood Banks and Transfusion Services*, 16th ed, Bethesda, MD: American Association of Blood Banks, 1994, 3-8.

Nousbaum JB, Pol S, Nalpas B, et al, "Hepatitis C Virus Type 1b (II) Infection in France and Italy," *Ann Intern Med*, 1995, 122(3):161-8.

Prince AM, Brotman B, Inchauspé G, et al, "Patterns and Prevalence of Hepatitis C Virus Infection in Post-Transfusion Non-A, Non-B Hepatitis," *J Infect Dis*, 1993, 167(6):1296-301.

Seeff LB, Buskell-Bales Z, Wright EC, et al, "Long-Term Mortality After Transfusion-Associated Non-A, Non-B Hepatitis," *N Engl J Med*, 1992, 327(27):1906-11.

Shakil AO, Conry-Cantilena C, Alter HJ, et al, "Volunteer Blood Donors With Antibody to Hepatitis C Virus: Clinical, Biochemical, Virologic, and Histologic Features, the Hepatitis C Study Group" *Ann Intern Med*, 1995, 123(5):330-7.

Weiss JB Jr and Persing DH, "Hepatitis C: Advances in Diagnosis," *Mayo Clin Proc*, 1995, 70(3):296-7.

Hepatitis D Serology

CPT 86306 (antigen); 86692 (antibody)

Related Information

Hepatitis B Core Antibody *on page 396*
Hepatitis B DNA Detection *on page 513*
Hepatitis B$_e$ Antibody *on page 397*
Hepatitis B$_e$ Antigen *on page 397*
Hepatitis B Surface Antibody *on page 398*
Hepatitis B Surface Antigen *on previous page*
Polymerase Chain Reaction *on page 523*

Synonyms Delta Agent Serology; Delta Hepatitis Serology

Abstract Hepatitis D virus (HDV) was first described in 1977. HDV always occurs simultaneously with hepatitis B (HBV). Patients coinfected with HDV and HBV have fulminant hepatitis more often than patients infected with HBV alone.[1]

Patient Preparation Avoid recent administration of radioisotopes if assay performed by RIA.

Specimen Serum

Container Red top tube

Reference Range Negative

Use Differential diagnosis of chronic, recurrent, and acute viral hepatitis. Testing for serological markers of HDV should be considered when a patient shows clinical signs of acute or fulminant hepatitis, or when deterioration takes place in chronic hepatitis B infection.

Limitations False-positive EIA results have been reported in patients with lipemia or high titer rheumatoid factor.

Methodology Radioimmunoassay (RIA), enzyme-linked immunosorbent assay (ELISA)

Additional Information Hepatitis D virus ("delta" agent) is an incomplete RNA virus, or viroid, that can infect livers already infected by hepatitis B virus. It may occur, therefore, as coinfection with acute HBV hepatitis or superimposed on chronic HBV infection. It cannot occur in an HB$_s$Ag-negative individual. It uses HBV surface antigen as its viral envelope. IgG and IgM antibodies to HDV develop 5-7 weeks after infection. IgM antibody is most useful in distinguishing those patients with active liver disease. IgM anti-HDV is transient and is rapidly replaced by IgG anti-HDV, which persists and is associated with hepatitis. Generally, laboratories use total anti-HDV ELISAs containing both IgM and IgG for diagnostic purposes. HDAg can be detected in serum or liver biopsies but is technically demanding and offers little to diagnosis. Studies of liver transplants in patients with end-stage liver disease due to hepatitis B/D have shown, through serial biopsies post-transplant, that HDV viral reinfection occurs within 1 week but without damage. Not until HBV proliferation occurs several weeks to months later does one find histologic and clinical changes.[2,3]

Transmission of this defective virus is mostly by injection drug use, and less commonly through sexual transmission. Among HBV-infected users of injection drugs, seroprevalence of HDV is 20% to 53%.[4]

Footnotes

1. Polish LB, Gallagher M, Fields HA, et al, "Delta Hepatitis: Molecular Biology and Clinical and Epidemiological Features," *Clin Microbiol Rev*, 1993, 6(3):211-29.
2. Craig JR, "Hepatitis Delta Virus - No Longer A Defective Virus," *Am J Clin Pathol*, 1992, 98(6):552-3.
3. Davies SE, Lau JY, O'Grady JG, et al, "Evidence That Hepatitis D Virus Needs Hepatitis B Virus to Cause Hepatocellular Damage," *Am J Clin Pathol*, 1992, 98(6):554-8.
4. Shapiro CN, "Transmission of Hepatitis Viruses," *Ann Intern Med*, 1994, 120(1):82-4 (editorial).

Hepatitis D Superinfection

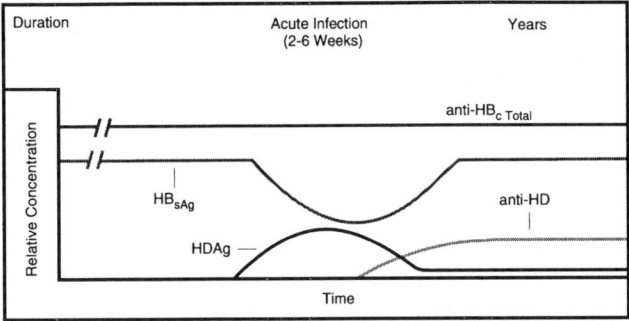

Reprinted from Abbott Diagnostics

Hepatitis D Coinfection

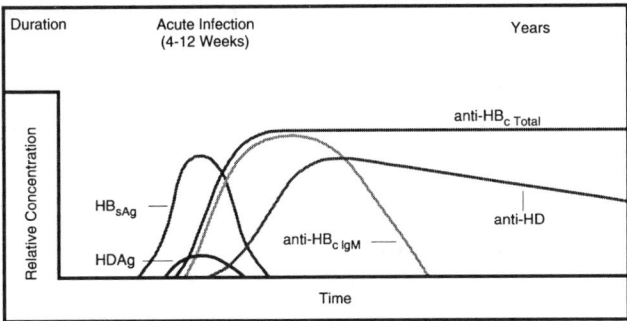

Reprinted from Abbott Diagnostics

References

Alter MJ and Hedler SE, "Delta Hepatitis Infection in North America," *Hepatitis Delta Virus, Molecular Biology, Pathogenesis, and Clinical Aspects*, Hadziyannis SJ, Tyler JM, and Bonino F, eds, New York, NY: Wiley-Liss, 1993.

Govindarajan S, Valinluck B, Lake-Bakkar G, "Evaluation of a Commercial Antidelta EIA Test for Detection of Antibodies to Hepatitis Delta Virus," *Am J Clin Pathol*, 1991, 95(2):240-1.

Gupta S, Govindarajan S, Cassidy WM, et al, "Acute Delta Hepatitis: Serological Diagnosis With Particular Reference to Hepatitis Delta Virus RNA," *Am J Gastroenterol*, 1991, 86(9):1227-31.

Pohl C, Baroudy BM, Bergmann KF, et al, "A Human Monoclonal Antibody that Recognizes Viral Polypeptides and *In Vitro* Translation Products of the Genome of the Hepatitis D Virus," *J Infect Dis*, 1987, 156(4):622-9.

Hepatitis Vaccine *see* Hepatitis B Surface Antibody *on page 398*

Hereditary Angioneurotic Edema Test *see* C1 Esterase Inhibitor, Serum *on page 372*

Herpes 1 and 2 *see* Herpes Simplex Antibody *on this page*

Herpes Hominis 1 and 2 *see* Herpes Simplex Antibody *on this page*

Herpes Simplex Antibody

CPT 86694 (nonspecific type); 86695 (type 1)

Related Information

Herpes Cytology *on page 296*
Herpes Simplex Virus Antigen Detection *on page 667*
Herpes Simplex Virus Culture *on page 668*
Herpes Simplex Virus DNA Detection *on page 514*
TORCH *on page 435*
Viral Culture *on page 675*

Synonyms Herpes 1 and 2; Herpes Hominis 1 and 2; HSV Antibodies

Test Commonly Includes IgG and IgM antibodies

Specimen Serum, cerebrospinal fluid

Container Red top tube, sterile CSF tube

Sampling Time Most useful after the fourth day of illness in herpes simplex virus encephalitis.[1] (However, other laboratory procedures are preferred for encephalitis; *vide infra*.)

Reference Range Interpretation depends on whether episode is initial or reinfection. Generally, IgG: <1:5; IgM: <1:10.

Critical Values Increased IgM antibodies or a fourfold rise in titer may indicate recent infection.

Use Determine a patient's exposure to herpes simplex virus 1 or 2, mostly in identification of seropositive organ transplant recipients.

Limitations Extensive background antibody in the population, and cross reaction of HSV 1 and HSV 2 responses make test useful only in epidemiology. False-negatives occur. PCR is more sensitive for early herpes simplex virus encephalitis than is detection of antibody in CSF.[1]

Methodology Indirect fluorescent antibody (IFA), hemagglutination, complement fixation (CF), enzyme immunoassay (EIA), Western blot assay

Additional Information A primary HSV 1 or HSV 2 infection will produce a classical rising antibody titer. However, because exposure to herpesvirus is almost universal, approximately 90% of adults have antibodies. The presence of antibodies to HSV is usually not helpful. The antibody to one virus type may be stimulated by infection with the heterologous virus type. Both false-positives and false-negatives are common with currently licensed enzyme immunoassays. Collecting the requisite paired sera to delineate which titers are rising or stable generally adds nothing to clinical management, and thus **herpes serology cannot be recommended in routine clinical cases.** Herpes serology has not been proved clinically useful in determining whether caesarean delivery should be undertaken in pregnant patients with questionably active herpes. Pap smear or immunochemical demonstration of viral antigen is more useful for this. Nor is herpes serology usually helpful in the differential of a very sick infant with possible congenital herpes. Because of the fulminant course, even early IgM antibody may not be demonstrable in time to contribute to care. See listing Herpes Simplex Virus DNA Detection *on page 514.*

Footnotes

1. Uren EC, Johnson PD, Montanaro J, et al, "Herpes Simplex Virus Encephalitis in Pediatrics: Diagnosis by Detection of Antibodies and DNA in Cerebrospinal Fluid," *Pediatr Infect Dis J*, 1993, 12(12):1001-6.

References

ARUP Laboratories, *Herpes Simplex Virus: New PCR Test vs Culture, Antigen Detection, and Antibody Titers*, April, 1996.

Ashley R, Cent A, Maggs U, et al, "Inability of Enzyme Immunoassays to Discriminate Between Infections With Herpes Simplex Virus Types 1 and 2," *Ann Intern Med*, 1991, 115(7):520-6.

Erlich KS, "Laboratory Diagnosis of Herpesvirus Infections," *Clin Lab Med*, 1987, 7(4):759-76.

Frenkel LM, Garratty EM, Shen JP, et al, "Clinical Reactivation of Herpes Simplex Virus Type 2 Infection in Seropositive Pregnant Women With No History of Genital Herpes," *Ann Intern Med*, 1993, 118(6):414-8.

Johnson RE, Nahmias AJ, Magder LS, et al, "A Seroepidemiological Survey of the Prevalence of Herpes Simplex Virus Type 2 Infection in the United States," *N Engl J Med*, 1989, 321(1):7-12.

Prober CG, Corey L, Brown ZA, et al, "The Management of Pregnancies Complicated by Genital Infections With Herpes Simplex Virus," *Clin Infect Dis*, 1992, 15(6):1031-8.

Wald A, Zeh J, Selke S, et al, "Virologic Characteristics of Subclinical and Symptomatic Genital Herpes Infections," *N Engl J Med*, 1995, 333(12):770-5.

Whitley R, Arvin A, Prober C, et al, "Predictors of Morbidity and Mortality in Neonates With Herpes Simplex Virus Infections," *N Engl J Med*, 1991, 324(7):450-4.

Herpes Zoster Serology *see* Varicella-Zoster Virus Serology *on page 437*

Heterophil Agglutinins

CPT 86308

Related Information

Epstein-Barr Virus Culture *on page 666*
Epstein-Barr Virus Serology *on page 392*
Infectious Mononucleosis Screening Test *on page 410*

Test Commonly Includes Differentiation and quantitation of antibodies associated with infectious mononucleosis from the Forssman as well as other heterophil antibodies.

Specimen Serum

Container Red top tube

Reference Range Negative agglutination

Use Detect heterophil antibodies related to infectious mononucleosis. **This test has largely been superseded by rapid screening tests. See Infectious Mononucleosis Screening Test *on page 410.***

Limitations Rare patients may have positive heterophil agglutinins after a negative screening test. Ten percent of cases of true EBV mononucleosis may have negative heterophil agglutinins. These may be diagnosed with EBV specific tests.

Methodology Differential serum absorption and agglutination of sheep red blood cells

Additional Information Heterophil agglutinins clump sheep erythrocytes. They develop in infectious mononucleosis, other conditions, and in some normal individuals. To diagnose infectious mononucleosis, an absorption of serum is done, with guinea pig kidney (which does not bind IgM antibody) and bovine red cells (which do). This differential absorption procedure is the Paul-Bunnell-Davidsohn test. In present usage horse erythrocytes are used in place of sheep cells in many laboratories. In the presumptive test, a positive test in the presence of consistent clinical and/or hematologic findings confirms the diagnosis of infectious mononucleosis. Approximately 10% of mononucleosis syndromes are (Continued)

Heterophil Agglutinins (Continued)

heterophil-negative. In some of these, antibody to specific Epstein-Barr viral antigen can be demonstrated. See Epstein-Barr Virus Serology *on page 392*. Others may be due to CMV, HHV-6, or toxoplasmosis. Although this classic test has excellent specificity, its performance is time consuming. False-positive tests occur and may lead to diagnostic confusion.

References
Fleisher GR, Collins M, and Fager S, "Limitations of Available Tests for Diagnosis of Infectious Mononucleosis," *J Clin Microbiol*, 1983, 17:619-24.

Horwitz CA, Henle W, Henle G, et al, "Persistent Falsely Positive Rapid Tests for Infectious Mononucleosis. Report of Five Cases with 4-6 Year Follow-Up Data," *Am J Clin Pathol*, 1979, 72:807-11.

Ridker PM, Enders GH, and Lifton RP, "False-Positive Mononucleosis Screening Test Results Associated With *Klebsiella* Hepatic Abscess," *Am J Clin Pathol*, 1990, 94(2):222-3.

Heterophil Antibody *see* Infectious Mononucleosis Screening Test *on page 410*

HHV-6, IgM, IgG *see* Human Herpesvirus 6, IgG and IgM Antibodies, Quantitative *on page 406*

Histocompatibility Testing *see* Tissue Typing *on page 434*

***Histoplasma* Antibodies** *see* Histoplasmosis Antibody *on this page*

***Histoplasma capsulatum* Antigen** *see* Histoplasmosis Antigen *on this page*

Histoplasmosis Antibody

CPT 86698

Related Information
Bronchoalveolar Lavage Cytology *on page 288*
Fungal Culture, Biopsy or Body Fluid *on page 476*
Fungal Culture, Blood *on page 477*
Fungal Culture, Sputum *on page 479*
Fungus Smear, Stain *on page 481*
Histoplasmosis Antigen *on this page*

Synonyms *Histoplasma* Antibodies

Test Commonly Includes Reaction with yeast and mycelial antigens

Abstract Serological diagnosis of histoplasmosis is **not always reliable** but is positive in 98% of cases of **self-limited** disease. Serologic testing is indicated in instances of chronic disease, but utilization of antibody response should only be used in conjunction with other tests.

Specimen Serum, cerebrospinal fluid

Container Red top tube, sterile CSF tube, plastic urine container

Collection Acute and convalescent sera are recommended, especially when acute titers are only presumptive.

Reference Range Less than a fourfold change in titer between acute and convalescent samples; titer: <1:4; CF titer: <1:8; CSF titer: negative

Use Diagnose chronic/self-limited histoplasmosis. Fungal stains and cultures of sputum are also needed for such patients.

Limitations Other diagnostic approaches are preferable. A negative result does not rule out histoplasmosis. False-negatives occur in immunosuppressed individuals.[1] Histoplasmin skin testing may interfere with results. Testing with both antigens must be performed. There are cross reactions with other fungi. Anticomplementary sera cannot be tested for complement fixing antibodies. The latex agglutination test gives some false-positives, and must be confirmed with another procedure.

Contraindications Previous skin testing

Methodology Immunodiffusion (ID), complement fixation (CF), latex agglutination (LA), radioimmunoassay (RIA), enzyme immunoassay (EIA)

Additional Information CF titers of 1:8 or 1:16 are presumptive evidence of histoplasmosis. Titers ≥1:32 are highly suggestive of *H. capsulatum* infection, but cannot be relied on as the sole means of diagnosis. Complement fixation and immunodiffusion each detect about 85% of disease. H and M bands on immunodiffusion indicate active disease. Complement fixation is less sensitive to disseminated or chronic disease. The latex agglutination test detects IgM antibodies and is positive early in disease, but not in late, chronic, or recurrent infection.

Histoplasmosis immunodiffusion: "H" and "M" precipitin bands are of diagnostic significance and if both are present indicate active infection. "H" identity bands alone are rarely seen; they are always associated with active infection. "M" identity bands alone indicate active infection, recent past infection (within the past year), or recent positive histoplasmin skin test (within past 2 months). The absence of precipitin antibodies does not rule out histoplasmosis.

Unfortunately, because of poorly standardized reagents and inherent biologic cross reactivity, and interference from complement, the general clinical utility of measuring or detecting fungal antibodies is low.

However, serologic tests for antibodies were found in all subjects with chronic pulmonary histoplasmosis and in 98% of those with self-limited disease.[1]

In addition to histoplasmosis in immunologically intact individuals, this fungal infection is a serious opportunistic infection in patients with AIDS (occasionally as its first manifestation). It can sometimes be found in leukocytes in Wright-stained peripheral blood films in patients with AIDS.

Giemsa or methenamine silver preparations of bone marrow, mucosal ulcers, biopsies of liver, lung, skin, lymph nodes, or bronchoalveolar lavage may provide rapid diagnosis; and cultures are required as well, especially of blood, bone marrow, sputum, urine and portions of biopsies. Isolates can be identified by DNA probe.[2]

Footnotes
1. Williams B, Fojtasek M, Connolly-Stringfield P, et al, "Diagnosis of Histoplasmosis by Antigen Detection During an Outbreak in Indianapolis, Ind," *Arch Pathol Lab Med*, 1994, 118(12):1205-8.

2. "Case Records of the Massachusetts General Hospital. Weekly Clinicopathological Exercises. Case 4-1994. A 38-Year-Old Man With AIDS and the Recent Onset of Diarrhea, Hematochezia, Fever, and Pulmonary Infiltrates," *N Engl J Med*, 1994, 330(4):273-80.

References
Kaufman L and Reiss E, "Serodiagnosis of Fungal Diseases," *Manual of Clinical Laboratory Immunology*, 4th ed, Vol 2, Chapter 78, Rose NR, Conway de Macario E, Fahey JL, et al, eds, Washington, DC: American Society for Microbiology, 1992, 506-28.

Wheat LJ, Connolly-Stringfield PA, Baker RL, et al, "Disseminated Histoplasmosis in the Acquired Immune Deficiency Syndrome: Clinical Findings, Diagnosis and Treatment, and Review of the Literature," *Medicine (Baltimore)*, 1990, 69(6):361-74.

Wheat LJ, Connolly-Stringfield PA, Blair R, et al, "Histoplasmosis Relapse in Patients With AIDS: Detection Using *Histoplasma capsulatum* Variety *capsulatum* Antigen Levels," *Ann Intern Med*, 1991, 115(12):936-41.

Zimmerman SE, Stringfield PC, Wheat LJ, et al, "Comparison of Sandwich Solid-Phase Radioimmunoassay and Two Enzyme-Linked Immunosorbent Assays for Detection of *Histoplasma capsulatum* Polysaccharide Antigen," *J Infect Dis*, 1989, 160(4):678-85.

Histoplasmosis Antigen

Related Information
Fungal Culture, Biopsy or Body Fluid *on page 476*
Fungal Culture, Blood *on page 477*
Fungal Culture, Sputum *on page 479*
Fungus Smear, Stain *on page 481*
Histoplasmosis Antibody *on this page*

Applies to *Histoplasma capsulatum* Antigen

Abstract Less helpful in chronic pulmonary or self-limited forms of histoplasmosis, in which cultures and serologic tests are needed. Antigen tests are useful in subjects with severe disease including disseminated histoplasmosis.

Patient Preparation Avoid recent administration of radioisotopes if assay performed by RIA.

Specimen Serum, urine, cerebrospinal fluid

Container Red top tube, urine container, sterile CSF tube

Reference Range <1.0 EIA or RIA units

Use This test has a specificity of greater than 98% and a sensitivity of 92% in disseminated histoplasmosis.[1] The immunoassay for *Histoplasma* polysaccharide antigen has proven diagnostically useful in a variety of clinical settings (particularly in AIDS patients), and is also useful for monitoring response to therapy. Biopsies, examination of peripheral blood smears for organisms, blood cultures, and serology are also indicated for investigation of disseminated histoplasmosis.[1]

Limitations The test currently is not widely performed. It frequently produces false-negative results with less severe forms of histoplasmosis, and even may give false-negative results in patients with proven disseminated disease.[1]

Methodology Microtiter plates with anti-*H. capsulatum* antibody;[1] enzyme immunoassay (EIA) or radioimmunoassay (RIA) for *Histoplasma* polysaccharide antigen

Additional Information In Indianapolis, almost half of culture-proven cases were found in AIDS patients.[1]

Footnotes
1. Williams B, Fojtasek M, Connolly-Stringfield P, et al, "Diagnosis of Histoplasmosis by Antigen Detection During an Outbreak in Indianapolis, Ind," *Arch Pathol Lab Med*, 1994, 118(12):1205-8.

References
"Case Records of the Massachusetts General Hospital. Weekly Clinicopathological Exercises. Case 4-1994. A 38 Year-Old Man With AIDS and the Recent Onset of Diarrhea, Hematochezia, Fever, and Pulmonary Infiltrates," *N Engl J Med*, 1994, 330(4):273-80.

Wheat LJ, Connolly-Stringfield PA, Baker RL, et al, "Disseminated Histoplasmosis in the Acquired Immune Deficiency Syndrome: Clinical Findings, Diagnosis and Treatment, and Review of the Literature," *Medicine (Baltimore)*, 1990, 69(6):361-74.

Wheat LJ, Connolly-Stringfield P, Blair R, et al, "Effect of Successful Treatment With Amphotericin B on *Histoplasma capsulatum* Variety *capsulatum* Polysaccharide Antigen Levels in Patients With AIDS and Histoplasmosis," *Am J Med*, 1992, 92:153-60.

Wheat LJ, Connolly-Stringfield P, Blair R, et al, "Histoplasmosis Relapse in Patients With AIDS: Detection Using *Histoplasma capsulatum* Variety *capsulatum* Antigen Levels," *Ann Intern Med*, 1991, 115(12):936-41.

Zimmerman SE, Stringfield PC, Wheat LJ, et al, "Comparison of Sandwich Solid-Phase Radioimmunoassay and Two Enzyme-Linked Immunosorbent Assays for Detection of *Histoplasma capsulatum* Polysaccharide Antigen," *J Infect Dis*, 1989, 160(4):678-85.

HIV-1/HIV-2 Serology

CPT 86701 (HIV-1); 86702 (HIV-2); 86703 (HIV-1 and HIV-2, single assay)

Related Information

Synonyms Acquired Immune Deficiency Syndrome Serology; AIDS Screen; HIV Antibody; Human Immunodeficiency Virus Serology; RIBA Test for HIV Antibody; Western Blot Test for HIV Antibody

Applies to Recombinant Antigen Immunoblot Assay; RIBA; Western Blot

Test Commonly Includes Detection of antibody to HIV by ELISA and confirmation by Western blot

Patient Preparation In some states test may not be done or results revealed without express written or informed consent of the patient or guardian.

Specimen Serum or plasma

Container Red top tube or lavender top (EDTA) tube

Special Instructions Blood and body fluid precautions must be observed.

Reference Range Negative

Use Document exposure to HIV-1 and HIV-2; screen blood and blood products for transfusion; screen organ transplant donors; test patients after documented needlestick exposure of healthcare personnel

Limitations Positive screening tests must be confirmed by more specific follow-up procedures (Western blot or immunofluorescent antibody). If the Western blot or immunofluorescent antibody for HIV-1 is negative or indeterminate with a positive HIV-1/HIV-2 serology, further testing is required for HIV-2. This may include HIV-2 EIA and HIV-2 Western blot. Antibody is not protective against disease. There are some cross reactions in some test systems due to histocompatibility antigen mismatches (in particular, antibodies to HLA-DR4). Cross reactions have been observed to other viral antigens as well. A recent influenza vaccine can result in reactivity against p24 antigen and give a false-positive enzyme-linked immunosorbent assay.

Because screening tests are neither 100% sensitive nor specific, alone or in combination, a positive result must be interpreted cautiously, considering the prevalence of AIDS in the population being tested. As prevalence decreases compared to high risk groups, false-positives increase, and the predictive value of a positive result decreases.

Contraindications Some states require informed consent.

Methodology Enzyme-linked immunosorbent assay (ELISA), Western blot, indirect fluorescent antibody (IFA); radioimmunoprecipitation assay (RIPA)

Additional Information Human immunodeficiency virus (HIV-1, formerly HTLV-III) is the etiologic agent of AIDS. Acute infection, spread by blood or sexual contact, is usually followed within days by a flu-like illness, or no symptoms. Generally, following infection with the virus, there is local replication of the virus in regional lymph nodes for 2 weeks before spilling into the blood. Within 11 days of entering the blood, the RNA virion can be detected by reverse transcriptase PCR. By 17 days after the virus enters the blood, the infection can be detected by p24 antigen test or by PCR for genomic DNA. On average, by 23 days, the antibody to the HIV virus can be detected in the serum or plasma.

HIV preferentially binds to and infects CD4 (T4, helper) lymphocytes. HIV also binds to monocytes and macrophages, and infection of bronchial macrophages may explain the frequency of *Pneumocystis* infections in AIDS patients. HIV probably enters the CNS by means of infected monocytes crossing the blood-brain barrier.

Ancillary tests for AIDS include quantitation of CD4 (helper) and CD8 (suppressor) lymphocytes. In AIDS (but **not** diagnostic for it), T4 cells are severely reduced, and the CD4:CD8 ratio is <1. An absolute CD4 count <300/mm^3 is used as an indication for AZT.

Present screening tests for HIV antibodies are ELISA procedures which use recombinant antigen products. Different antibodies are detected. Both the sensitivity and specificity of these tests are extremely high, but positive results on a screen should be repeated; if positive a second time they should be confirmed with a Western blot procedure. Because of the grave implications of a positive result, it is recommended that a second sample be assayed to eliminate false-positives due to switched samples or sample contamination. Before patients develop antibody (window phase), p24 antigen, HIV DNA amplification or RNA amplification or branched DNA (b-DNA) assays can be used for diagnosis. b-DNA assays can also be used to follow therapy (HIV viral load) and conversion to clinical AIDS.[1]

Some individuals may have reactive screening tests, restricted to one test system, and completely negative Western blots. This may be due to HLA antibodies reacting with residual human cell surface proteins incorporated in the test kit. False-positives have been reported in individuals who have received intravenous gamma globulin. Since these positives are due to antibodies in the transfused gamma globulin, repeat analysis in 3 months (half-life for IgG is about 3 weeks), will show a negative or much weaker EIA result. Sera which test positive by ELISA twice consecutively are subject to confirmatory testing by Western blot or immunofluorescent antibody technique.

In the Western blot procedure, electrophoretically separated HIV proteins and glycoproteins are overlaid with serum. Antibodies present will bind to the appropriate antigen, which is spatially separated by molecular weight from other viral components. The bound antibody is then visualized by reaction with a labeled (radioisotope or enzyme) antibody to human immunoglobulin or protein A (which binds to the Fc portion of the antibody). Although, early on, several different patterns were used for a positive interpretation, since 1988 two major patterns are used. The Consortium for Retrovirus Serology Standardization recommended that a positive blot have the following bands: p24 or p31 plus gp41 or gp160/120. The standard of the Association of State and Territorial Public Health Laboratory was adopted by the Centers for Disease Control in 1989 and is now the most widely accepted definition of a positive Western blot. This criteria requires the Western blot to contain at least two of the following three bands: p24, gp41, and gp 160/120. The presence of other band patterns is termed indeterminate and should be followed up with subsequent testing. The Western blot is a complex procedure, requiring great technical expertise and informed interpretation. False-positive rates may be in the range of 1% to 2%. False-negative rates are not well established. A disadvantage of WB is the high percentage of "indeterminate" patterns - neither positive nor negative. As many as 40% of repeat reactive specimens will have an indeterminate pattern. IFA, in contrast, reveals a <5% indeterminate pattern. Thus, for confirmatory testing IFA is more specific. On the other hand, it is more difficult and expensive than WB.

Another virus that causes AIDS, HIV-2, was recognized in 1986. HIV-2 is very closely related to HIV-1 with 40% nucleic acid homology. HIV-2 is endemic in West Africa, however, it has spread to other countries. As of September, 1991, 31 cases had been confirmed in the United States.[3] It produces the same clinical disease as HIV-1, although the incubation period before clinical AIDS develops in HIV-2 may be longer than in HIV-1.

The most recent EIA kits allow detection of both HIV-1 and HIV-2 antibodies. Further, recombinant antigens from HIV-1: p24 (gag), p17 (gag), and endonuclease p31 (pol) have been combined with two synthetic peptides from the env genes of HIV-1 and the env gene of HIV-2 to provide a strip-based confirmation assay similar to the Western blot. A similar recombinant antigen immunoblot assay (RIBA) confirmation assay employing HIV-1 p24, p31, p41, and gp120 has been proposed as an alternative confirmation method for HIV-1.

Prolonged latency of HIV has been suggested by several studies. Viral antigens and antibodies can be demonstrated by polymerase chain reaction for as long as 35 months before individuals seroconverted by ELISA testing. Such individuals may have normal numbers of CD4 lymphocytes.

Screening for AIDS infection in low risk populations will be hampered by false-positive results. Although the combined false-positive rate of sequential ELISA and Western blot testing may be very low (0.005% estimated in one article) testing large numbers of individuals in a population with a very low prevalence of disease will generate unmanageable numbers of false-positive results. The predictive value of a positive test will be low, and many individuals will be unnecessarily alarmed. Mass screening is not recommended with tests presently available.

For patients who received blood transfusions or blood products between 1978 and 1985, especially in California, New York City, or Miami, testing with currently available ELISA methodology is satisfactory as an initial procedure to exclude accidental infection via transfusion. (Continued)

HIV-1/HIV-2 Serology *(Continued)*

Patients who received only Rh immune globulin, or other gamma globulin products, need not be tested unless they fall into some other risk group. "Look back" programs, retrospectively testing blood recipients, and assessing risk of transfusion-associated AIDS, have been undertaken. Now that donor blood is screened for antibodies to HIV-1 (and HTLV-I) the blood supply is acceptably safe; risk is as low as one unit in 435,000. In 1992, testing of blood bank samples by HIV-1 and HIV-2 ELISA became the standard.

Patients in high risk groups (homosexual or bisexual men, I.V. drug abusers and their sexual contacts, male and female prostitutes, hemophiliacs exposed to large amounts of nonheat processed factor VIII) should be tested for diagnosis. This should include an initial ELISA test, and tests for HIV antigen. Repeated testing may be necessary.

There are no patterns of serologic response to HIV yet known to indicate resolution of disease or loss of infectivity (unlike the situation for hepatitis B virus). About 5% of HIV-infected individuals have nonprogressive courses with no secondary infections for up to 10 years after infection.[2] A patient in a risk group who has demonstrable antigen or antibody should be assumed to be infected and infectious. See chart.

Although **central nervous system involvement** is extremely common in AIDS, testing CSF for HIV antigen or antibody lacks both sensitivity and specificity. These tests do not help in differentiating neurologic symptoms secondary to HIV infection from those due to CNS neoplasm or opportunistic infection.

The October 1988 issue of *Scientific American* and July 1993 *Journal of NIH Research* are entirely devoted to a thorough consideration of social, biological and the medical aspects of the AIDS epidemic. An excellent position paper from the American College of Physicians should be consulted.[4]

TYPICAL SEROLOGICAL PROFILE IN HIV INFECTION

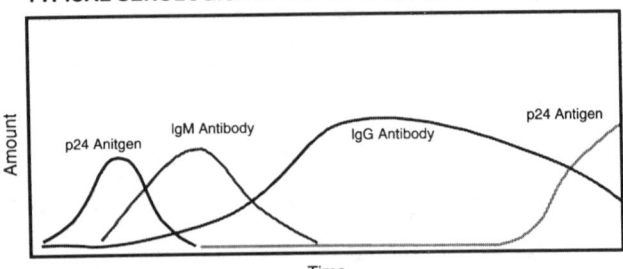

From Van de Peere P, Lepage P, and Simonon A, "Biological Markers Associated With Prolonged Survival in African Children Maternally Infected By the Human Immunodeficiency Virus Type 1," *AIDS Res Hum Retroviruses*, 1992, 8(4):435, with permission.

HUMAN RETROVIRUSES

HIV-1   HIV-2

Polymerase Gene Products (p66/51; p31)
Reverse Transcriptase
Gag Proteins — p17, p24
Envelope Proteins — gp41, gp120

Lipid Membrane
p16, p26 — Gag Proteins
gp36, gp105 — Envelope Proteins
(p68), (p34) — Polymerase Gene Products
RNA

Reprinted from Abbott Diagnostics

HUMAN RETROVIRUSES
HIV-1 Genome

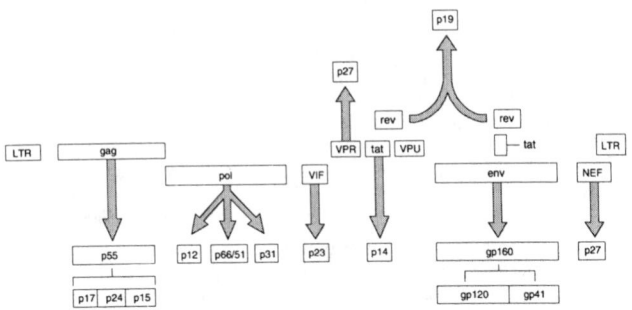

Footnotes

1. Mellors JW, Kingsley LA, Rinaldo CR Jr, et al, "Quantitation of HIV-1 RNA in Plasma Predicts Outcome After Seroconversion," *Ann Intern Med*, 1995, 122(8):573-9.
2. Cao Y, Qin L, Zhang L, et al, "Virologic and Immunologic Characterization of Long-Term Survivors of Human Immunodeficiency Virus Type 1 Infection," *N Engl J Med*, 1995, 332(4):201-8.
3. Kloser PC, Mangia AJ, Leonard J, et al, "HIV-2-Associated AIDS in the United States. The First Case," *Arch Intern Med*, 1989, 149(8):1875-7.
4. "Human Immunodeficiency Virus (HIV) Infection. American College of Physicians and Infectious Diseases Society of America," *Ann Intern Med*, 1994, 120(4):310-9.

References

Belshe RB, Clements ML, Keefer MC, et al, "Interpreting HIV Serodiagnostic Test Results in the 1990s: Social Risks of HIV Vaccine Studies in Uninfected Volunteers," *Ann Intern Med*, 1994, 121(8):584-9.

Burke DS, Brundage JF, Redfield RR, et al, "Measurement of the False Positive Rate in a Screening Program for Human Immunodeficiency Virus Infections," *N Engl J Med*, 1988, 319(15):961-4.

Centers for Disease Control, "Interpretation and Use of the Western Blot Assay for Serodiagnosis of Human Immunodeficiency Virus Type 1 Infections," *MMWR Morb Mortal Wkly Rep*, 1989, 38(Suppl 7):1-7.

Consortium for Retrovirus Serology Standardization, "Serologic Diagnosis of Human Immunodeficiency Virus Infection by Western Blot Testing," *JAMA*, 1988, 260(5):674-9.

Craven DE, Steger KA, La Chapelle R, et al, "Factitious HIV Infection: The Importance of Documenting Infection," *Ann Intern Med*, 1994, 121(10):763-6.

Cumming PD, Wallace EL, Schorr JB, et al, "Exposure of Patients to Human Immunodeficiency Virus Through the Transfusion of Blood Components That Test Antibody-Negative," *N Engl J Med*, 1989, 321(14):941-6.

Davey RT and Vasudevachari MB, "Serologic Evaluation of Patients With Human Immunodeficiency Virus Infection," *Manual of Clinical Laboratory Immunology*, 4th ed, Vol 2, Rose NR, Conway de Macario E, Fahey JL, et al, eds, Washington DC: American Society for Microbiology, 1992, 364-70.

De Cock KM, Porter A, Kouadio J, et al, "Cross-Reactivity on Western Blots in HIV-1 and HIV-2 Infections," *AIDS*, 1991, 5(7):859-63.

Dodd RY, "The Risk of Transfusion-Transmiteed Infection," *N Engl J Med*, 1992, 327(6):419-21.

Fauci AS and Lane HC, "Human Immunodeficiency Virus (HIV) Disease: AIDS and Related Disorders," *Harrison's Principles of Internal Medicine*, 13th ed, Isselbacher KJ, Braunwald E, Wilson JD, et al, eds, New York, NY: McGraw-Hill Inc, 1994, 1566-611.

Hollander H, "Cerebrospinal Fluid Normalities and Abnormalities in Individuals Infected With Human Immunodeficiency Virus," *J Infect Dis*, 1988, 158(4):855-8.

Imagawa DT, Lee MH, Wolinsky SM, et al, "Human Immunodeficiency Virus Type 1 Infection in Homosexual Men Who Remain Seronegative for Prolonged Periods," *N Engl J Med*, 1989, 320(22):1458-62.

Krieger JN, "Acquired Immunodeficiency Syndrome Antibody Testing and Precautions," *J Urol*, 1992, 147(3):713-6.

Leitman SF, Klein HG, Melpolder JJ, et al, "Clinical Implications of Positive Tests for Antibodies to Human Immunodeficiency Virus Type 1 in Asymptomatic Blood Donors," *N Engl J Med*, 1989, 321(14):917-24.

MacDonald KL, Jackson JB, Bowman RJ, et al, "Performance Characteristics of Serologic Tests for Human Immunodeficiency Virus Type 1 (HIV-1) Antibody Among Minnesota Blood Donors," *Ann Intern Med*, 1989, 110(8):617-21.

O'Gorman MR, Weber D, Landis SE, et al, "Interpretive Criteria of the Western Blot Assay for Serodiagnosis of Human Immunodeficiency Virus Type 1 Infection," *Arch Pathol Lab Med*, 1991, 115(1):26-30.

Pomerantz RJ, "HIV/AIDS," *Clin Lab Med*, 1994, 14(2).

Quinn TC, "Screening for HIV Infection - Benefits and Costs," *N Engl J Med*, 1992, 327(7):486-8.

HIV Antibody *see* HIV-1/HIV-2 Serology *on previous page*

HIV Core Antigen *see* p24 Antigen *on page 420*

HLA-Antigen B27 *see* HLA-B27 *on this page*

HLA-B8 *see* Smooth Muscle Antibody *on page 431*

HLA-B27

CPT 86812

Related Information
HLA Typing, Single Human Leukocyte Antigen *on next page*
Rheumatoid Factor *on page 427*
Tissue Typing *on page 434*

Synonyms B27; HLA-Antigen B27

Applies to Human Leukocyte Antigen

Test Commonly Includes Human leukocyte antigen testing for locus B27

Abstract HLA-B27 is an allele of the human HLA-B locus. Found at the major histocompatibility complex, HLA antigens are gene products.

Specimen Leukocytes

Container Green top (heparin) tube

Storage Instructions Store at room temperature; do not refrigerate

Special Instructions Sample must be tested as soon as possible; testing should be prearranged

Reference Range Requires clinical correlation

Use Evaluate spondyloarthritis, juvenile rheumatoid arthritis, Reiter's syndrome, psoriatic arthritis and anterior uveitis

Limitations An adequate test requires the presence of viable lymphocytes at the time of testing unless other testing methodology is used (eg, flow cytometry, molecular, ELISA). Even taking appropriate precautions, an occasional specimen will not be satisfactory for testing. In such cases, fresh blood should be drawn for retesting. False-positives may occur.

Methodology Incubation of lymphocyte suspensions with antisera to specific B27 locus. If lymphocytes bind the antisera (are B27 positive), they will be killed when complement is added. Live cells can be differentiated from dead ones by supravital dye (eosin, trypan blue) exclusion. Direct immunofluorescence and flow cytometry methods are in use.

Additional Information HLA-B27 bears a strong association with but is not found in all patients with ankylosing spondylitis (Marie-Strumpell disease); over 90% of such patients are positive. HLA-B27 antigen shares homology with a *Klebsiella* protein, which may imply a bacterial pathogenesis to ankylosing spondylitis. A B27-positive patient with consistent clinical and radiographic findings has approximately 100 times greater chance of having or developing ankylosing spondylitis than has a negative patient. However, the antigen is not causative, and 10% of normal subjects are B27 positive. **This test should not be considered a screening procedure for ankylosing spondylitis.** The antigen is less strongly associated with Reiter's syndrome and other arthritides than with ankylosing spondylitis. Other associations include psoriatic arthritis and juvenile rheumatoid arthritis. It has been linked with congenital deficiency of C4 and C2, adrenal hyperplasia, and with inflammatory bowel disease.

References

Braun WE and Zachary AA, "The HLA Histocompatibility System in Autoimmune States," *Clin Lab Med*, 1988, 8(2):351-72.

Keat A, "Reiter's Syndrome and Reactive Arthritis in Perspective," *N Engl J Med*, 1983, 309:1606-15.

Khan MA and Khan MK, "Diagnostic Value of HLA-B27 Testing in Ankylosing Spondylitis and Reiter's Syndrome," *Ann Intern Med*, 1982, 96:70-5.

Lipsky PE and Taurog JD, "The Second International Simmons Center Conference on HLA-B27-Related Disorders," *Arthritis Rheum*, 1991, 34(11):1476-82.

Yu DT, Choo SY, and Schaack T, "Molecular Mimicry in HLA-B27 Related Arthritis," *Ann Intern Med*, 1989, 111(7):581-91.

HLA Class II Antigens *see* Mixed Lymphocyte Culture *on page 418*

HLA-DP *see* Mixed Lymphocyte Culture *on page 418*

HLA-DQ *see* Mixed Lymphocyte Culture *on page 418*

HLA-DR *see* Mixed Lymphocyte Culture *on page 418*

HLA DR3 *see* Sjögren's Antibodies *on page 430*

HLA DRw52 *see* Sjögren's Antibodies *on page 430*

HLA Typing *see* Tissue Typing *on page 434*

HLA Typing, Crossmatch *see* Tissue Typing *on page 434*

HLA Typing, Single Human Leukocyte Antigen

CPT 86812

Related Information

HLA-B27 *on previous page*
Identification DNA Testing *on page 517*
Mixed Lymphocyte Culture *on page 418*
Paternity Studies *on page 613*
Rheumatoid Factor *on page 427*
Tissue Typing *on page 434*

Applies to Adhesion Molecule CD31; Major Histocompatibility Coded Antigens; Major Histocompatibility Complex (MHC)

Test Commonly Includes Identification of human leukocyte antigens (HLA) antigens

Abstract The major histocompatibility complex (MHC) exists as a group of genes which are closely linked. They encode the HLA antigens, which are the major histocompatibility antigens. They determine compatibility between donor and recipient in transplantation, and therefore are expressed as "major." The HLA antigen captures foreign peptides, to present to antigen-binding T-cell receptors.[1]

Specimen Leukocytes

Container Green top (heparin) tube

Collection Deliver immediately to the laboratory.

Storage Instructions Maintain at room temperature. Do not refrigerate.

Special Instructions Schedule in advance, since the test requires viable lymphocytes.

Reference Range Identification of specific leukocyte antigens

Use Epidemiologic marker, correlation with disease syndromes, paternity exclusion testing, transplantation candidate matching to diminish likelihood of rejection, eg, attempt to avoid graft-versus-host disease (GVHD)

or graft rejection, following major organ or bone marrow transplantation. The risk of GVHD exists even when donor and recipient share major antigens. Recently, mismatch of HA-1, a minor antigen, was recognized as a cause of GVHD in allogeneic bone marrow grafts from otherwise HLA-identical donors. Mismatches of HA-2, -4, and -5 in HLA-A2 positive donor-recipient pairs also correlate with GVHD.[2] Typing of the adhesion molecule CD31 may further diminish risk of acute GVHD.[3]

HLA matching of platelets may be indicated.

Limitations The clinical significance of many of the marker antigens is not well defined. HLA typing is not inexpensive.

Methodology HLA class I typing (A, B, and C loci) usually is done by use of a dye exclusion (eosin, trypan blue) method to assess lymphocyte viability after reaction with various HLA-directed antisera and complement (serology); molecular methods also used.

HLA class II typing (DR, DQ, and DP) by serological methods similar to those described above and may use B cells since T cells lack class II antigens. More HLA typing laboratories are moving toward using molecular methods for DR, DQ, and DP typing. Examples are PCR with sequence-specific primers, sequence-specific oligonucleotide probes and even DNA sequencing.

Peripheral blood leukocytes isolated by Ficoll-Isopaque density-gradient centrifugation, washed, and resuspended in RPMI-1640 medium were used for matching for marrow transplantation. Ten percent dimethyl sulfoxide was utilized for cryopreservation in liquid nitrogen.[2]

Additional Information The HLA system has been generally categorized into class I, class II, and class III gene regions. HLA class I genes including the A, B, and C locus genes and their respective antigens are expressed on most nucleated cells. The HLA class II genes encode a glycoprotein with two noncovalently associated chains (alpha and beta). The class II region encodes the complement proteins, C2, C4, and factor B of the alternative complement pathway. HLA class I and II molecules act as receptors for processed self and foreign peptides for presentation to CD8- and CD4-positive T cells, respectively. Most HLA genes are highly polymorphic, which accounts for their recognition in transplantation. Many of the alleles of these genes are in linkage disequilibrium. Many of these antigens have been more or less closely associated statistically with a wide ranging variety of illness, both physical and mental. The most striking association is that of HLA-B27 with ankylosing spondylitis. Another significant association is HLA-B8 and sarcoidosis. Many associations with SLE are known, as well as with other autoimmune disorders. However, none of these is an aid to diagnosis. Hereditary hemochromatosis is associated with HLA-A3, B7, and B14. HLA-A3 is found in about 70% of subjects with hemochromatosis, but the expense of HLA typing favors use of transferrin saturation and serum ferritin. Hemochromatosis is inherited as an autosomal recessive[4] and is HLA-linked.

HLA typing is also performed for cadaveric renal transplantation, in conjunction with ABO typing and crossmatching, since the degree of HLA mismatch between the recipient and donor is one component of the kidney allocation algorithm. These HLA molecules are the targets of rejection in GVHD.

The system is useful in exclusion of paternity and in forensic medicine, since the HLA system includes many alleles which can be identified in addition to the many red cell antigenic systems.

MHC antigens are a portion of the HLA system, a cluster of genes which encode HLA molecules on chromosome 6. Rheumatoid arthritis is associated with MHC class II molecules in many patients (eg, DR). Protective haplotypes exist as well. Rheumatoid arthritis is a polygenic process.[5]

Footnotes

1. Kernan NA and DuPont B, "Minor Histocompatibility Antigens and Marrow Transplantation," *N Engl J Med*, 1996, 334(5):323-4 (editorial).

2. Goulmy E, Schipper R, Pool J, et al, "Mismatches of Minor Histocompatibility Antigens Between HLA-Identical Donors and Recipients and the Development of Graft-Versus-Host Disease After Bone Marrow Transplantation," *N Engl J Med*, 1996, 334(5):281-5.

3. Behar E, Chao NJ, Hiraki DD, et al, "Polymorphism of Adhesion Molecule CD31 and Its Role in Acute Graft-Versus-Host Disease," *N Engl J Med*, 1996, 334(5):286-91.

4. Edwards CQ and Kushner JP, "Screening for Hemochromatosis," *N Engl J Med*, 1993, 328(22):1616-20.

5. Harris ED Jr, "Excitement and Confusion About HLA and Rheumatoid Arthritis," *Ann Intern Med*, 1995, 123(3):232-3 (editorial).

References

Bodmer JG, Albert ED, Bodmer WF, et al, "Nomenclature for Factors of the HLA System, 1990," *Immunogenetics*, 1991, 33:301-9.

Braun WE and Zachary AA, "The HLA Histocompatibility System in Autoimmune States," *Clin Lab Med*, 1988, 8(2):351-72.

Colvin RB, Bhan AK, and McCluskey RT, *Diagnostic Immunopathology*, New York, NY: Raven Press, 1988, 159.

Hansen TH, Carreno BM, and Sachs DH, "The Major Histocompatibility Complex," *Fundamental Immunology*, 3rd ed, Chapter 16, Paul WE, ed, New York, NY: Raven Press, 1993, 577.

Marsh SG and Bodmer JG, "HLA Class II Nucleotide Sequences, 1991," *Immunogenetics*, 1991, 33(5-6):321-34.

Peter JB and Hawkins BR, "The New HLA," *Arch Pathol Lab Med*, 1992, 116(1):11-5.

(Continued)

HLA Typing, Single Human Leukocyte Antigen
(Continued)

Sanfilippo F, "The Influence of HLA and ABO Antigens on Graft Rejection and Survival," *Clin Lab Med*, 1991, 11(3):537-50.

Zemmour J and Parham P, "HLA Class I Nucleotide Sequences, 1991," *Immunogenetics*, 1991, 33(3-5):310-20.

HSV Antibodies *see* Herpes Simplex Antibody *on page 401*

HTLV-I/II Antibody

CPT 86687 (HTLV-I); 86688 (HTLV-II)

Related Information

Donation, Blood *on page 607*

HIV-1/HIV-2 Serology *on page 403*

Human Immunodeficiency Virus DNA Amplification *on page 515*

Polymerase Chain Reaction *on page 523*

Risks of Transfusion *on page 623*

Synonyms Human T-Cell Leukemia Virus Type I and Type II; Human T-Lymphotropic Virus Type I Antibody

Test Commonly Includes Screening test with confirmation of positives

Abstract Human T-lymphotropic virus type I (HTLV-I) and type II (HTLV-II) are two closely related retroviruses discovered by Dr Robert Gallo in the 1970s. The viruses can cause, after lengthy incubation periods, leukemia and neuromuscular disease.

Specimen Serum

Container Red top tube

Reference Range Negative

Use Screen blood and blood products for transfusion; differential diagnosis of spastic myelopathy for HTLV-I. HTLV-I is also the causative virus for adult T-cell acute lymphoblastic leukemia (ALL). HTLV-II has been associated with chronic neuromuscular diseases.

Limitations The combined assay for Anti HTLV-I/II is used mainly to screen blood donors. The assay cross reacts with only 80% of patients with antibody to HTLV-II.[1] The 20% of blood donors who are not detected by the assay for HTLV-II are not at sufficiently high risk to transmit the disease to warrant a separate assay.

Methodology Screen: enzyme immunoassay (EIA); confirmation: Western blot (WB) or radioimmunoprecipitation (RIPA). Western blot is associated with a large number of indeterminate results, neither positive nor negative.[2]

Additional Information HTLV-I is a pathogenic retrovirus which is irregularly distributed in the world. Infection is generally uncommon in the U.S. and Europe. The virus is most common in Japan and the Carribean. The virus can be asymptomatic for prolonged periods (20 years) but is strongly associated with myelopathies and adult T-cell leukemia. Less than 5% of those infected with HTLV-I develop myelopathies or leukemia even after 20 years. Adult T-cell leukemia is an aggressive malignancy of T lymphocytes often associated with skin infiltrates and hypercalcemia. The virus is tropic for T4 lymphocytes and is passed by sexual contact, blood products, from mother to fetus, and by breast milk. Pretransfusion testing for antibody to HTLV-I is now mandated by blood banks, in order to avoid transfusion transmitted HTLV-I infection from asymptomatic infected donors. Retrospective studies from the American Red Cross have concluded that about 700 individuals per year received HTLV-I/II blood prior to 1988 when donor testing began. The risk of this is extremely low (0.024% per unit). Early seroconverters have antibodies to the C-terminal region of gp46 (envelope protein) and to gag p19 and p24. The clinical course of HTLV-I infection, and the meaning of a positive serology are not yet well understood. Indeed, a recent study of hemophiliacs who were transfused regularly with plasma or its derivatives found no evidence of HTLV-I/II antibody in 179 patients.

Footnotes

1. CDCP and USPHS Working Group, "Guidelines for Counseling Persons Infected With Human T-Lymphotropic Virus Type I (HTLV-I) and Type II (HTLV-II)," *Ann Intern Med*, 1993, 118(6):448-54.

2. Zaaijer HL, Cuypers HT, Dudok de Wit C, et al, "Results of 1-Year Screening of Donors in the Netherlands for Human T-Lymphotropic Virus (HTLV) Type I: Significance of Western Blot Patterns for Confirmation of HTLV Infection," *Transfusion*, 1994, 34(10):877-80.

References

Blattner WA, "Human T-Lymphotropic Viruses and Diseases of Long Latency," *Ann Intern Med*, 1989, 111(1):4-6.

Canavaggio M, Leckie G, Allain JP, et al, "The Prevalence of Antibody to HTLV I/II in United States Plasma Donors and in United States and French Hemophiliacs," *Transfusion*, 1990, 30(9):780-2.

Chen YM, Gomez-Lucia E, Okayama A, et al, "Antibody Profile of Early HTLV-I Infection," *Lancet*, 1990, 336(8725):1214-6.

Gessain A and Gout O, "Chronic Myelopathy Associated With Human T-Lymphotropic Virus Type I (HTLV-I)," *Ann Intern Med*, 1992, 117(11):933-46.

Sullivan MT, Williams AE, Fang CT, et al, "Transmission of Human T-Lymphotropic Virus Types I and II by Blood Transfusion," *Arch Intern Med*, 1991, 151(10):2043-8.

Washitani Y, Kuroda N, Shiraki H, et al, "Serological Discrimination Between HTLV-I and HTLV-II Antibodies by ELISA Using Synthetic Peptides as Antigens," *Int J Cancer*, 1991, 49(2):173-7.

Human Herpesvirus 6, IgG and IgM Antibodies, Quantitative

CPT 86790

Related Information

Human Herpesvirus 6 Culture *on page 669*

Human Herpesvirus 6 DNA Detection *on page 515*

Infectious Mononucleosis Screening Test *on page 410*

Synonyms HHV-6, IgM, IgG

Test Commonly Includes Detection and quantitation of antibodies to human herpesvirus 6 (HHV-6)

Abstract HHV-6 causes exanthem subitum, an acute febrile illness in children usually occurring in the first 2 years of life. It has caused fatal encephalitis in a bone marrow transplant recipient and has been implicated in interstitial pneumonitis and bone marrow suppression following transplantation.[1]

Specimen Serum

Container Red top tube or serum separator tube

Collection Acute and convalescent specimens are recommended. Specimens should be free from bacterial contamination and hemolysis.

Storage Instructions Refrigerate serum.

Causes for Rejection Gross lipemia

Critical Values An increase in IgG HHV-6 (fourfold increase in titer) between acute and convalescent samples is evidence of a recent HHV-6 infection.

Use IgM HHV-6 may aid in the diagnosis of acute or recent infection with HHV-6.

Methodology Indirect fluorescent antibody (IFA)

Additional Information Human herpesvirus 6 (HHV-6) has recently been identified as an agent associated with both pediatric and adult infections. Most infections are asymptomatic and usually children have been infected by 3 years of age. The illness in children is characterized clinically by an acute febrile illness, irritability, inflammation of tympanic membranes, and (uncommonly) a rash characteristic of roseola. When acute and convalescent (4-6 weeks later) serum samples are compared, a fourfold rise in HHV-6 IgG titer is typical. In adults, HHV-6 has been associated with spontaneously resolving fever resembling a mononucleosis-like illness. HHV-6 has also been implicated in post-transplant infections.[1] During the acute episode an elevated IgM HHV-6 is useful. An increase in IgG HHV-6 between acute and convalescent serum sample is consistent with a recent HHV-6 infection.

Footnotes

1. Drobyski WR, Knox KK, Majewski D, et al, "Brief Report: Fatal Encephalitis Due to Variant B Human Herpesvirus-6 Infection in a Bone Marrow Transplant Recipient," *N Engl J Med*, 1994, 330(19):1356-60.

References

Buchwald D, Cheney PR, Peterson DL, et al, "A Chronic Illness Characterized by Fatigue, Neurologic and Immunologic Disorders, and Active Human Herpesvirus Type 6 Infection," *Ann Intern Med*, 1992, 116(2):103-13.

Hall CB, Long CE, Schnabel KC, et al, "Human Herpesvirus-6 Infection in Children. A Prospective Study of Complications and Reactivation," *N Engl J Med*, 1994, 331(7):432-8.

Irving WL and Cunningham AL, "Serological Diagnosis of Infection With Human Herpesvirus Type 6," *BMJ*, 1990, 300(6718):156-9.

Pruksananonda P, Hall CB, Insel RA, et al, "Primary Human Herpesvirus 6 Infection in Young Children," *N Engl J Med*, 1992, 326(22):1445-50.

Steeper TA, Horwitz CA, Ablashi DV, et al, "The Spectrum of Clinical and Laboratory Findings Resulting From Human Herpesvirus-6 (HHV-6) in Patients With Mononucleosis-Like Illnesses Not Resulting From Epstein-Barr Virus or Cytomegalovirus," *Am J Clin Pathol*, 1990, 93(6):776-83.

Human Immunodeficiency Virus Serology *see* HIV-1/HIV-2 Serology *on page 403*

Human Leukocyte Antigen *see* HLA-B27 *on page 404*

Human Leukocyte Antigens *see* Tissue Typing *on page 434*

Human T-Cell Leukemia Virus Type I and Type II *see* HTLV-I/II Antibody *on this page*

Human T-Lymphotropic Virus Type I Antibody *see* HTLV-I/II Antibody *on this page*

Hydatid Disease Serological Test *see* Echinococcosis Serological Test *on page 390*

Hypersensitivity Pneumonitis Serology

CPT 86329

Related Information

Bacterial Culture, Sputum *on page 465*

Synonyms Extrinsic Allergic Alveolitis Serology; Farmer's Lung Disease Serology

Applies to *Aspergillus fumigatus* Precipitating Antibodies; *Aspergillus niger* Precipitating Antibodies; *Micropolyspora faeni* Precipitating Antibodies; *Thermoactinomyces vulgaris* Precipitating Antibodies; *Thermolospora viridis* Precipitating Antibodies

Replaces *Thermoactinomyces* Precipitating Antibodies

Test Commonly Includes *Micropolyspora faeni*, *Aspergillus fumigatus*, *Alternaria* sp, *Aspergillus niger*, *Thermoactinomyces vulgaris*, *Thermolospora viridis* antigen testing by immunodiffusion of combined antigenic extract.

Abstract The diagnostic expression **hypersensitivity pneumonitis** (extrinsic allergic alveolitis) applies to types of acute, subacute, or chronic interstitial lung disease which are caused by inhaled organic dusts derived from living sources: *vide supra*.

Specimen Serum

Container Red top tube

Reference Range Negative

Use Support the clinical diagnosis of hypersensitivity pneumonitis in those, following repeated exposure to moist hay or grains, developing fever, chills, and dyspnea.

Limitations A positive test does not establish the diagnosis of hypersensitivity pneumonitis, nor does the absence of precipitins eliminate the diagnosis. Open lung biopsy may be needed to establish the diagnosis. T cells participate in the alveolitis.

Methodology Immunodiffusion (ID)

Additional Information Some individuals become sensitized to inhaled antigens and develop acute bronchospastic symptoms 4-6 hours following exposure to them. Many of these have been diagnosed with disease names indicating the nature of the exposure (ie, bird-fancier's disease, farmer's lung, mushroom-picker's disease, silo-filler's disease, maple bark-stripper's disease, paprika-slicer's lung, sauna-taker's lung). The antigen material is usually an *Aspergillus* sp or one of the thermophilic actinomycetes. Individuals with precipitating antibodies may have no symptoms, and patients with severe symptoms may not show antibody while their disease is inactive. Thus, there must be careful correlation of clinical and laboratory results.

References
Colby TV, Lombard C, Yousen SA, et al, *Atlas of Pulmonary Surgical Pathology*, Philadelphia, PA: WB Saunders Co, 1991, 260-3.
Sharma OP, "Hypersensitivity Pneumonitis," *Dis Mon*, 1991, 37(7):409-71.

i Antigen *see* Cold Agglutinin Titer *on page 384*

I Antigen of Red Cell Membranes *see* Cold Agglutinin Titer *on page 384*

IEP, Serum or Urine *see* Immunoelectrophoresis, Serum or Urine *on next page*

IF Antibody *see* Intrinsic Factor Antibody *on page 411*

IFE *see* Immunofixation Electrophoresis *on next page*

IgA *see* Immunoglobulin A *on next page*

IgA Antibodies

CPT 86329

Related Information
Immunoglobulin A *on next page*
Risks of Transfusion *on page 623*

Synonyms Anti-immunoglobulin A

Abstract IgA deficient patients may suffer from hypersensitivity reactions to transfused IgA in blood fractions. Although immunoglobulins including IgA are assayed to evaluate immunity and disease entities such as myeloma, this test measures an antibody to an immunoglobulin antigen.

Specimen Serum

Container Red top tube

Sampling Time Ideally, prior to transfusion of blood or blood fractions in persons with history of anaphylaxis following exposure to small amounts of plasma, blood, or blood fractions

Reference Range Antibody not present

Use Evaluate transfusion reaction symptoms or history of such symptoms as dyspnea, laryngeal edema, bronchospasm, nausea, chills, stridor, sweating, substernal pain, abdominal cramps, emesis, diarrhea, flushing, hypotension, and collapse following infusion of very small quantities of blood[1]

Limitations Unfortunately, laboratory methods to detect IgE and IgG anti-IgA are not standardized. A negative assay does not rule out the possibility of an IgE-mediated anaphylactic event.

Of individuals subject to anaphylaxis on exposure to IgA, some have deficiency only to certain subclasses of IgA.

Methodology Immunodiffusion (ID)

Additional Information Approximately 1 in 500-1000 individuals is IgA deficient. Such individuals can develop antibodies to IgA, which they recognize as a foreign protein. If such a patient, with antibody to IgA, is transfused with blood or plasma containing IgA, he/she may experience an anaphylactic reaction. Patients with a history of anaphylactic reaction to blood transfusion should be tested for IgG and IgE antibody to IgA. Saline-washed or frozen, deglycerolized red cells with premedication or autologous transfusion should be used for such patients. Some workers have recommended that all IgA-deficient patients receive blood fractions lacking IgA. Such blood may be available although generally not on a stat basis. At the least, one should have epinephrine and hydrocortisone ready if signs of anaphylaxis appear. Injection of immunoglobulin can cause such reaction because immunoglobulin preparations contain some IgA.[1]

Footnotes
1. Mollison PL, Engelfriet CP, and Contreras M, "Some Unfavorable Effects of Transfusion," *Blood Transfusion in Clinical Medicine*, 9th ed, Oxford, UK: Blackwell Scientific Publications, 1993, 691-3.

References
Keren DF and Warren JS, "Immunodeficiency," *Diagnostic Immunology*, Baltimore, MD: Williams & Wilkins, 1992, 107-8.

IgD *see* Immunoglobulin D *on page 409*

IgE *see* Immunoglobulin E *on page 409*

IgG *see* Immunoglobulin G *on page 409*

IgG₁ *see* Immunoglobulin G Subclasses *on page 410*

IgG₂ *see* Immunoglobulin G Subclasses *on page 410*

IgG₃ *see* Immunoglobulin G Subclasses *on page 410*

IgG₄ *see* Immunoglobulin G Subclasses *on page 410*

IgG Antibodies to Rubella *see* Rubella Serology *on page 428*

IgG, CSF *see* Cerebrospinal Fluid Immunoglobulin G *on page 378*

IgG Ratios and IgG Index, Cerebrospinal Fluid *see* Cerebrospinal Fluid IgG Ratios and IgG Index *on page 377*

IgG Subclasses *see* Immunoglobulin G Subclasses *on page 410*

IgG Synthesis Rate, Cerebrospinal Fluid *see* Cerebrospinal Fluid IgG Synthesis Rate *on page 378*

IgM *see* Immunoglobulin M *on page 410*

IgM Antibodies to Rubella *see* Rubella Serology *on page 428*

Immune Complex Assay

CPT 86332

Applies to Conglutinin Solid-Phase Assay; Immune Complex by C1q Binding; Monoclonal Rheumatoid Factor Inhibition

Specimen Serum

Container Red top tube

Storage Instructions If immune complex by Raji cell is requested, serum must be frozen within 2 hours.

Reference Range Complexes not detected

Use These are nonspecific assays used in the past for monitoring some autoimmune diseases.

Limitations Certain cryoglobulins, cold agglutinins, rheumatoid factors, and paraproteins may cause false-positive results. Immune complex assays were once thought to be promising assays to follow patients with autoimmune disease. Due to their lack of specificity and poor correlation with each other, they no longer have diagnostic use. They may be useful in research and epidemiologic settings. **As these tests are expensive, rule nothing in or out, and are poorly standardized, we do not recommend they be used.**

Methodology C1q and monoclonal rheumatoid factor can bind to immunoglobulins in complexes and then be precipitated and quantitated. Raji cells and conglutinin bind the complement components of the complexes.

References
Colvin RB, Bhan AK, and McCluskey RT, *Diagnostic Immunopathology*, New York, NY: Raven Press, 1988, 27-9.
Keren DF, "Assays for Circulating Immune Complexes," *Clinical Laboratory Annual*, Batsakis JG and Homburger HA, eds, New York, NY: Appleton-Century-Crofts, 1985, 105-23.
Keren DF and Warren JS, "Agglutination, Precipitation, and Hemolytic Reactions," *Diagnostic Immunology*, Baltimore, MD: Williams & Wilkins, 1992, 288-90.

Immune Complex by C1q Binding *see* Immune Complex Assay *on this page*

Immune Complex Detection by C1q *see* C1q Immune Complex Detection *on page 373*

Immunodeficiency Profile *see* CD4/CD8 Enumeration *on page 375*

Immunoelectrophoresis see Protein Electrophoresis, Urine *on page 425*

Immunoelectrophoresis, Serum see Protein Electrophoresis, Serum *on page 424*

Immunoelectrophoresis, Serum or Urine

CPT 86320 (serum); 86325 (other fluids)

Related Information

Immunofixation Electrophoresis *on this page*
Protein Electrophoresis, Serum *on page 424*
Protein Electrophoresis, Urine *on page 425*
Protein, Quantitative, Urine *on page 649*
Protein, Total, Serum *on page 194*

Synonyms IEP, Serum or Urine

Applies to Dysgammaglobulinemia; Kappa and Lambda Light Chains Detection; Light Chains; Monoclonal Gammopathy; Paraproteinemia

Replaces Bence Jones Protein Test

Test Commonly Includes Typing of monoclonal proteins for light and heavy chain specificity

Specimen Serum or urine

Container Red top tube or plastic urine container

Reference Range Interpretation by pathologist

Use Recognize monoclonal gammopathy; diagnose myeloma, macroglobulinemia of Waldenström; evaluate monoclonal gammopathy (M spot or M spike) found in serum protein electrophoresis; evaluate amyloidosis; application to the evaluation of lymphoproliferative diseases (malignant lymphoma and others) and connective tissue diseases in general; diagnose and characterize immune-deficient and dysgammaglobulinemic states.

Limitations Immunoelectrophoresis is not quantitative. It is being replaced by immunofixation, which is more sensitive and easier to interpret. In most laboratories IgD and IgE specific reagents are not used routinely. Monoclonal gammopathies <300 mg/dL are difficult to detect with IEP. Large molecular weight monoclonal gammopathies (eg, Waldenström's macroglobulinemia) often require treatment with 2-mercaptoethanol prior to IEP or false-negatives will occur.

Methodology Electrophoresis of specimen, followed by immunodiffusion (ID) against monospecific antisera to immunoglobulin and individual heavy and light chains

Additional Information Immunoelectrophoresis of serum or urine is most often ordered to evaluate a monoclonal globulin detected in a protein electrophoresis or to delineate a possible lymphoproliferative process, particularly myeloma. This procedure will characterize the specific light and heavy chain components of a monoclonal protein. It may be useful in defining deficiencies of specific immunoglobulins or other serum proteins, however, it is not a quantitative technique and nephelometry of specific immunoglobulins is preferred for detection of immunodeficiencies. Specific identification of abnormal proteins is performed in an increasing number of clinical laboratories by immunofixation (IF). IF combines high resolution electrophoresis with immunoprecipitation. This method is more rapid and sensitive than immunoelectrophoresis.

References

Gochman N and Burke MA, "Electrophoretic Techniques in Today's Clinical Laboratory," *Clin Lab Med*, 1986, 6(3):403-26.

Keren DF, "Immunofixation Techniques," *High-Resolution Electrophoresis and Immunofixation: Techniques and Interpretation*, Boston, MA: Butterworth's Publishers, 1987, 107-130.

Sun T, *Interpretation of Protein and Isoenzyme Patterns in Body Fluids*, New York, NY: Igaku-Shoin, 1991.

Immunofixation Electrophoresis

CPT 86334

Related Information

Bone Marrow *on page 307*
Immunoelectrophoresis, Serum or Urine *on this page*
Immunoglobulin A *on this page*
Immunoglobulin G *on next page*
Immunoglobulin M *on page 410*
Lymph Node Biopsy *on page 50*
Protein Electrophoresis, Serum *on page 424*
Protein Electrophoresis, Urine *on page 425*
Protein, Quantitative, Urine *on page 649*
Protein, Total, Serum *on page 194*
Urine Collection, 24-Hour *on page 30*
Viscosity, Serum/Plasma *on page 350*

Synonyms IFE

Applies to Dysgammaglobulinemia Evaluation; Isotypes, Light Chains; Kappa Chains; Lambda Chains; Light Chains; Monoclonal Gammopathy; M Protein; Paraprotein Evaluation

Replaces Bence Jones Protein Test

Test Commonly Includes Identification of monoclonal gammopathies, pathologist interpretation

Abstract Immunofixation electrophoresis (IFE) has become the assay of choice to characterize monoclonal gammopathies.

Specimen Serum, 24-hour urine

Container Red top tube, plastic urine container

Collection Urine: See procedure for collection of a 24-hour urine. No preservative required.

Storage Instructions Separate serum from cells, centrifuge and/or filter urine.

Reference Range Interpretation by pathologist

Use Immunofixation electrophoresis of serum or urine is used to evaluate a monoclonal globulin (M spot or spike) detected in a protein electrophoresis or to delineate a possible lymphoproliferative process, particularly myeloma or macroglobulinemia, and amyloidosis. It is the assay of choice because it does not suffer from the false-negatives seen in serum immunoelectrophoresis. Especially helpful in recognition of biclonal gammopathies, small monoclonal gammopathies, and when results of immunoelectrophoresis are not definitive.

This procedure will characterize the specific light and heavy chain components of a monoclonal protein. **Bence Jones proteins** are homogeneous urinary light chain proteins of kappa or lambda type, monoclonal fragments which include a monoclonal light chain component. (Kappa and lambda are the two light chain isotypes.) IFE is the assay of choice for examination of urine for Bence Jones protein. Conventional electrophoresis is sometimes too insensitive.

Methodology High resolution electrophoresis combined with immunoprecipitation

Additional Information Although quantification of kappa and lambda chains in urine by nephelometry has been suggested as an alternative, it is too insensitive at the present to be practical. Urinary light chain ladder patterns may be confused with Bence Jones protein.[1]

Monoclonal Ig light chains, usually kappa, deposited in glomerular and tubular basement membranes cause light chain nephropathy. Such light chains are found in urine.

Footnotes

1. Bailey EM, McDermott TJ, and Bloch KJ, "The Urinary Light-Chain Ladder Pattern. A Product of Improved Methodology That May Complicate the Recognition of Bence Jones Proteinuria," *Arch Pathol Lab Med*, 1993, 117(7):707-10.

References

Keren DF, "Immunofixation Techniques," *High-Resolution Electrophoresis and Immunofixation: Techniques and Interpretation*, Boston, MA: Butterworth's Publishers, 1987, 107-30.

Keren DF, Warren JS, and Lowe JB, "Strategy to Diagnose Monoclonal Gammopathies in Serum: High-Resolution Electrophoresis, Immunofixation, and Kappa/Lambda Quantification," *Clin Chem*, 1988, 34(11):2196-201.

Levinson SS, "Studies of Bence Jones Proteins by Immunonephelometry," *Ann Clin Lab Sci*, 1992, 22(2):100-9.

Immunoglobulin A

CPT 82784

Related Information

Ataxia-Telangiectasia, Chromosome Breakage Study *on page 274*
IgA Antibodies *on previous page*
Immunofixation Electrophoresis *on this page*
Immunoglobulin G Subclasses *on page 410*
Kidney Profile *on page 153*
Protein, Total, Serum *on page 194*
Risks of Transfusion *on page 623*

Synonyms IgA, Quantitative

Applies to Isotypes

Abstract Five heavy chain isotypes are known: G, M, A, D, and E.

The physiologic role of IgA includes mucosal immunity. IgA is about 13% of serum gamma globulin.

Specimen Serum

Container Red top tube

Storage Instructions Samples suspected of having macroglobulins or cryoglobulins should be drawn and held at 37°C. Samples suspected of containing cold agglutinins should not be refrigerated prior to serum separation from clot.

Reference Range Adults: 85-385 mg/dL. Pediatrics: cord blood 0 mg/dL; 1-3 months 0-30 mg/dL; 3-6 months 4-55 mg/dL; 6-12 months 10-70 mg/dL; 12-24 months 18-111 mg/dL; 24-36 months 21-98 mg/dL; 3-5 years 30-178 mg/dL; 5-8 years 74-265 mg/dL; 8-12 years 68-333 mg/dL; 12-16 years 68-250 mg/dL. Ranges may vary among laboratories. IgA is about 13% of gamma globulin.

Critical Values In IgA monoclonal gammopathy, concentrations as high as 6.0 g/dL occur.

Use Evaluate humoral immunity; diagnose multiple myeloma; monitor therapy in IgA myeloma; evaluate anaphylaxis associated with transfusion of blood and blood components. Association of IgA deficiency with sprue is recognized.

Limitations If samples containing macroglobulins, cryoglobulins, or cold agglutinins are handled at incorrect temperatures, false low values may result. Of individuals subject to anaphylaxis on exposure to IgA, some have deficiency only to certain subclasses of IgA.

Methodology Radial immunodiffusion (RID), rate nephelometry

Additional Information Increased monoclonal IgA may be produced in lymphoproliferative disorders, especially multiple myeloma and "Mediterranean" lymphoma involving bowel. An IgA monoclonal peak >2 g/dL is a major criterion for myeloma. Of subjects with myeloma, about 20% have monoclonal IgA.[1] It may be elevated in a wide range of conditions affecting mucosal surfaces, where IgA is largely produced. Some clinically significant IgA deficiencies have concomitant deficiencies of IgG_2 and IgG_4. IgA may be decreased in patients with chronic sinopulmonary disease, in ataxia-telangiectasia, or congenitally. Patients with congenital IgA deficiency are prone to autoimmune diseases, and may develop antibody to IgA and anaphylaxis if transfused; see listings IgA Antibodies *on page 407* and Risks of Transfusion *on page 623*. IgA levels may rise with exercise and fall during pregnancy.

IgA deficiency bears association with respiratory and other bacterial infection, especially with IgG_2 deficiency. IgA deficiency relates also to giardiasis and severe viral hepatitis.[2]

Footnotes

1. Barlogie B, "Plasma Cell Myeloma," *Williams Hematology*, 5th ed, Chapter 114, Beutler E, Lichtman MA, Colller S, et al, eds, New York, NY: McGraw-Hill Inc, 1995, 1109-26.
2. Masur H and Fauci AS, "Infections in Patients With Inflammatory and Immunologic Defects," *Harrison's Principles of Internal Medicine*, 13th ed, Chapter 81, Isselbacher KJ, Braunwald E, Wilson JD, et al, eds, New York, NY: McGraw-Hill Inc, 1994, 494-8.

Immunoglobulin D

CPT 82784

Synonyms IgD, Quantitative

Abstract This is a vastly overused test. It provides clinically useful information only in characterizing monoclonal gammopathies.

Specimen Serum

Container Red top tube or two microbilirubin tubes

Storage Instructions Store serum at 4°C.

Reference Range 0-14 mg/dL (SI: 0-140 mg/L); IgD is about 0.2% of gamma globulin

Use Investigation of monoclonal gammopathy for diagnosis of IgD myeloma

Limitations Not a screening test

Methodology Radial immunodiffusion (RID), rate nephelometry

Additional Information The significance of IgD in health and disease remains largely obscure. When looking for myeloma, initial investigation usually includes serum protein electrophoresis and quantification of IgG, IgA, IgM, kappa and lambda. In cases in which an unexplained restriction is seen which is not explained by the heavy chain studies obtained, an IgD assay should be performed. Rare IgD-producing myelomas are reported, <1% of reported cases.

References

Bianchi P, MacNamara E, Bergami MR, et al, "Immunochemical Evaluation of Monoclonal Gammopathies: Heavy Chain to Light Chain Ratio Is of Little Practical Value for Detecting IgD Myelomas and Free Light Chains," *Clin Chem*, 1992, 38(2):317-9.

Immunoglobulin E

CPT 82785

Related Information

Aspergillus Serology *on page 369*
Ataxia-Telangiectasia, Chromosome Breakage Study *on page 274*

Synonyms IgE, Quantitative

Patient Preparation Avoid exposure to radioisotopes when assay method is RIA.

Specimen Serum

Container Red top tube

Reference Range Newborn: <12 IU/mL; younger than 1 year: <50 IU/mL; 2-4 years: <100 IU/mL; 5 years and older: <300 IU/mL. One unit equals 2.4 ng of IgE protein.

Use Initial evaluation of atopic/allergic disorders, eosinophilic enteritis. Increases are found with helminthic infestations and with types of angioedema.

Limitations Normal IgE levels do not exclude allergic phenomena.

Methodology Radioimmunosorbent assay, nephelometry

Additional Information IgE antibodies do not fix complement, but can bind to basophils and mast cells. When an allergen is then encountered the cells release a variety of bioactive materials, including histamine,

prostaglandin D_2, leukotrienes C, D and E, and kallikrein, which can produce symptoms as severe as anaphylaxis. The protective role of such antibodies is not clear. IgE is frequently increased in parasitic infestations and atopic individuals. IgE myeloma is extremely rare and should be sought after abnormal protein electrophoresis (restriction) and/or abnormal kappa/lambda ratio unexplained by IgG, IgA, or IgM.

A trait for serum total IgE increase is coinherited with a trait for bronchial hyperresponsiveness. The latter is recognized as a risk factor in asthma.[1]

Footnotes

1. Postma DS, Bleecker ER, Amelung PJ, et al, "Genetic Susceptibility to Asthma - Bronchial Hyperresponsiveness Coinherited With a Major Gene for Atopy," *N Engl J Med*, 1995, 333(14):894-900.

References

Ownby DR, "Allergy Testing: *In Vivo* Versus *In Vitro*," *Pediatr Clin North Am*, 1988, 35(5):995-1009.
Van Arsdel PP Jr and Larson EB, "Diagnostic Tests for Patients With Suspected Allergic Disease," *Ann Intern Med*, 1989, 110(4):304-12.
Williams PB, Dolen WK, Koepke JW, "Comparison of Skin Testing and Three *In Vitro* Assays for Specific IgE in the Clinical Evaluation of Immediate Hypersensitivity," *Ann Allergy*, 1992, 68(1):35-45.

Immunoglobulin G

CPT 82784

Related Information

Ataxia-Telangiectasia, Chromosome Breakage Study *on page 274*
Immunofixation Electrophoresis *on previous page*
Immunoglobulin G Subclasses *on next page*
Protein Electrophoresis, Urine *on page 425*
Protein, Total, Serum *on page 194*

Synonyms IgG, Quantitative

Abstract Criteria for diagnosis of plasma cell myeloma include atypias of plasma cells, marrow plasmacytosis with >30% plasma cells, monoclonal globulin spike ("M spot") on electrophoresis, anemia, and often, lytic bone lesions.

Specimen Serum

Container Red top tube

Storage Instructions Samples suspected of having macroglobulins or cryoglobulins should be drawn and held at 37°C. Samples suspected of containing cold agglutinins should not be refrigerated prior to serum separation from clot.

Special Instructions Requisition must state patient's age.

Reference Range Adults: 564-1765 mg/dL; pediatrics: cord: 662-1793 mg/dL, 1-3 months: 161-713 mg/dL, 3-6 months: 88-563 mg/dL, 6-12 months: 296-1004 mg/dL, 12-24 months: 135-1106 mg/dL, 24-36 months: 517-1346 mg/dL, 3-5 years: 570-1592 mg/dL, 5-8 years: 757-1686 mg/dL, 8-12 years: 851-1805 mg/dL, 12-16 years: 767-1752 mg/dL

Critical Values In plasma cell myeloma, monoclonal IgG is usually >3.5 g/dL.

Use Quantitate IgG in patient's serum to evaluate humoral immunity; establish diagnosis and monitor therapy in IgG myeloma; evaluate patients, especially children and those with lymphoma, with propensity to infections. Reduction of IgG, usually <300 mg/dL, leads to susceptibility to infection due to encapsulated bacteria.[1]

Limitations If samples containing macroglobulins, cryoglobulins, or cold agglutinins are handled at incorrect temperatures, false low values may result.

Methodology Radial immunodiffusion (RID), rate nephelometry

Additional Information Immunoglobulin G is the major antibody containing protein fraction of blood. There are four subtypes, of which IgG_1 and IgG_2 comprise 85% of the total. IgG_1 and IgG_3 fix complement best; IgG_3 is hyperaggregable and effects serum viscosity disproportionately. With significant decreases in IgG level, on either a congenital or acquired basis, there is an increased susceptibility to infectious processes ordinarily dealt with by humoral antibody (ie, bacterial infection). Thus, patients with repeated infection should have their immunoglobulins, and specifically IgG, measured. Therapy with exogenous gamma globulins may be efficacious in such patients. Conversely, IgG levels will be increased in immunocompetent individuals responding to a wide variety of infections or inflammatory insults (indeed, this represents the basis of the serologic diagnosis of infectious diseases). IgG specific antibody can now be demonstrated for numerous organisms, and when coupled with IgM specific antibody, can give an accurate diagnosis of acute or chronic infection. Today, a major cause for a polyclonal increase in IgG is the acquired immunodeficiency syndrome. Monoclonal IgG can be demonstrated in approximately 60% of cases of multiple myeloma. 3 g/dL of monoclonal IgG is a major diagnostic criterion for myeloma. Oligoclonal IgG can be seen in multiple sclerosis and some instances of chronic hepatitis. Some of these are characterized by
(Continued)

Immunoglobulin G *(Continued)*

features of autoimmune hepatitis. In that entity, hypergammaglobulin-emia[2] with increased IgG concentration is recognized as a classical laboratory finding.[3]

A monoclonal gammopathy may be present when the total IgG value is in the normal range. While many of these patients do not have multiple myeloma, evaluation of these patients for such gammopathy and the presence of Bence Jones protein in urine is important. The differential diagnosis of myeloma includes essential monoclonal gammopathy, which is characterized by lack of symptoms, lack of anemia, lack of bone lesions, monoclonal gammopathy with M component <3.5 g/dL IgG or <2.5 g/dL IgA and marrow plasma cells <10%.

Other relevant disease entities include indolent myeloma and solitary plasmacytoma.

The four subclasses of IgG differ in the constant regions of their heavy chains. A patient may have a normal total IgG yet still have a significant decrease in one subclass. IgG_1 deficiencies are associated with EBV infections, IgG_2 with sinorespiratory infections and infections with encapsulated bacteria, IgG_3 with sinusitis and otitis media, and IgG_4 with allergies, ataxia telangiectasia, and sinorespiratory infections.

Footnotes

1. Masur H and Fauci AS, "Infections in Patients With Inflammatory and Immunologic Defects," *Harrison's Principles of Internal Medicine*, 13th ed, Chapter 81, Isselbacher KJ, Braunwald E, Wilson JD, et al, eds, New York, NY: McGraw-Hill Inc, 1994, 494-8.
2. Krawitt EL, "Autoimmune Hepatitis," *N Engl J Med*, 1996, 334(14):897-903.
3. Meyer zum Büschenfelde KH and Lohse AW, "Autoimmune Hepatitis," *N Engl J Med*, 1995, 333(15):1004-5 (letter).

References

Barlogie B, "Plasma Cell Myeloma," *Williams Hematology*, 5th ed, Chapter 114, Beutler E, Lichtman MA, Coller S, et al, eds, New York, NY: McGraw-Hill Inc, 1995, 1109-26.

Jacobson DL, McCutchan JA, Spechko PL, et al, "The Evaluation of Lymphadenopathy and Hypergammaglobulinemia are Evidence for Early and Sustained Polyclonal B Lymphocyte Activation During Human Immunodeficiency Virus Infection," *J Infect Dis*, 1991, 163(2):240-6.

Immunoglobulin G, Cerebrospinal Fluid *see* Cerebrospinal Fluid Immunoglobulin G *on page 378*

Immunoglobulin G Subclasses

CPT 82787

Related Information

Ataxia-Telangiectasia, Chromosome Breakage Study *on page 274*
Immunoglobulin A *on page 408*
Immunoglobulin G *on previous page*
Protein, Total, Serum *on page 194*

Synonyms IgG Subclasses

Applies to IgG_1; IgG_2; IgG_3; IgG_4

Abstract Each of the four subclasses of IgG mediates different functions. IgG_1 is found in highest concentration.

Specimen Serum

Container Red top tube

Storage Instructions Store at 4°C.

Reference Range See table.

IgG Subclass Levels (mg/dL)

Age	IgG_1	IgG_2	IgG_3	IgG_4
0-1 y	190-620	30-140	9-62	6-63
1-2 y	230-710	30-170	11-98	4-43
2-3 y	280-830	40-240	6-130	3-120
3-6 y	350-810	50-310	9-160	5-180
>6 y	270-1740	30-630	13-320	11-620

Use Study of patients with recurrent bacterial infections. Selective deficiencies may be found among the subclasses in some individuals who suffer repeated infections, especially IgG_1.

Methodology Radial immunodiffusion (RID), enzyme-linked immunosorbent assay (ELISA)

Additional Information IgG antibody responses to certain antigens occur to a greater extent in one type of IgG subclass than another. Therefore, some patients with normal total IgG levels may have problems with pyogenic infections because they do not produce IgG_2 or combinations of IgG_2, IgG_3, and/or IgG_4. Some clinically significant IgG subclass deficiencies occur in patients who have IgA deficiency.

References

Keren DF and Warren JS, *Diagnostic Immunology*, Baltimore, MD: Williams & Wilkins, 1992, 109-10.

Shield JP, Strobel S, Levinsky RJ, et al, "Immunodeficiency Presenting as Hypergammaglobulinemia With IgG_2 Subclass Deficiency," *Lancet*, 1992, 340(8817):448-50.

Immunoglobulin M

CPT 82784

Related Information

Ataxia-Telangiectasia, Chromosome Breakage Study *on page 274*
Immunofixation Electrophoresis *on page 408*
Protein, Total, Serum *on page 194*
Viscosity, Blood *on page 350*

Synonyms IgM, Quantitative

Replaces Macroglobulins, Ultracentrifuge Determination

Specimen Serum, cerebrospinal fluid

Container Red top tube, sterile CSF tube

Storage Instructions Samples suspected of having macroglobulins or cryoglobulins should be drawn and held at 37°C. Samples suspected of containing cold agglutinins should not be refrigerated prior to serum separation from clot.

Reference Range Adults: 53-375 mg/dL; pediatrics: cord: 0-19 mg/dL, 1-3 months: 7-78 mg/dL, 3-6 months: 19-72 mg/dL, 6-12 months: 21-104 mg/dL, 12-24 months: 19-148 mg/dL, 24-36 months: 40-151 mg/dL, 3-5 years: 28-142 mg/dL, 5-8 years: 30-162 mg/dL, 8-12 years: 24-161 mg/dL, 12-16 years: 26-221 mg/dL

Use Evaluate humoral immunity; establish the diagnosis and monitor therapy in macroglobulinemia of Waldenström and other lymphoid and lymphoplasmacytic neoplasms. Differential diagnosis includes plasma cell myeloma (the rare IgM myeloma), essential macroglobulinemia, and other entities. IgM levels are used to evaluate likelihood of *in utero* infections or acuteness of infection. IgM deficiency is associated especially with gram-negative infections.

Limitations If samples containing macroglobulins, cryoglobulins, or cold agglutinins are handled at incorrect temperatures, false low values may result.

Methodology Radial immunodiffusion (RID), rate nephelometry

Additional Information Immunoglobulin M is a pentamer of 7S gamma globulin, and is an efficient complement binder. It is the antibody type produced initially in the immune response and the first immunoglobulin class to be synthesized by a fetus or newborn. IgM antibodies do not cross the placenta. For these reasons the demonstration of IgM-specific antibody is useful in assessing whether a particular infection is acute (in which case IgM antibodies will be present) or chronic (IgG antibodies will predominate) and whether a newborn has a congenital infection (a newborn with IgM antibody is infected; a newborn with IgG antibody has passively acquired maternal antibody, which crossed the placenta). In the hyper-IgM immunodeficiency syndrome, there is an absence of IgG and IgA in serum and a marked increase in IgM. Macroglobulins produced in Waldenström's disease are IgM, and may produce hyperviscosity syndrome. In contrast, monoclonal IgG or IgA are found in most cases of myeloma. Increased IgM (with other immunoglobulins) may develop in inflammatory/infectious conditions. IgM is characteristically elevated in primary biliary cirrhosis. The majority of rheumatoid factors are IgM. IgM will be decreased in congenital or acquired hypogammaglobulinemia, and this will be associated with increased, recurrent infection. In patients with bacterial meningitis, CSF IgM is usually elevated along with C-reactive protein.

In Waldenström's macroglobulinemia, weight loss and epistaxis are found, in contrast to essential macroglobulinemia. In the former, hepatosplenomegaly, purpura, and lymphadenopathy occur; IgM is >3 g/dL; and anemia and hyperviscosity are seen.[1]

Footnotes

1. Kipps TJ, "Macroglobulinemia," *Williams Hematology*, 5th ed, Chapter 115, Beutler E, Lichtman MA, Coller BS, et al, eds, New York, NY: McGraw-Hill Inc, 1995, 1127-32.

References

Gougeon ML, Morelet L, Doussau M, et al, "Hyper-IgM Immunodeficiency Syndrome: Influence of Lymphokines on *In Vitro* Maturation of Peripheral B Cells," *J Clin Immunol*, 1992, 12(2):92-100.

Jeske DJ and Capra JD, "Immunoglobulins: Structure and Function," *Fundamental Immunology*, Paul WE, ed, New York, NY: Raven Press, 1984, 131-65.

Jones RG, Aguzzi F, Bienvenu J, et al, "Use of Immunoglobulin Heavy-Chain and Light-Chain Measurements in a Multicenter Trial to Investigate Monoclonal Components: I. Detection," *Clin Chem*, 1991, 37(11):1917-21.

Ribeiro MA, Kimura RT, Irulegui I, et al, "Cerebrospinal Fluid Levels of Lysozyme, IgM, and C-Reactive Protein in the Identification of Bacterial Meningitis," *J Trop Med Hyg*, 1992, 95(2):87-94.

Immunoglobulins *see* Protein Electrophoresis, Serum *on page 424*

IM Serology *see* Infectious Mononucleosis Screening Test *on this page*

Infectious Mononucleosis Screening Test

CPT 86309 (titer); 86408 (screen)

Related Information

Epstein-Barr Virus Culture *on page 666*

Epstein-Barr Virus Serology *on page 392*
Heterophil Agglutinins *on page 401*
Human Herpesvirus 6, IgG and IgM Antibodies, Quantitative *on page 406*
Lymph Node Biopsy *on page 50*
Peripheral Blood: Differential Leukocyte Count *on page 336*

Synonyms Davidsohn Slide Test; Heterophil Antibody; IM Serology; Monospot™ Test; Monosticon® Dri-Dot® Test

Replaces Davidsohn Differential; Paul-Bunnell Davidsohn Test

Test Commonly Includes Screening for the presence of heterophil antibodies

Specimen Serum

Container Red top tube

Reference Range Negative

Use Infectious mononucleosis (IM) is the major entity within the mononucleosis syndromes. It is a self-limiting disease caused by the Epstein-Barr virus (EBV), characterized clinically by fever, cervical lymphadenitis, tonsillopharyngitis, and not infrequently, hepatosplenomegaly.

Limitations Correlation with clinical findings is imperative since false-positive and negative results have been reported. About 10% of the adult population with IM will not develop heterophil antibodies. Failure to develop heterophil antibodies occurs even more frequently in younger children. In such instances, the presence of EBV antibodies is relevant. Less than 2% false-positives have been reported with Hodgkin's disease, lymphoma, acute lymphocytic leukemia, infectious hepatitis, pancreatic carcinoma, cytomegalovirus, Burkitt's lymphoma, rheumatoid arthritis, malaria, and rubella. Rare unexplained positive horse cell screening tests have been reported with negative differential absorptions. Overall, the Monospot™ test has 99% specificity and 86% sensitivity.

Methodology Heterophil antibodies are IgM. They can agglutinate sheep or horse red blood cells. In IM, heterophil antibodies can be absorbed by beef erythrocytes but not by guinea pig kidney. The classical tests were introduced by Dr Israel Davidsohn. The rapid slide test is widely used.[1] It has essentially replaced the older Paul-Bunnel-Davidsohn technique, which is more sensitive but time consuming.

Additional Information The IM heterophil antibody appears in the serum of patients by the sixth to tenth day of illness. Highest titers are usually found in the second to third week. Antibody levels may remain detectable for as little as 1 week or persist up to a year; usual persistence is 4-8 weeks. The level of antibody activity is not correlated with the severity of disease or the degree of lymphocytosis. A positive test with the appropriate clinical and hematologic setting is sufficient to make the diagnosis of IM. If there is clinically a mononucleosis syndrome, but the screening test is negative, consider tests for EBV specific antibodies, CMV, HHV-6, and toxoplasmosis antibodies. Consider especially repeating this test after a short delay. Laboratory criteria for IM include peripheral blood lymphocytosis, >50% of WBCs with at least 10% of lymphocytes appearing reactive ("reactive lymphs") ie, virocytes. Serologic, hematologic, and clinical criteria all ideally should be met for diagnosis. The peripheral blood smear should be carefully examined.

Other tests often elevated in IM include aminotransferase with disproportionately greater elevations of LDH and alkaline phosphatase. The isomorphic pattern is found with LDH isoenzyme separation. Hemoglobin and platelets are usually normal in IM, usually not in leukemia. Complications occur in some individuals.

Footnotes
1. Lee CL, Davidsohn I, and Slaby R, "Horse Agglutinins in Infectious Mononucleosis," *Am J Clin Pathol*, 1968, 49:3-11.

References
Fleisher GR, Collins M, and Fager S, "Limitations of Available Tests for Diagnosis of Infectious Mononucleosis," *J Clin Microbiol*, 1983, 17(4):619-24.

Horwitz CA, Henle W, Henle G, et al, "Persistent Falsely Positive Rapid Tests for Infectious Mononucleosis. Report of Five Cases with 4-6 Year Follow-Up Data," *Am J Clin Pathol*, 1979, 72:807-11.

Lennette ET, "Epstein-Barr Virus," *Manual of Clinical Microbiology*, 6th ed, Chapter 34, Murray PR, Baron EJ, Pfaller MA, et al, eds, Washington, DC: American Society for Microbiology, 1995, 905-10.

Vahlne A, Uertborn M, and Iwarson S, "Mumps Occurring as a Mononucleosis-Like Syndrome With Positive Monospot™ Test," *JAMA*, 1979, 242:711.

Influenza A and B Antibodies *see* Influenza A and B Titer *on this page*

Influenza A and B Titer

CPT 86710 (each)

Related Information
Influenza Virus Culture *on page 670*
Virus, Direct Detection by Fluorescent Antibody *on page 682*

Synonyms Influenza A and B Antibodies

Test Commonly Includes IgG and IgM antibody titers to influenza A and/or B

Abstract Influenza affects the upper and lower respiratory tracts, often brings systemic illness and may be complicated by primary viral pneumonia, secondary bacterial pneumonia, or mixed pneumonitis. A serious complication especially of influenza B is Reye's syndrome.

Specimen Serum

Container Red top tube

Collection Acute and convalescent sera drawn 10-14 days apart are required.

Reference Range Less than a fourfold increase in titer in paired sera; IgG <1:10, IgM <1:10

Use Although serologic diagnosis is seldom practical (or necessary) during an influenza epidemic, serologic typing is valuable for epidemiology and for planning therapy. Since type A influenza can be treated with amantadine but type B cannot, this distinction may need to be made. Presence of specific IgM antibody indicates acute infection.

Methodology Complement fixation (CF), hemagglutination inhibition (HAI), single radial immunodiffusion (RID), enzyme-linked immunosorbent assay (ELISA)

Additional Information Virus can be detected by culture; see listing Influenza Virus Culture *on page 670*.

References
Bryan JA, "The Serologic Diagnosis of Viral Infections," *Arch Pathol Lab Med*, 1987, 111(11):1015-23.

Dolan R, "Influenza," *Harrison's Principles of Internal Medicine*, 13th ed, Isselbacher KJ, Braunwald E, and Wilson JD, eds, New York, NY: McGraw-Hill Inc, 1994.

Walls HH, Harmon MW, Slagle JJ, et al, "Characterization and Evaluation of Monoclonal Antibodies Developed for Typing Influenza A and Influenza B Viruses," *J Clin Microbiol*, 1986, 23(2):240-5.

Intrinsic Factor *see* Parietal Cell Antibody *on page 421*

Intrinsic Factor Antibody

CPT 86340

Related Information
Folic Acid, Serum *on page 317*
Gastric Analysis *on page 133*
Parietal Cell Antibody *on page 421*
Schilling Test *on page 346*
Vitamin B_{12} *on page 351*
Vitamin B_{12} Unsaturated Binding Capacity *on page 352*

Synonyms IF Antibody

Abstract A glycoprotein, intrinsic factor (IF), is generated in gastric parietal cells. It tightly binds cyanocobalamin (vitamin B_{12}) and facilitates its absorption. About half of patients with pernicious anemia (PA) develop antibodies to intrinsic factor. Secretion of IF parallels that of gastric HCl.

Patient Preparation Avoid recent radioactive scan, B_{12} injection within the past 48 hours.

Specimen Serum

Container Red top tube

Reference Range None detected

Use Differentiate pernicious anemia (PA) from other megaloblastic anemias; investigate patients with low vitamin B_{12} levels

Limitations Negative results do not rule out PA.

Methodology Radioimmunoassay (RIA)

Additional Information Antibodies to intrinsic factor (IF) are found in very high percentage of children with juvenile pernicious anemia (PA). Approximately 50% to 75% of adult patients have IF antibodies. There are two types of antibody. **Type I, blocking antibody**, the more common, prevents the binding of B_{12} and intrinsic factor, but will not react with complexed intrinsic factor. **Type II antibody**, or **binding antibody**, reacts with either free or complexed IF. Blocking antibody is extremely specific for PA. Type II antibodies are rarely found without Type I. A proportion of patients have IgA IF antibody in gastric juice (serum antibody is IgG). IF antibody may be especially useful as an adjunct to serum vitamin B_{12} levels to detect vitamin B_{12} malabsorption in the elderly.

References
Bunting RW, Bitzer AM, Kenney RM, et al, "Prevalence of Intrinsic Factor Antibodies and Vitamin B_{12} Malabsorption in Older Patients Admitted to a Rehabilitation Hospital," *J Am Geriatr Soc*, 1990, 38(7):743-7.

Harty RF and Leibach JR, "Immune Disorders of the Gastrointestinal Tract and Liver," *Med Clin North Am*, 1985, 69(4):675-704.

Isotypes *see* Immunoglobulin A *on page 408*

Isotypes, Light Chains *see* Immunofixation Electrophoresis *on page 408*

Jo-1 Antibody

CPT 86235

Related Information
Antinuclear Antibody *on page 368*
(Continued)

Jo-1 Antibody *(Continued)*

Muscle Biopsy *on page 53*
Myositis-Specific Autoantibody *on page 420*
Scleroderma Antibody *on page 430*
Sjögren's Antibodies *on page 430*

Synonyms Antihistidyl Transfer tRNA Synthase

Applies to Antisynthetases

Abstract An autoantibody identifiable in ANA-positive sera, Jo-1 is more common than the other antisynthetases.[1] It is the only myositis-specific antibody presently available for clinical use.[2]

Specimen Serum

Container Red top tube

Storage Instructions Refrigerate; freeze in the summer.

Reference Range Negative

Use Marker for idiopathic inflammatory myopathies, including polymyositis and dermatomyositis. Jo-1 antibody is found in approximately 30% to 50% of patients with myositis. Its presence suggests that an aggressive disease course may take place with decreased survival.[2]

Methodology Immunoblot assay, polyacrylamide gel electrophoresis

Additional Information Diffuse cytoplasmic staining of HEp-2 cells in the ANA suggests anti-Jo-1, which bears association with increased incidence of lung fibrosis and interstitial lung disease in subjects with polymyositis. More than 50% of patients with myositis have positive ANA.

The role of T lymphocytes in myositis may be that of primary determinants of pathogenesis. Environmental agents reported associated with myositis include infectious agents (eg, *Borrelia*), foods, drugs, occupational exposure and medical devices, and genetic factors play a role.[1] SLE shares some features of myositis.

The clinical effects of antisynthetases including anti-Jo-1 are characterized by relatively acute onset, fever, Raynaud's phenomenon, and arthritis, as well as interstitial lung disease and dry cracked skin on patient's hands.

Footnotes
1. Plotz PH, Rider LG, Targoff IN, et al, "Myositis: Immunologic Contributions to Understanding Cause, Pathogenesis, and Therapy," *Ann Intern Med*, 1995, 122(9):715-24.
2. Moder KG, "Use and Interpretation of Rheumatologic Tests: A Guide for Clinicians," *Mayo Clin Proc*, 1996, 71(4):391-6.

References
Homburger HA, "Cascade Testing for Autoantibodies in Connective Tissue Diseases," *Mayo Clin Proc*, 1995, 70(2):183-4.

Kahn Test *replaced by RPR on page 428*

Kahn Test *replaced by VDRL, Serum on page 438*

Kala-azar Serological Test *see Leishmaniasis Serological Test on next page*

Kappa and Lambda Light Chains Detection *see Immunoelectrophoresis, Serum or Urine on page 408*

Kappa Chains *see Immunofixation Electrophoresis on page 408*

Kline Test *replaced by RPR on page 428*

Kline Test *replaced by VDRL, Serum on page 438*

La Antibodies *see Sjögren's Antibodies on page 430*

LaCrosse Virus Titer *see California Encephalitis Virus Titer on page 374*

Lambda Chains *see Immunofixation Electrophoresis on page 408*

LATS *see Thyrotropin Receptor Antibody on page 434*

LATS Protector *see Thyrotropin Receptor Antibody on page 434*

L. bosemanii *see Legionnaires' Disease Antibodies on this page*

L. bosemanii *see Legionnaires' Disease Direct Fluorescent Antibody Smear on next page*

L. dumoffii *see Legionnaires' Disease Antibodies on this page*

L. dumoffii *see Legionnaires' Disease Direct Fluorescent Antibody Smear on next page*

Legionella Antigen, Urine *see Legionnaires' Disease Urine Antigen on next page*

Legionella bosemanii Antigen, Urine *see Legionnaires' Disease Urine Antigen on next page*

Legionella dumoffii Antigen, Urine *see Legionnaires' Disease Urine Antigen on next page*

Legionella gormanii Antigen, Urine *see Legionnaires' Disease Urine Antigen on next page*

Legionella jordanis Antigen, Urine *see Legionnaires' Disease Urine Antigen on next page*

Legionella longbeachae Antigen, Urine *see Legionnaires' Disease Urine Antigen on next page*

Legionella micdadei Antigen, Urine *see Legionnaires' Disease Urine Antigen on next page*

Legionella pneumophila Antibodies *see Legionnaires' Disease Antibodies on this page*

Legionella pneumophila Antigen, Urine *see Legionnaires' Disease Urine Antigen on next page*

Legionella pneumophila Direct FA Smear *see Legionnaires' Disease Direct Fluorescent Antibody Smear on next page*

Legionella pneumophila Titer *see Legionnaires' Disease Antibodies on this page*

Legionnaires' Disease Antibodies

CPT 86713

Related Information

Bacterial Culture, Sputum *on page 465*
Legionella Culture *on page 485*
Legionnaires' Disease Direct Fluorescent Antibody Smear *on next page*
Legionnaires' Disease Urine Antigen *on next page*

Synonyms *Legionella pneumophila* Antibodies; *Legionella pneumophila* Titer; Legionnaires', Indirect Fluorescent Antibody

Applies to *L. bosemanii*; *L. dumoffii*; *L. gormanii*; *L. jordanis*; *L. longbeachae*; *L. micdadei*; Pneumonia, Atypical Agents

Test Commonly Includes Detection of antibody (IgG or IgA) to *Legionella pneumophila*

Abstract The differential diagnosis of the atypical pneumonias includes *Chlamydia pneumoniae*, Legionnaires' disease, *Mycoplasma* pneumonia, and rickettsial pneumonia.[1] *Legionella*, *Mycoplasma pneumoniae*, and *Chlamydia pneumoniae* collectively cause 10% to 20% of cases of pneumonia. Antibody detection for Legionnaires' disease from a random sample is unlikely to be useful. *Legionella* is found especially in immunosuppressed patients who do not respond to beta-lactam antibiotics.

Specimen Serum, acute and convalescent

Container Red top tube

Collection A convalescent sample is recommended to be drawn 10-14 days after acute sample

Reference Range Less than a fourfold change in titer between acute and convalescent samples; <1:256 in a single sample

Use Support for the clinical diagnosis of Legionnaires' disease

Limitations It is important to test for both IgG and IgM; when this is done, overall sensitivity is approximately 80%. Specificity is fairly high (approaching 95%), but predictive values may be low in low prevalence populations. Serologic diagnosis is often retrospective and should be considered presumptive. Antibody may persist for years. False-positives are found.

Methodology Indirect fluorescent antibody (IFA) assay using serogroup 1: Philadelphia, Knoxville, serogroup 2: Togus, serogroup 3: Los Angeles, serogroup 4: Bloomington. When available a polyvalent antigen, which includes serogroup 1-6, is utilized. Latex agglutination (LA).

Additional Information A fourfold rise in titer to >1:128 provides evidence of recent infection. A single titer ≥1:256 is evidence of infection at an undetermined time. However, due to the relatively high prevalence of antibodies to *Legionella pneumophila*, acute and convalescent titers are preferred to a single sample. Most seroconversions can be documented within 3 weeks of onset. Demonstration of IgM antibody to serogroup I may allow rapid diagnosis. Serologic study is also valuable in evaluation of epidemic disease. The presence of IgM in high titer is presumptive evidence for acute infection, but this test is not definitive, as IgM antibody to *L. pneumophila* may persist for months.

Features of *Legionella pneumoniae* may include bradycardia, increased transaminases and/or hypophosphatemia.[1]

Footnotes
1. Johnson DH and Cunha BA, "Atypical Pneumonias. Clinical and Extrapulmonary Features of *Chlamydia*, *Mycoplasma*, and *Legionella* Infections," *Postgrad Med*, 1993, 93(7):69-72, 75-6, 79-82.

References
Bartlett JG and Mundy LM, "Community-Acquired Pneumonia," *N Engl J Med*, 1995, 333(24):1618-24.
"Case Records of the Massachusetts General Hospital. Weeky Clinicopathological Exercises. Case 8-1994. An 84-Year-Old Woman With Lymphomas Fever, and Pulmonary Infiltrate," *N Engl J Med*, 1994, 330(8):557-64.
Holliday MG, "Use of Latex Agglutination Technique for Detecting *Legionella pneumophila* (Serogroup 1) Antibodies," *J Clin Pathol*, 1990, 43(10):860-2.

Roig J, Domingo C, and Morera J, "Legionnaires' Disease," *Chest*, 1994, 105(6):1817-25.

Winn WC Jr, "*Legionella* and the Clinical Microbiologist," *Infect Dis Clin North Am*, 1993, 7(2):377-92.

Legionnaires' Disease Direct Fluorescent Antibody Smear

CPT 87206

Related Information

Bacterial Culture, Sputum *on page 465*

Legionella Culture *on page 485*

Legionnaires' Disease Antibodies *on previous page*

Legionnaires' Disease Urine Antigen *on this page*

Synonyms FA Smear for *Legionella pneumophila*; *Legionella pneumophila* Direct FA Smear

Applies to *L. bosemanii*; *L. dumoffii*; *L. gormanii*; *L. jordanis*; *L. long-beachae*; *L. micdadei*

Abstract Direct fluorescent antibody (DFA) used to screen for organisms for rapid diagnosis.

Specimen Lung tissue, pleural fluid, other body fluid, transtracheal aspirate, sputum, bronchial washing or bronchoalveolar lavage

Container Sterile container

Reference Range No *Legionella pneumophila*

Use Determine the presence of *Legionella pneumophila* organisms in direct smear of specimen by fluorescent antibody, providing rapid diagnosis. Monoclonal antibody is available.

Limitations DFA is not as sensitive as culture and false-positive results occur with other bacterial infections and with environmental *Legionella* sp. False-positive reaction has been reported in a case of pleuropulmonary tularemia and in cases of *Campylobacter* infection.[1,2] Sensitivity ranges for various respiratory specimens are as follows: sputum - 18% to 33%, tracheal aspirates - 33% to 40%, bronchoalveolar lavage - 66%. Culture is needed as well.

Methodology Direct fluorescent antibody (DFA)

Additional Information Community-acquired and nosocomial infections caused by multiple serogroups of *Legionella* are increasingly recognized. Culture is now possible on buffered charcoal yeast extract agar. However, the demonstration of organisms in sputum, tissue, or brushings is a rapid means to make a diagnosis. It also has the advantage of applicability to specimens contaminated with other bacteria. Development of monoclonal antibodies has increased sensitivity and specificity. A combination of both culture and antigen detection is recommended. A direct FA should not be ordered alone; it should always be accompanied by a request for *Legionella* culture. Direct fluorescence antibody staining can be done on tissue specimens as well. *Legionella* species can be cultured, requiring 3-5 days.

Footnotes

1. Andersen LP and Bangsborg J, "Cross Reactions Between *Legionella* and *Campylobacter* Species," *Lancet*, 1992, 340(8813):245.
2. Roy TM, Fleming D, and Anderson WH, "Tularemic Pneumonia Mimicking Legionnaires' Disease With False-Positive Direct Fluorescent Antibody Stains for *Legionella*," *South Med J*, 1989, 82:1429-31.

References

Blatt SP, et al, "Nosocomial Legionnaires' Disease: Aspiration as a Primary Mode of Disease Acquisition," *JAMA*, 1994, 271(4):264D.

"Case Records of the Massachusetts General Hospital. Weekly Clinocopathological Exercises. Case 8-1994. An 84-Year-Old Woman With Lymphomas, Fever, and Pulmonary Infiltrate," *N Engl J Med*, 1994, 330(8):557-64.

Hart CA and Makin T, "*Legionella* in Hospitals: A Review," *J Hosp Infect*, 1991, 18(Suppl A):481-9.

Roig J, Domingo C, and Morera J, "Legionnaires' Disease," *Chest*, 1994, 105(6):1817-25.

Winn WC Jr, "*Legionella* and the Clinical Microbiologist," *Infect Dis Clin North Am*, 1993, 7(2):377-92.

Legionnaires' Disease Urine Antigen

Related Information

Legionnaires' Disease Antibodies *on previous page*

Legionnaires' Disease Direct Fluorescent Antibody Smear *on this page*

Synonyms *Legionella* Antigen, Urine

Applies to *Legionella bosemanii* Antigen, Urine; *Legionella dumoffii* Antigen, Urine; *Legionella gormanii* Antigen, Urine; *Legionella jordanis* Antigen, Urine; *Legionella longbeachae* Antigen, Urine; *Legionella micdadei* Antigen, Urine; *Legionella pneumophila* Antigen, Urine

Test Commonly Includes Detection of excreted *Legionella* antigen in urine

Patient Preparation Avoid recent administration of radioisotopes if assay performed by RIA.

Specimen Urine

Container Sterile urine container

Reference Range Negative

Use Antigen detection in urine is an additional approach to diagnosis of *Legionella* infection.

Limitations A commercially available RIA is designed to detect *L. pneumophila* serogroup 1 antigen; it is highly sensitive and specific for *L. pneumophila* serogroup 1 infections, but is negative in patients infected with other serogroups of *L. pneumophila* or other *Legionella* species. *L. pneumophila* serogroup 1 accounts for 70% to 90% of cases.[1] Antigen excretion in urine may persist for months after recovery from infection. Commercially available latex agglutination tests have not proven clinically useful due to unacceptably low sensitivity and specificity. This test should only be ordered in conjunction with other, more proven, laboratory tests such as *Legionella* culture and/or antibody assays.

Methodology Radioimmunoassay (RIA), enzyme immunoassay (EIA), or latex agglutination

Additional Information The reliability of this test is highly method dependent; consequently, it is important to consider the method used before choice of a reference laboratory for this test.

Footnotes

1. Bartlett JG and Mundy LM, "Community-Acquired Pneumonia," *N Engl J Med*, 1995, 333(24):1618-24.

References

Roig J, Domingo C, and Morera J, "Legionnaires' Disease," *Chest*, 1994, 105(6):1817-25.

Winn WC Jr, "*Legionella* and the Clinical Microbiologist," *Infect Dis Clin North Am*, 1993, 7(2):377-92.

Legionnaires', Indirect Fluorescent Antibody *see* Legionnaires' Disease Antibodies *on previous page*

***Leishmania braziliensis* Serological Test** *see* Leishmaniasis Serological Test *on this page*

***Leishmania donovani* Serological Test** *see* Leishmaniasis Serological Test *on this page*

Leishmaniasis Serological Test

CPT 86717

Related Information

Bone Marrow *on page 307*

Lymph Node Biopsy *on page 50*

Parasite Antibodies *on page 421*

Protein Electrophoresis, Serum *on page 424*

Skin Biopsy *on page 54*

Synonyms Espundia Serological Test; Kala-azar Serological Test; *Leishmania braziliensis* Serological Test; *Leishmania donovani* Serological Test; *Leishmania tropica* Serological Test; Oriental Sore Serological Test

Abstract Visceral leishmaniasis (kala-azar) is typically caused by *Leishmania donovani*. It parasitizes monocytic cells (eg, macrophages) and is found in spleen, bone marrow, liver, and lymph nodes. Other types include cutaneous leishmaniasis (*L. tropica*, *L. major*, *L. aethiopica*) and new world cutaneous leishmaniasis (*L. mexicana*, *L. braziliensis*, *L. venezuelensis*, *L. peruviana*). Mucocutaneous leishmaniasis (espundia) is caused primarily by *L. braziliensis*.

Specimen Serum

Container Red top tube

Reference Range Negative

Use Support the clinical diagnosis of visceral, cutaneous, and mucocutaneous leishmaniasis. Antibodies are most helpful in visceral leishmaniasis.

Limitations Cross reactivity with Chagas' disease; false-positives in malaria. Sensitivity of serologic tests for cutaneous leishmaniasis is poor. Serologic diagnosis often is insufficient in subjects infected with HIV virus.[1]

Methodology Indirect hemagglutination (IHA), indirect fluorescent antibody (IFA), complement fixation (CF), enzyme-linked immunosorbent assay (ELISA), immunodot assay. Of these, the enzyme-linked immunosorbent assay (ELISA) presently is considered the most sensitive.[1] Direct agglutination detecting IgM is a sensitive test for acute disease. The gp63 ELISA may distinguish a current from a prior infection.[2]

Additional Information Serodiagnosis of visceral leishmaniasis is more reliable than serodiagnosis of cutaneous disease, although this has been improved by the use of direct agglutination tests. An ELISA test is positive in 85% of cases. Visceral leishmaniasis is atypical in patients with AIDS.[1] Splenomegaly, a major feature in other patients is often absent in AIDS patients.

Massive polyclonal IgG gammopathy on serum protein electrophoresis is characteristic of kala-azar. Leukopenia, thrombocytopenia, and anemia are found. **Bone marrow aspiration** provides diagnostic organisms in kala-azar. **Skin biopsies** for stains, culture, and histopathology are useful in cutaneous and mucocutaneous leishmaniasis. *L. tropica*, which usually causes cutaneous disease, produced visceral infection in
(Continued)

Leishmaniasis Serological Test *(Continued)*

soldiers returning from Desert Storm.[3] Transmission is by phlebotomine sand flies.

The differential diagnosis of nodular lymphangitis includes *L. braziliensis*, as well as *Sporothrix schenckii*, *Nocardia brasiliensis*, *Mycobacterium marinum*, and *Francisella tularensis*.[4]

Diagnosis of visceral leishmaniasis remains dependent on detection of *L. donovani* in specimens in some settings.

Footnotes

1. Albrecht H, Sobottka I, Emminger C, et al, "Visceral Leishmaniasis Emerging as an Important Opportunistic Infection in HIV-Infected Persons Living in Areas Nonendemic for *Leishmania donovani*," *Arch Pathol Lab Med*, 1996, 120:189-98.
2. Okong'o-Odera EA, Kurtzhals JA, Hey AS, et al, "Measurement of Serum Antibodies Against Native *Leishmania* gp63 Distinguishes Between Ongoing and Previous *L. donovani* Infection," *APMIS*, 1993, 101(8):642-6.
3. Magill AJ, Grögl M, Gasser RA Jr, et al, "Visceral Infection Caused by *Leishmania tropica* in Veterans of Operation Desert Storm," *N Engl J Med*, 1993, 328(19):1383-7.
4. Kostman JR and Di Nubile MJ, "Nodular Lymphangitis: A Distinctive but Often Unrecognized Syndrome," *Ann Intern Med*, 1993, 118(11):883-8.

References

Borowy NK, Schell D, Schafer C, et al, "Diagnosis of African Trypanosomiasis and Visceral Leishmaniasis Based on the Detection of Antiparasite-Enzyme Antibodies," *J Infect Dis*, 1991, 164(2):422-5.

Grimaldi G Jr and Tesh RB, "Leishmaniases of the New World: Current Concepts and Implications for Future Research," *Clin Microbiol Rev*, 1993, 6(3):230-50.

Gupta S, Srivastava JK, Ray S, et al, "Evaluation of Enzyme-Linked Immunosorbent Assay in the Diagnosis of Kala-Azar in Malda District (West Bengal)," *Indian J Med Res*, 1993, 97:242-6.

Kagan IG and Maddison SE, "Serodiagnosis of Parasitic Diseases," *Manual of Clinical Laboratory Immunology*, 4th ed, Vol 2, Chapter 79, Rose NR, Conway de Macario E, Fahey JL, et al, eds, Washington, DC: American Society for Microbiology, 1992, 529-43.

Locksley RM, "Leishmaniasis," *Harrison's Principles of Internal Medicine*, 13th ed, Isselbacher KJ, Braunwald E, Wilson JD, et al, eds, New York, NY: McGraw-Hill Inc, 1994, 896-9.

Peters BS, Fish D, Golden R, et al, "Visceral Leishmaniasis in HIV Infection and AIDS: Clinical Features and Response to Therapy," *Q J Med*, 1990, 77(283):1101-11.

***Leishmania tropica* Serological Test** *see* Leishmaniasis Serological Test *on previous page*

***Leptospira* Antibodies** *see Leptospira* Serodiagnosis *on this page*

Leptospira Serodiagnosis

CPT 86720

Related Information

Darkfield Examination, Leptospirosis *on page 475*
Leptospira Culture *on page 486*

Synonyms *Leptospira* Antibodies

Test Commonly Includes Testing of patient's serum for antibodies against *Leptospira biflexa* serovar *L. patoc*, and the following serovars of *Leptospira interrogans*: *L. copenhageni*, *L. canicola*, *L. pomona*, *L. autumnalis*, *L. grippotyphosa*, *L. wolffi*, and *L. djatzi*. Supplemental testing may be needed against serovars: *L. poi*, *L. castellonis*, *L. pyrogenes*, *L. borincana*, *L. szwajizak*, *L. bratislava*, *L. tarassovi*, *L. shermani*, *L. panama*, *L. celledoni*, *L. djasiman*, *L. cynopteri*, and *L. louisiana*.

Abstract Occurring in all parts of the world, leptospirosis can present as a mild or as a severe fatal disease with general symptoms of fever, malaise, muscle aches, hemorrhages, jaundice, gastroenteritis, pulmonary abnormalities, and headache. Weil's syndrome is hepatorenal leptospirosis. Culture of blood and urine for organisms is strongly recommended. Cerebrospinal fluid may be cultured.

Specimen Serum

Container Red top tube

Sampling Time Acute and convalescent sera drawn 10-14 days apart are suggested.

Reference Range Negative. A fourfold increase in titer in paired sera is diagnostic of infection.

Critical Values IgM titer ≥1:100 provides evidence of recent or active disease

Use Leptospirosis is an acute febrile zoonotic illness caused primarily by *Leptospira interrogans*, a large spirochete with over 180 serologic variants. Patients with extensive animal contact, either in the wild or with carcasses or excrement, are particularly at risk. Although leptospires can be cultured from blood or urine during the first week of illness, this interval is often missed, and diagnosis must be based on the demonstration of rising antibody titers. Antibody appears at the end of the first week of illness and peaks at 3-4 weeks, after which it slowly disappears.

Limitations The antigens used in the test are the ones most commonly causing disease, but there are many other serovars which might not be detected. A battery of antigens should be used.

Methodology Microscopic agglutination test, macroagglutination, complement fixation (CF), hemagglutination, enzyme-linked immunosorbent assay (ELISA); IgM: enzyme-linked immunosorbent assay (ELISA)

Additional Information An association between patients with leptospirosis and anticardiolipin antibodies exists which may induce vascular endothelial injury in severe cases.[1]

Footnotes

1. Rugman FP, Pinn G, Palmer MF, et al, "Anticardiolipin Antibodies in Leptospirosis," *J Clin Pathol*, 1991, 44(6):517-9.

References

Larsen SA, Pope V, and Quan TJ, "Immunologic Methods for the Diagnosis of Spirochetal Diseases," *Manual of Clinical Laboratory Immunology*, 4th ed, Vol 2, Chapter 73, Rose NR, Conway de Macario E, Fahey JL, et al, eds, Washington, DC: American Society for Microbiology, 1992, 467-81.

Raoult D, Bres P, and Baranton G, "Serologic Diagnosis of Leptospirosis: Comparison of Line Blot and Immunofluorescence Techniques With the Genus-Specific Microscopic Agglutination Test," *J Infect Dis*, 1989, 160(4):734-5.

Ribeiro MA, Sakata EE, Silva MV, et al, "Antigens Involved in the Human Antibody Response to Natural Infections With *Leptospira interrogans* serovar *copenhageni*," *J Trop Med Hyg*, 1992, 95(4):239-45.

Leukemia/Lymphoma Immunophenotyping Panel *see* Leukocyte Immunophenotyping *on this page*

Leukocyte Immunophenotyping

CPT 88180

Related Information

Ataxia-Telangiectasia, Chromosome Breakage Study *on page 274*
bcl-2 Gene Rearrangement *on page 503*
CD4/CD8 Enumeration *on page 375*
Gene Rearrangement for Leukemia and Lymphoma *on page 512*
HIV-1/HIV-2 Serology *on page 403*
Human Immunodeficiency Virus DNA Amplification *on page 515*
Immunoperoxidase Procedures *on page 43*
Immunophenotypic Analysis of Tissues by Flow Cytometry *on page 45*
Lymph Node Biopsy *on page 50*
Lymphocyte Transformation Test *on page 416*
Mantle Cell Lymphoma *on page 51*
p24 Antigen *on page 420*
Polymerase Chain Reaction *on page 523*

Synonyms Leukemia/Lymphoma Immunophenotyping Panel; Lymphocyte Receptor Studies; Lymphocyte Subset Identification; Lymphocyte Surface Immunoglobulin Analysis; T and B Lymphocyte Subset Assay

Applies to Cluster Designations; Flow Cytometry

Replaces T- and B-Cell Rosettes Studies

Test Commonly Includes Currently extremely variable. Contact your laboratory to determine what is available on a local and/or referred basis.

Specimen Most procedures call for heparinized whole blood. Methods are available for obtaining suspensions of lymph node, spleen (see listings Immunophenotypic Analysis of Tissue by Flow Cytometry *on page 45* and Lymph Node Biopsy *on page 50*), or bone marrow cells for analysis. Fresh tissue fragments are minced/homogenized to release individual cells into suspension for cell by cell analysis. Fresh tissue may be required to prepare frozen sections for immunofluorescence analysis. Immunoperoxidase methods have been applied with variable results to sections of formalin-fixed, paraffin-imbedded material. Arrangements must be made with your laboratory preparatory to obtaining material for these specialized studies.

Container Green top (heparin) tube

Storage Instructions Maintain specimen at room temperature. Process within 2-3 hours. There is evidence that delay and exposure to refrigerator temperatures is related to significant loss of the T4 (inducer/helper) T-lymphocyte subset marker.[1]

Special Instructions Consult laboratory for special arrangements or instructions before collecting specimen.

Reference Range T cells: 60% to 80%; B cells: 5% to 15%; B-cell surface immunoglobulins FITC polyvalent: 5% to 15%

Use Quantitate T and B lymphocytes and lymphocyte subsets; type and classify lymphocytic leukemias (see table) and lymphomas; define immunodeficiency states including AIDS; monitor immunosuppressive therapy

Limitations Method related variables and their effect on normal values are not entirely defined. A lymphocyte subset defined by a monoclonal antibody identified antigen may not be all-inclusive of one functional subset (eg, lymphocytes with T4 antigens are inducer/helper cells but additional cells of this functional class may exist in the same individual that are T4-negative). Steroid and immunosuppressive drug therapy may significantly change (usually decreasing) lymphocyte populations.

Methodology Flow cytometers and fluorescence-activated cell sorter analyzers for which there are currently three major commercial sources. These devices can identify, count, and/or physically separate individual

Antigenic Profiles of Subtypes of Acute and Chronic Forms of Leukemia

Type of Leukemia	Immunologic Categories With Usual Antigenic Profile	Comments
ALL	Null cell ALL: HLA-DR, TdT, variable CD19	10% of non-T ALL
	Common ALL: HLA-DR, TdT, CD19, CD10, CD20	Most frequent type of ALL (70% of non-T ALL)
	Pre-B ALL: HLA-DR, TdT, CD19, CD10, CD20, cytoplasmic mu	15% to 20% of non-T ALL
	B ALL: HLA-DR, CD19, CD20, SIg	<1% of ALL
	Early thymocyte T ALL: CD7, CD5, T9, CD38, CD2, TdT	15% to 20% of ALL is of T-cell origin
	Common thymocyte T ALL: CD7, CD5, CD38, CD2, CD1, CD3, CD4, CD8, TdT	
	Mature thymocyte T ALL: CD7, CD5, CD38, CD2, CD3, CD4, or CD8	
Chronic lymphoid leukemias	B CLL: weak SIg (often IgM and D), CIg in some cases, HLA-DR, mouse erythrocyte receptor, CD5, CD19, CD20, CD21, CD23	CLL phenotype may correlate with prognosis
	T CLL: variable; pan T (E rosette), may have helper or suppressor phenotype	2% CLL of T-cell origin
	B PLL: moderate to strong SIg, HLA-DR, CD19, CD20	80% PLL of B-cell origin
	T PLL: variable; pan T (E rosette), may have helper or suppressor phenotype	20% PLL of T-cell origin
	HCL: SIg, CD11, CD19, CD20, CD25, HLA-DR	Rare cases of T HCL described
ANLL M1, M2	HLA-DR, CD13, CD33 (variable expression of My8, CD11, CD13)	Some association between phenotype and prognosis
M3	CD13, CD33, My8, CD11	Loss of HLA-Dr common
M4	HLA-DR, CD13, CD33, CD14, CD11, My8	
M5	HLA-DR, CD13, CD14, CD11, variable CD33	
M6	Glycophorin A (myeloid precursors react with monoclonals listed for M1, M2)	
M7	Platelet glycoprotein IIb/IIIa, variable Ib	
CML	Blast crisis cells similar in phenotype to corresponding type of acute leukemia	Blast crisis can be of various cell types, although myeloid and lymphoid are most common

cells that bear a fluorescent labeled immunologically identified antigen. The flow cytometer has become the standard method for immunophenotyping cells with monoclonal antibodies.

Additional Information A table in the Immunology Appendix lists current CD and cellular expression of antigen. See table Antigen Expression With Cluster Designation *on page 441.*

See listing Immunophenotypic Analysis of Tissues by Flow Cytometry *on page 45.*

Footnotes
1. Weiblen BJ, Debell K, and Valeri CR, "Acquired Immunodeficiency of Blood Stored Overnight," *N Engl J Med*, 1983, 309:793.

References
"Guidelines for the Performance of CD4+ T-Cell Determinations in Persons With Human Immunodeficiency Virus Infection," *MMWR Morb Mortal Wkly Rep*, 1992, 41(RR-8):1-17.

Kagan J, Calvelli T, Denny TN, et al, "Guideline for Flow Cytometric Immunophenotyping, a Report From the National Institute of Allergy and Infectious Diseases, Division of AIDS," *Cytometry*, 1993, 14(7):702-15.

Keren DF, Hanson CA, and Hurtubise PE, *Flow Cytometry and Clinical Diagnosis*, Chicago, IL: American Society of Clinical Pathologists, 1994.

Landay A, Ohlsson-Wilhelm B, and Giorgi JV, "Application of Flow Cytometry to the Study of HIV Infection," *AIDS*, 1990, 4(6):479-9.

Laurence J, "T-Cell Subsets in Health, Infectious Disease, and Idiopathic CD4+ T Lymphocytopenia," *Ann Intern Med*, 1993, 119(1):55-62.

Nicholson JK, "Use of Flow Cytometry in the Evaluation and Diagnosis of Primary and Secondary Immunodeficiency Diseases," *Arch Pathol Lab Med*, 1989, 113(6):598-605.

Schmidt RE, "Monoclonal Antibodies for Diagnosis of Immunodeficiencies," *Blut*, 1989, 59(3):200-6.

Schroeder TJ, First MR, Hurtubise PE, et al, "Immunologic Monitoring With Orthoclone OKT3 Therapy," *J Heart Transplant*, 1989, 8(5):371-80.

Stein DS, Korvick JA, and Vermund SH, "CD4+ Lymphocyte Cell Enumeration for Prediction of Clinical Course of Human Immmunodeficiency Virus Disease: A Review," *J Infect Dis*, 1992, 165(2):352-63.

L. gormanii *see* Legionnaires' Disease Antibodies *on page 412*

L. gormanii *see* Legionnaires' Disease Direct Fluorescent Antibody Smear *on page 413*

LGV Titer *see* Lymphogranuloma Venereum Titer *on page 417*

Light Chains *see* Immunoelectrophoresis, Serum or Urine *on page 408*

Light Chains *see* Immunofixation Electrophoresis *on page 408*

Light Chains *see* Protein Electrophoresis, Serum *on page 424*

Light Chains, Urine *see* Protein Electrophoresis, Urine *on page 425*

Liver/Kidney Microsomal Type 1 Antibodies
Related Information
Antimitochondrial Antibody *on page 366*
Liver Biopsy *on page 48*
Liver Profile *on page 161*
Smooth Muscle Antibody *on page 431*

Synonyms Anti-ER Antibodies; Antiliver/Kidney Microsomal Antibodies; Anti-LKM1

Applies to Antiliver Cytosol 1 Antibodies

Specimen Serum

Container Red top tube

Reference Range Negative

Critical Values 1:10 or more considered positive

Use One of three major immunologic tests for autoimmune liver disease, especially in children.

Methodology Indirect immunofluorescence

Additional Information A portion of cases of autoimmune/chronic active hepatitis, autoimmune hepatitis type 2, found especially in girls and young women, are positive for these antibodies. This reactive subset includes a number with related immunologic disorders. Such patients are characterized as well by the presence of antiliver cytosol 1 antibodies.[1]

In a recent publication, only two of 26 cases of recent onset autoimmune hepatitis were reactive with LKM1, while 22 were reactive with smooth muscle antibodies. Each of the two was reported to have titer of 1:320, and one was negative to smooth muscle antibody.[2]

Footnotes
1. Krawitt EL, "Autoimmune Hepatitis," *N Engl J Med*, 1996, 334(14):897-903.
2. Burgart LJ, Batts KP, Ludwig J, et al, "Recent-Onset Autoimmune Hepatitis. Biopsy Findings and Clinical Correlations," *Am J Surg Pathol*, 1995, 19(6):699-708.

Liver/Kidney Microsomes (LKM) Antibody *see* Smooth Muscle Antibody *on page 431*

L. jordanis *see* Legionnaires' Disease Antibodies *on page 412*

L. jordanis *see* Legionnaires' Disease Direct Fluorescent Antibody Smear *on page 413*

L. longbeachae *see* Legionnaires' Disease Antibodies *on page 412*

L. longbeachae *see* Legionnaires' Disease Direct Fluorescent Antibody Smear *on page 413*

L. micdadei *see* Legionnaires' Disease Antibodies *on page 412*

L. micdadei *see* Legionnaires' Disease Direct Fluorescent Antibody Smear *on page 413*

***Loa loa* Serology** *see* Filariasis Serological Test *on page 393*

Long-Acting Thyroid Stimulator *see* Thyrotropin Receptor Antibody *on page 434*

Lupus Anticoagulant (LA) *see* Anticardiolipin Antibody *on page 364*

Lyme Borreliosis Serology *see* Lyme Disease Serology *on this page*

Lyme Disease Serology
CPT 86617 (Western blot); 86618 (antibody)
Related Information
Arthropod Identification *on page 453*
Babesiosis Serological Test *on page 370*
Ehrlichiosis Serology *on page 390*
Lyme Disease DNA Detection *on page 518*
Synovial Fluid Analysis *on page 656*

Synonyms *Borrelia burgdorferi* Serology; Lyme Borreliosis Serology

(Continued)

Lyme Disease Serology (Continued)

Test Commonly Includes Detection of serological response to *Borrelia burgdorferi*

Abstract *Borrelia burgdorferi* infection is often characterized by fever and migratory arthralgia with arthritis appearing much later. There are neurologic complications, and carditis occurs in some patients. Without a reliable laboratory method for recovery of *Borrelia burgdorferi*, diagnosis of Lyme borreliosis is difficult for the clinician and presents problems as well for the clinical laboratory. The clinical presentation and exposure in an endemic area support clinical and laboratory integration.[1] Early, clinical identification of erythema migrans is helpful. Therapy may be appropriate in seronegative individuals with clinical evidence of Lyme disease.

Specimen Serum or cerebrospinal fluid

Container Red top tube, sterile CSF tube

Reference Range Values vary among laboratories

Use Diagnose Lyme disease; investigate arthritis, rash, encephalopathy, polyneuropathy, carditis

Limitations False-positives occur, and seronegative results are frequent, early. Sensitivity bears a relationship to disease duration.[2] Positives remain so for years after treatment.[3] There are cross reactions with antibodies to EB virus, *Rickettsia*, syphilis. There is significant inter- and intra-laboratory variation in this assay, poor standardization and variation in sensitivity and specificity. Even the Western blot is not considered a definitive assay; Western blot is not recommended for chronic stage or for neuroborreliosis. Consequently serologic evidence should not be the sole criterion for a diagnosis of Lyme disease. Positive serologic results in apparently healthy subjects are likely to be false-positives. Positive results must be considered critically.[1]

Methodology The least sensitive and least specific is indirect immunofluorescent antibody (IFA). Enzyme-linked immunosorbent assay (ELISA) is better but can be insensitive and nonspecific. Specific IgM, IgG, and IgA by antibody capture is described as optimal. Western blot is useful for patients with late disease.[4] Enzyme immunoassay (EIA) followed by Western blot of positive specimens has been recommended.[5]

Additional Information Lyme disease is a multisystem disorder, with rash and arthritis conspicuous symptoms. It is widespread in the U.S. and is caused by *Borrelia burgdorferi*, a spirochete transmitted by the bite of the tick *Ixodes dammini*, which also transmits *Babesia*. The disease has protean manifestation, can become chronic, and responds to antibiotics; prompt proper diagnosis is therefore important. Assay is available for IgG and IgM antibody in both serum and CSF. In early disease, a negative assay does not exclude the diagnosis because sensitivity is 40% to 60% and response may be blunted by antibiotics. Most patients with chronic disease will have positive assays. Recent studies using recombinant outer surface protein A and B and flagellin hold out promise for better serologic testing in the near future.[6,7] Patients may harbor *B. burgdorferi* asymptomatically and have positive serology. Such individuals may have symptoms of some other illness incorrectly attributed to Lyme disease and be given inappropriate and ineffective treatment. Antibodies against Lyme disease antigens can interfere with the ANA test.

Cultivation of *B. burgdorferi* from skin lesions suggestive of erythema migrans is described as a practical and clinically relevant procedure,[8] and culture of biopsy or aspiration is described.[9] However, culture is difficult, not reproducible and not done in a routine clinical laboratory.

Neurologic manifestations are found in about 15% of subjects. CSF pleocytosis is found in many but not all patients who have cranial nerve or meningeal involvement.[10] Increased lymphocytes may be found in cerebrospinal fluid.[2] *Borrelia*-specific DNA using PCR assay has been compared to conventional serologic testing.[11] An intrathecal antibody response is found with acute meningitis associated with Lyme disease.[12] See listing Lyme Disease DNA Detection *on page 518*.

B. burgdorferi may cause some cases of diffuse fasciitis with peripheral eosinophilia.[13]

Footnotes
1. Golightly MG, "Laboratory Considerations in the Diagnosis and Management of Lyme Borreliosis," *Am J Clin Pathol*, 1993, 99(2):168-74.
2. Berglund J, Eitrem R, Ornstein K, et al, "An Epidemiologic Study of Lyme Disease in Southern Sweden," *N Engl J Med*, 1995, 333(20):1319-27.
3. Steere AC, Taylor E, McHugh GL, et al, "The Overdiagnosis of Lyme Disease," *JAMA*, 1993, 269(14):1812-6.
4. Berardi VP and Seder RH, "Test for Lyme Disease in a Prepaid Health Plan," *JAMA*, 1994, 272(3):203.
5. Ley C, Reingold AL, and Le C, "The Use of Serologic Tests for Lyme Disease in a Prepaid Health Plan," *JAMA*, 1994, 272(3):203 (reply).
6. Fikrig E, Huguenel ED, Berland R, et al, "Serological Diagnosis of Lyme Disease Using Recombinant Outer Surface Proteins A and B and Flagellin," *J Infect Dis*, 1992, 165(6):1127-32.
7. Robinson JM, Pilot-Matias TJ, Pratt SD, et al, "Analysis of the Humoral Response to the Flagellin Protein of *Borrelia burgdorferi*: Cloning of Regions Capable of Differentiating Lyme Disease From Syphilis," *J Clin Microbiol*, 1993, 31(3):629-35.
8. Mitchell PD, Reed KD, Vandermause MF, et al, "Isolation of *Borrelia burgdorferi* From Skin Biopsy Specimens of Patients With Erythema Migrans," *Am J Clin Pathol*, 1993, 99(1):104-7.
9. Campbell GL, Piesman J, Mitchell PD, et al, "An Evaluation of Media for Transport of Tissues Infected With *Borrelia burgdorferi*," *Am J Clin Pathol*, 1994, 101(2):154-6.
10. Kaslow RA, "Current Perspective on Lyme Borreliosis," *JAMA*, 1992, 267(10):1381-3.
11. Luft BJ, Steinman CR, Neimark HC, et al, "Invasion of the Central Nervous System by *Borrelia burgdorferi* in Acute Disseminated Infection," *JAMA*, 1992, 267(10):1364-7.
12. "Case Records of the Massachusetts General Hospital. Weekly Clinicopathological Exercises. Case 42-1994. A 19-Year-Old Man With Rapidly Progressive Lower-Extremity Weakness and Dysesthesias After a Respiratory Tract Infection," *N Engl J Med*, 1994, 331(21):1437-44.
13. Granter SR, Barnhill RL, Hewins ME, et al, "Identification of *Borrelia burgdorferi* in Diffuse Facsiitis With Peripheral Eosinophilia: Borrelial Fasciitis," *JAMA*, 1994, 272(16):1283-5.

References
Bakken LL, Case KL, Callister SM, et al, "Performance of 45 Laboratories Participating in a Proficiency Testing Program for Lyme Disease Serology," *JAMA*, 1992, 268(7):891-5.

Kaell AT, Redecha PR, Elkon KB, et al, "Occurrence of Antibodies to *Borrelia burgdorferi* in Patients With Nonspirochetal Subacute Bacterial Endocarditis," *Ann Intern Med*, 1993, 119(11):1079-83.

Lovece S, Stern R, and Kagen LJ, "Effects of Rheumatoid Factor, Antinuclear Antibodies and Plasma Reagin on the Serologic Assay for Lyme Disease," *J Rheumatol*, 1991, 18(12):1813-8.

Magid D, Schwartz B, Craft J, et al, "Prevention of Lyme Disease After Tick Bites: A Cost-Effectiveness Analysis," *N Engl J Med*, 1992, 327(8):534-41.

Magnarelli LA, Anderson JF, and Johnson RC, "Cross-Reactivity in Serological Tests for Lyme Disease and Other Spirochetal Infections," *J Infect Dis*, 1987, 156(1):183-8.

Nocton JJ, Dressler F, Rutledge BJ, et al, "Detection of *Borrelia burgdorferi* DNA by Polymerase Chain Reaction in Synovial Fluid From Patients With Lyme Arthritis," *N Engl J Med*, 1994, 330(4):229-34.

Pinals RS, "Polyarthritis and Fever," *N Engl J Med*, 1994, 330(11):769-74.

Rahn DW, "Lyme Disease - Where's the Bug?" *N Engl J Med*, 1994, 330(4):282-3.

Spach DH, Liles WC, Campbell GL, et al, "Tick-Borne Diseases in the United States," *N Engl J Med*, 1993, 329(13):936-47.

Lymphocyte CD4 Counts *see* CD4/CD8 Enumeration *on page 375*

Lymphocyte Crossmatch *see* Tissue Typing *on page 434*

Lymphocyte Mitogen Response Test *see* Lymphocyte Transformation Test *on this page*

Lymphocyte Receptor Studies *see* Leukocyte Immunophenotyping *on page 414*

Lymphocyte Subset Identification *see* Leukocyte Immunophenotyping *on page 414*

Lymphocyte Surface Immunoglobulin Analysis *see* Leukocyte Immunophenotyping *on page 414*

Lymphocyte Transformation Test

CPT 86353

Related Information
Ataxia-Telangiectasia, Chromosome Breakage Study *on page 274*
Fanconi's Anemia, Chromosome Breakage Study *on page 282*
Leukocyte Immunophenotyping *on page 414*
Mixed Lymphocyte Culture *on page 418*
Tumor Aneuploidy by Flow Cytometry *on page 57*

Synonyms Lymphocyte Mitogen Response Test; PHA Stimulation

Applies to Mitogens

Abstract Lymphocyte proliferation normally occurs early in an immune response. Lymphocyte transformation assays test the integrity of the early proliferative response using either nonspecific mitogens or specific antigens to induce blastogenesis. Antigen induced lymphocyte proliferation also correlates with previous exposure and acquisition of cellular immunity.

Specimen Whole blood

Container Yellow top (ACD) tube or green top (heparin) tube. Check with the laboratory performing the assay for special instructions.

Causes for Rejection Old specimen, specimen without viable lymphocytes, specimen refrigerated or frozen

Special Instructions Schedule procedure in advance with laboratory. Specimens to evaluate therapy should include three baseline samples.

Reference Range Mitogen: phytohemagglutinin (PHA), stimulation index >130; mitogen: pokeweed mitogen (PWM), stimulation index >20; mitogen: concanavalin A (con A), stimulation index >40

Use Detect and classify congenital or acquired immunodeficiency disorders, study the integrity of lymphokine production, monitor immunosuppressive or immunoenhancing therapy. Document cellular hypersensitivity reactions to environmental allergens or antigens. Similar methods are used to predict allograft compatibility in the transplantation setting. See listing Mixed Lymphocyte Culture *on page 418*.

Methodology Most commonly, lymphocyte transformation is measured by the incorporation of tritiated thymidine into lymphocytes. Lymphocytes are isolated from peripheral blood and set up in microtiter plate cultures for a period of 3-7 days with and without mitogen or antigen. Commonly, cell density and mitogen or antigen concentration is varied to establish a dose-response curve. Approximately 6-18 hours prior to harvest, lymphocytes are pulsed with tritiated thymidine. Incorporated thymidine is measured and a stimulation index calculated based on control values.

Flow cytometric assays have also been developed. In these procedures, measurement of S-phase fraction or incorporation of bromodeoxyuridine correlates with blastogenesis. Multiparameter analysis allows assessment of blastogenic response within lymphocyte subpopulations co-labeled with selected monoclonal antibodies.

Additional Information PHA and con A are potent T-cell mitogens while PWM, lipopolysaccharide and staphylococcal protein A are selective B-cell mitogens. Patients with DiGeorge anomaly, Nezelof's syndrome, and severe combined immunodeficiency syndrome typically show selectively impaired blastogenic responses to T-cell mitogens, while patients with pure humoral immunodeficiencies generally show normal responses. Humoral immunodeficiency disorders show variable blastogenic responses to B-cell selective mitogens.

Patients with chronic mucocutaneous candidiasis may show relatively normal mitogenic responses with T- and B-cell selective mitogens but will have impaired blastogenesis to *Candida* antigen.

Patients with pulmonary berylliosis show beryllium induced lymphocyte blastogenesis. Evidence suggests that blastogenic responses of lymphocytes isolated from bronchoalveolar washings are more closely related to active lung disease than blastogenesis measured in peripheral blood lymphocytes.[1]

Footnotes
1. Newman LS, Bobka C, Schumacher B, et al, "Compartmentalized Immune Response Reflects Clinical Severity of Beryllium Disease," *Am J Respir Crit Care Med*, 1994, 150(1):135-42.

References
Fletcher MA, Klimas N, Morgan R, et al, "Lymphocyte Proliferation," *Manual of Clinical Laboratory Immunology*, 4th ed, Vol 2, Rose NR, Conway de Macario E, Fahey JL, et al, eds, Washington, DC: American Society for Microbiology, 1992, 213-9.
Pacheco SE and Shearer WT, "Laboratory Aspects of Immunology," *Pediatr Clin North Am*, 1994, 41(4):623-55.
Shearer WT, Paul ME, Smith CW, et al, "Laboratory Assessment of Immune Deficiency Disorders," *Immunol Allerg Clin North Am*, 1994, 14(2):265-99.

Lymphogranuloma Venereum Titer
CPT 86729
Related Information
Chlamydia Group Titer *on page 383*
Chlamydia trachomatis Culture *on page 662*
Chlamydia trachomatis Direct FA Test *on page 663*
Chlamydia trachomatis Genome Detection *on page 505*
Synonyms LGV Titer
Replaces Frei Test
Abstract LGV is a sexually transmitted disease which causes pronounced regional lymphadenopathy and systemic symptoms.
Specimen Serum
Container Red top tube
Sampling Time Acute and convalescent specimens should be collected 10-14 days apart.
Reference Range A fourfold increase in titer in paired sera is usually indicative of acute chlamydial infection. However, patients commonly seek care after the acute stage, precluding collection of paired sera; unpaired sera: <1:64.
Use Support the clinical diagnosis of lymphogranuloma venereum, investigation of inguinal lymphadenopathy, rectal stricture, urethritis, pelvic inflammatory disease, epididymitis, proctitis, proctocolitis, neonatal pneumonia, and conjunctivitis
Limitations While a rising titer of antibody supports the diagnosis of LGV, the period of rise is usually missed. Because of the prevalence of antibodies to *Chlamydia*, demonstration of antibody in itself is insufficient to diagnose acute infection.
Methodology The microimmunofluorescence test is technically difficult to perform properly but can be useful for identifying the infecting serovar. Complement fixation tests identify antibody to an antigen common to all members of the genus but do not provide information on the species or serovar involved. Consequently, a fourfold rise in CF antibody titer provides evidence that a chlamydial infection occurred, but it cannot distinguish LGV from other chlamydial infections. Interpretation of complement fixation test results performed on unpaired sera is complicated by high "background" levels of antibody in the general population. CF antibody titers ≥1:64 are rarely seen in less invasive chlamydial infections in the general population or in sexually active males but may be seen in sexually active females, veterinarians, and patients with Reiter's syndrome.
Additional Information LGV is a sexually transmitted disease caused by the L1, L2, and L3 serovars of *Chlamydia trachomatis*. When infants

are exposed during delivery, they become vulnerable to pneumonia and conjunctivitis. Serologic study is particularly useful to screen for asymptomatic cases that may act as a reservoir for the disease. The presence of complement fixing antibodies **in the proper clinical setting (lymphadenopathy/rectal strictures)** supports the diagnosis of LGV. However, the increasing prevalence of chlamydial genital infections and the attendant increase in "background" antibody titers are vitiating the role of serology in diagnosis of acute illnesses. Tests for IgM antibody are not as useful as in some other infectious diseases because LGV is chronic, and short-lived IgM may no longer be detectable when the diagnosis is considered. Patients being evaluated for LGV should also have serologic testing for other sexually transmitted diseases. A commercial PCR kit has become available for the detection of *Chlamydia* in asymptomatic individuals.

References
Buntin DM, Rosen T, Lesher JL Jr, et al, "Sexually Transmitted Diseases: Bacterial Infections," *J Am Acad Dermatol*, 1991, 25(2 Pt 1):287-99.
Martin DH, "Chlamydial Infections," *Med Clin North Am*, 1990, 74(6):1367-87.
Schachter J, "Chlamydiae," *Manual of Clinical Laboratory Immunology*, 4th ed, Chapter 96, Rose NR, Conway de Macario E, Fahey JL, et al, eds, Washington, DC: American Society for Microbiology, 1992, 661-6.

MA Antibody *see* Antinuclear Antibody *on page 368*

Macroglobulins, Ultracentrifuge Determination *replaced by* Immunoglobulin M *on page 410*

Major Histocompatibility Coded Antigens *see* HLA Typing, Single Human Leukocyte Antigen *on page 405*

Major Histocompatibility Complex (MHC) *see* HLA Typing, Single Human Leukocyte Antigen *on page 405*

***Mansonella ozzardi* Serology** *see* Filariasis Serological Test *on page 393*

***Mansonella perstans* Serology** *see* Filariasis Serological Test *on page 393*

***Mansonella streptocerca* Serology** *see* Filariasis Serological Test *on page 393*

Mazzini *replaced by* RPR *on page 428*

Mazzini *replaced by* VDRL, Serum *on page 438*

β₂-M *see* Beta₂-Microglobulin *on page 371*

MBP Assay *see* Cerebrospinal Fluid Myelin Basic Protein *on page 379*

Measles Antibody
CPT 86765
Related Information
Virus, Direct Detection by Fluorescent Antibody *on page 682*
Synonyms Rubeola Antibodies
Applies to Rubeola Serology, CSF
Test Commonly Includes Antibodies specific for rubella, IgG and IgM levels, in patient's serum or cerebrospinal fluid
Abstract Measles is a viral disease which involves the respiratory tract and lymphoreticular tissues. It includes a papular eruption, lymphadenopathy, cough, and fever.
Specimen Serum or cerebrospinal fluid
Container Red top tube, sterile CSF tube
Reference Range Less than fourfold rise in IgG titer, absent IgM titer; IgG: <1:5; IgM: <1:10; hemagglutination inhibition >1:10, neutralization >1:20 indicates immunity
Use Differential diagnosis of viral exanthems, particularly in pregnant women; diagnosis of subacute sclerosing panencephalitis; document measles immunization
Limitations Antibody sometimes present in multiple sclerosis
Methodology Hemagglutination inhibition (HAI), viral neutralization (NT), enzyme-linked immunosorbent assay (ELISA)
Additional Information Measles (rubeola) is caused by a paramyxovirus, and despite vaccination programs has caused several recent epidemics. Revaccination appears to be of value; no cases have been reported in people who have received two doses of vaccine.[1] Serologic study can be useful in establishing that an individual has immunity subsequent to vaccination. In many individuals **detectable** immunity does not persist. In acute illness, hemagglutinating and neutralizing antibody peak 2 weeks after the rash appears. It is necessary to demonstrate rising titers over 2 weeks, or identify IgM antibody to establish diagnosis. Very high serum titers in the absence of acute illness, or high CSF titer, are seen in subacute sclerosing panencephalitis. Protective antibody levels of antibodies to measles, mumps, and rubella have been assessed by oral fluid sampling.[2]
(Continued)

Measles Antibody *(Continued)*

Footnotes

1. Centers for Disease Control and Prevention, "Measles - United States, First 26 Weeks, 1993," *JAMA*, 1993, 270(20):2423-4.
2. Thieme T, Piacentini S, Davidson S, et al, "Determination of Measles, Mumps, and Rubella Immunization Status Using Oral Fluid Samples," *JAMA*, 1994, 272(3):219-21.

References

Bellini WJ, Rota JS, and Rota PA, "Virology of Measles Virus," *J Infect Dis*, 1994, 170(Suppl 1):S15-23.
Black FL, "Measles and Mumps," *Manual of Clinical Laboratory Immunology*, 4th ed, Vol 2, Chapter 89, Rose NR, Conway de Macario E, Fahey JL, et al, eds, Washington, DC: American Society for Microbiology, 1992, 596-9.
Condorelli F and Ziegler T, "Dot Immunobinding Assay for Simultaneous Detection of Specific Immunoglobulin G Antibodies to Measles Virus, Mumps Virus, and Rubella Virus," *J Clin Microbiol*, 1993, 31(3):717-9.
Markowitz LE, Albrecht P, Orenstein WA, et al, "Persistence of Measles Antibody After Revaccination," *J Infect Dis*, 1992, 166(1):205-8.
Osterhaus AD, de Vries P, and van Binnendijk RS, "Measles Vaccines: Novel Generations and New Strategies," *J Infect Dis*, 1994, 170(Suppl 1):S42-55.
Wittler RR, Veit BC, McIntyre S, et al, "Measles Revaccination Response in a School-Age Population," *Pediatrics*, 1991, 88(5):1024-30.

MHA-TP

CPT 86781

Related Information

Automated Reagin Test *on page 370*
FTA-ABS, Serum *on page 394*
RPR *on page 428*
VDRL, Cerebrospinal Fluid *on page 438*
VDRL, Serum *on page 438*

Synonyms Microhemagglutination-*Treponema pallidum*

Applies to EIA for Syphilis, IgG and IgM; Syphilis Serology

Test Commonly Includes Detection of serologic response to *Treponema pallidum*

Abstract A treponemal (confirmatory) test for syphilis, more specific but less sensitive than the FTA-ABS. The FTA-ABS and the MHA-TP are the standard treponemal tests. A reactive treponemal test in a subject also reactive in a nontreponemal test is highly specific.[1]

Patient Preparation Patient should be fasting if possible.

Specimen Serum

Container Red top tube

Storage Instructions Freeze to ship.

Causes for Rejection Plasma collected

Reference Range Nonreactive

Critical Values Results reported as nonreactive, inconclusive, or reactive

Possible Panic Range Serodiagnosis of syphilis in pregnancy

Use Confirmatory serologic test for syphilis, used also in evaluation of equivocal FTA-ABS result. In addition to verification of reactivity of the nontreponemal tests, the treponemal tests may be used to confirm a clinical impression of syphilis when nontreponemal testing is nonreactive.

Limitations Moderate sensitivity in early (primary) stages of syphilis. False-positives may occur in systemic lupus, infectious mononucleosis, and lepromatous leprosy. More technically demanding and costly than the nontreponemal tests. Potential causes of false-positive serologic tests for syphilis are tabulated in the listing VDRL, Serum *on page 438*.

Methodology Hemagglutination - sensitized sheep cells are coated with *T. pallidum* antigen

Additional Information This is a *Treponema*-specific test and probably should not be used as a screening test. It is as sensitive and specific as FTA-ABS in all stages of syphilis except primary, in which it is less sensitive. It provides fewer false-positives than the FTA-ABS.[1] It will be positive with treponemal infections other than syphilis (bejel, pinta, yaws). Like FTA-ABS, MHA-TP once positive remains so, and cannot be used to judge effect of treatment. The test is not applicable to CSF. The reaginic (nontreponemal) tests for syphilis include RPR and VDRL.

A TPHA index is described.[2]

EIA, IgG and IgM, is a recently available method. IgM EIA is reported to be useful for diagnosis of congenital syphilis. IgG EIA is reported to be a reliable test which can replace the MHA-TP or FTA-ABS. However, it is insufficiently sensitive for diagnosis of primary lues. It does not reflect disease activity.[2]

PCR may be useful for congenital syphilis but is not presently commercially available.

Footnotes

1. Larsen SA, Steiner BM, and Rudolph AH, "Laboratory Diagnosis and Interpretation of Tests for Syphilis," *Clin Microbiol Rev*, 1995, 8(1):1-21.
2. Woods GL, "Update on Laboratory Diagnosis of Sexually Transmitted Diseases," *Clin Lab Med*, 1995, 15(3):665-84.

References

Romanowski B, Sutherland R, Fick GH, et al, "Serologic Response to Treatment of Infectious Syphilis," *Ann Intern Med*, 1991, 114(12):1005-9.

Microfilariae Serological Test *see* Filariasis Serological Test *on page 393*

β₂-Microglobulin *see* Beta₂-Microglobulin *on page 371*

Microhemagglutination-*Treponema pallidum* *see* MHA-TP *on this page*

***Micropolyspora faeni* Precipitating Antibodies** *see* Hypersensitivity Pneumonitis Serology *on page 406*

Microsomal Antibody *see* Thyroid Antimicrosomal Antibody *on page 433*

Mitochondrial Antibody *see* Antimitochondrial Antibody *on page 366*

Mitogens *see* Lymphocyte Transformation Test *on page 416*

Mixed Lymphocyte Culture

CPT 86821

Related Information

HLA Typing, Single Human Leukocyte Antigen *on page 405*
Lymphocyte Transformation Test *on page 416*
Polymerase Chain Reaction *on page 523*
Tissue Typing *on page 434*

Synonyms Mixed Lymphocyte Culture Reaction; MLC; MLR

Applies to Blood Mononuclear Cells; HLA Class II Antigens; HLA-DP; HLA-DQ; HLA-DR

Test Commonly Includes Blood lymphocytes (and some monocytes) from potential donors and the recipient are cultured together and tested for reactivity against each other.

Abstract Mixed lymphocyte culture (MLC) is used primarily to predict histocompatibility in the transplantation setting.

Specimen Leukocytes

Container Green top (heparin) tube

Collection Blood must be delivered to the laboratory immediately.

Causes for Rejection Lack of sterile collection, specimen not collected in heparin, specimen without viable lymphocytes, specimen refrigerated or frozen

Special Instructions Blood specimen must be collected fresh on day of test. Check with the laboratory performing the assay for special instructions.

Reference Range Response compared with that of simultaneously evaluated normal control; requires interpretation

Use Tissue matching for transplantation; evaluate cellular immunocompetence

Limitations Test will be negative if donor or responder cells have a severe cellular immunodeficiency. Test depends on viability of lymphocytes.

Methodology Lymphocytes from two individuals are typically co-cultured to measure unidirectional lymphocyte blastogenesis. Lymphocytes from the allograft donor are typically rendered nonresponsive by treating with mitomycin-C or radiation. Responder lymphocytes are derived from the prospective allograft recipient. After several days in culture, proliferating cells are pulsed with tritiated thymidine approximately 6-18 hours prior to harvest. Therefore, measurement of incorporated thymidine is a function of responder (allograft recipient) lymphocyte blastogenesis. See listing Lymphocyte Transformation Test *on page 416*. In the setting of bone marrow transplantation when graft versus host response is of concern, lymphocytes from the prospective allograft recipient may be rendered unresponsive in order to measure blastogenesis of donor lymphocytes.

Additional Information MLC measure the ability of CD4 positive lymphocytes to recognize HLA class II antigens encoded by the HLA-DR, DQ, and DP loci. Incompatibility of these antigens are among the most potent of blastogenic stimuli. Unidirectional or bidirectional histocompatibility is reflected by little or no blastogenesis. Prominent blastogenic responses predict tissue incompatibility and poor graft survival. Recent advances in molecular genetic typing has also shown high predictive value and may eventually supplant the need for MLC.

References

Hansen JA, Mickelson EM, Choo SY, et al, "Clinical Bone Marrow Transplantation: Donor Selection and Recipient Monitoring," *Manual of Clinical Laboratory Immunology*, 4th ed, Vol 2, Chapter 129, Rose NR, Conway de Macario E, Fahey JL, et al, eds, Washington, DC: American Society for Microbiology, 1992, 850-66.
Hansen TH, Carreno BM, and Sachs DH, "The Major Histocompatibility Complex," *Fundamental Immunology*, 3rd ed, Chapter 16, Paul WE, ed, New York, NY: Raven Press, 1993, 577.

Mixed Lymphocyte Culture Reaction *see* Mixed Lymphocyte Culture *on this page*

MLC *see* Mixed Lymphocyte Culture *on this page*

MLR *see* Mixed Lymphocyte Culture *on this page*

Monoclonal Gammopathies *see* Protein Electrophoresis, Serum *on page 424*

Monoclonal Gammopathy *see* Immunoelectrophoresis, Serum or Urine *on page 408*

Monoclonal Gammopathy *see* Immunofixation Electrophoresis *on page 408*

Monoclonal Gammopathy Work-up *see* Protein Electrophoresis, Urine *on page 425*

Monoclonal Rheumatoid Factor Inhibition *see* Immune Complex Assay *on page 407*

Monospot™ Test *see* Infectious Mononucleosis Screening Test *on page 410*

Monosticon® Dri-Dot® Test *see* Infectious Mononucleosis Screening Test *on page 410*

***M. pneumoniae* Titer** *see* Mycoplasma Serology *on this page*

M Protein *see* Immunofixation Electrophoresis *on page 408*

Muerto Canyon Strain Virus *see* Hantavirus Serology *on page 395*

Mumps Antibodies *see* Mumps Serology *on this page*

Mumps Serology

CPT 86735

Related Information
Mumps Virus Culture *on page 670*
Viral Culture, Central Nervous System Symptoms *on page 677*
Virus, Direct Detection by Fluorescent Antibody *on page 682*

Synonyms Mumps Antibodies

Test Commonly Includes Detection of serologic response to mumps infection or vaccination

Abstract Mumps is caused by a paramyxovirus and man is the only known reservoir.

Specimen Serum

Container Red top tube

Sampling Time Acute and convalescent sera drawn 10-14 days apart are required.

Reference Range A fourfold or greater increase in titer is indicative of recent mumps infection in complement fixation test; normal IgG is <1:5 and IgM is <1:10; a positive (≥1:10) IgM indirect fluorescent test and IgG ≥1:5 are indicative of recent infection; demonstrable IgG usually provides indication of immunity and prior exposure

Use Support for the diagnosis of mumps virus infection; document previous exposure to mumps virus; document immunity

Limitations Several test systems are not specific for mumps and may cross react with another paramyxovirus.

Methodology Complement fixation (CF), enzyme-linked immunosorbent assay (ELISA), indirect fluorescent antibody (IFA), hemagglutination inhibition (HAI), hemolysis-in-gel, virus neutralization

Additional Information Complications include aseptic meningitis, encephalitis, and inflammation of the testes, pancreas, and ovaries. Serologic study may be undertaken to confirm a diagnosis in acute disease or to demonstrate established immunity. For diagnosis in an acute illness, measuring IgM antibody is simplest and fastest.

References
Black FL, "Measles and Mumps," *Manual of Clinical Laboratory Immunology*, 4th ed, Chapter 89, Rose NR, Conway de Macario E, Fahey JL, et al, eds, Washington, DC: American Society for Microbiology, 1992, 596-9.

Condorelli F and Ziegler T, "Dot Immunobinding Assay for Simultaneous Detection of Specific Immunoglobulin G Antibodies to Measles Virus, Mumps Virus, and Rubella Virus," *J Clin Microbiol*, 1993, 31(3):717-9.

Costello MJ, Smernoff NT, and Yungbluth M, "Laboratory Diagnosis of Viral Respiratory Tract Infections," *Lab Med*, 1993, 24(3):150.

Harmsen T, Jongerius MC, van der Zwan CW, et al, "Comparison of a Neutralization Enzyme Immunoassay and an Enzyme-Linked Immunosorbent Assay for Evaluation of Immune Status of Children Vaccinated for Mumps," *J Clin Microbiol*, 1992, 30(8):2139-44.

***Mycoplasma* Antibodies** *see* Mycoplasma Serology *on this page*

***Mycoplasma pneumoniae* Titer** *see* Mycoplasma Serology *on this page*

Mycoplasma Serology

CPT 86738

Related Information
Bacterial Culture, Sputum *on page 465*
Cold Agglutinin Titer *on page 384*
Mycoplasma pneumoniae Diagnostic Procedures *on page 671*

Mycoplasma pneumoniae DNA Probe Test *on page 520*

Synonyms Eaton Agent Titer; *M. pneumoniae* Titer; *Mycoplasma* Antibodies; *Mycoplasma pneumoniae* Titer; Pleuropneumonia-like Organism (PPLO) Titer; Walking Pneumonia Titer

Test Commonly Includes Detection of serologic response to *Mycoplasma pneumoniae* infection

Abstract *Mycoplasmas* lack the rigid cell walls of other bacteria. Thus, they do not react with Gram's stain. They are fastidious and smaller than some viruses. *Mycoplasma pneumoniae* accounts for up to 8% of hospitalized adults with community-acquired pneumonia, and a larger percentage of those treated as outpatients.[1] Pneumonias caused by atypical organisms include chlamydial and mycoplasmal pneumonia, Legionnaires' disease, and rickettsial pneumonias.

Specimen Serum

Container Red top tube

Sampling Time Acute and convalescent sera drawn 10-14 days apart are desirable.

Reference Range Negative. IgG <1:10, IgM <1:10. A fourfold increase in titer in paired sera, drawn 2-3 weeks apart, is a definitive diagnosis. Increase in IgG titer in paired sera may be helpful, but high IgG titer usually is evidence of prior exposure. IgM titer is needed for evaluation in community-acquired pneumonia.

Use Support the diagnosis of *Mycoplasma pneumoniae* infection, investigate atypical pneumonia. Although the most common agent which causes croup is the parainfluenza virus, *M. pneumoniae* and a number of viruses can be etiologic.

Limitations False-positives occur when antibody from prior infection is detected. The complement fixation procedures are based on lipid extracts of the organism, which cross react with antigens in streptococci and chloroplasts.[2] False-positives in patients with pancreatitis are described. False-negatives are found when testing is done too early and may be found in immunocompromised individuals.[3] Rational implementation requires interprocedure comparisons, as well as understanding of the population served.[4]

Methodology Complement fixation (CF), indirect fluorescent antibody (IFA), enzyme immunoassay (EIA), nucleic acid hybridization, polymerase chain reaction (PCR), specific IgM antibody by agglutination, IgM anti-P1 immunoblotting, microtiter procedure utilizing anti-*M. pneumoniae* IgM[4]

Additional Information *Mycoplasma pneumoniae* is a cause of "primary atypical pneumonia." *Mycoplasma* is more difficult to culture than ordinary bacteria and thus serologic confirmation of the diagnosis is often desirable. A fourfold or greater rise in titer occurs in about 80% of cases. Serologic tests for antibody to *M. pneumoniae* are more specific and more sensitive than the cold agglutinin titer. Demonstration of specific IgG and IgM antibody by immunofluorescence is rapid, sensitive, and specific. IgM antibody indicates acute infection.

ESR and C-reactive protein are often abnormal. Cold agglutinins are elevated, IgM antibodies against the I antigen of red cells.

See also the listings *Mycoplasma pneumoniae* DNA Probe Test *on page 520* and *Mycoplasma pneumoniae* Diagnostic Procedures *on page 671*.

Footnotes
1. Bartlett JG and Mundy LM, "Community-Acquired Pneumonia," *N Engl J Med*, 1995, 333(24):1618-24.
2. "Case Records of the Massachusetts General Hospital. Weekly Clinocopathological Exercises. Case 42-1994. A 19-Year-Old Man With Rapidly Progressive Lower-Extremity Weakness and Dysesthesias After a Respiratory Tract Infection," *N Engl J Med*, 1994, 331(2):1437-44.
3. Jacobs E, "Serological Diagnosis of *Mycoplasma pneumoniae* Infections: A Critical Review of Current Procedures," *Clin Infect Dis*, 1993, 17(Suppl 1):S79-82.
4. Cimolai N and Cheong AC, "An Assessment of a New Diagnostic Indirect Enzyme Immunoassay for the Detection of Anti-*Mycoplasma pneumoniae* IgM," *Am J Clin Pathol*, 1996, 105:205-9.

References
Clyde WA Jr, "*Mycoplasma* Infections," *Harrison's Principles of Internal Medicine*, 13th ed, Isselbacher KJ, Braunwald E, Wilson JD, et al, eds, New York, NY: McGraw-Hill Inc, 1994, 757-9.

"From the Centers for Disease Control and Prevention. Outbreaks of *Mycoplasma pneumoniae* Respiratory Infection - Ohio, Texas, and New York, 1993," *JAMA*, 1994, 271(5):338-9.

Johnson DH and Cunha BA, "Atypical Pneumonias. Clinical and Extrapulmonary Features of *Chlamydia, Mycoplasma*, and *Legionella* Infections," *Postgrad Med*, 1993, 93(7):69-72, 75-6, 79-82.

Kleemola SR, Karjalainen JE, and Raty RK, "Rapid Diagnosis of *Mycoplasma pneumoniae* Infection: Clinical Evaluation of a Commercial Probe Test," *J Infect Dis*, 1990, 162(1):70-5.

Smith TF, "*Mycoplasma pneumoniae* Infections: Diagnosis Based on Immunofluorescence Titer of IgG and IgM Antibodies," *Mayo Clin Proc*, 1986, 61(10):830-1.

Myelin Basic Protein, Cerebrospinal Fluid *see* Cerebrospinal Fluid Myelin Basic Protein *on page 379*

Myositis-Specific Autoantibody

CPT 86255 (screen); 86256 (titer)

Related Information

Creatine Kinase *on page 115*
Jo-1 Antibody *on page 411*
Muscle Biopsy *on page 53*
Scleroderma Antibody *on page 430*
Striational Antibodies *on page 432*

Applies to Antihistidyl-Transfer RNA (tRNA) Synthetase; Anti-Ku Autoantibodies; Anti-Mi-2 Autoantibodies; Anti-PM-Scl Autoantibodies; Antisignal Recognition (Anti-SRP) Autoantibodies; Anti-SRP Autoantibodies; Anti-U1-Ribonucleoprotein Autoantibodies

Test Commonly Includes Anti Jo-1 Antibodies

Abstract The most common forms of the inflammatory myopathies are polymyositis and dermatomyositis. Several types of myositis-specific antibodies have been described. Myositis-specific autoantibodies are found almost exclusively in myositis.[1]

Specimen Serum

Container Red top tube

Reference Range Negative. Titers correlate with disease activity.

Use Diagnose inflammatory myopathies and the differential diagnosis of dermatomyositis, systemic sclerosis, SLE, polymyositis, arthritis, antisynthetase syndrome, antisignal recognition particle syndrome, Raynaud's phenomenon, Gottron's papules, shawl sign rashes, and other findings.

Methodology Indirect fluorescent antibody (IFA)

Additional Information Abnormalities in serum immunoglobulin levels occur. Immunoglobulins reacting to, or deposited in, muscle can be demonstrated in numerous rheumatic disorders. Sarcolemmal basement membrane, fibers, and vessels may all be involved, individually or in combination. Unfortunately, variability and inconsistency of patterns exist. Creatine kinase, aldolase, lactate dehydrogenase, AST, ALT, and muscle biopsy are relevant.

Patients with antisynthetase autoantibodies have **antisynthetase syndrome**, characterized by arthritis, lung disease, Raynaud's phenomenon, photosensitive facial rashes, and fever. They may be misdiagnosed as systemic sclerosis.

Antisignal recognition particle syndrome is characterized by acute onset of polymyositis in the fall, often with cardiac involvement, with palpitation and death from cardiac complications. Patients with this antibody (anti-SRP) always have polymyositis.[1]

Subjects with **anti-Mi-2 autoantibodies** have a good prognosis.

A number of types of myositis and myopathies exist.

Other relevant antibodies include **antihistidyl-transfer RNA (tRNA) synthetase**, found only in myositis; **anti-Mi-2 autoantibodies**, found almost always in patients with dermatomyositis; **anti-U1-ribonucleoprotein autoantibodies**, associated with mixed connective tissue disease; **anti-PM-Scl autoantibodies**; and **anti-Ku autoantibodies**.

Footnotes

1. Plotz PH, Rider LG, Targoff IN, et al, "Myositis: Immunologic Contributions to Understanding Cause, Pathogenesis, and Therapy," *Ann Intern Med*, 1995, 122(9):715-24.

References

Miller FW, "Myositis-Specific Autoantibodies - Touchstones for Understanding the Inflammatory Myopathies," *JAMA*, 1993, 270(15):1846-9.

Nantucket Fever Serological Test *see* Babesiosis Serological Test *on page 370*

Nasopharyngeal Smear for *Bordetella pertussis* *see* Bordetella pertussis *Direct Fluorescent Antibody on page 371*

n-DNA *see* Anti-DNA *on page 365*

Neutrophil Antibody *see* Antineutrophil Antibody *on page 366*

Non-A, non-B Hepatitis *see* Hepatitis C Serology *on page 399*

Nucleolar Antibody *see* Antinuclear Antibody *on page 368*

Oligoclonal Bands, Cerebrospinal Fluid *see* Cerebrospinal Fluid Oligoclonal Bands *on page 379*

***Onchocerca volvulus* Serology** *see* Filariasis Serological Test *on page 393*

Organ Donor Tissue Typing *see* Tissue Typing *on page 434*

Oriental Sore Serological Test *see* Leishmaniasis Serological Test *on page 413*

p24 Antigen

CPT 86311

Related Information

HIV-1/HIV-2 Serology *on page 403*
Human Immunodeficiency Virus Culture *on page 669*

Human Immunodeficiency Virus DNA Amplification *on page 515*
Leukocyte Immunophenotyping *on page 414*
Risks of Transfusion *on page 623*

Synonyms HIV Core Antigen

Applies to Gag Gene of HIV

Test Commonly Includes Detection of HIV p24 antigen in serum or cerebrospinal fluid

Specimen Serum or cerebrospinal fluid

Container Red top tube, sterile CSF tube

Special Instructions In some states written or informed patient consent is a prerequisite for the test. Results may need to be kept confidential.

Reference Range Negative

Use Diagnose recent acute infection with HIV; may also be of prognostic significance in AIDS, if antigen becomes positive during infection, after having been negative. (Can also be used to test viral culture supernatants.)

Limitations Test is not as sensitive as culture or reverse transcriptase polymerase chain reaction for detecting HIV infection.

Methodology Enzyme immunoassay (EIA)

Additional Information p24 antigen is a 24 kD protein product of the **gag** gene of HIV. As a viral rather than host product, it appears concomitant with initial infection, and then generally becomes undetectable during periods of viral latency. It reappears with renewed viral replication; the reappearance of p24 antigen in serum generally heralds progression of clinical disease in AIDS. Measuring antigen may also be useful in assessing therapy. Recent studies indicate that an acid dissociation procedure that disrupts the p24 antigen-antibody complexes can increase the sensitivity of the procedure up to fivefold. This may improve its diagnostic utility,[1] especially for neonate testing. It has been suggested that AIDS patients being treated with dideoxyinosine be followed with p24 levels to determine efficacy of treatment.[2] The p24 EIA does appear to precede seroconversion by a few days.[3] In July, 1995, the FDA's Blood Product Advisory Committee (BPAC) had advised against the test for several reasons. First, the cost of the additional test would be about $80 million nationally and would prevent as few as 10 HIV transmissions. Second, until 1996 there was not an FDA-licensed test that could be automated or performed in the time the other seven infectious disease tests were completed. Finally, the p24 test could cause a magnet effect. That is, high-risk groups might come to the blood donor centers for a free test that is more sensitive than the tests available at health departments. This may actually increase the number of HIV transmissions through blood transfusion. Despite all the above arguments, in early 1996, the FDA required all blood for transfusion be screened for the HIV p24 antigen.

Footnotes

1. Bollinger RC Jr, Kline RL, Francis HL, et al, "Acid Dissociation Increases the Sensitivity of p24 Antigen Detection for the Evaluation of Antiviral Therapy and Disease Progression in Asymptomatic HIV-Infected Persons," *J Infect Dis*, 1992, 165(5):913-6.
2. Drusano GL, Yuen GJ, Lambert JS, et al, "Relationship Between Dideoxyinosine Exposure, CD4 Counts, and p24 Antigen Levels in Human Immunodeficiency Virus Infection: A Phase I Trial," *Ann Intern Med*, 1992, 116(7):562-6.
3. Busch MP, Lee LL, Satten GA, et al, "Time Course of Detection of Viral and Serologic Markers Preceding Human Immunodeficiency Virus Type 1 Seroconversion: Implications for Screening of Blood and Tissue Donors," *Transfusion*, 1995, 35:91-7.

References

Goudsmit J, Lange JM, Paul DA, et al, "Antigenemia and Antibody Titers to Core and Envelope Antigens in AIDS, AIDS-Related Complex, and Subclinical Human Immunodeficiency Virus Infection," *J Infect Dis*, 1987, 155(3):558-60.
Le Pont F, Costagliola D, Rouzioux C, et al, "How Much Would the Safety of Blood Transfusion be Improved by Including p24 Antigen in the Battery of Tests?" *Transfusion*, 1995, 35(7):542-7.
Phair JP and Wolinsky S, "Diagnosis of Infection With the Human Immunodeficiency Virus," *Clin Infect Dis*, 1992, 15(1):13-6.
Wilber JC, "Serologic Testing of Human Immunodeficiency Virus Infection," *Clin Lab Med*, 1987, 7(4):777-91.
Wittek AE, Phelan MA, Wells MA, et al, "Detection of Human Immunodeficiency Virus Core Protein in Plasma by Enzyme Immunoassay," *Ann Intern Med*, 1987, 107(3):286-92.

PA *see* Parietal Cell Antibody *on next page*

p-ANCA *see* Antineutrophil Cytoplasmic Antibody *on page 367*

Parainfluenza Viral Serology

CPT 86710

Related Information

Parainfluenza Virus Culture *on page 671*
Viral Culture *on page 675*
Viral Culture, Respiratory Symptoms *on page 680*
Virus, Direct Detection by Fluorescent Antibody *on page 682*

Test Commonly Includes Antibody titers to parainfluenza virus types 1, 2, 3, and 4

Specimen Serum

Container Red top tube; capillary puncture: minimum eight full blue tip capillary tubes

Sampling Time Acute and convalescent sera drawn 10-14 days apart are recommended.

Reference Range A single low titer or less than a fourfold change in titer in paired sera

Use Support the diagnosis of parainfluenza virus infection. Serologic studies are of value in epidemiology.

Limitations Need for convalescent specimen delays diagnosis. Heterotypic rises in parainfluenza titers may occur in infections with other viruses. Infant antibody response may be undetectable. Parainfluenza viral serology is not recommended for clinical diagnostic purposes.

Methodology Complement fixation (CF), hemagglutination inhibition (HAI), enzyme-linked immunosorbent assay (ELISA)

Additional Information Since the demonstration of a fourfold rise in antibody titer requires testing a convalescent specimen, serologic diagnosis is seldom useful in clinical management of an acute illness. This is especially so since the rise may occur even in an infection caused by some other virus such as mumps. **Rapid diagnosis during acute illness may be accomplished by demonstrating viral antigen in smears or tissue by immunofluorescence.** Parainfluenza culture is available; see listing Parainfluenza Virus Culture *on page 671.* Since parainfluenza virus may respond to ribavirin, prompt accurate diagnosis could become important, particularly in the immunocompromised host.

References

Fedova D, Novotny J, and Kubinova I, "Serological Diagnosis of Parainfluenza Virus Infections: Verification of the Sensitivity and Specificity of the Haemagglutination-Inhibition (HI), Complement Fixation (CF), Immunofluorescence (IFA) Tests, and Enzyme Immunoassay (ELISA)," *Acta Virol*, 1992, 36(3):304-12.

Mufson MA and Belshe RB, "Respiratory Syncytial Virus and the Parainfluenza Viruses," *Manual of Clinical Laboratory Immunology*, 4th ed, Vol 2, Chapter 87, Rose NR, Conway de Macario E, Fahey JL, et al, eds, Washington, DC: American Society for Microbiology, 1992, 582-9.

Sperber SJ and Hayden FG, "Antiviral Chemotherapy and Prophylaxis of Viral Respiratory Disease," *Clin Lab Med*, 1987, 7(4):869-96.

Paraproteinemia *see* Immunoelectrophoresis, Serum or Urine *on page 408*

Paraprotein Evaluation *see* Immunofixation Electrophoresis *on page 408*

Parasite Antibodies

CPT 86171 (complement fixation); 86280 (hemagglutination inhibition); 86329 (immunodiffusion)

Related Information

Babesiosis Serological Test *on page 370*
Chagas' Disease Serological Test *on page 383*
Cysticercosis Titer *on page 388*
Echinococcosis Serological Test *on page 390*
Entamoeba histolytica Serological Test *on page 391*
Eosinophil Count *on page 315*
Filariasis Serological Test *on page 393*
Leishmaniasis Serological Test *on page 413*
Malaria Smear *on page 332*
Ova and Parasites, Stool *on page 494*
Ova and Parasites, Urine *on page 495*
Schistosomiasis Serological Test *on page 429*
Toxoplasmosis Serology *on page 435*
Trichinosis Serology *on page 436*

Synonyms Parasite Screen; Parasite Titer

Applies to *Toxocara* Excretory-Secretory ELISA (TES)

Test Commonly Includes *Echinococcus, Entamoeba histolytica, Paragonimus,* Toxoplasmosis, Chagas' Disease, Malaria, Filaria, *Schistosoma,* Trichinosis, *Fasciola hepatica, Leishmania,* Visceral Larva Migrans (VLM) (hyper-*Ascaris* and *Toxocara*), *Strongyloides,* cysticercosis, *Taenia solium* and *Taenia saginata,* Trypanosomiasis, *Giardia, Onchocerca volvulus*

Specimen Serum

Container Red top tube

Sampling Time Acute and convalescent specimens drawn 10-14 days apart are recommended

Reference Range Negative. A fourfold increase in titer in paired sera is usually indicative of acute infestation. For TES-ELISA for VLM, titer ≥1:32 is regarded as significant.

Use Support diagnosis of suspected parasitic infestation

Limitations Cross reactions occur. Serologic diagnosis does not replace demonstration of the parasite itself or its eggs as a definitive diagnostic procedure in many instances. False-positive reactions for toxocariasis were found in 25% of subjects with schistosomiasis and filariasis by ELISA technology.[1]

Methodology *Toxocara* excretory-secretory (TES) enzyme-linked immunosorbent assay (ELISA) is the serologic test of choice for visceral larva

migrans. Other tests for other entities include complement fixation (CF), immunodiffusion (ID), and hemagglutination inhibition (HAI).

Additional Information "Parasite Screen" is not a specific test as such, but is a service offered by some laboratories, consisting of a battery of procedures to detect antibodies to specific parasites. Antibodies will rarely be present unless tissue invasion has taken place.

VLM is one of two entities caused by the dog roundworm, *Toxocara canis,* in the United States. It is found in humans mainly between ages 1 and 4 years. Its characteristics include leukocytosis with eosinophilia, hyperglobulinemia, fever, pulmonary infiltrates, hepatomegaly, and often, rashes. An enzyme-linked immunosorbent assay (ELISA) has confirmed the diagnosis in an adult with bronchospasm.[2] Elevated isohemagglutinins (anti-A, anti-B) are found since *T. canis* larvae expresses surface antigens cross reacting with ABO epitopes.

The second entity caused by dog roundworm is ocular toxocariasis (ocular larva migrans).

Footnotes

1. Gillespie SH, Bidwell D, Voller A, et al, "Diagnosis of Human Toxocariasis by Antigen Capture Enzyme-Linked Immunosorbent Assay," *J Clin Pathol*, 1993, 46(6):551-4.
2. Feldman GJ and Parker HW, "Visceral Larva Migrans Associated With the Hypereosinophilic Syndrome and the Onset of Severe Asthma," *Ann Intern Med*, 1992, 116(10):838-40.

References

English BK, "Toxocariasis," *Principles and Practice of Pediatrics*, 2nd ed, Oski FA, DeAngelis CD, Feigin RD, et al, eds, Philadelphia, PA: JB Lippincott Co, 1994, 1405-8.

Kagan IG and Maddison SE, "Serodiagnosis of Parasitic Diseases," *Manual of Clinical Laboratory Immunology*, 4th ed, Vol 2, Chapter 79, Rose NR, Conway de Macario E, Fahey JL, et al, eds, Washington, DC: American Society for Microbiology, 1992, 529-43.

Orihel TC and Ash LR, *Parasites in Human Tissues*, Chicago, IL: ASCP Press, 1995.

Parasite Screen *see* Parasite Antibodies *on this page*

Parasite Titer *see* Parasite Antibodies *on this page*

Parietal Cell Antibody

CPT 86255 (screen); 86256 (titer)

Related Information

Folic Acid, RBC *on page 317*
Folic Acid, Serum *on page 317*
Gastric Analysis *on page 133*
Intrinsic Factor Antibody *on page 411*
Phosphorus, Urine *on page 183*
Schilling Test *on page 346*
Vitamin B_{12} *on page 351*
Vitamin B_{12} Unsaturated Binding Capacity *on page 352*

Synonyms Antiparietal Cell Antibody; PA

Applies to Intrinsic Factor

Abstract The gastric parietal (oxyntic) cell secretes intrinsic factor which combines with ingested vitamin B_{12} to permit absorption in the ileum. Parietal cells also secrete HCl and blood group substances.

Specimen Serum

Container Red top tube

Reference Range Negative

Use Occasionally used in the differential diagnosis of pernicious anemia and atrophic gastritis

Limitations Nonspecific: found in 20% to 30% of patients with a variety of autoimmune disorders and 16% of asymptomatic people older than 60 years of age. In a study of autoantibodies in presumably healthy blood donors, two with antiparietal cell and others with other antibodies were detected. On follow up, no increase in the incidence of autoimmune diseases in such healthy subjects was elicited.[1]

Methodology Indirect fluorescent antibody (IFA)

Additional Information Antibodies to parietal cells are present in 90% of adults with pernicious anemia and in up to 60% of subjects with atrophic gastritis; they do not correlate with malabsorption of vitamin B_{12}. However, they may participate in the early pathogenesis of parietal cell destruction. They are also present in occasional patients with gastric ulcer or gastric cancer. There is cross positivity of parietal cell and thyroid antibodies in patients with thyroiditis and pernicious anemia. With time, the titer of parietal cell antibodies will decline in some patients with pernicious anemia (possibly related to loss of parietal cells) whereas intrinsic factor antibodies persist.

Footnotes

1. Vrethem M, Skogh T, Berlin G, et al, "Autoantibodies Versus Clinical Symptoms in Blood Donors," *J Rheumatol*, 1992, 19(12):1919-21.

References

Burman P, Kampe O, Kraaz W, et al, "A Study of Autoimmune Gastritis in the Postpartum Period and at a 5-Year Follow-up," *Gastroenterology*, 1992, 103(3):934-42.

Davidson RJ, Atrah HI, and Sewell HF, "Longitudinal Study of Circulating Gastric Antibodies in Pernicious Anemia," *J Clin Pathol*, 1989, 42(10):1092-5.

Harty RF and Leibach JR, "Immune Disorders of the Gastrointestinal Tract and Liver," *Med Clin North Am*, 1985, 69(4):675-704.

Parvovirus B19 DNA

CPT 83898

Related Information

Parvovirus B19 Serology *on this page*

Test Commonly Includes Detection of parvovirus B19 by DNA hybridization using polymerase chain reaction (PCR)

Abstract Parvovirus B19 clinical manifestations include arthralgias, erythema infectiosum, flu-like symptoms with fever. Replication is in erythroid progenitor cells in marrow.

Specimen Serum, amniotic fluid

Container Red top tube

Use Parvovirus B19 infection is associated with stillbirth, arthritis, aplastic crisis and fifth disease. This test may be positive in immunocompromised patients who do not produce antibodies against parvovirus B19.

Methodology Polymerase chain reaction (PCR) to detect parvovirus B19 DNA

Additional Information Parvovirus B19 is a DNA virus which can cause a wide spectrum of disease including self-limited erythema infectiosum (fifth disease), which includes facial rash in half or more patients. It causes bone marrow failure and fetal death. In most people, the low titer viremia which begins about 1 week after exposure and persists for 7-10 days is associated with mild symptoms and a subclinical red cell aplasia. Because the virus destroys red blood cell precursors, there is a reduction in erythrocyte production. This transient aplastic crisis may be particularly severe clinically in patients with hemoglobinopathies associated with decreased erythrocyte lifespan (sickle cell disease, spherocytosis, and β-thalassemia). The presence of parvovirus DNA provides definite evidence of recent infection.

References

Koch WC, Massey G, Russell CE, et al, "Manifestations and Treatment of Human Parvovirus B19 Infections in Immunocompromised Patients," *J Pediatr*, 1990, 116(3):355-9.

Kovacs BW, Carlson DE, Shahbahrami B, et al, "Prenatal Diagnosis of Human Parvovirus B19 in Nonimmune Hydrops Fetalis by Polymerase Chain Reaction," *Am J Obstet Gynecol*, 1992, 167(2):461-6.

McOmish F, Yap PL, Jordan A, et al, "Detection of Parvovirus B19 in Donated Blood: A Model System for Screening by Polymerase Chain Reaction," *J Clin Microbiol*, 1993, 31(2):323-8.

Patou G, Pillay D, Myint S, et al, "Characterization of a Nested Polymerase Chain Reaction Assay for Detection of Parvovirus B19," *J Clin Microbiol*, 1993, 31(3):540-6.

Parvovirus B19 Serology

CPT 86747

Related Information

Parvovirus B19 DNA *on this page*

Synonyms Anti-B19 IgG Antibodies; Anti-B19 IgM Antibodies

Test Commonly Includes Assays for parvovirus B19 may include IgM and IgG antibodies

Specimen Serum, amniotic fluid for IgM antibody. In the presence of hydrops, amniocentesis and fetal blood sampling are advocated.[1]

Container Red top tube

Sampling Time B19-specific IgM antibodies appear in 3 days after onset and persist for only 30-60 days. Collect acute and convalescent sera for IgG antibodies.

Storage Instructions Separate serum and freeze.

Reference Range <0.80 is usually negative for IgG and IgM.

Use The mainstay of diagnosis of parvovirus B19 infection is serologic. Such serologic testing is employed in investigation of maculopapular rash with fever, arthralgias, red cell aplastic crisis in subjects with hemolytic anemias; work-up of fetal hydrops and spontaneous abortion

Limitations Immunocompromised patients show poor antibody response. Unpaired sera tested for IgG are of little use for diagnosing infection, as 2% to 15% of children younger than 5 years of age, 15% to 60% of 5-19 years of age and up to 60% of adults have circulating IgG antibodies. IgM antibodies rise rapidly after infection and remain elevated for 2-3 months, though occasional patients may remain positive for up to 6 months. Detection of IgM antibodies provides strong evidence for recent infection. Once positive, IgG antibodies remain elevated for life and probably confer life-long immunity. Fetal blood sampling prior to 22 weeks of gestation often produces false-negative IgM results. Some cross reactions with patient sera containing rubella virus-specific IgM.

Methodology Radioimmunoassay (RIA), indirect enzyme immunoassay for IgG, or immunoblot assay (Western blot) for the detection of IgM antibodies to parvovirus B19. IgM detects recent infection. Serologic methods are preferable to electron microscopy, which can detect the virus.[2]

Additional Information Parvovirus B19 is a DNA virus and can cause a wide spectrum of disease, ranging form outbreaks of self-limiting erythema infectiosum (fifth disease) to bone marrow failure and to fetal death. Intrauterine transfusion has been suggested when there is evidence of B19 parvovirus-associated anemia and hydrops. The low-

titer parvovirus B19 viremia, which begins approximately 1 week after exposure and lasts 7-10 days, is usually associated with mild symptoms and subclinical red cell aplasia. Because the virus destroys erythroid precursors, which leads to a reduction in normal red blood cell production, infection with parvovirus B19 can cause aplastic crisis in patients already at maximum red cell production and in those with increased red cell destruction (sickle cell disease, β-thalassemia, and spherocytosis). In immunocompromised patients, parvovirus B19 infection can cause life-threatening anemia. IgG antibody production usually occurs 18-24 days after exposure and is probably immune-complex mediated. The presence of IgM antibodies to parvovirus B19 provide definite evidence of recent infection.

Footnotes

1. Ghidini A and Lynch L, "Prenatal Diagnosis and Significance of Fetal Infections," *West J Med*, 1993, 159(3):366-73.

2. Jones MF, Wold AD, Espy MJ, "Serologic Diagnosis of Parvovirus B19 Infections," *Mayo Clin Proc*, 1993, 68(11):1107-8.

References

Brown KE, Hibbs JR, Gallinella G, et al, "Resistance to Parvovirus B19 Infection Due to Lack of Virus Receptor (Erythrocyte P Antigen)," *N Engl J Med*, 1994, 330(17):1192-6.

Kerr JR, McQuaid S, and Coyle PV, "Expression of P Antigen in Parvovirus B19-Infected Bone Marrow," *N Engl J Med*, 1995, 332(2):128.

Patou G and Ayliffe U, "Evaluation of Commercial Enzyme-Linked Immunosorbent Assay for Detection of B19 Parvovirus IgM and IgG," *J Clin Pathol*, 1991, 44(10):831-4.

Rodis JF, Quinn DL, Gary GW Jr, et al, "Management and Outcome of Pregnancies Complicated by Human B19 Parvovirus Infection: A Prospective Study," *Am J Obstet Gynecol*, 1991, 164(4 Pt 1):1363-4.

Paul-Bunnell Davidsohn Test *replaced by* Infectious Mononucleosis Screening Test *on page 410*

PCR Assay for *Bartonella* *see* Cat Scratch Disease Serology *on page 375*

PCR Assay for *Rochalimaea* *see* Cat Scratch Disease Serology *on page 375*

Pemphigoid Antibodies *see* Pemphigus-Like Antibodies *on this page*

Pemphigus-Like Antibodies

CPT 86255 (screen); 86256 (titer)

Related Information

Skin Biopsy *on page 54*

Skin Biopsy, Immunofluorescence *on page 56*

Viral Culture *on page 675*

Synonyms Pemphigoid Antibodies

Abstract IgG antibasement membrane zone antibodies are found in patients with pemphigoid, epidermolysis bullosa acquisita, and bullous eruption of lupus erythematosus. Subjects with pemphigus have IgG anti-intercellular substance antibodies.[1]

Specimen Serum

Container Red top tube

Reference Range Negative

Use Differential diagnosis of pemphigus, pemphigoid, epidermolysis bullosa acquisita, bullous eruption of lupus erythematosus; evaluate response to therapy in subjects with pemphigus

Limitations False-positives may be seen in lupus, burns, and drug reactions, but these are usually weak. These observations require correlation with clinical findings, skin biopsy patterns, and if needed, direct immunofluorescence.

Methodology Indirect fluorescent antibody (IFA) on frozen section of monkey esophagus and NaCl - split human skin[1]

Additional Information Pemphigus vulgaris (and its variants) and bullous pemphigoid are blistering diseases of the skin. Although often diagnosed on clinical presentation and conventional histologic examination, such diseases may require skin immunofluorescence for differentiation. In pemphigus, IgG antibodies are directed against intercellular material within the epithelium and C3 are found on cell surfaces. Patients with oral lesions may not have circulating antibody. In pemphigoid, antibody is directed against the basement membrane. Circulating antibody is present in 70% of patients, and 25% will show IgG and C3 basement membrane deposits on skin biopsy. These antibodies correlate with disease activity, and are present in 60% of patients with pemphigoid and 80% of patients with pemphigus.

Footnotes

1. Leavelle DE, *Mayo Medical Laboratories Interpretive Handbook*, Rochester, MN: Mayo Medical Laboratories, 1994.

References

Harrist TJ and Mihm MC, "Cutaneous Immunopathology. The Diagnostic Use of Direct and Indirect Immunofluorescence Techniques in Dermatologic Disease," *Hum Pathol*, 1979, 10:625-53.

Izuno GT, "Cutaneous Immunofluorescence," *Clin Lab Med*, 1986, 6(1):95-102.

Stanley JR, "Pemphigus. Skin Failure Mediated by Autoantibodies," *JAMA*, 1990, 264(13):1714-7.

Pertussis DFA see *Bordetella pertussis* Direct Fluorescent Antibody on page 371

Pertussis Serology see *Bordetella pertussis* Serology on page 372

PHA Stimulation see Lymphocyte Transformation Test on page 416

Pi Phenotype see Alpha₁-Antitrypsin Phenotyping on page 362

Pleuropneumonia-like Organism (PPLO) Titer see Mycoplasma Serology on page 419

Pneumocystis carinii Serology see Pneumocystis Immunofluorescence on this page

Pneumocystis Immunofluorescence

CPT 86255 (screen); 86256 (titer); 87206 (smear, fluorescent)

Related Information

Bacterial Culture, Bronchoscopy Specimen *on page 459*
Bacterial Culture, Sputum *on page 465*
Bronchial Washings Cytology *on page 287*
Bronchoalveolar Lavage Cytology *on page 288*
Pneumocystis carinii Preparation *on page 299*
Polymerase Chain Reaction *on page 523*
Sputum Cytology *on page 300*

Synonyms *Pneumocystis carinii* Serology

Test Commonly Includes Direct and indirect immunofluorescence for detection of antibody to *Pneumocystis carinii* or to detect the organism in clinical specimens

Abstract The most common lung complication in AIDS is pneumonia caused by *Pneumocystis carinii*, but *P. carinii* causes diseases in other patients as well. Many are immunocompromised, but some do not present identifiable risk factors. Systemic corticosteroid therapy was given to most patients without HIV infection prior to onset of *P. carinii* pneumonia.[1]

Specimen Tissue, sputum, bronchoalveolar lavage

Container Sterile container

Special Instructions Tissue specimens should be received fresh or snap-frozen.

Reference Range No organisms observed

Possible Panic Range Organisms seen

Use Diagnose *Pneumocystis carinii* pneumonia

Limitations A negative result does not exclude the diagnosis.

Methodology Indirect (IFA) and direct fluorescent antibody (DFA)

Additional Information With the onslaught of the AIDS epidemic *Pneumocystis*, previously an obscure and infrequent pathogen of immunosuppressed cancer and transplant patients, become a common, treatable pathogen. Diagnosis depends primarily on seeing either cysts or trophozoites in tissue or cytology preparations. Silver impregnations (eg, methenamine silver) have been the gold standard (to mix metals if not metaphors) to bring out the cyst wall in tissue sections. Direct immunofluorescence is more sensitive than silver stain and rapid, although Wright-Giemsa stain for sporozoites/trophozoites is probably even better and faster for imprints and cytologic specimens. Other advantages of silver stains include detection of various fungal infections. Studies in PCR detection of *P. carinii* show that it is more sensitive than cytology or immunofluorescence.[2] Newer, more sensitive PCR technology is able to detect PCP in symptom-free carriers, patients on anti-PCP prophylaxis and subclinical infection.[2,3]

Extrapulmonary infection in patients with AIDS has involved liver, spleen, eyes, ears, lymph nodes, thymus, skin, omentum, mastoids, ascitic fluid, stomach and duodenum, kidneys, bone marrow, pancreas, and adrenals and has caused vasculitis.[4] Osteomyelitis has been described.[5]

Footnotes

1. Yale SH and Limper AH, "*Pneumocystis carinii* Pneumonia in Patients Without Acquired Immunodeficiency Syndrome: Associated Illness and Prior Corticosteroid Therapy," *Mayo Clin Proc*, 1996, 71(1):5-13.
2. Leibovitz E, Pollack H, Moore T, et al, "Comparison of PCR and Standard Cytological Staining for Detection of *Pneumocystis carinii* From Respiratory Specimens From Patients With or at High Risk for Infection by Human Immunodeficiency Virus," *J Clin Microbiol*, 1995, 33(11):3004-7.
3. Lipschik GY, Gill VJ, Lundgren JD, et al, "Improved Diagnosis of *Pneumocystis carinii* Infection by Polymerase Chain Reaction on Induced Sputum and Blood," *Lancet*, 1992, 340(8813):203-6.
4. "Case Records of the Massachusetts General Hospital. Weekly Clinicopathological Exercises. Case 3-1995. A 29-Year-Old Man With AIDS and Multiple Splenic Abscesses," *N Engl J Med*, 1995, 332(4):249-57.
5. Esolen LM, Fasano MB, Flynn J, et al, "*Pneumocystis carinii* Osteomyelitis in a Patient With Common Variable Immunodeficiency," *N Engl J Med*, 1992, 326(15):999-1001.

References

Amin MB, Mezger E, and Zarbo RJ, "Detection of *Pneumocystis carinii*. Comparative Study of Monoclonal Antibody and Silver Impregnation," *Am J Clin Pathol*, 1992, 98(1):13-8

Bédos JP, Hignette C, Lucet JC, et al, "Serum Carcinoembryonic Antigen: A Prognostic Marker in HIV-Related *Pneumocystis carinii* Pneumonia," *Scand J Infect Dis*, 1992, 24(3):309-15.

Blumenfeld W, Miller CN, Chew KL, et al, "Correlation of *Pneumocystis carinii* Cyst Density With Mortality in Patients With Acquired Immunodeficiency Syndrome and *Pneumocystis* pneumonia," *Hum Pathol*, 1992, 23(6):612-8.

Coulman CU, Greene I, and Archibald RW, "Cutaneous Pneumocystosis," *Ann Intern Med*, 1987, 106(3):396-8.

Homer KS, Wiley EL, Smith AL, et al, "Monoclonal Antibody to *Pneumocystis carinii*: Comparison With Silver Stain in Bronchial Lavage Specimens," *Am J Clin Pathol*, 1992, 97(5):619-24.

Jacobs JL, Libby DM, Winters RA, et al, "A Cluster of *Pneumocystis carinii* Pneumonia in Adults Without Predisposing Illnesses," *N Engl J Med*, 1991, 324(4):246-50.

Kovacs JA, Ng VL, Masur H, et al, "Diagnosis of *Pneumocystis carinii* Pneumonia: Improved Detection in Sputum With Use of Monoclonal Antibodies," *N Engl J Med*, 1988, 318(10):589-93.

Martin WJ 2d, "Diagnostic Bronchoalveolar Lavage in Immunosuppressed Patients With New Pulmonary Infiltrates," *Mayo Clin Proc*, 1992, 67(3):296-8.

Sepkowitz KA, Brown AE, Telzak EE, et al, "*Pneumocystis carinii* Pneumonia Among Patients Without AIDS at a Cancer Hospital," *JAMA*, 1992, 267(6):832-7.

Watts JC and Chandler FW, "Evolving Concepts of Infection by *Pneumocystis carinii*," *Pathol Annu*, 1991, 26(Pt 1):93-138.

Pneumonia, Atypical Agents see Legionnaires' Disease Antibodies on page 412

Poliomyelitis I, II, III Titer

CPT 86658

Related Information

Enterovirus Culture *on page 666*
Viral Culture *on page 675*
Viral Culture, Stool *on page 680*

Synonyms Poliovirus Titer

Test Commonly Includes Detection of antibodies to poliovirus in patient's serum

Abstract Individuals with acute aseptic meningitis with or without paralysis should be considered for poliomyelitis if they have not been immunized. Three antigenic types exist.

Specimen Serum

Container Red top tube

Sampling Time Acute and convalescent sera drawn 10-14 days apart are required to test for neutralizing antibody for each of the three poliovial types.

Reference Range Presence of neutralizing antibody indicates adequate immunization; normal <1:8

Possible Panic Range A fourfold increase in neutralizing antibody titer in paired sera is diagnostic of poliomyelitis. Specific IgM neutralizing antibody is diagnostic as well.

Use Support for the diagnosis of acute poliovirus infection, documentation of previous exposure to poliovirus (complement fixing antibodies); documentation of immunization (neutralizing antibodies)

Limitations Complement-fixing antibodies can be broadly cross-reactive with other enteroviruses.

Methodology Viral neutralization, complement fixation (CF)

Additional Information Poliovirus, an enterovirus, may also be cultured, producing a characteristic cytopathic effect in tissue culture. Culture is more suitable than serology for diagnosis of acute infection. Amplification of poliovirus genome has also been investigated and may soon be used to diagnose poliovirus versus nonpoliovirus enteroviruses.[1]

Footnotes

1. Abraham R, Chonmaitree T, McCombs J, et al, "Rapid Detection of Poliovirus by Reverse Transcription and Polymerase Chain Amplification: Application for Differentiation Between Poliovirus and Nonpoliovirus Enteroviruses," *J Clin Microbiol*, 1993, 31(2):395-9.

References

Melnick JL, "Enteroviruses," *Manual of Clinical Laboratory Immunology*, 4th ed, Vol 2, Chapter 93, Rose NR, de Macario EC, Fahey JL, et al, eds, Washington, DC: American Society for Microbiology, 1992, 631-3.

Poliovirus Titer see Poliomyelitis I, II, III Titer on this page

Progressive Systemic Sclerosis Antibody see Scleroderma Antibody on page 430

Properdin see Factor B on page 393

Prostigmin® Test see Acetylcholine Receptor Antibody on page 362

Protease Inhibitors see Alpha₁-Antitrypsin Phenotyping on page 362

Protease Inhibitors see Alpha₁-Antitrypsin, Serum on page 363

Proteinase 3 (PR3) see Antineutrophil Cytoplasmic Antibody on page 367

Protein, Cerebrospinal Fluid see Cerebrospinal Fluid Protein on page 380

Protein Electrophoresis, Serum

CPT 84165

Related Information

Albumin, Serum *on page 66*
Alpha$_1$-Antitrypsin Phenotyping *on page 362*
Alpha$_1$-Antitrypsin, Serum *on page 363*
Cerebrospinal Fluid Protein Electrophoresis *on page 381*
Immunoelectrophoresis, Serum or Urine *on page 408*
Immunofixation Electrophoresis *on page 408*
Leishmaniasis Serological Test *on page 413*
Protein Electrophoresis, Urine *on next page*
Protein, Total, Serum *on page 194*
Smooth Muscle Antibody *on page 431*
Viscosity, Serum/Plasma *on page 350*

Synonyms Electrophoresis, Serum; Immunoelectrophoresis, Serum; Serum Protein Electrophoresis; SPE

Applies to Beta-Gamma Bridging; Globulin, Serum; Immunoglobulins; Light Chains; Monoclonal Gammopathies

Test Commonly Includes Serum electrophoresis for quantitation of albumin, alpha$_1$, alpha$_2$, beta, and gamma globulins. A total protein value is needed, since the fractions are otherwise available only as percentages. Used with total protein, the fractions can be expressed as absolute quantities.

Abstract A variable number of the over 100 proteins present in human serum can be separated by an electric field and quantitated.

Specimen Serum

Container Red top tube

Storage Instructions Refrigerate separated serum.

Reference Range Values in the table are representative, but variation between methods and laboratories exists. The figures in the table are based on an agarose system. Values in infancy and early childhood are not identical to adult reference ranges.

Protein Electrophoresis, Serum

Component	Relative (%) Normal Range	Absolute (g/dL) Normal Range
Total protein		5.90-8.00
Albumin	58.0-74.0	4.00-5.50
Alpha$_1$	2.0-3.5	0.15-0.25
Alpha$_2$	5.4-10.6	0.43-0.75
Beta	7.0-14.0	0.50-1.00
Gamma	8.0-18.0	0.60-1.30
A/G ratio	1.4-2.6	

Use The principal use is in detection of monoclonal gammopathies. These are usually found in association with hematopoietic neoplasms, especially multiple myeloma and macroglobulinemia of Waldenström. They also occur in other benign and malignant conditions. Such proteins should be identified by an alternative technique, such as immunofixation or immunoelectrophoresis.

Other applications of serum protein electrophoresis include the following:

- Serum protein evaluation, nutritional status.
- Work-up for **liver disease**, including cirrhosis and autoimmune (chronic active) hepatitis. (More information about autoimmune hepatitis is provided in the listing Smooth Muscle Antibody *on page 431*.) In liver disease, albumin is apt to be decreased and alpha$_2$ may be low. Gamma is often polyclonal (ie, dome-shaped) in many cases of autoimmune/chronic active hepatitis[1] and cirrhosis. The normal depression between beta and gamma area may be missing in hepatic cirrhosis; this is called beta-gamma bridging. No one of these findings is pathognomonic. All rarely are found together, even in patients who have obvious hepatic cirrhosis. Polyclonal gammopathy occurs in a wide range of entities which have in common chronic immunologic stimulation (eg, sarcoidosis, visceral leishmaniasis, and other entities: *vide infra*).
- The **gamma globulin** may present an isolated increase. The gamma globulin fraction includes IgG, IgA, IgM, IgD, and IgE. Diffuse polyclonal elevation indicates a chronic immunologic process such as that found with liver disease (eg, autoimmune hepatitis, cirrhosis), connective tissue diseases (eg, systemic LE, rheumatoid arthritis), infectious diseases (eg, osteomyelitis, bronchiectasis, visceral leishmaniasis, leprosy), other inflammatory states (eg, sarcoidosis), neoplasms (eg, some instances of Hodgkin's disease), and chronic myelomonocytic leukemia. Several small bands (oligoclonal) are seen in patients with hepatitis, immune complex diseases, acquired immunodeficiency syndrome, and angioimmunoblastic lymphoadenopathy.
- **Monoclonal gammopathy (M protein) (M spot)** patterns may be benign, especially when small and not increasing, but monoclonal gammopathies relate especially to myeloma, primary amyloidosis, macroglobulinemia of Waldenström, and occasional malignant lymphomas. These are tall, narrow, spire-shaped formations as seen in densitometer tracings. Although small monoclonal gammopathies ("M spots") may be found with benign diseases, they may also be detected with early or evolving plasma cell dyscrasias or malignant lymphoproliferative diseases. Therefore, such small monoclonal gammopathies are regarded as "monoclonal gammopathies of undetermined significance." All patients with monoclonal gammopathies should be followed with periodic serum protein electrophoresis to differentiate stable from increasing M spikes. Increasing M proteins require further evaluation (bone marrow examination, skeletal x-ray studies, urinary protein electrophoresis, immunoelectrophoretic or immunofixation studies and so forth).

- **Low gamma globulin:** Although gamma globulins may decrease slightly with advancing age, any decrease below the normal range if unexplained by obvious causes of protein loss (such as known renal disease), should be further evaluated with urine immunofixation to detect possible monoclonal free light chains (Bence Jones protein) in the urine. Hypogammaglobulinemia is also seen in many patients with B-cell lymphoproliferative disorders such as chronic lymphocytic leukemia. They may be decreased with cytotoxic or immunosuppressive drug therapy (long-term steroid use, antineoplastic chemotherapy), malignant lymphoproliferative diseases, and plasma cell dyscrasias (multiple myeloma), and adult common variable immunodeficiency syndrome. If there is clinical history of susceptibility to infection in the patient or the family, then quantitative immunodiffusion or nephelometric assay for IgG, IgA, and IgM may prove helpful. Attention to lymphocytes in the peripheral blood film, presence or absence of hepatosplenomegaly and in patients older than age 40, presence or absence of light chains in urine immunoelectrophoresis or immunofixation may be relevant (eg, light chain disease).

- **High alpha$_2$:** Alpha$_2$ includes inflammation-reactive fractions, and may be increased with neoplasms (eg, renal cell carcinomas), acute infections, rheumatic fever, arteritis, nephrotic syndromes, and other inflammatory states. Alpha$_2$-macroglobulin is increased in pregnancy and with diabetes mellitus. Healthy children may have higher levels of alpha$_2$-macroglobulin than adults.

- **Low alpha$_2$:** One of the important fractions of alpha$_2$ is haptoglobin. Depression of haptoglobin may indicate hemolysis. Alpha$_2$ globulins may be decreased in hepatocellular damage. Trauma and transfusions may cause a drop in alpha$_2$.

- **Alpha$_1$ globulins** are increased in active inflammatory or neoplastic diseases.

- **Low alpha$_1$ or flat alpha$_1$ curve:** Alpha$_1$-antitrypsin is responsible for 90% of serine antiprotease activity in serum. Its deficiency is due to a genetic abnormality which must be investigated because it leads to emphysema and cirrhosis. If the patient has emphysema, a family history of emphysema, or liver disease of uncertain type, alpha$_1$-antitrypsin assay and phenotype may be indicated. See listings Alpha$_1$-Antitrypsin Phenotyping *on page 362* and Alpha$_1$-Antitrypsin, Serum *on page 363*.

- **Albumin** is better measured by electrophoresis than by chemical methods when it is relevant to do so. Electrophoresis permits diagnosis of rare entities such as analbuminemia and bisalbuminemia. Albumin is increased in dehydration and decreased in a wide variety of subacute, subchronic, and chronic diseases including liver, renal, and gastrointestinal diseases, malnutrition, and cachexia.

- **Decreased total protein with essentially normal pattern** might indicate dietary deficiency or hemodilution (eg, I.V. fluid running at time of venipuncture).

- **Significantly elevated total protein with essentially normal pattern** is likely to be secondary to dehydration.

- **Significantly low total protein and albumin, increased alpha$_2$ and low gamma** is prototypical of the nephrotic syndrome.

Limitations Serum protein electrophoresis detects some but not all liver disease. Protein electrophoresis and immunoelectrophoresis or immunofixation of urine as well as serum are useful when one is working up a patient for myeloma or macroglobulinemia of Waldenström. Such urine studies may be helpful even if serum protein electrophoresis is unremarkable. Light chain disease is found by urine immunoelectrophoresis or immunofixation for light chains (kappa and lambda).

Alpha and beta lipoproteins may be slurred anodally in sera of heparinized patients on high resolution electrophoresis.[2]

Methodology Cellulose acetate and agarose electrophoresis are widely used methods. Negatively charged particles migrate toward the positive electrode.

Additional Information Detection of a significant monoclonal gammopathy should be followed by more specific examinations (serum quantitative immunoglobulins, immunoelectrophoresis, or immunofixation). Further information is provided in listings addressing each immunoglobulin.

Footnotes

1. Krawitt EL, "Autoimmune Hepatitis," *N Engl J Med*, 1996, 334(14):897-903.
2. Pearson JP and Keren DF, "The Effects of Heparin on Lipoproteins in High-Resolution Electrophoresis of Serum," *Am J Clin Pathol*, 1995, 104(4):468-71.

References

Bernett A, Allerhand J, Efremides AP, et al, "Long-Term Study of Gammopathies. Clinically Benign Cases Showing Transition to Malignant Plasmacytomas After Long Periods of Observation," *Clin Biochem*, 1986, 19(4):244-9.

Filomena CA, Filomena AP, Hudock J, et al, "Evaluation of Serum Immunoglobulins by Protein Electrophoresis and Rate Nephelometry Before and After Therapeutic Plasma Exchange," *Am J Clin Pathol*, 1992, 98(2):243-8.

Gandara DR and MacKenzie MR, "Differential Diagnosis of Monoclonal Gammopathy," *Med Clin North Am*, 1988, 72(5):1155-67.

Gerard SK, Chen KH, and Khayam-Bashi H, "Immunofixation Compared With Immunoelectrophoresis for the Routine Characterization of Paraprotein Disorders," *Am J Clin Pathol*, 1987, 88(2):198-203.

Gertz MA and Kyle RA, "Hepatic Amyloidosis (Primary [AL], Immunoglobulin Light Chain): The Natural History in 80 Patients," *Am J Med*, 1988, 85(1):73-80.

Heer M, Joller-Jemelka H, Fontana A, et al, "Monoclonal Gammopathy in Chronic Active Hepatitis," *Liver*, 1984, 4(4):255-63.

Keren DF, "Interpretation of High-Resolution Electrophoresis Patterns in Serum, Urine, and Cerebrospinal Fluid," *High Resolution Electrophoresis and Immunofixation: Techniques and Interpretation*, Boston, MA: Butterworth's Publishers, 1987, 67-106.

Kyle RA, "Benign Monoclonal Gammopathy. A Misnomer?" *JAMA*, 1984, 251(4):1849-54.

McManamon TG and Lott JA, "Serum Protein Electrophoresis," *Clinical Chemistry - Theory, Analysis, and Correlation*, 2nd ed, Kaplan LA and Pesce AJ, eds, St Louis, MO: Mosby-Year Book Inc, 1989, 1054-7.

Miller RH, Linet MS, Van Natta ML, et al, "Serum Protein Electrophoresis Patterns in Chronic Lymphocytic Leukemia. Clinical and Epidemiologic Correlations," *Arch Intern Med*, 1987, 147(9):1614-7.

Ng VL, Hwang KM, Reyes GR, et al, "High Titer Anti-HIV Antibody Reactivity Associated With a Paraprotein Spike in a Homosexual Male With AIDS Related Complex," *Blood*, 1988, 71(5):1397-401.

Tefferi A, Hoagland HC, Therneau TM, et al, "Chronic Myelomonocytic Leukemia: Natural History and Prognostic Determinants," *Mayo Clin Proc*, 1989, 64(10):1246-54.

Tsianos EV, Di Bisceglie AM, Papadopoulos NM, et al, "Oligoclonal Immunoglobulin Bands in Serum in Association With Chronic Viral Hepatitis," *Am J Gastroenterol*, 1990, 85(8):1005-8.

Vladutiu AO, "Prevalence of M-Proteins in Serum of Hospitalized Patients. Physicians' Response to Finding M-Proteins in Serum Protein Electrophoresis," *Ann Clin Lab Sci*, 1987, 17(3):157-61.

Protein Electrophoresis, Spinal Fluid *see* Cerebrospinal Fluid
Protein Electrophoresis *on page 381*

Protein Electrophoresis, Urine

CPT 84165

Related Information

Immunoelectrophoresis, Serum or Urine *on page 408*
Immunofixation Electrophoresis *on page 408*
Immunoglobulin G *on page 409*
Microalbuminuria *on page 643*
Protein Electrophoresis, Serum *on previous page*
Protein, Quantitative, Urine *on page 649*
Protein, Semiquantitative, Urine *on page 650*
Urine Collection, 24-Hour *on page 30*
Viscosity, Serum/Plasma *on page 350*

Synonyms Electrophoresis, Protein, Urine; Globulins, Urine; Urine Electrophoresis; Urine Protein Electrophoresis

Applies to Immunoelectrophoresis; Light Chains, Urine; Monoclonal Gammopathy Work-up

Replaces Bence Jones Protein

Test Commonly Includes Quantitative total urine protein, urine albumin, urine alpha$_1$, urine alpha$_2$, urine beta, and urine gamma globulin fractions

Abstract Electrophoresis provides separation of proteins, which then can be quantified.

Specimen Urine, early morning or 24-hour

Storage Instructions Refrigerate

Causes for Rejection Total protein too low to measure or to yield usable electrophoretic pattern

Reference Range No monoclonal gammopathy detected.

Use Evaluate patients for myeloma, macroglobulinemia of Waldenström, lymphoma, amyloidosis, search for free monoclonal light chain (Bence Jones protein); for further investigation following recognition of monoclonal protein in serum.

The types of proteins excreted may be evaluated in patients who have proteinuria. In minimal change disease there is mostly albumin in urine, while in disorders of renal tubules or interstitium, albumin is not as prominent.[1]

Limitations May not detect pathologic light chains due to insufficient sensitivity of this method. Immunoelectrophoretic or immunofixation study performed on concentrated urine, in particular utilizing antisera against kappa and lambda light chain protein is more sensitive.

Microalbuminuria is defined as albumin excretion in the range of 30-300 mg/24 hours. The sensitivity of dipstick protein estimation is 150-300 mg/L. Following sample concentration, electrophoresis is not sufficiently sensitive to detect clinically relevant but low concentrations of albumin.[2] More sensitive methods are described in the listing Microalbuminuria *on page 643*.

Methodology Electrophoresis, cellulose acetate, and agarose substrates are most commonly used. High resolution techniques are available in some laboratory settings.

Additional Information A serum protein electrophoresis should be reviewed concurrently if one has not been recently studied. In nonselective glomerular proteinuria, the urine electrophoretic pattern is often a nonspecific one which may be called "mirror image" to that of the serum. Contamination of the urine with blood can give a similar pattern. With selective glomerular permeability, albumin, alpha$_1$ proteins, and transferrin are the predominant proteins identified on the urine protein electrophoresis, with a relative absence of heavier molecular weight proteins (ie, alpha$_2$-macroglobulin and immunoglobulins). With tubular proteinuria, low molecular weight proteins (alpha$_2$- and beta$_2$-microglobulins) are predominant, with trace amounts of albumin. So called "overflow proteinuria" occurs when low molecular weight proteins are filtered through the glomerulus in increased amounts.

Duplicate prealbumin bands have been reported in a case of hepatorenal failure.[3]

Footnotes

1. Larson TS, "Evaluation of Proteinuria," *Mayo Clin Proc*, 1994, 69(12):1154-8.
2. Shihabi ZK, Konen JC, and O'Connor ML, "Albuminuria vs Urinary Total Protein for Detecting Chronic Renal Disorders," *Clin Chem*, 1991, 37(5):621-4.
3. Castaneda L and Ruiz P, "Duplicate Prealbumin Bands in Urine - Association With Hepatorenal Failure," *Am J Clin Pathol*, 1994, 101(4):475-7.

References

Brigden ML, Neal ED, McNeely MD, et al, "The Optimum Urine Collections for the Detection and Monitoring of Bence Jones Proteinuria," *Am J Clin Pathol*, 1990, 93(5):689-93.

Deegan MJ, Abraham JP, Sawdyk M, et al, "High Incidence of Monoclonal Proteins in the Serum and Urine of Chronic Lymphocytic Leukemia Patients," *Blood*, 1984, 64(6):1207-11.

Keren DF, "Interpretation of High-Resolution Electrophoresis Patterns in Serum, Urine, and Cerebrospinal Fluid," *High Resolution Electrophoresis and Immunofixation: Techniques and Interpretation*, Boston, MA: Butterworth's Publishers, 1987, 67-106.

Sifuentes AA, "Electrophoretic Profile of Proteinuria in Normal Pregnancy and in Gestational Hypertension," *Ginecol Obstet Mex*, 1995, 63:147-51.

Proteus OX-19 *replaced by* Rocky Mountain Spotted Fever Serology *on page 427*

Psittacosis Titer

CPT 86631; 86632 (IgM)

Related Information

Chlamydia Group Titer *on page 383*

Synonyms *Chlamydia psittaci* Antibodies; *Chlamydia psittaci* Titer

Applies to *Chlamydia psittaci* Direct Immunofluorescent Antibody; *Chlamydia psittaci* PCR

Test Commonly Includes Detection of antibody specific for *Chlamydia psittaci*

Abstract Usually presenting as a pneumonia, psittacosis exists in birds including domestic fowl. Infected birds are the source of human psittacosis. It occurs in epidemic and sporadic forms.[1] Employment history may be relevant. *C. psittaci* is a prevalent zoonotic infection in which a wide host range is recognized.

Specimen Serum

Container Red top tube

Collection Acute and convalescent samples are needed.

Reference Range Less than a fourfold increase in titer in paired sera

Use Diagnose psittacosis for which the best presently available laboratory means of diagnosis is serologic. A broad clinical differential diagnosis exists.

Limitations The microimmunofluorescence test is technically difficult to perform properly but can be useful for identifying the infecting species or serovar. Complement fixation tests identify antibody to an antigen common to all members of the genus but do not provide information on the species or serovar involved. Consequently, a fourfold rise in CF antibody titer provides evidence that a chlamydial infection occurred, but it cannot distinguish psittacosis from other chlamydial infections. Interpretation of complement fixation test results performed on unpaired sera is complicated by high "background" levels of antibody in the general population. The presence of IgG titer may indicate prior exposure.

Methodology Complement fixation (CF), enzyme immunoassay (EIA), microimmunofluorescence which has been improved with application of monoclonal antibodies.[2] Direct immunofluorescent antibody can be applied to respiratory secretions.[3] PCR can be useful.[2,4]

Additional Information Ornithosis is a disease of birds and fowl caused by *C. psittaci*.

Most patients with psittacosis develop high titers of complement fixing antibody and in the appropriate clinical setting a single very high titer *(Continued)*

Psittacosis Titer *(Continued)*

may be strongly supportive of the diagnosis. Specific IgM antibody can sometimes be demonstrated.

Direct detection of *Chlamydia psittaci* can be accomplished by direct immunofluorescent antibody staining of respiratory secretions with monoclonal antibodies or by PCR.

Culture for *C. psittaci* is not widely available. The organism is difficult to isolate and is dangerous.

Footnotes

1. Schlossberg D, Delgado J, Moore MM, et al, "An Epidemic of Avian and Human Psittacosis," *Arch Intern Med*, 1993, 153(22):2594-6.
2. Herring AJ, "Typing *Chlamydia psittaci* - A Review of Methods and Recent Findings," *Br Vet J*, 149(5):455-75.
3. Oldach DW, Gaydos CA, Mundy LM, et al, "Rapid Diagnosis of *Chlamydia psittaci* Pneumonia," *Clin Infect Dis*, 1993, 17(3):338-43.
4. Tong CY and Sillis M, "Detection of *Chlamydia pneumoniae* and *Chlamydia psittaci* in Sputum Samples by PCR," *J Clin Pathol*, 1993, 46(4):313-7.

References

Blanchard TJ and Mabey DC, "Chlamydial Infections," *Br J Clin Pract*, 1994, 48(4):201-5.
Hedberg K, White KE, Hedberg CW, et al, "Persistence of *Chlamydia* Complement-Fixation Antibody After an Outbreak of Psittacosis," *J Infect Dis*, 1993, 167(2):502-3.
Schachter J, "Chlamydiae," *Manual of Clinical Laboratory Immunology*, 4th ed, Vol 2, Chapter 96, Rose NR, Conway de Macario E, Fahey JL, et al, eds, Washington, DC: American Society for Microbiology, 1992, 661-6.

Q Fever Titer

CPT 86638

Related Information

Arthropod Identification *on page 453*
Liver Biopsy *on page 48*

Synonyms *Coxiella burnetii* Titer

Abstract *Coxiella burnetii*, originally called *Rickettsia burneti*, is a member of the family Rickettsiaceae. It is an obligate intracellular pathogen. The primary reservoirs for Q fever are cattle, sheep, and goats. Exposure to ruminants and to raw milk is relevant for this zoonosis. Originally described in Australia, its distribution is worldwide. It is also called Balkan grippe. Its clinical characteristics include fever with interstitial pneumonitis but not an exanthem. Its complications include granulomatous hepatitis, osteomyelitis, endocarditis, and lymphocytic meningitis. It infects vascular aneurysms and prostheses. A broad clinical spectrum exists, from subclinical to fatal. The organism is extremely infectious. Transmission is by inhalation, handling, and ticks, but not between humans. Mortality rate may be >65%.[1]

Specimen Serum

Container Red top tube

Sampling Time Acute and convalescent samples are recommended, the latter 2-4 weeks from onset. CF antibodies to phase-1 antigen are found in 7-10 days.

Reference Range Titer: <1:10; comparison of acute and convalescent titers is of greatest diagnostic value

Critical Values Titer ≥1:10; fourfold or greater increase in titer provides evidence of recent infection

Possible Panic Range Titer ≥1:160 indicates active infection

Use Support the diagnosis of Q fever, a disease in which respiratory abnormalities are most common. Consider Q fever in the presence of fever with negative blood culture, especially in the presence of cardiovascular disease.[2]

Limitations Reagents prepared from fresh isolates (phase I organisms) react differently from those from multiply-passaged organism, a laboratory artifact (phase II). Sera drawn early may be negative.

Methodology Complement fixation (CF), indirect immunofluorescent antibody (IFA); enzyme-linked immunosorbent assays; monoclonal antibodies can detect *C. burnetii* in paraffin tissue blocks[3,4]

Additional Information Sera from patients with Q fever do not react in the archaic Weil-Felix test with *Proteus* antigen. Convalescent sera react best with phase II organism (see above), but sera from chronic persistent infection react best with phase I organisms. Chronic Q fever is uncommon and tends to affect patients with valvular heart disease. Cross reactions with *Legionella* have been described.

Footnotes

1. Dumler JS and Walker DH, "Diagnostic Tests for Rocky Mountain Spotted Fever and Other Rickettsial Diseases," *Dermatol Clin*, 1994, 12(1):25-36.
2. Brouqui P, Dupont HT, Drancourt M, et al, "Chronic Q Fever. Ninety-two Cases From France, Including 27 Cases Without Endocarditis," *Arch Intern Med*, 1993, 153(5):642-8.
3. Raoult D, Laurent JC, and Mutillod M, "Monoclonal Antibodies to *Coxiella burnetii* for Antigenic Detection in Cell Cultures and In Paraffin-Embedded Tissues," *Am J Clin Pathol*, 1994, 101(3):318-20.

References

Anguita M, Ciudad M, Gallardo A, et al, "Infectious Endocarditis Due to Q Fever. A Report of 4 New Cases," *Rev Esp Cardiol*, 1993, 46(8):506-8.
Guigno D, Coupland B, Smith EG, et al, "Primary Humoral Antibody Response to *Coxiella burnetii*, the Causative Agent of Q Fever," *J Clin Microbiol*, 1992, 30(8):1958-67.

Hechemy KE, "The Immunoserology of Rickettsiae," *Manual of Clinical Laboratory Immunology*, 4th ed, Vol 2, Chapter 97, Rose NR, Conway de Macario E, Fahey JL, et al, eds, Washington, DC: American Society for Microbiology, 1992, 667-75.
Htwe KK, Yoshida T, Hayashi S, et al, "Prevalence of Antibodies to *Coxiella burnetii* in Japan," *J Clin Microbiol*, 1993, 31(3):722-3.
Ordi-Ros J, Selva-O'Callaghan A, Monegal-Ferran F, et al, "Prevalence, Significance, and Specificity of Antibodies to Phospholipids in Q Fever," *Clin Infect Dis*, 1994, 18(2):213-8.
Reimer LG, "Q Fever," *Clin Microbiol Rev*, 1993, 6(3):193-8.
Rice PS, Kudesia G, McKendrick MW, et al, "*Coxiella burnetii* Serology in Granulomatous Hepatitis," *J Infect*, 1993, 27(1):63-6.
Schattner A, Kushnir M, Zhornicky T, et al, "Lymphocytic Meningitis as the Sole Manifestation of Q Fever," *Postgrad Med J*, 1993, 69(814):636-7.
Soriano F, Camacho MT, Ponte C, et al, "Serological Differentiation Between Acute (Late Control) and Endocarditis Q Fever," *J Clin Pathol*, 1993, 46(5):411-4.

Quantitative IgA *see Immunoglobulin A on page 408*

Quantitative IgD *see Immunoglobulin D on page 409*

Quantitative IgE *see Immunoglobulin E on page 409*

Quantitative IgG *see Immunoglobulin G on page 409*

Quantitative IgM *see Immunoglobulin M on page 410*

Rabbit Fever Antibodies *see Tularemia Agglutinins on page 436*

Rapid Nerve Stimulation Test *see Acetylcholine Receptor Antibody on page 362*

Rapid Plasma Reagin Test *see RPR on page 428*

Receptor Blocking Antibody *see Acetylcholine Receptor Antibody on page 362*

Receptor Modulating Antibody *see Acetylcholine Receptor Antibody on page 362*

Recombinant Antigen Immunoblot Assay *see HIV-1/HIV-2 Serology on page 403*

Respiratory Syncytial Virus Serology

CPT 86756

Related Information

Respiratory Syncytial Virus Antigen Detection *on page 673*
Respiratory Syncytial Virus Culture *on page 673*
Viral Culture, Respiratory Symptoms *on page 680*
Virus, Direct Detection by Fluorescent Antibody *on page 682*

Synonyms RSV Antibodies

Test Commonly Includes Detection of antibodies specific for RSV

Abstract Antigen detection from nasopharyngeal washings is better for patient care.

Specimen Serum

Container Red top tube

Special Instructions Acute and convalescent specimens are recommended.

Reference Range IgG: less than fourfold rise in titer; IgM: negative

Use Respiratory syncytial virus (RSV) is a common cause of winter acute respiratory disease, including serious disease among older persons. Complications, especially in infants, children with underlying cardiopulmonary disease, and the immunocompromised, include bronchiolitis and pneumonia. Nosocomial outbreaks occur. Death may follow outbreaks among immunocompromised individuals.[1]

Limitations Young infants have maternal IgG antibody. A fourfold rise in IgG titers cannot be detected in half of the children younger than 6 months of age. IgM antibody is not detected in about 50% of patients with documented infection.

Methodology Complement fixation (CF), enzyme-linked immunosorbent assay (ELISA)

Additional Information RSV and parainfluenza viruses are the most common etiologic agents of viral acute lower respiratory disease. Diagnosis by CF depends on demonstration of a rise in antibody titer over a 2- to 3-week period. As such, the test is seldom useful in planning clinical care in an acute illness or in control of nosocomial infections.

For rapid diagnosis, the demonstration of viral antigen in nasopharyngeal washings is more useful; EIA is readily available. Immunofluorescence is comparable to EIA. See listings Respiratory Syncytial Virus Antigen Detection *on page 673* and Respiratory Syncytial Virus Culture *on page 673*.

Footnotes

1. "From the Centers for Disease Control and Prevention. Update: Respiratory Syncytial Virus Activity - United States, 1994-95 Season," *JAMA*, 1995, 273(4):282

References

Costello MJ, Smernoff NT, and Yungbluth M, "Laboratory Diagnosis of Viral Respiratory Tract Infections," *Lab Med*, 1993, 24(3):150-1.
Falsey AR, Cunningham CK, Barker WH, et al, "Respiratory Syncytial Virus and Influenza A Infections in the Hospitalized Elderly," *J Infect Dis*, 1995, 172(2):389-94.
Hemming VG, "Viral Respiratory Diseases in Children: Classification, Etiology, Epidemiology, and Risk Factors," *J Pediatr*, 1994, 124(5 Pt 2):S13-6.

Meddens MJ, Herbrink P, Lindeman J, et al, "Serodiagnosis of Respiratory Syncytial Virus (RSV) Infection in Children as Measured by Detection of RSV-Specific Immunoglobulins G, M, and A With Enzyme-Linked Immunosorbent Assay," *J Clin Microbiol*, 1990, 28(1):152-5.

Walker TA, Khurana S, and Tilden SJ, "Viral Respiratory Infections," *Pediatr Clin North Am*, 1994, 41(6):1365-81.

RF *see* Rheumatoid Factor *on this page*

Rheumatoid Factor

CPT 86430

Related Information
Acetylcholine Receptor Antibody *on page 362*
Antinuclear Antibody *on page 368*
Body Fluid Glucose *on page 91*
Cryoglobulin, Qualitative, Serum *on page 388*
HLA-B27 *on page 404*
HLA Typing, Single Human Leukocyte Antigen *on page 405*
Synovial Fluid Analysis *on page 656*

Synonyms RF

Applies to Rheumatoid Factor, Synovial Fluid

Replaces Rose-Waaler Test; Singer-Plotz Test

Abstract A clinical syndrome, rheumatoid arthritis (RA) is characterized by pain and swelling in joints. Rheumatoid factor (RF) is an autoantibody, a marker of immune activation, and is not specific.[1]

Specimen Serum

Container Red top tube

Reference Range Negative

Critical Values At ≥80 IU/mL; sensitivity for RA is 61% with 97% specificity[2]

Use Differential diagnosis and prognosis of rheumatoid arthritis (RA) and related entities

Limitations There are numerous interlaboratory and intermethod variations. IgG and IgA rheumatoid factors are not distinguished by most commercial test kits. About 20% of patients with RA are negative,[1] and about 33% of patients with juvenile RA are RF negative. Some RF negative patients subsequently become positive. After treatment, RF reactivity may disappear.

Many rheumatic conditions and chronic inflammatory processes additional to connective tissue diseases also may produce rheumatoid factors. An incomplete list includes Sjögren's syndrome, SLE, scleroderma, dermatomyositis, infectious mononucleosis, syphilis, tuberculosis, viral hepatitis, bacterial endocarditis, and entities characterized by gammopathies which include leprosy, leishmaniasis, sarcoidosis, malaria, and Waldenström's macroglobulinemia. Thus, the presence of RF, especially in low titer, is far from diagnostic for RA. False-positives are found in about 5% of people with no clinical illness.[1]

Methodology Latex-human IgG agglutination; sheep RBC-rabbit IgG agglutination; rate nephelometry in which international units are reported.

Additional Information Rheumatoid factors (RF) are autoantibodies directed against the Fc fragment of IgG. These are usually IgM antibodies, but may be IgG or IgA. RF is present in the serum of a majority of patients with RA, depending in part on the method used. Latex beads coated with human IgG are positive in 70% to 85% (and have significant numbers of false-positives). Sheep RBCs coated with rabbit IgG will be positive in 60% to 70% (and have fewer false-positives). RF can also be measured quantitatively by laser nephelometry, which has good interlaboratory reproducibility.

Statistically, patients with RA who have high titer RF are more likely to have severe disease and systemic involvement than other patients. High titers correlate with presence of rheumatoid nodules, and low synovial fluid complement. However, RF is not recognized as useful to assess activity (ESR provides a better index of activity).[3]

RF can be detected in synovial fluid, but contributes little more than a positive serum test. Some rheumatoid factors may behave as cryoglobulins.

Factors predictive of outcome include HLA-DR4, as well as joint swelling, Ritchie score, radiological assessment, and positive IgM and IgG RF.[4]

The production of RF may be regulated by anti-idiotypic antibodies, IgG antibodies directed against specific sites on Fab fragments.

Footnotes
1. Lisse JR, "Does Rheumatoid Factor Always Mean Arthritis?" *Postgrad Med*, 1993, 94(6):133-4, 139.
2. Leavelle DE, *Mayo Medical Laboratories Interpretive Handbook*, Rochester, MN: Mayo Medical Laboratories, 1994.
3. Moder KG, "Use and Interpretation of Rheumatologic Tests: A Guide for Clinicians," *Mayo Clin Proc*, 1996, 71(4):391-6.
4. van Zeben D, Hazes JM, Zwinderman AH, et al, "Factors Predicting Outcome of Rheumatoid Arthritis: Results of a Follow-Up Study," *J Rheumatol*, 1993, 20(8):1288-96.

References
Bauman GP and Hurtubise P, "Anti-idiotypes and Autoimmune Disease," *Clin Lab Med*, 1988, 8(2):399-407.

Chandor SB, "Autoimmune Phenomena in Lymphoid Malignancies," *Clin Lab Med*, 1988, 8(2):373-84.

Kalsi J and Isenberg D, "Rheumatoid Factor: Primary or Secondary Event in the Pathogenesis of RA?" *Int Arch Allergy Immunol*, 1993, 102(3):209-15.

Ota T and Kobayashi T, "Rheumatoid Factors - Recent Advances in Measurement Techniques, Their Fine Specificities and Mechanisms of Their Production," *Rinsho Byori*, 1993, 41(1):26-35.

Shmerling RH and Delbanco TL, "How Useful Is the Rheumatoid Factor? An Analysis of Sensitivity, Specificity, and Predictive Value," *Arch Intern Med*, 1992, 152(12):2417-20.

van Schaardenburg D, Lagaay AM, Otten HG, et al, "The Relation Between Class-Specific Serum Rheumatoid Factors and Age in the Gerneral Population," *Br J Rheumatol*, 1993, 32(7):546-9.

Wolfe F, Cathey MA, and Roberts FK, "The Latex Test Revisited Rheumatoid Factor Testing in 8287 Rheumatic Disease Products," *Arthritis Rheum*, 1991, 34(8):951-60.

Rheumatoid Factor, Synovial Fluid *see* Rheumatoid Factor *on this page*

RIBA *see* HIV-1/HIV-2 Serology *on page 403*

RIBA Test for HIV Antibody *see* HIV-1/HIV-2 Serology *on page 403*

Rickettsial Disease Agglutinins *see* Weil-Felix Agglutinins *on page 439*

***Rickettsia rickettsii* Serology** *see* Rocky Mountain Spotted Fever Serology *on this page*

RNA Polymerase III *see* Scleroderma Antibody *on page 430*

RNP Antibody *see* Antinuclear Antibody *on page 368*

Ro Antibodies *see* Sjögren's Antibodies *on page 430*

***Rochalimaea* Antibodies** *see* Cat Scratch Disease Serology *on page 375*

Rocky Mountain Spotted Fever Serology

CPT 86255 (fluorescent screen); 86256 (titer)

Related Information
Arthropod Identification *on page 453*
Ehrlichiosis Serology *on page 390*
Febrile Agglutinins, Serum *on page 393*
Weil-Felix Agglutinins *on page 439*

Synonyms *Rickettsia rickettsii* Serology

Replaces *Proteus* OX-19

Abstract Transmitted by ticks, this acute, febrile disease is characterized by headache, fever, weakness, and a centipetal macular eruption beginning on wrists and ankles. Rocky Mountain spotted fever (RMSF) is caused by *Rickettsia rickettsii*, obligate intracellular bacteria that cannot be detected by routine microbiological culture. In the United States, RMSF is seen most frequently in a narrow geographic band from North Carolina to Oklahoma. Serologic diagnosis may be accomplished in one of two ways. The archaic Weil-Felix test (discussed elsewhere) utilizes several strains of *Proteus* that cross react with *Rickettsia* to detect serologic responses. The assays which rely on cultivated *R. rickettsii* as the antigen source detect specific rather than cross reacting antibodies. Untreated, the case fatality rate has reached 20% to 25%.[1]

Specimen Serum

Container Red top tube

Sampling Time Paired sera 7 or more days apart is recommended.[1]

Special Instructions Acute and convalescent specimens are recommended.

Reference Range Less than a fourfold increase in titer in paired sera; IgG <1:32, IgM <1:8

Critical Values Fourfold increase to specific rickettsial antigen is diagnostic

Possible Panic Range IgG: ≥1:128

Use Diagnose Rocky Mountain spotted fever

Limitations Diagnostic IgG titers may persist for years and IgM titers as high as 1:64 have occasionally been demonstrated a year after infection. IgG titer may be negative early in disease. Consequently, convincing serologic diagnosis can only be demonstrated with increasing titers or an IgM titer ≥1:128; the threshold for therapeutic intervention is often considerably less than that which is required for a convincing serologic diagnosis. False-positive reactions occur during pregnancy, particularly in the last two trimesters. False-positives are also occasionally seen with other Rickettsias in the spotted fever group.

Methodology Indirect immunofluorescent antibody (IFA) and enzyme-linked immunosorbent assay (ELISA) are highly sensitive. Complement fixation (CF) and microagglutination methods are more specific than the Weil-Felix, but they lack sensitivity. Latex agglutination (LA) is helpful in early convalescence. Solid phase immunoassays have become available.

(Continued)

Rocky Mountain Spotted Fever Serology
(Continued)

The complement fixation test can be used with different concentration of antigen to minimize cross reactions. Hemagglutination and immunofluorescent tests are least subject to cross reactions with other *Rickettsia*. Tests for IgM specific antibody are helpful in early disease, since they appear in 3-8 days. Patients treated with antibiotics early in illness may not develop serologic responses. Immunohistologic methods are in use.[1] A direct fluorescent test is available to demonstrate the *Rickettsia* in tissue. As many as 71% of patients with Rocky Mountain spotted fever also develop antibodies against cardiolipin and endothelial cells.

More recently, PCR techniques have been used to detect *R. rickettsii* DNA in patients' specimens. These studies showed that the technique is highly specific but lacks sensitivity, likely due to inhibitors of the PCR assay.

Additional Information Rocky Mountain spotted fever occurs primarily from April through October. It is a disease of variable clinical manifestation (indeed some cases present with few or no "spots"), and since there is good specific therapy, and serious outcome if untreated, all aids to diagnosis are important. Renal shutdown may occur. Serologic diagnosis may be made promptly enough to direct therapy.

The differential diagnosis includes ehrlichiosis.[2]

Clinically, the rash may be confused with those of meningococcemia, typhus, and measles.

Footnotes
1. Dumler JS and Walker DH, "Diagnostic Tests for Rocky Mountain Spotted Fever and Other Rickettsial Diseases," *Dermatol Clin*, 1994, 12(1):25-36.
2. Silberg SL, Bisonni R, Parker DE, et al, "Human Ehrlichiosis - An Overview," *J Okla State Med Assoc*, 1993, 86(3):124-7.

References
Jones D, Anderson B, Olson J, et al, "Enzyme-linked Immunosorbent Assay for Detection of Human Immunoglobulin G to Lipopolysaccharide of Spotted Fever Group Rickettsiae," *J Clin Microbiol*, 1993, 31(1):138-41.
Radulovic S, Speed R, Feng HM, et al, "EIA With Species-Specific Monoclonal Antibodies: A Novel Seroepidemiologic Tool for Determination of the Etiologic Agent of Spotted Fever Rickettsiosis," *J Infect Dis*, 1993, 168(5):1292-5.
Sexton DJ and Corey GR, "Rocky Mountain "Spotless" and "Almost Spotless" Fever: A Wolf in Sheep's Clothing," *Clin Infect Dis*, 1992, 15(3):439-48.
Spach DH, Liles WC, Campbell GL, et al, "Tick-Borne Diseases in the United States," *N Engl J Med*, 1993, 329(13):936-47.
Walker TS and Triplett DA, "Serologic Characterization of Rocky Mountain Spotted Fever. Appearance of Antibodies Reactive With Endothelial Cells and Phospholipids, and Factors That Alter Protein C Activation and Prostacyclin Secretion," *Am J Clin Pathol*, 1991, 95(5):725-32.
Welch KJ, Rumley RL, and Levine JA, "False-Positive Results in Serologic Tests for Rocky Mountain Spotted Fever During Pregnancy," *South Med J*, 1991, 84(3):307-11.

Rose-Waaler Test *replaced by* Rheumatoid Factor *on previous page*

Rotavirus Serology
CPT 86759
Related Information
Electron Microscopic Examination for Viruses, Stool *on page 665*
Rotavirus, Direct Detection *on page 674*
Use Rotavirus serology is used only as a research tool. See Rotavirus, Direct Detection *on page 674*.

RPR
CPT 86592
Related Information
Anticardiolipin Antibody *on page 364*
Antinuclear Antibody *on page 368*
Automated Reagin Test *on page 370*
Bacterial Culture, Genital Specimen *on page 463*
Darkfield Examination, Syphilis *on page 475*
Donation, Blood *on page 607*
FTA-ABS, Serum *on page 394*
MHA-TP *on page 418*
Neisseria gonorrhoeae Culture and Smear *on page 492*
Risks of Transfusion *on page 623*
VDRL, Cerebrospinal Fluid *on page 438*
VDRL, Serum *on page 438*
Synonyms Rapid Plasma Reagin Test
Applies to Syphilis Serology
Replaces ART Test; Kahn Test; Kline Test; Mazzini; Wassermann
Test Commonly Includes Reactive specimens may be titered and/or an FTA-ABS test performed
Abstract The two major screening (reaginic) (nontreponemal) tests for syphilis are VDRL and RPR. Positive screening tests must be confirmed.
Specimen Serum
Container Red top tube
Reference Range Negative

Use Screening test for syphilis
Limitations This is a nontreponemal test and is associated with false-positive reactions due to intercurrent infections, pregnancy, drug addiction, autoimmune disease, increased age, autoimmunity, Gaucher's disease, and a number of other entities.[1] Potential causes of false-positive serologic tests for syphilis are tabulated in the listing VDRL, Serum *on page 438*.
Methodology Agglutination test with reagin antibody
Additional Information RPR is a screening test for syphilis and detects antibodies to reagin. Such antibodies usually develop within 4-6 weeks of inoculation, peak during the secondary phase of disease, and then decrease. They also decrease and usually disappear with treatment. The RPR is more sensitive than the VDRL and the ART. Ninety-three percent of patients with primary syphilis have positive tests. RPR titers are usually higher in HIV-infected patients than in those who do not have HIV infection.

Because of the many causes of false-positive tests, any reactive serum should be tested by a treponemal-specific test, preferably MHA-TP or FTA-ABS. The RPR should not be done on cerebrospinal fluid. False-negative tests may occur at birth in some infants with recently acquired congenital syphilis. Therefore, especially in areas where the disease is prevalent, a serologic test for syphilis should be included in evaluation of febrile infants even if they had a negative screen at birth. False-negatives have also been due to the prozone effect. Therefore, dilution should be performed on serum of pregnant women in areas with high syphilis prevalence when screening tests are negative.

The number of cases of syphilis has been increasing since 1987. The increase seems to be associated with HIV infection and prostitution associated with drug abuse. Because most infants with congenital syphilis lack signs of infection, serology for both nontreponemal and treponemal antibodies is needed for diagnosis. "Reagin" is an antibody which cross reacts with extracts of cardiac muscle and treponemal cell wall components. Such nontreponemal tests are subject to false-positives. Serial serologic testing during pregnancy with maternal and neonatal serologic studies at delivery is desirable for detection of neonates at risk. In instances of negative tests even following dilutions, serology should be repeated within several weeks when suspicion of congenital syphilis exists.[2]

The RPR card test has become the most widely used nontreponemal test in the U.S.[3]

In a series of 291 inpatients, of reactive RPR in 19%, 66% were confirmed with FTA-ABS. In an additional 5.5%, reactive FTA-ABS with nonreactive RPR was found.[4]

Footnotes
1. Hook EW 3d and Marra CM, "Acquired Syphilis in Adults," *N Engl J Med*, 1992, 326(16):1060-9.
2. Chhabra RS, Brion LP, Castro M, et al, "Comparison of Maternal Sera, Cord Blood, and Neonatal Sera for Detecting Presumptive Congenital Syphilis: Relationship With Maternal Treatment," *Pediatrics*, 1993, 91(1):88-91.
3. Larsen SA, Steiner BM, and Rudolph AH, "Laboratory Diagnosis and Interpretation of Tests for Syphilis," *Clin Microbiol Rev*, 1995, 8(1):1-21.
4. Burton AA, Flynn JA, Neumann TM, et al, "Routine Serologic Screening for Syphilis in Hospitalized Patients: High Prevalence of Unsuspected Infection in the Elderly," *Sex Transm Dis*, 1994, 21:133-6.

References
Berkowitz K, Baxi L, and Fox HE, "False-Negative Syphilis Serology: The Prozone Phenomenon, Nonimmune Hydrops, and Diagnosis of Syphilis During Pregnancy," *Am J Obstet Gynecol*, 1990, 163(3):975-7.
Desforges JF, "Infectious Disease Testing for Blood Transfusions," *NIH Consensus Statement*, 1995, 13(1):1-27.
Dorfman DH and Glaser JH, "Congenital Syphilis Presenting in Infants After the Newborn Period," *N Engl J Med*, 1990, 323(19):1299-302.
Hart G, "Syphilis Tests in Diagnostic and Therapeutic Decision Making," *Ann Intern Med*, 1986, 104(3):368-76.
Huber TW, Storms S, Young P, et al, "Reactivity of Microhemagglutination, Fluorescent Treponemal Antibody Absorption, Venereal Disease Research Laboratory, and Rapid Plasma Reagin Tests in Primary Syphilis," *J Clin Microbiol*, 1983, 17:405-9.
Hutchinson CM, Rompalo AM, Reichart CA, et al, "Characteristics of Patients With Syphilis Attending Baltimore STD Clinics. Multiple High-Risk Groups and Interactions With Human Immunodeficiency Virus Infection," *Arch Intern Med*, 1991, 151(3):511-6.
Kirchner JT, "Syphilis - An STD on the Increase," *Am Fam Physician*, 1991, 44(3):843-54.
Klein HG, *Standards for Blood Banks and Transfusion Services*, 16th ed, Bethesda, MD: American Association of Blood Banks, 1994, 3-8.
Thomas DL and Quinn TC, "Serologic Testing for Sexually Transmitted Diseases," *Infect Dis Clin North Am*, 1993, 7(4):793-824.
Young H, Moyes A, McMillan A, et al, "Enzyme Immunoassay for Antitreponemal IgG: Screening or Confirmatory Test?" *J Clin Pathol*, 1992, 45(1):37-41.

RSV Antibodies *see* Respiratory Syncytial Virus Serology *on page 426*

Rubella Serology
CPT 86762
Related Information
Rubella Virus Culture *on page 674*
TORCH *on page 435*

Synonyms German Measles Serology

Applies to IgG Antibodies to Rubella; IgM Antibodies to Rubella

Test Commonly Includes Detection of serologic response to rubella infection or vaccination

Abstract German measles is an RNA viral infection usually characterized by a macular exanthem, an incubation period of 14-21 days and lymphadenopathy, pharyngitis, and conjunctivitis. Severe transplacental infections occur in the first trimester. The presence of specific IgG antibodies bears correlation with protective immunity.

Specimen Serum, fetal blood

Container Red top tube

Collection Acute and convalescent samples for IgG.

Reference Range Absence of antibody indicates susceptibility to rubella. IgG: less than a fourfold titer increase; IgM: negative. **Postvaccination:** positive.

Critical Values Presence of IgM antibody indicates acute infection or vaccination. Fourfold increase in IgG titer may indicate acute infection.

Possible Panic Range Evidence of susceptibility in a pregnant woman recently exposed to rubella

Use Prenatal diagnosis of congenital rubella infection (IgM); evaluate immune status

Limitations Most laboratories perform rubella serologies as a qualitative test (to determine susceptibility to infection) and do not determine titers. This presents a problem when trying to diagnose infection by increasing IgG titers; special arrangements need to be made with the laboratory.

In an attempt to gain market share, some commercial sources have provided a "more sensitive" test for rubella antibodies. Such assays may detect antibody titers lower than the 1:8 hemagglutination inhibition titer to which classical assays are calibrated. Unfortunately, it is unclear whether titers <1:8 confer protective immunity, and use of these assays to assess susceptibility to infection may occasionally be misleading.

Methodology Indirect fluorescent antibody (IFA), hemagglutination, enzyme-linked immunosorbent assay (ELISA), radioimmunoassay (RIA), hemolysis-in-gel, complement fixation (CF), latex agglutination (LA), enzyme immunoassay (EIA)

Additional Information Rubella virus is the cause of German measles, usually a mild exanthem, often subclinical. However, when acquired *in utero*, rubella virus can lead to fetal demise, cataracts, malformation, deafness, and mental retardation. For this reason the federal government and many states support programs to immunize women against rubella before they have children. There has been a resurgence of congenital rubella in the early 1990s and more widespread screening for rubella serology is recommended.

The role of serologic testing for antibodies to rubella is different in different clinical settings. The simplest and most straight forward application is in assessment of immunity. If a woman has antibodies against rubella, even of low titer, demonstrated by any of multiple methods, she need not worry about infection during subsequent pregnancy. If she is not immune, and is not pregnant, she can receive rubella vaccine.

This test may also be used in the management of a pregnant woman who has been exposed to rubella. In this situation, it must be determined if the patient is susceptible, has an acute infection, and evaluate the risk to the fetus. Several flowcharts are available to assess these possibilities, utilizing antibody titers, class of antibody, and changes in titer over time. Management of such a case requires individualized expert consultation.

An infant born with an illness which may be congenital rubella should also be evaluated for rubella titers. Problems here include evaluation of whether antibody represents passively acquired immunity by transplacental passage or is indicative of true neonatal infection. In this setting, determination of the immunoglobulin class is particularly important; the presence of IgM antibody strongly supports congenital infection.

References

Boyd AS, "Laboratory Testing in Patients With Morbilliform Viral Eruptions," *Dermatol Clin*, 1994, 12(1):69-82.
Condorelli F and Ziegler T, "Dot Immunobinding Assay for Simultaneous Detection of Specific Immunoglobulin G Antibodies to Measles Virus, Mumps Virus, and Rubella Virus," *J Clin Microbiol*, 1993, 31(3):717-9.
"Consensus Conference on Measles," *Can Commun Dis Rep*, 1993, 19(10):72-9.
Duverlie G, Roussel C, Driencourt M, et al, "Latex Enzyme Immunoassay for Measuring IgG Antibodies to Rubella Virus," *J Clin Pathol*, 1990, 43(9):766-70.
Ghidini A and Lynch L, "Prenatal Diagnosis and Significance of Fetal Infections," *West J Med*, 1993, 159(3):366-73.
Lee SH, Ewert DF, Frederick PD, et al, "Resurgence of Congenital Rubella Syndrome in the 1990s. Report on Missed Opportunities and Failed Prevention Policies Among Women of Childbearing Age," *JAMA*, 1992, 267(19):2616-20.
Valente P and Sever JL, "*In Utero* Diagnosis of Congenital Infections by Direct Fetal Sampling," *Ir J Med Sci*, 1994, 35(5-6):414-20.
Zhang T, Mauracher CA, Mitchell LA, et al, "Detection of Rubella Virus-Specific Immunoglobulin G (IgG), IgM, and IgA Antibodies by Immunoblot Assays," *J Clin Microbiol*, 1992, 30(4):824-30.

Rubeola Antibodies *see* Measles Antibody *on page 417*

Rubeola Serology, CSF *see* Measles Antibody *on page 417*

sAβ *see* Cerebrospinal Fluid Amyloid Precursor Protein and Amyloid β-Protein *on page 376*

Sabin-Feldman Dye Test *replaced by* Toxoplasmosis Serology *on page 435*

***Salmonella* Agglutinins** *see Salmonella* Titer *on this page*

Salmonella Titer

CPT 86768

Related Information

Bacterial Culture, Blood *on page 457*
Bacterial Culture, Stool *on page 466*
Febrile Agglutinins, Serum *on page 393*

Synonyms *Salmonella* Agglutinins; Typhoid Agglutinins

Applies to Widal Agglutination Test

Test Commonly Includes Agglutination of "O" and/or "H" *Salmonella* antigens for groups A, B, C, or D

Abstract The genus *Salmonella* are gram-negative organisms which fail to ferment lactose. It includes typhoid/paratyphoid bacilli.

Specimen Serum

Container Red top tube

Collection Acute and convalescent specimens are recommended

Reference Range Less than a fourfold increase in titer

Use Detect antibodies to specific *Salmonella* antigens. Serologic study may be useful to detect chronic carriers of *S. typhi*.

Limitations Numerous false-positives due to cross reacting bacterial antigens and heterospecific anamnestic responses. Clinical correlation is mandatory. **Single determinations are without value. Stool cultures should be obtained.** Misleading titers due to infection with some other organism, false low titers because of partial treatment with antibiotics, and uninterpretable low titers make this a poor test.

Methodology Agglutination, enzyme-linked immunosorbent assay (ELISA)

Additional Information Salmonellosis may cause infections requiring surgical intervention. It may involve the hepatobiliary system and cause other intra-abdominal infections, infections of bones and joints, and soft tissues.[1] *Salmonella* possess "H" ("Hauch") or flagellar antigens and "O" ("ohne Hauch") or somatic cell wall antigens. The diversity of these is staggering, and screening agglutination tests, even of restricted antigen batteries, are too insensitive and nonspecific to be useful. Agglutinating titers can only be interpreted if a series of tests are obtained over time, and a single group shows a clear, significant rise. Some of the recently developed EIA techniques may prove more useful than the older agglutination assays. **The practice of obtaining a single set of agglutinations with no follow-up is condemned. Stool culture remains the definitive technique for diagnosis of bacterial diarrheal disease, supplemented by blood culture.**

Footnotes

1. Lalitha MK and John R, "Unusual Manifestations of Salmonellosis - A Surgical Problem," *Q J Med*, 1994, 87(5):301-9.

References

Isomaki O, Vuento R, and Granfors K, "Serological Diagnosis of *Salmonella* Infections by Enzyme Immunoassay," *Lancet*, 1989, 1(8652):1411-4.
Mandal BK, "*Salmonella typhi* and Other Salmonellas," *Gut*, 1994, 35(6):726-8
Sack RB and Sack DA, "Immunologic Methods for the Diagnosis of Infections by Enterobacteriaceae and Vibrionaceae," *Manual of Clinical Laboratory Immunology*, 4th ed, Chapter 74, Rose NR, Conway de Macario E, Fahey JL, et al, eds, Washington, DC: American Society for Microbiology, 1992, 482-8.

Schistosomiasis Serological Test

CPT 86317 (immunoassay, quantitative); 86318 (immunoassay, qualitative or semiqualitative); 88347 (indirect immunofluorescence)

Related Information

Ova and Parasites, Stool *on page 494*
Ova and Parasites, Urine *on page 495*
Parasite Antibodies *on page 421*

Synonyms Bilharziasis

Applies to Flukes

Abstract In excess of 200 million people have schistosomiasis (bilharziasis). The three major species of these blood flukes are *Schistosoma haematobium*, *S. mansoni*, and *S. japonicum*. **Identification of ova on rectal or vesical biopsy is definitive.**

Specimen Serum

Container Red top tube

Reference Range Negative

Use Support a clinical diagnosis of schistosomiasis in selected cases

Limitations Test does not differentiate between recently acquired infection and chronic multiple exposures and so is simply reported as positive or negative. Test does not differentiate between intestinal and vesical (Continued)

429

Schistosomiasis Serological Test *(Continued)*

schistosomiasis. Serologic diagnosis is now sensitive and specific, but its present role in clinical decision making appears limited to instances in which ova cannot be found in fecal or urine specimens, or rectal or vesical biopsy.

Methodology Indirect fluorescent antibody (IFA) using sections of adult worms; enzyme-linked immunosorbent assay (ELISA) with egg antigen; indirect hemagglutination (IHA). An ELISA test has recently been used to differentiate acute from chronic schistosomiasis from *Schistosoma mansoni*.[1]

Additional Information Schistosomiasis worldwide represents one of our greatest public health challenges, and one of the most common diseases (the most common cause of hematuria, for example). **Demonstration of eggs in bladder or bowel biopsy is definitive, and the examination of stool and urine for eggs is a mainstay of diagnosis.**

Eosinophil counts add little to screening and are inferior to stool examination and serology.[2]

Footnotes
1. Lambertucci JR, "Acute Schistosomiasis: Clinical, Diagnostic and Therapeutic Features," *Rev Inst Med Trop Sao Paulo*, 1993, 35(5):399-404.
2. Libman MD, Mac Lean JD, and Gyorkos TW, "Screening for Schistosomiasis, Filariasis, and Stronglyioidiasis Among Expatriates Returning From the Tropics," *Clin Infect Dis*, 1993, 17(3):353-9.

References
Ash LR and Orihel TC, *Atlas of Human Parasitology*, 3rd ed, Chicago, IL: American Society of Clinical Pathologists, 1990, 206-11.

Kagan IG and Maddison SE, "Serodiagnosis of Parasitic Diseases," *Manual of Clinical Laboratory Immunology*, 4th ed, Vol 2, Chapter 79, Rose NR, Conway de Macario E, Fahey JL, et al, eds, Washington, DC: American Society for Microbiology, 1992, 529-43.

Kamal KA, Shaheen HI, and el-Said AA, "Applicability of ELISA on Buffer-Eluates of Capillary Blood Spotted on Filter Papers for the Diagnosis and Clinical Staging of Human Schistosomiasis," *Trop Geogr Med*, 1994, 46(3):138-41.

Khalil HM, Azab ME, Abdel Ghaffar FM, et al, "Evaluation of Different Serological Tests in Mansonian Schistosomiasis and Correlation to Hepatitis B Virus Infection," *J Egypt Soc Parasitol*, 1994, 24(1):1-12.

Li Y, Rabello AL, Simpson AJ, et al, "The Serological Differentiation of Acute and Chronic *Schistosoma japonicum* Infection by ELISA Using Keyhole Limpet Haemocyanin as Antigen," *Trans R Soc Trop Med Hyg*, 1994, 88(2):249-51.

Maddison SE, "The Present Status of Serodiagnosis and Seroepidemiology of Schistosomiasis," *Diagn Microbiol Infect Dis*, 1987, 7(2):93-105.

Scl-70 *see* Antinuclear Antibody *on page 368*

Scl-70 Antibody *see* Scleroderma Antibody *on this page*

Scleroderma Antibody

CPT 86235

Related Information
Anti-DNA *on page 365*
Antinuclear Antibody *on page 368*
Centromere/Kinetochore Antibody *on page 376*
Jo-1 Antibody *on page 411*
Kidney Biopsy *on page 47*
LE Cell Test *on page 330*
Myositis-Specific Autoantibody *on page 420*
Sjögren's Antibodies *on this page*
Skin Biopsy *on page 54*

Synonyms Progressive Systemic Sclerosis Antibody; Scl-70 Antibody

Applies to RNA Polymerase III; Topoisomerase I

Abstract Progressive systemic sclerosis (diffuse scleroderma) (PSS) is a multisystem disease which includes sclerosis (fibrosis) of skin, gastrointestinal tract, lungs, vessels, heart, and renal parenchyma. Scleroderma may be localized. This antibody often is related to more widespread skin and internal organ disease than is anticentromere antibody. Both antibodies are useful to confirm the diagnosis of scleroderma.[1]

Specimen Serum

Container Red top tube

Storage Instructions Refrigerate separated serum.

Reference Range Negative; titers are not usually offered.

Use Aid the diagnosis of diffuse scleroderma (progressive systemic sclerosis) and CREST syndrome. The antibody is found in up to a quarter of individuals who have idiopathic Raynaud's phenomenon.

Limitations Absence of scleroderma antibody does not exclude diagnosis either of PSS or of CREST syndrome.

Contraindications Once demonstrated, this test need not be repeated.

Methodology Indirect fluorescent antibody (IFA)

Additional Information The antigen for the systemic sclerosis autoantibody is the nuclear enzyme DNA **topoisomerase I** (an enzyme responsible for unwinding supercoiled DNA and creating single-stranded nicks in DNA). In older literature it was referred to as Scl-1. **Scl-70** antibody is specific but seen in only 26% to 76% of patients with scleroderma[1] and in some patients with a limited variant, CREST syndrome (**c**alcinosis cutis, **R**aynaud's, **e**sophageal dysfunction, **s**clerodactyly, **t**elangiectasia).

These syndromes are also associated with a high frequency of speckled pattern using immunofluorescent antinuclear antibody tests. Scl-70 may identify a subset of scleroderma patients with severe skin, joint, and lung disease. ANA by indirect immunofluorescence on HEp-2 cells is positive in almost all subjects with scleroderma. Predominant patterns are speckled (anticentromere) and nucleolar. Testing for anti-Scl-70 antibody is indicated with positive ANA with anticentromere pattern and with nucleolar pattern.[2]

Patients with antisynthetase syndrome may be misdiagnosed as systemic sclerosis; see listing Myositis-Specific Autoantibody *on page 420*. **RNA polymerase III** autoantibody by immunoprecipitation, immunoblotting, and immunodepletion was reactive in 57 of 252 patients with scleroderma, without reactivity in 170 controls.[3]

In scleroderma, positive ANA with nucleolar and speckled patterns are found. Centromere pattern is found with CREST syndrome.

Footnotes
1. Moder KG, "Use and Interpretation of Rheumatologic Tests: A Guide for Clinicians," *Mayo Clin Proc*, 1996, 71(4):391-6.
2. Homburger HA, "Cascade Testing for Autoantibodies in Connective Tissue Diseases," *Mayo Clin Proc*, 1995, 70(2):183-4.
3. Okano Y, Steen VD, and Medsger TA Jr, "Autoantibody Reactive With RNA Polymerase III in Systemic Sclerosis," *Ann Intern Med*, 1993, 119(10):1005-13.

References
Gilliland BC, "Systemic Sclerosis (Scleroderma)," *Harrison's Principles of Internal Medicine*, 13th ed, Vol 2, Isselbacher KJ, Braunwald E, Wilson E, et al, eds, New York, NY: McGraw-Hill Inc, 1994, 1655-62.

Keren DF and Warren JS, *Diagnostic Immunology*, Baltimore, MD: Williams & Wilkins, 1992, 154.

Plotz PH, Rider LG, Targoff IN, et al, "Myositis: Immunologic Contributions to Understanding Cause, Pathogenesis, and Therapy," *Ann Intern Med*, 1995, 122(9):715-24.

Serologic Test for Syphilis *see* Automated Reagin Test *on page 370*

Serum Hepatitis Marker *replaced by* Hepatitis B Surface Antigen *on page 399*

Serum Protein Electrophoresis *see* Protein Electrophoresis, Serum *on page 424*

Serum VDRL *see* VDRL, Serum *on page 438*

Singer-Plotz Test *replaced by* Rheumatoid Factor *on page 427*

Single-Fiber Electromyographic Test *see* Acetylcholine Receptor Antibody *on page 362*

Sjögren's Antibodies

CPT 86235

Related Information
Anticardiolipin Antibody *on page 364*
Anti-DNA *on page 365*
Antinuclear Antibody *on page 368*
Jo-1 Antibody *on page 411*
LE Cell Test *on page 330*
Scleroderma Antibody *on this page*

Synonyms La Antibodies; Ro Antibodies; SS-A Antibodies; SS-B Antibodies

Applies to ENA; Extractable Nuclear Antibodies/Antigens; HLA DR3; HLA DRw52; Sm; SS-A/Ro; SS-B/La; U₁RNP Antibody

Abstract Sjögren's syndrome (SS) is a complex immunologic, autoimmune entity. It includes keratoconjunctivitis, pharyngitis sicca, xerostomia, parotid enlargement, and arthritis. A secondary form is found in patients with other diseases regarded as autoimmune. Lymphoproliferative processes occur. Renal involvement is found in about 40% of those with primary Sjögren's syndrome. Antibodies to double-stranded DNA are not found in Sjögren's syndrome.

Extractable nuclear antigens (**ENA**) include nuclear ribonuclear protein (**RNP**), Smith (**Sm**), Sjögren's syndrome A (**SS-A/Ro**), and Sjögren's syndrome B (**SS-B/La**).

Specimen Serum

Container Red top tube

Reference Range Negative

Use Useful in diagnosis of Sjögren's syndrome (especially with vasculitis) and some forms of lupus; may be present in antiphospholipid antibody syndrome

Methodology Immunoassay

Additional Information Anti-Sm antibodies have specificity for SLE but have poor sensitivity. They are found in about 30% of SLE patients.[1]

SS-A(Ro) (anti-SS-A/Ro) is found in 60% to 70% of patients with Sjögren's syndrome and 25% to 40% of patients with SLE. **SS-B(La)** (anti-SS-B/La) is found in 50% to 60% of Sjögren's syndrome and 10% to 15% of SLE. **SS-A** may be weak or negative by immunofluorescence (it is soluble in the buffers used), but **SS-B** may be seen as a speckled antinuclear pattern. **SS-A** and **SS-B** are particularly useful in "**ANA**

negative" cases of SLE, being present in a majority of such cases. Patients who are ANA positive and who have SS-A but not SS-B are very likely to have nephritis. A majority of patients positive for anti-Ro/SS-A antibodies have photosensitivity.[2] Antibodies to SS-A are also associated with **HLA loci DR3 and DRw52** and with hereditary deficiency of C2. Anti-SS-A and anti-SS-B are found in almost all children with neonatal lupus. Patients with SS-A may also have antibodies to cardiolipin, lupus anticoagulant, and clinical thromboses. This is the antiphospholipid antibody syndrome.

Anti-SS-A/Ro predicts congenital heart block in neonates born to mothers with SLE. Also an ENA antibody, it is found in Sjögren's patients who have extraglandular manifestations including vasculitis, purpura, cytopenias, and adenopathy. A third antibody to ENA, **anti-SS-B/La**, occurs with primary Sjögren's, as well as in subjects with Sjögren's syndrome associated with SLE.[3]

Antibody to **RNP (U_1RNP)**, an extractable nuclear antigen (ENA), is found in mixed connective tissue disease and in up to 40% of subjects with SLE, as well as in Sjögren's syndrome. Alone, in high concentration, it suggests mixed connective tissue disease (MCTD).

Biopsy of the lower lip provides minor salivary gland tissue for histopathologic evaluation for Sjögren's syndrome.

Footnotes
1. Moder KG, "Use and Interpretation of Rheumatologic Tests: A Guide for Clinicians," *Mayo Clin Proc*, 1996, 71(4):391-6.
2. Boumpas DT, Fessler BJ, Austin HA 3d, et al, "Systemic Lupus Erythematosus: Emerging Concepts. Part 2: Dermatologic and Joint Disease, the Antiphospholipid Antibody Syndrome, Pregnancy and Hormonal Therapy, Morbidity and Mortality, and Pathogenesis," *Ann Intern Med*, 1995, 123(1):42-53.
3. Homburger HA, "Cascade Testing for Autoantibodies in Connective Tissue Diseases," *Mayo Clin Proc*, 1995, 70(2):183-4.

References
Arnett FC, Hamilton RG, Reveille JD, et al, "Genetic Studies of Ro (SS-A) and La (SS-B) Autoantibodies in Families With Systemic Lupus Erythematosus and Primary Sjögren's Syndrome," *Arthritis Rheum*, 1989, 32(4):413-9.

"Case Records of the Massachusetts General Hospital. Weekly Clinicopathological Exercises. Case 37-1988. A 35-Year-Old Woman With Recurrent Strokes, an Intracardiac Lesion, Anemia, and Thrombocytopenia," *N Engl J Med*, 1988, 319(11):699-712.

Fox RI, Chan EK, and Kang HI, "Laboratory Evaluation of Patients With Sjögren's Syndrome," *Clin Biochem*, 1992, 25(3):213-22.

Sm *see* Sjögren's Antibodies *on previous page*

SMA *see* Smooth Muscle Antibody *on this page*

Sm Antibody *see* Antinuclear Antibody *on page 368*

Smooth Muscle Antibody
CPT 86255 (screen); 86256 (titer)

Related Information
Antimitochondrial Antibody *on page 366*
Hepatitis C RNA Detection *on page 513*
LE Cell Test *on page 330*
Liver Biopsy *on page 48*
Liver/Kidney Microsomal Type 1 Antibodies *on page 415*
Liver Profile *on page 161*
Protein Electrophoresis, Serum *on page 424*

Synonyms Antismooth Muscle Antibody; SMA

Applies to Antiactin Antibodies; Anti-F Actin; Asialoglycoprotein Receptor Antibodies; DR-3; DR-4; DR52a; HLA-B8; Liver/Kidney Microsomes (LKM) Antibody; Soluble Liver Antigen (SLA) Antibody

Abstract Autoantibodies are found in almost all subjects with autoimmune hepatitis but one of the two classic markers (antinuclear or antismooth muscle antibodies) are only found in about 66%. The serum of about 10% of subjects with viral hepatitis contains autoantibodies and about 5% of sera of patients who have autoimmune hepatitis has antibodies to hepatitis C. About 20% of patients who have chronic hepatitis have autoimmune hepatitis.[1]

Specimen Serum

Container Red top tube

Reference Range Negative

Critical Values Titers ≥1:320 often reflect the presence of antibodies to actin.[2]

Use Useful in the differential diagnosis of liver disease. Antismooth muscle antibodies (SMA) are found mainly in chronic active (autoimmune) hepatitis (CAH) (40% to 70% of cases), type 1 autoimmune hepatitis.

Limitations Presence of antinuclear antibody may interfere with the interpretation of smooth muscle antibody. Less than 2% of normal patients have low titer antibody. Antismooth muscle antibody is present, usually at titers <1:80, in 50% of patients with primary biliary cirrhosis, and in occasional cases of cryptogenic cirrhosis, infectious mononucleosis, asthma, and neoplasm.

Methodology Indirect immunofluorescent antibody (IFA)

Additional Information Titers of 1:80-1:320 are characteristic of the entity which has been called autoimmune or chronic active hepatitis. When the antibody is present in other conditions it is almost always at titers <1:80. Other laboratory findings suggesting autoimmune hepatitis include increased serum transaminases, antinuclear and antiactin antibodies, positive LE preparation with negative anti-DNA test. Other tests likely to be abnormal include serum bilirubin, alkaline phosphatase, prothrombin time, and protein electrophoresis, in which hypergammaglobulinemia is found with selective elevation of IgG. Most patients with autoimmune hepatitis are positive for HLA-B8, DR3, DR52a, or DR4.[1] Many patients with chronic hepatitis (HB_sAg negative) have high titers of antibody to measles, which are not cross reactive with antibody to smooth muscle. SMA are reactive with F-actin. For the best delineation of autoimmune liver disease, SMA should not be done alone, but with assays of antibodies against liver/kidney microsomes (LKM) and soluble liver antigen (SLA). Patients reactive with antinuclear antibody and SMA rarely demonstrate anti-LKM1. Reactivity for SLA may characterize a third patient subgroup.[3] For diagnosis of autoimmune chronic active hepatitis, liver biopsy is desirable. The entity previously called "lupoid hepatitis", and presently expressed as "type 1 autoimmune hepatitis", is the most common form of autoimmune hepatitis and bears SMA and ANA reactivity, polyclonal or oligoclonal gammopathy, and antiactin antibodies including especially anti-F actin.[3]

Antibodies against the liver-specific asialoglycoprotein receptors are often found with autoimmune hepatitis.[2]

Footnotes
1. Meyer zum Büschenfelde KH and Lohse AW, "Autoimmune Hepatitis," *N Engl J Med*, 1995, 333(15):1004-5.
2. Krawitt EL, "Autoimmune Hepatitis," *N Engl J Med*, 1996, 334(14):897-903.
3. Czaja AJ, "Chronic Active Hepatitis: The Challenge for a New Nomenclature," *Ann Intern Med*, 1993, 119(6):510-7.

References
Colvin RB, Bhan AK, and McCluskey RT, *Diagnostic Immunopathology*, New York, NY: Raven Press, 1988, 108-10.

Manns MP and Nakamura RM, "Autoimmune Liver Diseases," *Clin Lab Med*, 1988, 8(2):281-301.

Nakamura RM and Deodhar S, *Laboratory Tests in the Diagnosis of Autoimmune Disorders*, Chicago, IL: American Society of Clinical Pathologists, 1976.

Sommer AI and Haukenes G, "Lack of Cross Reactivity Between Antibody Against Smooth Muscle and Antibodies to Measles Virus in Sera From Patients With Chronic Active Hepatitis," *J Clin Pathol*, 1982, 35:1388-91.

Vrethem M, Skogh T, Berlin G, et al, "Autoantibodies Versus Clinical Symptoms in Blood Donors," *J Rheumatol*, 1992, 19(12):1919-21.

Wands JR and Isselbacher KJ, "Chronic Hepatitis," *Harrison's Principles of Internal Medicine*, 12th ed, Vol 1, Wilson JD, Braunwald E, Isselbacher KJ, et al, eds, New York, NY: McGraw-Hill Inc, 1991, 1337-40.

Soluble Amyloid Beta *see* Cerebrospinal Fluid Amyloid Precursor Protein and Amyloid β-Protein *on page 376*

Soluble Liver Antigen (SLA) Antibody *see* Smooth Muscle Antibody *on this page*

SPE *see* Protein Electrophoresis, Serum *on page 424*

Spherulin® *see* Coccidioidomycosis Antibodies *on page 384*

Spinal Fluid Electrophoresis *see* Cerebrospinal Fluid Protein Electrophoresis *on page 381*

Spinal Fluid Globulin *see* Cerebrospinal Fluid Immunoglobulin G *on page 378*

Spinal Fluid Immunoglobulin *see* Cerebrospinal Fluid Immunoglobulin G *on page 378*

Spinal Fluid Myelin Basic Protein *see* Cerebrospinal Fluid Myelin Basic Protein *on page 379*

Spinal Fluid Oligoclonal Bands *see* Cerebrospinal Fluid Oligoclonal Bands *on page 379*

Spinal Fluid Protein *see* Cerebrospinal Fluid Protein *on page 380*

Spinal Fluid Tau Protein *see* Cerebrospinal Fluid Tau Protein *on page 382*

Spinal Fluid VDRL *see* VDRL, Cerebrospinal Fluid *on page 438*

Sporothrix Antibodies *see* Sporotrichosis Serology *on this page*

Sporothrix schenckii *see* Sporotrichosis Serology *on this page*

Sporotrichosis Serology
CPT 86609

Related Information
Fungal Culture, Biopsy or Body Fluid *on page 476*
Fungal Culture, Sputum *on page 479*
Fungus Smear, Stain *on page 481*

Synonyms *Sporothrix* Antibodies

(Continued)

Sporotrichosis Serology *(Continued)*

Applies to *Sporothrix schenckii*

Abstract Sporotrichosis is a fungal disease classically beginning in the distal extremity, often at a site of inoculation as a painless papule. It spreads proximally, involving lymphatics (lymphangitic sporotrichosis). The organisms in tissue and in 37°C culture exist as small structures. They are often difficult or impossible to see in tissue sections. Extracutaneous disease includes monarticular arthritis. Pulmonary sporotrichosis is much less frequently found than osteoarticular infection. **Optimally, diagnosis is made by culture of biopsy material, rather than by culture of drainage or by serology.**

Specimen Serum or cerebrospinal fluid

Container Red top tube; sterile CSF tube

Reference Range Latex agglutinating titer: <1:4; ELISA: <1:16 in serum, <1:8 in CSF. Depending upon laboratory and method, titers up to 1:40 may be found in normal subjects.

Critical Values Titer ≥1:4 may provide evidence for sporotrichosis. Titers greater than 1:128, rising titers, and persistent elevation are common with pulmonary or systemic disease. Positive reaction in CSF is diagnostic, and is particularly useful in chronic meningitis caused by this organism, which is difficult to culture.

Use Support the diagnosis of sporotrichosis, especially extracutaneous disease

Limitations A negative test result does not rule out infection. Serial titers are not prognostically useful. There are occasional low titer false-positives from nonfungal disease. This test is not widely available and is not standardized.

Methodology Tube agglutination, latex agglutination (LA), enzyme-linked immunosorbent assay (ELISA)

Additional Information Sporotrichosis is usually acquired by traumatic implantation of the dimorphic fungus *Sporothrix schenckii*, a plant saprophyte. Rose gardening is involved in some cases. The disease is found in gardeners and florists, among others. The first signs of infection appear after an average incubation period of 3 weeks; the initial lesion may appear as a small ulcer or a small, hard movable, nontender and nonattached subcutaneous nodule. Disease progresses along lymphatic channels that drain the area of the initial lesion. Less frequent forms of sporotrichosis include pulmonary , osteoarticular, central nervous system, and disseminated disease. Immunosuppression, including the acquired immunodeficiency syndrome (AIDS), increases the probability of hematogenous dissemination, particularly to skin and bone.

The clinical differential diagnosis of **nodular lymphangitis** includes sporotrichosis, as well as *Nocardia brasiliensis, Mycobacterium kansasii, Mycobacterium marinum, Leishmania braziliensis*, and *Francisella tularensis*.[1]

Footnotes

1. Kostman JR and Di Nubile MJ, "Nodular Lymphangitis: A Distinctive but Often Unrecognized Syndrome," *Ann Intern Med*, 1993, 118(11):883-8.

References

Bennett JE, "*Sporothrix schenckii*," *Principles and Practice of Infectious Diseases*, 3rd ed, Mandell GL, Douglas RG Jr, and Bennett JE, eds, New York, NY: Churchill Livingstone, 1990, 1972-5.

Purvis RS, Diven DG, Drechsel RD, et al, "Sporotrichosis Presenting as Arthritis and Subcutaneous Nodules," *J Am Acad Dermatol*, 1993, 28(5 Pt 2):879-84.

Scott EN, Kaufman L, Brown AC, et al, "Serologic Studies in the Diagnosis and Management of Meningitis Due to *Sporothrix schenckii*," *N Engl J Med*, 1987, 317(15):935-40.

Werner AH and Werner BE, "Sporotrichosis in Man and Animal," *Int J Dermatol*, 1994, 33(10):692-700.

Squamous Cancer *see TA-4 on next page*

SS-A Antibodies *see Sjögren's Antibodies on page 430*

SS-A/Ro *see Antinuclear Antibody on page 368*

SS-A/Ro *see Sjögren's Antibodies on page 430*

SS-B Antibodies *see Sjögren's Antibodies on page 430*

SS-B/La *see Antinuclear Antibody on page 368*

SS-B/La *see Sjögren's Antibodies on page 430*

ss-DNA *see Anti-DNA on page 365*

St Louis Encephalitis Virus *see Encephalitis Viral Serology on page 391*

St Louis Encephalitis Virus Serology

CPT 86653

Related Information

California Encephalitis Virus Titer *on page 374*
Eastern Equine Encephalitis Virus Serology *on page 389*
Viral Culture, Central Nervous System Symptoms *on page 677*
Western Equine Encephalitis Virus Serology *on page 439*

Abstract St Louis encephalitis virus causes fever with headache, aseptic meningitis, and encephalitis. Viral transmission includes birds and mosquitoes. Severity of illness increases with age. Patients older than 60 years of age have the highest frequency of encephalitis.

Specimen Serum or cerebrospinal fluid

Container Red top tube, sterile CSF tube

Sampling Time Acute and convalescent sera drawn 10-14 days apart are recommended.

Reference Range Less than a fourfold increase in titer in paired sera; HI titer: <1:10; CF titer: <1:8; plaque reduction: <70%; no IgM antibody in CSF

Use Used to support the diagnosis of St Louis encephalitis virus infection in individuals with CSF pleocytosis. The patient's age, season of the year, place of residence, and exposure are important in the differential diagnosis.

Limitations Cross reactivity between alphavirus group and flavivirus group; false reactions from yellow fever vaccination. (Yellow fever is found in the family Flaviviridae, as is St Louis encephalitis.)

Methodology Complement fixation (CF), hemagglutination inhibition (HAI), plaque reduction neutralization, indirect immunofluorescent antibody; enzyme-linked immunosorbent assay (ELISA) for IgM in CSF or serum antibodies

Additional Information Epidemics occur. In the elderly, the disease may be confused with a cerebrovascular accident. Demonstration of IgM antibody in CSF rapidly establishes a diagnosis of arboviral encephalitis.

References

Monath TP, "Flavivirus (Yellow Fever, Dengue, and St Louis Encephalitis)," *Principles and Practice of Infectious Diseases*, 3rd ed, Mandell GL, Douglas RG Jr, and Bennett JE, eds, New York, NY: Churchill Livingstone, 1990, 1248-51.

Tsai TF, "Arboviruses," *Manual of Clinical Laboratory Immunology*, 4th ed, Vol 2, Chapter 91, Rose NR, Conway de Macario E, Fahey JL, et al eds, Washington, DC: American Society for Microbiology, 1992, 606-18.

Tsai TF, "Arboviruses and Related Zoonotic Viruses," *Principles and Practice of Pediatrics*, 2nd ed, Oski FJ, DeAngelis CD, Feigin RD, et al, eds, Philadelphia, PA: JB Lippincott Co, 1994, 1266-88.

Streptodornase *see Antideoxyribonuclease-B Titer, Serum on page 365*

Streptozyme

CPT 86403 (agglutination, screen); 86406 (agglutination, titer)

Related Information

Antideoxyribonuclease-B Titer, Serum *on page 365*
Antihyaluronidase Titer *on page 365*
Antistreptolysin O Titer, Serum *on page 369*
Bacterial Culture, Throat *on page 468*
Kidney Profile *on page 153*

Specimen Serum

Container Red top tube

Reference Range <100 streptozyme units

Use Screening for antibodies to streptococcal antigens NADase, DNase, streptokinase, streptolysin O, and hyaluronidase This test is most useful for evaluating patients suspected of having poststreptococcal sequelae following *Streptococcus pyogenes* infection, such as rheumatic fever.

Limitations A single determination is less useful than a series. May not be as sensitive in children as in adults. A disadvantage of the test is that borderline antibody elevations, which could be clinically significant particularly in children, may not be detected.

Methodology Hemagglutination

Additional Information Streptozyme is a screening test for antibodies to several streptococcal antigens. It has the advantages of detecting several antibodies in a single assay (although which one has been detected cannot be ascertained), of being technically quick and easy, and of being unaffected by several factors producing false-positives in the ASO test. A serially rising titer is more significant than a single determination.

References

Bisno AL, "Group A Streptococcal Infections and Acute Rheumatic Fever," *N Engl J Med*, 1991, 325(11):783-93.

el-Kholy A, Hafez K, and Krause RM, "Specificity and Sensitivity of the Streptozyme Test for the Detection of Streptococcal Antibodies," *Appl Microbiol*, 1974, 27(4):748-52.

Washington JA, "Medical Microbiology," *Todd-Sanford-Davidsohn Clinical Diagnosis and Management by Laboratory Methods*, 18th ed, Henry JB, ed, Philadelphia, PA: WB Saunders Co, 1991, 1025-74.

Striational Antibodies

Related Information

Acetylcholine Receptor Antibody *on page 362*
Muscle Biopsy *on page 53*
Myositis-Specific Autoantibody *on page 420*

Abstract Striational autoantibodies, like acetylcholine receptor antibody, are markers for acquired myasthenia gravis.[1]

Specimen Serum

Container Red top tube

Reference Range A titer represents the reciprocal of the highest serum dilution reactive.

Use Work up for myasthenia gravis (MG), especially in older subjects and in those with thymoma

Limitations Reactive in only 30% of subjects with autoimmune myasthenia gravis, but it is reported reactive in 80% of those with MG related to thymoma. It is reactive in 24% of subjects who have thymoma without MG and in about 25% of patients who have rheumatoid arthritis treated by D-penicillamine.

Methodology Enzyme immunoassay (EIA)

Additional Information Such antibodies may be IgG, IgA, or IgM class. Correlation between striational and antiacetylcholine receptor autoantibodies is reported.[1]

Footnotes

1. Sano M and Lennon VA, "Enzyme Immunoassay of Anti-Human Acetylcholine Receptor Autoantibodies in Patients With Myasthenia Gravis Reveals Correlation With Striational Autoantibodies," *Neurology*, 1993, 43(3 Pt 1):573-8.

Surrogate Tests see Hepatitis C Serology on page 399

Synovial Fluid C1q Immune Complexes Detection see C1q Immune Complex Detection on page 373

Syphilis Screening Test see Automated Reagin Test on page 370

Syphilis Serology see FTA-ABS, Cerebrospinal Fluid on page 394

Syphilis Serology see FTA-ABS, Serum on page 394

Syphilis Serology see MHA-TP on page 418

Syphilis Serology see RPR on page 428

Syphilis Serology see VDRL, Cerebrospinal Fluid on page 438

Syphilis Serology see VDRL, Serum on page 438

TA-4

CPT 86316

Synonyms Tumor-Antigen 4

Applies to Squamous Cancer

Specimen Serum

Container Red top tube

Reference Range ≤2.6 ng/mL

Use May be useful in diagnosis and management of patients with squamous carcinoma of lung, cervix, or other sites.

Limitations TA-4 is **not** a screening test. Little current literature addresses it.

Methodology Radioimmunoassay (RIA), immunoradiometric assay (IRMA)

Additional Information TA-4 is a protein (MW 48,000) purified from a cervical squamous carcinoma. Patients with squamous carcinomas, particularly those with advanced disease, may have elevated levels of TA-4. Elevation correlates with stage of disease, and rising levels after operation indicate recurrence.

References

Mino N, Iio A, and Hamamoto K, "Availability of Tumor-Antigen 4 as a Marker of Squamous Cell Carcinoma of the Lung and Other Organs," *Cancer*, 1988, 62(4):730-4.

Mino-Miyagawa N, Kimura Y, and Hamamoto K, "Tumor-Antigen 4. Its Immunohistochemical Distribution and Tissue and Serum Concentrations in Squamous Cell Carcinoma of the Lung and Esophagus," *Cancer*, 1990, 66(7):1505-12.

Taenia solium see Cysticercosis Titer on page 388

T- and B-Cell Rosettes Studies replaced by Leukocyte Immunophenotyping on page 414

T and B Lymphocyte Subset Assay see Leukocyte Immunophenotyping on page 414

Tau Fraction see Cerebrospinal Fluid Protein Electrophoresis on page 381

Tetanus Antibody

CPT 86774

Synonyms Tetanus Immunostatus

Specimen Serum

Container Red top tube

Reference Range Hemagglutinating antibody present

Use Assess immunocompetence. Immunity against tetanus can be evaluated in populations.

Contraindications Not valid in an unimmunized individual

Methodology Hemagglutination, enzyme-linked immunosorbent assay (ELISA)

Additional Information Since most individuals have been immunized against tetanus, assessing whether they have antibody to tetanus antigen is a way to document intact humoral immunity. Serologic studies have no place in management of clinical tetanus. The tests are too slow, too insensitive, and do not correlate with the course of disease or response to treatment. Indeed, clinical tetanus has been reported in patients with high antitetanus titers. Only 12% of individuals over age 49 years were considered immune in a survey done in Spain.[1]

Footnotes

1. Cilla G, Saenz-Dominguez JR, Montes M, et al, "Immunity Against Tetanus in Adults Over the Age of 49 Years," *Med Clin*, 1994, 103(15):571-3.

References

Arreaza EE, Gibbons JJ Jr, Siskind GW, et al, "Lower Antibody Response to Tetanus Toxoid Associated With Higher Autoanti-idiotypic Antibody in Old Compared With Young Humans," *Clin Exp Immunol*, 1993, 92(1):169-73.

Craig JP, "Immune Response to *Corynebacterium diphtheriae* and *Clostridium tetani*: Diagnostic Methods," *Manual of Clinical Laboratory Immunology*, 4th ed, Vol 2, Chapter 69, Rose NR, Conway de Macario E, Fahey JL, et al, eds, Washington, DC: American Society for Microbiology, 1992, 435-9.

Crone NE and Reder AT, "Severe Tetanus in Immunized Patients With High Antitetanus Titers," *Neurology*, 1992, 42(4):761-4.

Hazlewood M, Nusrat R, Kumararatne DS, Goodall M, et al, "The Acquisition of Antipneumococcal Capsular Polysaccharide *Haemophilus influenzae* Type b and Tetanus Toxoid Antibodies, With Age, in the UK," *Clin Exp Immunol*, 1993, 93(2):157-64.

Tetanus Immunostatus see Tetanus Antibody on this page

***Thermoactinomyces* Precipitating Antibodies** replaced by Hypersensitivity Pneumonitis Serology on page 406

***Thermoactinomyces vulgaris* Precipitating Antibodies** see Hypersensitivity Pneumonitis Serology on page 406

***Thermolospora viridis* Precipitating Antibodies** see Hypersensitivity Pneumonitis Serology on page 406

Thyroglobulin Antibody see Thyroid Antithyroglobulin Antibody on next page

Thyroid Antimicrosomal Antibody

CPT 86376

Related Information

Acetylcholine Receptor Antibody on page 362
Free Thyroxine Index on page 129
T_3 Uptake on page 201
Thyroid Antithyroglobulin Antibody on next page
Thyroid Stimulating Hormone on page 204
Thyroxine on page 206
Thyroxine, Free on page 208

Synonyms Antithyroid Peroxidase Antibody; Anti-TPO; Microsomal Antibody

Applies to Thyroid Autoantibodies

Abstract Antimicrosomal and antithyroglobulin antibodies are detectable in most subjects who have Hashimoto's thyroiditis and many who have Graves' disease. The most common cause of spontaneous hypothyroidism is chronic autoimmune thyroiditis (Hashimoto's disease).

Specimen Serum

Container Red top tube

Storage Instructions Separated serum stable for 5 days at room temperature

Reference Range Passive hemagglutination: <1:100; IFA: negative

Use Used in differential diagnosis of hypothyroidism, Hashimoto's thyroiditis, and primary myxedema

Limitations Should be used in conjunction with antithyroglobulin test, since autoimmune thyroiditis may demonstrate a response to antigens other than thyroid microsomes. Patients who have autoimmune disorders such as Sjögren's syndrome, lupus erythematosus, rheumatoid arthritis, pernicious anemia, and others may be positive for antimicrosomal and/or antithyroglobulin antibodies. Patients with myxedema, granulomatous thyroiditis, nontoxic nodular goiter and thyroid carcinoma may occasionally produce thyroid antibodies. Thyroid microsomal antibodies have been reported in drug-induced hypersensitivity reactions to anticonvulsants and sulfonamides resulting in hypothyroidism.

Methodology Passive hemagglutination, indirect fluorescent antibody (IFA), enzyme-linked immunosorbent assay (ELISA)

Additional Information Antibodies to thyroid microsomes (thyroid peroxidase) are present in 70% to 90% of patients with chronic thyroiditis and about 40% of patients with Graves' disease. They are also present in smaller percentages of patients with other thyroid diseases and with pernicious anemia. Antibody production may be confined to lymphocytes within the thyroid, and serum may be negative. Small numbers (3%) of people with no evidence of disease may have antibody, more frequently in females and increasing with age. The possible role of infectious (Continued)

Thyroid Antimicrosomal Antibody *(Continued)*

agents in autoimmune thyroid disease has been discussed.[1] Thyroid status may modulate expression of thyroid autoimmunity in subjects who have euthyroid or hypothyroid goitrous Hashimoto's thyroiditis.[2]

The roles of CD8[+] and CD4[+] T cells, thyroid-associated lymphoid tissue (TALT) and other facets of autoimmune thyroid disease, are addressed in a paper which recognizes three autoimmune thyroid diseases. They are Hashimoto goiter, primary myxedema, and Graves' disease, with autoimmune reactions known in additional entities.[3]

Euthyroid individuals with increased levels of sensitive TSH and marginally decreased free thyroxine concentration, with associated positive antimicrosomal antibodies, are at risk for development of hypothyroidism in the future.[4]

Footnotes

1. Tomer Y and Davies TF, "Infection, Thyroid Disease, and Autoimmunity," *Endocr Rev*, 1993, 14(1):107-20.
2. Rieu M, Richard A, Rosilio M, et al, "Effects of Thryoid Status on thyroid Autoimmunity Expression in Euthyroid and Hypothyroid Patients With Hashimoto's Thyroiditis," *Clin Endocrinol*, 1994, 40(4):529-35.
3. Mooij P and Drexhage HA, "Autoimmune Thyroid Disease," *Clin Lab Med*, 1993, 13(3):683-97.
4. Klee GG and Hay ID, "Biochemical Thyroid Function Testing," *Mayo Clin Proc*, 1994, 69(5):469-70.

References

Baker JR Jr, Saunders NB, Wartofsky L, et al, "Seronegative Hashimoto Thyroiditis With Thyroid Autoantibody Production Localized to the Thyroid," *Ann Intern Med*, 1988, 108(1):26-30.

Gupta A, Eggo MC, Uetrecht JF, et al, "Drug-Induced Hypothyroidism: The Thyroid as a Target Organ in Hypersensitivity Reactions to Anticonvulsants and Sulfonamides," *Clin Pharmacol Ther*, 1992, 51(1):56-67.

Takasu N, Yamada T, Takasu M, et al, "Disappearance of Thyrotropin-Blocking Antibodies and Spontaneous Recovery From Hypothyroidism in Autoimmune Thyroiditis," *N Engl J Med*, 1992, 326(8):513-8.

Tandon N and Weetman AP, "T Cells and Thyroid Autoimmunity," *J R Coll Physicians Lond*, 1994, 28(1):10-8.

Thyroid Antithyroglobulin Antibody

CPT 86800

Related Information

Acetylcholine Receptor Antibody *on page 362*
Thyroid Antimicrosomal Antibody *on previous page*
Thyrotropin Receptor Antibody *on this page*

Synonyms Antithyroglobulin Antibody; Thyroglobulin Antibody

Applies to CA2; Thyroid Autoantibodies

Test Commonly Includes Titers on positive specimens

Specimen Serum

Container Red top tube

Reference Range Hemagglutination: <1:400; IFA: negative; values vary with technology used

Use Useful in detection and confirmation of autoimmune thyroiditis, Hashimoto's thyroiditis and primary myxedema

Limitations Must be used in conjunction with antimicrosomal test, since autoimmune thyroiditis may demonstrate a response to antigen other than thyroglobulin. Other autoimmune disorders such as Sjögren's syndrome, SLE, RA, autoimmune hemolytic anemia, may be positive for thyroid antibodies, as may patients with myxedema, granulomatosis thyroiditis, thyrotoxicosis, nontoxic nodular goiter and thyroid carcinoma.

Methodology Passive hemagglutination, indirect fluorescent antibody (IFA), enzyme-linked immunosorbent assay (ELISA)

Additional Information Antibodies to thyroglobulin can be detected in 40% to 70% of patients with chronic thyroiditis. Antibodies may also be present in 70% of hypothyroid patients, 40% of patients with Graves' disease, and smaller numbers of patients with other autoimmune conditions, particularly pernicious anemia. Normal individuals, especially elderly females, may have antibody. The immunofluorescent test can detect an additional antibody, to CA2, the "second colloid antigen." A small fraction of patients with thyroiditis will have only antibody to CA2. Rare patients may have antibody production confined to the thyroid gland.

Patients with thyroid autoantibodies may develop hypothyroidism without recognized Hashimoto's goiter, a disorder called primary thyroid atrophy.[1]

Footnotes

1. Mooij P and Drexhage HA, "Autoimmune Thyroid Disease," *Clin Lab Med*, 1993, 13(3):683-97.

References

Baker JR Jr, Saunders NB, Wartofsky L, et al, "Seronegative Hashimoto Thyroiditis With Thyroid Autoantibody Production Localized to the Thyroid," *Ann Intern Med*, 1988, 108(1):26-30.

Harchali AA, Montagne P, Cuilliere ML, et al, "Detection of Antithyroglobulin Autoantibodies With Defined Epitopic Specificity by a Microparticle-Enhanced Nephelometric Immunoassay," *Clin Chem*, 1992, 38(9):1859-64.

Mizukami Y, Michigishi T, Nonomura A, et al, "Pathology of Chronic Thyroiditis: A New Clinically Relevant Classification," *Pathol Annu*, 1994, 29(Pt 1):135-58.

Takaichi Y, Tamai H, Honda K, et al, "The Significance of Antithyroglobulin and Antithyroidal Microsomal Antibodies in Patients With Hyperthyroidism Due to Graves' Disease Treated With Antithyroid Drugs," *J Clin Endocrinol Metab*, 1989, 68(6):1097-100.

Thyroid Autoantibodies *see* Thyroid Antimicrosomal Antibody *on previous page*

Thyroid Autoantibodies *see* Thyroid Antithyroglobulin Antibody *on this page*

Thyroid Stimulating Autoantibody *see* Thyrotropin Receptor Antibody *on this page*

Thyroid Stimulating Immunoglobulins *see* Thyrotropin Receptor Antibody *on this page*

Thyrotropin Receptor Antibody

CPT 80439 (TSH); 80440 (prolactin)

Related Information

Free Thyroxine Index *on page 129*
T$_3$ Uptake *on page 201*
Thyroid Antithyroglobulin Antibody *on this page*
Thyroid Stimulating Hormone *on page 204*
Thyroxine *on page 206*
Thyroxine, Free *on page 208*

Synonyms Thyroid Stimulating Autoantibody; Thyroid Stimulating Immunoglobulins; TRAb; Ts Antibodies; TSH-Receptor Antibodies; TSIG

Applies to LATS; LATS Protector; Long-Acting Thyroid Stimulator

Abstract The group of endocrinologically active antireceptor antibodies includes TRAb. TRAb are a group of diverse autoantibodies which recognize cell surface antigens of thyroid epithelium in the environs of the TSH receptor. They play a role in the pathogenesis of thyrotoxicosis in Graves' disease.[1] Graves' disease is recognized as an autoimmune endocrine disorder.[2]

Specimen Serum

Container Red top tube

Reference Range Negative; results depend on the laboratory method.

Use Used to understand the pathogenesis of hyperthyroidism in Graves' disease and evaluate response to therapy; may be especially helpful when clinical suspicion of Graves' disease is unsupported by standard thyroid testing protocols. High TRAb levels may indicate relapse.

Limitations Four percent false-positive rate in normals. Occasionally, TRAb are inhibitory rather than stimulatory and can cause hypothyroidism.[3]

Methodology Bioassay, radioreceptor assay

Additional Information Thyrotropin receptor antibody is an autoantibody to the thyroid cell receptor for thyroid stimulating hormone. It can be demonstrated in 90% of patients with Graves' disease, and is the cause of the hyperthyroidism of that condition. The characterization of TRAb resolved much confusion about long-acting thyroid stimulator (LATS) and LATS protector, which are both, in fact, thyroid stimulating autoantibodies which simply behaved differently in animal test systems. These antibodies are present in 50% of euthyroid Graves' disease as well as hyperthyroid patients. They play a major role in the pathogenesis of Graves' disease. Detection of such antibodies is useful in prediction of neonatal hyperthyroidism and prediction of relapse of Graves' hyperthyroidism.

Footnotes

1. Kahn CR, Smith RJ, and Chin WW, "Mechanism of Action of Hormones That Act at the Cell Surface," *Williams Textbook of Endocrinology*, Chapter 4, Wilson JD and Foster DW, eds, Philadelphia, PA: WB Saunders Co, 1992, 91-134.
2. Mooij P and Drexhage HA, "Autoimmune Thyroid Disease," *Clin Lab Med*, 1993, 13(3):683-97.
3. Takasu N, Yamada T, Takasu M, et al, "Disappearance of Thyrotropin-Blocking Antibodies and Spontaneous Recovery From Hypothyroidism in Autoimmune Thyroiditis," *N Engl J Med*, 1992, 326(8):513-8.

References

Gupta MK, "Thyrotropin Receptor Antibodies: Advances and Importance of Detection Techniques in Thyroid Disease," *Clin Biochem*, 1992, 25(3):193-9.

Rieu M, Richard A, Rosilio M, et al, "Effects of Thyroid Status on Thyroid Autoimmunity Expression in Euthyroid and Hypothyroid Patients With Hashimoto's Thyroiditis," *Clin Endocrinol*, 1994, 40(4):529-35.

Whitley RJ, Meikle AW, and Watts NB, "Endocrinology," *Textbook of Clinical Chemistry*, 2nd ed, Chapter 35, Teitz NW, Bortis CA, and Ashwood ER, eds, Philadelphia, PA: WB Saunders Co, 1994, 1645-739.

Tickborne Diseases *see* Ehrlichiosis Serology *on page 390*

Tissue Typing

CPT 86805 (with titration); 86821 (without titration)

Related Information

HLA-B27 *on page 404*
HLA Typing, Single Human Leukocyte Antigen *on page 405*
Identification DNA Testing *on page 517*
Mixed Lymphocyte Culture *on page 418*

Paternity Studies *on page 613*

Synonyms Crossmatch, Lymphocyte; Histocompatibility Testing; HLA Typing; HLA Typing, Crossmatch; Human Leukocyte Antigens; Lymphocyte Crossmatch; Organ Donor Tissue Typing; Tissue Typing, Donor; Transplant Tissue Typing; White Cell Crossmatch

Test Commonly Includes Determination of compatibility between recipient and donors for organ or bone marrow transplant

Specimen Heparinized blood from donor, serum from recipient for kidney or bone marrow transplantation

Container Donor: green top (heparin) tube; recipient: red top tube

Storage Instructions Should be tested immediately. Do **not** refrigerate or freeze.

Use Tissue typing aids in determination of compatibility of kidney or bone marrow transplant. HLA-B27 is addressed in a separate listing. HLA-B8 is found in diseases with immune associations. Addison's disease is strongly associated with B8. Juvenile diabetes mellitus, myasthenia gravis and Graves' disease also show association with B8, as does gluten-sensitive enteropathy.

Methodology Lymphocytotoxicity assay, mixed lymphocyte culture (MLC), polymerase chain reaction (PCR)

Additional Information HLA antigens are glycoproteins, the product of four closely linked genes on chromosome 6, usually inherited as an intact unit. HLA antigens are the primary determinants of tissue graft acceptance, and thus, the histocompatibility complex. This same HLA region contains genes of importance to complement and immune responses. The HLA loci are HLA-A, B, C (class I) and DR, DQ, DP, and DW (class II). A, B, and C antigens are expressed on nearly all nucleated human cells, D antigens are restricted to B lymphocytes, monocytes, and possibly endothelial cells. HLA antigens are inherited as two sets of six antigens, one set from each parent and are codominantly expressed. These antigens show linkage disequilibrium, that is certain pairs or triplets occur more frequently than expected by chance.

Associations with HLA-A and C are rare. Multiple sclerosis is associated with HLA-DRw2 and is an example of linkage disequilibrium being earlier reported to be associated with A3, then B7, and then Dw2, with highest association with DRw2. This has become a quite detailed and complex area of medicine.

Tissue typing is usually undertaken to assess the "match" between donor and recipient of an organ for transplantation. Since these antigens are widely expressed in tissue, mismatches result in graft rejection, or graft-vs-host disease.

References
Braun WE and Zachary AA, "The HLA Histocompatibility System in Autoimmune States," *Clin Lab Med*, 1988, 8(2):351-72.

Olerup O and Zetterquist H, "HLA-DR Typing by PCR Amplification With Sequence-Specific Primers in 2 Hours: An Alternative to Serological DR Typing in Clinical Practice Including Donor-Recipient Matching in Cadaveric Transplantation," *Tissue Antigens*, 1992, 39(5):225-35.

Perkins HA, "Clinical Applications of HLA Typing," *Clin Lab Med*, 1982, 2:123-35.

Tissue Typing, Donor *see* Tissue Typing *on previous page*

Topoisomerase I *see* Scleroderma Antibody *on page 430*

TORCH

CPT 80090

Related Information

Cytomegalovirus Antibody *on page 389*
Herpes Simplex Antibody *on page 401*
Rubella Serology *on page 428*
Toxoplasmosis Serology *on this page*

Synonyms TORCH Battery; TORCH Screen; TORCH Titer

Test Commonly Includes Toxoplasmosis, rubella, cytomegalovirus, and herpesvirus serology

Abstract Although the acronym TORCH serves to enhance awareness of congenital infections, the disease entities must be considered separately rather than collectively.[1] The entities are **T**oxoplasmosis, **O**ther, **R**ubella, **C**ytomegalovirus, **H**erpes.

Specimen Serum

Container Red top tube

Collection Paired specimens drawn 2-4 weeks apart.

Reference Range IgG: less than a fourfold increase in titer; IgM: negative

Use Screen for serologic response to toxoplasmosis, rubella, cytomegalovirus, and herpesvirus infection, important in newborn infants for evaluation of possible congenital infection

Limitations The presence of IgG antibodies in maternal blood indicates prior exposure to that specific agent through natural infection or immunization (rubella). Since the prevalence of antibodies to HSV and CMV is very high in the general population, a single positive IgG antibody to these agents is of little diagnostic value regardless of titer. Fetal or neonatal IgG antibodies merely indicate transplacental transfer of maternal antibodies. Negative serologic results do not exclude infection.

Methodology Indirect fluorescent antibody (IFA), enzyme-linked immunosorbent assay (ELISA), IgG and IgM specificity

Additional Information *Toxoplasma*, rubella, cytomegalovirus, and herpes are all causes of potentially catastrophic congenital infections, which can be quickly fatal or lead to chronic sequelae including hepatitis, encephalitis, and failure to thrive. In the fulminant case serologic diagnosis is of little use since the disease outstrips the immune response and even IgM antibody cannot be demonstrated in time to be clinically useful. However, in the disease which becomes manifest weeks to months after birth, demonstration of IgM antibody or rising titers of IgG antibody can confirm a diagnosis of specific infection. The presence of IgM-specific antibody in cord, fetal, or neonatal blood indicates congenital infection. **It should be emphasized that TORCH testing is of very limited usefulness. Results must be interpreted in conjunction with complete clinical information, and such testing in no way substitutes for careful clinical examination and judgment. TORCH testing should not be applied indiscriminately to pregnant women or infants with nondescript illnesses.** See individual listings.

Footnotes
1. Stamos JK and Rowley AH, "Timely Diagnosis of Congenital Infections," *Pediatr Clin North Am*, 1994, 41(5):1017-33.

References
Chiodo F, Verucchi G, Mori F, et al, "Infective Diseases During Pregnancy and Their Teratogenic Effects," *Ann Ist Super Sanita*, 1993, 29(1):57-67.

Donley DK, "TORCH Infections in the Newborn," *Semin Neurol*, 1993, 13(1):106-15.

Ghidini A and Lynch L, "Prenatal Diagnosis and Significance of Fetal Infections," *West J Med*, 1993, 159(3):366-73.

Gonik B, *Viral Diseases in Pregnancy*, New York, NY: Springer-Verlag, 1994.

Greenough A, "The TORCH Screen and Intrauterine Infections," *Arch Dis Child*, 1994, 70(3 Spec No):163-5

TORCH Battery *see* TORCH *on this page*

TORCH Screen *see* TORCH *on this page*

TORCH Titer *see* TORCH *on this page*

Total Hemolytic Complement *see* Complement, Total, Serum *on page 386*

***Toxocara* Excretory-Secretory ELISA (TES)** *see* Parasite Antibodies *on page 421*

***Toxoplasma* Antibodies** *see* Toxoplasmosis Serology *on this page*

Toxoplasmosis Serology

CPT 86777; 86778 (IgM)

Related Information

HIV-1/HIV-2 Serology *on page 403*
Ova and Parasites, Stool *on page 494*
Parasite Antibodies *on page 421*
TORCH *on this page*

Synonyms *Toxoplasma* Antibodies; Toxoplasmosis Titer

Replaces Sabin-Feldman Dye Test

Test Commonly Includes IgG and IgM antibody specific for *Toxoplasma gondii*

Abstract *Toxoplasma gondii* is an intracellular protozoan parasite that infects both humans and animals. The organism has a worldwide distribution and human infections are very common; serologic studies indicate that approximately half of the United States population has been infected with *T. gondii*. Most human infections follow an asymptomatic chronic course, however, severe disseminated infections occur, particularly in immunocompromised hosts. Human infection is most commonly acquired by ingestion of oocysts in undercooked meat, but contamination of food or drink with oocysts from cat feces is also an important mode of human infection.

Toxoplasmosis infection is especially important in two clinical situations: infections transmitted to the fetus and as the most common opportunistic infection of the central nervous system in patients with acquired immunodeficiency syndrome (AIDS).[1]

Specimen Serum, amniotic fluid. Amniocentesis with ultrasonography and fetal blood sampling can lead to correct diagnosis in approximately 92% of patients.[2]

Container Red top tube

Collection Acute and convalescent serum specimens are recommended at 3-week interval

Reference Range IgG: less than a fourfold increase in titer; IgM: negative

Use Support the diagnosis of toxoplasmosis; document past exposure and/or immunity to *Toxoplasma gondii*

Limitations Diagnosis of neonatal infection may be difficult because infection outstrips demonstrable antibody response. Toxoplasmosis
(Continued)

Toxoplasmosis Serology *(Continued)*

occurs in advanced AIDS. The absence in such patients of anti-*Toxo-plasma* antibodies on immunofluorescence assay does not exclude the diagnosis.[1] There is a high prevalence of antibody to *Toxoplasma* in most populations. Although a single high titer is frequently used to suggest active infection, it is unreliable because titers may persist at high levels for years in healthy people. Distinction between chronic active, inactive, and past infection may be obscure. Many different tests are available and false-positive and false-negative results are seen with these tests to varying degrees. Serologic responses in the presence of immunodeficiency lack reliability.

Methodology Indirect fluorescent antibody (IFA), indirect hemagglutination (IHA), direct agglutination test with 2-mercaptoethanol IgM capture test,[3] enzyme-linked immunosorbent assay (ELISA). The Sabin Feldman dye test remains in use. PCR used for prenatal diagnosis of congenital *T. gondii* infection is reported as safe, rapid, and accurate.[4]

Additional Information *Toxoplasma gondii* is a protozoan parasite endemic in cats and excreted by them. Humans are easily exposed to oocysts, either in caring for pets or in casual environmental contact. The majority of individuals develop antibody without any clinical disease, and a self-limited lymphadenitis is the most common clinical presentation in symptomatic infection.

Congenital toxoplasmosis and infection in immunocompromised hosts (especially AIDS patients) are more serious, and can produce a fatal cerebritis or disseminated illness. **Congenital toxoplasmosis** can now be diagnosed *in utero* by detection of IgM antibody in fetal blood. Diagnosis is supported by high or rising IgG antibody titer, or the demonstration of IgM antibody. The recent availability of IgA anti-*Toxoplasma* may be useful in detection of congenital toxoplasmosis. However, IgM is still the established technique. Neonatal screening by IgM capture immunoassay, with confirmation by specific IgG and IgM antibodies in neonatal and maternal serum is described.[5] The median CD4 cell count in subjects with AIDS and toxoplasmosis, at presentation, was 50/mm^3.[1]

IgG antibodies usually appear within 1-2 weeks of infection, peak within 1-2 months, fall at variable rates, and persist for life. Diagnosis of congenital infection is made by demonstrating specific IgM or IgA in serum obtained by periumbilical blood sampling or at birth; contamination with maternal blood can be excluded by assaying for β-hCG and coagulation factors, as well as by the Kleihauer test. IgG in neonatal of fetal blood merely indicates transplacental transfer of maternal antibody.

Intrathecal production suggesting CNS infection can be determined as follows: C = (antibody titer in CSF x IgG concentration in serum) / (antibody titer in serum x IgG concentration in CSF). Intrathecal production is probable when C is ≥8.

Footnotes

1. Porter SB and Sande MA, "Toxoplasmosis of the Central Nervous System in the Acquired Immunodeficiency Syndrome," *N Engl J Med*, 1992, 327(23):1643-8.
2. Stamos JK and Rowley AH, "Timely Diagnosis of Congenital Infections," *Pediatr Clin North Am*, 1994, 41(5):1017-33.
3. Bertoli F, Espino M, Arosemena JR 5th, et al, "A Spectrum in the Pathology of Toxoplasmosis in Patients With Acquired Immunodeficiency Syndrome," *Arch Pathol Lab Med*, 1995, 119(3):214-24.
4. Hohlfeld P, Daffos F, Costa JM, et al, "Prenatal Diagnosis of Congenital Toxoplasmosis With a Polymerase-Chain-Reaction Test on Amniotic Fluid," *N Engl J Med*, 1994, 331(11):695-9.
5. Guerina NG, Hsu HW, Meissner HC, et al, "Neonatal Serologic Screening and Early Treatment for Congenital *Toxoplasma gondii* Infection," *N Engl J Med*, 1994, 330(26):1858-63.

References

Cesbron MF, Dubremetz JF, and Sher A, "The Immunobiology of Toxoplasmosis," *Res Immunol*, 1993, 144(1):7-8.
Decker CF and Tauzon CU, "Toxoplasmosis: An Update on Clinical and Therapeutic Aspects," *Prog Clin Parasitol*, 1993, 3:21-41.
Griffith BP and Booss J, "Neurologic Infections of the Fetus and Newborn," *Neurol Clin*, 1994, 12(3):541-64.
Guerina NG, "Congenital Infection With *Toxoplasma gondii*," *Pediatr Ann*, 1994, 23(3):138-42, 147-51.
Herwaldt BL and Juranek DD, "Laboratory-Acquired Malaria, Leishmaniasis, Trypanosomiasis, and Toxoplasmosis," *Am J Trop Med Hyg*, 1993, 48(3):313-23.
Hunter CA and Remington JS, "Immunopathogenesis of Toxoplasmic Encephalitis," *J Infect Dis*, 1994, 170(5):1057-67.
Israelski DM and Remington JS, "Toxoplasmosis in the Non-AIDS Immunocompromised Host," *Curr Clin Top Infect Dis*, 1993, 13:322-56.
Joiner KA and Dubremetz JF, "*Toxoplasma gondii*: A Protozoan for the Nineties," *Infect Immun*, 1993, 61(4):1169-72.
Mariuz P, Bosler EM, and Luft BJ, "Toxoplasmosis in Individuals With AIDS," *Infect Dis Clin North Am*, 1994, 8(2):365-81.
Matsui D, "Prevention, Diagnosis, and Treatment of Fetal Toxoplasmosis," *Clin Perinatol*, 1994, 21(3):675-89.
McCabe R and Chirurgi V, "Issues in Toxoplasmosis," *Infect Dis Clin North Am*, 1993, 7(3):587-604.
New LC and Holliman RE, "Toxoplasmosis and Human Immunodeficiency Virus (HIV) Disease," *J Antimicrob Chemother*, 1994, 33(6):1079-82.
Nussenblatt RB and Belfort R Jr, "Ocular Toxoplasmosis. An Old Disease Revisited," *JAMA*, 1994, 271(4):304-7.
Subauste CS and Remington JS, "Immunity to *Toxoplasma gondii*," *Curr Opin Immmunol*, 1993, 5(4):532-7.
Valente P and Sever JL, "*In Utero* Diagnosis of Congenital Infections by Direct Fetal Sampling," *Isr J Med Sci*, 1994, 30(5-6):414-20.

Wong SY and Remington JS, "Toxoplasmosis in Pregnancy," *Clin Infect Dis*, 1994, 18(6):853-61.

Toxoplasmosis Titer *see* Toxoplasmosis Serology *on previous page*

TRAb *see* Thyrotropin Receptor Antibody *on page 434*

Transplant Tissue Typing *see* Tissue Typing *on page 434*

Transthyretin *see* Cerebrospinal Fluid Protein Electrophoresis *on page 381*

***Treponema pallidum* Antibodies, CSF** *see* FTA-ABS, Cerebrospinal Fluid *on page 394*

***Trichinella spiralis* Antibodies** *see* Trichinosis Serology *on this page*

Trichinosis Serology

CPT 86784

Related Information

Muscle Biopsy *on page 53*
Ova and Parasites, Stool *on page 494*
Parasite Antibodies *on page 421*

Synonyms *Trichinella spiralis* Antibodies

Specimen Serum

Container Red top tube

Sampling Time Measurable antibody titers are not usually reached until 2-3 weeks after infestation. Paired specimens are recommended.

Reference Range Negative; <1:16 by ELISA; less than a fourfold increase in paired titer; dependent upon laboratory and method

Use Screen for antibodies to *Trichinella spiralis* to establish the diagnosis of trichinosis. Ingestion of undercooked pork, bear, or walrus meat containing larvae may lead to myalgias, fever, myocardial infestation, neurological symptoms, and peripheral blood eosinophilia.

Limitations Low titers may represent antibody from previous rather than current infection. Antibody remains detectable for 2-3 years. The test may have a high false-negative rate of 15% to 22% during the first period of the infection.

Methodology Bentonite flocculation test (BFT), indirect fluorescent antibody (IFA), complement fixation (CF), latex agglutination (LA), enzyme-linked immunosorbent assay (ELISA)

Additional Information The bentonite flocculation test is sensitive and specific. Antibody becomes detectable 3 weeks after infection, rises for several weeks, and then declines slowly so that most individuals will test negative in 2-3 years. Immunofluorescence is more sensitive for light infection in pigs.

In humans, diagnosis can also be made by finding cysts in a muscle biopsy. As an incidental finding, trichinosis was not infrequently found in pharyngeal striated muscle adhering to tonsillectomy specimens.

References

Mawhorter SD and Kazura JW, "Trichinosis of the Central Nervous System," *Semin Neurol*, 1993, 13(2):148-52.
Murrell KD and Bruschi F, "Clinical Trichinellosis," *Prog Clin Parasitol*, 1994, 4:117-50.
Wakelin D, "*Trichinella spiralis*: Immunity, Ecology, and Evolution," *J Parasitol*, 1993, 79(4):488-94.
Wassom DL, "Immunoecological Succession in Host-Parasite Communities," *J Parasitol*, 1993, 79(4):483-7.

Trypanosoma cruzi *see* Chagas' Disease Serological Test *on page 383*

Ts Antibodies *see* Thyrotropin Receptor Antibody *on page 434*

TSH-Receptor Antibodies *see* Thyrotropin Receptor Antibody *on page 434*

TSIG *see* Thyrotropin Receptor Antibody *on page 434*

Tularemia Agglutinins

CPT 86668

Related Information

Bacterial Culture, Blood *on page 457*
Febrile Agglutinins, Serum *on page 393*
Lymph Node Biopsy *on page 50*

Synonyms *Francisella tularensis* Antibodies; Rabbit Fever Antibodies

Applies to *Francisella tularensis* Culture

Abstract *Francisella tularensis*, found in wild rabbits and in a number of other animals, may be transmitted to man by direct contact and by ticks and deer flies.

Specimen Serum

Container Red top tube

Sampling Time Paired sera collected 2-3 weeks apart are recommended.

Reference Range Agglutination titer: <1:40; ELISA: <1:500; less than a fourfold increase in paired titer

Critical Values A single serologic result with a titer ≥1:160 in a subject having clinical tularemia or a fourfold rise in titer is diagnostic.

Use Investigation of illness characterized by an ulcerative lesion at a site of inoculation, with regional lymphadenopathy, fever, and pneumonia. Liver and spleen are affected. Conjunctivitis may occur. **Agglutinins represent the key laboratory evaluation in many cases.**

Limitations There is serologic cross reactivity with *Brucella* sp, *Proteus* OX-19, and *Yersinia* sp. IgM and IgG titers may remain elevated for over a decade after infection, limiting the value of unpaired specimens; single titers may be misleading. Cell-mediated immunity is also important in host response to *F. tularensis*.

Methodology Agglutination, hemagglutination, enzyme-linked immunosorbent assay (ELISA)

Additional Information Antibodies to *F. tularensis* develop 2-3 weeks after infection and peak in 4-5 weeks. Although antibodies may cross react with *Brucella* those titers will generally be much lower. Rising titers over a 2-week interval are the best indicator of recent infection.

Although laboratory diagnosis of tularemia is often established by serologic methods, *F. tularensis* may be recovered in culture from a variety of clinical specimens. Blood cultures are often negative. *F. tularensis* is an extremely hazardous infectious agent responsible for several laboratory acquired infections. **If tularemia is clinically suspected, please contact the laboratory so that appropriate precautions can be taken.**

Nodular lymphangitis occurs with sporotrichosis. *Nocardia braziliensis*, *Mycobacterium marinum*, *Leishmania braziliensis*, and *Francisella tularensis*. A painful ulcer at the initial site is suggestive of tularemia in such cases.[1]

Footnotes

1. Kostman JR and Di Nubile MJ, "Nodular Lymphangitis: A Distinctive but Often Unrecognized Syndrome," *Ann Intern Med*, 1993, 118(11):883-8.

References

Fortier AH, Green SJ, Polsinelli T, et al, "Life and Death of an Intracellular Pathogen: *Francisella tularensis* and the Macrophage," *Immunol Ser*, 1994, 60:349-61.

Spach DH, Liles WC, Campbell GL, et al, "Tick-Borne Diseases in the United States," *N Engl J Med*, 1993, 329(13):936-47.

Stewart SJ, "*Francisella*," *Manual of Clinical Microbiology*, 6th ed, Chapter 43, Murray PR, Baron EJ, Pfaller MA, et al, eds, Washington, DC: American Society for Microbiology, 1995, 545-55.

Tumor-Antigen 4 *see TA-4 on page 433*

Typhoid Agglutinins *see Salmonella Titer on page 429*

U₁RNP *see Antinuclear Antibody on page 368*

U₁RNP Antibody *see Sjögren's Antibodies on page 430*

Ubiquitin *see Cerebrospinal Fluid Tau Protein on page 382*

Undulant Fever *see Brucellosis Agglutinins on page 372*

Urine Electrophoresis *see Protein Electrophoresis, Urine on page 425*

Urine Protein Electrophoresis *see Protein Electrophoresis, Urine on page 425*

Valley Fever *see Coccidioidomycosis Antibodies on page 384*

Varicella-Zoster Virus Serology

CPT 86787

Related Information

Herpes Cytology *on page 296*
Skin Biopsy *on page 54*
Varicella-Zoster Virus Culture *on page 675*
Viral Culture *on page 675*
Virus, Direct Detection by Fluorescent Antibody *on page 682*

Synonyms Chickenpox Titer; VZV Serology; Zoster Titer

Applies to Herpes Zoster Serology

Abstract Varicella-zoster is a herpes virus that produces two clinical syndromes. **Chickenpox**, the manifestation of primary exposure, is usually benign in immunocompetent children but may have severe complications in adults and the immunosuppressed. Following primary infection, it is presumed that VZV establishes latency with the dorsal root ganglia. **Shingles** or **herpes zoster** occurs when VZV infection is reactivated.

Diagnosis of chickenpox and shingles is usually based upon history and physical examination. In cases in which VZV infection cannot be clinically distinguished from similar infections (eg, disseminated herpes simplex infection vs disseminated zoster), the diagnostic test of choice is viral culture.[1] Serologic tests are used primarily to confirm recent or past infections that are unlikely to produce positive culture results.

Specimen Serum

Container Red top tube

Sampling Time Acute and convalescent sera drawn 10-14 days apart are recommended. A single specimen is satisfactory to establish immune status.

Reference Range Diagnosis of infection: A single low titer or less than a fourfold increase in IgG titer in paired sera; undetectable antibody by fluorescent antibody to membrane antigen test. **Immune status:** IgG alone is sufficient. Reactive result indicates immunity (either from infection or vaccination) but does not assure protection from shingles.

Critical Values Negative serology in an adult exposed to varicella-zoster virus

Use Occasionally, to establish diagnosis of varicella-zoster infection; more often used to determine adult susceptibility or immunity to infection. Some seronegative women may have primary infection while pregnant. The risk of fetal damage in the presence of maternal varicella infection in the first 20 weeks of pregnancy is approximately 2%, and life-threatening illness may develop in the mother. Neonatal infection is possible if the mother contracts the infection in the last 3 weeks of gestation.[2] Varicella pneumonia in adults is the most frequent severe complication.[3] Viral myocarditis occurs[4] and may progress to dilated cardiomyopathy experimentally[5] and clinically. Pregnant and postpartum women are at increased risk of VZV pneumonia.[3]

IgM antibodies are used to identify congenital infection.

Limitations Complement fixation test is insensitive and has heterologous reactions with herpesvirus. Primary or secondary infections with other herpes viruses may produce significant VZV titer increases in individuals who have previously had chickenpox. A positive low titer may not correlate with protection.

Methodology Fluorescent antibody to membrane antigen (FAMA), hemagglutination, anticomplement immunofluorescence, enzyme-linked immunosorbent assay (ELISA). Molecular techniques (eg, PCR) will become methods of choice for VZV when methods become widely available.[1] Detection of viral DNA in amniotic fluid by PCR may prove to be useful.[7]

Additional Information More than 85% of adults who do not recall having chickenpox are seropositive for this virus.[1] Although most cases of varicella or zoster are clinically unambiguous, serology may be occasionally useful in the differential diagnosis of other blistering illnesses or when infection shows an unusual complication, such as hepatitis. It may also be important to establish whether an individual is susceptible when clinical history is unclear, or when varicella immune globulin may be needed, as in the immunocompromised host or cancer patient on toxic chemotherapy. Zoster is more common with aging and may occur in the face of significant antibody titers, demonstrating that cell-mediated immunity is also significant. A vaccine consisting of live-attenuated varicella is now available. Patients who are immunocompromised (eg, childhood leukemics) and other susceptible individuals may now be immunized. Positive serology should be indicative of protection.

See listing Varicella-Zoster Virus Culture *on page 675*.

Footnotes

1. Cohen PR, "Tests for Detecting Herpes Simplex Virus and Varicella-Zoster Virus Infections," *Dermatol Clin*, 1994, 12(1):51-68.
2. Pastuszak AL, Levy M, Schick B, et al, "Outcome After Maternal Varicella Infection in the First 20 Weeks of Pregnancy," *N Engl J Med*, 1994, 330(13):901-5.
3. Feldman S, "Varicella-Zoster Virus Pneumonitis," *Chest*, 1994, 106(Suppl 1):22S-7S.
4. Tsintsof A, Delprado WJ, and Keogh AM, "Varcella Zoster Myocarditis Progressing to Cardiomyopathy and Cardiac Transplantation," *Br Heart J*, 1993, 70(1):93-5.
5. Rich R and McErlean M, "Complete Heart Block in a Child With Varicella," *Am J Emerg Med*, 1993, 11(6):602-5.
6. Schnitt SJ, Stillman IE, Owings DV, et al, "Myocardial Fibrin Deposition in Experimental Viral Myocarditis That Progresses to Dilated Cardiomyopathy," *Circ Res*, 1993, 72(4):914-20.
7. Ghidini A and Lynch L, "Management Strategies for Congenital Infections," *Mt Sinai J Med*, 1994, 61(5):376-88.

References

Brunell PA, Novelli VM, Keller PM, et al, "Antibodies to the Three Major Glycoproteins of Varicella-Zoster Virus: Search for the Relevant Host Immune Response," *J Infect Dis*, 1987, 156(3):430-5.
Escalante M, Franco-Vicario R, Cisterna R, et al, "Varicella Pneumonia in the Adult," *An Med Interna*, 1994, 11(5):244-6.
Gilden DH, Wright RR, Schneck SA, et al, "Zoster Sine Herpete, a Clinical Variant," *Ann Neurol*, 1994, 35(5):530-3.
Landry ML, Cohen SD, Mayo DR, et al, "Comparison of Fluorescent Antibody to Membrane Antigen Test, Indirect Immunofluorescence Assay, and a Commercial Enzyme-Linked Immunosorbent Assay for Determination of Antibody to Varicella-Zoster Virus," *J Clin Microbiol*, 1987, 25(5):832-5.
Ljungman P, "Herpes Virus Infections in Immunocompromised Patients: Problems and Therapeutic Interventions," *Ann Med*, 1993, 25(4):329-33.
Qureshi F and Jacques SM, "Maternal Varicella During Pregnancy: Correlation of Maternal History and Fetal Outcome With Placental Histopathology," *Hum Pathol*, 1996, 27(2):191-5.
Smith TF, Wold AD, Espy MJ, et al, "New Developments in the Diagnosis of Viral Diseases," *Infect Dis Clin North Am*, 1993, 7(2):183-201.
Straus SE, "Overview: The Biology of Varicella-Zoster Virus Infection," *Ann Neurol*, 1994, 35(Suppl):4-8.
Weller TH, "Varicella and Herpes Zoster: Changing Concepts of the Natural History, Control, and Importance of a Not-So-Benign Virus," *N Engl J Med*, 1983, 309(22):1362-8.

VCA *see* Epstein-Barr Virus Serology *on page 392*

VCA Titer *see* Epstein-Barr Virus Serology *on page 392*

VDRL, Cerebrospinal Fluid

CPT 86592 (qualitative); 86593 (quantitative titer)

Related Information

Antinuclear Antibody *on page 368*
Automated Reagin Test *on page 370*
Bacterial Culture, Cerebrospinal Fluid *on page 460*
Cerebrospinal Fluid Protein *on page 380*
Darkfield Examination, Syphilis *on page 475*
FTA-ABS, Cerebrospinal Fluid *on page 394*
MHA-TP *on page 418*
RPR *on page 428*
VDRL, Serum *on this page*

Synonyms Cerebrospinal Fluid VDRL; CSF; Spinal Fluid VDRL

Applies to Syphilis Serology

Test Commonly Includes Titer of reactive specimens

Abstract A reactive CSF VDRL is acceptable to establish the diagnosis of neurosyphilis, but a nonreactive test is inconclusive.

Specimen Cerebrospinal fluid

Container Clean, sterile CSF container

Special Instructions Do not heat inactivate the CSF.

Reference Range Nonreactive

Use Test for syphilis, neurosyphilis; VDRL, CSF is the only laboratory test for neurosyphilis approved by the Centers for Disease Control. It is very specific. The sensitivity of the CSF VDRL for the diagnosis of neurosyphilis is approximately 30% to 70%.[1]

Limitations CSF VDRL is insensitive.[2]

Methodology Flocculation test detects reagin, antibody to nontreponemal antigen

Additional Information Central nervous system syphilis may be asymptomatic. Neurosyphilis includes **meningeal syphilis**, which is usually found within a year of infection. Its characteristics include headache, stiff neck, nausea and vomiting, sometimes with cranial nerve involvement. **Syphilitic meningitis** can be localized (**gumma**). **Meningovascular syphilis** is found 4-7 years after infection. **General paresis** or **tabes dorsalis** occur late, frequently decades after infection. Uveitis, retinitis, luetic optic neuritis may occur with or without syphilitic meningitis. Optic atrophy is usually found with tabes dorsalis.[1]

A positive VDRL in a spinal fluid uncontaminated by serum is essentially diagnostic of neurosyphilis. However, a negative test may occur in 30% of patients with tabes dorsalis, and was positive in only 22% to 69% of patients who had active neurosyphilis.[2] The CSF VDRL may take years to become nonreactive after adequate therapy.

Criteria for neurosyphilis include CSF cell count >5 mononuclear cells/mm^3 and CSF total protein >40 mg/dL.[3]

Subjects with HIV, following therapy for syphilis that is usually considered adequate, may develop neurosyphilis. In AIDS patients, serial CSF VDRL determinations may be needed when neurosyphilis is suspected. By requiring either a positive serum RPR or FTA-ABS, seropositivity of CSF VDRL could increase to 90%.

Footnotes

1. Hook EW 3d and Marra CM, "Acquired Syphilis in Adults," *N Engl J Med*, 1992, 326:1060-9.
2. Woods GL, "Update on Laboratory Diagnosis of Sexually Transmitted Diseases," *Clin Lab Med*, 1995, 15(3):665-84.
3. Larsen SA, Steiner BM, and Rudolph AH, "Laboratory Diagnosis and Interpretation of Tests for Syphilis," *Clin Microbiol Rev*, 1995, 8(1):1-21.

References

Albright RE Jr, Christenson RH, Emlet JL, et al, "Issues in Cerebrospinal Fluid Management. CSF Venereal Disease Research Laboratory Testing," *Am J Clin Pathol*, 1991, 95(3):397-401.

Davis LE and Schmitt JW, "Clinical Significance of Cerebrospinal Fluid Tests for Neurosyphilis," *Ann Neurol*, 1989, 25(1):50-5.

Desforges JF, "Infectious Disease Testing for Blood Transfusions," *NIH Consensus Statement*, 1995, 13(1):1-27.

Feraru ER, Aronow HA, and Lipton RB, "Neurosyphilis in AIDS Patients: Initial CSF VDRL May Be Negative," *Neurology*, 1990, 40(3 Pt 1):541-3.

Horowitz HW, Valsamis MP, Wicher V, et al, "Brief Report: Cerebral Syphilitic Gumma Confirmed by the Polymerase Chain Reaction in a Man With Human Immunodeficiency Virus Infection," *N Engl J Med*, 1994, 331(22):1488-91.

Klein HG, *Standards for Blood Banks and Transfusion Services*, 16th ed, Bethesda, MD: American Association of Blood Banks, 1994, 3-8.

VDRL, Serum

CPT 86592 (qualitative); 86593 (quantitative)

Related Information

Anticardiolipin Antibody *on page 364*
Anticoagulant, Circulating *on page 229*
Antinuclear Antibody *on page 368*
Automated Reagin Test *on page 370*

Bacterial Culture, Genital Specimen *on page 463*
Darkfield Examination, Syphilis *on page 475*
Donation, Blood *on page 607*
FTA-ABS, Serum *on page 394*
MHA-TP *on page 418*
Neisseria gonorrhoeae Culture and Smear *on page 492*
Risks of Transfusion *on page 623*
RPR *on page 428*
VDRL, Cerebrospinal Fluid *on this page*

Synonyms Serum VDRL; Venereal Disease Research Laboratory Test, Serum

Applies to Syphilis Serology

Replaces Kahn Test; Kline Test; Mazzini; Wassermann

Test Commonly Includes Determination of serologic response to *Treponema* infection

Abstract Sexually transmitted diseases include chancroid, gonorrhea, certain chlamydial infections, AIDS, instances of viral hepatitis, herpes simplex, and syphilis.

Specimen Serum

Container Red top tube

Collection The CDC recommends that when screening for congenital syphilis the mother's serum should be tested rather than cord blood.

Causes for Rejection Plasma cannot be used

Reference Range Nonreactive

Possible Panic Range Positive results in pregnancy should be confirmed by a treponemal test.

Use VDRL is a reaginic (nontreponemal) test for syphilis. It is a screening test for syphilis which may be used to assess adequacy of treatment.

Limitations Nonspecific positive reactions may be found in advancing age, malaria, infectious mononucleosis, infectious hepatitis, leprosy, brucellosis, SLE, atypical pneumonia, typhus, and other entities.[1] See table. Reactive tests due to related treponemal infections also occur. Other pathogens include *T. pallidum* subspecies *pertenue*, which causes yaws; *T. carateum* which causes pinta and *T. pallidum* subspecies *endemicum*, the cause of nonvenereal or endemic syphilis.

False-positive results may occur in the first few days of postnatal life.

False-negative tests due to prozone phenomenon indicates that repeat testing with diluted serum should be performed in individuals who test negative despite high clinical suspicion.

The serum VDRL may be negative in as many as 25% of subjects who have late neurosyphilis. The specific tests (eg, FTA-ABS) remain reactive.[1] Treponemal tests (eg, FTA-ABS) become reactive before nontreponemal (reaginic) tests such as VDRL.[1] Positive result in cord blood may be due to passive transfer from mother's blood.

Methodology Flocculation procedure detecting the presence of reagin, antibody to nontreponemal cardiolipin antigen

Additional Information Despite false-positive results due to now well known causes, VDRL remains an extremely useful screening test for syphilis. VDRL becomes positive starting 2 weeks after the chancre appears, and by 6 weeks, 90% of cases will be positive. By 9-12 weeks, the secondary stage, 100% of patients should be reactive. With therapy the VDRL reverts to negative. Even without treatment the VDRL may become negative years after infection. Thus, in tertiary syphilis, the VDRL may be negative. The VDRL test can be done on CSF and is useful in diagnosis of CNS syphilis (see VDRL, Cerebrospinal Fluid *on page 438*). Positive VDRL tests should have confirmatory testing with a *Treponema*-specific test. The VDRL test is recommended as a screen for uveitis or unexplained ocular inflammation.

The diagnosis of syphilis in persons infected with HIV may be difficult: lack of serologic response in a patient with confirmed syphilis and rapid progression in spite of treatment.[2]

Current reviews of syphilis in the fetus and newborn are available.[2,3]

Footnotes

1. Hook EW 3d and Marra CM, "Acquired Syphilis in Adults," *N Engl J Med*, 1992, 326:1060-9.
2. Larsen SA, Steiner BM, and Rudolph AH, "Laboratory Diagnosis and Interpretation of Tests for Syphilis," *Clin Microbiol Rev*, 1995, 8(1):1-21.
3. Ingall D, Sánchez PJ, and Musher DM, "Syphilis," *Infectious Diseases of the Fetus and Newborn Infant*, 4th ed, Chapter 12, Remington JS and Klein JO, eds, Philadelphia, PA: WB Saunders Co, 1995, 529-64.

References

Berkowitz K, Baxi L, and Fox HE, "False-Negative Syphilis Screening: The Prozone Phenomenon, Nonimmune Hydrops, and Diagnosis of Syphilis During Pregnancy," *Am J Obstet Gynecol*, 1990, 163(3):975-7.

Desforges JF, "Infectious Disease Testing for Blood Transfusions," *NIH Consensus Statement*, 1995, 13(1):1-27.

Horowitz HW, Valsamis MP, Wicher V, et al, "Brief Report: Cerebral Syphilitic Gumma Confirmed by the Polymerase Chain Reaction in a Man With Human Immunodeficiency Virus Infection," *N Engl J Med*, 1994, 331(22):1488-91.

Klein HG, *Standards for Blood Banks and Transfusion Services*, 16th ed, Bethesda, MD: American Association of Blood Banks, 1994, 3-8.

Potential Causes of False-Positive Serologic Tests for Syphilis

	Infectious Causes	Noninfectious Causes
Reaginic or nontreponemal tests (RPR, VDRL) Bacterial	Pneumococcal pneumonia	Pregnancy
	Scarlet fever	Chronic liver disease
	Leprosy	Advanced cancer
	Lymphogranuloma venereum	Intravenous drug use
	Relapsing fever	Multiple myeloma, other types of malignancy, other entities causing immunoglobulin abnormalities
	Bacterial endocarditis	Advancing age
	Malaria	Connective tissue diseases, (eg, SLE)
	Rickettsial disease	Multiple blood transfusions
	Psittacosis	Narcotic addiction
	Leptospirosis	Technical error
	Chancroid	
	Tuberculosis	
	Mycoplasmal pneumonia	
	Trypanosomiasis	
Viral	Vaccinia (vaccination)	
	Chickenpox	
	HIV	
	Measles	
	Infectious mononucleosis	
	Mumps	
	Viral hepatitis	
Treponemal tests (FTA-ABS, MHA-TP)	Lyme disease	Systemic lupus erythematosus
	Leprosy	
	Malaria	
	Infectious mononucleosis	
	Relapsing fever	
	Leptospirosis	

Modified from Hook EW 3d and Marra CM, "Acquired Syphilis in Adults," *N Engl J Med*, 1992, 326:1060-9, with permission.

Musher DM and Baughn RE, "Neurosyphilis in HIV-Infected Persons," *N Engl J Med*, 1994, 331(22):1516-7.

Tamesis RR and Foster CS, "Ocular Syphilis," *Ophthalmology*, 1990, 97(10):1281-7.

Thomas DL and Quinn TC, "Serologic Testing for Sexually Transmitted Diseases," *Infect Dis Clin North Am*, 1993, 7(4):793-824.

Venereal Disease Research Laboratory Test, Serum *see*
VDRL, Serum *on previous page*

Viral Capsid Antigen *see* Epstein-Barr Virus Serology *on page 392*

VZV Serology *see* Varicella-Zoster Virus Serology *on page 437*

WA1-Antibody *see* Babesiosis Serological Test *on page 370*

Walking Pneumonia Titer *see* Mycoplasma Serology *on page 419*

Wassermann *replaced by* RPR *on page 428*

Wassermann *replaced by* VDRL, Serum *on previous page*

Weil-Felix Agglutinins
CPT 86000

Related Information
Febrile Agglutinins, Serum *on page 393*
Rocky Mountain Spotted Fever Serology *on page 427*

Synonyms Rickettsial Disease Agglutinins

Test Commonly Includes Titer of serum against *Proteus* OX-19, OX-2, and OX-K antigens

Abstract An archaic test which is nonspecific and insensitive. It uses no rickettsial antigen. This method is best relegated to the ranks of long forgotten and ineffective laboratory methods.[1]

Specimen Serum

Container Red top tube

Sampling Time Acute and convalescent specimens drawn 10-14 days apart are recommended.

Reference Range Titer ≤1:160

Interpretation of Weil-Felix Reaction

Rickettsial Infection	*Proteus* Antigen		
	OX-19	OX-2	OX-K
Rocky Mountain spotted fever	++++ or +	+ or ++++	–
Epidemic typhus	++++	+	–
Murine typhus	++++	+	–
Brill-Zinsser disease*	–	–	–
Scrub typhus	–	–	++++
Rickettsialpox	–	–	–
Q fever	–	–	–

* = A positive OX-19 reaction is occasionally observed.

++++ = Fourfold or greater rise in titer; – = no reaction.

From *Gradwohl's Clinical Laboratory Methods and Diagnosis*, 8th ed, Sonnenwirth AC and Jarett L, eds, Mosby-Year Book Inc, St Louis, MO: 1980, 2311, with permission.

Use Attempt to support the clinical diagnosis of rickettsial infection

Limitations The absence of agglutinins does not rule out rickettsial disease. False-positives occur in patients with leptospirosis, severe liver disease, *Borrelia* and *Proteus* infections. Some normal sera may possess a titer to *Proteus* antigens. Rickettsial vaccination will result in an antibody titer. Rickettsialpox, Q fever or trench fever do not demonstrate titers when tested. Partial or early treatment with antibiotics may thwart antibody response.

Contraindications Intercurrent infection with *Proteus*

Methodology Agglutination

Additional Information This test is based on cross reaction of antibodies to *Rickettsia* with *Proteus* antigens. Rocky Mountain spotted fever, epidemic typhus, and scrub typhus may be distinguished (see table). Antibodies appear 4-5 days after infection and peak a week later. Titers >1:160 are significant, but a fourfold rise in titer is more diagnostic. Specific tests for IgG and IgM rickettsial antibodies may be confirmatory. Polymerase chain reaction is insensitive for detection of *R. rickettsii* in blood, and serum antibodies are diagnostic in <20% of subjects in the acute phase of illness. Skin biopsy of the eschar examined by indirect or direct fluorescent antibody provides improved diagnosis for *R. rickettsii*.[2,3]

Footnotes
1. Dumler JS and Walker DH, "Diagnostic Tests for Rocky Mountain Spotted Fever and Other Rickettsial Diseases," *Dermatol Clin*, 1994, 12(1):25-36.
2. Kass EM, Szaniawski WK, Levy H, et al, "Rickettsialpox in a New York City Hospital, 1980 to 1989," *N Engl J Med*, 1994, 331(24):1612-7.
3. Walker DH and Dumler JS, "Emerging and Reemerging Rickettsial Diseases," *N Engl J Med*, 1994, 331(24):1651-2.

References
Hechemy KE, "The Immunoserology of Rickettsiae," *Manual of Clinical Laboratory Immunology*, 4th ed, Vol 2, Chapter 97, Rose NR, Conway de Macario E, Fahey JL, et al, eds, Washington, DC: American Society for Microbiology, 1992, 667-75.

Western Blot *see* HIV-1/HIV-2 Serology *on page 403*

Western Blot Test for HIV Antibody *see* HIV-1/HIV-2 Serology *on page 403*

Western Equine Encephalitis *see* Encephalitis Viral Serology *on page 391*

Western Equine Encephalitis Virus Serology
CPT 86654

Related Information
California Encephalitis Virus Titer *on page 374*
Eastern Equine Encephalitis Virus Serology *on page 389*
St Louis Encephalitis Virus Serology *on page 432*
Viral Culture, Central Nervous System Symptoms *on page 677*

Synonyms Encephalitis Virus Titer, Western Equine

Abstract Western equine encephalitis (WEE) is a disease of summer. Its geographic predominance is the entire United States. Infants are susceptible and are at risk for sequelae. WEE often causes infantile convulsions. Its case fatality rate is 3% to 5%. Transmission is via the mosquito vector *Culex tarsalis*. The pathogenesis of WEE resembles that of Eastern equine encephalitis (EEE). Clinical features are similar to those of St Louis encephalitis.

Specimen Serum or cerebrospinal fluid

Container Red top tube, sterile CSF tube

Collection Acute and convalescent specimens are recommended.

Reference Range Less than a fourfold increase in titer in paired sera; HAI titer: <1:10; CF titer: <1:8; **no IgM antibody in serum or CSF**
(Continued)

Western Equine Encephalitis Virus Serology
(Continued)

Use Establish the diagnosis of Western equine encephalitis virus infection; differential diagnosis includes St Louis encephalitis (SLE). Generally an encephalitis antibody panel is tested that includes WEE, EEE, SLE, and California encephalitis virus.

Limitations Cross reactions can occur to Eastern equine encephalitis (EEE) virus.

Methodology Diagnosis is best established by detection of specific IgM antibody, particularly in CSF. Complement fixation (CF), hemagglutination inhibition (HAI), neutralization, indirect fluorescent antibody (IFA), enzyme-linked immunosorbent assay (ELISA) are available. Alphaviruses share antigenic relationships.

Additional Information Symptoms of this arbovirus infection include fever, aseptic meningitis, and meningoencephalitis. CSF pleocytosis includes CSF WBC of 10-300 /mm^3. Virus has been recovered from CSF, blood, and brain. This alphavirus disease is usually most severe in infants and children.

References

Monath TP, "Alphavirus (Eastern, Western, and Venezuelan Equine Encephalitis)," *Principles and Practice of Infectious Diseases*, 3rd ed, Mandell GL, Douglas RG Jr, and Bennett JE, eds, New York, NY: Churchill Livingstone, 1990, 1241-2.

Tsai TF, "Arboviruses," *Manual of Clinical Laboratory Immunology*, 4th ed, Vol 2, Chapter 91, Rose NR, Conway de Macario E, Fahey JL, et al, eds, Washington, DC: American Society for Microbiology, 1992, 606-18.

White Cell Crossmatch see Tissue Typing *on page 434*

Widal Agglutination Test see *Salmonella* Titer *on page 429*

***Wuchereria bancrofti* Serology** see Filariasis Serological Test *on page 393*

Yersinia enterocolitica Antibody

CPT 86793

Related Information

Bacterial Culture, Blood *on page 457*

Bacterial Culture, Stool *on page 466*

Risks of Transfusion *on page 623*

Viral Culture, Stool *on page 680*

Abstract Reservoirs of *Y. enterocolitica* include pigs, goats, dogs, and cats. Transmission may include milk, pork, and water. Organisms are ingested, but the infection can be acquired by transfusion (of platelets). Often the differential diagnosis includes appendicitis. *Y. enterocolitica* and *Y. pseudotuberculosis* may cause similar clinical presentations.[1]

Specimen Serum

Container Red top tube

Collection Acute and convalescent specimens are recommended.

Reference Range Titer <1:160

Critical Values Antibodies may not be detectable for the first week of symptoms, but then rise rapidly to high titers (1:1280 is diagnostic).

Use Useful in diagnosis of *Yersinia enterocolitica* infection, which is characterized by mesenteric lymphadenitis and/or terminal ileitis with abdominal pain, gastroenteritis, and diarrhea. It manifests often as enterocolitis in children younger than 5 years of age. Arthritis and other extraintestinal complications may occur; yersiniosis is considered within the differential diagnosis of rheumatic and collagen diseases.[1] It is a cause of liver abscesses; 60% of such patients were associated with hemochromatosis.[2] Most infections are self-limited.

Limitations Present serodiagnostic techniques are described as having only limited value.[1]

Methodology Agglutination with serotypes 03, 08, and 09; newer techniques such as immunoblotting and indirect immunofluorescence may prove to enhance diagnosis.

Additional Information This test should be used in conjunction with culture to confirm a diagnosis of yersiniosis. After recovery, low titers (1:40 or 1:80) may persist for years. **When stool is sent to the laboratory for culture, request for culture of this organism is usually needed so that an enrichment technique can be utilized.**

Yersinia enterocolitica is a cause of liver abscesses.

Footnotes

1. Baert F, Peetermans W, and Knockaert D, "Yersiniosis: The Clinical Spectrum," *Acta Clin Belg*, 1994, 49(2):76-85.

2. Vadillo M, Corbella X, Pac V, et al, "Multiple Liver Abscesses Due to *Yersinia enterocolitica* Discloses Primary Hemochromatosis: Three Cases Reports and Reviews," *Clin Infect Dis*, 1994, 18(6):938-41.

References

Gilchrist MJ, "Enterobacteriaceae: Opportunistic Pathogens and Other Genera," *Manual of Clinical Microbiology*, 6th ed, Chapter 34, Murray PR, ed, Washington, DC: American Society for Microbiology, 1995, 457-64.

Kohlstrom E, Foberg U, Bengtsson A, et al, "Intestinal Symptoms and Serological Response in Patients With Complicated and Uncomplicated *Yersinia enterocolitica* Infections," *Scand J Infect Dis*, 1993, 24:57-63.

Tiddia F, Cherchi GB, Pacifico L, et al, "*Yersinia enterocolitica* Causing Suppurative Arthritis of the Shoulder," *J Clin Pathol*, 1994, 47(8):760-1.

Yersinia pestis Antibody

CPT 86793

Related Information

Bacterial Culture, Blood *on page 457*

Gram's Stain *on page 481*

Viral Culture, Stool *on page 680*

Applies to *Yersinia pestis* Culture

Abstract The forms of plague include lymphadenitis (bubonic plague), septicemic, pneumonic, cutaneous, and meningeal. This is the disease which caused historical pandemics, including the black death of the fourteenth century. An infection of humans and animals, it is caused by *Yersinia pestis* (*Pasteurella pestis* until 1970). A zoonotic infection, cases continue to appear in a number of areas including portions of the southwestern United States.

Specimen Serum

Container Red top tube

Storage Instructions Acidified serum may be stored in a refrigerator

Special Instructions In cases of suspected plague, the Centers for Disease Control and Prevention, Atlanta, should be contacted at once. Sera must be inactivated and absorbed with sheep erythrocytes prior to testing.

Reference Range Titer <1:16

Use Used to confirm diagnosis of plague

Methodology Passive hemagglutination on acute and convalescent serum

Additional Information A hemagglutination titer ≥1:256 is presumptive evidence of an immunologic response to *Yersinia pestis*, the plague bacillus. Diagnosis can also be made by seeing the stained organism in clinical material. Blood, bubo (lymph node) aspiration, and other materials can be cultured on special request.

References

Kelly JD, Fritz DL, Pitt ML, et al, "Pathology of Experimental Pneumonic Plague Produced by Fraction 1-Positive and Fraction 1-Negative *Yersinia pestis* in African Green Monkeys (*Cercopithecus aethiops*)," *Arch Pathol Lab Med*, 1996, 120(2):156-63.

Gilchrist MJ, "Enterobacteriaceae: Opportunistic Pathogens and Other Genera," *Manual of Clinical Microbiology*, 6th ed, Chapter 34, Murray PR, ed, Washington, DC: American Society for Microbiology, 1995, 457-64.

***Yersinia pestis* Culture** see *Yersinia pestis* Antibody *on this page*

Zoster Titer see Varicella-Zoster Virus Serology *on page 437*

Antigen Expression With Cluster Designation

Cluster Designation	Main Cellular Expression of Antigen	Other Names	Antigen Molecular Weight (kDa)
CD1a	Cortical thymocytes (strong), Langerhans cells, B-cell subset, dendritic cells		49, 12
CD1b	Cortical thymocytes (moderate), Langerhans cells, B-cell subset, dendritic cells		45, 12
CD1c	Cortical thymocytes (weak), Langerhans cells, B-cell subset, dendritic cells		43, 12
CD2	T cells, thymocytes, NK cells	E rosette receptor, leucocyte function antigen-2 (LFA-2)	50
CD2R	Activated T cells, NK cells		50
CD3	Thymocytes, mature T cells (associated with T-cell receptor antigens)		16, 20, 25-28
CD4	T-helper/inducer cells, monocytes, macrophages	Receptor for MHC class II and HIV antigens	56
CD5	Thymocytes, T cells, B-cell subset		67
CD6	Thymocytes, T-cell subset, B-cell subset		105
CD7	Majority of T cells		40
CD8	T-Cytotoxic/Suppressor cells	MHC class I receptor	32-34
CD9	Pre-B cells, monocytes, platelets		24
CD10	Lymphoid progenitor cells, granulocytes	CALLA (common acute lymphoblastic leukemia antigen)	100
CD11a	Leucocytes	Leucocyte function antigen (LFA-I) integrin α^L subunit	180
CD11b	Granulocytes, monocytes, NK cells	Integrin α^M subunit Mac-1, CR3, C3biR	170
CD11c	Granulocytes, monocytes, NK cells, B-cell subset T-cell subset	Integrin α^X subunit	150
CDw12	Granulocytes, monocytes		90-120
CD13	Myeloid monocytes, granulocytes	Aminopeptidase N	130
CD14	Monocytes, some granulocytes and macrophages		55
CD15	Granulocytes, monocytes		Mulitple
CD15s	Neutrophils	sialyl-Lewis x(sLe-x), ligand for CD62 structures	Multiple
CD16a	Macrophage, NK cells (neutrophils)	Transmembrane form, FcγRIIIA/FcγRIIIB	50-65
CD16b	Granulocyte form only	GPI-linked form, FcγRIIIβ	48
CDw17	Granulocytes, monocytes, platelets	Lactosylceramide	Not determined
CD18	Leucocytes, platelets negative	Integrin β2 subunit	95
CD19	Pan B cell		90
CD20	Pan B cell		33, 35, 37
CD21	Mature B cells, follicular dendritic cells	C3d/EBV-receptor (CR2)	145
CD22	Mature B cells, hairy cell leukemia cells		140
CD23	Activated B cells, activated macrophages, eosinophils, platelets	IgE Fc low affinity receptor (RII)	50-45
CD24	B cells, granulocytes		41/38
CD25	Activated T cells, B cells, and macrophages	IL-2 receptor, Tac	55
CD26	Activate T cells and B cells, macrophages		110
CD27	Thymocyte subset, mature T cells, EBV transformed B cells		55
CD28	T-cell subset, activated B cells		44
CD29	Ubiquitous (but not on erythrocytes)		130
CD30	Activated T and B cells, Reed-Sternberg cells	Ki-1 antigen	105
CD31	Platelets, monocytes, macrophages, granulocytes, B cells	Platelet GPIIa, PECAM-1 (platelet endothelial cell adhesion molecule-1)	140
CD32	Monocytes, granulocytes, B cells, eosinophils	IgG Fc receptor II	40
CD33	Myeloid progenitor cells, monocytes		67
CD34	Hematopoietic precursor cells, capillary endothelial cells		105-120
CD35	Granulocytes (basophil-negative), monocytes, B cells, erythrocytes, some NK cells	CR1, C3b receptor	160, 190, 220, 250
CD36	Monocytes, macrophages, platelets, B cells (weakly)	Platelet GPIV (IIIb)	88
CD37	Mature B cells, T cells, and myeloid cells (weakly)	gp52-40	52-40
CD38	Plasma cells, thymocytes, activated T cells	T10	45
CD39	Mature B cells, monocytes, some macrophages, vascular endothelium	gp80	100-70
CD40	B cells, monocytes (weakly), carcinoma cells	gp50	48/44
CD40L	T cells	CD40 ligand, T-BAM	
CD41a	Platelets, megakaryocytes	GPIIb/IIIa	23/110/120
CD41b	Platelets, megakaryocytes	GPIIb	23/120
CD42a	Platelets, megakaryocytes	GPIX	23
CD42b	Platelets, megakaryocytes	GPIbα	135, 23
CD42c	Platelets, megakaryocytes	GPIbβ	22
CD42d	Platelets, megakaryocytes	GPV	85
CD43	Leucocytes but not peripheral B cells	Leukosialin, sialophorin	90-100

(continued)

Cluster Designation	Main Cellular Expression of Antigen	Other Names	Antigen Molecular Weight (kDa)
CD44	Leucocytes, erythrocytes, platelets (weakly), brain cells	Pgp-1, H-CAM	80-90
CD44R	Recognizes alternatively spliced form of molecule	eg, exon 9, V9	
CD45	Pan leucocyte	T200, LCA	180, 190, 205, 220
CD45RA	B cells, T-cell subset, monocytes	T200 restricted	220, 205
CD45RB	B cells, T-cell subset, monocytes, macrophages, granulocytes (weakly)	T200	190, 205, 220
CD45RO	T cells, B-cell subset, monocytes, macrophages	T200 restricted	180
CD46	Hematopoietic and nonhematopoietic cells (erythrocytes negative)	MCP (membrane cofactor protein)	66/56
CD47	All cell types	Rh group associated	47-52
CD48	Leucocytes	Blast-1	43
CD49a	Activated T cells, monocytes	VLA-1	210
CD49b	B cells, monocytes, platelets	VLA-2	160
CD49c	B cells	VLA-3	125
CD49d	Thymocytes, B cells	VLA-4	150, 80, 70
CD49e	Memory T cells, monocytes, platelets	VLA-5	135/25
CD49f	Memory T cells, thymocytes, monocytes	VLA-6	120/25
CD50	Leucocytes (platelets and erythrocytes negative)		124
CD51	Platelets	VNRα (vitronectin receptor)	125, 25
CD51/61 complex	Platelets, endothelial cells	Vitronectin receptor, integrin αVβ3	
CDw52	Leucocytes (platelets and erythrocytes negative)	CAMPATH-1	21-28
CD53	Pan leucocytes		32-40
CD54	Endothelial cells, many activated cell types	ICAM-1	90
CD55	Many hematopoietic and nonhematopoietic cells	DAF (decay accelerating factor)	75
CD56	NK cells	NKH1, isoform of N-CAM	220/135
CD57	NK cells, T cells, B-cell subsets	HNK-1	110
CD58	Many hematopoietic and nonhematopoietic cells	LFA-3	65-70
CD59	Many hematopoietic and nonhematopoietic cells	P18, gP18, Mac inhibitor	18-20
CDw60	Platelets, T-cell subset		carbohydrate
CD61	Platelets, megakaryocytes	Integrin β3, GPIIIa, vitronectin receptor β	110
CD62E	Endothelium	E-selectin, ELAM-1, LECAM-2	140
CD62L	B and T cells, monocytes, NK cells	L-selectin, LECAM-1, LAM-1	150
CD62P	Platelets, endothelial cells, megakaryocytes	P-selectin, GMP-140, PADGEM, LECAM-3	75-80
CD63	Activated platelets, monocytes, macrophages	Platelet activation antigen	53
CD64	Monocytes	High affinity IgG Fc receptor 1, FCR1	75
CDw65	Granulocytes, monocytes	Fucoganglioside	Not confirmed
CD66a	Neutrophil lineage cells	Biliary glycoprotein (BGP-1)	160-180
CD66b	Granulocytes	CEA gene member 6 (CGM6) previously CD67	95-100
CD66c	Neutrophils, colon carcinoma	Nonspecific cross-reacting antigen (NCA)	90
CD66d	Neutrophils	CEA gene member 1 (CGM1)	30
CD66e	Adult colon epithelia, colon carcinoma	Carcinoembryonic antigen (CEA)	180-200
CD68	Monocytes, macrophages		110
CD69	Activated T and B cells, activated macrophages, NK cells	gp34/28, AIM (activation inducer molecule)	34/28
CD70	Activated T and B cells, Reed-Sternberg cells, macrophages (weakly)	Ki-24	75, 95, 170
CD71	Activated T and B cells, macrophages, proliferating cells	T9, transferrin receptor	95
CD72	Pan B cell		43/39
CD73	B- and T-cell subsets	Ecto-5′-NT	69
CD74	B cells, macrophages, monocytes	gp41/35/33, Ii	41, 35, 33
CDw75	Mature B cells, T-cell subset (weak expression)		Not confirmed
CDw76	Mature B cells, T-cell subset		Not confirmed
CD77	Activated B cells, follicular centre B cells, endothelial cells	BLA, Gb3, p^k	Not confirmed
CDw78	B cells	Ba	Not confirmed
CD79α	B cell specific	mb.1, BPC#1 alpha, Ig alpha	33, 40
CD79β	B cell specific	B29, BPC#1 beta, Ig beta	33, 40
CD80	B-cell subset *in vivo*, most activated B cells *in vitro*	B7, BB1, BPC#2	60
CD81	B cells (broad expression including lymphocytes)	TAPA-1 (target of an antiproliferative antibody)	22
CD82	Broad expression on leucocytes (weak) not erythrocytes	R2	50-53
CD83	Specific marker for circulating dendritic cells, activated B and T cells, germinal centre cells	HB15, BPC#5	43
CDw84	Platelets and monocytes (strong), circulating B cells (weak)	GR6, BPC#6	73
CD85	Circulating B cells (weak), monocytes (strong)	BO31, BO32, BPC#7, GR4	120, 83
CD86	Circulating monocytes, germinal centre cells (histol), activated B cells	FUN-1, GR65	80
CD87	Granulocytes, monocytes, macrophage, activated T cells	UPA-R (urokinase plasminogen activator receptor)	50-65

(continued)

Cluster Designation	Main Cellular Expression of Antigen	Other Names	Antigen Molecular Weight (kDa)
CD88	Polymorphonuclear leucocytes, mast cells, macrophage, smooth muscle	C5a receptor, GR10	40
CD89	Neutrophils, monocytes, macrophage, T- and B-cell subpopulation	FCαR, IgA receptor	55-70
CDw90	CD34 positive, subset on bone marrow, cord blood, fetal liver	Human thy-1	25-35
CD91	Monocytes and some nonhematopoietic cell lines	α2 macroglobulin receptor	600
CDw92	Neutrophils, monocytes, endothelial cells, platelets	"Group 9", GR9	70
CD93	Neutrophils, monocytes, endothelial cells	"Group 11", GR11	120
CD94	NK cells, α/β,γ/δ, T-celll subsets	KP43	43
CD95	Variety of cell lines including myeloid and T lymphoblastoid	APO-1, FAS	42
CD96	Activated T cells	TACTILE (T-cell activation increased late expression)	160
CD97	Activated cells	GR1, BL-KDD/F12	74, 80, 89
CD98	T cells and B cells (weak), monocytes (strong), most human cell lines	4F2	80, 40
CD99	Peripheral blood lymphocytes, thymocytes	MIC2, E2	32
CD99R	B and T lymphocytes, some leukemias	MIC2, E2	
CD100	Broad expression on hemopoietic cells	5T-005, 5T-003, 5T-039, GR3	150
CDw101	Granulocytes, macrophage	5T-004, 5T-040, GR14, BPC#4	140
CD102	Resting lymphocytes, monocytes, vascular endothelial cells (strongest)	ICAM-2	60
CD103	Intraepithelial lymphocytes, 2-6%, PBL	αE integrin, α6, HML-1	150, 25
CD104	Epithelia, Schwann cells, some tumor cells	β4 integrin chain, beta4	220
CD105	Endothelial cells, bone marrow cell subset, *in vitro* activated macrophage	Endoglin, TGF B1 and β3 receptor, GR7	95
CD106	Endothelial cells	VCAM-1, INCAM-110	100, 110
CD107a	Activated platelets	LAMP 1 (lysosomal associated membrane protein)	110
CD107b	Activated platelets	LAMP 2	120
CDw108	Activated T cells in spleen, some stromal cells	GR2	80
CDw109	Activated T cells, platelets, endothelial cells	Platelet activation factor, GR56	170/150
CD110-CD114	Nothing yet assigned to these numbers		
CD115	Monocytes, macrophage, placenta	M-CSFR (macrophage colony stimulating factor receptor)	150
CDw116	Monocytes, neutrophils, eosinophils, fibroblasts, endothelial cells	GM-CSFR (granulocyte, macrophage colony stimulating factor receptor)	75-85
CD117	Bone marrow progenitor cells	Stem cell factor receptor (SCFR), c-KIT	145
CD118*	Broad cellular expression	IFN α,β receptor	
CD119	Macrophage, monocyte, B cells, epithelial cells	IFNγR (interferon γ receptor)	90
CD120a	Most cell types, higher levels on epithelial cell lines	TNF (tumor necrosis factor receptor) R type 1	55
CD120b	Most cell types, higher levels on myeloid cell lines	TNFR type 2	75
CDw121a	T cells, thymocytes, fibroblasts, endothelial cells	IL-1R (interleukin-1 receptor), type I	80
CDw121b	B cells, macrophages, monocytes	IL-1R, type II	68
CD122	NK cells, resting T-cell subpopulation, some B-cell lines	IL-2Rβ	75
CD123*	Bone marrow stem cells, granulocytes, monocytes, megakaryocytes	IL-3R	
CDw124	Mature B and T cells, hemopoietic precursor cells	IL-4R	140
CD125*	Eosinophils and basophils	IL-5R	
CD126	Activated B cells and plasma cells (strong), most leucocytes (weak)	IL-6R	80 (α subunit)
CDw127	Bone marrow lymphoid precursors, pro-B cells, mature T cells, monocytes	IL-7R	75
CDw128	Neutrophils, basophils, T-cell subset	IL-8R	58-67
CD129	Nothing yet assigned to this number		
CDw130	Acitvated B cells and plasma cells (strong), most leucocytes (weak), endothelial cells	IL-6R-gp 130SIG	130

From Schlossman SF, Bournsell L, Gilk W, et al, "CD Antigens 1993," *Blood*, 1994, 83(4):879-80, with permission.

MICROBIOLOGY

Rebecca T. Horvat, PhD

Christopher J. Papasian, PhD

David S. Jacobs, MD

Bernard L. Kasten, Jr, MD

Even in the age of antibiotics, infectious diseases continue to pose significant problems. Such problems have been magnified in recent years by increased numbers of immunosuppressed individuals including those with AIDS, transplant patients, and cancer patients. The morbidity and mortality of infectious agents can be greatly reduced if the physician has information to provide proper treatment early. Thus, the function of the clinical microbiology laboratory is to culture and identify microorganisms associated with the infectious process and to assess *in vitro* antibiotic susceptibility in a quick, efficient, and accurate manner.

The most important step in obtaining a useful microbiology report is the acquisition and transport of an appropriate specimen. Material submitted for culture should be collected at the site of infection with minimal contamination from indigenous flora. All specimens should be collected in a sterile container and properly labeled with the patient's name, identification number, body site, and date and time of collection with provision of suspected clinical diagnosis (pneumonia, urinary tract infection, meningitis, etc). Finally, specimens should be promptly transported to the laboratory (less than 1 hour) to prevent overgrowth of normal microorganisms, or they must be refrigerated for storage.

A rapid result for infectious diseases is essential in patient management, especially for life-threatening diseases such as meningitis. In such instances, microscopy is invaluable. The Gram's stain in microbiology sometimes provides the first indication of the etiology of an infectious process. Other rapid methods are also available, including antigen detection assays. The new DNA technology currently being introduced will also provide more rapid detection and accurate identification of infectious agents. (See Molecular Pathology chapter.) Currently, however, a complete bacteriology result is usually not available until 48 hours after submission. Certain fastidious organisms, mycobacteria, and fungal cultures require longer culture times, and results may often take as long as 4-8 weeks.

Acid-Fast Stain

CPT 87206

Related Information

Acid-Fast Stain, Modified, *Nocardia* Species *on this page*
Mycobacteria by DNA Probe *on page 520*
Mycobacterial Culture, Biopsy or Body Fluid *on page 487*
Mycobacterial Culture, Cerebrospinal Fluid *on page 489*
Mycobacterial Culture, Cutaneous and Subcutaneous Tissue *on page 489*
Mycobacterial Culture, Sputum *on page 490*
Mycobacterial Culture, Stool *on page 491*
Mycobacterial Culture, Urine *on page 491*

Synonyms AFB Smear; Atypical *Mycobacterium* Smear; Kinyoun Stain; *Mycobacterium* Smear; TB Smear; Ziehl-Neelsen Stain

Applies to Auramine-Rhodamine Stain; Fluorochrome Stain

Test Commonly Includes Acid-fast stain and culture are usually ordered together.

Abstract Acid-fast bacilli are so called because they are surrounded by a waxy cell wall that is resistant to destaining by acid alcohol. Heat (classic Ziehl-Neelsen), prolonged exposure, or detergent (Tergitol™ Kinyoun method) is required to allow carbol-fuchsin stain to penetrate the cell wall. Once stained, acid-fast bacteria resist decolorization with acid alcohol.[1] The acid-fast smear is inexpensive, has high specificity (which is <100%), but it has low sensitivity. New developments are becoming available to provide more sensitive and rapid detection and evaluation.[2]

Patient Preparation Same as for mycobacteria culture of given site

Specimen The appropriate specimen for an acid-fast smear is the same as for culture. Specimens may include sputum, bronchopulmonary lavage, tissue including liver biopsy and endometrium, material from fine needle aspiration, bone marrow, CSF, gastric aspiration, urine, and stool. In neonates, smears and cultures of gastric and endotracheal aspirates are useful.[3]

Such specimens should be cultured as well. See mycobacteria culture listings for details.

Causes for Rejection Specimen received on a dry swab

Reference Range No acid-fast organisms. Positive smears are quantitated and reported as 1+ (3-9 bacilli in entire smear), 2+ (≥10 in entire smear), or 3+ (1 or more bacilli per field) acid-fast bacilli seen.

Use Determine the presence of mycobacteria

Limitations Cultures are more sensitive than smears, therefore, negative acid-fast smears do not exclude a diagnosis of mycobacterial disease. Acid-fast stains are not specific for *M. tuberculosis*; other species in the genus *Mycobacterium* will stain acid-fast, and other organisms will occasionally stain acid-fast (eg, *Nocardia* sp, *Legionella micdadei*, *Rhodococcus equi*).[4,5] Immunocompromised individuals (eg, those who are HIV positive) may have infection by organisms of the *Mycobacterium avium-intracellulare* complex (MAC). Some laboratories may guess an organism's identity (eg, *M. tuberculosis* vs atypical *Mycobacterium* sp) by its staining characteristics and morphology, but definitive identification can only be accomplished by culture and subsequent phenotypic or genotypic characterization.[6] Occasional strains of rapidly growing mycobacteria may not be acid-fast by fluorochrome stains.[7]

Methodology Acid-fast stain of concentrated or unconcentrated specimen (Ziehl-Neelsen, Kinyoun, or fluorochrome stain).[1] See diagram. Use of the cytocentrifuge to concentrate organisms in sputum enhances sensitivity of smears.[8]

Carbolfuchsin
(triaminotriphenylmethane)

Additional Information In a large prospective study of **pulmonary tuberculosis**, the sensitivity and specificity of acid-fast staining was 53.1% and 99.8%, respectively; the sensitivity and specificity of culture was 81.5% and 98.4%, respectively.[9] The sensitivity of acid-fast stains performed on nonrespiratory specimens was recently reported at 67% for CSF, 80% for lymph node biopsies, 75% for peritoneal biopsies, and 80% for urine.[10,11]

At least 5 mL of **CSF** is needed for proper acid-fast staining and evaluation.[8]

Molecular target amplification techniques are currently being used with significant success for rapid detection and identification of *Mycobacterium tuberculosis* in clinical specimens.[12,13] Certain laboratories may use these techniques as an adjunct to, AFB smears.

Occasionally request for stat AFB stains are performed without prior digestion and concentration, which compromises sensitivity. Discontinuing AFB or respiratory isolation on the basis of a negative stat result is inappropriate. Identification of positive AFB smear 12-18 hours earlier than routine smears may be useful for controlling exposure of healthcare workers.

Footnotes

1. Koneman EW, Allen SD, Janda WM, et al, *Color Atlas and Textbook of Diagnostic Microbiology*, 4th ed, Philadelphia, PA: JB Lippincott Co, 1992, 713-4.
2. Pfaller MA, "Application of New Technology to the Detection, Identification, and Antimicrobial Susceptibility Testing of Mycobacteria," *Am J Clin Pathol*, 1994, 101(3):329-37.
3. Cantwell MF, Shehab ZM, Costello AM, et al, "Brief Report: Congenital Tuberculosis," *N Engl J Med*, 1994, 330(15):1051-4.
4. Hilton E, Freedman RA, Clintron F, et al, "Acid-Fast Bacilli in Sputum: A Case of *Legionella micdadei* Pneumonia," *J Clin Microbiol*, 1986, 24(6):1102-3.
5. Harvey RL and Sunstrum JC, "*Rhodococcus equi* Infection in Patients With and Without Human Immunodeficiency Virus Infection," *Rev Infect Dis*, 1991, 13(1):139-45.
6. Scott B, Schmid M, and Nettleman MD, "Early Identification and Isolation of Inpatients at High Risk for Tuberculosis," *Arch Intern Med*, 1994, 154(3):326-30.
7. Joseph S, Vaichulis E, and Houk V, "Lack of Auramine-Rhodamine Fluorescence of Runyon Group IV Mycobacteria," *Am Rev Respir Dis*, 1967, 95:114.
8. Christie JD and Callihan DR, "The Laboratory Diagnosis of Mycobacterial Diseases. Challenges and Common Sense," *Clin Lab Med*, 1995, 15(2):279-306.
9. Alvarez S and McCabe WR, "Extrapulmonary Tuberculosis Revisited: A Review of Experience of Boston City and Other Hospitals," *Medicine (Baltimore)*, 1984, 63(1):25-55.
10. Klotz SA and Penn RL, "Acid-Fast Staining of Urine and Gastric Contents is an Excellent Indicator of Mycobacterial Disease," *Am Rev Respir Dis*, 1987, 136(5):1197-8.
11. Saceanu CA, Pfeiffer NC, and McLean T, "Evaluation of Sputum Smears Concentrated by Cytocentrifugation for Detection of Acid-Fast Bacilli," *J Clin Microbiol*, 1993, 31(9):2371-4.
12. Miller N, Hernandez SG, and Cleary TJ, "Evaluation of Gen-Probe® Amplified *Mycobacterium tuberculosis* Direct Test and PCR for Direct Detection of *Mycobacterium tuberculosis* in Clinical Specimens," *J Clin Microbiol*, 1994, 32(2):393-7.
13. Clarridge JE 3d, Shawar RM, Shinnick TM, et al, "Large-Scale Use of Polymerase Chain Reaction for Detection of *Mycobacterium tuberculosis* in a Routine Mycobacteriology Laboratory," *J Clin Microbiol*, 1993, 31(8):2049-56.

References

Dutt AK and Stead WW, "Smear-Negative Pulmonary Tuberculosis," *Semin Respir Infect*, 1994, 9(2):113-9.
Gordin F and Slutkin G, "The Validity of Acid-Fast Smears in the Diagnosis of Pulmonary Tuberculosis," *Arch Pathol Lab Med*, 1990, 114(10):1025-7.
Menzies D, Fanning A, Yuan L, et al, "Tuberculosis Among Health Care Workers," *N Engl J Med*, 1995, 332(2):92-8.
Smith RL, Yew K, Berkowitz KA, et al, "Factors Affecting the Yield of Acid-Fast Sputum Smears in Patients With HIV and Tuberculosis," *Chest*, 1994, 106(3):684-6.
"Diagnosis and Treatment of Disease Caused by Nontuberculous Mycobacteria," *Am Rev Respir Dis*, 1990, 142(4):940-53.

Acid-Fast Stain, Modified, *Cryptosporidium* see Cryptosporidium Diagnostic Procedures *on page 474*

Acid-Fast Stain, Modified, *Nocardia* Species

CPT 87206

Related Information

Acid-Fast Stain *on this page*
Actinomyces Culture *on next page*
Cryptosporidium Diagnostic Procedures *on page 474*
Fungus Smear, Stain *on page 481*
Gram's Stain *on page 481*
Nocardia Culture *on page 493*

Synonyms Hank's Stain; *Nocardia* Species Modified Acid-Fast Stain

Test Commonly Includes Modified acid-fast stain. Culture must be ordered specifically as such. The recovery of *Nocardia* sp frequently requires special culture techniques.

Abstract Infections with *Nocardia* sp resemble other more common diseases. Because therapy differs, it is important to establish a definitive diagnosis, preferably by culture. The diagnosis of nocardiosis should be considered in unexplained cavitary lung disease, granulomatous lung disease of established cause not responsive to appropriate therapy, brain abscess particularly in the presence of cavitary lung disease, alveolar proteinosis, with mycetoma, and in any patient in whom a disseminated granulomatous disease is considered.

Specimen Appropriate specimen for smear is the same as for culture

Causes for Rejection Specimen received on a dry swab

Reference Range No acid-fast organisms seen

Use Determine the presence or absence of *Nocardia* sp which can be acid-fast when stained by the modified acid-fast stain. *Actinomyces* and *Streptomyces* sp which may be microscopically similar to *Nocardia* on Gram's stain, are negative with the modified acid-fast stain. Establish the etiology of maduromycosis and of fever of unknown origin in patients with suspected defects of cellular immunity (eg, AIDS, Hodgkin's disease, lymphoma, and so forth).

Limitations *Nocardia* sp do not always stain acid-fast by this method, consequently, the presence of branching, gram-positive bacilli on Gram's stain may have greater sensitivity. *Nocardia* sp, however, cannot be distinguished from *Actinomyces* sp and other closely related organisms by Gram's stain.

Methodology Kinyoun stain followed by light decolorization with 3% acid alcohol (940 mL of 95% ethanol and 60 mL of concentrated HCl)[1]

Additional Information *Nocardia* sp can cause a spectrum of disease that varies from a self-limited infection to a progressive disease that results in death. Nocardiosis has also been reported with lupus, rheumatoid arthritis, and liver disease. Aggressive diagnostic procedures are often necessary to obtain an appropriate specimen for definitive diagnosis. Elements consistent with *Nocardia* sp can be identified presumptively on Gram's stain and modified acid-fast stain pending more definitive diagnosis by culture.[2] Examination of sputum with *Nocardia* may show thin, crooked, weakly to strongly gram-positive, modified acid-fast positive, irregularly staining or beaded filaments. Opaque or pigmented sulfur granules may occasionally be present in direct smear of pus. Colonization without apparent infection may occur.

Footnotes

1. Koneman EW, Allen SD, Janda WM, et al, *Color Atlas and Textbook of Diagnostic Microbiology*, 4th ed, Philadelphia, PA: JB Lippincott Co, 1992, 505.
2. Osoagbaka OU and Njoku-Obi AN, "Presumptive Diagnosis of Pulmonary Nocardiosis: Value of Sputum Microscopy," *J Appl Bacteriol*, 1987, 63(1):27-38.

References

Ashdown LR, "An Improved Screening Technique for Isolation of *Nocardia* Species From Sputum Specimens," *Pathology*, 1990, 22(3):157-61.

Beaman BL and Beaman L, "*Nocardia* Species: Host Parasite Relationships," *Clin Microbiol Rev*, 1994, 7(2):213-64.

Chazen G, "*Nocardia*," *Infect Control*, 1987, 8(6):260-3.

Javaly K, Horowitz HW, and Wormser GP, "Nocardiosis in Patients With Human Immunodeficiency Virus Infection. Report of 2 Cases and Review of the Literature," *Medicine (Baltimore)*, 1992, 71(3):128-38.

McNeil MM and Brown JM, "The Medically Important Aerobic Actinomycetes: Epidemiology and Microbiology," *Clin Microbiol Rev*, 1994, 7(3):357-417.

Actinomyces Culture

CPT 87081

Related Information

Acid-Fast Stain, Modified, *Nocardia* Species *on previous page*
Bacterial Culture, Anaerobes *on page 456*
Bacterial Culture, Biopsy or Body Fluid *on page 456*
Bacterial Culture, Endometrium *on page 462*
Nocardia Culture *on page 493*

Synonyms Wound *Actinomyces* Culture

Applies to Intrauterine Device Culture; IUD Culture; Sulfur Granule, Culture

Test Commonly Includes Anaerobic culture for *Actinomyces* sp and direct microscopic examination of Gram's stain for sulfur granules and gram-positive branching bacilli

Abstract Actinomycosis is a chronic progressive suppurative disease characterized by the formation of multiple abscesses, draining sinuses, and dense fibrosis. The classic presentations include cervicofacial, thoracic, abdominal, and pelvic infections.

Patient Preparation Cleanse the skin around the opening of a draining sinus or lesion with an alcohol swab, allow to dry, and obtain the specimen from as deep within the sinus or lesion as possible.

Specimen Exudate, material from draining sinus, tissue

Container Anaerobic specimen transport medium or needle and syringe

Collection *Actinomyces* sp are fastidious anaerobic organisms. It is, therefore, essential that the specimen be placed into the appropriate anaerobic transport tube and delivered to the laboratory as quickly as possible. All air should be expelled from syringes before transport or transfer. Swabs, if used, should be transported in anaerobic transport medium. With a draining sinus, obtain the specimen by aspirating with needle and syringe as far up the sinus or lesion as possible.

Storage Instructions Specimens should be transported immediately to the laboratory and processed as soon as possible.

Causes for Rejection Specimens exposed to air, specimens which have been refrigerated or have an excessive delay in transit; specimens from sites which have anaerobic bacteria as normal flora (eg, throat, feces, colostomy stoma, rectal swabs, bronchial washes, cervical-vaginal mucosal swabs, sputums, skin and superficial wounds, voided or catheterized urine).

Turnaround Time Cultures with no growth may be reported after 14 days.

Special Instructions Inform the laboratory that actinomycosis is clinically suspected to ensure that cultures will be incubated sufficiently long to permit recovery of *Actinomyces* sp. The specific site of specimen, current antibiotic therapy, and clinical diagnosis should be provided.

Reference Range No *Actinomyces* isolated. *A. israelii* is a normal inhabitant of the mouth, oropharynx, and gastrointestinal tract.

Use Detect infections due to *Actinomyces* sp; establish the etiology of granulomatous disease, chronic draining sinus, and fever of unknown origin (FUO) particularly in immunocompromised patients

Limitations *Actinomyces* sp are relatively slow growing and will often fail to grow in the period in which most laboratories incubate routine cultures. Additionally, even when incubated appropriately, recovery of *Actinomyces* sp may be hindered by overgrowth with obligate and facultative anaerobic bacteria.

Methodology Anaerobic culture including thioglycolate broth media

Additional Information In tissues, *Actinomyces* sp produce chronic suppuration, commonly with formation of multiple draining sinuses. Microscopic examination of material from such sinuses often reveals tangled masses of filamentous elements and granules called **sulfur granules**. The presence of sulfur granules is highly suggestive of *Actinomyces* infection. The differential diagnosis between actinomycosis and nocardiosis is relevant because treatment of each is different.

If granules are detected on the gauze pad covering a draining sinus, submit the granules to the laboratory for Gram's stain and culture; on smear, branching gram-positive rods may be found. They may be similar in appearance to other actinomycetes including species of *Nocardia*, *Streptomyces*, and also *Mycobacterium*.[1] Actinomycetes are not acid-fast by the modified acid-fast stain used for *Nocardia* sp. Several species of *Actinomyces* are responsible for human infection. *Actinomyces israelii* is the most significant. *A. naeslundii*, *A. odontolyticus*, *A. viscosus*, and *Arachnia propionica* also have been reported as human pathogens. Pelvic and perirectal infections have been associated with intrauterine devices (IUDs). A classic presentation of actinomycosis is as a painless lump in the jaw.[2] *Actinomyces* may be found in rare instances of recurrent ventral hernia following appendectomy for appendicitis. The diagnosis of actinomycosis often requires clinical consideration of this possibility, communication to the laboratory, and persistence on the part of laboratory personnel.

Footnotes

1. Berd D, "Laboratory Identification of Clinically Important Actinomycetes," *Appl Microbiol*, 1973, 25(4):665-81.
2. Feder HM Jr, "Actinomycosis Manifesting as an Acute Painless Lump of the Jaw," *Pediatrics*, 1990, 85(5):858-64.

References

Allen SD, Siders JA, and Marler LM, "Current Issues and Problems in Dealing With Anaerobes in the Clinical Laboratory," *Clin Lab Med*, 1995, 15(2):333-64.

Bellingan GJ, "Disseminated Actinomycosis," *BMJ*, 1990, 301(6764):1323-4.

Holtz HA, Lavery DP, and Kapila R, "Actinomycetales Infection in the Acquired Immunodeficiency Syndrome," *Ann Intern Med*, 1985, 102(2):203-5.

Levine LA and Doyle CJ, "Retroperitoneal Actinomycosis: A Case Report and Review of the Literature," *J Urol*, 1988, 140(2):367-9.

McNeil MM and Brown JM, "The Medically Important Aerobic Actinomycetes: Epidemiology and Microbiology," *Clin Microbiol Rev*, 1994, 7(3):357-417.

Persson E, "Genital Actinomycosis and *Actinomyces israelii* in the Female Genital Tract," *Adv Contracept*, 1987, 3(2):115-23.

Stewart MG and Sulek M, "Pediatric Actinomycosis of the Head and Neck," *Ear Nose Throat J*, 1993, 72(9):614-6, 618-9.

Aerobic Bacterial Culture *see* Bacterial Culture, Aerobes *on page 455*

Aerobic Culture, Abscess *see* Bacterial Culture, Abscess *on page 454*

Aerobic Culture, Blood *see* Bacterial Culture, Blood *on page 457*

AFB Culture, Biopsy *see* Mycobacterial Culture, Biopsy or Body Fluid *on page 487*

AFB Culture, Body Fluid *see* Mycobacterial Culture, Biopsy or Body Fluid *on page 487*

AFB Culture, Sputum *see* Mycobacterial Culture, Sputum *on page 490*

AFB Culture, Stool *see* Mycobacterial Culture, Stool *on page 491*

AFB Culture, Urine *see* Mycobacterial Culture, Urine *on page 491*

AFB Smear *see* Acid-Fast Stain *on previous page*

Amebiasis *see* Ova and Parasites, Stool *on page 494*

Amniotic Fluid Anaerobic Culture *see* Bacterial Culture, Endometrium *on page 462*

Anaerobic Bacterial Culture *see* Bacterial Culture, Anaerobes *on page 456*

Anaerobic Bacterial Susceptibility *see* Antimicrobial Susceptibility Testing, Anaerobic Bacteria *on page 449*

Anaerobic Culture, Abscess *see* Bacterial Culture, Abscess *on page 454*

Anaerobic Culture, Blood *see* Bacterial Culture, Blood *on page 457*

Antibacterial Activity, Serum *see* Serum Bactericidal Test *on page 496*

Antibiotic-Associated Colitis Toxin Test *see* Clostridium difficile Toxin Assay *on page 473*

Antimicrobial Combinations - Test for Synergism and Antagonism *see* Antimicrobial Susceptibility Testing, Antimicrobial Combinations *on next page*

Antimicrobial Drugs *see* Antimicrobial Susceptibility Testing, Aerobic and Facultatively Anaerobic Bacteria *on this page*

Antimicrobial Removal Device (ARD) Blood Culture *see* Bacterial Culture, Blood *on page 457*

Antimicrobial Susceptibility Testing, Aerobic and Facultatively Anaerobic Bacteria

CPT 87181 (agar diffusion, each antibiotic); 87184 (disk method, each antibiotic); 87186 (MIC microtiter); 87188 (macrotube dilution, each antibiotic)

Related Information
Aminoglycosides *on page 531*
Antimicrobial Susceptibility Testing, Antimicrobial Combinations *on next page*
Antimicrobial Susceptibility Testing, Fungi *on page 450*
Antimicrobial Susceptibility Testing, Minimum Bactericidal Concentration *on page 451*
Antimicrobial Susceptibility Testing, Mycobacteria *on page 452*
Antimicrobial Susceptibility Testing, Unusual Isolates/Fastidious Organisms *on page 452*
Bacterial Culture, Abscess *on page 454*
Bacterial Culture, Aerobes *on page 455*
Beta-Lactamase Test *on page 470*
Chloramphenicol *on page 542*
Serum Bactericidal Test *on page 496*
Vancomycin *on page 578*

Synonyms Kirby-Bauer Susceptibility Test; MIC; Minimum Inhibitory Concentration Susceptibility Test; Sensitivity Testing, Aerobic and Facultatively Anaerobic Organisms; Susceptibility Testing Aerobic and Facultatively Anaerobic Organisms

Applies to Antimicrobial Drugs; Beta-Lactam Ring; Penicillinase

Test Commonly Includes Qualitative or quantitative determination of antimicrobial susceptibility of an isolated organism

Abstract The purpose of antimicrobial susceptibility testing is to determine the antibacterial activity of antimicrobial agents against specific pathogens. These susceptibility assays have been standardized for use in clinical laboratories by the National Committee for Clinical Laboratory Standards (NCCLS).[1,2] Standards include the use of quality control microorganisms to ensure that results are reliable and the use of standard agar and broth media to diminish variability between laboratories.

Specimen Viable pure culture of a rapidly growing aerobic or facultatively anaerobic organism

Turnaround Time Usually 1 day after recovering an organism from a clinical specimen

Reference Range Minimal inhibitory concentration (MIC) reported. Results may be qualitatively reported as susceptible (S), intermediate (I), or resistant (R).

Use Determine antimicrobial susceptibility of organisms involved in infectious processes when the susceptibility of the organism cannot be predicted from its identity. The pattern of antibiotic susceptibility is sometimes used to monitor nosocomial infections such as methicillin-resistant *Staphylococcus aureus* and to evaluate or follow the development of resistance to new antimicrobial drugs.[3,4,5]

Limitations Interpretive guidelines developed for antimicrobial susceptibility tests are applicable to most nonfastidious, rapidly growing bacteria (*Staphylococcus* sp, *Pseudomonas aeruginosa*, and members of the Enterobacteriaceae); additionally, common fastidious pathogens (eg, *Streptococcus pneumoniae*, *Haemophilus influenzae*, *Neisseria gonorrhoeae*) have been studied sufficiently to produce reasonable interpretive criteria. Interpretive criteria for less common pathogens (eg, *Corynebacterium* sp, *Nocardia* sp, rapidly growing mycobacteria, *Bacillus* sp) are much more vague.

Methodology Disk diffusion (qualitative) broth dilution, microbroth dilution, or agar dilution (quantitative), or antimicrobial concentrations are selected to correspond to therapeutically relevant levels. Several automated instruments have been developed to perform routine susceptibility testing of microorganisms.[6]

Additional Information Effective antimicrobial therapy is usually selected with intent to achieve a peak level two to four times the MIC at the site of infection. An antimicrobial level 10 times the MIC is usually sought in urinary tract infections. The "breakpoints" indicate MICs above which organisms are moderately or very resistant and would not be expected to respond to readily achievable levels of antimicrobial therapy.

Susceptible: This category implies that an infection due to the strain may be appropriately treated with the dosage of antimicrobial agent recommended for that type of infection and infecting species, unless otherwise contraindicated.

Intermediate: This category provides a "buffer zone," which should prevent small, uncontrolled, technical factors from causing major discrepancies in interpretations (eg, species that should have few or no endpoints in this range, or drugs with *in vitro* results affected by media variation or drugs with narrow pharmacotoxicity margins).

Antimicrobial agents that are excreted via the kidneys can usually be used to treat uncomplicated cystitis due to an organism with intermediate susceptibility. For systemic infections, antimicrobials with intermediate activity should be avoided unless used in combination with a nonantagonistic agent with greater activity against the infecting organism; if such an agent does not exist, use maximal nontoxic dosing of the agent with intermediate activity.

Resistant: Strains falling in this category are not inhibited by the usually achievable systemic concentrations of the agent with normal dosage schedules and/or fall in the range where specific microbial resistance mechanisms are likely (eg, beta-lactamases), and clinical efficacy has not been reliable in treatment studies. See table.

Major Mechanisms of Bacterial Antimicrobial Resistance

Enzymatic inactivation or modification of drug
- β-lactamase hydrolysis of β-lactam ring with subsequent inactivation of β-lactam antibiotics
- Modification of aminoglycosides by acetylating, adenylating, or phosphorylating enzymes
- Modification of chloramphenicol by chloramphenicol acetyltransferase

Decreased drug uptake or accumulation
- Intrinsic or acquired lack of outer membrane permeability
- Faulty or lacking antibiotic uptake and transport system
- Antibiotic efflux system (eg, tetracycline resistance)

Altered or lacking antimicrobial target
- Altered penicillin-binding proteins (β-lactam resistance)
- Altered ribosomal target (eg, aminoglycoside, macrolide, and lincomycin resistance)
- Altered enzymatic target (eg, sulfonamide, trimethoprim, rifampin, and quinolone resistance)

Circumvention of drug action consequences
- Hyperproduction of drug targets or competitive substrates (eg, sulfonamide and trimethoprim resistance)

Uncoupling of antibiotic attack and cell death
- Bacterial tolerance and survival in presence of usually bactericidal drugs (eg, β-lactams and vancomycin)

A MIC to penicillin >0.1 µg/mL for *S. aureus* indicates resistance due to penicillinase production.

Footnotes
1. National Committee for Clinical Laboratory Standards, "Performance Standards for Antimicrobial Disk Susceptibility Tests," Approved Standard M2-A5, Villanova, PA: National Committee for Clinical Laboratory Standards, 1993.
2. National Committee for Clinical Laboratory Standards, "Methods for Dilution Susceptibility Tests for Bacteria That Grow Aerobically." Approved Standard M7-A3, Villanova, PA: National Committee for Clinical Laboratory Standards, 1993.
3. Grayson ML and Eliopoulos GM, "Antimicrobial Resistance in the Intensive Care Unit," *Semin Respir Infect*, 1990, 5(3):204-14.
4. Georgopapadakou NH, "Penicillin-Binding Proteins and Bacterial Resistance to β-Lactams," *Antimicrob Agents Chemother*, 1993, 37(10):2045-53.
5. Speer BS, Shoemaker NB, and Salyers AA, "Bacterial Resistance to Tetracycline: Mechanisms, Transfer, and Clinical Significance," *Clin Microbiol Rev*, 1992, 5(4):387-99.
6. Stager CE and Davis JR, "Automated Systems for Identification of Microorganisms," *Clin Microbiol Rev*, 1992, 5(3):302-27.

References
Jorgensen JH, "Antimicrobial Susceptibility Testing of Bacteria That Grow Aerobically," *Infect Dis Clin North Am*, 1993, 7(2):393-409.
National Committee for Clinical Laboratory Standards, *Performance Standards for Antimicrobial Susceptibility Testing*, Fifth Information Supplement NCCLS Document M100-S5, Villanova, PA: National Committee for Clinical Laboratory Standards, 1994.
Rosenblatt JE, "Laboratory Tests Used to Guide Antimicrobial Therapy," *Mayo Clin Proc*, 1991, 66(9):942-8.
Sherris JC, "Antimicrobic Susceptibility Testing. A Personal Perspective," *Clin Lab Med*, 1989, 9(2):191-202.

Silver LL and Bostian KA, "Discovery and Development of New Antibiotics: The Problem of Antibiotic Resistance," *Antimicrob Agents Chemother*, 1993, 37(3):377-83.

Wilkowske CJ, "General Principles of Antimicrobial Therapy," *Mayo Clin Proc*, 1991, 66(9):931-41.

Antimicrobial Susceptibility Testing, Anaerobic Bacteria

CPT 87181 (agar dilution, each antibiotic); 87188 (tube dilution, each antibiotic)

Related Information

Antimicrobial Susceptibility Testing, Antimicrobial Combinations *on this page*

Antimicrobial Susceptibility Testing, Unusual Isolates/Fastidious Organisms *on page 452*

Bacterial Culture, Abscess *on page 454*

Bacterial Culture, Anaerobes *on page 456*

Beta-Lactamase Test *on page 470*

Synonyms Anaerobic Bacterial Susceptibility; MIC, Anaerobic Bacteria; Susceptibility Testing, Anaerobic Bacteria

Applies to E Test

Specimen A pure culture of the isolated organism to be tested, prepared by the laboratory

Turnaround Time 2-5 days from time organism is isolated and identified

Special Instructions Appropriateness and scope of anaerobic susceptibility testing in a particular clinical setting requires laboratory consultation.

Reference Range See table.

Use Antimicrobial susceptibility testing of individual anaerobic isolates rarely contributes significantly to patient management. Antimicrobial therapy of anaerobic infections is usually empiric. Restrict testing to unusual circumstances such as anaerobic brain abscess, endocarditis, osteomyelitis, and prosthetic device or vascular graft infections.[1] Additionally, periodic surveillance may be useful to establish institutional or regional susceptibility patterns which can be used to guide future empiric therapy.

Limitations The broth disk-elution method, which has been used for years by many laboratories, produces unreliable results and should not be used to determine the antimicrobial susceptibility of anaerobic bacteria.[2]

Anaerobic infections are often polymicrobial (involving aerobic and anaerobic organisms), and are associated with tissue necrosis and abscess formation resulting in impaired delivery of antimicrobial agents to the infection site. Additionally, methods for recovering and identifying anaerobic bacteria are cumbersome and time consuming resulting in elapsed periods of nearly a week before susceptibility test results are available. These factors, in conjunction with the fact that standardized methods for testing anaerobes are not always reliable and often produce growth patterns that are difficult to interpret, make the usefulness of susceptibility testing of anaerobic bacteria questionable.

Contraindications Anaerobic bacterial isolate from patient is not available or fails to give adequate growth for susceptibility testing.

Methodology Broth microdilution, macrobroth dilution, and agar dilution technique; beta-lactamase testing

Additional Information At present, routine susceptibility testing of anaerobic isolates is not recommended.[3] Infections involving anaerobes frequently contain mixed flora, and appropriate drainage rather than antimicrobial therapy seems to be the most crucial factor in the successful treatment of these infections.

Indications for anaerobic susceptibility testing include:
- determination of susceptibility of anaerobes to new antimicrobial agents
- monitoring susceptibility patterns by geographic area
- monitoring susceptibility patterns in local hospitals
- assisting in the management of selected individual patients; *vide supra, vide infra*

Some anaerobes have predictable *in vitro* susceptibility patterns but grow so slowly that by the time isolation and susceptibility testing are completed (6-14 days), such results are of little clinical value. Thus, susceptibility testing is generally performed only on anaerobic isolates from blood, pleural fluid, peritoneal fluid, and CSF. In cases of chronic anaerobic infections (septic arthritis, osteomyelitis, etc), susceptibility testing may be done by special request. The physician should contact the laboratory regarding the specific antibiotic(s) to be tested and the testing method available.

Organisms that are recognized as virulent such as *Bacteroides fragilis* group, pigmented *Prevotella* sp, *Porphyromonas* sp (formerly *Bacteroides gracilis*), certain *Fusobacterium*, *Clostridium perfringens*, and *Clostridium ramosus*, may also be considered for testing.[4]

The E test is a new method under investigation for testing antimicrobial susceptibility of anaerobic organisms. It has recently been approved by the FDA, and initial studies show that it correlates well with the reference methods.[5] The advantages of the E test would be to provide a quick, reliable susceptibility test that is not labor intensive.

Footnotes

1. Finegold SM, "Susceptibility Testing of Anaerobic Bacteria," *J Clin Microbiol*, 1988, 26(7):1253-6.
2. Wexler HM and Doern GV, "Susceptibility Testing of Anaerobic Bacteria," *Manual of Clinical Microbiology*, 6th ed, Murray PR, Baron EJ, Pfaller MA, et al, eds, Washington, DC: American Society for Microbiology, 1995, 379-99.
3. National Committee for Clinical Laboratory Standards, "Methods for Antimicrobial Susceptibility Testing of Anaerobic Bacteria," Approved Standard, M11-A3, Villanova, PA: National Committee for Clinical Laboratory Standards, 1993.
4. Styrt B and Gorbach SL, "Recent Developments in the Understanding of the Pathogenesis and Treatment of Anaerobic Infections," *N Engl J Med*, 1989, 321(5):298-302.
5. Citron DM, Ostovari MI, Karlsson A, et al, "Evaluation of the E Test for Susceptibility Testing of Anaerobic Bacteria," *J Clin Microbiol*, 1991, 29(10):2197-203.

References

Bolmstrom A, "Susceptibility Testing of Anaerobes With Etest," *Clin Infect Dis*, 1993, 16(Suppl 4):S367-70.

Johnson CC, "Susceptibility of Anaerobic Bacteria to Beta-Lactam Antibiotics in the United States," *Clin Infect Dis*, 1993, 16(Suppl 4):S371-6.

Johnson MJ, Thatcher E, and Cox ME, "Antimicrobial Susceptibility Tests for Anaerobic Bacteria With Use of the Disk Diffusion Method," *Clin Infect Dis*, 1995, 20(S2):334-6.

Rosenblatt JE, "Susceptibility Testing of Anaerobic Bacteria," *Clin Lab Med*, 1989, 9(2):239-54.

Wexler HM, "Susceptibility Testing of Anaerobic Bacteria - The State of the Art," *Clin Infect Dis*, 1993, 16(Suppl 4):S328-33.

Antimicrobial Susceptibility Testing, Antimicrobial Combinations

CPT 87184 (disk method, each antibiotic); 87186 (MIC, any number of antibiotics)

Related Information

Antimicrobial Susceptibility Testing, Aerobic and Facultatively Anaerobic Bacteria *on previous page*

Antimicrobial Susceptibility Testing, Anaerobic Bacteria *on this page*

Typical Sensitivities of Important Anaerobic Pathogens to Major Classes of Antibiotics

Antibiotic	B. fragilis Group	B. melaninogenicus Group	Fusobacterium	Clostridium	Propionibacterium	Actinomyces	Peptostreptococcus
Penicillin G	– to +	– to +++	++	+ to ++	+++	+++	+++
Antipseudomonal penicillins	++ to +++	+ to +++	+++	+++	+++	+++	+++
Cefoxitin	++	+++	++ to +++	– to ++	+++	+++	+++
Imipenem-cilastatin	+++	+++	++	+++	+++	+++	+++
Combinations of beta-lactam and beta-lactamase inhibitor	+++	+++	+++	+++	+++	+++	+++
Clindamycin	++ to +++	+++	+++	++	+++	+++	+++
Chloramphenicol	+++	+++	+++	+++	+++	+++	+++
Metronidazole	+++	+++	+++	+++	–	–	++ to +++

From Styrt B and Gorbach SL, "Recent Developments in the Understanding of the Pathogenesis and Treatment of Anaerobic Infections," *N Engl J Med*, 1989, Part I, 321:240-6 and Part II, 321:298-302 (review), with permission.

– denotes that <50% of the strains were susceptible.

+ denotes that 50% to 70% of the strains were susceptible.

++ denote that 70% to 90% of the strains were susceptible.

+++ denote that >90% of the strains were susceptible.

(Continued)

Antimicrobial Susceptibility Testing, Antimicrobial Combinations (Continued)

Antimicrobial Susceptibility Testing, Unusual Isolates/Fastidious Organisms *on page 452*

Serum Bactericidal Test *on page 496*

Synonyms Antimicrobial Combinations - Test for Synergism and Antagonism; Susceptibility Testing, Antimicrobial Combinations; Synergistic Studies, Antimicrobial

Applies to Fractional Bactericidal Concentration (FBC); Fractional Inhibitory Concentration (FIC); Minimal Bactericidal Concentration (MBC); Minimal Inhibitory Concentration (MIC); Schlichter Test

Test Commonly Includes MICs of both antibiotics against patient's organism, determination of synergistic or antagonistic antimicrobial effect of drug combination

Specimen A pure culture of the isolated organism to be tested, prepared by the laboratory

Causes for Rejection Organism discarded prior to request for test by physician, organism fails to grow on subculture or is too fastidious to grow under usual conditions of testing

Turnaround Time 2-4 days (depends on antimicrobials assayed and procedure used)

Special Instructions Notify the laboratory to retain organism needed for test.

Reference Range Additive effect, synergism or antagonism

Use Determine whether the addition of a second antibiotic (B) will increase or decrease the known sensitivity of an organism to antibiotic (A). Some antibiotics have well established synergistic activity such as a cell wall active agent (ie, penicillin and vancomycin) and an aminoglycoside.[1,2] This is recommended for serious infections due to enterococci. Other antibacterial agents are tested for their ability to inhibit each other, usually done for experimental purposes during development of new antibiotics.

Limitations This test procedure is usually available only from specialized laboratories, predicated upon availability of antibiotic standard for testing. Test cannot be run if organism fails to grow. The clinical relevance of synergy studies and standardized methods is still being defined.

Methodology Checkerboard titration, time-kill technique, double diffusion testing

Additional Information Laboratory should be notified 24 hours in advance of time when test is to be performed. Patient's organism must be saved at request of physician. Physician must specify antimicrobials to be tested in combination culture, site of isolated organism, and culture date. The MICs of antibiotics to be tested must be known or performed.

Combinations of antimicrobials are often used with intent of achieving a synergistic effect (ie, a demonstrated inhibitory or bactericidal activity that is greater than the sum of the activities of the agents alone). The use of combination therapy is also often undertaken to reduce potential toxicity. A lower dose of each agent may be used (eg, aminoglycosides and a cephalosporin or penicillin). The use of combinations prevents or minimizes the emergence of resistant strains.

Several methods, checkerboard titration, time-kill technique, and diffusion tests, are used in research settings. In usual clinical practice, testing of enterococci and viridans streptococci isolated from patients with serious infections for high level aminoglycoside resistance is adequate to predict the potential presence or absence of synergism, when these agents are combined with cell wall active agents (eg, cephalosporins, penicillins). Fixed-dose combinations, trimethoprim-sulfamethoxazole and beta-lactam/beta-lactamase inhibitor combinations (eg, amoxicillin-clavulanate or ticarcillin-clavulanate) can be tested because of the standard availability of combination disks and commercially prepared microtiter susceptibility panels which include the combinations. A clear consensus regarding the usefulness of synergy studies has not yet emerged, primarily because of organism strain differences in response and lack of consensus on choice of laboratory methods. The greatest potential for clinical usefulness exists in patients with sustained profound neutropenia and in patients with endocarditis. The **serum bactericidal test (Schlichter test)** has efficacy to determine potential clinical effects of antimicrobial combinations, particularly in endocarditis and osteomyelitis.

Definition of Technical Terms

• **Minimal Inhibitory Concentration (MIC)**: The lowest concentration of drug that **inhibits** growth >99% of the bacterial population.

• **Minimal Bactericidal Concentration (MBC)**: The lowest concentration of drug that **kills** >99.9% of the bacterial population in a broth culture. The MIC/MBC ratio is the standard for expressing the bactericidal potency of the drug.

• **Fractional Inhibitory Concentration (FIC)**: An interaction coefficient indicating whether the combined inhibitory (bacteriostatic) effect of drugs is synergistic (FIC ≤0.5), additive (FIC = 1), or antagonistic (FIC ≥4) ("a" and "b" are drugs):

$$FIC = \frac{MIC_a \text{ in combination}}{MIC_a \text{ alone}} + \frac{MIC_b \text{ in combination}}{MIC_b \text{ alone}}$$

• **Fractional Bactericidal Concentration (FBC)**: An interaction coefficient indicating whether the combined bactericidal effect of drugs is synergistic, additive, or antagonistic:[3]

$$FBC = \frac{MBC_a \text{ in combination}}{MBC_a \text{ alone}} + \frac{MBC_b \text{ in combination}}{MBC_b \text{ alone}}$$

Footnotes

1. Sahm DF and Torres C, "High-Content Aminoglycoside Disks for Determining Aminoglycoside-Penicillin Synergy Against *Enterococcus faecalis*," *J Clin Microbiol*, 1988, 26(2):257-60.
2. Winstanley TG and Hastings JG, "Penicillin-Aminoglycoside Synergy and Postantibiotic Effect for Enterococci," *J Antimicrob Chemother*, 1989, 23(2):189-99.
3. Heifets L, "Qualitative and Quantitative Drug Susceptibility Test in Mycobacteriology," *Am Rev Respir Dis*, 1988, 137(5):1217-22.

References

Amsterdam D, "Evaluating the *In Vitro* Efficacy of Antimicrobic Combination," *Antimicrob Newslet*, 1989, 6:41-3.

Edberg SC, "Antibiotic Interaction Tests Should They Be Performed," *Clin Microbiol Newslet*, 1988, 10:77-8.

Eliopoulos GM and Eliopoulos CT, "Antibiotic Combinations Should They Be Tested," *Clin Microbiol Rev*, 1988, 1(2):139-56.

Peterson LR and Shanholtzer CJ, "Tests for Bactericidal Effects of Antimicrobial Agents: Technical Performance and Clinical Relevance," *Clin Microbiol Rev*, 1992, 5(4):420-32.

Rand KH, Houck HJ, Brown P, et al, "Reproducibility of the Microdilution Checkerboard Method for Antibiotic Synergy," *Antimicrob Agents Chemother*, 1993, 37(3):613-5.

Antimicrobial Susceptibility Testing, Fungi

CPT 87192 (each drug)

Related Information

Amphotericin B *on page 535*

Antimicrobial Susceptibility Testing, Aerobic and Facultatively Anaerobic Bacteria *on page 448*

Fungal Culture, Biopsy or Body Fluid *on page 476*

Fungal Culture, Blood *on page 477*

Fungal Culture, Skin *on page 478*

Fungal Culture, Sputum *on page 479*

Fungus Smear, Stain *on page 481*

Itraconazole *on page 555*

Ketoconazole *on page 556*

Synonyms Fungi Susceptibility Testing; Susceptibility Testing, Fungi

Test Commonly Includes Broth dilution, agar dilution and disk diffusion testing of antifungal agents. Results may be quantitative or qualitative.

Abstract Fungi have emerged in the last ten years as important nosocomial pathogens. As the incidence of serious fungal infections has increased a number of new antifungal agents have been introduced, thus the need for *in vitro* antifungal susceptibility tests. Unfortunately, the results of antifungal susceptibility tests show little clinical correlation.

Specimen A pure culture of the isolated organism to be tested, prepared by the laboratory

Causes for Rejection Organism disposed of prior to request for testing.

Special Instructions Consult the laboratory to determine availability and choice of methods.

Reference Range See table.

Use Routine antifungal susceptibility testing is clearly unwarranted. In certain clinical circumstances it may be appropriate to test amphotericin B against *Candida* sp, the zygomycetes, and *Pseudoallescheria boydii*; other fungi need not be tested since they are almost always susceptible to amphotericin B.[1] Several yeasts have demonstrated resistance to the azoles (eg, ketoconazole, itraconazole, fluconazole) and susceptibility testing may occasionally be warranted; the dimorphic fungi need not be tested since they are virtually always susceptible.[1]

Limitations Although susceptibility testing of yeasts has recently been standardized, the relationship between test results and patient response to therapy has not been established. In fact, there is little correlation between *in vitro* susceptibility results and clinical results.[1] Susceptibility testing of yeasts against the azoles often produces variable results.[1] Susceptibility testing of filamentous fungi has not been standardized and is quite variable; isolates should be sent to a well respected reference laboratory for testing.

Methodology Standardized methods are proposed for the susceptibility testing of yeasts.[2] The availability of a choice of therapeutic agents will

In vitro Antifungal Activities of Four Antifungal Agents Against Pathogenic Fungi*

Organism	Amphotericin B		Flucytosine (5-FC)		Miconazole		Ketoconazole
	MIC (µg/mL)	MFC (µg/mL)	MIC (µg/mL)	MFC (µg/mL)	MIC (µg/mL)	MFC (µg/mL)	MIC (µg/mL)
Pathogenic yeasts							
Cryptococcus neoformans	0.05-0.78†	0.1-12.5	0.10-100#	0.39->100	0.05-3.13	0.05-25	0.1-32
Candida albicans	0.2-0.78•	0.39-0.78	0.05-12.5#	0.10->100	0.1-2.0•	0.1-10	<0.1-128
Candida sp not *C. albicans*	0.2-1.56•	0.39-6.25	0.10-50#	0.20->100	<0.1-2.0	0.1->10	<0.1-64
Torulopsis glabrata	0.1-0.4	0.2-0.78	0.05-1.56	0.4->100	0.5-10	2-10	1-64
Trichosporon sp	0.78-3.13	1.56-3.13	25-100	>100	0.2-25	0.2->100	
Geotrichum sp	0.4-1.56	0.78-3.13	1.56-12.5	25->100	0.1-2	0.5->10	
Filamentous fungi							
Pseudallescheria (Petrillidium) boydii	1.56->100#	>100	Resistant		0.5§	0.05	0.1-4#
Aspergillus sp including *A. fumigatus*	0.05-8	6.25->100	0.2-1.56#	>100	0.4->100	0.8->100	0.1-100
Blastomyces dermatitidis	0.05-0.2	0.1-0.4	Resistant		≤0.25	ND	0.1-2
Xylohypha bautiano	3.13->100	3.13->100	3.13-12.5#	12.5->100	0.5->64	ND	0.1-64
Coccidioides immitis	0.1-0.78	0.70-1.56	Resistant		0.25-1.0	ND	0.1-0.8
Histoplasma capsulatum	0.05-1.0	0.05-0.2	Resistant		≤0.25	ND	0.1-0.5
Phialophora sp and other dematiaceous fungi	0.05->128	6.25->128	Variable susceptibility	Resistant	0.05-32	ND	0.1-64
Sporothrix schenckii	1.56-12.5	3.13->100	Resistant		1-2	ND	0.1-16
Zygomycetes	0.78-1.56	1.56->100	Variable susceptibility	Resistant			
Control organisms							
S. cerevisiae ATCC 36375, etc	0.1	0.2	0.05	0.10	0.20	0.39	0.20
C. pseudotropicalis ATCC 28838			0.05	0.10	0.10	0.20	0.05

From Shadomy S and Pfaller MA, "Laboratory Studies With Antifungal Agents: Susceptibility Tests and Quantitation in Body Fluids," *Manual of Clinical Microbiology*, 5th ed, Washington, DC, American Society for Microbiology, 1991, 1173-83, with permission.

*Based upon both data obtained at the Medical College of Virginia, Virginia Commonwealth University, Richmond, and a review of the literature. *In vitro* data for nystatin is not included because of the narrow clinical spectrum of this agent; however, most isolates of *Candida* species and *Torulopsis* species should be clinically susceptible (MIC of ≤10 µg/mL) to nystatin. MFC, minimal fungicidal concentration; ND, not determined.

†Expected ranges of MICs and MFCs.

#Resistance not uncommon.

•Resistance reported but rare.

§Only limited data available.

‡ *In vitro* susceptibility of *Aspergillus* sp to ketoconazole is highly species dependent.

continue to cause laboratories to attempt to provide susceptibility data with useful predictive value for clinicians.

Additional Information Interpretation of *in vitro* susceptibility data for antifungal drugs has been hindered by the absence of standardized test criteria. Thus, it has been extremely difficult to identify a clear relation between *in vitro* minimal inhibitory concentrations and clinical outcome. However, some recent reports suggest that clinically significant resistance exists in some important fungal strains.[3,4] The situation appears more readily resolvable for yeast-like than for filamentous fungi since the former are more easily quantified by standardized microbiologic techniques.[5,6]

Footnotes

1. Espinel-Ingroff A and Pfaller MA, "Antifungal Agents and Susceptibility Testing," *Manual of Clinical Microbiology*, 6th ed, Murray PR, Baron EJ, Pfaller MA, et al, eds, Washington, DC: American Society for Microbiology, 1995, 1405-14.
2. National Committee for Clinical Laboratory Standards, "Reference Method for Broth Dilution Antifungal Susceptibility Testing for Yeasts," Proposed Standard Document M-27-P, Villanova, PA: National Committee for Clinical Laboratory Standards, 1992.
3. McIlroy MA, "Failure of Fluconazole to Suppress Fungemia in a Patient With Fever, Neutropenia, and Typhlitis," *J Infect Dis*, 1991, 163(2):420-1.
4. Willocks L, Leen CL, Brettle RP, et al, "Fluconazole Resistance in AIDS Patient," *J Antimicrob Chemother*, 1991, 28(6):937-9.
5. Hector RF and Schaller K, "Positive Interaction of Nikkomycins and Azoles Against *Candida albicans In Vitro* and *In Vivo*," *Antimicrob Agents Chemother*, 1992, 36(6):1284-9.
6. Espinel-Ingroff A, Kish CW Jr, Kerkering TM, et al, "Collaborative Comparison of Broth Macrodilution and Microdilution Antifungal Susceptibility Tests," *J Clin Microbiol*, 1992, 30(12):3138-45.

References

Fromtling RA, Galgiani JN, Pfaller MA, et al, "Multicenter Evaluation of a Broth Macrodilution Antifungal Susceptibility Test for Yeasts," *Antimicrob Agents Chemother*, 1993, 37(1):39-45.

Hector RF, "Compounds Active Against Cell Walls of Medically Important Fungi," *Clin Microbiol Rev*, 1993, 6(1):1-21.

Pfaller MA and Rinaldi MG, "Antifungal Susceptibility Testing. Current State of Technology, Limitations, and Standardizations," *Infect Dis Clin North Am*, 1993, 7(2):435-44.

Rex JH, Pfaller MA, Rinaldi MG, et al, "Antifungal Susceptibility Testing," *Clin Microbiol Rev*, 1993, 6(4):367-81.

Antimicrobial Susceptibility Testing, Minimum Bactericidal Concentration

CPT 87187 (MBC); 87188 (macrotube dilution)

Related Information

Antimicrobial Susceptibility Testing, Aerobic and Facultatively Anaerobic Bacteria *on page 448*

Synonyms MBC; Minimum Bactericidal Concentration; Minimum Lethal Concentration; MLC; Susceptibility Testing, Minimum Bactericidal Concentration

Applies to Tolerance Testing, Antimicrobial

Abstract The minimum bactericidal concentration (MBC) is the concentration of an antibiotic that kills 99%, 99.9%, or 100% of a standardized bacterial inoculum.

Specimen A pure culture of the isolated organism to be tested, prepared by the laboratory

Causes for Rejection Organism discarded prior to request by physician to save the organism for MBC, organism fails to grow on subculture from original plates

Turnaround Time 48 hours after isolation of bacterium to be tested

Special Instructions In order to perform an MBC test, an isolate of the organism of interest must be saved at the request of the physician often within 48 hours of submission of specimen for initial culture. If the isolate has not been saved, the test cannot be performed. The laboratory should be informed by the physician of the specific source of the culture, culture date, as well as the specific bacterial isolate to be tested and the antimicrobial agent to be tested.

Reference Range End points are generally reported as µg/mL of antimicrobial agent required to kill 99.9% of colonies.

Use Determine minimum bactericidal concentration, MBC, of an antimicrobial agent. Frequently utilized in endocarditis and osteomyelitis in immunocompromised hosts.

Limitations Results are accurate to plus or minus one dilution. However, technical factors including inoculum, medium, incubation, growth phase, tube type, mixing, etc, are a significant influence on results.

Contraindications Bacterium isolated from patient is not available or fails to grow for susceptibility testing.

Methodology Macrodilution or microdilution technique with subculture. Twofold dilutions of antibiotics are added to broth media that is then inoculated with a standard number of bacteria. After incubation, bacterial growth is monitored. The MIC of the isolate is determined by visually inspecting broth media, while the MBC is determined by plating a portion (Continued)

Antimicrobial Susceptibility Testing, Minimum Bactericidal Concentration (Continued)

of each well/tube onto solid media and performing colony counts to determine the percent survival.

Additional Information Tolerance, defined as inhibition of growth without killing, is manifested in the laboratory as an MBC (minimum bactericidal concentration) 32 or more times the MIC (minimum inhibitory concentration). Tolerance is most frequently observed with vancomycin and beta-lactam antibiotics against gram-positive organisms. Although tolerance is frequently observed in the laboratory, it is not often associated with clinical treatment failure. The selection of an endpoint of 99.9% killing is used to avoid the problem of the "persistent phenomenon" where a few highly resistant organisms persist regardless of the concentration of the antimicrobial agent.

References

James PA, "Comparison of Four Methods for the Determination of MIC and MBC of Penicillin for Viridans Streptococci and the Implications for Penicillin Tolerance," *J Antimicrob Chemother*, 1990, 25(2):209-16.

National Committee for Clinical Laboratory Standards, "Methods for Determining Bactericidal Activity of Antimicrobial Agents," Tentative Guideline M26-T, 1992.

Peterson LR and Shanholtzer CJ, "Tests for Bactericidal Effects of Antimicrobial Agents: Technical Performance and Clinical Relevance," *Clin Microbiol Rev*, 1992, 5(4):420-32.

Sherris JC, "Problems in the *In Vitro* Determination of Antibiotic Tolerance in Clinical Isolates," *Antimicrob Agents Chemother*, 1986, 30(5):633-7.

Antimicrobial Susceptibility Testing, Mycobacteria

CPT 87190 (each drug)

Related Information

Antimicrobial Susceptibility Testing, Aerobic and Facultatively Anaerobic Bacteria *on page 448*

Mycobacterial Culture, Biopsy or Body Fluid *on page 487*

Mycobacterial Culture, Cutaneous and Subcutaneous Tissue *on page 489*

Mycobacterial Culture, Sputum *on page 490*

Mycobacterial Culture, Stool *on page 491*

Mycobacterial Culture, Urine *on page 491*

Synonyms Mycobacteria Susceptibility Testing; Susceptibility Testing, Mycobacteria

Test Commonly Includes Panel of antimycobacterial agents tested against clinical isolates at appropriate concentrations

Specimen A pure culture of the isolated organism to be tested, prepared by the laboratory

Causes for Rejection Specimen not available for testing.

Turnaround Time 4-6 weeks after organism is isolated

Use Determine the susceptibility of the isolated organism to a panel of antimycobacterial agents

Limitations Methodology and interpretive criteria for *M. tuberculosis* is well standardized. Methodology and interpretive criteria for *Mycobacterium* sp other than *M. tuberculosis* have not been standardized; consequently, the distinction between susceptible and resistant isolates is often unclear.[1]

Methodology Disk diffusion, agar containing antibiotic, or broth containing antibiotic. Quantitative methods may be required to accurately assess the clinical value of susceptibility data provided when atypical species, particularly *M. avium*, is tested. See table.

Additional Information Susceptibilities are performed on the first organism isolated from a patient and at 3- to 6-month intervals if that organism continues to be isolated while the patient is on therapy. Susceptibility tests should be performed in patients with recurrent tuberculosis as resistant strains are common in recurrent infection. In the United States, the rate of newly diagnosed tuberculosis cases has increased since 1985.[2] More alarming is the increased number of nosocomial outbreaks of multidrug-resistant tuberculosis (MDR-TB). Since 1990, over 200 patients have been reported to CDC. These outbreaks have occurred in healthcare workers, prison inmates, and prison employees.[3,4] Failure to take all drugs in a multidrug regimen can lead to a shift toward resistant organisms and treatment failure. Atypical or environmental mycobacteria, particularly strains of the *M. avium* complex, demonstrate variable susceptibility within species. They are frequently resistant to oral therapy.[5]

Footnotes

1. Inderfield CB and Salfinger M, "Antimicrobial Agents and Susceptibility Tests: Mycobacteria," *Manual of Clinical Microbiology*, 6th ed, Murray PR, Baron EJ, Pfaller MA, et al, eds, Washington, DC: American Society for Microbiology, 1995, 1385-1404.

2. Centers for Disease Control, "Tuberculosis Morbidity - United States, 1991," *MMWR Morb Mortal Wkly Rep*, 1992, 41:240.

3. Beck-Sague C, Dooley Sw, Hutton MD, et al, "Hospital Outbreak of Multidrug-Resistant *Mycobacterium tuberculosis* Infections. Factors in Transmission to Staff and HIV-Infected Patients," *JAMA*, 1992, 268(10):1280-6.

Antimicrobials Commonly Used for Mycobacterial Susceptibility Testing

Antituberculosis Drugs	
Primary	**Secondary**
Ethambutol	Capreomycin
Isoniazid	Ciprofloxacin
Pyrazinamide	Cycloserine
Rifampin	Ethionamide
Streptomycin	Kanamycin
Other Mycobacterial Isolates*	
Primary	**Secondary**
Amikacin	Azithromycin
Ciprofloxacin	Clarithromycin
Ethambutol	Clofazimine
Isoniazid	Doxycycline
Rifampin	
Streptomycin	
Sulfonamides	
Tobramycin	

From Wolinsky E, "Mycobacterial Diseases Other Then Tuberculosis," *Clin Infect Dis*, 1992, 15:1-12, with permission.

*Drug regimens will depend on the mycobacterial species identified.

4. Dooley SW, Villarino ME, Lawrence M, et al, "Nosocomial Transmission of Tuberculosis in a Hospital Unit for HIV-Infected Patients," *JAMA*, 1992, 267(19):2632-4.

5. Wolinsky E, "Mycobacterial Diseases Other Than Tuberculosis," *Clin Infect Dis*, 1992, 15(1):1-10.

References

Heifets LB, "Antimycobacterial Drugs," *Semin Respir Infect*, 1994, 9(2):84-103.

Mor N and Heifets L, "MICs and MBCs of Clarithromycin Against *Mycobacterium avium* Within Human Macrophages," *Antimicrob Agents Chemother*, 1993, 37(1):111-4.

Neville K, Bromberg A, Bromberg R, et al, "The Third Epidemic - Multidrug-Resistant Tuberculosis," *Chest*, 1994, 105(1):45-8.

Rastogi N and Goh KS, "Effect of pH on Radiometric MICs of Clarithromycin Against 18 Species of Mycobacteria," *Antimicrob Agents Chemother*, 1992, 36(12):2841-2.

Siddiqi SH, Heifets LB, Cynamon MH, et al, "Rapid Broth Macrodilution Method for Determination of MICs for *Mycobacterium avium* Isolates," *J Clin Microbiol*, 1993, 31(9):2332-8.

Van Scoy RE and Wilkowske CJ, "Antituberculous Agents," *Mayo Clin Proc*, 1992, 67(2):179-87.

Antimicrobial Susceptibility Testing, Unusual Isolates/Fastidious Organisms

CPT 87181 (agar dilution, each antibiotic); 87184 (disk method, each antibiotic); 87186 (microtiter); 87188 (tube dilution, each antibiotic)

Related Information

Antimicrobial Susceptibility Testing, Aerobic and Facultatively Anaerobic Bacteria *on page 448*

Antimicrobial Susceptibility Testing, Anaerobic Bacteria *on page 449*

Antimicrobial Susceptibility Testing, Antimicrobial Combinations *on page 449*

Synonyms MIC, Fastidious Organisms, Unusual Isolates; Minimum Inhibitory Concentration, Unusual Isolates; Susceptibility Testing, Unusual Isolates/Fastidious Organisms

Applies to E-Test

Specimen A pure culture of the isolated organism to be tested, prepared by the laboratory

Causes for Rejection Organism disposed of prior to request by physician to save the organism for susceptibility testing. Certain isolates are too fastidious (eg, some anaerobes, some streptococci) to perform susceptibility testing.

Turnaround Time 24-48 hours after isolation of bacterium

Special Instructions An isolate of the organism of interest must be saved at the request of the physician. The request usually must be received by the laboratory within 48 hours of submission of specimen for initial culture in order to perform an MIC test. Broth dilution minimum inhibitory concentration (MIC) susceptibility can be requested for drugs not in the routine panels. The laboratory should be informed by the physician of the specific source of the culture, culture date, the specific bacterial isolate to be tested, and the antimicrobial agent to be tested.

Reference Range Minimal inhibitory concentration reported in μg/mL of antimicrobial agent. Results may be qualitatively reported as susceptible (S), intermediate (I), and resistant (R).

Use Determine minimum inhibitory concentration (MIC) of a given organism to an antimicrobial agent

Limitations The organism may fail to grow in media used for testing. A disk diffusion susceptibility test (Kirby-Bauer susceptibility) is usually reported (susceptible, intermediate, resistant) if interpretive criteria exist. If interpretive criteria do not exist, the MIC or zone size will be reported.

Methodology Microtiter or macrotiter broth dilution technique, disk diffusion. Special methods are required for individual species. These generally include addition of supplement and/or alteration of incubation atmosphere.

Additional Information The terms "fastidious or unusual isolates" refer to organisms which do not grow well on Mueller-Hinton medium or are unusual in that there is insufficient data to document that reliable susceptibility testing can be performed by routine methods. Organisms such as *Haemophilus influenzae* and *Neisseria gonorrhoeae* have developed resistance to beta-lactam antibiotics by plasmid or chromosomal genes mediating the production of beta-lactamase.[1,2] Other organisms, such as *Streptococcus pneumoniae*, have developed chromosomal gene mediated alteration of the penicillin-binding proteins. Because of the emergence of resistance, empiric therapy with penicillin or ampicillin can no longer be relied upon, and susceptibility testing for those "fastidious" organisms may be necessary. Susceptibility testing for group A streptococci is still not necessary because the organism remains highly susceptible to penicillin, which is the drug of choice. Rare resistant strains have been reported.

The following organisms generally require special susceptibility testing procedures: anaerobes, *Moraxella* (*Branhamella*) *catarrhalis*, *Helicobacter* sp, *Corynebacterium* sp, *Francisella tularensis*, *Haemophilus influenzae*, *Legionella* sp, *Listeria monocytogenes*, *Neisseria meningitidis*, *Neisseria gonorrhoeae*, *Nocardia* sp, nonfermentative bacteria, *Streptococcus pneumoniae*, *Streptococcus* sp, *Streptococcus* sp peridoxal dependent, *Enterococcus* sp.

Methods for susceptibility testing of the above organisms are reasonably well defined and are designed to vary as little as possible from the well established methods used for rapidly growing "nonfastidious" aerobic organisms.[3]

The **E test** is a new *in vitro* susceptibility testing method now being used for quantitative determination of susceptibility to antimicrobial agents.[4,5] This test uses a defined continuous antimicrobial gradient on a thin plastic strip. When the E-strip is placed on a confluent lawn of bacteria on agar media, the antimicrobial agent diffuses producing an organism inhibition ellipse. The intercept of the ellipse with the graded test strip indicates MICs. This testing procedure provides a reliable method to assess antimicrobial sensitivity of fastidious isolates.

Footnotes

1. Barry AL, Fuchs PC, and Pfaller MA, "Susceptibilities of β-Lactamase-Producing and - Nonproducing Ampicillin-Resistant Strains of *Haemophilus influenzae* to Ceftibuten, Cefaclor, Cefuroxine, Cefixime, Cefotaxime, and Amoxicillin-Clavulanic Acid," *Antimicrob Agents Chemother*, 1993, 37(1):14-8.
2. Fuchs PC, Barry AL, Baker CN, et al, "Proposed Interpretive Criteria and Quality Control Parameters for Testing Susceptibility of *Neisseria gonorrhoeae* to β-Lactam-Clavulanate Combinations," *J Clin Microbiol*, 1992, 30(8):2191-4.
3. National Committee for Clinical Laboratory Standards, "Performance Standards for Antimicrobial Testing," Fifth Information Supplement NCCLS Document M100-S5 (M7-A2 Aerobic Dilution), Villanova, PA: National Committee for Clinical Laboratory Standards, 1994.
4. Sanchez ML, Barrett MS, and Jones RN, "The E-Test Applied to Susceptibility Tests for Gonococci, Multiply Resistant Enterococci and *Enterobacterioceae* Producing Potent Beta-Lactamases," *Diagn Microbiol Infect Dis*, 1992, 15(5):459-64.
5. Sanchez ML, Barrett MS, and Jones RN, "Use of the E-Test to Predict High-Level Resistance to Aminoglycosides Among Enterococci," *J Clin Microbiol*, 1992, 30(11):3030-2.

References

Doern GV, "*In Vitro* Susceptibility Testing of *Haemophilus influenzae*: Review of New National Committee for Clinical Laboratory Standards Recommendations," *J Clin Microbiol*, 1992, 30(12):3035-8.

Doern GV, "Susceptibility Tests of Fastidious Bacteria," *Manual of Clinical Microbiology*, 6th ed, Murray PR, Baron EJ, Pfaller MA, et al, eds, Washington, DC: American Society for Microbiology, 1995, 1342-9.

Fekete T, "Antimicrobial Susceptibility Testing of *Neisseria gonorrhoea* and Implications for Epidemiology and Therapy," *Clin Microbiol Rev*, 1993, 6(1):22-3.

Jorgensen JH, Doern GV, Maher LA, et al, "Antimicrobial Resistance Among Respiratory Isolates of *Haemophilus influenzae*, *Moraxella catarrhalis*, and *Streptococcus pneumoniae* in the United States," *Antimicrob Agents Chemother*, 1990, 34(11):2075-80.

Powell MD, McVey MH, Kassim MH, et al, "Antimicrobial Susceptibility of *Streptococcus pneumoniae*, *Haemophilus influenzae*, and *Moraxella* (*Branhamella catarrhalis*) Isolated in the UK From Sputa," *J Antimicrob Chemother*, 1991, 28(2):249-59.

ARD, Blood Culture *see* Bacterial Culture, Blood *on page 457*

Arthropod Identification

CPT 88300 (surgical pathology gross examination)

Related Information

Babesiosis Serological Test *on page 370*
Ehrlichiosis Serology *on page 390*
Lyme Disease Serology *on page 415*
Q Fever Titer *on page 426*
Rocky Mountain Spotted Fever Serology *on page 427*

Synonyms Ectoparasite Identification; Insect Identification

Applies to *Cimex* Identification; Flea Identification; *Ixodes dammini* Identification; Lice Identification; Mite Identification; Nits Identification; *Pediculus humanus* Identification; *Phthirus pubis* Identification; Rocky Mountain Spotted Fever, *Dermacentor andersoni*; *Sarcoptes scabiei* Skin Scrapings Identification; Skin Scrapings for *Sarcoptes scabiei* Identification; Tick Identification

Abstract Arthropoda is a phylum which includes Arachnida and Insecta, among other classes. Species include parasites and vectors. Arachnida includes spiders, ticks, mites, and scorpions.

Specimen Gross arthropod, skin scrapings

Container Screw-cap tube or screw-cap jar

Collection Arthropods (gross) are to be submitted in alcohol (70%) or formaldehyde in tube or container with secure closure. To establish the diagnosis of scabies, skin scrapings may be collected with a scalpel and a drop of mineral oil. The liquid may be examined directly or alternatively the organism may be teased away from its burrow or papule with a needle or scalpel.

Storage Instructions Maintain specimen at room temperature. Fill the container with preservative as completely as possible to avoid damage to the specimen by air bubbles in the container.

Use Identify arthropods affecting man; establish the presence of ectoparasite infestation

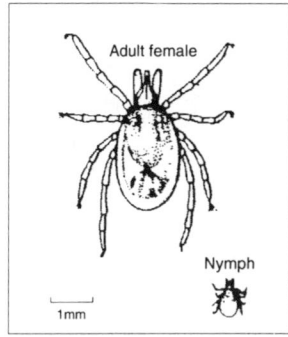

Deer tick (*Ixodes dammini*)

Methodology Macroscopic evaluation

Additional Information **Lyme disease** and **babesiosis** may be transmitted to humans by two species of ticks. *Ixodes scapularis* (or *I. dammini*) has been implicated along the eastern seaboard, and in southern and north central states. *I. pacificus* is the most common vector in western states. In Europe, **Lyme disease** is most often transmitted to humans by *I. ricinus*. *Ehrlichia* sp known to cause human **ehrlichiosis** are carried by the tick *Amblyomma americanum*. Several other infectious diseases are known to be transmitted by arthropods; **Rocky Mountain spotted fever, tick typhus, Q fever, tularemia, rickettsialpox, and babesiosis**.

The only vector of louseborne **relapsing fever** is the body louse. The other variety of relapsing fever is tickborne.

References

Agger W, Case KL, Bryant GL, et al, "Lyme Disease: Clinical Features, Classification, and Epidemiology in the Upper Midwest," *Medicine (Baltimore)*, 1991, 70(2):83-90.

Dalton MT and Haldane DJ, "Unusual Dermal Arthropod Infestations," *Can Med Assoc J*, 1990, 143(2):113-4.

Fritsche TR and Pfaller MA, "Arthropods of Medical Importance," *Manual of Clinical Microbiology*, 6th ed, Murray PR, Baron EJ, Pfaller MA, et al, eds, Washington, DC: American Society of Microbiology, 1995, 379-99.

Goddard J, *Physician's Guide to Arthropods of Medical Importance*, Boca Raton, FL: CRC Press, 1993.

Hobbs GD and Harrell RE Jr, "Brown Recluse Spider Bites: A Common Cause of Necrotic Arachnidism," *Am J Emerg Med*, 1989, 7(3):309-12.

Honig PJ, "Bites and Parasites," *Pediatr Clin North Am*, 1983, 30:563-81.

Kaslow RA, "Current Perspective on Lyme Borreliosis," *JAMA*, 1992, 267(10):1381-3.

Moffitt JE, Yates AB, and Stafford CT, "Allergy to Insect Stings. A Need for Improved Preventive Management," *Postgrad Med*, 1993, 93(8):197-9, 203-4, 207-8.

Moran ME, Ehreth JT, and Drach GW, "Venomous Bites to the External Genitalia: An Unusual Cause of Acute Scrotum," *J Urol*, 1992, 147(4):1085-6.

Reisman RE, "Venom Hypersensitivity," *J Allergy Clin Immunol*, 1994, 94(4):651-8.

Spach DH, Liles WC, Campbell GL, et al, "Tick-Borne Diseases in the United States," *N Engl J Med*, 1993, 329(13):936-47.

White DJ, Chang H-G, Benach JL, et al, "The Geographic Spread and Temporal Increase of the Lyme Disease Epidemic," *JAMA*, 1991, 266(9):1230-6.

Atypical *Mycobacterium* Smear *see* Acid-Fast Stain *on page 446*

Auramine-Rhodamine Stain *see* Acid-Fast Stain *on page 446*

Autoclave Sterility Check *see* Sterility Culture *on page 497*

Bactec® *see* Bacterial Culture, Blood *on page 457*

Bacterial Antigens by Coagglutination *replaced by* Bacterial Antigens, Rapid Detection Methods *on next page*

Bacterial Antigens by Counterimmunoelectrophoresis *replaced by* Bacterial Antigens, Rapid Detection Methods *on next page*

Bacterial Antigens, CSF *see* Bacterial Antigens, Rapid Detection Methods *on this page*

Bacterial Antigens, Rapid Detection Methods

CPT 86313 (immunoassay, multiple step); 86315 (immunoassay, single step)

Related Information

Bacteremia Detection, Buffy Coat Micromethod *on page 305*
Bacterial Culture, Cerebrospinal Fluid *on page 460*
Cerebrospinal Fluid Analysis *on page 309*
Cerebrospinal Fluid Glucose *on page 105*
Cerebrospinal Fluid Protein *on page 380*
Cryptococcal Antigen Titer *on page 388*
Fungal Culture, Cerebrospinal Fluid *on page 477*
Group A *Streptococcus* Screen, Rapid *on page 483*
Group B *Streptococcus* Screen, Rapid *on page 483*
Mycobacterial Culture, Cerebrospinal Fluid *on page 489*
Viral Culture, Central Nervous System Symptoms *on page 677*

Synonyms Latex Agglutination for Bacterial Antigens

Applies to Bacterial Antigens, CSF; Bacterial Antigens, Urine; Cerebrospinal Fluid Bacterial Antigen Testing

Replaces Bacterial Antigens by Coagglutination; Bacterial Antigens by Counterimmunoelectrophoresis

Test Commonly Includes Qualitative determination of the presence of antigens of *H. influenzae, S. pneumoniae, N. meningitidis.* Test may also identify subgroups of above organisms and may include testing for group B *Streptococcus* and *E. coli* K1 antigen in neonates. Gram's staining and culture take precedence over bacterial antigen testing,[1] and results of Gram's staining must be coordinated with antigen testing by knowledgeable laboratory workers.[2]

Abstract Rapid bacterial antigen tests on CSF is done by latex agglutination.[1,3] The newer antigen detection systems have a reported sensitivity similar to that of the Gram's stain; about 80% of cases have been diagnosed with either technique.[1] However, a study reports that all latex agglutination true-positive CSF specimens show the causative microorganisms in Gram's stain as well. Of 57 latex agglutination positives, 31 were false-positives (54%), 22 were true-positive (38%), and four were indeterminant (7%). There was no change in therapy on the basis of any true-positive result. Results of the 31 false-positives included prolonged hospitalization, clinical complications, and charges of $175,000 without detected benefit.[4] In addition, false-negative results occur.[2] It is recommended that **these latex agglutination tests are not intended as a substitute for bacterial culture. Confirmatory diagnosis of bacterial meningitis infection is possible only with appropriate culture procedures.**[3,5] Concentration of antigen depends on variables including the number of bacteria, the duration of infection, and the presence or absence of specific antibodies which may prevent antigen detection.[5] This controversial test may be done also on urine, pleural fluid, or synovial fluid.

Patient Preparation Usual aseptic aspiration

Specimen Cerebrospinal fluid, serum, urine

Container Sterile CSF tube, red top tube, sterile urine container

Storage Instructions Keep refrigerated. **If culture is requested on the same specimen do not refrigerate.**

Reference Range Negative

Use Although the test is intended to detect bacterial antigens in CSF for the rapid diagnosis of meningitis, its specific indications remain to be elucidated.

Limitations Antigen detection does not replace Gram's stain and culture. May be negative in early meningitis. *Staphylococcus aureus* and *Pseudomonas aeruginosa* are not detected by these methods. Most members of the Enterobacteriaceae also fail to react. Group B *Streptococcus* and the *E. coli* K1 antigen are frequently not tested on patients older than 6 months of age. Antigenic cross reactions are seen. The sensitivity of commercial antigen detection kits remains imperfect.[2] False-negative results occur[1,2] with low antigen load. Pneumococcal and *Haemophilus* strains not possessing capsular antigens may not be detected by immunological techniques. Pneumococcal antigen is not detected in urine. False-positives cause expense and complications.[4] Latex agglutination testing is reported to be least accurate when applied to urine specimens, in which false-positives were often detected.[4]

Methodology Latex agglutination (LA) of capsular polysaccharide bacterial antigen provides rapid laboratory response. Excellent performance and characteristics are recognized.[4]

Additional Information The CSF white blood cell count and differential are the best predictors of meningitis.[6] When discussing the differential diagnosis of meningitis, many authors do not include latex agglutination testing in discussion of laboratory results.[5,7,8,9,10] Granoff et al observed that the test had no measurable impact on patient care in patients with bacterial meningitis. In this series, the role of rapid antigen testing was confirmation of positive Gram's stain results. Culture results rather than antigen testing were used for pivotal decisions. The study noted in discussion that one must await the results of culture and concluded that the test may be helpful only in selected situations.[11]

Antigen detection methods should never be substituted for culture and Gram's stain. Culture and Gram's stain must always have priority when limited quantities of CSF are available.[11]

Bacterial antigens may be detected despite previous antibiotic therapy. Immunologic methods should have an advantage over Gram's stain in partially treated cases, but positive latex agglutination in patients with negative cultures caused by prior antimicrobial treatment were not found in a recent study.[4] The sensitivity ranges for each of the three commercial assays are published for *H. influenzae* type b, *S. pneumoniae, Streptococcus* group B, and *N. meningitidis.*[12] They are variable between manufacturers and with differing organisms, but fall substantially short of 100%.[1,12]

The rapid diagnosis of group A and group B *Streptococcus* infection is discussed specifically in the listings Group A *Streptococcus* Screen, Rapid *on page 483* and Group B *Streptococcus* Screen, Rapid *on page 483.*

Footnotes

1. Fishman RA, *Cerebrospinal Fluid in Diseases of the Nervous System,* 2nd ed, Philadelphia, PA: WB Saunders Co, 1992, 267.
2. Connolly KJ and Hammer SM, "The Acute Aseptic Meningitis Syndrome," *Infect Dis Clin North Am,* 1990, 4(4):599-622.
3. Smith AL, "Bacterial Meningitis," *Pediatr Rev,* 1993, 14(1):11-8.
4. Perkins MD, Mirrett S, and Reller LB, "Rapid Bacterial Antigen Detection Is Not Clinically Useful," *J Clin Microbiol,* 1995, 33(6):1486-91.
5. Rodewald LE, Woodin KA, Szilágyi PG, et al, "Relevance of Common Tests of Cerebrospinal Fluid in Screening for Bacterial Meningitis," *J Pediatr,* 1991, 119(3):363-9.
6. Feuerborn SA, Capps WI, and Jones JC, "Use of Latex Agglutination Testing in Diagnosing Pediatric Meningitis," *J Fam Pract,* 1992, 34(2):176-9..
7. Durand ML, Calderwood SB, Weber DJ, et al, "Acute Bacterial Meningitis in Adults - A Review of 493 Episodes," *N Engl J Med,* 1993, 328(1):21-8.
8. Schaad UB, Suter S, Gianella-Borradori A, et al, "A Comparison of Ceftriazone and Cefuroxime for the Treatment of Bacterial Meningitis in Children," *N Engl J Med,* 1990, 322(3):141-7.
9. Kilpi T, Anttila M, Kallio MJ, et al, "Severity of Childhood Bacterial Meningitis and Duration of Illness Before Diagnosis," *Lancet,* 1991, 338(8764):406-9.
10. Phillips SE and Millan JC, "Reassessment of Microbiology Protocol for Cerebrospinal Fluid Specimens," *Lab Med,* 1991, 22:619-22.
11. Granoff DM, Murphy TV, Ingram DL, et al, "Use of Rapidly Generated Results in Patient Management," *Diagn Microbiol Infect Dis,* 1986, 4(3 Suppl):157S-66S.
12. Gray LD and Fedorko DP, "Laboratory Diagnosis of Bacterial Meningitis," *Clin Microbiol Rev,* 1992, 5(2):130-45.

References

Greenlee JE, "Approach to Diagnosis of Meningitis. Cerebrospinal Fluid Evaluation," *Infect Dis Clin North Am,* 1990, 4(4):583-98.
Spanos A, Harrell FE Jr, and Durack DT, "Differential Diagnosis of Acute Meningitis. An Analysis of the Predictive Value of Initial Observations," *JAMA,* 1989, 262(19):2700-7.

Bacterial Antigens, Urine *see* Bacterial Antigens, Rapid Detection Methods *on this page*

Bacterial Culture, Abscess

CPT 87070 (aerobic); 87075 (anaerobic)

Related Information

Antimicrobial Susceptibility Testing, Aerobic and Facultatively Anaerobic Bacteria *on page 448*
Antimicrobial Susceptibility Testing, Anaerobic Bacteria *on page 449*
Bacterial Culture, Biopsy or Body Fluid *on page 456*
Bacterial Culture, Endometrium *on page 462*
Bacterial Culture, Wound *on page 470*
Fine Needle Aspiration, Deep Seated Lesions *on page 294*
Fine Needle Aspiration, Superficial Palpable Masses *on page 294*

Applies to Aerobic Culture, Abscess; Anaerobic Culture, Abscess

Test Commonly Includes A request for bacterial culture on a specimen of this type will result in a Gram's stain and aerobic and anaerobic bacterial cultures. At some institutions, culture for anaerobic bacteria must be specifically requested, especially if specimens are submitted on swabs.

Patient Preparation The aspiration site is prepared aseptically. The overlying and adjacent areas must be carefully prepared to eliminate potentially contaminating aerobic and anaerobic bacteria which colonize the skin surfaces.

Specimen Fluid, pus, or other material properly obtained from an abscess for optimal yield. This material should suffice for both aerobic and anaerobic cultures.

Container Specimen may be aspirated into a syringe and capped with an airtight stopper; all air should be expelled from the syringe prior to transport. Alternatively, clinical material may be transferred from the syringe to commercially available vials that contain anaerobic indicators and maintain anaerobic conditions. Specimens may also be transferred to sterile containers that do not maintain anaerobic conditions, but transport to the laboratory should be expedited to maximize survival of anaerobes. Submission of specimens in syringes with needles are not acceptable because of concerns about needlestick injuries. Swabs (even anaerobic swabs) provide inferior specimens.

Collection Contamination with normal flora must be avoided. Some anaerobes will be killed by contact with oxygen for only a few seconds. Ideally, pus obtained by needle aspiration through an intact surface, which has been aseptically prepared, is put directly into an anaerobic transport device or transported directly to the laboratory in the original syringe. Sampling of open lesions is enhanced by deep aspiration using a sterile needle and syringe. Curettings of the base of an open lesion may also provide a good yield. Irrigation should be done with nonbacteriostatic sterile saline. Pulmonary samples are obtained by transtracheal percutaneous needle aspiration by trained physicians or by use of a special sheathed catheter. If swabs must be used, two should be collected; one for culture and one for Gram's stain. Specimens collected and transported in syringes should be transported to the laboratory within 30 minutes of collection.

Storage Instructions Syringes should have air expelled and needles removed.

Causes for Rejection Specimens exposed to air, specimens which have been refrigerated, or have an excessive delay in transit have a less than optimal yield.

Clinical Observations Suggestive of Anaerobic Infection

Foul-smelling discharge
Location of infection in proximity to a mucosal surface
Necrotic tissue, gangrene, pseudomembrane formation
Gas in tissues or discharges
Endocarditis with negative routine blood cultures
Infection associated with malignancy or other process producing tissue destruction
Infection related to the use of aminoglycosides (oral, parenteral, or topical)
Septic thrombophlebitis
Bacteremic picture with jaundice
Infection resulting from human or other bites
Black discoloration of blood-containing exudates (may fluoresce red under ultraviolet light in *B. melaninogenicus* infections)
Presence of "sulfur granules" in discharges (actinomycosis)
Classical clinical features of gas gangrene
Clinical setting suggestive for anaerobic infection (septic abortion, infection after gastrointestinal surgery, genitourinary surgery, etc)

From Bartlett JG," Anaerobic Bacterial Infections of the Lung," *Chest*, 1987, 91:901-9, with permission.

Use Define the microbial etiology of the abscess and provide a guide for therapy

Limitations Fastidious anaerobes may not be recovered despite significant efforts to collect and properly submit a specimen. Any specimen submitted for microbial culture can be contaminated with colonizing organisms that are not contributing to disease. Organisms most likely to contaminate specimens of this type include, but are not limited to, *Corynebacterium* sp and coagulase-negative staphylococci. These organisms are not invariably contaminants, however, and may be pathogenic in certain settings. A Gram's stain should always be performed, if sufficient material is obtained, to provide early presumptive information and to help interpret culture results.

The only sources for specimens with established validity for meaningful anaerobic culture in patients with pleuropulmonary infections are blood, pleural fluid, transtracheal aspirates, transthoracic pulmonary aspirates, specimens obtained at thoracotomy, and fiberoptic bronchoscopic aspirates using the protected brush or sheathed catheter. Pleural fluid is preferred for patients with empyema[1]. Blood cultures yield positive results in <5% of cases of anaerobic pulmonary infection. Specimens received in anaerobic transport containers are not optimal for aerobic fungus cultures.

Usual laboratory procedure includes screening only for aerobic bacteria and rapidly growing anaerobes (*Bacteroides fragilis*, *Clostridium perfringens*, *Fusobacterium*, and anaerobic gram-positive cocci). Slow-growing *Mycobacterium* sp or *Nocardia* sp which may cause abscesses will **not** be recovered in routine bacterial cultures even if present, since extended

incubation periods or special media are necessary for their isolation. Cultures for these organisms should be specifically requested.

Contraindications Bronchoscopically-obtained specimens are not ideal as the instrument becomes contaminated by organisms normally contaminating the oropharynx during insertion. Culture of specimens from sites harboring endogenous anaerobic organisms or contaminated by endogenous organisms may be misleading with regard to etiology and selection of appropriate therapy. Special sheathed catheters are available to reduce oropharyngeal flora contamination of bronchial aspirate cultures.

Methodology Aerobic and anaerobic culture, usually with broth and solid media. Special handling to maintain anaerobic conditions is required.

Additional Information Serious anaerobic infections are often due to mixed flora which are pathologic synergists. Anaerobes frequently recovered from closed postoperative wound infections include *Bacteroides fragilis*, approximately 50%; *Prevotella melaninogenica* (previously *Bacteroides melaninogenicus*), approximately 25%; *Peptostreptococcus prevotii*, approximately 15%; and *Fusobacterium* sp, approximately 25%. Anaerobes are seldom recovered in pure culture (10% to 15% of cultures). Aerobes and facultative bacteria when present are frequently found in lesser numbers than the anaerobes. Anaerobic infection is most commonly associated with operations involving opening or manipulating the bowel or a hollow viscus (eg, appendectomy, cholecystectomy, colectomy, gastrectomy, bile duct exploration, etc). The ratio of anaerobes to facultative species is normally about 10:1 in the mouth, vagina, and sebaceous glands and at least 1000:1 in the colon.

Footnotes
1. Bartlett JG, "Anaerobic Bacterial Infections of the Lung," *Chest*, 1987, 91(6):901-9.

References
Brook I, "The Effect of Antimicrobial Therapy on Mixed Infections With *Bacteroides* Species. Is Eradication of the Anaerobes Important?" *J Infect*, 1991, 22(1):27-35.
Brook I and Frazier EH, "Significant Recovery of Nonsporulating Anaerobic Rods From Clinical Specimens," *Clin Infect Dis*, 1993, 16(4):476-80.
Finegold SM, Jousimies-Somer HR, and Wexler HM, "Current Perspectives on Anaerobic Infections: Diagnostic Approaches," *Infect Dis Clin North Am*, 1993, 7(2):257-75.
Hill MK and Sanders CV, "Anaerobic Disease of the Lung," *Infect Dis Clin North Am*, 1991, 5(3):453-66.
Holden J, "Collection and Transport of Clinical Specimens for Anaerobic Culture," *Clinical Microbiology Procedures Handbook*, Isenberg HD, ed, Washington, DC: American Society of Microbiology.
Nichols RL and Smith JW, "Anaerobes From a Surgical Perspective," *Clin Infect Dis*, 1994, 18(Suppl 4):S280-6.

Bacterial Culture, Aerobes

Related Information
Antimicrobial Susceptibility Testing, Aerobic and Facultatively Anaerobic Bacteria *on page 448*
Bacterial Culture, Anaerobes *on next page*
Bacterial Culture, Ear *on page 462*
Bacterial Culture, Intravascular Device *on page 463*
Gram's Stain *on page 481*

Synonyms Aerobic Bacterial Culture

Applies to Enterobacteriaceae; Enterococci; *Haemophilus*; *Neisseria*; *Pseudomonas*; Staphylococci; Streptococci

Test Commonly Includes Culture of aerobic or facultative anaerobes contributing to an infectious process. May also include antimicrobial susceptibility testing.

Abstract Culture for aerobic bacteria utilizes methods capable of detecting obligately aerobic (those incapable of reproducing in the absence of oxygen) and facultatively anaerobic (those capable of reproducing in the presence or absence of oxygen) organisms. Obligately anaerobic organisms (those incapable of reproducing in the presence of oxygen) will not be recovered in aerobic cultures.

Patient Preparation Varies with source.

Specimen Body site, tissue, or fluid associated with infection

Container Sterile container or swab; varies with source

Collection Varies with source.

Turnaround Time Varies with specimen. Negative results are typically reported as follows: blood and CSF: 5-7 days; urine: 1 day; sputum and wounds: 2 days; aseptically obtained body fluids: 5 days. Preliminary morphologic information for positive cultures (for specimens other than blood and aseptically obtained body fluids) is usually available within 24 hours; speciation and antimicrobial susceptibility is usually available 24 hours later.

Use Recover, identify, and determine antimicrobial susceptibility for obligately aerobic and facultatively anaerobic bacteria suspected of causing infections

Limitations Routine aerobic bacterial cultures are designed to recover most potential bacterial pathogens; however, obligate anaerobes (eg, *Clostridium*, *Bacteroides*, *Peptostreptococcus*, *Actinomyces*, *Fusobacterium*, *Prevotella*, *Porphyromonas* spp) and unusual or difficult to grow (Continued)

Bacterial Culture, Aerobes *(Continued)*

aerobic organisms (eg, *Nocardia*, *Legionella*, *Mycobacterium*, *Rhodococcus*, *Corynebacterium diphtheriae*, *Bordetella pertussis*, *Brucella*, *Francisella tularensis*) may not be recovered using routine methods. Recovery of aerobic bacteria from clinical specimens may represent contamination; it is often very challenging to distinguish contaminating organisms from etiologic agents of infection (see table). Occasionally, organisms may grow slowly, be difficult to isolate in pure culture, be difficult to identify, or present technical challenges in performing antimicrobial susceptibility tests; these organisms will result in delayed reporting. Initial recovery of organisms from blood and body fluids may take several days.

Possible Sources of Contamination With Normal Bacterial Flora

Body Sites	Specimens Contaminated
Skin	Blood culture, abscess, wound, eye, middle ear
Oralpharyngeal	Sputum, gastric biopsy, oral lesion or abscess
Vagina	Urine, endometrial, genital
Gastrointestinal tract	Urine

Methodology Inoculation of microbiological media, incubation of media at temperatures varying from 25°C to 42°C (usually 35°C) in ambient or CO_2-enhanced atmospheric conditions

Additional Information The overwhelming majority of bacterial pathogens are facultatively anaerobic organisms (eg, all streptococci, enterococci, staphylococci, members of the family Enterobacteriaceae, *Haemophilus influenzae*, *Pasteurella multicida*, *Vibrio* spp). There are relatively few obligately aerobic bacteria that are human pathogens; those that are commonly encountered include *Pseudomonas* spp and most *Neisseria* spp.

Streptococcal infections include erysipelas, acute cellulitis, necrotizing infections, and **streptococcal toxic shock syndrome**. Characteristics of the last include pain at the infection site, fever, impaired renal function preceding hypotension. Laboratory studies include marked left shift in granulocytes, uremia, hypocalcemia, hypoalbuminemia, thrombocytopenia, hematuria, and increased CK.[1]

Footnotes

1. Bisno AL and Stevens DL, "Streptococcal Infections of Skin and Soft Tissues," *N Engl J Med*, 1996, 334(4):240-5.

References

Isenberg HD and D'Amato RF, "Indigenous and Pathogenic Microorganisms of Humans," *Manual of Clinical Microbiology*, 6th ed, Murray PR, Baron EJ, Pfaller MA, et al, eds, Washington, DC: American Society for Microbiology, 1995, 5-18.

Miller JM and Holmes HT, "Specimen Collection, Transport, and Storage," *Manual of Clinical Microbiology*, 6th ed, Murray PR, Baron EJ, Pfaller MA, et al, eds, Washington, DC: American Society for Microbiology, 1995, 19-32.

Tuomanen EI, Austrian R, and Masure HR, "Pathogenesis of Pneumococcal Infection," *N Engl J Med*, 1995, 332(19):1280-4.

Bacterial Culture, Anaerobes

Related Information

Actinomyces Culture *on page 447*

Antimicrobial Susceptibility Testing, Anaerobic Bacteria *on page 449*

Bacterial Culture, Aerobes *on previous page*

Gram's Stain *on page 481*

Synonyms Anaerobic Bacterial Culture

Test Commonly Includes Culture for anaerobic bacteria

Abstract Culture for anaerobic bacteria utilizes methods capable of detecting obligate anaerobes (those incapable of reproducing in the absence of oxygen). Facultatively anaerobic (those capable of reproducing in the presence of oxygen) organisms are also recovered in these cultures, but the primary purpose of anaerobic cultures is to recover obligate anaerobes. Only 20-25 species are clinically relevant.

Specimen Abscess, blood, aseptically obtained body fluid (eg, pleural, peritoneal, synovial), wounds, etc

Container Needle and syringe; biopsy; anaerobic transport media, blood culture media

Collection Swabs usually cause unacceptable exposure of anaerobes to oxygen and have a propensity to dry out.

Causes for Rejection Specimens from sites in which anaerobic bacteria are normal flora (eg, throat, rectal swabs, urine, bronchial washes, cervico-vaginal mucosal swabs, sputums) are unacceptable for anaerobic culture.

Turnaround Time Negative cultures are typically reported as follows: blood cultures: 5-7 days; aseptically obtained body fluids: 5 days; swab specimen: 2-5 days. Prolonged turnaround times present a problem for clinical care.

Use Recover and identify obligately anaerobic bacteria suspected of causing infections

Limitations Anaerobic bacterial cultures are designed to recover most common obligately anaerobic bacterial pathogens. Some obligate anaerobes die after brief exposure to oxygen and are very difficult to recover in culture. Anaerobic bacteria may contaminate clinical specimens that are not collected aseptically; it is often very challenging to distinguish contaminants from etiologic agents of infection.

Contraindications It is usually not relevant to seek anaerobes in acute cholecystitis, acute osteomyelitis, acute otitis media, acute sinusitis, appendicitis, bronchitis, cystitis, meningitis, pharyngitis, primary peritonitis, pyelonephritis, or superficial skin lesions.[1]

Methodology Inoculation of microbiological media suitable for recovering anaerobes and incubation of media at 35°C in an atmosphere lacking oxygen. Gas-liquid chromatography (GLC), DNA hybridization, and RNA homology and sequencing define anaerobic genera.

Additional Information Common obligately anaerobic potential pathogens include *Bacteroides*, *Prevotella*, *Porphyromonas*, *Peptostreptococcus*, and *Fusobacterium* spp. These organisms have been associated with a wide variety of infections outlined in the table.

Principle Types of Anaerobic Infections

Location	Type of Infection
Head and neck	Brain abscess
	Gingivitis
	Chronic sinusitis
	Chronic otitis
	Odontogenic and oropharyngeal space infections
Respiratory tract	Aspiration pneumonia
	Necrotizing pneumonia
	Lung abscess
	Empyema (adults)
Gastrointestinal tract	Peritonitis
	Intra-abdominal abscess
	Liver abscess
Female genital tract	Tubo-ovarian abscess
	Salpingitis (30% to 50% of cases)
	Septic abortion and endometritis
	Bartholin's gland abscess
	Bacterial vaginosis
Skin and soft tissue	Crepitant cellulitis
	Necrotizing fasciitis
	Myonecrosis (gas gangrene)
	Decubitus ulcer
	Diabetic foot ulcer
	Bite wounds

From Styrt B and Gorbach SL, "Recent Developments in the Understanding of the Pathogenesis and Treatment of Anaerobic Infections," *N Engl J Med*, 1989, 321:240-6, with permission.

Clostridia are the only gram-positive spore-forming anaerobic bacilli. Other anaerobes include both gram-positive and negative cocci and bacilli. Exogenous clostridial infections are much less common than endogenous infections.

Footnotes

1. Allen SD, Siders JA, and Marler LM, "Current Issues and Problems in Dealing With Anaerobes in the Clinical Laboratory," *Clin Lab Med*, 1995, 15(2):333-64.

References

Isenberg HD and D'Amato RF, "Indigenous and Pathogenic Microorganisms of Humans," *Manual of Clinical Microbiology*, 6th ed, Murray PR, Baron EJ, Pfaller MA, et al, eds, Washington, DC: American Society for Microbiology, 1995, 5-18.

Miller JM and Holmes HT, "Specimen Collection, Transport, and Storage," *Manual of Clinical Microbiology*, 6th ed, Murray PR, Baron EJ, Pfaller MA, et al, eds, Washington, DC: American Society for Microbiology, 1995, 19-32.

Bacterial Culture, Biopsy or Body Fluid

CPT 87070

Related Information

Actinomyces Culture *on page 447*

Bacterial Culture, Abscess *on page 454*

Bacterial Culture, Endometrium *on page 462*

Bacterial Culture, Wound *on page 470*

Body Fluid *on page 89*

Body Fluid Analysis, Cell Count *on page 306*

Body Fluid Cytology *on page 286*

Body Fluid pH *on page 92*

Bone Marrow *on page 307*
Fine Needle Aspiration, Deep Seated Lesions *on page 294*
Fine Needle Aspiration, Superficial Palpable Masses *on page 294*
Fungal Culture, Biopsy or Body Fluid *on page 476*
Gram's Stain *on page 481*
Histopathology *on page 42*
Lymph Node Biopsy *on page 50*
Mycobacterial Culture, Biopsy or Body Fluid *on page 487*
Synovial Fluid Analysis *on page 656*

Synonyms Biopsy Aerobic Culture; Body Fluid Aerobic Culture

Applies to Bone Marrow Culture; Synovial Fluid Culture; Tissue Culture

Test Commonly Includes Aerobic and anaerobic culture of biopsy or body fluid; may include Gram's stain and susceptibility testing on selected pathogens.

Patient Preparation Aseptic preparation of biopsy site or site of body fluid.

Specimen Aseptically aspirated body fluid (excludes cerebrospinal fluid, blood, and urine) or biopsy from normally sterile site. A single specimen will usually suffice for both aerobic and anaerobic cultures.

Container Sterile container with lid, Petri dish, no preservative. Bone marrow aspirates and body fluids may be directly inoculated into blood culture media.

Collection Do not submit swab, it is rarely productive. The portion of the biopsy specimen submitted for culture should be separated from the portion submitted for histopathology by the surgeon or pathologist, utilizing sterile technique. Bedside inoculation of blood culture bottles with ascitic fluid improves sensitivity.[1]

Causes for Rejection Specimens in fixative, biopsy specimens from sites which have anaerobic bacteria as normal flora

Turnaround Time Preliminary negative reports can be generated for aerobic bacteria within 1 day and for anaerobic bacteria within 2 days. Final negative results are usually provided after 4-5 days of incubation; if actinomycosis is suspected, however, the specimen may be held for 2 weeks. Positive results may be generated by 18-24 hours (preliminary results for aerobic culture), but final positive results for anaerobic cultures take at least 4 days, and often take considerably longer if speciation and antimicrobial susceptibilities are required (7-14 days).

Use Isolate and identify aerobic and anaerobic bacteria before causing infections in tissue

Limitations Any specimen submitted for bacterial culture can be contaminated with colonizing organisms that are not contributing to disease. *Corynebacterium* spp, *Propionibacterium acnes*, and coagulase-negative staphylococci are usually contaminants and should only be considered pathogens if there is substantial evidence that they are clinically significant (eg, repeated isolation, present in large numbers on Gram's stain, more likely pathogens absent). Typical pathogens (such as *E. coli, P. aeruginosa, Enterococcus* spp, *Bacteroides*, and *Peptostreptococcus* spp) may also contaminate clinical specimens (eg, biopsy specimens of chronically-infected wounds); in order to enhance the value of cultures of this type, it is necessary to carefully debride the site prior to specimen collection and collect viable infected tissue. A Gram's stain should always be performed if sufficient material is obtained to provide early presumptive information and to help interpret culture results.

Specimens collected on swabs, exposed to air, or have had excessive travel time to the laboratory may have less than optimal yield of obligate anaerobes.

Methodology Aerobic and anaerobic culture

Additional Information Whenever possible, the specimen should be obtained before empiric antimicrobial therapy is started.

The organisms recovered from ascitic fluid of patients with spontaneous **bacterial peritonitis** are usually portions of normal intestinal flora; 92% are monomicrobial.[2]

Footnotes
1. Runyon BA, "Care of Patients With Ascites," *N Engl J Med*, 1994, 330(5):337-42.
2. Gilbert JA and Kamath PS, "Spontaneous Bacterial Peritonitis: An Update," *Mayo Clin Proc*, 1995, 70(4):365-70.

References
Chapin-Robertson K, Dahlberg SE, and Edberg SC, "Clinical and Laboratory Analysis of Cytospin-Prepared Gram Stains for Recovery and Diagnosis of Bacteria From Sterile Body Fluids," *J Clin Microbiol*, 1992, 30(2):377-80.
Simor AE, Roberts FJ, and Smith JA, "Infections of the Skin and Subcutaneous Tissues," *Cumitech 23*, Smith JA, ed, Washington, DC: American Society for Microbiology, 1988.

Bacterial Culture, Blood

CPT 87040

Related Information
Bacteremia Detection, Buffy Coat Micromethod *on page 305*
Bacterial Culture, Cerebrospinal Fluid *on page 460*
Bacterial Culture, Intravascular Device *on page 463*

Bacterial Culture, Sputum *on page 465*
Bacterial Culture, Stool *on page 466*
Brucella Culture *on page 472*
Brucellosis Agglutinins *on page 372*
Buffy Coat Smear Study of Peripheral Blood *on page 309*
Entamoeba histolytica Serological Test *on page 391*
Fungal Culture, Blood *on page 477*
Leptospira Culture *on page 486*
Salmonella Titer *on page 429*
Tularemia Agglutinins *on page 436*
Viral Culture *on page 675*
Viral Culture, Blood *on page 677*
Yersinia enterocolitica Antibody *on page 440*
Yersinia pestis Antibody *on page 440*

Synonyms Aerobic Culture, Blood; Anaerobic Culture, Blood; Culture, Blood

Applies to Antimicrobial Removal Device (ARD) Blood Culture; ARD, Blood Culture; Bactec®; Blood Culture, BactAlert®; Blood Culture, Isolator™; Blood Culture, Lysis Centrifugation; Blood Culture With Antimicrobial Removal Device (ARD); *Francisella tularensis* Culture; Isolator™ Blood Culture

Test Commonly Includes Isolation of both aerobic and anaerobic microorganisms and antimicrobial susceptibility testing on all significant isolates

Abstract Factors relevant to detection of microbial pathogens in blood include the volume of blood cultured, the number of separate cultures, the extent of dilution, the types of media, devices selected, and the presence of antibiotics.

Patient Preparation Blood cultures are often contaminated by skin flora. This contamination can be markedly reduced by careful attention to skin preparation and antisepsis **prior** to collection of the specimen.

After location of the vein by palpation, the venipuncture site should be cleansed with 70% alcohol (isopropyl or ethyl) and then swabbed in a circular motion concentrically from the center outward using tincture of iodine or a povidone iodine solution. **The iodine should be allowed to dry before the venipuncture is undertaken.** If palpation is required during the venipuncture, the glove covering the palpating finger tip should be disinfected. In iodine-sensitive patients, a double alcohol, green soap, or acetone alcohol preparation may be substituted.

Aftercare Iodine used in the skin preparation should be carefully removed from the skin after venipuncture.

Specimen Venous blood. The yield of positives is not increased by culturing arterial blood even in endocarditis.

Container Bottles of trypticase soy broth or other standard medium. Recovery may be enhanced by lysis filtration or concentration.[1]

Sampling Time Ideally, three sets of blood cultures should be collected per febrile episode; collection of each set should be temporally separated (by at least 1 hour) from the previous specimen. This provides maximum recovery of microorganisms in patients with intermittent bacteremia, and documentation of persistent bacteremia in patients with intravascular infections (eg, endocarditis, intravenous catheter site infections). If multiple sets must be collected simultaneously, draw two sets initially from separate sites, and collect a third set at least 1 hour later. Although three blood culture sets provide optimal yield, the cost effectiveness of this approach has been challenged and some individuals propose collecting only two sets per febrile episode. **More than three sets of blood cultures per day do not add significantly to the rate of pathogen recovery.**

Collection Blood cultures should be drawn prior to initiation of antimicrobial therapy. If more than one culture is ordered, the specimens should be drawn from separately prepared sites. A syringe and needle, transfer set, or pre-evacuated set of tubes containing culture media may be used to collect blood. Collection tubes should be held below the level of the venipuncture to avoid reflux. A sample volume of 10-20 mL in adults or 1-5 mL in pediatric patients is collected for each set. The likelihood of recovering a pathogen increases as the volume of blood sampled increases;[1] however, collecting more than three blood culture sets per bacteremia episode rarely increases yield. If a syringe and needle or transfer set is used, the top of the blood culture bottles should also be aseptically prepared. See table.

Transient bacteremia caused by brushing teeth, bowel movements, etc or by local irritations caused by scratching of the skin may cause positive blood cultures as can contamination by skin flora at the time of collection. Interpretation of results can be enhanced by collecting blood cultures from more than one site and after a time interval (1 hour). Cultures should be taken as early as possible in the course of a febrile episode.

Storage Instructions Specimens collected in tubes with SPS (sodium polyanetholesulfonate) should be processed without delay. The specimen should be transferred to appropriate culture media to avoid any (Continued)

Bacterial Culture, Blood (Continued)

Blood Culture Collection

Clinical Disease Suspected	Culture Recommendation	Rational
Sepsis, meningitis osteomyelitis, septic arthritis, bacterial pneumonia	Two sets of cultures - one from each of two prepared sites, the second drawn after a brief time interval, then begin therapy.	Assure sufficient sampling in cases of intermittent or low level bacteremia. Minimize the confusion caused by a positive culture resulting from transient bacteremia or skin contamination.
Fever of unknown origin (eg, occult abscess, empyema, typhoid fever, etc)	Two sets of cultures - one from each of two prepared sites, the second drawn after a brief time interval (30 minutes). If cultures are negative after 24-48 hours obtain two more sets, preferably prior to an anticipated temperature rise.	The yield after four sets of cultures is minimal. A maximum of three sets per patient per day for 3 consecutive days is recommended.
Endocarditis:		
Acute	Obtain three blood culture sets within 2 hours, then begin therapy.	95% to 99% of acute endocarditis patients (untreated) will yield a positive in one of the first three cultures.
Subacute	Obtain three blood culture sets on day 1, repeat if negative after 24 hours. If still negative or if the patient had prior antibiotic therapy, repeat again.	Adequate sample volume despite low level bacteremia or previous therapy should result in a positive yield.
Immunocompromised host (eg, AIDS):		
Septicemia, fungemia mycobacteremia	Obtain two sets of cultures from each of two prepared sites; consider lysis concentration technique to enhance recovery for fungi and mycobacteria.	Low levels of fungemia and mycobacteremia frequently encountered.
Previous antimicrobial therapy:		
Septicemia, bacteremia; monitor effect of antimicrobial therapy	Obtain two sets of cultures from each of two prepared sites; consider use of antimicrobial removal device (ARD) or increased volume >10 mL/set.	Recovery of organisms is enhanced by dilution, increased sample volume, and removal of inhibiting antimicrobials.

possible decrease in yield due to storage or prolonged contact with SPS. Culture bottles from some automated systems can sit at room temperature for several hours.

Turnaround Time Common laboratory procedure is to issue a final negative culture report after 5-7 days. A preliminary positive culture report based upon Gram's stain and primary subculture is usually available at 24-72 hours.

Special Instructions The requisition should indicate current antibiotic therapy and clinical diagnosis.

Reference Range Negative

Critical Values Positive cultures are immediately phoned to the physician.

Interpretation of Positive Blood Cultures

Virtually *any* organism, including normal flora, **can** cause bacteremia.

A negative culture result does not necessarily rule out bacteremia; false-negative results occur when pathogens fail to grow.

A positive culture result does not necessarily indicate bacteremia; false-positive results occur when contaminants grow.

Gram-negative bacilli, anaerobes, and fungi should be considered pathogens until proven otherwise.

The most difficult interpretation problem is to determine whether an organism that is usually considered normal skin flora is a true pathogen.

From Flournoy DJ and Adkins L, "Understanding the Blood Culture Report," *Am J Infect Control*, 1986,14:41-6, with permission.

Use Isolate, identify, and determine antimicrobial susceptibility of potentially pathogenic organisms causing bacteremia. Blood culture is indicated in community-acquired pneumonia; 67% of positive cultures are *Streptococcus pneumoniae* with that entity.[2]

The most important single test for diagnosis of infective endocarditis is the blood culture. In the absence of antibiotic therapy, negative blood cultures are found in experienced laboratories in <5% of cases.

Limitations Three sets of blood cultures in the absence of antimicrobial therapy provide optimal yield for detection of bacteremia.[3] Prior antibiotic therapy may cause negative blood cultures or delayed growth. The detection of such therapy is important. Blood cultures from patients suspected of having *Brucella*, tularemia, or *Leptospira* must be requested as special cultures. Consultation with the laboratory for the recovery of these organisms prior to collection of the specimen is recommended. When patients with infective endocarditis have negative blood cultures, the differential diagnosis includes fungi. Yeast often are isolated from routine blood cultures. However, if yeast or other fungi are specifically suspected, a separate fungal blood culture should be drawn along with each of the routine blood culture specimens. See separate listing Fungal Culture, Blood *on page 477* for proper collection of specimen. *Mycobacterium avium-intracellulare* (MAI) is recovered from blood of immunocompromised patients, particularly those with acquired immunodeficiency syndrome (AIDS). Special procedures are required for the recovery of these organisms (ie, lysis filtration concentration or use of a special mycobacteria blood culture medium). Radiometric methods facilitate the recovery of mycobacteria from blood.

A substantial fraction of blood culture isolates are not clinically significant. Many of the false-positives involve coagulase-negative staphylococci, however, such organisms can cause serious infections.

Blood culture contamination (ie, false-positives) cause substantial negative financial impact that include laboratory costs, hospital stay, pharmaceutical costs, and associated side effects of inappropriate therapy.

Although a relationship between the volume of blood cultured and detection of pathogens is relevant for low-level bacteremia,[4] the volume of blood removed can be important in children and especially in neonates, whose blood volumes are limited.

Contraindications Use of a 2% iodine preparation is contraindicated in patients sensitive to iodine. Green soap may be substituted for the iodine or alcohol acetone alone may be used.

Methodology Aerobic and anaerobic culture in broth media with detection of bacterial growth by a variety of methods including visual, radiometric, or infrared monitoring, or blind subculture to solid media. The antimicrobial removal device procedure (ARD) includes use of an adsorbent resin in the aerobic bottle. Resin-containing bottles are also available for several automated detection systems. In the lysis centrifugation procedure, blood is lysed and centrifuged using a Wampole Isolator™ tube or similar method. The sediment is inoculated to media appropriate for growing aerobic and anaerobic bacteria, fungi, and mycobacteria. A new method of continuously monitoring media for increased CO_2 content is available.

Additional Information Sequential blood cultures in nonendocarditis patients using a 20 mL sample resulted in an 80% positive yield after the first set, a 93% yield after the second set, and a 98% yield after the third set. Volume of blood cultured seems to be more important than the specific culture technique being employed by the laboratory. The isolation of coagulase-negative staphylococci (CNS) poses a critical and difficult clinical dilemma. Although CNS are the most commonly isolated organism from blood cultures, only a few (6.3%) of the isolates represent "true" clinically significant bacteremia.[5] Conversely, CNS are well recognized as a cause of infections involving prosthetic devices, cardiac valves, CSF shunts, dialysis catheters, and indwelling vascular catheters.[5] Ultimately, the physician is responsible for determination of whether an organism is a contaminant or a pathogen. The decision is based on both laboratory and clinical data. Patient data including patient history, physical examination, body temperatures, clinical course, and laboratory data (ie, culture results, white blood cell count, and differential) are relevant. Clinical experience and judgment may play a significant role in resolution of this clinical dilemma.[6] Various sources of contamination include the patient's own skin flora, transient benign bacteremias, and perhaps, disinfection materials.

The use of a lysis centrifugation system has been reported to increase the recovery rate and decrease the time of fungal recovery compared to traditional or biphasic blood culture systems.[7] Recovery of mycobacteria, atypical mycobacteria, and *Legionella* may also be enhanced by lysis filtration.

The use of antimicrobial removal devices (ARD) or resin bottles to attempt to increase the yield of blood cultures drawn from patients on antimicrobial therapy is controversial. Some microorganisms are occasionally not recovered with the use of ARD blood cultures. It is, therefore, advised that at least one culture in a series of three be requested without the use of the ARD bottles. ARD blood cultures are substantially more expensive than routine blood cultures. There is no consensus as to the effectiveness of the ARD cultures in enhancing recovery of organisms. A recent study reports no significant increase in recovery of organisms with the device.[8] Selective use of the ARD with consideration of the clinical setting has been recommended.[9]

The diagnosis of bacterial meningitis is accomplished by blood culture as well as culture and examination of the cerebrospinal fluid.[10] Most children with bacterial meningitis are initially bacteremic.[11,12] Any organism isolated from the blood is usually tested for susceptibility.

The special problems of *Bartonella* infections (*Rochalimaea henselae*) have been addressed by culture with immunofluorescent confirmation.[13,14]

Footnotes

1. Mermel LA and Maki DG, "Detection of Bacteremia in Adults: Consequences of Culturing an Inadequate Volume of Blood," *Ann Intern Med*, 1993, 119(4):270-2.
2. Bartlett JG and Mundy LM, "Community-Acquired Pneumonia," *N Engl J Med*, 1995, 333(24):1618-24.
3. Ellis CJ, "The Use and Abuse of Blood Cultures," *Infect Dis Newslet*, 1991, 10:27-30.
4. Kellogg JA, Bankert DA, Manzella JP, et al, "Occurrence and Documentation of Low-Level Bacteremia in a Community Hospital's Patient Population," *Am J Clin Pathol*, 1995, 104(5):524-9.
5. Goldmann DA and Pier GB, "Pathogenesis of Infections Related to Intravascular Catheterization," *Clin Microbiol Rev*, 1993, 6(2):176-92.
6. Riley JA and Weinstein MP, "Laboratory Diagnosis of Bacteremia and Endocarditis," *Infect Dis Newslet*, 1991, 10:4-6.
7. Bille J, Stockman L, Roberts GD, et al, "Evaluation of a Lysis Centrifugation System for Recovery of Yeast and Filamentous Fungi From Blood," *J Clin Microbiol*, 1983, 18:469-74.
8. Weinstein MP, Mirrett S, Reimer LG, et al, "Controlled Evaluation of BacT/Alert® Standard Aerobic and FAN Aerobic Blood Culture Bottles for Detection of Bacteremia and Fungemia," *J Clin Microbiol*, 1995, 33(4):978-81.
9. Schwabe LD, Thomson RB Jr, Flint KK, et al, "Evaluation of Bactec® 9240 Blood Culture System by Using High-Volume Aerobic Resin Media," *J Clin Microbiol*, 1995, 33(9):2451-3.
10. Francke E, "The Many Causes of Meningitis," *Postgrad Med*, 1987, 82(2):175-8, 181-3, 187-8.
11. Klein JO, Feigin RD, and McCracken GH Jr, "Report of the Task Force on Diagnosis and Management of Meningitis," *Pediatrics*, 1986, 78(5 Pt 2):959-82.
12. Feigin RD, McCracken GH Jr, and Klein JO, "Diagnosis and Management of Meningitis," *Pediatr Infect Dis J*, 1992, 11(9):785-814.
13. Tierno PM Jr, Inglima K, and Parisi MT, "Detection of *Bartonella* (*Rochalimaea*) *henselae* Bacteremia Using BacT/Alert Blood Culture System," *Am J Clin Pathol*, 1995, 104(5):530-6.
14. Cockerell CJ and Bottone EJ, "*Bartonella* Infections. Evolution From the Esoteric," *Am J Clin Pathol*, 1995, 104(5):487-90.

References

Bannister ER and Woods GL, "Evaluation of Routine Anaerobic Blood Cultures in the BacT/Alert Blood Culture System," *Am J Clin Pathol*, 1995, 104(3):279-82.
Murray PR, Traynor P, and Hopson D, "Critical Assessment of Blood Culture Techniques: Analysis of Recovery of Obligate and Facultative Anaerobes, Strict Aerobic Bacteria, and Fungi in Aerobic and Anaerobic Blood Culture Bottles," *J Clin Microbiol*, 1992, 30(6):462-8.
Ram S, Mylotte JM, and Pisano M, "Rapid Classification of Positive Blood Cultures: Validation and Modification of a Prediction Model," *J Gen Intern Med*, 1995, 10(12):82-8.
Ryan MR and Murray PR, "Laboratory Detection of Anaerobic Bacteremia," *Clin Lab Med*, 1994, 14(1):107-17.
Schifman RB and Pindur A, "The Effect of Skin Disinfection Materials on Reducing Blood Culture Contamination," *Am J Clin Pathol*, 1993, 99(5):536-8.
Sharp SE, McLaughlin JC, Goodman JM, et al, "Clinical Assessment of Anaerobic Isolates From Blood Cultures," *Diagn Microbiol Infect Dis*, 1993, 17(1):19-22.
Tunkel AR and Kaye D, "Endocarditis With Negative Blood Cultures," *N Engl J Med*, 1992, 326(18):1215-7.
Wilson ML, Weinstein MP, Reimer LG, et al, "Controlled Comparison of the BacT/Alert® and Bactec® 660/730 Nonradiometric Blood Culture Systems," *J Clin Microbiol*, 1992, 30(2):323-9.

Bacterial Culture, Bronchoscopy Specimen

CPT 89051 (cell count with differential)

Related Information

Bacterial Culture, Sputum *on page 465*
Bronchial Washings Cytology *on page 287*
Bronchoalveolar Lavage Cytology *on page 288*
Cytomegalic Inclusion Disease Cytology *on page 293*
Cytomegalovirus Antibody *on page 389*
Fungal Culture, Sputum *on page 479*
Mycobacterial Culture, Sputum *on page 490*
Pneumocystis carinii Preparation *on page 299*
Pneumocystis Immunofluorescence *on page 423*
Viral Culture, Respiratory Symptoms *on page 680*

Synonyms Bronchoscopy Specimen Bacterial Culture

Applies to BAL, Culture; Bronchoalveolar Lavage Culture

Test Commonly Includes Semiquantitative aerobic bacterial culture; anaerobic bacterial cultures also performed on Bartlett catheters

Abstract Defining the bacterial etiology of lower respiratory infections occasionally requires collection of specimens at bronchoscopy. The type of specimen collected impacts the information that can be obtained and the way it should be processed in the laboratory.

Specimen Bronchoscopically obtained specimens for bacterial culture fall into three distinct categories:
- bronchial washes
- bronchoalveolar lavages
- specimens obtained using a protected catheter brush (PCB), also called a Bartlett catheter

Container Bartlett catheters should be submitted in 1 mL of sterile nonbacteriostatic saline in a sterile container. Bronchial washes or bronchoalveolar lavages should be submitted in tightly sealed, sterile containers.

Collection Collected at bronchoscopy by a physician skilled in the procedure. Transport the specimen to the laboratory within 1 hour of collection.

Causes for Rejection Bronchial wash specimens can be heavily contaminated with normal oral flora.

Turnaround Time Complete reports of cultures with anaerobic bacteria may require as long as 2 weeks after receipt of culture depending upon the nature of the organisms isolated.

Reference Range Bartlett catheters (in 1 mL saline): $<10^3$ CFU/mL is within the expected level of contamination

Bronchoalveolar lavages: bacteria: $<10^4$ CFU/mL aerobic bacteria; normal total cell count: $4-23 \times 10^6$; differential; 95% alveolar macrophages; 3% lymphocytes; 1% polymorphonuclear cells, 0.2% eosinophils

Bronchial washes: cannot be established; often contaminated heavily with oral flora

Use Identify the etiology of pulmonary infections

Limitations Contamination with oral pharyngeal secretions causes false-positive aerobic and anaerobic bacterial cultures; quantitative or semiquantitative cultures on bronchoalveolar lavage and Bartlett catheter specimens circumvent this problem. The use of bronchoalveolar lavage for defining the etiology of anaerobic pulmonary infections has not been established. Differentiation of colonization versus infection may be difficult with agents such as *Aspergillus* or *Candida* species which occasionally grow in bacterial cultures.

Methodology Semiquantitative or quantitative aerobic bacterial culture for BALs. Semiquantitative aerobic and anaerobic bacterial cultures on solid media for protected catheter brushes.

Additional Information Bronchoalveolar lavage (BAL) has become an established procedure for defining the etiology of pulmonary infections. It is particularly useful for recovering opportunistic pathogens (eg, *Pneumocystis, Histoplasma capsulatum, Candida* spp, *Aspergillus* spp, *Mycobacterium* spp) from immunocompromised individuals and in defining the etiology of nosocomial pneumonia in patients undergoing mechanical ventilation.[1,2,3] It has a role for evaluation of *Legionella, Nocardia, T. gondii*, viruses including CMV and RSV, adenovirus and herpes simplex virus. The procedure has an acceptable morbidity in immunocompromised and thrombocytopenic patients and is often an initial diagnostic procedure in the immunosuppressed. BAL is performed with a catheter wedged into a segmented bronchus. Bronchial washings or airway washings are collected with a nonwedged, more proximally positioned scope tip. Bronchial washings, therefore, preferentially sample airways. Lavage is preferred for the diagnosis of *Pneumocystis* pneumonia, which is primarily an alveolar process. Limiting lavage to one segment reduces the risk of postprocedural respiratory compromise. Quantitative bacterial cultures of BAL specimens have also proven useful for defining the etiology of acute bacterial pneumonia.[4,5]

The abundant normal anaerobic flora of the mouth makes **anaerobic cultures** of any specimen contaminated by oral secretions (eg, bronchial washes, sputums) essentially useless for defining the anaerobic bacterial etiology of lower respiratory infection.[6] Only specimens that bypass the mouth should be cultured anaerobically. Transtracheal aspirates meet this need, but in most hospital settings, they are rarely, if ever, collected. They have been replaced by bronchoscopically obtained specimens using a PCB.[7] Specimens obtained by PCB are subject to low level contamination with normal oral flora, however, this can be accounted for by semiquantitative culture.[8,9]

Footnotes

1. Martin WJ II, Smith TF, Sanderson DR, et al, "Role of Bronchoalveolar Lavage in the Assessment of Opportunistic Pulmonary Infections: Utility and Complications," *Mayo Clin Proc*, 1987, 62(7):549-57.
2. Birriel JA Jr, Adams JA, Saldana MA, et al, "Role of Flexible Bronchoscopy and Bronchoalveolar Lavage in the Diagnosis of Pediatric Acquired Immunodeficiency Syndrome-Related Pulmonary Diseases," *Pediatrics*, 1991, 87(6):897-9.
3. Guerra LF and Baughman RP, "Use of Bronchoalveolar Lavage to Diagnose Bacterial Pneumonia in Mechanically Ventilated Patients," *Crit Care Med*, 1990, 18(2):169-73.
4. Baselski VS, El-Torky M, Coalson JJ, et al, "The Standardization of Criteria for Processing and Interpreting Laboratory Specimens in Patients With Suspected Ventilator-Associated Pneumonia," *Chest*, 1992, 102(5 Suppl 1):571S-9S.
5. Thorpe JE, Baughman RP, Frame PT, et al, "Bronchoalveolar Lavage for Diagnosing Acute Bacterial Pneumonia," *J Infect Dis*, 1987, 155(5):855-61.
6. Bartlett JG, Alexander J, Mayhew J, et al, "Should Fiberoptic Bronchoscopy Aspirates Be Cultured?" *Am Rev Respir Dis*, 1976, 114:73-8.
7. Kirkpatrick MB and Bass JB Jr, "Quantitative Bacterial Cultures of Bronchoalveolar Lavage Fluids and Protected Brush Catheter Specimens From Normal Subjects," *Am Rev Respir Dis*, 1989, 139(2):546-8.
8. Broughton WA, Bass JB, and Kirkpatrick MB, "The Technique of Protected Brush Catheter Bronchoscopy," *J Crit Illness*, 1987, 2:63-70.

(Continued)

Bacterial Culture, Bronchoscopy Specimen
(Continued)

9. Pollock HM, Hawkins EL, Bonner JB, et al, "Diagnosis of Bacterial Pulmonary Infections With Quantitative Protected Catheter Cultures Obtained During Bronchoscopy," *J Clin Microbiol*, 1983, 17:255-9.

References

Henderson AJ, "Bronchoalveolar Lavage," *Arch Dis Child*, 1994, 70(3):167-9.

Matusiewicz SP, Fergusson RJ, Greening AP, et al, "*Pneumocystis carinii* in Bronchoalveolar Lavage Fluid and Bronchial Washings," *BMJ*, 1994, 308(6938):1206-7.

Rankin JA, Collman R, and Daniele RP, "Acquired Immune Deficiency Syndrome and the Lung," *Chest*, 1988, 94(1):155-64.

Xaubet A, Torres A, Marco F, et al, "Pulmonary Infiltrates in Immunocompromised Patients. Diagnostic Value of Telescoping Plugged Catheter and Bronchoalveolar Lavage," *Chest*, 1989, 95(1):130-5.

Yungbluth M, "The Laboratory Diagnosis of Pneumonia. The Role of the Community Hospital Pathologist," *Clin Lab Med*, 1995, 15(2):209-34.

Bacterial Culture, Burn Sites

CPT 87070 (aerobic culture); 87999 (unlisted procedure for quantitation)

Related Information

Bacterial Culture, Wound *on page 470*
Gram's Stain *on page 481*
Zeta Sedimentation Ratio *on page 354*

Synonyms Burn Culture, Quantitative; Quantitative Burn Culture; Skin Burn Culture, Quantitative

Applies to Biopsy Specimen Culture, Quantitative; Quantitative Culture, Biopsy Specimen

Test Commonly Includes Quantitative bacterial counts (colonies/g of tissue) of skin and tissue specimens from burn patients. Identification of bacterial isolates and susceptibility testing when indicated. May also include direct Gram's stain smear and histopathology.

Specimen Viable tissue, **not** eschar

Container Sterile container, no fixative

Collection Aseptic technique

Storage Instructions Transport to the laboratory as soon as possible.

Causes for Rejection Eschar specimen rather than viable tissue, specimen <0.1 g, specimen in fixative

Turnaround Time Quantitative bacterial counts are usually available in 24 hours. Identification of bacterial isolates is usually available in 48 hours.

Special Instructions The laboratory should be informed of the specific site of specimen. The laboratory should be contacted prior to collection of the specimens to ascertain availability and specific procedures required.

Reference Range No growth to <10^5 colonies/g of tissue

Use Determine bacterial identity and quantity of organism present (colonies/g) in tissue or skin specimen from burn patient

Limitations Predictive value for sepsis is limited.

Methodology Culture is performed after weighing the specimen and disruption in a glass homogenizer. Trypticase soy broth is the diluent. Colony counts are reported after 24 and 48 hours of incubation (35°C with CO_2). Fungus cultures are planted on Sabouraud's agar or supplemented Sabouraud's agar and held at 30°C for 4 weeks.

Additional Information Major thermal injuries often precipitate a profound multicentric immunologic depression that may predispose

Histopathologic Findings and Organisms Cultured

Histopathologic Finding	Organism Cultured	No. of Cases
Gram-negative rods	*Pseudomonas aeruginosa*	22
	Klebsiella pneumoniae	4
	Pseudomonas fluorescens	1
	Providencia stuartii	1
	Serratia marcescens	1
	Total	29
Gram-positive cocci	*Staphylococcus aureus*	2
Filamentous fungi	*Aspergillus* species	2
	Fusarium species	2
	Rhizopus species	1
	None*	3
	Total	8

From McManus AT, "Opportunistic Infections in Severely Burned Patients," *Am J Med*, 1984, 75:146-54, with permission.

* Not diagnosed by culture.

patients to sepsis. Impairment of immune function is almost universal in patients with greater than 40% total body surface area burns and in very young or very old patients with far smaller burns.[1] The principal value of quantitative burn-wound biopsies is the demonstration of the predominant burn-wound flora. Agreement of 96% was found between negative culture (<10^5 colonies/g of tissue) and the absence of histopathologic invasive infection. Histopathologic invasion was documented in only 36% of cases with positive cultures.[2] Thus, the use of quantitative burn cultures has little value in identifying patients with invasive infection and in differentiating those patients likely to develop burn-wound sepsis. The organism most frequently recovered from burn wounds is *Pseudomonas aeruginosa*.

Quantitative cultures taken from the center and advancing edge of involved areas from patients with untreated cellulitis had a low yield both in terms of positive (18% of 50) and density of microorganisms recovered except from next to the edges of ulcers. Lymphatic compromise was suspected as a major factor contributing to the intensity of inflammation.[3] See tables.

Potential Mediators of Immunosuppression Following Thermal Injuries

Arachidonic acid metabolites (prostaglandins, leukotrienes)
Interferon
Bacterial endotoxin
Cutaneous burn toxin
Denatured protein
Corticosteroids
Neutrophil products
Histamine
Anaphylatoxins
Suppressive serum proteins
Immunoglobulins (autoantibody)
Immune complexes
Alpha globulin
Alpha fetoprotein
Iatrogenic
Antibiotics
Topical agents
Pain medication (opiates)
Anesthetics
Blood products

From Ninneman JL, "Trauma, Sepsis, and the Immune Response," *J Burn Care Rehabil*, 1987, 8:462-8, with permission.

Footnotes

1. Ninnemann JL, "Trauma, Sepsis, and The Immune Response," *J Burn Care Rehabil*, 1987, 8(6):462-8.
2. McManus AT, Kim SH, McManus WF, et al, "Comparison of Quantitative Microbiology and Histopathology in Divided Burn-Wound Biopsy Specimens," *Arch Surg*, 1987, 122(1):74-6.
3. Duvanel T, Auckenthaler R, and Rohner P, "Quantitative Cultures of Biopsy Specimens From Cutaneous Cellulitis," *Arch Intern Med*, 1989, 149(2):293-6.

References

Kagan RJ and Warden GD, "Management of the Burn Wound," *Clin Dermatol*, 1994, 12(1):47-56.

Ninnemann JL, "Clinical and Immune Status of Burn Patients," *Antibiot Chemother*, 1987, 39:16-25.

Pruitt BA Jr and McManus AT, "Opportunistic Infections in Severely Burned Patients," *Am J Med*, 1984, 76(3A):146-54.

Robson MC, "Quantitative Bacteriology and the Burned Patient," *Quantitative Bacteriology: Its Role in the Armamentarium of the Surgeon*, Heggers JP and Robson MC, eds, Boca Raton, FL: CRC Press Inc, 1991, 97-108.

Bacterial Culture, Cerebrospinal Fluid

CPT 87070

Related Information

Bacterial Antigens, Rapid Detection Methods *on page 454*
Bacterial Culture, Blood *on page 457*
Cerebrospinal Fluid Analysis *on page 309*
Cerebrospinal Fluid Cytology *on page 290*
Cerebrospinal Fluid Glucose *on page 105*
Cerebrospinal Fluid Lactic Acid *on page 106*
Cerebrospinal Fluid LD *on page 106*
Cerebrospinal Fluid Protein *on page 380*
Enterovirus Genome Detection *on page 510*
FTA-ABS, Cerebrospinal Fluid *on page 394*
Fungal Culture, Cerebrospinal Fluid *on page 477*
Gram's Stain *on page 481*
India Ink Preparation *on page 484*

Mycobacterial Culture, Cerebrospinal Fluid *on page 489*
VDRL, Cerebrospinal Fluid *on page 438*
Viral Culture, Central Nervous System Symptoms *on page 677*

Synonyms Cerebrospinal Fluid Culture; CSF Culture; Culture, Cerebrospinal Fluid; Spinal Fluid Culture

Applies to Ventricular Fluid Culture

Test Commonly Includes Aerobic culture and Gram's stain. Many laboratories inoculate specimens onto broth media that can support growth of anaerobic bacteria.

Abstract The major test to be performed on the CNS for meningitis is the bacteriologic culture. The "gold standard" for the diagnosis of bacterial meningitis is the isolation of a bacterium from the cerebrospinal fluid.[1] Diagnosis of meningitis is made by examination and culture of CSF. Nucleated blood cell count, differential and Gram's stain, CSF glucose and CSF protein are needed. Blood cultures are often positive with meningitis.

Patient Preparation Aseptic preparation of the aspiration site

Specimen Cerebrospinal fluid

Container Sterile CSF tube

Collection Contamination with normal flora from skin or other body surfaces must be avoided. Risks to the patient of lumbar puncture are described.[2,3] Since blood cultures are often positive in subjects with bacterial meningitis,[1] they should be requested as well. Peripheral blood white cell count and differential are usually abnormal in patients with meningitis and represent an important part of the clinical investigation.

Tubes should be numbered 1, 2, 3 with tube #1 representing the first portion of the sample collected. Contamination with normal flora from skin or other body surfaces must be avoided. The third tube collected is most suitable for culture, as skin contaminants from the puncture usually are washed out with fluid collected in the first two tubes.

Storage Instructions The specimen should be transported immediately to the laboratory. If the specimen cannot be processed immediately, it should be kept at room temperature or placed in an incubator. Refrigeration inhibits viability of certain anaerobic organisms and may prevent the recovery of common aerobic pathogens, *Neisseria meningitidis* and *Haemophilus influenzae*.

Turnaround Time Gram's stain results can be reported within 1 hour. Preliminary culture results are usually available at 24 hours. Identification of pathogens may require 48 hours.

Special Instructions The laboratory should be informed of the specific source of specimen, age of patient, current antibiotic therapy, clinical diagnosis, and time of collection.

Reference Range No growth

Critical Values Positive Gram's stain result

Use Isolate and identify pathogenic organisms causing meningitis, shunt infection, brain abscess, subdural empyema, cerebral or spinal epidural abscess, bacterial endocarditis with embolism. Gram's stain with cultures of CSF in suspected bacterial meningitis are fundamental to appropriate diagnosis and treatment.[3]

Limitations Cultures may be negative in partially treated cases of meningitis. Microorganisms such as *Neisseria meningitidis* and *Haemophilus influenzae* are sensitive to temperature shifts. Refrigeration can inhibit their isolation from the specimen. Gram's stains should be interpreted with care. Gram-positive organisms may decolorize (ie, stain gram-negative in partially treated cases).

Methodology Aerobic culture

Additional Information *Haemophilus influenzae, Neisseria meningitidis*, and *Streptococcus pneumoniae*, commonly isolated organisms, can be serotyped if requested. Infections of cerebrospinal fluid shunts pose a difficult clinical problem. Organisms most commonly cultured from shunts include *S. epidermidis*, other coagulase-negative staphylococci, *S. aureus, S. viridans*, streptococci, enterococci, and *H. influenzae*. Culture of CSF or shunt fluid is diagnostic. Removal of the catheter and later replacement are frequently required to eradicate infection.[4]

Bacterial meningitis remains a diagnostic problem. Symptoms suggestive of the diagnosis are those associated with febrile illness (eg, fever, lethargy, and anorexia); meningeal inflammation giving rise to nausea, vomiting, photophobia, and nuchal rigidity, leading to apathy; and encephalopathy with headache, confusion, and seizures. Stupor, coma, and focal neurologic signs indicate a poor prognosis if present before start of therapy.[5] **Mortality of bacterial meningitis** reaches 30%. Prognosis is worse in the very young, very old, in the presence of sickle cell disease, asplenia, and with endocarditis. Complications occur in survivors despite early diagnosis and appropriate use of antimicrobial drugs.[6] Developmental or neurologic sequelae were found in 33% to 40% of survivors.[7,8,9]

Anaerobic culture on solid media is indicated only if brain abscess, subdural empyema, or epidural abscess is suspected or in the presence of an anaerobic infection at another site. Cerebrospinal fluid is not the specimen of choice in this setting, collection of cerebrospinal fluid may be contraindicated, and anaerobic bacteria are rarely recovered from spinal fluid.[10] Common underlying conditions associated with central nervous system anaerobic infections include otitis media, lung and pleural infections, sinusitis, oral infections (ie, tonsillitis, paratonsillar abscess, dental infections), and congenital heart disease.

Factors of bacterial virulence and impaired host defense are relevant to septicemia. Susceptibility to bacterial meningitis is affected by deficiencies in host defense. Susceptibility relates to age as well.[11,12]

Footnotes

1. Smith AL, "Bacterial Meningitis," *Pediatr Rev*, 1993, 14(1):11-8.
2. Greenlee JE, "Approach to Diagnosis of Meningitis - Cerebrospinal Fluid Evaluation," *Infect Dis Clin North Am*, 1990, 4(4):583-98.
3. Fishman RA, *Cerebrospinal Fluid in Diseases of the Nervous System*, 2nd ed, Philadelphia, PA: WB Saunders Co, 1992, 266-7.
4. McLaurin RL and Frame PT, "Treatment of Infections of Cerebrospinal Fluid Shunts," *Rev Infect Dis*, 1987, 9(3):595-603.
5. Dagbjartsson A and Ludvigsson P, "Bacterial Meningitis: Diagnosis and Initial Antibiotic Therapy," *Pediatr Clin North Am*, 1987, 34(1):219-30.
6. Feigin RD, McCracken GH Jr, and Klein JO, "Diagnosis and Management of Meningitis," *Pediatr Infect Dis J*, 1992, 11(9):785-814.
7. Sáez-Llorens X, Ramilo O, Mustafa MM, et al, "Molecular Pathophysiology of Bacterial Meningitis: Current Concepts and Therapeutic Implications," *J Pediatr*, 1990, 116(5):671-84.
8. McCracken GH Jr, "Current Management of Bacterial Meningitis in Infants and Children," *Pediatr Infect Dis J*, 1992, 11(2):169-74.
9. Franco SM, Cornelius VE, and Andrews BF, "Long-Term Outcome of Neonatal Meningitis," *Am J Dis Child*, 1992, 146(5):567-71.
10. Gray LD and Fedorko DP, "Laboratory Diagnosis of Bacterial Meningitis," *Clin Microbiol Rev*, 1992, 5(2):130-45.
11. Kilpi T, Anttila M, Kallio MJ, et al, "Severity of Childhood Bacterial Meningitis and Duration of Illness Before Diagnosis," *Lancet*, 1991, 338(8764):406-9.
12. Tullus K, Brauner A, Fryklund B, et al, "Host Factors Versus Virulence-Associated Bacterial Characteristics in Neonatal and Infantile Bacteraemia and Meningitis Caused by *Escherichia coli*," *J Med Microbiol*, 1992, 36(3):203-8.

References

Bell WE, "Bacterial Meningitis in Children - Selected Aspects," *Pediatr Clin North Am*, 1992, 39(4):651-68.
Sáez-Llorens X and McCracken GH Jr, "Bacterial Meningitis in Neonates and Children," *Infect Dis Clin North Am*, 1990, 4(4):623-44.
Scheld WM, Whitley RJ, and Durack DT, *Infections of the Central Nervous System*, New York, NY: Raven Press, 1991.
Tunkel AR and Scheld WM, "Pathogenesis and Pathophysiology of Bacterial Meningitis," *Clin Microbiol Rev*, 1993, 6(2):118-36.

Bacterial Culture, Conjunctiva

CPT 87070

Related Information

Adenovirus Antibody Titer *on page 362*
Adenovirus Culture *on page 662*
Chlamydia trachomatis Culture *on page 662*
Chlamydia trachomatis Direct FA Test *on page 663*
Chlamydia trachomatis Genome Detection *on page 505*
Fungal Culture, Ocular Infections *on page 478*
Fungus Smear, Stain *on page 481*
Gram's Stain *on page 481*
Herpes Simplex Virus Antigen Detection *on page 667*
Herpes Simplex Virus Culture *on page 668*
Neisseria gonorrhoeae Genome Detection *on page 521*
Ocular Cytology *on page 298*
Viral Culture *on page 675*
Viral Culture, Eye or Ocular Symptoms *on page 679*

Synonyms Conjunctival Culture

Applies to Corneal Culture; Eye Culture; Ocular Culture

Test Commonly Includes Aerobic bacterial culture and smears (Gram's and Giemsa) if specifically requested

Patient Preparation Cleanse skin around eye with mild antiseptic. Gently remove make-up and ointment with sterile cotton and saline.

Specimen Eye swab

Container Swab with transport media

Collection The specimen should be transported to the laboratory immediately. Collect the specimen by swabbing; pass moistened swab two times over lower inferior tarsal conjunctival fornix. Avoid eyelid border and lashes. (Culture these separately in a similar fashion if indicated.) Scrapings: Use local anesthetic and platinum spatula. Rub the spatula with scrapings gently over small area on slide. If the specimen is too dry, use a very small amount of nonbacteriostatic sterile water. Scraping should be done by a physician. Swab collection has a better yield for bacteria, while scraping enhances yield of filamentous organisms.[1] The laboratory and the referring physician should consult to avoid misunderstanding regarding the collection, labeling, or handling of specimens (OD=right eye, OS=left eye). Inoculation of prewarmed plates at the time of collection of the specimen (C-streak) is a useful adjunct to optimal culture yield because of the low numbers of organisms usually present.

(Continued)

Bacterial Culture, Conjunctiva *(Continued)*

Storage Instructions Handle carefully; transport to the laboratory immediately.

Special Instructions The laboratory should be informed of the specific source of the specimen, current antibiotic therapy, and suspected clinical diagnosis. If orbital cellulitis is present or suspected, this should be communicated to the laboratory as well.

Reference Range Normal flora of the eye may include *Corynebacterium* sp (diphtheroids), *Staphylococcus epidermidis*, saprophytic fungi, *Moraxella catarrhalis*, *Moraxella* sp, *Streptococcus* sp (nonhemolytic), and gram-negative rods (rare). Abnormal ocular flora include *Haemophilus influenzae*, *Haemophilus aegyptius*, *Streptococcus pneumoniae*, *Staphylococcus aureus*, *Pseudomonas aeruginosa*, *Noguchia granulosus*, *Bacillus subtilis*, *Neisseria gonorrhoeae*, and *Mycobacterium chelonei*.

Use Isolate and identify potentially pathogenic organisms

Limitations The procedure will not detect *Chlamydia*, viruses, fungal agents, or mycobacteria which may cause conjunctivitis and/or keratitis. Scrapings are a more useful specimen than a swab for Gram's stain.

Methodology Aerobic culture on blood and chocolate agar, incubation at 37°C with CO_2

Additional Information The major modes of transmission of disease to the conjunctiva include the hands, airborne fomites, and spread for adjacent adnexal infections. Eye infections include eyelid infections, blepharitis, dacryocystitis, orbital cellulitis, conjunctivitis, keratitis, endophthalmitis retinitis, and chorioretinitis. Pinkeye is caused by adenovirus. It presents as bilateral conjunctivitis with a sudden onset. Herpes simplex and varicella zoster present as periorbital or corneal infections. Nontuberculous mycobacterial keratitis may occur following trauma or surgery accompanied by the use of local corticosteroids.[2]

Giemsa and Gram's stains must specifically be requested. If gonorrhea is suspected, a Thayer-Martin plate should be inoculated. *Acanthamoeba* may be detected with the Calcofluor white stain (see test listing Fungus Smear, Stain *on page 481* for a description of the stain) and grown on nutrient agar overlaid with a lawn of *E. coli*; cultures for *Acanthamoeba* are not available at many institutions.

Footnotes

1. Benson WH and Lanier JD, "Comparison of Techniques for Culturing Corneal Ulcers," *Ophthalmology*, 1992, 99(5):800-4.
2. Bullington RH Jr, Lanier JD, and Font RL, "Nontuberculous Mycobacterial Keratitis. Report of Two Cases and Review of the Literature," *Arch Ophthalmol*, 1992, 110(4):519-24.

References

Baum J, "Infections of the Eye," *Clin Infect Dis*, 1995, 21:479-88.

Jones DB, Leisegang TJ, and Robinson NM, *Laboratory Diagnosis of Ocular Infections*, Washington JA, coordinating ed, Cumitech 13, Washington, DC: American Society for Microbiology, 1981.

Peake JE and Slaughter BD, "Hemorrhagic Conjunctivitis and Invasive *Haemophilus influenzae* Tybe b Infection," *Pediatr Infect Dis J*, 1994, 13(3):230-1.

Pellerano RA, Bishop V, and Silber TJ, "Gonococcal Conjunctivitis in Adolescents. Recognition and Management," *Clin Pediatr (Phila)*, 1994, 33(2):114-6.

Bacterial Culture, Ear

CPT 87070 (aerobic)

Related Information

Bacterial Culture, Aerobes *on page 455*

Gram's Stain *on page 481*

Synonyms Culture, Ear; Ear Culture

Applies to Middle Ear Culture; Outer Ear Culture; Tympanocentesis Culture

Test Commonly Includes Gram's stain and culture for aerobic bacteria

Patient Preparation Cleanse the site to reduce the background contamination level

Specimen Aspirate (tympanocentesis) for otitis media; moist swab for otitis externa. In cases of otitis media in which the eardrum has ruptured, a swab may be used to collect the exudate.

Container Sterile tube or Culturette®

Collection Specimen should be transported to the laboratory as soon as possible.

Special Instructions When ear cultures for obligate anaerobic bacteria are needed, consultation with the laboratory may be helpful. If a specific agent such as *Pseudomonas*, *Haemophilus*, or *Candida* is suspected, the laboratory should be informed.

Reference Range Normal flora of the skin of the healthy ear includes *Staphylococcus epidermidis*, *Corynebacterium* sp, and *Staphylococcus aureus*

Use Determine the etiologic agent of otitis externa or otitis media

Limitations Superficial swab specimens are insensitive and nonspecific for defining the etiology of otitis media; their use for this purpose should be discouraged. Initial therapy of this condition should be empiric.

Contraindications The presence of topical ointments or drugs in or on the site to be cultured

Methodology Aerobic and anaerobic bacterial culture of specimens obtained by tympanocentesis; aerobic cultures, only, of swab specimens

Additional Information Correlation of nasopharyngeal cultures with results of tympanocentesis culture is poor; nasopharyngeal cultures lack predictive value in identification of the causative agent of otitis media. Bodor[1,2] and associates have described a good correlation between conjunctival cultures and cultures obtained by tympanocentesis and have described the simultaneous occurrence of conjunctivitis and otitis as a clinical syndrome in children. In decreasing order of frequency, the following organisms have been recovered from tympanocentesis: *S. pneumoniae* (50% to 75%), *H. influenzae* (10% to 30%), *Moraxella (Branhamella) catarrhalis* (5% to 10%), *Streptococcus pyogenes* (5% to 10%), *Staphylococcus aureus* (1% to 5%), *Pseudomonas aeruginosa* (0.1% to 1%). *E. coli*, *Klebsiella pneumoniae*, *Pseudomonas aeruginosa* may be isolated from neonates. In therapeutic failures, *S. aureus*, and *P. aeruginosa* are most frequently recovered.[3] In a series of 908 cases, *H. influenzae* made up 49.7% of them. The incidence of *H. influenzae* peaked at 2 years of age and fell off markedly after 6 years of age.[4] Tympanocentesis is not usually required in primary infections. It should be reserved for complicated, recurrent, or chronic otitis media. *Candida* superinfection may complicate therapy for recurring ear infections and may be a cause of persistent otorrhea.[5] Otitis externa is frequently caused by *P. aeruginosa* and less frequently by *Candida* sp, *Proteus* sp, *S. aureus*, and *Trichophyton* sp.

Footnotes

1. Bodor FF, Marchant CD, and Shurin PA, "Bacterial Etiology of Conjunctivitis-Otitis Media Syndrome," *Pediatrics*, 1985, 76(1):26-8.
2. Bodor FF, "Conjunctivitis-Otitis Syndrome," *Pediatrics*, 1982, 69:695-8.
3. Bland RD, "Otitis Media in the First Six Weeks of Life. Diagnosis Bacteriology and Management," *Pediatrics*, 1972, 187-97.
4. Calhoun KH, Norris WB, and Hokanson JA, "Bacteriology of Middle Ear Effusions," *South Med J*, 1988, 81(3):332-6.
5. Cohen SR and Thompson JW, "Otitic Candidiasis in Children: An Evaluation of the Problem and Effectiveness of Ketoconazole in 10 Patients," *Ann Otol Rhinol Laryngol*, 1990, 99(6 Pt 1):427-31.

References

Kligman EW, "Treatment of Otitis Media," *Am Fam Physician*, 1992, 45(1):242-50.

Macknin ML, "Respiratory Infections in Children. What Helps and What Doesn't?" *Postgrad Med*, 1992, 92(2):235-8, 243, 247-50.

Randall DA, Fornadley JA, and Kennedy KS, "Management of Recurrent Otitis Media," *Am Fam Physician*, 1992, 45(5):2117-23.

Bacterial Culture, Endometrium

CPT 87070 (aerobic); 87075 (anaerobic isolation); 87076 (definitive identification, each anaerobic organism)

Related Information

Actinomyces Culture *on page 447*

Bacterial Culture, Abscess *on page 454*

Bacterial Culture, Biopsy or Body Fluid *on page 456*

Chlamydia trachomatis Culture *on page 662*

Chlamydia trachomatis Genome Detection *on page 505*

Genital Culture for *Ureaplasma urealyticum* *on page 667*

Synonyms Endometrium Culture

Applies to Amniotic Fluid Anaerobic Culture; Cul-de-sac Anaerobic Culture; Endocervical Anaerobic Culture; Genitourinary Anaerobic Culture, Female; Intrauterine Device Culture; IUD Culture; Uterus Anaerobic Culture

Test Commonly Includes Aerobic and anaerobic bacterial culture and direct smear if requested

Patient Preparation Aseptic preparation of the aspiration site

Specimen Scrapings, aspirates, or swabs taken from endometrium or endocervix without contamination with vaginal or exocervical flora. Protected or sheathed swabs are useful in reducing contamination. Use of an unprotected swab is reported to significantly increase the recovery of both aerobic and anaerobic bacteria commonly regarded as potential pathogens.[1] Specimens for anaerobic culture should be accompanied by a specimen for routine culture from the same site.

Container Anaerobic transport tube; sterile tube or swab

Collection Disinfect cervix and attempt to aspirate material through the cervical os, expel air bubbles from the syringe, and inject into an anaerobic transport vial. Transport the specimen to the laboratory as soon as possible after collection.

Storage Instructions Do not refrigerate or incubate.

Causes for Rejection Specimens which have been refrigerated or have an excessive delay in transit have suboptimal yield

Special Instructions The laboratory should be informed of current antibiotic therapy and clinical diagnosis.

Reference Range No growth

Use Isolate and identify aerobic and anaerobic organisms

Anaerobic Infections of the Female Genital Tract

Abscesses in glands	Peritonitis
Abscesses in soft tissues	Postoperative infections
Endocervicitis	Pyometra
Endometritis	Salpingitis
IUD (intrauterine device) associated infections	Septic abortion
Pelvic abscess	Tubo-ovarian abscess
Pelvic actinomycosis	Vaginitis, nonspecific

Limitations Unprotected swab cultures are invariably contaminated with cervicovaginal flora. Specimens received in anaerobic transport containers are not optimal for routine or fungus culture.

Additional Information Actinomycosis has been reported in association with endometritis and pelvic infection associated with intrauterine devices.[2]

Clinical findings associated with anaerobic infections include proximity of the infection to a mucosal surface, foul-smelling discharge, gas in the tissues, and abscess formation. Infections are frequently polymicrobic. Aggressive antimicrobial therapy including beta-lactamase resistant antimicrobials[3] and surgical procedures (curettage, incision, and drainage) are frequently required. *Chlamydia* and *Ureaplasma* are often implicated in endometrial and pelvic infections and require separate culture techniques.[4]

In a large series of patients with obstetric and gynecologic infections, the most frequently isolated aerobic and facultative organisms were *Lactobacillus* sp, *E. coli*, *N. gonorrhoeae*, *S. aureus*, and group B *Streptococcus*. The most commonly isolated anaerobic organisms were *Bacteroides* sp; anaerobic gram-positive cocci, and *Fusobacterium* sp were also recovered. Eighteen percent of the isolates were beta-lactamase producing.[4]

Footnotes
1. Martens MG, Faro S, Hammill HA, et al, "Transcervical Uterine Cultures With a New Endometrial Suction Curette: A Comparison of Three Sampling Methods in Postpartum Endometritis," *Obstet Gynecol*, 1989, 74(2):273-6.
2. Evans DTP, "*Actinomyces israelii* in the Female Genital Tract: A Review," *Genitourin Med*, 1993, 69(1):54-9.
3. Brook I, Frazier EH, and Thomas RL, "Aerobic and Anaerobic Microbiologic Factors and Recovery of Beta-Lactamase Producing Bacteria From Obstetric and Gynecologic Infection," *Surg Gynecol Obstet*, 1991, 172(2):138-44.
4. Watts DH, Eschenbach DA, and Kenny GE, "Early Postpartum Endometritis: The Role of Bacteria, Genital *Mycoplasmas*, and *Chlamydia trachomatis*," *Obstet Gynecol*, 1989, 73(1):52-60.

References
Gibbs RS, "Severe Infections in Pregnancy," *Med Clin North Am*, 1989, 73(3):713-21.

Bacterial Culture, Genital Specimen

CPT 87070
Related Information
Chlamydia trachomatis Culture *on page 662*
Chlamydia trachomatis Direct FA Test *on page 663*
Chlamydia trachomatis Genome Detection *on page 505*
Genital Culture for *Ureaplasma urealyticum* on page 667
Group B *Streptococcus* Screen, Rapid *on page 483*
Herpes Simplex Virus Antigen Detection *on page 667*
Herpes Simplex Virus Culture *on page 668*
Neisseria gonorrhoeae Culture and Smear *on page 492*
Neisseria gonorrhoeae Genome Detection *on page 521*
RPR *on page 428*
Trichomonas Preparation *on page 498*
VDRL, Serum *on page 438*
Viral Culture *on page 675*
Viral Culture, Urogenital *on page 681*

Synonyms Genital Culture

Applies to *Candida* Culture, Genital; Cervical Culture; Clue Cells; Endocervical Culture; Prostatic Fluid Culture; Vaginal Culture

Test Commonly Includes Culture for *Neisseria gonorrhoeae*, other aerobic bacteria, and *Candida* sp. *Gardnerella* and *Mobiluncus*, Gram's stain, and fungal stain may require separate requests.

Specimen Swab of vagina, cervix, discharge, aspirated endocervical, endometrial, prostatic fluid, or urethral discharge

Container Sterile tube or Culturette®

Collection The specimen should be transported to the laboratory within 2 hours of collection. Do not refrigerate.

Special Instructions Recovery of *N. gonorrhoeae* is enhanced by cultures taken at the bedside (onto special medium at room temperature) and delivery to the laboratory within 30 minutes. The laboratory should be informed of the specific source of specimen, current antibiotic therapy, clinical diagnosis, and time of collection.

Reference Range Normal flora; properly collected prostatic fluid and endocervical cultures are normally sterile.

Critical Values Recovery of *Neisseria gonorrhoeae* and perhaps *Streptococcus agalactiae* (beta-hemolytic group B strep) during pregnancy

Use Isolate and identify *Neisseria gonorrhoeae* and to screen for genital carriage of *Streptococcus agalactiae* during pregnancy. Upon special request, a culture for the presence of *Staphylococcus aureus* in cases of suspected toxic shock syndrome will be done.

Limitations Herpes simplex virus, *Chlamydia*, and *Ureaplasma urealyticum* are not recovered by this procedure.

Methodology Aerobic culture with selective (Thayer-Martin) and nonselective media incubated at 35°C to 37°C with CO_2

Additional Information Susceptibility testing can be performed if indicated. Routine cultures include screening for *N. gonorrhoeae* and group B streptococci. Normal flora of the vagina is dependent upon age, glycogen content, pH, exogenous hormone therapy, etc. Normal vaginal flora includes numerous anaerobes, corynebacteria, enteric gram-negative rods, enterococci, lactobacilli, *Moraxella* sp, staphylococci, streptococci (alpha and nonhemolytic), *Mycobacterium smegmatis*. The laboratory should be consulted to arrange for special toxin identification procedures if toxic shock syndrome is suspected and *Staphylococcus aureus* is recovered.

Vaginitis is one of the most commonly encountered complaints of female patients. A significant portion of these appear to be due to specific etiologic agents such as *Candida* sp or *Trichomonas vaginalis*. Nonspecific vaginitis, also called bacterial vaginosis, is characterized by an excessive malodorous vaginal discharge associated with a decrease in the number of lactobacilli and an increase in the number of *Gardnerella vaginalis* and other bacteria such as *Bacteroides* sp, *Prevotella* sp, and *Peptostreptococcus* sp.[1] Additionally, curved, motile, anaerobic gram-negative bacilli identified as *Mobiluncus* sp have been associated with bacterial vaginosis. **Presently, bacterial cultures contribute little to the diagnosis of bacterial vaginosis.** Minimum diagnostic requirements for bacterial vaginosis include three of the following signs:[2]

- excessive vaginal discharge
- vaginal pH >4.5
- "clue" cells (vaginal epithelial cells covered by small gram-negative rods)
- a fishy amine-like odor in the KOH test (10% KOH added to vaginal discharge)

Candida sp are frequently present as normal flora in vagina. A saline wet mount may demonstrate yeast cells or pseudohyphae and may provide rapid diagnostic information. The most common clinical presentation is a characteristic clumpy white cottage cheese appearance with vaginal or vulvar itching. Vaginitis and balanitis caused by *Candida albicans* are more common than is generally perceived. Vaginitis frequently complicates pregnancy and diabetes and is seen with broad spectrum antibiotic therapy, as well as, in conditions which lower host resistance (AIDS).[3]

Footnotes
1. Catlin BW, "*Gardnerella vaginalis*: Characteristics, Clinical Considerations, and Controversies," *Clin Microbiol Rev*, 1992, 5(3):213-37.
2. Joesoef MR and Schmid GP, "Bacterial Vaginosis: Review of Treatment Options and Potential Clinical Indications for Therapy," *Clin Infect Dis*, 1995, 20(Suppl 1):S72-9.
3. Kinghorn GR, "Vulvovaginal Candidosis," *J Antimicrob Chemother*, 1991, 28(Suppl A):59-66.

References
Faro S, "Bacterial Vaginitis," *Clin Obstet Gynecol*, 1991, 34(3):582-6.
Moran JS and Levine WC, "Drugs of Choice for the Treatment of Uncomplicated Gonococcal Infections," *Clin Infect Dis*, 1995, 20(S1):47-65.
Sobel JD, "Vaginal Infections in Adult Women," *Med Clin North Am*, 1990, 74(6):1573-602.
Thomason JL, Gelbart SM, and Scaglione NJ, "Bacterial Vaginosis: Current Review With Indications for Asymptomatic Therapy," *Am J Obstet Gynecol*, 1991, 165(4 Pt 2):1210-7.

Bacterial Culture, Intravascular Device

CPT 87070 (aerobic); 87075 (anaerobic); 87076 (definitive ID); 87102 (fungi isolation); 87106 (fungi definitive identification)
Related Information
Bacterial Culture, Aerobes *on page 455*
Bacterial Culture, Blood *on page 457*

Synonyms Intravascular Device Culture

Applies to Catheter Tip Culture; Hemovac® Tip Culture; Hyperalimentation Line Culture; Intravenous Catheter Culture; Quantitative Tip Culture (QTC); Swan-Ganz Tip Culture

Test Commonly Includes Quantitative or semiquantitative culture of an intravascular catheter or blood specimen collected through the catheter; organism identification, and antimicrobial susceptibilities if appropriate

Abstract Intravascular devices are used to provide continuous vascular access for a variety of therapeutic and diagnostic purposes. Their use in individuals with serious underlying illness and the fact that they penetrate the integument places patients at risk for infection.
(Continued)

Bacterial Culture, Intravascular Device

(Continued)

Specimen I.V. catheter tip, foreign body, blood collected through catheter

Container Sterile container

Collection Clean the insertion site with an iodophor and alcohol, and aseptically remove the cannula after the alcohol has dried. If purulent material is present at the exit site, it should be submitted for culture and Gram's stain. If the catheter is short, the entire cannula should be submitted following removal of the hub with sterile scissors or other sterile device. For longer catheters, two 2-3 cm segments should be submitted, one from the proximal transcutaneous segment and the other from the distal intravascular tip. Alternatively, blood for comparative quantitative cultures may be collected simultaneously from a peripheral vein and from the central venous catheter. A procedure for accomplishing this is as follows:

A blood sample, 0.5-1 mL, is drawn from a peripheral blood vessel and from the central catheter. Aseptic technique at the peripheral site includes three applications of povidone-iodine followed by one application of 70% isopropyl alcohol to the skin. A butterfly needle and a sterile syringe are used for phlebotomy. Aseptic technique at the catheter is as follows.

- The catheter is clamped and the needle adapter removed.
- The end of the catheter is swabbed three times with povidone-iodine and once with 70% isopropyl alcohol.
- A sterile needle adapter is inserted into the end of the catheter.
- The clamp is removed and 2 mL of blood is drawn through a sterile syringe to clear the catheter.
- The blood for culture is then subsequently obtained in a separate sterile syringe.
- The catheter adapter is reattached to the intravenous tubing.

The paired blood specimens are placed in separate lysis centrifugation tubes after the stopper is swabbed three times with povidone-iodine.[1] See also listing Bacterial Culture, Blood *on page 457*.

Storage Instructions Specimens should be transported to the laboratory within 1 hour of collection for optimal results. However, if specimens cannot be collected and delivered to the laboratory during regular hours, specimen may be refrigerated overnight.

Causes for Rejection Foley catheters are unacceptable specimens because they are invariably contaminated with environmental flora.

Reference Range Roll plate semiquantitative cultures yielding <15 colonies, sonicated specimens yielding <10^4 colonies of coagulase-negative staphylococci (cutoffs for other organisms are less clear), and comparative quantitative cultures yielding a ratio <10:1 (central venous catheter vs peripheral vein cultures) or <100 CFU/mL (central venous catheter only) suggests that the catheter should not be strongly considered as the cause of sepsis.[1]

Use Culture of intravascular devices should be limited to patients who have laboratory confirmed bacteremia or who appear clinically septic but have no apparent source of infection. In this situation, the intravascular device is investigated as the possible origin of infection by the methods described. Randomly culturing patients who are not bacteremic or who are not clinically septic is unwarranted.

Limitations Results of intravascular device cultures contribute to the work-up of patients with bloodstream infections who lack an obvious source. These results do not stand alone, however, and all methods described give a significant number of false-positive and false-negative results. The sonication and comparative quantitative culture methods are still evolving.

Methodology Roll plate semiquantitative cultures: Aseptically roll the catheter tip on a blood and/or chocolate agar plate.

Quantitative sonication method: Place catheter segment in 10 mL of tryptic soy broth, sonicate for 1 minute, then vortex for 15 seconds (original specimen). Add 0.1 mL of this specimen to 9.9 mL of saline (diluted specimen) and inoculate separate blood agar plates with 0.1 mL of the original and diluted specimens. Perform colony counts and multiply by 10^2 (original specimen) or 10^4 (diluted specimen) to determine the number of organisms on the catheter.

Comparative quantitative cultures: Follow procedures for collection listed above and process as you would blood cultures using the lysis centrifugation method. Perform colony counts on both specimens.

Sonication technique is considered useful.[2]

Additional Information Infections complicating therapy with indwelling central venous catheters pose a difficult problem. Catheter-related sepsis is defined when:

- positive blood cultures collected through the central venous catheter show a tenfold or greater colony count compared with peripheral quantitative blood culture or >100 CFU/mL if only central venous catheter blood culture is available

- no obvious clinical or microbiologic source for the infection is apparent

Exit site infections are defined as purulent drainage or erythema at the catheter exit site. Tunnel infection is defined as spreading cellulitis with erythema, tenderness, and swelling of the skin surrounding the subcutaneous tunnel tract of the catheter. Successful therapy of catheter-related infection with antibiotics and local care was reported by Benezra et al. However, they noted that catheter removal was required to achieve cure particularly in *Pseudomonas* tunnel infections. *Staphylococcus aureus* and polymicrobial infections also were more difficult to eradicate. Intraluminal cultures correlate well with catheter tip cultures (87.5% identical) while skin puncture sites were less frequently identical (37.5%).[3] See table.

Summary of Results of Prospective Studies Using Semiquantitative Techniques to Diagnose Vascular-Access Infections

Organism	No. With Same Organism in Semiquantitative Catheter Culture and Blood Culture
Coagulase-negative staphylococci	27
Staphylococcus aureus	26
Yeast	17
Enterobacter	7
Serratia	5
Enterococcus	5
Klebsiella	4
Streptococcus viridans group	3
Pseudomonas species	2
Proteus	2
Others: *Pseudomonas aeruginosa, Yersinia*	1 each

From Hampton A and Sheretz RJ, "Vascular-Access Infections in Hospitalized Patients," *Surg Clin North Am*, 1988, 68:57-72, with permission.

Footnotes

1. Sherertz RJ, Raad II, Belani A, et al, "Three-Year Experience With Sonicated Vascular Catheter Cultures in a Clinical Microbiology Laboratory," *J Clin Microbiol*, 1990, 28(1):76-82.
2. Kelly M, Wunderlich Wciorka LR, McConico S, et al, "Sonicated Vascular Catheter Tip Cultures: Quantitative Association With Catheter-Related Sepsis and the Non-Utility of an Adjuvant Cytocentrifuge Gram Stain," *Am J Clin Pathol*, 1996, 105:210-5.
3. Jakobsen CJ, Hansen V, Jensen JJ, et al, "Contamination of Subclavian Vein Catheters: An Intraluminal Culture Method," *J Hosp Infect*, 1989, 13(3):253-60.

References

Fry DE, Fry RV, and Borzotta AP, "Nosocomial Blood-Borne Infection Secondary to Intravascular Devices," *Am J Surg*, 1994, 167(2):268-72.
Garrison RN and Wilson MA, "Intravenous and Central Catheter Infections," *Surg Clin North Am*, 1994, 74(3):557-70.
Goldmann DA and Pier GB, "Pathogenesis of Infections Related to Intravascular Catheterization," *Clin Microbiol Rev*, 1993, 6(2):176-87.
Raad II and Bodey GP, "Infectious Complications of Indwelling Vascular Catheters," *Clin Infect Dis*, 1992, 15(2):197-208.
Reimer LG, "Catheter-Related Infections and Blood Cultures," *Clin Lab Med*, 1994, 14(1):51-8.

Bacterial Culture, Nasopharynx

CPT 87060

Related Information

Bordetella pertussis Culture *on page 471*

Synonyms Nasopharyngeal Culture

Specimen Nasopharyngeal swab

Container Sterile wire swab expressed into transport medium or transported directly to the laboratory

Collection Use special nasopharyngeal wire swabs/Calgiswab®. Gently insert swab through nose to posterior nasopharynx; allow to remain for a few seconds and gently remove wire. The specimen should be transported to the laboratory as soon as possible. Swabs must be collected carefully, taking care not to touch the skin.

Special Instructions The laboratory should be informed of current antibiotic therapy. Also, the laboratory should be informed of the specimen request to screen for *Staphylococcus aureus*. Objectives of the program should be clearly defined because of the relatively high frequency of carriers in the normal population.

Reference Range Normal nasopharyngeal flora

Use Isolate and identify potentially pathogenic organisms. Nasopharyngeal culture may reflect infection of tonsils, oropharynx, nasopharynx, and sinuses. Useful in identifying carriers of *S. aureus* and *N. meningitidis*.

Limitations Results suggesting primary nasopharyngeal infection must be interpreted with caution, because of the variety of potentially pathogenic normal flora and the potential presence of infection in adjacent sites.

Methodology Aerobic culture

Additional Information Presence or absence of normal flora is usually reported. Normal flora of the nose includes *S. epidermidis* (coagulase-negative *Staphylococcus*), *S. aureus*, *S. pneumoniae*, *H. influenzae*, *S. pyogenes*, *M. catarrhalis*, and *Neisseria* sp. Consequently, nasal cultures for bacteria rarely provide useful clinical information.

References

Gittelman PD, Jacobs JB, Lebowitz AS, et al, "*Staphylococcus aureus* Nasal Carriage in Patients With Rhinosinusitis," *Laryngoscope*, 1991, 101(7 Pt 1):733-7.

Godley FA, "Chronic Sinusitis: An Update," *Am Fam Physician*, 1992, 45(5):2190-9.

Oppenheimer RW, "Sinusitis. How to Recognize and Treat It," *Postgrad Med*, 1992, 91(5):281-6, 289-92.

Wald ER, "Sinusitis in Children," *N Engl J Med*, 1992, 326(5):319-23.

Bacterial Culture, Sputum

CPT 87070 (culture); 87205 (Gram's stain)

Related Information

Bacterial Culture, Blood *on page 457*
Bacterial Culture, Bronchoscopy Specimen *on page 459*
Bordetella pertussis Serology *on page 372*
Bronchial Washings Cytology *on page 287*
Bronchoalveolar Lavage Cytology *on page 288*
Fungal Culture, Blood *on page 477*
Fungal Culture, Sputum *on page 479*
Gram's Stain *on page 481*
Hypersensitivity Pneumonitis Serology *on page 406*
Legionella Culture *on page 485*
Legionnaires' Disease Antibodies *on page 412*
Legionnaires' Disease Direct Fluorescent Antibody Smear *on page 413*
Mycobacterial Culture, Sputum *on page 490*
Mycoplasma pneumoniae Diagnostic Procedures *on page 671*
Mycoplasma Serology *on page 419*
Pneumocystis Immunofluorescence *on page 423*
Sputum Cytology *on page 300*
Viral Culture, Respiratory Symptoms *on page 680*

Synonyms Sputum Culture

Applies to Bronchial Washings Culture; Bronchoscopy Culture; Percutaneous Transtracheal Culture; Tracheal Aspirate Culture

Test Commonly Includes Culture of aerobic organisms and usually Gram's stain

Abstract Pneumonia is the sixth leading cause of death in the United States. It is the most common cause of death from infectious disease. Laboratory evaluation includes Gram's staining and culture of sputum, with culture and staining if appropriate for mycobacteria; culture for *Legionella* with direct FA smear, antibodies, and urine antigen; *Mycoplasma* serology; pleural fluid analysis if thoracentesis is done; chemistry profile, CBC, arterial blood gas analysis, and HIV serology for patients 15-54 years of age. Blood culture may be helpful.[1]

Patient Preparation The patient should be instructed to remove dentures, rinse mouth, and gargle with water. The patient should then be instructed to cough deeply and expectorate sputum into proper container.

Specimen Sputum, first morning specimen preferred; tracheal aspiration, bronchoscopy specimen, or transtracheal aspirate

Container Sterile sputum container, sputum trap, sterile tracheal aspirate or bronchoscopy aspirate tube

Collection Collect expectorated sputum under direct supervision of nurse or physician. Specimen collected, at time of bronchoscopy, by aspiration or by transtracheal aspiration by a physician skilled in the procedure. The specimen should be transported to the laboratory within 1 hour of collection for processing.

Storage Instructions Refrigerate if the specimen cannot be promptly processed.

Causes for Rejection Specimens contaminated on the outside of the container pose excessive risk.

Turnaround Time Stat Gram's stain results usually are available in 15-30 minutes. Identification of pathogens usually requires at least 48 hours for completion.

Reference Range Normal upper respiratory flora. Tracheal aspirate and bronchoscopy specimens can be contaminated with normal oral flora. Transtracheal aspiration should have no growth.

Use Isolate and identify potentially pathogenic organisms present in the lower respiratory tract. Presence or absence of normal upper respiratory flora is often reported.

Limitations The primary limitation associated with expectorated sputum specimens submitted for bacterial culture is the difficulty in distinguishing organisms infecting the lower respiratory tract from potentially pathogenic organisms colonizing (but not infecting) the upper respiratory tract. The most important tool for making this distinction is Gram's stain of a representative portion of the specimen examined initially at low power (100x total magnification) for the presence of squamous epithelial cells and polymorphonuclear leukocytes; several fields should be examined.[2,3,4] The presence of ≥25 squamous epithelial cells per low power field indicates excessive oral contamination and mandates specimen rejection for bacterial culture; no useful information about lower respiratory bacterial pathogens can be gleaned from such a specimen. Stricter criteria suggest that specimens with ≥10 squamous epithelial cells should be rejected; while this may be administratively disadvantageous at many institutions, it is clear that such specimens often provide confusing results. The presence of polymorphonuclear neutrophils is used to indicate specimen collection from an area of active inflammation, presumably the infected lung or bronchus. Consequently, the best expectorated sputum specimens have many PMNs and few to no squamous epithelial cells. Such specimens are likely to include the etiologic agent of the infection in relatively high numbers and comparatively few contaminating organisms from the upper respiratory tract. Microscopic examination of these specimens under oil (1000x total magnification) often provides preliminary morphologic information about the etiologic agent that can be used to guide empiric therapy. Organisms are especially important in Gram's stain when phagocytosis is seen. Interpretation of results of bacterial sputum cultures without considering specimen quality (determined by Gram's stain) is essentially impossible.

The yield from sputum culture in patients with bacteremic *Streptococcus pneumoniae* pneumonia is only about 50%.[1]

Methodology Aerobic culture following appropriate specimen selection. The most important step in the evaluation is to be certain that the secretions that are examined are the product of the inflammatory process in the bronchi and not oropharyngeal material. This can be accomplished by a simple microscopic evaluation of the sputum specimen. A promising (thick) portion should be separated from the sputum sample and placed on a microscopic slide. This selection is easier if the sputum is poured into one-half of a Petri dish and viewed against a dark background so that a likely plug can be identified. The specimen placed on the slide is scanned under low magnification. The most productive material is that which represents bronchial secretions. Frequently, they are present as a plug or cast of the infected bronchus. The identified portions are selected and inoculated on selective and nonselective media.

Additional Information See table. Potential pathogens recovered by usual sputum culture methods include *Staphylococcus aureus*, *Haemophilus influenzae*, *Streptococcus pneumoniae*, *Neisseria meningitidis*, *Pseudomonas aeruginosa*, *Escherichia coli*, *Proteus* sp, *Moraxella* (*Branhamella*) *catarrhalis*, and rarely many other organisms. *Haemophilus* sp and *Neisseria* sp may not be routinely isolated and identified. Thus, if their presence is clinically suspected, they should be specifically requested.

Bacterial Species Recovered From Sputa in 103 Acute Bronchitic Exacerbations

	Number	Percent of All Types Cultured	Percent of Sputa Cultured
H. influenzae	41	24.0	39.8
H. parainfluenzae	29	17.0	28.2
S. pneumoniae	34	19.9	33.0
M. catarrhalis	19	11.1	18.4
N. meningitidis	5	2.9	4.9
K. pneumoniae	8	4.7	7.8
P. aeruginosa	4	2.3	3.9
Other possible pathogens	14	8.2	13.6
Unlikely pathogens	17	9.9	16.5

From Chodosh S, "Acute Bacterial Exacerbations in Bronchitis and Asthma," *Am J Med*, 1987, 82(Suppl 4A):154-63, with permission.

Agents such as *Bordetella pertussis*, *Chlamydia pneumoniae* TWAR strain, *Corynebacterium diphtheriae*, *Legionella pneumophila*, *Mycoplasma pneumoniae*, and *Mycobacterium tuberculosis* require special laboratory measures for isolation. Clinical suspicion of involvement by these agents should be communicated to the laboratory. See also listings for the specific agents.

The critical criteria for the diagnosis of acute bacterial infection of the bronchi are obtained from examination and culture of the sputum. The
(Continued)

Bacterial Culture, Sputum *(Continued)*

presence of bacteria in numbers greater than when the patient's condition is stable and a significant increase (ie, doubling) in the numbers of neutrophils present are essential laboratory criteria for the diagnosis of an acute bronchitic exacerbation. Gram's stain results more closely reflect the clinical outcome and along with the criterion of the number of neutrophils in the sputum should be laboratory basis for determination of success.[5] Other commonly recognized agents causing pneumonia are reviewed in the tables.

Community-Acquired Bacterial Pneumonias: Frequency of Various Pathogens	%
Streptococcus pneumoniae	40-60
Haemophilus influenzae	2.5-20
Gram-negative bacilli	6-37
Staphylococcus aureus	2-10
Anaerobic infections	5-10
Legionella	0-22.5
Mycoplasma pneumoniae	5-15
Nosocomial Pneumonias: Frequency of Various Pathogens	**%**
Klebsiella	13
Pseudomonas aeruginosa	10-12
Staphylococcus aureus	3-10.6
Escherichia coli	4-7.2
Enterobacter	6.2
Group D *Streptococcus*	1.3
Proteus and *Providencia*	6
Serratia	3.5
Pneumococcus	10-20
Aspiration pneumonia anaerobic pneumonia*	5-25
*Legionella**	0-15

From Verghese A and Berk SL, "Bacterial Pneumonia in the Elderly Medicine," 1983, 62:271-85, with permission.

* The specific incidence of pneumonias caused by *Mycoplasma*, *Legionella*, and anaerobes is difficult to document because of the technical problems in isolating the organisms.

Spectrum of Frequent Etiologic Agents in Pneumonia

Aerobic Bacteria	Anaerobes	Fungi
Gram-positive aerobes	*Bacteroides melaninogenicus*	*Aspergillus*
Streptococcus pneumoniae	*Fusobacterium*	*Coccidioides immitis*
Staphylococcus aureus	*Peptostreptococcus*	*Histoplasma capsulatum*
Streptococcus pyogenes	*Bacteroides fragilis*	*Blastomyces dermatitidis*
Gram-negative aerobes	*Actinomyces israelii*	*Cryptococcus neoformans*
Haemophilus influenzae		Zygomycetes
Legionella pneumophila		
Escherichia coli		
Klebsiella pneumoniae		
Pseudomonas aeruginosa		
Viruses	**Parasites**	**Other**
Respiratory syncytial virus	*Pneumocystis carinii*	*Mycoplasma pneumoniae*
Parainfluenza virus	*Ascaris lumbricoides*	*Chlamydia trachomatis*
Influenza virus	*Toxocara canis* and *catis*	*Chlamydia psittaci*
Adenovirus	Filaria	*Mycobacterium tuberculosis*
Enterovirus	*Strongyloides stercoralis*	*Chlamydia* TWAR strains
Rhinovirus	Hookworms	*Nocardia*
Measles virus	*Paragonimus*	
Varicella-zoster virus	*Echinococcus*	
Rickettsia	Schistosomes	
Coxiella burnetii		
Cytomegalovirus		
Hantavirus		

From Cohen GJ, "Management of Infections of the Lower Respiratory Tract in Children," *Pediatr Infect Dis*, 1987, 6:317-23, with permission.

The risk of bacterial pneumonia is greater in HIV-positive individuals and is highest with CD4 lymphocyte counts <200/mm^3 and in intravenous drug abusers.[6]

Footnotes
1. Bartlett JG and Mundy L, "Community-Acquired Pneumonia," *N Engl J Med*, 1995, 333(24):1618-24.
2. Murray PR and Washington JA, "Microscopic and Bacteriologic Analysis of Expectorated Sputum," *Mayo Clin Proc*, 1975, 50:339-44.
3. Van Scoy RE, "Bacterial Sputum Cultures," *Mayo Clin Proc*, 1977, 52:39-41.
4. Geckler RW, Gremillion DH, McAllister CK, et al, "Microscopic and Bacteriological Comparison of Paired Sputa and Transtracheal Aspirates," *J Clin Microbiol*, 1977, 6:396-9.
5. Chodosh S, "Acute Bacterial Exacerbations in Bronchitis and Asthma," *Am J Med*, 1987, 82(4A):154-63.
6. Hirschtick RE, Glassroth J, Jordan MC, et al, "Bacterial Pneumonia in Persons Infected With the Human Immunodeficiency Virus," *N Engl J Med*, 1995, 333(13):845-51.

References
"Case Records of the Massachusetts General Hospital. Weekly Clinicopathological Exercises. Case 25-1994. A 58-Year-Old Woman With Bloody Diarrhea After Chemotherapy for Carcinoma of the Tongue," *N Engl J Med*, 1994, 330(25):1811-7.

Stratton CW, "Bacterial Pneumonias - An Overview With Emphasis on Pathogenesis, Diagnosis, and Treatment," *Heart Lung*, 1986, 15(3):226-44.

Tuomanen EI, Austrian R, and Masure HR, "Pathogenesis of Pneumococcal Infection," *N Engl J Med*, 1995, 332(19):1280-4.

Wijnands GJ, "Diagnosis and Interventions in Lower Respiratory Tract Infections," *Am J Med*, 1992, 92(4SA):91S-7S.

Yungbluth M, "The Laboratory Diagnosis of Pneumonia. The Role of the Community Hospital Pathologist," *Clin Lab Med*, 1995, 15(2):209-34.

Bacterial Culture, Stool

CPT 87045

Related Information
Bacterial Culture, Blood *on page 457*
Botulism Diagnostic Procedure *on page 472*
Clostridium difficile Toxin Assay *on page 473*
Cryptosporidium Diagnostic Procedures *on page 474*
Electron Microscopic Examination for Viruses, Stool *on page 665*
Entamoeba histolytica Serological Test *on page 391*
Enterovirus Culture *on page 666*
Fungal Culture, Stool *on page 480*
Methylene Blue Stain, Stool *on page 642*
Microsporidia Diagnostic Procedures *on page 487*
Mycobacterial Culture, Stool *on page 491*
Ova and Parasites, Stool *on page 494*
Rotavirus, Direct Detection *on page 674*
Salmonella Titer *on page 429*
Viral Culture, Stool *on page 680*
Yersinia enterocolitica Antibody *on page 440*

Synonyms Enteric Pathogens Culture, Routine; Rectal Swab Culture; Stool Culture

Applies to *Clostridium difficile*; Enterohemorrhagic *E. coli*

Test Commonly Includes Screening culture for bacterial pathogens. Most laboratories routinely look for *Salmonella*, *Shigella*, and *Campylobacter* sp. Specific requests may be required for less common pathogens such as *Escherichia coli* 0157:H7, *Yersinia enterocolitica*, *Vibrio* sp, *Aeromonas hydrophila*, and *Plesiomonas shigelloides*.

Abstract In general, the presence of stool leukocytes provides indication for stool culture. *Escherichia coli* O157:H7, *Salmonella* sp, and *Campylobacter jejuni* are most often cultured from stools in summer months. *Aeromonas* sp, *Shigella* sp, and *Yersinia enterocolitica* occurred less often in one series.[1]

Specimen Fresh random stool, rectal swab

Container Stool container, Culturette®

Collection If stool is collected in a clean bedpan, it must not be contaminated with urine, residual soap, or disinfectants. Swabs of lesions of the rectal wall during proctoscopy or sigmoidoscopy are preferred.

Rectal swab: Insert the swab past the anal sphincter, move the swab circumferentially around the rectum. Allow 15-30 seconds for organisms to adsorb onto the swab. Withdraw swab, place in Culturette® tube, and crush media compartment.

Storage Instructions Fresh specimens should be promptly delivered to the laboratory and processed within 1-2 hours. If specimen transport or processing will be delayed, the specimen may be preserved in modified Cary-Blair or buffered glycerol-saline media and refrigerated.

Causes for Rejection A study at the University of Pennsylvania School of Medicine showed that patients who develop diarrhea 3 or more days after hospitalization virtually never have bacteria or parasites identified by routine examination; the only etiologic agent implicated with any frequency in this setting is *Clostridium difficile*.[2] During a 3-year period, only 1 of 191 positive stool cultures was from a patient who had been hospitalized for 3 or more days, while over half of the 3000 specimens submitted per year were from such patients. A College of American Pathologists study found only 0.6% of specimens positive for enteric pathogens that had not previously been recovered from stools.[3] Based on these studies, it is strongly recommended that stool specimens should not be worked up for routine bacterial pathogens when collected from patients hospitalized for 3 or more days before the onset of diarrhea; *C. difficile* should be tested for using toxin assays.

Because of risk to laboratory personnel, specimens sent on diaper or tissue paper, or specimen contaminating outside of transport container may not be acceptable. Specimen containing interfering substances (eg, castor oil, bismuth, Metamucil®, barium), specimens delayed in transit and those contaminated with urine may not have optimal yield.

Turnaround Time Minimum 48 hours if negative; 72 hours if identification of *Yersinia* is required

Special Instructions The laboratory should be informed of the specific pathogen suspected if not *Salmonella*, *Shigella*, or *Campylobacter*.

Reference Range Negative for *Campylobacter*, *Salmonella*, and *Shigella*. In endemic areas the isolation of a pathogen may not indicate the cause or only cause of diarrhea.

Use Screen for pathogenic bacterial organisms in the stool; diagnose typhoid fever, enteric fever, bacillary dysentery, *Salmonella* infection, *Escherichia coli* 0157:H7 infection.

Indications for stool culture include:[4]
- bloody diarrhea
- fever
- tenesmus
- severe or persistent symptoms
- recent travel to a third world country
- known exposure to a bacterial agent
- presence of fecal leukocytes

Limitations An enormous variety of microorganisms have been proven to cause diarrhea, and many others have been associated with diarrhea. Still, even with the most extensive work-ups, a substantial proportion of patients with gastrointestinal disorders fail to yield an etiologic agent. Routine bacterial stool cultures are designed to recover only a few specific organisms; these vary with the laboratory, but usually includes *Salmonella*, *Shigella*, *Campylobacter* sp, and may include *E. coli* 0157:H7. Culture for the last may require special request, unless the stool is bloody.[5] The laboratory should be consulted if other etiologic agents are suspected (eg, *Vibrio* or *Yersinia*), or a more extensive work-up is required. Rectal swab cultures may not be as effective as stool cultures for identifying individuals with small numbers of organisms. *Clostridium difficile* infection is usually diagnosed by toxin assays rather than culture.

Contraindications A rectal swab culture is not as effective as a stool culture for detection of the carrier state.

Methodology Aerobic culture on selective media

Additional Information Stool cultures on patients hospitalized ≥3 days are not productive and should not be ordered unless special circumstances exist. In enteric fever caused by *Salmonella typhi*, *S. choleraesuis*, or *S. enteritidis*, blood culture may be positive before stool cultures.

Diarrhea is common in patients with the acquired immunodeficiency syndrome (AIDS). It may be caused by classic bacterial pathogens or unusual opportunistic bacteria viral or parasites (eg, *Giardia*, microsporidia, *Cryptosporidium*, and *Entamoeba histolytica*).[6] Rectal swabs are useful for the diagnosis of *Neisseria gonorrhoeae* and *Chlamydia* infections.

In acute or subacute diarrhea, three common syndromes are recognized: gastroenteritis, enteritis, and colitis (dysenteric syndrome). With colitis, patients have fecal urgency and tenesmus. Stools are frequently small in volume and contain blood, mucus, and leukocytes. External hemorrhoids are common and painful. Diarrhea of small bowel origin is indicated by the passage of few large volume stools. This is due to accumulation of fluid in the large bowel before passage. **Leukocytes** usually indicate bacterial colonic inflammation or ulcerative colitis rather than a specific pathogen; see listing Methylene Blue Stain, Stool *on page 642*. Bacterial diarrhea may be present in the absence of fecal leukocytes, and fecal leukocytes may be present in the absence of bacterial or parasitic agents (ie, idiopathic inflammatory bowel disease).[7] See table. Although most bacterial diarrhea is transient (1-30 days), cases of persistent symptoms (10 months) have been reported.[8] Infants younger than 1 year of age with a history of blood in the stool, more than 10 stools in 24 hours, and temperature greater than 39°C have a high probability of having bacterial diarrhea.[9,10] Diarrhea is also a common side effect of long-term antibiotic treatment. Although often associated with ***Clostridium difficile***, other bacteria and yeasts have been implicated.[11]

Escherichia coli 0157:H7 infection (enterohemorrhagic *E. coli*) presents a wide clinical spectrum which includes hemolytic uremic syndrome, thrombotic thrombocytopenic purpura as well as bacterial diarrhea. It causes up to 36% of cases of hemorrhagic colitis. It produces at least two toxins, including verotoxins (Shiga-like toxins). Its most common symptom is bloody diarrhea.[5] Revisions of laboratory protocols are described for organism recognition and verotoxin assay.[12,13]

Yersinia enterocolitica may cause inflammation of the distal ileum and show with mesenteric lymphadenitis and with marked lymphoid hyperplasia. There is necrosis of germinal centers and a clinical presentation which may resemble that of acute appendicitis. Culture may miss identification of the colonies unless the laboratory is aware of clinical suspicion for the organisms. Incubation at cooler temperature and use of selective media are useful.[14] See listing *Yersinia enterocolitica* Antibody *on page 440*.

Footnotes
1. Church DL, Cadrain G, Kabani A, et al, "Practice Guidelines for Ordering Stool Cultures in a Pediatric Population. Alberta Children's Hospital, Calgary, Alberta, Canada," *Am J Clin Pathol*, 1995, 103(2):149-53.
2. Siegel DL, Edelstein PH, and Nachamkin I, "Inappropriate Testing for Diarrheal Diseases in the Hospital," *JAMA*, 1990, 263(7):979-82.
3. Valenstein P, Pfaller M, and Yungbluth M, "The Use and Abuse of Routine Stool Microbiology: A College of American Pathologists Q-Probes Study of 601 Institutions," *Arch Pathol Lab Med*, 1996, 120:206-11.
4. Bishop WP and Ulshen MH, "Bacterial Gastroenteritis," *Pediatr Clin North Am*, 1988, 35(1):69-87.
5. Su C and Brandt LJ, "*Escherichia coli* 0157:H7 Infection in Humans," *Ann Intern Med*, 1995, 123(9):698-714.
6. Angulo FJ and Swerdlow DL, "Bacterial Enteric Infections in Persons Infected With Human Immunodeficiency Virus," *Clin Infect Dis*, 1995, 21(Suppl 1):S84-93.
7. DuPont HL, "Subacute Diarrhea to Treat or to Wait?" *Hosp Pract (Off Ed)*, 1989, 24(3A)111-8.
8. Clements D, Ellis CJ, and Allan RN, "Persistent Shigellosis - Case Report," *Gut*, 1988, 29(9):1277-8.
9. Finkelstein JA, Schwartz JS, Torrey S, et al, "Common Clinical Features as Predictors of Bacterial Diarrhea in Infants," *Am J Emerg Med*, 1989, 7(5):469-73.
10. Cohen MB, "Etiology and Mechanisms of Acute Infectious Diarrhea in Infants in the United States," *J Pediatr*, 1991, 118(4 Pt 2):S34-9.
11. Bartlett JG, "Antibiotic-Associated Diarrhea," *Clin Infect Dis*, 1992, 15(4):573-81.
12. Yungbluth M, "The Laboratory's Role in Diagnosing Enterohemorrhagic *Escherichia coli* Infections: Helping the Doctor Out," editorial, *Am J Clin Pathol*, 1994, 101(1):3-4.
13. Park CH, Hixon DL, Morrison WL, et al, "Rapid Diagnosis of Enterohemorrhagic *Escherichia coli* O157:H7 Directly From Fecal Specimens Using Immunofluorescence Stain," *Am J Clin Pathol*, 1994, 101(1):91-4.
14. Ashkenazi S and Cleary TG, "*Yersinia enterocolitica*," *Principles and Practice of Pediatrics*, Oski FA, DeAngelis CD, Feigin RD, et al, eds, Philadelphia, PA: JB Lippincott Co, 1994, 1259-61.

References
DeWitt TG, "Acute Diarrhea in Children," *Pediatr Rev*, 1989, 11(1):6-13.
Farmer RG, "Infectious Causes of Diarrhea in the Differential Diagnosis of Inflammatory Bowel Disease," *Med Clin North Am*, 1990, 74(1):29-38.
Griffin PM, Ostroff SM, and Tauxe RV, "Illness Associated With *Escherichia coli* 0157:H7 Infections. A Broad Clinical Spectrum," *Ann Intern Med*, 1988, 109(9):705-12.
Kao YS and Liu FJ, "Laboratory Diagnosis of Gastrointestinal Tract and Exocrine Pancreatic Disorders," *Clinical Diagnosis and Management by Laboratory Methods*, 18th ed, Chapter 23, Henry JB, ed, Philadelphia, PA: WB Saunders Co, 1991, 519-49.
Persaud CA and Eykyn SJ, "Stool Culture: Are You Getting Value for Money?" *J Clin Pathol*, 1994, 47(9):790-2.
Pickering LK, "Therapy for Acute Infectious Diarrhea in Children," *J Pediatr*, 1991, 118(4 Pt 2):S118-28.
Sanchez-Mejorada G and Ponce de Leon S, "Clinical Patterns of Diarrhea in AIDS: Etiology and Prognosis," *Rev Invest Clin*, 1994, 46(3):187-96.
Talal AH and Murray JA, "Acute and Chronic Diarrhea. How to Keep Laboratory Testing to a Minimum," *Postgrad Med*, 1994, 96(3):30-2, 35-8, 43.

Diarrhea Syndromes Classified by Predominant Features

Syndrome (anatomic site)	Features	Characteristic Etiologies
Gastroenteritis (stomach)	Vomiting	Rotavirus
		Norwalk virus
		Staphylococcal food poisoning
		Bacillus cereus food poisoning
Enteritis (small bowel)	Watery diarrhea Large-volume stools, few in number	Enterotoxigenic *Escherichia coli*
		Vibrio cholerae
		Any enteric microbe
		Inflammatory bowel disease
Dysentery, colitis (colon)	Small-volume stools containing blood and/or mucus and many leukocytes	*Shigella*
		Campylobacter
		Salmonella
		Invasive *E. coli*
		Plesiomonas shigelloides
		Aeromonas hydrophila
		Vibrio parahaemolyticus
		Clostridium difficile
		Entamoeba histolytica
		Inflammatory bowel disease

Bacterial Culture, Throat

CPT 87060

Related Information

Antideoxyribonuclease-B Titer, Serum *on page 365*
Antihyaluronidase Titer *on page 365*
Antistreptolysin O Titer, Serum *on page 369*
Corynebacterium diphtheriae Throat Culture *on page 474*
Gram's Stain *on page 481*
Group A *Streptococcus* Screen, Rapid *on page 483*
Streptozyme *on page 432*

Synonyms Throat Culture

Applies to Beta-Hemolytic Strep Culture, Throat; Group A Beta-Hemolytic *Streptococcus* Culture, Throat; Strep Throat Screening Culture; *Streptococcus pyogenes* Culture; Throat Culture, *Candida albicans*; Throat Culture for Group A Beta-Hemolytic *Streptococcus*

Test Commonly Includes Screening for group A beta-hemolytic streptococci

Patient Preparation Do not swab throat in cases of acute epiglottitis unless provisions to establish an alternate airway are readily available.

Specimen Throat swab

Container Sterile Culturette®; cotton, dacron, or alginate swabs are acceptable.

Collection The specimen should be transported to the laboratory promptly. Both tonsillar pillars and the oropharynx should be swabbed. The tongue should be depressed while the tonsillar pillars and the oropharynx are swabbed. Exudates should be swabbed, and the tongue and uvula should be avoided.

Storage Instructions Refrigerate

Turnaround Time Reports on specimens from which beta-hemolytic streptococci group A have been isolated usually require 24-48 hours for completion. Cultures with no growth are usually reported after 48 hours.

Special Instructions The laboratory should be informed of the specific site of the specimen, the age of patient, current antibiotic therapy, and clinical diagnosis.

Reference Range See table.

Throat Culture

Organisms Implicated in Infections of the Oropharynx	Organisms Commonly Present in the Normal Oropharynx	
Bordetella pertussis *†	*Actinomyces israelii* (tonsils)	*Haemophilus parainfluenzae*
Candida albicans	*Bacteroides* sp (tonsils)	*Klebsiella* sp
Corynebacterium diphtheriae†	*Candida albicans*	*Neisseria meningitidis*
Leptotrichia buccalis†	*Candida* sp	Nonhemolytic streptococci
Neisseria gonorrhoeae†	*Corynebacterium* sp (diphtheroids)	*Proteus* sp
Respiratory viruses:†	*E. coli*	*Staphylococcus aureus*
Adenovirus	Enterococci	*Staphylococcus epidermidis*
Enterovirus	*Fusobacterium* sp (tonsils)	*Streptococcus pneumoniae*
Epstein-Barr virus	*Haemophilus influenzae*	*Streptococcus pyogenes*
Parainfluenza virus		*Veillonella* sp
Reovirus		
Rhinovirus		
Streptococcus pyogenes		

* Rare because of vaccination.

† Not recovered by routine culture.

Use Isolate and identify beta-hemolytic group A *Streptococcus*

Limitations Beta-hemolytic streptococci are the only bacteria that should be routinely reported on throat culture.[1] Many other etiologic agents not isolated by routine bacterial culture can be responsible for pharyngitis (see table).[2] **This procedure does not usually include screening for Neisseria gonorrhoeae or Corynebacterium diphtheriae.** See listing *Corynebacterium diphtheriae* Throat Culture *on page 474*. Cultures for *Candida albicans* are usually held for about 1 week; thus, fungi other than *Candida albicans* will not be recovered. *Candida* sp frequently do not adhere well to swabs, therefore, scraping may have a higher yield.[3] Anaerobic organisms which are frequently implicated in chronic infection of the tonsils and adenoids are not recovered by aerobic culture methods.

Methodology Aerobic culture including blood agar medium

Additional Information A saline wet preparation, Gram's stain, or KOH preparation demonstrating yeast cells or pseudohyphae may also be useful in rapidly establishing the diagnosis of oral or mucocutaneous candidiasis. Thrush, oral candidiasis, and *Candida* esophagitis frequently complicate antineoplastic therapy, hyperalimentation, transplantation immunosuppression, pregnancy, and the acquired immunodeficiency syndrome (AIDS). Routine throat cultures will detect group A *Streptococcus*, however, in some settings a specific culture can be requested for detection of beta-hemolytic *Streptococcus* only.

Streptococcus pyogenes (group A beta-hemolytic strep) is generally susceptible to penicillin and its derivatives, therefore, susceptibility need not be routinely determined. The principal reason for considering an alternative drug for individual patients is allergy to penicillin. Erythromycin, a cephalosporin, or clindamycin might be substituted in these cases. Patients allergic to penicillins may also be allergic to cephalosporins.

Use of latex agglutination screening tests and enzyme-linked immunoassay tests provide rapid confirmation of the presence of group A streptococci.[4] The sensitivity of the rapid methods is as high as 96% in overt clinical pharyngitis and/or scarlet fever. Confirmation of negatives by culture is recommended.[4] Lieu et al recommend both antigen testing and culture as the most clinically effective strategy giving consideration to the complications of therapy for those who do not have streptococcal infection and the relative lack of sensitivity of antigen tests as compared to culture.[5]

In the late 1980s, a resurgence of serious *Streptococcus pyogenes* infection was observed. Complications including rheumatic fever, sepsis, severe soft tissue invasion, and toxic shock-like syndrome (TSLS) are reported to be most common with the M1 serotype and that a unique invasive clone has become the predominant cause of severe streptococcal infections.[6]

Footnotes

1. Welch DF, Hensel D, Pickett D, et al, "Comparative Evaluation of Selective and Nonselective Culture Techniques for Isolation of Group A Beta-Hemolytic Streptococci," *Am J Clin Pathol*, 1991, 95(4):587-90.
2. Lang SD and Singh K, "The Sore Throat, When to Investigate and When to Prescribe," *Drugs*, 1990, 40(6):854-62.
3. Gray LD and Roberts GD, "Laboratory Diagnosis of Systemic Fungal Diseases," *Infect Dis Clin North Am*, 1988, 2(4):779-803.
4. Tenjarla G, Kumar A, and Dyke JW, "TestPack Strep A Kit for the Rapid Detection of Group A Streptococci on 11,088 Throat Swabs in a Clinical Pathology Laboratory," *Am J Clin Pathol*, 1991, 96(6):759-61.
5. Lieu TA, Fleisher GR, and Schwartz JS, "Cost-Effectiveness of Rapid Latex Agglutination Testing and Throat Culture for Streptococcal Pharyngitis," *Pediatrics*, 1990, 85(3):246-56.
6. Cleary PP, Kaplan EL, Handley JP, et al, "Clonal Basis for Resurgence of Serious *Streptococcus pyogenes* Disease in the 1980s," *Lancet*, 1992, 339(8792):518-21.

References

Bisno AL, "Group A Streptococcal Infections and Acute Rheumatic Fever," *N Engl J Med*, 1991, 325(11):783-93.
Givner LB, Abramson JS, and Wasilauskas B, "Apparent Increase in the Incidence of Invasive Group A Beta-Hemolytic Streptococcal Disease in Children," *J Pediatr*, 1991, 118(3):341-6.
Kiselica D, "Group A Beta-Hemolytic Streptococcal Pharyngitis: Current Clinical Concepts," *Am Fam Physician*, 1994, 49(5):1147-54.
Wheeler MC, Roe MH, Kaplan EL, et al, "Outbreak of Group A *Streptococcus* Septicemia in Children: Clinical, Epidemiologic, and Microbiological Correlates," *JAMA*, 1991, 266(4):533-7.

Bacterial Culture, Urine, Clean Catch

CPT 87086 (quantitative culture); 87088 (identification)

Related Information

Bacterial Culture, Urine, Suprapubic Puncture *on next page*
Chlamydia trachomatis Culture *on page 662*
Fungal Culture, Urine *on page 480*
Gram's Stain *on page 481*
Kidney Stone Analysis *on page 640*
Leukocyte Esterase, Urine *on page 641*
Mycobacterial Culture, Urine *on page 491*
Nitrite, Urine *on page 645*
Urinalysis *on page 658*
Viral Culture *on page 675*
Viral Culture, Urine *on page 681*

Synonyms CMVS Culture; Midstream Urine Culture; Urine Culture, Clean Catch

Applies to Urine Culture, Foley Catheter

Abstract Urinary tract infections (UTI) cause seven million patient visits annually. They include acute urethral syndrome, acute cystitis, and pyelonephritis. Evaluation of UTI includes use of leukocyte esterase and nitrite on reagent strips, microscopy, methylene blue and Gram's stain, culture and an enzyme-based test for bacteriuria, URISCREEN.[1]

Patient Preparation Instruct patient for proper collection of "clean catch" specimen. Wash hands thoroughly. Wash penis or vulva using downward strokes four times with four soapy sponges, then once with sponge wet with warm water. Urethral meatus and perineum must be washed. Each sponge must be discarded after one use. Urinate about 30 mL (1 ounce) of urine directly into toilet or bedpan **- stop -** position container and take middle portion of urine sample. Screw cap securely on container without touching the inside rim. Apply the completed patient label to the specimen cup. Most patients, with instruction, do better with privacy than with an attendant.

Specimen Random urine

Container Plastic urine container or sterile tube

Collection Early morning specimens yield highest bacterial counts from overnight incubation in the bladder. Forced fluids dilute the urine and may cause reduced colony counts. Hair from perineum will contaminate the specimen. The stream from a male may be contaminated by bacteria from beneath the prepuce. Bacteria from vaginal secretions, vulva, or distal urethra may also contaminate the specimen as may organisms from hands or clothing. Receptacle must be sterile. Provide time and date of urine collection.

Storage Instructions Refrigerate the specimen if it cannot be promptly processed. A transport stabilizer may be used to preserve the specimen if refrigeration is not available.[2]

Causes for Rejection Unrefrigerated specimen more than 2 hours old is subject to overgrowth of bacteria and may yield false-positive results.

Reference Range <10^4 CFU/mL. Quantitative culture is in global use. Significant bacteriuria is usually considered to be 10^5 CFU/mL (colony forming units). A break point of 10^2 maximizes diagnostic sensitivity,[3] but produces numerous false-positive results.

Use Isolate and identify potentially pathogenic organisms causing urinary tract infection

Limitations Bacteria present in numbers <1000 organisms/mL may not be detected by routine methods. Contamination during collection (particularly in women) may cause colony counts of 10^3 or 10^4; thus, a breakpoint of 10^2 CFU/mL causes inclusion of a large number of normal women without significant bacteriuria.[4] The first few drops of urine pick up unimportant organisms from periurethral or perineal sources. Contamination from nonurinary sources remains a problem.[5] So-called "low-count bacteriuria" has been considered a possible early phase of urinary tract infection.[6] When more than two organisms are recovered, the likelihood of contamination is high; thus, the significance of definitive identification of the organisms and susceptibility testing in this situation is severely limited. A repeat culture with proper specimen collection including patient preparation is often indicated.

Failure to recover aerobic organisms from patients with pyuria or positive Gram's stains of urinary sediment may indicate the presence of mycobacteria or anaerobes.

Methodology Quantitative aerobic culture; usually plated at a 0.001 dilution, allowing detection of organisms in enumeration of 10^3 CFU/mL or greater

Additional Information A single culture is about 80% accurate in the female; two containing the same organism with count of 10^5 or more represents 95% chance of true bacteriuria; three such specimens mean virtual certainty of true bacteriuria. Recent studies have shown that a Gram's stain from 0.2 mL of urine cytocentrifuged onto a slide is a very sensitive method of screening for bacteriuria.[7] Rapid detection of bacteriuria is helpful in the early treatment of patients. Several other methods have also been described for the rapid detection of bacteriuria, growth-photometric, bioluminescence, measurement of bacterial adenosine triphosphate, and acridine orange stain.

Urinary tract infection is significantly higher in women who use diaphragm-spermicide contraception, perhaps secondary to increased vaginal pH and a higher frequency of vaginal colonization with *E. coli*.[8] A single, clean-voided specimen from an adult male may be considered diagnostic with proper preparation and care in specimen collection. If the patient is receiving antimicrobial therapy at the time the specimen is collected, any level of bacteriuria may be significant.

Periodic screening of diabetics and pregnant women for asymptomatic bacteriuria has been recommended.[9] Institutionalized patients, especially elderly individuals, are prone to urinary tract infections which can be severe.[10] Cultures of specimens from Foley catheters yielding multiple organisms with high colony counts may represent colonization of the catheter and not true significant bacteriuria. Most laboratories limit the number of organisms which will be identified when recovered from urine to two. Similarly, most do not routinely perform susceptibility tests on isolates from presumably contaminated specimens.

The acute urethral syndrome occurs in women. It includes symptoms of urinary tract infection with low bacterial counts and >8-10 WBC/hpf urine.[11]

Detection of bacteriuria can be accomplished by slide centrifuge Gram's stained smear and by other means as well.[12] In elderly women, screening for asymptomatic bacteriuria did not appear warranted in a study using clean catch urine specimens.[13] The practice of not treating asymptomatic bacteriuria in nursing home residents was supported in another study.[14]

Footnotes

1. Carroll KC, Hale DC, Von Boerum DH, et al, "Laboratory Evaluation of Urinary Tract Infections in an Ambulatory Clinic," *Am J Clin Pathol*, 1994, 101(1):100-3.
2. Williams JD, "Criteria for Diagnosis of Urinary Tract Infection and Evaluation of Therapy," *Infection*, 1992, 4(20 Suppl 4):S257-60.
3. Johnson JR and Stamm WE, "Urinary Tract Infections in Women: Diagnosis and Treatment," *Ann Intern Med*, 1989, 111(11):906-17.
4. Hooton TM and Stamm WE, "Management of Acute Uncomplicated Urinary Tract Infection in Adults," *Med Clin North Am*, 1991, 75(2):339-57.
5. Jaffe JS, "Collection of Urine for Culture," *N Engl J Med*, 1994, 331(9):617-8.
6. Kunin CM, White LV, and Hua TH, "A Reassessment of the Importance of 'Low-Count' Bacteriuria in Young Women With Acute Urinary Symptoms," *Ann Intern Med*, 1993, 119(6):454-60.
7. Olson ML, Shanholtzer CJ, Willard KE, et al, "The Slide Centrifuge Gram Stain as a Urine Screening Method," *Am J Clin Pathol*, 1991, 96(4):454-8.
8. Stamm WE, Hooton TM, Johnson JR, et al, "Urinary Tract Infections: From Pathogenesis to Treatment," *J Infect Dis*, 1989, 159(3):400-6.
9. Andriole VT, "Urinary Tract Infections in the 90s: Pathogenesis and Management," *Infection*, 1992, 4(20 Suppl 4):S251-6.
10. Nicolle LE, "Urinary Tract Infection in the Elderly: How to Treat and When?" *Infection*, 1992, 4(20 Suppl 4):S261-5.
11. Sodeman TM, "A Practical Strategy for Diagnosis of Urinary Tract Infections," *Clin Lab Med*, 1995, 15(2):235-50.
12. Rippin KP, Stinson WC, Eisenstadt J, et al, "Clinical Evaluation of the Slide Centrifuge (Cytospin) Gram's Stained Smear for the Detection of Bacteriuria and Comparison With the Filtracheck-UTI and UTIscreen," *Am J Clin Pathol*, 1995, 103(3):316-9.
13. Abrutyn E, Mossey J, Berlin JA, et al, "Does Asymptomatic Bacteriuria Predict Mortality and Does Antimicrobial Treatment Reduce Mortality in Elderly Ambulatory Women?" *Ann Intern Med*, 1994, 120(10):827-33.
14. Ouslander JG, Schapira M, Schnelle JF, et al, "Does Eradicating Bacteriuria Affect the Severity of Chronic Urinary Incontinence in Nursing Home Residents?" *Ann Intern Med*, 1995, 122(10):749-54.

References

Rippin KP, Stinson WC, Eisenstadt J, et al, "Clinical Evaluation of the Slide Centrifuge (Cytospin) Gram's Stained Smear for the Detection of Bacteriuria and Comparison With the Filtracheck-UTI and UTIscreen," *Am J Clin Pathol*, 1995, 103(3):316-9.
Ronald AR, Nicolle LE, and Harding GK, "Standards of Therapy for Urinary Tract Infections in Adults," *Infection*, 1992, 20(Suppl 3):S164-70.
Stamm WE, "Criteria for the Diagnosis of Urinary Tract Infection and for the Assessment of Therapeutic Effectiveness," *Infection*, 1992, 20(Suppl 3):S151-9.
Stamm WE and Hooton TM, "Management of Urinary Tract Infections in Adults," *N Engl J Med*, 1993, 392(18):1328-34.
Zhanel GG, Nicolle LE, Harding GK, et al, "Prevalence of Asymptomatic Bacteriuria and Associated Host Factors in Women With Diabetes Mellitus," *Clin Infect Dis*, 1995, 21:316-22.

Bacterial Culture, Urine, Suprapubic Puncture

CPT 87086 (quantitative culture); 87088 (identification)

Related Information

Bacterial Culture, Urine, Clean Catch *on previous page*
Fungal Culture, Urine *on page 480*
Gram's Stain *on page 481*
Mycobacterial Culture, Urine *on page 491*

Synonyms Suprapubic Puncture Culture; Urine Culture, Suprapubic Puncture

Applies to Urine Anaerobic Culture, Suprapubic Puncture; Urine Culture, Straight Catheter

Test Commonly Includes Leukocyte esterase may be included.[1]

Abstract Suprapubic aspiration of the urinary bladder is only indicated infrequently.

Patient Preparation Aseptic preparation of the aspiration site. Collect the specimen to avoid contamination with normal skin flora. Fluids should be forced prior to collection of the specimen to distend the bladder. Successful suprapubic collection requires a distended bladder; 6-10 hours may be required for the bladder to fill.

Specimen Label the specimen as urine obtained by suprapubic puncture

Container Sterile, plastic urine container

Collection After aseptic preparation of the skin, the specimen is aspirated in a sterile syringe by a physician skilled in the technique.

Storage Instructions **To optimize the recovery of fastidious organisms, the specimen should be transported to the laboratory as soon as possible after collection.** Refrigerate the specimen if it cannot be promptly processed.

Causes for Rejection Unrefrigerated specimen more than 2 hours old is subject to overgrowth of microorganisms.

Turnaround Time Reports on specimens from which an organism or organisms have been isolated usually require 48 hours for completion.

Special Instructions The laboratory should be informed that the specimen is a "suprapubic puncture," current antibiotic therapy, and time of collection.

Reference Range No growth. Any organisms so recovered are considered significant if the specimen has been properly obtained.

Use Isolate and identify pathogenic organisms causing urinary tract infection; obtain sterile urine specimens on newborns. Suprapubic aspiration may allow isolation of organisms which are too fastidious to be recovered by culture of voided urine and markedly reduces the probability of contamination during collection.
(Continued)

Bacterial Culture, Urine, Suprapubic Puncture
(Continued)

Limitations Bacteria present in numbers <1000 organisms/mL may not be detected by routine methods.

Methodology Quantitative aerobic culture. All rapid-growing, nonfastidious aerobic bacteria will usually be isolated and identified. Antimicrobial susceptibility testing is usually performed if indicated, regardless of colony count when obtained by suprapubic puncture. This is the only acceptable urine specimen for isolation of anaerobic organisms. Anaerobic organisms may be recovered if anaerobic culture is requested. Special culture procedures must be undertaken to recover *Ureaplasma urealyticum*, *Gardnerella vaginalis*, and *Mycoplasma hominis*, which are the most frequently encountered fastidious species.[2] The cultures are usually plated at a 0.01 dilution, allowing detection of organisms in a concentration of 10^2 CFU/mL or greater.

Additional Information Fairley and Birch, studying male and female patients with acute urinary tract symptoms, found 31% (561/1817) females and 12% (36/300) males culture positive.[3] Seventy percent of the isolates were "fastidious" bacteria which are not usually recovered by conventional techniques. The organisms recovered were frequently (67%) present in $<10^5$ CFU/mL. Thirty-four percent of females but none of the males had polymicrobic isolates which usually included a fastidious organism. Many cases of negative culture in females with acute urinary symptoms may represent cases of low count 10^2 to 10^4 CFU/mL cystitis. Suprapubic puncture can be used to document ascending infection (ie, cystitis) due to *Neisseria gonorrhoeae*.[4] Specimens for *N. gonorrhoeae* culture should not be refrigerated and should be transported to the laboratory quickly.

The **acute urethral syndrome** presents with urgency, frequency, and dysuria but may include low bacterial counts. More than 8-10 WBC/hpf are found. Suprapubic puncture urine specimens for culture may be indicated.[1]

Footnotes
1. Sodeman TM, "A Practical Strategy for Diagnosis of Urinary Tract Infections," *Clin Lab Med*, 1995, 15(2):235-50.
2. Gilbert GL, Garland SM, and Fairley KF, "Bacteriuria Due to *Ureaplasma* and Other Fastidious Organisms During Pregnancy," *Pediatr Infect Dis*, 1986, 5(6 Suppl):S239-43.
3. Fairley KF and Birch DF, "Detection of Bladder Bacteriuria in Patients With Acute Urinary Symptoms," *J Infect Dis*, 1989, 159:226-31.
4. Péc J Jr, Moravčík P, Kliment J, et al, "Isolation of *Neisseria gonorrhoeae* from Urine Obtained by Suprapubic Puncture of Bladders of Men With Gonococcal Urethritis," *Genitourin Med*, 1988, 64(3):156-8.

References
Komaroff AL, "Urinalysis and Urine Culture in Women With Dysuria," *Ann Intern Med*, 1986, 104(2):212-8.
Stamm WE, Hooton TM, Johnson JR, et al, "Urinary Tract Infections: From Pathogenesis to Treatment," *J Infect Dis*, 1989, 159(3):400-6.

Bacterial Culture, Wound
CPT 87070

Related Information
Bacterial Culture, Abscess *on page 454*
Bacterial Culture, Biopsy or Body Fluid *on page 456*
Bacterial Culture, Burn Sites *on page 460*

Synonyms Wound Culture

Applies to Gunshot Wound Culture; Puncture Wound, Foreign Body, Culture

Test Commonly Includes Culture for aerobic organisms and usually Gram's stain; anaerobic cultures may be indicated.

Patient Preparation Sterile preparation of the aspiration site

Specimen Pus or other material properly obtained from a wound site or abscess

Container Syringe, sterile tube, or Culturette® swab

Collection Drainage cultured by aspiration away from a sinus tract may provide more useful information. Contamination with normal flora from skin, rectum, vaginal tract, or other body surfaces should be avoided. If anaerobes are suspected, a properly collected specimen for anaerobic culture should also be submitted.

Causes for Rejection Specimens delayed in transit to the laboratory may have suboptimal yields.

Special Instructions Procedures for laboratory work-up of wound cultures which may contain contamination from the skin surface are different than those from sterile sites.

Reference Range No growth. A simultaneous Gram's stain should always be performed to facilitate interpretation. Gram-negative organisms frequently colonize wounds, and mixed culture results are common.

Use Isolate and identify potentially pathogenic organisms from wounds or biopsy/aspiration material

Limitations Unless specifically requested by the physician or mandated by the specimen source (ie, genital specimen), fastidious organisms such as *N. gonorrhoeae* may not be isolated. Anaerobic, fungal, and mycobacterial pathogens should be considered, and appropriate cultures requested if indicated.

Contraindications Culture of contaminated open wounds which have not been cleansed or debrided may prove suboptimal.

Additional Information See table. The majority of bacteria infecting surgical wounds are common airborne microorganisms.[1] Effective treatment of wound infection usually includes drainage, removal of foreign bodies, infected prosthetic devices, and retained foreign objects such as grass or suture material. Suction irrigation may be helpful in resolving wound infections. Species commonly recovered from wounds include *Escherichia coli*, *Proteus* sp, *Klebsiella* sp, *Pseudomonas* sp, *Enterobacter* sp, enterococci, other streptococci, *Bacteroides* sp, *Prevotella* sp, *Clostridium* sp, *Staphylococcus aureus*, and *Staphylococcus epidermidis* (coagulase-negative *Staphylococcus*).

Classification of Soft-Tissue Infections

Tissue Level	Common Surgical Pathogens				
	S. pyogenes	*S. aureus*	*C. perfringens*	Mixed Bacteria	
				Staph & Strep	Enteric
Epidermis	Ecthyma contagiosum	Scalded-skin syndrome		Possibly impetigo	
Dermis and sub-dermis	Erysipelas/cellulitis	Folliculitis/abscess	Abscess/cellulitis	Meleny's ulcer (synergistic gangrene)	Tropical ulcer
Fascial planes	Strep gangrene	Carbuncle	Fasciitis	Necrotizing fasciitis	
Muscle tissue	Strep myositis	Muscular abscess/pyomyositis	Myonecrosis	Nonclostridial myonecrosis	

From Ahrenholz DH, 'Necrotizing Soft Tissue Infections,' *Surg Clin North Am*, 1988, 68:198-214, with permission.

Footnotes
1. Whyte W, Hambraeus A, Laurell G, et al, "The Relative Importance of the Routes and Sources of Wound Contamination During General Surgery. II. Airborne," *J Hosp Infect*, 1992, 22(1):41-54.

References
Burdette-Taylor S and Taylor TG, "Wound Culture: What, When and Why," *Ostomy Wound Manage*, 1993, 39(8):26-7, 30, 32.
Cheadle WG, "Current Perspectives on Antibiotic Use in the Treatment of Surgical Infections," *Am J Surg*, 1992, 164(4A Suppl):44S-47S.
Cuzzell JZ, "The Right Way to Culture a Wound," *Am J Nurs*, 1993, 93(5):48-50.
Garibaldi RA, Cushing D, and Lerer T, "Risk Factors for Postoperative Infection," *Am J Med*, 1991, 91(3B):158S-163S.
Goldstein EJ, "Management of Human and Animal Bite Wounds," *J Am Acad Dermatol*, 1989, 21(6):1275-9.
McConnell EA, "Obtaining an Aerobic Wound Culture Specimen," *Nursing*, 1991, 21(5):21.
Pollock AV and Evans M, "Microbiologic Prediction of Abdominal Surgical Wound Infection," *Arch Surg*, 1987, 122(1):33-7.

Bacterial Inhibitory Level, Serum *see* Serum Bactericidal Test *on page 496*

BAL, Culture *see* Bacterial Culture, Bronchoscopy Specimen *on page 459*

Beta-Hemolytic Strep Culture, Throat *see* Bacterial Culture, Throat *on page 468*

Beta-Lactamase Test
CPT 87999

Related Information
Antimicrobial Susceptibility Testing, Aerobic and Facultatively Anaerobic Bacteria *on page 448*
Antimicrobial Susceptibility Testing, Anaerobic Bacteria *on page 449*
Neisseria gonorrhoeae Culture and Smear *on page 492*

Synonyms Cefinase (Nitrocefin) Testing; Cephalosporinase Production Testing; Penicillinase-Producing Organisms Susceptibility Testing; Penicillinase Test

Applies to Beta-Lactam Ring; Cephalosporinases; *Haemophilus influenzae* Susceptibility Testing; *Neisseria gonorrhoeae* Susceptibility Testing; Penicillinases

Test Commonly Includes Rapid testing of isolated bacterial colonies for the production of beta-lactamase

Abstract Certain bacteria produce enzymes that inactivate beta-lactam antibiotics. Some enzymes can hydrolyze penicillin (penicillinases);

others hydrolyze cephalosporins (cephalosporinases). In either case the detection of enzyme production by bacterial isolates is essential in determination of appropriate therapy.

Specimen Isolated colonies of *Haemophilus influenzae*, *Moraxella* (*Branhamella*) *catarrhalis*, *Neisseria gonorrhoeae*, enterococci, *Staphylococcus aureus*, or gram-negative anaerobic rods including *Bacteroides fragilis*

Use Rapid detection of beta-lactamase production from isolated colonies of *Haemophilus influenzae*, *Neisseria gonorrhoeae*, *Moraxella catarrhalis*, and *Enterococcus* sp. This test can be used to predict resistance to penicillins and some cephalosporins.

Limitations Beta-lactamase negative strains may be resistant to penicillins or cephalosporins by other mechanisms. This is rare for the organisms listed above, except enterococci.

Methodology The acidimetric method uses pH color indicators to detect increased acidity that results when the beta-lactam ring of penicillin is cleaved to yield a penicilloic acid. Penicilloic acid can also reduce iodine that can be detected as the decolorization of a starch-iodine mixture. This method is referred to as the iodometric method. The most commonly used method is the use of a chromogenic cephalosporin reagent. The hydrolysis of the beta-lactam ring results in a color change that is quickly detected. The chromogenic assay can detect both penicillinases and cephalosporinases.

Additional Information The beta-lactamase test can provide clinically useful information when used for organisms in which the primary mechanism of resistance to beta-lactam antibiotics is by means of beta-lactamase enzymes, and in which resistance patterns to other antimicrobial agents is predictable. Consequently, beta-lactamase testing is restricted to a few specific circumstances that meet such criteria. *H. influenzae* and *M. catarrhalis* isolates that produce beta-lactamase are resistant to ampicillin, but resistance to other agents is predictable (ie, virtually all isolates are presently susceptible to most second and third generation cephalosporins, beta-lactamase inhibitor combinations, azithromycin, and clarithromycin).[1] *N. gonorrhoeae* isolates that are beta-lactamase positive are resistant to penicillin, but uniformly susceptible to ceftriaxone.[1] Beta-lactamase testing of anaerobic gram-negative bacilli (eg, *Bacteroides*, *Porphyromonas*, and *Prevotella* sp) is of limited clinical utility due to low sensitivity.[2]

Footnotes

1. Doern GV, "Susceptibility Tests of Fastidious Bacteria," *Manual of Clinical Microbiology*, 6th ed, Murray PR, Baron EJ, Pfaller MA, eds, et al, Washington, DC: American Society for Microbiology, 1995, 1342-9.
2. Wexler HM and Doern GV, "Susceptibility Testing of Anaerobic Bacteria," *Manual of Clinical Microbiology*, 6th ed, Murray PR, Baron EJ, Pfaller MA, eds, et al, Washington, DC: American Society for Microbiology, 1995, 379-99.

References

Jones RN and Edson DC, "Antimicrobial Susceptibility Testing Trends and Accuracy in the United States. A Review of the College of American Pathologists Microbiology Surveys, 1972-1989. Microbiology Resource Committee of the College of American Pathologists," *Arch Pathol Lab Med*, 1991, 115(5):429-36.
Jorgensen JH, "Update on Mechanisms and Prevalence of Antimicrobial Resistance in *Haemophilus influenzae*," *Clin Infect Dis*, 1992, 14(5):1119-23.

Beta-Lactam Ring *see* Antimicrobial Susceptibility Testing, Aerobic and Facultatively Anaerobic Bacteria *on page 448*

Beta-Lactam Ring *see* Beta-Lactamase Test *on previous page*

Biopsy Aerobic Culture *see* Bacterial Culture, Biopsy or Body Fluid *on page 456*

Biopsy *Legionella* Culture *see* Legionella Culture *on page 485*

Biopsy or Body Fluid Fungus Culture *see* Fungal Culture, Biopsy or Body Fluid *on page 476*

Biopsy Specimen Culture, Quantitative *see* Bacterial Culture, Burn Sites *on page 460*

Blastocystis hominis *see* Ova and Parasites, Stool *on page 494*

Blood Culture, BactAlert® *see* Bacterial Culture, Blood *on page 457*

Blood Culture, *Brucella* *see* Brucella Culture *on next page*

Blood Culture, Isolator™ *see* Bacterial Culture, Blood *on page 457*

Blood Culture, *Leptospira* *see* Leptospira Culture *on page 486*

Blood Culture, Lysis Centrifugation *see* Bacterial Culture, Blood *on page 457*

Blood Culture With Antimicrobial Removal Device (ARD) *see* Bacterial Culture, Blood *on page 457*

Blood Fungus Culture *see* Fungal Culture, Blood *on page 477*

Body Fluid Aerobic Culture *see* Bacterial Culture, Biopsy or Body Fluid *on page 456*

Body Fluid Fungus Culture *see* Fungal Culture, Biopsy or Body Fluid *on page 476*

Body Fluid Mycobacteria Culture *see* Mycobacterial Culture, Biopsy or Body Fluid *on page 487*

Bone Marrow Culture *see* Bacterial Culture, Biopsy or Body Fluid *on page 456*

Bone Marrow Culture for *Brucella* *see* Brucella Culture *on next page*

Bone Marrow Fungus Culture *see* Fungal Culture, Biopsy or Body Fluid *on page 476*

Bone Marrow Mycobacteria Culture *see* Mycobacterial Culture, Biopsy or Body Fluid *on page 487*

Bordetella pertussis Culture

CPT 87081 (culture, single organism); 87206 (fluorescent smear)

Related Information

Bacterial Culture, Nasopharynx *on page 464*
Bordetella pertussis Direct Fluorescent Antibody *on page 371*
Bordetella pertussis Serology *on page 372*

Synonyms Nasopharyngeal Culture for *Bordetella pertussis*; Pertussis Culture; Whooping Cough Culture

Replaces Cough Plate Culture for Pertussis; Throat Culture for *Bordetella pertussis*

Patient Preparation Patient should not be on antimicrobial therapy prior to the collection of the specimen.

Specimen Nasopharyngeal swab, cough plate optional

Container Flexible calcium alginate swab (Calgiswab®) and Bordet Gengou plate. Transport medium composed of half strength Oxoid charcoal agar CM19 supplemented with 40 µg/mL cephalexin and 10% hemolyzed defibrinated horse blood may be used.[1]

Collection Shape the flexible swab into the contour of the nares. Pass the swab gently through the nose. Leave swab in place near septum and floor of nose for 15-30 seconds. Rotate and remove. The recovery of the organism depends on collecting an adequate specimen. Inoculate the plate or transport medium directly at the bedside.

The following procedure optimizes the laboratory diagnosis of pertussis.

- Collect nasopharyngeal specimens in the early stage of illness. Provision of specimen collection kits facilitates appropriate specimen collection and transportation.
- For swab collected specimens, use a transport medium consisting of half strength Oxoid charcoal agar supplemented with 10% hemolyzed, defibrinated horse blood, and 40 µg/mL cephalexin.
- Inoculate a selective primary plating medium composed of Oxoid charcoal agar, 10% defibrinated horse blood, and 40 µg/mL cephalexin. A nonselective medium without cephalexin may be used in addition to the selective medium.
- Perform direct fluorescent antibody (DFA) tests on appropriately collected nasopharyngeal secretions with *B. pertussis*- and *B. parapertussis*-conjugated antisera to facilitate an earlier diagnosis.
- After inoculation of primary plating media, retain swabs in the original transport medium at room temperature. If cultures become overgrown with indigenous bacterial flora or fungi, use swabs to inoculate additional media.
- Identify suspicious isolates with appropriate cultural and biochemical tests. The DFA test performed on growth from isolated colonies is an excellent procedure for confirmatory or definitive identification.

Storage Instructions The specimen should not be refrigerated. It should be transported to the laboratory as soon as possible.

Causes for Rejection Excessive delay in transit to the laboratory results in less than optimal yield.

Turnaround Time Growth of *Bordetella pertussis* takes at least 72 hours to be detected.

Special Instructions Consult the laboratory prior to collection of the specimen so that the special isolation medium can be obtained. The laboratory should be made aware of the specific request to screen for *Bordetella pertussis* with information relevant to current antibiotic therapy.

Reference Range No *B. pertussis* or *B. parapertussis* isolated

Use Isolate and identify *B. pertussis*, and *B. parapertussis*; establish the diagnosis of whooping cough

Limitations Isolation of *Bordetella* sp probably has sensitivity of <50% compared to comprehensive serologic testing.

Contraindications Current antibiotic therapy; history of vaccination is a relative contraindication

Methodology Culture on selective medium (selective chocolate agar with 10% defibrinated horse blood and 40 µg/mL cephalexin), presumptive

(Continued)

Bordetella pertussis Culture *(Continued)*

confirmation by direct fluorescent antibody (DFA). Culture after enrichment in transport medium for 48 hours increases yield. Detection by DNA amplification is currently in development.[1,2]

Additional Information Direct fluorescent antibody (DFA) procedures provide more rapid results and have been increasingly used in the diagnosis of *B. pertussis* infection. The DFA procedures are most useful in the first 2-3 weeks of the illness. DFA test detected 42 of 164 (26%) of patients who proved culture positive for *B. pertussis* and 8 of 38 (21%) of patients who proved culture positive for *B. parapertussis*. False-negatives may be caused by inadequate specimens having little cellular material (leukocytes and brush border epithelial cells).[3]

Footnotes

1. He Q, Mertsola J, Soini H, et al, "Comparison of Polymerase Chain Reaction With Culture and Enzyme Immunoassay for Diagnosis of Pertussis," *J Clin Microbiol*, 1993, 31(3):642-5.
2. van der Zee A, Agterberg C, Peeters M, et al, "Polymerase Chain Reaction Assay for Pertussis: Simultaneous Detection and Discrimination of *Bordetella pertussis* and *Bordetella parapertussis*," *J Clin Microbiol*, 1993, 31(8):2134-40.
3. Young SA, Anderson GL, and Mitchell PD, "Laboratory Observations During an Outbreak of Pertussis," *Clin Microbiol Newslet*, 1987, 9:22, 176-9.

References

Hallander HO, Reizenstein E, Renemar B, et al, "Comparison of Nasopharyngeal Aspirates With Swabs for Culture of *Bordetella pertussis*," *J Clin Microbiol*, 1993, 31(1):50-2.
Halperin SA, "Interpretation of Pertussis Serologic Tests," *Pediatr Infect Dis J*, 1991, 10(10):791-2.
Halperin SA, Bortolussi R, and Wort AJ, "Evaluation of Culture, Immunofluorescence, and Serology for the Diagnosis of Pertussis," *J Clin Microbiol*, 1989, 27(4):752-7.
Herwaldt LA, "Pertussis is Adults. What Physicians Need to Know," *Arch Intern Med*, 1991, 151(8):1510-2.
Marchant CD, Loughlin AM, Lett SM, et al, "Pertussis in Massachusetts, 1981-1991: Incidence, Serologic Diagnosis, and Vaccine Effectiveness," *J Infect Dis*, 1994, 169(6):1297-305.

Botulism Diagnostic Procedure

CPT 87001 (animal inoculation); 87081 (culture, single organism)

Related Information

Bacterial Culture, Stool *on page 466*

Synonyms *Clostridium botulinum* Toxin Identification Procedure; Infant Botulism, Toxin Identification; Sudden Death Syndrome

Abstract *Clostridium botulinum* produces a potent neurotoxic protein which effects the nervous system without direct bacterial invasion of the CNS. The clinical manifestations of such intoxication include diplopia and dysphagia with descending progression of paralysis, leading to respiratory embarrassment. Gastrointestinal tract complaints occur.

Specimen Vomitus, serum, stool, gastric washings, cerebrospinal fluid or autopsy tissue; food samples

Container Sterile wide-mouth, leakproof, screw-cap jar; red top tube

Storage Instructions Keep refrigerated at $4^\circ C$ except for unopened food samples.

Turnaround Time 3-7 days

Special Instructions The laboratory must be notified prior to obtaining specimen in order to prepare for transport of the specimen to the State Health Laboratory or Centers for Disease Control.

Reference Range No toxin identified, no *Clostridium botulinum* isolated

Use Diagnose classic foodborne botulism, wound botulism (rare), infant botulism, sudden death syndrome, or floppy baby syndrome

Limitations The toxin from *C. botulinum* binds almost irreversibly to individual nerve terminals; thus, serum and cerebrospinal fluid specimens can yield false-negative results.

Contraindications Due to the difficulty in performance of the diagnostic test and because of the extensive epidemiological studies initiated upon receipt of the specimen, State Department of Health Laboratories require specific clinical symptomatology for botulism. Clinician may be asked to submit specific forms before test is submitted to the State Department of Health or CDC. Therefore, they should be consulted early to optimize handling of the suspect case.

Methodology Toxin neutralization test in mice, isolation of *Clostridium botulinum* from feces

Additional Information *C. botulinum* is an obligate anaerobic, spore-forming, gram-positive bacillus that can be recovered from a wide variety of environmental sources. Infant botulism occurs most commonly in the second and third postnatal months and is rarely seen after the sixth month of life. The disease occurs when infants ingest *C. botulinum* spores that germinate and produce botulinum toxin (usually serotypes A or B) within the gastrointestinal tract. The toxin is disseminated hematogenously, enters nerve cells, and irreversibly interferes with release of acetylcholine. Infants seem particularly susceptible to colonization with *C. botulinum* because their gastrointestinal flora is not fully established. By 12 months of age, the human gastrointestinal tract is more resistant to colonization with *C. botulinum*; foodborne disease is usually a result of ingestion of toxin (rather than organisms) in food. The

spectrum of disease in infants varies from mild constipation to sudden death. Infant botulism has in fact been implicated as a cause of sudden infant death syndrome (SIDS). The typical course of infant botulism is constipation followed, within 1-3 weeks, by lethargy and listlessness, decreased gag reflex, and poor feeding. Ptosis may develop, and the child may have difficulty keeping his head up.[1,2]

Foodborne botulism usually develops 12-36 hours after toxin ingestion. Initial complaints consist of nausea, dry mouth, and diarrhea followed by evidence of cranial nerve dysfunction.[3]

In wound botulism, spores are introduced into a wound where they germinate and produce toxin. Clinically, wound botulism lacks the prodromal gastrointestinal disorder of foodborne botulism but is otherwise similar.

Footnotes

1. Schmidt RD and Schmidt TW, "Infant Botulism: A Case Series and Review of the Literature," *J Emerg Med*, 1992, 10(6):713-8.
2. Mygrant BI and Renaud MT, "Infant Botulism," *Heart Lung*, 1994, 23(2):164-8.
3. Chia JK, Clark JB, Ryan CA, et al, "Botulism in an Adult Associated With Foodborne Intestinal Infection With *Clostridium botulinum*," *N Engl J Med*, 1986, 315(4):239-41.

References

Mechem CC and Walter FG, "Wound Botulism," *Vet Hum Toxicol*, 1994, 36(3):233-7.
Fred HL, "Case in Point. Wound Botulism," *Hosp Pract (Off Ed)*, 1994, 29(1):39
Hatheway CL, "Toxigenic Clostridia," *Clin Microbiol Rev*, 1990, 3(1):66-98.
Wigginton JM and Thill P, "Infant Botulism. A Review of the Literature," *Clin Pediatr (Phila)*, 1993, 32(11):669-74.

Bronchial Washings Culture *see Bacterial Culture, Sputum on page 465*

Bronchoalveolar Lavage Culture *see Bacterial Culture, Bronchoscopy Specimen on page 459*

Bronchoscopic Legionella Culture *see Legionella Culture on page 485*

Bronchoscopy Culture *see Bacterial Culture, Sputum on page 465*

Bronchoscopy Fungus Culture *see Fungal Culture, Sputum on page 479*

Bronchoscopy Specimen Bacterial Culture *see Bacterial Culture, Bronchoscopy Specimen on page 459*

Brucella Culture

CPT 87040; 87163 (addition identification methods)

Related Information

Bacterial Culture, Blood *on page 457*
Brucellosis Agglutinins *on page 372*

Synonyms Blood Culture, *Brucella*; Undulant Fever, Culture

Applies to Bone Marrow Culture for *Brucella*

Abstract *Brucella* spp are intracellular bacteria that cause epizootic abortions in animals and localized or septicemic febrile illness in humans.

Specimen Blood, bone marrow, infected tissues, spleen, liver biopsies; rarely, cerebrospinal fluid, urine, pleural or peritoneal fluid are submitted for *Brucella* culture.

Container Ideally, blood should be collected in biphasic blood culture bottles; if these are not available, blood may be collected in routine blood culture bottles or lysis centrifugation tubes. Specimens other than blood should be collected in a sterile tightly closed container.

Collection Prior to antimicrobial therapy, when possible.

Turnaround Time Blood cultures may be held for up to 6 weeks before reporting out negatives.

Special Instructions *Brucella* spp pose a significant infection control hazard to laboratorians and require special procedures for recovery. In order to ensure that proper precautions and methods are used, **the laboratory must be informed when brucellosis is suspected.**

Reference Range No growth

Use Establish the diagnosis of brucellosis

Limitations Diagnosis of brucellosis in the United States is hampered by failure to consider the diagnosis in early acute phases, and laboratorians who have little experience with this fastidious organism. Blood cultures for *Brucella* are useful in acute infection but are rarely positive in subacute or chronic brucellosis; bone marrow should always be cultured when subacute or chronic brucellosis is suspected. It is also reasonable to collect bone marrow in suspected acute brucellosis since it produces positive results faster and with greater frequency than blood cultures.[1]

Methodology Extended incubation in an atmosphere of 5% to 10% CO_2 on media capable of supporting *Brucella* growth. For culture of blood or other body fluids, a biphasic medium is recommended. If biphasic media is not available, commercial blood culture bottles can be vented and incubated at $35^\circ C$ to $37^\circ C$ with subculture to solid media every 4-5 days for 30 days. Lysis centrifugation techniques have also been used with success. Solid media usually available in the laboratory that is capable of supporting growth of *Brucella* spp includes selective buffered charcoal yeast extract agar, Thayer-Martin agar, and chocolate agar containing VCNT.[2]

Additional Information Brucellosis is common worldwide, particularly in the USSR, Mediterranean, Latin America, and Spain. It is rare in the United States with approximately 100 cases reported annually, primarily in persons who have traveled to endemic areas or have been exposed to animals or laboratory cultures. Clinical suspicion in low prevalence populations is complicated by the fact that human *Brucella* infections have variable incubation periods, insidious or abrupt onset, and no pathognomonic symptoms or signs.[1,3] Clinical suspicion is often based merely on risk factors such as travel to endemic areas or occupational exposure to animals.

Footnotes
1. Moyer NP and Holcomb LA, "*Brucella*," *Manual of Clinical Microbiology*, 6th ed, Murray PR, Baron EJ, Pfaller MA, et al, eds, Washington, DC: American Society for Microbiology, 1995, 549-55.
2. Kolman S, Maayan MC, Gotesman G, et al, "Comparison of the Bactec® and Lysis Concentration Methods for Recovery of *Brucella* Species From Clinical Specimens," *Eur J Clin Microbiol Infect Dis*, 1991, 10(8):647-8.
3. Georghiou PR and Young EJ, "Prolonged Incubation in Brucellosis," *Lancet*, 1991, 337(8756):1543.

References
Etemadi H, Raissadt A, Pickett MJ, et al, "Isolation of *Brucella* spp. From Clinical Specimens," *J Clin Microbiol*, 1984, 20(3):586.
Olle-Goig JE, Canela-Soler J, "An Outbreak of *Brucella melitensis* Infection by Airborne Transmission Among Laboratory Workers," *Am J Public Health*, 1987, 77(3):335-8.
Peiris V, Fraser S, Fairhurst M, et al, "Laboratory Diagnosis of *Brucella* Infection: Some Pitfalls," *Lancet*, 1992, 339(8806):1415-6.
Wilson ML and Mirrett S, "Recovery of Select Rare and Fastidious Microorganisms From Blood Cultures," *Clin Lab Med*, 1994, 14(1):119-31.

Burn Culture, Quantitative *see* Bacterial Culture, Burn Sites *on page 460*

Calcofluor White *see* Fungus Smear, Stain *on page 481*

***Campylobacter pylori* Urease Test and Culture** *see* Helicobacter pylori Urease Test and Culture *on page 484*

***Candida* Culture, Genital** *see* Bacterial Culture, Genital Specimen *on page 463*

Catheter Tip Culture *see* Bacterial Culture, Intravascular Device *on page 463*

Cefinase (Nitrocefin) Testing *see* Beta-Lactamase Test *on page 470*

Cephalosporinase Production Testing *see* Beta-Lactamase Test *on page 470*

Cephalosporinases *see* Beta-Lactamase Test *on page 470*

Cerebrospinal Fluid Bacterial Antigen Testing *see* Bacterial Antigens, Rapid Detection Methods *on page 454*

Cerebrospinal Fluid Culture *see* Bacterial Culture, Cerebrospinal Fluid *on page 460*

Cerebrospinal Fluid Fungus Culture *see* Fungal Culture, Cerebrospinal Fluid *on page 477*

Cerebrospinal Fluid India Ink Preparation *see* India Ink Preparation *on page 484*

Cerebrospinal Fluid Mycobacteria Culture *see* Mycobacterial Culture, Cerebrospinal Fluid *on page 489*

Cervical Culture *see* Bacterial Culture, Genital Specimen *on page 463*

***Cimex* Identification** *see* Arthropod Identification *on page 453*

***Clostridium botulinum* Toxin Identification Procedure** *see* Botulism Diagnostic Procedure *on previous page*

Clostridium difficile *see* Bacterial Culture, Stool *on page 466*

Clostridium difficile Toxin Assay

CPT 87081 (culture); 87230 (toxin)

Related Information
Bacterial Culture, Stool *on page 466*
Fungal Culture, Stool *on page 480*
Methylene Blue Stain, Stool *on page 642*
Ova and Parasites, Stool *on page 494*
pH, Stool *on page 648*

Synonyms Antibiotic-Associated Colitis Toxin Test; Pseudomembranous Colitis Toxin Assay; Toxin Assay, *Clostridium difficile*

Applies to Toxin A

Abstract Plaques of exudate seen endoscopically on the colonic mucosa bear characteristic features on biopsy, designated pseudomembranous colitis.

Specimen Stool or proctoscopic specimen

Container Plastic stool container (swabs are inadequate because of small volume)

Collection Keep specimen **cold** and transport immediately. Specimens can be frozen if transportation will be delayed.

Storage Instructions If the specimen cannot be processed immediately, it should be refrigerated or frozen.

Turnaround Time 1-2 days

Special Instructions When antibiotic-associated colitis is suspected, a toxin assay rather than a *C. difficile* stool culture should initially be ordered.

Reference Range Presence of toxin is suggestive of disease. Isolation of organism (*C. difficile*) may occur in normal adults (5% to 21%) and in normal newborns.[1] Isolation of the organism without demonstration of toxin production is a nonspecific finding.

Use Diagnose antibiotic-related, pseudomembranous colitis caused by *C. difficile* toxin

Limitations Results given as titers are not significant as such because size/amounts of original specimens are usually not standardized. Titer result should be interpreted as simply positive.

The latex agglutination test is simple and rapid, but it does not detect (is not specific for) toxin A, the protein thought to be primarily responsible for pseudomembranous colitis, and thus provides unreliable results. Cytotoxin assays or immunoassays for toxin A are specific but usually have sensitivities <90%.

Methodology Latex agglutination (LA) test to detect toxin, neutralization test in tissue culture (toxin), selective anaerobic culture (organism), enzyme immunoassay (EIA) (toxin), fluorogenic immunoassay (toxin)

Additional Information Antibiotic-associated pseudomembranous colitis is produced primarily by toxigenic *C. difficile*. Toxigenic strains usually produce two toxins: toxin A, an enterotoxin and toxin B, a cytotoxin which is detected by cell culture. Not all *C. difficile* strains are toxigenic, and even toxigenic strains may not produce disease if present in insufficient numbers; consequently, culture for *C. difficile*, often produces false-positive results. The most accurate clinical laboratory test for diagnosis of pseudomembranous colitis appears to be enzyme immunoassays for toxin A.[2] These assays are more rapid and accessible than cytotoxin assays and are highly specific (99%) and fairly sensitive (87%).[2] Latex agglutination has been widely utilized because it is fast and easy to use.[3] Unfortunately, the assay detects an antigen produced by many microorganisms other than *C. difficile* and probably should not be relied upon to diagnose *C. difficile* disease.[1]

Pseudomembranous colitis attributable to *C. difficile* is usually associated with antimicrobial therapy,[4] anti-AIDS or antineoplastic drugs.[5] *C. difficile* is an important nosocomial pathogen that may be treated by discontinuing antimicrobial therapy, if possible, or initiating oral metronidazole or vancomycin therapy.[6]

Complications of pseudomembranous colitis include the hemolytic-uremic syndrome.[5]

Interrelationships of pseudomembranous colitis, antibiotic-associated diarrhea, and *C. difficile* toxin are addressed.[7]

Footnotes
1. Wilson KH, "The Microecology of *Clostridium difficile*," *Clin Infect Dis*, 1993, 16(Suppl 4):S214-8.
2. De Girolami PC, Hanff PA, Eichelberger K, et al, "Multicenter Evaluation of a New Enzyme Immunoassay for Detection of *Clostridium difficile* Enterotoxin A," *J Clin Microbiol*, 1992, 30(5):1085-8.
3. Kelly MT, Champagne SG, Sherlock CH, et al, "Commercial Latex Agglutination Test for Detection of *Clostridium difficile* Associated Diarrhea," *J Clin Microbiol*, 1987, 25(7):1244-7.
4. Lyerly DM, "Epidemiology of *Clostridium difficile* Disease," *Clin Microbiol Newslet*, 1993, 15:49-52.
5. Sommers SC, "Large Intestine: Appendix, Colon, and Rectum," *Biopsy Diagnosis of the Digestive Tract*, 2nd ed, Chapter 6, Rotterdam H, Sheahan DG, and Sommers SC, eds, New York, NY: Raven Press, 1993, 576-782.
6. Clabots CR, Johnson S, Olson MM, et al, "Acquisition of *Clostridium difficile* by Hospitalized Patients: Evidence for Colonized New Admission as a Source of Infection," *J Infect Dis*, 1992, 166(3):561-7.
7. Talbot IC and Price AB, *Biopsy Pathology in Colorectal Disease*, London: Chapman and Hall, 1987, 173-85.

References
Bartlett JG, "*Clostridium difficile*: History of Its Role as an Enteric Pathogen and the Current State of Knowledge About the Organism," *Clin Infect Dis*, 1994, 18(Suppl 4):S265-72.
Fekety R and Shah AB, "Diagnosis and Treatment of *Clostridium difficile* Colitis," *JAMA*, 1993, 269(1):71-5.
Gerding DN and Brazier JS, "Optimal Methods for Identifying *Clostridium difficile* Infections," *Clin Infect Dis*, 1993, 16(Suppl 4):S439-42.
Gilligan PH, Janda JM, Karmali MA, et al, "Laboratory Diagnosis of Bacterial Diarrhea," *Cumitech 12A*, Nolte FS, ed, Washington, DC: American Society for Microbiology, 1992.
Knoop FC, Owens M, and Crocker IC, "*Clostridium difficile*: Clinical Disease and Diagnosis," *Clin Microbiol Rev*, 1993, 6(3):251-65.

Clue Cells *see* Bacterial Culture, Genital Specimen *on page 463*

CMVS Culture *see* Bacterial Culture, Urine, Clean Catch *on page 468*

Coagglutination Test for Group A Streptococci *replaced by* Group A *Streptococcus* Screen, Rapid *on page 483*

Coccidia *see Cryptosporidium* Diagnostic Procedures *on this page*

Conjunctival Culture *see* Bacterial Culture, Conjunctiva *on page 461*

Conjunctival Fungus Culture *see* Fungal Culture, Ocular Infections *on page 478*

Corneal Culture *see* Bacterial Culture, Conjunctiva *on page 461*

Corynebacterium diphtheriae Throat Culture

CPT 87060 (culture); 87163 (additional identification methods)

Related Information

Bacterial Culture, Throat *on page 468*

Synonyms Diphtheria Culture; Throat Culture for *Corynebacterium diphtheriae*

Applies to Nasopharyngeal Culture for *Corynebacterium diphtheriae*

Abstract Diphtheria causes pseudomembranes. It may be found in the anterior nasal mucosa (nasal diphtheria) or larynx (resembling infectious croup), but classically it is a disease of the oropharynx, pharynx, and tonsils. It may spread to or begin in the larynx and can involve the tracheobronchial tree. The major effects of the exotoxin include damage to the heart, kidneys, and nervous system. It can cause circulatory collapse, respiratory failure, myocarditis, and neuritis.

Aftercare Observe for laryngospasm following collection of specimen.

Specimen Throat swab, nasopharyngeal swab; culture nose or larynx if clinically appropriate

Container Sterile Mini-Tip Culturette® or flexible calcium alginate swab, Calgiswab®, is recommended for obtaining nasopharyngeal culture.

Collection The tongue should be depressed while both the tonsillar crypts and nasopharynx and throat lesions are swabbed. If a pseudomembrane is present, the swab should be taken from beneath the membrane or a part of the membrane should be cultured if possible.

Turnaround Time Final reports on specimens from which *C. diphtheriae* has been isolated usually take at least 4 days.

Special Instructions The laboratory should be notified before collection of specimens so that special isolation media can be made available.

Reference Range No *C. diphtheriae* isolated

Use Isolate *C. diphtheriae* from patients suspected of having diphtheria. The organisms remain superficial in the respiratory tract and skin, but the potent exotoxin is responsible for the virulence of the disease. The differential diagnosis of pharyngeal diphtheria includes streptococcal pharyngitis, infectious mononucleosis, and candidiasis.

Limitations Cultures should be taken from nasopharynx, as well as, the throat; culture of both sites increases the chance of recovery of the organism. Stain results are presumptive and are commonly reported out as "gram-positive pleomorphic bacilli suggestive of *C. diphtheriae*". Definitive diagnosis depends on isolation of the organism because of the similar appearance of other organisms commonly found in the oropharynx.

Contraindications Lack of clinical symptoms or signs of diphtheria, valid history of immunization

Methodology Culture on selective medium (Löeffler's), cystine tellurite agar, and blood agar smear stained with Löeffler's methylene blue stain and/or Gram's stain. *C. diphtheriae* may appear as V, Y, or L figures. Metachromatic granules which stain deep blue may also be seen.

Additional Information Conventional throat culture should be ordered in addition. *C. diphtheriae* may occasionally cause skin infections, wound infections, pulmonary infections, and endocarditis and may be recovered from the oropharynx of healthy carriers. *C. diphtheriae* is spread through respiratory secretions by convalescent and healthy carriers. The clinical presentation includes a grayish pseudomembrane, overlying superficial ulcers in the oropharynx. The organism is noninvasive, however, the exotoxin elaborated in the throat affects primarily the heart, kidneys, and nervous system. Mortality is 10% to 30%. Only strains of *C. diphtheriae* infected by B-phage are capable of producing toxin, a protein metabolite. Nontoxigenic strains are commonly recovered and are capable of producing pharyngitis. Confirmation of exotoxin production requires animal testing and is rarely done for clinical testing. *C. ulcerans* may also produce a diphtheria-like disease.

Group A beta-hemolytic streptococcal and other secondary infections occur. Hypoglycemia may be seen secondary to hepatotoxicity.[1]

Footnotes

1. Feigin RD, "Diphtheria," *Principles and Practice of Pediatrics*, 2nd ed, Oski FA, DeAngelis CD, Feigin RD, et al, eds, Philadelphia, PA: JB Lippincott Co, 1994, 1180-3.

References

Coyle MB and Lipsky BA, "Coryneform Bacteria in Infectious Disease: Clinical and Laboratory Aspects," *Clin Microbiol Rev*, 1990, 3(3):227-46.

Efstratiou A, Tiley SM, Sangrador A, et al, "Invasive Disease Caused by Multiple Clones of *Corynebacterium diphtheriae*," *Clin Infect Dis*, 1993, 17(1):136.

Farizo KM, Strebel PM, Chen RT, et al, "Fatal Respiratory Disease Due to *Corynebacterium diphtheriae*: Case Report and Review of Guidelines for Management, Investigation, and Control," *Clin Infect Dis*, 1993, 16(1):59-68.

MacGregor RR, "*Corynebacterium diphtheriae*," *Principles and Practice of Infectious Diseases*, 3rd ed, Mandell GL, Douglas RG Jr, and Bennett JE, eds, New York, NY: Churchill Livingstone, 1990, 1574-81.

Wilson AP, Matthews S, Bahl M, et al, "Screening for *Corynebacterium diphtheriae*," *J Clin Pathol*, 1992, 45(11):1036-7.

Cough Plate Culture for Pertussis *replaced by Bordetella pertussis* Culture *on page 471*

Counterimmunoelectrophoresis for Group B Streptococcal Antigen *replaced by* Group B *Streptococcus* Screen, Rapid *on page 483*

Cryptosporidium Diagnostic Procedures

CPT 87015 (concentration); 87206 (fluorescent stain); 87207 (special stain)

Related Information

Acid-Fast Stain, Modified, *Nocardia* Species *on page 446*
Bacterial Culture, Stool *on page 466*
Fungus Smear, Stain *on page 481*
Methylene Blue Stain, Stool *on page 642*
Microsporidia Diagnostic Procedures *on page 487*
Ova and Parasites, Stool *on page 494*

Synonyms Coccidia; Stool Examination for *Cryptosporidium*

Applies to Acid-Fast Stain, Modified, *Cryptosporidium*; *Cryptosporidium parvum*; *Cyclospora cayetensis*; *Isospora belli*; *S. bovihominis*; *S. suihominis*

Test Commonly Includes Examination of stool for the presence of *Cryptosporidium* by phase contrast microscopy, modified acid-fast stain, or fluorescent-labeled antibody

Abstract Human infections caused by the intracellular *Coccidia* parasites, including ***Cryptosporidium parvum***, are manifest as diarrhea in both normal and immunocompromised subjects. Disease in immunocompromised individuals is more severe and prolonged. Some cause traveler's diarrhea.[1]

Specimen Fresh stool; stool preserved with 10% formalin or sodium acetate-acetic acid formalin preservative

Reference Range Negative

Use A part of the differential work-up of diarrhea, particularly in immunocompromised hosts and suspected AIDS patients; establish the diagnosis of cryptosporidiosis by demonstration of the oocysts. An outbreak in healthy individuals from a contaminated water supply was noted. *I. belli* causes eosinophilic enteritis.

Limitations *Cryptosporidium* is not detected by standard methods used to examine stool specimens for other ova and parasites; special stains are required for its detection, and in many laboratories, must be specifically requested. The organisms are most readily demonstrated in watery diarrheal stools. Forms of *Blastocystis hominis* may cause confusion if Giemsa stain is used. Most recommended procedures cannot be performed on polyvinyl alcohol (PVA) preserved specimens.

Methodology Phase contrast microscopy after floatation or sedimentation concentration techniques; modified acid-fast stain on air-dried, methanol-fixed smears (decolorization with 1% H_2SO_4).[2] A technique utilizing formalin-ethyl acetate and floatation over hypertonic saline is reported to enhance detection of *Cryptosporidium* oocysts.[3] Fluorescent-labeled anti-*Cryptosporidium* antibodies are commercially available and provide excellent sensitivity and specificity.[4]

Additional Information *Cryptosporidium* is a coccidian parasite of the intestines and respiratory tract of many animals including mice, sheep, snakes, turkeys, chickens, cows, monkeys, and domestic cats. It is a cause of severe and chronic diarrhea in patients with hypogammaglobulinemia and the acquired immune deficiency syndrome.[5] HIV-infected patients with CD4 counts ≤50/mm^3 are especially at risk when exposed to *Cryptosporidium*.[6] Although the organism is widely recognized as a disease of the immunocompromised patient, it can also cause disease in immunocompetent subjects. Animal contact, travel to endemic areas, living in a rural environment, day care attendance by toddlers, and exposure to contaminated public water have been recognized as risk factors for the development of cryptosporidiosis.[7] Children are more prone to develop infection than are adults. In these patients, the disease is a self-limited gastroenteritis, but in immunocompromised patients, a profound enteropathy results. A seasonal variation in incidence exists with the highest frequency reported in summer and autumn. The organism can be demonstrated in biopsies of small bowel and colon, adherent to surface of the epithelial cells (Giemsa stain) and by demonstration in feces with modified acid-fast stain or smear. Most therapeutic regimens for cryptosporidiosis are not successful unless immunosuppression is reversed. In HIV-positive patients, the prognosis of *C. parvum* correlates with CD4 cell counts; the disease is self-limited when CD4 counts exceed 80/mm^3.[1]

Footnotes

1. Long EG and Christie JD, "The Diagnosis of Old and New Gastrointestinal Parasites," *Clin Lab Med*, 1995, 15(2):307-31.
2. Koneman EW, Allen SD, Janda WM, et al, *Color Atlas and Textbook of Diagnostic Microbiology*, 4th ed, Philadelphia, PA: JB Lippincott Co, 1992.
3. Weber R, Bryan RT, and Juranek DD, "Improved Stool Concentration Procedure for Detection of *Cryptosporidium* Oocysts in Fecal Specimens," *J Clin Microbiol*, 1992, 30(11):2869-73.
4. Garcia LS, Shum AC, and Bruckner DA, "Evaluation of a New Monoclonal Antibody Combination Reagent for Direct Fluorescence Detection of *Giardia* Cysts and *Cryptosporidium* Oocysts in Human Fecal Specimens," *J Clin Microbiol*, 1992, 30(12):3255-7.
5. Koch KL, et al, "Cryptosporidiosis in a Patient With Hemophilia, Common Variable Hypogammaglobulinemia and the Acquired Immunodeficiency Syndrome," *Ann Intern Med*, 1983, 99:337-40.
6. Vakil NB, Schwartz SM, Buggy BP, et al, "Biliary Cryptosporidiosis in HIV-Infected People After the Waterborne Outbreak of Cryptosporidiosis in Milwaukee," *N Engl J Med*, 1996, 334(1):19-23.
7. Mackenzie WR, Hoxie NJ, Proctor ME, et al, "A Massive Outbreak in Milwaukee of *Cryptosporidium* Infection Transmitted Through the Public Water Supply," *N Engl J Med*, 1994, 331(3):161-7.

References

Baron EJ, Schenone C, and Tanenbaum B, "Comparison of Three Methods for Detection of *Cryptosporidium* Oocysts in a Low-Prevalence Population," *J Clin Microbiol*, 1989, 27(1):223-4.
Clayton F, Heller T, and Kotler DP, "Variation in the Enteric Distribution of Cryptosporidia in Acquired Immunodeficiency Syndrome," *Am J Clin Pathol*, 1994, 102(4):420-5.
Current WL and Garcia LS, "Cryptosporidiosis," *Clin Microbiol Rev*, 1991, 4(3):325-58.
Garcia LS, Brewer TC, and Bruckner DA, "Incidence of *Cryptosporidium* in All Patients Submitting Stool Specimens for Ova and Parasite Examination: Monoclonal Antibody IFA Method," *Diagn Microbiol Infect Dis*, 1989, 11(1):25-7.
Petersen C, "Cryptosporidiosis in Patients Infected With the Human Immunodeficiency Virus," *Clin Infect Dis*, 1992, 15(6):903-9.

Cryptosporidium parvum see *Cryptosporidium* Diagnostic Procedures *on previous page*

Crystal Violet see Gram's Stain *on page 481*

CSF Culture see Bacterial Culture, Cerebrospinal Fluid *on page 460*

CSF Fungus Culture see Fungal Culture, Cerebrospinal Fluid *on page 477*

CSF Mycobacteria Culture see Mycobacterial Culture, Cerebrospinal Fluid *on page 489*

Cul-de-sac Anaerobic Culture see Bacterial Culture, Endometrium *on page 462*

Culture, Blood see Bacterial Culture, Blood *on page 457*

Culture, Cerebrospinal Fluid see Bacterial Culture, Cerebrospinal Fluid *on page 460*

Culture, Ear see Bacterial Culture, Ear *on page 462*

Cyclospora cayetensis see *Cryptosporidium* Diagnostic Procedures *on previous page*

***Cyclospora* Species** see Ova and Parasites, Stool *on page 494*

Darkfield Examination, Leptospirosis

CPT 87164

Related Information
Leptospira Culture *on page 486*
Leptospira Serodiagnosis *on page 414*

Synonyms Darkfield Microscopy, *Leptospira*; Leptospirosis, Darkfield Examination

Test Commonly Includes Examination of serum, urine, or CSF for organisms

Abstract The general term leptospirosis is preferred to the synonyms, **Weil's disease** and **canicola fever**. It is a widespread zoonosis. Culture and serology are recommended for diagnosis; darkfield examination is not. Darkfield microscopic examination of specimens for leptospires can be useful in establishing a rapid diagnosis, but culture and serology are recommended for confirmation of diagnosis.

Specimen Urine, serum, cerebrospinal fluid

Container Sterile plastic urine container, red top tube, or sterile CSF tube

Use Determine the presence of *Leptospira* for the diagnosis of Weil's syndrome, hemorrhagic fever with renal syndrome, atypical pneumonia syndrome, aseptic meningitis, and myocarditis including cardiac arrhythmias.

Limitations The concentration of leptospires in blood and CSF is low. Therefore, concentration by centrifugation with sodium oxalate or heparin can be useful. The incidence of false-positives is increased because fibrils and cellular extrusions can be mistaken for organisms.

Failure to detect leptospires does not rule out their presence. **Direct examination of blood or urine by darkfield methods frequently results in failure or misdiagnosis.**[1]

Methodology A very small drop of fluid is distributed in a thin layer between a glass coverslip and slide. The typical morphology helicoidal, flexible organisms 6-12 µm long and 0.1 µm in diameter usually with semicircular hooked ends should be observed before a presumptive diagnosis is made.

Additional Information *Leptospira* are present in blood early in course of disease (first week only). After 10-14 days, they may be found in the urine. Urine must be neutral or alkaline. If the urine is acidic, it should be neutralized by diluting with 1% bovine serum albumin.[1] Culture has much greater value for diagnosis. Saprophytic strains as well as pathogenic ones exist. Darkfield microscopy is best used to demonstrate leptospires in specimens in which a high concentration of organisms is present, ie, tissue from animals (guinea pig or hamster), inoculation including blood, peritoneal fluid, or liver suspensions. Urine or kidney suspensions from swine, dogs, and domestic animals may also yield positive darkfield examination.

Recently, a DNA amplification method has been used to detect leptospires in clinical specimens.[2] This assay seems to be more sensitive and specific than microscopic examination or culture. Currently, this test is not widely available.

Footnotes

1. Kaufmann AF and Weyant RS, "Leptospiraceae," *Manual of Clinical Microbiology*, 6th ed, Murray PR, Baron EJ, Pfaller MA, et al, eds, Washington, DC: American Society for Microbiology, 1995, 621-5.
2. Merien F, Amouriax P, Perolat P, et al, "Polymerase Chain Reaction for Detection of *Leptospira* spp in Clinical Samples," *J Clin Microbiol*, 1992, 30(9):2219-24.

References

Farr RW, "Leptospirosis," *Clin Infect Dis*, 1995, 21(1):1-8.
Jackson LA, Kaufmann AF, Adams WG, et al, "Outbreak of Leptospirosis Associated With Swimming," *Pediatr Infect Dis J*, 1993, 12(1):48-54.

Darkfield Examination, Syphilis

CPT 87164

Related Information
Automated Reagin Test *on page 370*
FTA-ABS, Cerebrospinal Fluid *on page 394*
FTA-ABS, Serum *on page 394*
RPR *on page 428*
VDRL, Cerebrospinal Fluid *on page 438*
VDRL, Serum *on page 438*

Synonyms Darkfield Microscopy, Syphilis; Syphilis, Darkfield Examination; *Treponema pallidum* Darkfield Examination

Abstract *Treponema pallidum* is a thin organism that cannot be visualized by conventional light microscopy. Darkfield examination is appropriate for the evaluation of chancre (primary lues) and condylomata lata (secondary syphilis)

Patient Preparation The surface of the chancre or condyloma is cleansed by the physician with a swab moistened with saline. This removes exudate and excess bacteria contamination. Serous fluid is then collected from the surface of the chancre using a small pipette. The fluid is placed on a slide or coverslip. Alternatively, the specimen can be collected by directly touching the slide to the lesion. The objective is to obtain clear exudate from the subsurface of the lesion. It is then examined by darkfield microscopy.

Specimen Moist serous fluid from the base of a cleansed, unhealed chancre or condyloma. The youngest lesion available is best. The chance of identification of treponemes decreases with the age of the lesion as it dries and locally heals. *Treponema pallidum* can be found by lymph node aspiration in the secondary stage of lues.

Collection Collect with a pipette and put directly on a glass slide.

Causes for Rejection Healed chancre, previous treatment, ointment, dried-up specimen

Reference Range Negative

Critical Values Positive darkfield examination

Use Determine the presence of characteristic spirochetes to support diagnosis of primary or secondary syphilis

Limitations Darkfield examination is of limited value in oral and rectal lesions because of the normal presence of other, nonpathogenic spirochetes. Dry or bloody specimens render this examination worthless. The specimen should be examined within 15 minutes of collection because the organisms lose motility with decrease in temperature, exposure to oxygen and desiccation.
(Continued)

Darkfield Examination, Syphilis *(Continued)*

Contraindications Antibiotic therapy prior to the darkfield examination. The organisms are rapidly cleared following therapy.

Methodology Darkfield microscopy. Motile organisms are observed to rotate around their long axis and to bend, snap, and flex along their length at 90 degree angles. A smooth translational back and forth directed movement is also apparent. Nonpathogenic mucosal treponemes are often irregularly coiled, longer than *T. pallidum*, and are characterized by a different kind of motility.[1]

Additional Information *Treponema pallidum* has a rapid and purposeful motion as it travels across the microscopic field. The organisms appear as a tight corkscrew characterized by 6-14 coils. The organisms are 1 to 1.5 times the diameter of an RBC in length (0.10-0.18 μm by 6-20 μm).[1]

T. pallidum can be found in skin lesions and lymph nodes in secondary syphilis but are more plentiful in primary chancres. They cannot be grown in culture. The Centers for Disease Control (CDC) and others use fluorescent microscopy with monoclonal or polyclonal anti-*T. pallidum* antibodies for examination of exudates.[1]

A technique for direct detection of *T. pallidum* is specific amplification of DNA.[2] This test is currently only available as a research tool and further studies of its use as a diagnostic test are needed before it is universally available.

Footnotes
1. Hook EW 3d and Marra CM, "Acquired Syphilis in Adults," *N Engl J Med*, 1992, 326(16):1060-9.
2. Wicher K, Noordhoek GT, Abbruscato F, et al, "Detection of *Treponema pallidum* in Early Syphilis by DNA Amplification," *J Clin Microbiol*, 1992, 30(2):497-500.

References
Larsen SA, "Syphilis," *Clin Lab Med*, 1989, 9(3):545-57.
Larsen SA, Steiner BM, and Rudolph AH, "Laboratory Diagnosis and Interpretation of Tests From Syphilis," *Clin Microbiol Rev*, 1995, 8(1):1-21.
Marra CM, "Syphilis and Human Immunodeficiency Virus Infection," *Semin Neurol*, 1992, 12(1):43-50.
Norris SJ and Larsen SA, "*Treponema* and Other Host-Associated Spirochetes," *Manual of Clinical Microbiology*, 6th ed, Murray PR, Baron EJ, Pfaller MA, et al, eds, Washington, DC: American Society for Microbiology, 1995, 636-51.

Darkfield Microscopy, *Leptospira* *see* Darkfield Examination, Leptospirosis *on previous page*

Darkfield Microscopy, Syphilis *see* Darkfield Examination, Syphilis *on previous page*

Dermatophyte Fungus Culture *see* Fungal Culture, Skin *on page 478*

Diphtheria Culture *see Corynebacterium diphtheriae* Throat Culture *on page 474*

DNA Probe *Legionella* *see Legionella* Culture *on page 485*

Ear Culture *see* Bacterial Culture, Ear *on page 462*

Ectoparasite Identification *see* Arthropod Identification *on page 453*

Endocervical Anaerobic Culture *see* Bacterial Culture, Endometrium *on page 462*

Endocervical Culture *see* Bacterial Culture, Genital Specimen *on page 463*

Endometrium Culture *see* Bacterial Culture, Endometrium *on page 462*

Enteric Pathogens Culture, Routine *see* Bacterial Culture, Stool *on page 466*

Enterobacteriaceae *see* Bacterial Culture, Aerobes *on page 455*

Enterobius vermicularis Preparation *see* Pinworm Preparation *on page 496*

Enterococci *see* Bacterial Culture, Aerobes *on page 455*

Enterohemorrhagic *E. coli* *see* Bacterial Culture, Stool *on page 466*

Enzyme Immunoassay for Group A *Streptococcus* Antigen *see* Group A *Streptococcus* Screen, Rapid *on page 483*

E Test *see* Antimicrobial Susceptibility Testing, Anaerobic Bacteria *on page 449*

E-Test *see* Antimicrobial Susceptibility Testing, Unusual Isolates/Fastidious Organisms *on page 452*

Eye Culture *see* Bacterial Culture, Conjunctiva *on page 461*

Eye Fungus Culture *see* Fungal Culture, Ocular Infections *on page 478*

Flagellates *see* Ova and Parasites, Stool *on page 494*

Flea Identification *see* Arthropod Identification *on page 453*

Fluorochrome Stain *see* Acid-Fast Stain *on page 446*

Fractional Bactericidal Concentration (FBC) *see* Antimicrobial Susceptibility Testing, Antimicrobial Combinations *on page 449*

Fractional Inhibitory Concentration (FIC) *see* Antimicrobial Susceptibility Testing, Antimicrobial Combinations *on page 449*

Francisella tularensis Culture *see* Bacterial Culture, Blood *on page 457*

Fungal Culture, Biopsy or Body Fluid

CPT 87102 (isolation); 87106 (definitive identification)

Related Information
Amphotericin B *on page 535*
Antimicrobial Susceptibility Testing, Fungi *on page 450*
Aspergillus Serology *on page 369*
Bacterial Culture, Biopsy or Body Fluid *on page 456*
Blastomycosis Serology *on page 371*
Body Fluid *on page 89*
Body Fluid Analysis, Cell Count *on page 306*
Body Fluid Cytology *on page 286*
Body Fluid pH *on page 92*
Bone Marrow *on page 307*
Candida Antigen *on page 374*
Candidiasis Serologic Test *on page 375*
Coccidioidomycosis Antibodies *on page 384*
Fine Needle Aspiration, Deep Seated Lesions *on page 294*
Fine Needle Aspiration, Superficial Palpable Masses *on page 294*
Fungal Culture, Blood *on next page*
Fungal Culture, Cerebrospinal Fluid *on next page*
Fungal Culture, Skin *on page 478*
Fungal Culture, Sputum *on page 479*
Fungus Smear, Stain *on page 481*
Histopathology *on page 42*
Histoplasmosis Antibody *on page 402*
Histoplasmosis Antigen *on page 402*
Sporotrichosis Serology *on page 431*
Synovial Fluid Analysis *on page 656*

Synonyms Biopsy or Body Fluid Fungus Culture; Body Fluid Fungus Culture

Applies to Bone Marrow Fungus Culture; Synovial Fluid Fungus Culture; Tissue Fungus Culture

Abstract Cultures of biopsy material are desirable. They are superior to cultures from drainage.

Patient Preparation Aseptic preparation of biopsy site or site of body fluid aspiration

Specimen Surgical tissue, bone marrow, biopsy material, sterile body fluid (synovial fluid, peritoneal fluid, pleural fluid, ascites, etc). See also the table in Fungal Culture, Sputum *on page 479*.

Collection The portion of the biopsy specimen submitted for culture should be separated from the portion submitted for histopathology by the surgeon, pathologist, or microbiologist utilizing sterile technique.

Causes for Rejection Culture specimen in fixative

Reference Range No growth

Use Establish the diagnosis of localized or disseminated mycosis; isolate and identify fungi

Methodology Culture under aerobic conditions on several media, usually including Sabouraud's and brain heart infusion (BHI), biphasic media with or without lysis concentration technique, frequently incubation at room temperature or at both 30°C and 37°C

Additional Information Optimal isolation of fungi from tissue is accomplished by processing as much tissue as possible. Swabs should be submitted only when adequate tissue is not available. Specimen selection tables are provided in the listings Fungal Culture, Sputum *on page 479* and Fungal Culture, Skin *on page 478*. Depending upon the geographic area, *Histoplasma capsulatum*, *Blastomyces dermatitidis*, and *Coccidioides immitis* are the most frequently isolated deep pathogenic fungi. *Candida* sp are common opportunistic pathogens in all geographic locations and are the most common opportunistic fungal infections related to the gastrointestinal tract. Immunocompromised patients, transplant patients, and patients with acquired immunodeficiency syndrome (AIDS) are at increased risk for opportunistic mycoses.[1] Isolates such as *Aspergillus* sp or zygomycetes may be environmental in origin and must be interpreted in clinical context.

Fungal peritonitis is clinically similar to bacterial peritonitis with pain, fever, and abdominal tenderness. Fungal infections due to *Candida* sp (mostly *Candida albicans* and *Candida parapsilosis*), and rare cases of *Aspergillus fumigatus*, *Fusarium*, and *Nocardia asteroides*, have been reported in patients undergoing chronic dialysis. In a series of AIDS patients, bone marrow biopsy detected opportunistic fungal or mycobacterial infections in 20%. Eighty percent of the positive biopsies were associated with bone marrow granulomas. Fever, anemia, and neutropenia were often correlated with a positive biopsy.[2] Neutrophil count <1000/µL is associated with infection by *Candida*, *Aspergillus*, *Mucor*, *Rhizopus*, *Trichosporon*, and *Fusarium* sp. T-cell defects and/or impaired cell-mediated immunity are associated with infection by *Candida*, *Cryptococcus neoformans*, *Histoplasma capsulatum*, *Coccidioides immitis*, and *Aspergillus* sp. Catheterization (arterial, venous, or urinary) and mechanical disruption of the skin are associated with *Candida* and *Rhodotorula* sp infections. Disruption of the natural barrier of the GI tract and respiratory tree by cytotoxic chemotherapy predispose to *Candida* sp infections.[3]

Footnotes
1. Bodey GP, "Overview of the Problems of Infections in the Immunocompromised Host," *Am J Med*, 1985, 79(5B):56-61.
2. Nichols L, Florentine B, Lewis W, et al, "Bone Marrow Examination for the Diagnosis of Mycobacterial and Fungal Infections in the Acquired Immunodeficiency Syndrome," *Arch Pathol Lab Med*, 1991, 115(11):1125-32.
3. Brown AE, "Overview of Fungal Infections in Cancer Patients," *Semin Oncol*, 1990, 17(3 Suppl 6):2-5.

References
Moyana TN, Kulaga A, and Xiang J, "Granulomatous Appendicitis in Acute Myeloblastic Leukemia: Expanding the Clinicopathologic Spectrum of Invasive Candidiasis," *Arch Pathol Lab Med*, 1996, 120:203-5.
Musial CE, Cockerill FR 3d, and Roberts GD, "Fungal Infections of the Immunocompromised Host: Clinical and Laboratory Aspects," *Clin Microbiol Rev*, 1988, 1(4):349-64.
Pappas PG, Threlkeld MG, Bedsole GD, et al, "Blastomycosis in Immunocompromised Patients," *Medicine*, 1993, 72(5):311-25.
Sarosi GA and Johnson PC, "Disseminated Histoplasmosis in Patients Infected With Human Immunodeficiency Virus," *Clin Infect Dis*, 1992, 14(Suppl 1):S60-7.
Schell WA, "New Aspects of Emerging Fungal Pathogens. A Multifaceted Challenge," *Clin Lab Med*, 1995, 15(2):365-87.

Fungal Culture, Blood

CPT 87103 (isolation); 87106 (definitive identification)

Related Information
Amphotericin B *on page 535*
Antimicrobial Susceptibility Testing, Fungi *on page 450*
Aspergillus Serology *on page 369*
Bacterial Culture, Blood *on page 457*
Bacterial Culture, Sputum *on page 465*
Candida Antigen *on page 374*
Candidiasis Serologic Test *on page 375*
Coccidioidomycosis Antibodies *on page 384*
Fungal Culture, Biopsy or Body Fluid *on previous page*
Fungal Culture, Stool *on page 480*
Fungal Culture, Urine *on page 480*
Fungus Smear, Stain *on page 481*
Histoplasmosis Antibody *on page 402*
Histoplasmosis Antigen *on page 402*
Itraconazole *on page 555*

Synonyms Blood Fungus Culture

Abstract One of the needs for fungal blood culture is evaluation of patients with AIDS, in whom disseminated histoplasmosis was diagnosed in 27% in a study in Indianapolis.[1]

Patient Preparation See preparation in Bacterial Culture, Blood *on page 457*.

Specimen Blood

Container Fungal blood culture media (eg, biphasic blood culture media) or lysis centrifugation collecting tubes (Wampole Isolator™)

Collection Remove plastic cap from biphasic bottle, cleanse stoppers with acetone alcohol and 2% iodine. Collect 8 mL blood in a yellow Vacutainer® tube containing 0.35% sodium polyanethol sulfonate as an anticoagulant. Transfer appropriate volume of blood to biphasic medium to achieve an approximate 1:10 dilution of blood in the broth medium. Alternatively, 10 mL of blood is directly collected in an Isolator™ tube.

Special Instructions The laboratory should be informed of current antifungal therapy and clinical diagnosis.

Reference Range No growth

Use Isolate and identify fungi; establish the diagnosis of fungemia, fungal endocarditis, and disseminated mycosis. Certain yeasts such as *Candida* sp and *Candida glabrata* (*Torulopsis glabrata*) can be isolated from conventional bacterial blood cultures; for other agents of systemic mycoses, however, it is essential to perform blood fungal cultures as outlined above.

Limitations Negative fungal blood culture does not exclude disseminated fungal infection. If disseminated or deep fungal infection is strongly suspected, biopsy of the appropriate tissue and/or bone marrow aspiration for sections and fungus culture should be considered.

Methodology Biphasic (broth and agar) blood culture medium, or broth alone with early subculture to solid media, or lysis centrifugation with prompt subculture to solid media are appropriate methodologies. Lysis centrifugation appears to produce higher yields and more rapid detection

than other methods.[2,3] Fungal cultures should be held not less than 4 weeks.

Additional Information Fungemia can be a complication of venous or arterial catheterization, hyperalimentation, the acquired immunodeficiency syndrome (AIDS), and therapy with steroids, antineoplastic drugs, radiation, or broad spectrum antimicrobial agents. Intravenous drug abusers are prone to *Candida* endocarditis.

Fungemia represents a failure of the host defense system. Although many fungal species including *Histoplasma capsulatum*, *Coccidioides immitis*, and *Cryptococcus neoformans* are recoverable from blood cultures, the most common cause of fungemia is *Candida albicans* followed by other *Candida* sp including *Candida glabrata* (*Torulopsis glabrata*). Most *Candida* sp will also grow in routine aerobic bacterial blood cultures. Fungemia may be precipitated by contamination of an indwelling catheter or, in the critically ill and immunocompromised patient, invasion from the gastrointestinal and less frequently the urinary tract.[4]

Rarely, blastospores (budding yeast structures) and pseudohyphae can be seen by examination of Wright's stained venous peripheral blood smears.

See other listings including Histoplasmosis Antigen *on page 402*, Histoplasmosis Antibody *on page 402*, Coccidioidomycosis Antibodies *on page 384*, Candidiasis Serologic Test *on page 375*, and *Candida* Antigen *on page 374*.

Footnotes
1. Williams B, Fojtasek M, Connolly-Stringfield P, et al, "Diagnosis of Histoplasmosis by Antigen Detection During an Outbreak in Indianapolis, Ind," *Arch Pathol Lab Med*, 1994, 118(12):1205-8.
2. Bille J, Stockman L, Roberts GD, et al, "Evaluation of a Lysis-Centrifugation System for Recovery of Yeasts and Filamentous Fungi From Blood," *J Clin Microbiol*, 1983, 18:469-71.
3. Paya CV, Roberts GD, and Cockerill FR 3d, "Laboratory Methods for the Diagnosis of Disseminated Histoplasmosis: Clinical Importance of the Lysis-Centrifugation Blood Culture Technique," *Mayo Clin Proc*, 1987, 62(6):480-5.
4. Edwards JE Jr and Filler SG, "Current Strategies for Treating Invasive Candidiasis: Emphasis on Infections in Non-Neutropenic Patients," *Clin Infect Dis*, 1992, 14(Suppl 1):S106-13.

References
Geha DJ and Roberts GD, "Laboratory Detection of Fungemia," *Clin Lab Med*, 1994, 14(1):83-97.
Telenti A, Steckelberg JM, Stockman L, et al, "Quantitative Blood Cultures in Candidemia," *Mayo Clin Proc*, 1991, 66(11):1120-3.
Weinstein MP, "Clinical Importance of Blood Cultures," *Clin Lab Med*, 1994, 14(1):9-16.
Wilson ML and Weinstein MP, "General Principles in the Laboratory Detection of Bacteremia and Fungemia," *Clin Lab Med*, 1994, 14(1):69-82.

Fungal Culture, Cerebrospinal Fluid

CPT 87102 (isolation); 87106 (definitive identification)

Related Information
Amphotericin B *on page 535*
Bacterial Antigens, Rapid Detection Methods *on page 454*
Bacterial Culture, Cerebrospinal Fluid *on page 460*
Cerebrospinal Fluid Analysis *on page 309*
Cerebrospinal Fluid Cytology *on page 290*
Cerebrospinal Fluid Glucose *on page 105*
Cerebrospinal Fluid Protein *on page 380*
Cryptococcal Antigen Titer *on page 388*
Flucytosine *on page 551*
Fungal Culture, Biopsy or Body Fluid *on previous page*
Fungus Smear, Stain *on page 481*
India Ink Preparation *on page 484*
Itraconazole *on page 555*
Mycobacterial Culture, Cerebrospinal Fluid *on page 489*
Viral Culture, Central Nervous System Symptoms *on page 677*

Synonyms Cerebrospinal Fluid Fungus Culture; CSF Fungus Culture; Spinal Fluid Fungus Culture

Abstract Fungal infections that have disseminated or localized to the CNS are seen primarily in patients with underlying immunosuppression. Fungi that are yeasts at body temperatures, such as *Histoplasma capsulatum*, *Cryptococcus neoformans*, and *Blastomyces dermatitidis*, have access to the cerebral microcirculation, enabling such organisms to invade the subarachnoid space to produce acute and chronic leptomeningitis. *Candida* sp, which exists as both yeasts and pseudofungi at body temperatures, are also common meningeal pathogens.

Patient Preparation Aseptic preparation of aspiration site

Specimen Cerebrospinal fluid (see also the table in Fungal Culture, Sputum *on page 479*)

Collection Sterile tubes should be numbered 1, 2, 3 with tube #1 representing the first portion of the sample collected. Contamination from skin or other body surfaces must be avoided. The third tube collected during lumbar puncture is most suitable for culture, as skin contaminants from the puncture usually are washed out with fluid collected in the first two tubes.

(Continued)

Fungal Culture, Cerebrospinal Fluid *(Continued)*

Reference Range No growth

Use Diagnosis and etiology of fungal meningitis

Limitations Recovery of fungi from cerebrospinal fluid is directly related to the volume of cerebrospinal fluid available. A minimum of 10 mL is recommended. *Cryptococcus* can be mistaken for small lymphocytes in the counting chamber. Culture of additional specimens increases the chance for recovery.

Methodology Aerobic culture of centrifuged sediment on noninhibitory media usually including Sabouraud's, brain heart infusion agar (BHI) with blood agar at 25°C to 30°C and also frequently at 37°C.

Additional Information The diagnosis of central nervous system fungal infections is frequently complicated by the overlapping array of signs and symptoms which may accompany other clinical entities such as tuberculous meningitis, pyogenic abscess, brain tumor, hypersensitivity or allergic reactions, collagen vascular disease, leptomeningeal malignancy, chemical meningitis, meningeal inflammation secondary to contiguous suppuration, Behçet's disease, Mollaret's meningitis, and the uveomeningitic syndromes.[1]

Cryptococcosis may be indolent to fulminant, terminating in death within 2 weeks.[2] The India ink preparation is positive in 50% to 90% of cases, and the latex agglutination is positive in >95% of cases. Latex agglutination tests performed on serum are often positive in AIDS patients with cryptococcal meningitis.

The diagnosis of cryptococcal meningitis is sometimes recognized in CSF cytologic studies.

Footnotes
1. Reik L Jr, "Disorders That Mimic CNS Infections" *Neurol Clin*, 1986, 4(1):223-48.
2. Fishman RA, *Cerebrospinal Fluid in Diseases of the Nervous System*, 2nd ed, Philadelphia, PA: WB Saunders Co, 1992, 273-7.

References
Gripshover BM and Ellner JJ, "Chronic Meningitis," *Principles and Practice of Infectious Diseases*, 4th ed, Mandell GL, Bennett JE, and Dolin R, eds, New York, NY: Churchill Livingstone, 1995.
Greenlee JE, "Approach to Diagnosis of Meningitis - Cerebrospinal Fluid Evaluation," *Infect Dis Clin North Am*, 1990, 4(4):583-98.
Pappas PG, Pottage JC, Powderly WG, et al, "Blastomycosis in Patients With the Acquired Immunodeficiency Syndrome," *Ann Intern Med*, 1992, 116(10):847-53.
Tunkel AR, Wispelwey B, and Scheld WM, "Pathogenesis and Pathophysiology of Meningitis," *Infect Dis Clin North Am*, 1990, 4(4):555-81.

Fungal Culture, Ocular Infections

CPT 87102 (isolation); 87106 (definitive identification)

Related Information
Bacterial Culture, Conjunctiva *on page 461*
Fungus Smear, Stain *on page 481*

Synonyms Conjunctival Fungus Culture

Applies to Eye Fungus Culture

Test Commonly Includes Culture, and if specimen is adequate, KOH preparation and PAS smear

Patient Preparation Avoid contamination with skin flora.

Specimen Scrapings of corneal ulcer, washings of lacrimal duct, wet swabs of conjunctiva

Collection The physician should collect corneal fragments from the edge and base of the ulcer. Swabs are often insufficient.

Reference Range No growth; normal eye flora can have *Candida* sp

Use Establish the presence of keratomycosis

Limitations A single negative culture does not rule out the presence of fungal infection.

Methodology Culture on appropriate media usually including Sabouraud's medium, brain heart infusion (BHI), and blood agar incubation at 37°C and 25°C to 30°C

Additional Information The more common causes of keratomycosis include *Fusarium* sp, *Candida albicans*, *Aspergillus fumigatus*, *Curvularia* sp, *Aspergillus flavus*, other species of *Aspergillus*, *Penicillium*, and *Paecilomyces*. Many of these fungi cause other types of infection as well, eg, the subcutaneum. A keratomycosis-like clinical presentation may also be caused by *Nocardia asteroides* and *Mycobacterium fortuitum*. Keratomycosis is a rare complication of contact lens use.[1] Direct microscopic observation provides a higher yield than culture for the diagnosis of keratomycosis.[2]

Footnotes
1. White GL Jr, Thiese SM, and Lundergan MK, "Contact Lens Care and Complications," *Am Fam Physician*, 1988, 37(4):187-92.
2. Ishibashi Y, Hommura S, and Matsumoto Y, "Direct Examination vs Culture of Biopsy Specimens for the Diagnosis of Keratomycosis," *Am J Ophthalmol*, 1987, 103(5):636-40.

References
Baum J, "Infections of the Eye," *Clin Infect Dis*, 1995, 21:479-88.
Isenberg HD and D'Amato RF, "Indigenous and Pathogenic Microorganisms of Humans," *Manual of Clinical Microbiology*, 6th ed, Murray PR, Baron EJ, Pfaller MA, et al, eds, Washington, DC: American Society for Microbiology, 1995, 5-18.

Schell WA, "New Aspects of Emerging Fungal Pathogens. A Multifaceted Challenge," *Clin Lab Med*, 1995, 15(2):365-87.

Fungal Culture, Skin

CPT 87101 (isolation); 87106 (definitive identification)

Related Information
Amphotericin B *on page 535*
Antimicrobial Susceptibility Testing, Fungi *on page 450*
Fungal Culture, Biopsy or Body Fluid *on page 476*
Fungal Culture, Stool *on page 480*
Fungus Smear, Stain *on page 481*
HIV-1/HIV-2 Serology *on page 403*
Itraconazole *on page 555*
KOH Preparation *on page 485*
Mycobacterial Culture, Cutaneous and Subcutaneous Tissue *on page 489*
Skin Biopsy *on page 54*

Synonyms Dermatophyte Fungus Culture; Skin Fungus Culture

Applies to Fungus Culture, Hair and Nails

Test Commonly Includes Detection of superficial fungal infections of the skin or hair

Patient Preparation Select hairs which are broken off and appear diseased, and pluck them with sterile forceps. If diseased hair stubs are not apparent, scrape the edges of a scalp lesion with a sterile scalpel. Cleanse skin lesions first with 70% alcohol to reduce bacteria and saprophytic fungi. Scrape from the outer edges of skin lesions. In infections of the nails, scrape out the friable material beneath the edge of the nails, or scrape or clip off portions of abnormal appearing nail and submit for examination and culture.

Specimen Skin scrapings, exudates, nail clippings, whole nail, debris under nail, hair

Selection of Specimens for the Diagnosis of Superficial Mycosis and Dermatomycosis

Diagnosis	Specimen of Choice
Superficial mycoses	
Piedra	Hair
Tinea nigra	Skin scraping
Tinea versicolor	Skin scraping
Dermatomycoses (cutaneous mycoses)	
Onychomycosis	Nail scraping
Tinea capitis	Hair (black dot)
Tinea corporis	Skin scraping
Tinea pedis	Skin scraping
Tinea cruris	Skin scraping
Candidiasis	
Thrush	Scraping of oral white patches
Diaper dermatitis	Scraping of pustules at margin
Paronychia	Scraping skin around nail
Cutaneous candidiasis	Scraping of pustules at margin
Erosio interdigitalis blastomycetia (coinfection with gram-negative rods)	Scrapings of interdigital space (routine culture also)
Congenital candidiasis	Scraping of scales, pustules and cutaneous debris, cultures of umbilical stump, mouth, urine and stool
Mucocutaneous candidiasis	Scraping of affected area

Collection Enclose hair specimens, skin scrapings, or nail clippings or scrapings in clean paper envelopes, sterile urine container, or Petri dish. Do not put specimens in cotton-plugged tubes, because the specimen may become trapped among the cotton fibers and lost. Do not put specimen into closed containers, such as rubber-stoppered tubes, because this keeps the specimen moist and allows overgrowth of bacteria and saprophytic fungi. The laboratory should be informed of the fungal species suspected.

Turnaround Time Cultures in which suspicion of systemic fungal infection has been indicated are usually reported upon becoming positive or negative after 4 weeks.

Special Instructions Careful choice of specimens for laboratory study is important. See table. A Wood's lamp is useful in the collection of specimens in tinea capitis infections, since hairs infected by some members of the genus *Microsporum* exhibit fluorescence under a Wood's lamp.

However, in tinea capitis due to *Trichophyton* sp, infected hairs usually do not fluoresce.

Reference Range No growth

Use Isolate and identify fungi

Limitations A single negative specimen does not rule out fungal infections. *Malassezia furfur*, which causes pityriasis (formerly tinea) versicolor, frequently fails to grow in culture.

Methodology Aerobic culture on selective media usually including nonselective Sabouraud's agar incubated at 25°C to 30°C; some laboratories also incubate these cultures at 35°C to 37°C.

Additional Information Tissues that contain keratin (hair, nails, skin, etc) can become infected with dermatophytes, which are a group of related keratinophilic fungi. Infections are generally mild but may be severe as a consequence of the reaction of the patient to products made by the fungus. Cutaneous infections that resemble dermatophytoses may be caused by yeasts or certain filamentous fungi. *Candida* sp may colonize skin. Clinical diagnosis of *Candida* infection involves consideration of predisposing factors such as occlusion, maceration altered cutaneous barrier function. Signs of *Candida* infection include bright erythema, fragile papulopustules, and satellite lesions.[1] Patients with defects in T-lymphocyte responses, such as AIDS patients or individuals being treated with antineoplastic drugs, are especially susceptible to many fungal infections including superficial mycoses.[2,3] Most cutaneous fungal infections can be treated with the antifungal azole drugs like ketoconazole, itraconazole, and fluconazole. Severe infections should be treated with intravenous amphotericin B.[4]

Footnotes

1. McKay M, "Cutaneous Manifestations of Candidiasis," *Am J Obstet Gynecol*, 1988, 158(4):991-3.
2. Herrod HG, "Chronic Mucocutaneous Candidiasis in Childhood and Complications of Non-*Candida* Infection: A Report of the Pediatric Immunodeficiency Collaborative Group," *J Pediatr*, 1990, 116(3):377-82.
3. Diamond RD, "The Growing Problem of Mycoses in Patients Infected With the Human Immunodeficiency Virus," *Rev Infect Dis*, 1991, 13(3):480-6.
4. Hector RF, "Compounds Active Against Cell Walls of Medically Important Fungi," *Clin Microbiol Rev*, 1993, 6(1):1-21.

References

Chang P and Logemann H, "Onychomycosis in Children," *Int J Dermatol*, 1994, 33(8):550-1.

Cohn MS, "Superficial Fungal Infections. Topical and Oral Treatment of Common Types," *Postgrad Med*, 1992, 91(2):239-44, 249-52.

Frieden IJ and Howard R, "Tinea Capitis: Epidemiology, Diagnosis, Treatment, and Control," *J Am Acad Dermatol*, 1994, 31(3 Pt 2):S42-6.

Ginsburg CM, "Tinea capitis," *Pediatr Infect Dis J*, 1991, 10(1):48-9.

Hay RJ, "Fungal Skin Infections," *Arch Dis Child*, 1992, 67(9):1065-7.

Rasmussen JE, "Cutaneous Fungus Infections in Children," *Pediatr Rev*, 1992, 13(4):152-6.

Rezabek GH and Friedman AD, "Superficial Fungal Infections of the Skin Diagnosis and Current Treatment Recommendations," *Drugs*, 1992, 43(5):674-82.

Fungal Culture, Sputum

CPT 87102 (isolation); 87106 (definitive identification)

Related Information

Amphotericin B *on page 535*
Antimicrobial Susceptibility Testing, Fungi *on page 450*
Aspergillus Serology *on page 369*
Bacterial Culture, Bronchoscopy Specimen *on page 459*
Bacterial Culture, Sputum *on page 465*
Blastomycosis Serology *on page 371*
Bronchial Washings Cytology *on page 287*
Bronchoalveolar Lavage Cytology *on page 288*
Candidiasis Serologic Test *on page 375*
Coccidioidomycosis Antibodies *on page 384*
Cryptococcal Antigen Titer *on page 388*
Fungal Culture, Biopsy or Body Fluid *on page 476*
Fungal Culture, Stool *on next page*
Fungal Culture, Urine *on next page*
Fungus Smear, Stain *on page 481*
Histoplasmosis Antibody *on page 402*
Histoplasmosis Antigen *on page 402*
Itraconazole *on page 555*
KOH Preparation *on page 485*
Mycobacterial Culture, Sputum *on page 490*
Nocardia Culture *on page 493*
Sporotrichosis Serology *on page 431*
Sputum Cytology *on page 300*
Viral Culture, Respiratory Symptoms *on page 680*

Synonyms Sputum Fungus Culture

Applies to Bronchoscopy Fungus Culture; Fungus Culture, Gastric Aspirate

Patient Preparation The patient should be instructed to remove dentures, rinse mouth with water, and cough deeply expectorating sputum into the sputum collection cup.

Specimen First morning sputum, gastric aspirate, induced sputum, aspirated sputum, bronchial aspirate, tracheal aspirate, transtracheal aspirate. See table.

Selection of Specimens for the Diagnosis of Systemic and Subcutaneous Mycosis

Diagnosis	Specimen of Choice in Order of Usefulness	Diagnosis	Specimen of Choice in Order of Usefulness
Systemic Mycoses		**Systemic Mycoses** *(continued)*	
Aspergillosis	Sputum	Mycomycosis/ phycomycosis	Sputum
	Bronchial aspirate		Bronchial aspirate
	Biopsy (lung)		Biopsy (lung)
Blastomycosis	Skin scrapings	Paracoccidioido-mycosis	Skin scrapings
	Abscess drainage (pus)	(South American	Mucosal scrapings
	Urine		Biopsy (lymph nodes)
	Sputum	blastomycosis)	Sputum
	Bronchial aspirate		Bronchial aspirate
Candidiasis	Sputum		
	Bronchial aspirate	**Subcutaneous Mycoses**	
	Blood		
	Cerebrospinal fluid	Chromoblasto-mycosis	Skin scrapings
	Urine		Biopsy (skin)
	Stool		Drainage (pus)
Coccidioido-mycosis	Sputum	Maduromycosis	Drainage (pus)
	Bronchial aspirate	(mycetoma)	Abscess drainage
	Cerebrospinal fluid		Biopsy (lesion)
	Urine		
	Skin scrapings	Sporotrichosis	Drainage (pus)
	Abscess drainage (pus)		Abscess drainage
			Biopsy (skin, lymph node)
Cryptococcosis	Cerebrospinal fluid		
	Sputum		
	Abscess drainage (pus)		
	Skin scraping		
	Urine		

Container Sterile sputum cup, sputum trap, sterile tracheal aspirate or bronchoscopy tube

Collection A recommended screening procedure is three first morning specimens submitted on successive days. The specimen can be divided for fungus culture and KOH preparation, mycobacteria culture and smear, and routine bacterial culture and Gram's stain if the specimen is of adequate volume. Deeply coughed sputum, transtracheal aspirate, bronchial washing or brushing, or deep tracheal aspirate are preferred specimens.

Turnaround Time Negative cultures are reported after 4 weeks

Reference Range No growth; normal flora such as yeast from the oropharynx may be present.

Use Oncology patients, transplant patients, and patients with the acquired immunodeficiency syndrome (AIDS) are particularly prone to infection with fungi,[1] including histoplasmosis, for which cultures of respiratory secretions as well as blood fungal cultures and immunologic methods are useful.[2]

Limitations The yield may be reduced by bacterial overgrowth during storage or on standing; therefore, fresh sputum is preferred. A single negative culture does not rule out the presence of fungal infection. Simultaneously received specimens may be pooled.

Methodology Culture on selective media usually including supplemented Sabouraud's agar and brain heart infusion (BHI) with antibiotics to reduce bacterial overgrowth

Additional Information Primary fungal pulmonary infections include *Histoplasma capsulatum*, *Coccidioides immitis*, *Cryptococcus neoformans*, and *Blastomyces dermatitidis*. The incidence is largely related to geographic exposure and cases can occur in seemingly normal hosts. Numbers of reports of opportunistic fungal pulmonary infections due to a variety of etiologic agents which are ubiquitous in the environment are being published. Definitive diagnosis depends upon the presence of clinical signs of pulmonary infection, a chest x-ray revealing abnormality (Continued)

Fungal Culture, Sputum (Continued)

such as granuloma; laboratory isolation of a potentially significant organism from a suitable specimen; histologic documentation of tissue invasion by the isolated organism. A list of etiologic agents of pulmonary fungal disease has been compiled.[3] See table. In practice a diagnosis sufficient for therapy can frequently be established by observation of hyphae, pseudohyphae, or yeast cells in tissue sections using Gomori methenamine silver or other methods; recovery of the organism from a normally sterile site; repeated isolation of the same suspect organism from the same or different sites; seroconversion (ie, the development of an immune response to the suspected organism).[4] *Candida* and *Aspergillus* sp are the most frequently isolated, however, they are frequently present as the result of contamination from the patient's normal flora or airborne sources. Their presence may represent colonization rather than invasion. Recovery of *Candida* from blood (see Fungal Culture, Blood on page 477) is a major adjunct to definitive diagnosis. Even without invasion **Aspergillus** may cause IgE mediated asthma, allergic alveolitis cell mediated hypersensitivity, mucoid impaction, and bronchocentric granulomatosis.[5] The differential diagnosis between **chronic necrotizing pulmonary aspergillosis** and **Aspergillus fungus ball** is relevant, because in the former symptoms are present, cavitation is found secondary to lung necrosis, and medical therapy is available.[6] Fungal tracheobronchitis has recently been recognized as a pseudomembranous form involving the circumference of the bronchial wall or as multiple or discrete plaques. The plaques or pseudomembranes are composed of necrotic tissue exudate and fungal hyphae.[7]

Common Pulmonary Fungal Infections

Endemic Fungi	Opportunistic Fungi
Histoplasma capsulatum	Candida albicans
Blastomyces dermatitidis	Candida tropicalis
Coccidioides immitis	Aspergillus niger
Paracoccidioides brasiliensis	Aspergillus fumigatus
	Mucor
	Rhizopus
	Absidia
	Cryptococcus neoformans

From Haque AK, "Pathology of Common Pulmonary Fungal Infections," *J Thorac Imaging*, 1992, 7:1-11, with permission.

Sporotrichosis, widely recognized as a plant saprophyte which infects skin and subcutaneous tissue, causes pulmonary infection as well. It may be acquired from animal handling and exposure, and may be transmitted by domestic cats.[8]

Footnotes

1. Stansell JD, "Pulmonary Fungal Infections in HIV-Infected Persons," *Semin Respir Infect*, 1993, 8(2):116-23.
2. Williams B, Fojtasek M, Connolly-Stringfield P, et al, "Diagnosis of Histoplasmosis By Antigen Detection During an Outbreak in Indianapolis, Ind," *Arch Pathol Lab Med*, 1994, 118(12):1205-8.
3. Haque AK, "Pathology of Common Pulmonary Fungal Infections," *J Thorac Imaging*, 1992, 7(4):1-11.
4. Boyars MC, Zwischenberger JB, and Cox CS Jr, "Clinical Manifestations of Pulmonary Fungal Infections," *J Thorac Imaging*, 1992, 7(4):12-22.
5. Fraser RS, "Pulmonary Aspergillosis: Pathologic and Pathogenetic Features," *Pathol Annu*, 1993, 28(Pt 1):231-77.
6. Caras WE and Pluss JL, "Chronic Necrotizing Pulmonary Aspergillosis: Pathologic Outcome After Itraconazole Therapy," *Mayo Clin Proc*, 1996, 71(1):25-30.
7. Clarke A, Skelton J, and Fraser RS, "Fungal Tracheobronchitis. Report of 9 Cases and Review of the Literature," *Medicine (Baltimore)*, 1991, 70(1):1-14.
8. Schell WA, "New Aspects of Emerging Fungal Pathogens. A Multifaceted Challenge," *Clin Lab Med*, 1995, 15(2):365-87.

References

Batra P, "Pulmonary Coccidioidomycosis," *J Thorac Imaging*, 1992, 7(4):29-38.
Gray LD and Roberts GD, "Laboratory Diagnosis of Systemic Fungal Diseases," *Infect Dis Clin North Am*, 1988, 2(4):779-803.
Saral R, "*Candida* and *Aspergillus* Infections in Immunocompromised Patients: An Overview," *Rev Infect Dis*, 1991, 13(3):487-92.
Schuyler MR, "Allergic Bronchopulmonary Aspergillosis," *Clin Chest Med*, 1983, 4:15-22.
Tang CM and Cohen J, "Diagnosing Fungal Infections in Immunocompromised Hosts," *J Clin Pathol*, 1992, 45(1):1-5.
Temeck BK, Venzon DJ, Moskaluk CA, et al, "Thoracotomy for Pulmonary Mycoses in Non-HIV-Immunosuppressed Patients," *Ann Thorac Surg*, 1994, 58(2):333-8.
Wheat LJ, "Systemic Fungal Infections: Diagnosis and Treatment. I. Histoplasmosis," *Infect Dis Clin North Am*, 1988, 2(4):841-59.

Fungal Culture, Stool

CPT 87102 (isolation); 87106 (definitive identification)

Related Information

Amphotericin B on page 535
Bacterial Culture, Stool on page 466
Candida Antigen on page 374
Candidiasis Serologic Test on page 375
Clostridium difficile Toxin Assay on page 473

Fungal Culture, Blood on page 477
Fungal Culture, Skin on page 478
Fungal Culture, Sputum on previous page
Fungus Smear, Stain on next page
Methylene Blue Stain, Stool on page 642

Synonyms Stool Fungus Culture

Specimen Stool (see also the table in Fungal Culture, Sputum on page 479)

Container Plastic stool container or Culturette®

Collection The specimen can be divided for fungus culture and KOH preparation if the specimen is of adequate volume.

Storage Instructions Caution: Refrigeration will impede recovery of *H. capsulatum.*

Causes for Rejection Specimen containing interfering substances (eg, castor oil, bismuth, Metamucil®, barium) and those contaminated with urine may not have optimal yield.

Reference Range No growth

Use Establish the presence of fungi, particularly *Candida* sp in debilitated hosts, patients receiving antimicrobial chemotherapeutic agents and hyperalimentation

Limitations Use of this test is generally limited to screening for *Candida*. Stool cultures have a low yield and are not recommended for the isolation of systemic fungi, however, *Histoplasma capsulatum* is recovered from the stool of AIDS patients with disseminated infection. See listings Fungal Culture, Sputum on page 479 and Fungal Culture, Skin on page 478 for fungus culture specimen selection and Fungal Culture, Blood on page 477 for additional discussion of appropriate specimens.

Methodology Culture on selective media usually including Sabouraud's agar with antibiotics

Additional Information *Candida* can be isolated in up to 65% of stool cultures. Neonates and adults may develop watery diarrhea due to intestinal overgrowth by yeast which readily responds to specific therapy. *Candida* may become disseminated in patients with leukopenia, immunosuppressive therapy, AIDS, corticosteroid therapy, phagocytic defects, hyperalimentation, use of broad spectrum antibiotics, and oral contraceptives. Travelers in endemic areas with poor sanitation have also experienced intestinal overgrowth with *Candida*, although the specific mechanism causing diarrhea is unknown.

Candida-associated diarrhea is predominantly of the secretory type, characterized by frequent watery stools, usually without blood, mucus, tenesmus, or abdominal pain.[1] Overgrowth of *Candida* sp should be considered when evaluating *Clostridium difficile* negative cases of antibiotic-associated colitis.[2]

Footnotes

1. Gupta TP and Ehrinpreis MN, "*Candida*-Associated Diarrhea in Hospitalized Patients," *Gastroenterology*, 1990, 98(3):780-5.
2. Sanderson PJ and Bukhari SS, "*Candida* spp and *Clostridium difficile* Toxin-Negative Antibiotic-Associated Diarrhoea," *J Hosp Infect*, 1991, 19(2):142-3.

References

Anaissie EJ, Bodey GP, and Kantarjian H, "A New Spectrum of Fungal Infections in Patients With Cancer," *Rev Infect Dis*, 1989, 11(3):369-78.
Danna PL, Urban C, Bellin E, et al, "Role of *Candida* in Pathogenesis of Antibiotic-Associated Diarrhoea in Elderly Inpatients," *Lancet*, 1991, 337(8740):511-4.
Ullrich R, Heise W, Bergs C, et al, "Gastrointestinal Symptoms in Patients Infected With Human Immunodeficiency Virus: Relevance of Infective Agents Isolated From Gastrointestinal Tract," *Gut*, 1992, 33(8):1080-4.

Fungal Culture, Urine

CPT 87102 (isolation); 87106 (definitive identification)

Related Information

Bacterial Culture, Urine, Clean Catch on page 468
Bacterial Culture, Urine, Suprapubic Puncture on page 469
Blastomycosis Serology on page 371
Candidiasis Serologic Test on page 375
Fungal Culture, Blood on page 477
Fungal Culture, Sputum on previous page
Fungus Smear, Stain on next page
Itraconazole on page 555
Mycobacterial Culture, Urine on page 491
Urine Cytology on page 301

Synonyms Urine Fungus Culture

Abstract Use of antibacterial, antineoplastic, and immunosuppressive drugs, corticosteroids, urinary indwelling catheters, urinary tract obstruction, or the presence of diseases such as diabetes mellitus predispose to funguria. *C. albicans* is reported to cause up to 59% of positive urinary fungal cultures. *Torulopsis glabrata* and other *Candida* species account for many of the remainder.[1]

Patient Preparation Usual preparation for clean catch midvoid urine specimen collection. See listing Bacterial Culture, Urine, Clean Catch on page 468.

Specimen Urine. See table for fungus culture specimen selection in the listing Fungal Culture, Sputum *on page 479.*

Collection The patient must be instructed to thoroughly cleanse skin and collect midstream specimen.

Causes for Rejection Unrefrigerated specimen more than 2 hours old is subject to overgrowth of microorganisms.

Reference Range $<10^4$ CFU/mL

Use Detect and identify yeasts and fungi in urine specimens. Candiduria associated with hematogenous infections is observed in patients with granulocytopenia, corticosteroid therapy, and with immunosuppression. The source is frequently the gastrointestinal tract or indwelling catheters particular with hyperalimentation.[1] Urine is a useful specimen for culture in cryptococcosis, blastomycosis, and candidiasis. In addition to *Candida*, opportunistic pathogens in the genitourinary tract include *Aspergillus* and *Cryptococcus.* Endemic pathogens such as *Histoplasma, Blastomyces,* and *Coccidioides* are also encountered.[2]

Limitations A single negative culture does not rule out the presence of fungal infection.

Methodology Specimen is cultured on selective media such as supplemented Sabouraud's agar and/or brain heart infusion (BHI) with antibiotics.

Additional Information Asymptomatic funguria often ultimately clears spontaneously. However, candiduria with >15,000 colony forming units/mL of urine and with such evidence of dissemination as elevated serum precipitin antibody titers, is associated with increased mortality.[3] Patients with candiduria may or may not have candidemia; positive urine culture for fungi often may be followed by positive blood culture for fungi. Ascending infections occur in patients with diabetes, prolonged antimicrobial therapy, or following instrumentation. Urinary obstruction due to "fungus balls" may occur in diabetes and following renal transplantation.

A blood fungus culture is useful to define invasive disease. However, proof of invasive *Candida* infection requires direct cystoscopic or operative visualization, fungus balls, pyelonephritis, or histological evidence of mucosa invasion. The incidence of genitourinary fungal infections is increasing. They are usually associated with broad spectrum antibiotic therapy, corticosteroid therapy, underlying general debility, and AIDS.

Footnotes
1. Kunin CM, and Lipsky BA, "Treatment of Candiduria," *JAMA,* 1989, 262:691-2.
2. Frangos DN and Nyberg LM Jr, "Genitourinary Fungal Infections," *South Med J,* 1986, 79(4):455-9.
3. Wong-Beringer A, Jacobs RA, and Guglielmo BJ, "Treatment of Funguria," *JAMA,* 1992, 267(20):2780-5.

References
Leu HS and Huang CT, "Clearance of Funguria With Short-Course Antifungal Regimens: A Prospective, Randomized, Controlled Study," *Clin Infect Dis,* 1995, 20(5):1152-7.
Korzeniowsky OM, "Urinary Tract Infection in the Impaired Host," *Med Clin North Am,* 1991, 75(2):391-404.

Fungi Susceptibility Testing *see* Antimicrobial Susceptibility Testing, Fungi *on page 450*

Fungus Culture, Gastric Aspirate *see* Fungal Culture, Sputum *on page 479*

Fungus Culture, Hair and Nails *see* Fungal Culture, Skin *on page 478*

Fungus Smear, Stain
CPT 87205
Related Information
Acid-Fast Stain, Modified, *Nocardia* Species *on page 446*
Antimicrobial Susceptibility Testing, Fungi *on page 450*
Bacterial Culture, Conjunctiva *on page 461*
Blastomycosis Serology *on page 371*
Candida Antigen *on page 374*
Candidiasis Serologic Test *on page 375*
Coccidioidomycosis Antibodies *on page 384*
Cryptococcal Antigen Titer *on page 388*
Cryptosporidium Diagnostic Procedures *on page 474*
Fungal Culture, Biopsy or Body Fluid *on page 476*
Fungal Culture, Blood *on page 477*
Fungal Culture, Cerebrospinal Fluid *on page 477*
Fungal Culture, Ocular Infections *on page 478*
Fungal Culture, Skin *on page 478*
Fungal Culture, Sputum *on page 479*
Fungal Culture, Stool *on previous page*
Fungal Culture, Urine *on previous page*
Gram's Stain *on this page*
Histoplasmosis Antibody *on page 402*
Histoplasmosis Antigen *on page 402*
India Ink Preparation *on page 484*
KOH Preparation *on page 485*
Skin Biopsy *on page 54*

Sporotrichosis Serology *on page 431*

Applies to Calcofluor White; GMS Stain; Gomori Methenamine Silver Stain; Periodic Acid Schiff (PAS)

Test Commonly Includes Smear only; fungus culture and KOH preparation must usually be ordered separately

Patient Preparation Avoid contamination with skin flora.

Specimen The same specimen as required for fungal culture of the specific site. For conjunctiva or cornea, scrapings of corneal ulcer or wet swabs of conjunctiva. Specimen from conjunctiva or cornea should be obtained by physician only.

Reference Range No yeast or hyphal elements seen

Use Aid in the diagnosis of fungal disease; used in combination with fungus culture. Calcofluor white stain and KOH preparation may be more sensitive than culture in detecting keratomycosis.

Limitations A negative smear does not rule out the presence of fungal infection.

Methodology Periodic acid Schiff (PAS) stain, Calcofluor white, and Gomori methenamine silver stain (GMS) are used to identify fungal structures.

Additional Information Calcofluor white dye binds to cellulose and chitin and fluoresces with longwave UV light and shortwave visible light. Fungal elements viewed under UV light demonstrate a brilliant fluorescence that stands out from cells, tissue debris, and background. The preparations can subsequently be overstained with PAS or GMS. Calcofluor white is useful to screen stool specimens for **Microsporidia** spores.[1] ***Acanthamoeba*** keratitis can be documented by use of Calcofluor white stain.[2] **Caution:** Do not fix with ethanol as *Acanthamoeba* cysts will be desiccated and will not adhere adequately to the direct preparation slides. The PAS stain with a light green counterstain demonstrates the yeast forms, spores and the hyphae of fungi as pinkish red on a green background. The filaments of *Actinomyces* and *Nocardia* are not satisfactorily shown but do stain with Gram's stain. *Nocardia* is modified acid-fast positive.

Footnotes
1. Luna VA, Stewart BK, Bergeron DL, et al, "Use of the Fluorochrome Calcofluor White in the Screening of Stool Specimens for Spores of Microsporidia," *Am J Clin Pathol,* 1995, 103(5):656-9.
2. Marines HM, Osato MS, and Font RL, "The Value of Calcofluor White in the Diagnosis of Mycotic and *Acanthamoeba* Infections of the Eye and Ocular Adnexa," *Ophthalmology,* 1987, 94(1):23-6.

References
Gray LD and Roberts GD, "Laboratory Diagnosis of Systemic Fungal Diseases," *Infect Dis Clin North Am,* 1988, 2(4):779-803.
Kim YK, Parulekar S, Yu PK, et al, "Evaluation of Calcofluor White Stain for Detection of *Pneumocystis carinii,*" *Diagn Microbiol Infect Dis,* 1990, 13(4):307-10.
St Germain G and Summerbell R, "Identifying Filamentous Fungi," *A Clinical Laboratory Handbook,* Belmont, CA: Star Publishing, 1996.

Gastric Biopsy Culture for *Helicobacter pylori* *see Helicobacter pylori* Urease Test and Culture *on page 484*

GC Culture *see Neisseria gonorrhoeae* Culture and Smear *on page 492*

Genital Culture *see* Bacterial Culture, Genital Specimen *on page 463*

Genitourinary Anaerobic Culture, Female *see* Bacterial Culture, Endometrium *on page 462*

Giardia *see* Ova and Parasites, Stool *on page 494*

Giardia Immunosorbent Assay *see* Ova and Parasites, Stool *on page 494*

GMS Stain *see* Fungus Smear, Stain *on this page*

Gomori Methenamine Silver Stain *see* Fungus Smear, Stain *on this page*

Gonorrhea Culture *see Neisseria gonorrhoeae* Culture and Smear *on page 492*

Gram's Stain
CPT 87205
Related Information
Acid-Fast Stain, Modified, *Nocardia* Species *on page 446*
Bacterial Culture, Aerobes *on page 455*
Bacterial Culture, Anaerobes *on page 456*
Bacterial Culture, Biopsy or Body Fluid *on page 456*
Bacterial Culture, Burn Sites *on page 460*
Bacterial Culture, Cerebrospinal Fluid *on page 460*
Bacterial Culture, Conjunctiva *on page 461*
Bacterial Culture, Ear *on page 462*
Bacterial Culture, Sputum *on page 465*
Bacterial Culture, Throat *on page 468*
Bacterial Culture, Urine, Clean Catch *on page 468*
Bacterial Culture, Urine, Suprapubic Puncture *on page 469*
(Continued)

Gram's Stain *(Continued)*

Applies to Crystal Violet; Safranin

Abstract Gram's stain is a differential stain used to demonstrate the staining properties of bacteria. Gram-positive bacteria retain crystal violet after decolorization and appear deep blue to purple. Gram-negative bacteria do not retain crystal violet after decolorization and are counterstained red by safranin. Gram's staining characteristics may be atypical in very young, old, dead, or degenerating cultures.[1]

Patient Preparation Same as for routine culture of specific site

Specimen Duplicate of specimen appropriate for routine culture of the specific site

Collection Collection procedure same as for routine culture of the specific site. Specimen must be collected to avoid contamination with skin, adjacent structures, and nonsterile surfaces.

Critical Values Organisms detected in aseptically obtained specimens

Possible Panic Range Organisms detected in cerebrospinal fluid

Use For many clinical specimens, a specimen Gram's stain is performed upon specimen receipt. The specimen Gram's stain reveals information about specimen quality (eg, by comparing numbers of squamous epithelial cells and polymorphonuclear neutrophils in sputum specimens), presence or absence of potential pathogens, and initial presumptive morphologic categorization of potential pathogens (eg, yeasts, gram-positive cocci vs gram-negative bacilli, etc). Gram's stain results can provide a guide for initial empiric therapy, and should be correlated with subsequent culture results to help determine the significance of organisms isolated from clinical specimens.

Limitations Although Gram's stain results can provide important information shortly after specimen collection, the information provided is presumptive. Organism detection with specimen Gram's stain requires that large numbers of potential pathogens be present; consequently, sensitivity with many specimens is substantially <100% and direct Gram's stain of blood is unwarranted because organisms are almost never present in sufficient numbers for detection. Additionally, clinical specimens that are heavily contaminated with normal flora rarely provide diagnostically useful information unless probable pathogens are morphologically distinct from normal flora. Thus, direct Gram's stain of throat swabs, stool, and rectal swabs is usually unwarranted. Certain organisms (eg, *Rickettsia* spp, *Treponema pallidum*, *Legionella* spp, *Mycobacterium* spp) stain poorly, or not at all with Gram's stain.

Methodology Gram's stain technique:

- Make a thin smear of the material for study and allow to air dry.
- Fix the material to the slide by passing the slide three or four times through the flame of a Bunsen burner so that the material does not wash off during the staining procedure. Some workers now recommend the use of alcohol for the fixation of material to be Gram's stained (flood the smear with methanol or ethanol for a few minutes or warm for 10 minutes at 60°C on a slide warmer).
- Place the smear on a staining rack and overlay the surface with crystal violet solution.
- After 1 minute (less time may be used with some solutions) of exposure to the crystal violet stain, wash thoroughly with distilled water or buffer.
- Overlay the smear with Gram's iodine solution for 1 minute. Wash again with water.
- Hold the smear between the thumb and forefinger and flood the surface with a few drops of the acetone-alcohol decolorizer until no violet color washes off. This usually takes 10 seconds or less.
- Wash with running water and again place the smear on the staining rack. Overlay the surface with safranin counterstain for 1 minute. Wash with running water.
- Place the smear in an upright position in a staining rack, allowing the excess water to drain off and the smear to dry.
- Examine the stained smear under the 100x (oil) immersion objective of the microscope. Gram-positive bacteria stain dark blue; gram-negative bacteria appear pink-red.[1] See diagram.

Crystal Violet
(hexamethylpararosanilin)

Safranin
(dimethyl phenosafranin)

Additional Information Culture results, including organism identification and antimicrobial susceptibility, need to be reviewed to confirm and enhance the initial information provided by Gram's stain. The choice of initial empiric antimicrobial therapy should be re-evaluated; and an equally effective, less expensive, narrower spectrum antimicrobial agent should be substituted whenever possible.

Gram's stains are usually scanned for the presence or absence of white blood cells (indicative of infection) and squamous epithelial cells (indicative of mucosal contamination). A **sputum specimen** showing >25 squamous epithelial cells per low power field, regardless of the number of white blood cells, indicates that the specimen is grossly contaminated with saliva and bacterial culture should not be performed. Additional sputum specimens should be submitted to the laboratory if evidence of contamination by saliva is revealed. The Gram's stain can be a reliable indicator to guide initial antibiotic therapy. Substantial numbers of neutrophils and bacteria consistent with a pulmonary pathogen are appropriate for initial clinical therapeutic decision making, especially when phagocytosis of the organisms is found.[2] Typically a 90% correlation between Gram's stain and culture can be achieved.[3] It is imperative that a valid sputum specimen be obtained for Gram's stain.

Gram's stains revealing an occasional bacterium per high powered field in an uncentrifuged **urine specimen** suggest a colony count of 10,000 bacteria/mL. Bacteria in the majority of fields suggests >100,000 bacteria/mL, a level associated with significant bacteriuria. Gram staining was the only test which provided sensitivity and specificity of 80% or better simultaneously in detection of asymptomatic urinary tract infection in obstetric patients.[4] Detection of bacteriuria can be accomplished by slide centrifuge Gram's stained smear.[5]

Gram's stain is the most valuable diagnostic test in **bacterial meningitis** that is immediately available.[6] Organisms are detectable in 60% to 80% of patients who have not been treated and in 40% to 60% of those who have been given antibiotics.[6] Its sensitivity relates to the number of organisms present. The sensitivity of the Gram's stain is greater in gram-positive infections and is only positive in half of the instances of gram-negative meningitis. It is positive even less frequently with listeriosis meningitis or with anaerobic infections.[6] Culture and Gram's stain must have priority over antigen detection methods if only a small volume of CSF is available.[7]

Footnotes

1. Koneman EW, Allen SD, Janda WM, et al, *Color Atlas and Textbook of Diagnostic Microbiology*, 4th ed, Philadelphia, PA: JB Lippincott Co, 1992, 21, 24.
2. Yungbluth M, "The Laboratory Diagnosis of Pneumonia. The Role of the Community Hospital Pathologist," *Clin Lab Med*, 1995, 15(2):209-34.
3. Bartlett JG and Mundy LM, "Community-Acquired Pneumonia," *N Engl J Med*, 1995, 333(24):1618-24.
4. Bachman JW, Heise RH, Naessens JM, et al, "A Study of Various Tests to Detect Asymptomatic Urinary Tract Infections in an Obstetric Population," *JAMA*, 1993, 270(16):1971-4.
5. Rippin KP, Stinson WC, Eisenstadt J, et al, "Clinical Evaluation of the Slide Centrifuge (Cytospin) Gram's Stained Smear for the Detection of Bacteriuria and Comparison With the Filtracheck-UTI and UTIscreen," *Am J Clin Pathol*, 1995, 103(3):316-9.
6. Greenlee JE, "Approach to Diagnosis of Meningitis - Cerebrospinal Fluid Evaluation," *Infect Dis Clin North Am*, 1990, 4(4):583-98.
7. Gray LD and Fedorko DP, "Laboratory Diagnosis of Bacterial Meningitis," *Clin Microbiol Rev*, 1992, 5(2):130-45.

References

Chapin-Robertson K, Dahlberg SE, and Edberg SC, "Clinical and Laboratory Analyses of Cytospin-Prepared Gram Stains for Recovery and Diagnosis of Bacteria From Sterile Body Fluids," *J Clin Microbiol*, 1992, 30(2):377-80.

Morris AJ, Tanner DC, and Reller LB, "Rejection Criteria for Endotracheal Aspirates From Adults," *J Clin Microbiol*, 1993, 31(5):1027-9.

Riccardi NB and Felman YM, "Laboratory Diagnosis in the Problem of Suspected Gonococcal Infection," *JAMA*, 1979, 242(24):2703-5.

Smith AL, "Bacterial Meningitis," *Pediatr Rev*, 1993, 14(1):11-8.

Group A Beta-Hemolytic *Streptococcus* Culture, Throat *see* Bacterial Culture, Throat *on page 468*

Group A *Streptococcus* Screen, Rapid

CPT 86588 (direct)

Related Information

Antideoxyribonuclease-B Titer, Serum *on page 365*
Antistreptolysin O Titer, Serum *on page 369*
Bacterial Antigens, Rapid Detection Methods *on page 454*
Bacterial Culture, Throat *on page 468*
Group B *Streptococcus* Screen, Rapid *on this page*

Synonyms *Streptococcus* Group A Latex Screen; Throat Swab for Group A Streptococcal Antigen

Applies to Enzyme Immunoassay for Group A *Streptococcus* Antigen

Replaces Coagglutination Test for Group A Streptococci

Specimen Throat swab; many laboratories request two swabs, one for culture if the rapid screen is negative

Container Rayon or dacron swabs rather than cotton swabs enhance the chance of detection.

Collection Rigorous swabbing of the tonsillar pillars and posterior throat increases the probability of detection of streptococcal antigen.

Special Instructions Some laboratories favor submission of dry swabs for antigen testing. Consult the laboratory for their specific recommendations.

Use Rapidly screen for the presence of group A streptococci using culture independent methods

Limitations Many reviews have indicated a sensitivity of 75% to 80% and a specificity of 95% to 98% for the rapid methods. Sensitivity varies between manufacturers. Some kits are capable of detecting 10^5 colony forming units (CFUs) while others require 10^6-10^7 CFU/mL. Specimens which yield less than 10 colonies on culture usually are negative by rapid method. Adequate specimen collection on younger patients may be difficult, and thus, contribute to the false-negative rate. A positive result can be relied upon as a rational basis to begin therapy. **A negative result is only presumptive, and a culture should be performed to reasonably exclude the diagnosis of group A streptococcal infection.** Careful attention to the details of the method and the use of appropriate controls are required to assume adequate performance. Group A streptococcal antigen disappears rapidly following antibiotic therapy. Thus, a history of prior therapy should be sought when assessing pharyngitis.[1]

Contraindications This test should not be ordered unless results available within 1-2 hours of specimen collection will impact therapeutic decisions.

Methodology The streptococcal group carbohydrate antigen is extracted from the swab used for collection by use of acid or enzyme reagents. The group A antigen is detected by enzyme immunoassay (EIA) or latex agglutination (LA). A nucleic acid based test has been developed.[2]

Additional Information Rheumatic fever remains a concern in the United States and serious complications including sepsis, soft tissue invasion, and toxic shock-like syndrome have been reported to be increasing in frequency.[1] Therefore, timely diagnosis and early institution of appropriate therapy remains important. Timely therapy may reduce the acute symptoms and overall duration of streptococcal pharyngitis. The sequelae of poststreptococcal glomerulonephritis and rheumatic fever are diminished by early therapy.

Footnotes

1. Givner LB, Abramson JS, and Wasilauskas B, "Apparent Increase in the Incidence of Invasive Group A Beta-Hemolytic Streptococcal Disease in Children," *J Pediatr*, 1991, 118(3):341-6.
2. Heiter BJ and Bourbeau PP, "Comparison of the Gen-Probe® Group A *Streptococcus* Test With Culture and a Rapid Streptococcal Antigen Detection Assay for Diagnosis of Streptococcal Pharyngitis," *J Clin Microbiol*, 1993, 31(8):2070-3.

References

Harbeck RJ, Teague J, Crossen GR, et al, "Novel, Rapid Optical Immunoassay Technique for Detection of Group A Streptococci From Pharyngeal Specimens: Comparison With Standard Culture Methods," *J Clin Microbiol*, 1993, 31(4):839-44.
Hoffmann S, "Detection of Group A Streptococcal Antigen From Throat Swabs With Five Diagnostic Kits in General Practice," *Diagn Microbiol Infect Dis*, 1990, 13(3):209-15.
"Rapid Diagnostic Tests for Group A Streptococcal Pharyngitis," *Med Lett Drugs Ther*, 1991, 33(843):40-1.
Schwartz B, Fries S, Fitzgibbon AM, et al, "Pediatricians' Diagnostic Approach to Pharyngitis and Impact of CLIA 1988 on Office Diagnostic Tests," *JAMA*, 1994, 271(3):234-8.

Group B *Streptococcus* Screen, Rapid

CPT 86588 (direct)

Related Information

Bacterial Antigens, Rapid Detection Methods *on page 454*
Bacterial Culture, Genital Specimen *on page 463*
Group A *Streptococcus* Screen, Rapid *on this page*

Synonyms *Streptococcus agalactiae* Latex Screen; *Streptococcus* Group B Latex Screen

Replaces Counterimmunoelectrophoresis for Group B Streptococcal Antigen

Test Commonly Includes Culture-independent detection of group B beta *Streptococcus* antigen

Specimen Cerebrospinal fluid, blood, urine, endocervical, vaginal, rectal, or amniotic fluid

Container Sterile container, red top tube

Storage Instructions Set up cultures. If a specimen for antigen detection cannot be tested immediately, it may be stored at 2°C to 8°C for 1 day or frozen at -20°C for longer storage. Storage is inconsistent with the role of the test for rapid diagnosis.

Turnaround Time About 1 hour stat

Critical Values Positive intrapartum test

Possible Panic Range Positive neonatal test

Use Culture-independent detection of group B *Streptococcus* is used in two settings. First, it is used to diagnose patients (usually in the neonatal period) suspected of group B *Streptococcus* sepsis and/or meningitis. Secondly, it is used as a rapid intrapartum test to identify maternal group B *Streptococcus* carriers who might transmit the organism to their newborn.

Limitations Rapid group B *Streptococcus* detection has a sensitivity range of 70% to 90% in neonatal meningitis. Identification of maternal group B *Streptococcus* carriers using rapid group B *Streptococcus* tests often fails to identify women colonized with low numbers of organisms; the significance of this insensitivity is unclear.

Methodology Polystyrene latex particles coated with antibodies specific for the group B *Streptococcus* antigen agglutinate in the presence of the homologous antigen. Controls for nonspecific agglutination of latex particles are generally used. See package insert directions relevant to heat inactivation. Urine may be concentrated to increase sensitivity of the method. Infection can be diagnosed by detection of group B specific carbohydrate antigen of bacterial cell wall, which may be present in body fluids, serum and cerebrospinal fluid and which is excreted in urine. Counterimmunoelectrophoresis (CIE) has been a method for detection of the group B *Streptococcus* antigen. Alternatively, swab specimens collected during antepartum visits may be cultured on appropriate media.

Additional Information Group B *Streptococcus* is one of the most common human pathogens in the neonatal period.[1] Neonatal infection follows exposure to maternal genital flora *in utero* through ruptured membranes, or by colonization during passage through the birth canal. Neonatal infection presents as either early or late onset disease (EOD or LOD, respectively). EOD, which occurs within 5 days of birth (mean period to onset of symptoms is 20 hours), manifests as pneumonia and sepsis, occasionally accompanied by meningitis. LOD, which occurs 7 days to 3 months after birth (mean period to onset is 24 days) usually presents as meningitis.

Intrapartum antimicrobial therapy has been shown to be an effective means of reducing the incidence of EOD. It is currently not clear how best to identify individuals who should be treated.[1,2,3,4] Several options have been proposed; treat all pregnant women, treat pregnant women who have specific risk factors (eg, premature rupture of membranes, prolonged rupture of membranes, fever), treat pregnant women who are colonized with group B *Streptococcus*, or treat pregnant women who are colonized with group B *Streptococcus* and have other risk factors.

Footnotes

1. Noya FJ and Baker CJ, "Prevention of Group B Streptococcal Infection," *Infect Dis Clin North Am*, 1992, 6(1):41-55.
2. Larsen JW and Dooley SL, "Group B Streptococcal Infections: An Obstetrical Viewpoint," *Pediatrics*, 1993, 91(1):148-9.
3. Rouse DJ, Goldenberg RL, Cliver SP, et al, "Strategies for the Prevention of Early-Onset Neonatal Group B Streptococcal Sepsis: A Decision Analysis," *Obstet Gynecol*, 1994, 83(4):483-94.
4. "American Academy of Pediatrics Committee on Infectious Diseases and Committee on Fetus and Newborn: Guidelines for Prevention of Group B Streptococcal (GBS) Infection by Chemoprophylaxis," *Pediatrics*, 1992, 90(5):775-8.

References

Agnoli FL, "Group B *Streptococcus*: Perinatal Considerations," *J Fam Pract*, 1994, 39(2):171-7.
Green M, Dashefsky B, Wald ER, et al, "Comparison of Two Antigen Assays for Rapid Intrapartum Detection of Vaginal Group B Streptococcal Colonization," *J Clin Microbiol*, 1993, 31(1):78-82.
Patel DM, Leblanc MH, Morrison JC, et al, "Postnatal Penicillin Prophylaxis and the Incidence of Group B Streptococcal Sepsis in Neonates," *South Med J*, 1994, 87(11):1117-20.
Simpson AJ, Mawn JA, and Heard SR, "Assessment of Two Methods for Rapid Intrapartum Detection of Vaginal Group B Streptococcal Colonisation," *J Clin Pathol*, 1994, 47(8):752-5.
Wust J, Hebisch G, and Peters K, "Evaluation of Two Enzyme Immunoassays for Rapid Detection of Group B Streptococci in Pregnant Women," *Eur J Clin Microbiol Infect Dis*, 1993, 12(2):124-7.

Gunshot Wound Culture *see* Bacterial Culture, Wound *on page 470*

Haemophilus *see* Bacterial Culture, Aerobes *on page 455*

Haemophilus influenzae Susceptibility Testing *see* Beta-Lactamase Test *on page 470*

Hanging Drop Mount for Trichomonas *see* Trichomonas Preparation *on page 498*

Hank's Stain *see* Acid-Fast Stain, Modified, *Nocardia* Species *on page 446*

Helicobacter pylori Urease Test and Culture

CPT 43600 (gastric biopsy); 87081 (culture single organism); 87205 (Gram's stain); 88104 (cytopathology smears with interpretation)

Related Information
Gastric Analysis *on page 133*
Gastrin, Serum *on page 135*
Helicobacter pylori Serology *on page 395*

Synonyms *Campylobacter pylori* Urease Test and Culture; Gastric Biopsy Culture for *Helicobacter pylori*; Urease Test and Culture, *Helicobacter pylori*

Test Commonly Includes Screening for the presence of urease activity indirectly indicating the presence of *Helicobacter pylori*; culture of the organism from gastric biopsy specimens

Abstract *H. pylori* is a gram-negative motile microaerophilic spiral-shaped bacillus which is a frequent cause of gastritis.[1] It plays a major role in pathogenesis of peptic ulcer disease. *H. pylori* infection is an independent risk factor for gastric cancer, adenocarcinoma, and primary gastric malignant lymphoma.

Its urease activity is important in detection and identification. Culture with biopsy is the gold standard for identification of *H. pylori*[1] (formerly, *Campylobacter pylori*).

Specimen Gastric mucosal biopsy

Container Sterile container, **no fixative** for these microbiologic tests

Storage Instructions If specimen cannot be transported immediately to the laboratory, it should be placed in 0.5 mL transport medium (normal saline).

Reference Range Negative for urease activity, negative culture, biopsy negative for gastritis and negative for *H. pylori*

Use Establish the presence and possible etiologic role of *Helicobacter pylori* in cases of chronic gastric ulcer, chronic active gastritis, and a relationship with duodenal ulcers

Limitations Culture and urease testing alone, without biopsies, may allow occult neoplasms to go undetected.

Methodology Urease test: Gastric biopsies are incubated on slightly buffered medium. A change of phenol red to alkaline (pink color) persisting more than 5 minutes is considered positive and presumptively indicative of the presence of *Helicobacter pylori* even if the organism cannot be grown in culture. Specimens negative at 30 minutes should be re-examined periodically up to 24 hours. The sensitivity of urease testing leaves something to be desired. It was only 62% at 24 hours in a 1991 report. It also is characterized by false-positive results.[2]

Culture: Culture media may include enriched chocolate, Thayer-Martin with antibiotics, brain heart infusion (BHI) with 7% horse blood, and Mueller-Hinton with 5% sheep blood. Nichols et al describe horse blood agar plate (Columbia agar base), then a 5% sheep blood agar plate (trypticase soy base), and finally a plate of Skirrow medium.[2] The organism is microaerophilic and grows best in a reduced O_2 atmosphere or in a Campy-Pak™ system at 35°C. Cultures are usually observed for 7 days before being reported as negative.

Cytology: Touch cytology preparations (ie, imprints from biopsies) may provide rapid diagnosis and preserve the biopsy specimen for histopathology or culture.

Smear: A direct smear can be Gram's stained.[2]

Sensitivity of methods for detection of *H. pylori*:
- 24-hour urease: 62%
- direct Gram's stain: 69%
- culture: 90%
- histology: 93%[2]

Additional Information *Helicobacter pylori* is a major cause of chronic active gastritis. Its association with duodenal ulcer is strong. It is known that more than 90% of subjects who have duodenal ulcer have *H. pylori* infection, but 3% to 70% of patients without duodenal ulcer have *H. pylori* as well.[3,4] Only 50% of patients with Zollinger-Ellison syndrome with duodenal ulcer have *H. pylori*, thus, Zollinger-Ellison syndrome may be suspected when *H. pylori* is absent in subjects with duodenal ulcer.[5] Of patients with gastric ulcers, 75% to 80% have *H. pylori*. The organism may be seen in biopsies stained with Gram's stain,[2] hematoxylin-eosin (H & E), Giemsa or Warthin-Starry silver stain. It is most often recognized in biopsies from the antrum but may also be seen in the fundic mucosa, metaplastic gastric mucosa of esophagus (Barrett's esophagus), or duodenum.[1] Biopsy may also establish the diagnosis of carcinoma or lymphoma. *H. pylori* was not found in the gastric mucosa of Meckel's diverticula.[6] Gram's stains performed by a reuse imprint technique on biopsies from both the antrum and fundus yielded positives in 100% of 32 culture positive cases.[7]

Most peptic ulcers related to *H. pylori* infection can be treated with antibiotics and medication to suppress gastric acid.[4,8,9]

Breath isotope methods measuring bacterial urease by detection of labeled CO_2 and serologic tests for the detection of antibody are also useful if available. The breath test is preferred as a means of documenting presence of active infection and eradication of infection after therapy in the absence of endoscopy. Target amplification techniques such as polymerase chain reaction have shown promising results.[10] Serologic tests are also seeing increased usage in many settings.

Past *H. pylori* infection increases risk of carcinoma of stomach. Chronic atrophic gastritis and intestinal metaplasia are related to *H. pylori* infection, which induces as well development of lymphoid tissue in the gastric mucosa. The role of *H. pylori* in development of primary malignant lymphoma of stomach was recently discussed.[11,12,13]

Footnotes
1. Peterson WL, "*Helicobacter pylori* and Peptic Ulcer Disease," *N Engl J Med*, 1991, 324(15):1043-8.
2. Nichols L, Sughayer M, DeGirolami PC, et al, "Evaluation of Diagnostic Methods for *Helicobacter pylori* Gastritis," *Am J Clin Pathol*, 1991, 95(6):769-73.
3. Shocket ID, "*Helicobacter pylori* and Duodenal Ulcer: A Review," *Ann Intern Med*, 1992, 116(Suppl 2):61.
4. Graham DY, "Treatment of Peptic Ulcers Caused by *Helicobacter pylori*," *N Engl J Med*, 1993, 328(5):349-50.
5. Jensen RT and Fraker DL, "Zollinger-Ellison Syndrome. Advances in Treatment of Gastric Hypersecretion and the Gastrinoma," *JAMA*, 1994, 271(18):1429-35.
6. Fich A, Talley NJ, Shorter RG, et al, "Does *Helicobacter pylori* Colonize the Gastric Mucosa of Meckel's Diverticulum?" *Mayo Clin Proc*, 1990, 65(2):187-91.
7. Parsonnet J, Welch K, Compton C, et al, "Simple Microbiologic Detection of *Campylobacter pylori*," *J Clin Microbiol*, 1988, 26(5):948-9.
8. Sung JJ, Chung SC, Ling TK, et al, "Antimicrobial Treatment of Gastric Ulcers Associated With *Helicobacter pylori*," *N Engl J Med*, 1995, 332(3):139-42.
9. Hentschel E, Brandstätter G, Dragosics B, et al, "Effect of Ranitidine and Amoxicillin Plus Metronidazole on the Eradication of *Helicobacter pylori* and the Recurrence of Duodenal Ulcer," *N Engl J Med*, 1993, 328(5):308-12.
10. Fabre R, Sobhani I, Laurent-Puig P, et al, "Polymerase Chain Reaction Assay for the Detection of *Helicobacter pylori* in Gastric Biopsy Specimens: Comparison With Culture, Rapid Urease Test, and Histopathological Tests," *Gut*, 1994, 35(7):905-8.
11. Isaacson PG and Spencer J, "Is Gastric Lymphoma an Infectious Disease?" *Hum Pathol*, 1993, 24(6):569-70.
12. Genta RM, Hamner HW, and Graham DY, "Gastric Lymphoid Follicles in *Helicobacter pylori* Infection: Frequency, Distribution, and Response to Triple Therapy," *Hum Pathol*, 1993, 24(6):577-83.
13. Parsonnet J, Hansen S, Rodriguez L, et al, "*Helicobacter pylori* Infection and Gastric Lymphoma," *N Engl J Med*, 1994, 330(18):1267-71.

References
Atherton JC and Spiller RC, "The Urea Breath Test for *Helicobacter pylori*," *Gut*, 1994, 35(6):723-5.

"Case Records of the Massachusetts General Hospital. Weekly Clinicopathological Exercises. Case 13-1995. A 35-Year-Old Woman With Recurrent Bleeding From a Gastric Ulcer After Treatment for *Helicobacter pylori* Infection," *N Engl J Med*, 1995, 332(17):1153-9.

Chan WY, Hui PK, Leung KM, et al, "Coccoid Forms of *Helicobacter pylori* in the Human Stomach," *Am J Clin Pathol*, 1994, 102:503-7.

Chan WY, Hui PK, Chan JK, et al, "Epithelial Damage by *Helicobacter pylori* in Gastric Ulcers," *Histopathology*, 1991, 19(1):47-53.

Clearfield HR, "*Helicobacter pylori*: Aggressor or Innocent Bystander?" *Med Clin North Am*, 1991, 75(4):815-29.

Debongnie JC, Delmee M, Mainguet P, et al, "Cytology: A Simple, Rapid, Sensitive Method in the Diagnosis of *Helicobacter pylori*," *Am J Gastroenterol*, 1992, 87(1):20-3.

Debongnie JC, Mairesse J, Donnay M, et al, "Touch Cytology. A Quick, Simple, Sensitive Screening Test in the Diagnosis of Infections of the Gastrointestinal Mucosa," *Arch Pathol Lab Med*, 1994, 118(11):1115-8.

"*Helicobacter pylori* in Peptic Ulcer Disease," *NIH Consens Statement*, 1994, 12(1):1-23.

Hilzenrat N, Lamoureux E, Weintrub I, et al, "*Helicobacter heilmannii*-Like Spiral Bacteria in Gastric Mucosal Biopsies, Prevalence and Clinical Significance," *Arch Pathol Lab Med*, 1995, 119(12):1149-53.

Laine L and Peterson WL, "Bleeding Peptic Ulcer," *N Engl J Med*, 1994, 331(11):717-27.

Popovic-Uroic T, Patton CM, Wachsmuth IK, et al, "Evaluation of an Oligonucleotide Probe for Identification of *Campylobacter* Species," *Lab Med*, 1991, 22:533-9.

Ruiz B, Correa P, Fontham ET, et al, "Antral Atrophy, *Helicobacter pylori* Colonization, and Gastric pH," *Am J Clin Pathol*, 1996, 105:96-101.

Taylor DN and Blaser MJ, "The Epidemiology of *Helicobacter pylori* Infection," *Epidemiol Rev*, 1991, 13:42-59.

Veenendaal RA, Pena AS, Meijer JL, et al, "Long-Term Serological Surveillance After Treatment of *Helicobacter pylori* Infection," *Gut*, 1991, 32(11):1291-4.

Helminths *see* Ova and Parasites, Stool *on page 494*

Hemovac® Tip Culture *see* Bacterial Culture, Intravascular Device *on page 463*

Hyperalimentation Line Culture *see* Bacterial Culture, Intravascular Device *on page 463*

India Ink Preparation

CPT 87210

Related Information
Bacterial Culture, Cerebrospinal Fluid *on page 460*

Cryptococcal Antigen Titer *on page 388*
Fungal Culture, Cerebrospinal Fluid *on page 477*
Fungus Smear, Stain *on page 481*
KOH Preparation *on this page*

Synonyms Cerebrospinal Fluid India Ink Preparation

Test Commonly Includes Staining of CSF sediment with India ink to detect the polysaccharide capsule surrounding the yeast

Patient Preparation Same as for culture of specific site

Specimen Cerebrospinal fluid

Storage Instructions Do **not** refrigerate.

Reference Range No *Cryptococcus* identified

Critical Values Presence of encapsulated yeast

Use Establish a diagnosis of cryptococcal meningitis

Limitations This technique is only 30% to 50% sensitive in cases of cryptococcal meningitis. Cultures and rapid latex agglutination (LA) methods are more sensitive than direct preparations; therefore, the India ink preparation may be negative when the culture or LA test is positive. Many laboratories have abandoned the use of the India ink preparation in favor of LA.

Methodology Wet mount with India ink (nigrosin) for contrast. Centrifugation may concentrate organisms and improve sensitivity (10-20 minutes at 1500 g). Some sources of India ink are better than others for this purpose. Finer particles are desirable.

Additional Information *Cryptococcus neoformans* is the most common central nervous system fungal disease in both normal hosts and patients with the acquired immunodeficiency syndrome (AIDS). Skin, lungs, spleen, kidneys, liver, and/or bone may also be infected. Pigeon droppings act as a year-round vector for dispersion of encapsulated yeast cells.

References
Berlin L and Pincus JH, "Cryptococcal Meningitis. False-Negative Antigen Test Results and Cultures in Nonimmunosuppressed Patients," *Arch Neurol*, 1989, 46(12):1312-6.
Ellis DH and Pfeiffer TJ, "Ecology, Life Cycle, and Infectious Propagule of *Cryptococcus neoformans*," *Lancet*, 1990, 336(8720):923-5.

Infant Botulism, Toxin Identification *see* Botulism Diagnostic Procedure *on page 472*

Insect Identification *see* Arthropod Identification *on page 453*

Intrauterine Device Culture *see Actinomyces* Culture *on page 447*

Intrauterine Device Culture *see* Bacterial Culture, Endometrium *on page 462*

Intravascular Device Culture *see* Bacterial Culture, Intravascular Device *on page 463*

Intravenous Catheter Culture *see* Bacterial Culture, Intravascular Device *on page 463*

Isolator™ Blood Culture *see* Bacterial Culture, Blood *on page 457*

Isospora belli *see Cryptosporidium* Diagnostic Procedures *on page 474*

IUD Culture *see Actinomyces* Culture *on page 447*

IUD Culture *see* Bacterial Culture, Endometrium *on page 462*

Ixodes dammini Identification *see* Arthropod Identification *on page 453*

Kinyoun Stain *see* Acid-Fast Stain *on page 446*

Kirby-Bauer Susceptibility Test *see* Antimicrobial Susceptibility Testing, Aerobic and Facultatively Anaerobic Bacteria *on page 448*

KOH Preparation

CPT 87220

Related Information
Fungal Culture, Skin *on page 478*
Fungal Culture, Sputum *on page 479*
Fungus Smear, Stain *on page 481*
Gram's Stain *on page 481*
India Ink Preparation *on previous page*
Skin Biopsy *on page 54*

Synonyms Potassium Hydroxide Preparation

Test Commonly Includes Potassium hydroxide (KOH) hydrolysis of proteinaceous debris, cells, etc; microscopic examination under 10x and 40x objectives

Specimen Appropriate specimen for KOH preparation is the same as for culture. See specific site fungus culture listing for details. See the specimen selection tables provided in the listings Fungal Culture, Skin *on page 478* and Fungal Culture, Sputum *on page 479*.

Special Instructions The laboratory should be informed of the specific source of the specimen and the clinical diagnosis.

Reference Range No fungus elements identified

Use Determine the presence of fungi in skin, nails, or hair. Exudates from abscesses, sinus tracts, aspirates, etc, can be examined by KOH preparation and also smeared for Gram's stain. For the diagnosis of keratomycosis, direct examination may have a higher yield than culture because of the presence of dead organisms in the corneal tissue.[1]

Limitations Cultures are usually more sensitive than KOH preparations. The test may require overnight incubation for complete disintegration of hair, nail, or skin debris.

Methodology 10% KOH with gentle heat, alternately 10% to 20% KOH and 40% dimethyl sulfoxide (DMSO)[2]

Additional Information Recent reports have emphasized the changing pattern of tinea capitis, particularly the fact that infection due to *Trichophyton tonsurans* has become increasingly common. When present it causes a less discrete, more diffuse pattern of alopecia. It is negative by Wood's light examination. The "black dot", a remnant of a broken infected hair shaft, is a good source for diagnostic material which should be sought with a magnifying glass and collected with forceps. Scale and pulled hairs are also useful specimens.[3] Diagnostic specimens should be collected before antifungal therapy is instituted. Topical steroids should not be prescribed until fungal infection is excluded.[4]

Footnotes
1. Ishibashi Y, Hommura S, and Matsumoto Y, "Direct Examination vs Culture of Biopsy Specimens for the Diagnosis of Keratomycosis," *Am J Ophthalmol*, 1987, 103(5):636-40.
2. Stein DH, "Superficial Fungal Infections," *Pediatr Clin North Am*, 1983, 30(3):545-61.
3. Krowchuk DP, Lucky AW, Primmer SI, et al, "Current Status of the Identification and Management of Tinea Capitis," *Pediatrics*, 1983, 72:625-31.
4. Pariser DM, "Superficial Fungal Infections. A Practical Guide for Primary Care Physicians," *Postgrad Med*, 1990, 87(5):205-14.

References
Chang P and Logemann H, "Onychomycosis in Children," *Int J Dermatol*, 1994, 33(8):550-1.
Cohn MS, "Superficial Fungal Infections. Topical and Oral Treatment of Common Types," *Postgrad Med*, 1992, 91(2):239-44, 249-52.
Gray LD and Roberts GD, "Laboratory Diagnosis of Systemic Fungal Diseases," *Infect Dis Clin North Am*, 1988, 2(4):779-803.
St Germain G and Summerbell R, "Identifying Filamentous Fungi," *A Clinical Laboratory Handbook*, Belmont, CA: Star Publishing, 1996.

Latex Agglutination for Bacterial Antigens *see* Bacterial Antigens, Rapid Detection Methods *on page 454*

Latex Agglutination *Legionella pneumophila* *see* Legionella Culture *on this page*

Legionella Culture

CPT 87081 (culture single organism); 87163 (additional identification methods)

Related Information
Bacterial Culture, Sputum *on page 465*
Legionnaires' Disease Antibodies *on page 412*
Legionnaires' Disease Direct Fluorescent Antibody Smear *on page 413*

Synonyms Legionnaires' Disease Agent

Applies to Biopsy *Legionella* Culture; Bronchoscopic *Legionella* Culture; DNA Probe *Legionella*; Latex Agglutination *Legionella pneumophila*; Pleural Fluid, *Legionella* Culture; Transtracheal Aspiration *Legionella* Culture

Test Commonly Includes Culture and frequently direct fluorescent antibody (DFA) smear for *Legionella* spp

Abstract The family Legionellaceae are ubiquitous, gram-negative, motile, fastidious, aerobic bacilli. During an American Legion Convention in Philadelphia in 1976, an epidemic of pneumonia caused 34 deaths. Sputum characterized by acute inflammatory features, without a classical pattern of bacteria, may represent *Legionella*, influenza, or respiratory syncytial virus.

Specimen Lung tissue, other body tissue, pleural fluid, other body fluid, transtracheal aspiration, bronchoalveolar lavage, bronchial brushing, sputum

Turnaround Time Positive results are usually generated between 2-5 days. Primary plates are often held for 7-14 days before a final negative report is issued.

Reference Range No *Legionella* recovered

Use Isolate and identify *Legionella pneumophila*

Limitations Sputum (expectorated), bronchial aspirates, and other specimens having normal flora are subject to bacterial overgrowth and are not as desirable as transtracheal aspirates, pleural fluid, and biopsy material for culture. Sensitivity of cultures is relatively low (50% to 80%), however, specificity approaches 100%.[1,2]

(Continued)

Legionella Culture *(Continued)*

Methodology Culture on selective and nonselective media (buffered charcoal yeast extract). *Legionella* requires L-cysteine and ferric salt supplementation of growth media

Additional Information Laboratory diagnosis of *Legionella* infection can be attempted with three distinct methodological approaches.[1,2,3] Firstly, a rapid diagnosis can be attained by culture-independent methods that detect bacterial products in clinical specimens (eg, direct fluorescent antibody tests on respiratory specimens, DNA amplification, radioimmunoassay or enzyme immunoassays on urine specimens). The sensitivity of these methods is usually between 70% and 90%, and specificity exceeds 95%. Secondly, indirect fluorescence antibody methods can be used to detect the patient's antibody response to *Legionella* spp. Serologic methods have sensitivities of 70% to 80% and specificities exceeding 95%, but their clinical utility is limited by the retrospective nature of most serologic methods. Finally, *Legionella* cultures can be performed; *Legionella* cultures have sensitivities and specificities of approximately 70% and 100%, respectively. The low sensitivity of each of the methods for diagnosing legionellosis mandates that multiple methods be used in most situations; culture should be one of these methods.

Nosocomial infections have been recognized with reservoirs, water distribution systems, cooling systems, and hot water systems. Over 34 species in the Legionellaceae family of bacteria have been discovered since *Legionella pneumophila* was first recognized. Thirteen species have been implicated as causes of human pneumonia. See tables.

Infections Caused by *Legionella*

Culture proven
Pneumonia
Empyema
Sinusitis
Prosthetic valve endocarditis
Wound infection
Associated with pneumonia
Bowel abscesses
Brain abscesses
Empyema
Lung abscesses
Myocarditis
Pericarditis
Peritonitis
Renal abscesses/pyelonephritis
Vascular graft infections
Strong seroepidemiological evidence
Pontiac fever
Weak seroepidemiological evidence
Encephalopathy without pneumonia
Myocarditis without pneumonia
Pericarditis without pneumonia

From Edelstein PH, "Laboratory Diagnosis of Infections Caused by *Legionella*," *Eur J Clin Microbiol*, 1987, 6:4-10, with permission.

Clinical Clues to the Diagnosis of Legionnaires' Disease

- Gram's stain of respiratory secretions reveals numerous neutrophils, but few organisms
- Presence of hyponatremia (serum sodium ≤130 mmol/L)
- Failure to respond to β-lactam and aminoglycoside antibiotics
- Occurrence in hospital where potable water system is known to be contaminated with *Legionella*
- History of smoking and alcohol use
- Pleuritic chest pain
- Fever malaise, myalgia, headache

From Harrison TG and Taylor AG, "Timing of Seroconversion in Legionnaires' Disease," *Lancet*, Oct 1988, 795, with permission.

Footnotes

1. Winn WC Jr, "*Legionella* and the Clinical Microbiologist," *Infect Dis Clin North Am*, 1993, 7(2):377-92.
2. Roig J, Domingo C, and Morera J, "Legionnaires' Disease," *Chest*, 1994, 105(6):1817-25.
3. Koide M and Saito A, "Diagnosis of *Legionella pneumophila* Infection by Polymerase Chain Reaction," *Clin Infect Dis*, 1995, 21(1):199-201.

References

Plouffe JF, File TM, Breiman RF, et al, "Reevaluation of the Definition of Legionnaire's Disease; Use of the Urinary Antigen Assay. Community Based Pneumonia Incidence Study Group," *Clin Infect Dis*, 1995, 20(5):1286-91.

Winn WC, "*Legionella*," *Manual of Clinical Microbiology*, 6th ed, Murray PR, Baron EJ, Pfaller MA, et al, eds, Washington, DC: American Society for Microbiology, 1995, 533-44.

Yungbluth M, "The Laboratory Diagnosis of Pneumonia. The Role of the Community Hospital Pathologist," *Clin Lab Med*, 1995, 15(2):209-34.

Legionnaires' Disease Agent *see Legionella* Culture *on previous page*

Leptospira Culture

CPT 87081 (culture single organism); 87163 (additional identification methods)

Related Information

Bacterial Culture, Blood *on page 457*
Darkfield Examination, Leptospirosis *on page 475*
Leptospira Serodiagnosis *on page 414*

Applies to Blood Culture, *Leptospira*

Abstract Weil's disease (leptospirosis) is best worked up with culture and serology. Special culture media is needed.

Patient Preparation Thoroughly instruct the patient in the proper collection technique for a midvoid urine specimen; avoid contamination with skin flora. See also test listings Bacterial Culture, Urine, Clean Catch *on page 468* and Bacterial Culture, Blood *on page 457* for detailed instructions.

Specimen Urine, indicate midvoid, catheter or suprapubic puncture specimen; **blood** and **cerebrospinal fluid** may also be cultured

Container Sterile, urine container; for blood, lavender top (EDTA) Vacutainer® or green top (heparin) Vacutainer®

Collection Specimen should be transported to the laboratory within 1 hour of collection. For midvoid urine culture, patient should be instructed to clean skin thoroughly, do not collect first portion of stream, collect midportion of stream, and do not collect final portion of stream. Catheter or suprapubic puncture specimen may also be used.

Storage Instructions Specimens should not be refrigerated. They should be left at room temperature. Urine with an acid pH should be alkalinized if it cannot be set up immediately.

Turnaround Time 4-8 weeks

Special Instructions The laboratory should be informed of the specific request for *Leptospira* culture, collection time, current antibiotic therapy, and date of onset of illness. Urine must be alkaline; *Leptospira* do not survive in acid urine. Repeated cultures may be required.

Reference Range No *Leptospira* isolated

Use Investigate possible leptospirosis (Weil's disease)

Limitations Other organisms are not isolated or identified.

Contraindications Leptospiremia occurs during the septicemic acute phase of infection. This phase last 4-7 days after which organisms are not recoverable from blood.

Methodology Urine or blood is inoculated onto specially prepared media containing rabbit serum or albumin and fatty acids. Incubation is for 4-6 weeks in the dark at 28°C to 29°C. Cultures are examined with darkfield or phase microscopy for motile leptospires at weekly intervals; growth occurs 1-3 cm below the surface.

Additional Information Leptospirosis in humans is usually associated with occupational exposure. Veterinarians, dairymen, swineherds, abattoir workers, miners, fish and poultry processors, and those who work in a rat-infested environment are at increased risk. During the first week of disease, the most reliable means of detecting leptospires is by direct culture of blood or spinal fluid on appropriate media.[1,2] Urine does not become positive for *Leptospira* until the second week of disease and then can remain positive for several months. Concentration of *Leptospira* in human urine is low and shedding may be intermittent. Therefore, repeated isolation attempts should be made. Serology (acute and early convalescent) is recommended. Darkfield examination is no longer recommended.

Footnotes

1. Sperber SJ and Schleupner CJ, "Leptospirosis: A Forgotten Cause of Aseptic Meningitis and Multisystem Febrile Illness," *South Med J*, 1989, 82(10):1285-8.
2. Kaufmann AF and Weyant RS, "Leptospiraceae," *Manual of Clinical Microbiology*, 6th ed, Murray PR, Baron EJ, Pfaller MA, et al, eds, Washington, DC: American Society for Microbiology, 1995, 621-5.

References

Farr RW, "Leptospirosis," *Clin Infect Dis*, 1995, 21(1):1-8.

Raoult D, Bres P, and Baranton G, "Serologic Diagnosis of Leptospirosis: Comparison of Line Blot and Immunofluorescence Techniques With the Genus-Specific Microscopic Agglutination Test," *J Infect Dis*, 1989, 160:734-5.

Leptospirosis, Darkfield Examination *see* Darkfield Examination, Leptospirosis *on page 475*

Lice Identification *see* Arthropod Identification *on page 453*

Maximum Bactericidal Dilution see Serum Bactericidal Test on page 496

MBC see Antimicrobial Susceptibility Testing, Minimum Bactericidal Concentration on page 451

MBD see Serum Bactericidal Test on page 496

MIC see Antimicrobial Susceptibility Testing, Aerobic and Facultatively Anaerobic Bacteria on page 448

MIC, Anaerobic Bacteria see Antimicrobial Susceptibility Testing, Anaerobic Bacteria on page 449

MIC, Fastidious Organisms, Unusual Isolates see Antimicrobial Susceptibility Testing, Unusual Isolates/Fastidious Organisms on page 452

Microsporidia Diagnostic Procedures

Related Information
Bacterial Culture, Stool on page 466
Cryptosporidium Diagnostic Procedures on page 474
Electron Microscopy on page 37
Ova and Parasites, Stool on page 494
Ova and Parasites, Urine on page 495

Synonyms Stool Examination for Microsporidia

Test Commonly Includes Examination of stool, body fluids, or biopsy for microsporidia using special stains or electron microscopy

Abstract Microsporidiosis refers to diseases produced by microsporidia, a group of primitive, obligate intracellular protozoan parasites belonging to the phylum Microspora. Five different genera (Enterocytozoon, Encephalitozoon, Nosema, Septata, Pleistophora) have been implicated in human infections. They are best known as causes of diarrhea in patients with AIDS and also cause acute bilateral keratoconjunctivitis, sinonasal disease, bronchiolitis, pneumonia, infection of biliary and pancreatic ducts, acalculus, cholecystitis, and other disease states.[1]

Specimen Feces, urine, sputum, corneal or conjunctival scrapings, muscle or other tissue, gastrointestinal biopsy, bronchial biopsy

Collection Biopsies should be fixed in formalin as soon as possible.

Special Instructions If microsporidiosis is suspected, consult with the laboratory. These organisms may not be detected with usual stains.

Use A part of the differential diagnostic work-up of diarrhea and other microsporidia-associated diseases in immunocompromised patients, particularly AIDS patients; establish the diagnosis of microsporidiosis. Microsporidia have been demonstrated in immunocompetent persons.

Limitations Detection of microsporidia is entirely dependent on the adequacy of the specimen, staining and preparation of the specimen, and experience of the person who examines the specimen. They are small and easily missed in biopsies and cytology specimens as well as in stool specimens by light microscopy. Positive controls are needed, and microsporidiosis can appear from ingested food. Conventional H & E and Papanicolaou stains do not lend themselves to recognition of these organisms.

Methodology Microsporidia do not stain well with either hematoxylin, eosin, or the Papanicolaou stains. There are several good stains for microsporidia; however, not all of these stains stain the five major species of microsporidia. Microsporidia in paraffin-embedded tissues stain with a tissue Gram's stain (Brown and Hopps stain, Brown and Brenn stain, Steiner stains, chromotrope methods). Microsporidia in plastic-embedded tissues stain well with toluidine blue and with methylene blue-azure II-basic fuchsin. Electron microscopy remains the standard for tissue diagnosis. Microsporidia in cytologic centrifugation, smears, and scrapings preparations usually stain well with Gram's stain for specimens with little or no bacterial contamination. In these preparations, most microsporidia and bacteria are dark purple; some microsporidia are gram-negative or gram-variable. Weber's modified trichrome (chromotrope-based) stain works well with specimens with bacterial contamination; microsporidia are magenta-pink and the background (including bacteria) is blue-green. When large numbers of bacteria are present, the Weber chromotrope stain is also useful.[1] Some laboratories use Giemsa stain to stain stool smears and body fluids. Calcofluor white is useful for screening stools for microsporidia spores.[2] Gram's stain is useful for demonstration of spores in sputum.[3] Most stains cause microsporidia to appear as extremely fat bacteria which have a uniform oval shape, do not show budding, contain polar densities, and have a central clear band or area. Positive controls are needed for each of the methods.[3] The identification of microsporidia to species is very important in the selection of treatment. Speciation is accomplished most commonly by electron microscopy and, where available, molecular biology techniques. Cross reactions between the antibodies to the different types of microsporidia prevent serology from being clinically useful. Immunofluorescence staining techniques which include labeled antibody to specific microsporidia appear to work well in detecting microsporidia in clinical

specimens and to be able to differentiate infections due to certain microsporidia. Some microsporidia have been cultured in vitro, but routine culture for microsporidia is not yet practical. PCR has been successfully utilized.[1]

Additional Information Before the AIDS epidemic, microsporidiosis was an unusual cause of infections in immunocompromised patients. Since that time it has now been recognized as one of the major causes of AIDS enteropathy, especially in homosexual patients.[4] The diarrhea in these patients is of gradual onset and persists for at least 1 month. The stools are usually watery and blood and mucus are not present. Undigested food may be seen in feces. The diarrhea may lead to dehydration, hypokalemia, and hypomagnesemia.[5]

Footnotes
1. Schwartz DA, Sobottka I, Leitch GJ, et al, "Pathology of Microsporidiosis: Emerging Parasitic Infections in Patients With Acquired Immunodeficiency Syndrome," Arch Pathol Lab Med, 1996, 120(2):173-88.
2. Luna VA, Stewart BK, Bergeron DL, et al, "Use of the Fluorochrome Calcofluor White in the Screening of Stool Specimens for Spores of Microsporidia," Am J Clin Pathol, 1995, 103(5):656-9.
3. Long EG and Christie JD, "The Diagnosis of Old and New Gastrointestinal Parasites," Clin Lab Med, 1995, 15(2):307-31.
4. Molina JM, Sarfati C, Beauvais B, et al, "Intestinal Microsporidiosis in Human Immunodeficiency Virus-Infected Patients With Chronic Unexplained Diarrhea: Prevalence and Clinical and Biologic Features," J Infect Dis, 1993, 167(1):217-21.
5. Asmuth DM, De Girolami PC, Federman M, et al, "Clinical Features of Microsporidiosis in Patients With AIDS," Clin Infect Dis, 1994, 18(5):819-25.

References
Bryan RT and Weber R, "Microsporidia, Emerging Pathogens in Immunodeficient Persons," Arch Pathol Lab Med, 1993, 117(12):1243-5.
Garcia LS, Shimizu RY, and Bruckner DA, "Detection of Microsporidial Spores in Fecal Specimens From Patients Diagnosed With Cryptosporidiosis," J Clin Microbiol, 1994, 32(7):1739-41.
Joste NE, Rich JD, Busam KJ, et al, "Autopsy Verification of Encephalitozoon intestinalis (Microsporidiosis) Eradication Following Albendazole Therapy," Arch Pathol Lab Med, 1996, 120:199-203.
Pol S, Romana CA, Richard S, et al, "Microsporidia Infection in Patients With the Human Immunodeficiency Virus and Unexplained Cholangitis," N Engl J Med, 1993, 328(2):95-9.
Ryan NJ, Sutherland G, Coughlan K, et al, "A New Trichrome-Blue Stain for Detection of Microsporidial Species in Urine, Stool, and Nasopharyngeal Specimens," J Clin Microbiol, 1993, 31(12):3264-9.
Shadduck JA and Orenstein JM, "Comparative Pathology of Microsporidiosis," Arch Pathol Lab Med, 1993, 117(12):1215-9.
Sun T, "Microsporidiosis in the Acquired Immunodeficiency Syndrome," Infect Dis Newslet, 1993, 12:20-2.
Weber R and Bryan RT, "Microsporidial Infections in Immunodeficient and Immunocompetent Patients," Clin Infect Dis, 1994, 19(3):517-21.
Weber R, Bryan RT, Owen RL, et al, "Improved Light-Microscopical Detection of Microsporidia Spores in Stool and Duodenal Aspirates. The Enteric Opportunistic Infections Working Group," N Engl J Med, 1992, 326(3):161-6.
Wittner M, Tanowitz HB, and Weiss LM, "Parasitic Infections in AIDS Patients," Infect Dis Clin North Am, 1993, 7(3):569-86.

Middle Ear Culture see Bacterial Culture, Ear on page 462

Midstream Urine Culture see Bacterial Culture, Urine, Clean Catch on page 468

Minimal Bactericidal Concentration (MBC) see Antimicrobial Susceptibility Testing, Antimicrobial Combinations on page 449

Minimal Inhibitory Concentration (MIC) see Antimicrobial Susceptibility Testing, Antimicrobial Combinations on page 449

Minimum Bactericidal Concentration see Antimicrobial Susceptibility Testing, Minimum Bactericidal Concentration on page 451

Minimum Inhibitory Concentration Susceptibility Test see Antimicrobial Susceptibility Testing, Aerobic and Facultatively Anaerobic Bacteria on page 448

Minimum Inhibitory Concentration, Unusual Isolates see Antimicrobial Susceptibility Testing, Unusual Isolates/Fastidious Organisms on page 452

Minimum Lethal Concentration see Antimicrobial Susceptibility Testing, Minimum Bactericidal Concentration on page 451

Mite Identification see Arthropod Identification on page 453

MLC see Antimicrobial Susceptibility Testing, Minimum Bactericidal Concentration on page 451

Mycobacteria Culture, Bronchial Aspirate see Mycobacterial Culture, Sputum on page 490

Mycobacteria Culture, Gastric Aspirate see Mycobacterial Culture, Sputum on page 490

Mycobacteria, DNA Probe see Mycobacterial Culture, Sputum on page 490

Mycobacterial Culture, Biopsy or Body Fluid

CPT 87116 (isolation); 87118 (definitive identification)

Related Information
Acid-Fast Stain on page 446
(Continued)

Mycobacterial Culture, Biopsy or Body Fluid
(Continued)

Antimicrobial Susceptibility Testing, Mycobacteria *on page 452*
Bacterial Culture, Biopsy or Body Fluid *on page 456*
Body Fluid *on page 89*
Body Fluid Analysis, Cell Count *on page 306*
Body Fluid Cytology *on page 286*
Body Fluid pH *on page 92*
Bone Marrow *on page 307*
Fine Needle Aspiration, Deep Seated Lesions *on page 294*
Fine Needle Aspiration, Superficial Palpable Masses *on page 294*
Histopathology *on page 42*
Mycobacteria by DNA Probe *on page 520*
Mycobacterial Culture, Cutaneous and Subcutaneous Tissue *on next page*
Mycobacterial Culture, Sputum *on page 490*
Synovial Fluid Analysis *on page 656*

Synonyms AFB Culture, Biopsy; AFB Culture, Body Fluid; TB Culture, Biopsy; TB Culture, Body Fluid

Applies to Body Fluid Mycobacteria Culture; Bone Marrow Mycobacteria Culture; Tissue Mycobacteria Culture

Specimen Surgical tissue, bone marrow, biopsy material, endometrial curettings, aspirated fluid; **swab specimens are never adequate.**

Container Sterile container

Collection The portion of the surgical specimen submitted for culture should be separated from the portion submitted for histopathology by the surgeon, pathologist, or microbiologist utilizing sterile technique.

Turnaround Time Negative cultures are reported after 8 weeks.

Reference Range No growth

Use Isolate and identify mycobacteria; establish the etiology of granulomatous disease, fever of unknown origin (FUO) particularly in immunocompromised patients

Limitations Transbronchial biopsy cultures may be of assistance in diagnosing tuberculosis in sputum smear negative cases; however, sputum and bronchial washing cultures have a higher yield.[1,2] In one study, only 2 out of 12 (16%) transbronchial biopsies were positive and in those cases the biopsy was not the only source of culture positive material.[1]

Mycobacterium marinum may cause a localized cutaneous lesion that may be nodular, verrucous, ulcerative, or sporotrichoid, and which may rarely involve deeper structures. If it is suspected, the laboratory must be notified so that the culture may be incubated at an appropriate temperature (30°C).[3] *Mycobacterium marinum* infection occurs in patients who have been exposed to the organism following cutaneous abrasion or penetrating injury while cleaning aquariums, clearing barnacles, use of heated swimming pools, and with other aquatic exposures. *M. marinum* infections have followed alligator or crocodile bites. *M. haemophilum*, which has been recovered in a variety of biopsy specimens from immunosuppressed patients, also requires special media and conditions to grow; inform the laboratory if this organism is suspected.

Methodology Culture on specialized selective media, usually including Löwenstein-Jensen (LJ) and Middlebrook 7H11, incubated at 35°C with 5% to 10% CO_2. Cutaneous and subcutaneous tissues are incubated at room temperature to enhance recovery of *M. marinum* and *M. ulcerans*. If *M. haemophilum* is suspected, blood containing medium is inoculated and incubated at room temperature in 10% CO_2.[4] Mycobacteria are usually definitively identified and may be tested for antimicrobial susceptibility. Radiometric (Bactec®) and DNA probe methods are utilized by some laboratories to provide rapid detection and identification of mycobacteria.

With the emergence of multidrug-resistant *Mycobacterium tuberculosis* strains, most isolates are submitted for antimicrobial susceptibility testing. A specific request may be required by some laboratories (see Antimicrobial Susceptibility Testing, Mycobacteria *on page 452*). Susceptibility testing of mycobacteria is frequently referred to specialized laboratories.

Additional Information Occult infections with **atypical mycobacteria**, particularly *Mycobacterium avium* and *Mycobacterium intracellulare*, occur in patients with acquired immune deficiency syndrome (AIDS).[5] In some institutions, the incidence of isolation of non-*Mycobacterium tuberculosis* species, specifically *M. avium-intracellulare* (*M. avium* complex), may exceed the rate of isolation of *M. tuberculosis*. Mycobacteria have been recovered from several types of tissue, in which the characteristic granulomatous reaction has been absent.[6,7] Optimal isolation of mycobacteria from tissue is accomplished by processing as much tissue as possible for culture.

Rapidly growing mycobacteria have been implicated in cases of sternal wound infection, early prosthetic valve endocarditis, infections complicating mammary augmentation surgery, and other cutaneous/ subcutaneous infections.[8,9] *M. fortuitum* is most commonly implicated in these infections. Rapidly growing mycobacteria grow on routine bacterial culture media within incubation periods used in routine bacterial cultures. Such organisms can be misidentified as "diphtheroids" and disregarded as contaminants.

Tuberculous spondylitis represents 50% to 60% of all cases of skeletal tuberculosis. It is seen in children in developing countries and adults older than 50 years of age in the United States and Europe. Frequently, several vertebrae are involved and adjacent psoas muscle abscesses or paravertebral abscesses are not uncommon ("cold abscesses"). Colony counts obtained from bone biopsies are low; however, >90% are culture positive. The diagnosis of vertebral tuberculosis should be considered in all cases of unexplained spondylitis.

Pleural effusions frequently yield positive cultures in cases of pulmonary tuberculosis. The diagnosis of peritoneal tuberculosis is difficult and is usually made at laparotomy or after a considerable delay. Tuberculosis should be considered in any patient with **ascitic fluid** and chronic abdominal pain.[10] Peritoneal tuberculosis accounted for 11% of a series of cases of extrapulmonary tuberculosis reported by Alvarez and McCabe.[11] Pericardial tuberculosis accounts for <5% of extrapulmonary tuberculosis and frequently requires biopsy for diagnosis. See table.

Predisposing Clinical Conditions and Site of Involvement of Non-*M. tuberculosis* Mycobacterial Infections

Site	Predisposing Clinical Conditions	Species
Disseminated	Immunodeficiency/ malignancy	*M. avium-intracellulare* *M. kansasii*
Gastrointestinal tract/ disseminated	Acquired immunodeficiency syndrome	*M. avium-intracellulare*
Lung	Chronic pulmonary disease	*M. avium-intracellulare* *M. kansasii*
Lymph nodes	Pediatric age group	*M. avium-intracellulare* *M. scrofulaceum*
Peritonitis	Chronic ambulatory peritoneal dialysis	*M. fortuitum* *M. chelonae*
Skeleton	Immunodeficiency/ malignancy	*M. avium-intracellulare* *M. kansasii*
Skin and soft tissue	Percutaneous trauma/ abrasion	*M. fortuitum* *M. chelonae*
	Immunodeficiency/ malignancy	*M. haemophilum*

Mycobacterium avium-intracellulare complex (MAC) bacteremia develops in approximately 43% of AIDS patients who survive 2 years following diagnosis. A single blood culture is recommended; if it is negative in 7 days, another is indicated in subjects perceived as having disseminated MAC.[12]

Footnotes

1. Stenson W, Aranda C, and Bevelagua FA, "Transbronchial Biopsy Culture in Pulmonary Tuberculosis," *Chest*, 1983, 83:883-4.
2. Saceanu C, Pfeiffer N, and McLean T, "Evaluation of Sputum Smears Concentrated by Cytocentrifugation for Detection of Acid-Fast Bacilli," *J Clin Microbiol*, 1993, 31(9):2371-4.
3. Brown JW 3d and Sanders CV, "*Mycobacterium marinum* Infections: A Problem of Recognition, Not Therapy?" *Arch Intern Med*, 1987, 147(5):817-8.
4. Straus WL, Ostroff SM, Jerrigan DB, et al, "Clinical and Epidemiologic Characteristics of *Mycobacterium haemophilus*, an Emerging Pathogen in Immunocompromised Patients," *Ann Intern Med*, 1994, 120(2):118-25.
5. Ellner JJ, Goldberger MJ, and Parenti DM, "*Mycobacterium avium* Infection and AIDS: A Therapeutic Dilemma in Rapid Evaluation," *J Infect Dis*, 1991, 163(6):1326-35.
6. Horsburgh CR Jr, Metchock BG, McGowan JE Jr, et al, "Clinical Implications of Recovery of *Mycobacterium avium* Complex From the Stool or Respiratory Tract of HIV-Infected Individuals," *AIDS*, 1992, 6(5):512-4.
7. Inderlied CB, Kemper C, and Bermudez LE, "The *Mycobacterium avium* Complex," *Clin Microbiol Rev*, 1993, 6(3):266-310.
8. Wallace RJ, Musser JM, Hull SI, et al, "Diversity and Sources of Rapidly Growing Mycobacteria Associated With Infections Following Cardiac Surgery," *J Infect Dis*, 1989, 159(4):708-16.
9. Wallace RJ, Steele LC, Labidi A, et al, "Heterogeneity Among Isolates of Rapidly Growing Mycobacteria Responsible for Infections Following Augmentation Mammoplasty Despite Case Clustering in Texas and Other Southern Coastal States," *J Infect Dis*, 1989, 160(2):281-8.
10. Martin RE and Bradsher RW, "Elusive Diagnosis of Tuberculosis Peritonitis," *South Med J*, 1986, 79(9):1076-9.
11. Alvarez S and McCabe WR, "Extrapulmonary Tuberculosis Revisited: A Review of Experience at Boston City and Other Hospitals," *Medicine (Baltimore)*, 1984, 63(1):25-55.
12. Christie JD and Callihan DR, "The Laboratory Diagnosis of Mycobacterial Diseases. Challenges and Common Sense," *Clin Lab Med*, 1995, 15(2):279-306.

References
Holland SM, Eisenstein EM, Kuhns DB, et al, "Treatment of Refractory Disseminated Nontuberculous Mycobacterial Infection With Interferon Gamma. A Preliminary Report," *N Engl J Med*, 1994, 330(19):1348-55.
Wayne LG and Sramek HA, "Agents of Newly Recognized or Infrequently Encountered Mycobacterial Diseases," *Clin Microbiol Rev*, 1992, 5(1):1-25.
Wolinsky E, "Mycobacterial Diseases Other Than Tuberculosis," *Clin Infect Dis*, 1992, 15(1):1-10.

Mycobacterial Culture, Cerebrospinal Fluid

CPT 87116 (isolation only); 87118 (definitive identification)

Related Information

Acid-Fast Stain *on page 446*
Bacterial Antigens, Rapid Detection Methods *on page 454*
Bacterial Culture, Cerebrospinal Fluid *on page 460*
Cerebrospinal Fluid Analysis *on page 309*
Cerebrospinal Fluid Cytology *on page 290*
Cerebrospinal Fluid Glucose *on page 105*
Cerebrospinal Fluid Protein *on page 380*
Cryptococcal Antigen Titer *on page 388*
Fungal Culture, Cerebrospinal Fluid *on page 477*
Mycobacteria by DNA Probe *on page 520*
Viral Culture, Central Nervous System Symptoms *on page 677*

Synonyms Cerebrospinal Fluid Mycobacteria Culture; CSF Mycobacteria Culture; Spinal Fluid Mycobacteria Culture

Test Commonly Includes Culture for mycobacteria and acid-fast stain if requested

Patient Preparation Usual sterile preparation

Specimen Cerebrospinal fluid; 10 mL is optimum, 5 mL the minimum volume to achieve acceptable sensitivity

Reference Range No growth

Use Investigate cases of meningitis with subacute/subchronic or chronic onset, cases in which a history of contact with tuberculosis, or cases in which abnormal CSF findings suggest mycobacterial meningitis.

Limitations Recovery of mycobacteria is directly related to the volume of specimen available for culture; 5-10 mL is recommended for optimal yield. Recovery of organisms can require 4-6 weeks.[1] Usually CSF glucose ≤60 mg/dL (3.3 mmol/L) and CSF WBC is increased; if not, culture is unlikely to be useful.[2]

Methodology Culture on selective media usually including Löwenstein-Jensen (LJ) and Middlebrook 7H11. Broth media is also used with or without radiometric monitoring.

Additional Information Early in the course, neutrophils may predominate in the CSF. Lymphocytes, mononuclear cells, and granulocytes are found later. Rarely does the cell count exceed 1000 cells/mm³. The CSF is clear and colorless early; later, a pellicle forms on standing.[1] Low CSF glucose, <40 mg/dL, is frequently observed. Increased protein, almost always, is often >300 mg/dL. Measured CSF parameters may differ markedly from those anticipated for a given clinical entity for patients incapable of mounting a "normal" inflammatory response (eg, neonates, HIV-infected individuals). Other factors raising the index of suspicion include subacute or chronic onset, positive tuberculin skin test, previous active tuberculosis, significant recent exposure to tuberculosis, and suspicion of tuberculosis on imaging procedures. Acid-fast organisms can be identified on centrifuged sediments in 60% to 80% of cases.[1]

Untreated tuberculous meningitis is fatal, usually within 3 weeks of presentation. African-Americans, Hispanics, and the elderly are most frequently affected. Alcohol abuse, drug abuse, steroid therapy, head trauma, pregnancy, and AIDS all may increase risk. Despite therapy, mortality is high, approximately 30%.[3] Evaluation of contacts is recommended. Atypical mycobacteria species can also cause meningitis, primarily in immunosuppressed and elderly patients.[4]

Footnotes
1. Fishman RA, *Cerebrospinal Fluid in Diseases of the Nervous System*, 2nd ed, Philadelphia, PA: WB Saunders Co, 1992, 271-2.
2. Christie JD and Callihan DR, "The Laboratory Diagnosis of Mycobacterial Diseases. Challenges and Common Sense," *Clin Lab Med*, 1995, 15(2):279-306.
3. Ogawa SK, Smith MA, Brennessel DJ, et al, "Tuberculous Meningitis in an Urban Medical Center," *Medicine (Baltimore)*, 1987, 66:317-26.
4. Wayne LG and Sramek HA, "Agents of Newly Recognized or Infrequently Encountered Mycobacterial Diseases," *Clin Microbiol Rev*, 1992, 5(1):1-25.

References
Behrman RE, Kliegman RM, Nelson WE, et al, "Acute Aseptic Meningitis," *Nelson Textbook of Pediatrics*, 14th ed, Philadelphia, PA: WB Saunders Co, 1992, 664-6.
Bell WE, "Bacterial Meningitis in Children - Selected Aspects," *Pediatr Clin North Am*, 1992, 39(4):651-68.
Berenguer J, Moreno S, Laguna F, et al, "Tuberculous Meningitis in Patients Infected With the Human Immunodeficiency Virus," *N Engl J Med*, 1992, 326(10):668-72.
Wolinsky E, "Mycobacterial Diseases Other Than Tuberculosis," *Clin Infect Dis*, 1992, 15(1):1-10.

Mycobacterial Culture, Cutaneous and Subcutaneous Tissue

CPT 87116 (isolation); 87118 (definitive identification)

Related Information

Acid-Fast Stain *on page 446*
Antimicrobial Susceptibility Testing, Mycobacteria *on page 452*
Fungal Culture, Skin *on page 478*
Mycobacteria by DNA Probe *on page 520*
Mycobacterial Culture, Biopsy or Body Fluid *on page 487*
Mycobacterial Culture, Sputum *on next page*
Mycobacterial Culture, Stool *on page 491*
Mycobacterial Culture, Urine *on page 491*
Skin Biopsy *on page 54*

Synonyms Skin Mycobacteria Culture; TB Culture, Skin

Test Commonly Includes Culture and identification of acid-fast bacteria. This may include a direct acid-fast smear of specimen.

Abstract Cutaneous or subcutaneous manifestations of mycobacterial infection may result from either direct inoculation or hematogenous dissemination of infecting organisms. A variety of *Mycobacterium* spp may cause infections of this type; they are most likely to occur in patients at risk due to immunosuppression (eg, *M. tuberculosis*, *M. haemophilum*, *M. kansasii*), poverty and geographic exposure (eg, *M. leprae*), prior surgical treatment (eg, *M. fortuitum*), or hobbies or occupational exposure (eg, *M. marinum*).

Container Sterile tube containing 0.5 mL sterile saline

Turnaround Time Negative cultures are usually reported after 6-8 weeks.

Reference Range No growth

Use Isolate and identify mycobacteria

Limitations For optimal yield, scrapings, curettings, or biopsy tissue rather than swabs of lesions should be submitted to the laboratory. The yield on cultures is proportional to the volume of specimen submitted. *M. leprae* does not grow in culture.

Methodology Acid-fast stain of smear prepared from clinical specimen, culture of specimen on appropriate media (eg, Lowenstein-Jensen, Middlebrook 7H11 solid media, or 7H12 liquid media). Incubation at both 35°C and 25°C to 30°C. Hemin-containing media such as chocolate agar incubated at 25°C to 30°C is required to recover *M. haemophilum*.[1] Identification is based on growth rate, colony morphology (rough vs smooth), development of pigment, color of pigment, and whether or not the pigment is induced by light. Other biochemical and nucleic acid tests can be used to confirm the identification.

Additional Information Diagnosis of *Mycobacterium marinum* infection is frequently delayed. A careful clinical history addressing occupational or recreational activities usually yields important clues to the diagnosis, eg, swimming pool or seawall abrasions, barnacle scrapes, fish fin punctures, and exposure to tropical fish tanks (salt water).[2]

Mycobacterium marinum causes granulomatous cutaneous lesions. Lesions are similar to those seen with sporotrichosis and follow lymphatics; see listing Mycobacterial Culture, Biopsy or Body Fluid *on page 487*. Members of the *Mycobacterium fortuitum* complex can cause surgical wound infections and cutaneous abscesses and osteomyelitis in trauma victims and debilitated hosts. The organisms are not fastidious and may grow well on usual blood or chocolate agar. The key clinical feature is that symptoms of infection, localized cellulitis, or abscess formation appear 4-6 weeks after traumatic injury. *Mycobacterium ulcerans* causes a chronic granulomatous skin lesion called Buruli ulcer. *M. ulcerans* may also be saprophytic, colonizing cutaneous ulcers associated with circulatory insufficiency and diabetes. *M. ulcerans* is uncommon in North America. It is most frequently isolated in Australia and Africa. Isolates of *Mycobacterium avium-intracellulare* (MAI) have been reported from skin and Kaposi's sarcoma lesions of patients with the acquired immunodeficiency syndrome (AIDS).[3,4] Cutaneous tuberculosis has been found in patients with neoplastic disease.[5,6] *M. haemophilum* produces disseminated cutaneous disease and infections of the bones, joints, and lymphatics in immunocompromised individuals.[7]

The atypical or environmental mycobacteria are frequently resistant to oral antituberculosis therapy. There is wide variation in susceptibility within species. Susceptibility testing should be considered.

Footnotes
1. Nolte FS and Metchcock B, "*Mycobacterium*," *Manual of Clinical Microbiology*, 6th ed, Murray PR, Baron EJ, Pfaller MA, et al, eds, Washington, DC: American Society for Microbiology, 1995, 400-37.
2. Brown JW 3d and Sanders CV, "*Mycobacterium marinum* Infections: A Problem of Recognition, Not Therapy?" *Arch Intern Med*, 1987, 147(5):817-8.
3. Croxson TS, Ebanks D, and Mildvan D, "Atypical Mycobacteria and Kaposi's Sarcoma in the Same Biopsy Specimens," *N Engl J Med*, 1983, 308:1476.
4. Hawkins CC, Gold JW, Whimbey E, et al, "*Mycobacterium avium* Complex Infections in Patients With the Acquired Immunodeficiency Syndrome," *Ann Intern Med*, 1986, 105(2):184-8.
5. Asnis DS and Bresciani AR, "Cutaneous Tuberculosis: A Rare Presentation of Malignancy," *Clin Infect Dis*, 1992, 15(1):158-60.
6. Beyt BE, Ortbals DW, Santa Cruz DJ, et al, "Cutaneous Mycobacteriosis: Analysis of 34 Cases With a New Classification of the Disease," *Med*, 1980, 60:95-109.
7. Straus WL, Ostroff SM, Jernigan DB, et al, "Clinical and Epidemiologic Characteristics of *Mycobacterium haemophilum*, an Emerging Pathogen in Immunocompromised Patients," *Ann Intern Med*, 1994, 120(2):118-25.

(Continued)

Mycobacterial Culture, Cutaneous and Subcutaneous Tissue (Continued)

References
Wayne LG and Sramek HA, "Agents of Newly Recognized or Infrequently Encountered Mycobacterial Diseases," *Clin Microbiol Rev*, 1992, 5(1):1-25.
Wolinsky E, "Mycobacterial Diseases Other Than Tuberculosis," *Clin Infect Dis*, 1992, 15(1):1-10.

Mycobacterial Culture, Sputum

CPT 87116 (isolation); 87117 (concentration plus isolation); 87118 (definitive identification)

Related Information

Acid-Fast Stain *on page 446*
Antimicrobial Susceptibility Testing, Mycobacteria *on page 452*
Bacterial Culture, Bronchoscopy Specimen *on page 459*
Bacterial Culture, Sputum *on page 465*
Bronchial Washings Cytology *on page 287*
Bronchoalveolar Lavage Cytology *on page 288*
Fungal Culture, Sputum *on page 479*
Mycobacteria by DNA Probe *on page 520*
Mycobacterial Culture, Biopsy or Body Fluid *on page 487*
Mycobacterial Culture, Cutaneous and Subcutaneous Tissue *on previous page*
Mycobacterial Culture, Stool *on next page*
Mycobacterial Culture, Urine *on next page*
Nocardia Culture *on page 493*
Sputum Cytology *on page 300*
Viral Culture, Respiratory Symptoms *on page 680*

Synonyms AFB Culture, Sputum; Sputum Mycobacteria Culture; TB Culture, Sputum

Applies to Mycobacteria Culture, Bronchial Aspirate; Mycobacteria Culture, Gastric Aspirate; Mycobacteria, DNA Probe

Test Commonly Includes Mycobacteria (AFB) stain, culture, and identification

Abstract Increased morbidity in the U.S. from tuberculosis is concentrated in minorities, individuals who have human immunodeficiency virus infection, and the foreign born.

Diagnosis of *M. tuberculosis* by DNA probe and polymerase chain reaction permits rapid diagnosis.[1,2]

DNA fingerprinting enhances delineation of transmission.[1,2,3,4,5] A significant fraction of cases of active tuberculosis in San Francisco and the City of New York derive from person-to-person transmission.[4,5]

Patient Preparation The patient should be instructed to remove dentures, rinse mouth with water, and then cough deeply expectorating sputum into the sputum collection cup.

Specimen First morning sputum or induced sputum, fasting gastric aspirate, bronchial aspirate, tracheal aspirate, transtracheal aspirate. In neonates, gastric and endotracheal aspirates may be used.[6]

Container Sputum cup, sputum trap, sterile tracheal aspirate or bronchoscopy tube

Sampling Time In children, gastric aspiration should be done early in the morning as the child awakens before the stomach empties, on three separate mornings.

Collection A recommended screening procedure is three first morning specimens submitted on successive days. The patient should be instructed to brush his/her teeth and/or rinse their mouth well with water before attempting to collect the specimen, to reduce the possibility of contamination of the specimen with food particles, oropharyngeal secretions, etc. After the specimen has been collected, it should be examined to make sure it contains a sufficient quantity (at least 5 mL) of thick mucus (**not saliva**). If a two-part collection system has been used, only the screw-cap tube should be submitted to the laboratory. (The outer container is considered contaminated and its transport through the hospital constitutes a health hazard!) The specimen should be properly labeled and accompanied by properly completed requisition. The specimen can be divided in the laboratory for fungal, mycobacterial, and routine cultures.

Storage Instructions The specimen should be refrigerated if it cannot be promptly processed. If a gastric aspirate cannot be processed immediately, its pH should be neutralized for storage.

Turnaround Time Negative cultures are reported after 6-8 weeks; *vide infra*.

Special Instructions Early morning specimen is preferred. Since at least 5 mL of sputum (**not saliva**) is required, the specimen may be collected over a 1- to 2-hour period in order to obtain sufficient quantity.

Reference Range No growth

Use Diagnose pulmonary tuberculosis or other *Mycobacterium* sp from expectorated sputum, induced sputum, nasotracheal aspiration, or, if necessary, gastric aspiration, bronchoscopy, or bronchoalveolar lavage.

Tuberculosis must be considered in patients who have chronic cough and fever, regardless of results of tuberculin testing, especially in the presence of HIV infection.[5] Sputum for AFB smear and culture should be available to healthcare workers.[7]

Limitations Bronchial washings are frequently diluted with topical anesthetics and irrigating fluids, but bronchoscopy still provides a high yield of positive specimens. Postbronchoscopy expectorated specimens may provide a better yield of organisms than those obtained during the procedure. Gastric aspirates yield organisms in <50% of cases of *M. tuberculosis* infection in children. Acid-fast stain of gastric aspirate has a sensitivity of 30% and provides a useful clinical diagnosis if positive.[8] Bronchoscopy can be an important adjunct to serial sputum collection in the definitive diagnosis of pulmonary infection due to mycobacteria. The relative yield of mycobacteria from clinical specimens is prebronchoscopy sputum > bronchial washings > postbronchoscopy sputum > bronchial biopsy.

Severe limitations are recognized with traditional diagnostic approaches for mycobacteria. Poor sensitivity of smears and prolonged intervals for culture have complicated emerging problems of immunocompromised individuals and of multidrug-resistant organisms;[9] *vide infra*.

Methodology Concentration and decontamination by exposure to acid or alkaline agents, mycolytic agents, and centrifugation. Culture on selective media usually including Löwenstein-Jensen (LJ) and Middlebrook 7H11 with and without antibiotics. DNA probe technology using chemiluminescent-labeled DNA probes complementary to the ribosomal RNA of the *M. tuberculosis* complex which includes *M. tuberculosis*, *M. bovis*, BCG, *M. africanum*, and *M. microti* are available for culture confirmation. Probes are also available for *M. avium-intracellulare* complex, *M. gordonae*, and *M. kansasii*. The probes can provide more rapid confirmation of the species of mycobacteria isolated. Mycobacteria in clinical specimens can be detected by the radiometric Bactec® system which detects production of $^{14}CO_2$ from ^{14}C-labeled palmitic acid supplemented Middlebrook 7H12 medium.[10] Detection times are more rapid than with conventional culture methods. Gas-liquid chromatography (GLC) can also be used to rapidly speciate mycobacterial colonies. The detection and identification of mycobacterial organisms directly in clinical specimens is improving with the development of a test that amplifies specific mycobacterial DNA.[11]

Additional Information Tuberculosis decreased in incidence in the United States in the 1970s and 1980s, but the incidence of tuberculosis in the United States has increased since 1986. High incidence populations exist in depressed inner city areas, some rural areas, amongst new immigrants, in prison inmates, and in HIV-positive patients. The emergence of *M. tuberculosis* and *M. avium-intracellulare* infections complicating the acquired immunodeficiency syndrome has been striking. When tuberculosis occurs as a first or case-defining opportunistic infection, 75% to 100% of HIV-positive patients have pulmonary disease. After the diagnosis of AIDS has been made, 25% to 70% of HIV-associated tuberculosis patients have an extrapulmonary site of infection.[12]

In an ambulatory inner city population, two specimens processed for acid-fast stain and culture identified all cases of active tuberculosis within the time required for culture. The most infective cases were identified immediately by the acid-fast stain. Tuberculin tests and chest x-rays were also performed but did not significantly increase the number of cases identified in this population.[13]

M. kansasii is uncommon as an environmental contaminant. Implication of *M. avium-intracellulare* as a pathogen usually requires at least one of the following criteria:

- clinical evidence of a disease process that can be explained by atypical mycobacterial infection
- repeated isolation of the same mycobacterial species from sputum over a period of weeks to months
- exclusion of other possible etiologies
- biopsy demonstrating acid-fast bacilli or diagnostic histopathologic changes[14]

Nosocomial transmission of multidrug-resistant *Mycobacterium tuberculosis* has been noted to occur from patient to patient and from patient to healthcare worker. Acid-fast bacilli isolation precautions and adherence to appropriate infection control procedures is recommended.[15,16]

While *M. tuberculosis* is contagious and is usually transmitted from person to person, most of the other disease-causing mycobacteria are not characterized by person-to-person spread, are found in the environment, and are considered opportunistic pathogens. They include *M. avium*, *M. intracellulare*, *M. asiaticum*, *M. flavescens*, *M. fortuitum* complex, *M. gordonae*, *M. haemophilum*, *M. kansasii*, *M. malmoense*, *M. marinum*, *M. scrofulaceum*, *M. simiae*, *M. smegmatis*, and *M. xenopi*.

See listing Mycobacteria by DNA Probe *on page 520*.

Footnotes
1. Barnes PF and Barrows SA, "Tuberculosis in the 1990s," *Ann Intern Med*, 1993, 119(5):400-10.

2. Woods GL, "Tuberculosis. Role of the Clinical Laboratory in Providing Rapid Diagnosis and Assessment of Disease Activity," *Am J Clin Pathol*, 1994, 101(6):679-80.

3. Small PM, Hopewell PC, Singh SP, et al, "The Epidemiology of Tuberculosis in San Francisco. A Population-Based Study Using Conventional and Molecular Methods," *N Engl J Med*, 1994, 330(24):1703-9.

4. Alland D, Kalkut GE, Moss AR, et al, "Transmission of Tuberculosis in New York City. An Analysis by DNA Fingerprinting and Conventional Epidemiologic Methods," *N Engl J Med*, 1994, 330(24):1710-6.

5. Hamburg MA and Frieden TR, "Tuberculosis Transmission in the 1990s," *N Engl J Med*, 1994, 330(24):1750-1.

6. Cantwell MF, Shehab ZM, Costello AM, et al, "Brief Report: Congenital Tuberculosis," *N Engl J Med*, 1994, 330(15):1051-4.

7. Menzies D, Fanning A, Yuan L, et al, "Tuberculosis Among Health Care Workers," *N Engl J Med*, 1995, 332(2):92-8.

8. Klotz SA and Penn RL, "Acid-Fast Staining of Urine and Gastric Contents Is An Excellent Indicator of Mycobacterial Disease," *Am Rev Respir Dis*, 1987, 136(5):1197-8.

9. Haas DW, "Current and Future Applications of Polymerase Chain Reaction for *Mycobacterium tuberculosis*," *Mayo Clin Proc*, 1996, 71(3):311-3.

10. Stager CE, Libonati JP, Siddiqi SH, et al, "Role of Solid Media When Using in Conjunction With the Bactec® System for Mycobacterial Isolation and Identification," *J Clin Microbiol*, 1991, 29(1):154-7.

11. Kolk AH, Schuitema AR, Kuijper S, et al, "Detection of *Mycobacterium tuberculosis* in Clinical Samples by Using Polymerase Chain Reaction and a Nonradioactive Detection System," *J Clin Microbiol*, 1992, 30(10):2567-75.

12. Chaisson RE and Slutkin G, "Tuberculosis and Human Immunodeficiency Virus Infection," *J Infect Dis*, 1989, 159(1):96-100.

13. Tenover FC, Crawford JT, Huebner RE, et al, "The Resurgence of Tuberculosis: Is Your Laboratory Ready?" *J Clin Microbiol*, 1993, 31(4):767-70.

14. Wayne LG and Sramek HA, "Agents of Newly Recognized or Infrequently Encountered Mycobacterial Diseases," *Clin Microbiol Rev*, 1992, 5(1):1-25.

15. Pearson ML, Jereb JA, Frieden TR, et al, "Nosocomial Transmission of Multidrug-Resistant *Mycobacterium tuberculosis*. A Risk to Patients and Healthcare Workers," *Ann Intern Med*, 1992, 117(3):191-6.

16. Iseman MD, "A Leap of Faith. What Can We Do to Curtail Intrainstitutional Transmission of Tuberculosis?" *Ann Intern Med*, 1992, 117(3):251-3.

References

Beck-Sague C, Dooley SW, Hutton MD, et al, "Hospital Outbreak of Multidrug-Resistant *Mycobacterium tuberculosis* Infections. Factors in Transmission to Staff and HIV-Infected Patients," *JAMA*, 1992, 268(10):1280-6.

"Case Records of the Massachusetts General Hospital. Weekly Clinicopathological Exercises. Case 6-1996. A 40-Year-Old Man With a Cough, Increasing Dyspnea, and Bilateral Nodular Lung Opacities," *N Engl J Med*, 1996, 334(8):521-6.

Frieden TR, Fujiwara PI, Washko RM, et al, "Tuberculosis in New York City - Turning the Tide," *N Engl J Med*, 1995, 333(4):229-33.

Mehta JB and Morris F, "Impact of HIV Infection on Mycobacterial Disease," *Am Fam Physician*, 1992, 45(5):2203-11.

Raviglione MC, Snider DE Jr, and Kochi A, "Global Epidemiology of Tuberculosis. Prevalence and Mortality of a Worldwide Epidemic," *JAMA*, 1995, 273(3):220-6.

Telzak EE, Sepkowitz K, Alpert P, et al, "Multidrug-Resistant Tuberculosis in Patients Without HIV Infection," *N Engl J Med*, 1995, 333(14):907-11.

Weis SE, Slocum PC, Blais FX, et al, "The Effect of Directly Observed Therapy on the Rates of Drug Resistance and Relapse in Tuberculosis," *N Engl J Med*, 1994, 330(17):1179-84.

Witebsky FG and Conville PS, "The Laboratory Diagnosis of Mycobacterial Diseases," *Infect Dis Clin North Am*, 1993, 7(2):359-76.

Wolinsky E, "Mycobacterial Diseases Other Than Tuberculosis," *Clin Infect Dis*, 1992, 15(1):1-10.

Mycobacterial Culture, Stool

CPT 87116 (isolation); 87118 (definitive identification)

Related Information

Acid-Fast Stain *on page 446*

Antimicrobial Susceptibility Testing, Mycobacteria *on page 452*

Bacterial Culture, Stool *on page 466*

Mycobacteria by DNA Probe *on page 520*

Mycobacterial Culture, Cutaneous and Subcutaneous Tissue *on page 489*

Mycobacterial Culture, Sputum *on previous page*

Mycobacterial Culture, Urine *on this page*

Synonyms AFB Culture, Stool; Stool Mycobacterial Culture; TB Culture, Stool

Storage Instructions If the specimen cannot be processed immediately by the laboratory, it should be refrigerated.

Turnaround Time Negative cultures are usually reported after 8 weeks.

Reference Range No growth

Use Isolate and identify mycobacteria

Limitations Isolation of *M. tuberculosis* from feces does not necessarily imply intestinal tuberculosis. Mycobacteria in feces are most likely from sputum swallowed by patient with pulmonary disease. The recovery of *M. gordonae*, "the tap water bacillus," from stool occurs occasionally. The recovery of mycobacteria from stool is technically limited by the rapid overgrowth of normal intestinal bacterial flora. **Stool is rarely the specimen of choice** for the primary diagnosis of mycobacterial infection.

Methodology Culture on selective media usually including Löwenstein-Jensen (LJ) and Middlebrook 7H11 media with antibiotics after decontamination of the specimen by a procedure similar to that used for sputum cultures. Many laboratories screen by smear before culturing. In such circumstances, if the smear is negative, culture is not performed.

Additional Information The increasing recognition of mycobacterial infections in patients with the acquired immunodeficiency syndrome (AIDS) has resulted in increased awareness of the potential to recover clinically significant mycobacteria from stool. Patients with AIDS are often found to be colonized with *M. avium-intracellulare*.[1] If a stool culture is positive for *Mycobacterium* spp, dissemination often follows.[2] Isolation of mycobacteria from stool indicates disseminated disease, and cultures from blood, bone marrow, and lymph nodes are usually also positive for the same mycobacterial isolate.[3]

Footnotes

1. Havlik JA Jr, Metchock B, Thompson SE, et al, "A Prospective Evaluation of *Mycobacterium avium* Complex Colonization of the Respiratory and Gastrointestinal Tracts of Persons With Human Immunodeficiency Virus Infection," *J Infect Dis*, 1993, 168(4):1045-8.

2. Horsburgh CR Jr, Metchock B, McGowan JE Jr, et al, "Clinical Implications G of Recovery of *Mycobacterium avium* Complex From the Stool or Respiratory Tract of HIV-Infected Individuals," *AIDS*, 1992, 6(5):512-4.

3. Wolinsky E, "Mycobacterial Diseases Other Than Tuberculosis," *Clin Infect Dis*, 1992, 15(1):1-10.

References

Claydon EJ, Coker RJ, and Harris JR, "*Mycobacterium malmoense* Infection in HIV Positive Patients," *J Infect*, 1991, 23(2):191-4.

Gradon JD, Timpone JG, and Schnittman SM, "Emergence of Unusual Opportunistic Pathogens in AIDS: A Review," *Clin Infect Dis*, 1992, 15(1):134-57.

Yajko DM, Nassos PS, Sanders CA, et al, "Comparison of Four Decontamination Methods for Recovery of *Mycobacterium avium* Complex From Stools," *J Clin Microbiol*, 1993, 31(2):302-6.

Mycobacterial Culture, Urine

CPT 87116 (isolation); 87117 (concentration plus isolation); 87118 (definitive identification)

Related Information

Acid-Fast Stain *on page 446*

Antimicrobial Susceptibility Testing, Mycobacteria *on page 452*

Bacterial Culture, Urine, Clean Catch *on page 468*

Bacterial Culture, Urine, Suprapubic Puncture *on page 469*

Fungal Culture, Urine *on page 480*

Mycobacteria by DNA Probe *on page 520*

Mycobacterial Culture, Cutaneous and Subcutaneous Tissue *on page 489*

Mycobacterial Culture, Sputum *on previous page*

Mycobacterial Culture, Stool *on this page*

Synonyms AFB Culture, Urine; TB Culture, Urine; Urine Mycobacteria Culture

Abstract Active extragenitourinary tuberculosis is found in fewer than 10% of subjects who have genitourinary tuberculosis.

Patient Preparation Usual preparation for clean catch midvoid urine specimen collection. See Bacterial Culture, Urine, Clean Catch *on page 468* for detailed information.

Specimen First morning voided urine

Collection Three first morning voided urine specimens should be submitted. The specimen may be divided for fungus culture and KOH preparation, mycobacteria culture and AFB stain, and routine bacterial culture and Gram's stain if the specimen is of adequate volume for all tests requested.

Turnaround Time Negatives are reported after 6-8 weeks.

Reference Range No growth

Use Isolate and identify mycobacteria from the urinary tract. Most patients with genitourinary tuberculosis have symptoms of urinary tract disease, but some are asymptomatic.

Limitations Positive acid-fast stained smears are not diagnostic, because of the presence of *Mycobacterium smegmatis* in genital secretions of normal patients.

Contraindications A 24-hour urine collection is less valuable because of increased chance of bacterial contamination.

Additional Information If mycobacteria are cultured, isolates can be definitively identified, and susceptibility testing performed on request. Although it has been thought that tuberculosis of the urinary tract should be suspected when hematuria and pyuria (sterile pyuria) occur without recovery by routine culture of usual urinary tract pathogens, concomitant infections with ordinary pathogens are not rare. Mycobacteria cultures of the urine are approximately 90% sensitive. The kidney is the most frequent site of infection; prostate, salpinx, and endometrial involvement also occurs. Continuing tuberculous bacilluria may cause cystitis with frequency. Genitourinary infections with atypical mycobacteria, particularly *M. kansasii* and *M. avium-intracellulare*, occur.[1] Mycobacterial genitourinary tract infections represented about 20% of extrapulmonary tuberculosis cases.[2] This proportion will probably increase as more infections with *M. tuberculosis* and *M. avium-intracellulare* are identified in patients with the acquired immunodeficiency syndrome (AIDS). Urine cultures were reported positive in 77% of HIV-positive patients with extrapulmonary tuberculosis.[3] The direct detection of mycobacterial DNA in urine is being investigated. Specific DNA sequences can be amplified from patient specimens.[4]

(Continued)

Mycobacterial Culture, Urine *(Continued)*

Footnotes

1. Wayne LG and Sramek HA, "Agents of Newly Recognized or Infrequently Encountered Mycobacterial Diseases," *Clin Microbiol Rev*, 1992, 5(1):1-25.
2. Alvarez S and McCabe WR, "Extrapulmonary Tuberculosis Revisited: A Review of Experience at Boston City and Other Hospitals," *Medicine*, 1984, 63(1):25-55.
3. Shafer RW, Kim DS, Weiss JP, et al, "Extrapulmonary Tuberculosis in Patients With Human Immunodeficiency Virus Infection," *Medicine (Baltimore)*, 1991, 70(6):384-97.
4. Kolk AH, Schuitema AR, Kuijper S, et al, "Detection of *Mycobacterium tuberculosis* in Clinical Samples by Using Polymerase Chain Reaction and a Nonradioactive Detection System," *J Clin Microbiol*, 1992, 30(10):2567-75.

References

Des Prez RM and Heim CR, "Mycobacterium Tuberculosis," *Principles and Practice of Infectious Diseases*, 3rd ed, Mandell GL, Douglas RG Jr, and Bennett JE, eds, New York, NY: Churchill Livingstone, 1990, 1877-906.

Mycobacteria Susceptibility Testing *see* Antimicrobial Susceptibility Testing, Mycobacteria *on page 452*

Mycobacterium Smear *see* Acid-Fast Stain *on page 446*

Nasopharyngeal Culture *see* Bacterial Culture, Nasopharynx *on page 464*

Nasopharyngeal Culture for *Bordetella pertussis see* Bordetella pertussis Culture *on page 471*

Nasopharyngeal Culture for *Corynebacterium diphtheriae see* Corynebacterium diphtheriae Throat Culture *on page 474*

Neisseria see Bacterial Culture, Aerobes *on page 455*

Neisseria gonorrhoeae Culture and Smear

CPT 87081 (culture, single organism); 87082 (commercial kit)

Related Information

Bacterial Culture, Genital Specimen *on page 463*
Beta-Lactamase Test *on page 470*
Cervical/Vaginal Cytology *on page 290*
Chlamydia trachomatis Genome Detection *on page 505*
Genital Culture for *Ureaplasma urealyticum on page 667*
Gram's Stain *on page 481*
Herpes Simplex Virus Culture *on page 668*
HIV-1/HIV-2 Serology *on page 403*
Neisseria gonorrhoeae Genome Detection *on page 521*
RPR *on page 428*
VDRL, Serum *on page 438*

Synonyms GC Culture; Gonorrhea Culture

Test Commonly Includes Selective culture for *Neisseria gonorrhoeae*; Gram's stain of specimen from normally sterile site and male urethral swabs

Patient Preparation Preparation same as for clean catch urine. See Bacterial Culture, Urine, Clean Catch *on page 468* for detailed information. *Neisseria gonorrhoeae* is very sensitive to lubricants and disinfectants. If possible, avoid collecting urethral specimens until at least 1 hour after urination.

Specimen Body fluid, discharge, pus, swab of genital lesions, urethral discharge (best when available for men); endocervix (best when available for female); throat swab, rectal swab; sediment of first 10 mL of centrifuged urine collected at least 2 hours after last micturition, or first few drops of urine voided into a sterile cup for "first voided urine specimen" for asymptomatic males, or first void overnight urine, centrifuged.

Container Swab with transport medium, sterile container, direct plating on Transgrow, Jembec™, or Thayer-Martin medium

Collection

Urethral discharge: Collect male urethral discharge by endourethral swab after stripping toward the orifice to express exudate.

Rectal swab: Collect anorectal specimens from the crypts just inside the anal ring. Direct visualization with anoscopy is useful. Insert the swab past the anal sphincter. Move the swab circumferentially around the anal crypts. Allow 15-30 seconds for organisms to adsorb onto the swab.

Prostatic fluid yields fewer positives than does culture of urethral discharge.

Urethral or vaginal cultures are indicated from females when endocervical culture is not possible.

Urethra in women: Massage the urethra against the pubic symphysis to express discharge or use endourethral swab.

Vagina: Obtain the specimen from the vaginal vault. Allow 15-30 seconds for organisms to adsorb onto the swab.

Endocervical/cervical: Gently compress cervix between speculum blades to express any endocervical exudate. Swab in a circular pattern.

Bartholin gland: Express exudate from duct. Abscesses should be aspirated with needle and syringe.

Specimens should be transported to the laboratory within 1 hour of collection.

Storage Instructions Specimen should not be refrigerated or exposed to a cold environment. Growth of the organism is less likely following refrigeration. If the specimen is directly inoculated on Thayer-Martin medium, it should be transported to the laboratory as soon as possible and placed directly in CO_2 incubator or candle jar.

Turnaround Time Gram's stain results are usually available in less than 1 hour. Cultures from which *N. gonorrhoeae* is isolated usually require 48 hours for completion.

Reference Range Gram's stain: no intracellular gram-negative diplococci seen; no *Neisseria gonorrhoeae* isolated

Critical Values Positive culture for *Neisseria gonorrhoeae* during pregnancy

Use Isolate and identify *Neisseria gonorrhoeae*; establish the diagnosis of gonorrhea

Limitations Cultures are usually screened only for *Neisseria gonorrhoeae*. No other organisms are usually identified. Overgrowth by *Proteus* and yeast may make it impossible to rule out presence of *N. gonorrhoeae*. The vancomycin in Thayer-Martin media may inhibit some strains of *N. gonorrhoeae*. See table.

Selection of Culture Sites for the Isolation of *Neisseria gonorrhoeae*

Culture Site	Diagnostic Sensitivity (%)
Female (nonhysterectomized)	
Primary site	
Endocervical canal	86-96
Secondary sites	
Vagina	55-90
Urethra	60-86
Anal canal	70-85
Oropharynx	50-70
Female (hysterectomized)	
Primary site	
Urethra	88.9
Secondary sites	
Vagina	55.7
Anal canal	40.7
Male (heterosexuals)	
Primary site	
Urethra	94-98 (symptomatic) 84 (asymptomatic)
Male (homosexuals)	
Primary sites	
Urethra	60-98
Anal canal	40-85
Oropharynx	50-70

From Ehret JM and Knapp JS, "Gonorrhea," *Clin Lab Med*, 1989, 9:445-80, with permission.

Methodology Culture on selective medium, Thayer-Martin, or NYC. DNA probes, monoclonal antibodies, enzyme immunoassays (EIA), and chromogenic substrate assays are used as alternatives or adjuncts to culture in some laboratories. Advantages of the newer methods over traditional culture and smear techniques are not universally recognized.

Additional Information Gram's stain smear has a high sensitivity in a symptomatic male with urethral discharge (95% to 99%). Endocervical Gram's stain is of little value in the female as the sensitivity is lower (50%), and endemic normal flora have a similar morphologic appearance causing false-positives. The Gram's stain smear will detect 75% of gonococcal conjunctivitis and 10% to 20% of gonococcal skin lesions. It is of no value in pharyngitis. Cervical and/or anal and throat cultures are recommended for female patients. Cervical cultures have a sensitivity of 80% to 90%. Although demonstration of gram-negative diplococci in leukocytes in a urethral smear from a symptomatic male is presumptive evidence of gonorrhea and is sufficiently diagnostic to initiate therapy, cultural confirmation should be considered if available.

Serologic tests for syphilis (VDRL, RPR, or ART), and HIV, Cervical/Vaginal Cytology, and a diagnostic test for *Chlamydia* should be performed in patients suspected of having gonorrhea. As many as 45% of women with gonorrheal infection have chlamydial infection as well.[1]

Sensitivity and Specificity of Gram's Stains for Diagnosis of Gonorrhea

Specimen Source	Sensitivity (%)	Specificity (%)
Female		
Endocervical canal	45-65	90-97
Vagina	Not studied	–
Urethra	16	–
Anal canal	Not recommended	–
Pharynx	Not recommended	–
Male		
Urethra (symptomatic)	95-99	97-98
Urethra (asymptomatic)	50-70	86
Anal canal (with mucopurulent discharge)	40-80	87-100
Pharynx	Not recommended	–

From Ehret JM and Knapp JS, "Gonorrhea," *Clin Lab Med*, 1989, 9:445-80, with permission.

Thayer-Martin medium and transport systems are available in most laboratories. Aseptically obtained body fluids from patients with suspected gonococcal arthritis should be inoculated to chocolate agar; isolates may fail to grow on selective media.

Laboratories may presumptively identify *Neisseria gonorrhoeae* from clinical specimens if the following criteria are met:
- specimen is from a genital source
- patient is presumed to be sexually active
- organism grows on selective medium, is oxidase positive, and is morphologically consistent with *Neisseria gonorrhoeae* (ie, gram-negative diplococci with adjacent sides flattened)

If any of these criteria are not met, the organism must be definitively identified using stricter definitions. **Thus, organisms from the throat or rectum, or isolates from nonsexually active (eg, infants or young children) individuals should never be presumptively identified using the criteria listed above.**[2,3] Similarly, many of the rapid biochemical methods for identifying *Neisseria gonorrhoeae* based on three or four biochemical reactions and a very limited database are only acceptable for genital specimens from sexually active patients.

Nongonococcal urethritis may be caused by *Ureaplasma urealyticum*, *Corynebacterium genitalium* type 1, *Trichomonas vaginalis*, *Chlamydia trachomatis*, herpes simplex virus, and rarely, *Candida albicans*.

Footnotes
1. "Gonorrhea and Chlamydial Infections. ACOG Technical Bulletin Number 190-March 1994," *Int J Gynaecol Obstet*, 1994, 45(2):169-74.
2. Knapp JS, "Historical Perspectives and Identification of *Neisseria* and Related Species," *Clin Microbiol Rev*, 1988, 1(4):415-31.
3. Whittington WL, Rice RJ, Biddle JW, et al, "Incorrect Identification of *Neisseria gonorrhoeae* From Infants and Children," *Pediatr Infect Dis J*, 1988, 7(1):3-10.

References
Baron EJ, Cassell GH, Duffy LB, et al, "Cumitech 17A: Laboratory Diagnosis of Female Genital Tract Infections," Baron EJ, ed, Washington, DC: American Society for Microbiology, 1993.
Bowie WR, "Approach to Men With Urethritis and Urologic Complications of Sexually Transmitted Diseases," *Med Clin North Am*, 1990, 74(6):1543-57.
Evangelista AT and Beilstein HR, "Cumitech 4A: Laboratory Diagnosis of Gonorrhea," Abramson C, ed, Washington, DC: American Society for Microbiology, 1993.
Judson FN, "Gonorrhea," *Med Clin North Am*, 1990, 74(6):1353-66.

Neisseria gonorrhoeae Susceptibility Testing *see* Beta-Lactamase Test *on page 470*

Nits Identification *see* Arthropod Identification *on page 453*

Nocardia Culture
CPT 87081

Related Information
Acid-Fast Stain, Modified, *Nocardia* Species *on page 446*
Actinomyces Culture *on page 447*
Fungal Culture, Sputum *on page 479*
Mycobacterial Culture, Sputum *on page 490*

Applies to Sputum *Nocardia* Culture

Test Commonly Includes Culture for *Nocardia* spp and direct microscopic examination of clinical specimens by Gram's stain and/or modified acid-fast stains

Abstract Nocardial infections may be divided into six categories based on body site involved, and clinical and pathological characteristics: 1. pulmonary nocardiosis; 2. systemic nocardiosis; 3. central nervous system nocardiosis; 4. extrapulmonary, localized nocardiosis; 5. cutaneous, subcutaneous, and lymphocutaneous nocardioses; and 6. mycetoma.

Specimen Pus, tissue, cerebrospinal fluid or other body fluid, aspirate, sputum. The usual portal of entry is the lung.

Turnaround Time Negative cultures are reported after 2-4 weeks.

Special Instructions Consultation with laboratory prior to collection of the specimen is recommended when nocardiosis is suspected clinically. **Culture should be specifically ordered as Culture for *Nocardia*.**

Reference Range No *Nocardia* sp isolated

Critical Values *Nocardia* sp recovered from a central nervous system specimen

Use Establish the diagnosis of nocardiosis or mycetoma; identify its etiologic agent

Limitations *Nocardia* spp will not be recovered by routine bacterial culture techniques because of its relatively slow growth. Growth of *Nocardia* may be obscured by overgrowth of other organisms in mixed culture (ie, sputum). The diagnosis may not be made unless the laboratory is advised of the clinical suspicion of nocardiosis. *Nocardia* spp are not strongly gram-positive, but their branching pattern when visible is helpful. A modified acid-fast stain (see Acid-Fast Stain, Modified, *Nocardia* Species *on page 446*) is needed, since *Nocardia* are weakly acid-fast and may not be found with conventional acid-fast staining. Staining may be positive when cultures fail.

Methodology Aerobic culture on various bacterial culture media including blood and chocolate agars. Recent data supports the use of *Legionella* culture media (selective and nonselective buffered charcoal yeast agar) for recovery of *Nocardia*.[1,2] *Nocardia* spp can also be cultured on noninhibitory fungal media. Cultures are usually held for 10-30 days, when the laboratory is aware of clinical suspicion of nocardiosis.

Additional Information *Nocardia* spp are aerobic, gram-positive bacteria which are filamentous, relatively slow growing, and variably acid-fast. *N. asteroides*, *N. brasiliensis*, *N. farcinica*, *N. nova*, *N. otitidiscaviarum* (formerly *N. caviae*), and *N. transvalensis* are human pathogens.[3] Many laboratories do not distinguish organisms in the *N. asteroides* complex (ie, *N. asteroides*, *N. nova*, *N. farcinica*) from one another, and identify all these organisms as *N. asteroides*. Human infection is seen most frequently in patients whose immune systems are suppressed by HIV infection, lymphoreticular malignancy, or chemotherapy.[4] The clinical picture may be similar to that observed with systemic mycobacterial or fungal infections. Infections may be acute, subacute, or chronic; and they may be disseminated or localized to cutaneous sites or the respiratory tract.[4] Metastatic infection in brain, bone, skin, or subcutaneous infection in the presence of pulmonary involvement is suggestive of nocardiosis. Organisms in the *N. asteroides* complex are the species most commonly recovered from clinical specimens; they are usually associated with respiratory infections. *N. brasiliensis* is the species usually associated with mycetoma.[5]

Nocardia sp are variably acid-fast and may be frequently confused with *Actinomyces* sp or saprophytic fungi in Gram's stains of clinical specimens. Prognosis is dependent on early diagnosis, treatment with appropriate antimicrobials, and the course of the underlying disease.

Footnotes
1. Vickers RM, Rihs JD, and Yu VL, "Clinical Demonstration of Isolation of *Nocardia asteroides* on Buffered Charcoal-Yeast Extract Media," *J Clin Microbiol*, 1992, 30(1):227-8.
2. Kerr E, Snell H, Black BL, et al, "Isolation of *Nocardia asteroides* From Respiratory Specimens by Using Selective Buffered Charcoal-Yeast Extract Agar," *J Clin Microbiol*, 1992, 30(5):1320-2.
3. Beaman BL, Saubolle MA, and Wallace RJ, "*Nocardia, Rhodococcus, Streptomyces, Oerskovia*, and Other Aerobic Actinomycetes of Medical Importance," *Manual of Clinical Microbiology*, 6th ed, Murray PR, Baron EJ, Pfaller MA, et al, eds, Washington, DC: American Society for Microbiology, 1995, 379-99.
4. Beaman BL and Beaman L, "*Nocardia* Species: Host-Parasite Relationships," *Clin Microbiol Rev*, 1994, 7(2):213-64.
5. McNeil MM, Brown JM, Jarvis WR, et al, "Comparison of Species Distribution and Antimicrobial Susceptibility of Aerobic Actinomycetes From Clinical Specimens," *Rev Infect Dis*, 1990, 12(5):778-83.

References
Javaly K, Horowitz HW, and Wormser GP, "Nocardiosis in Patients With Human Immunodeficiency Virus Infection. Report of 2 Cases and Review of the Literature," *Medicine (Baltimore)*, 1992, 71(3):128-38.
McNeil MM and Brown JM, "The Medically Important Aerobic Actinomycetes: Epidemiology and Microbiology," *Clin Microbiol Rev*, 1994, 7(3):357-417.
Wilson JP, Turner HR, Kirchner KA, et al, "Nocardial Infections in Renal Transplant Recipients," *Medicine (Baltimore)*, 1989, 68(1):38-57.

Nocardia Species Modified Acid-Fast Stain *see* Acid-Fast Stain, Modified, *Nocardia* Species *on page 446*

Ocular Culture *see* Bacterial Culture, Conjunctiva *on page 461*

Outer Ear Culture *see* Bacterial Culture, Ear *on page 462*

Ova and Parasites, Stool

CPT 87177

Related Information

Synonyms Parasites, Stool; Parasitology Examination, Stool; Stool for Ova and Parasites

Applies to Amebiasis; *Blastocystis hominis*; *Cyclospora* Species; Flagellates; *Giardia*; *Giardia* Immunosorbent Assay; Helminths

Test Commonly Includes Gross appearance, direct wet mounts, saline and iodine, concentration procedure, hematoxylin smear or trichrome smear

Patient Preparation Specimens obtained with a warm saline enema or Fleet Phospho®-Soda are acceptable. Specimens obtained with mineral oil, bismuth, or magnesium compounds are unsatisfactory. Wait 1 week or more after barium procedures or laxative administration before collecting stools for examination.

Aftercare Warning: Any stool collected by or from the patient may harbor pathogens which are **immediately infective.** Use extreme caution when *Entamoeba histolytica*, *Hymenolepis nana*, *Cryptosporidium*, and *Taenia* sp are suspected or reported.

Specimen Fresh or preserved random stool or duodenal aspirate. If pinworm is suspected, a Scotch® Tape preparation should be submitted to the laboratory instead of stool.

Container Plastic stool container. The collection procedure of choice is to provide patients with containers with polyvinyl alcohol (PVA) and formalin into which they can place stool. Zinc sulfate can replace mercuric chloride in PVA. Sodium acetate-acetic acid-formalin (SAF) fixative also avoids use of mercury.[1] This procedure assures that the specimen will be well preserved for examination.

Collection Unpreserved specimen should be delivered within 1 hour of collection to the laboratory. Direct wet preparation exams for motile trophozoite observation can only be performed on fresh stools. The recommendation is the examination of a single specimen and after obtaining its result; then the examination of additional specimens if indicated. If specimen delivery will be delayed, specimens may be preserved in polyvinyl alcohol (PVA) fixative which is suitable for the preparation of permanent stains and formalin or merthiolate-iodine-formalin (MIF).

Storage Instructions Liquid specimens should be brought directly to the laboratory. Wet mounts should be performed immediately, and the specimen placed in PVA and/or MIF preservatives to maintain ova and trophozoite states.

Causes for Rejection Patients who develop diarrhea 3 or more days after hospitalization virtually never have bacteria or parasites identified by routine examination; the only etiologic agent implicated with any frequency in this setting is *Clostridium difficile*.[2] The third specimen detects 98.8% of pathogens. Parasitology specimens are unlikely to include a pathogen after 4 days of hospitalization.[3]

Because of risk to laboratory personnel, specimens sent on diaper or tissue paper, specimen contaminating outside of transport container may not be acceptable. Specimen containing interfering substances (eg, castor oil, bismuth, Metamucil®, barium, specimens delayed in transit, and those contaminated with urine) will not have optimal yield.

Special Instructions Geographic history is needed by the Parasitology Laboratory.

Reference Range No parasites seen

Use Establish the diagnosis of parasitic infestation. Watery or bloody stools with variable numbers of fecal leukocytes may harbor amebae.

Limitations One negative result does not rule out the possibility of parasitic infestation. Stool examination for *Giardia* may be negative in early stages of infection, in patients who shed organisms cyclically, and in chronic infections.[4] The sensitivity of microscopic methods for the detection of *Giardia* range from 46% to 95%.[5] *Giardia* are found predominantly in the upper small intestine. Tests for *Giardia* antigen may have a much higher yield.[6] An enzyme-linked immunosorbent assay is available for detection of *Giardia* antigen in stool. Its sensitivity is 92%, specificity 98%.[7]

Contraindications Parasite exams on stool from patients hospitalized ≥3 days are not productive and should not be ordered unless special circumstances exist. Administration of barium, bismuth, Metamucil®, castor oil, mineral oil, tetracycline therapy, administration of antiamebic drugs within 1 week prior to test. Purgation contraindicated for pregnancy, ulcerative colitis, cardiovascular disease, child younger than 5 years of age, appendicitis or possible appendicitis.

Stool must be collected directly into a dry container or into fixative. Urine and water destroy amebae.[7]

Methodology Wet mount and trichrome stain after concentration, immunofluorescence (IF), counterimmunoelectrophoresis (CIE), or enzyme-linked immunosorbent assay (ELISA) for the detection of *Giardia* antigens. Immunologic techniques are helpful for *Cryptosporidium* sp. A role for the iron hematoxylin stain continues to exist.[1] The use of pooled preserved specimens to contain costs is warranted.[8]

Additional Information Amebas and certain other parasites cannot be seen in stools containing barium. Optimal diagnostic yield is obtained by the examination of fresh, warm stool by an experienced technologist. Amebic cysts, *Giardia* cysts, and helminth eggs can be recovered from formed stools. Mushy or liquid stools (either normally passed or obtained by purgation) often yield trophozoites. Purgation does not enhance the yield of *Giardia*. Stools which can be processed by the laboratory in less than 1 hour need not be preserved. Mushy, loose, or watery stools which cannot reach the laboratory within 1 hour should be preserved in formalin or merthiolate-iodine-formalin (MIF) and/or polyvinyl alcohol (PVA). Formalin will preserve protozoan cysts and larvae and the eggs of helminths. It is used for concentration procedures. PVA will preserve the trophozoite stage of protozoa. A trichrome-stained smear may be prepared from PVA fixed material. Specimens submitted in PVA cannot be concentrated; therefore, they should always be accompanied by a portion of the specimen in formalin. Formed stools may be preserved in formalin or refrigerated in a secure container until they can be transported to the laboratory. The MIF kit will preserve protozoan cysts, helminth eggs and larvae. It is intended to be sent home with the patient and mailed back to the laboratory.

Parasites identified in the stool of **immunocompromised subjects** (eg, AIDS patients) include *Cryptosporidium*, microsporidia, *Entamoeba histolytica*, *Giardia lamblia*, *Isospora belli*, and *Strongyloides stercoralis*.[9,10] Microsporidia are obligate intracellular spore-forming protozoa. *Enterocytozoon bieneusi*, a microsporidia sp, is a common cause of chronic diarrhea in HIV-positive persons.[11] Its diagnosis is facilitated by duodenal pinch biopsies.[12]

The pathogenic potential of *Blastocystis hominis* which is commonly observed in stool of healthy and symptomatic patients, is currently being debated. A review of the literature by Miller and Minshew indicated that there was no convincing proof of a causal relationship between *B. hominis* and symptoms, that there was no correlation between resolution of symptoms with therapy or with the disappearance of the organism from stool, and that treatment directed at the indication of *B. hominis* is not indicated.[13] Doyle et al observed a role for *Blastocystis* in acute and chronic gastroenteritis but were unable to conclude whether the role is one of association or causation.[14]

In a large children's hospital study of nosocomial diarrhea, rotavirus, *C. difficile*, and enteric adenovirus were recovered. Stool for ova and parasites and bacterial stool cultures yielded no pathogens.[15]

The observation of erythrophagocytic trophozoites in bloody, mucoid stools provides optimal evidence of the presence of invasive **amebiasis**. Such forms are best examined from fresh, warm stool. A smear stained by trichrome or iron hematotoxylin is confirmatory. *E. histolytica* is recognized in endoscopic biopsies in only half of the cases. Amebae are not always present in the stools of patients who have amebic abscess of liver.[1] In such patients, serologic tests are more reliable: see listing *Entamoeba histolytica* Serological Test *on page 391*. It is needed for the critical differential diagnosis between pyogenic and amebic liver abscess.[16]

Footnotes

1. Long EG and Christie JD, "The Diagnosis of Old and New Gastrointestinal Parasites," *Clin Lab Med*, 1995, 15(2):307-31.
2. Siegel DL, Edelstein PH, and Nachamkin I, "Inappropriate Testing for Diarrheal Diseases in the Hospital," *JAMA*, 1990, 263(7):979-82.
3. Valenstein P, Pfaller M, and Yungbluth M, "The Use and Abuse of Routine Stool Microbiology," *Arch Pathol Lab Med*, 1996, 120:206-11.
4. Brooke MM and Melvin DM, *Morphology of Diagnostic Stages of Intestinal Parasites of Humans*, 2nd ed, U.S. Department of Health and Human Services, Publication No 84-8116, Atlanta, GA: Centers for Disease Control, 1984.

OVA AND PARASITES, AMEBAE

¹Rare, probably of animal origin Scale: 0 5 10µm
²Flagellate

Amebae found in human stool specimens.

OVA AND PARASITES, COCCIDIA

Ciliate, coccidia, and *B. hominis* found in human stool specimens.

OVA AND PARASITES, FLAGELLATES

Flagellates found in human stool specimens.

5. Janoff EN, Craft CJ, and Pickering LK, "Diagnosis of *Giardia lamblia* Infections by Detection of Parasite-Specific Antigens," *J Clin Microbiol*, 1989, 27(3):431-5.
6. Chappell CL and Matson CC, "*Giardia* Antigen Detection in Patients With Chronic Gastrointestinal Disturbances," *J Fam Pract*, 1992, 35(1):49-53.
7. Donowitz M, Kokke FT, and Saidi R, "Evaluation of Patients With Chronic Diarrhea," *N Engl J Med*, 1995, 332(11):725-9.
8. Peters CS, Hernandez L, Sheffield N, et al, "Cost Containment of Formalin-Preserved Stool Specimens for Ova and Parasites From Outpatients," *J Clin Microbiol*, 1988, 26(8):1584-5.
9. Garcia LS and Shimizu R, "Diagnostic Parasitology: Parasitic Infections and the Compromised Host," *Lab Med*, 1993, 24:205-15.
10. Curry A, Turner AJ, and Lucas S, "Opportunistic Protozoan Infections in Human Immunodeficiency Virus Disease: Review Highlighting Diagnostic and Therapeutic Aspects," *J Clin Pathol*, 1991, 44(3):182-93.
11. Asmuth DM, De Girolami PC, Federman M, et al, "Clinical Features of Microsporidiosis in Patients With AIDS," *Clin Infect Dis*, 1994, 18(5):819-25.
12. Peacock CS, Blanshard C, Tovey DG, et al, "Histological Diagnosis of Intestinal Microsporidiosis in Patients With AIDS," *J Clin Pathol*, 1991, 44(7):558-63.
13. Miller RA and Minshew BH, "*Blastocystis hominis*: An Organism in Search of a Disease," *Rev Infect Dis*, 1988, 10(5):930-8.
14. Doyle PW, Helgason MM, Mathias RG, et al, "Epidemiology and Pathogenicity of *Blastocystis hominis*," *J Clin Microbiol*, 1990, 28(1):116-21.
15. Brady MT, Pacini DL, Budde CT, et al, "Diagnostic Studies of Nosocomial Diarrhea in Children: Assessing Their Use and Value," *Am J Infect Control*, 1989, 17(2):77-82.
16. Pitt HA, "Surgical Management of Hepatic Abscesses," *World J Surg*, 1990, 14(4):498-504.

References
Kabani A, Cadrain G, Trevenen C, et al, "Practice Guidelines for Ordering Stool Ova and Parasite Testing in a Pediatric Population," *Am J Clin Pathol*, 1995, 104(3):272-8.
Orihel TC and Ash LR, *Parasites in Human Tissues*, Chicago, IL: ASCP Press, 1995.
Reed SL, "Amebiasis: An Update," *Clin Infect Dis*, 1992, 14(2):385-93.
Reitano M, Masci JR, and Bottone EJ, "Amebiasis: Clinical and Laboratory Perspective," *Crit Rev Clin Lab Sci*, 1991, 28(5-6):357-85.
Senay H and MacPherson D, "Parasitology: Diagnostic Yield of Stool Examination," *Can Med Assoc J*, 1989, 140(11):1329-31.
Sun T, "Current Topics in Protozoal Diseases," *Am J Clin Pathol*, 1994, 102(1):16-29.
Sun T, Ilardi CF, Asnis D, "Light and Electron Microscopic Identification of *Cyclospora* Species in the Small Intestine: Evidence of the Presence of Asexual Life Cycle in Human Host ," *Am J Clin Pathol*, 1996, 105:216-20.
Walker JC, "Parasitology. Diagnostic Techniques in the Laboratory," *Med J Aust*, 1993, 158(12):824-9.
Wolfe MS, "Giardiasis," *Clin Microbiol Rev*, 1992, 5(1):93-100.

Ova and Parasites, Urine
CPT 87177

Related Information
Blood, Urine *on page 631*
Eosinophil Count *on page 315*
Eosinophils, Urine *on page 634*
Filariasis Serological Test *on page 393*
Hemoglobin, Qualitative, Urine *on page 637*
Microsporidia Diagnostic Procedures *on page 487*
Ova and Parasites, Stool *on previous page*
Parasite Antibodies *on page 421*
Pinworm Preparation *on next page*
Schistosomiasis Serological Test *on page 429*
Urine Cytology *on page 301*

Synonyms Parasites, Urine; Urine for Parasites; Urine for *Schistosoma haematobium*

Applies to Schistosomiasis

Test Commonly Includes Wet preparation and concentration procedure

Abstract The two parasites for which urine specimens are most likely to be submitted to the laboratory include *Schistosoma haematobium* and *Trichomonas vaginalis*.

Specimen Freshly voided urine; whole specimen, not midstream void

Container Sterile, plastic urine container

Collection For *Trichomonas vaginalis*, collect freshly passed urine and immediately transport to the laboratory without refrigeration so that the sediment can be examined for motile trophozoites. For *Schistosoma haematobium*, the terminal portion of the urine specimen may contain numerous eggs trapped in mucus and pus. Peak egg excretion occurs between noon and 3 PM; samples collected during this time, or during a 24-hour urine collection (without preservatives) may be obtained for examination.

Storage Instructions Do not refrigerate.

Special Instructions The laboratory should be informed of the parasite clinically suspected. Geographic history may be useful.

Reference Range No parasites identified

Use Detect parasitic infestation, particularly *Trichomonas* or *Schistosoma haematobium*. Eggs of *Enterobius vermicularis* are sometimes present in urine as the result of fecal contamination, but are best investigated as described under the listing Pinworm Preparation *on page 496*.

Limitations A single negative result does not rule out the possibility of parasitic infestation.

Additional Information Immunodiagnostic tests including enzyme-linked immunosorbent assay and immunoblot tests have been used to diagnose schistosomiasis in some centers.[1] Patient should have a geographic history consistent with schistosomiasis to warrant undertaking screening the urine. A direct DNA-based diagnostic kit is being developed for detection of *Trichomonas vaginalis*.[2]

Footnotes
1. Tsang VC and Wilkins PP, "Immunodiagnosis of Schistosomiasis. Screen With FAST-ELISA and Confirm With Immunoblot," *Clin Lab Med*, 1991, 11(4):1029-39.
2. Briselden AM and Hillier SL, "Evaluation of Affirm VP Microbial Identification Test for *Gardnerella vaginalis* and *Trichomonas vaginalis*," *J Clin Microbiol*, 1994, 32(1):148-52.

References
Ash LR and Orihel TC, *Atlas of Human Parasitology*, 3rd ed, Chicago, IL: American Society of Clinical Pathologists, 1990.
Ash LR and Orihel TC, *A Guide to Laboratory Procedures and Identification*, Chicago, IL: ASCP Press, 1991.

Parasites, Stool *see* Ova and Parasites, Stool *on previous page*

Parasites, Urine *see* Ova and Parasites, Urine *on this page*

Parasitology Examination, Stool *see* Ova and Parasites, Stool *on previous page*

***Pediculus humanus* Identification** *see* Arthropod Identification *on page 453*

Penicillinase *see* Antimicrobial Susceptibility Testing, Aerobic and Facultatively Anaerobic Bacteria *on page 448*

Penicillinase-Producing Organisms Susceptibility Testing *see* Beta-Lactamase Test *on page 470*

Penicillinases *see* Beta-Lactamase Test *on page 470*

Penicillinase Test *see* Beta-Lactamase Test *on page 470*

Percutaneous Transtracheal Culture *see* Bacterial Culture, Sputum *on page 465*

Periodic Acid Schiff (PAS) *see* Fungus Smear, Stain *on page 481*

Pertussis Culture *see* Bordetella pertussis Culture *on page 471*

***Phthirus pubis* Identification** *see* Arthropod Identification *on page 453*

Pinworm Preparation
CPT 87208
Related Information
Ova and Parasites, Stool *on page 494*
Ova and Parasites, Urine *on previous page*

Synonyms *Enterobius vermicularis* Preparation; Scotch® Tape Test

Test Commonly Includes Detection of pinworm eggs from the perianal region

Specimen Scotch® Tape slide preparation of perianal region

Container Scotch® Tape slide must be submitted in a covered container. Commercial kit products are also available for collection of pinworm specimens. **Caution:** Pinworm eggs are very infectious.

Collection The specimen is best obtained a few hours after the patient has retired (ie, 10 or 11 PM), or early in the morning before a bowel movement or bath. This collection procedure is essential if valid results are expected. Clear Scotch® Tape should be used; the nontransparent type is unsatisfactory. An 8 cm (3 in) piece of cellophane tape is placed over the end of a glass slide sticky side out. The anal folds are spread apart and the mucocutaneous junction is firmly pressed in all four quadrants. The tape is then pressed over the slide and the specimen is transported to the laboratory in a carefully sealed container. Refer to diagram. It is important to provide clear instructions, because these specimens are often collected at home.

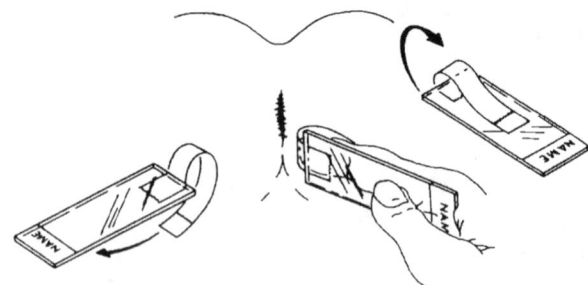

Cellophane tape slide preparation. Attach 3" piece of cellophane tape to undersurface of clear end of microscope slide, which has previously been identified (ground-glass end). Press sticky surface of tape against perianal skin. Then roll back tape onto slide, sticky surface down. Wash hands and nails well. From Bauer JD, *Clinical Laboratory Methods*, 9th ed, Mosby-Year Book Inc, St Louis, MO: 1982 , 989, with permission.

Causes for Rejection Use of nontransparent Scotch® Tape, Scotch® Tape on both sides of the slide, specimen which is not inside a covered container, use of frosted slide, tape sent sticky side up. Specimens which are not properly contained pose excessive risk to laboratory personnel.

Reference Range No pinworm eggs (*Enterobius vermicularis*) identified. Positives reported as few, moderate, or many eggs identified.

Use Detect cases of pinworm infestation (enterobiasis), *Enterobius vermicularis* parasitic infestation

Limitations Examination for pinworm only. One negative result does not rule out possibility of parasitic infestation. Examinations on multiple days may be required to diagnose infection. Stool specimens are not usually satisfactory for pinworm studies.

Contraindications Specimen collection at improper time

Methodology Microscopy

Additional Information The most satisfactory means of diagnosing pinworm infection is by the recovery of eggs or female worms from the perianal region. Only 5% to 10% of infected persons have demonstrable eggs in their stools. If fecal material is submitted for examination, only the surface should be sampled. Enterobiasis often is present in multiple family members. Therefore, it is recommended that all members of the family be tested. The responsible parent should be instructed how to collect samples, using one kit per individual. Female worms or parts of them may be demonstrated on the tape by microscopic examination.

The proportion of positive specimens correlate with severity of disease. Eggs, if present, may be immature, embryonated (with viable or dead larvae), or (if the specimen is several days or more old) empty egg shells will be present. *Enterobius vermicularis* has been reported as a rare cause of appendicitis, salpingitis, epididymitis, and hepatic granuloma. Diagnosis at colonoscopy has been reported.

References
Mondou EN and Gnepp DR, "Hepatic Granuloma Resulting From *Enterobius vermicularis*," *Am J Clin Pathol*, 1989, 91(1):97-100.
Russell LJ, "The Pinworm, *Enterobius vermicularis*," *Prim Care*, 1991, 18(1):13-24.
Schnell VL, Yandell R, Van Zandt S, et al, "*Enterobius vermicularis* Salpingitis: A Distant Episode From Precipitating Appendicitis," *Obstet Gynecol*, 1992, 80(3 Pt 2):553-5.
Sun T, Schwartz NS, Sewell C, et al, "*Enterobius* Egg Granuloma of the Vulva and Peritoneum: Review of the Literature," *Am J Trop Med Hyg*, 1991, 45(2):249-53.

Pleural Fluid, *Legionella* Culture *see Legionella* Culture *on page 485*

Potassium Hydroxide Preparation *see* KOH Preparation *on page 485*

Prostatic Fluid Culture *see* Bacterial Culture, Genital Specimen *on page 463*

Pseudomembranous Colitis Toxin Assay *see Clostridium difficile* Toxin Assay *on page 473*

Pseudomonas *see* Bacterial Culture, Aerobes *on page 455*

Puncture Wound, Foreign Body, Culture *see* Bacterial Culture, Wound *on page 470*

Quantitative Burn Culture *see* Bacterial Culture, Burn Sites *on page 460*

Quantitative Culture, Biopsy Specimen *see* Bacterial Culture, Burn Sites *on page 460*

Quantitative Tip Culture (QTC) *see* Bacterial Culture, Intravascular Device *on page 463*

Rectal Swab Culture *see* Bacterial Culture, Stool *on page 466*

Rocky Mountain Spotted Fever, *Dermacentor andersoni* *see* Arthropod Identification *on page 453*

Safranin *see* Gram's Stain *on page 481*

***Sarcoptes scabiei* Skin Scrapings Identification** *see* Arthropod Identification *on page 453*

SBD *see* Serum Bactericidal Test *on this page*

S. bovihominis *see Cryptosporidium* Diagnostic Procedures *on page 474*

Schistosomiasis *see* Ova and Parasites, Urine *on previous page*

Schlichter Test *see* Serum Bactericidal Test *on this page*

Schlichter Test *see* Antimicrobial Susceptibility Testing, Antimicrobial Combinations *on page 449*

Scotch® Tape Test *see* Pinworm Preparation *on this page*

Sensitivity Testing, Aerobic and Facultatively Anaerobic Organisms *see* Antimicrobial Susceptibility Testing, Aerobic and Facultatively Anaerobic Bacteria *on page 448*

Serum Antibacterial Titer *see* Serum Bactericidal Test *on this page*

Serum Bactericidal Dilution *see* Serum Bactericidal Test *on this page*

Serum Bactericidal Level *see* Serum Bactericidal Test *on this page*

Serum Bactericidal Test
CPT 87197
Related Information
Aminoglycosides *on page 531*
Antimicrobial Susceptibility Testing, Aerobic and Facultatively Anaerobic Bacteria *on page 448*
Antimicrobial Susceptibility Testing, Antimicrobial Combinations *on page 449*
Chloramphenicol *on page 542*
Vancomycin *on page 578*

Synonyms Antibacterial Activity, Serum; Bacterial Inhibitory Level, Serum; Maximum Bactericidal Dilution; MBD; Schlichter Test; Serum Antibacterial Titer; Serum Bactericidal Level; Serum Inhibitory Titer; Susceptibility Testing, Serum Bactericidal Dilution Method

Applies to SBD; Serum Bactericidal Dilution; Serum Inhibitory Dilution; SID

Test Commonly Includes Assay of serum or body fluid for antimicrobial activity

Patient Preparation Sterile aspiration of body fluid

Specimen Peak and trough serum from patient and bacterial isolate causing infection (prepared by laboratory)

Container Red top tube; sterile tube for body fluid

Sampling Time Both peak and trough levels should be obtained. The peak level is the level 60 minutes after completing an intravenous or intramuscular dose and 90 minutes after an oral dose.[1] With vancomycin, the peak occurs 2 hours after an I.V. dose. Trough levels are obtained immediately before the next dose. If more than one antibiotic is administered, an attempt should be made to draw the peak and trough specimens around a dose when antibiotics are administered simultaneously. If this is not feasible, draw the specimens around the dose of the more frequently administered agent.

Collection Specimen should be transported to the laboratory within 1 hour of collection. Label specimens with time and date collected, time of last antimicrobial infusion (start and completion of infusion), and whether the specimen is a peak or trough.

Storage Instructions Separate serum from cells and freeze if test will not be performed within 2 hours.

Causes for Rejection Isolate discarded before request for testing, serum specimen allowed to sit at room temperature for more than 2 hours

Turnaround Time 2-3 days

Special Instructions If a serum bactericidal test is desired, the physician should request that the laboratory save the patient's isolate within 48 hours of submission of the specimen for initial culture. **If the isolate has not been saved, the test cannot be performed.** The laboratory should be informed of current antibiotic therapy including date and time of last dosage, route of administration on all antimicrobial agents patient is receiving, and clinical diagnosis. Time of specimen collection should be indicated on requisition.

Reference Range Peak and trough titers ≥1:32 and ≥1:8, respectively, are considered adequate. Peak and trough titers ≤1:2 are considered inadequate. Titers between these ranges are considered intermediate.[1]

Use Determine the maximum bactericidal dilution (MBD) or serum bactericidal dilution (SBD) of serum or body fluid after administration of antibiotic(s). This is the last serum/body fluid dilution which is bactericidal for the patient's infecting organism. This titer is useful in monitoring total therapeutic effect. Frequently it is used to evaluate therapy in endocarditis, osteomyelitis, and suppurative arthritis.

Limitations Technical and biological variables affecting test performance make interpretation of test results difficult. There is probably insufficient data to support standardized interpretation at this time.[2]

Contraindications The bacterium isolated from patient is not available or fails to grow for the serum bactericidal test.

Methodology Serial dilution of patient's serum with Mueller-Hinton broth, 1:1 final ratio recommended, supplemented if necessary. Each dilution is incubated with a standard inoculum of the patient's isolate.[1]

Additional Information Results will reflect the combined *in vitro* effect of all antimicrobial agents present in the patient's serum or body fluid on his/her infecting organism(s). Results are accurate to ±1 dilution and are not necessarily equivalent to a serum assay. Maximum inhibitory dilution (MID) or serum inhibitory dilution (SID) may also be reported. An apparently adequate ratio may represent a highly susceptible organism responding to a relatively low blood level or a moderately resistant organism responding to an unexpectedly high blood level. A serum inhibitory titer might suggest an adequate therapeutic level but would give no clue to potential toxicity, when an extremely narrow margin exists between a therapeutically adequate dose and a possibly toxic one (eg, aminoglycosides).

The serum bactericidal test has been applied experimentally to detect antimicrobial activity in cerebrospinal fluid, joint fluid, and amniotic fluid.[3,4] It is also useful in determining whether serum antimicrobial activity remains adequate after a shift from parenteral to oral therapy. Serum bactericidal titers are useful in evaluating synergy between antibiotics after administration of the drugs.[5]

Footnotes

1. National Committee for Clinical Laboratory Standards, *Methodology for the Serum Bactericidal Test, Tentative Standard M21-T*, Villanova, PA: National Committee for Clinical Laboratory Standards, 1992.
2. Peterson LR and Shanholtzer CJ, "Tests for Bacterial Effects of Antimicrobial Agents: Technical Performance and Clinical Relevance," *Clin Microbiol Rev*, 1992, 5(4):420-32.
3. Viladrich PF, Gudiol F, Liñares J, et al, "Evaluation of Vancomycin for Therapy of Adult Pneumococcal Meningitis," *Antimicrob Agents Chemother*, 1991, 35(12):2467-72.
4. Nix DE, Goodwin SD, Peloquin CA, et al, "Antibiotic Tissue Penetration and Its Relevance: Impact of Tissue Penetration on Infection Response," *Antimicrob Agents Chemother*, 1991, 35(10):1953-9.
5. Van der Auwera P, "*Ex Vivo* Study of Serum Bactericidal Titers and Killing Rates of Daptomycin (LY 146032) Combined or Not Combined With Amikacin Compared With Those of Vancomycin," *Antimicrob Agents Chemother*, 1989, 33(10):1783-90.

References
MacLowry JD, "Perspective: The Serum Dilution Test," *J Infect Dis*, 1989, 160(4):624-6.
Rosenblatt JE, "Laboratory Tests Used to Guide Antimicrobial Therapy," *Mayo Clin Proc*, 1991, 66(9):942-8.
Stratton CW, "Serum Bactericidal Test," *Clin Microbiol Rev*, Jan 1988, 1(1):19-26.

Serum Inhibitory Dilution *see* Serum Bactericidal Test *on previous page*

Serum Inhibitory Titer *see* Serum Bactericidal Test *on previous page*

SID *see* Serum Bactericidal Test *on previous page*

Skin Burn Culture, Quantitative *see* Bacterial Culture, Burn Sites *on page 460*

Skin Fungus Culture *see* Fungal Culture, Skin *on page 478*

Skin Mycobacteria Culture *see* Mycobacterial Culture, Cutaneous and Subcutaneous Tissue *on page 489*

Skin Scrapings for *Sarcoptes scabiei* Identification *see* Arthropod Identification *on page 453*

Spinal Fluid Culture *see* Bacterial Culture, Cerebrospinal Fluid *on page 460*

Spinal Fluid Fungus Culture *see* Fungal Culture, Cerebrospinal Fluid *on page 477*

Spinal Fluid Mycobacteria Culture *see* Mycobacterial Culture, Cerebrospinal Fluid *on page 489*

Sputum Culture *see* Bacterial Culture, Sputum *on page 465*

Sputum Fungus Culture *see* Fungal Culture, Sputum *on page 479*

Sputum Mycobacteria Culture *see* Mycobacterial Culture, Sputum *on page 490*

Sputum *Nocardia* Culture *see* Nocardia Culture *on page 493*

S. suihominis *see* Cryptosporidium Diagnostic Procedures *on page 474*

Staphylococci *see* Bacterial Culture, Aerobes *on page 455*

Sterility Culture

CPT 87070

Synonyms Autoclave Sterility Check; Sterilizer Function Check

Specimen Three strips (one control and two test strips)

Container Sterility test envelope

Collection The two test strips should be placed separately in the center of the two largest packs, in the largest loads or in areas of the load that is least likely to come up to sterilizing temperature. Do not place the strips on open shelves, on the peripheral, or the exterior surface of a pack.

Special Instructions One strip (control strip) must not be autoclaved or steam sterilized. The two other strips (test strips) must be sterilized.

Reference Range No growth in test strips; growth in control strip

Use Confirm that adequate sterilization conditions have been attained

Limitations Manufacturers instructions should be followed carefully. It may be necessary to add water (500 mL) to sealed plastic biohazard bags. See bag manufacturer's instructions.

Methodology Indicator strips impregnated with spores of *Bacillus stearothermophilus* are used with steam autoclaves, and *Bacillus subtilis* variety *niger* are used for ethylene oxide sterilizers.

Additional Information Biological indicators must be used at least once weekly with the steam autoclaves and with every load with the ethylene oxide sterilizer.

References
Association of Operating Room Nurses, "Proposed Recommended Practices: Sterilization," *AORN J*, 1991, 54(1):82-9, 92-6.
Kaczmarek RG, Moore RM Jr, McCrohan J, et al, "Multistate Investigation of the Actual Disinfection/Sterilization of Endoscopes in Health Care Facilities," *Am J Med*, 1992, 92(3):257-61.
Rutala WA, "Disinfection, Sterilization, and Waste Disposal," *Prevention and Control of Nosocomial Infections*, 2nd ed, Wenzel RP, ed, Baltimore, MD: Williams and Wilkins Co, 1993, 460-95.

Sterilizer Function Check *see* Sterility Culture *on this page*

Stool Culture *see* Bacterial Culture, Stool *on page 466*

Stool Examination for *Cryptosporidium* *see* Cryptosporidium Diagnostic Procedures *on page 474*

Stool Examination for Microsporidia *see* Microsporidia Diagnostic Procedures *on page 487*

Stool for Ova and Parasites *see* Ova and Parasites, Stool *on page 494*

Stool Fungus Culture *see* Fungal Culture, Stool *on page 480*

Stool Mycobacterial Culture *see* Mycobacterial Culture, Stool *on page 491*

Strep Throat Screening Culture *see* Bacterial Culture, Throat *on page 468*

Streptococci *see* Bacterial Culture, Aerobes *on page 455*

***Streptococcus agalactiae* Latex Screen** *see* Group B *Streptococcus* Screen, Rapid *on page 483*

***Streptococcus* Group A Latex Screen** *see* Group A *Streptococcus* Screen, Rapid *on page 483*

***Streptococcus* Group B Latex Screen** *see* Group B *Streptococcus* Screen, Rapid *on page 483*

***Streptococcus pyogenes* Culture** *see* Bacterial Culture, Throat *on page 468*

Sudden Death Syndrome *see* Botulism Diagnostic Procedure *on page 472*

Sulfur Granule, Culture *see Actinomyces* Culture *on page 447*

Suprapubic Puncture Culture *see* Bacterial Culture, Urine, Suprapubic Puncture *on page 469*

Susceptibility Testing Aerobic and Facultatively Anaerobic Organisms *see* Antimicrobial Susceptibility Testing, Aerobic and Facultatively Anaerobic Bacteria *on page 448*

Susceptibility Testing, Anaerobic Bacteria *see* Antimicrobial Susceptibility Testing, Anaerobic Bacteria *on page 449*

Susceptibility Testing, Antimicrobial Combinations *see* Antimicrobial Susceptibility Testing, Antimicrobial Combinations *on page 449*

Susceptibility Testing, Fungi *see* Antimicrobial Susceptibility Testing, Fungi *on page 450*

Susceptibility Testing, Minimum Bactericidal Concentration *see* Antimicrobial Susceptibility Testing, Minimum Bactericidal Concentration *on page 451*

Susceptibility Testing, Mycobacteria *see* Antimicrobial Susceptibility Testing, Mycobacteria *on page 452*

Susceptibility Testing, Serum Bactericidal Dilution Method *see* Serum Bactericidal Test *on page 496*

Susceptibility Testing, Unusual Isolates/Fastidious Organisms *see* Antimicrobial Susceptibility Testing, Unusual Isolates/Fastidious Organisms *on page 452*

Swan-Ganz Tip Culture *see* Bacterial Culture, Intravascular Device *on page 463*

Synergistic Studies, Antimicrobial *see* Antimicrobial Susceptibility Testing, Antimicrobial Combinations *on page 449*

Synovial Fluid Culture *see* Bacterial Culture, Biopsy or Body Fluid *on page 456*

Synovial Fluid Fungus Culture *see* Fungal Culture, Biopsy or Body Fluid *on page 476*

Syphilis, Darkfield Examination *see* Darkfield Examination, Syphilis *on page 475*

TB Culture, Biopsy *see* Mycobacterial Culture, Biopsy or Body Fluid *on page 487*

TB Culture, Body Fluid *see* Mycobacterial Culture, Biopsy or Body Fluid *on page 487*

TB Culture, Skin *see* Mycobacterial Culture, Cutaneous and Subcutaneous Tissue *on page 489*

TB Culture, Sputum *see* Mycobacterial Culture, Sputum *on page 490*

TB Culture, Stool *see* Mycobacterial Culture, Stool *on page 491*

TB Culture, Urine *see* Mycobacterial Culture, Urine *on page 491*

TB Smear *see* Acid-Fast Stain *on page 446*

Throat Culture *see* Bacterial Culture, Throat *on page 468*

Throat Culture, *Candida albicans* *see* Bacterial Culture, Throat *on page 468*

Throat Culture for *Bordetella pertussis* *replaced by Bordetella pertussis* Culture *on page 471*

Throat Culture for *Corynebacterium diphtheriae* *see* Corynebacterium diphtheriae Throat Culture *on page 474*

Throat Culture for Group A Beta-Hemolytic *Streptococcus* *see* Bacterial Culture, Throat *on page 468*

Throat Swab for Group A Streptococcal Antigen *see* Group A *Streptococcus* Screen, Rapid *on page 483*

Tick Identification *see* Arthropod Identification *on page 453*

Tissue Culture *see* Bacterial Culture, Biopsy or Body Fluid *on page 456*

Tissue Fungus Culture *see* Fungal Culture, Biopsy or Body Fluid *on page 476*

Tissue Mycobacteria Culture *see* Mycobacterial Culture, Biopsy or Body Fluid *on page 487*

Tolerance Testing, Antimicrobial *see* Antimicrobial Susceptibility Testing, Minimum Bactericidal Concentration *on page 451*

Toxin A *see Clostridium difficile* Toxin Assay *on page 473*

Toxin Assay, *Clostridium difficile* *see Clostridium difficile* Toxin Assay *on page 473*

Tracheal Aspirate Culture *see* Bacterial Culture, Sputum *on page 465*

Transtracheal Aspiration *Legionella* Culture *see Legionella* Culture *on page 485*

***Treponema pallidum* Darkfield Examination** *see* Darkfield Examination, Syphilis *on page 475*

***Trichomonas* Culture** *see Trichomonas* Preparation *on this page*

***Trichomonas* Pap Smear** *see Trichomonas* Preparation *on this page*

Trichomonas Preparation

CPT 87210 (wet mount); 87211 (wet and dry mount)

Related Information
Bacterial Culture, Genital Specimen *on page 463*
Cervical/Vaginal Cytology *on page 290*

Synonyms Hanging Drop Mount for *Trichomonas*; *Trichomonas vaginalis* Wet Preparation

Applies to *Trichomonas* Culture; *Trichomonas* Pap Smear; Urethral *Trichomonas* Smear; Urine *Trichomonas* Wet Mount

Test Commonly Includes Wet mount and microscopic examination. Pap smear and/or culture may also be performed.

Specimen Vaginal, cervical, or urethral swabs, prostatic fluid, urine sediment

Container Sterile tube containing 1 mL of sterile nonbacteriostatic saline

Collection The specimen should be collected using a speculum without lubricant. The mucosa of the posterior vagina may be swabbed, or the secretions may be collected with a pipette. The swab should be expressed into saline for transport. The specimen should be examined as soon as possible.

Storage Instructions Do not refrigerate. Transport immediately to the laboratory so that viable motile organisms may be obtained.

Turnaround Time Same day; 48 hours if culture in Kupferberg's medium

Special Instructions Provide the specific source of the specimen to the laboratory.

Reference Range Negative: no trichomonads identified; positive: demonstration of actively motile flagellates, positive culture

Use Establish the presence of *Trichomonas vaginalis*

Limitations The specimen is examined for *Trichomonas vaginalis* only. A separate swab (Culturette®) must be collected for culture of bacteria or fungus cultures, if required. One negative result does not rule out the possibility of *Trichomonas vaginalis* infection. The wet mount is negative in 30% to 50%[1] of women with trichomoniasis. Culture is not available in many laboratories.

Contraindications Douching within 3 days prior to specimen collection

Methodology Wet mount microscopic examination, Pap smear, culture in Kupferberg's liquid medium or Hirsch charcoal agar, direct immunofluorescent technique with monoclonal antibody

Additional Information The absence of the classical yellow, frothy discharge does not exclude trichomoniasis. Culture may yield positive results when wet preparations are negative. Cultures are expensive and have limited availability.[2] The high rate of false-negatives, 48.4%, and false-positives observed with stained preparations (Pap smears) requires that confirmation by wet mount or culture be considered when the reported results are inconsistent with the clinical findings.[3] Culture provides similar sensitivity to wet mount methods,[4] although other studies have reported wet mount/cytology sensitivity of about 60%.[5] Immunofluorescence tests are being adopted which have increased sensitivity. The false-positives observed when immunofluorescent methods are compared to culture may represent failure of culture in patients with few organisms.

In a series of 600 "high risk" women, 88 *Trichomonas* infected patients were observed. Co-infection was noted as follows: *Ureaplasma urealyticum* 96%, *Gardnerella vaginalis* 91%, *Mycoplasma hominis* 89%, bacterial vaginosis 57%, *Neisseria gonorrhoeae* 29%, and *Chlamydia trachomatis* 15%. *Candida albicans* and other *Candida* sp are frequently implicated in vulvovaginitis.[1] A vaginal pH >5 is suggestive of *Trichomonas*.

In males, a milky white fluid discharge and urethral irritation present for more than 4 weeks is frequently associated with urethritis caused by *T. vaginalis*.

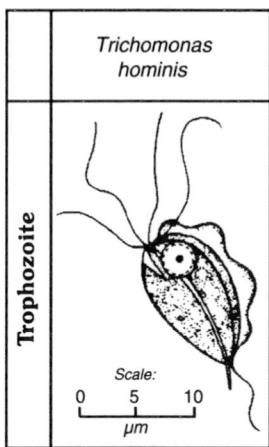

Trichomonas hominis — Trophozoite

Scale: 0 5 10 µm

From Brooks MM and Melvin DM, *Morphology of Diagnostic Stages of Intestinal Parasites of Humans*, 2nd ed, Atlanta, GA: U.S. Department of Health and Human Services, Publication No. 84-8116, Centers for Disease Control, 1984, with permission.

Footnotes

1. Bennett JR, "The Emergency Department Diagnosis of *Trichomonas vaginalis*," *Ann Emerg Med*, 1989, 18(5):564-6.
2. Beal C, Goldsmith R, Kotby M, et al, "The Plastic Envelope Method, A Simplified Technique for Culture Diagnosis of Trichomoniasis," *J Clin Microbiol*, 1992, 30(9):2265-8.
3. Borchardt KA, Hernandez V, Miller S, et al, "A Clinical Evaluation of Trichomoniasis in San Jose, Costa Rica Using the In Pouch TV Test," *Genitourin Med*, 1992, 68(5):328-30.
4. Bickley LS, Krisher KK, Ponsalang A Jr, et al, "Comparison of Direct Fluorescent Antibody, Acridine Orange, Wet Mount, and Culture for Detection of *Trichomonas vaginalis* in Women Attending a Public Sexually Transmitted Diseases Clinic," *Sex Transm Dis*, 1989, 16(3):127-31.
5. Krieger JN, Tam MR, Stevens CE, et al, "Diagnosis of Trichomoniasis. Comparison of Conventional Wet-Mount Examination With Cytologic Studies, Cultures, and Monoclonal Antibody Staining of Direct Specimens," *JAMA*, 1988, 259(8):1223-7.

References

Clay JC, Veeravahu M, and Smyth RW, "Practical Problems of Diagnosing Trichomoniasis in Women," *Genitourin Med*, 1988, 64(2):115-7.

Lossick JG, "The Diagnosis of Vaginal Trichomoniasis," *JAMA*, 1988, 259(8):1230.

Moldwin RM, "Sexually Transmitted Protozoal Infections. *Trichomonas vaginalis*, *Entamoeba histolytica*, and *Giardia lamblia*," *Urol Clin North Am*, 1992, 19(1):93-101.

Wolner-Hanssen P, Krieger JN, Stevens CE, et al, "Clinical Manifestations of Vaginal Trichomoniasis," *JAMA*, 1989, 261:571-6.

Trichomonas vaginalis Wet Preparation *see Trichomonas* Preparation *on previous page*

Tympanocentesis Culture *see* Bacterial Culture, Ear *on page 462*

Undulant Fever, Culture *see Brucella* Culture *on page 472*

Urease Test and Culture, Helicobacter pylori *see Helicobacter pylori* Urease Test and Culture *on page 484*

Urethral Trichomonas Smear *see Trichomonas* Preparation *on previous page*

Urine Anaerobic Culture, Suprapubic Puncture *see* Bacterial Culture, Urine, Suprapubic Puncture *on page 469*

Urine Culture, Clean Catch *see* Bacterial Culture, Urine, Clean Catch *on page 468*

Urine Culture, Foley Catheter *see* Bacterial Culture, Urine, Clean Catch *on page 468*

Urine Culture, Straight Catheter *see* Bacterial Culture, Urine, Suprapubic Puncture *on page 469*

Urine Culture, Suprapubic Puncture *see* Bacterial Culture, Urine, Suprapubic Puncture *on page 469*

Urine for Parasites *see* Ova and Parasites, Urine *on page 495*

Urine for Schistosoma haematobium *see* Ova and Parasites, Urine *on page 495*

Urine Fungus Culture *see* Fungal Culture, Urine *on page 480*

Urine Mycobacteria Culture *see* Mycobacterial Culture, Urine *on page 491*

Urine Trichomonas Wet Mount *see Trichomonas* Preparation *on previous page*

Uterus Anaerobic Culture *see* Bacterial Culture, Endometrium *on page 462*

Vaginal Culture *see* Bacterial Culture, Genital Specimen *on page 463*

Ventricular Fluid Culture *see* Bacterial Culture, Cerebrospinal Fluid *on page 460*

Whooping Cough Culture *see Bordetella pertussis* Culture *on page 471*

Wound Actinomyces Culture *see Actinomyces* Culture *on page 447*

Wound Culture *see* Bacterial Culture, Wound *on page 470*

Ziehl-Neelsen Stain *see* Acid-Fast Stain *on page 446*

MOLECULAR PATHOLOGY

Rebecca T. Horvat, PhD

Steven H. Hinrichs, MD

Lowell L. Tilzer, MD, PhD

Contributors:
Julia Bridge, MD
Diane Persons, MD
Patricia D. Murphy, PhD

Over the past few decades remarkable progress has been made in the field of molecular biology. This new technology is rapidly being translated into new diagnostic tests. Molecular biology has revealed much about the nature of the mechanisms involved in cancer and genetic diseases. Nucleic acid analysis has also aided in the identification of infectious microorganisms, especially those microorganisms that require tedious isolation or cannot be cultured. The progress in this area of diagnostic testing continues to grow with the advent of nucleic acid amplification technology. The most frequently used amplification procedure is the polymerase chain reaction (PCR), which is able to amplify a specific DNA target sequence in a short period of time. Several other amplification techniques have been developed that include amplification of the probe (ligase chain reaction (LCR)) or amplification of the signal detection method (bDNA). In addition, molecular probes have been developed that detect naturally amplified targets such as ribosomal RNA. These new amplification methods will allow greater usage of molecular detection in the clinical laboratory.

The cytogenetic analysis of cancer cells has lead to the identification of translocations, amplifications, deletions, and insertions associated with certain cancers. This has lead to the identification of oncogenes, antioncogenes, and genetic aberrations that are central to the process of malignant transformation. Genetic analysis is now used to study the DNA abnormalities associated with human tumors. Used diagnostically, these DNA studies can detect amplified oncogenes, translocations, mutations, deletions, and clonal rearrangements that can aid in the diagnosis and prognosis of several types of tumors. Likewise, cytogenetic analysis has identified certain mutations associated with inherited diseases such as fragile X syndrome and muscular dystrophy. These observations eventually led to the identification of the genes involved in these genetic abnormalities. These genetic diseases can now be detected by using DNA analysis. Several other genetic diseases can currently be detected by molecular analysis while many others are under investigation. Molecular biology will become a major facet in the future detection of inherited defects and analysis of tumors.

Another major area of diagnostic testing that has benefited from molecular technology is the identification of infectious microorganisms. Most infectious agents, both bacterial and viral, are present in specimens in very limited quantities unless they are first cultured. Some infectious microorganisms cannot be cultured or require long tedious incubations before they can be identified. The use of nucleic acid-based detection tests provide a distinct advantage in the diagnosis of infectious agents in that it provides a quick, accurate result. Molecular techniques in infectious disease are used for detection of antibiotic resistance, epidemiology, rapid assessment of bacteremia and meningitis, detection of bacteriuria, and rapid detection of viral infections. Nucleic acid-based tests have become automated and are displacing or supplementing many current methods of detecting infectious agents.

Adult Polycystic Kidney Disease DNA Detection

CPT 83890 (molecular isolation or extraction); 83894 (separation); 83896 (nucleic acid probe, each)

Related Information

Kidney Biopsy *on page 47*

Synonyms Adult Polycystic Kidney Disease Inheritance Determination With DNA Restriction Fragment Length Polymorphism Probes; Genetic Detection of Presymptomatic Adult Polycystic Kidney Disease; Molecular Diagnosis of Polycystic Kidney Disease; Polycystic Kidney Disease, Prenatal Diagnosis

Test Commonly Includes This test can detect DNA linkage association with the major genetic mutation (autosomal dominant polycystic kidney disease locus 1, ADPKD1) on chromosome 16. This gene is tightly linked with adult polycystic kidney disease, presently designated autosomal dominant PKD.

Abstract Autosomal dominant polycystic kidney disease (adult PKD) is a disorder characterized by the development of myriads of renal cysts. Although the biochemical nature of this disease is not known, DNA technology has been applied to families affected with this progressive disease. A linkage has been established in a large number of families with a gene on chromosome 16. The abnormal gene on the short arm of chromosome 16 is found in >95% of individuals with adult (autosomal dominant) polycystic disease. Individuals in families affected with this entity can now have genetic studies performed to determine their risk for developing the disease. Patients at high risk can then be followed closely. Such testing must be done only with genetic counseling.

Specimen Blood, amniotic fluid, chorionic villus, or tissue

Container Blood should be collected in yellow top (ACD) Vacutainer® tube; amniotic fluid and chorionic villus should be collected in a sterile manner and transferred to a sterile tube for transport or to a T25 culture flask; amniotic cells can be sent after culturing or can be sent directly to the laboratory.

Sampling Time Amniotic fluid should be collected between the 17th and 18th week of pregnancy. Chorionic villus specimens should be collected between the 8th and 12th week of gestation.

Storage Instructions All specimens should be sent to the laboratory **immediately** after collection, preferably by overnight delivery. All specimens should be kept at room temperature or refrigerated, never frozen.

Causes for Rejection Any amniotic fluid specimen that is bloody may be contaminated with maternal blood and is unsuitable for this test, any specimen that has been frozen before processing cannot be tested, specimens unlabeled or mislabeled

Turnaround Time Results are usually available after 3 weeks.

Reference Range The laboratory generally provides an interpretive report that includes a risk analysis.

Use This test is indicated for a family with history of autosomal dominant polycystic disease. For this purpose it is necessary to have a family pedigree that includes all medical histories. Test is also indicated for prenatal diagnosis in couples known to be carriers of the much less common recessive form of polycystic kidney disease, which has been called infantile PKD and is strongly associated with hepatic fibrosis and pulmonary maldevelopment. This test requires genetic testing of several family members (often as many as seven or eight) to determine the characteristic of the mutation.

Limitations DNA linkage analysis for polycystic kidney disease can detect the inheritance pattern associated with one of the major genes responsible for the disease. However, a negative result does not rule out the possibility that an individual may carry another mutation causing polycystic kidney disease or even be affected with polycystic kidney disease. However, the test can greatly lower that probability. Such testing is available only in a few reference laboratories.

Methodology DNA is isolated from the specimen. Several regions on chromosome 16 close to and flanking the ADPKD1 gene are examined using Southern blotting techniques. Restriction enzyme sites on the DNA close to the disease gene are examined. Genetic linkage analysis uses specific DNA probes to follow the inheritance of a gene associated with disease. This requires testing several members of a family, including both affected and unaffected individuals, preferably from several generations. The DNA probes used to follow the gene must be located very close to the disease gene and must show differences in the size of DNA that results from restriction enzyme digestion (polymorphic) between individuals from the same family (see figure). This allows for distinction between all the possible different chromosomes 16 that an individual could inherit; it can be determined from this information which chromosome is associated with disease. If these polymorphic sites are located very close to the disease gene then they are called "informative". The accuracy of genetic linkage analysis is greater if DNA probes on both sides of the disease gene are informative. The genetic linkage analysis

for polycystic kidney disease uses flanking markers very closely associated with ADPKD1, the gene associated with the disease.[1] Thus, in families in which this mutation is found, linkage analysis can very accurately predict inheritance of the disease gene (ADPKD1).

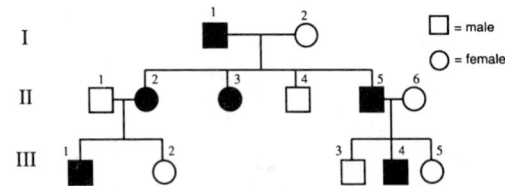

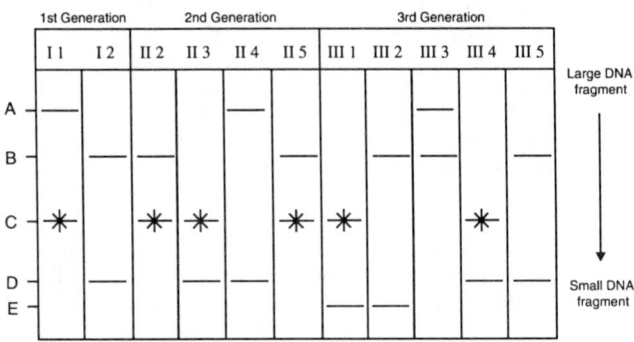

DNA is digested with restriction enzymes to make smaller pieces of DNA. This DNA is then electrophoresed in an agarose gel to separate DNA of different sizes (large to small). After transfer to a membrane, the DNA is hybridized with a radioactive DNA probe and hybridized DNA bands are visible with autoradiography. Inheritance patterns are noted that associate with disease (—✱—). Open symbols are normal individuals and shaded symbols are affected individuals.

Additional Information Autosomal dominant polycystic kidney disease is a common fatal inherited disorder which affects approximately 1 in 1000 people. Thus, each child born of an affected parent has a 50% chance of inheritance of the disease gene. Polycystic kidney disease is characterized by progressive increase and enlargement of numerous fluid-filled renal cysts. The growth of such cysts causes progressive impairment which usually leads to irreversible renal failure in middle age. In 40% to 70% of patients, cysts are also present in the liver. They are encountered sporadically in the pancreas, spleen, subarachnoid space, and pineal gland, and other abnormalities are described as well. The mechanism of cyst formation and the biochemical defect of the disease are currently not known. Genetic linkage studies with a large number of families (more than 50) have localized a disease-associated gene to the short arm of chromosome 16. The gene was designated autosomal dominant polycystic kidney disease locus 1 (ADPKD1).[2] Because the ADPKD1 gene has not been cloned, the nature of the exact genetic mutation is not known. Therefore, genetic analysis depends on indirect inference from linkage analysis. Individuals within a family with a history of autosomal dominant PKD must be analyzed in the context of the entire family to determine linkage. The family should be referred to a genetic counselor for advice in this regard. Several affected families have been described that show no linkage to this gene and no diagnosis would be possible using this test.[3,4]. Therefore, patients should be made aware that this test is not indicated for all affected families. A review of autosomal dominant polycystic kidney disease has recently been published.[5]

Footnotes

1. Reeders ST, Keith T, Green P, et al, "Regional Localization of the Autosomal Dominant Polycystic Kidney Disease Locus," *Genomics*, 1988, 3(3):150-5.
2. Reeders ST, Breuning MH, Davies KE, et al, "A Highly Polymorphic DNA Marker Linked to Adult Polycystic Kidney Disease on Chromosome 16," *Nature*, 1985, 317(6037):542-4.
3. Kimberling WJ, Fain PR, Kenyon JB, et al, "Linkage Heterogeneity of Autosomal Dominant Polycystic Kidney Disease," *N Engl J Med*, 1988, 319(14):913-8.
4. Romeo G, Costa G, Catizone L, et al, "A Second Genetic Locus for Autosomal Dominant Polycystic Kidney Disease," *Lancet*, 1988, 2(8601):8-11.
5. Gabow PA, "Autosomal Dominant Polycystic Kidney Disease," *Am J Kidney Dis*, 1993, 22(4):511-2.

References

Bear JC, Parfrey PS, Morgan JM, et al, "Autosomal Dominant Polycystic Kidney Disease: New Information for Genetic Counseling," *Am J Med Genet*, 1992, 43(3):548-53.

Grantham JJ, "Polycystic Kidney Disease," *The Principles and Practice of Nephrology*, Jacobson HR, Striker GE, and Klahr S, eds, Philadelphia, PA: BC Decker Inc, 1991, 370-3.

Kimberling WJ, Pieke-Dahl SA, and Kumar S, "The Genetics of Cystic Diseases of the Kidney," *Semin Nephrol*, 1991, 11(6):596-606.

Reeders ST, Germino GG, and Gillespie GA, "Mapping the Locus of Autosomal Dominant Polycystic Kidney Disease: Diagnostic Application," *Clin Chem*, 1989, 35(7 Suppl):B13-6.

Ye M and Grantham JJ, "The Secretion of Fluid by Renal Cysts From Patients With Autosomal Dominant Polycystic Kidney Disease," *N Engl J Med*, 1993, 329(5):310-3.

Adult Polycystic Kidney Disease Inheritance Determination With DNA Restriction Fragment Length Polymorphism Probes *see* Adult Polycystic Kidney Disease DNA Detection *on previous page*

B-Cell Lymphomas *see* bcl-2 Gene Rearrangement *on this page*

bcl-2 Gene Analysis *see* bcl-2 Gene Rearrangement *on this page*

bcl-2 Gene Rearrangement

CPT 83890 (molecular isolation or extraction); 83892 (enzymatic digestion); 83894 (separation); 83896 (nucleic acid probe, each)

Related Information
Gene Rearrangement for Leukemia and Lymphoma *on page 512*
Leukocyte Immunophenotyping *on page 414*
Lymph Node Biopsy *on page 50*
Polymerase Chain Reaction *on page 523*

Synonyms *bcl-2* Gene Analysis; Southern Blot of *bcl-2* Gene Rearrangement

Applies to B-Cell Lymphomas; Oncogenes

Test Commonly Includes Identification of unique DNA bands associated with the *bcl-2* oncogene rearrangement in B-cell lymphomas

Abstract Three types of oncogenes are recognized. Those which act as growth and proliferation regulatory genes include *myc*, *ras*, and *abl*. Those which inhibit growth and proliferation include Rb and *p53*. The *bcl-2* oncogene is among the third group. It codes for a protein that is located in the mitochondria of the cell. The *bcl-2* protein regulates cell death and when it is overexpressed the cell is resistant to the "natural" death cycle, called apoptosis. The rearrangement of the *bcl-2* gene with the B-cell receptor genes are found in a number of different B-cell lymphomas. This translocation can be identified cytogenetically as t(14;18) in follicular lymphomas, its original relationship, or large diffuse lymphomas.[1]

Specimen 0.1 g or more of frozen tissue, specifically from the involved area of the lymph node or tumor

Container Tissue must be shipped on dry ice or in 95% ethanol.

Collection Tissue must be carefully cut from the surgically removed tumor and contain at least 10% of tumor cells from the involved area.

Storage Instructions Tissue can be stored in a -70°C freezer until shipped.

Causes for Rejection Tissue samples that have thawed during transit cannot be used for DNA analysis. DNA cannot be isolated from tissue that has been fixed in formalin or paraffin.

Turnaround Time Results are usually available 10 days to 2 weeks.

Reference Range No rearrangement of *bcl-2* is normal.

Use Detect *bcl-2* rearrangement in B-cell lymphomas, in both frozen and paraffin sections. It is used most to distinguish follicular lymphoma from follicular hyperplasia in lymphoid tissue. Reactive follicles are negative to *bcl-2*. The *bcl-2* rearrangement is found in follicular lymphomas, large diffuse B-cell lymphomas, and undifferentiated lymphomas. Usually this rearrangement also involves a reciprocal translocation with the J_H region on chromosome 14, thus forming t(14;18). Abnormal expression of *bcl-2* has been found in solid malignant neoplasms as well. With HPV, it may play a role in early stages of tumorigenesis in the uterine cervix.[2]

Limitations Rearrangement will not be found if the tissue is not from the involved tumor. Tissue samples that are too small will not yield enough DNA to do an accurate Southern blot analysis. The method is not useful to distinguish follicular lymphomas from other lymphoma cell types.

Methodology DNA is extracted from the clinical sample and digested with restriction enzymes. The digested fragments of DNA are electrophoresed in an agarose gel and then transferred to a nylon membrane by Southern blotting. The DNA on the membrane is hybridized with a labeled DNA probe specific for the *bcl-2* gene. Hybridization of the *bcl-2* probe is detected using autoradiography or enzymatic color development. Clinical samples are always compared to a normal control sample that does not have a *bcl-2* rearrangement. Hybridization to a DNA fragment different from the control sample typically indicates a rearranged *bcl-2* gene. PCR with conventional gel electrophoresis is now commonly used.

In immunohistochemical application, *bcl-2* is best in B5 and Bouin fixed tissues, unless microwaved.

Additional Information The protein coded for by the oncogene, *bcl-2*, acts by suppressing the cell death program or apoptosis.[3] Its role involves control of cell growth. Apoptosis occurs in all cells but is especially important in immune and hematopoietic cells, which have a high cell turnover rate. When the *bcl-2* gene is overexpressed, it will act to

prevent apoptosis and possibly may render cells resistant to cell death by irradiation and certain chemotherapeutic agents.[4,5] A translocation between immunoglobulin genes (heavy chain or light chain genes) and *bcl-2* results in the overexpression of *bcl-2* protein and thus the expansion of B cells due to halting cell death. This type of translocation is found in 100% in small cleaved type, 76% to 85% in mixed cell and 59% to 75% in large cell types. It is found in some cases of chronic lymphocytic leukemia, acute lymphoblastic leukemia, and small noncleaved cell lymphoma as well as cases of Hodgkin's lymphoma[6] and myeloid neoplasms. The t(14;18) is rarely detected in monocytoid B-cell lymphoma and MALT lymphomas. *bcl-2* is not pathognomic for lymphomas. It is found in 10% of reactive lymph nodes, and in some normal cells (eg, lymphoid and myeloid precursors, medullary thymocytes, most T cells, nongerminal center B cells, and plasma cells). It is not expressed in reactive germinal centers.

Increased *bcl-2* protein is reported in some carcinomas of prostate.[7]

Footnotes
1. Weiss LM, Warnke RA, Sklar J, et al, "Molecular Analysis of the t(14;18) Chromosomal Translocation in Malignant Lymphomas," *N Engl J Med*, 1987, 317(19):1185-9.
2. Saegusa M, Takano Y, Hashimura M, et al, "The Possible Role of *bcl-2* Expression in the Progression of Tumors of the Uterine Cervix," *Cancer*, 1995, 76(11):2297-303.
3. Cohen JJ, "Programmed Cell Death in the Immune System," *Adv Immunol*, 1991, 50:55-85.
4. Strasser A, Harris AW, and Cory S, "*bcl-2* Transgene Inhibits T-Cell Death and Perturbs Thymic Self-Censorship," *Cell*, 1992, 67(5):889-99.
5. Sentman CL, Shutter JR, Hockenbery D, et al, "*bcl-2* Inhibits Multiple Forms of Apoptosis but Not Negative Selection in Thymocytes," *Cell*, 1992, 67(5):879-88.
6. Lones MA, Pinkus GS, Shintaku IP, et al, "*bcl-2* Oncogene Protein Is Preferentially Expressed in Reed-Sternberg Cells in Hodgkin's Disease of the Nodular Sclerosis Subtype," *Am J Clin Pathol*, 1994, 102(4):464-7.
7. Kalakury BVS, Figge J, Leibovich B, et al, "Increased *bcl-2* Protein Levels in Prostatic Adenocarcinomas Are Not Associated With Rearrangements in the 2.8 kb Major Breakpoint Region or With *p53* Protein Accumulation," *Mod Pathol*, 1996, 9(1):41-7.

References
Chaganti RSK, Doucette LA, Offit K, et al, "Specific Translocations in non-Hodgkin's Lymphoma: Incidence, Molecular Detection, and Histological and Clinical Correlations," *Cancer Cells*, Vol 7, Furth ME and Greaves MF, eds, 1989, 33-6.
Corbally N, Grogan L, Keane MM, et al, "*Bcl-2* Rearrangement in Hodgkin's Disease and Reactive Lymph Nodes," *Am J Clin Pathol*, 1994, 101(6):756-60.
Crisan D, "*bcl-2* Gene Rearrangements in Lymphoid Malignancies," *Clin Lab Med*, 1996, 16(1):23-47.
Inghirami G and Frizzera G, "Role of the *bcl-2* Oncogene in Hodgkin's Disease," editorial, *Am J Clin Pathol*, 1994, 101(6):681-3.
Mies C, "Molecular Biological Analysis of Paraffin-Embedded Tissues," *Hum Pathol*, 1994, 25(6):555-60.
Pezzella F and Gatter K, "What Is the Value of *bcl-2* Protein Detection for Histopathologists?" *Histopathology*, 1995, 26(1):89-93.
Warnke RA, Weiss LM, Chan JK, et al, "Tumors of the Lymph Nodes and Spleen," *Atlas of Tumor Pathology*, 3rd Series, Fascicle 14, Washington, DC: Armed Forces Institute of Pathology, 1995.
Yanis JJ, "*bcl-2* Oncogene Rearrangement in Follicular and Diffuse Large-Cell and Mixed-Cell Lymphoma," *Cancer Cells*, Vol 7, Furth ME and Greaves MF, eds, 1989, 37-40.

Borrelia burgdorferi DNA Assay *see* Lyme Disease DNA Detection *on page 518*

Borrelia burgdorferi DNA Probe Test *see* Lyme Disease DNA Detection *on page 518*

BRCA1 Gene Testing *see* Breast Cancer, Hereditary (BRCA1) *on next page*

Breakpoint Cluster Rearrangement *see* Breakpoint Cluster Region Rearrangement in CML *on this page*

Breakpoint Cluster Region Rearrangement in CML

CPT 83890 (molecular isolation or extraction); 83892 (enzymatic digestion); 83894 (separation); 83896 (nucleic acid probe, each)

Related Information
Bone Marrow *on page 307*
Chromosome Analysis, Blood *on page 276*
Chromosome Analysis, Bone Marrow *on page 277*
Leukocyte Alkaline Phosphatase *on page 330*
Leukocyte Cytochemistry *on page 331*
Polymerase Chain Reaction *on page 523*

Synonyms Breakpoint Cluster Rearrangement; Chronic Myelogenous Leukemia; Gene Rearrangement, *bcr*

Applies to Oncogenes; Philadelphia Chromosome

Test Commonly Includes DNA detection of chromosomal translocation associated with chronic myelogenous leukemia (CML)

Abstract Chronic myelogenous leukemia (CML) is a myeloproliferative disorder characterized by the transformation of pluripotent hematopoietic stem cells. Ninety percent to 95% of the CML cases have a translocation between chromosome 9 and chromosome 22. This chromosomal translocation results in an abnormal gene rearrangement that can be detected (Continued)

Breakpoint Cluster Region Rearrangement in CML (Continued)

using nucleic acid technology. The translocation involves a rearrangement of the breakpoint cluster region (bcr) gene located on chromosome 22 with the c-abl oncogene on chromosome 9. The hybrid bcr/c-abl gene is transcribed into an abnormal messenger RNA which is translated into an abnormal tyrosine kinase of 210,000 molecular weight instead of the normal 160,000 molecular weight protein. Most patients with clinically documented CML that lack the Philadelphia chromosome still have the bcr/c-abl rearrangement. A small number of patients do not have the Philadelphia chromosome as the bcr/c-abl rearrangement. During reassessment many of these patients have a myelodysplastic syndrome, usually chronic myelomonocytic leukemia. A very small number of patients with clinical CML remain both Philadelphia chromosome negative and bcr/c-abl negative.

Specimen Blood or bone marrow

Container Blood should be collected in a lavender top (EDTA) Vacutainer® tube; bone marrow should be collected in a syringe with heparin or transferred to a green top (heparin) tube or lavender top (EDTA) tube.

Turnaround Time 1-2 weeks

Reference Range No rearrangement observed

Use This test is used for the confirmation of CML along with bone marrow examination, cytogenetics, and leukocyte alkaline phosphatase score.

The bcr/c-abl rearrangement assay is clinically useful for:
- confirmation of Philadelphia chromosome-positive CML
- diagnosis of Philadelphia-negative CML
- diagnosis and monitoring of CML blast crisis during and after chemotherapy as bone marrow transplantation
- detection of remission or early detection of relapse Characterize and monitor chronic myelogenous leukemia (CML)

Methodology Leukocyte DNA is extracted, cut with restriction enzymes, electrophoresed in agarose, and then transferred to membranes using the Southern blot method. The membrane is hybridized with a gene probe that will bind only to the target bcr gene on the membrane. The banding pattern is developed by autoradiography or color detection methods. Detection of this translocation is also accomplished by reverse transcription polymerase chain reaction (RT-PCR). The RNA from patients' cells is extracted and transcribed into copy DNA (cDNA). The cDNA is then amplified by PCR with specific primers to detect the bcr-abl translocation.[1]

Additional Information Chronic myelogenous leukemia (CML) is characterized by a reciprocal translocation between chromosomes 9 and 22 producing the Philadelphia chromosome. The translocation involves a gene rearrangement of the breakpoint cluster region (bcr) gene located on chromosome 22 with the c-abl oncogene on chromosome 9.[2] The hybrid bcr/c-abl gene is transcribed into an abnormal messenger RNA which is translated into an abnormal tyrosine kinase of 210,000 molecular weight instead of the normal 160,000 molecular weight protein. More than 90% of patients with CML have the Philadelphia chromosome by cytogenetic analysis as well as the rearrangement of the bcr/c-abl. Most patients with clinically documented CML that lack the Philadelphia chromosome still have the bcr/c-abl rearrangement. A small number of patients do not have the Philadelphia chromosome as the bcr/c-abl rearrangement. During reassessment many of these patients have a myelodysplastic syndrome, usually chronic myelomonocytic leukemia. A very small number of patients with clinical CML remain both Philadelphia chromosome negative and bcr/c-abl negative.

Cytogenetically the Philadelphia chromosome has been found in 20% to 25% of patients with acute lymphoblastic leukemia (ALL) and 2% of patients with acute myelogenous leukemia (AML).[3] The Philadelphia chromosome from ALL cases appears similar to CML Philadelphia chromosomes in cytogenetic analysis. However, the two chromosomes result from distinct molecular rearrangements that can be analyzed and detected with DNA analysis. Some ALL Philadelphia chromosomes have been found to be identical to the CML Philadelphia chromosome even at the molecular level. These ALL cases are generally regarded as the blast crisis of CML.[4]

Some laboratories now provide a DNA amplification assay (PCR) for detection of this translocation. This is helpful in the detection of minimal residual disease.[5]

Footnotes
1. Tilzer LL and Concepcion EG, "Detection of the Gene Rearrangement in Chronic Myelogenous Leukemia With Biotinylated Gene Probes," Am J Clin Pathol, 1989, 91(4):464-7.
2. Groffen J, Stephenson JR, Heisterkamp N, et al, "Philadelphia Chromosome Breakpoints Are Clustered Within a Limited Region, bcr, on Chromosome 22," Cell, 1984, 36(1):93-9.
3. Kurzrock R, Gutterman J, and Talpaz M, "The Molecular Genetics of Philadelphia Chromosome-Positive Leukemias," N Engl J Med, 1988, 319(15):990-8.

4. Saikevych I, Timson L, Denny C, et al, "Philadelphia Chromosome Positive (Ph⁺) Leukemias With p210 bcr-abl and p185 bcr-abl May Be Distinct Disorders," Blood, 1989, 74:79a.
5. Lee MS, Chang KS, Freireich EJ, et al, "Detection of Minimal Residual bcr/abl Transcripts by a Modified Polymerase Chain Reaction," Blood, 1988, 72(3):893-7.

References
Brunning RD and McKenna RW, "Tumors of the Bone Marrow," Atlas of Tumor Pathology, 3rd Series, Fascicle 9, Washington, DC: Armed Forces Institute of Pathology, 1994.
Crisan D and Carr ER, "bcr/abl Gene Rearrangement in Chronic Myelogenous Leukemia and Acute Leukemias," Lab Med, 1992, 23:730-6.
Groffen J, Hermans A, Grosveld G, et al, "Molecular Analysis of Chromosome Breakpoints," Prog Nucleic Acid Res Mol Biol, 1989, 36:281-300.
McClure JS and Litz CE, "Chronic Myelogenous Leukemia: Molecular Diagnostic Considerations," Hum Pathol, 1994, 25(6):594-7.
Watson JD, Hopkin NA, Roberts JW, et al, Molecular Biology of the Gene, 4th ed, Menlo Park, CA: Benjamin/Cummings, 1987, 1058-94.

Breast Cancer, Hereditary (BRCA1)

CPT 83890 (nuclear molecular diagnostics, molecular isolation or extraction); 83894 (enzymatic digestion); 83898 (nucleic acid probe with amplification); 83912 (interpretation and report)

Related Information
Ataxia-Telangiectasia, Chromosome Breakage Study on page 274
Breast Biopsy on page 35
CA 15-3 on page 93
Chromosome Analysis, Lymph Node and Solid Tumor on page 279
p53, Functional Assay/Sequencing on page 522

Synonyms BRCA1 Gene Testing; Familial Breast/Ovarian Cancer

Test Commonly Includes This molecular test involves end-to-end sequencing and/or protein truncation assay to detect carriers of mutations in the gene.

Abstract BRCA1 maps to 17q and was cloned in 1994.[1] A second gene on 13q also conferring an increased risk for breast cancer, BRCA2, has recently been cloned[2] but is not yet clinically available. A database of known mutations in these two genes is available on the Internet.[3] Sequencing is considered the most accurate method of mutation detection.

Specimen Whole blood

Container Blue top (sodium citrate) tube or yellow top (ACD) tube

Storage Instructions All specimens should be sent to the laboratory **immediately** after collection, preferably by overnight delivery. All specimens should be kept at room temperature or refrigerated, never frozen.

Causes for Rejection Lysed or frozen blood sample

Turnaround Time Results are available in phases: top three mutations: 2-3 weeks; exon 11: 8 additional weeks; rest of the gene: 6-10 weeks

Use The laboratory generally provides an interpretive report based upon direct sequencing analysis and/or the protein truncation assay. This test is indicated for families with a history of autosomal dominant early-onset breast/ovarian cancer (ie, identification of those with high risk).

Limitations While the methods for detection of BRCA1 mutations are extremely accurate, BRCA1 testing is currently available only in investigational settings. In part, this is because such settings provide the necessary structure to ensure that the patient is informed of the risks and benefits of testing and to orchestrate the provision of appropriate genetic counseling. In addition, clinical interpretation of the results of BRCA1 testing can be complex. Once a BRCA1 mutation is identified in an affected family member, testing of asymptomatic at-risk relatives is virtually 100% sensitive and specific. However, since there are multiple genes associated with breast cancer, if a high-risk affected woman tests negative for BRCA1 mutation, an inherited form of breast cancer may still exist, and she should be counseled accordingly.

This detection method is costly.

Methodology DNA and/or RNA are isolated from the specimen. A protein truncation assay will detect mutations that cause shortened protein products.[4] Regions within the BRCA1 gene are amplified by PCR and sequenced in entirety.

Additional Information Breast cancer is one of the most common diseases in women. The lifetime risk for a woman in the United States to develop breast cancer is 1 in 9 (11%). A positive family history of breast cancer increases risk. The empiric risk increases with the strength of the family history and with earlier ages of onset (premenopausal). Although the occurrence of breast cancer **in families** may be due to chance alone or shared environment, the inheritance of a gene mutation increasing susceptibility to breast cancer is the most common reason. About 10% of all breast cancer is believed to be due to an autosomal dominant gene mutation. In October of 1994, BRCA1, the first gene conferring an increased risk for the development of breast and ovarian cancer, was cloned.[1] It is estimated that 1 in 200 to 1 in 400 women carry BRCA1 mutations. Mutations in BRCA1 are thought to be responsible for about 50% of all inherited breast cancer and about 85% to 90% of breast/ovarian family histories.[5] The lifetime risk for breast cancer in a woman who has inherited a mutation in BRCA1 is about 85% by age 85 as opposed to 11% for women in the general population, and the risk for ovarian cancer is about 45% compared to 1% in the general population.[6] Once breast cancer has been diagnosed, the risk for carcinoma in the contralateral breast is about 60%. Breast and ovarian cancer survival rates are significantly better when diagnosis occurs in an early, localized stage.

When a BRCA1 mutation is identified in a family, asymptomatic, at-risk women should be offered testing. Women found to carry the mutation should be encouraged to undergo earlier and more intensive surveillance for breast cancer, which is expected to lead to earlier detection and improved outcome. Some women may consider the option of prophylactic surgery (mastectomy and/or oophorectomy). BRCA1 testing can help rule out family members who, because they do not carry the mutation, do not require increased surveillance. Men who carry a BRCA1 mutation appear not to be at great risk for breast cancer but are at increased risk for prostate and colon cancer. (Women are also at greater risk of colon cancer.)

See listing Breast Biopsy *on page 35.*

Footnotes
1. Miki Y, Swensen J, Shattuck-Eidens D, et al, "A Strong Candidate for the Breast and Ovarian Cancer Susceptibility Gene BRCA1," *Science*, 1994, 266(5182):66-71.
2. Wooster R, Bignell G, Lancaster J, et al, "Identification of the Breast Cancer Susceptibility Gene BRCA2," *Nature*, 1995, 378(6559):789-92.
3. Friend S, Borresen AL, Brody L, et al, "Breast Cancer Information on the Web," *Nat Genet*, 1995, 11(3):238-9.
4. Hogervorst FB, Cornelis RS, Bout M, et al, "Rapid Detection of BRCA1 Mutations by the Protein Truncation Test," *Nat Genet*, 1995, 10(2):208-12.
5. Narod SA, Ford D Devilee P, et al, "An Evaluatio of Genetic Heterogeneity in 145 Breast-Ovarian Cancer Families. Breast Cancer Linkage Consortium," *Am J Hum Genet*, 1995, 56(1):254-64.
6. Easton DF, Ford D, and Bishop DT, "Breast and Ovarian Cancer Incidence in BRCA1-Mutation Carriers. Breast Cancer Linkage Consortium," *Am J Hum Genet*, 1995, 56(1):265-71.

References
Castilla LH, Couch FJ, Erdos MR, et al, "Mutations in the BRCA1 Gene in Families With Early-Onset Breast and Ovarian Cancer," *Nat Genet*, 1994, 8(4):387-91.
Friedman LS, Ostermeyer EA, Szabo CI, et al, "Confirmation of BRCA1 by Analysis of Germline Mutations Linked to Breast and Ovarian Cancer in Ten Families," *Nat Genet*, 1994, 8(4):399-404.
Lerman C, Daly M, Masny A, et al, "Attitudes About Genetic Testing for Breast-Ovarian Cancer Susceptibility," *J Clin Oncol*, 1994, 12(4):843-50.
National Advisory Council for Human Genome Research, "Statement on Use of DNA Testing for Presymptomatic Identification of Cancer Risk," *JAMA*, 1994, 271(10):785.
Shattuck-Eidens D, McClure M, Simard J, et al, "A Collaborative Survey of 80 Mutations in the BRCA1 Breast and Ovarian Cancer Susceptibility Gene. Implications for Presymptomatic Testing and Screening," *JAMA*, 1995, 273(7):535-41.
Simard J, Tonin P, Durocher F, et al, "Common Origins of BRCA1 Mutations in Canadian Breast and Ovarian Cancer Families," *Nat Genet*, 1994, 8(4):392-8.
Wooster R, Neuhausen SL, Mangion J, et al, "Localization of a Breast Cancer Susceptibility Gene, BRCA2, to Chromosome 13q12-13," *Science*, 1994, 265(5181):2088-90.

***Chlamydia* Ligase Chain Reaction (LCR)** *see Chlamydia trachomatis* Genome Detection *on this page*

***Chlamydia* PCR** *see Chlamydia trachomatis* Genome Detection *on this page*

***Chlamydia trachomatis* DNA Detection Test** *see Chlamydia trachomatis* Genome Detection *on this page*

Chlamydia trachomatis Genome Detection
CPT 87179

Related Information
Bacterial Culture, Conjunctiva *on page 461*
Bacterial Culture, Endometrium *on page 462*
Bacterial Culture, Genital Specimen *on page 463*
Chlamydia Group Titer *on page 383*
Chlamydia trachomatis Culture *on page 662*
Chlamydia trachomatis Direct FA Test *on page 663*
Lymphogranuloma Venereum Titer *on page 417*
Neisseria gonorrhoeae Culture and Smear *on page 492*
Neisseria gonorrhoeae Genome Detection *on page 521*
Polymerase Chain Reaction *on page 523*
Synovial Fluid Analysis *on page 656*
Viral Culture *on page 675*
Viral Culture, Eye or Ocular Symptoms *on page 679*
Viral Culture, Urogenital *on page 681*

Synonyms *Chlamydia* Ligase Chain Reaction (LCR); *Chlamydia* PCR; *Chlamydia trachomatis* DNA Detection Test; *Chlamydia trachomatis* Molecular Probe Assay; DNA Hybridization Test for *Chlamydia trachomatis*; DNA Test for *Chlamydia trachomatis*; PACE2®

Test Commonly Includes Detection of *Chlamydia trachomatis* nucleic acid in clinical specimens

Abstract *Chlamydia trachomatis* is the most common sexually transmitted bacterial infection. Between 60 and 70 million new cases occur annually worldwide. *Chlamydia* infections may be asymptomatic in up to 70% of women and 30% of men. Disease and infection is associated with a high rate of tubal pregnancies, pelvic inflammatory disease, and infertility. *Chlamydia* also causes a severe infection of the eye which, if untreated, may lead to blindness. While in the past, *Chlamydia trachomatis* had been principally diagnosed by culture or immunoassay, the commercial availability of two assays employing molecular approaches has significantly altered the standard approach for detection of this agent. The Roche Amplicor assay utilizes the PCR technique for amplification of the bacterial genome, whereas the GenProbe Pace II assay detects ribosomal RNA of the organism (rRNA). A third recently developed clinical assay, Abbott LCx, utilizes the ligase chain reaction technique for amplification of the chlamydial genome. In addition to their use on swab specimens of eye, cervix, and urethra, the new assays are sufficiently sensitive to detect organism in the urine of infected individuals.

Specimen Either direct swabs of a potentially infected site or urine may be used depending on the assay. A swab specimen may be collected from the genital/urinary tract of males or females or a specimen may consist of a swab of the conjunctiva and sclera. Commercial assays have also been approved for detection of *Chlamydia* from urine. Although rectum and the nasal pharynx are also sites that may be infected by *Chlamydia*, swabs of these sites have not been approved for use with molecular assays.

Container Special collection and transport kits are an integral component of the assay and must be used with the appropriate commercial detection assay. A commercial kit typically contains a swab and a transport media or device.

Collection Two swabs are provided in the typical commercial kit for use in females. The cervix or endocervix is first cleaned with one swab and the second swab is used to collect the specimen. The swab is inserted into the endocervical canal and rotated to collect epithelial cells from the infected site. The swab is then placed into transport media and sent to the laboratory. In males, the swab is inserted into the urethral meatus and rotated to collect epithelial cells. The swab is then placed into transport media and sent to the laboratory.

Storage Instructions These specimens may be contained at room temperature and sent without freezing to the laboratory. Specimens collected for commercial molecular assays are typically stable for up to 1 week after collection.

Causes for Rejection Collection of a specimen from a nonapproved site; some assays cannot detect genomic material if the specimen contains excess blood.

Turnaround Time Results are usually available within 24 hours.

Reference Range Negative for *Chlamydia trachomatis*

Use The rapid detection of *C. trachomatis* in clinical specimens. The sensitivity of the test exceeds that for culture and other nonmolecular assays.

Limitations Results by molecular assays have not been accepted as evidence by the courts and legal system.

Methodology Three separate molecular assays have been approved or are under review by the Food and Drug Administration. An assay for *Chlamydia* was the first PCR test licensed by the FDA in 1993. The PCR detects the presence of *Chlamydia* DNA following extraction, denaturation, and hybridization with a specific DNA probe. The presence of bound probe is detected using an immunochemical technique. The ligase chain reaction procedure incorporates the extraction and denaturation of DNA followed by specific amplification through the ligation of two segments of the target. Detection is similar to that for PCR. The GenProbe assay detects the presence of ribosomal RNA which is in vast excess to single copy genes of an organism. The probe incorporates a chemiluminescent chemical which upon activation emits light. Various instrumentation is utilized by each of the three methodologies and various aspects of the assay have been automated.

Additional Information The molecular probe assays provide several advantages over traditional culture assays or antibody-based tests. One of the most significant advantages is the ability to detect nonviable organisms since only the presence of nucleic acids is necessary. This latter property also minimizes the need to rapidly transfer the specimen to culture media or cells. The sensitivity of molecular assays may either equal or significantly exceed that of culture techniques depending upon the prevalence of disease and the site of collection. The ability to detect organisms in urine provides an additional advantage over alternative methods and may have a significant impact on public health attempts at limiting the spread of disease. A major disadvantage to molecular assays is the lack of acceptance by the legal community and court system, and currently the results of molecular assays have not been accepted as evidence.

Footnotes
1. Thomson SE and Washington AE, "Epidemiology of Sexually Transmitted *Chlamydia trachomatis* Infections," *Epidemiol Rev*, 1983, 5:96-123.

(Continued)

Chlamydia trachomatis Genome Detection

(Continued)

2. Limberger RJ, Biega R, Evancoe A, et al, "Evaluation of Culture and the GenProbe PACE2 Assay for Detection of *Neisseria gonorrhoeae* and *Chlamydia trachomatis* in Endocervical Specimens Transported to a State Health Laboratory," *J Clin Microbiol*, 1992, 30(5):1162-6.
3. "*Chlamydia trachomatis* Infections. Policy Guidelines for Prevention and Control," *MMWR Morb Mortal Wkly Rep*, 1985, 34(Suppl 3):53S-74S.
4. Dean D, Palmer L, Pant CR, et al, "Use of a *Chlamydia trachomatis* DNA Probe for Detection of Ocular Chlamydiae," *J Clin Microbiol*, 1989, 27(5):1062-7.
5. Iwen PC, Blair TM, and Woods GL, "Comparison of the GenProbe PACE2 System, Direct Fluorescent Antibody, and Cell Culture for Detecting *Chlamydia trachomatis* in Cervical Specimens," *Am J Clin Pathol*, 1991, 95(4):578-82.
6. LeBar W, Herschman B, Jemal C, et al, "Comparison of DNA Probe, Monoclonal Antibody Enzyme Immunoassay and Cell Culture for the Detection of *Chlamydia trachomatis*," *J Clin Microbiol*, 1989, 27(5):826-8.

References

Barnes RC, "Laboratory Diagnosis of Human Chlamydial Infections," *Clin Microbiol Rev*, 1989, 2(2):119-36.

Dembry LM and Zervos MJ, "Molecular Biologic Techniques: Applications to the Clinical Microbiology Laboratory," *Lab Med*, 1992, 23:743-51.

Ehret JM and Judson FN, "Genital *Chlamydia* Infections," *Clin Lab Med*, 1989, 9(3):481-500.

Mahony JB, "Multiplex Polymerase Chain Reaction for the Diagnosis of Sexually Transmitted Diseases," *Clin Lab Med*, 1996, 16(1):61-71.

Peterson EM, Oda R, Alexander R, et al, "Molecular Techniques for the Detection of *Chlamydia trachomatis*," *J Clin Microbiol*, 1989, 27(10):2359-63.

Chlamydia trachomatis Molecular Probe Assay *see Chlamydia trachomatis* Genome Detection *on previous page*

Chronic Myelogenous Leukemia *see* Breakpoint Cluster Region Rearrangement in CML *on page 503*

CMV DNA Detection *see* Cytomegalovirus DNA Detection *on page 508*

CMV Quantitation *see* Cytomegalovirus DNA Detection *on page 508*

Colon Cancer, Hereditary Nonpolyposis Type

CPT 83890 (nuclear molecular diagnostics, molecular isolation or extraction); 83894 (enzymatic digestion); 83898 (nucleic acid probe with amplification); 83912 (interpretation and report)

Related Information
Carcinoembryonic Antigen *on page 100*
Chromosome Analysis, Lymph Node and Solid Tumor *on page 279*
Occult Blood, Stool *on page 645*

Synonyms Hereditary Nonpolyposis Colon Cancer; HNPCC Gene Testing; Nonpolyposis Type Colon Cancer

Test Commonly Includes This molecular test involves end-to-end sequencing of four genes in a sequential fashion: MSH2, MLH1, PMS1, and PMS2.

Abstract Polyposis and nonpolyposis syndromes include HNPCC types I and II, as well as other entities.

Mutations in at least four genes (MSH2[1], MLH1[2], PMS1, PMS2) are known to cause hereditary nonpolyposis colon cancer (HNPCC). Sequencing is the most accurate method for detection of mutations. Ninety percent of HNPCC mutations are found in MSH2 and MLH1.

Specimen Whole blood

Container Blue top (sodium citrate) tube or yellow top (ACD) tube

Storage Instructions All specimens should be sent to the laboratory **immediately** after collection, preferably by overnight delivery. All specimens should be kept at room temperature or refrigerated, never frozen.

Causes for Rejection Lysed or frozen blood sample

Turnaround Time Results are available in phases: MSH2: 6 weeks; MLH1: 6 additional weeks; PMS1 and PMS2 together: 4 additional weeks

Use The laboratory generally provides an interpretive report based upon direct sequencing analysis and/or the protein truncation assay. This test is indicated for families with a history of nonpolyposis colon cancer in an autosomal dominant pattern.

Limitations Because the genes for HNPCC have only recently been identified, HNPCC testing is much newer and is generally available only in investigational settings. Such settings provide the structure needed to assure that patients are adequately informed of the risks and benefits of testing and orchestrate the provision of genetic counseling. Such testing is costly. The cost of detecting gene mutations associated with HNPCC in a family depends on the number of genes which need to be sequenced.

Methodology DNA is isolated from the specimen. Regions within the MSH2, MLH1, PMS1, and PMS2 genes are amplified by PCR and sequenced in entirety.

Additional Information Colorectal carcinoma (CRC) ranks second as a cause of cancer deaths in the United States. Approximately 56,000

deaths are presently projected annually. A positive family history of CRC increases risk. The empiric risk increases with the strength of the family history and with earlier ages of onset. As a result, increased surveillance in first degree relatives of an individual with CRC is currently recommended for early detection of CRC. Five-year survival rates are substantially higher for localized CRC. Survival in asymptomatic patients is greater. About 15% to 20% of CRC may be due to an autosomal dominant mutation. Two of the types of inherited CRC are hereditary nonpolyposis colon cancer (HNPCC) and familial adenomatous polyposis coli (FAP). HNPCC is characterized by CRC in the absence of large numbers of polyps, early age of onset (mean 40-45 years of age), mucinous and poorly differentiated tumors, and an excess of tumors in the proximal colon. (Carcinoma develops early in polyps associated with HNPCC.) The lifetime risk for CRC in individuals who inherit a mutation associated with HNPCC is >90%. In addition, individuals with type II HNPCC are at increased risk for extracolonic cancers including tumors of endometrium, stomach, pancreaticobiliary system, ovary, small intestine, skin, bone marrow, larynx, and upper urological tract.[3,4] Because there are no distinguishing characteristics of HNPCC, historically the diagnosis has been made on the basis of the family history. The "Amsterdam Criteria" were developed to provide a uniform clinical method of diagnosis.[5] These criteria include histologically-verified CRC in three or more relatives, one of whom is a first-degree relative of the other two; CRC in at least two generations; and at least one CRC diagnosed before the age of 50. The limitations of the Amsterdam Criteria as a means of diagnosis became apparent upon the identification of the genes responsible for HNPCC. Mutations have been found in families that do not meet the Amsterdam Criteria. In addition, since these criteria were established, studies have shown that the presence of other cancers in the family including endometrial, ovarian, and ureteral tumors provides a strong indicator of HNPCC. In 1993, the first HNPCC gene (MSH2)[1] was cloned, with the second gene (MLH1) cloned shortly thereafter in 1994.[2] Mutations of MSH2 and MLH1 account for 90% of HNPCC. Two additional HNPCC genes (PMS1 and PMS2) were cloned in 1994.[6] The identification of mutations in any of these genes permits accurate diagnosis of HNPCC. Once a mutation has been identified in a family, at-risk presymptomatic relatives should be offered testing. If a relative is found to carry the mutation, annual colonoscopy is recommended. Colonoscopy is recommended over sigmoidoscopy especially in these individuals because of the predilection for right-sided tumors in HNPCC. Due to the high incidence of multiple synchronous and metachronous cancers, subtotal colectomy is recommended in affected individuals. In an individual who has already had partial resection, aggressive surveillance of the remaining colon is warranted.

An excellent review of the hereditary polyposis and nonpolyposis syndromes of the gastrointestinal tract has recently been published.[4]

Footnotes

1. Fishel R, Lescoe MK, Rao MR, et al, "The Human Mutator Gene Homolog MSH2 and Its Association With Hereditary Nonpolyposis Colon Cancer," *Cell*, 1993, 75(5):1027-38.
2. Papadopoulos N, Nicolaides NC, and Wei YF, "Mutation of a mutL Homolog in Hereditary Colon Cancer," *Science*, 1994, 263(5153):1625-9.
3. Marra G and Boland CR, "Hereditary Nonpolyposis Colorectal Cancer. The Syndrome, the Genes, and Historical Perspectives," *J Natl Cancer Inst*, 1995, 87(15):1114-25.
4. Rustgi AK, "Hereditary Gastrointestinal Polyposis and Nonpolyposis Syndromes," *N Engl J Med*, 1994, 331(25):1694-702.
5. Vasen HF, Mecklin JP, Khan PM, et al, "The International Collaborative Group on Hereditary Non-Polyposis Colorectal Cancer (ICG-HNPCC)," *Dis Colon Rectum*, 1991, 34(5):424-5.
6. Nicolaides NC, Papadopoulos N, Liu B, et al, "Mutations of Two PMS Homologues in Hereditary Nonpolyposis Colon Cancer," *Nature*, 1994, 371(6492):75-80.

References

Bronner CE, Baker SM, Morrison PT, et al, "Mutation in the DNA Mismatch Repair Gene Homologue hMLH1 is Associated With Hereditary Nonpolyposis Colon Cancer," *Nature*, 1994, 368(6468):258-61.

Jen J, Kim H, Piantadosi S, et al, "Allelic Loss of Chromosome 18q and Prognosis in Colorectal Cancer," *N Engl J Med*, 1994, 331(4):213-21.

Leach FS, Nicolaides NC, Papadopoulos N, et al, "Mutations of a mutS Homolog in Hereditary Nonpolyposis Colorectal Cancer," *Cell*, 1993, 75(6):8:1215-25.

Lynch HT, Smyrk TC, Watson P, et al, "Genetics, Natural History, Tumor Spectrum, and Pathology of Hereditary Nonpolyposis Colorectal Cancer: An Updated Review," *Gastroenterology*, 1993, 104(5):1535-49.

Peltomaki P, Aaltonen LA, Sistonen P, et al, "Genetic Mapping of a Locus Predisposing to Human Colorectal Cancer," *Science*, 1993, 260(5109):810-2.

Tempero M and Anderson J, "Progress in Colon Cancer - Do Molecular Markers Matter?" *N Engl J Med*, 1994, 331(4):267-8.

Wijnen J, Vasen H, Khan PM, et al, "Seven New Mutations in hMSH2, and HNPCC Gene, Identified by Denaturing Gradient-Gel Electrophoresis," *Am J Hum Genet*, 1995, 56(5):1060-6.

Constant Region of T-Cell Receptor *see* Gene Rearrangement for Leukemia and Lymphoma *on page 512*

Cystic Fibrosis Carrier Detection *see* Cystic Fibrosis DNA Detection *on next page*

Cystic Fibrosis DNA Detection

CPT 83890 (molecular isolation or extraction); 83892 (enzymatic digestion); 83894 (separation); 83898 (nucleic acid probe with amplification)

Related Information

Alpha₁-Fetoprotein, Amniotic Fluid *on page 71*
Amniotic Fluid, Chromosome and Genetic Abnormality Analysis *on page 273*
Amniotic Fluid Pulmonary Surfactant *on page 78*
Chloride, Sweat *on page 108*
Chorionic Villus Sampling (CVS), Chromosome and Genetic Abnormality Analysis *on page 275*
d-Xylose Absorption Test *on page 122*
Polymerase Chain Reaction *on page 523*

Synonyms Cystic Fibrosis Carrier Detection; Cystic Fibrosis, Prenatal Diagnosis; Genetic Detection of Cystic Fibrosis; Molecular Diagnosis of Cystic Fibrosis; Mutation Test for Cystic Fibrosis

Test Commonly Includes Detection of the major genetic mutations responsible for causing cystic fibrosis

Abstract Recent developments have identified the gene defects responsible for cystic fibrosis (CF).[1,2,3] The defective gene was discovered in 1989. Until the cystic fibrosis gene was identified there was no information on the biochemical basis of CF. Since the discovery of the gene numerous studies have clarified the function of both the normal CF gene product and the defective gene product responsible for disease. Genetic studies can be done on both carriers and patients to identify the defect and risk of disease. A list of common mutations can be found in the table. Some mutations are associated with milder forms of cystic fibrosis. This information will be useful in the management of disease and as a diagnostic tool.

Mutations Identified With the Cystic Fibrosis Disease Gene

Name	Mutation	Location	Footnote	Frequency
delF508	3 bp deletion	Exon 10	5	70%-73%
D110H	G →C (460)	Exon 4	10	NA
R117H	G →A (482)	Exon 4	10	0.4%
621+1	G →T (621)	Exon 4	15	0.6%
R347P	C →G (1173)	Exon 7	10	1.1%
A455E	C →A (1496)	Exon 9	7	NA*
Q493X	C →T (1609)	Exon 10	7	NA
dell5O7	3 bp deletion	Exon 10	7	0.4%
1717-1	G →A (1717-1)	Intron 10	7	0.6%
G542X	G →T (1756)	Exon 11	7	2.2%
S549N	G →A (1778)	Exon 11	6	0.1%
S549I	G →T (1778)	Exon 11	7	NA
S549R	T →G (1779)	Exon 11	7	NA
G551D	G →A (1784)	Exon 11	6	2.4%
R553X	C →T (1789)	Exon 11	6	1.1%
A559T	G →A (1807)	Exon 11	6	NA
R560T	G →C (1811)	Exon 11	7	1.0%
Y563N	T →A (1819)	Exon 12	7	NA
P574H	C →A (1853)	Exon 12	7	NA
2566insAT	AT insertion (2566)	Exon 13	11	NA
W846X	G →A (2670)	Exon 14a	12	NA
Y913C	A →G (2870)	Exon 15	12	NA
3659delC	C deletion (3659)	Exon 19	7	NA
S1255X	C →A (3896)	Exon 20	13	NA
W1282X	G →A (3978)	Exon 20	12	1.6%
N1303K	C →G (4041)	Exon 21	14	1.7%

*NA means that this information is not available on the mutation.

Specimen 10-20 mL amniotic fluid, 10-15 mL whole blood, 30-50 mg wet chorionic villus

Container Blood should be collected in a yellow top (ACD) Vacutainer® tube; blood collected in a lavender top (EDTA) Vacutainer® tube is also acceptable. Amniotic fluid and chorionic villus should be collected in a sterile manner and transferred to a sterile tube for transport or to a T25 culture flask.

Sampling Time Amniotic fluid should be collected between the 17th and 18th week of pregnancy. Chorionic villus specimens should be collected between the 8th and 12th week of gestation.

Collection All specimens should be sent to the laboratory **immediately** after collection preferably by overnight delivery.

Storage Instructions All specimens should be maintained at room temperature or refrigerated, never frozen.

Causes for Rejection Any amniotic fluid specimen that is bloody may be contaminated with maternal blood and is unsuitable for this test. Specimens that are unlabeled or mislabeled are not acceptable.

Turnaround Time 10-21 days

Special Instructions It is helpful to have a complete family pedigree that includes all medical histories.

Reference Range The laboratory usually provides an interpretive report which includes a risk analysis.

Use This test is indicated for a family with history of cystic fibrosis. For this purpose it is helpful to have a complete family pedigree that includes all medical histories. This test is also indicated for prenatal diagnosis in couples known to be carriers. It is helpful in diagnosing neonates in whom cystic fibrosis is suspected, but who have had equivocal sweat tests. The American Society of Human Genetics has recently published guidelines for the use of genetic testing of cystic fibrosis carriers.

Recommendations: Although the sensitivity of carrier testing for CF has improved and pilot studies are under way, CF testing is not recommended, at this time, for individuals or couples who do not have a family history of CF. Individuals with a positive family history of CF or who have a blood relative identified as a CF carrier should be offered CF testing with appropriate education and counseling. Optimally, carrier testing should be offered prior to conception, to provide a couple the broadest range of reproductive options.

When indicated, CF counseling and testing should adhere to the following guidelines.
- Screening should be voluntary, and confidentiality must be ensured.
- Screening requires informed consent. Pretest education should explain the benefits and hazards (eg, stigmatization and possible loss of insurability).
- Providers of screening services have the obligation to ensure that adequate post-test counseling is provided.
- Quality control of all aspects of laboratory testing, including systemic proficiency testing, is required.
- As with all indicated healthcare services, there should be equal access to testing.

Efforts should be expanded to educate healthcare providers and the public, regarding the complexities of CF screening in particular and issues involved in genetic healthcare services in general.[4]

Limitations The estimated carrier rate for cystic fibrosis in the United States is 1 in 25. Current technology will detect 10-20 of the most common cystic fibrosis mutations, however, other mutations are also responsible for this disease. An extensive list can be found in footnote 15. Individuals found to be negative for the known mutations reduce their chance of being cystic fibrosis carriers to 1 in 250. Thus, a negative result does not rule out the possibility that an individual is a cystic fibrosis carrier but can lower that probability.

Methodology DNA is isolated from the specimen and several regions on chromosome 7 are amplified using the polymerase chain reaction. Several of the most common cystic fibrosis mutations are detected within the amplified regions of DNA. The presence of these mutations results in a smaller amplified DNA product or a DNA product which reflects a change in restriction enzyme sites. These changes can be detected visually after digestion with appropriate restriction enzymes and gel electrophoresis. Some laboratories will assay for cystic fibrosis mutations by directly examining the specimen DNA using Southern blot techniques. These assays require a longer turnaround time and are rapidly being replaced by the amplification technique.

Additional Information Cystic fibrosis is inherited as an autosomal recessive disorder and affects approximately 1 in 2500 Caucasians.[5] The disease locus was initially mapped to chromosome 7q31.[6] The gene responsible for the disease has recently been identified and was found to have over 250 kilobases and codes for a protein that contains 1480 amino acids called the cystic fibrosis transmembrane conductance regulator (CFTR). This protein was found to be a transmembrane protein that regulated the conduction of ions across epithelial cell membranes.[1,2] The most common mutation causing the disease has been identified in the tenth exon of this gene as a deletion of three nucleotides. The loss of these nucleotides removes a phenylalanine codon at position 508 (delF508) in the first ATP binding domain.[3] This mutation accounts for approximately 70% of all cystic fibrosis chromosomes, while the remaining 30% of cystic fibrosis chromosomes are made up of numerous heterogeneous mutations.[7,8] Over 150 of these less common mutations have now been identified. Several of these mutations occur with reasonable frequency, while the others are rare (see table). A special NIH Workshop on Population Screening for the Cystic Fibrosis Gene in March 1990 recommended that the delF508 test "be offered to all individuals and couples with a family history of cystic fibrosis".[9] Currently these tests have a total detection rate >84% in Caucasian North American populations with European ancestry.[10]
(Continued)

Cystic Fibrosis DNA Detection *(Continued)*

The CFTR is a cAMP-activated chloride channel. The CFTR appears to be involved in transport of molecules across cell membranes.

Footnotes

1. Rommens JM, Iannuzzi MC, Kerem B-S, et al, "Identification of the Cystic Fibrosis Gene: Chromosome Walking and Jumping," *Science*, 1989, 245(4922):1059-65.
2. Riordan JR, Rommens JM, Kerem B-S, et al, "Identification of the Cystic Fibrosis Gene: Cloning and Characterization of Complementary DNA," *Science*, 1989, 245(4922):1066-73.
3. Kerem B-S, Rommens JM, Buchanan JA, et al, "Identification of the Cystic Fibrosis Gene: Genetic Analysis," *Science*, 1989, 245(4922):1073-80.
4. ASHG Ad Hoc Committee on Cystic Fibrosis Carrier Screening, "Statement of the American Society of Human Genetics on Cystic Fibrosis Carrier Screening," *Am J Hum Genet*, 1992, 51(6):1443-4.
5. Boat TF, Welsh MJ, and Beaudet AL, "Cystic Fibrosis," *The Metabolic Basis of Inherited Disease*, 6th ed, Scriver CR, Beaudet AL, Sly WS, et al, eds, New York, NY: McGraw-Hill Inc, 1989, 2649-80.
6. Tsui L-C, Buchwald M, Barker D, et al, "Cystic Fibrosis Locus Defined by a Genetically Linked Polymorphic DNA Marker," *Science*, 1985, 230(4729):1054-7.
7. Cutting GR, Kasch LM, Rosenstein BJ, et al, "A Cluster of Cystic Fibrosis Mutations in the First Nucleotide-Binding Fold of the Cystic Fibrosis Conductance Regulator Protein," *Nature*, 1990, 346(6282):366-9.
8. Kerem B-S, Zielenski J, Markiewicz D, et al, "Identification of Mutations in Regions Corresponding to the Two Putative Nucleotide (ATP)-Binding Folds of the Cystic Fibrosis Gene," *Proc Natl Acad Sci U S A*, 1990, 87(21):8447-51.
9. Workshop on Population Screening for the Cystic Fibrosis Gene, "Statement From the National Institutes of Health Workshop on Population Screening for the Cystic Fibrosis Gene," *N Engl J Med*, 1990, 323(1):70-1.
10. "Population Analysis of the Major Mutation in Cystic Fibrosis," *Hum Genet*, 1990, 85(4):391-445.
11. Dean M, White MB, Amos J, et al, "Multiple Mutations in Highly Conserved Residues Are Found in Mildly Affected Cystic Fibrosis," *Cell*, 1990, 61(5):863-70.
12. White MB, Amos J, Hsu JMC, et al, "A Frame-Shift Mutation in the Cystic Fibrosis Gene," *Nature*, 1990, 344(6267):665-7.
13. Vidaud M, Fanen P, Martin J, et al, "Three Point Mutations in the CFTR Gene in French Cystic Fibrosis Patients: Identification by Denaturing Gradient Gel Electrophoresis," *Hum Genet*, 1990, 85(4):446-9.
14. Cutting GR, Kasch LM, Rosenstein BJ, et al, "Two Patients With Cystic Fibrosis, Nonsense Mutations in Each Cystic Fibrosis Gene and Mild Pulmonary Disease," *N Engl J Med*, 1990, 323(24):1685-9.
15. Tsui L-C and Buchwald M, "Biochemical and Molecular Genetics of Cystic Fibrosis," *Adv Hum Genet* , 1991, 20:153-266, 311-2.

References

Beaudet AL, "Carrier Screening for Cystic Fibrosis," *Am J Hum Genet*, 1990, 47(14):603-5.

Davies K, "Cystic Fibrosis. Complementary Endeavours," *Nature*, 1990, 348(6297):110-1.

Nishimi RY, "Cystic Fibrosis and DNA Tests - The Implications of Carrier Screening," *JAMA*, 1993, 269(15):1921.

Rosenstein BJ, "Cystic Fibrosis," *Principles and Practice of Pediatrics*, 2nd ed, Chapter 72, Oski FA, DeAngelis CD, Feigin RD, et al, eds, Philadelphia, PA: JB Lippincott Co, 1994, 1490-501.

Smith DR, Fulton TR, Swain P, et al, "Cystic Fibrosis: Diagnostic Testing and the Search for the Gene," *Clin Chem*, 1989, 35(7 Suppl):B17-20.

"Correlation Between Genotype and Phenotype in Patients With Cystic Fibrosis. The Cystic Fibrosis Genotype-Phenotype Consortium," *N Engl J Med*, 1993, 329(18):1308-13.

Weinberger SE, "Recent Advances in Pulmonary Medicine," *N Engl J Med*, 1993, 328(19):1389-97.

Cystic Fibrosis, Prenatal Diagnosis *see* Cystic Fibrosis DNA Detection *on previous page*

Cytomegalovirus DNA Detection

CPT 83890 (molecular extraction); 83894 (separation); 83896 (nucleic acid probe); 83898 (molecular amplification)

Related Information

Cytomegalic Inclusion Disease Cytology *on page 293*
Cytomegalovirus Antibody *on page 389*
Cytomegalovirus Antigen Detection *on page 664*
Cytomegalovirus Culture *on page 664*
Polymerase Chain Reaction *on page 523*

Synonyms CMV DNA Detection; CMV Quantitation; Molecular Assay for CMV Detection

Test Commonly Includes Direct detection of cytomegalovirus nucleic acid in white blood cells, plasma, serum, urine, CSF, and bronchial alveolar lavage fluid. CMV may also be detected in tissue samples.

Abstract Cytomegalovirus (CMV) disease is one of the major risks for immunosuppressed individuals. The number of patients who are immunosuppressed as result of therapeutic intervention (bone marrow transplant, solid organ transplant, and/or cancer chemotherapy) has greatly increased in addition to the number of individuals with altered immune functions due to HIV infection. CMV disease in the nonimmunosuppressed is typically limited to a mononucleosis-like syndrome with fever, pharyngitis, and lymphadenitis. The detection of CMV disease at an early stage is critical for beginning intervention, and several different assays have been developed using culture or antigen detection techniques. Molecular assays for detection of CMV DNA involve the extraction of viral genome from a variety of sources followed by amplification using oligonucleotide primers to specific regions. A number of targets

have been described, such as the polymerase gene or immediate early antigen gene. Detection of CMV DNA by amplification procedures has been shown to have a higher sensitivity than either culture techniques or the antigenemia assay.[1] However, problems related to the predictive value of a positive or negative test are being investigated to establish correlation with disease and therapeutic decision making. Newer techniques that incorporate quantitation appear to be useful for establishing significance for detecting CMV DNA by PCR.

Specimen CMV DNA may be extracted from peripheral blood lymphocytes, plasma, serum, bronchial alveolar lavage fluid, urine, cerebrospinal fluid, and various tissues including lung and brain

Container Glass or plastic containers are acceptable; anticoagulants may be used with the exception of heparin

Storage Instructions While freezing is known to reduce the viability of CMV and its isolation by culture techniques, freezing does not impair detection by amplification procedures. Any of the above fluid samples should be rapidly transported to the laboratory, however if transportation is expected to exceed 2 hours, the sample should be refrigerated, and if transportation exceeds 8 hours, a specimen should be frozen. All tissue samples should be frozen as soon as possible after the biopsy procedure.

Causes for Rejection Collection of blood in heparinized tubes may result in inhibition of amplification.

Turnaround Time 1-3 days

Special Instructions Specimen should **not** be obtained utilizing heparin as an anticoagulant.

Reference Range An interpretative report usually accompanies results. CMV may be excreted in urine and saliva or be present in blood without clinical symptoms.

Use The detection of CMV DNA is useful for identifying patients in whom appropriate therapy could be instituted, including ganciclovir, immune globulin, or high dose acyclovir. Quantitative assays may be useful in establishing disease.

Limitations A negative result does not rule out the presence of CMV in all tissues of the body. CMV detection by PCR has shown a relatively low specificity when compared with viral culture and a lower predictive value for disease.

Methodology DNA is extracted from fluids or tissues using a standard lysis buffer followed by phenochloroform extraction and amplification. Alternatively, protocols exist for the direct amplification of CMV DNA following the lysis of cells by boiling or detergent without phenol extraction.

Additional Information Greater than 80% of adults have been exposed to CMV as evidenced by the presence of antibodies. Although in most nonimmunosuppressed individuals infection by CMV is self-limited, one important exception is found in neonates who are infected *in utero*. Infection of the fetus during the early stages of pregnancy may result in multiorgan failure, CNS abnormalities or paradoxically, continuous CMV excretion in the urine without disease.[2] The development of solid organ transplantation and bone marrow or stem cell transplantation has accelerated the need for early CMV detection. When detected early, CMV infection may be effectively treated with ganciclovir or high acyclovir and immunoglobulin. Amplification assays for the detection of CMV have been developed because of the increased sensitivity that these assays provide. The standard assays for CMV detection in the transplant setting, include the shell vial assay and the antigenemia assay. In comparison studies, PCR of CMV DNA has shown a higher sensitivity, however a lower specificity and a lower positive predictive value for disease. These findings emphasize the importance of correlating the detection of CMV DNA with clinical symptoms.[3] Recent studies have confirmed the ability of CMV DNA detection to detect CMV earlier than reference assays.[4] Quantitative CMV DNA detection assays have been used to demonstrate viral load and correlate with the progression of CMV disease, as well as response to therapy. Another approach to improve the correlation of a positive test by PCR with CMV disease has been to use plasma rather than DNA extracted from peripheral blood lymphocytes. The most appropriate use of a PCR assay for CMV may be in determining the appropriate duration of ganciclovir therapy as well as correlation with progression of disease. At the present time, commercial assays for CMV detection by PCR are not available, and its specific utility is therefore dependent upon institutional modifications of the assay and should be correlated with clinical findings before being used to alter therapeutic protocols.

Footnotes

1. Boeckh M, Myerson M, and Bowden RA, "Early Detection and Treatment of Cytomegalovirus Infections in Marrow Transplant Patients: Methodological Aspects and Implications for Therapeutic Interventions," *Bone Marrow Transplant*, 1994, 14(Suppl 4):S66-70.
2. Fowler KB, Stagno S, Pass RF, et al, "The Outcome of Congenital Cytomegalovirus Infection in Relation to Maternal Antibody Status," *N Engl J Med*, 1992, 326(10):663-7.

3. Einsele H, Ehninger G, Hebart H, et al, "Polymerase Chain Reaction Monitoring Reduces the Incidence of Cytomegalovirus Disease and the Duration and Side Effects of Antiviral Therapy After Bone Marrow Transplantation," *Blood*, 1995, 86(7):2815-20.
4. Storch GA, Bullei RS, Bailey TC, et al, "Comparison of PCR and PP65 Antigenemia Assay With Quantitative Shell Vial Culture for Detection of Cytomegalovirus in Blood Leukocytes From Solid Organ Transplant Recipients," *J Clin Microbiol*, 1994, 32(4):997-1003.

References

Woods GL, "Herpesvirus," *Diagnostic Pathology of Infectious Disease*, Chapter 5, Malvern, PA: Lea & Febiger, 1993, 51-3.

DNA Amplification see Polymerase Chain Reaction on page 523

DNA Amplification Assay see Mycobacteria by DNA Probe on page 520

DNA Amplification of N-*myc* see N-*myc* Amplification on page 522

DNA Analysis for Parentage Evaluation see Identification DNA Testing on page 517

DNA Banking

CPT 83890

Synonyms DNA Storage

Test Commonly Includes Isolation and storage of DNA specimens for future diagnostic testing

Abstract Understanding of the molecular basis of disease is proceeding at a rapid rate and will continue to progress into the next century. The sequencing of human genes has largely been due to the federally-supported Human Genome Project. One of the greatest advances expected from this project is the increase in diagnostic tests for inherited diseases and genetic abnormalities associated with cancers. This information will also elucidate the influence of the environment on genetic material. Thus, the storage of DNA from individuals or tumors will be invaluable both to scientists and to individuals interested in their family history of disease.

Specimen Whole blood, tissue, or cultured cells

Container Blood should be collected in yellow top (ACD) tubes; tissue should be frozen at -70°C; amniotic cells, fibroblasts, or lymphocytes should be grown in appropriate media in T25 tissue culture flasks.

Collection A 0.1-1 g of tissue should be obtained. The specimen should then be put into a sealable plastic freezer bag and frozen at -70°C. The specimen should be kept frozen until shipped to the laboratory. Cell cultures should be grown to confluency and tightly sealed before shipping.

Storage Instructions Store tissue at -70°C or on dry ice. Peripheral blood should be stored and shipped at 4°C. Do **not** freeze blood.

Causes for Rejection If the tissue specimen thaws out during transport to the laboratory or before shipping, DNA may not be obtained from the specimen; if less than 0.1 g of tissue is sent to the laboratory, it may not yield enough DNA for analysis; blood samples that have been frozen and thawed will yield low quality DNA.

Turnaround Time Samples can be stored for an unlimited amount of time.

Use The storage of DNA isolated from individuals provides purified genetic material that can be used either for identification or for future diagnostic testing.

Limitations Failure to obtain DNA from the blood, tissue, or cultured cells due to inappropriate shipping or processing (as mentioned above)

Methodology DNA is released and isolated from the white blood cells, tissue, or cultured cells by lysing the cells and extracting the cell lysate with phenol and chloroform. Purified, intact DNA is precipitated with salt in the presence of alcohol. The DNA is then stored indefinitely at -70°C usually at two separate facilities.

Additional Information There has been remarkable progress recently in the field of diagnostic molecular biology. Rapid advances are expected to continue. The new tests currently being developed will analyze DNA for the diagnosis of genetic diseases and may facilitate the genetic testing of future generations.[1] This enables individuals to have access to their genetic heritage which could be crucial to future family testing. Some of the other tests being developed will be able to diagnose certain cancers;[2] thus, it can sometimes be prudent to bank DNA from certain unusual cancers. Tissue from such cancers can be used to isolate DNA that can be stored for years at -70°C. This would allow investigation of the genetics of these cancers in the future. Stored DNA is always the property of the person from whom it was isolated. When family testing for either a genetic disease or cancer diagnosis is desired, signed permission is usually required before the sample is released. If the person owning the DNA is deceased then its disposition is under the control of a legal guardian or heir. All information received from DNA tests performed on any DNA sample is completely confidential and is released only to the individual requesting the test (through an appropriate medical professional).

Footnotes

1. Katayama S, "Molecular Biological Approaches to Genetic Disorders in Prenatal Diagnosis," *Early Hum Dev*, 1992, 29(1-3):149-53.
2. Bishop JM, "The Molecular Genetics of Cancer," *Science*, 1987, 235(4786):305-11.

References

Antonarakis SE, "Recombinant DNA Technology in the Diagnosis of Human Genetic Disorders," *Clin Chem*, 1989, 35(7 Suppl):B4-6.
Caskey CT, "Disease Diagnosis by Recombinant DNA Methods," *Science*, 1987, 236(4806):1223-4.
Housman D, "Human DNA Polymorphism," *N Engl J Med*, 1995, 332(5):318-20.
Landegren U, Kaiser R, Caskey CT, et al, "DNA Diagnostic: Molecular Techniques and Automation," *Science*, 1988, 242(4876):229-37.
Lederberg J, "What the Double Helix (1953) Has Meant for Basic Biomedical Science. A Personal Commentary," *JAMA*, 1993, 269(15):1981-5.

DNA Detection for *Neisseria gonorrhoeae* see Neisseria gonorrhoeae Genome Detection on page 521

DNA Fingerprinting see Identification DNA Testing on page 517

DNA Hybridization Test for *Borrelia burgdorferi* see Lyme Disease DNA Detection on page 518

DNA Hybridization Test for *Chlamydia trachomatis* see Chlamydia trachomatis Genome Detection on page 505

DNA Hybridization Test for HBV see Hepatitis B DNA Detection on page 513

DNA Hybridization Test for HPV see Human Papillomavirus DNA Probe Test on page 516

DNA Hybridization Test for Mycobacteria see Mycobacteria by DNA Probe on page 520

DNA Hybridization Test for *Mycoplasma pneumoniae* see Mycoplasma pneumoniae DNA Probe Test on page 520

DNA Probe Test for HBV see Hepatitis B DNA Detection on page 513

DNA Probe Test for HPV see Human Papillomavirus DNA Probe Test on page 516

DNA Probe Test for Lyme Disease see Lyme Disease DNA Detection on page 518

DNA Storage see DNA Banking on this page

DNA Test for *Chlamydia trachomatis* see Chlamydia trachomatis Genome Detection on page 505

DNA Test for Mycobacteria see Mycobacteria by DNA Probe on page 520

DNA Test for *Mycoplasma pneumoniae* see Mycoplasma pneumoniae DNA Probe Test on page 520

Duchenne/Becker Muscular Dystrophy Carrier Detection see Duchenne/Becker Muscular Dystrophy DNA Detection on this page

Duchenne/Becker Muscular Dystrophy DNA Detection

CPT 83890 (molecular isolation or extraction); 83892 (enzymatic digestion); 83894 (separation); 83896 (nucleic acid probe, each)

Related Information

Aldolase, Serum on page 66

Alpha$_1$-Fetoprotein, Amniotic Fluid on page 71

Amniotic Fluid, Chromosome and Genetic Abnormality Analysis on page 273

Chorionic Villus Sampling (CVS), Chromosome and Genetic Abnormality Analysis on page 275

Creatine Kinase on page 115

Muscle Biopsy on page 53

Polymerase Chain Reaction on page 523

Synonyms Duchenne/Becker Muscular Dystrophy Carrier Detection; Duchenne/Becker Muscular Dystrophy, Prenatal Diagnosis; Genetic Detection of Duchenne/Becker Muscular Dystrophy; Molecular Diagnosis of Duchenne/Becker Muscular Dystrophy; Mutation Test for Duchenne/Becker Muscular Dystrophy

Applies to Dystrophin Protein

Abstract Duchenne and Becker progressive muscular dystrophies are X-linked recessive mutations. Both familial and sporadic cases are seen. About 33% of patients have new mutations.[1,2] Molecular biology advances have identified the muscular dystrophy gene on the short arm of the X chromosome. This information showed for the first time that Duchenne muscular dystrophy (DMD) and Becker muscular dystrophy (BMD) are actually allelic disorders. Allelic disorders are diseases caused by different mutation on the same gene. They are locus
(Continued)

Duchenne/Becker Muscular Dystrophy DNA Detection *(Continued)*

diseases. These molecular advances have increased the understanding of the biochemical defect in DMD and BMD and permit diagnosis based on molecular analysis.

Patient Preparation Consultation with a medical geneticist is desirable.

Specimen Whole blood, amniotic fluid, chorionic villus

Container Blood should be collected in yellow top (ACD) Vacutainer® tubes, blood collected in lavender top (EDTA) Vacutainer® tubes is also acceptable; amniotic fluid and chorionic villus should be collected in a sterile manner and transferred to a sterile tube for transport or to a T25 culture flask.

Sampling Time Amniotic fluid should be collected between the 14th and 17th week of pregnancy. Chorionic villus specimens should be dissected free of maternal tissue and blood clot. Transport medium is needed.

Storage Instructions All specimens should be sent to the laboratory **immediately** after collection, preferably by overnight delivery. All specimens should be kept at room temperature or refrigerated, never frozen.

Causes for Rejection Amniotic fluid specimens that are bloody may be unsuitable.

Turnaround Time 10-21 days

Special Instructions A complete family pedigree and clinical information are needed.

Reference Range An interpretive report which includes a risk analysis is usually provided.

Use This test is indicated for patients and families with history of Duchenne or Becker muscular dystrophy. This test is also indicated for prenatal diagnosis in females known to be carriers. It is helpful for diagnosis of neonates suspected of Duchenne or Becker muscular dystrophy.

Limitations DNA analysis for Duchenne or Becker muscular dystrophy can only detect ~65% of the abnormalities responsible for the disease. Thus, a negative result does not rule out the possibility that an individual is a muscular dystrophy carrier or affected, but it can lower that probability. Gonadal mosaicism occurs in about 10% of cases.

Methodology DNA is isolated from the specimen and several regions within the dystrophin gene are detected using Southern blotting techniques. The DNA in each exon can be examined. Because of the large size of the gene, as many as seven different Southern blots are required. Multiplex polymerase chain reaction (PCR) is used to detect many of the most common deletions found at the 5′ end of the gene. Several of the DNA regions can be amplified in the same PCR and a change (either loss or varied mobility) in the DNA fragments indicates an abnormality. Such changes can be detected visually after gel electrophoresis and staining with ethidium bromide. In affected families in which there is no detectable deletion, linkage analysis can be done using Southern blotting to detect linkage to several known mutations.[3,4]

Additional Information **Duchenne's muscular dystrophy**, the most common of the childhood dystrophies, is the most severe type of progressive primary muscular degeneration. A crippling muscle disorder, it is associated with an abnormality in band 1 of region 2 of the short arm on the X chromosome, a locus designated Xp2.1. It is clinically evident by 5 years. CK is very high during its early phase. Cardiac involvement leads to ECG abnormalities; heart failure and arrhythmias may occur. Cardiomyopathy may be severe.[1]

Becker muscular dystrophy is a milder form with a similar clinical course followed at a much slower rate.[5] CK bears a less marked increase. These are inherited as X-linked recessive disorders with an incidence of approximately 1 in 3500 male births.

The gene responsible for these disorders has been cloned and the protein product has been identified as the dystrophin protein, a muscle cytoskeletal protein. This protein was found to be 427 kilodalton (kDa) and the gene identified was very large, with a 14 kilobase (kb) transcript encoding more than 70 exons spread over 2500 kb of genomic DNA.[6,7] The polymerase chain reaction (PCR) and Southern blotting can both be used to detect alterations of the dystrophin gene. Approximately 65% of muscular dystrophy patients have detectable deletions that can be detected using molecular methods. In these families, females can be tested to detect carrier status and prenatal diagnosis can be done on either chorionic villus sampling or amniotic cells.[3,4] Many of the deletions in the dystrophin gene are found within two "hotspot" regions at the 5′ end of the gene.[8] Taking advantage of the clustering of deletions, the multiplex PCR analysis amplifies such particular DNA regions and compares them with normal DNA. Genetic deletions are detected as specimens missing one or more DNA bands when compared with DNA bands amplified from normal DNA.[9] Advantages of the PCR test over Southern blotting include decreased turnaround time (1-2 days versus 1-2 weeks) and increased sensitivity (as little as 0.5 mL of blood) which may be useful in prenatal diagnosis.

When deletion is not identified, linkage analysis is usually successful in provision of risk assessment. In cases with a positive family history but with no detectable mutation, a more intensive search using restriction fragment length polymorphism (RFLP)-linkage analysis can be done to determine the existence of known point mutations or alterations not detected by the other assay. This requires the participation of several family members both affected and unaffected, to correlate the inheritance pattern of the RFLPs with inheritance of disease.[10]

Muscle biopsy with dystrophin analysis may be needed in selected patients.[11]

Footnotes

1. Oldfors A, Eriksson BO, Kyllerman M, et al, "Dilated Cardiomyopathy and the Dystrophin Gene: An Illustrated Review," *Br Heart J*, 1994, 72(4):344-8.
2. Tsukamoto H, Inui K, and Okada S, "Carrier and Prenatal Diagnosis of Duchenne and Becker Muscular Dystrophy by PCR Methods," *Nippon Rinsho*, 1993, 51(9):2428-34.
3. Davies KE, Pearson PL, Harper PS, et al, "Linkage Analysis of Two Cloned DNA Sequences Flanking the Duchenne Muscular Dystrophy Locus on the Short Arm of the Human X Chromosome," *Nucleic Acids Res*, 1983, 11:2303-12.
4. Kingston HM, Sarfarazi M, Thomas NS, et al, "Localisation of the Becker Muscular Dystrophy Gene on the Short Arm of the X Chromosome by Linkage to Cloned DNA Sequences," *Hum Genet*, 1984, 67(1):6-17.
5. Koenig M, Beggs AH, Moyer M, et al, "The Molecular Basis for Duchenne Versus Becker Muscular Dystrophy: Correlation of Severity With Type of Deletion," *Am J Hum Genet*, 1989, 45(4):498-506.
6. Monaco AP, Neve RL, Colletti-Feener C, et al, "Isolation of Candidate cDNAs for Portions of the Duchenne Muscular Dystrophy Gene," *Nature*, 1986, 323(6089):646-50.
7. Burghes AH, Logan C, Hu X, et al, "A cDNA Clone From the Duchenne/Becker Muscular Dystrophy Gene," *Nature*, 1987, 328(6129):434-7.
8. Forrest SM, Cross GS, Speer A, et al, "Preferential Deletion of Exons in Duchenne and Becker Muscular Dystrophies," *Nature*, 1987, 329(6140):638-40.
9. Chamberlain JS, Gibbs RA, Ranier JE, et al, "Deletion Screening of the Duchenne Muscular Dystrophy Locus Via Multiplex DNA Amplification," *Nucleic Acids Res*, 1988, 16(23):11141-56.
10. Fassati A, Tedeschi S, Bordoni A, et al, "Rapid Direct Diagnosis of Deletions Carriers of Duchenne and Becker Muscular Dystrophies," *Lancet*, 1994, 344(8918):302-3.
11. Richards S and Iannaccone ST, "Dystrophin and DNA Diagnosis in a Large Pediatric Muscle Clinic," *J Child Neurol*, 1994, 9(2):162-6.

References

Ballo R, Viljoen D, and Beighton P, "Duchenne and Becker Muscular Dystrophy Prevalence in South Africa and Molecular Findings in 128 Persons Affected," *S Afr Med J*, 1994, 84(8 Pt 1):494-7.

Beggs AH and Kunkel LM, "Improved Diagnosis of Duchenne/Becker Muscular Dystrophy," *J Clin Invest*, 1990, 85(3):613-9.

Bushby KM, "The Muscular Dystrophies," *Baillieres Clin Neurol*, 1994, 3(2):407-30.

Clemens PR, Fenwick RG, Chamberlain JS, et al, "Carrier Detection and Prenatal Diagnosis in Duchenne and Becker Muscular Dystrophy Families, Using Dinucleotide Repeat Polymorphisms," *Am J Hum Genet*, 1991, 49(5):951-60.

Darras BT, "Molecular Genetics of Duchenne and Becker Muscular Dystrophy," *J Pediatr*, 1990, 117(1 Pt 1):1-15.

De Vivo DC and DiMauro S, "Hereditary and Acquired Types of Myopathy," *Principles and Practice of Pediatrics*, 2nd ed, Chapter 159, Oski FA, DeAngelis CD, Feigin RD, et al, eds, Philadelphia, PA: JB Lippincott Co, 1994, 2082-96.

Mansfield ES, Robertson JM, Lebo RV, et al, "Duchenne/Becker Muscular Dystrophy Carrier Detection Using Quantitative PCR and Fluorescence-Based Strategies," *Am J Med Genet*, 1993, 48(4):200-8.

Rininsland F and Reiss J, "Microlesions and Polymorphisms in the Duchenne/Becker Muscular Dystrophy Gene," *Hum Genet*, 1994, 94(2):111-6.

Shomrat R, Gluck E, Legum C, et al, "Relatively Low Proportion of Dystrophin Gene Deletions in Israeli Duchenne and Becker Muscular Dystrophy Patients," *Am J Med Genet*, 1994, 49(4):369-73.

Sjoberg G, Edstrom L, Lendahl U, et al, "Myofibers From Duchenne/Becker Muscular Dystrophy and Myositis Express the Intermediate Filament Nestin," *J Neuropathol Exp Neurol*, 1994, 53(4):416-23.

Duchenne/Becker Muscular Dystrophy, Prenatal Diagnosis

see Duchenne/Becker Muscular Dystrophy DNA Detection *on previous page*

Dystrophin Protein

see Duchenne/Becker Muscular Dystrophy DNA Detection *on previous page*

Eaton Agent Pneumonia

see Mycoplasma pneumoniae DNA Probe Test *on page 520*

Enterovirus Genome Detection

CPT 83890 (molecular extraction); 83894 (separation); 83896 (nucleic acid probe); 83898 (molecular amplification)

Related Information

Bacterial Culture, Cerebrospinal Fluid *on page 460*
Cerebrospinal Fluid Analysis *on page 309*
Enterovirus Culture *on page 666*
Polymerase Chain Reaction *on page 523*

Synonyms Enterovirus Molecular Probe Assay; Enterovirus RNA Detection; Molecular Probe for Enterovirus

Test Commonly Includes Indirect detection of enterovirus RNA through the generation of a DNA complement followed by amplification

Abstract Enteroviruses cause a wide variety of clinical disease, including upper respiratory tract infection, aseptic meningitis, myocarditis, conjunctivitis, herpangina, and pleurodynia. Enteroviruses are the most common cause of meningitis in the United States and account for over 80% of aseptic meningitis. The differential of meningitis is a difficult clinical problem and principally involves either bacterial infection or viral infection and requires the discrimination between herpes viruses and enteroviruses. Rapid antigen assays have not been useful due to the large number of serotypes. The enterovirus genome detection assay provides for the recovery of enterovirus RNA with its subsequent conversion to complementary DNA, which then enters the polymerase chain reaction for amplification. The amplification steps are followed by specific hybridization with an oligonucleotide probe which may be identified in a variety of formats, including radiography or an enzymatic reaction. The ability to detect enterovirus genome is based on the presence of a highly conserved 5′ noncoding region to which specific primers may hybridize.[1] The value of the enterovirus genome assay lies in the ability to identify the likely etiologic agent and allow for conservative management and cessation of other antivirals and antibiotics.[2] Several research assays have been developed that show excellent sensitivity and specificity as compared to culture. Commercial assays are anticipated in the near future.

Specimen Blood, cerebrospinal fluid, and selected tissues including lymph nodes and myocardial tissue

Container Blood: lavender top (EDTA) tube; CSF: plastic or glass tube is acceptable

Collection Tissue samples should be snap-frozen immediately and stored at -80°C.

Storage Instructions Specimens should be transported to the laboratory as soon as they become available. If specimens cannot be processed immediately, they should be frozen and maintained at -80°C.

Causes for Rejection Specimens collected using heparin

Turnaround Time 1-3 days

Reference Range No enterovirus genome detected

Use Identify an etiologic agent associated with meningitis, myocarditis, or other enterovirus-related diseases

Limitations A negative result does not rule out the presence of enterovirus genome. Inhibitors of the assay may be present, and the specimen may not have been transported in a timely fashion or handled appropriately. Limited cross-reactivity and amplification of other viruses within the Picornavirus family has been described, including amplification of some rhinovirus serotypes.

Methodology Enterovirus RNA is extracted from the specimen and a homologous DNA strand is generated using reverse transcriptase. Specific product is amplified using primers that anneal to the conserved 5′ nontranslated region of most enteroviruses.

Additional Information The enterovirus genus includes 67 serotypes, including poliovirus 1-3, coxsackievirus A1-A22, A24, B1-B6, echovirus 1-9, 11-27, 29-33, and enterovirus 68-71, all of which are members of the large Picornaviridae family. To date no specific disease has been accepted to be uniquely associated with any one enterovirus serotype.[2] Many nonpolio enteroviruses are capable of causing the paralytic disease particularly associated with polio viruses. Although enteroviruses are responsible for a wide-spectrum of clinical diseases, neonatal sepsis, aseptic meningitis, poliomyelitis, and myocarditis represent the most significant entities. Enteroviruses are believed to be the most common cause of meningitis in the U.S. and, in some studies, have accounted for approximately 80% of cases of meningitis for which an etiology can be found. Meningitis due to enteroviral infections has a classic pattern of appearance in the late summer and fall in the northern hemisphere.

The detection of enteroviruses by standard cell culture techniques has several limitations including cellular and viral restrictions which prevent the recovery of certain enteroviral strains in cell culture systems.[3] In addition, detection of enterovirus by serologic techniques or the detection of antigen has been limited by the lack of common antigens for all of enteroviruses. Prior to the development of the RT PCR assay, alternative molecular methods for the identification of enteroviruses included the use of specific nucleic acid probes using a Northern blot technique.

Although it is possible to utilize a serotype-specific or group-specific method of detecting enteroviruses, the absence of a disease-specific correlation argues for the use of a general method capable of detecting most enterovirus serotypes. Several strategies have been successful based on the sequence similarity found in the 5′ nontranslated region (NTR) and the development of primers that bind to this region. It should be recognized, however, that even the most generic approach based on the many enterovirus serotypes that have been sequenced to date are not likely to detect all serotypes. For example, the primers designed by Chapman and associates which have an overall homology of 90% to 100% with the NTR of enteroviruses were able to detect 40 of 41 tested serotypes but were unable to amplify echovirus serotype 22.[4] Similar results have been experienced by others.

Footnotes

1. Rotbart HA, "Nucleic Acid Detection Systems for Enteroviruses," *Clin Microbiol Rev*, 1991, 4(2):156-68.

2. Romero JR and Rotbart HA, "Polymerase Chain Reaction Strategies for the Detection of the Human Enteroviruses," *J Pediatr Infect Dis*, 1996.
3. Wildin S and Chonmaitree T, "The Importance of the Virology Laboratory in the Diagnosis and Management of Viral Meningitis," *Am J Dis Child*, 1987, 141(4):454-7.
4. Chapman NM, Tracy S, Gauntt CJ, et al, "Molecular Detection and Identification of Enteroviruses Using Enzymatic Amplification and Nucleic Acid Hybridization," *J Clin Microbiol*, 1990, 28(5):843-50.

References

Woods GL, "Picornaviruses," *Diagnostic Pathology of Infectious Disease*, Chapter 13, Malvern, PA: Lea & Febiger, 1993, 105-15.

Enterovirus Molecular Probe Assay *see* Enterovirus Genome Detection *on previous page*

Enterovirus RNA Detection *see* Enterovirus Genome Detection *on previous page*

Familial Breast/Ovarian Cancer *see* Breast Cancer, Hereditary (BRCA1) *on page 504*

Familial Medullary Thyroid Carcinoma/Multiple Endocrine Neoplasia *see* Multiple Endocrine Neoplasia/Familial Medullary Thyroid Carcinoma *on page 519*

Fragile X, Carrier Detection *see* Fragile X DNA Detection *on this page*

Fragile X DNA Detection

CPT 83890 (molecular isolation or extraction); 83892 (enzymatic digestion, each); 83894 (separation); 83896 (nucleic acid probe, each); 83898 (nucleic acid probe with amplification); 83912 (interpretation and report)

Related Information

Amniotic Fluid, Chromosome and Genetic Abnormality Analysis *on page 273*

Chorionic Villus Sampling (CVS), Chromosome and Genetic Abnormality Analysis *on page 275*

Chromosome Analysis, Blood *on page 276*

Synonyms Fragile X, Carrier Detection; Fragile X, Premutation and/or Full Mutation Analysis; Fragile X, Prenatal Diagnosis; Genetic Detection of Fragile X Syndrome; Molecular Diagnosis of Fragile X; Mutation Test for Fragile X; Mutation Test for Trinucleotide Repeat Disorder, Fragile X

Test Commonly Includes Polymerase chain reaction and Southern blot analysis are used to measure the size of the trinucleotide repeat region (CGG) within the FMR1 (fragile X mental retardation-1 gene) and the methylation status of both the CGG repeats and a closely associated CpG island 5′ to the repeats.

Abstract Fragile X syndrome is the most common cause of inherited mental retardation, occurring in 1 in every 1200 males and 1 in every 2500 females. Early diagnosis based on clinical findings is difficult. Males with fragile X syndrome usually have mental retardation, characteristic physical features, developmental and speech delays combined with behavioral abnormalities, attention deficit and hyperactivity. Affected females exhibit a similar but usually less severe phenotype.

Until recently, the only laboratory test available for diagnosis of fragile X syndrome was the cytogenetic detection of the folate-sensitive fragile site of Xq27.3 (FRAXA). Cytogenetic testing for the diagnosis of fragile X syndrome is laborious, requires considerable expertise, varies greatly between individuals and laboratories, and is not sensitive for carrier detection. Cytogenetic analysis, however, is necessary to detect other chromosomal abnormalities which may be found in a patient suspected of having fragile X syndrome.

Individuals with fragile X syndrome exhibit full mutations consisting of expansion of a tandemly repeated trinucleotide sequence (CGG) within the FMR1 gene (greater than 200 repeats) and methylation of the promoter region of the gene and associated gene inactivation. The number of repeats in the FMR1 gene in the normal population varies from six to approximately 50. Females with premutation show a moderate CGG repeat expansion (50-200 repeats) and no methylation and are capable of transmitting full mutations to offspring.

Specimen Whole blood, amniotic fluid, chorionic villus sample

Container Blood should be collected in lavender top (EDTA) tube or a yellow top (ACD) tube; amniotic fluid and chorionic villus samples should be collected in a sterile manner and transferred to a sterile tube for transport

Sampling Time Amniotic fluid: at or after 14 weeks of gestation; chorionic villus sample: 8-12 weeks gestation

Storage Instructions All specimens should be sent to the laboratory immediately after collection, preferably by overnight delivery. Specimens should be kept at room temperature or refrigerated but not frozen.

Causes for Rejection Whole blood submitted in a sodium heparin (green top) or other type of tube; amniotic fluid specimen that is bloody may be contaminated with maternal blood and may be cause for erroneous results

Turnaround Time 10-21 days

(Continued)

Fragile X DNA Detection (Continued)

Reference Range The laboratory usually provides an interpretive report which includes a risk analysis. The number of CGG repeats in the FMR1 gene in the normal population ranges from six to approximately 50. Individuals with premutations show a CGG repeat expansion ranging from 50-200, and individuals with full mutations show greater than 200 CGG repeats and abnormal methylation.

Use This test is indicated for individuals of either sex with mental retardation, developmental delay, or autism, especially if they have any physical or behavioral characteristics of fragile X syndrome, a family history of fragile X syndrome, or male or female relatives with undiagnosed mental retardation. Additionally, individuals seeking reproductive counseling who have a family history of fragile X syndrome or a family history of undiagnosed mental retardation should be tested. Also, fetuses of known carrier mothers should be considered for testing, as well as patients who have a cytogenetic fragile X test result that is discordant with their phenotype. The latter includes patients who have a strong clinical indication (including risk of being a carrier) and who have had a negative or ambiguous test result, and patients with an atypical phenotype who have had a positive test result.

Limitations In a small number of fragile X patients, mechanisms other than trinucleotide expansion, such as deletion or point mutation, are responsible for the syndrome. In these cases, linkage studies and/or studies for rare mutations may be useful for relatives. PCR analysis may not detect large mutations and does not provide information with respect to methylation status, however, Southern blot analysis will.

Methodology PCR analysis utilizes flanking primers to amplify a fragment of DNA spanning the CGG repeat region. The sizes of the PCR products are indicative of the approximate number of repeats present in each allele of the individual being tested. For Southern blot analysis, extracted DNA is subjected to restriction enzymes and hybridized with a radiolabeled probe to the fragile X region of the X chromosome (Xq27.3). This form of analysis allows for detection of alleles of all sizes and methylated and unmethylated alleles can be distinguished.

Additional Information Molecular diagnostic studies for fragile X syndrome have also recently uncovered distinctive findings for a small group of fragile X males who are "high-functioning" (IQ greater than 70). This group of males shows a mosaic pattern or incomplete methylation of a fully expanded mutation. Additionally, the presence of FMR1 protein can be demonstrated in these individuals but not in retarded fragile X males. Cytogenetic studies cannot distinguish "high-functioning" fragile X males from retarded fragile X males.

References

"Fragile X Syndrome: Diagnostic and Carrier Testing. Working Group of the Genetic Screening Subcommittee of the Clinical Practice Committee. American College of Medical Genetics," *Am J Med Genet*, 1994, 53(4):380-1.

Hagerman RJ, Hull CE, Safanda JF, et al, "High Functioning Fragile X Males: Demonstration of an Unmethylated Fully Expanded FMR-1 Mutation Associated With Protein Expression," *Am J Med Genet*, 1994, 51(4):298-308.

Wang Z, Taylor A, and Bridge JA, "FMR1 Fully Expanded Mutation With Minimal Methylation in a High Functioning Fragile X Male," *J Med Genet*, 1996.

Warren ST and Nelson DL, "Advances in Molecular Analysis of Fragile X Syndrome," *JAMA*, 1994, 271(7):536-42.

Fragile X, Premutation and/or Full Mutation Analysis see
Fragile X DNA Detection *on previous page*

Fragile X, Prenatal Diagnosis see Fragile X DNA Detection *on previous page*

Gene Rearrangement, bcr see Breakpoint Cluster Region Rearrangement in CML *on page 503*

Gene Rearrangement for Leukemia and Lymphoma

CPT 83890 (molecular isolation or extraction); 83892 (enzymatic digestion); 83894 (separation); 83896 (nucleic acid probe, each)

Related Information

bcl-2 Gene Rearrangement *on page 503*
Body Fluid Cytology *on page 286*
Bone Marrow *on page 307*
Chromosome Analysis, Lymph Node and Solid Tumor *on page 279*
Histopathology *on page 42*
Immunoperoxidase Procedures *on page 43*
Immunophenotypic Analysis of Tissues by Flow Cytometry *on page 45*
Leukocyte Immunophenotyping *on page 414*
Lymph Node Biopsy *on page 50*
Skin Biopsy *on page 54*

Synonyms Leukemia Gene Rearrangement; Lymphocyte T-Cell Receptor Gene Rearrangement; Lymphoma Gene Rearrangement

Applies to Constant Region of T-Cell Receptor; Joining Region of B-Cell Receptor; Kappa Light Chains; Lambda Light Chains

Test Commonly Includes Detection of unique DNA rearrangements associated with T- and B-cell leukemias and lymphomas

Abstract Molecular biology techniques allow for detection of receptor genes rearrange from germline DNA to that in maturing T or B cells. As lymphoid cells mature they go through rearrangements of variable, joining, and constant DNA coding regions of immunoglobulin or T-cell receptors. Such recombinations allow for almost unlimited diversity of immune responses allowing response to literally millions of antigens. Lymphoma and lymphocytic leukemia are neoplastic disorders, diagnosis of which sometimes requires demonstration of clonal expansion of lymphoid cells. In the typical case, demonstration of clonality may be satisfied immunophenotypically by demonstration of surface T- and B-cell markers. When immunophenotypic methods fail to demonstrate clonality, the detection of T-cell and B-cell receptor gene rearrangements may be an invaluable test in cases in which morphologic diagnosis is difficult.

Specimen Peripheral whole blood for leukemia or lymphoma cells. **Unfixed, fresh or frozen lymph node biopsy** of suspected lymphoma is obtained during surgery for histopathologic diagnosis, immunophenotyping, and gene rearrangement assay. Other tissue such as skin biopsies, gastrointestinal tissue, and bone marrow may also be studied for gene rearrangement. Use of paraffin-embedded tissue is possible in some laboratories.

Container Lavender top (EDTA) tube

Storage Instructions Isolated white cells, lymph nodes, or tissue can be frozen at -70°C until DNA is extracted.

Causes for Rejection Insufficient DNA isolated. Muscle tissue yields little DNA for analysis.

Turnaround Time 10 days to 3 weeks

Reference Range No unique rearrangement of T- and B-cell receptors is found in normal white blood cells. An interpretive report is usually included with results.

Use Gene rearrangement may be used to supplement and complement conventional histopathology and immunophenotyping in difficult cases in the diagnosis of lymphoid leukemia and lymphoma. Gene rearrangement studies have revealed that most lymphoid leukemias are pre-B cells and not non-B, non-T. Such leukemic cells have rearrangements of genes coding for B-cell receptors, but are too immature to express cytoplasmic or surface immunoglobulins. Occasionally, lymphoid leukemia and lymphoma are of T-cell phenotype, which may be confirmed using probes designed to detect rearrangements of genes coding for T-cell receptors. Rarely, lymphoid neoplasms may have rearrangements of both T- and B-cell genes.[1,2]

Lymphoproliferative Disease and Gene Rearrangements*

Lymphoproliferative Disease	Rearrangement, % of Cases				
	Immunoglobulin			T-Cell Receptor	
	Ig H	κ	λ	β	γ
B-cell					
Precursor B ALL	100	40	20	10-30	40
B CLL; B follicular lymphoma	100	100	30	<20	<10
Diffuse lymphoma — large cell, Burkitt's, and undifferentiated	100	100	30	0	0
Hairy cell leukemia	100	100	75	–	–
T-cell					
Precursor T ALL	10-20	0	0	90	95
Diffuse lymphoma	0	0	0	100	–
MF/Sèzary syndrome	2	0	0	100	–
T CLL	0	0	0	100	–
Tλ LPD	0	0	0	60	–
ATL	0	0	0	100	–
Lymphomatoid papulosis	0	0	0	66	–
Other					
Hodgkin's disease	30-60	30-60	–	50	–
AILD	40	40	–	100	–
AML	5	–	–	10	30

From Crossman J, Uppenkamp M, Sundeen J, et al, 'Molecular Genetics and the Diagnosis of Lymphoma,' *Arch Pathol Lab Med*, 1988, 112:120, with permission.

*ALL = acute lymphocytic leukemia

CLL = chronic lymphocytic leukemia

MF = mycosis fungoides LPD, lymphoproliferative disorder

ATL = adult T-cell leukemia/lymphoma

AILD = angioimmunoblastic lymphadenopathy with dysproteinemia

AML = acute myelogenous leukemia

Limitations Some tissue yield little DNA or DNA that is degraded. Lymph nodes with <1% tumor cells cannot provide evidence of gene rearrangements when the Southern blotting method is used.

Methodology Genomic DNA is extracted and then digested with restriction endonucleases. Digested DNA is electrophoresed in agarose gel and then transferred to nitrocellulose or nylon filters by Southern blotting. DNA is exposed to labeled gene probes. Specificity of most probes **is nearly perfect**. Detection of rearrangements thus may help to demonstrate clonality (neoplastic nature) of an atypical lymphoid lesion. Filters containing hybridized DNA-probe complexes are examined for bands after autoradiography or color detection to ascertain if germline or unique gene rearrangements are present. Recently, detection of unique rearrangements of the B-cell receptor gene has been found using PCR. In many laboratories PCR serves as the first test followed by Southern blotting if results are negative or uninterpretable. Guidelines for interpretation and use of gene rearrangements in the diagnosis of lymphomas and leukemias have recently been published.[3]

Additional Information This procedure is useful to determine whether T- or B-cell gene rearrangements exist in lymphoid neoplasms. A list of various tumors and gene rearrangements can be seen in the table. Most commonly used probes are for the joining region of B-cell receptors (J_H) and the constant region of the T-cell receptor (C_BT). B-cell maturation may be further categorized by determining if kappa and/or lambda light chain genes have undergone rearrangement, using probes directed against their constant or joining DNA regions. Gene rearrangements may be detected in minute quantities of tissue, sometimes as little as 200 mg. The assay is so sensitive that gene rearrangements may be detected in larger specimens even if the percentage of cancer cells is 1%. Gene rearrangement studies are invaluable adjunctive tests that may provide evidence of clonality in an atypical lymphoid infiltrate when other methods fail. They may become a standardized diagnostic modality, should results of these studies with greater experience be found useful for therapeutic or prognostic purposes.

Footnotes

1. Farkas DH, "The Southern Blot: Application to the B- and T-Cell Gene Rearrangement Test," *Lab Med*, 1992, 23:723-9.
2. Cossman J, Uppenkamp M, Sundeen J, et al, "Molecular Genetics and the Diagnosis of Lymphoma" *Arch Pathol Lab Med*, 1988, 112(2):117-27.
3. Cossman J, Zehnbauer B, Garrett CT, et al, "Gene Rearrangements in the Diagnosis of Lymphoma/Leukemia: Guidelines for Use Based on a Multi-Institutional Study," *Am J Clin Pathol*, 1991, 95(3):347-54.

References

Harrington DS, "Molecular Gene Rearrangement Analysis in Hematopathology," *Am J Clin Pathol*, 1990, 93(4 Suppl 1):S38-43.

Korsmeyer SJ, Arnold A, Bakhshi A, et al, "Immunoglobulin Gene Rearrangement and Cell Surface Antigen Expression in Acute Lymphocytic Leukemias of T-Cell and B-Cell Precursor Origins," *J Clin Invest*, 1983, 71:301-13.

Krause JR, "Clinical Use of B- and T-Cell Gene Rearrangement Analysis in Hematopoietic Disorders," *Clin Lab Med*, 1996, 16:1-21.

Genetic Detection of Cystic Fibrosis *see* Cystic Fibrosis DNA Detection *on page 507*

Genetic Detection of Duchenne/Becker Muscular Dystrophy *see* Duchenne/Becker Muscular Dystrophy DNA Detection *on page 509*

Genetic Detection of Fragile X Syndrome *see* Fragile X DNA Detection *on page 511*

Genetic Detection of Presymptomatic Adult Polycystic Kidney Disease *see* Adult Polycystic Kidney Disease DNA Detection *on page 502*

Genetic Identification by DNA Fingerprinting *see* Identification DNA Testing *on page 517*

Gonorrhea DNA Detection *see* Neisseria gonorrhoeae Genome Detection *on page 521*

Growth Suppressor/Oncoprotein p53 *see* p53, Functional Assay/Sequencing *on page 522*

HBV DNA Probe Test *see* Hepatitis B DNA Detection *on this page*

Hepatitis B DNA Detection

CPT 83890 (molecular isolation or extraction); 83892 (enzymatic digestion); 83894 (separation); 83896 (nucleic acid probe, each)

Related Information

Hepatitis A Antibody, IgM *on page 396*
Hepatitis B Core Antibody *on page 396*
Hepatitis B$_e$ Antibody *on page 397*
Hepatitis B$_e$ Antigen *on page 397*
Hepatitis B Surface Antibody *on page 398*
Hepatitis B Surface Antigen *on page 399*
Hepatitis C Serology *on page 399*

Hepatitis D Serology *on page 400*
Liver Profile *on page 161*

Synonyms DNA Hybridization Test for HBV; DNA Probe Test for HBV; HBV DNA Probe Test; Hepatitis B Viral DNA Assay

Test Commonly Includes Use of an HBV specific DNA probe for the detection of HBV viral DNA in serum samples or tissue. Sometimes the HBV DNA is amplified by polymerase chain reaction (PCR).

Abstract Chronic viral hepatitis is due to infection with the human hepadnavirus, hepatitis B (HBV). Infection may result in a long-term carrier state of either mild to severe chronic liver disease. Two weeks after infection with hepatitis B a large excess of viral protein can be detected in serum (surface antigen of HBV) and is followed by an antibody response to the viral proteins (anti-HB$_s$). The antihepatitis B response will persist in most patients for life. However, about 10% of HBV infections result in a chronic carrier state marked by a lack of seroconversion. Diagnosis in these cases should be supplemented by additional analysis. Hepatitis B viral DNA can be detected in the serum or liver tissue from these individuals. Recent studies on symptomatic individuals with chronic liver disease of unknown etiology show that >90% are positive when tested for HBV DNA;[1] indicating that current serological testing does not detect all infections due to HBV. With the rapid growth of technology in this area, it is expected that DNA testing for HBV will soon be done in routine clinical laboratories.

Specimen Serum or plasma, liver tissue

Container Red top tube or lavender top (EDTA) tube, sterile container

Storage Instructions Serum or plasma should be transferred to a plastic tube and kept frozen at -20°C. Tissue should be frozen at -70°C.

Causes for Rejection Samples containing sodium azide cannot be used in this test.

Turnaround Time 4-7 days; turnaround time may vary with individual laboratories.

Reference Range No HBV viral DNA detected

Use Aids in the diagnosis of HBV versus the other non-B hepatitis entities; help to establish the stage of disease.[2]

Methodology A slot-blot DNA hybridization based assay or amplification by polymerase chain reaction (PCR) is used. Quantitation of HBV DNA is also available for monitoring HBV infection.[3,4]

Additional Information The DNA probe assay provides a direct measure of HBV in serum or plasma and correlates with infectivity titers. The information provided from this test should be used in conjunction with serologic tests and HBV antigen detection. DNA detection should not replace serologic testing.

Footnotes

1. Overby LR and Houghton M, "Hepatitis Viruses," *Laboratory Diagnosis of Viral Infections*, 2nd ed, Chapter 19, Lennette EH, ed, New York, NY: Marcel Dekker Inc, 1992, 403-41.
2. Brechot C, Degos F, Lugassy C, et al, "Hepatitis B Virus DNA in Patients With Chronic Liver Disease and Negative Tests for Hepatitis B Surface Antigen," *N Engl J Med*, 1985, 312(5):270-6.
3. Larzul D, Guigue F, Sninsky JJ, et al, "Detection of Hepatitis B Virus Sequences in Serum by Using *In Vitro* Enzymatic Amplification," *J Virol Methods*, 1988, 20(3):227-37.
4. Kaneko S, Feinstone SM, and Miller RH, "Rapid and Sensitive Method for the Detection of Serum Hepatitis B Virus DNA Using the Polymerase Chain Reaction Technique," *J Clin Microbiol*, 1989, 27(9):1930-3.

References

Desmet VJ, Gerber M, Hoofnagle JH, et al, "Classification of Chronic Hepatitis: Diagnosis, Grading and Staging," *Hepatology*, 1994, 19(6):1513-20.

Hytiroglou P, Dash S, Haruna Y, et al, "Detection of Hepatitis B and Hepatitis C Viral Sequences in Fulminant Hepatic Failure of Unknown Etiology," *Am J Clin Pathol*, 1995, 104(5):588-93.

Weller IVD, Fowler MJ, Monjardino J, et al, "The Detection of HBV DNA in Serum by Molecular Hybridization: A More Sensitive Method for the Detection of Complete HBV Particles," *J Med Virol*, 1982, 9:273-80.

Wu P-C, Fang JW, Lai C-L, et al, "Hepatic Expression of Hepatitis B Virus Genome in Chronic Hepatitis B Virus Infection," *Am J Clin Pathol*, 1996, 105:87-95.

Hepatitis B Viral DNA Assay *see* Hepatitis B DNA Detection *on this page*

Hepatitis C Amplification *see* Hepatitis C RNA Detection *on this page*

Hepatitis C PCR *see* Hepatitis C RNA Detection *on this page*

Hepatitis C RNA Detection

CPT 83890 (molecular isolation or extraction); 83892 (enzymatic digestion); 83894 (separation); 83896 (nucleic acid probe, each)

Related Information

Hepatitis C Serology *on page 399*
Liver Biopsy *on page 48*
Liver Profile *on page 161*
Smooth Muscle Antibody *on page 431*

Synonyms Hepatitis C Amplification; Hepatitis C PCR

(Continued)

Hepatitis C RNA Detection *(Continued)*

Abstract Hepatitis C virus (HCV) is responsible for the majority of cases of non-A, non-B post-transfusion hepatitis, as well as a significant proportion of community-acquired hepatitis. Since this virus can not be cultivated in tissue culture, liver biopsy and the detection of antibodies to HCV has provided the only evidence of infection. However, antibodies are only detectable after an undetermined time following infection and the low titer of HCV in patients does not allow for detection of HCV antigens. Thus, the only method of detection of viremia is the specific amplification of the HCV RNA genome.

Specimen Serum or liver tissue

Container Red top tube; tissue in a sterile container or sealed plastic bag

Storage Instructions Serum should be collected within 2 hours of specimen collection. Store or ship serum a -20°C. Tissue should be stored or shipped a t -70°C.

Causes for Rejection Serum samples not separated within 2 hours of collection; tissue specimens that have thawed during storage or shipping

Turnaround Time 4-7 days; may vary between different laboratories

Reference Range No HCV viral RNA detected

Use Aid in the diagnosis of HCV infection and monitor therapy; needed in the differential diagnosis between severe autoimmune hepatitis and hepatitis C.[1]

Limitations HCV RNA degrades quickly and may cause a false-negative result if specimens are not handled properly. False-positives are a problem.[2]

Methodology Viral RNA is extracted from serum or tissue and transcribed into cDNA using a reverse transcriptase (RT) enzyme. The highly conserved 5′ region of the HCV genome sequences are then amplified by polymerase chain reaction (PCR). The product of the HCV RT-PCR is then detected with an HCV-specific probe. Quantitation of the HCV RNA is also available either by direct binding with detection by branched chain DNA probes or by quantitation of the RT-PCR product.

Additional Information Occasionally, cases characterized by profound jaundice, prolonged prothrombin time, and marked AST and ALT increases present a differential diagnosis between severe viral hepatitis and autoimmune hepatitis. Antibodies against hepatitis C are not consistently found early.[1]

HCV is a single-stranded RNA virus that has been classified as belonging to the Flaviviridae family. Since the discovery of HCV in 1989, serologic testing and now molecular testing has developed to aid in the diagnosis of infected individuals. The HCV RNA detection assays will provide information on the viremic stage of infection.

Footnotes
1. Krawitt EL, "Autoimmune Hepatitis," *N Engl J Med*, 1996, 334(14):897-903.
2. Finkelstein SD, Sayegh R, Uchman S, et al, "Disease Activity of Hepatitis C Correlates With Single-Stage Polymerase Chain Reaction Detection of Hepatitis C Virus," *Am J Clin Pathol*, 1994, 101(3):321-6.

References
Bresters D, Cuypers HT, Reesink HW, et al, "Comparison of Quantitative cDNA-PCR With the Branched DNA Hybridization Assay for Monitoring Plasma Hepatitis C Virus RNA Levels in Haemophilia Patients Participating in a Controlled Interferon Trial," *J Med Virol*, 1994, 43(3):247-8.

Cuthbert JA, "Hepatitis C: Progress and Problems," *Clin Microbiol Rev*, 1994, 7(4):505-32.

Desmet VJ, Gerber M, Hoofnagle JH, et al, "Classification of Chronic Hepatitis: Diagnosis, Grading and Staging," *Hepatology*, 1994, 19(6):1513-20.

Hytiroglou P, Dash S, Haruna Y, et al, "Detection of Hepatitis B and Hepatitis C Viral Sequences in Fulminant Hepatic Failure of Unknown Etiology," *Am J Clin Pathol*, 1995, 104(5):588-93.

van Doorn LJ, "Review: Molecular Biology of the Hepatitis C Virus," *J Med Virol*, 1994, 43(4):345-56.

Hereditary Nonpolyposis Colon Cancer *see Colon Cancer, Hereditary Nonpolyposis Type on page 506*

Herpes Simplex Virus DNA Detection

CPT 83890 (molecular extraction); 83894 (separation); 83896 (nucleic acid probe); 83898 (molecular amplification)

Related Information
Herpes Cytology *on page 296*
Herpes Simplex Antibody *on page 401*
Herpes Simplex Virus Antigen Detection *on page 667*
Herpes Simplex Virus Culture *on page 668*
Polymerase Chain Reaction *on page 523*
Viral Culture *on page 675*

Synonyms HSV DNA Detection; Molecular Assay for HSV Detection

Test Commonly Includes Direct detection of herpes simplex virus nucleic acid in cells, blood, or CSF. HSV may also be detected in swabs of lesions or tissue samples obtained by biopsy. Depending on the target sequence of the primers, it is possible to detect varicella zoster virus (VZV) as well as CMV by PCR.

Abstract Herpes simplex virus (HSV) type 1 and 2 are distinct from other members of the Herpesviridae family, VZV, CMV, EBV, HHV-6, and HHV-7. HSV is capable of infecting epithelial cells and is responsible for vesicular lesions of the mouth, intestinal tract, and genital tract. HSV is able to establish a latent infection of nerve ganglion cells from which it reactivates, travels through neuronal axons, and reinfects epithelial cells. Transmission is through direct contact and may be spread to the newborn.[1,2] HSV is a common sexually transmitted disease. Infection may cause a wide variety of clinical diseases including encephalitis, for which timely diagnosis and treatment is critical. Differentiation from other viral, bacterial, or treponemal causes of CNS disease is important for appropriate therapy which includes the antiviral agent acyclovir. Detection of HSV may be accomplished by a variety of molecular techniques including amplification, such as by PCR, or through *in situ* hybridization. HSV may be detected by culture in only 40% to 70% of genital lesions and in only 25% to 40% of neonates with encephalitis. Detection of HSV by PCR has been shown to have greater sensitivity than routine culture methods.[1] As with culture techniques, it is possible to distinguish HSV 1 from HSV 2. Molecular assays such as *in situ* hybridization have been used to establish the presence of latent infection, when the virus is not replicating.

Culture is the method of choice for many acute clinical presentations.

Specimen Bronchial alveolar lavage fluid, cerebrospinal fluid, vesicle fluid, blood or serum, and various tissues including lung and brain

Container Glass or plastic containers are acceptable; lavender top (EDTA) tube for blood

Storage Instructions While freezing may reduce the viability of HSV and its isolation by culture techniques, freezing does not impair detection by amplification procedures. Any of the above fluid samples should be rapidly transported to the laboratory, however, if transportation is expected to exceed 2 hours, the sample should be refrigerated and if transportation exceeds 8 hours, a specimen should be frozen. All tissue samples should be frozen as soon as possible after the biopsy procedure.

Causes for Rejection Blood collected in heparinized tubes results in inhibition of amplification

Turnaround Time 1-3 days

Reference Range Most laboratories provide an interpretative report.

Critical Values Detection of HSV DNA in CSF

Use Useful for rapidly identifying active infection with HSV. Herpes encephalitis and neonatal herpes are fatal in a majority of patients, and neurologic sequellae are common.

Limitations A negative result does not rule out the presence of HSV in all tissues of the body or even in the sample submitted for analysis, since factors such as degradation of the nucleic acid or interference with amplification by substances that may be present. HSV detection by PCR has shown a relatively low specificity when compared with viral culture. False-positive results are possible.

Methodology Two different techniques are in common use, either PCR or *in situ* hybridization. However, the application of these techniques may be limited to reference laboratories. The molecular amplification assay utilizes specific primers which may be to a variety of viral gene sequences including polymerase, capsid antigen, or nonstructural genes such as VP-16. For the PCR assay, DNA is extracted from fluids or tissues using a standard lysis buffer followed by phenol-chloroform extraction and amplification. Alternatively, protocols exist for the direct amplification of HSV DNA following the lysis of cells by boiling or detergent without phenol extraction. For *in situ* hybridization, sections of tissue are cut and placed on glass slides, followed by incubation with a labeled probe. The target of *in situ* hybridization may be either DNA or RNA, the latter allowing for the study of the state of activity of the virus.

Additional Information Greater than 80% of adults have been exposed to HSV, as evidenced by the presence of antibodies in the serum. Although in most nonimmunosuppressed individuals infection by HSV is self-limited, one important exception is found in individuals who develop encephalitis. Although all risk factors are not known, individuals who experience multiple recurrences of oral herpes are at risk for infection of the CNS, possibly through a retrograde infection through nerves. Neonates who are infected by passage through the birth canal may have overwhelming infection with multiorgan failure or encephalitis. Amplification assays for the detection of HSV have been developed because of the increased sensitivity that these assays provide. The standard assays for HSV detection include culture on appropriate cell lines. In comparison settings, PCR of HSV DNA has shown a higher sensitivity than culture but did not detect viral genome in all cases of HSV encephalitis.[3] These findings emphasize the importance of correlating the detection of HSV DNA with clinical symptoms. Studies have confirmed the ability of PCR to detect HSV DNA when culture results are negative.[2,3] At the present time, commercial assays for HSV detection by PCR are not available and reference laboratories provide assays developed in-house, using local expertise. The specific utility of these assays is therefore dependent upon institutional modifications, and results should be correlated with clinical findings before being used to alter therapeutic protocols.

Immunocompromised patients may suffer severe infections.

Footnotes
1. Hardy DA, Arvin AM, Yasukawa LL, et al, "Use of Polymerase Chain Reaction for Successful Identification of Asymptomatic Genital Infection With Herpes Simplex Virus in Pregnant Women," *J Infect Dis*, 1990, 162(5):1031-5.
2. Cone RW, Hobson AC, Palmer J, et al, "Extended Duration of Herpes Simplex Virus DNA in Genital Lesions Detected by the Polymerase Chain Reaction," *J Infect Dis*, 1991, 164(4):757-60.
3. Kimura H, Futamura M, Kito H, et al, "Detection of Viral DNA in Neonatal Herpes Simplex Virus Infections: Frequent and Prolonged Presence in Serum and Cerebral Spinal Fluid," *J Infect Dis*, 1991, 164(2):289-93.

References
Whitley RJ, "Herpes Simplex Virus Infection," *Infectious Disease of the Fetus and Newborn Infant*, Remington JS and Klein JO, eds, Philadelphia, PA: WB Saunders Co, 1990, 282-305.
Woods GL, "Herpesviruses," *Diagnostic Pathology of Infectious Disease*, Chapter 5, Malvern, PA: Lea & Febiger, 1993, 51-3.

Herpesvirus 6 DNA Detection *see* Human Herpesvirus 6 DNA Detection *on this page*

HHV-6 DNA Detection *see* Human Herpesvirus 6 DNA Detection *on this page*

HIV DNA Amplification Assay *see* Human Immunodeficiency Virus DNA Amplification *on this page*

HIV DNA PCR Test *see* Human Immunodeficiency Virus DNA Amplification *on this page*

HNPCC Gene Testing *see* Colon Cancer, Hereditary Nonpolyposis Type *on page 506*

HPV DNA Probe Test *see* Human Papillomavirus DNA Probe Test *on next page*

HPV Screen *see* Human Papillomavirus DNA Probe Test *on next page*

HPV Type *see* Human Papillomavirus DNA Probe Test *on next page*

HSV DNA Detection *see* Herpes Simplex Virus DNA Detection *on previous page*

Human Herpesvirus 6 DNA Detection

CPT 83890 (molecular extraction); 83894 (separation); 83896 (nucleic acid probe); 83898 (molecular amplification)

Related Information
Human Herpesvirus 6 Culture *on page 669*
Human Herpesvirus 6, IgG and IgM Antibodies, Quantitative *on page 406*
Polymerase Chain Reaction *on page 523*

Synonyms Herpesvirus 6 DNA Detection; HHV-6 DNA Detection

Test Commonly Includes Direct detection of human herpesvirus type 6 nucleic acid in peripheral blood mononuclear cells or CSF. HHV-6 may also be detected in tissue samples obtained by biopsy or in bronchial lavage fluids.

Abstract Human herpesvirus 6 (HHV-6) is antigenetically and genetically distinct from other members of the Herpesviridae family, including HSV 1 and 2, VZV, CMV, and EBV, but it is related genetically to CMV. HHV-6 is the causative agent of a characteristic rash and fever in children known as roseola, or exanthem subitum, and is associated with several other conditions in immunosuppressed individuals including interstitial pneumonitis, encephalitis, and hepatitis.[1,2] Recently, another member of the herpes family, HHV-7 may also cause a clinical syndrome indistinguishable from roseola.[3] Primary infection occurs in the first 2 years of life, and most adults have antibodies to the virus with some population variation.[4] Primary infection may also occur without clinical symptoms. The virus may be isolated from peripheral blood mononuclear cells, although culture procedures are limited to research institutions. The most common means for directly detecting HHV-6 is through amplification procedures.

Specimen Bronchial alveolar lavage fluid, cerebrospinal fluid, lymphocytes and monocytes, and various tissues including liver and lung

Container Glass or plastic containers are acceptable; lavender top (EDTA) tube for blood sample

Storage Instructions Freezing does not impair detection by amplification procedures. Samples should be rapidly transported to the laboratory, however if transportation is expected to exceed 2 hours, the sample should be refrigerated, and if transportation exceeds 8 hours, a specimen should be frozen. All tissue samples should be frozen as soon as possible after the biopsy procedure.

Causes for Rejection Collection of blood in heparinized tubes result in inhibition of amplification

Turnaround Time 1-3 days

Special Instructions Specimens should **not** be obtained utilizing heparin as an anticoagulant.

Reference Range Most laboratories provide an interpretative report. It should be recognized that detection of HHV-6 in a tissue may reflect latently infected cells and not active infection.

Critical Values Detection of HHV-6 DNA in CSF is a critical value.

Use Rapid identification of a causative agent for clinical symptoms which may indicate need for appropriate therapy.

Limitations A negative result does not rule out the presence of HHV-6 in all tissues of the body or even in the sample submitted for analysis since factors such as degradation of the nucleic acid or interference with amplification by substances that may be present. False-positive results are possible. The most simple, usual diagnostic approach is measurement of antibody titers.

Methodology The molecular amplification assay utilizes specific primers which may be to a variety of viral gene sequences. DNA is extracted from fluids or tissues using a standard lysis buffer followed by phenol-chloroform extraction and amplification. Alternatively, protocols exist for the direct amplification of HHV-6 DNA following the lysis of cells by boiling or detergent without phenol extraction.

Additional Information Primary infection by HHV-6 is self-limited in most nonimmunosuppressed individuals. However, encephalitis has been reported as a complication. In bone marrow transplant patients, pneumonitis may occur associated with HHV-6.[5,6] Amplification assays for the detection of HHV-6 have been developed because of the difficulty of isolating the virus and the high sensitivity that these assays provide. As a result, CSF has been found to be positive for HHV-6 by PCR from patients with exanthem subitum and evidence of encephalitis.[2] The full clinical spectrum of disease may not yet be known, and in addition to encephalitis and pneumonitis, infection is also associated with lymphadenopathy and the mononucleosis syndrome.[7] HHV-6 shares other features with EBV and CMV, including latency and reactivation. Transmission is thought to occur through close contact since the virus can be detected in the saliva of asymptomatic individuals. The knowledge that HHV-6 may be found in asymptomatic individuals emphasizes the importance of correlating the detection of HHV-6 DNA with clinical symptoms. Detection of the virus does not necessarily provide evidence of causation of disease. At the present time, commercial assays for HHV-6 detection by PCR are not available, and reference laboratories provide assays developed in-house. The specific utility of such assays is therefore dependent upon institutional experience.

Footnotes
1. Tajiri H, Nose O, Baba K, et al, "Human Herpesvirus 6 Infection With Liver Injury in Neonatal Hepatitis," *Lancet*, 1990, 335(8693):863.
2. Kondo K, Nagafuji H, Hata A, et al, "Association of Human Herpesvirus 6 Infection of the Central Nervous System With Recurrence of Febrile Convulsions," *J Infect Dis*, 1993, 167(5):1197-200.
3. Tanaka K, Kondo T, Torigoe S, et al, "Human Herpesvirus 7: Another Causal Agent for Roseola (Exanthem Subitum)," *J Pediatr*, 1994, 125(1):1-5.
4. Ueda K, Kusuhara K, Hirose M, et al, "Exanthem Subitum and Antibody to Human Herpesvirus 6," *J Infect Dis*, 1989, 159(4):750-2.
5. Carrigan DR, Drobyski WR, Russlor SK, et al, "Interstitial Pneumonitis Associated With Human Herpesvirus-6 Infection After Marrow Transplantation," *Lancet*, 1991, 338(8760):147-9.
6. Cone RW, Hackman RC, Huang ML, et al, "Human Herpesvirus 6 in Lung Tissue From Patients With Pneumonitis After Bone Marrow Transplantation," *N Engl J Med*, 1993, 329(3):156-61.
7. Steeper TA, Horwitz CA, Ablashi DV, et al, "The Spectrum of Clinical and Laboratory Findings Resulting From Human Herpesvirus 6 (HHV-6) in Patients With Mononucleosis-like Illness Not Resulting From Epstein-Barr Virus or Cytomegalovirus," *Am J Clin Pathol*, 1990, 93(6):776-83.

References
Hinrichs SH, "Viral Diseases," *Anderson's Pathology*, 10th ed, Vol 1:Part 3 Infectious Diseases, Damjanov I, Linder J, eds, Philadelphia, PA: Mosby, 1995.

Human Immunodeficiency Virus DNA Amplification

CPT 83890 (molecular isolation or extraction); 83898 (nucleic acid probe with amplification)

Related Information
HIV-1/HIV-2 Serology *on page 403*
HTLV-I/II Antibody *on page 406*
Human Immunodeficiency Virus Culture *on page 669*
Leukocyte Immunophenotyping *on page 414*
p24 Antigen *on page 420*
Polymerase Chain Reaction *on page 523*
Viral Culture, Tissue *on page 680*

Synonyms HIV DNA Amplification Assay; HIV DNA PCR Test; Human Immunodeficiency Virus (HIV) Proviral DNA by Polymerase Chain Reaction Amplification; PCR for HIV DNA
(Continued)

Human Immunodeficiency Virus DNA Amplification *(Continued)*

Test Commonly Includes HIV DNA is detected by amplifying specific proviral DNA sequences from peripheral blood lymphocytes and subsequent hybridization with a specific HIV DNA probe.

Abstract Human immunodeficiency virus (HIV) is the causative agent of acquired immune deficiency syndrome (AIDS). Currently, testing for HIV is based on evidence of circulating antibody to the viral proteins. Commercially available tests are remarkably accurate with a low false-positive rate (1:135,000).[1] However, accuracy of the test is compromised during the time interval between infection and the development of antibody to HIV. The exact time to seroconversion is controversial but certain cases of accidental exposure have shown seroconversion to occur within 2-3 months.[2] Babies born to HIV-infected mothers will be seropositive for HIV due to transplacental antibodies. Studies have shown that only 30% to 50% of babies born to HIV infected mothers are actually infected with the virus.[1] Thus, the serologic test is unreliable for assessing HIV infection in these populations.

This virus contains an RNA genome that will incorporate into host DNA as proviral DNA. The target cells of this virus are the CD4 (T4) T-lymphocytes (helper T cells) and monocytes/macrophage populations; however, during infection, few such peripheral blood cells contain HIV.[3] To detect the incorporated viral genome, the DNA must be amplified. This procedure specifically increases the amount of DNA within the HIV genome, and the amplified DNA product is detected by specific binding to an HIV probe. The DNA detection assay has been useful for the diagnosis of HIV in infants and for monitoring individuals with a known exposure to HIV.

Specimen Peripheral blood lymphocytes from 10-20 mL whole blood

Container Two yellow top (ACD), lavender top (EDTA), or green top (sodium heparin) tubes should be collected. Type of tube is dependent on the laboratory performing the test.

Storage Instructions Tubes of blood can be sent directly to the laboratory at ambient temperature and should arrive within 48 hours of collection.

Causes for Rejection Specimens with inadequate volume or more than 48 hours old may be rejected.

Turnaround Time 2 weeks is usually required. Turnaround time may vary with individual laboratories.

Reference Range No HIV viral DNA detected in peripheral blood lymphocytes.

Use HIV detection in patients with unusual or indeterminant HIV serology.[4] It may also be useful in patients with immunodeficiency syndromes characterized by a negative HIV serology and Western blot tests.

Methodology DNA amplification is used, polymerase chain reaction (PCR).[5] DNA is extracted from peripheral blood lymphocytes. The proviral HIV DNA is exponentially amplified by using specific primers that bind to regions of the HIV genome. Using a series of denaturation, annealing, and polymerization steps the original proviral DNA can be amplified 10^5 to 10^6 fold (see figure in the listing Polymerase Chain Reaction *on page 524*). The amplified HIV DNA is confirmed by hybridization with an HIV-specific DNA probe. Hybridization with the HIV DNA probe can be detected using autoradiography or enzymatic detection procedures.

Additional Information Currently, the diagnosis of HIV infection is dependent on the detection of specific antibodies.[4] The antibody screening test commonly used is the enzyme linked immunosorbent assay (ELISA) with a confirmatory Western blot or immunoblot. These serologic assays will identify individuals with prior exposure to HIV or passively obtained antibody such as babies born to HIV-positive mothers. In addition, serologic tests may not identify patients with recent active infection. Due to this problem, other tests have also been used to document the presence of HIV, such as viral antigen assays, viral culture, and the detection of viral DNA.[3,5,6] Viral culture of HIV is a prolonged procedure taking 3-4 weeks; it suffers from a lack of sensitivity in that HIV cannot be consistently isolated from seropositive patients.[7] Studies using *in situ* hybridization have shown that few peripheral blood mononuclear cells may actually harbor HIV proviral DNA (1 in 10,000).[3] This makes it difficult to directly assay for HIV proviral DNA. Thus, DNA amplification assays have been developed to detect HIV DNA. The assay most commonly used is the polymerase chain reaction (PCR), which can amplify a single copy of DNA by 10^5 to 10^6 fold.[8] The PCR test for HIV DNA is useful in resolution of unsatisfactory HIV antibody test results and in determination of the status of children born to mothers with positive HIV serology[9,10] without the need for viral culture.

Footnotes

1. Wilber JC, "Human Immunodeficiency Viruses: HIV-1 and HIV-2," *Laboratory Diagnosis of Viral Infections*, 2nd ed, Chapter 22, Lennette EH, ed, New York, NY: Marcel Dekker Inc, 1992, 477-94.
2. Bowen PA, Lobel SA, Caruana RJ, et al, "Transmission of Human Immunodeficiency Virus (HIV) by Transplantation: Clinical Aspects and Time Course Analysis of Viral Antigenemia and Antibody Production," *Ann Intern Med*, 1988, 108(1):46-8.
3. Harper ME, Marselle LM, Gallo RC, et al, "Detection of Lymphocytes Expressing Human T-Lymphotropic Virus Type III in Lymph Nodes and Peripheral Blood From Infected Individuals by *In Situ* Hybridization," *Proc Natl Acad Sci U S A*, 1986, 83(3):772-6.
4. Burke DS, Brundage JF, Redfield RR, et al, "Measurement of False-Positive Rate in a Screening Program for Human Immunodeficiency Virus Infections," *N Engl J Med*, 1988, 319(15):961-4.
5. Jackson JB, Sannerud KJ, Hopsicker JS, et al, "Hemophiliacs With the HIV Antibody Are Actively Infected," *JAMA*, 1988, 260(15):2236-9.
6. Goudsmit J, Wolfe F, Paul DA, et al, "Expression of Human Immunodeficiency Virus Antigen (HIV-Ag) in Serum and Cerebrospinal Fluid During Acute and Chronic Infection," *Lancet*, 1986, 2(8500):177-80.
7. Feorino PM, Kalyanaraman VS, Haverkos HW, et al, "Lymphadenopathy Associated Virus Infection of a Blood Donor-Recipient Pair With Acquired Immunodeficiency Syndrome," *Science*, 1984, 225(4657):69-72.
8. Saiki RK, Gelfand DH, Stoffel S, et al, "Primer-Directed Enzymatic Amplification of DNA With a Thermostable DNA Polymerase," *Science*, 1988, 239(4839):487-91.
9. Rogers MF, Ou C-Y, Rayfield M, et al, "Use of the Polymerase Chain Reaction for Early Detection of the Proviral Sequences of Human Immunodeficiency Virus in Infants Born to Seropositive Mothers," *N Engl J Med*, 1989, 320(25):1649-54.
10. Imagawa DT, Lee MH, Wolinsky SM, et al, "Human Immunodeficiency Virus Type 1 Infection in Homosexual Men Who Remain Seronegative for Prolonged Periods," *N Engl J Med*, 1989, 320(22):1458-62.

References

Loche M and Mach B, "Identification of HIV-Infected Seronegative Individuals by a Direct Diagnostic Test Based on Hybridisation to Amplified DNA," *Lancet*, 1988, 2(8608):418-21.

Phair JP and Wolinsky S, "Diagnosis of Infection With the Human Immunodeficiency Virus," *Clin Infect Dis*, 1992, 15(1):13-6.

Romano JW, van Gemen B, and Kievits T, "A Novel, Isothermal Detection Technology for Qualitative and Quantitative HIV-1 RNA Measurements," *Clin Lab Med*, 1996, 16(1):89-103.

Sheppard HW, Dondero D, Arnon J, et al, "An Evaluation of the Polymerase Chain Reaction in HIV-1 Seronegative Men," *J Acquir Immune Defic Syndr*, 1991, 4(8):819-23.

Human Immunodeficiency Virus (HIV) Proviral DNA by Polymerase Chain Reaction Amplification *see* Human Immunodeficiency Virus DNA Amplification *on previous page*

Human Papillomavirus DNA Probe Test

CPT 83890 (molecular isolation or extraction); 83892 (enzymatic digestion); 83894 (separation); 83896 (nucleic acid probe, each)

Related Information

Cervical/Vaginal Cytology *on page 290*
Histopathology *on page 42*
p53, Functional Assay/Sequencing *on page 522*
Viral Culture, Tissue *on page 680*
Viral Culture, Urogenital *on page 681*

Synonyms DNA Hybridization Test for HPV; DNA Probe Test for HPV; HPV DNA Probe Test; HPV Screen; HPV Type; ViraPap®; ViraType®

Test Commonly Includes Screening specimens for the presence of HPV and optional determination of the specific type(s) of HPV present in positive specimens

Abstract Papillomaviruses are nonencapsulated icosahedral viruses which belong to the papovavirus family. The life cycle of HPV is linked to squamous cell differentiation. HPV infection of the uterine cervix is venereally transmitted. It causes koilocytosis, condyloma acuminatum, and cervical intraepithelial neoplasia. See listing Cervical/Vaginal Cytology *on page 290*. Squamous intraepithelial lesion (SIL) is defined, *vide infra*. HPV infections of the cervix frequently cause low-grade SIL and are commonplace in young, sexually active women. Such infections often resolve spontaneously, but some progress. Risk factors which support progression are thought to include cell-mediated immunity and reproduction factors, as well as HPV type and intensity.[1]

HPV has been detected in certain tumors of the upper airway. Many other such viral infections probably have little oncogenic potential.

Patient Preparation At least 2 days must elapse between the time acetic acid or iodine preparations are used and the time swab specimens are taken. Biopsies can be taken immediately after the use of acetic acid or iodine.

Specimen Cervical swab, cervical biopsy, vulvar biopsy

Container Specific tubed transport medium provided by the laboratory. Do **not** substitute.

Sampling Time At the time of clinical suspicion of HPV infection

Collection Use **specific** swab provided by the laboratory to collect endocervical and ectocervical cells similar to the manner in which Pap smear cells are taken. Obtain biopsy in usual manner. Biopsies **must** be ≤3 mm. Cervical cells also can be taken by **scraping** the cervix with an appropriate spatula. Place swabs, scrapings, and biopsies into specific transport medium. **Important:** Collection of a sufficiently large number of epithelial cells is mandatory. However, scraping/removal of cells to the point of bleeding should not be done, because visible blood in specimen might reduce the chance of detection of HPV.

Storage Instructions Freeze biopsies in transport medium immediately. Swab or scrape specimens can be stored at room temperature for several days, but for simplicity, can be frozen immediately.

Causes for Rejection Some laboratories reject visibly bloody specimens.

Turnaround Time Usually 4 days to 2 weeks, but depends on laboratory protocol and lability of radioactive reagents

Reference Range HPV has been found in genital lesions of both normal and symptomatic persons.[2,3] HPV has been detected in patients whose exfoliative cytology smears are morphologically normal.[4]

Use Possible aid in making decisions regarding treatment, follow-up visits and tests, management, and prognosis of patients with HPV infections, including proliferative, atypical lesions of the uterine cervix and the anorectal mucosa. Such lesions include carcinomas and their precursors.

Limitations

- Detects only 7 of the approximately 57 genotypes of HPV, of which 20 have been isolated from the female genital tract
- Can be negative with accompanying cytological changes
- Can be positive without accompanying cytological changes; by Southern blot hybridization, HPV DNA is found in approximately 15% of morphologically normal cervices
- Viral integration is not always found in invasive carcinoma of uterine cervix
- Can give false-negative results if specimens are visibly bloody or if an insufficient sample of HPV-infected cells is obtained
- Latent viral infection does not cause morphologic abnormalities
- A fraction of patients with high-risk HPV infection have only low-grade lesions when biopsied.
- A wide variety of HPV types is found in CIN 1
- Can give borderline results
- Expensive

Recognizing that HPV plays an important role in the development of SIL, Kurman observes that identification of HPV DNA in the uterine cervix by Southern blot hybridization, in situ hybridization, or PCR for clinical diagnosis and management of the preinvasive squamous proliferative lesions represent technologic advances for which the value has not been determined. He has indicated (1993) that **the routine use of this test at present is not recommended**. This recommendation continues in 1996.[4]

Methodology Disruption and digestion of specimen, attachment of specimen DNA to filters, and probing denatured (HPV) DNA with commercially available nucleic acid probes which are specific for HPV types 6, 11, 16, 18, 31, 33, and 35. Amplification by polymerase chain reaction is also used to detect HPV types in cervical and anorectal specimens. In situ hybridization, as well as PCR, is used.[5]

Additional Information The presence of HPV types 6/11, 16/18, and 31/33/35 has been associated with "low" (condyloma), "high," and "moderate" risk of development of cervical cancer, respectively.[4,6,7] HPV 16 is found in 20% of CIN 1, 40% of CIN 2, and 66% of CIN 3 and is found in about 50% of the invasive squamous cell carcinomas of the cervix. HPV 18 is found in about 20% of invasive cervical squamous cell carcinomas. HPV detection in intraepithelial proliferative lesions of the cervix segregate into two morphologic groups. The **Bethesda System** provides **low grade and high grade squamous intraepithelial lesion** (SIL) classifications, in which low grade corresponds to CIN 1. High grade lesions are CIN 2, and 3, moderate and severe dysplasia and carcinoma in situ.

The utility of HPV typing continues to be studied. All HPV-infected subjects do not develop cervical carcinoma, even when infected with oncogene types 16, 18, 31, 33, or 35.[4] The screening test is FDA-approved, and the typing test is currently pending FDA approval.

HPV may exert a role in development of laryngeal squamous papilloma and nasal inverted papilloma.[8]

Tumor suppressor proteins *p53* and Rb inhibit cell cycle progression. They are inactivated by viral proteins E6 and E7 that are produced by high-risk HPV types, leading to dysregulated entry of cells into S phase. *p53* may be inactivated by mutation as well.[9]

Early phases of carcinogenesis of the cervix uteri include other factors as well; *bcl-2* expression may be among them.[10]

Footnotes
1. Schiffman MH and Brinton LA, "The Epidemiology of Cervical Carcinogenesis," *Cancer*, 1995, 76(Suppl 10):1888-901.
2. Meanwell CA, Cox MF, Blackledge G, et al, "HPV 16 DNA in Normal and Malignant Cervical Epithelium: Implications for the Aetiology and Behavior of Cervical Neoplasia," *Lancet*, 1987, 1(8535):703-7.
3. de Villiers EM, Wagner D, Schneider A, et al, "Human Papillomavirus Infections in Women With and Without Abnormal Cervical Cytology," *Lancet*, 1987, 2(8561):703-6.
4. Chua KL and Hjerpe A, "Persistence of Human Papillomavirus (HPV) Infections Preceding Cervical Carcinoma," *Cancer*, 1996, 97(1):121-7.
5. Shroyer KR, Brookes CG, Markham NE, et al, "Detection of Human Papillomavirus in Anorectal Squamous Cell Carcinoma. Correlation With Basaloid Pattern of Differentiation," *Am J Clin Pathol*, 1995, 104(3):299-305.
6. zurHausen H and Schneider A, "The Role of Papillomaviruses in Human Anogenital Cancer," *The Papoviridae*, Vol 2, Salzmann NP and Howley PM, eds, New York, NY: Plenum, 1987, 245-63.
7. Shah KV and Buscema J, "Genital Warts, Papillomaviruses, and Genital Malignancies," *Annu Rev Med*, 1988, 39:371-9.
8. Shen J, Tate JE, Crum CP, et al, "Prevalence of Human Papillomaviruses (HPV) in Benign and Malignant Tumors of the Upper Respiratory Tract," *Mod Pathol*, 1996, 9(1):15-20.
9. Cannistra SA and Niloff JM, "Cancer of the Uterine Cervix," *N Engl J Med*, 1996, 334(16):1030-8.
10. Saegusa M, Takano Y, Hashimura M, et al, "The Possible Role of bcr-2 Expression in the Progression of Tumors of the Uterine Cervix," *Cancer*, 1995, 76:2297-303.

References

Bauer HM, Ting Y, Greer CE, et al, "Genital Human Papillomavirus Infection in Female University Students as Determined by A PCR-Based Method," *JAMA*, 1991, 265(4):472-7.

Chang F, "Role of Papillomaviruses," *J Clin Pathol*, 1990, 43(4):269-76.

Crum CP and Roche JK, "Molecular Pathology of the Lower Female Genital Tract - The Papillomavirus Model," *Am J Surg Pathol*, 1990, 14(Suppl 1):26-33.

Herrington CS, Evans MF, Gray W, et al, "Morphological Correlation of Human Papillomavirus Infection of Matched Cervical Smears and Biopsies From Patients With Persistent Mild Cervical Cytological Abnormalities," *Hum Pathol*, 1995, 26(9):951-5.

Howley PM and Schlegel R, "The Human Papillomaviruses. An Overview," *Am J Med*, 1988, 85(2A):155-8.

Kurman RJ, "Current Concepts in the Relationship of HPV Infection to the Pathogenesis and Classification of Precancerous Squamous Lesions of the Cervix," (discussion), *Current Issues in Surgical Pathology*, XII, University of Texas Southwestern Medical Center at Dallas, May, 1993.

Lungu O, Sun XW, Felix J, et al, "Relationship of Human Papillomavirus Type to Grade of Cervical Intraepithelial Neoplasia," *JAMA*, 1992, 267(18):2493-6.

Milde-Langosch K, Schreiber C, Becker G, et al, "Human Papillomavirus Detection in Cervical Adenocarcinoma by Polymerase Chain Reaction," *Hum Pathol*, 1993, 24(6):590-4.

Reid R, "Human Papillomaviral Infection. The Key to Rational Triage of Cervical Neoplasia," *Obstet Gynecol Clin North Am*, 1987, 14(2):407-29.

Roman A and Fife KH, "Human Papillomaviruses: Are We Ready to Type?" *Clin Microbiol Rev*, 1989, 2(2):166-90.

Shroyer KR, Brookes CG, Markham NE, et al, "Detection of Human Papillomavirus in Anorectal Squamous Cell Carcinoma. Correlation With Basaloid Pattern of Differentiation," *Am J Clin Pathol*, 1995, 104(3):299-305.

Identification DNA Testing

CPT 83890 (molecular isolation or extraction); 83892 (enzymatic digestion); 83894 (separation); 83896 (nucleic acid probe, each)

Related Information

Chain-of-Custody Protocol *on page 542*
HLA Typing, Single Human Leukocyte Antigen *on page 405*
Paternity Studies *on page 613*
Tissue Typing *on page 434*

Synonyms DNA Analysis for Parentage Evaluation; DNA Fingerprinting; Genetic Identification by DNA Fingerprinting; Parentage Studies; Paternity Testing by DNA Testing; RFLP Analysis for Parentage Evaluation

Test Commonly Includes Identification of individuals by using DNA polymorphic regions

Abstract The progress in the field of DNA technology and the ongoing Human Genome Project has resulted in a tremendous store of information about the genetic material that makes each individual unique. The human genome is made up of about 120 million base pairs organized into 46 different chromosomes. Half of an individual's genetic material is "donated" by their mother while the other half is "donated" by their father. The DNA from both maternal and paternal sources may be normal, but will have slight variations in character. These variations can be detected and used to map heredity much like the variations in blood group antigens and the human leukocyte antigen (HLA) system. By using between 20-30 different polymorphic sites on different chromosomes, identity or parentage can be established with up to 99.99% exclusion probability.[1,2]

Patient Preparation Patient should receive no transfusions 90 days prior to testing.

Specimen Peripheral whole blood, tissue, amniotic fluid, semen, or cultured cells

Container Blood should be collected in a yellow top (ACD) tube or lavender top (EDTA) tube; tissue should be frozen at -70°C; amniotic cells, fibroblasts, or lymphocytes should be grown in appropriate media in T25 tissue culture flasks.

Collection A 0.1-1 g of tissue should be obtained. The specimen should then be put into a sealable plastic freezer bag and frozen at -70°C. The specimen should be kept frozen until shipped to the laboratory. Cell cultures should be grown to confluency and tightly sealed before shipping.

Storage Instructions Store tissue at -70°C or on dry ice. Peripheral blood should be stored and shipped at 4°C. Do **not** freeze blood.

Causes for Rejection If the tissue specimen thaws out during transport to the laboratory or before shipping, DNA may not be obtained from the specimen; if less than 0.1 g of tissue is sent to the laboratory, it may not
(Continued)

Identification DNA Testing (Continued)

yield enough DNA for analysis; blood samples that have been frozen and thawed will yield low quality DNA; specimens inadequately identified will be rejected.

Turnaround Time 2-4 weeks. Samples of DNA can be stored for an unlimited amount of time.

Reference Range The laboratory bears an obligation to communicate results in confidence. The test provides a 99.99% exclusion probability.

Use The analysis of highly polymorphic regions of human DNA can clarify the relationships between individuals and verify the identify of unknown individuals (such as suspects in criminal investigations or unidentified victims of murder).

Limitations Failure to obtain DNA from the blood, tissue, or cultured cells due to inappropriate shipping or processing

Methodology DNA is released and isolated from the white blood cells, tissue, or cultured cells by lysing the cells and extracting the cell lysate with phenol and chloroform. Purified, intact DNA is precipitated with salt in the presence of alcohol. The DNA is then digested with various restriction enzymes and electrophoresed through an agarose gel. DNA is then transferred to a solid support such as a nylon membrane and hybridized with a radioactive DNA probe. After washing the unhybridized DNA probe off the membrane, the target DNA is exposed to x-ray film to detect the polymorphic regions of DNA. All autosomal genes are inherited as a pair. One gene copy is of maternal origin and one copy is of paternal origin. Certain regions of the human genome show a high degree of polymorphism in that >85% of the population show heterogeneity.[3] These regions are highly informative in determining DNA identification. When human DNA in these regions is digested with different restriction enzymes, the size and pattern of the DNA fragments will vary with each individual. This pattern is an inherited trait and if the appropriate family members are tested, the inheritance pattern can be established. This is important in determining the paternity of a child or if a set of twins is heterozygous or monozygous. This can also help establish the identity of an unknown criminal or victim.

Additional Information The genetic material of humans is highly polymorphic, and an individual's genotype represents a unique pattern which determines that person's identity and heredity. The only exception to this rule is identical twins, since they are derived from a single fertilized egg and hence have the same DNA profile.[4] As a general rule, DNA is constant in all tissues of the body (even prenatal samples such as amniotic cells and chorionic villi specimens). DNA isolated from any specimen from an individual will be identical, which can prove to be very valuable in forensic evidence.[5]

DNA typing provides a valuable tool for establishing family relationships and associations between forensic specimens (dried blood, semen, hair, skin scrapings, etc) and criminal suspects. Southern blots using a panel of DNA probes specific for several polymorphic DNA regions can produce a composite profile which is unique to an individual and can be traced through families to establish relationships.[1,6] DNA identification can be used for many applications such as paternity identification, identification of military casualties, clarifying parentage of infants possibly switched at birth or abducted, immigration disputes dealing with relationships, determination of sexual abuse and rape, as well as other criminal investigations.[2,7]

Healthcare professionals are often involved in collecting specimens. Great care should be taken in the collection and storage of these specimens to prevent contamination and to preserve the evidence which may be crucial to any legal case.[7]

Footnotes

1. Honma M and Ishiyama I, "Application of DNA Fingerprinting to Parentage and Extended Family Relationship Testing," *Hum Hered*, 1990, 40(6):356-62.
2. Jeffreys AJ, Turner M, and Debenham P, "The Efficiency of Multilocus DNA Fingerprint Probes for Individualization and Establishment of Family Relationships, Determined From Extensive Casework," *Am J Hum Genet*, 1991, 48(5):824-40.
3. Nakamura Y, Leppert M, O'Connell P, et al, "Variable Number of Tandem Repeat (VNTR) Markers For Human Gene Mapping," *Science*, 1987, 253(4796):1616-22.
4. Jones L, Thein SL, Jefferys AJ, et al, "Identical Twin Marrow Transplantation for 5 Patients With Chronic Myeloid Leukaemia: Role of DNA Finger-Printing to Confirm Monozygosity in 3 Cases," *Eur J Haematol*, 1987, 39(2):144-7.
5. Gill P, Jeffreys AJ, and Werret DJ, "An Evaluation of DNA Fingerprinting for Forensic Purposes," *Electrophoresis*, 1987, 8:38-44.
6. Balazs I, Baird M, Clyne M, et al, "Human Population Genetics Studies of Five Hypervariable DNA Loci," *Am J Hum Genet*, 1989, 44(2):182-90.
7. Lander ES, "Research on DNA Typing Catching Up With Courtroom Application [Invited Editorial]," *Am J Hum Genet*, 1991, 48(5):819-23.

References

McCabe ER, "Application of DNA Fingerprinting in Pediatric Practice," *J Pediatr*, 1992, 120(4 Pt 1):499-509.

Walker RH, "Molecular Biology in Paternity Testing," *Lab Med*, 1992, 23:752-7.

Wolff RK, Nakamura Y, and White R, "Molecular Characterization of a Spontaneously Generated New Allele at VNTR Locus: No Exchange of Flanking DNA Sequences," *Genomics*, 1988, 3(4):347-51.

Wong Z, Wilson V, Jeffreys AJ, et al, "Cloning a Selected Fragment From a Human DNA Fingerprint: Isolation of an Extremely Polymorphic Minisatellite," *Nucleic Acids Res*, 1986, 14(11):4605-16.

Joining Region of B-Cell Receptor see Gene Rearrangement for Leukemia and Lymphoma on page 512

Kappa Light Chains see Gene Rearrangement for Leukemia and Lymphoma on page 512

Lambda Light Chains see Gene Rearrangement for Leukemia and Lymphoma on page 512

Leukemia Gene Rearrangement see Gene Rearrangement for Leukemia and Lymphoma on page 512

Li-Fraumeni Syndrome see p53, Functional Assay/Sequencing on page 522

Lyme Disease DNA Detection

CPT 87179

Related Information

Lyme Disease Serology on page 415
Polymerase Chain Reaction on page 523
Synovial Fluid Analysis on page 656

Synonyms *Borrelia burgdorferi* DNA Assay; *Borrelia burgdorferi* DNA Probe Test; DNA Hybridization Test for *Borrelia burgdorferi*; DNA Probe Test for Lyme Disease

Test Commonly Includes DNA from the spirochete *Borrelia burgdorferi* is amplified from a patient specimen and specific DNA hybridization is used to detect the amplified product.

Abstract Lyme disease was first recognized in the U.S. in Wisconsin in 1969. Since that time sporadic epidemics of Lyme disease have been reported primarily in the northeastern and upper midwestern United States, California, Georgia, and Texas. Isolated reports have occurred in 46 states. The disease is caused by the spirochete *Borrelia burgdorferi*. Epidemics tend to occur in the spring and fall when the tick vector, *Ixodes ricinus*, is proliferating. Ticks transmit the spirochete to humans through bites. The diagnosis of Lyme disease is difficult due to the insensitivity and unreliability of serological tests. Thus, recent developments have made available a DNA based test that can detect *Borrelia burgdorferi* in body fluids such as serum, spinal fluid, synovial fluid, and urine. This test can often establish the diagnosis of Lyme disease when serologic tests are equivocal.

Specimen Serum or plasma, cerebrospinal fluid, synovial fluid, urine

Container Red top tube or lavender top (EDTA) tube for blood samples. Spinal fluid and synovial fluid should be collected in a sterile container. Plastic container is used for urine.

Sampling Time Urine should be collected before antibiotic therapy is initiated.

Storage Instructions All specimens should be sent to the laboratory immediately or kept at 4°C until shipped to the laboratory. Once in the laboratory, serum or plasma should be transferred to a sealed plastic tube.

Causes for Rejection Samples containing sodium azide cannot be used in this test; samples left at extreme temperature will yield suboptimal results.

Turnaround Time 1 week

Reference Range No *Borrelia burgdorferi* DNA detection

Use Detect the presence of DNA from the spirochete *Borrelia burgdorferi* in patients with signs and symptoms of Lyme disease, providing improved sensitivity for diagnosis

Methodology Patient specimens are treated to isolate DNA and rid the sample of substances that inhibit amplification of DNA. The DNA is then amplified using specific primers for *Borrelia burgdorferi* sequences. The amplified DNA is then confirmed to be *B. burgdorferi* by hybridization with a DNA probe.

Additional Information Transmission of *Borrelia burgdorferi*, a pathogenic spirochete, to humans occurs primarily by way of infected *Ixodid* ticks, including *I. dammini*, *I. pacificus*, and others, the *Ixodes ricinus* complex. The signs and symptoms of Lyme disease vary, but the most common clinical manifestation following the bite of an infected tick is a distinctive skin lesion, erythema chronicum migrans. This initial stage of Lyme disease is benign and is usually successfully treated with oral antibiotics. Symptoms sometimes persist or reappear after antibiotic treatment and the later stage disease may include chronic progressive encephalomyelitis, chronic severe arthritis, as well as various cardiac manifestations.[1,2,3] Direct microscopic detection of *Borrelia burgdorferi* is difficult; therefore the most widely used indicator of infection is *Borrelia burgdorferi* serologic study. Serologic work-up provides limited sensitivity, and antibody can be detected in only 40% to 60% of infected patients.[4] Serological testing also suffers from lack of specificity and reproducibility when examined in a trial proficiency testing program.[5]

Thus, a more direct and sensitive method to diagnosis Lyme disease has been needed. Infected patients appear to have spirochetes in their tissues, serum, or spinal fluids. Amplification of *Borrelia burgdorferi* DNA supports detection of the organism in a specific and sensitive assay from patient specimens. A test for direct detection of *Borrelia burgdorferi* DNA would enable detection of dissemination of the spirochete early in the course of infection.[2,3,6] Thus, appropriate antibiotic therapy can be initiated. It also allows for monitoring of patients during and after chemotherapy. This is a valuable diagnostic tool since recognition of Lyme disease is often complicated by the variety of clinical signs and presentation.

Footnotes

1. Steere AC, Schoen RT, and Taylor E, "The Clinical Evolution of Lyme Arthritis," *Ann Intern Med*, 1987, 107(5):725-31.
2. Reik L, Steere AC, Bartenhagen NH, et al, "Neurologic Abnormalities of Lyme Disease," *Medicine (Baltimore)*, 1979, 58:281-94.
3. Steere AC, Batsford WP, Weinberg M, et al, "Lyme Carditis: Cardiac Abnormalities of Lyme Disease," *Ann Intern Med*, 1980, 93:8-16.
4. Grodzicki RL and Steere AC, "Comparison of Immunoblotting and Indirect Enzyme-Linked Immunosorbent Assay Using Different Antigen Preparations for Diagnosing Early Lyme Diseases," *J Infect Dis*, 1988, 157(4):790-7.
5. Bakker LL, Case KL, Callister SM, et al, "Performance of 45 Laboratories Participating in a Proficiency Testing Program for Lyme Disease Serology," *JAMA*, 1992, 268(7):891-5.
6. Luft BJ, Steinman CR, Neimark HC, et al, "Invasion of the Central Nervous System by *Borrelia burgdorferi* in Acute Disseminated Infection," *JAMA*, 1992, 267(10):1364-7.

References

Guy EC and Stanek G, "Detection of *Borrelia burgdorferi* in Patients With Lyme Disease by the Polymerase Chain Reaction," *J Clin Pathol*, 1991, 44(7):610-1.

Kaslow RA, "Current Perspective on Lyme Borreliosis," *JAMA*, 1992, 267(10):1381-3.

Malloy DC, Nauman RK, and Paxton H, "Detection of *Borrelia burgdorferi* Using the Polymerase Chain Reaction," *J Clin Microbiol*, 1990, 28(6):1089-93.

Nocton JJ, Dressler F, Rutledge BJ, et al, "Polymerase Chain Reaction *Borrelia burgdorferi* Synovial Fluid," *N Engl J Med*, 1994, 330(4):229-34.

Rosa PA and Schwan TG, "A Specific and Sensitive Assay for the Lyme Disease Spirochete *Borrelia burgdorferi* Using the Polymerase Chain Reaction," *J Infect Dis*, 1989, 160(6):1018-29.

Steere AC, "*Borrelia burgdorferi* (Lyme Disease, Lyme Borreliosis)," *Principles and Practice of Infectious Diseases*, 3rd ed, Mandell GL, Douglas RG Jr, and Bennett JE, eds, New York, NY: Churchill Livingstone, 1990, 1819-27.

Lymphocyte T-Cell Receptor Gene Rearrangement *see* Gene Rearrangement for Leukemia and Lymphoma *on page 512*

Lymphoma Gene Rearrangement *see* Gene Rearrangement for Leukemia and Lymphoma *on page 512*

MEN 2A *see* Multiple Endocrine Neoplasia/Familial Medullary Thyroid Carcinoma *on this page*

MEN 2B *see* Multiple Endocrine Neoplasia/Familial Medullary Thyroid Carcinoma *on this page*

MEN2/FMTC *see* Multiple Endocrine Neoplasia/Familial Medullary Thyroid Carcinoma *on this page*

Molecular Assay for CMV Detection *see* Cytomegalovirus DNA Detection *on page 508*

Molecular Assay for HSV Detection *see* Herpes Simplex Virus DNA Detection *on page 514*

Molecular Diagnosis of Cystic Fibrosis *see* Cystic Fibrosis DNA Detection *on page 507*

Molecular Diagnosis of Duchenne/Becker Muscular Dystrophy *see* Duchenne/Becker Muscular Dystrophy DNA Detection *on page 509*

Molecular Diagnosis of Fragile X *see* Fragile X DNA Detection *on page 511*

Molecular Diagnosis of Polycystic Kidney Disease *see* Adult Polycystic Kidney Disease DNA Detection *on page 502*

Molecular Probe for Enterovirus *see* Enterovirus Genome Detection *on page 510*

Multiple Endocrine Neoplasia/Familial Medullary Thyroid Carcinoma

CPT 83890 (nuclear molecular diagnostics, molecular isolation or extraction); 83894 (enzymatic digestion); 83898 (nucleic acid probe with amplification); 83912 (interpretation and report)

Related Information

Calcitonin *on page 96*
Calcium, Serum *on page 97*
Metanephrines *on page 165*

Synonyms Familial Medullary Thyroid Carcinoma/Multiple Endocrine Neoplasia; MEN 2A; MEN 2B; MEN2/FMTC; RET Gene Testing

Test Commonly Includes This molecular test can detect point mutations in the RET gene.

Abstract Medullary thyroid carcinoma is an entity distinct from papillary or follicular carcinoma of thyroid. It may be sporadic as well as familial.

Mutations in the RET proto-oncogene associated with familial medullary thyroid carcinoma (FMTC) and multiple endocrine neoplasia (type II A and B) (MEN 2A and 2B) were first described in 1993.[1] Mutations are detected by sequencing the DNA of the RET gene. Testing for RET mutations in all individuals with MTC has been recommended since September of 1994[2] and has become the clinically accepted approach to the diagnosis of MEN 2 and FMTC.

Specimen Whole blood

Container Blue top (sodium citrate) tube or yellow top (ACD) tube

Storage Instructions All specimens should be sent to the laboratory **immediately** after collection, preferably by overnight delivery. All specimens should be kept at room temperature or refrigerated, never frozen.

Causes for Rejection Lysed or frozen blood sample

Turnaround Time Results are usually available in 3 weeks.

Use The laboratory generally provides an interpretive report based upon direct sequencing analysis. This test is indicated for families with a history of MEN 2A or MEN 2B or FMTC (autosomal dominant).

Limitations If a high-risk affected individual tests negative for RET mutations, an inherited form of cancer may still exist and appropriate genetic counseling should be provided. This evaluation is costly.

Methodology DNA is isolated from the specimen. Regions within the RET gene (exons 10, 11, 13, 14, and 16) are amplified by PCR and sequenced in entirety.

Additional Information Medullary thyroid carcinoma (MTC) is a malignancy of the calcitonin-secreting cells (C-cells) of the thyroid and accounts for about 10% of thyroid cancer. One in 5000 individuals is affected with MTC each year; about 50% of patients have metastases at the time of diagnosis. The historical 10-year survival is about 50%. About 20% of MTC occurs as part of one of three familial syndromes: multiple endocrine neoplasia type 2A (MEN 2A) characterized by MTC, pheochromocytoma (~50%), and hyperparathyroidism (~10%); multiple endocrine neoplasia type 2B (MEN 2B) consisting of MTC, pheochromocytoma (-50%), and ganglioneuromatosis; and familial medullary thyroid carcinoma syndrome (FMTC) characterized by MTC alone. All are autosomal dominantly inherited. Virtually everyone who inherits a mutation in RET will develop MTC. Prior to the identification of the RET gene in 1993, it was the standard of practice to perform annual biochemical screening on all individuals in definite or suspected FMTC, MEN 2A, and MEN 2B families. Because it is not possible to distinguish sporadic from familial tumors histopathologically and because the family history is often unreliable, biochemical screening has been performed on first-degree relatives of many individuals affected with apparently sporadic MTC. Such screening has been performed annually from 5 years of age to about 40 years to detect C-cell hyperplasia (the precursor of medullary thyroid carcinoma) as early as possible, followed by total thyroidectomy. Pentagastrin stimulation testing yields false-positives, false-negatives, and equivocal results requiring test repetition.[3] The majority of cases of MTC are **not** familial, and in those families in which it is inherited, 50% of first-degree relatives would be expected not to have inherited the gene. DNA testing for mutations in the RET gene in all individuals with MTC accurately diagnoses a heritable form of MTC in >90% of cases and identifies family members who have inherited the mutation.[4] Family members who have not inherited the mutation require no further screening. It is recommended that those family members who do inherit the mutation undergo thyroidectomy. Additionally, with the knowledge that such individuals are at risk for other MEN 2-associated tumors, biochemical screening for premorbid detection of pheochromocytoma and hyperparathyroidism can be initiated.

Footnotes

1. Donis-Keller H, Dou S, Chi D, et al, "Mutations in the RET Proto-Oncogene Are Associated With MEN 2A and FMTC," *Hum Mol Genet*, 1993, 2(7):851-6.
2. Utiger RD, "Medullary Thyroid Carcinoma, Genes, and the Prevention of Cancer," *N Engl J Med*, 1994, 331(13):870-1.
3. Lips CJ, Landsvater RM, Höppener JW, et al, "Clinical Screening as Compared With DNA Analysis in Families With Multiple Endocrine Neoplasia Type 2A," *N Engl J Med*, 1994, 331(13):828-35.
4. Chi DD, Toshima K, Donis-Keller H, et al, "Predictive Testing for Multiple Endocrine Neoplasia Type 2A (MEN 2A) Based on the Detection of Mutations in the RET Proto-Oncogene," *Surgery*, 1994, 116(2):124-33.

References

Xue F, Yu H, Maurer LH, et al, "Germline RET Mutations in MEN 2A and FMTC and Their Detection by Simple DNA Diagnostic Tests," *Hum Mol Genet*, 1994, 3(4):635-8.

Zedenius J, Wallin G, and Hamberger B, "Somatic and MEN 2A De Novo Mutations Identified in the RET Proto-Oncogene by Screening of Sporadic MTCs," *Hum Mol Genet*, 1994, 3(8):1259-62.

Mutation Test for Cystic Fibrosis *see* Cystic Fibrosis DNA Detection *on page 507*

Mutation Test for Duchenne/Becker Muscular Dystrophy *see* Duchenne/Becker Muscular Dystrophy DNA Detection *on page 509*

Mutation Test for Fragile X *see* Fragile X DNA Detection *on page 511*

Mutation Test for Trinucleotide Repeat Disorder, Fragile X *see* Fragile X DNA Detection *on page 511*

Mycobacteria by DNA Probe

CPT 87179

Related Information

Acid-Fast Stain *on page 446*
Mycobacterial Culture, Biopsy or Body Fluid *on page 487*
Mycobacterial Culture, Cerebrospinal Fluid *on page 489*
Mycobacterial Culture, Cutaneous and Subcutaneous Tissue *on page 489*
Mycobacterial Culture, Sputum *on page 490*
Mycobacterial Culture, Stool *on page 491*
Mycobacterial Culture, Urine *on page 491*

Synonyms DNA Hybridization Test for Mycobacteria; DNA Test for Mycobacteria; Mycobacteria DNA Detection Test; Mycobacterial Accuprobe®

Applies to DNA Amplification Assay

Test Commonly Includes Direct detection of mycobacterial DNA in patient specimens or after primary culture

Abstract The number of infections due to *Mycobacterium tuberculosis* (TB) has risen dramatically in the last few years. This increased frequency of infection includes patients with acquired immune deficiency syndrome, patients with malignant disorders and immunosuppression, I.V. drug users, prison inmates, refugees and immigrants, nursing home residents, and the homeless population.[1,2] The lack of a rapid and unequivocal means of detecting *M. tuberculosis* has been a major obstacle in establishing effective infection control. Following exposure, baseline and 12-week follow-up tuberculin skin tests (PPD) are included in standard assessment protocols. However, tuberculin testing is unreliable in immunocompromised individuals (eg, those with HIV infection). Culture and identification of this organism can take up to 8 weeks and direct staining procedures are insensitive.

Delay in diagnosis may be catastrophic in those with HIV and TB coinfection. Multidrug-resistant tuberculosis has become a major concern in those with and without immunodeficiency and in healthcare workers as well. Thus, the ability to detect specific mycobacterial DNA directly from the patient specimen with provision of early diagnosis has great advantages in diagnosis, treatment, and prevention of spread to others. Detection of paucibacillary TB cases by these means supports early recognition of outbreaks, especially those involving multidrug resistance.[3] Nucleic acid tests are also available to determine the species of *Mycobacterium* after isolation by culture. Many of the culture confirmation DNA tests for *Mycobacterium* are available in larger clinical laboratories.

Specimen Whole blood, sputum, pleural fluid, cerebrospinal fluid, bronchial aspirates, urine, and tissue biopsy

Container Blood requires a yellow top (ACD) Vacutainer® tube. Sputum, pleural fluid, and cerebrospinal fluid should be collected and transported in a tightly sealed plastic container such as a sputum cup or a sterile bronchoscopy tube. This container should be transferred into a secondary sealed container for transport.

Collection Samples should be collected as for mycobacteria culture. Sputum should be collected as early in the morning as possible, preferably before the morning meal. Urine should be collected in midvoid as for culture.

Storage Instructions The specimens should be kept refrigerated if not immediately processed. Do not freeze.

Causes for Rejection External contamination of containers poses a risk to laboratory personnel. Samples that are left at room temperature for more than 12 hours may be rejected due to overgrowth of other bacteria.

Turnaround Time Approximately 4-7 days

Reference Range No *M. tuberculosis* DNA detected

Use Rapid detection and identification of *Mycobacterium tuberculosis* in clinical specimens. Use of PCR in search of mycobacterial DNA is superior to the Ziehl-Neelsen and auramine-rhodamine stains for acid-fast bacilli and is helpful to distinguish TB from sarcoidosis in paraffin-embedded tissue.

Limitations A potential for false-positive results exists with molecular assays for TB,[3] and false-negatives may occur as well. Since nonviable mycobacterial DNA can lead to positive PCR, positives may not always represent active infection.[4]

Methodology DNA is isolated from the patient specimen or from cultured acid-fast bacteria. A specific *Mycobacterium* DNA probe is then hybridized to the denatured specimen DNA. After hybridization the excess probe is removed and the bound probe is detected by chemiluminescence, color detection, or autoradiography. Specific amplification of *Mycobacterium tuberculosis* nucleic acid by polymerase chain reaction (PCR) or transcription-based amplification is currently available.

Additional Information Mycobacteria are aerobic rod-shaped bacteria noted for their very slow growth. The laboratory diagnosis of mycobacterial disease is currently based on a positive acid-fast stain and on laboratory culture of the mycobacterial organism. The most common isolates in the United States are *Mycobacterium tuberculosis* and species within the *Mycobacterium avium* complex.[5] Because of the long culture periods required and the difficulty of isolation, detection and identification of mycobacteria to the species level has been difficult. Often clinical and therapeutic decisions are made before a laboratory diagnosis is available. To improve upon the detection of mycobacteria, DNA detection assays have been developed that have increased sensitivity and specificity when compared with culture assays and have a decreased turnaround time.[6,7] Specimens may be smear negative, culture negative, but PCR positive. Recently, several studies have shown that amplification of mycobacterial DNA in patient specimens is feasible and can provide a rapid and sensitive diagnosis.[8,9] Because of its increased sensitivity, DNA amplification assay for mycobacteria may soon replace DNA detection assay.

Footnotes

1. Centers for Disease Control, "A Strategic Plan for the Elimination of Tuberculosis in the United States," *MMWR Morb Mortal Wkly Rep*, 1989, 38(16):269-72.
2. Rieder HL, Cauthen GM, Kelly GD, et al, "Tuberculosis in the United States," *JAMA*, 1989, 262(3):385-9.
3. Cockerill FR 3d, Williams DE, Eisenach KD, et al, "Prospective Evaluation of the Utility of Molecular Techniques for Diagnosing Nosocomial Transmission of Multidrug-Resistant Tuberculosis," *Mayo Clin Proc*, 1996, 71(3):221-9.
4. Choi YJ, Hu Y, and Mahmood A, "Clinical Significance of a Polymerase Chain Reaction Assay for the Detection of *Mycobacterium tuberculosis*," *Am J Clin Pathol*, 1996, 105:200-4.
5. Good RC, "Opportunistic Pathogens in the Genus *Mycobacterium*," *Annu Rev Microbiol*, 1985, 39:347-69.
6. Eisenach KD, Crawford JT, and Bates JH, "Repetitive DNA Sequences as Probes for *Mycobacterium tuberculosis*," *J Clin Microbiol*, 1988, 26(11):2240-5.
7. Pao CC, Lin SS, Wu SY, et al, "The Detection of Mycobacterial DNA Sequences in Uncultured Clinical Specimens With Cloned *Mycobacterium tuberculosis* DNA as Probes," *Tubercle*, 1988, 69(1):27-36.
8. DeWit D, Steyn L, Shoemaker S, et al, "Direct Detection of *Mycobacterium tuberculosis* in Clinical Specimens by DNA Amplification," *J Clin Microbiol*, 1990, 28(11):2437-41.
9. Hance AJ, Grandchamp B, Levy-Frebault V, et al, "Detection and Identification of Mycobacteria by Amplification of Mycobacterial DNA," *Mol Microbiol*, 1989, 3(7):843-9.

References

Alland D, Kalkut GE, Moss AR, et al, "Transmission of Tuberculosis in New York City. An Analysis by DNA Fingerprinting and Conventional Epidemiologic Methods," *N Engl J Med*, 1994, 330(24):1710-6.
Barnes PF and Barrows SA, "Tuberculosis in the 1990s," *Ann Intern Med*, 1993, 119(5):400-10.
Brisson-Noel A, Aznar C, Chureau C, et al, "Diagnosis of Tuberculosis by DNA Amplification in Clinical Practice Evaluation," *Lancet*, 1991, 338(8763):364-6.
Centers for Disease Control, "Diagnosis of Tuberculosis by Nucleic Acid Amplification Methods Applied to Clinical Specimens," *MMWR Morb Mortal Wkly Rep*, 1993, 42:686.
Forbes BA and Hicks KE, "Direct Detection of *Mycobacterium tuberculosis* in Respiratory Specimens in a Clinical Laboratory by Polymerase Chain Reaction," *J Clin Microbiol*, 1993, 31(7):1688-94.
Ghossein RA, Ross DG, Salomon RN, et al, "A Search for Mycobacterial DNA in Sarcoidosis Using the Polymerase Chain Reaction," *Am J Clin Pathol*, 1994, 101(6):733-7.
Haas DW, "Current and Future Applications of Polymerase Chain Reaction for *Mycobacterium tuberculosis*," *Mayo Clin Proc*, 1996, 71(3):311-3.
Jonas V, Alden MJ, Curry JI, et al, "Detection and Identification of *Mycobacterium tuberculosis* Directly From Sputum Sediments by Amplification of RNA," *J Clin Microbiol*, 1993, 31(9):2410-6.
Noordhoek GT, Kolk AH, Bjune G, et al, "Sensitivity and Specificity of PCR for Detection of *Mycobacterium tuberculosis*: A Blind Comparison Study Among Seven Laboratories," *J Clin Microbiol*, 1994, 32(2):277-84.
Patel RJ, Piessens WF, David JR, et al, "A Cloned DNA Fragment for Identification of *Mycobacterium tuberculosis*," *Rev Infect Dis*, 1989, 11(Suppl 2):411-9.
Popper HH, Winter E, and Höfler G, "DNA of *Mycobacterium tuberculosis* in Formalin-Fixed, Paraffin-Embedded Tissue in Tuberculosis and Sarcoidosis Detected by Polymerase Chain Reaction," *Am J Clin Pathol*, 1994, 101(6):738-41.
Roberts MC, McMillan C, and Coyle MB, "Whole Chromosomal DNA Probes for Rapid Identification of *Mycobacterium tuberculosis* and *Mycobacterium avium* Complex," *J Clin Microbiol*, 1987, 25(7):1239-43.

Mycobacteria DNA Detection Test *see* Mycobacteria by DNA Probe *on this page*

Mycobacterial Accuprobe® *see* Mycobacteria by DNA Probe *on this page*

Mycoplasma pneumoniae **DNA Detection Test** *see Mycoplasma pneumoniae* DNA Probe Test *on this page*

Mycoplasma pneumoniae DNA Probe Test

CPT 87179

Related Information

Cold Agglutinin Titer *on page 384*
Mycoplasma pneumoniae Diagnostic Procedures *on page 671*
Mycoplasma Serology *on page 419*

Synonyms DNA Hybridization Test for *Mycoplasma pneumoniae*; DNA Test for *Mycoplasma pneumoniae*; Eaton Agent Pneumonia; *Mycoplasma pneumoniae* DNA Detection Test; Primary Atypical Pneumonia

Test Commonly Includes Direct detection of *Mycoplasma pneumoniae* nucleic acids in clinical specimens

Abstract Synonyms for this agent include atypical or primary atypical pneumonia and Eaton agent pneumonia. Respiratory infections due to *Mycoplasma pneumoniae* are difficult to assess because current laboratory techniques lack sensitivity or require long periods of time (3 weeks) for results. Serological procedures are the most widely used but require paired acute and convalescent sera to confirm diagnosis.[1] Cold agglutinins are also used to diagnose *M. pneumoniae*; however, only 50% of infected patients become positive.[2] Culture of this microorganism is rarely done due to the difficulty of recovery and the long incubation time required for growth. A rapid and sensitive laboratory diagnosis of *M. pneumoniae* infection is important since effective antibiotic therapy is available. The nucleic acid based test is a sensitive and promising method for rapid diagnosis of respiratory infections of *M. pneumoniae*.

Specimen Sputum, throat swab, bronchial wash, lung biopsy

Container Special DNA transport medium is usually provided by the laboratory. If this is not available, a sterile container is acceptable. Sterile viral swabs can be used to collect throat specimens.

Collection Sputum specimens should be collected early in the day so they can be sent directly to the laboratory.

Storage Instructions The specimens should be maintained at room temperature or refrigerated. Do not freeze.

Turnaround Time 1-2 days

Reference Range Negative for *Mycoplasma pneumoniae*

Use Rapid detection of *Mycoplasma pneumoniae* in clinical specimens from respiratory sites. *M. pneumoniae* causes an influenza-like illness.

Limitations This assay cannot determine whether the microorganism is viable or not. Antibiotic susceptibility cannot be established. Costs and the potential for intralaboratory contamination must be controlled.[3]

Methodology This test detects *Mycoplasma pneumoniae* rRNA directly from respiratory specimens. It requires lysis of the cells in the specimen and release of the *Mycoplasma pneumoniae*-specific rRNA. The lysed specimens are then hybridized with a specific DNA probe. Detection of the bound probe is assessed after several washing steps. Detection can be done by use of a radioactive DNA probe, but positive samples are now commonly detected with chemiluminescence.

Additional Information There is a wide range of clinical manifestations of *Mycoplasma pneumoniae* respiratory infections, from mild infection to severe pneumonia. This microorganism causes approximately 1% to 8% of pneumonias in patients with community-acquired lower respiratory infection, but mortality is rare.[4] It is usually self-limited. Laboratory diagnosis of *Mycoplasma pneumoniae* is usually based on serology of paired sera and/or isolation of the organism by culture. Culture isolation of the fastidious *Mycoplasma pneumoniae* is tedious, labor intensive, and usually requires several weeks.[3] Serological assays are the most commonly used tests. However, they lack sensitivity and specificity and require acute- and convalescent-phase sera, which also may require 2-3 weeks.[1] The DNA detection assay for *Mycoplasma pneumoniae* has been found to have a specificity and sensitivity which match culture and serology assays.[2,5] The advantage of this test is the rapid turnaround time, which facilitates the treatment with appropriate antibiotics.

Footnotes

1. Hirschberg L, Krook A, Pettersson CA, et al, "Enzyme-Linked Immunosorbent Assay for Detection of *Mycoplasma pneumoniae* Specific Immunoglobulin M," *Eur J Clin Microbiol Infect Dis*, 1988, 7(3):420-3.
2. Kleemola SR, Karjalainen JE, and Raty RK, "Rapid Diagnosis of *Mycoplasma pneumoniae* Infection: Clinical Evaluation of a Commercial Probe Test," *J Infect Dis*, 1990, 162(1):70-5.
3. Clyde WA Jr, "*Mycoplasma* Infections," *Harrison's Principles of Internal Medicine*, 13th ed, Isselbacher KJ, Braunwald E, Wilson JD, et al, eds, New York, NY: McGraw-Hill Inc, 1994, 757-9.
4. Yungbluth M, "The Laboratory Diagnosis of Pneumonia. The Role of the Community Hospital Pathologist," *Clin Lab Med*, 1995, 15(2):209-34.
5. Dular R, Kajioka R, and Kasatiya S, "Comparison of Gen-Probe® Commercial Kit and Culture Technique for the Diagnosis of *Mycoplasma pneumoniae* Infection," *J Clin Microbiol*, 1988, 26(5):1068-9.

References

Harris R, Marmion BP, Varkanis G, et al, "Laboratory Diagnosis of *Mycoplasma pneumoniae* Infection," *Epidemiol Infect*, 1988, 101(3):685-94.
Hata D, Kuze F, Mochizuki Y, et al, "Evaluation of DNA Probe Test for Rapid Diagnosis of *Mycoplasma pneumoniae* Infections," *J Pediatr*, 1990, 116(2):273-6.
Hyman HC, Yogev D, and Razin S, "DNA Probes for Detection and Identification of *Mycoplasma pneumoniae* and *Mycoplasma genitalium*," *J Clin Microbiol*, 1987, 25(4):726-8.
Marmion BP, Williamson J, Worswick DA, et al, "Experience With Newer Techniques for the Laboratory Detection of *Mycoplasma pneumoniae* Infection," *Clin Infect Dis*, 1993, 17(Suppl 1):S90-9.

Neisseria gonorrhoeae DNA Detection Test see *Neisseria gonorrhoeae* Genome Detection *on this page*

Neisseria gonorrhoeae Genome Detection

CPT 87179

Related Information

Bacterial Culture, Conjunctiva *on page 461*
Bacterial Culture, Genital Specimen *on page 463*
Chlamydia trachomatis Genome Detection *on page 505*
Gram's Stain *on page 481*
Neisseria gonorrhoeae Culture and Smear *on page 492*

Synonyms DNA Detection for *Neisseria gonorrhoeae*; Gonorrhea DNA Detection; *Neisseria gonorrhoeae* DNA Detection Test; *Neisseria gonorrhoeae* Molecular Probe Assay

Test Commonly Includes Detection of *Neisseria gonorrhoeae* nucleic acid in clinical specimens

Abstract *Neisseria gonorrhoeae* is one of the most common sexually transmitted infections after *Chlamydia* and papillomavirus. Gonorrhea infections are commonly asymptomatic in women. Disease and infection is associated with a high rate of tubal pregnancies, pelvic inflammatory disease, infertility, and tubal pregnancy. While in the past, *Neisseria gonorrhoeae* was principally diagnosed by culture, the commercial availability of two assays employing molecular approaches has significantly altered the standard approach for detection of this agent and have greatly decreased the time for identification of this organism. *N. gonorrhoeae* is fastidious, and optimal growth conditions must be maintained for its recovery. Although the cost of molecular assays is typically greater than that of culture, the molecular probe is recommended for situations where specimens must be transported to an off-site laboratory for testing.[1] In recognition of the common dual infection by *Chlamydia* and gonorrhea, commercial assays have been developed that allow detection of these organisms with a single swab or specimen. The Roche Amplicor assay utilizes PCR technique for amplification of the bacterial genome, whereas the GenProbe Pace II assay detects ribosomal RNA of the organism (rRNA).[2,3] A third recently developed clinical assay, Abbott LCx, utilizes the ligase chain reaction technique for amplification of the bacterial genome. In addition to their use on swab specimens of cervix and urethra, the new assays are sufficiently sensitive to detect organisms in the urine of infected individuals.

Patient Preparation For urethral specimens, the patient should not have urinated for 1 hour prior to collection.

Specimen Either direct swabs of a potentially infected site or urine may be used depending on the assay. A swab specimen may be collected from the genital/urinary tract of males or females. Commercial assays have also been approved for detection of gonorrhea from urine. Although rectum and the nasopharynx are also sites that may be infected by gonorrhea, swabs of these sites have not been approved for use with molecular assays.

Container Special collection and transport kits are an integral component of the assay and must be used with the appropriate commercial detection assay. A commercial kit typically contains a swab and transport media or device.

Collection Two swabs are provided in the typical commercial kit for use in females. The cervix or endocervix is first cleaned with one swab and the second swab is used to collect the specimen. The swab is inserted into the endocervical canal and rotated to collect epithelial cells from the infected site. The swab is then placed into transport media and sent to the laboratory. In males, the swab is inserted into the urethral meatus and rotated to collect epithelial cells. The swab is then placed into transport media and sent to the laboratory.

Storage Instructions These specimens may be contained at room temperature and sent without freezing to the laboratory. Specimens collected for commercial molecular assays are typically stable for up to 1 week after collection.

Causes for Rejection Collection of a specimen from a nonapproved site, excessively bloody specimens

Turnaround Time Results are typically available within 24 hours of receipt of the specimen.

Reference Range Negative for *Neisseria gonorrhoeae*

Use This test provides for the rapid detection of *N. gonorrhoeae* in a wide variety of clinical specimens. The sensitivity of the test exceeds that for culture and other nonmolecular assays.

Limitations Results by molecular assays have not been accepted as evidence by the courts and legal system. For these purposes, a culture is required.

Methodology Three separate molecular assays have been approved or are under review by the Food and Drug Administration. The PCR detects the presence of gonorrhea DNA following extraction, denaturation, and hybridization with a specific DNA probe. The presence of bound probe is detected using an immunochemical technique. The ligase chain reaction procedure incorporates the extraction and denaturation of DNA followed by specific amplification through the ligation of two segments of the
(Continued)

Neisseria gonorrhoeae Genome Detection
(Continued)

target. Detection is similar to that for PCR. The GenProbe assay detects the presence of ribosomal RNA which is in vast excess to single copy genes of an organism. The probe incorporates a chemiluminescent chemical which upon activation emits light. Various instrumentation is utilized by each of the three methodologies, and various aspects of the assay have been automated.

Additional Information Gonorrhea is one of the most important sexually transmitted diseases in the United States. Infection is characterized by acute urethritis in males and as cervicitis in females. The molecular probe assays provide several advantages over traditional culture assays or antibody-based tests. One of the most significant advantages is the ability to detect nonviable organisms since only the presence of nucleic acids is necessary. This latter property also minimizes the need to rapidly transfer the specimen to culture media or cells.[1] The sensitivity of molecular assays may either equal or significantly exceed that of culture techniques depending upon the prevalence of disease and the site of collection.[3] Detection of organisms in urine provides an additional advantage over alternative methods, and may have a significant impact on public health attempts at limiting the spread of disease. A major disadvantage to molecular assays is the lack of acceptance by the legal community and court system, and currently the results of molecular assays have not been accepted as evidence.

Footnotes
1. Limberger RJ, Biega R, Evancoe A, et al, "Evaluation of Culture and Gen-Probe PACE2 Assay for Detection of *Neisseria gonorrhoeae* and *Chlamydia trachomatis* in Endocervical Specimens Transported to a State Health Laboratory," *J Clin Microbiol*, 1992, 30(5):1162-6.
2. Mahony JB, "Multiplex Polymerase Chain Reaction for the Diagnosis of Sexually Transmitted Diseases," *Clin Lab Med*, 1996, 16(1):61-71.
3. Panke ES, Yang LI, Leist PA, et al, "Comparison of Gen-Probe DNA Probe Test and Culture for the Detection of *Neisseria gonorrhoeae* in Endocervical Specimen," *J Clin Microbiol*, 1991, 29(5):883-8.

References
"DNA Probe Confirmatory Test for *Neisseria gonorrhoeae*," *J Clin Microbiol*, 1990, 28(10):2349-50.
Knapp JS, Holmes KK, Bonin P, et al, "Epidemiology of Gonorrhea: Distribution and Temporal Changes in Auxotype/Serovar Classes of *Neisseria gonorrhoeae*," *J Clin Microbiol*, 1990, 28:2340-50.
Lind I, "Epidemiology of Antibiotic Resistant *Neisseria gonorrhoeae* in Industrialized and Developing Countries," *Scand J Infect Dis Suppl*, 1990, 69:77-82.
Putnam SD, Lavin BS, Stone JR, et al, "Evaluation of the Standardized Disk Diffusion and Agar Dilution Antibiotic Susceptibility Test Methods by Using Strains of *Neisseria gonorrhoeae* From the United States and Southeast Asia," *J Clin Microbiol*, 1992, 30(4):974-80.

Neisseria gonorrhoeae **Molecular Probe Assay** *see Neisseria gonorrhoeae* Genome Detection *on previous page*

N-*myc* Amplification

CPT 83890 (molecular isolation or extraction); 83896 (nucleic acid probe, each)

Related Information
Chromosome Analysis, Lymph Node and Solid Tumor *on page 279*
Histopathology *on page 42*
Homovanillic Acid, Urine *on page 145*
Immunoperoxidase Procedures *on page 43*

Synonyms DNA Amplification of N-*myc*; N-*myc* Gene Amplification

Test Commonly Includes Detection of increased N-*myc* oncogene copy number

Abstract The role of oncogenes in the progression of tumor development has been clarified by recent advances in molecular biology. Neuroblastoma was the first human tumor in which an increased number of copies of a specific oncogene (N-*myc*) correlated with progression of disease. Patients with amplification of the N-*myc* oncogene have a worse prognosis than patients whose tumors have a single copy of N-*myc* gene.

The neuroectodermal tumors, neuroepitheliomas, lack amplification of the N-*myc* oncogene. This is useful in distinguishing between neuroblastomas and neuroepitheliomas. Thus, detection of N-*myc* amplification in immature tumors is helpful in establishing both diagnosis and prognosis.

Specimen Tissue from neuroblastoma or other "small round cell tumors"

Container The specimen should be immediately frozen and then shipped to the laboratory on dry ice.

Collection A 0.1-1 g of neuroblastoma tissue should be cut from the biopsy. The specimen is then put into a sealable plastic freezer bag and frozen at -70°C. The specimen should be kept frozen until shipped to the laboratory.

Storage Instructions Store tissue at -70°C or on dry ice.

Causes for Rejection If the specimen thaws out during transport to the laboratory or before shipping then the specimen must be rejected. If less than 0.1 g of tissue is sent to the laboratory for evaluation it may not yield enough DNA for analysis.

Turnaround Time Results require about 3 weeks.

Special Instructions Tumor specimen should be frozen immediately at -70°C or in liquid nitrogen.

Reference Range An interpretive report usually is included with the results of analysis.

Use In neuroblastomas, N-*myc* amplification is an established prognostic indicator. It is associated with poor prognosis and rapid tumor progression. The poor clinical outcome in these patients seems to be independent of tumor stage. N-*myc* copy numbers greater than five indicate a poor prognosis, but about half of aggressive neuroblastomas lack N-*myc* amplification. High levels of N-*myc* amplification have been found in aggressive medulloblastoma. Abnormal DNA content is associated with better prognosis. Evaluations then of N-*myc* gene amplification and DNA ploidy are complementary.

Limitations Failure to obtain DNA from the tissue sample due to inappropriate shipping or processing (such as freeze/thaw series)

Methodology DNA is released and isolated from the tumor tissue by lysing the cells and extracting cell lysate with phenol and chloroform. Several dilutions of the DNA is then suctioned onto a solid support and hybridized with a specific radioactive N-*myc* probe. After hybridization, the copy number of N-*myc* is calculated by extrapolation to a standard curve. The standard curve is generated by using various dilutions of a known N-*myc* DNA sample, such as a plasmid containing the N-*myc* gene. After hybridization of the standard dilutions, the hybridized dots of DNA are counted in a beta scintillation counter and plotted as cpm vs copy number.

Formalin-fixed, paraffin-embedded tissue can be immunostained for N-*myc* gene product. Polyclonal antibody OA-11-803 has been used.[1]

Additional Information A number of studies have shown that an increased copy number of N-*myc* in neuroblastoma is predictive of a poor prognosis.[2,3,4] Thus, the determination of N-*myc* copy number provides information that has prognostic significance. This information may direct a more appropriate choice of treatment since N-*myc* amplification is associated with poor prognosis regardless of clinical stage.[3]

Immunoreactivity to N-*myc* provides an adjunct for prediction of clinical behavior of medullary thyroid carcinoma.[1]

Footnotes
1. Roncalli M, Viale G, Grimelius L, et al, "Prognostic Value of N-*myc* Immunoreactivity in Medullary Thyroid Carcinoma," *Cancer*, 1994, 74(1):134-41.
2. Brodeur GM, Seeger RC, Schwab M, et al, "Amplification of N-*myc* in Untreated Human Neuroblastomas Correlates With Advanced Disease Stage," *Science*, 1984, 224(4653):1121-4.
3. Nakagawara A, Ikeda K, Tsuda T, et al, "Amplification of N-*myc* Oncogene in Stage II and IVS Neuroblastomas May Be a Prognostic Indicator," *J Pediatr Surg*, 1987, 22(5):415-8.
4. Seeger RC, Brodeur GM, Sather H, et al, "Association of Multiple Copies of the N-*myc* Oncogene With Rapid Progression of Neuroblastomas," *N Engl J Med*, 1985, 313(18):1111-6.

References
Bordow SB, Haber M, Madafiglio J, et al, "Expression of the Multidrug Resistance-Associated Protein (MRP) Gene Correlates With Amplification and Overexpression of the N-*myc* Oncogene in Childhood Neuroblastoma," *Cancer Res*, 1994, 54(19):5036-40.
Brodeur GM, "Clinical Significance of Genetic Rearrangements in Human Neuroblastoma," *Clin Chem*, 1989, 35(7 Suppl):B38-42.
Brodeur GM and Fong CT, "Molecular Biology and Genetics of Human Neuroblastoma," *Cancer Genet Cytogenet*, 1989, 41(2):153-74.
Muraji T, Okamoto E, Fujimoto J, et al, "Combined Determination of N-*myc* Oncogene Amplification and DNA Ploidy in Neuroblastoma. Complementary Prognostic Indicators," *Cancer*, 1993, 72(9):2763-8.
Tomlinson FH, Jenkins RB, Scheithauer BW, et al, "Aggressive Medulloblastoma With High-Level N-*myc* Amplification," *Mayo Clin Proc*, 1994, 69(4):359-65.
Wada RK, Seeger RC, Brodeur GM, et al, "Human Neuroblastoma Cell Lines That Express N-*myc* Without Gene Amplification," *Cancer*, 1993, 72(11):3346-54.

N-*myc* **Gene Amplification** *see* N-*myc* Amplification *on this page*

Nonpolyposis Type Colon Cancer *see* Colon Cancer, Hereditary Nonpolyposis Type *on page 506*

Nuclear Phosphoprotein p53 *see* p53, Functional Assay/Sequencing *on this page*

Oncogenes *see* bcl-2 Gene Rearrangement *on page 503*

Oncogenes *see* Breakpoint Cluster Region Rearrangement in CML *on page 503*

p11O[RB1] *see* Retinoblastoma Gene DNA Detection *on page 524*

p53, Functional Assay/Sequencing
Related Information
Breast Biopsy *on page 35*
Breast Cancer, Hereditary (BRCA1) *on page 504*
Histopathology *on page 42*
Human Papillomavirus DNA Probe Test *on page 516*
Immunoperoxidase Procedures *on page 43*

Polymerase Chain Reaction *on this page*
Retinoblastoma Gene DNA Detection *on next page*

Synonyms Growth Suppressor/Oncoprotein *p53*; Nuclear Phosphoprotein *p53*; *p53* Tumor Suppressor Gene

Applies to Li-Fraumeni Syndrome

Test Commonly Includes Functional gene assay of *p53* and sequencing of the gene for ascertainment of mutations.

Abstract The *p53* gene is located on the short arm of chromosome 17 and codes for a nuclear protein that plays a role in the regulation of cell growth and division. The *p53* gene is classified as a tumor suppressor gene because mutation or loss of its normal regulatory function is associated with uncontrolled cellular proliferation and tumor growth. Mutations of *p53* have been implicated in many inherited and sporadic forms of cancer and are particularly common in bladder, breast, colorectal, lung cancer, brain tumors, and adrenocorticocarcinoma in children.[1] Li-Fraumeni syndrome, a rare autosomal dominant disorder, is characterized by a germline mutation of *p53* and high incidence of malignancies of the breast, soft tissue, and brain. Functional and sequencing assays are available to assess *p53* mutations providing information which can be used to monitor and manage disease.

Specimen 30 mL whole blood; 100 mg solid tumor, frozen or paraffin-embedded

Container Yellow top (ACD) tube for blood

Storage Instructions Transport whole blood at ambient temperature to the laboratory immediately. Fresh solid tumor should be frozen and transported with 10 lbs dry ice.

Turnaround Time 3-4 weeks

Reference Range The *p53* functional assay will detect mutations located within codons 67 and 347 of the *p53* gene, where >95% of *p53* mutations have been found. Sequence analysis will provide a complete analysis of the *p53* sequence. Interpretative reports are usually provided by laboratories.

Use Detection of *p53* mutations in families at high risk of developing cancer (Li-Fraumeni syndrome) and as a prognostic parameter in patients with cancer (particularly breast, colon, lung,[2] bladder, ovary,[3] and prostate). *p53* has been detected in a variety of gynecologic tumors.[4]

Limitations The functional assay cannot detect mutations outside of codons 67 and 347 including mutations in the regulatory domains. Association of *p53* mutations with *in situ* bladder tumors which bear a propensity for progression and with high grade or advanced bladder neoplasms is recognized, but *p53* mutations may occur late in the natural history of some tumors. About 40% of carcinomas of bladder lack *p53* mutations.[5]

Methodology RNA is extracted and converted back to its DNA blueprint in the functional assay. The DNA is inserted into yeast cells where the yeast will grow if the DNA is coding for normal protein. If there is a mutation within codons 67 and 347 of *p53* gene, yeast will not grow. Sequencing of the complete *p53* gene may also be performed.

Monoclonal antibodies PAb1801 and PAb421 may be used for immunohistochemistry. They react with the *p53* gene product. Frozen sections[2] and paraffin-embedded tissues[3,4] are used.

Additional Information Reactivity of *p53* is variable in immunocytochemistry, bearing association with subtypes (small cell and squamous carcinomas).[2]

Association with tumor progression is reported with immunocytochemistry in mucinous borderline tumors of ovary. *p53* accumulation was found in some but not most mucinous, serous, and endometrioid carcinomas.[3]

Footnotes

1. King MC, Rowell S, and Love SM, "Inherited Breast and Ovarian Cancer - What Are the Risks? What Are the Choices?" *JAMA*, 1993, 269(15):1975-80.
2. Dosaka-Akita H, Shindoh M, Fjuino M, et al, "Abnormal *p53* Expression in Human Lung Cancer Is Associated With Histologic Subtypes and Patient Smoking History," *Am J Clin Pathol*, 1994, 102(5):660-4.
3. Kupryjańczyk, Bell DA, Yandell DW, et al, "*p53* Expression in Ovarian Borderline Tumors and Stage I Carcinomas," *Am J Clin Pathol*, 1994, 102(5):671-6.
4. Inoue M, Fujita M, Enomoto T, et al, "Immunohistochemical Analysis of *p53* in Gynecologic Tumors," *Am J Clin Pathol*, 1994, 102(5):665-70.
5. Hruban RH, van der Riet P, Erozan YS, et al, "Brief Report: Molecular Biology and the Early Detection of Carcinoma of the Bladder - the Case of Hubert H. Humphrey," *N Engl J Med*, 1994, 330(18):1276-8.

References

Eguchi S, Kohara N, Komuta K, et al, "Mutations of the *p53* Gene in the Stool of Patients With Resectable Colorectal Cancer," *Cancer*, 1996, 77(8):1707-10.
Harris CC and Hollstein M, "Clinical Implications of the *p53* Tumor-Suppressor Gene," *N Engl J Med*, 1993, 329(18):1318-27.
Hollstein M, Sidransky D, Vogelstein B, et al, "*p53* Mutations in Human Cancers," *Science*, 1991, 253(5015):49-53.
Ishioka C, Frebourg T, Yan YX, et al, "Screening Patients for Heterozygous *p53* Mutations Using a Functional Assay in Yeast," *Nat Genet*, 1993, 5(2):124-9.
Kinzler KW and Vogelstein B, "Cancer Therapy Meets *p53*," *N Engl J Med*, 1994, 331(1):49-50.

p53 Tumor Suppressor Gene *see p53, Functional Assay/Sequencing on previous page*

PACE2® *see Chlamydia trachomatis Genome Detection on page 505*

Parentage Studies *see Identification DNA Testing on page 517*

Paternity Testing by DNA Testing *see Identification DNA Testing on page 517*

PCR *see Polymerase Chain Reaction on this page*

PCR for HIV DNA *see Human Immunodeficiency Virus DNA Amplification on page 515*

Philadelphia Chromosome *see Breakpoint Cluster Region Rearrangement in CML on page 503*

Polycystic Kidney Disease, Prenatal Diagnosis *see Adult Polycystic Kidney Disease DNA Detection on page 502*

Polymerase Chain Reaction

CPT 83898 (nuclear molecular diagnostics); 87179 (microbial identification by PCR)

Synonyms DNA Amplification; PCR

Test Commonly Includes Amplification of target DNA sequences as much as a millionfold

Abstract The polymerase chain reaction is a technique developed in molecular biology with unlimited potential use in the medical laboratory. It was developed at the Cetus Corporation in Emeryville, California, and was first described for use in the prenatal diagnosis of sickle cell anemia. The technique may become as important as gene cloning itself. The PCR technique permits a millionfold amplification of small pieces of DNA in several hours. The amplification is performed by multiple cycles of DNA polymerizing enzyme in the presence of known sequences, of primer DNA sequences, flanking the region of DNA to be amplified. (See figure.) Thus, the nucleotide sequence of the gene to be amplified must be known so oligonucleotide primers can be constructed on oligonucleotide synthesizers. The method has continually expanding applications not only in prenatal diagnosis, but also for cancer and infectious disease detection and diagnosis.

Specimen The specimen for the PCR assay will depend on the type of analysis. For example, prenatal diagnosis will require amniotic fluid or chorionic villus biopsy (see Amniotic Fluid, Chromosome and Genetic Abnormality Analysis *on page 273*), whole blood will be required for human immunodeficiency virus (HIV) detection, other specimens such as cerebrospinal fluid, sputum, serum, biopsies, or discharge from wounds for other infectious agents, or solid tissue by biopsy for cancer diagnosis.

Collection Varies with type of specimen

Use The use of the technique to amplify short fragments of DNA is limited only by one's imagination. The uses in the laboratory include prenatal diagnosis of sickle cell anemia, hemophilia, cystic fibrosis, and muscular dystrophy, as well as oncogene activation in the case of lymphoma and chronic myelogenous leukemia. Numerous infectious agents such as *Mycobacterium* species, the agent of Lyme disease, and viruses, have been detected using this amplification technique.

Limitations The tests must be carefully monitored with appropriate controls (especially negative controls) due to the great sensitivity of the amplification technique.

Methodology The PCR technique requires knowledge of the base sequence of the gene of interest to be amplified. From the sequence data, oligonucleotide primers 25 nucleotides in length can be constructed using oligonucleotide synthesizers. These primers flank a 100-2000 base sequence of the gene of interest. The primers are constructed so that the primers bind (anneal) to opposite strands of the target double helix. A special DNA polymerase, purified from *Thermus aquaticus (Taq)*, is used because it can withstand the many denaturing, reannealing, and polymerizing cycles without the need for replenishment. The reaction requires the target DNA, the primers, *Taq* polymerase, and the four deoxynucleotide triphosphates. The mixture is heated several minutes to 95°C to separate the target DNA double strands. The primers are then allowed to bind to the target DNA at 50°C to 60°C and the polymerase reaction allowed to proceed for several minutes at 72°C. This cycle of denaturation, annealing, polymerization is repeated over and over as many as 25-35 times amplifying the sequence between the primers hundreds of thousands to millions of times (see figure). The amplified DNA can then be detected by agarose electrophoresis followed by ethidium bromide staining. The amplified bands can be seen with a UV light and photographed for analysis. The PCR technique requires knowledge of the base sequence of the target gene. From the sequence data, oligonucleotide primers, 25 nucleotides in length, can be constructed using oligonucleotide synthesizers. These primers flank a (Continued)

Polymerase Chain Reaction *(Continued)*

100-2000 base sequence in the gene of interest. The primers are constructed so that the primers bind (anneal) to opposite strands of the target double helix. A special DNA polymerase, purified from *Thermus aquaticus* (*Taq*), is used because it can withstand the many denaturing, reannealing, and polymerizing cycles without the need for replenishment. The reaction requires the target DNA, the primers, *Taq* polymerase, and the four deoxynucleotide triphosphates. The mixture is heated several minutes to 95°C to separate the target DNA double strands. The primers are then allowed to bind to the target DNA at 50°C to 60°C and the polymerase reaction allowed to proceed for several minutes at 72°C. This cycle of denaturation, annealing, polymerization is repeated over and over as many as 25-35 times amplifying the sequence between the primers hundreds of thousands to millions of times (see figure). The amplified DNA can then be detected by agarose electrophoresis followed by ethidium bromide staining. The amplified bands can be seen with a UV light and photographed for analysis.

DNA can be extracted from paraffin-embedded tissue for PCR analysis. Such tissue is best fixed in 10% formalin. Genotype can be ascertained by selective ultraviolet radiation fractionation.

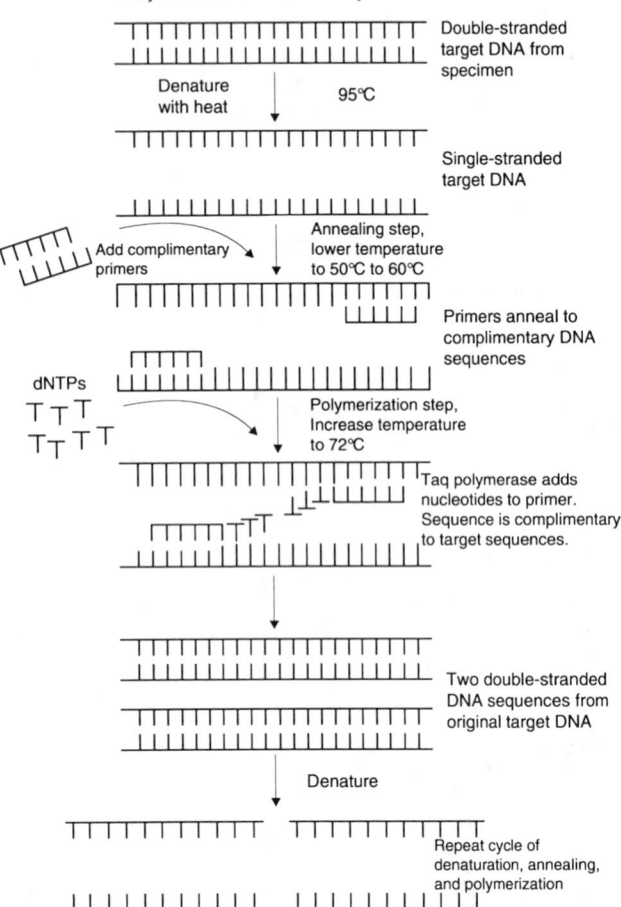

Polymerase Chain Reaction Cycles

Double-stranded target DNA from specimen

Denature with heat — 95°C

Single-stranded target DNA

Add complimentary primers — Annealing step, lower temperature to 50°C to 60°C

Primers anneal to complimentary DNA sequences

dNTPs — Polymerization step, Increase temperature to 72°C

Taq polymerase adds nucleotides to primer. Sequence is complimentary to target sequences.

Two double-stranded DNA sequences from original target DNA

Denature

Repeat cycle of denaturation, annealing, and polymerization

Additional Information The technique is being expanded and refined. The procedure is automated with programmable heating blocks to cycle the reaction automatically. The technique has unprecedented sensitivity, being able to use nanogram quantities of target DNA and could theoretically be used to amplify the DNA from a single cell. Other amplification reactions are also being developed for use in the diagnostic laboratory.

References

Crotty PL, Staggs RA, Porter PT, et al, "Quantitative Analysis in Molecular Diagnostics," *Hum Pathol*, 1994, 25(6):572-9.

Embury SH, Scharf SJ, Saiki RK, et al, "Rapid Prenatal Diagnosis of Sickle Cell Anemia by a New Method of DNA Analysis," *N Engl J Med*, 1987, 316(11):656-61.

Erlich HA, ed, *PCR Technology: Principles and Applications for DNA Amplification*, New York, NY: Stockton Press, 1989.

Kogan SC, Doherty M, and Gitschier J, "An Improved Method for Prenatal Diagnosis of Genetic Diseases by Analysis of Amplified DNA Sequences. Application to Hemophilia A," *N Engl J Med*, 1987, 317(16):985-90.

Loda M, "Polymerase Chain Reaction-Based Methods for the Detection of Mutations in Oncogenes and Tumor Suppressor Genes," *Hum Pathol*, 1994, 25(6):564-71.

Mies C, "Molecular Biological Analysis of Paraffin-Embedded Tissues," *Hum Pathol*, 1994, 25(6):555-60.

Ou C, Kwok S, Mitchell SW, et al, "DNA Amplification for Direct Detection of HIV-1 in DNA of Peripheral Blood Mononuclear Cells," *Science*, 1988, 239(4867):295-7.

Rogers BB, "Nucleic Acid Amplification and Infectious Disease," *Hum Pathol*, 1994, 25(6):590-3.

Saiki RK, Chang, CA, Levenson CH, et al, "Diagnosis of Sickle Cell Anemia and β-Thalassemia With Enzymatically Amplified DNA and Nonradioactive Allele-Specific Oligonucleotide Probes," *N Engl J Med*, 1988, 319(9):537-41.

Saiki RK, Gelfand DH, Stoffel S, et al, "Primer-Directed Enzymatic Amplification of DNA With Thermostable DNA Polymerase," *Science*, 1988, 239(4839):487-9.

Saiki RK, Scharf S, and Faloona F, "Enzymatic Amplification of β-Globin Genomic Sequences and Restriction Site Analysis for Diagnosis of Sickle Cell Anemia," *Science*, 1985, 230(4732):1350-4.

Shibata D, "Extraction of DNA From Paraffin-Embedded Tissue for Analysis by Polymerase Chain Reaction: New Tricks From an Old Friend," *Hum Pathol*, 1994, 25(6):561-3.

Shibata D and Klatt EC, "Analysis of Human Immunodeficiency Virus and Cytomegalovirus Infection by Polymerase Chain Reaction in the Acquired Immunodeficiency Syndrome," *Arch Pathol Lab Med*, 1989, 113(11):1239-44.

Primary Atypical Pneumonia *see Mycoplasma pneumoniae* DNA Probe Test *on page 520*

RB1 Gene *see* Retinoblastoma Gene DNA Detection *on this page*

RB Tumor Suppressor Gene *see* Retinoblastoma Gene DNA Detection *on this page*

RET Gene Testing *see* Multiple Endocrine Neoplasia/Familial Medullary Thyroid Carcinoma *on page 519*

Retinoblastoma Gene DNA Detection

Related Information

Histopathology *on page 42*

p53, Functional Assay/Sequencing *on page 522*

Polymerase Chain Reaction *on previous page*

Synonyms p110^RB1; RB1 Gene; RB Tumor Suppressor Gene

Test Commonly Includes Restriction fragment length polymorphism (RBLP) analysis and/or polymerase chain reaction (PCR) amplification followed by sequencing of the gene for ascertainment of mutations.

Abstract The retinoblastoma (RB1) gene is the prototype tumor suppressor gene. Located on chromosome 13, the gene encodes a nuclear protein that participates in the control of cell proliferation and progression through the cell cycle. Deletion or inactivation of both RB alleles plays an essential role in the development of retinoblastoma, a tumor of retinoblasts affecting newborns and young children. Retinoblastoma occurs in either a hereditary (40% of cases) or a nonhereditary (sporadic) form (60% of cases). Hereditary predisposition to retinoblastoma is caused by a germline mutation at the RB1 locus. The germline mutation is transmitted in an autosomal dominant fashion with 90% penetrance. Retinoblastoma develops following a somatic mutation or deletion affecting the remaining RB allele. Bilateral disease occurs in the majority of hereditary cases and patients have an increased risk for developing nonocular tumors (mainly osteosarcoma) in later life. In nonhereditary retinoblastoma, the tumor is usually unilateral and arises following successive somatic mutations affecting the two RB alleles. Somatic inactivation of the RB gene is also found in other tumors not associated with retinoblastoma, including astrocytomas, several sarcomas, small cell and squamous cell carcinoma of lung, and carcinomas of breast, bladder, prostate, and parathyroid.[1]

Specimen 30 mL whole blood; 100 mg solid tumor, frozen; amniotic cells grown in appropriate media

Container Blood: Yellow top (ACD) tube; amniotic cells: T25 tissue culture flask

Storage Instructions Transport whole blood at ambient temperature to the laboratory immediately. Store solid tumor at -70°C.

Turnaround Time 3-4 weeks

Reference Range The laboratory usually provides an interpretive report.

Use DNA tests make it possible to predict the occurrence of tumors in offspring and siblings of patients with retinoblastoma. DNA testing is useful in several settings. Identification of unaffected relatives of patients with retinoblastoma who are carriers of the germline defect aids in accurate risk assessment. DNA testing can be performed in newborns of affected or carrier parents to determine if the newborn carries the mutation. If a mutation is present, more frequent examination for detection of the tumor is warranted. Although successful treatment is available for early diagnosed retinoblastomas, patients remain at risk for nonocular tumors. Because of these risks, prenatal diagnosis can be offered to families with germline mutations.

Limitations Failure to obtain DNA from the blood, tissue, or cultured cells due to inappropriate shipping or processing.

Methodology Southern blot analysis with restriction fragment length polymorphism (RFLP) is used to detect loss of an RB allele. Amplification by polymerase chain reaction followed by RFLP, single-strand conformation polymorphism analysis, and/or sequencing to detect loss of an RB allele and/or function mutation.[1,2]

Expression of the retinoblastoma gene product can also be studied by immunochemistry.

Additional Information The role of the RB tumor suppressor gene in tumor initiation and progression is currently being studied in numerous tumors unrelated to retinoblastoma. Such studies may in the future produce prognostic information useful in tumors other than retinoblastoma.

Footnotes

1. Cryns VL, Thor A, Xu HJ, et al, "Loss of the Retinoblastoma Tumor-Suppressor Gene in Parathyroid Carcinoma," *N Engl J Med*, 1994, 330(11):757-61.
2. Shimizu T, Toguchida J, Kato MV, et al, "Detection of Mutations of the RB1 Gene in Retinoblastoma Patients by Using Exon-by-Exon PCR-SSCP Analysis," *Am J Hum Genet*, 1994, 54(5):793-800.

References

Bernstam VA, "Gene Level Evaluation of Selected Neurologic and Connective Tissue Disorders," *Handbook of Gene Level Diagnostics in Clinical Practice*, Chapter 5, Boca Raton, FL: CRC Press, Inc, 1992, 413-8.

Hamel PA, Phillips RA, Muncaster M, et al, "Speculations on the Roles of RB1 in Tissue-Specific Differentiation, Tumor Initiation, and Tumor Progression," *FASEB J*, 1993, 7(10):846-54.

Horsthemke B, "Genetics and Cytogenetics of Retinoblastoma," *Cancer Genet Cytogenet*, 1992, 63(1):1-7.

RFLP Analysis for Parentage Evaluation *see* Identification DNA Testing *on page 517*

Southern Blot of *bcl-2* Gene Rearrangement *see bcl-2* Gene Rearrangement *on page 503*

ViraPap® *see* Human Papillomavirus DNA Probe Test *on page 516*

ViraType® *see* Human Papillomavirus DNA Probe Test *on page 516*

THERAPEUTIC DRUG MONITORING / TOXICOLOGY / DRUGS OF ABUSE

David S. Jacobs, MD

Harold J. Grady, PhD

Sandra B. Earle, PharmD

Daniel H. Jacobs, MD

Christopher J. Papasian, PhD

Contributors:
Wayne R. DeMott, MD
Charles W. Gorodetzky, MD, PhD

Therapeutic Drug Monitoring

It has been established that for many drugs, drug dosage regulated through the measurement of serum/plasma drug levels (therapeutic drug monitoring - TDM) is more likely to produce the desired therapeutic effect without toxicity than when empiric dosing is used. This observation is consistent with three common assumptions concerning the pharmacological effects of drugs.

- Therapeutic and dose-related toxic effects are initiated through interaction of the drug with specific receptors on the cells of the target tissue.
- Therapeutic/toxic effects are proportional to drug concentration at the receptor site which is represented by the free or unbound concentration at that site.
- Concentration of free drug at the receptor site is directly proportional to the free drug concentration in the serum and, in most cases, to the total drug concentration. Exceptions to this relationship occur when the drug is highly protein bound and changes in the fraction bound are produced by various physiological or pathological processes.

Although many drugs are safely and effectively administered without TDM, it is useful to monitor serum/plasma levels when one or more of the following conditions apply.

- The drug has a narrow therapeutic range.
- The drug exhibits large intra- or interindividual variation.
- The drug does not produce the desired therapeutic effect or produces toxicity when empiric dosing is used.
- Secondary disease alters drug utilization.
- Noncompliance is suspected.
- Drug interactions may have taken place.
- Medicolegal verification is desired.
- Bioavailability of the drug is suspect.
- Therapeutic or toxic effect cannot be easily measured clinically.

The availability of a rapid and accurate assay method is necessary for TDM. For the most part, current laboratory methods meet these requirements. It is common practice to use TDM to monitor many of the drugs in the following classes:

- antibiotics
- antiasthmatics
- anticonvulsants
- antipsychotics and antidepressants
- antiarrhythmics

The serum drug concentration achieved is a consequence of a wide variety of processes. The study of the interrelationships of such processes and their consequences is **pharmacokinetics**. An appreciation of some pharmacokinetic principles helps in interpretation of serum drug levels. The aim of TDM is to achieve a steady-state drug concentration within the therapeutic range. This is achieved by controlling a dosage regimen which consists of two parts, the **dose rate** (amount of drug given per dose) and the **dose interval** (how often this amount is given). When starting (or changing) a dosage regimen, it is necessary to wait a period of time to allow for establishment of a stable concentration (**steady-state**). To do so without the use of a loading dose usually requires about five half-lives ($t_{1/2}$). The **elimination half-life** is the time required for the serum level to change from one value to half that value. Increasing the dose rate will increase the steady-state concentration while increasing the dose interval will increase the peak/trough ratio. The **peak value** is the highest value obtained after a given dose, and the **trough** is the lowest value. Blood samples for TDM are normally drawn at either peak or trough or both. For proper interpretation of TDM values, the sampling time must be known and recorded. Trough samples (used for most drugs) are usually drawn just before the next dose. Peak samples are drawn at various times depending upon the route of administration or the formulation of the oral dose. For I.V. administration, peak samples are drawn 30-60 minutes after completion of the infusion. For I.M. administration, the peak time is 2-4 hours after dosing. For oral dosing, 2-3 hours following administration can usually be used for peak sampling except for sustained-release products, which require 4-5 hours. Exceptions to the use of only trough samples are aminoglycoside antibiotics and theophylline, which are sampled at both peak and trough. Any of the following factors may influence the serum level achieved after a given dosage regimen.

- patient age
- genetic variability
- disease processes
- compliance
- absorption
- distribution

- metabolism
- excretion
- drug tolerance
- toxicity

In the drug listings in this chapter, therapeutic ranges are given when TDM is applicable. Separate ranges apply to peak and trough values and are so labeled. At the beginning of the Additional Information section of each listing, the following pharmacokinetic parameters are listed when applicable.

- $t_{1/2}$ (elimination half-life)
- V_d (volume of distribution)
- PB (protein binding)

In the text of that section, special information concerning toxicity, sampling time, drug-drug interactions, and other helpful clinical data is presented. Tables summarizing some of the above information for several classes of drugs can be found in the **Therapeutic Drug Monitoring/Toxicology/Drugs of Abuse Appendix** *on page 581.*

A number of drugs are highly protein bound by serum albumin and an alpha$_1$ globulin (80% to 90%). It is the **"free" or unbound concentration** of the drug that is in equilibrium with intracellular free drug. It determines the pharmacological effect, the rate of liver metabolism, and the amount of parent drug presented to the kidney for excretion. Decreases in binding can occur because of competition for protein binding sites by bilirubin and metabolites accumulating because of renal insufficiency. Momentary increase in free drug will result but increased liver metabolism and/or renal excretion will bring levels down to near the previous level. The total drug concentration will, however, decrease and may be deceptively low. Increasing drug level by changing dosage regimen under such circumstances could cause toxicity. Analysis of free or unbound drug level would be the ideal solution, and this is available in some laboratories for a number of drugs. It is not a common practice because it is somewhat labor-intensive. In situations not involving changes in protein binding, total drug concentration is useful and almost always proportional to the free value.

Certain classes of drugs may require specialized knowledge concerning drug interactions and level of efficacy of the individual members of that group, as illustrated by the following discussion of **antiepileptics**. Antiepileptic drugs (AED) are titrated clinically to prevent seizures and to avoid adverse effects. Some patients require drug levels outside the classical therapeutic range. Thus, some dosing may be empiric, based on patient weight rather than on the AED level. With drugs of this class, changes in serum levels may not always be related to efficacy or toxicity. For example, **phenytoin** and **carbamazepine** may mutually lower the level of the other drug without decrease in efficacy. It is also true that undesirable side effects can occur with drug levels in the therapeutic range. We have included in this edition information about recently developed antiepileptic drugs including **lamotrigene, gabapentin, vigabatrin,** and **felbamate**.

Both desktop and large automated laboratory systems are available for TDM analysis; essentially all provide acceptable accuracy and precision.

Toxicology

Modern toxicology has three divisions: environmental, clinical, and forensic. All are concerned with poisons and their effect on living organisms. They differ with respect to the types of samples involved and the use to which the results will be put. Most hospital laboratory toxicology is concerned with clinical toxicology, namely, the identification of substances involved in acute or chronic poisoning of man. When little or no clue is available concerning the toxin from the history and physical, the laboratory is frequently asked to perform a comprehensive drug screen. The term "comprehensive" is a relative one since no hospital laboratory can truly screen for all possible toxic substances. Two available systems, a thin-layer chromatographic method from Toxi-Lab, Inc, called Toxi-Lab® and an automated high performance liquid chromatographic instrument from Biorad Inc, called Remedi®, can each screen for several hundred drugs. However, they must be supplemented with individual methods to detect the drugs not measured such as salicylates, and for one of the systems, acetaminophen and marijuana. Most of the time qualitative identification of the toxin in a timely manner (1-2 hours) is the most useful, although in a few cases a quantitative response is of value. Quantitative measurement is usually carried out on serum/plasma and is most often used for the following drugs:

- acetaminophen
- salicylate
- carboxyhemoglobin
- digoxin (usually from TDM)
- ethanol
- heavy metals
- iron
- theophylline (usually from TDM)
- phenytoin (usually from TDM)
  Of the other anticonvulsants, carbamazepine, primidone, phenobarbital, and valproic acid are most commonly monitored, although others may also be measured.

The laboratory can be most helpful when it has all the information available concerning possible substances involved. The dialogue between the laboratory and the treating physician should be reciprocal and ongoing as the situation develops. Forms designed by the laboratory for requesting toxicological analyses should require as much of this detail as possible to be submitted along with the sample. Toxicology and TDM overlap when drug levels significantly above the therapeutic range are involved. It should be noted that at such levels the usual values for elimination rates (half-lives) may not apply because enzyme systems can become saturated and then the typical first-order kinetics are not valid.

Drugs of Abuse

The drugs or drug classes most commonly listed as drugs of abuse are the following:

- amphetamine/methamphetamine
- barbiturates
- benzodiazepines
- cannabinoids (marijuana or THC)

- cocaine
- opiates (heroin, morphine, codeine)
- phencyclidine (PCP)
- methadone
- methaqualone
- propoxyphene

These drugs are measured under one of two circumstances: one, in the overdose situation in which the analysis is treated as any toxicological sample, and two, in testing for the presence of the drug in clinically well persons. Most of the following discussion applies to the latter situation. Analysis for these drugs in clinically-well subjects frequently involves two sequential tests, the first a screening test and the second a confirmatory test performed only on positive screens. The screening test must have good sensitivity but may lack some specificity, while the confirmatory test must be both sensitive and specific and involve a different chemical principle than the screen. When used strictly for clinical purposes, the screening test result may be used without confirmation if an occasional false-positive will do no serious harm. However, when medicolegal or forensic application is a possibility, confirmation is essential. It is also extremely important for forensic applications that the sample be accompanied by a chain-of-custody document which will assure the integrity of the sample through the process of collection, delivery, receipt, and analysis. Samples without such a document have no forensic value, regardless of the quality of the analysis.

The sample for analysis of drugs of abuse is urine because of the ease of collection and because concentrations of drugs and metabolites are usually higher than in serum/plasma or saliva. Laboratory reports for detection of drugs of abuse in well persons are not quantitative and are usually expressed as "positive" or "negative." For each drug a predetermined threshold or cutoff value has been agreed upon by scientific and regulatory groups and results equal to the cutoff or above are considered positive and all other values negative. Thus, a report of "negative" does not necessarily mean absence of the drug but rather a result less than the cutoff. Cutoff values for a given drug are often different for the screening test than for the confirmatory test. For a few drugs (eg, marijuana) several different cutoff values are in current use. When such specimens are sent to reference laboratories, one must verify that the cutoff they use will satisfy needs. A sample having either a negative screening test or negative confirmatory test is reported as negative. When screening in the overdose situation, quantitative estimates are sometimes given when values are well above the cutoff. In a number of cases metabolites, rather than the parent drug, are the substances actually measured in the screening and confirmatory tests.

The federal agency responsible for regulation of laboratories involved in analysis of drugs of abuse for federal employees and for companies operating under federal control is the **Substance Abuse and Mental Health Services Administration (SAMHSA)**. This agency has set up strict guidelines for sample handling, measurement, and reporting of drugs of abuse in urine. This aspect of federal control of drugs-of-abuse testing was formerly under the **National Institute for Drug Abuse (NIDA)**, which continues to perform other functions in this area. SAMHSA certifies laboratories following a rigorous proficiency testing and inspection procedure. Only SAMHSA-certified laboratories may perform drugs-of-abuse testing for federal agencies or for firms contracting with federal agencies. Only five drugs are on the SAMHSA panel: amphetamine/methamphetamine, cannabinoids, cocaine, opiates, and phencyclidine. Other drugs are measured by SAMHSA laboratories but are not part of the certification. The College of American Pathologists (CAP) also certifies laboratories for toxicology and drugs-of-abuse testing using similar proficiency testing and inspection procedures. SAMHSA and CAP guidelines for all aspects of drugs-of-abuse testing are goals to which all good drug laboratories aspire. A majority of the laboratories screening for drugs of abuse employ enzyme immunoassay (EIA) methodology, which has adequate sensitivity and reasonable specificity in most cases. The amphetamine/methamphetamine class produces the most problems with false-positives. They, of course, will give negative confirmatory tests. Thin-layer chromatography (TLC) is occasionally used to screen (and rarely to confirm), but it is inferior because of borderline sensitivity for some drugs. Confirmatory testing is frequently done by gas chromatography/mass spectrometry (GC/MS) which is clearly the method of choice and is considered the "gold standard". For drugs-of-abuse entries, the cutoff values for screening and confirmation are listed.

Urine collection procedures for drugs-of-abuse testing should incorporate certain checks and precautions to preserve sample integrity. The collection room should not have warm water available, and the stool water should be colored with a dye. If the specimen is to be used for forensic purposes, witnessed voiding is preferred. The temperature within 4 minutes of collection should be between 90°F and 99°F. Later measurement of pH should be between 5 and 9 and the specific gravity (refractometer) >1.002. Any unusual colors, odors, or physical appearance should be noted.

Serum collection tubes for drugs: Silicones and plasticizers used on stoppers of standard red top tubes interfere with some drug assay procedures. Silicones and plasticizers also interfere with GC assays. Some drugs adsorb to the silicone in the red tops and to tops with plasticizers. Gel separator tubes should not be utilized. Use of navy top Vacutainer® tubes avoids this problem since they are free of these interferants. When a drug screen on serum is contemplated, use of a navy top tube rather than a red top tube is suggested.

Please see the chain-of-custody protocol and related information in the Therapeutic Drug Monitoring/Toxicology/Drugs of Abuse Appendix *on page 581.*

See also the **Trace Elements introduction** *on page 585.*

References

Amdur MO, Doull J, and Klaasen CD, *Cararett and Doull's Toxicology*, 4th ed, New York, NY: Pergammon Press, 1991.
Baer DM and Dito WR, *Interpretations in Therapeutic Drug Monitoring*, Chicago, IL: ASCP Press, 1981.
Baselt RC and Cravey RH, *Disposition of Toxic Drugs and Chemicals in Man*, 3rd ed, Littleton, MA: Year Book Medical Publishers, 1989.
Bryson PD, *Comprehensive Review in Toxicology*, Rockville, MD: Aspen Publishers, Inc., 1989.
Burtis CA and Ashwood ER, *TietzTextbook of Clinical Chemistry*, Philadelphia, PA: WB Saunders Co, 1994.
Journal of Analytical Toxicology, Niles, IL: Preston Publications, Inc, 1977.
Journal of Clinical Toxicology, New York, NY: Marcel Dekker Journals, 1968.
Kaplan LA and Pesce AJ, *Clinical Chemistry: Theory, Analysis, and Correlation*, St Louis, MO: Mosby-Year Book Inc, 1996.
Therapeutic Drug Monitoring, New York, NY: Raven Press, 1979.
Toxicology and Applied Pharmacology, New York NY: Academic Press, 1959.
Toxicology Methods, New York, NY: Raven Press, 1991.

Abuse Screen *see* Drugs of Abuse Testing, Urine *on page 548*

Accenon *see* Ethotoin *on page 550*

Acephen® *see* Acetaminophen, Serum *on this page*

Aceta® *see* Acetaminophen, Serum *on this page*

Acetaminophen, Serum

CPT 82003

Related Information
Alanine Aminotransferase *on page 65*
Aspartate Aminotransferase *on page 84*
Lactic Acid, Blood *on page 156*
Liver Biopsy *on page 48*
Liver Profile *on page 161*

Synonyms Acephen®; Aceta®; Anacin-3®; Apacet®; Banesin®; Dapa®; Datril®; Dorcol®; Feverall™; Genapap®; Halenol®; Liquiprin®; Meda-Cap®; Myapap® Drops; Neopap®; Panadol®; Redutemp®; Snaplets-FR® Granules; Tempra®; Tylenol®; Ty-Pap; Uni-Ace®

Applies to Acetanilide; Phenacetin

Abstract Acetaminophen is an analgesic-antipyretic. It is frequently seen in the deliberate overdose situation. In addition to suicidal overdose, acetaminophen-related hepatic necrosis is recognized in a "therapeutic misadventure" scenario. This alcohol-acetaminophen syndrome, in which an alcoholic uses acetaminophen in doses exceeding those recommended (4 g/24 hours), is characterized by a direct toxic reaction. It may be the most common form of acute liver failure.[1]

Specimen Serum

Container Red top tube

Sampling Time Trough

Reference Range Acetaminophen, serum: 20-110 ng/mL (SI: 43-240 nmol)

Critical Values Toxic: >150 µg/mL (SI: >990 µmol/L) (within 4 hours); >50 µg/mL (SI: >330 µmol/L) (within 12 hours)

Use Evaluation of possible toxicity, therapeutic monitoring, or compliance assessment. Acetaminophen causes dose-related hepatic centrilobular necrosis. Its toxic effect is predictable when quantities exceeding recommended doses are taken.[1]

Methodology UV spectrophotometry, immunoassay, gas-liquid chromatography (GLC), or high performance liquid chromatography (HPLC)

Additional Information
- Half-life: 1-3 hours
- Volume of distribution: 0.95 L/kg
- Protein binding: 20% to 50%

Acetaminophen is an analgesic and antipyretic with limited anti-inflammatory properties. It is used for headache, fever, and relief of pain in patients who cannot tolerate aspirin or those with bleeding disorders, peptic ulcer disease, or for those at high risk of bleeding or morbidity from bleeding. Acetaminophen is the analgesic/antipyretic of choice in children 13 years of age or younger due to the association of aspirin with possible development of Reye's syndrome.

Acetaminophen is rapidly absorbed from the GI tract. Peak plasma concentrations are reached in 30-60 minutes after a therapeutic dose. However, following overdose the peak plasma concentration may not be reached for 4 hours or more. Acetaminophen is metabolized to several inactive conjugated forms. There is an intermediate metabolite, N-acetyl-p-benzoquinonemine, that may be responsible for the hepatic toxicity seen with high doses and prolonged use of acetaminophen. Acetanilide and phenacetin owe much of their analgesic effect to their metabolite, acetaminophen.

Acetaminophen is called a "silent" killer because symptoms can appear 24-48 hours after ingestion and unfortunately, well after the time that an antidote can be effective. The main site of toxicity is the liver, in which damage can occur with untreated ingestion of 140 mg/kg (7.5 g in an adult). In an acute overdose situation, the Rumack nomogram will help to determine if acetylcysteine treatment is necessary and if hepatotoxicity is likely. The first concentration should not be drawn until at least 4 hours after ingestion. This allows for complete absorption, but a longer interval may be required in a patient with alcoholic liver disease or other underlying hepatic disease. Acetaminophen toxicity can be underestimated in such patients.[2] Using the Rumack nomogram, if the concentration of acetaminophen at 4 hours postingestion, is above the broken line, an entire course of the antidote, acetylcysteine, is necessary. If the concentration at that time falls below the broken line, treatment with acetylcysteine is not needed and can be discontinued if it has been started. If a patient presents within 6 hours of ingestion, gastrointestinal decontamination procedures can be started while awaiting the results of the acetaminophen concentration. If the patient presents more than 6 hours after ingestion, a loading dose of acetylcysteine should be given empirically if the patient has ingested more than 140 mg/kg of acetaminophen. Chronic ingestion is more difficult to evaluate. If a patient has been

consuming more than 140 mg/kg/24 hours for more than 1-2 days, treatment with acetylcysteine should be started. Early treatment is especially recommended in pregnant subjects.[3] See nomogram.

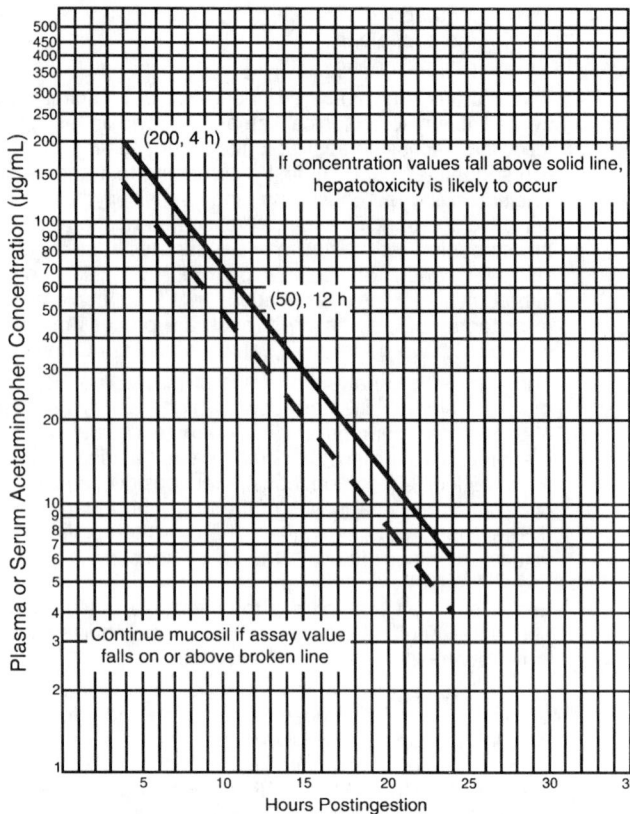

From Rumack BH and Matthews H, "Acetaminophen Poisoning and Toxicity," *Pediatrics*, 1975, 55:871-6, with permission.

Hepatic toxicity may appear 3-5 days after ingestion of a toxic dose. Toxic levels require monitoring liver function with AST (SGOT), ALT (SGPT), and bilirubin with study also of glucose, creatinine, prothrombin time, PTT, CBC, and electrolytes, as well as acetaminophen concentrations for at least 4 days. Extreme increases in AST and ALT distinguish alcohol-acetaminophen syndrome or intentional overdose from alcoholic or viral hepatitis.[1] Serum levels drawn before 4 hours may not represent peak levels. The hepatotoxicity of acetaminophen is related to the formation of one or more highly reactive metabolites in the liver. Impaired hepatic metabolism may be found in the elderly. Orally administered N-acetylcysteine (Mucomyst®) given through a nasogastric tube immediately and for 48 hours has been shown to provide dramatic protection against acetaminophen hepatotoxicity by replenishment of glutathione.

Footnotes
1. Lee WM, "Drug-Induced Hepatotoxicity," *N Engl J Med*, 1995, 333(17):1118-27.
2. Cheung L, Potts RG, and Meyer KC, "Acetaminophen Treatment Nomogram," *N Engl J Med*, 1994, 330(26):1907-8.
3. Riggs BS, Bronstein AC, Kulig K, et al, "Acute Acetaminophen Overdose During Pregnancy," *Obstet Gynecol*, 1989, 74(2):247-53.

References
Ashbourne JF, Olson KR, and Khayam-Bashi H, "Value of Rapid Screening for Acetaminophen in All Patients With Intentional Drug Overdose," *Ann Emerg Med*, 1989, 18(10):1035-8.
Baselt RC and Cravey RH, "Acetaminophen," *Disposition of Toxic Drugs and Chemicals in Man*, 3rd ed, Chicago, IL: Year Book Medical Publishers Inc, 1989, 2-5.
Janes J and Routledge PA, "Recent Developments in the Management of Paracetamol (Acetaminophen) Poisoning," *Drug Saf*, 1992, 7(3):170-7.
Kumar S and Rex DK, "Failure of Physicians to Recognize Acetaminophen Hepatotoxicity in Chronic Alcoholics," *Arch Intern Med*, 1991, 151(6):1189-91.
Lewis RK and Paloucek FP, "Assessment and Treatment of Acetaminophen Overdose," *Clin Pharm*, 1991, 10(10):765-74.
Lieber CS, "Medical Disorders of Alcoholism," *N Engl J Med*, 1995, 333(16):1058-65.
Montamat SC, Cusack BJ, and Vestal RE, "Management of Drug Therapy in the Elderly," *N Engl J Med*, 1989, 321(5):303-9.
Rumack BH and Matthew H, "Acetaminophen Poisoning and Toxicity," *Pediatrics*, 1975, 55:871-6.
Smilkstein MJ, Knapp GL, Kulig KW, et al, "Efficacy of Oral N-Acetylcysteine in the Treatment of Acetaminophen Overdose. Analysis of the National Multicenter Study (1976 to 1985)," *N Engl J Med*, 1988, 319(24):1557-62.
Tighe TV and Walter FG, "Delayed Toxic Acetaminophen Level After Initial Four Hour Nontoxic Level," *J Toxicol Clin Toxicol*, 1994, 32(4):431-4.

Acetanilide *see* Acetaminophen, Serum *on this page*

Acetone *see* Volatile Screen *on page 579*

Acetylsalicylic Acid, Blood *see* Salicylate *on page 573*

ACT® *see* Fluoride, Serum *on page 551*

Actacode *see* Codeine, Urine *on page 544*

Adapin® *see* Doxepin *on page 548*

Adapin® *see* Antidepressants, Cyclic *on page 535*

Adumbran® *see* Oxazepam, Serum *on page 566*

Alcohol, Blood or Urine

CPT 82055 (chemical)

Related Information

Anion Gap *on page 81*
Cocaine (Cocaine Metabolite), Qualitative, Urine *on page 543*
Diazepam, Blood *on page 546*
Drugs of Abuse Testing, Urine *on page 548*
Glucose, Fasting *on page 137*
High Density Lipoprotein Cholesterol *on page 143*
Ketone Bodies, Blood *on page 152*
Lactic Acid, Blood *on page 156*
Liver Biopsy *on page 48*
Liver Profile *on page 161*
Osmolality, Calculated *on page 172*
Osmolality, Serum *on page 172*
Phosphorus, Serum *on page 182*
Uric Acid, Serum *on page 213*
Urine Collection, 24-Hour *on page 30*
Venous Blood Collection *on page 30*
Volatile Screen *on page 579*

Synonyms Ethanol, Blood; Ethyl Alcohol, Blood; EtOH

Abstract Ethyl alcohol is a central nervous system depressant. The most abused drugs in the United States are nicotine and ethyl alcohol. Whole blood alcohol values are required for legal use.

Patient Preparation Do not use alcohol wipe to clean venipuncture site. Hexachlorophene-based, iodine-based, or mercury-based antiseptics not containing alcohol may be used.

Specimen Serum or plasma, urine

Container Red top tube, gray top (sodium fluoride) tube recommended for medicolegal specimens and prolonged storage; plastic urine container

Collection Do not prepare venipuncture site with an alcohol swab. When police agencies bring an individual in for blood alcohol levels, medical and laboratory people should at all times be aware of their state statutes.[1]

Storage Instructions Refrigerate in a tightly stoppered tube.

Special Instructions Concentrations of ethanol are 10% to 15% higher in serum and plasma versus whole blood. For forensic purposes, only whole blood values are used.

Reference Range Blood: negative. In most laboratories, values <10 mg/dL (SI: <2 mmol/L) are considered negative. Signs of intoxication or impairment can be observed at levels of 50-100 mg/dL (SI: 10.9-21.7 mmol/L). Urine: negative. Less than 10 mg/dL is considered negative. Presence of any level of urine alcohol cannot be used to determine impairment.

Critical Values Fatal concentration is usually considered to be >400 mg/dL (SI: >86.8 mmol/L). Lethal blood levels vary greatly and may be substantially lower when ingested with hypnotics or tranquilizers. Whole blood levels of 300 mg/dL (SI: 65.1 mmol/L) are associated with coma and can be associated with fatalities. In most states, levels ≥100 mg/dL are considered evidence of impairment for driving.

Possible Panic Range ≥300 mg/dL (SI: ≥65.1 mmol/L)

Use Quantitation of alcohol level for medical or legal purposes; screen unconscious patients; used to diagnose alcohol intoxication and determine appropriate therapy; screen for alcoholism and monitor I.V. ethanol treatment for methanol and ethylene glycol intoxication. Must be tested as possible cause of coma of unknown etiology, since alcohol intoxication may mimic diabetic coma, cerebral trauma, and drug overdose.

Limitations Certain other alcohols (in high concentration) can interfere with enzymatic methods. The rate of dehydrogenation of isopropanol (2-propanol) is 6%, of methanol and ethylene glycol about 3% to 4%, and that of n-propanol (1-propanol) is 36% of that of ethanol. However, manufacturers of kits for alcohol determination indicate interference is less than these values (about 1%). Gas chromatography is the most specific methodology because it can separate, identify, and quantitate each type of alcohol present. Freezing point osmometry and enzymatic analysis can together determine the presence of volatile intoxicants and can determine causes of metabolic intoxication.

Methodology Enzymatic analysis (alcohol dehydrogenase), freezing point osmometry, gas chromatography (GC)

Additional Information Ethanol is absorbed rapidly from the GI tract. Peak blood levels usually occur within 40-70 minutes on an empty stomach. Food in the stomach can decrease the absorption of alcohol. Ethanol is metabolized by the liver to acetaldehyde. Once peak blood ethanol levels are reached, disappearance is linear; a 70 kg man metabolizes 7-10 g of alcohol/hour (15±5 mg/dL/hour). The plasma/whole blood ratio varies from 1.10 to 1.35 with an average of about 1.20. The urine/blood ratio is considered to be about 1.3 but is quite variable. The average saliva/blood ratio is 1.2. Symptoms of intoxication in the presence of low alcohol levels could indicate a serious acute medical problem requiring immediate attention. The half-lives and effectiveness of certain drugs (eg, barbiturates, etc) are increased in the presence of ethanol. Urine alcohol can be measured by immunoassay and gas chromatography and is tested for in abused drug screening programs. Only in Europe are urine ethanol levels accepted as legal evidence. Alcohol ingestions are discussed in the listings Osmolality, Serum *on page 172;* Anion Gap *on page 81*; and Ketones Bodies, Blood *on page 152.* Breath alcohol analyzers are used by law enforcement personnel; its results are accepted as legal evidence of intoxication. They must not be used less than 15 minutes after the last alcohol ingestion.[2] The blood/breath ratio has a mean value of about 2200.

Electrolyte and acid base problems found with alcohol abuse include hypophosphatemia, hypomagnesemia, hypocalcemia, hypokalemia, hypoglycemia, metabolic acidosis, hypoglycemia, and compensatory respiratory alkalosis.[3] See listing Liver Profile *on page 161.* The alcohol-acetaminophen syndrome is addressed in the Acetaminophen, Serum listing.

Moderate ingestion of alcohol may be beneficial. A letter recites its use by the grandfather of a physician who survived to 111 years of age.[4,5]

Footnotes

1. Gerson B, "Alcohol," *Clin Lab Med*, 1990, 10(2):355-74.
2. Simpson G, "Accuracy and Precision of Breath Alcohol Measurements for a Random Subject in the Postabsorptive State," *Clin Chem*, 1987, 33(2 Pt 1):261-8.
3. De Marchi S, Cecchin E, Basile A, et al, "Renal Tubular Dysfunction in Chronic Alcohol Abuse - Effects of Abstinence," *N Engl J Med*, 1993, 329(26):1927-34.
4. Clarfield AM, "Alcohol Intake and Risk of Myocardial Infarction," *N Engl J Med*, 1994, 330(17):1241-2.
5. Gaziano JM, Buring JE, Breslow JL, et al, "Moderate Alcohol Intake, Increased Levels of High Density Lipoprotein and Its Subfractions, and Decreased Risk of Myocardial Infarction," *N Engl J Med*, 1993, 329(25):1829-34.

References

Blume SB, "Women and Alcohol," *JAMA*, 1986, 256(11):1467-70.
Burtis CA and Ashwood ER, *Tietz Textbook of Clinical Chemistry*, Philadelphia, PA: WB Saunders Co, 1994, 1170-4.
Gadsden RH and Terry CS, "Alcohols in Biological Fluids by Gas Chromatography," *Selected Methods of Emergency Toxicology*, Frings CS and Faulkner WR, eds, Washington, DC: American Association of Clinical Chemistry Press, 1986, 40-3.
Lieber CS, "Medical Disorders of Alcoholism," *N Engl J Med*, 1995, 333(16):1058-65.
Lovejoy FH, "Ethanol Intoxication," *Clin Toxicol Rev*, 1981, 4:1-2.
Rainey PM, "Relation Between Serum and Whole Blood Ethanol Concentrations," *Clin Chem*, 1993, 39(11 Pt 1): 2288-92.
Wilkinson PK, "Pharmacokinetics of Ethanol," *Alcohol Clin Exp Res*, 1980, 4:6-21.

Aliseum® *see* Diazepam, Blood *on page 546*

Allegron® *see* Nortriptyline *on page 565*

Allocar® *see* Digoxin *on page 546*

Almartyn® *see* Flecainide *on page 551*

Alupram® *see* Diazepam, Blood *on page 546*

Alurate® *see* Barbiturates, Quantitative, Blood *on page 537*

Amazin® *see* Chlorpromazine, Serum or Urine *on page 543*

Amethopterin *see* Methotrexate *on page 563*

Amikacin, Serum *see* Aminoglycosides *on this page*

Aminoglycosides

Related Information

Antimicrobial Susceptibility Testing, Aerobic and Facultatively Anaerobic Bacteria *on page 448*
Beta$_2$-Microglobulin *on page 371*
Creatinine, Serum *on page 118*
Magnesium, Serum *on page 164*
Magnesium, Urine *on page 165*
Serum Bactericidal Test *on page 496*
Vancomycin *on page 578*

Applies to Amikacin, Serum; Gentamicin, Serum; Tobramycin, Serum

Abstract Aminoglycoside antibiotics are used primarily to treat infections caused by aerobic gram-negative bacilli. Additionally, when used in combination with penicillins, aminoglycosides may have synergistic bactericidal activity against gram-positive cocci such as *Staphylococcus aureus* and *Enterococcus faecalis*. Aminoglycosides have a narrow therapeutic window, and their use in life-threatening infections makes it mandatory that effective levels be achieved without overdose.
(Continued)

Aminoglycosides (Continued)

Specimen Serum

Container Red top tube

Sampling Time Peak: 30-60 minutes after end of 30-minute I.V. infusion or 60 minutes post I.M. dose; trough: immediately prior to next dose. Specimens should be drawn at steady-state, usually after fifth dose, if drug given every 8 hours, or after third dose, if drug given every 12 hours.

Collection Obtain culture before the first dose. Aminoglycosides are inactivated in vitro by extended-spectrum penicillins such as carbenicillin and piperacillin. Amikacin is the least affected. Aminoglycosides may also be affected by antineoplastics like daunorubicin, bleomycin, and doxorubicin. This will give a falsely low measured concentration.

Storage Instructions Separate within 1 hour of collection and refrigerate or freeze until assayed. Must be frozen if a β-lactam antibiotic is also present, because of potential inactivation of aminoglycosides.

Reference Range See table.

Aminoglycosides

Drug	Therapeutic Range (μg/mL)	Possible Panic Range (μg/mL)	Half-life (h)	Time to Sample (After Starting) (h)
Amikacin Peak	20-30 (SI: 34-52 μmol/L)			
Trough	4-8 (SI: 7-14 μmol/L)	>10 (SI: >17 μmol/L)		
Gentamicin Peak	6-10 (SI: 12-21 μmol/L)		2-3	15
Trough	<2 (SI: <4 μmol/L)	>2 (SI: >4 μmol/L)		
Tobramycin Peak	6-10 (SI: 8-21 μmol/L)			
Trough	<2 (SI: <4 μmol/L)	>2 (SI: >4 μmol/L)		

Possible Panic Range Amikacin: toxic: trough: >8 μg/mL (SI: >17 μmol/L); gentamicin or tobramycin: trough: >2 μg/mL (SI: >4 μmol/L)

Use Peak levels are necessary to assure adequate therapeutic level for the organism being treated. Trough levels are necessary to diminish the likelihood of nephrotoxicity.

Limitations High peak levels may not have strong correlation with toxicity. Therapeutic peak levels depend in part on the minimal inhibitory concentration of the drug against the organism being treated. Blood taken from Silastic® central catheters can give misleading high results.

Additional Information

- Half-life: 4-8 hours
- Volume of distribution: 0.4-1.3 L/kg
- Protein binding: 50%

Aminoglycosides are cleared by the kidney and accumulate in renal tubular cells. Nephrotoxicity is most closely related to the length of time that trough levels exceed 2 μg/mL (SI: >4 μmol/L) for gentamicin and tobramycin, and 10 μg/mL (SI: >17 μmol/L) for amikacin. Creatinine levels should be monitored every 2-3 days as an indicator of impending renal toxicity. The initial toxic result is nonoliguric renal failure, which is usually reversible if the drug is discontinued. Continued administration of gentamicin may cause oliguric renal failure. Nephrotoxicity may occur in as many as 10% to 25% of patients receiving aminoglycosides; most of this toxicity can be avoided by monitoring levels and adjusting dosing schedules accordingly.

Aminoglycosides may also cause irreversible ototoxicity that is manifested clinically as hearing loss. Aminoglycoside ototoxicity is relatively uncommon. Clinical trials in which levels were carefully monitored and dosing adjusted failed to show correlation between auditory toxicity and plasma aminoglycoside levels. In situations in which dosing is not monitored and adjusted, however, sustained high levels may be associated with ototoxicity. The association is not clear and once daily dosing regimens that produce high peak concentrations do not seem to enhance toxicity.

References

Edson RS and Terrell CL, "The Aminoglycosides," Mayo Clin Proc, 1991, 66(11):1158-64.

Gilbert DN, "Once-Daily Aminoglycoside Therapy," Antimicrob Agents Chemother, 1991, 35(3):399-405.

Lortholary O, Tod M, Cohen Y, et al, "Aminoglycosides," Med Clin North Am, 1995, 79(4):761-87.

Aminophylline see Theophylline on page 575

Amiodarone, Serum

CPT 80299

Related Information

Cyclosporine on page 545
Digoxin on page 546
Flecainide on page 551
Lidocaine on page 558
Liver Biopsy on page 48
Liver Profile on page 161
Phenytoin on page 569
Procainamide on page 570
Quinidine, Serum on page 572
Theophylline on page 575
Thyroid Stimulating Hormone on page 204
Thyroxine on page 206
Warfarin on page 579

Synonyms Cordarone®

Test Commonly Includes Desethylamiodarone

Abstract Amiodarone is an antiarrhythmic characterized by substantial toxicity. Some of its adverse effects are potentially fatal. Its level should be monitored. It is used for life-threatening recurrent ventricular arrhythmias which have not responded to alternative therapy in patients at risk for sudden death. Aggravation of arrhythmia has usually taken place in subjects with hypokalemia or those receiving another antiarrhythmic agent. Close monitoring of chest films, liver, thyroid, and cardiac status is recommended.

Specimen Serum

Container Red top tube

Sampling Time Steady-state plasma concentrations are reached in 50-300 days. Time to peak serum concentrations is 4-7 hours after an oral dose.[1] Use trough levels for monitoring.

Reference Range 1.0-2.5 μg/mL (SI: 1.6-3.9 μmol/L) (parent); desethyl metabolite is active and is present in equal concentration to parent drug.

Possible Panic Range Adverse effects at >2.5 μg/mL (SI: >4.0 μmol/L) (parent) and >5.0 μg/mL (SI: >7.0 μmol/L) (both)

Use Compliance and toxicity assessment; used for rhythm abnormalities

Limitations Life-threatening side effects and management difficulties occur, but unlike other antiarrhythmic agents amiodarone has not been shown to increase mortality. Wide interpatient variability in dose concentration relationships limits usefulness of serum concentrations.[1]

Contraindications Amiodarone decreases the hepatic enzyme activity needed to metabolize many drugs. This results in a decrease in clearance and therefore an increase in concentration, which may result in toxicity. Serum concentrations and pharmacologic effects of the following drugs may be increased by amiodarone: cyclosporine, digitalis, flecainide, lidocaine, phenytoin, procainamide, quinidine, theophylline, and warfarin type oral anticoagulants.

Methodology High performance liquid chromatography (HPLC)

Additional Information

- Half-life: 250-1200 hours
- Volume of distribution: 20-100 L/kg
- Protein binding: 95% to 97%

Amiodarone is a class III antiarrhythmic agent approved for the treatment of life-threatening ventricular tachyarrhythmias. Because of potential toxicity, the serum level of this drug should be monitored.[2] Its major elimination is by hepatic metabolism. Negligible renal excretion occurs. Use of the drug is restricted because of its many side effects, including pulmonary fibrosis (hypersensitivity pneumonitis or interstitial/alveolar pneumonitis), adult respiratory distress syndrome (ARDS), neuromuscular weakness, exacerbation of arrhythmia, tremor, thyroid dysfunction and interaction with other drugs. It contains 37% iodine by weight. Up to 5% to 10% of patients on the drug develop hypothyroidism or hyperthyroidism. It may cause increased thyroxine levels and decreased T_3. TSH levels may be useful for diagnosis of thyroid complications. Potassium or magnesium deficiency should be corrected. AST and ALT should be monitored on a regular basis, because side effects of amiodarone include liver complications, and it is cleared by hepatic metabolism. Increased aminotransferase and alkaline phosphatase levels are found in 25% of subjects. Increased serum concentrations of AST and ALT may be three times normal. If serum AST or ALT concentrations go beyond normal or double in a patient with an elevated baseline, then reduction of dosage or withdrawal should be considered. When liver biopsy has been performed, the histopathological appearance of the liver has been that of nonalcoholic steatohepatitis. Cirrhosis can evolve in only a few months. The biopsy is characterized by microvesicular fat resembling the hepatic abnormalities related to pregnancy, tetracyclines, and Reye's syndrome.[3] The drug is embryotoxic. Skin complications are recognized.[4] Cardiac rate, rhythm, and ECG also should be monitored regularly.

Because pulmonary toxicity is the most serious noncardiac complication, chest radiographs are recommended for screening.[1]

Amiodarone can potentiate effects of warfarin, elevating prothrombin time. It can elevate serum digoxin level, levels of other antiarrhythmic drugs including quinidine, procainamide, mexiletine, and propafenone. There are effects with anesthetics, β-blockers, or calcium channel blockers.[1]

Footnotes
1. Podrid PJ, "Amiodarone: Reevaluation of an Old Drug," *Ann Intern Med*, 1995, 122(9):689-700.
2. Vrobel TR, Miller PE, Mostow ND, et al, "A General Overview of Amiodarone Toxicity: Its Prevention, Detection, and Management," *Prog Cardiovasc Dis*, 1989, 31(6):393-426.
3. Lee WM, "Drug-Induced Hepatotoxicity," *N Engl J Med*, 1995, 333(17):1118-27.
4. Primka EJ 3rd, Liranzo MO, Bergfeld WF, et al, "Amiodarone-Induced Linear IgA Disease," *J Am Acad Dermatol*, 1994, 31(5 Pt 1):809-11.

References
Breithardt G, "Amiodarone in Patients With Heart Failure," editorial, *N Engl J Med*, 1995, 333(2):121-2.
Disch DL, Greenberg ML, Holzberger PT, et al, "Managing Chronic Atrial Fibrillation: A Markov Decision Analysis Comparing Warfarin, Quinidine, and Low-Dose Amiodarone," *Ann Intern Med*, 1994, 120(6):449-57.
Evans SJ, Myers M, Zaher C, et al, "High Dose Oral Amiodarone Loading: Electrophysiologic Effects and Clinical Tolerance," *J Am Coll Cardiol*, 1992, 19(1):169-73.
Falik R, Flores BT, Shaw L, et al, "Relationship of Steady-State Serum Concentrations of Amiodarone and Desethylamiodarone to Therapeutic Efficacy and Adverse Effects," *Am J Med*, 1987, 82(6):1102-8.
Mason JW, "Amiodarone," *N Engl J Med*, 1987, 316(8):455-66.
Physicians' Desk Reference (PDR), 48th ed, Mont Vale, NJ: Medical Economics Data, 1994, 2528-31.
Roden DM, "Pharmacokinetics of Amiodarone: Implications for Drug Therapy," *Am J Cardiol*, 1993, 72(16):45F-50F.

Amitriptyline, Blood
CPT 80152

Related Information
Antidepressants, Cyclic *on page 535*
Nortriptyline *on page 565*

Synonyms Elavil®; Endep®; Etrafon®; Limbitrol®; Triavil®

Applies to Pamelor®

Test Commonly Includes Nortriptyline levels

Abstract Amitriptyline is a tricyclic antidepressant. Nortriptyline is a major active metabolite.

Specimen Serum or plasma

Container Red top tube, green top (heparin) tube

Sampling Time Trough levels at steady-state

Reference Range Amitriptyline: 80-250 ng/mL (SI: 289-903 nmol/L); nortriptyline: 50-150 ng/mL (SI: 190-570 nmol/L)

Critical Values >300 ng/mL (SI: >1080 nmol/L)

Possible Panic Range ≥1000 ng/mL

Use Therapeutic monitoring and toxicity assessment. Amitriptyline is a tricyclic antidepressant that blocks the re-uptake of serotonin and norepinephrine at nerve endings. It possesses high anticholinergic activity, sedation and cardiovascular toxicity. It has quinidine-like effects on cardiac conduction.

Limitations Use of therapeutic drug monitoring is controversial. Some data indicate no definite correlation of concentration and clinical outcome and/or severity of side effects. Nortriptyline to amitriptyline ratio may be useful.[1]

Methodology Immunoassay, high performance liquid chromatography (HPLC), gas chromatography (GC)

Additional Information
- Half-life: 17-40 hours
- Volume of distribution: 10-36 L/kg
- Protein binding: 85% to 95%

It is cleared by the liver alone and is extensively metabolized to many polar compounds. The most important metabolite is the N-desmethyl metabolite, nortriptyline, which is an important antidepressant itself. Please see the nortriptyline section for more information. A second active metabolite is 10-hydroxynortriptyline.

Amitriptyline is completely absorbed but undergoes some first-pass elimination. The bioavailability of amitriptyline is 40% to 60% with a peak concentration 2-6 hours after an oral dose.

Anticholinergic side effects are common with this drug. They are not severe and may diminish with continued therapy or can be treated with other pharmacologic and nonpharmacologic therapies. Anticholinergic side effects are more troublesome in the elderly. Sedation may also decrease with continued use. Amitriptyline can lower the seizure threshold and cause orthostasis and arrhythmias. Its cardiovascular effects are more common in patients with underlying cardiovascular disorders.

Drug interactions are common with the cyclic antidepressants. Since they are cleared by the liver, they are susceptible to decreases in enzyme activity caused by cimetidine, fluoxetine, and antipsychotics resulting in increased concentrations of amitriptyline. Enzyme inducers like phenytoin, chloral hydrate, smoking, and the barbiturates will decrease amitriptyline concentrations. Additive anticholinergic side effects occur when cyclics are combined with antihistamines, anti-Parkinson drugs, and antipsychotics. The cardiovascular effects of the cyclics will be additive with any of the class IA antiarrhythmics (quinidine, procainamide, disopyramide). Direct-acting sympathomimetics (epinephrine, norepinephrine, phenylephrine) will be potentiated by cyclics. Monoamine oxidase (MAO) inhibitors and thyroid hormones will potentiate the toxicity of cyclics. Hyperthermia, delirium, convulsions, coma, and fatalities have occurred with the combination of MAOIs and cyclics. These drugs have been used in combination in refractory cases of depression. The cyclics can also affect other drugs. The antihypertensive effects of the central α-agonists (clonidine, methyldopa, guanethidine) are reversed when combined with cyclics. Anticoagulation effects of warfarin may be potentiated by the cyclics.

Cyclic antidepressants should be avoided in pregnant and lactating women because these drugs have not been established to be safe. Geriatric patients are especially susceptible to orthostasis, urinary retention, constipation, and sedation. The cyclic antidepressants are commonly seen in overdose situations. Cardiovascular, anticholinergic, and central nervous system toxicities can be lethal.

References
Hulten BA, Heath A, Knudsen K, et al, "Amitriptyline and Amitriptyline Metabolites in Blood and Cerebrospinal Fluid Following Human Overdose," *J Toxicol Clin Toxicol*, 1992, 30(2):181-201.
Katz IR, Curlik S, and Lesher EL, "Use of Antidepressants in the Frail Elderly. When, Why and How," *Clin Geriatr Med*, 1988, 4(1):203-22.
Katz MM, Koslow SH, Maas JW, et al, "Identifying the Specific Clinical Actions of Amitriptyline: Interrelationships of Behavior, Affect, and Plasma Levels in Depression," *Psychol Med*, 1991, 21(3):599-611.
Knudsen K, Ricksten SE, and Heath A, "Clonidine Interaction in Amitriptyline Poisoning," *J Toxicol Clin Toxicol*, 1988, 26(3-4):223-32.
Lukey BJ, Jones DR, Wright JH, et al, "Relationships Among Nortriptyline, 10-OH (E) Nortriptyline and 10-OH (Z) Nortriptyline Steady-State Plasma Levels and Nortriptyline Dosage," *Ther Drug Monit*, 1989, 11(3):221-7.
Preskorn SH, Dorey RC, and Jerkovich GS, "Therapeutic Drug Monitoring of Tricyclic Antidepressants," *Clin Chem*, 1988, 34(5):822-8.
Wong SH, "Measurement of Antidepressants by Liquid Chromatography: A Review of Current Methodology," *Clin Chem*, 1988, 34(5):848-55.

Amobarb *see* Barbiturates, Qualitative, Urine *on page 537*

Amobarbital *see* Barbiturates, Quantitative, Blood *on page 537*

Amoxapine, Blood
CPT 80299

Related Information
Antidepressants, Cyclic *on page 535*
Disopyramide *on page 547*
Fluoxetine *on page 551*
Phenytoin *on page 569*
Procainamide *on page 570*
Quinidine, Serum *on page 572*

Synonyms Asendin®; Demolox®; Moxadil®; Omnipres®

Applies to Loxapine

Test Commonly Includes 8-OH-amoxapine

Abstract Amoxapine is a tricyclic antidepressant.

Specimen Serum or plasma

Container Red top tube or green top (heparin) tube

Sampling Time Trough level at steady-state. Time to steady-state is 35-50 hours.

Reference Range Amoxapine 20-100 ng/mL (SI: 64-319 nmol/L); 8-OH-amoxapine 150-400 ng/mL (SI: 478-1275 nmol/L); both 200-500 ng/mL (SI: 637-1594 nmol/L)

Critical Values >500 ng/mL (SI: >1594 nmol/L) (both)

Possible Panic Range ≥1000 ng/mL

Use Toxicity assessment. Amoxapine is a heterocyclic antidepressant that blocks the reuptake of serotonin and norepinephrine at nerve endings.

Limitations Use of therapeutic drug monitoring is probably not warranted at this time. There is no data that successfully describes a relationship between concentration and effect.

Methodology High performance liquid chromatography (HPLC), gas chromatography (GC)

Additional Information
- Half-life: 8-15 hours
- Volume of distribution: 1.0-1.2 L/kg
- Protein binding: 80% to 90%; highly bound to tissues also

The drug is a demethylated derivative of loxapine, a neuroleptic used to treat schizophrenia. It possesses anticholinergic activity, sedation, and (Continued)

Amoxapine, Blood *(Continued)*

cardiovascular toxicity. It has quinidine-like effects on cardiac conduction. It is cleared by the liver alone and is hydroxylated to form two active metabolites: 7-hydroxy and 8-hydroxy-amoxapine. The 7-OH metabolite has dopamine-blocking activity giving it a neuroleptic effect similar to haloperidol.

Amoxapine is completely and quickly absorbed. The peak concentration occurs 1-4 hours after an oral dose, with a bioavailability of 46% to 82%.

Anticholinergic side effects are common with this drug. They are not severe and may diminish with continued therapy or can be treated with other pharmacologic and nonpharmacologic therapies. Anticholinergic side effects are more troublesome in the elderly. Sedation may also decrease with continued use. Amoxapine can lower the seizure threshold and cause orthostasis and arrhythmias. Its cardiovascular effects are more common in patients with underlying cardiovascular disorders.

Drug interactions are common with the cyclic antidepressants. Since they are cleared by the liver, they are susceptible to decreases in enzyme activity caused by cimetidine, fluoxetine, and antipsychotics resulting in increased concentrations of amoxapine. Enzyme inducers like phenytoin, chloral hydrate, smoking, and the barbiturates will decrease amoxapine concentrations. Additive anticholinergic side effects occur when cyclics are combined with antihistamines, anti-Parkinson drugs, and antipsychotics. The cardiovascular effects of the cyclics are additive with any of the class IA antiarrhythmics (quinidine, procainamide, disopyramide). Direct-acting sympathomimetics (epinephrine, norepinephrine, phenylephrine) will be potentiated by cyclics. Monoamine oxidase inhibitors (MAOIs) and thyroid hormones potentiate the toxicity of cyclics. Hyperthermia, delirium, convulsions, coma, and fatalities have occurred with the combination of MAOIs and cyclics. These drugs have been used in combination in refractory cases of depression. The cyclics can also effect other drugs. The antihypertensive effects of the central α-agonists (clonidine, methyldopa, guanethidine) are reversed when combined with cyclics. Anticoagulation effects of warfarin may be potentiated by the cyclics.

Cyclic antidepressants should be avoided in pregnant and lactating women because these drugs have not been established to be safe. The 7-OH metabolite has been detected in the breast milk of nursing mothers. Geriatric patients are especially susceptible to orthostasis, urinary retention, constipation, and sedation. The cyclic antidepressants are commonly seen in overdose situations. Cardiovascular, anticholinergic, and central nervous system toxicities can be lethal.

Adverse reactions of amoxapine:

- Anticholinergic: extrapyramidal effects, tardive dyskinesia, blurred vision
- Cardiovascular: hypotension, sinus tachycardia; relatively low cardiac toxicity as compared to other tricyclic antidepressants
- Central nervous system: drowsiness, dizziness/vertigo, nervousness, insomnia, seizures, Parkinson's-like symptoms, chorea (extrapyramidal), tardive dyskinesia, fever
- Dermatologic: rash, toxic epidermal necrolysis
- Endocrine & metabolic: amenorrhea, galactorrhea
- Gastrointestinal: constipation, dry mouth
- Hematologic: leukopenia/neutropenia (agranulocytosis, granulocytopenia)
- Ocular: oculogyric crisis (extrapyramidal)
- Miscellaneous: neuroleptic malignant syndrome, pancreatitis

Signs and symptoms of acute overdose include grand mal convulsions, photosensitivity, insomnia, hyperprolactinemia, cognitive dysfunction, nystagmus, acidosis, coma, supraventricular arrhythmias, hematuria, incomplete right bundle-branch block, renal failure (acute) (neurotoxic effects may be permanent), myoglobinuria, hematuria.

References

Anton RF Jr and Burch EA Jr, "Amoxapine Versus Amitriptyline Combined With Perphenazine in the Treatment of Psychotic Depression," *Am J Psychiatry*, 1990, 147(9):1203-8.

Coccaro EF and Siever LJ, "Second Generation Antidepressants: A Comparative Review," *J Clin Pharmacol*, 1985, 25(4):241-60.

Osiewicz RJ and Middleburg R, "Detection of a Novel Compound After Overdoses of Aspirin and Amoxapine," *J Anal Toxicol*, 1989, 13(2):97-9.

Amphetamine, Qualitative, Urine

CPT 80101 (screen); 80102 (confirmation); 82145 (quantitative)

Related Information

Drugs of Abuse Testing, Urine *on page 548*
Haloperidol *on page 553*
Methamphetamine, Qualitative, Urine *on page 562*

Synonyms Bennies; Crystal; Dexies; Ice; Speed; Uppers

Test Commonly Includes Amphetamine, methamphetamine

Abstract Amphetamine is a sympathomimetic agent that is used as a central nervous system stimulant for the management of hyperkinetic

syndromes and narcolepsy. Due to euphoric effects, it has a high potential for abuse and the use of amphetamine for weight reduction has been curtailed. It is a DEA schedule II drug.

Specimen Random urine

Collection If forensic, observe precautions (see the Therapeutic Drug Monitoring/Toxicology/Drugs of Abuse Introduction *on page 527*).

Storage Instructions Refrigerate

Causes for Rejection If forensic, failure to meet temperature requirements and/or tests for unusual urine dilution (specific gravity or creatinine) or alteration

Turnaround Time Usually 1-2 hours for screen if done in-house. Confirmation, 1 day.

Special Instructions If forensic, use chain-of-custody form. See the Therapeutic Drug Monitoring/Toxicology/Drugs of Abuse Appendix *on page 581*.

Reference Range Negative (less than cutoff)

Critical Values Cutoff: screen: 1000 ng/mL; confirmation: 500 ng/mL (SAMHSA). For methamphetamine, a positive report requires methamphetamine >500 ng/mL and amphetamine (a metabolite) >200 ng/mL in the same sample.

Use Drug abuse evaluation, toxicity assessment

Limitations Some over-the-counter cold and antiallergy medications may cross react in certain immunoassay screens; confirmation by a different, more sensitive method (eg, GC/MS) is necessary.

Methodology Screen: fluorescence polarization immunoassay (FPIA),[1] radioimmunoassay (RIA), enzyme immunoassay (EIA), gas chromatography (GC), thin-layer chromatography (TLC), high performance liquid chromatography (HPLC); confirmation: gas chromatography/mass spectrometry (GC/MS)

Additional Information

- Half-life: 10-20 hours
- Volume of distribution: 3-4 L/kg
- Protein binding: 10% to 40%

For the amphetamine class, the material detected is the parent drug. Amphetamines are stimulants that tend to increase alertness and physical activity. Methamphetamine is more frequently the abused drug because its more pronounced central effects are preferred. See listing Metamphetamine, Qualitative, Urine *on page 562*. Some drivers use amphetamines to counteract the drowsiness or "down" feeling caused by sleeping pills or alcohol. In pure form, they are yellowish crystals that are manufactured into tablets or capsules. Abusers also sniff the crystals, make a solution and inject it, or smoke the form known as "ice." Can be detected in urine as early as 3 hours after use and persists for as long as 24-48 hours.

Amphetamines increase heart and breathing rate and blood pressure, dilate pupils, and decrease appetite. The user can experience a dry mouth, sweating, headache, blurred vision, dizziness, sleeplessness, and anxiety. Extremely high doses can cause people to flush or become pale; they can cause a rapid or irregular heartbeat, tremors, loss of coordination, and even physical collapse. Individuals who use a large dose over a long period of time may develop an amphetamine psychosis: seeing, hearing, and feeling things that do not exist, having irrational thoughts or beliefs and feeling that people are out to get them. People in this extremely suspicious state frequently exhibit bizarre and sometimes violent behavior. Tolerance to the drug is developed after repeated use. Life-threatening overdoses are rare.

Footnotes

1. Turner GJ, Colbert DL, and Chowdry BZ, "A Broad Spectrum Immunoassay Using Fluorescence Polarization for the Detection of Amphetamines in Urine," *Ann Clin Biochem*, 1991, 28(Pt 6):588-94.

References

Bost RO, "3,4 Methylenedioxymethamphetamine (MDMA) and Other Amphetamine Derivatives," *J Forensic Sci*, 1988, 33(2):576-87.

Ellenhorn MJ and Barceloux DG, "Amphetamines," *Medical Toxicology*, New York, NY: Elsevier, 1988, 625-42.

Gillogley KM, Evans AT, Hansen RL, et al, "The Perinatal Impact of Cocaine, Amphetamine, and Opiate Use Detected by Universal Intrapartum Screening," *Am J Obstet Gynecol*, 1990, 163(5 Pt 1):1535-42.

Grinstead GF, "Ranitidine and High Concentrations of Phenylpropanolamine Cross React in the EMIT Monoclonal Amphetamine/Methamphetamine Assay," *Clin Chem*, 1989, 35(9):1998-9.

Hughes R, Hughes A, Levine B, et al, "Stability of Phencyclidine and Amphetamines in Urine Specimens," *Clin Chem*, 1991, 37(12):2141-2.

Jones AL, Jarvie DR, McDermid G, et al, "Hepatocellular Damage Following Amphetamine Intoxication," *J Toxicol Clin Toxicol*, 1994, 32(4):435-44.

Martz W and Schutz HW, "Synthetic Sweetener Cyclamate as a Potential Source of False-Positive Amphetamine Results in the TDx System," *Clin Chem*, 1991, 37(11):2016-7.

Amphetamines, Urine *see* Methamphetamine, Qualitative, Urine *on page 562*

Amphotericin B

CPT 80299

Related Information

Antimicrobial Susceptibility Testing, Fungi *on page 450*
Creatinine, Serum *on page 118*
Flucytosine *on page 551*
Fungal Culture, Biopsy or Body Fluid *on page 476*
Fungal Culture, Blood *on page 477*
Fungal Culture, Cerebrospinal Fluid *on page 477*
Fungal Culture, Skin *on page 478*
Fungal Culture, Sputum *on page 479*
Fungal Culture, Stool *on page 480*
Itraconazole *on page 555*
Ketoconazole *on page 556*
Magnesium, Serum *on page 164*
Magnesium, Urine *on page 165*

Synonyms Fungizone®

Abstract Amphotericin B is a clinically useful but highly toxic antifungal agent available for intravenous or intrathecal administration. It is used for histoplasmosis, blastomycosis, paracoccidioidomycosis (*Blastomyces brasiliensis*), candidiasis, and cryptococcosis. Less responsive fungi diseases include coccidioidomycosis, extra-articular sporotrichosis, aspergillosis, and mucomycosis. Newer, less toxic agents are available. However, for many serious fungal infections, amphotericin B is the drug of choice despite its toxicity.

Specimen Serum

Container Red top tube

Reference Range Therapeutic: peak serum concentrations of 0.5-2 µg/mL are seen after a dose of 0.4-0.6

Use Monitor serum levels for potential toxicity and correlation with *in vitro* susceptibility data

Limitations Poor penetration of the drug into CSF is recognized.

Routine monitoring of amphotericin B concentrations is not indicated. Studies have not been able to correlate serum concentrations and efficacy or toxicity. In usual clinical use, it is probably more prudent to follow serum creatinine, potassium, bicarbonate, and magnesium concentrations and CBC than to perform amphotericin B assays. Assays for amphotericin B are performed only in a few reference laboratories.

Methodology High performance liquid chromatography (HPLC), bioassay

Additional Information

- Half-life: 15 days
- Volume of distribution: 4 L/kg

Amphotericin B irreversibly binds to sterols in fungal cell membranes, disrupting the permeability and fluidity of the cell membrane. It is not significantly absorbed after oral administration. Amphotericin is not by the kidneys but its metabolism is not clearly described.

Amphotericin B therapy frequently induces fever, chills, nausea, and reversible bone marrow suppression. Approximately 80% of patients develop increased creatinine concentrations, and occasional patients suffer acute deterioration in **renal function**; when creatinine levels exceed 3.0 µg/mL it is advisable to withhold amphotericin B for several days and resume therapy at a lower dose. Because the pharmacokinetics and biodistribution of the drug are not clearly defined, it may be useful to correlate serum levels with desired concentrations determined by *in vitro* susceptibility testing. Susceptibility testing, however, is not widely available, not well standardized, and may not accurately predict clinical response. Amphotericin B can increase digitalis toxicity and decrease the anti-*Candida* effect of miconazole. Its toxicities are additive with those of the aminoglycosides.

References

Bennett JE, "Diagnosis and Therapy of Fungal Infections," *Harrison's Principles of Internal Medicine*, 13th ed, Isselbacher KJ, Braunwald E, Wilson JD, et al, eds, New York, NY: McGraw-Hill Inc, 1994, 854-6.
Bodey GP, "Topical and Systemic Antifungal Agents," *Med Clin North Am*, 1988, 72(3):637-59.
Branch RA, "Prevention of Amphotericin B Induced Renal Impairment," *Arch Intern Med*, 1988, 148(11):2389-94.
Chabot GG, Pazdur R, Valeriote FA, et al, "Pharmacokinetics and Toxicity of Continuous Infusion Amphotericin B in Cancer Patients," *J Pharm Sci*, 1989, 78(4):307-10.
Christiansen KJ, Bernard EM, Gold JW, et al, "Distribution and Activity of Amphotericin B in Humans," *J Infect Dis*, 1985, 152(5):1037-43.
Dugoni BM, Gugliemo BJ, and Hollander H, "Amphotericin B Concentration in Cerebrospinal Fluid of Patients With AIDS and Cryptococcal Meningitis," *Clin Pharm*, 1989, 8(3):220-1.
Edmonds LC, Davidson L, and Bertino JS Jr, "Solubility and Stability of Amphotericin B in Human Serum," *Ther Drug Monit*, 1989, 11(3):323-6.
Starke JR, Mason EO Jr, Kramer WG, et al, "Pharmacokinetics of Amphotericin B in Infants and Children," *J Infect Dis*, 1987, 155(4):766-74.
Terrell CL and Hughes CE, "Antifungal Agents Used for Deep-Seated Mycotic Infections," *Mayo Clin Proc*, 1992, 67(1):69-91.

Amytal® *see* Barbiturates, Quantitative, Blood *on page 537*

Anacin® *see* Salicylate *on page 573*

Anacin-3® *see* Acetaminophen, Serum *on page 530*

Ancobon® *see* Flucytosine *on page 551*

Anestacon® *see* Lidocaine *on page 558*

Angel Dust *see* Phencyclidine, Qualitative, Urine *on page 567*

Angilol® *see* Propranolol *on page 571*

Anticoagulants, Oral *see* Warfarin *on page 579*

Antidepressants, Cyclic

CPT 80101 (screen); 80102 (confirmation, each procedure)

Related Information

Amitriptyline, Blood *on page 533*
Amoxapine, Blood *on page 533*
Diazepam, Blood *on page 546*
Doxepin *on page 548*
Fluoxetine *on page 551*
Imipramine *on page 554*
Maprotiline *on page 559*
Nortriptyline *on page 565*
Phenobarbital, Blood *on page 568*
Phenytoin *on page 569*
Trazodone *on page 577*

Synonyms CAD; Cyclic Antidepressants

Applies to Adapin®; Aventyl®; Desipramine; Etrafon®; Norpramin®; Pamelor®; Pertofrane®; Presamine®; Protriptyline; Sinequan®; TAD; TCA; Tetracyclic Antidepressants; Tofranil®; Tricyclic Antidepressants; Vivactil®

Abstract Drugs in this class are widely used as antidepressants. They are frequently involved in suicidal ingestion and responsible for a large percentage of drug-related deaths.

Specimen Serum or plasma

Container Red top tube, green top (heparin) tube; avoid serum separator tubes and the plasticizer, TBEP

Sampling Time Steady-state specimen after 1 week of dose schedule; draw specimen 12 hours after the last dose.

Storage Instructions Remove serum within 2 hours of drawing; refrigerate or freeze if not analyzed immediately.

Special Instructions Order individual drug level or tricyclic overdose screen

Reference Range See table.

Cyclic Antidepressants Therapeutic Levels

Drug	Reference Range (ng/mL)	Half-life (h)
Amitriptyline	80-250	20-40
Amoxapine	20-100	8-15
8-Hydroxyamoxapine	150-400	
Amoxapine and 8-hydroxyamoxapine	200-500	
Desipramine	75-300	20-90
Doxepin	150-250	10-25
Fluoxetine	100-800	26-220
Imipramine	150-250	5-25
Maprotiline	200-600	25-30
Nortriptyline	50-150	20-90
Protriptyline	70-250	60-90
Trazodone	800-1600	6-15

Possible Panic Range >500 ng/mL; toxicity observed at ≥300 ng/mL

Use Therapeutic monitoring and toxicity assessment

Limitations Immunoassays for cyclic antidepressants (toxic overdose) do not distinguish between parent compounds and active metabolites. Immunoassays are available for amitriptyline, nortriptyline, desipramine, and imipramine. Drug-drug interactions occur; hydrocortisone, neuroleptics, methylphenidate, cimetidine, and oral contraceptives produce higher levels by inhibiting metabolism of tricyclics by the liver. Barbiturates, chloral hydrate, and glutethimide lower plasma tricyclic levels by stimulating liver microsomal activity. Interactions with fluoxetine are recognized. Cigarette smoking also lowers steady-state plasma levels, apparently by a similar hepatic enzyme induction mechanism. Plasma levels do not always correlate with clinical effectiveness.

Contraindications Patient taking more than one cyclic antidepressant, patient taking phenothiazines or monoamine oxidase inhibitors (Continued)

Antidepressants, Cyclic (Continued)

Methodology Immunoassay, gas chromatography (GC), gas chromatography/mass spectrometry (GC/MS), high performance liquid chromatography (HPLC)

Additional Information Cyclic antidepressants are metabolized to secondary active compounds. These agents are useful in treating clinical depression, and enuresis (imipramine). However, they show a narrow therapeutic window, and great individual variations in blood levels associated with dosage. African-Americans usually have 50% greater blood level than whites for same dose schedule. Symptoms of overdose may mimic those of condition for which agent was prescribed. The most important of the more serious or toxic effects of CADs is cardiotoxicity. Arrhythmias and conduction defects with precipitation of congestive heart failure and possibly myocardial infarction are common at combined levels >1000 ng/mL. Widening of the QRS interval to >100 msec is highly suggestive of a TAD overdose.

Cyclic antidepressant drugs represent a frequent and serious problem in both unintentional and intentional overdosage. Reports of poor correlations between plasma levels and toxic clinical manifestations indicate that QRS duration >100 msec may provide the most reliable indicator of toxicity. It has been reported that levels of parent to metabolite (P/M) ratios >2 are associated with acute overdosage. In contrast, P/M ratios <2 are more consistent with high steady-state plasma levels following "therapeutic" dosages although ECG or other clinical evidence of toxicity may be present. Variations in blood levels between doses are comparatively small. Peak levels occur 4-8 hours after oral ingestion. A level dose of medication should be prescribed for at least 2 weeks to obtain steady plasma levels. Monitoring of cyclic antidepressant plasma levels is useful in a number of situations. Older patients may develop higher steady-state plasma levels than younger individuals. In geriatric patients, conventional doses may lead to toxic levels. Toxic plasma levels of cyclic drugs may be dangerous in cardiac disease patients. Recommended lower and higher plasma levels for the different cyclic drugs are evolving and are discussed in the literature. A recent study of cyclic levels in children and adolescents has emphasized the lack of correlation between oral dose and plasma concentration and has found that the incidence of side effects and therapeutic effect in treatment of enuresis relates to concentration of circulating drug.

References

Beaumont G, "The Toxicity of Antidepressants," *Br J Psychiatry*, 1989, 154:454-8.

Bergstrom RF, Peyton AL, and Lemberger L, "Quantification and Mechanism of the Fluoxetine and Tricyclic Antidepressant Interaction," *Clin Pharmacol Ther*, 1992, 51(3):239-48.

Brasfield KH, "Practical Psychopharmacologic Considerations in Depression," *Nurs Clin North Am*, 1991, 26(3):651-63.

Frommer DA, Kulig KW, Marx JA, et al, "Tricyclic Antidepressant Overdose: A Review," *JAMA*, 1987, 257(4):521-6.

Hulten BA, Adams R, Askenasi R, et al, "Predicting Severity of Tricyclic Antidepressant Overdose," *J Toxicol Clin Toxicol*, 1992, 30(12):161-70.

Krishel S and Jackimczyk K, "Cyclic Antidepressants, Lithium, and Neuroleptic Agents. Pharmacology and Toxicology," *Emerg Med Clin North Am*, 1991, 9(1):53-86.

Lavoie FW, Gansert GG, and Weiss RE, "Value of Initial ECG Findings and Plasma Drug Levels in Cyclic Antidepressant Overdose," *Ann Emerg Med*, 1990, 19(6):696-700.

Newton EH, Shih RD, and Hoffman RS, "Cyclic Antidepressant Overdose: A Review of Current Management Strategies," *Am J Emerg Med*, 1994, 12(3):376-9.

Antifreeze see Ethylene Glycol on page 550

Antisacer® see Phenytoin on page 569

Apacet® see Acetaminophen, Serum on page 530

A-Poxide® see Chlordiazepoxide, Blood on page 542

Aprobarbital see Barbiturates, Quantitative, Blood on next page

Apsolol® see Propranolol on page 571

Arsenic, Blood

CPT 82175

Related Information

Arsenic, Hair, Nails on this page
Heavy Metal Screen, Blood on page 554
Heavy Metal Screen, Urine on page 554
Semen Analysis on page 652

Synonyms Heavy Metal Screen, Arsenic

Applies to Hair Analysis

Abstract Arsenic is a toxic heavy metal. The largest source of human exposure is arsenic in food resulting from broad use of arsenical pesticides. Acute arsenic toxicity follows accidental ingestion, industrial accidents, suicide or homicide. For children, 2 mg/kg body weight can cause lethal arsenic poisoning.

Specimen Blood, oxalated

Container Trace metal-free container

Collection See Blood Collection Methods for Trace Elements in the Trace Elements Introduction on page 585.

Causes for Rejection Containers not metal-free

Reference Range <23 µg/L (SI: <0.31 µmol/L)

Critical Values Chronic poisoning: 100-500 µg/L (SI: 1.3-6.6 µmol/L); acute poisoning: 600-9300 µg/L (SI: 8-124 µmol/L)

Use Blood arsenic is for diagnosis of acute poisoning only

Limitations Short half-life in blood

Methodology Electrothermal atomic absorption spectrometry (AA)

Additional Information Whole blood and serum have been used for arsenic determination. Blood levels of arsenic have a short half-life and are useful only within a few days of exposure. Urine arsenic concentration is a better measure of arsenic poisoning. In addition to pesticides, rodenticides, weed killers, paint, and wood preservatives contain inorganic arsenic. See Arsenic, Hair, Nails on page 536.

Arsene gas, combining with the globin chain in red cells, causes hemolysis with hemoglobinuria and hematuria. Acute renal failure may cause death.

References

Campbell JP and Alvarez JA, "Acute Arsenic Intoxication," *Am Fam Physician*, 1989, 40(6):93-7.

Goyer RA, "Toxic Effects of Metals," *Casarett and Doull's Toxicology*, 4th ed, Klassen CD, Amdur MO, and Doull J, eds, New York, NY: Macmillan Publishing, 1991, 623-80.

Graef JW, "Heavy Metal Poisoning," *Harrison's Principles of Internal Medicine*, 13th ed, Isselbacher KJ, Braunwald E, Wilson JD, et al, eds, New York, NY: McGraw-Hill Inc, 1994, 2461-6.

Mathieu D, Mathieu-Nolf M, Germain-Alonso M, et al, "Massive Arsenic Poisoning - Effect of Hemodialysis and Dimercaprol on Arsenic Kinetics," *Intensive Care Med*, 1992, 18(1):47-50.

Arsenic, Gastric Content see Arsenic, Urine on next page

Arsenic, Hair see Arsenic, Hair, Nails on this page

Arsenic, Hair, Nails

CPT 82175

Related Information

Arsenic, Blood on this page
Arsenic, Urine on next page
Heavy Metal Screen, Blood on page 554
Heavy Metal Screen, Urine on page 554

Synonyms Arsenic, Hair; Arsenic, Nails; As, Quantitative

Applies to Hair Analysis

Abstract This is a toxic heavy metal that is incorporated into hair and nails. Its presence there in abnormal concentrations is evidence of chronic poisoning. Chronic exposure to arsenic commonly involves industrial sources or contamination of food, water, or medications. Evidence of chronic arsenic poisoning is manifested 2-8 weeks after ingestion. In addition to hyperkeratosis and hyperpigmentation, transverse striae of fingernails (Aldrich-Mees lines) may be seen.[1]

Specimen Clean hair or nails

Container Clean envelope or heavy metal-free screw top plastic container

Collection Extreme care is necessary to avoid surface contamination; pubic hair and toenails are preferable.

Special Instructions Hair should be clean, free of oil and tonic; clip close. Nails should be thoroughly washed, dried, and clipped close to cuticle.

Reference Range Hair: up to 65 µg/100 g (SI: 8.7 nmol/g); nail: <180 µg/100 g (SI: <24 nmol/g)

Critical Values Values >100 µg/100 g (SI: >13.4 nmol/g) of hair are considered toxic

Use Diagnose chronic arsenic exposure and intoxication; accumulation of arsenic takes place in bones, hair, and nails since arsenic is laid down in keratin soon after ingestion.

Limitations Urine arsenic concentration is a better indication of recent exposure.

Methodology Electrothermal atomic absorption spectrometry (AA), neutron activation analysis

Additional Information Arsenic binds to protein sulfhydryl groups. Variations in arsenic hair levels may be due to geographic location and exposure to industrial waste and drinking water. Complications of chronic arsenic exposure include basal and squamous carcinomas of skin and Bowen's disease. An association with carcinoma of lung is recognized.[1]

Footnotes

1. Graef JW, "Heavy Metal Poisoning," *Harrison's Principles of Internal Medicine*, 13th ed, Isselbacher KJ, Braunwald E, Wilson JD, et al, eds, New York, NY: McGraw-Hill Inc, 1994, 2461-6.

References

Bryson PD, "Arsenic," *Comprehensive Review in Toxicology*, 2nd ed, Rockville, MD: Aspen Publishers Inc, 1989, 501-8.

Robertson WO, "Arsenic and Other Heavy Metals," *Clinical Management of Poisoning and Drug Overdose*, Haddad LM and Winchester JF, eds, Philadelphia, PA: WB Saunders Co, 1983, 656-64.

Arsenic, Nails *see* Arsenic, Hair, Nails *on previous page*

Arsenic, Urine

CPT 82175

Related Information

Arsenic, Hair, Nails *on previous page*

Heavy Metal Screen, Blood *on page 554*

Heavy Metal Screen, Urine *on page 554*

Semen Analysis *on page 652*

Urine Collection, 24-Hour *on page 30*

Synonyms As, Quantitative, Urine

Applies to Arsenic, Gastric Content; Hair Analysis

Abstract This toxic heavy metal appears in urine, and its excretion rate is used to determine toxicity.

Specimen 24-hour urine

Container Acid-washed plastic container, no preservative

Collection Collect a 24-hour urine specimen, on ice, with care to avoid specimen contact with metal.

Storage Instructions Refrigerate

Reference Range Ranges for urine arsenic levels can be variable among different laboratories. A general guideline[1] is given: normal: 0-50 µg/L (SI: 0-0.65 µmol/L); chronic industrial exposure: >100 µg/L (SI: >1.3 µmol/L). The 24-hour urinary excretion rate should be <50 µg/24 hours.

Critical Values Toxic: >850 µg/L (SI: >11.3 µmol/L).

Use Evaluate recent exposure to arsenic, arsenic toxicity

Methodology Atomic absorption spectrometry (AA)

Additional Information 25 mL acidified gastric washing is acceptable for arsenic analysis; gastric content normally contains no arsenic. Random urine samples are acceptable.

Footnotes

1. Bryson PD, "Arsenic," *Comprehensive Review in Toxicology*, 2nd ed, Rockville, MD: Aspen Publishers, 1989, 501-8.

References

Amdur MO, Doull J, and Klaasen CD, eds, *Casarett and Doull's Toxicology*, 4th ed, New York, NY: Pergammon Press, 1991, 623-80.

Nixon DE, Mussmann GV, Eckdahl SJ, et al, "Total Arsenic in Urine: Palladium-Persulfate vs Nickel as a Matrix Modifier for Graphite Furnace Atomic Absorption Spectrophotometry," *Clin Chem*, 1991, 37(9):1575-9.

ASA, Blood *see* Salicylate *on page 573*

Ascriptin® *see* Salicylate *on page 573*

Asendin® *see* Amoxapine, Blood *on page 533*

Aspergum® *see* Salicylate *on page 573*

Aspirin, Blood *see* Salicylate *on page 573*

As, Quantitative *see* Arsenic, Hair, Nails *on previous page*

As, Quantitative, Urine *see* Arsenic, Urine *on this page*

Astramorph™ PF *see* Morphine, Urine *on page 564*

Atensine® *see* Diazepam, Blood *on page 546*

Athrombin-K® *see* Warfarin *on page 579*

Auranofin *see* Gold *on page 553*

Aurothioglucose *see* Gold *on page 553*

Aventyl® *see* Antidepressants, Cyclic *on page 535*

Aventyl® Hydrochloride *see* Nortriptyline *on page 565*

Azidothymidine *see* Zidovudine *on page 580*

AZT *see* Zidovudine *on page 580*

Azupamil® *see* Verapamil *on page 578*

Banesin® *see* Acetaminophen, Serum *on page 530*

Barbita® *see* Phenobarbital, Blood *on page 568*

Barbiturate Screen, Urine *see* Barbiturates, Quantitative, Blood *on this page*

Barbiturates, Qualitative, Urine

CPT 80101

Synonyms Amobarb; Butalbital; Mephobarb; Pentobarb; Phenobarb; Secobarb

Test Commonly Includes Identification and confirmation of barbiturates in urine

Abstract Barbiturates are sedative hypnotics which are also drugs of abuse.

Specimen Random urine

Collection If forensic, observe precautions (see the Therapeutic Drug Monitoring/Toxicology/Drugs of Abuse Introduction *on page 527*).

Storage Instructions Refrigerate specimen.

Causes for Rejection If forensic, failure to meet temperature requirements or test for unusual urine dilution

Special Instructions Chain-of-custody documentation required for samples submitted for pre-employment, random employee testing, and forensic purposes. See the Therapeutic Drug Monitoring/Toxicology/Drugs of Abuse Appendix *on page 581*.

Reference Range Less than cutoff

Critical Values Cutoff: screen: 300 ng/mL, confirmation: 300 ng/mL

Use Urine drugs-of-abuse testing, pre-employment screens, random drug testing.

Limitations Short- and intermediate-acting barbiturates can be detected in urine 24-72 hours following ingestion, longer-acting drugs up to 7 days.

Methodology Enzyme immunoassay (EIA), gas chromatography/mass spectrometry (GC/MS)

Additional Information Barbiturates are nonselective CNS depressants that may be used as sedative-hypnotics or anticonvulsants. They are capable of producing all levels of CNS mood effects from sedation to hypnosis to deep coma and anesthesia. Sensory cortex functions, cerebellar functions, and motor activity are decreased. Secobarbital and pentobarbital are short-term hypnotics and lose effectiveness after about 2 weeks of continued usage. Withdrawal symptoms from any barbiturate may be severe and may include convulsions and delirium. The presence of barbiturates in urine is presumptively positive at a level >300 ng/mL using secobarbital as a standard and can indicate prescribed or abused intake of this class of drugs. The presence of these drugs should be confirmed.

References

Burtis CA and Ashwood ER, *Tietz Textbook of Clinical Chemistry*, Philadelphia, PA: WB Saunders Co, 1994, 1176-8.

Coudore F, Alazard JM, Paire M, et al, "Rapid Toxicological Screening of Barbiturates in Plasma by Wide-Base Capillary Gas Chromatography and Nitrogen-Phosphorous Detection," *J Anal Toxicol*, 1993, 17(2):109-13.

Maurer HH, "Identification and Differentiation of Barbiturates and Their Metabolites in Urine," *J Chromatogr*, 1990, 530:307-26.

Barbiturates, Quantitative, Blood

CPT 80102

Related Information

Diazepam, Blood *on page 546*

Phenobarbital, Blood *on page 568*

Applies to Alurate®; Amobarbital; Amytal®; Aprobarbital; Barbiturate Screen, Urine; Blue Angels; Butabarbital; Butalbital; Butisol Sodium®; Fiorinal®; Gemonil®; Lotusate®; Luminal®; Mebaral®; Mephobarbital; Metharbital; Nembutal®; Pentobarbital; Phenobarbital; Red Devils; Secobarbital; Seconal™; Talbutal; Yellow Jackets

Abstract Measurement of barbiturates as a class is usually used for drug-of-abuse testing or as evidence for toxicity.

Specimen Plasma or serum

Container Lavender top (EDTA) tube; green top (heparin) tube; red top tube (avoid serum separator tube)

Sampling Time Trough

Reference Range Negative. Therapeutic: short-acting (secobarbital): 1-5 µg/mL (SI: 4.2-21.0 µmol/L); intermediate-acting (amobarbital): 5-15 µg/mL (SI: 22-66 µmol/L); long-acting (phenobarbital): 15-40 µg/mL (SI: 65-172 µmol/L); for seizure control, phenobarbital therapeutic levels: 10-30 µg/mL (SI: 43-129 µmol/L)

Critical Values Toxic: short-acting: >10 µg/mL (SI: >43 µmol/L); intermediate-acting: >20 µg/mL (SI: >86 µmol/L); long-acting: >40 µg/mL (SI: >172 µmol/L)

Use Evaluate barbiturate toxicity, drug abuse, therapeutic levels; if barbiturates are suspected in a drug overdose, determination of long-, medium-, or short-acting may influence treatment

Limitations Only barbiturates will be identified and quantitated; individual agents cannot be identified by screening tests, particularly if there has been a mixed ingestion

Methodology Gas chromatography (GC), high performance liquid chromatography (HPLC), immunoassay

Additional Information To monitor therapeutic phenobarbital level see listing Phenobarbital, Blood *on page 568*. Barbiturates are sedative hypnotics and frequent drugs of abuse, alone and in combination with alcohol and/or amphetamines. If overdosage occurs, coma and death may result. The implication of any concentration is more serious for short-acting barbiturates than for phenobarbital. The toxic or lethal blood level varies with many factors and cannot be provided with certainty. Lethal blood levels determined at autopsy may be as low as 60 µg/mL (SI: 258 µmol/L) for long-acting (barbital and phenobarbital) and 10 µg/mL (SI: 43 µmol/L) for intermediate- and short-acting barbiturates (amobarbital, butabarbital, butalbital, pentobarbital, secobarbital). In presence of alcohol or other depressant drugs, the lethal concentrations (Continued)

Barbiturates, Quantitative, Blood *(Continued)*

may be lower. Addicts, however, may tolerate levels which would be acutely toxic to a nonaddicted individual with no ill effect. The long-acting drugs are metabolized slowly and depend primarily on the kidney for elimination. The short- and intermediate-acting drugs are metabolized primarily by the liver and are much less dependent on the kidney for excretion. Only barbital is dependent mainly on renal excretion for termination of its pharmacological action. Individual barbiturates can be identified and separated from each other by HPLC.

Barbiturates can be assayed in **urine** or **gastric contents**. The presence of barbiturates in urine is presumptively positive at a level ≥300 ng/mL. Levels above this cutoff can occur from medical use of these drugs as well as from abuse. The presence of these drugs should be confirmed. The most commonly abused barbiturates are secobarbital (red devils), pentobarbital (yellow jackets), and amobarbital (blue angels). Short and intermediate acting barbiturates can be detected in urine 24-72 hours following ingestion, longer-acting drugs up to 7 days.

References
Burtis CA and Ashwood ER, *Tietz Textbook of Clinical Chemistry*, 2nd ed, Philadelphia, PA: WB Saunders Co, 1994, 1176-8.

Chen XH, "Solid-Phase Extraction for Screening of Acidic, Neutral, and Basic Drugs in Plasma Using a Single-Column Procedure on Bond Elut Certify," *J Chromatogr*, 1990, 529:161-6.

Bay Clor® *see* Chlorpromazine, Serum or Urine *on page 543*

Baylocaine® *see* Lidocaine *on page 558*

Beaden® *see* Propranolol *on page 571*

Bedranol® *see* Propranolol *on page 571*

Bennies *see* Amphetamine, Qualitative, Urine *on page 534*

Benozil® *see* Flurazepam *on page 552*

Benzodiazepine, Serum *see* Benzodiazepines, Qualitative, Urine *on this page*

Benzodiazepines, Qualitative, Urine

CPT 80101 (screen); 80102 (confirmation)

Related Information
Chlordiazepoxide, Blood *on page 542*
Clonazepam *on page 543*
Diazepam, Blood *on page 546*
Oxazepam, Serum *on page 566*
Phenobarbital, Blood *on page 568*

Synonyms Tranquilizers (Valium®, Librium®, etc)

Applies to Benzodiazepine, Serum

Abstract This group of drugs is used as antianxiety agents (tranquilizers). They are used by more Americans than any other single prescription drug. Suicidal overdoses are not uncommon.

Specimen Random urine

Storage Instructions Refrigerate or freeze if not analyzing immediately

Reference Range None present unless prescribed. When used as drug-of-abuse screen, negative (less than cutoff).

Critical Values Cutoff: screen: 300 ng/mL (as oxazepam); confirmation: 200 ng/mL

Use Drug abuse evaluation, toxicity assessment

Methodology Immunoassay, thin-layer chromatography (TLC), high performance liquid chromatography (HPLC), gas chromatography (GC), gas chromatography/mass spectrometry (GC/MS)

Additional Information
• Half-life: 4-5 hours
• Volume of distribution: 2-5 L/kg
• Protein binding: 90% to 95%

This benzodiazepines are a class of chemically-related central nervous depressants used as sedative-hypnotics to treat sleep disorders, anxiety, alcohol withdrawal, and seizure disorders. This drug class in low doses can cause sedation, drowsiness, blurred vision, fatigue, mental depression, and loss of coordination. In higher doses or used chronically, they can cause confusion, slurred speech, hypotension, and diminished reflexes. Chronic use may produce a physical dependence and a withdrawal syndrome which can last for weeks. Urine should be screened for benzodiazepines in suspected overdose cases, or as part of an abused drug program. These drugs have a relatively low potential for abuse.[1] They are, however, frequently found with other drugs in emergency room drug screens. Immunoassay screens detect a broad range of drugs and their metabolites in this class using either oxazepam or nordiazepam as positive controls. Using the latter, the test is more specific and more sensitive for detection of flurazepam. Positive screen results (usually >300 ng/mL of urine metabolites) should be confirmed by an alternate technique.

A radioreceptor assay for benzodiazepine concentrations in serum is described.[2]

Footnotes
1. Cole JO and Chiarello RJ, "The Benzodiazepines as Drugs of Abuse," *J Psychiatr Res*, 1990, 24(Suppl 2):135-44.
2. Nishikawa T, Suzuki S, Ohtani H, et al, "Benzodiazepine Concentrations in Sera Determined by Radioreceptor Assay for Therapeutic-Dose Recipients," *Am J Clin Pathol*, 1994, 102(5):605-10.

References
Baker MI and Oleen MA, "The Use of Benzodiazepines Hypnotics in the Elderly," *Pharmacotherapy*, 1988, 8(4):241-7.

Beck O, Lafolie P, Hjemdahl P, et al, "Detection of Benzodiazepine Intake in Therapeutic Doses by Immunoanalysis of Urine: Two Techniques Evaluated and Modified for Improved Performance," *Clin Chem*, 1992, 38(2):271-5.

Fitzgerald RL, Rexin DA, and Herold DA, "Detecting Benzodiazepines: Immunoassays Compared With Negative Chemical Ionization Gas Chromatography/Mass Spectrometry," *Clin Chem*, 1994, 40(3):373-80.

Jones CE, Wians FH Jr, Martinez LA, et al, "Benzodiazepines Identified by Capillary Gas Chromatography-Mass Spectrometry With Specific Ion Screening Used to Detect Benzophenone Derivatives," *Clin Chem*, 1989, 35(7):1394-8.

Montamat SC, Cusack BJ, and Vestal RE, "Management of Drug Therapy in the Elderly," *N Engl J Med*, 1989, 321(5):303-9.

Report of a Committee of the Institute for Behavior and Health, Inc., "Abuse of Benzodiazepines: The Problem and the Solutions," *Am J Drug Alcohol Abuse*, 1988, 14(Suppl 1):1-69.

Smith DE and Landry MJ, "Benzodiazepine Dependency Discontinuation: Focus on the Chemical Dependency Detoxification Setting and Benzodiazepine-Polydrug Abuse," *J Psychiatr Res*, 1990, 24(Suppl 2):145-56.

Benzoylecgonine *see* Cocaine (Cocaine Metabolite), Qualitative, Urine *on page 543*

Berkolol® *see* Propranolol *on page 571*

Berkomine® *see* Imipramine *on page 554*

Biocoryl® *see* Procainamide *on page 570*

Biquin® *see* Quinidine, Serum *on page 572*

Blue Angels *see* Barbiturates, Quantitative, Blood *on previous page*

Bromide, Serum

CPT 84311

Related Information
Chloride, Serum *on page 108*

Abstract Inorganic bromide salts were formerly used as antiepileptics. They are no longer available as nonprescription items in the United States.

Specimen Serum

Container Red top tube

Reference Range Normal: <20 mg/dL (SI: <2.5 mmol/L); therapeutic: 20-120 mg/dL (SI: 2.5-15.0 mmol/L)

Critical Values Toxic: >120 mg/dL (SI: >15.0 mmol/L)

Use Evaluate bromide toxicity. Bromism may be suspected in the presence of a history of ingestion of proprietary bromide preparations, fever, skin rash, and neurologic symptoms.

This test is seldom ordered.

Limitations Patients on iodide therapy will have falsely elevated serum bromide levels. A high level of bromide in the serum will falsely elevate the chloride level.

Methodology Reaction of bromide in a protein-free filtrate with gold chloride

Additional Information
• Half-life: 9-15 days
• Volume of distribution: 0.3-0.5 L/kg
• Protein binding: 0%

In order to convert mg/dL to mEq/L (the same units in which serum or plasma chlorides are reported), multiply the bromide values in mg/dL by 0.125. Both chloride and bromide react identically to titrimetric chloride methods (chloridometer). Many ion selective chloride electrodes give a response to bromide which is double that for chloride. A reported "chloride" value will equal the true sum of chloride and bromide. Over-the-counter former bromide-containing preparations such as Bromo-Seltzer® and Nervine® have not contained bromide in the U.S. since 1971.

References
Burtis CA and Ashwood ER, *Tietz Textbook of Clinical Chemistry*, 2nd ed, Philadelphia, PA: WB Saunders Co, 1994, 1118.

Goldfrank LR, Kirstein RH, and Howland MA, "Bromides," *Toxicological Emergencies*, Goldfrank LR, et al, eds, Norwalk, CT: Appleton-Century-Crofts, 1986, 398-403.

Bufferin® *see* Salicylate *on page 573*

Butabarbital *see* Barbiturates, Quantitative, Blood *on previous page*

Butalbital *see* Barbiturates, Qualitative, Urine *on previous page*

Butalbital *see* Barbiturates, Quantitative, Blood *on previous page*

Butisol Sodium® *see* Barbiturates, Quantitative, Blood *on previous page*

CAD *see* Antidepressants, Cyclic *on page 535*

Cadmium, Urine

CPT 82300

Related Information

Beta$_2$-Microglobulin *on page 371*

Heavy Metal Screen, Blood *on page 554*

Heavy Metal Screen, Urine *on page 554*

Protein, Quantitative, Urine *on page 649*

Urine Collection, 24-Hour *on page 30*

Synonyms Cd, Blood; Cd, Urine

Abstract This toxic heavy metal is used in industry in alloys and metal platings. Exposure is predominantly occupational, involving mining and smelting. A byproduct of lead, copper, and zinc smelting, cadmium is used in batteries, ceramics, soldering, and electroplating, and as a pigment.

Specimen 24-hour urine is recommended for chronic exposure

Container Plastic (preferably polycarbonate) urine container

Collection A 24-hour urine specimen must be collected in a metal-free container and be properly labeled, capped, and sealed.

Storage Instructions Refrigerate urine.

Causes for Rejection Specimen allowed to contact metal

Reference Range Nonsmokers: urine: <1 µg/L (SI: <8.9 nmol/L), <1 µg/g creatinine; whole blood: <1 µg/L, but blood cadmium measurement is reported not to be useful.

Possible Panic Range Levels >10 µg/L (SI: >88.97 µmol/L) in whole blood and 10-20 µg/L (SI: 89-178 µmol/L) in urine probably reflect excessive exposure.

Use Evaluate cadmium toxicity in industrial exposure to cadmium fumes or cadmium ingestion. Dyspnea, cough, and chest pain may follow acute inhalation.

Methodology Flameless atomic absorption spectrophotometry (AA)

Additional Information Inhalation of cadmium fumes produces an acute chemical pneumonitis which can produce pulmonary edema and respiratory failure. Long-term exposure may lead to emphysema (with decreased α_1-antitrypsin). Increased cadmium is reported to be associated with hypertension, it may be a carcinogen for lung cancer and (perhaps) prostatic cancer. Cadmium ingestion may result from contact of acid foods with metal containers. There is exposure of the general populace to cadmium from food, water, and air contamination. Because of slow excretion and constant exposure cadmium values increase with age. Body cadmium elimination half-life may be greater than 20 years. Chronic cadmium exposure can cause proteinuria, increased beta$_2$ microglobulin excretion, and renal insufficiency. Microcytic hypochromic anemia not responsive to iron may be seen.

References

Baselt RC, *Disposition of Toxic Drugs and Chemicals in Man*, 2nd ed, Davis, CA: Biomedical Publications, 1982, 105-8.

Graef JW, "Heavy Metal Poisoning," *Harrison's Principles of Internal Medicine*, 13th ed, Isselbacher KJ, Braunwald E, Wilson JD, et al, eds, New York, NY: McGraw-Hill Inc, 1994, 2461-6.

Roels H, Bernard A, Cardenas A, et al, "Markers of Early Renal Changes Induced by Industrial Pollutants. III. Application to Workers Exposed to Cadmium," *Br J Ind Med*, 1993, 50(1):37-48.

Tonks DB, "Cadmium," *Methods in Clinical Chemistry*, Pesce AJ and Kaplan LA, eds, St Louis, MO: Mosby-Year Book Inc, 1987, 346-61.

Caffeine, Blood

CPT 82486 (chromatography, qualitative); 82491 (chromatography, quantitative)

Related Information

Theophylline *on page 575*

Synonyms Coffee Break®; Dexitac®; Durvitan®; Magnum®; Max Alert Magnum®; Mole®; No-Doz®; Pep Back®; Percoffedrinol N®; Percutafeine®; Pick-me-up®; Pro-Plus®; Stay Awake®; Vivarin®

Abstract Caffeine is a methylxanthine structurally related to theophylline. It is used clinically to treat neonatal apnea, as an aid in restoring mental alertness, and as an analgesic adjuvant. The principle intake is from drinking coffee and tea. Some soft drinks may also contain moderate amounts of caffeine. It is a metabolite of theophylline in infants.

Specimen Serum

Container Red top tube

Collection Indicate exact time blood drawn and relationship to last theophylline or caffeine dose on requisition.

Reference Range None present. The therapeutic range in the treatment of neonatal apnea is 8-14 µg/mL (SI: 41-72 µmol/L).

Possible Panic Range Toxic concentration: >50 µg/mL (SI: >155 µmol/L); fatal: >80 µg/mL (SI: >410 µmol/L)

Use Monitor total xanthine concentration in newborns receiving theophylline. Monitoring clinical endpoints (eg, cessation of apnea) should be used for therapeutic decision making.

Limitations Not often ordered

Methodology High performance liquid chromatography (HPLC)

Additional Information

- Half-life (adults): 3-5 hours; 100 hours in neonates
- Volume of distribution: 0.7 L/kg; 0.8 L/kg in neonates
- Protein binding: 35%

Caffeine is one of the most widely used mind-altering substances. It is found in numerous beverages (cocoa, coffee, cola, tea) and prescription and nonprescription medications. Xanthines, caffeine and theophylline, are used to treat neonatal apnea. Unlike its metabolism in adults, theophylline in neonates is extensively metabolized to caffeine. Caffeine is well absorbed in adults after oral administration with peak concentrations occurring in 15-45 minutes after administration. Theophylline is used to treat neonatal apnea. In neonates, theophylline has a half-life of 30 hours. Caffeine overdoses are rare. The clinical presentation is similar to that of theophylline.

References

Bryson PD, "Stimulants," *Comprehensive Review in Toxicology*, 2nd ed, Rockville, MD: Aspen Publishers, 1989, 374-9.

Dietrich AM and Mortensen ME, "Presentation and Management of an Acute Caffeine Overdose," *Pediatr Emerg Care*, 1990, 6(4):296-8.

Dobrocky P, Bennett PN, and Notarianni LJ, "Rapid Method for the Routine Determination of Caffeine and Its Metabolites by HPLC," *J Chromatogr*, 1994, 652(1):104-8.

Lewin NA, Goldfrank LR, Melinetz M, et al, "Caffeine," *Toxicological Emergencies*, Goldfrank LR, et al, eds, Norwalk, CT: Appleton-Century-Crofts, 1986, 537-44.

Calan® *see* Verapamil *on page 578*

Cannabinoid/Creatinine Ratio *see* Cannabinoids (Marijuana Metabolites), Qualitative, Urine *on this page*

Cannabinoids (Marijuana Metabolites), Qualitative, Urine

CPT 80101 (screen); 80102 (confirmation)

Related Information

Chain-of-Custody Protocol *on page 542*

Drugs of Abuse Testing, Urine *on page 548*

Semen Analysis *on page 652*

Synonyms Cannabis; Carboxy THC; Hashish; Hemp; Marijuana; 11-Nor-9-Carboxy-Delta-9-Tetrahydrocannabinol; Pot; THC (Delta-9-Tetrahydrocannabinol)

Applies to Cannabinoid/Creatinine Ratio

Abstract The main active ingredient of marijuana (cannabinoids) is tetrahydrocannabinol (THC). It is metabolized to THC-carboxylic acid, which is detected in the urine. The name comes from the source of marijuana, the plant *Cannabis sativa*. It is a DEA schedule I drug and a widely used drug of abuse.

Specimen Random urine

Collection For employee screening or forensic purpose, use precautions during collection (see the Therapeutic Drug Monitoring/Toxicology/Drugs of Abuse Introduction *on page 527*).

Causes for Rejection Evidence of urine dilution or alteration

Special Instructions If forensic, use chain-of-custody protocol and form. See test listing Chain-of-Custody Protocol *on page 542* and the Therapeutic Drug Monitoring/Toxicology/Drugs of Abuse Appendix *on page 581*.

Reference Range Negative (less than cutoff)

Critical Values Cutoff: screen: 50 ng/mL; confirmation: 15 ng/mL (SAMHSA guidelines). Some laboratories used 20 ng/mL as a screen cutoff.

Use Drug abuse evaluation, toxicity assessment

Limitations Cannabinoids are rapidly metabolized from blood. Urine is the best specimen for screening although blood (serum or plasma) and saliva have been used. Cannabinoids can adhere to plastic.

Methodology Enzyme immunoassay (EIA), fluorescence polarization immunoassay (FPIA), thin-layer chromatography (TLC), gas chromatography/mass spectrometry (GC/MS)

Additional Information

- Half-life: 20-40 hours
- Volume of distribution: 4-19 L/kg

A positive screen for cannabinoids indicates the presence of cannabinoid metabolites, 11-nor-9-carboxy-delta-9-THC is the major one (carboxy THC), in urine but is not related to source, time of exposure, amount, or impairment. Unless the screen is confirmed by GC/MS, a positive result is presumptive and an unconfirmed screen should not be used to test employees. Urine may contain carboxy THC for a week or 10 days after light or moderate use and as long as a month to 6 weeks after heavy use. Rapid storage of THC metabolites in body fat occurs after use. These substances are then released from storage sites slowly over time.

(Continued)

Cannabinoids (Marijuana Metabolites), Qualitative, Urine (Continued)

A marijuana cigarette is made form the dried particles of the plant, *Cannabis sativa*. The immediate effects of smoking marijuana include a faster heartbeat and pulse rate, bloodshot eyes, and a dry mouth and throat. The drug can impair or reduce short-term memory, alter sense of time, and reduce the ability to do things which require concentration, swift reactions and coordination, such as driving and operating machinery.

Driving experiments show that marijuana affects a wide range of skills needed for safe driving. Thinking and reflexes are slowed, making it hard for drivers to respond to sudden unexpected events. Furthermore, a driver's ability to "track" through curves, brake quickly, and maintain speed and proper distance between vehicles is affected. Research shows that these skills are impaired for at least 4-6 hours after smoking a single marijuana cigarette. If a driver drinks alcohol along with using marijuana, the risks of a vehicular collision greatly increase. When monitoring urine cannabinoids over time to determine continued user abstinence, using the cannabinoid/creatinine ratio eliminates substantial variation from changes in urine dilution.[1]

Footnotes

1. Lafoli P, Beck O, Hjemdahl P, et al, "Using Relation Between Urinary Cannabinoid and Creatinine Excretions to Improve Monitoring of Abuser Adherence to Abstinence," *Clin Chem*, 1994, 40(1):170-1.

References

Chiang CN and Barnett G, "Marijuana Pharmacokinetics and Pharmacodynamics," *Cocaine, Marijuana, Designer Drugs: Chemistry, Pharmacology and Behavior*, Redda KK, Walker CA, and Barnell G, eds, Boca Raton, FL: CRC Press, 1989, 113-26.

ElSohly MA and ElSohly HN, "Marijuana: Analysis and Detection of Use Through Urinalysis," *Cocaine, Marijuana, Designer Drugs: Chemistry, Pharmacology and Behavior*, Redda KK, Walker CA, and Barnett G, eds, Boca Raton, FL: CRC Press, 1989, 145-62.

Hawks RL and Chiang CN, "Examples of Specific Drug Assays: Marijuana/Cannabinoids," *Urine Testing for Drugs of Abuse*, NIDA Research Monograph 73, Rockville, MD, 1986, 85-92.

Huestis MA, Mitchell JM, and Cone EJ, "Lowering the Federally-Mandated Cannabinoid Immunoassay Cutoff Increases True-Positive Results," *Clin Chem*, 1994, 40(5):729-33.

Schucket MA, "Cannabinols," *Drug and Alcohol Abuse*, New York, NY: Plenum, 1989, 143-57.

Wells DJ and Barnhill MT Jr, "Comparative Results With Five Cannabinoid Immunoassay Systems at the Screening Threshold of 100 Micrograms/L," *Clin Chem*, 1989, 35(11):2241-3.

Zuckerman B, Frank DA, Hingson R, et al, "Effects of Maternal Marijuana and Cocaine Use on Fetal Growth," *N Engl J Med*, 1989, 320(12):762-8.

Cannabis see Cannabinoids (Marijuana Metabolites), Qualitative, Urine *on previous page*

Carbamazepine

CPT 80156

Related Information

Carbamazepine-10,11-Epoxide *on this page*
Lamotrigine *on page 556*
Phenytoin *on page 569*
Theophylline *on page 575*
Valproic Acid *on page 577*
Verapamil *on page 578*
Warfarin *on page 579*

Synonyms Carbamazepinum; Carbategretal®; Carbazep®; CBZ; Epitrol®; Tegretol®

Applies to P-450 System

Abstract Carbamazepine is a first-line antiepileptic drug for generalized and partial seizures. It is also used for control of neurogenic pain from trigeminal neuralgia and diabetic neuropathy. It has been successfully used in the treatment of bipolar disease and other psychiatric and neurologic illnesses. It has a distinctive pharmacokinetic property of inducing the hepatic enzymes responsible for its own clearance, called "autoinduction."

Patient Preparation Levels should be drawn before next oral dose with patient at steady-state.

Specimen Serum

Container Red top tube

Sampling Time A consistent sampling time, ideally a trough level, should be used to monitor patients on chronic therapy.

Reference Range 8-12 µg/mL (SI: 34-51 µmol/L). **Low level:** The most common cause of a low level is noncompliance. The addition of anticonvulsants which induce the P-450 system, such as phenytoin, primidone, and phenobarbital, may decrease carbamazepine levels without causing seizures. (The P-450 system is a liver enzymatic system which degrades drugs.) The withdrawal of phenytoin from the regimen of a patient on carbamazepine may increase the level and still cause seizures. Because of autoinduction of metabolism, patients in the first 2 months of therapy may have diminishing levels and be at risk for seizures. Occasionally,

patients may have toxicity when levels are within the reference range. **High level:** Drugs which inhibit the P-450 system, including isoniazid, fluoxetine, propoxyphene, verapamil, and stiripentol can cause a precipitous rise in carbamazepine levels and clinical toxicity, usually within 48 hours. Danazol may cause a delayed toxicity. The addition of cimetidine, erythromycin, lithium, triacetyloleandomycin, and valproic acid also can cause toxicity.

Possible Panic Range Central nervous system toxicity occurs progressively with levels near or above high end of reference range.

Use Monitor for compliance, efficacy, or possible toxicity. Carbamazepine has concentration-related toxicities and toxicities unrelated to concentration. Most of the concentration related side effects are neurosensory. Disturbances of vision (nystagmus, diplopia), gait (ataxia), along with drowsiness, dizziness, and headache are commonly seen at concentrations >10 µg/mL.

Limitations See listing Carbamazepine-10,11-Epoxide *on page 540*.

Contraindications Half-life of warfarin is shortened; monoamine oxidase inhibitors not recommended.

Methodology Enzyme immunoassay (EIA), gas-liquid chromatography (GLC), high performance liquid chromatography (HPLC)

Additional Information

- Half-life: 15-40 hours
- Volume of distribution: 0.8-1.8 L/kg
- Protein binding: 60% to 80%

Carbamazepine is only commercially available in oral formulations. It is absorbed slowly and is about 80% bioavailable. Plasma concentrations peak at about 6 hours after an oral dose. Carbamazepine is totally cleared hepatically and has one active metabolite, the 10,11-epoxide. Carbamazepine induces the hepatic enzymes that are responsible for its clearance. Clearance increases with time. The enzymes are fully "induced" within 4-6 weeks after starting the drug. Since clearance is increasing, half-life correspondingly decreases. The average half-life of carbamazepine before autoinduction is about 25-40 hours and 15-25 hours after autoinduction. Along with inducing the enzymes used to metabolize its own metabolism, it also increases the enzyme activity and therefore clearance of many other drugs, including many anticonvulsants. Side effects, principally nausea, prevent oral "loading" of carbamazepine.

Leukopenia is the most common hematologic side effect, with incidences as high as 10% being reported and may be dose-related. The most serious, blood dyscrasias, aplastic anemia, agranulocytosis, and hepatic damage, are rare and not concentration-related. In most patients leukopenia is transient in nature and may be dose-related. Clinically carbamazepine can be continued until the WBC <2500/mm³ and/or the absolute neutrophil count is <1000/mm³.[1] Hypersensitivity reactions including Stevens-Johnson syndrome, hyponatremia, osteomalacia, and cardiac conduction effects can also occur. Hyponatremia is more common in older patients. Patients in the first month of pregnancy are at increased risk of neural tube defects.

Carbamazepine may interfere with the actions of theophylline, oral contraceptives, oral anticoagulants, or doxycycline. Carbamazepine may induce the metabolism of phenytoin, benzodiazepines, ethosuximide, valproic acid, corticosteroids, and thyroid hormones; synergistic anticonvulsant effect with propranolol. See Table A in the Therapeutic Drug Monitoring/Toxicology/Drugs of Abuse Appendix *on page 582*.

Carbamazepine increases BUN, AST, ALT, ammonia, bilirubin, alkaline phosphatase and decreases calcium, sodium, T_3, and T_4 in test samples.

Footnotes

1. Engel J, *Seizures and Epilepsy*, Contemporary Neurology Series, Philadelphia, PA: FA Davis Co, 1989.

References

Bertilsson L and Tomson T, "Clinical Pharmacokinetics and Pharmacological Effects of Carbamazepine and Carbamazepine-10,11-Epoxide. An Update," *Clin Pharmacokinet*, 1986, 11(3):177-98.

Grimsley SR, Jann MW, Carter JG, et al, "Increased Carbamazepine Concentrations After Fluoxetine Coadministration," *Clin Pharmacol Ther*, 1991, 50(1):10-5.

Levy RH, Dreifuss FE, Mattson RH, et al, *Antiepileptic Drugs*, 3rd ed, New York, NY: Raven Press, 1989.

Liu H and Delgado MR, "A Comprehensive Study of the Relation Between Serum Concentrations, Concentration Ratios, and Level/Dose Ratios of Carbamazepine and Its Metabolite With Age, Weight, Dose, and Clearances in Epileptic Children," *Epilepsia*, 1994, 35(6):1221-9.

Tibballs J, "Acute Toxic Reaction to Carbamazepine: Clinical Effects and Serum Concentrations," *J Pediatr*, 1992, 121(2):295-9.

Carbamazepine-10,11-Epoxide

CPT 80156

Related Information

Carbamazepine *on this page*

Synonyms Carbamazepine Metabolite

Test Commonly Includes Carbamazepine and carbamazepine-10,11-epoxide

Abstract Occasional cases of carbamazepine toxicity occur with normal levels of carbamazepine due to accumulation of the active metabolite, 10,11-epoxide.[1,2]

Specimen Serum

Container Red top tube

Reference Range 0.8-3.2 mg/L. High level: In patients on chronic carbamazepine therapy, the addition of valpromide or progabide produces clinical toxicity with high levels of metabolite and normal levels of parent compound.[3]

Limitations Valproic acid, a compound chemically related to valpromide, may increase the epoxide/carbamazepine ratio by eliminating excretion of the epoxide. Since most cases of fatal valproate hepatotoxicity occur in young children on multiple anticonvulsants, the combination of valproate and carbamazepine is not recommended in the susceptible population. Phenytoin may also increase the ratio of epoxide/parent compound.[4]

Methodology High performance liquid chromatography (HPLC), fluorescence polarization immunoassay (FPIA)

Additional Information Carbamazepine-10,11-epoxide has been shown to be pharmacologically active in animals.[5]

Footnotes

1. Pisani F, Fazio A, Oteri G, et al, "Sodium Valproate and Valpromide: Differential Interaction With Carbamazepine in Epileptic Patients," *Epilepsia*, 1986, 27(5):548-52.
2. Kutt H, Solomon GE, Dhar AK, et al, "Effects of Progabide on Carbamazepine Epoxide and Carbamazepine Concentrations in Plasma," *Epilepsia*, 1984, 25:674.
3. Meijer JW, Binnie CD, Debets RM, et al, "Possible Hazard of Valpromide-Carbamazepine Combination Therapy in Epilepsy," *Lancet*, 1984, 1(8380):802.
4. Theodore WH, Narang PK, Holmes MD, et al, "Carbamazepine and its Epoxide: Relation of Plasma Levels to Toxicity and Seizure Control," *Ann Neurol*, 1989, 25:194-6.
5. Albright PS and Bruni J, "Effects of Carbamazepine and its Epoxide Metabolite on Amygdala-Kindled Seizures in Rats," *Neurology*, 1984, 34(10):1383-6.

References

So EL, Ruggles KH, Cascino GD, et al, "Seizure Exacerbation and Status Epilepticus Related to Carbamazepine-10,11-epoxide," *Ann Neurol*, 1994, 35(6):743-6.

Carbamazepine Metabolite see Carbamazepine-10,11-Epoxide *on previous page*

Carbamazepinum see Carbamazepine *on previous page*

Carbategretal® see Carbamazepine *on previous page*

Carbazep® see Carbamazepine *on previous page*

Carbon Monoxide see Carboxyhemoglobin *on this page*

Carboxyhemoglobin

CPT 82375

Related Information

Blood Gases, Arterial *on page 87*
Lactic Acid, Blood *on page 156*
Methemoglobin *on page 166*
P-50 Blood Gas *on page 176*
Phlebotomy, Therapeutic *on page 614*

Synonyms Carbon Monoxide; CO; COHb

Test Commonly Includes COHb is sometimes included in Blood Gases, but may be ordered as a separate test.

Abstract A byproduct of incomplete combustion, carbon monoxide (CO) is colorless, tasteless, and odorless. It binds tightly to hemoglobin to form COHb, reducing oxygen-carrying capacity.

This test measures hemoglobin-bound carbon monoxide. The binding affinity of hemoglobin for carbon monoxide is about 250 times greater than that for oxygen. The percent bound measures the extent of carbon monoxide toxicity.

Patient Preparation In suspected carbon monoxide poisoning, the specimen should be collected immediately.

Specimen Whole blood

Container Green top (heparin) tube or lavender top (EDTA) tube, depending upon laboratory methods

Sampling Time Draw before the patient is started on oxygen if possible.

Collection Keep tube capped

Storage Instructions Refrigerate immediately after collection. Do not remove cap. Carboxyhemoglobin is stable 4 months in filled, well-capped tube.

Reference Range Nonsmokers: <2%; **smokers**: 1-2 packs/day: 4% to 5%, >2 packs/day: 8% to 9%. Carboxyhemoglobin in the **newborn** may run to 10% to 12%. Carbon monoxide is a metabolic product of hemoglobin catabolism. The increased turnover of hemoglobin in the newborn together with decreased efficiency of the infant's respiratory system may and does lead to higher levels of carboxyhemoglobin.

Critical Values Exposure to CO concentrations 80-140 ppm for 1-2 hours can lead to COHb results of 3% to 6%; even these levels can

precipitate angina and cardiac arrhythmias.[1] Toxic concentration is 20%; lethal is >50%

Possible Panic Range Disturbance of judgment, headache, and dizziness occur at 10% to 30%; coma at 50% to 60%; fatality occurs at 30% to 60% or more, and rapid death at level of 80%.

Use Determine the extent of carbon monoxide poisoning, toxicity in individuals exposed to exhausts or indoor combustion including heating, cooking, or fumes of gasoline-powered motors and tools, or incomplete combustion of wood or natural gas. Check on effect of smoking on the patient; work up headache, irritability, mental impairment, nausea, vomiting, vertigo, dyspnea, collapse, coma, convulsions. Work up persons exposed to fires and smoke inhalation.

Limitations CO binds to cytochrome oxidase, interfering with cellular respiration. Thus, although COHb assays provide information on exposure to CO, they do not always consistently correlate with symptoms or prognosis.[1]

Carbon monoxide levels are of limited value in screening for smoking, since it is cleared rapidly. The half-life of carboxyhemoglobin in individuals with normal cardiopulmonary function is 1-2 hours. Urinary nicotine, if available, is preferable as a screening test for tobacco use. Arterial blood gases may be of limited value in treatment decisions for carbon monoxide poisoning.[2]

Methodology Spectrophotometric, gas-liquid chromatography (GLC), pulse oximetry[3]

Additional Information Carboxyhemoglobin is useful in judging the extent of carbon monoxide toxicity and in considering the effect of smoking on the patient. A direct correlation has been claimed between CO level and symptoms of atherosclerotic diseases, intermittent claudication, angina, and myocardial infarction. Exposure may occur not only from smoking but also from exposure to automobile exhaust gases and gases from various engines. Coal gas contains carbon monoxide. A solvent found in paint removers, methylene chloride, is metabolized to CO. This test may be included when blood gases are ordered, when there is sufficient sample, and when such instrumentation is available. Carboxyhemoglobin leads to hypoxia and lactic acidosis. Myoglobinuria may develop. Natural gas does not contain CO but after combustion CO is produced.

A danger of missed diagnosis of CO intoxication is continued exposure of the patient and others to a toxic environment.[4] The cherry red color of CO poisoning is not consistently seen.[5] CO intoxication may contribute to the risk of myocardial infarction.[5,6]

A strong correlation is present between carboxyhemoglobin levels and psychometric testing abnormalities.[2] Psychometric testing measures actual neurologic disability and may therefore better define carboxyhemoglobin poisoning severity than blood CO level. The half-life with O_2 administration is 80 minutes. With O_2 at three atmospheres, the half-life is 24 minutes.

Footnotes

1. From the Centers for Disease Control and Prevention, "Carbon Monoxide Poisoning - Weld County, Colorado, 1993," *JAMA*, 1994, 272(19):1489-90.
2. Myers RA and Britten JS, "Are Arterial Blood Gases of Value in Treatment Decisions for Carbon Monoxide Poisoning?" *Crit Care Med*, 1989, 17(2):139-42.
3. Vegfors M and Lennmarken C, "Carboxyhaemoglobinaemia and Pulse Oximetry," *Br J Anaesth*, 1991, 66(5):625-6.
4. Crawford R, Campbell DG, and Ross J, "Carbon Monoxide Poisoning in the Home: Recognition and Treatment," *BMJ*, 1990, 301(6758):1161.
5. Grace TW and Platt FW, "Subacute Carbon Monoxide Poisoning. Another Great Imitator," *JAMA*, 1981, 246:1698-700.
6. Kaufman DW, Helmrich SP, Rosenberg L, et al, "Nicotine and Carbon Monoxide Content of Cigarette Smoke and the Risk of Myocardial Infarction in Young Men," *N Engl J Med*, 1983, 308:409-13.

References

Dolan MC, Haltom TL, Barrows GH, et al, "Carboxyhemoglobin Levels in Patients With Flu-Like Symptoms," *Ann Emerg Med*, 1987, 16(7):782-6.
Fechner GG and Gee DJ, "Study on the Effects of Heat on Blood and on the Postmortem Estimation of Carboxyhemoglobin and Methaemoglobin," *Forensic Sci Int*, 1989, 40(1):63-7.
Heckerling PS, Leikin JB, Maturen A, et al, "Screening Hospital Admissions From the Emergency Department for Occult Carbon Monoxide Poisoning," *Am J Emerg Med*, 1990, 8(4):301-4.
Kales S, "Carbon Monoxide Intoxication," *Am Fam Physician*, 1993, 48(6):1100-4.
Krantz T, Thisted B, Strøm J, et al, "Acute Carbon Monoxide Poisoning," *Acta Anaesthesiol Scand*, 1988, 32(4):278-82.
Mahoney JJ, Vreman HJ, Stevenson DK, et al, "Measurement of Carboxyhemoglobin and Total Hemoglobin by Five Specialized Spectrophotometers (CO-oximeter) in Comparison With Reference Methods," *Clin Chem*, 1993, 39(8):1693-1700.
Thom SR and Keim LW, "Carbon Monoxide Poisoning: A Review Epidemiology, Pathophysiology, Clinical Findings, and Treatment Options Including Hyperbaric Oxygen Therapy," *J Toxicol Clin Toxicol*, 1989, 27(3):141-56.
Variend S and Forrest AR, "Carbon Monoxide Concentrations in Infant Deaths," *Arch Dis Child*, 1987, 62(4):417-8.
Zijlstra WG, Buursma A, and Meeuwsen-van-der-Roest WP, "Absorption Spectra of Human Fetal and Adult Oxyhemoglobin, Deoxyhemoglobin, Carboxyhemoglobin, and Methemoglobin," *Clin Chem*, 1991, 37(9):1633-8.

Carboxy THC see Cannabinoids (Marijuana Metabolites), Qualitative, Urine *on page 539*

Cardioquin® *see* Quinidine, Serum *on page 572*

Cardioreg® *see* Digoxin *on page 546*

CBZ *see* Carbamazepine *on page 540*

Cd, Blood *see* Cadmium, Urine *on page 539*

Cd, Urine *see* Cadmium, Urine *on page 539*

Centralgine® *see* Meperidine, Blood or Urine *on page 560*

Cerebrospinal Fluid Methotrexate *see* Methotrexate *on page 563*

Chain-of-Custody Protocol
Related Information
Meperidine, Blood or Urine *on page 560*
Morphine, Urine *on page 564*
Paternity Studies *on page 613*
Specimen Identification Requirements *on page 29*
Venous Blood Collection *on page 30*

Synonyms Chain-of-Evidence Form; Specimen Chain-of-Custody Protocol

Applies to Medical Legal Specimens

Abstract A procedure to ensure sample integrity from collection through transport, receipt, sampling, and analysis. It is associated with a chain-of-custody form. See the Therapeutic Drug Monitoring/Toxicology/Drugs of Abuse Appendix *on page 581*. Similar forms are used (chain-of-evidence) for other forensic materials such as guns, bullets, chemicals, etc.

Specimen Usually urine for drugs-of-abuse-related monitoring

Container Plastic urine cup with locking lid covered by seal which is signed or initialed (if for drugs of abuse)

Collection See the Therapeutic Drug Monitoring/Toxicology/Drugs of Abuse Introduction *on page 527* for collection precautions.

Causes for Rejection Sample container not sealed or labeled

Special Instructions Form requires signature of sample donor as well as that of the person receiving the sample at the collection site.

Reference Range Normal: all seals intact and chain-of-custody form completed.

Use Chain-of-custody is a legal term that describes a method to maintain sample integrity in the collection, handling, and storage of urine or other samples.

Additional Information The chain-of-custody protocol is a clerical and custodial service offered by the laboratory to document specimen transfer and provide for extended specimen storage. A written record of specimen transfer from patient, to analyst, to storage and disposal is maintained on all specimens covered by chain-of-custody. All drug screens, blood alcohols, or any other tests or objects that have medico-legal significance should be accompanied by chain-of-custody and a written release form.

References
Smith ML, Bronner WE, Shimomura ET, et al, "Quality Assurance in Drug Testing Laboratories," *Clin Lab Med*, 1990, 10(3):503-16.

Chain-of-Evidence Form *see* Chain-of-Custody Protocol *on this page*

Chloramphenicol
CPT 82415
Related Information
Antimicrobial Susceptibility Testing, Aerobic and Facultatively Anaerobic Bacteria *on page 448*
Phenobarbital, Blood *on page 568*
Phenytoin *on page 569*
Serum Bactericidal Test *on page 496*

Synonyms Chloromycetin®; Mychel-S®

Abstract The use of chloramphenicol has been greatly diminished in recent years because of the introduction of a wide variety of less toxic alternative agents. It is still appropriately used to treat certain rickettsial infections or penicillin-allergic patients with bacterial meningitis. Life-threatening bone marrow toxicity is not closely associated with high serum levels.

Specimen Serum

Container Red top tube

Sampling Time Collect for trough level immediately before next dose; for peak level about 2 hours after oral dose, 30 minutes after I.V. dose (time to peak can be variable)

Storage Instructions Freeze processed specimen

Reference Range Therapeutic: 10-25 µg/mL (SI: 31-77 µmol/L), trough <5 µg/mL (SI: <15 µmol/L)

Critical Values Toxic: >25 µg/mL (SI: >77 µmol/L)

Use Monitor drug therapy; monitoring for potential toxicity. See Table B in the Therapeutic Drug Monitoring/Toxicology/Drugs of Abuse Appendix *on page 582*.

Limitations There are no data that correlate serum concentrations with efficacy. Trough concentrations have not been associated with efficacy or toxicity. Reversible dose related bone marrow depression may occur with serum/plasma concentrations >25 µg/mL (SI: >77 µmol/L). Idiosyncratic bone marrow aplasia is a rare event that usually occurs weeks to months after completion of therapy, but approximately 25% occur during the course of therapy. Hematologic studies should be performed before and during therapy.

Methodology High performance liquid chromatography (HPLC), gas-liquid chromatography (GLC), immunoassay

Additional Information
- Half-life (adult): 2-3 hours
- Volume of distribution: 0.9 L/kg
- Protein binding: 50% to 60%

Chloramphenicol is an extremely effective antibacterial agent which unfortunately has both idiosyncratic and dose-related toxicities. Half-life is increased by 1.6-3.3 hours in infants and patients with hepatic and renal disease.

Hematologic toxicities of chloramphenicol have limited its use. They can be manifested as concentration-related, reversible bone marrow suppression or rare, irreversible idiosyncratic aplastic anemia. The concentration related bone marrow suppression has been seen with peak concentrations >25 µg/mL. The reversible bone marrow suppression begins with a reticulocytopenia and a decrease in hemoglobin. With continued use, thrombocytopenia and neutropenia may occur. The more feared aplastic anemia is not concentration related. The incidence averages 1:40,000. It is more common in children and females and may occur months after discontinuation of the drug. There may be a genetic predisposition to this adverse effect. Gray baby syndrome is the other dreaded adverse effect seen with chloramphenicol use. As the name implies it is most often seen in infants and has been associated with peak concentrations >50 µg/mL.

Chloramphenicol is a hepatic enzyme inhibitor. It decreases the clearance of many drugs, including warfarin, tolbutamide, chlorpropamide, and phenytoin. Chloramphenicol clearance is increased by some enzyme inducers including phenobarbital, phenytoin, and rifampin.

References
Miceli JN, "Chloramphenicol and Vancomycin," *Clin Lab Med*, 1987, 7(3):531-40.
Mulhall A, deLouvois J, and Hurley R, "Chloramphenicol Toxicity in Neonates; Its Incidence and Prevention," *Br Med J (Clin Res Ed)*, 1983, 287:1424-7.
Smilack JD, Wilson WR, and Cockerill FR 3d, "Tetracyclines, Chloramphenicol, Erythromycin, Clindamycin, and Metronidazole," *Mayo Clin Proc*, 1991, 66(12):1270-80.
Yunis AA, "Chloramphenicol: Relation of Structure to Activity and Toxicity," *Annu Rev Pharmacol Toxicol*, 1988, 28:83-100.

Chlordiazepoxide, Blood
CPT 80154
Related Information
Benzodiazepines, Qualitative, Urine *on page 538*

Synonyms A-Poxide®; Equibral®; Librax®; Libritabs®; Librium®; Methaminodiazepoxide Hydrochloride; Mitran®; Resposan-10®; SK-Lygen®; Smail®; Solium®; Tropium®

Abstract This is a benzodiazepine drug used as a sedative-hypnotic (tranquilizer). It is widely prescribed.

Specimen Serum

Container Red top tube

Sampling Time Collect for trough level prior to next dose; collect for peak level 4 hours after oral dosing.

Storage Instructions Process immediately; avoid exposure to light; freeze if not analyzed immediately.

Reference Range Therapeutic: 0.7-1.0 µg/mL (SI: 2.3-3.3 µmol/L)

Critical Values Toxic: >5 µg/mL (SI: >17 µmol/L)

Use Monitor therapeutic drug level for compliance; determine toxic level

Methodology High performance liquid chromatography (HPLC), thin-layer chromatography (TLC), gas chromatography (GC), fluorometry

Additional Information
- Half-life: 8-12 hours
- Volume of distribution: 0.2-0.4 L/kg
- Protein binding: 90% to 95%

This drug is an antianxiety agent commonly used in suicide attempts. Chlordiazepoxide is slowly absorbed and may take several hours to reach a peak plasma level. Distribution after intramuscular administration is poor. The drug is highly (90%) protein bound. Overdosage with the benzodiazepines is frequent, but serious sequelae are rare. However, there is an additive effect when used with other CNS depressants (eg, ethanol). If a patient is comatose after a drug ingestion, chlordiazepoxide **alone** is not a sufficient explanation. Metabolism results in the production of four active metabolites.

References

Baselt RC, *Disposition of Toxic Drugs and Chemicals in Man*, 3rd ed, Davis, CA: Biomedical Publications, 1989, 155.

Minder EI, "Toxicity in a Case of Acute and Massive Overdose of Chlordiazepoxide and its Correlation to Blood Concentration," *J Toxicol Clin Toxicol*, 1989, 27(1-2):117-27.

Chloromycetin® see Chloramphenicol *on previous page*

Chlorpromazine see Methamphetamine, Qualitative, Urine *on page 562*

Chlorpromazine see Phenothiazines, Serum *on page 568*

Chlorpromazine, Serum or Urine

CPT 84022

Synonyms Amazin®; Bay Clor®; Dozine®; Hibanil®; Largactil®; Ormazine®; Prozil®; Repazine®; Thorazine®

Applies to Phenothiazines

Abstract This is an aliphatic phenothiazine used as an antipsychotic and sedative.

Specimen Serum or urine

Container Red top Vacutainer® or urine container

Sampling Time Trough (serum)

Collection Serum or freshly voided random urine

Storage Instructions Refrigerate

Reference Range Serum concentration: therapeutic: 50-300 ng/mL (SI: 157-942 nmol/L); urine: negative unless on therapeutic regimen

Critical Values Serum: toxic: >750 ng/mL (SI: >2355 nmol/L)

Use Screen for chlorpromazine in urine; evaluate possibility of chlorpromazine poisoning or drug toxicity (serum)

Limitations Urine test is not always specific for chlorpromazine; it may detect other phenothiazines if present.

Methodology Gas-liquid chromatography (GLC); thin-layer chromatography (TLC)

Additional Information
- Half-life: 30 hours
- Volume of distribution: 20 L/kg
- Protein binding: 95% to 98%

Due to the complex metabolism of this drug, the pharmacokinetics are variable and follow a multiphasic pattern. Attempts to correlate drug levels with clinical responses have not been successful. Antipsychotic drugs are nonaddicting. Deaths from accidental poisonings are rare. Chlorpromazine may have endocrinopathic, hematologic, and hepatic consequences. Endocrinopathic consequences may include blocked ovulation with increased urinary estrogens and decreased urinary gonadotropins and progestins. Other endocrinopathic consequences may be associated with decreased serum growth hormone, increased metabolism by hepatic microsomes (decreased thyroxine, T_4), increased metabolism and decreased organ uptake of norepinephrine (increased VMA), altered steroid metabolism (increased 17-ketosteroids), or an inhibition of the hypothalamus and decreased ACTH secretion (decreased 17-ketosteroids and 17-OH corticosteroids). Hematologic consequences may be associated with hemolytic anemia (decreased serum haptoglobin and decreased blood hematocrit, hemoglobin, and red cell count) as well as occasional neutropenia, agranulocytosis, leukopenia, and granulocytopenia. Some patients on this drug have an increase in antiphospholipid antibodies. However, no predisposition to thromboembolism was noted.[1] Increase in antinuclear antibodies has been noted.[2] Hepatic sensitivity may occur in 2% of patients and may be associated with increased alkaline phosphatase, AST, bilirubin, and in increased eosinophils, often a precursor of jaundice. False-positive pregnancy tests may occur in patients on chlorpromazine. Chlorpromazine causes false-positives for phenylketonuria, amylase, uroporphyrins, urobilinogen. It may cause positive direct Coombs' reaction and may interfere with determinations of BUN and vitamin B_{12}.

Chlorpromazine has an additive effect with other CNS-depressing agents. Chlorpromazine may increase valproic acid serum concentrations; when given piperazine, seizures may occur. Antacids, cimetidine may interfere with chlorpromazine absorption. Nortriptyline or propranolol may increase chlorpromazine levels. Salicylamide and acetanilide may displace chlorpromazine from its protein binding. H_2-antagonists decrease absorption of chlorpromazine.

Footnotes
1. Lillicrap DP, Pinto M, Benford K, et al, "Heterogeneity of Laboratory Test Results for Antiphospholipid Antibodies in Patients Treated With Chlorpromazine and Other Phenothiazines," *Am J Clin Pathol*, 1990, 93(6):771-5.
2. Zucker S, Zarrabi HM, Schubach WH, et al, "Chlorpromazine-Induced Immunopathy: Progressive Increase in Serum IgM," *Medicine (Baltimore)*, 1990, 69(2):92-100.

References

Baselt RC and Cravey RH, *Disposition of Toxic Drugs and Chemicals in Man*, 3rd ed, Chicago, IL: Year Book Medical Publishers Inc, 1989, 177-82.

Chrysotherapy see Gold *on page 553*

Cibalith-S® see Lithium *on page 558*

Cin-Quin® see Quinidine, Serum *on page 572*

Citrovorum Factor see Methotrexate *on page 563*

Clonazepam

CPT 80154

Related Information

Benzodiazepines, Qualitative, Urine *on page 538*

Synonyms Iktorivil®; Klonopin™; Rivatril®

Abstract The drug is in the class of benzodiazepines which are used as tranquilizers. This drug is used as an anticonvulsant. It is useful in reducing tardive dyskinesia.[1]

Specimen Serum

Container Red top tube

Sampling Time Serum peak levels occur approximately 2 hours after oral administration. The apparent half-life after a single oral dose is 20-40 hours. Use trough for monitoring.

Storage Instructions Separate serum and freeze. Protect from sunlight.

Reference Range Therapeutic: 10-50 ng/mL (SI: 32-158 nmol/L)

Critical Values Serum values >80 ng/mL

Possible Panic Range Toxic: >100 ng/mL (SI: >317 nmol/L)

Use Monitor drug level and toxicity

Methodology Gas-liquid chromatography (GLC), high performance liquid chromatography (HPLC)

Additional Information
- Half-life: 20-60 hours; active metabolites have longer half-lives than the parent drug; half-lives are increased in the elderly
- Volume of distribution: 2-6 L/kg
- Protein binding: 80% to 90%.

Therapeutic effect is not well correlated with serum levels. Effect of CNS depressants may be augmented by concomitant use of this agent. See Table A in the Therapeutic Drug Monitoring/Toxicology/Drugs of Abuse Appendix *on page 582*.

Footnotes
1. Thaker GK, Nguyen JA, Strauss ME, et al, "Clonazepam Treatment of Tardive Dyskinesia: A Practical GABAmimetic Strategy," *Am J Psychiatry*, 1990, 147(4):445-51.

References

Baselt RC and Cravey RH, *Disposition of Toxic Drugs and Chemicals in Man*, 3rd ed, Chicago, IL: Year Book Medical Publishers Inc, 1989, 199-201.

Sallustio BC, Kassapidis C, and Morris RG, "High-Performance Liquid Chromatography Determination of Clonazepam in Plasma Using Solid-Phase Extraction," *Ther Drug Monit*, 1994, 16(2):174-8.

CN⁻ see Cyanide, Blood *on next page*

CO see Carboxyhemoglobin *on page 541*

Cocaine (Cocaine Metabolite), Qualitative, Urine

CPT 80101 (screen); 80102 (confirmation)

Related Information

Alcohol, Blood or Urine *on page 531*
Chain-of-Custody Protocol *on previous page*
Drugs of Abuse Testing, Urine *on page 548*
Myoglobin, Qualitative, Urine *on page 644*
Semen Analysis *on page 652*

Synonyms Coke; Crack; Dama Blanca; Erythroxylon Coca; Free Base; Gold Dust; Liquid Lady; Nose Candy; Rock; Snow; Toot; White Lady

Applies to Benzoylecgonine

Abstract A prominent metabolite of cocaine is benzoylecgonine, which is the substance measured in urine to detect the presence of cocaine. Cocaine is a heavily abused drug which has legitimate medical uses in some ENT procedures.

Specimen Urine

Collection If forensic, observe precautions concerning surreptitious dilution or alteration.

Storage Instructions Refrigerate

Causes for Rejection If forensic, failure to meet temperature requirements immediately after collection and/or tests for unusual dilution (specific gravity, urine creatinine) or alteration.

Special Instructions If forensic, use chain-of-custody protocol and form. See test listing Chain-of-Custody Protocol *on page 542* and the Therapeutic Drug Monitoring/Toxicology/Drugs of Abuse Appendix *on page 581*.

Reference Range Negative (less than cutoff); therapeutic: 100-500 ng/mL (SI: 330-1650 nmol/L)

Critical Values Cutoff: screen: 300 ng/mL; confirmation: 150 ng/mL; toxic: >1000 ng/mL (SI: >3300 nmol/L)

Use Evaluation of cocaine use; work up in young adults as part of a drug screen

(Continued)

Cocaine (Cocaine Metabolite), Qualitative, Urine
(Continued)

Methodology Screen: immunoassay, fluorescence polarization immuno-assay (FPIA), thin-layer chromatography (TLC); confirmation: gas chromatography/mass spectrometry (GC/MS)

Additional Information
- Half-life: cocaine: 1 hour, benzoylecgonine: 7-9 hours
- Volume of distribution: 3-5 L/kg

Cocaine is a highly abused drug which is most frequently detected in the urine as the metabolite, benzoylecgonine, and usually as part of a multiclass drug panel. In pre-employment drug screening, the presence of cocaine (benzoylecgonine) should be confirmed by GC/MS.

Cocaine is a central nervous system stimulant. It usually appears as a fine crystal-like powder which is the hydrochloride or sulfate salt and as such is "snorted" (inhaled through the nose). When mixed with sodium bicarbonate and converted to free base, it appears as hard pieces called "crack" which can be smoked. This is currently a very prevalent form of the drug.

The effects of the drug begin within minutes and peak within 15-20 minutes. These effects include dilated pupils, increase in blood pressure, heart rate, breathing rate and body temperature. The dangers of cocaine use vary, depending on how the drug is taken, the dose, and the individual. Some regular users report feelings of restlessness, irritability, anxiety, and sleeplessness. In some people even low doses of cocaine may create psychological problems. People who use high doses of cocaine over a long period of time may become paranoid or experience what is called a cocaine psychosis. This may include hallucinations of touch, sight, taste, and smell. Alcohol inhibits cocaine degradation, enhancing its hepatotoxicity.[1] Benzoylecgonine is detectable in urine within 2-3 hours and for a period of 36-48 hours.

Up to a third of all instances of stroke in young adults relate to drug use including amphetamines, phenylpropanolamine, phencyclidine, methylphenidate, and opiates, as well as cocaine, but cocaine has become the most common drug implicated in such events.

Reckless drivers not intoxicated with alcohol may be intoxicated with cocaine and/or marijuana. Appropriate toxicologic testing has been recommended.[2]

Complications of cocaine use may include shock, disseminated intravascular coagulation, and myonecrosis. Cocaine is considered hepatotoxic.[3]

Footnotes
1. "Case Records of the Massachusetts General Hospital. Weekly Clinicopathological Exercises. Case 27-1993. A 32-Year-Old Man With the Sudden Onset of a Right-Sided Headache and Left Hemiplegia and Hemianesthesia," *N Engl J Med*, 1993, 329(2):117-24.
2. Brookoff D, Cook CS, Williams C, et al, "Testing Reckless Drivers for Cocaine and Marijuana," *N Engl J Med*, 1994, 331(8):518-22.
3. Lee WM, "Drug-Induced Hepatotoxicity," *N Engl J Med*, 1995, 333(17):1118-27.

References
Angell M and Kassirer JP, "Alcohol and Other Drugs - Toward a More Rational and Consistent Policy," *N Engl J Med*, 1994, 331(8):537-9.

Brogan WC 3d, Lange RA, Glamann DB, et al, "Recurrent Coronary Vasoconstriction Caused by Intranasal Cocaine; Possible Role for Metabolites," *Ann Intern Med*, 1992, 116(7):556-61.

Casanova OQ, Lombardero N, Behnke M, et al, "Detection of Cocaine Exposure in the Neonate. Analysis of Urine, Meconium, and Amniotic Fluid From Mothers and Infants Exposed to Cocaine," *Arch Pathol Lab Med*, 1994, 118(10):988-93.

Chan KM, Matthews WS, Saxena S, et al, "Frequency of Cocaine and Phencyclidine Detection at a Large Urban Public Teaching Hospital," *J Anal Toxicol*, 1993, 17(5):299-303.

Gawin FH and Ellinwood EH Jr, "Cocaine and Other Stimulants. Actions, Abuse, and Treatment," *N Engl J Med*, 1988, 318(18):1173-82.

Hippenstiel MJ and Gerson B, "Optimazation of Storage Conditions for Cocaine and Benzoylecgonine in Urine: A Review," *J Anal Toxicol*, 1994, 18(2):104-9.

Kain ZN, Kain TS, and Scarpelli EM, "Cocaine Exposure in Utero: Perinatal Development and Neonatal Manifestations - Review," *Clin Toxicol*, 1992, 30:607-36.

Karch SB, "The History of Cocaine Toxicity," *Hum Pathol*, 1989, 20(11):1037-9.

Romberg RW and Past MR, "Reanalysis of Forensic Urine Specimens Containing Benzoylecgonine and THC-COOH," *J Forensic Sci*, 1994, 39(2):479-85.

Uszenski RT, Gillis RA, and Schaer GL, "Additive Myocardial Depressant Effects of Cocaine and Ethanol," *Am Heart J*, 1992, 124(5):1276-83.

Warner EA, "Cocaine Abuse," *Ann Intern Med*, 1993, 119(3):226-33.

Zuckerman B, Frank DA, Hingson R, et al, "Effects of Maternal Marijuana and Cocaine Use on Fetal Growth," *N Engl J Med*, 1989, 320(12):762-8.

Codate *see* Codeine, Urine *on this page*

Co-Dax® *see* Doxepin *on page 548*

Codeine Phosphate *see* Codeine, Urine *on this page*

Codeine Sulfate *see* Codeine, Urine *on this page*

Codeine, Urine

CPT 80101 (screen); 80102 (confirmation); 82101 (quantitative)

Related Information
Chain-of-Custody Protocol *on page 542*
Glutethimide *on page 553*

Opiates, Qualitative, Urine *on page 566*

Synonyms Actacode; Codate; Codeine Phosphate; Codeine Sulfate; Codlin; Methylmorphine; Paveral; Tricodein

Test Commonly Includes Part of opiate screen

Abstract Codeine occurs naturally in opium but is produced commercially by 3-O-methylation of morphine. It is used as a narcotic analgesic. It is present in numerous proprietary preparations combined with non-narcotic analgesics and antihistamines. It is a drug of abuse.

Specimen Urine

Sampling Time Random

Storage Instructions Refrigerate specimen

Special Instructions If forensic, use precautions in collection and chain-of-custody form. See test listing Chain-of-Custody Protocol *on page 542* and the Therapeutic Drug Monitoring/Toxicology/Drugs of Abuse Appendix *on page 581*.

Reference Range Negative (below cutoff)

Critical Values Cutoff: screen: 300 ng/mL (for drug-of-abuse screen), confirmation: 300 ng/mL

Use Evaluate codeine toxicity; detect drug-of-abuse

Methodology Enzyme immunoassay (EIA); thin-layer chromatography (TLC)

Additional Information
- Half-life: 2.5-4.0 hours
- Volume of distribution: 3-4 L/kg
- Protein binding: 10% to 30%

Codeine, made by the methylation of morphine, is similar to morphine in uses, actions, contraindications, and adverse reactions. About $1/6$ to $1/10$ as potent as morphine, it is used to manage mild to moderate pain. In low doses, it is an antitussive. After oral dose, the onset of action is 15-30 minutes, and peak levels are reached in 1-1.5 hours. Codeine is excreted mainly in the urine as norcodeine and free and conjugated morphine. Adverse effects of codeine include miosis, increased intracranial pressure, antidiuretic hormone release, and physical and psychological dependence.

References
Barson W, "Narcotic Agents," *Ann Emerg Med*, 1986, 15:1019-20.

Cone EJ, Dickerson S, Paul BD, et al, "Forensic Drug Testing for Opiates: Urine Testing for Heroin, Morphine, and Codeine With Commercial Opiate Immunoassays," *J Anal Toxicol*, 1993, 17(3):156-64.

Kaplan LA and Pesce AJ, *Clinical Chemistry: Theory, Analysis, and Correlation*, St Louis, MO: Mosby Co, 1995, 1205-8.

Lin Z, Lafolie P, and Beck O, "Evaluation of Analytical Procedures for Urinary Codeine and Morphine Measurements," *J Anal Toxicol*, 1994, 18(3):129-33.

Codlin *see* Codeine, Urine *on this page*

Coffee Break® *see* Caffeine, Blood *on page 539*

COHb *see* Carboxyhemoglobin *on page 541*

Coke *see* Cocaine (Cocaine Metabolite), Qualitative, Urine *on previous page*

Comatose Profile *see* Toxicology Drug Screen, Blood *on page 576*

Comizial® *see* Phenobarbital, Blood *on page 568*

Compazine® *see* Phenothiazines, Serum *on page 568*

Cordarone® *see* Amiodarone, Serum *on page 532*

Cordilox® *see* Verapamil *on page 578*

Corramedan® *see* Digitoxin *on page 546*

Coumadin® *see* Warfarin *on page 579*

Crack *see* Cocaine (Cocaine Metabolite), Qualitative, Urine *on previous page*

"Crank" *see* Methamphetamine, Qualitative, Urine *on page 562*

Crystal *see* Amphetamine, Qualitative, Urine *on page 534*

Crystal *see* Methamphetamine, Qualitative, Urine *on page 562*

Crystal Joint *see* Phencyclidine, Qualitative, Urine *on page 567*

Cyanide *see* Thiocyanate, Blood or Urine *on page 575*

Cyanide, Blood

CPT 82600

Related Information
Hemoglobin *on page 323*
Lactic Acid, Blood *on page 156*

Synonyms CN⁻; Hydrocyanic Acid; Potassium or Sodium Cyanide

Abstract This highly toxic substance is one of the oldest poisons known. It binds to cytochrome oxidase and prevents cellular respiration, causing an entity called *histotoxic hypoxia*, and causes lactic acidosis.

Specimen Whole blood, since cyanide is concentrated in erythrocytes. Venous blood may appear bright red.

Container Lavender top (EDTA) tube or red top tube

Sampling Time Stat

Storage Instructions Fill tube to capacity and keep tightly closed; analyze as soon as possible. Refrigerate whole blood, gastric contents or tissue.

Reference Range Whole blood: smoker: 40 ng/mL, nonsmoker: 16 ng/mL; serum: smoker: 6 ng/mL, nonsmoker: 4 ng/mL

Critical Values In whole blood, values >1.0 µg/mL are potentially fatal although subjects with higher values have survived. Serum: >0.1 µg/mL.

Possible Panic Range Lethal: whole blood: >2.0 µg/mL

Use Establish the diagnosis of cyanide poisoning. Fires involving polymers have poisoned firemen. Symptoms of toxicity include headache, agitation, vomiting, and confusion. A scent of bitter almonds is suggestive but not all individuals can detect it.

Methodology Conway diffusion, color reaction, ion specific potentiometry

Additional Information
- Half-life: 45-65 hours

Cyanide is present in insecticides, rodenticides, vermicides, metal polishes, and electroplating baths. Other sources include ore refining, laetrile, synthetic rubber manufacturing, and the seeds of cherries, plums, peaches, apricots, pears, apples, crabapples, chokeberries, and lima beans.

Treatment with nitrites is effective. Nitrites produce methemoglobin which binds cyanide ions and thus removes them from cytochrome oxidase. Cyanide is metabolized by rhodanase to thiocyanate. Thiosulfate is given along with nitrites to promote the conversion of cyanide to thiocyanate which is much less toxic and is excreted. Cyanide itself blocks cellular metabolism by inhibiting mitochondrial ferricytochrome oxidase. High anion gap metabolic acidosis develops.

References
Barillo DJ, Goode R, and Esch V, "Cyanide Poisoning in Victims of Fire: Analysis of 364 Cases and Review of the Literature," *J Burn Care Rehabil*, 1994, 15(1):46-57.

Hall AH and Rumack BH, "Clinical Toxicology of Cyanide," *Ann Emerg Med*, 1986, 15(9):1067-74.

Hall AH and Rumack BH, "Hydroxocobalamin/Sodium Thiosulfate as a Cyanide Antidote," *J Emerg Med*, 1987, 5(2):115-21.

Kruszyna R, Kruszyna HG, and Smith RP, "A Spectrophotometric Method for Estimating Methemoglobin Concentration in the Presence of Cyanide," *Am J Emerg Med*, 1993, 11(6):642-3.

Laforge M, Buneaux F, Houeto P, et al, "A Rapid Spectrophotometric Blood Cyanide Determination Applicable to Emergency Toxicology," *J Anal Toxicol*, 1994, 18(3):173-5.

Lundquist P and Sorbo B, "Rapid Determination of Toxic Cyanide Concentrations in Blood," *Clin Chem*, 1989, 35(4):617-9.

Moore SJ, Ho IK, and Hume AS, "Severe Hypoxia Produced by Concomitant Intoxication With Sublethal Doses of Carbon Monoxide and Cyanide," *Toxicol Appl Pharmacol*, 1991, 109(3):412-20.

Cyclic Antidepressants *see* Antidepressants, Cyclic *on page 535*

Cyclosporine

CPT 80158

Related Information

Amiodarone, Serum *on page 532*

Itraconazole *on page 555*

Ketoconazole *on page 556*

Magnesium, Serum *on page 164*

Magnesium, Urine *on page 165*

Phenobarbital, Blood *on page 568*

Phenytoin *on page 569*

Verapamil *on page 578*

Synonyms Sandimmune®

Applies to Cyclosporine A

Abstract This drug is widely used as an immunosuppressant, especially following organ transplants.

Specimen Whole blood

Container Lavender top (EDTA) tube (whole blood)

Sampling Time Trough levels should be obtained 12-18 hours after oral dose (chronic usage), 12 hours after intravenous dose, or immediately prior to next dose.

Reference Range Since cyclosporine binds to erythrocytes and lipoproteins, measuring whole blood concentrations is preferred. 150-400 ng/mL (12 hours after dose).

Critical Values >400 ng/mL

Use Monitor blood level in management of immunosuppression for organ transplant recipients. The agent is used extensively to control rejection of organ transplants, especially of liver, heart, or kidney.

Monitoring of blood levels is imperative because the pharmacokinetics of cyclosporine are not only complex, but vary over time in the same patient; thus, blood levels cannot be well predicted from dosing schedules. Furthermore, this drug has a narrow therapeutic window and significant toxicity at levels above that range.

Limitations Results are method dependent - some measure multiple metabolites as well as parent drug. Single assays are not as informative as a series over time.

Methodology Radioimmunoassay (RIA), high performance liquid chromatography (HPLC), fluorescence polarization immunoassay (FPIA)

Additional Information
- Half-life: 8-24 hours
- Volume of distribution: 4-6 L/kg
- Protein binding: 90%

Cyclosporine is an immunosuppressive agent derived from *Tolypocladium inflatum gams*, a fungus originally isolated from a Norwegian soil sample. The exact mechanism of action of the drug is not known, but it appears to interfere with T-helper cell function and secretion of lymphokines. It is not myelosuppressive.

Renal toxicity with eventual renal failure is the most severe complication. Other assays to assess renal function (ie, BUN, creatinine clearance) should be ordered along with cyclosporine level, since toxicity may begin even with "acceptable" blood levels. Other toxicities include hypertension, convulsions, tremors, pulmonary edema, and an increased risk of lymphoma.

Drugs which enhance the potential toxicity of cyclosporine, and which are also likely to be administered to a transplant recipient, include aminoglycoside antibiotics, cephalosporins, trimethoprim-sulfa, amphotericin B, acyclovir, ketoconazole, and furosemide. **Agents which raise cyclosporine levels** by decreasing biotransformation include methylprednisolone, amphotericin B, cimetidine, and erythromycin. Other drugs which lead to increased concentrations of cyclosporine include ketoconazole, androgens, diltiazem, methyltrexate, oral contraceptives, verapamil, and nicardipine. Drugs which increase hepatic metabolism and thus **lower cyclosporine levels** include phenobarbital, phenytoin, rifampin, intravenous trimethoprim-sulfa, carbamazepine, ethotoin, mephenytoin, and primidone.

Because results will vary depending on whether the assay is done on whole blood or serum/plasma and on the method and cyclosporine antibody employed (monospecific or polyspecific), it is best for a given patient's specimens to be analyzed at a single laboratory to eliminate as many assay-dependent variables as possible. If switching of laboratories is unavoidable, it is advisable to have a few specimens run in parallel in the second laboratory prior to changing.

The clinical use of cyclosporine is difficult and requires experience and judgment. A drug blood level is only one of many pieces in the puzzle of transplant medicine. Electrolytes including magnesium and measures of renal and hepatic function are also needed.

References
Burtis CA and Ashwood ER, *Tietz Textbook of Clinical Chemistry*, Philadelphia, PA: WB Saunders Co, 1994, 1146-8.

Frey FJ, Horber FF, and Frey BM, "Trough Levels and Concentration Time Curves of Cyclosporine in Patients Undergoing Renal Transplantation," *Clin Pharmacol Ther*, 1988, 43(1):55-62.

Giesbrecht, EE, Soldin SJ, and Wong PY, "A Rapid, Reliable High Performance Liquid Chromatographic Micromethod for the Measurement of Cyclosporine in Whole Blood," *Ther Drug Monit*, 1989, 11(3):332-36.

Hayashi Y, Shibata N, Minouchi T, et al, "Evaluation of Fluorescence Polarization Immunoassay for Determination of Cyclosporine in Plasma," *Ther Drug Monit*, 1989, 11(2):205-9.

Hooks MA, Millikan WJ, Henderson JM, et al, "Comparison of Whole-Blood Cyclosporine Levels Measured by Radioimmunoassay and Fluorescence Polarization in Patients Post Orthotropic Liver Transplant," *Ther Drug Monit*, 1989, 11(3):304-9.

Kahan BD, "Cyclosporine," *N Engl J Med*, 1989, 321(25):1725-38.

Lindholm A and Henricsson S, "Simultaneous Monitoring of Cyclosporine in Blood and Plasma With Four Analytical Methods: A Clinical Evaluation," *Transplant Proc*, 1989, 21(1 Pt 2):1472-4.

Martinez L, Foradori A, Vaccarezza A, et al, "Monitoring of Cyclosporine Blood Levels With Polyclonal and Monoclonal Assays During Episodes of Renal Graft Dysfunction," *Transplant Proc*, 1989, 21(1 Pt 2):1490-1.

McBride JH, Rodgerson DO, Allin RE, et al, "Comparison of Four Immunoassays for the Measurement of Cyclosporine and Metabolites in Plasma," *Clin Chem*, 1988, 34(6):1259.

Moyer TP, Johnson P, Faynor SM, et al, "Cyclosporine: A Review of Drug Monitoring Problems and Presentation of a Simple, Accurate Liquid Chromatographic Procedure That Solves These Problems," *Clin Biochem*, 1986, 19(2):83-9.

Sanghvi A, Diven W, Seltman H, et al, "Abbott's Fluorescence Polarization Immunoassay for Cyclosporine and Metabolites Compared With the Sandoz "Sandimmune®" RIA," *Clin Chem*, 1988, 34(9):1904-6.

Terreros DA and Coombs J, "Cyclosporine Nephropathy: Inhibition of Osmoregulatory Renal Cell Transport," *Ann Clin Lab Sci*, 1989, 19(5):337-44.

Cyclosporine A *see* Cyclosporine *on this page*

Cystodigin® *see* Digitoxin *on next page*

Dalcaine® *see* Lidocaine *on page 558*

Dalmane® *see* Flurazepam *on page 552*

Dama Blanca *see* Cocaine (Cocaine Metabolite), Qualitative, Urine *on page 543*

Dapa® *see* Acetaminophen, Serum *on page 530*

Darvocet-N® *see* Propoxyphene, Serum or Urine *on page 571*

Darvon® *see* Propoxyphene, Serum or Urine *on page 571*

Datril® *see* Acetaminophen, Serum *on page 530*

DAU *see* Drugs of Abuse Testing, Urine *on page 548*

DAU-10 *see* Drugs of Abuse Testing, Urine *on page 548*

Delta Aminolevulinic Acid Dehydratase *see* Lead, Blood *on page 556*

Demerol® *see* Meperidine, Blood or Urine *on page 560*

Demolox® *see* Amoxapine, Blood *on page 533*

Depakene® *see* Valproic Acid *on page 577*

Depakote® *see* Valproic Acid *on page 577*

Depamide® *see* Valproic Acid *on page 577*

Deprax® *see* Trazodone *on page 577*

Deralin® *see* Propranolol *on page 571*

Desipramine *see* Antidepressants, Cyclic *on page 535*

Desipramine *see* Imipramine *on page 554*

Desoxyephedrine Hydrochloride *see* Methamphetamine, Qualitative, Urine *on page 562*

Desoxyn® *see* Methamphetamine, Qualitative, Urine *on page 562*

Desoxyphenobarbital *see* Primidone *on page 570*

Desyrel® *see* Trazodone *on page 577*

Dexies *see* Amphetamine, Qualitative, Urine *on page 534*

Dexitac® *see* Caffeine, Blood *on page 539*

Diazemuls® *see* Diazepam, Blood *on this page*

Diazepam, Blood

CPT 80154

Related Information

Alcohol, Blood or Urine *on page 531*
Antidepressants, Cyclic *on page 535*
Barbiturates, Quantitative, Blood *on page 537*
Benzodiazepines, Qualitative, Urine *on page 538*

Synonyms Aliseum®; Alupram®; Atensine®; Diazemuls®; Lamra®; Solis®; Stesolid®; Tensium®; Valium®; Valrelease®; Vatran®; Vivol®; Zetran®

Abstract This is a benzodiazepine used as a sedative-hypnotic (tranquilizer).

Specimen Serum

Container Red top tube

Sampling Time For peak level, 1 hour after oral dose or 15 minutes after I.V.

Storage Instructions Do not freeze

Reference Range Diazepam: therapeutic: 0.2-1.0 μg/mL (SI: 0.7-3.5 μmol/L); N-desmethyldiazepam (nordiazepam): therapeutic: 0.1-0.5 μg/mL (SI: 0.35-1.8 μmol/L)

Critical Values Toxic: sum of diazepam plus N-desmethyldiazepam >3.0 μg/mL

Possible Panic Range Total of diazepam and nordiazepam >5 μg/mL (SI: >18 μmol/L) is toxic.

Use Therapeutic monitoring and toxicity assessment; diazepam is a muscle relaxant and antianxiety drug.

Methodology Enzyme immunoassay (EIA), high performance liquid chromatography (HPLC), UV spectrophotometry, gas-liquid chromatography (GLC)

Additional Information

- Half-life: 20-50 hours
- Volume of distribution: 1.0-1.5 L/kg
- Protein binding: 96% to 99%

Peak blood levels are achieved within an hour after oral dose. The major metabolite (N-desmethyldiazepam) has a half-life in adults of 50-99 hours. It is the major metabolite also of Tranxene® and prazepam. Diazepam may exhibit synergism with barbiturates, tricyclic antidepressants, and amine oxidase inhibitors. Toxicity may be additive with other central nervous system depressants, and ethanol enhances the absorption of diazepam itself. Many cases of overdose are seen but few fatalities result from use of this drug alone. A frequent finding is a combination of this drug and ethanol.

Diazepam may cause false-negative urinary glucose determinations when using Clinistix® or Diastix®; it may inhibit thyroxine binding and may increase plasma testosterone.

References

Greenblatt DJ, Ehrenberg BL, Gunderman J, et al, "Pharmacokinetic and Electroencephalographic Study of Intravenous Diazepam, Midazolam, and Placebo," *Clin Pharmacol Ther,* 1989, 45(4):356-65.

Iwase H, Gondo K, Koike T, et al, "Novel Precolumn Deproteinization Method Using a Hydroxyapatite Cartridge for the Determination of Theophylline and Diazepam in Human Plasma by High-Performance Liquid Chromatography With Ultraviolet Detection," *J Chromatogr B Biomed Appl,* 1994, 655(1):73-81.

Dicorynan® *see* Disopyramide *on next page*

Digacin *see* Digoxin *on this page*

Digitalis *see* Digitoxin *on this page*

Digitalis-like Immunoreactive Substances *see* Digoxin *on this page*

Digitoxin

CPT 80299

Synonyms Corramedan®; Cystodigin®; Digitalis; Digitoxine®; Digitrin®; Lanotoxin®; Nativelle®; Purodigin®; Tardigal®

Abstract One of a group of plant glycosides used in the treatment of congestive heart failure, digitoxin is infrequently used (compared to digoxin). It must not be confused with **digoxin** when serum levels are ordered.

Specimen Serum

Container Red top tube

Sampling Time 6-12 hours after dose

Storage Instructions Separate serum and store in refrigerator.

Reference Range Therapeutic: 18-35 ng/mL (SI: 24-46 nmol/L)

Critical Values Levels >35 ng/mL (SI: >46 nmol/L) are associated with clinical toxicity in 80% of patients.

Use Therapeutic monitoring and toxicity assessment. See Table C in the Therapeutic Drug Monitoring/Toxicology/Drugs of Abuse Appendix *on page 583.*

Limitations Do not order digitoxin level on a patient receiving digoxin. Digitoxin is not commonly used.

Contraindications Patient on **digoxin;** recent radioactive tracer

Methodology Radioimmunoassay (RIA), gas-liquid chromatography (GLC), high performance liquid chromatography (HPLC)

Additional Information

- Half-life: 150-250 hours
- Volume of distribution: 0.7 L/kg
- Protein binding: 90% to 95%

Optimal sampling time after dosage is 6 hours. Optimal resampling time after change in dosage is 48-96 hours. Be sure the patient is not on **digoxin** instead of **digitoxin.** There is cross reactivity between the two drugs and the levels reported will not be valid, and in fact could be misleading and catastrophic. Digitalis leaf has both digoxin and digitoxin as active components. Digitoxin is the best test for evaluation of toxicity in a patient taking **digitalis leaf,** but neither test is truly satisfactory. There is considerable overlap in the upper therapeutic ranges with levels which may be toxic. **Digitoxin levels must be correlated with clinical and other chemical data.** Numerous factors modify the effect of cardiac glycosides, including serum potassium, calcium, magnesium, and cardiac blood flow. Hypokalemia, hypomagnesemia, and hypercalcemia all potentiate toxicity from cardiac glycosides. Decreased GI absorption of digitoxin is seen with antacids, cholestyramine, colestipol; increased hepatic metabolism occurs with phenytoin, phenobarbital, phenylbutazone, isoniazid, ethambutol, rifampin, spironolactone, and aminoglycosides. Decreased protein binding occurs with phenylbutazone, sulfadimethoxine, phenobarbital, clofibrate, and tolbutamide. Digitoxin increases levels of verapamil. Digibind® will increase serum digitoxin level tenfold; digitoxin can interfere with urinary 17-hydroxycorticosteroid assay. Digoxin-like immunoreactive substance (DLIS), an endogenous natriuretic substance, may cause false elevation.

References

Bayer MJ, "Recognition and Management of Digitalis Intoxication: Implications for Emergency Medicine," *Am J Emerg Med,* 1991, 9(2 Suppl 1):29-34.

Kulick DL and Rahimtoola SH, "Current Role of Digitalis Therapy in Patients With Congestive Heart Failure," *JAMA,* 1991, 265(22):2995-7.

Taboulet P, Baud FJ, Bismuth C, et al, "Acute Digitalis Intoxication - Is Pacing Still Appropriate?" *Clin Toxicol,* 1993, 31:261-73.

Digitoxine® *see* Digitoxin *on this page*

Digitrin® *see* Digitoxin *on this page*

Digoxin

CPT 80162

Related Information

Amiodarone, Serum *on page 532*
Creatinine, Serum *on page 118*
Flecainide *on page 551*
Itraconazole *on page 555*

Magnesium, Serum *on page 164*
Magnesium, Urine *on page 165*
Quinidine, Serum *on page 572*
Verapamil *on page 578*

Synonyms Allocar®; Cardioreg®; Digacin; Lanocor; Lanoxicaps®; Lanoxin®; Lenoxin®; Purgoxin®

Applies to Digitalis-like Immunoreactive Substances

Abstract Digoxin is a widely used cardiac glycoside that should be monitored.

Patient Preparation Avoid radioactivity prior to collection of specimen if assay performed by RIA.

Specimen Serum

Container Red top tube

Sampling Time Blood specimen must be drawn at least 6 hours after the administration of the last dose; additionally, just before next dose if steady-state estimate is needed. The steady-state is usually attained in 5 days.

Storage Instructions Separate serum and refrigerate.

Causes for Rejection Patient on a cardiac glycoside other than digoxin, recently administered radioisotopes if RIA is used for assay

Special Instructions Be sure patient is not on DIGITOXIN.

Reference Range Therapeutic: 0.8-2.0 ng/mL (SI: 1.0-2.6 nmol/L)

Critical Values Toxic: >2.0 ng/mL (SI: >2.6 nmol/L). The lethal dose is about double the level causing minor toxic manifestations.[1]

Possible Panic Range >3.0 ng/mL (SI: >3.8 nmol/L). See Table C in the Therapeutic Drug Monitoring/Toxicology/Drugs of Abuse Appendix *on page 583*.

Use Digoxin levels are useful for diagnosis and prevention of digoxin toxicity; prevention of underdosage of cardiac arrhythmias; patients with implanted pacemaker, especially patients on digoxin who are elderly, and/or who have renal failure, and/or who have been given quinidine. See listing Quinidine, Serum *on page 572*.

Limitations Digitoxin should not be confused with **digoxin**. Since there is cross reactivity between the two drugs, **results will not be valid if digoxin is measured when the patient is taking digitoxin**. All other digitalis derivatives will also cross react with this test and give invalid results. Toxic levels of digitoxin when assayed as digoxin give low results. Falsely normal or low levels may occur in patients recently given radioactive isotopes, when the method used is radioimmunoassay (RIA). RIA was the predominant method only a few years ago, but it has been largely replaced by enzyme immunoassay (EIA) and fluorescence polarization immunoassay (FPIA) methods. Endogenous digitalis-like immunoreactive substances (DLIS) are found in digoxin-free patients with a variety of clinical states associated with salt and fluid retention, such as renal failure, hepatic failure, low renin hypertension, and pregnancy. They are also present at birth in neonates and infants. These compounds (DLIS) cross react with digoxin-specific immunoassays and give falsely elevated plasma digoxin concentrations.

Methodology Enzyme immunoassay (EIA), fluorescence polarization immunoassay (FPIA), radioimmunoassay (RIA)

Additional Information
- Half-life: 20-60 hours
- Volume of distribution: 7 L/kg
- Protein binding: 20% to 25%

Digoxin is indicated for systolic heart failure and control of supraventricular tachyarrhythmias. Approximately 75% of an oral dose is bioavailable. The average volume of distribution is 7 L/kg and is decreased in patients on quinidine, with renal failure, and hypothyroidism. Plasma concentrations do not accurately reflect pharmacologic effects of the drug until it is completely distributed. If obtained before complete distribution, concentration will be misleading. Digoxin is cleared primarily by the kidney. The average half-life is 48 hours for a patient whose renal function is normal.

Be sure the patient is not on digitoxin instead of digoxin. Digitoxin is also an active component of digitalis leaf. Ninety percent of nontoxic patients have levels ≤2.0 ng/mL (SI: ≤2.6 nmol/L), 87% of toxic patients have levels >2.0 ng/mL. Levels >3.0 ng/mL in adults are strongly suggestive of overdosage. However, **digitalis levels must always be interpreted in light of clinical and chemical data**. Older, smaller patients require less digoxin. Proportionally lower loading doses are advocated in the elderly.[1] The most common cause of digitalis intoxication is potassium depletion.[2] The primary cause of digoxin toxicity in the aged is decreased renal function. Maintenance doses should be adjusted to the glomerular filtration rate (GFR).[2] Renal failure, hypercalcemia, alkalosis, myxedema, hypomagnesemia, recent MI and other heart disease, hypokalemia, and hypoxia may increase sensitivity to the toxic effects of digoxin.

Quinidine may cause elevation of digoxin level by decreasing its excretion.[3,4] It is recommended that serum digoxin concentration be measured before initiation of quinidine therapy and again in 4-6 days. **Verapamil** and **amiodarone** cause increased digoxin levels, also by decrease in

clearance. (Clearance parallels GFR.) Other drugs which decrease its clearance include cyclosporine, spironolactone, and propafenone.

When confronted with unexpectedly low digoxin levels, consider thyroid disease, malabsorption, and reduced intestinal blood flow from mesenteric arteriosclerosis. Drugs which diminish its bioavailability include metoclopramide, cholestyramine, colestipol, kaolin-pectin, neomycin, and sulfasalazine. Consider, as well, congestive failure and anticholinergic drug effects when low digoxin levels are encountered.

Digibind® will increase total serum digoxin level about 50-fold. Digoxin-like immunoreactive substance (DLIS), an endogenous natriuretic substance, may cause false elevation. Other drug interactions include antacids, cathartics, neomycin, phenytoin, and metoclopramide which may decrease absorption of digoxin; indomethacin, diltiazem, erythromycin, tetracycline, and spironolactone may increase digoxin serum concentration; penicillamine may decrease pharmacologic effects of digoxin. Propantheline and atropine may increase digoxin absorption.

Patients with **digitalis resistance** may require larger doses and higher than usual serum levels (eg, patients with hyperthyroidism).

The probability that a patient will take a drug exactly as the physician has prescribed it (compliance) has been shown to be hardly better than half. Probability of compliance is further decreased in elderly patients treated with a large number of medications. Measure trough serum concentrations because of variability of peak interval.

FAB fragments of digoxin-specific sheep antibodies are available for the treatment of digoxin toxicities but should be limited to potentially life-threatening overdoses.

Footnotes
1. Montamat SC, Cusack BJ, and Vestal RE, "Management of Drug Therapy in the Elderly," *N Engl J Med*, 1989, 321(5):303-9.
2. Braunwald E, "Heart Failure," *Harrison's Principles of Internal Medicine*, 13th ed, Isselbacher KJ, Braunwald E, Wilson J, et al, eds, New York, NY: McGraw-Hill Inc, 1994, 998-1009.
3. Leakey EB, "Digoxin-Quinidine Interaction: Current Status," *Ann Intern Med*, 1980, 93:775-6.
4. Mungall DR, Robichaux RP, Perry W, et al, "Effects of Quinidine on Serum Digoxin Concentration: A Prospective Study," *Ann Intern Med*, 1980, 93:689-93.

References
Antman EM, Wenger TL, Butler VP Jr, et al, "Treatment of 150 Cases of Life-Threatening Digitalis Intoxication With Digoxin-Specific Fab Antibody Fragments. Final Report of a Multicenter Study," *Circulation*, 1990, 81(6):1744-52.
Cohen AF, Kroon R, Schoemaker R, et al, "Influence of Gastric Acidity on the Bioavailability of Digoxin," *Ann Intern Med*, 1991, 115(7):540-5.
Datta P and Larsen F, "Specificity of Digoxin Immunoassays Toward Digoxin Metabolites," *Clin Chem*, 1994, 40(7 Pt 1):172-3.
Haddy FJ, "Endogenous Digitalis-Like Factor or Factors," *N Engl J Med*, 1987, 316(10):621-3.
Howanitz PJ and Steindel SJ, "Digoxin Therapeutic Drug Monitoring Practices. A College of American Pathologists Q-Probes Study of 666 Institutions and 18,679 Toxic Levels," *Arch Pathol Lab Med*, 1993, 117(7):684-90.
Martin-Suarez A, Lanao JM, Calvo MV, et al, "Digoxin Pharmacokinetics in Patients With High Serum Digoxin Concentrations," *J Clin Pharm Ther*, 1993, 18(1):63-8.
Smith TW, "Digoxin in Heart Failure," *N Engl J Med*, 1993, 329(1):51-3.
Stone JA and Soldin SJ, "An Update on Digoxin," *Clin Chem*, 1989, 35(7):1326-31.
Tsang P and Gerson B, "Digoxin Monitoring in the Geriatric Patient," *Drug Monitoring and Toxicology*, 1991, 12.
Tsang P and Gerson B, "Understanding Digoxin Use in the Elderly Patient," *Clin Lab Med*, 1990, 10(3):479-92.
Vine DL, "What Is the Practical Value of Digitalis in CHF?" *Kans Med*, 1992, 93(7):231-2.
Withering W, "An Account of the Foxglove," London, England: Paternoster-Row, 1785.
Woolf A, "Revising the Management of Digitalis Poisoning," *J Toxicol Clin Toxicol*, 1993, 31(2):275-6.
Woolf AD, Wenger T, Smith TW, et al, "The Use of Digoxin-Specific Fab Fragments for Severe Digitalis Intoxication in Children," *N Engl J Med*, 1992, 326(26):1739-44.

Dilantin® see Phenytoin *on page 569*

Dilocaine® see Lidocaine *on page 558*

Dimipressin®, Iprogen® see Imipramine *on page 554*

Dintoina® see Phenytoin *on page 569*

Diphenylan Sodium® see Phenytoin *on page 569*

Diphenylhydantoin see Phenytoin *on page 569*

Dipropylacetic Acid see Valproic Acid *on page 577*

Disopyramide

CPT 80299

Related Information

Amoxapine, Blood *on page 533*
Imipramine *on page 554*
Nortriptyline *on page 565*
Phenytoin *on page 569*
Verapamil *on page 578*

Synonyms Dicorynan®; Napamide®; Norpace®; Rhythmodan®; Ritmilen®

Abstract Disopyramide is a class IA antiarrhythmic agent, which requires frequent monitoring.

Specimen Serum or plasma

(Continued)

Disopyramide *(Continued)*

Container Red top tube, green top (heparin) tube, or lavender top (EDTA) tube

Sampling Time Collect specimen 2-3 hours after an oral dose of disopyramide for peak. Draw trough just before next dose. Trough level is the best guide for dosing. Time to peak serum concentration is 30 minutes to 3 hours.

Special Instructions Other cardiac medications should be made known to the laboratory.

Reference Range Therapeutic: **atrial arrhythmias**: 2.8-3.2 µg/mL (SI: 8.3-9.4 µmol/L); **ventricular arrhythmias**: 3.3-7.5 µg/mL (SI: 9.7-22.0 µmol/L)

Critical Values Toxic: >7.0 µg/mL (SI: >20.6 µmol/L)

Possible Panic Range Fatalities are seen with concentrations >20.0 µg/mL.

Use Therapeutic monitoring. See Table C in the Therapeutic Drug Monitoring/Toxicology/Drugs of Abuse Appendix *on page 583.*

Limitations Arrhythmias may occur at low levels. Disopyramide exhibits nonlinear binding in the therapeutic range. This combined with the fact that disopyramide is administered as a racemic mixture, makes total concentration difficult to correlate with pharmacodynamic effects.

Methodology Enzyme immunoassay (EIA), high performance liquid chromatography (HPLC)

Additional Information
- Half-life: 4-10 hours
- Volume of distribution: 0.7-0.9 L/kg
- Protein binding: 50% to 80%

Disopyramide shares electrophysiologic properties with quinidine and procainamide. Up to 80% of oral dose is absorbed. Eighty percent of the drug is excreted in the urine. Dosage must be modified (dosage intervals prolonged) in patients with renal failure, and dosage interval relates to creatinine clearance. Serious toxic effects are depression of myocardial contractility and disturbances in myocardial conduction. Other effects include dry mouth, constipation, urinary hesitancy, and blurred vision. Metabolite N-desisopropyl disopyramide is also pharmacologically active. Concomitant treatment with phenytoin may lead to decreased serum levels of disopyramide. There may be cumulative effects with other class I antiarrhythmic drugs (lidocaine, procainamide).

Disopyramide may cause decrease in glucose levels in test samples.

References
Duff HJ, Mitchell LB, Nath CF, et al, "Concentration-Response Relationships of Disopyramide in Patients With Ventricular Tachycardia," *Clin Pharmacol Ther,* 1989, 45(5):542-7.

Ragosta M, Weihl AC, and Rosenfeld LE, "Potentially Fatal Interaction Between Erythromycin and Disopyramide," *Am J Med,* 1989, 86(4):465-6.

Witek A, Zawisza P, and Przyborowski L, "Determination of Disopyramide in Plasma by High Performance Liquid Chromatography," *J Pharm Biomed Anal,* 1994, 12(3):425-7.

Ditan® *see* Phenytoin *on page 569*

Divalproex Sodium *see* Valproic Acid *on page 577*

d-Methamphetamine *see* Methamphetamine, Qualitative, Urine *on page 562*

Doe *see* Methamphetamine, Qualitative, Urine *on page 562*

Dolantin® *see* Meperidine, Blood or Urine *on page 560*

Dolantina® *see* Meperidine, Blood or Urine *on page 560*

Dolantine® *see* Meperidine, Blood or Urine *on page 560*

Dolophine® *see* Methadone, Urine *on page 561*

Dolosal® *see* Meperidine, Blood or Urine *on page 560*

Dorcol® *see* Acetaminophen, Serum *on page 530*

Doriden® *see* Glutethimide *on page 553*

Doxepin

CPT 80166

Related Information

Antidepressants, Cyclic *on page 535*

Synonyms Adapin®; Co-Dax®; Novoxapin®; Sinequan®; Triadapin®

Test Commonly Includes Desmethyldoxepin

Abstract This is a tricyclic antidepressant. It is not a drug of abuse.

Specimen Serum or plasma

Container Red top tube or green top (heparin) tube

Sampling Time Trough levels at steady-state. Time to peak serum concentration is 2-4 hours.

Reference Range Sum of doxepin and desmethyldoxepin 150-250 ng/mL (SI: 540-900 nmol/L)

Critical Values Toxic: >500 ng/mL (SI: >1800 nmol/L). Fatal cases associated with values >10,000 ng/mL.

Use Therapeutic monitoring (compliance) and toxicity assessment

Methodology High performance liquid chromatography (HPLC), gas chromatography (GC)

Additional Information
- Half-life: 10-25 hours
- Volume of distribution: 10-30 L/kg
- Protein binding: 75% to 85%

Doxepin, a tricyclic antidepressant, is a tertiary amine structural analog of amitriptyline with similar but less potent neurotransmitter effects and considerably less cardiotoxicity. Doxepin is metabolized to the active metabolite desmethyldoxepin (nordoxepin). Doxepin serum levels peak at 2-6 hours after an oral dose. The parent drug has a low bioavailability and steady-state is reached in 2-8 days. Geriatric patients respond well to doxepin.

Doxepin increases glucose and catecholamine levels in test serum.

References
Ereshefsky L, Tran-Johnson T, Davis CM, et al, "Pharmacokinetic Factors Affecting Antidepressant Drug Clearance and Clinical Effect: Evaluation of Doxepin and Imipramine - New Data and Review," *Clin Chem,* 1988, 34(5):863-80.

Milstein S, Buetikofer J, Dunnigan A, et al, "Usefulness of Disopyramide for Prevention of Upright Tilt-Induced Hypotension-Bradycardia," *Am J Cardiol,* 1990, 65(20):1339-44.

Dozic® *see* Haloperidol *on page 553*

Dozine® *see* Chlorpromazine, Serum or Urine *on page 543*

Drug Screen, Comprehensive Panel or Analysis *see* Toxicology Drug Screen, Blood *on page 576*

Drug Screen, Comprehensive Panel or Analysis, Urine *see* Toxicology Drug Screen, Urine *on page 576*

Drugs of Abuse Testing, Urine

CPT 80100 (screen); 80102 (confirmation, each procedure)

Related Information

Alcohol, Blood or Urine *on page 531*

Amphetamine, Qualitative, Urine *on page 534*

Cannabinoids (Marijuana Metabolites), Qualitative, Urine *on page 539*

Chain-of-Custody Protocol *on page 542*

Cocaine (Cocaine Metabolite), Qualitative, Urine *on page 543*

Electrolytes, Serum or Plasma *on page 123*

Glucose, Random *on page 138*

Methadone, Urine *on page 561*

Methamphetamine, Qualitative, Urine *on page 562*

Methaqualone *on page 562*

Morphine, Urine *on page 564*

Opiates, Qualitative, Urine *on page 566*

Osmolality, Serum *on page 172*

Phencyclidine, Qualitative, Urine *on page 567*

Propoxyphene, Serum or Urine *on page 571*

Urine Collection, 24-Hour *on page 30*

Synonyms Abuse Screen; DAU; DAU-10; Pre-employment Drug Screen

Test Commonly Includes Screens for common classes of abused drugs - amphetamines, barbiturates, benzodiazepines, cannabinoids, cocaine, methadone, methaqualone, opiates, phencyclidine, propoxyphene. In some laboratories, urine ethanol is included.

Abstract The usual drug-of-abuse screening panel consists of the 10 drugs listed above under "test includes". SAMSHA screen includes only the following: marijuana metabolite, cocaine metabolite, opiates, phencyclidine, and amphetamines.

Specimen Urine

Collection If forensic, observe precautions.

Storage Instructions Refrigerate

Causes for Rejection If forensic, failure to meet temperature requirements and tests for unusual urine dilution or alteration

Turnaround Time Screen: 1-2 hours if done in-house; confirmation: 1-2 days

Special Instructions Specify the drug or drugs suspected in an emergency situation. If forensic, use chain-of-custody protocol and form. See test listing Chain-of-Custody Protocol *on page 542* and the Therapeutic Drug Monitoring/Toxicology/Drugs of Abuse Appendix *on page 581.*

Reference Range Negative (less than cutoff)

Critical Values See individual drug entries for cutoff values.

Use Screen for drug overdose and toxicity; screen for the presence of drugs of abuse

Limitations This test provides only **qualitative** detection of drugs. Quantitation of drug levels is not included and is not recommended because urine levels are time and clearance dependent and are not directly related to toxic symptoms seen clinically. In a nonclinical setting (eg, pre-employment drug screening, etc), the sample should be collected under chain-of-custody, and all positive screens must be confirmed by a different, more sensitive method, preferably GC/MS. The transportation industry [Department of Transportation (DOT)] tests certain employees by screening for five classes of drugs only (amphetamines, cannabinoids, cocaine, opiates, phencyclidine) and confirms all positive results with GC/MS. Substance Abuse and Mental Health Services Administration (SAMHSA) requires certification to perform tests for DOT. (See Federal Register 54(230), December 1, 1989.) Any agent identified in a screening test **should be confirmed** by a test specific for that drug (usually GC/MS).

Methodology Screen: immunoassay, gas chromatography (GC), thin-layer chromatography (TLC), high performance liquid chromatography (HPLC); confirmation: gas chromatography/mass spectrometry (GC/MS)

Additional Information For specific drug classes see the listing by specific drug name.

The Kulig reference provides a helpful clinical outline addressing a wide variety of agents. In addition to drug testing, glucose, electrolytes, and osmolality are often needed.

References

Bosomworth M, "Drugs of Abuse in Urine: Some Pitfalls in Testing," *Br J Biomed Sci*, 1993, 50(2):150-5.

Caplan YH, "Drug Testing in Urine," *J Forensic Sci*, 1989, 34:1417-21.

De Cresce R, Mazura A, Lifschitz M, et al, *Drug Testing in the Workplace*, Chicago, IL: American Society of Clinical Pathologists, 1989.

Frings CS, White RM, and Battaglia DJ, "Status of Drugs-of-Abuse Testing in Urine: An AACC Study," *Clin Chem*, 1987, 33(9):1683-6.

Hawks RL and Chiang CN, *Urine Testing for Drugs of Abuse*, NIDA Research Monograph 73, Rockville, MD, 1986.

Kulig K, "Initial Management of Ingestions of Toxic Substances," *N Engl J Med*, 1992, 326(25):1677-81.

Moriya F, Chan KM, Noguchi TT, et al, "Testing for Drugs of Abuse in Meconium of Newborn Infants," *J Anal Toxicol*, 1994, 18(1):41-5.

McBay AJ and Mason AP, "Forensic Science Identification of Drugs of Abuse," *J Forensic Sci*, 1989, 34:1471-6.

Paul BD, McKinley RM, Walsh JK Jr, et al, "Effect of Freezing on the Concentration of Drugs of Abuse in Urine," *J Anal Toxicol*, 1993, 17(6):378-80.

Schwartz RH, "Urine Testing in the Detection of Drugs of Abuse," *Arch Intern Med*, 1988, 148(11):2407-12.

Simpson D, Jarvie DR, and Heyworth R, "An Evaluation of Six Methods for the Detection of Drugs of Abuse in Urine," *Ann Clin Biochem*, 1989, 26(Pt 2):172-81.

Soderstoom CA, Dailey JT, and Kerns TJ, "Alcohol and Other Drugs: An Assessment of Testing and Clinical Practices in U.S. Trauma Centers," *J Trauma*, 1994, 36(1):68-73.

Wells VE, Halperin W, Thun M, "The Estimated Predictive Value of Screening for Illicit Drugs in the Workplace," *Am J Public Health*, 1988, 78(7):817-9.

Wu AH, Wong SS, Johnson KG, et al, "Evaluation of a Triage System for Emergency Drugs-of-Abuse Testing in Urine," *J Anal Toxicol*, 1993, 17(4):241-5.

Duo-Trach® *see* Lidocaine *on page 558*

Duramorph® *see* Morphine, Urine *on page 564*

Durvitan® *see* Caffeine, Blood *on page 539*

Easprin® *see* Salicylate *on page 573*

Ecotrin® *see* Salicylate *on page 573*

Elavil® *see* Amitriptyline, Blood *on page 533*

Elephant Tranquilizers *see* Phencyclidine, Qualitative, Urine *on page 567*

Elixophyllin® *see* Theophylline *on page 575*

E-Lor® *see* Propoxyphene, Serum or Urine *on page 571*

Empirin® *see* Salicylate *on page 573*

Endep® *see* Amitriptyline, Blood *on page 533*

Enphenemalum *see* Methylphenobarbital *on page 563*

Epanutin® *see* Phenytoin *on page 569*

Epilim® *see* Valproic Acid *on page 577*

Epimorph Dolcontin® *see* Morphine, Urine *on page 564*

Epinat® *see* Phenytoin *on page 569*

Epitrol® *see* Carbamazepine *on page 540*

Eptadone® *see* Methadone, Urine *on page 561*

Equagesic® *see* Meprobamate *on page 560*

Equanil® *see* Meprobamate *on page 560*

Equibral® *see* Chlordiazepoxide, Blood *on page 542*

Ergenyl® *see* Valproic Acid *on page 577*

Erythroxylon Coca *see* Cocaine (Cocaine Metabolite), Qualitative, Urine *on page 543*

Eskalith® *see* Lithium *on page 558*

1,2-Ethanediol *see* Ethylene Glycol *on next page*

Ethanol *see* Volatile Screen *on page 579*

Ethanol, Blood *see* Alcohol, Blood or Urine *on page 531*

Ethchlorvynol

CPT 82690

Synonyms Placidyl®

Abstract This is a sedative hypnotic which is considered dangerous if not carefully monitored.

Specimen Serum or plasma

Container Red top tube or green top (heparin) tube

Sampling Time The peak blood level is attained in 1.5 hours

Reference Range 2-8 µg/mL (SI: 14-55 µmol/L)

Possible Panic Range Toxic: levels >20 µg/mL (SI: >138 µmol/L) are associated with severe sedation, coma, respiratory depression, hypotension, bradycardia, and hypothermia

Use Monitor therapeutic drug level

Methodology High performance liquid chromatography (HPLC), gas chromatography (GC), spectrophotometry

Additional Information

- Half-life: 10-20 hours
- Volume of distribution: 4 L/kg
- Protein binding: 60%

Ethchlorvynol is a nonbarbiturate sedative-hypnotic drug. The peak blood level is attained in 1.5 hours. The half-life increases to 100 hours when high levels of drug are present. Most of the drug is metabolized in the liver. Exaggerated hypnotic effects occur if taken with ethanol. Can be detected in urine but only small amounts of the parent drug are present. Should be used cautiously in combination with oral anticoagulants. Effect is potentiated by alcohol.

References

Baselt RC, *Disposition of Toxic Drugs and Chemicals in Man*, 3rd ed, Davis, CA: Biomedical Publications, 1989, 326.

Gomolin I, "Ethchlorvynol," *Clin Toxicol Rev*, 1980, 2:1-2.

Winek CL, Wahba WW, and Winek CL Jr, "Body Distribution of Ethchlorvynol," *J Forensic Sci*, 1989, 34(3):687-90.

Yell RP, "Ethchlorvynol Overdose," *Am J Emerg Med*, 1990, 8(3):246-50.

Ethosuximide

CPT 80168

Related Information

Phenobarbital, Blood *on page 568*
Phenytoin *on page 569*

Synonyms Suxinutin®; Zarontin®; Zartalin®

Abstract Ethosuximide is a drug of choice for absence seizures not accompanied by other seizure types.

Specimen Serum or plasma

Container Red top tube or green top (heparin) tube

Sampling Time Peak or trough levels may be used to monitor therapy, because blood levels are fairly constant.

Reference Range 40-100 µg/mL (SI: 284-710 µmol/L)

Possible Panic Range >150 µg/mL (SI: >1062 µmol/L); toxicity may manifest with lethargy or psychotic behavior; significant drug interactions are uncommon. At steady-state, each 1 mg/kg will result in a serum rise of 2 µg/mL. See Table A in the Therapeutic Drug Monitoring/Toxicology/Drugs of Abuse Appendix *on page 582*.

Use Monitor for compliance, efficacy, or possible toxicity

Limitations Ethosuximide has relatively few serious adverse effects with chronic administration. Dose-related adverse effects, including photophobia and lethargy, sometimes may be avoided by slowly titrating the drug to effective levels. Other side effects include nausea, vomiting, anorexia, headache, and dizziness. Blood dyscrasias may occur and respond to decreasing the dose or stopping the drug. If patients have other seizure types in addition to absence seizures, ethosuximide may exacerbate the other seizure types. Therefore, valproic acid is the drug of choice in that situation.[1] Other succinimides, notably methsuximide and phensuximide, have been used adjunctively for absence seizures but are less effective and more toxic.[2]

Methodology Enzyme immunoassay (EIA), gas-liquid chromatography (GLC), high performance liquid chromatography (HPLC)

Additional Information

- Half-life: 25-70 hours
- Volume of distribution: 0.7 L/kg
- Protein binding: 0% to 5%

Footnotes

1. Engel J, *Seizures and Epilepsy*, Contemporary Neurology Series, Philadelphia, PA: FA Davis Co, 1989.
2. Chang T, "Ethosuximide: Chemistry and Methods of Determination," *Antiepileptic Drugs*, 3rd ed, Levy RH, Dreifuss FE, Mattson RH, et al, eds, New York, NY: Raven Press, 1989.

References

Baselt RC and Cravey RH, "Ethosuximide," *Disposition of Toxic Drugs and Chemicals in Man*, 3rd ed, Chicago, IL: Year Book Medical Publishers Inc, 1989, 332-4.

Ethotoin

CPT 80299

Synonyms Accenon; Ethylphenylhydantoin; Peganone®

Test Commonly Includes Ethotoin. Antiepileptic activity is due to parent compound.

Abstract Ethotoin is occasionally used as an adjunctive anticonvulsant. Patients suffer dose-related gingival hyperplasia and hirsutism less often than with phenytoin.

Specimen Serum

Container Red top tube

Reference Range 14-34 µg/mL

Additional Information Like phenytoin, ethotoin has zero-order kinetics and small dosage changes may produce large changes in clinical response. Teratogenicity may occur, particularly since ethotoin is usually combined with other anticonvulsants. The half-life of ethotoin is approximately 5-10 hours (dose dependent), necessitating four times daily dosing. Most common side effect is a bitter taste.

Test interactions include an increase in alkaline phosphatase and a decrease in calcium.

References

Carter CA, Helms RA, and Boehm R, "Ethotoin in Seizures of Childhood and Adolescence," *Neurology*, 1984, 34(6):791-5.

Kupferberg HJ, "Other Hydantoins: Mephenytoin and Ethotoin," *Antiepileptic Drugs*, 3rd ed, Levy RH, Dreifuss FE, Mattson RH, et al, eds, New York, NY: Raven Press, 1989, 257-65.

Ethyl Alcohol, Blood *see* Alcohol, Blood or Urine *on page 531*

Ethyl and Methyl Thiocyanate (Thanite® and Lethane®) *see* Thiocyanate, Blood or Urine *on page 575*

Ethylenediamine *see* Theophylline *on page 575*

Ethylene Glycol

CPT 82693

Related Information

Anion Gap *on page 81*
Osmolality, Calculated *on page 172*
Osmolality, Serum *on page 172*
Oxalate, Urine *on page 174*
Urinalysis *on page 658*

Synonyms 1,2-Ethanediol

Applies to Antifreeze

Test Commonly Includes Propylene glycol

Abstract A commercial chemical used as a radiator antifreeze and for commercial chemical synthesis.

Specimen Serum or plasma

Container Red top tube or green top (heparin) tube

Reference Range Negative

Critical Values Toxic: 50 mg/dL

Possible Panic Range Values between 0.3-4.0 g/L have been observed in fatal cases; levels at 50 mg/dL with metabolic acidosis not corrected with therapy or with renal failure indicate a need for hemodialysis, but survival has taken place with levels of 650 mg/dL (SI: 100 mmol/L).

Use Detect and quantitate ingestion of ethylene glycol

Methodology Gas-liquid chromatography (GLC), photometry, fluorometry, enzymatic assay (automated)[1]

Additional Information

- Half-life: 3-6 hours
- Volume of distribution: 0.8 L/kg

Ethylene glycol is a colorless, odorless, sweet tasting compound. It has been utilized in suicide attempts, as a substitute for ethanol, and in accidental poisonings in both children and domestic pets. 100 mL is lethal; rapid treatment can prevent damage. Toxicity is manifested by CNS depression (1-12 hours after ingestion), cardiopulmonary symptoms (12-24 hours after ingestion), and renal damage (24-72 hours after ingestion). Oxalate is a minor metabolite of ethylene glycol; and its crystals are commonly seen in urine and may be helpful for diagnosis. In addition to blood levels of ethylene glycol, hypocalcemia, severe anion gap metabolic acidosis (low chloride, low bicarbonate, low pH), and osmolal gap elevation are observed. Lactic acid production takes place. See the following listings, Anion Gap *on page 81*; Osmolality, Calculated *on page 172*, and Osmolality, Serum *on page 172*. **Precaution:** Toxicity may be manifested without osmolal gap changes and osmolal and anion gap increases can be present with very low levels of glycol.

When antifreeze contains sodium fluorescein (intended to support identification of radiator leakage), urine or gastric content can be screened with a Wood's lamp.

Footnotes

1. Standefer J and Blackwell N, "Enzymatic Method for Measuring Ethylene Glycol With a Centrifugal Analyzer," *Clin Chem*, 1991, 37(10 Pt 1):1734-6.

References

Burkhart KK and Kulig KW, "The Other Alcohols. Methanol, Ethylene Glycol, and Isopropanol," *Emerg Med Clin North Am*, 1990, 8(4):913-28.

Jarvie DR and Simpson D, "Simple Screening Tests for the Emergency Identification of Methanol and Ethylene Glycol in Poisoned Patients," *Clin Chem*, 1990, 36(11):1957-61.

Ochs ML, Glick MR, Ryder KW, et al, "Improved Method for Emergency Screening for Ethylene Glycol in Serum," *Clin Chem*, 1988, 34(7):1507-8.

Porter GA, "The Treatment of Ethylene Glycol Poisoning Simplified," *N Engl J Med*, 1988, 319(2):109-10.

Walder AD and Tyler CK, "Ethylene Glycol Antifreeze Poisoning," *Anaesthesia*, 1994, 49(11):964-7.

Ethylphenylhydantoin *see* Ethotoin *on this page*

EtOH *see* Alcohol, Blood or Urine *on page 531*

Etrafon® *see* Amitriptyline, Blood *on page 533*

Etrafon® *see* Antidepressants, Cyclic *on page 535*

Etrafon® *see* Phenothiazines, Serum *on page 568*

5-FC *see* Flucytosine *on next page*

Felbamate

CPT 80299

Related Information

Phenytoin *on page 569*
Valproic Acid *on page 577*

Synonyms Felbamyl; Felbatol™

Abstract Felbamate is an antiepileptic drug used as monotherapy and adjunctive therapy in adults with partial seizures and as adjunctive therapy in children with the Lennox-Gastaut syndrome (a syndrome of frequent seizures with multiple seizure types).

Specimen Serum

Container Red top tube; do not use serum separator tube

Sampling Time Consistent sampling point; 1 hour prior to next dose has been recommended.[1]

Storage Instructions Refrigerate serum.

Reference Range Levels of 20-100 µg/mL[1] have been obtained without serious toxicity.

Critical Values No critical value is established. Serum levels have varied considerably in published trials. ≥200 µg/mL may be noteworthy.

Use Evaluate efficacy, compliance, possible malabsorption, possible interactions with other agents, and possible toxicity

Limitations Relationships between serum levels and response are yet to be established.

Methodology High performance liquid chromatography (HPLC)

Additional Information

- Half-life: 20-23 hours
- Protein binding: 20% to 25%

Peak concentrations are reached 1-6 hours after administration of an oral dose of felbamate with 90% bioavailable. It is cleared by the liver and can decrease the hepatic enzyme activity of other drugs cleared by the liver.

The most common adverse effects, anorexia and headache, may respond to lowering the dose or stopping the drug. Toxicity is more common in patients on more than one anticonvulsant. Significant interactions: If felbamate is added to the regimen of patients taking either phenytoin or valproic acid, the dose of the other drug should be lowered to prevent toxicity. The blood level of carbamazepine may be lowered, but the level of its metabolite, 10,11-epoxide, is raised.

The risk of aplastic anemia in patients taking felbamate may be 1 in 2000 or greater, and there have been at least three fatalities associated with felbamate. There have been eight cases of acute liver failure and four deaths among patients taking Felbatol™. These have limited the use of the drug. In several cases, patients were taking combined therapy with other antiepileptic drugs or nonprescription drugs. The time for diagnosis of felbamate-related serious adverse reactions ranges from 14-257 days after initiation of felbamate treatment. Patients remaining on treatment should have complete blood counts and liver function tests monitored frequently.

Footnotes

1. *Mayo Medical Laboratories Communique*, December, 1994.

References

"Efficacy of Felbamate in Childhood Epileptic Encephalopathy (Lennox-Gastaut Syndrome)," *N Engl J Med*, 1993, 328(1):29-33.

Leppik IE, Dreifuss FE, Pledger GW, et al, "Felbamate for Partial Seizures: Results of a Controlled Clinical Trial," *Neurology*, 1991, 41(11):1785-9.

Theodore WH, Raubertas RF, Porter RJ, et al, "Felbamate: A Clinical Trial for Complex Partial Seizures," *Epilepsia*, 1991, 32(3):392-7.

Wagner ML, "Felbamate: A New Antiepileptic Drug," *Am J Hosp Pharm*, 1994, 51(13):1657-66.

Felbamyl *see* Felbamate *on this page*

Felbatol™ *see* Felbamate *on this page*

Fenilcal® *see Phenobarbital, Blood on page 568*

Fenitoina *see Phenytoin on page 569*

Fenytoin® *see Phenytoin on page 569*

Feverall™ *see Acetaminophen, Serum on page 530*

Fiorinal® *see Barbiturates, Quantitative, Blood on page 537*

Flecainide

CPT 80299

Related Information

Amiodarone, Serum *on page 532*

Digoxin *on page 546*

Propranolol *on page 571*

Synonyms Almartyn®; Tambocor®

Abstract Flecainide is a class IC antiarrhythmic drug. FDA recommends that the drug be reserved for life-threatening ventricular arrhythmias unresponsive to conventional therapy. When coadministered, flecainide can affect activity of other antiarrhythmic drugs, including digoxin and propranolol.

Specimen Serum or plasma

Container Red top tube (preferred) or green top (heparin) tube; do not use serum separator tube

Sampling Time Draw sample 3 hours after last dose.

Storage Instructions Separate serum or plasma within 2 hours of specimen draw.

Special Instructions Draw immediately prior to next dose for trough levels.

Reference Range Therapeutic (trough): 0.2-1.0 µg/mL (SI: 0.5-2.4 µmol/L)

Critical Values Levels >1.0 µg/mL (SI: >2.4 µmol/L) have been related to higher incidence of adverse experiences. Monitor with ECG as well as with serum concentrations.

Use Therapeutic monitoring and toxicity assessment (toxic effects - hypotension, asystole - proportional to dose and concentration). Monitoring is required in subjects with severe renal failure or severe hepatic disease, and is recommended strongly in patients on concurrent amiodarone. It may be helpful in persons with congestive heart failure and also in patients with moderate renal disease.

Methodology High performance liquid chromatography (HPLC), fluorescence polarization immunoassay (FPIA)

Additional Information

- Half-life (normal adult): 7-27 hours
- Volume of distribution: 5-13 L/kg
- Protein binding: 30% to 60%

Flecainide is a class IC antiarrhythmic drug approved for the suppression of ventricular arrhythmias. The drug is well absorbed orally. Plasma half-life averages 20 hours in adults although in children it has been reported to be 8 hours.[2] Steady-state concentrations are achieved in 3-5 days. Since 10% to 50% of the drug is eliminated in the urine as unchanged drug, impaired renal function will significantly prolong the plasma half-life. Half-life is also increased with congestive heart failure. Clearance of flecainide can be accelerated by phenobarbital and rifampin. There are no significant metabolites of flecainide. Coadministration with digoxin increases serum digoxin by 20%; coadministration with propranolol increases both by 20% in serum and creates an additive pharmacological effect. Elevations of serum alkaline phosphatase and also transaminases have been reported.

Footnotes

1. *Physicians' Desk Reference*, 48th ed, Montvale, NJ: Medical Economics Data Production Company, 1994.
2. Till JA, Shinebourne EA, Rowland E, et al, "Pediatric Use of Flecainide in Supraventricular Tachycardia: Clinical Efficacy and Pharmacokinetics," *Br Heart J*, 1989, 62(2):133-9.

References

Evers J, Eichelbaum M, and Kroemer HK, "Unpredictability of Flecainide Plasma Concentrations in Patients With Renal Failure: Relationship to Side Effects and Sudden Death," *Ther Drug Monit*, 1994, 16(4):349-51.

Perry JC, McQuinn RL, Smith RT Jr, et al, "Flecainide Acetate for Resistant Arrhythmias in the Young: Efficacy and Pharmacokinetics," *J Am Coll Cardiol*, 1989, 14(1):185-93.

Roden DM and Woosely RL, "Drug Therapy. Flecainide," *N Engl J Med*, 1986, 315(1):36-41.

Flucytosine

CPT 80299

Related Information

Amphotericin B *on page 535*

Fungal Culture, Cerebrospinal Fluid *on page 477*

Synonyms Ancobon®; 5-FC; 5-Fluorocytosine

Abstract Flucytosine is a synthetic antifungal agent often used in conjunction with amphotericin B, for treatment of fungal (primarily cryptococcal) meningitis, candidiasis, and chromoblastomycosis. Bone marrow toxicity is occasionally seen in patients being treated with flucytosine; neutropenia and thrombocytopenia are found.

Specimen Serum

Container Red top tube

Sampling Time 2 hours after dose

Reference Range Therapeutic: 25-100 µg/mL (SI: 194-775 µmol/L)

Possible Panic Range 100-125 µg/mL (SI: 775-970 µmol/L)

Use Monitor for bone marrow toxicity; evaluate weekly if patient has normal renal function, more often if renal function is abnormal. Diminution of renal function can cause toxic levels.

Limitations Serum levels do not correlate well with clinical toxicity

Methodology High performance liquid chromatography (HPLC), gas chromatography/mass spectrometry (GC/MS)

Additional Information

- Half-life: 3-8 hours
- Protein binding: 2% to 4%

Clinical use of flucytosine is associated with significant frequency of life-threatening bone marrow suppression which occurs most often when blood levels are >100 µg/mL (SI: >775 µmol/L) for 2 or more weeks. Bone marrow suppression is usually reversible and is most likely to occur in patients with underlying hematologic disorders or in patients undergoing myelosuppressive therapy.

Elevated drug levels may predispose to colitis.

References

Bennett JE, "Diagnosis and Therapy of Fungal Infections," *Harrison's Principles of Internal Medicine*, 13th ed, Isselbacher KJ, Braunwald E, Wilson JD, et al, eds, New York, NY: McGraw-Hill Inc, 1994, 854-6.

Bodey GP, "Topical and Systemic Antifungal Agents," *Med Clin North Am*, 1988, 72(3):637-59.

Gerson B, "Flucytosine (5-Fluorocytosine)," *Clin Lab Med*, 1987, 7(3):541-4.

Terrell CL and Hughes CE, "Antifungal Agents Used for Deep-Seated Mycotic Infections," *Mayo Clin Proc*, 1992, 67(1):69-91.

Fluoride, Serum

CPT 82735

Synonyms ACT®; Fluorigard®; Fluorinse®; Fluoritab®; Flura®; Flura-Drops®; Flura-Loz®; Gel Kam®; Gel-Tin®; Karidium®; Karigel®; Karigel®-N; Listermint® With Fluoride; Luride®; Luride® Lozi-Tab®; Luride®-SF Lozi-Tab®; Minute-Gel®; Pediaflor®; Pharmaflur®; Phos-Flur®; Point-Two®; Prevident®; Stop®

Abstract Fluoride is added at low levels to toothpaste and is added to drinking water in many areas at a level of 1 ppm. It is present in high concentrations in insecticides and rodenticides.

Specimen Serum

Container Red top tube

Reference Range Diet dependent, approximately 1.0-20 µg/dL (SI: 0.5-10.5 µmol/L)

Possible Panic Range Toxic concentration: >28.5 µg/dL (SI: >15 µmol/L)

Use Evaluate fluoride toxicity; work up ant poison, roach poison intoxication

Methodology Fluoride-specific electrode

Additional Information

- Half-life: 2-9 hours
- Volume of distribution: 0.5-0.7 L/kg

Fluoride poisoning can occur from ingestion of ant or roach poisons; death is usually from cardiovascular collapse. Fatal dose is 5-10 g orally.

References

Arnow PM, Bland LA, Garcia-Houchins S, et al, "An Outbreak of Fatal Fluoride Intoxication in a Long-Term Dialysis Unit," *Ann Intern Med*, 1994, 121(5):339-44.

Frink EJ Jr, Ghantous H, Malan TP, et al, "Plasma Inorganic Fluoride With Sevoflurane Anesthesia: Correlation With Indices of Hepatic and Renal Function," *Anesth Analg*, 1992, 74(2):231-5.

Gruber HE and Baylink DJ, "The Effects of Fluoride on Bone," *Clin Orthop*, 1991, 267:264-77.

Whitford GM, "The Physiological and Toxicological Characteristics of Fluoride," *J Dent Res*, 1990, 69:539-49.

Fluorigard® *see Fluoride, Serum on this page*

Fluorinse® *see Fluoride, Serum on this page*

Fluoritab® *see Fluoride, Serum on this page*

5-Fluorocytosine *see Flucytosine on this page*

Fluoxetine

CPT 80299

Related Information

Amoxapine, Blood *on page 533*

Antidepressants, Cyclic *on page 535*

Imipramine *on page 554*

Synonyms Fontex; Prozac®

Test Commonly Includes Fluoxetine and norfluoxetine

(Continued)

Fluoxetine *(Continued)*

Abstract This is a **nontricyclic** antidepressant with a long half-life and an active metabolite. It is the most widely prescribed antidepressant in the U.S.. Interactions with tricyclic antidepressants are well recognized.

Specimen Serum or plasma

Container Red top tube or green top (heparin) tube; do not use serum separator tube

Sampling Time Trough just prior to next dose

Reference Range Fluoxetine 100-800 ng/mL (SI: 289-2314 nmol/L); norfluoxetine 100-600 ng/mL (SI: 289-1735 nmol/L)

Critical Values >2000 ng/mL (SI: >5784 nmol/L) (fluoxetine and norfluoxetine). Although overdose of this drug alone is often not apt to be critical, overdose with a tricyclic antidepressant, or with lithium, carbamazepine, monoamine oxidase inhibitors, or other drugs may be significant.[1]

Use Therapeutic monitoring and toxicity assessment

Methodology High performance liquid chromatography (HPLC), gas chromatography (GC)

Additional Information
- Half-life: 26-220 hours
- Volume of distribution: 12-42 L/kg
- Protein binding: 90% to 98%

Fluoxetine is an antidepressant that is a potent, selective inhibitor of serotonin reuptake. It is metabolized via demethylation to the active norfluoxetine. Because of extensive tissue binding, the parent drug has an elimination half-life of 1-10 days and norfluoxetine, 3-20 days, which facilitate maintenance of steady-state concentrations (2-6 weeks to steady-state). Fluoxetine may be helpful for subjects with moderate depression treated as outpatients.[1] The overall toxicity of the drug is considerably less than that of the tricyclics.

Adverse effects, drug reactions and interactions, pharmacology, and indications have recently been reviewed.[1]

Footnotes

1. Gram LF, "Fluoxetine," *N Engl J Med* 1994, 331(20):1354-61.

References

Borys DJ, Setzer SC, Ling LJ, et al, "The Effects of Fluoxetine in the Overdose Patient," *J Toxicol Clin Toxicol*, 1990, 28(3):331-40.

Gidal BE, Anderson GD, Seaton TL, et al, "Evaluation of the Effect of Fluoxetine on the Formation of Carbamazepine Epoxide," *Ther Drug Monit*, 1993, 15(5):405-9.

Norman TR, Gupta RK, Burrows GD, et al, "Relationship Between Antidepressant Response and Plasma Concentrations of Fluoxetine and Norfluoxetine," *Int Clin Psychopharmacol*, 1993, 8(1):25-9.

Pary R, Tobias CR, and Lippmann S, "Fluoxetine: Prescribing Guidelines for the Newest Antidepressant," *South Med J*, 1989, 82(8):1005-9.

Tacke U, "Fluoxetine: An Alternative to the Tricyclics in the Treatment of Major Depression?" *Am J Med Sci*, 1989, 298(2):126-9.

Fluphenazine

CPT 80299

Related Information

Phenothiazines, Serum *on page 568*

Synonyms Moditen®; Permitil®; Prolixin®

Abstract Fluphenazine is a phenothiazine antipsychotic active at low dosage.

Specimen Serum

Container Red top tube

Reference Range 0.2-4.0 ng/mL (SI: 0.4-8.4 nmol/L)

Critical Values >50 ng/mL (SI: >98 nmol/L)

Use Therapeutic monitoring and toxicity assessment

Methodology High performance liquid chromatography (HPLC), gas chromatography (GC), radioimmunoassay (RIA)

Additional Information
- Half-life: the hydrochloride: 10-60 hours (*vide infra*), the decanoate: 5-12 days
- Protein binding: 99%

Fluphenazine is a phenothiazine derivative used in the treatment of psychotic disorders. Its dose in milligrams equivalent to 100 mg of chlorpromazine is 0.6-1.2 mg. As a high potency antipsychotic it may have a high potential for causing extrapyramidal side effects. This would be in addition to the usual adverse effects of antipsychotic drugs (neurologic, anticholinergic, hypotension). Elderly patients should be observed for these occurrences. The half-life of fluphenazine is formulation-dependent. Fluphenazine is also used to alleviate pain and in childhood development disorders.

Fluphenazine decreases barbiturate levels, increases cholesterol and glucose levels, and decreases uric acid in test samples.

References

Chouinard G, Annable L, and Campbell W, "A Randomized Clinical Trial of Haloperidol Decanoate and Fluphenazine Decanoate in the Outpatient Treatment of Schizophrenia," *J Clin Psychopharmacol*, 1989, 9(4):247-53.

Cooper JK, Hawes EM, Hubbard JW, et al, "An Ultrasensitive Method for the Measurement of Fluphenazine in Plasma by High Performance Liquid Chromatography With Coulometric Detection," *Ther Drug Monit*, 1989, 11(3):354-60.

Levinson DF, Simpson GM, Singh H, et al, "Fluphenazine Dose, Clinical Response, and Extrapyramidal Symptoms During Acute Treatment," *Arch Gen Psychiatry*, 1990, 47(8):761-8.

Marder SR, Midha KK, Van Putten T, et al, "Plasma Levels of Fluphenazine in Patients Receiving Fluphenazine Decanoate. Relationship to Clinical Response," *Br J Psychiatry*, 1991, 158:658-65.

Midha KK, Hubbard JW, Marder SR, et al, "Impact of Clinical Pharmacokinetics on Neuroleptic Therapy in Patients With Schizophrenia," *J Psychiatry Neurosci*, 1994, 19(4):254-64.

Midha KK, Marder SR, Jaworski TJ, et al, "Clinical Perspectives of Some Neuroleptics Through Development and Application of Their Assays," *Ther Drug Monit*, 1993, 15(3):179-89.

Flura® *see* Fluoride, Serum *on previous page*

Flura-Drops® *see* Fluoride, Serum *on previous page*

Flura-Loz® *see* Fluoride, Serum *on previous page*

Flurazepam

CPT 82742

Synonyms Benozil®; Dalmane®; Staurodorm®

Abstract This drug is a sedative-hypnotic of the benzodiazepine class with a rather wide therapeutic window.

Specimen Serum

Container Red top tube

Reference Range Therapeutic: 0-4 ng/mL (SI: 0-9 nmol/L); metabolite N-desalkylflurazepam: 20-110 ng/mL (SI: 43-240 nmol/L)

Possible Panic Range Toxic: 200 ng/mL (SI: 500 nmol/L)

Use Monitor therapeutic drug level (rarely), toxicity assessment

Methodology Thin-layer chromatography (TLC), high performance liquid chromatography (HPLC)

Additional Information
- Half-life: parent drug: 3-6 hours; metabolite (N-desalkylflurazepam): 50-100 hours
- Volume of distribution: 15-30 L/kg
- Protein binding: 96% to 98%

Most common side effect is daytime drowsiness. The major urinary metabolite is N-1-hydroxyethyl flurazepam.

References

Greenblatt DJ, Harmatz JS, Engelhardt N, et al, "Pharmacokinetic Determinants of Dynamic Differences Among Three Benzodiazepine Hypnotics. Flurazepam, Temazepam, and Triazolam," *Arch Gen Psychiatry*, 1989, 46(4):326-32.

Kales A, "Benzodiazepine Hypnotics and Insomnia," *Hosp Pract (Off Ed)*, 1990, 25(Suppl 3):7-23.

Folex® *see* Methotrexate *on page 563*

Fontex *see* Fluoxetine *on previous page*

Fortunan® *see* Haloperidol *on next page*

Free Base *see* Cocaine (Cocaine Metabolite), Qualitative, Urine *on page 543*

Free Phenytoin *see* Phenytoin, Free *on page 570*

Fungizone® *see* Amphotericin B *on page 535*

Gabapentin

CPT 80299

Synonyms Neurontin®

Abstract Gabapentin is a GABAergic anticonvulsant effective for partial and secondarily generalized seizures. Its lack of interactions with other anticonvulsants makes it useful as add-on therapy in refractory partial epilepsy.

Specimen Plasma

Container Green top (heparin) tube

Sampling Time Peak: 1.5-3 hours after a 200 mg dose

Storage Instructions Refrigerate

Reference Range Peak plasma level: 2 μg/mL 1.5-3 hours after a 200 mg dose

Additional Information
- Half-life: 5-7 hours
- Volume of distribution: 1.0 L/kg
- Protein binding: <3%

Therapeutic monitoring is not required with gabapentin. Absorption of gabapentin is dose related, with less absorption at doses >600 mg, resulting in less toxicity after large ingestions. Fifty percent to 60% is absorbed after an oral dose of gabapentin, with a peak concentration 1-3 hours after administration. A distinct advantage of gabapentin is that it is cleared totally by the kidneys so it is not subject to and does not cause changes in hepatic enzyme activity. Gabapentin has not been reported to interact with any other antiepileptic. Dosage adjustment may be necessary in renal impairment. Toxicities (not concentration related) include somnolence, dizziness, ataxia, headache, and diplopia.

References
Goa KL and Sorkin EM, "Gabapentin: A Review of Its Pharmacological Properties and Clinical Potential in Epilepsy," *Drugs*, 1993, 46(3):409-27.
Sivenius J, Kalviainen R, Ylinen A, et al, "Double Blind Study of Gabapentin in the Treatment of Partial Seizures," *Epilepsia*, 1991, 32(4):539-42.
UK Gabapentin Study Group, "Gabapentin in Partial Epilepsy," *Lancet*, 1990, 335(8698):1114-7.

Gamma Vinyl GABA *see* Vigabatrin *on page 579*

Gardenal® *see* Phenobarbital, Blood *on page 568*

Gel Kam® *see* Fluoride, Serum *on page 551*

Gel-Tin® *see* Fluoride, Serum *on page 551*

Gemonil® *see* Methylphenobarbital *on page 563*

Gemonil® *see* Barbiturates, Quantitative, Blood *on page 537*

Genagesic® *see* Propoxyphene, Serum or Urine *on page 571*

Genapap® *see* Acetaminophen, Serum *on page 530*

Gentamicin, Serum *see* Aminoglycosides *on page 531*

Glutethimide
CPT 82980
Related Information
Codeine, Urine *on page 544*
Synonyms Doriden®; Loads
Abstract This drug is a sedative hypnotic which has been in use since 1954. The pharmacological effect is similar to that of barbiturates.
Specimen Serum
Container Red top tube
Reference Range Therapeutic: 2-6 µg/mL (variable) (SI: 9-28 µmol/L)
Possible Panic Range Toxic: >6 µg/mL (SI: >28 µmol/L). Fatalities have occurred with serum levels between 10-100 µg/mL (average, 50 µg/mL).
Use Monitor therapeutic drug level, determine toxic level
Limitations Serum levels obtained during dialysis may not reflect tissue levels
Methodology Gas-liquid chromatography (GLC), high performance liquid chromatography (HPLC), thin-layer chromatography (TLC). A spot test is described.[1]
Additional Information
- Half-life: 5-22 hours (*vide infra*)
- Volume of distribution: 3 L/kg
- Protein binding: 50%

Glutethimide is a nonbarbiturate sedative-hypnotic. The drug is erratically absorbed from the gastrointestinal tract and undergoes extensive metabolism to pharmacologically active and inactive metabolites. An important active metabolite in 4-hydroxy-2-ethyl-2-phenylglutarimide. This metabolite has twice the potency of glutethimide and a longer half-life. Peak blood levels are at 2-3 hours postingestion. The average plasma half-life is 10 hours. Serious toxic effects are respiratory depression and circulatory collapse. Glutethimide and codeine ("packs" or "loads") in combination are frequently used by drug abusers. Glutethimide may cause a decreased effect of anticoagulants.

Footnotes
1. Wingard L, Brody T, Larner J, et al, *Human Pharmacology*, St Louis, MO: Mosby Yearbook Inc, 1991, 465-9.

References
Bailey DN and Shaw RF, "Blood Concentrations and Clinical Findings in Nonfatal and Fatal Intoxications Involving Glutethimide and Codeine," *J Toxicol Clin Toxicol*, 1985, 23(7-8):557-70.

Gold
CPT 80172
Synonyms Auranofin; Aurothioglucose; Chrysotherapy; Gold Sodium Thiomalate; Myochrysine®; Ridaura®; Solganal®
Abstract Gold is sometimes used as a treatment for rheumatoid arthritis, but its value is being questioned.
Specimen Serum, urine
Container Red top tube for blood, acid-washed polyethylene container for urine
Reference Range Normal: 0-0.1 µg/mL (SI: 0-0.5 µmol/L); therapeutic: 1.0-3.0 µg/mL (SI: 5.1-15.2 µmol/L); urine <0.1 µg/24 hours
Use Complex gold compounds are used in the treatment of severe, progressive rheumatoid arthritis which is not controlled by other medical therapy. It is also used selectively for juvenile rheumatoid arthritis and for psoriatic arthritis affecting peripheral joints.[1] The mechanism of action is not clear, but may be due to reticuloendothelial system blockade, and/or effects on lymphocyte proliferation and antibody production.

Limitations Blood levels do not correlate with therapeutic or toxic effects. No relationship between serum gold levels and efficacy is established. Serum gold concentrations have not been helpful in monitoring adverse reactions.[1] A relationship is not recognized between urinary gold and response to therapy. Hair and nail gold concentrations have not been helpful.[1]
Methodology Atomic absorption spectrometry (AA)
Additional Information Elimination is mainly renal and the half-life is 5.5 days. Gold toxicity may be manifested by dermatitis, pruritus, stomatitis, metallic taste, eosinophilia, leukopenia, anemia, thrombocytopenia, hematuria, proteinuria, nephrosis, and bone marrow suppression, among other possible effects. Discussing the pharmacokinetics and clinical-pharmacologic correlates, Gottlieb has provided recommendations for monitoring chrysotherapy.[1]

Footnotes
1. Gottlieb NL, "Gold Compounds," *Textbook of Rheumatology*, 2nd ed, Vol 1, Kelley WN, Harris ED, Ruddy S, et al, eds, Philadelphia, PA: WB Saunders Co, 1985, 789-809.

References
Bendix G and Bjelle A, "Outcome of Parenteral Gold Therapy in RA Patients: A Comparison Between Two Periods Using Life-Table Analysis," *Br J Rheumatol*, 1991, 30(6):407-12.
Epstein WV, Henke CJ, Yelin EH, et al, "Effect of Parenterally Administered Gold Therapy on the Course of Adult Rheumatoid Arthritis," *Ann Intern Med*, 1991, 114(6):437-44.

Gold Dust *see* Cocaine (Cocaine Metabolite), Qualitative, Urine *on page 543*

Gold Sodium Thiomalate *see* Gold *on this page*

Goon *see* Phencyclidine, Qualitative, Urine *on page 567*

GX *see* Lidocaine *on page 558*

Hair Analysis *see* Arsenic, Blood *on page 536*

Hair Analysis *see* Arsenic, Hair, Nails *on page 536*

Hair Analysis *see* Arsenic, Urine *on page 537*

Hair Analysis *see* Heavy Metal Screen, Urine *on next page*

Hair Analysis *see* Mercury, Blood *on page 561*

Haldol® *see* Haloperidol *on this page*

Haldol® Decanoate *see* Haloperidol *on this page*

Halenol® *see* Acetaminophen, Serum *on page 530*

Haloneural® *see* Haloperidol *on this page*

Haloperidol
CPT 80299
Related Information
Amphetamine, Qualitative, Urine *on page 534*
Lithium *on page 558*
Synonyms Dozic®; Fortunan®; Haldol®; Haldol® Decanoate; Haloneural®; Serenace®
Abstract This drug is an antipsychotic agent. It is used in the treatment of Tourette's syndrome, severe behavioral problems in children, and for emergency sedation. It is extensively metabolized and should be monitored.
Specimen Serum or plasma
Container Red top tube or green top (heparin) tube
Sampling Time Time to peak serum concentration: Oral: 3-6 hours; I.M.: 10-20 minutes; I.M. (long-acting): 3-9 days
Reference Range 5-20 ng/mL (SI: 10-43 nmol/L) (psychotic disorders - less for Tourette's and mania)
Critical Values >42 ng/mL (SI: >84 nmol/L) (variable)
Use Therapeutic monitoring and toxicity assessment. Haloperidol is an antipsychotic tranquilizer used to control acute and chronic psychotic disorders, for the control of Tourette's syndrome, and for the treatment of severe behavior problems in hyperactive children. Haloperidol should be monitored to assess and optimize dosing regimens and maintenance therapy since the relationship between dosage and serum levels at steady-state can be highly variable. The drug should also be monitored to assess adverse reactions and changes associated with coadministered drugs.
Methodology High performance liquid chromatography (HPLC), gas chromatography (GC)
Additional Information
- Half-life: 15-40 hours
- Volume of distribution: 18-30 L/kg
- Protein binding: 90%

Haloperidol is metabolized by dealkalization, oxidation, and conjugation; the hydroxy derivative is active but concentrations are very low. Haloperidol may increase serum tricyclic concentrations, increase the toxicity of
(Continued)

Haloperidol *(Continued)*

lithium, inhibit hypertensive action, and antagonize the stimulant effect of amphetamines.

References

Cannon DJ, McMillan DE, Newton JE, et al, "Serum Haloperidol and Neuroleptic Receptor Levels in Chronic Psychosis," *Ann Clin Lab Sci*, 1988, 18(5):378-83.

Derlet RW, Albertson TE, and Rice P, "The Effect of Haloperidol in Cocaine and Amphetamine Intoxication," *J Emerg Med*, 1989, 7(6):633-7.

Goff DC, Midha KK, Brotman AW, et al, "Elevation of Plasma Concentrations of Haloperidol After the Addition of Fluoxetine," *Am J Psychiatry*, 1991, 148(6):790-2.

Hemstrom CA, Evans RL, and Lobeck FG, "Haloperidol Decanoate: A Depot Antipsychotic," *Drug Intell Clin Pharm*, 1988, 22(4):290-5.

Lawson GM, "Monitoring of Serum Haloperidol," *Mayo Clin Proc*, 1994, 69(2):189-90.

Leroux JM, Jacquet M, Pommery J, et al, "Correlation of Clinical Response and Plasma Levels of Haloperidol and Reduced Haloperidol in Schizophrenia," *Prog Neuropsychopharmacol Biol Psychiatry*, 1994, 18(2):347-53.

Rifkin A, Doddi S, Karajgi B, et al, "Dosage of Haloperidol for Schizophrenia," *Arch Gen Psychiatry*, 1991, 48(2):166-70.

Volavka J and Cooper TB, "Review of Haloperidol Blood Levels and Clinical Response: Looking Through the Window," *J Clin Psychopharmacol*, 1987, 7(1):25-30.

Hashish *see* Cannabinoids (Marijuana Metabolites), Qualitative, Urine *on page 539*

Heavy Metal Screen, Arsenic *see* Arsenic, Blood *on page 536*

Heavy Metal Screen, Blood

CPT 83015 (screen); 83018 (quantitative, each)

Related Information

Aluminum, Serum *on page 586*
Arsenic, Blood *on page 536*
Arsenic, Hair, Nails *on page 536*
Arsenic, Urine *on page 537*
Cadmium, Urine *on page 539*
Chromium, Serum *on page 587*
Chromium, Urine *on page 588*
Copper, Serum *on page 589*
Copper, Urine *on page 590*
Heavy Metal Screen, Urine *on this page*
Lead, Blood *on page 556*
Lead, Urine *on page 557*
Manganese, Blood *on page 591*
Manganese, Urine *on page 592*
Mercury, Blood *on page 561*
Mercury, Urine *on page 561*
Molybdenum, Blood *on page 593*
Selenium, Serum *on page 593*
Selenium, Urine *on page 594*
Thallium, Urine or Blood *on page 574*
Zinc, Serum *on page 595*
Zinc, Urine *on page 596*

Synonyms Metals, Blood; Poisonous Metals, Blood; Toxic Metals, Blood

Test Commonly Includes Antimony, arsenic, bismuth, boron, cadmium, cobalt, copper, lead, mercury, selenium, tellurium, thallium, zinc

Abstract Used principally to detect arsenic, cadmium, mercury, and lead poisoning.

Specimen Whole blood (EDTA) plus serum

Container Special metal-free tube and red top tube

Storage Instructions Refrigerate; do not spin down.

Special Instructions Check with laboratory performing the assay to determine what elements will be detected and for special instructions.

Reference Range See individual test listings.

Use Screen for heavy metal poisoning

Methodology Atomic absorption spectrometry (AA)

Additional Information See individual test listings.

References

Gerson B, "Lead," *Clin Lab Med*, 1990, 10(3):441-73.

Malachowski ME, "An Update on Arsenic," *Clin Lab Med*, 1990, 10(3):459-72.

Heavy Metal Screen, Urine

CPT 83015 (screen); 83018 (quantitative, each)

Related Information

Aluminum, Serum *on page 586*
Arsenic, Blood *on page 536*
Arsenic, Hair, Nails *on page 536*
Arsenic, Urine *on page 537*
Cadmium, Urine *on page 539*
Chromium, Serum *on page 587*
Chromium, Urine *on page 588*
Copper, Serum *on page 589*
Copper, Urine *on page 590*
Heavy Metal Screen, Blood *on this page*
Lead, Blood *on page 556*
Lead, Urine *on page 557*
Manganese, Blood *on page 591*
Manganese, Urine *on page 592*
Mercury, Blood *on page 561*
Mercury, Urine *on page 561*
Molybdenum, Blood *on page 593*
Selenium, Serum *on page 593*
Selenium, Urine *on page 594*
Thallium, Urine or Blood *on page 574*
Urine Collection, 24-Hour *on page 30*
Zinc, Serum *on page 595*
Zinc, Urine *on page 596*

Synonyms Metal Screen; Metals, Toxic; Poisonous Metals, Urine; Toxic Metals, Urine

Applies to Hair Analysis

Test Commonly Includes Arsenic, mercury, lead (could also include nickel and cadmium)

Abstract Used to detect arsenic, mercury, lead, and cadmium poisoning

Specimen 24-hour urine

Container Plastic, acid-washed urine container (preferably polyethylene), no preservative, 20-25 mL 6N HCl (low metal content)

Storage Instructions Refrigerate

Reference Range Arsenic: <50 µg/L; lead: <80 µg/L; mercury: <20 µg/L; nickel: <25 µg/L; cadmium: <10 µg/L

Use Screen for heavy metal poisoning and toxic exposure; urine lead analysis is useful for organic lead exposure and to monitor chelation. Blood is preferred for inorganic lead exposure monitoring.

Limitations Hair analysis should be used for arsenic and mercury poisoning or exposure especially if one is interested in determining chronic exposure. Hair should be clean, free of oil, and clipped (0.5 g for As; 2 g for Hg) as close as possible. Recent ingestion of seafood can cause misleading increases of urine arsenic.

Methodology Atomic absorption spectrometry (AA)

Additional Information Please see the test listings Heavy Metal Screen, Blood *on page 554* for further information. See also the Trace Elements listings.

References

Malachowski ME, "An Update on Arsenic," *Clin Lab Med*, 1990, 10(3):459-72.

Philip AT and Gerson B, "Lead Poisoning - Part II. Effects and Assay," *Clin Lab Med*, 1994, 14(3):651-70.

Hemp *see* Cannabinoids (Marijuana Metabolites), Qualitative, Urine *on page 539*

Heroin *see* Opiates, Qualitative, Urine *on page 566*

Heroin Metabolite, Urine *see* Morphine, Urine *on page 564*

Hexamidinum *see* Primidone *on page 570*

Hg, Blood *see* Mercury, Blood *on page 561*

Hg, Urine *see* Mercury, Urine *on page 561*

Hibanil® *see* Chlorpromazine, Serum or Urine *on page 543*

Hog *see* Phencyclidine, Qualitative, Urine *on page 567*

Hydrocyanic Acid *see* Cyanide, Blood *on page 544*

Ice *see* Amphetamine, Qualitative, Urine *on page 534*

"Ice" *see* Methamphetamine, Qualitative, Urine *on page 562*

Ikacor® *see* Verapamil *on page 578*

Iktorivil® *see* Clonazepam *on page 543*

Imipramine

CPT 80174

Related Information

Antidepressants, Cyclic *on page 535*
Disopyramide *on page 547*
Fluoxetine *on page 551*
Phenytoin *on page 569*
Procainamide *on page 570*
Quinidine, Serum *on page 572*
Warfarin *on page 579*

Synonyms Berkomine®; Dimipressin®; Iprogen®; Janimine®; Presamine®; SK-Pramine®; Tofranil®

Applies to Desipramine; Norpramin®; Pertofrane®

Test Commonly Includes Desipramine levels

Abstract This drug is a cyclic antidepressant. It has an active metabolite which should also be monitored.

Specimen Serum or plasma

Container Red top tube or green top (heparin) tube

Sampling Time Trough levels at steady-state

Reference Range Imipramine and desipramine 150-250 ng/mL (SI: 530-890 nmol/L); desipramine 150-300 ng/mL (SI: 560-1125 nmol/L). Metabolism may be impaired in geriatric patients.[1]

Critical Values >300 ng/mL (SI: >1070 nmol/L)

Possible Panic Range 1000 ng/mL (SI: 3570 nmol/L)

Use Therapeutic monitoring and toxicity assessment of imipramine, a cyclic antidepressant that blocks the reuptake of serotonin and norepinephrine at nerve endings. It possesses high anticholinergic activity, sedation and cardiovascular toxicity. It has quinidine-like effects on cardiac conduction.

Contraindications Cyclic antidepressants should be avoided in pregnant and lactating women because these drugs have not been established to be safe. Geriatric patients are especially susceptible to orthostasis, urinary retention, constipation, and sedation. The cyclic antidepressants are commonly seen in overdose situations. Cardiovascular, anticholinergic, and central nervous system toxicities can be lethal.

Methodology Immunoassay, high performance liquid chromatography (HPLC), gas chromatography (GC)

Additional Information
- Half-life: 6-28 hours
- Volume of distribution: 9-23 L/kg
- Protein binding: 60% to 95%

Imipramine is cleared by the liver alone and is extensively metabolized to many polar compounds. The most important metabolite is desipramine, which is an important antidepressant itself.

Imipramine is completely absorbed but undergoes some first-pass elimination. The bioavailability is 22% to 77% with a peak concentration 2-6 hours after an oral dose. Imipramine takes about 2-6 days to reach steady-state.

Anticholinergic side effects are common with this drug. They are not severe and may diminish with continued therapy or can be treated with other pharmacologic and nonpharmacologic therapies. Anticholinergic side effects are more troublesome in the elderly. Sedation may also decrease with continued use. Imipramine can also lower the seizure threshold and cause orthostasis and arrhythmias. The cardiovascular effects are more common in patients with underlying cardiovascular disorders.

Drug interactions are common with the cyclic antidepressants. Since they are cleared by the liver, they are susceptible to decreases in enzyme activity caused by cimetidine, fluoxetine, and antipsychotics resulting in increased concentrations of imipramine. Enzyme inducers like phenytoin, chloral hydrate, smoking, and the barbiturates will decrease imipramine concentrations. Additive anticholinergic side effects occur when cyclics are combined with antihistamines, anti-Parkinson drugs, and antipsychotics. The cardiovascular effects of the cyclics will be additive with any of the class IA antiarrhythmics (quinidine, procainamide, disopyramide). Direct-acting sympathomimetics (epinephrine, norepinephrine, phenylephrine) will be potentiated by cyclics. Monoamine oxidase inhibitors (MAOIs) and thyroid hormones will potentiate the toxicities of cyclics. Hyperthermia, delirium, convulsions, coma, and fatalities have occurred with the combination of MAOIs and cyclics. These drugs have been used in combination in refractory cases of depression. The cyclics can also affect other drugs. The antihypertensive effects of the central α-agonists (clonidine, methyldopa, guanethidine) are reversed when combined with cyclics. Anticoagulation effects of warfarin may be potentiated by the cyclics.

Footnotes

1. Montamat SC, Cusack BJ, and Vestal RE, "Management of Drug Therapy in the Elderly," *N Engl J Med*, 1989, 321(5):303-9.

References

Amsterdam JD, Brunswick DJ, Potter L, et al, "Desipramine and 2-Hydroxydesipramine Plasma Levels in Endogenous Depressed Patients," *Arch Gen Psychiatry*, 1985, 42(4):361-4.

Ereshefsky L, Tran-Johnson T, Davis CM, et al, "Pharmacokinetic Factors Affecting Antidepressant Drug Clearance and Clinical Effect: Evaluation of Doxepin and Imipramine - New Data and Review," *Clin Chem*, 1988, 34(5):863-80.

Gawin FH, Kleber HD, Byck R, et al, "Desipramine Facilitation of Initial Cocaine Abstinence," *Arch Gen Psychiatry*, 1989, 46(2):117-21.

Kline JA, De Stefano AA, Schroeder JD, et al, "Magnesium Potentiates Imipramine Toxicity in the Isolated Rat Heart," *Ann Emerg Med*, 1994, 24(2):224-32.

Siegel DM, "Bulimia, Tricyclic Antidepressants and Mania," *Clin Pediatr (Phila)*, 1989, 28(3):123-6.

Spina E, Avenoso A, Campo GM, et al, "Decreased Plasma Concentrations of Imipramine and Desipramine Following Cholestyramine Intake in Depressed Patients," *Ther Drug Monit*, 1994, 16(4):432-4.

Inderal® see Propranolol *on page 571*

Iproveratril Hydrochloride see Verapamil *on page 578*

Isonipecaine Hydrochloride see Meperidine, Blood or Urine *on page 560*

Isopropanol see Volatile Screen *on page 579*

Isoptin® see Verapamil *on page 578*

Itraconazole

CPT 80299

Related Information

Amphotericin B *on page 535*
Antimicrobial Susceptibility Testing, Fungi *on page 450*
Cyclosporine *on page 545*
Digoxin *on page 546*
Fungal Culture, Blood *on page 477*
Fungal Culture, Cerebrospinal Fluid *on page 477*
Fungal Culture, Skin *on page 478*
Fungal Culture, Sputum *on page 479*
Fungal Culture, Urine *on page 480*
Ketoconazole *on next page*

Synonyms Sporanox

Abstract Itraconazole is a relatively new orally administered antifungal agent with a broad spectrum of activity, including most pathogenic fungi. Efficacy in candidiasis, blastomycosis, blastomycosis brasiliensis (paracoccidioidomycosis), chromoblastomycosis, coccidioidomycosis, cryptococcosis, histoplasmosis, sporotrichosis, maduramycotic mycetomas, many cases of phaeomycosis[1] and *Aspergillus* infections[2] is described. A triazole analogue of ketoconazole, it is described as superior to its parent compound. Similarly, its role in clinical medicine is still evolving. It appears likely that this agent will become widely accepted due to its low toxicity compared with other antifungal agents and its broad spectrum of activity. The role for monitoring of serum levels has not been established.

Specimen Serum

Container Red top tube

Sampling Time 4 hours after oral dose and approximately 1-2 weeks after therapy has begun so that a steady-state is achieved

Reference Range Therapeutic: varies with methodology; see Additional Information. Tissue levels are 3- to 20-fold higher than plasma concentrations. Only negligible concentrations were reported in CSF and urine.[3]

Use Serum therapeutic levels may be useful if poor absorption is suspected, or in cases of therapeutic failure or relapse.

Limitations *In vitro* susceptibility testing of fungi against itraconazole is method dependent and may not accurately predict clinical success. Consequently, monitoring levels and adjusting dosage to attain therapeutic concentrations as determined by minimum inhibitory concentrations may not be helpful. Itraconazole bioavailability is decreased when given with H_2 antagonists and DDI. Itraconazole is an important enzyme inhibitor. Oral hypoglycemics, cisapride, cyclosporine, digoxin, and terfenadine have been increased when itraconazole is added. Itraconazole is also influenced by enzyme inducers and inhibitors. Phenytoin, phenobarbital, and rifampin decrease enzyme activity resulting in increased itraconazole. Assays for itraconazole are performed only in a few reference laboratories.

Methodology Bioassay, high performance liquid chromatography (HPLC)

Additional Information Half-life ranges from 17 to 21 hours. 99.8% binds to plasma proteins, especially albumin. It is metabolized mainly in the liver. A metabolite, hydroxy-itraconazole, has antifungal activity. Serum levels as determined by bioassay are approximately 10 times the levels determined by HPLC, presumably because bioassay also detects an active metabolite. Consequently therapeutic levels vary with method. Concentrations >5 μg/mL (bioassay) were predictive of therapeutic success in invasive aspergillosis, whereas serum concentrations <1 μg/mL (bioassay) predicted therapeutic failure in cases of cryptococcal meningitis. Concentrations <0.25 μg/mL (HPLC) predicted failure to prevent aspergillosis in granulocytopenic patients. Absorption is often depressed in bone marrow transplant and in AIDS patients.

Footnotes

1. Odds FC, "Intraconazole - A New Oral Antifungal Agent With a Very Broad Spectrum of Activity in Superficial and Systemic Mycoses," *J Dermatol Sci*, 1993, 5(2):65-72.

2. Zuckerman JM and Tunkel AR, "Itraconazole: A New Triazole Antifungal Agent," *Infect Control Hosp Epidemiol*, 1994, 15(6):397-410.

3. Negroni R and Arechavala AI, "Itraconazole: Pharmacokinetics and Indications," *Arch Med Res*, 1993, 24(4):387-93.

References

Bennett JE, "Diagnosis and Therapy of Fungal Infections," *Harrison's Principles of Internal Medicine*, 13th ed, Isselbacher KJ, Braunwald E, Wilson JD, et al, eds, New York, NY: McGraw-Hill Inc, 1994, 854-6.

British Society for Antimicrobial Chemotherapy Working Party, "Laboratory Monitoring of Antifungal Chemotherapy," *Lancet*, 1991, 337(8769):1577-80.

Hostetler JS, Heykants J, Clemons KV, et al, "Discrepancies in Bioassay and Chromatography Determinations Explained by Metabolism of Itraconazole to Hydroxyitraconazole: Studies of Interpatient Variations in Concentrations," *Antimicrob Agents Chemother*, 1993, 37(10):2224-7.

Terrell CL and Hughes CE, "Antifungal Agents Used for Deep-Seated Mycotic Infections," *Mayo Clin Proc*, 1992, 67(1):69-91.

Tucker RM, Haq Y, Denning DW, et al, "Adverse Effects Associated With Itraconazole in 189 Patients on Chronic Therapy," *J Antimicrob Chemother*, 1990, 26(4):561-6.

Janimine® see Imipramine on page 554

Karidium® see Fluoride, Serum on page 551

Karigel® see Fluoride, Serum on page 551

Karigel®-**N** see Fluoride, Serum on page 551

Kay Jay see Phencyclidine, Qualitative, Urine on page 567

Ketoconazole
CPT 80299
Related Information
Amphotericin B on page 535
Antimicrobial Susceptibility Testing, Fungi on page 450
Cyclosporine on page 545
Itraconazole on previous page
Mexiletine on page 563
Phenytoin on page 569
Theophylline on page 575
Warfarin on page 579
Synonyms Nizoral
Abstract Ketoconazole is an orally administered antifungal agent that is appropriately used for a variety of fungal infections.
Specimen Serum
Container Red top tube
Sampling Time 2 hours after administration
Reference Range Therapeutic: peak: 1-10 µg/mL (mean 3.5 µg/mL); trough: ≤1 µg/mL
Use Monitoring is usually not necessary. May be useful to ensure therapeutic levels if poor absorption is suspected, or in cases of therapeutic failure or relapse.
Limitations Itraconazole, a triazole analogue of ketoconazole, is described as superior to its parent in safety and efficacy.[1] In vitro susceptibility testing of fungi against ketoconazole is method dependent and may not accurately predict clinical success. Consequently, monitoring levels and adjusting dosage to attain therapeutic concentrations as determined by minimum inhibitory concentrations may not be helpful. Assays for ketoconazole are performed only in a few reference laboratories.
Methodology Bioassay, high performance liquid chromatography (HPLC)
Additional Information
• Half-life: 2-8 hours
• Volume of distribution: 1-5 L/kg
• Protein binding: 90% to 95%

Approximately 5% to 10% of patients receiving ketoconazole develop abnormally elevated serum transaminases, a transient and reversible state. Testing with transaminases, GGT, alkaline phosphatase, and bilirubin before and during therapy is recommended. Rarely, patients develop symptomatic hepatitis which is idiosyncratic and not dependent upon serum concentrations. Absorption is often depressed in bone marrow transplant and AIDS patients.

Absorption is decreased in subjects with AIDS.

Drugs that affect absorption (raise gastric pH) such as antacids, H$_2$-receptor blockers; drugs that decrease serum concentrations of ketoconazole (rifampin, isoniazid); drug concentrations that are increased by ketoconazole (phenytoin, cyclosporine, theophylline, terfenadine, warfarin); and drugs that cause hepatotoxicity; terfenadine may cause life-threatening cardiac arrhythmias; concomitant use with phenytoin may effect the metabolism of one or both agents; when used together, levels of each should be monitored. Temporary, dose-related effects reported include diminished adrenal cortical reserve, gynecomastia; decreased testosterone and menstrual irregularities.[1]

Footnotes
1. Bennett JE, "Diagnosis and Therapy of Fungal Infections," *Harrison's Principles of Internal Medicine*, 13th ed, Isselbacher KJ, Braunwald E, Wilson JD, et al, eds, New York, NY: McGraw-Hill Inc, 1994, 854-6.

References
Bodey GP, "Topical and Systemic Antifungal Agents," *Med Clin North Am*, 1988, 72(3):637-59.
British Society for Antimicrobial Chemotherapy Working Party, "Laboratory Monitoring of Antifungal Chemotherapy," *Lancet*, 1991, 337(8769):1577-80.
Terrell CL and Hughes CE, "Antifungal Agents Used for Deep-Seated Mycotic Infections," *Mayo Clin Proc*, 1992, 67(1):69-91.

Kiditard® see Quinidine, Serum on page 572

Killer Weed see Phencyclidine, Qualitative, Urine on page 567

Kinidin® see Quinidine, Serum on page 572

Klonopin™ see Clonazepam on page 543

Lamictal® see Lamotrigine on this page

Lamotrigine
Related Information
Carbamazepine on page 540
Phenytoin on page 569
Synonyms Lamictal®
Abstract Lamotrigine is a newly approved antiepileptic drug that is thought to act by inhibiting the presynaptic release of the excitatory amino acid glutamate, due to its effect on voltage sensitive sodium channels.
Specimen Serum
Container Red top tube
Sampling Time Trough
Reference Range 2-4 µg/mL
Critical Values LD-50 in mice is >160 mg/kg
Limitations The most common adverse effects seen with lamotrigine have been dose-related central nervous system effects, including somnolence, dizziness, ataxia, and diplopia. Rash also occurs in 5% to 15%. While lamotrigine does not effect the serum concentrations of other antiepileptic drugs, lamotrigine pharmacokinetics are significantly altered by phenytoin, carbamazepine, and barbiturates.
Additional Information
• Half-life: 24-30 hours
• Volume of distribution: 0.9-1.4 L/kg
• Protein binding: 50% to 60%

Lamotrigine is a new antiepileptic used for partial and generalized seizures. It is 98% bioavailable and reaches peak concentrations 1-4 hours after oral administration. It is cleared by the liver but does not alter hepatic enzyme activity as many other antiepileptics do. It is, however, effected by some enzyme inducers and inhibitors. The long half-life permits once daily dosing in most patients, but that may not apply to patients receiving combined treatments with other antiepileptic drugs.
References
Loiseau P, Yuen AW, Duche B, et al, "A Randomized, Double-Blind, Placebo-Controlled Crossover Add-On Trial of Lamotrigine in Patients With Treatment-Resistant Partial Seizures," *Epilepsy Res*, 1990, 7(2):136-45.
Sander JW, Patsalos PN, Oxley JR, et al, "A Randomised Double-Blind Placebo-Controlled Add-On Trial of Lamotrigine in Patients With Severe Epilepsy," *Epilepsy Res*, 1990, 6(3):221-6.

Lamra® see Diazepam, Blood on page 546

Lanocor® see Digoxin on page 546

Lanotoxin® see Digitoxin on page 546

Lanoxicaps® see Digoxin on page 546

Lanoxin® see Digoxin on page 546

Largactil® see Chlorpromazine, Serum or Urine on page 543

Lead, Blood
CPT 83655
Related Information
Delta Aminolevulinic Acid, Urine on page 121
Heavy Metal Screen, Blood on page 554
Heavy Metal Screen, Urine on page 554
Porphobilinogen, Qualitative, Urine on page 185
Porphyrins, Quantitative, Urine on page 186
Protoporphyrin, Free Erythrocyte on page 195
Protoporphyrin, Zinc, Blood on page 196
Semen Analysis on page 652
Uric Acid, Serum on page 213
Synonyms Pb, Blood
Applies to Delta Aminolevulinic Acid Dehydratase
Abstract Blood lead concentrations are used to detect recent lead exposure but do not necessarily measure lead body burden from past chronic exposure. The hematopoietic system, nervous system, and kidneys are most effected.
Specimen Whole blood; venous blood is recommended
Container Special lead-free tube with heparin; trace metal Vacutainer® tubes containing lithium heparin can be used. EDTA is satisfactory.
Collection See Blood Collection Methods for Trace Elements in the Trace Elements Introduction on page 585.
Storage Instructions Do not separate red cells.
Causes for Rejection Improper draw
Special Instructions Avoid contact with leaded glass during collection
Reference Range <10 µg/dL (whole blood) (SI: <0.5 µmol/L). The blood lead level of preindustrial humans is estimated at about 0.016 µg/dL.[1] See accompanying CDC chart for evaluation of blood lead concentrations in children.

OSHA uses a lead level of 40 µg/dL for occupational exposure. Lead level >40 µg/dL requires the employer to notify the worker in writing

CDC Classification of Blood Lead in Children

Class	Blood Lead Level* (μg/dL)	Comment
I	≤9	Not lead-poisoned
IIA	10-14	Rescreen frequently and consider prevention activities
IIB	15-19	Institute nutritional and educational interventions and more frequent screening
III	20-44†	Evaluate environment and consider chelation therapy
IV	45-69†	Institute environmental intervention and chelation therapy
V	≥70	A medical emergency

From Roper WL, Centers for Disease Control, modified.

*Due to possible contamination during collection, elevated levels should be confirmed with a second specimen before action is instituted.

†Full medical evaluation indicated with history, examination, and investigation for iron deficiency.

within 5 days. The employee should be removed from work and enter a chelation program if lead level is >60 μg/dL, or with certain other circumstances.[1] Average levels in 1995 are 2.8 μg/dL.[2]

Possible Panic Range >80 μg/dL (SI: >3.86 μmol/L) in acute lead poisoning; toxicity at lower levels in chronic poisoning

Use Evaluate lead exposure, toxicity, and poisoning

Limitations Lead poisoning is not ruled out by normal blood levels; clinical findings and heme synthetic enzymes must also be evaluated. The EDTA lead mobilization test or x-ray fluorescence is needed for diagnosis of lead nephropathy.[3]

Methodology Electrothermal atomic absorption spectrometry (EAAS), photometry, anodic stripping voltammeter, inductively coupled plasma-atomic emission spectroscopy, x-ray fluorescence spectroscopy

Additional Information Great care is required to avoid contamination in the collection of specimens for lead analysis. Lead can be measured in tissue and urine. Another test that may be used to evaluate lead intoxication is **free erythrocyte protoporphyrin (FEP)**. FEP concentrations >35 μg/dL are consistent with undue absorption of lead. However, FEP is also elevated in iron deficiency, sickle cell anemia, and chronic infection. **Erythrocyte zinc protoporphyrin** is a more specific indicator of lead toxicity and, therefore, superior to FEP. Normal values for erythrocyte zinc protoporphyrin are <100 ng/dL. See listings Delta Aminolevulinic Acid, Urine *on page 121* and Porphyrins, Quantitative, Urine *on page 186*. Inhibition of erythrocyte **delta aminolevulinic acid dehydratase** is a very sensitive measure of lead toxicity. However, a blood lead assay is the definitive test for recent acute exposure if sample collection is meticulous. Blood lead concentrations are evidence of **recent** exposure but do not indicate the body burden from past exposure. See listing Lead, Urine *on page 557* for lead mobilization test.

Of sources of lead poisoning in children, paint is still the most important. A single paint chip can contain as much as 10,000 μg of lead.

Other sources of lead include air, soil, dust, drinking water, food (especially in lead-soldered cans), solder, storage batteries, ammunition, other metal objects, gasoline additives, other chemicals, and imported Asian products including third world cosmetics. Other sources including hobbies, folk remedies, and moonshine are published as well. Occupational exposure is important in adults.[1] A branch of the CDC, the National Institute for Occupational Safety and Health (NIOSH), provides recommendations for prevention of occupational lead poisoning.

Lead absorption is influenced by iron deficiency.[2] Greater than 90% of absorbed lead is deposited in the skeleton and in teeth. It crosses the placenta. Plumbism has been identified with lead poisoning in pets.[4] Bone lead concentration can be estimated with K x-ray fluorescence[5] or L x-ray fluorescence.[6]

Effects of lead are mediated by its ability to complex sulfhydryl groups and other ligands in enzyme systems. Lead toxicity occurs secondary to environmental, occupational, or recreational activities. Acute exposures are commonly associated with symptoms of anorexia, malaise, nausea, vomiting, and abdominal pain. Fecal discoloration (black or red) may occur. Constipation, anemia, tremor, headache, coma, motor neuropathy, paresthesia/peripheral neuropathy, hearing loss, tinnitus, alopecia, and bradycardia may be seen. Severe exposures can result in encephalopathy and death; chronic exposures manifest with microcytic, hypochromic anemia and basophilic stippling, hypertension, arthralgias, teratogenesis, and impotence. Fanconi syndrome (amino aciduria, glycosuria, hyperphosphaturia with hypophosphatemia, and proteinuria) may be found with renal dysfunction/failure. Nuclear inclusions in renal tubular cells are found.

Central nervous system effects include ataxia, neuropsychiatric symptoms, encephalopathy, headache, learning disabilities, lethargy, mood and/or mental status changes, and seizures. Lead causes peripheral neuropathy in which wrist drop and foot drop are characteristic. Gastrointestinal effects include abdominal colic, constipation, nausea, and vomiting. Saturnine gout is mentioned in the listing Uric Acid, Serum *on page 213*.

Footnotes

1. Philip AT and Gerson B, "Lead Poisoning. Part I. Incidence, Etiology, and Toxicokinetics," *Clin Lab Med*, 1994, 14(2):423-44.
2. *American Medical News*, Feb 1995, 15.
3. Batuman V, "Lead Nephropathy, Gout, and Hypertension," *Am J Med Sci*, 1993, 305(4):241-7.
4. Dowsett R and Shannon M, "Childhood Plumbism Identified After Lead Poisoning in Household Pets," *N Engl J Med*, 1994, 331(24):1661-2
5. Kosnett MJ, Becker CE, Osterich JD, et al, "Factors Influencing Bone Lead Concentration in a Suburban Community Assessed by Noninvasive K X-ray Fluorescence," *JAMA*, 1994, 271(3):197-203.
6. Landrigan PJ and Todd AC, "Direct Measurement of Lead in Bone: A Promising Biomarker," *JAMA*, 1994, 271(3):239-40.

References

Beritic T, "Misconceptions About Blood Lead Concentrations," *Br J Ind Med*, 1993, 50(12):1123-4.

Bernard BP and Becker CE, "Environmental Lead Exposure and the Kidney," *J Toxicol Clin Toxicol*, 1988, 26(1-2):1-34.

Braithwaite RA and Brown SS, "Clinical and Subclinical Lead Poisoning: A Laboratory Perspective," *Hum Toxicol*, 1988, 7(5):503-13.

Brody DJ, Pirkle JL, Kramer RA, et al, "Blood Lead Levels in the U.S. Population. Phase I of the Third National Health and Nutritional Examination Survey," *JAMA*, 1994, 272(4):277-83.

Markowitz ME and Rosen JF, "Need for the Lead Mobilization Test in Children With Lead Poisoning," *J Pediatr*, 1991, 119(2):305-10.

Mushak P, Davis JM, Crocetti AF, et al, "Prenatal and Postnatal Effects of Low-Level Lead Exposure: Integrated Summary of a Report to the U.S. Congress on Childhood Lead Poisoning," *Environ Res*, 1989, 50(1):11-36.

Piomelli S, "Childhood Lead Poisoning in the '90s," *Pediatrics*, 1994, 93(3):508-10.

Rempel D, "The Lead-Exposed Worker," *JAMA*, 1989, 262(4):532-4.

Staessen JA, Lauwerys RR, Buchet J-P, et al, "Impairment of Renal Function With Increasing Blood Lead Concentrations in the General Population," *N Engl J Med*, 1992, 327(3):151-6.

Lead Excretion Ratio *see* Lead, Urine *on this page*

Lead Mobilization Test *see* Lead, Urine *on this page*

Lead, Urine

CPT 83655

Related Information

Delta Aminolevulinic Acid, Urine *on page 121*
Ferritin, Serum *on page 127*
Heavy Metal Screen, Blood *on page 554*
Heavy Metal Screen, Urine *on page 554*
Iron and Total Iron Binding Capacity/Transferrin *on page 150*
Porphyrins, Quantitative, Urine *on page 186*
Protoporphyrin, Free Erythrocyte *on page 195*
Semen Analysis *on page 652*
Uric Acid, Urine *on page 215*
Urine Collection, 24-Hour *on page 30*

Synonyms Pb, Urine

Applies to Lead Excretion Ratio; Lead Mobilization Test

Abstract This test is used to assess lead body burden (lead mobilization test), not to diagnose lead poisoning. The kidneys represent the most important mechanism of lead excretion, but only slight loss through the kidneys takes place without BAL or EDTA chelation.

Patient Preparation Patient should be instructed to use a specially cleaned plastic urinal or bedpan

Specimen 24-hour urine is preferred; in an emergency, random specimens may be acceptable

Container Plastic (preferably polyethylene) acid-washed (nitric acid) urine container copiously rinsed with appropriate (non-tap) water

Collection Avoid a catheter if possible.

Storage Instructions Record total volume. Acidify to pH 2 with concentrated HCl or add 20 mL 6N HCl to the 24-hour volume.

Causes for Rejection Specimen allowed to contact glass or metal, specimen not collected in acid-washed containers

Special Instructions Indicate if a chelating agent has been administered

Reference Range ≤80 μg/24 hours (SI: ≤0.39 μmol/day)

Critical Values >125 μg/24 hours (SI: >0.60 μmol/day) is considered excessive and associated with toxicity; values of 80-125 μg/24 hours (SI: 0.39-0.60 μmol/day) are inconclusive

Use Evaluate lead toxicity and chelation therapy

Limitations The value of urinary lead levels without prior administration of a chelating agent is questionable.

Methodology Electrothermal atomic absorption (AA)
(Continued)

Lead, Urine (Continued)

Additional Information Lead is poorly excreted and is found in lower concentrations in urine versus blood. Urine is not the appropriate specimen for screening potential toxicity. Urine lead mobilization tests (postchelation therapy) are good indicators of lead body burden. Children with blood lead levels between 25-40 µg/dL should be evaluated by a lead mobilization test to determine need for chelation therapy. Those with levels >40 µg/dL should receive chelation therapy.[1] The **lead mobilization test (LMT)** is performed by administering 500 mg/m^2 of CaNa$_2$-ethylenediaminetetraacetic acid (EDTA) and then collecting urine for 8 hours; a positive result is defined as a ratio of urinary lead/dose EDTA >0.6 (µg lead/mg EDTA given) or a total urinary excretion >200 µg of lead. Details are published.[2]

The **lead excretion ratio (LER)** is calculated by dividing the amount of lead excreted (in µg/24 hours) by the amount of Ca EDTA given (in mg). A ratio >0.60 is considered positive for the LER. Blood for lead and free erythrocyte protoporphyrin should be obtained before chelation. Unstimulated urinary excretion at rates >0.19 µg lead/mg creatinine may also be used to indicate need for chelation therapy.[3]

Serum ferritin or serum iron and total iron binding capacity/transferrin are needed because iron deficiency enhances absorption and toxicity of lead.[2]

Footnotes

1. Markowitz ME and Rosen JF, "Need for the Lead Mobilization Test in Children With Lead Poisoning," *J Pediatr*, 1991, 119(2):305-10.
2. Philip AT and Gerson B, "Lead Poisoning. Part II. Effects and Assay," *Clin Lab Med*, 1994, 14(3):651-70.
3. Berger OG, Gregg DJ, and Succop PA, "Using Unstimulated Lead Excretion to Assess the Need for Chelation in the Treatment of Lead Poisoning," *J Pediatr*, 1990, 116(1):46-51.

References

Cory-Slechta DA, "Lead Exposure During Advanced Age: Alterations in Kinetics and Biochemical Effects," *Toxicol Appl Pharmacol*, 1990, 104(1):67-78.

D'Haese PC, Lamberts LV, Liang L, et al, "Elimination of Matrix and Spectral Interferences in the Measurement of Lead and Cadmium in Urine and Blood by Electrothermal Atomic Absorption Spectrometry With Deuterium Background Correction," *Clin Chem*, 1991, 37(9):1583-8.

Paloucek FP, "Lead Poisoning," *Am Pharm*, 1993, NS33(11):81-8, quiz 88-90.

Lenoxin® *see* Digoxin *on page 546*

Leptilan® *see* Valproic Acid *on page 577*

Librax® *see* Chlordiazepoxide, Blood *on page 542*

Libritabs® *see* Chlordiazepoxide, Blood *on page 542*

Librium® *see* Chlordiazepoxide, Blood *on page 542*

Lidocaine

CPT 80176

Related Information

Amiodarone, Serum *on page 532*
Monoethylglycinexylidide *on page 564*
Tocainide *on page 576*

Synonyms Anestacon®; Baylocaine®; Dalcaine®; Dilocaine®; Duo-Trach®; LidoPen®; Lignocaine; Nervocaine®; Norocaine®; Octocaine®; Xylocaine®

Applies to GX

Abstract Lidocaine is a class IB antiarrhythmic and a local anesthetic. It is extensively metabolized with two active metabolites, monoethylglycinexylidide **(MEGX)** and glycinexylidide **(GX)**.

Specimen Serum or plasma

Container Red top tube, green top (heparin) tube, or lavender top (EDTA) tube

Sampling Time Draw specimens 12 hours after initiating therapy for arrhythmia prophylaxis, then every 24 hours thereafter. Obtain specimens every 12 hours when cardiac or hepatic insufficiency exists.

Collection Avoid collection tubes with stoppers containing the plasticizer, TBEP.

Reference Range Therapeutic: 1.5-5.0 µg/mL (SI: 6.4-21.4 µmol/L), up to 6.0 µg/mL (SI: 25.6 µmol/L) if necessary.

Critical Values At levels >6.0 µg/mL (SI: >25.6 µmol/L), there may be seizure activity. See Table C in the Therapeutic Drug Monitoring/Toxicology/Drugs of Abuse Appendix *on page 583*.

Possible Panic Range Toxic: >8.0 µg/mL (SI: >34.2 µmol/L); levels >15.0 µg/mL (SI: 64.5 µmol/L) are associated with fatalities

Use Monitor therapeutic drug level. Lidocaine is used especially in acute arrhythmias.

Limitations Cross reactions with other drugs occur. Certain blood collection tubes have been shown to lead to falsely low results; see Collection. Serum levels are more useful as a gauge for toxicity rather than for efficacy.

Methodology Enzyme immunoassay (EIA), gas-liquid chromatography (GLC), high performance liquid chromatography (HPLC)

Additional Information

- Half-life: 1.5-2 hours
- Volume of distribution: 1.0-1.5 L/kg
- Protein binding: 60% to 80%

Lidocaine is used in therapy of ventricular but not supraventricular arrhythmias. It is unique as its activity is directed solely at the HIS-Purkinje network without affecting the S-A and A-V nodal conduction. Oral absorption is rapid, but it is a high extraction or "first-pass" drug; therefore lidocaine is not bioavailable when given orally. It is 60% to 80% serum protein bound and lidocaine becomes more highly bound after myocardial infarction. The volume of distribution is also variable. Lidocaine undergoes two compartment distribution. The initial volume is 0.5 L/kg; but as the drug distributes to the tissues, the eventual volume at steady-state is 1.3 L/kg. Volumes are increased in patients with cirrhosis and decreased in patients with congestive heart failure (CHF). Because of the two compartment distribution lidocaine exhibits, its loading dose is unique. The initial dose is based upon the initial volume of distribution. That first dose will distribute quickly into the tissues, therefore, subsequent mini loading doses are needed until the maintenance infusion produces the desired concentration. A high extraction/first-pass drug, lidocaine is totally cleared by the liver. Lidocaine is extensively metabolized. Two metabolites are active, monoethylglycinexylidide (MEGX) and glycinexylidide (GX). Since it is a high extraction drug, it is liver blood flow dependent for clearance; therefore, patients who have CHF, arrhythmias, acute myocardial infarction, or cirrhosis will have a decreased clearance. Impaired renal function should have little impact upon clearance. With clearance and volume being variable, half-life is variable as well.

Adverse effects can be concentration related in many cases. Central nervous system effects such as confusion, dizziness, or blurred vision can be seen at the high end of the therapeutic range. Seizures, cardiovascular depression, tremors, and coma are seen usually at levels >8 µg/mL. Such effects may be due to an accumulation of metabolites, particularly MEGX. Elderly patients with CHF or acute myocardial infarct are at highest risk for these toxicities.

Pharmacokinetic drug interactions occur with drugs that change liver blood flow or plasma protein binding. Beta-blockers and cimetidine decrease liver blood flow, causing increased lidocaine levels. Anticonvulsants, quinidine, and oral contraceptives can change the plasma protein binding of lidocaine, causing toxicity. Other cardiovascular drugs can potentiate the cardiovascular effects of lidocaine when given concomitantly.

Footnotes

1. Burtis CA and Ashwood ER, *Tietz Textbook of Clinical Chemistry*, Philadelphia, PA: WB Saunders Co, 1994, 1122-3.

References

Gumucio CA, Bennie JB, Fernando B, et al, "Plasma Lidocaine Levels During Augmentation Mammoplasty and Suction-Assisted Lipectomy," *Plast Reconstr Surg*, 1989, 84(4):624-7.

Klein J, Fernandes D, Gazarian M, et al, "Simultaneous Determination of Lidocaine, Prilocaine, and Prilocaine Metabolite O-Toluidine in Plasma by High Performance Liquid Chromatography," *J Chromatogr B Biomed Appl*, 1994, 655(1):83-8.

Montamat SC, Cusack BJ, and Vestal RE, "Management of Drug Therapy in the Elderly," *N Engl J Med*, 1989, 321(5):303-9.

Palmisano JM, Meliones JN, Crowley DC, et al, "Lidocaine Toxicity After Subcutaneous Infiltration in Children Undergoing Cardiac Catheterization," *Am J Cardiol*, 1991, 67(7):647-8.

Pieper JA and Johnson KE, "Lidocaine," *Appl Pharmacokinetics*.

Lidocaine Metabolite *see* Monoethylglycinexylidide *on page 564*

LidoPen® *see* Lidocaine *on this page*

Lignocaine *see* Lidocaine *on this page*

Limbitrol® *see* Amitriptyline, Blood *on page 533*

Liquid Lady *see* Cocaine (Cocaine Metabolite), Qualitative, Urine *on page 543*

Liquiprin® *see* Acetaminophen, Serum *on page 530*

Listermint® **With Fluoride** *see* Fluoride, Serum *on page 551*

Lithane® *see* Lithium *on this page*

Lithium

CPT 80178

Related Information

Haloperidol *on page 553*
Sodium, Blood *on page 199*
Theophylline *on page 575*
Thyroid Stimulating Hormone *on page 204*
Thyroxine *on page 206*
Verapamil *on page 578*

Synonyms Cibalith-S®; Eskalith®; Lithane®; Lithobid®; Lithonate®; Lithotabs®; PFI-Lith®; Phasal®

Abstract Lithium is used in the treatment of mania and particularly for manic-depressive psychosis. It should be monitored.

Aftercare Follow urine osmolality, ECGs, thyroid profile, BUN, creatinine, and sodium. Avoid sodium depletion.

Specimen Serum

Container Red top tube

Sampling Time Draw sample 12 hours after the last dose. This ensures that the concentration is not representing the initial distribution phase. It correlates with most of the published data.

Storage Instructions Refrigerate a minimum of 2 mL serum. Serum specimens are stable for 24 hours at room temperature. Separate serum immediately.

Causes for Rejection Specimen collected in tube containing lithium heparin, hemolysis

Reference Range Therapeutic: 0.6-1.2 mEq/L (SI: 0.6-1.2 mmol/L), for acute mania; 0.8-1.0 mEq/L (SI: 0.8-1.0 mmol/L) for protection against future episodes in most patients with bipolar disorder. A higher rate of relapse is described in subjects who are maintained at levels <0.4 mEq/L (SI: 0.4 mmol/L).[1]

Possible Panic Range Toxic: >1.5 mEq/L (SI: >1.5 mmol/L). Toxicity can become serious when levels rise to levels ≥2.0 mEq/L (SI: ≥2.0 mmol/L). Levels >4.0 mEq/L (SI: >4.0 mmol/L) are associated with coma, death. A narrow therapeutic index exists for lithium.[2] See table.

Lithium (Acute Ingestion)

Serum Level	Symptoms
1.5-2.5 mEq/L	Polyuria, blurred vision, weakness, lethargy, dizziness, increased reflexes, fasiculations
2.5-3.0 mEq/L	Myoclonic twitching, incontinence, stupor, restlessness, coma
>3.0 mEq/L	Seizures, hypotension, cardiac arrhythmias

Use Monitor therapeutic drug level, evaluate coma

Limitations Lithium toxicity, including severe neurotoxic effects, can occur with normal serum lithium levels. Instances of acute intoxication may be accompanied by high serum lithium levels without clinical evidence of neurotoxic effects. Lithium penetrates neurons slowly.[3] Thiazides can cause significant rise in serum lithium.

Methodology Flame photometry, atomic absorption spectrophotometry (AA), ion-selective electrode (ISE). Instruments have recently been evaluated.[4]

Additional Information
- Half-life: 18-24 hours
- Volume of distribution: 0.7-1.0 L/kg
- Protein binding: 0%

Lithium as lithium carbonate or citrate is used as a psychoactive agent in the treatment of manic depressive disorders. These oral products are completely absorbed and are completely bioavailable. It takes 1-2 hours and 4-5 hours for the regular versus the sustained release forms to reach their maximum concentration. Like lidocaine, lithium has two compartments. Concentrations measured during the initial phase do not correlate with efficacy or toxicity. Lithium is cleared by the kidney. It is filtered at the glomerulus and actively reabsorbed at the proximal tubule much like sodium and other electrolytes and vitamins. This is important for potential drug and food interactions. The clearance of lithium is increased in pregnancy and when sodium supplements are given. The clearance is decreased in renal impairment, dehydration, and when patients are hyponatremic. Patients should try to maintain a consistent intake of sodium while on this drug.

Acute lithium toxicity is neuro- and nephrotoxic. Concentration-related side effects include weakness, muscle weakness, tremor, and confusion. Gastrointestinal effects like nausea and vomiting can be lessened if given an extended release product.

There are many drugs that can alter the clearance of lithium. Drugs that decrease clearance of lithium include thiazide diuretics, ACE inhibitors, and some nonsteroidal anti-inflammatory agents. Drugs that can increase the clearance of lithium and decrease the concentration are acetazolamide, theophylline, caffeine, and osmotic diuretics. Lithium therapy demands daily monitoring of serum lithium levels until the proper dose schedule is determined.

A fully developed case of intoxication is characterized by coma to semi-coma, rigidity, hyperactive reflexes and seizures at times. There is a high incidence of pulmonary complications. It is advisable to perform periodic plasma sodium determinations. Low plasma sodium levels are associated with lithium retention; high levels with lithium elimination. Varying degrees of nephrogenic diabetes insipidus have been reported to occur

in 33% of lithium treated patients. Lithium significantly inhibits antidiuretic-hormone-induced water transport in kidney. Lithium interferes with solute and water absorption from the gastrointestinal system producing nausea, vomiting, diarrhea, and abdominal pain. These symptoms may occur at any time, at any serum level. They most commonly occur during early treatment stages and usually clear spontaneously or by adjustment of dosage. Chronic lithium administration has a goitrogenic effect on 4% of lithium-treated patients, with or without hypothyroidism. In general, lithium administration results in slightly decreased serum T_4 levels and transiently elevated levels of TSH in nearly 33% of these patients. Lithium affects the cardiac conduction system by incomplete substitution for other cations, especially sodium and potassium. These electrolyte changes account for the usually unimportant and reversible T-wave depressions observed in 10% to 20% of patients on lithium therapy. Other relevant interactions include possible effects upon calcium, glucose, magnesium, potassium, bicarbonate, BUN, and bromide levels, leukopenia, and thrombocytopenia.

Footnotes
1. Gelenberg AJ, Kane JM, Keller MB, et al, "Comparison of Standard and Low Serum Levels of Lithium for Maintenance Treatment of Bipolar Disorder," *N Engl J Med*, 1989, 321(22):1489-93.
2. Ritschel WA, "Therapeutic Drug Monitoring," *Clinical Chemistry Theory, Analysis, and Correlation*, Kaplan LA and Pesce AJ, eds, St Louis, MO: Mosby-Year Book Inc, 1989, 795-807.
3. Stern R, "Lithium in the Treatment of Mood Disorders," *N Engl J Med*, 1995, 332(2):127-8.
4. Sampson M, Ruddel M, and Elin RJ, "Lithium Determinations Evaluated in Eight Analyzers," *Clin Chem*, 1994, 40(6):869-72.

References
Chamberlain S, Hahn PM, Casson P, et al, "Effect of Menstrual Cycle Phase and Oral Contraceptive Use on Serum Lithium Levels After a Loading Dose of Lithium in Normal Women," *Am J Psychiatry*, 1990, 147(7):907-9.
De Maio D, Buffa G, Riva M, et al, "Lithium Ratio, Phospholipids and the Incidence of Side Effects," *Prog Neuropsychopharmacol Biol Psychiatry*, 1994, 18(2):285-93.
Gangadhar B, Subnash MN, Umapathy C, et al, "Lithium Toxicity at Therapeutic Serum Levels," *Br J Psychiatry*, 1993, 163:695.
Groleau G, "Lithium Toxicity," *Emerg Med Clin North Am*, 1994, 12(2):511-31.
Harvey NS and Merriman S, "Review of Clinically Important Drug Interactions With Lithium," *Drug Saf*, 1994, 10(6):455-63.
Krishel S and Jackimczyk K, "Cyclic Antidepressants, Lithium, and Neuroleptic Agents. Pharmacology and Toxicology," *Emerg Med Clin North Am*, 1991, 9(1):53-86.
Manji HK, Hsiao JK, Risby ED, et al, "The Mechanisms of Action of Lithium. I. Effects on Serotoninergic and Noradrenergic Systems in Normal Subjects," *Arch Gen Psychiatry*, 1991, 48(6):505-12.
Murray RL, "Lithium," *Clinical Chemistry - Theory Analysis, and Correlation*, 2nd ed, Kaplan LA and Pesce AJ, eds, St Louis, MO: Mosby-Year Book Inc, 1989, 1108-10.
Price LH and Heninger GR, "Lithium in the Treatment of Mood Disorders," *N Engl J Med*, 1994, 331(9):591-8.
Schweyen DH, Sporka MC, and Burnakis TG, "Evaluation of Serum Lithium Concentration Determinations," *Am J Hosp Pharm*, 1991, 48(7):1536-7.

Lithobid® see Lithium *on previous page*

Lithonate® see Lithium *on previous page*

Lithotabs® see Lithium *on previous page*

l-Methamphetamine see Methamphetamine, Qualitative, Urine *on page 562*

Loads see Glutethimide *on page 553*

Lotusate® see Barbiturates, Quantitative, Blood *on page 537*

Loxapine see Amoxapine, Blood *on page 533*

Lude® see Methaqualone *on page 562*

Ludes see Methaqualone *on page 562*

Ludiomil® see Maprotiline *on this page*

Luminal® see Phenobarbital, Blood *on page 568*

Luminal® see Barbiturates, Quantitative, Blood *on page 537*

Luride® see Fluoride, Serum *on page 551*

Luride® Lozi-Tab® see Fluoride, Serum *on page 551*

Luride®-SF Lozi-Tab® see Fluoride, Serum *on page 551*

Lyphocin® see Vancomycin *on page 578*

Magnum® see Caffeine, Blood *on page 539*

Majsolin® see Primidone *on page 570*

Maprotiline

CPT 80299

Related Information

Antidepressants, Cyclic *on page 535*

Synonyms Ludiomil®

Abstract Maprotiline is a tetracyclic antidepressant with a long half-life.

Specimen Serum

Container Red top tube

Sampling Time Peak serum values are reached in 12 hours and steady-state is achieved in 20-24 days; half-life is 27-58 hours.

(Continued)

Maprotiline *(Continued)*

Storage Instructions Separate serum from clot and refrigerate.

Reference Range 200-600 ng/mL (SI: 721-2163 nmol/L)

Critical Values >1000 ng/mL (SI: >3605 nmol/L)

Use Evaluate toxicity and therapeutic drug monitoring

Methodology High performance liquid chromatography (HPLC), gas chromatography (GC)

Additional Information
- Half-life: 25-30 hours
- Volume of distribution: 15-35 L/kg
- Protein binding: 80% to 90%

Maprotiline is a tetracyclic antidepressant prescribed for depression, chronic schizophrenia, idiopathic pain, and potentially for drug abuse withdrawal. It is metabolized to an active metabolite, desmethyl maprotiline. Maprotiline is often used in patients who do not respond to tricyclics. The drug is taken orally at an average adult dose of 75-300 mg/day (50-75 mg/day in elderly patients). Maprotiline is a very potent inhibitor of the reuptake of norepinephrine to the presynaptic nerve terminal. The drug possesses moderate anticholinergic activity and cardiovascular toxicity. It also may lower seizure control. It has a higher incidence of seizures than tricyclic antidepressants. It should not be given in combination with MAO inhibitor.[1] Overdoses (coma, convulsions, dysrhythmias, hypotension) are exacerbated by its long half-life.

Footnotes

1. Craig CR and Stitzel RE, *Modern Pharmacology*, 3rd ed, Boston, MA: Little, Brown and Co, 1990, 479-81.

References

Drebit R, Baker GB, and Dewhurst WG, "Determination of Maprotiline and Desmethylmaprotiline in Plasma and Urine by Gas Chromatography With Nitrogen-Phosphorus Detection," *J Chromatogr*, 1988, 432:334-9.

Fukuchi H, Kitaura T, Miyake K, et al, "Association Between Dosage and Serum Concentration of Antidepressants," *Clin Pharm*, 1990, 9(1):45-9.

Tollefson GD, Montaque-Clouse J, Lesan T, et al, "Pharmacokinetic Properties of Maprotiline in Geriatric Depression," *J Clin Psychopharmacol*, 1989, 9(4):313-5.

Yamagami S and Soejima K, "Effect of Maprotiline Combined With Conventional Neuroleptics Against Negative Symptoms of Chronic Schizophrenia," *Drugs Exp Clin Res*, 1989, 15(4):171-6.

Marijuana *see* Cannabinoids (Marijuana Metabolites), Qualitative, Urine *on page 539*

Max Alert Magnum® *see* Caffeine, Blood *on page 539*

MDMA *see* Methamphetamine, Qualitative, Urine *on page 562*

Measurin® *see* Salicylate *on page 573*

Mebaral® *see* Methylphenobarbital *on page 563*

Mebaral® *see* Barbiturates, Quantitative, Blood *on page 537*

Meda-Cap® *see* Acetaminophen, Serum *on page 530*

Medical Legal Specimens *see* Chain-of-Custody Protocol *on page 542*

MEGX *see* Monoethylglycinexylidide *on page 564*

Mellaril® *see* Phenothiazines, Serum *on page 568*

Meperidine, Blood or Urine

CPT 83925

Related Information

Chain-of-Custody Protocol *on page 542*

Synonyms Centralgine®; Demerol®; Dolantin®; Dolantina®; Dolantine®; Dolosal®; Isonipecaine Hydrochloride; Pethidine Hydrochloride

Test Commonly Includes This test is included in the comprehensive Urine Drug Screen.

Abstract Meperidine is a synthetic narcotic analgesic with about one-tenth the potency of morphine. It is a drug of abuse.

Specimen Serum or urine

Container Red top tube, plastic urine container

Sampling Time Trough for serum

Storage Instructions Refrigerate

Special Instructions If forensic, use chain-of-custody protocol and form. See test listing Chain-of-Custody Protocol *on page 542* and the Therapeutic Drug Monitoring/Toxicology/Drugs of Abuse Appendix *on page 581*. When evaluating drug of abuse, order Toxicology Drug Screen, Blood.

Reference Range Serum: 400-700 ng/mL (SI: 1.6-2.8 µmol/L); urine: negative when not on therapy. Patients with therapeutic blood levels can have up to 10 µg/mL in urine.

Use Evaluate toxicity; detect an abused drug. Meperidine is a synthetic morphine-like compound used in the management of moderate to severe pain and as an adjunct to anesthesia and preoperative sedation.

Limitations Therapeutic levels not detected by enzyme-multiplied immunoassay technique (EMIT), thin-layer chromatography, and enzyme immunoassay. Use HPLC methods to detect therapeutic concentrations.

Methodology Thin-layer chromatography (TLC) and enzyme immunoassay (EIA); gas chromatography (GC), high performance liquid chromatography (HPLC)

Additional Information
- Half-life: 2-4 hours
- Volume of distribution: 3-4 L/kg
- Protein binding: 40% to 60%

Analgesic effects after oral ingestion or I.M. injection peak in 1 hour. Adverse effects include tachycardia, CNS and respiratory depression, nausea and vomiting, hypotension, bradycardia, miosis, increased intracranial pressure, and physical and psychological dependence. When evaluating therapeutic levels, order Meperidine, Blood.

References

Belgrade MJ, Ling LJ, Schleevogt MB, et al, "Comparison of Single-Dose Meperidine, Butorphanol, and Dihydroergotamine in the Treatment of Vascular Headache," *Neurology*, 1989, 39(4):590-2.

Johnson MD, Hurley RJ, Gilbertson LI, et al, "Continuous Microcatheter Spinal Anesthesia With Subarachnoid Meperidine for Labor and Delivery," *Anesth Analg*, 1990, 70(6):658-61.

Mephenytoin

CPT 80299

Related Information

Phenytoin *on page 569*

Synonyms Mesantoin®; Methoin; Methylphenylethylhydantoin; Phenantoin; Sedantoinal®

Applies to 5-Phenyl-5-Ethylhydantoin (Nirvanol®)

Abstract Mephenytoin has a pharmacologic effect similar to that of phenytoin. Mephenytoin has serious toxicity but less dose-related effects compared to phenytoin.

Specimen Serum

Container Red top tube

Sampling Time Consistent sampling time

Reference Range 25-40 µg/mL for the sum of the parent drug and 5-phenyl-5-ethylhydantoin metabolite, which is usually present at a higher level than the parent compound

Possible Panic Range Toxic level about 50 µg/mL (SI: 230 µmol/L). See Table A in the Therapeutic Drug Monitoring/Toxicology/Drugs of Abuse Appendix *on page 582*.

Use Monitor for compliance, efficacy, and possible toxicity. Mephenytoin may be suited for patients who respond to phenytoin but who cannot tolerate dose-related side effects.

Limitations Unlike phenytoin, cognitive side effects, cerebellar symptoms, gingival hypertrophy, and hirsutism do not occur as commonly with increasing dosage. The main active metabolite, 5-ethyl-5-phenylhydantoin, is a biologically active anticonvulsant with a half-life of 100 hours.

Methodology Gas chromatography (GC)

Additional Information
- Half-life: parent compound: 8 hours, metabolite: >100 hours
- Protein binding: 20% to 50%

Mephenytoin, like phenytoin, has zero-order kinetics so that small changes in dosage may produce large changes in clinical response. Acute overdosage results in sedation and eventually coma. Most adverse effects are not dose-related, but are due to the accumulation of arene-oxide intermediates. They include rash, hepatotoxicity, blood dyscrasias, systemic lupus erythematosus, periarteritis nodosa, and fever. The drug is considered more highly toxic than other hydantoins.

Test interactions include increased serum alkaline phosphatase and decreased calcium.

References

Engel J, *Seizures and Epilepsy*, Contemporary Neurology Series, Philadelphia, PA: FA Davis Co, 1989.

Kupferberg HJ, "Other Hydantoins: Mephenytoin and Ethotoin," *Antiepileptic Drugs*, 3rd ed, Levy RH, Dreifuss FE, Mattson RH, et al, eds, New York, NY: Raven Press, 1989, 257-65.

Mephobarb *see* Barbiturates, Qualitative, Urine *on page 537*

Mephobarbital *see* Methylphenobarbital *on page 563*

Mephobarbital *see* Barbiturates, Quantitative, Blood *on page 537*

Mephobarbitone *see* Methylphenobarbital *on page 563*

Meprobamate

CPT 83805

Synonyms Equagesic®; Equanil®; Meprospan®; Miltown®; Neuramate®; Tenavoid®

Abstract Meprobamate is a sedative-anxiolytic, producing effects similar to those of the benzodiazepines and barbiturates.

Specimen Serum

Container Red top tube

Reference Range Sedative dose: 6-12 µg/mL (SI: 28-55 µmol/L)

Critical Values Toxic: >60 µg/mL (SI: >275 µmol/L)

Possible Panic Range Coma is associated with levels >70 µg/mL (SI: >321 µmol/L); fatalities can occur at >142 µg/mL (SI: >650 µmol/L); lethal: 200 µg/mL (SI: 916 µmol/L)

Use Therapeutic monitoring and toxicity assessment. Meprobamate is a propanediol carbamate sedative and tranquilizer, having pharmacological effects similar to barbiturates. Respiratory depression, coma, and cardiovascular collapse characterize overdosage.

Methodology Gas-liquid chromatography (GLC)

Additional Information
- Half-life: 6-15 hours
- Volume of distribution: 0.5-1.0 L/kg

Meprobamate is well absorbed from the gastrointestinal tract and reaches its peak concentration in 2-3 hours. It may also be detected in urine or gastric juice.

References

Bertran F, de la Sayette V, Lacotte J, et al, "Acute Rhabdomyolysis and Meprobamate Poisoning," *Therapie*, 1992, 47(5):444.

Dennison J, Edwards JN, and Volans GN, "Meprobamate Overdosage," *Hum Toxicol*, 1985, 4(2):215-7.

Kintz P and Mangin P, "Determination of Meprobamate in Human Plasma, Urine, and Hair by Gas Chromatography and Electron Impact Mass Spectrometry," *J Anal Toxicol*, 1993, 17(7):408-10.

Lambert WE, De Leenheer AP, Van Bocxlaer JF, et al, "Meprobamate Intoxication: Rare and Difficult to Find," *J Toxicol Clin Toxicol*, 1992, 30(4):683-4.

Trenque T, Lamiable D, Millart H, et al, "Gas Chromatographic Determination of Meprobamate in Human Plasma," *J Chromatogr*, 1993, 615(2):343-6.

Meprospan® see Meprobamate *on previous page*

Mercury, Blood

CPT 83825

Related Information

Fat, Urine *on page 635*

Heavy Metal Screen, Blood *on page 554*

Heavy Metal Screen, Urine *on page 554*

Synonyms Hg, Blood; Organic Mercury

Applies to Hair Analysis

Abstract This metal is toxic in any of its three forms: elemental, inorganic, and organic. The mode of entry into the body varies among the three forms. **Blood** analysis for mercury is used principally for evaluation of toxicity from **organic** mercury. Organic mercury is found in wood preservatives, paints, fungicides, cosmetics, foods and seeds. The mercury catastrophe in Minamata Bay, Japan, involved methyl mercury from methylation of mercuric salt wastes.

Specimen Whole blood

Container Special metal-free EDTA tube

Collection See Blood Collection Methods for Trace Elements in the Trace Elements Introduction *on page 585*.

Special Instructions Whole blood is analyzed.

Reference Range Whole blood: <0.06 µg/mL (SI: 0.3 nmol/L)

Critical Values 0.6-60.0 µg/L (SI: 3-300 nmol/L)

Possible Panic Range >100.0 µg/L (SI: 500 nmol/L)

Use Evaluate for mercury toxicity, neurological findings related to organic mercurials, inhalation of mercury vapors. Such vapors are efficiently absorbed. Useful principally for organic mercury.

Limitations Methyl mercury must be measured in whole blood or erythrocytes. Inorganic mercury is best evaluated by urine mercury levels.

Methodology Electrothermal atomic absorption (AA), gold electrode deposition, gas chromatography (GC)

Additional Information Organic methyl mercury is a new important environmental mercurial contaminant. It was discovered that inorganic mercurial industrial wastes dumped into Minimata Bay (Japan) could be organified by plankton and incorporated into fish, and thus, the human food chain. Ingestion of mercury-laden fish leads to severe neurologic deficits. Inhalation of mercury vapors can lead to pneumonitis. Inorganic mercurials deposit in kidneys, liver, heart, striated muscle, marrow, brain, and lungs. Gastrointestinal symptoms, stomatitis, colitis, anemia, and peripheral neuritis can relate to mercury poisoning. Ingestion of inorganic mercurials results in a serious medical emergency. Mercury exposure from a brand of interior latex paint has been described.[1] Half-life of inorganic mercury is 24 days and of methyl mercury (organic mercury) is 54 days. Long-term consequences of methylmercury poisoning from pork are described.[2] Hair analysis can be used for poisoning or exposure. It should be clean and clipped as close to the scalp as possible. Mercurial salts can cause renal failure.

Footnotes

1. Agocs MM, Etzel RA, Parrish RG, et al, "Mercury Exposure From Interior Latex Paint," *N Engl J Med*, 1990, 323(16):1096-101.
2. Davis LE, Kornfeld M, Mooney HS, et al, "Methylmercury Poisoning: Long-Term Clinical, Radiological, Toxicological, and Pathological Studies of an Affected Family," *Ann Neurol*, 1994, 35(6):680-8.

References

Florentine MJ and San Filippo DJ 2nd, "Elemental Mercury Poisoning," *Clin Pharm*, 1991, 10(3):213-21.

Graef JW, "Heavy Metal Poisoning," *Harrison's Principles of Internal Medicine*, 13th ed, Isselbacher KJ, Braunwald E, Wilson JD, et al, eds, New York, NY: McGraw-Hill Inc, 1994, 2461-6.

Mason HJ and Calder IM, "The Correction of Mercury Concentrations in Untimed, Random Samples," *Occup Environ Med*, 1994, 51(4):287.

Snapp KR, Boyer DB, Peterson LC, et al, "The Contribution of Dental Amalgam to Mercury in Blood," *J Dent Res*, 1989, 68(5):780-5.

Mercury, Urine

CPT 83825

Related Information

Fat, Urine *on page 635*

Heavy Metal Screen, Blood *on page 554*

Heavy Metal Screen, Urine *on page 554*

Urine Collection, 24-Hour *on page 30*

Synonyms Hg, Urine

Abstract This metal is toxic in inorganic salt and elemental and organic forms. **Urine mercury** is used for evaluation of **inorganic** forms. Use of elemental mercury includes thermometers and other instruments, some batteries and dental amalgams. Mercuric salts are present in some cathartics such as calomel, topically applied medicines, plastics, and some foods.

Specimen 24-hour urine

Container Plastic (preferably polyethylene) acid-washed container, no preservative

Storage Instructions Store in special metal-free container

Reference Range 10-50 µg/24 hours (SI: 0.05-0.25 µmol/day)

Possible Panic Range >100 µg/24 hours (SI: >0.50 µmol/day); >150 µg/L (0.7 µmol/L). Symptoms are found with levels >600 µg/L (>3 µmol/L).

Use Inorganic mercury toxicity is best evaluated by urine mercury levels. Neurologic sequelae of mercury poisoning include intention tremor and clinical features which led to the expression "mad as a hatter," applied to workers making felt hats who were exposed to mercury vapor and mercuric salts.

Limitations Organic mercury is found mostly in red cells; see listing Mercury, Blood *on page 561*. Urine mercury is not useful for organic mercury poisoning.

Methodology Electrothermal atomic absorption (AA), gold electrode deposition, gas chromatography (GC)

Additional Information
- Half-life of inorganic mercury: about 20-25 days

Industrial and agricultural exposure usually includes inhalation of vapor, which is efficiently absorbed, oxidized to mercuric form and excreted in urine and feces. Ingestion is the major route for mercuric salts, with urine excretion.

References

Aikoh H and Shibahara T, "Determination of Mercury Levels in Human Urine and Blood by Ultraviolet-Visible Spectrophotometry," *Analyst*, 1993, 118(10):1329-32.

Gothe CJ, Langworth S, Carleson R, et al, "Biological Monitoring of Exposure to Metallic Mercury," *J Toxicol Clin Toxicol*, 1985, 23(4-6):381-9.

Graef JW, "Heavy Metal Poisoning," *Harrison's Principles of Internal Medicine*, 13th ed, Isselbacher KJ, Braunwald E, Wilson JD, et al, eds, New York, NY: McGraw-Hill Inc, 1994, 2461-6.

Piikivi L and Ruokonen A, "Renal Function and Long-Term Low Mercury Vapor Exposure," *Arch Environ Health*, 1989, 44(3):146-9.

Mesantoin® see Mephenytoin *on previous page*

Mesoridazine see Phenothiazines, Serum *on page 568*

Metabolites of Primidone see Primidone *on page 570*

Metals, Blood see Heavy Metal Screen, Blood *on page 554*

Metal Screen see Heavy Metal Screen, Urine *on page 554*

Metals, Toxic see Heavy Metal Screen, Urine *on page 554*

Metasedin® see Methadone, Urine *on this page*

"Meth" see Methamphetamine, Qualitative, Urine *on next page*

Methadone, Urine

CPT 83840

Related Information

Chain-of-Custody Protocol *on page 542*

Drugs of Abuse Testing, Urine *on page 548*

Synonyms Dolophine®; Eptadone®; Metasedin®; Physeptone®; Symoron®

(Continued)

Methadone, Urine *(Continued)*

Abstract This drug is a synthetic opiate agonist used during World War II as a morphine substitute. It is used for detoxification of opiate addicts. It is a drug of abuse.

Specimen Urine

Storage Instructions Refrigerate

Special Instructions If forensic, use chain-of-custody protocol and form. See test listing Chain-of-Custody Protocol *on page 542* and the Therapeutic Drug Monitoring/Toxicology/Drugs of Abuse Appendix *on page 581*.

Reference Range Negative (less than cutoff); when used therapeutically for pain, plasma levels are in the range of 0.10-0.40 µg/mL (SI: 0.32-1.29 µmol/L).

Critical Values Cutoff for urine screening: 300 ng/mL; confirmation: 200 ng/mL

Use Evaluate toxicity and detection as drug of abuse. Methadone is a drug of abuse and is included in most drug-of-abuse screening panels.

Limitations Patients on methadone maintenance protocols will test above cutoff in urine drug screens.

Methodology Thin-layer chromatography (TLC) and enzyme immunoassay (EIA) for screening; gas chromatography/mass spectrometry (GC/MS) for confirmation

Additional Information
- Half-life: 15-25 hours
- Volume of distribution: 4-6 L/kg
- Protein binding: 85% to 95%

Methadone is a synthetic diphenylheptane derivative. It produces less sedation and euphoria than morphine and its effects are cumulative. Methadone is highly addictive, but the withdrawal symptoms are less intense. This drug is used in the management of severe pain and in narcotic detoxification maintenance programs. Onset of action is 30-60 minutes after oral dose and 10-20 minutes following parenteral administration. Adverse effects include marked sedation after repeated administration, CNS and respiratory depression, nausea and vomiting, bradycardia, hypotension, increased intracranial pressure, miosis, antidiuretic hormone release, and physical and psychological dependence.

References

Calsyn DA, Saxon AJ, and Barndt DC, "Urine Screening Practices in Methadone Maintenance Clinics. A Survey of How the Results Are Used," *J Nerv Ment Dis*, 1991, 179(4):222-7.

Gayle MO, Ryan CA, and Nazarali S, "Unusual Cause of Methadone Poisoning," *Acta Paediatr Scand*, 1991, 80(4):486-7.

Molyneux E, Ahern R, and Baldwin B, "Accidental Ingestion of Methadone," *BMJ*, 1991, 303(6807):922-3.

Schmidt N, Brune K, Sittl R, et al, "Rapid Determination of Methadone in Plasma, Cerebrospinal Fluid, and Urine by Gas Chromatography and Its Application to Routine Drug Monitoring," *Pharm Res*, 1993, 10(3):441-4.

Wolff K, Hay AW, and Raistrick D, "Plasma Methadone Measurements and Their Role in Methadone Detoxification Programs," *Clin Chem*, 1992, 38(3):420-5.

Wolff K, Sanderson M, Hay AW, et al, "Methadone Concentrations in Plasma and Their Relationship to Drug Dosage," *Clin Chem*, 1991, 37(2):205-9.

Wu CH and Henry JA, "Deaths of Heroin Addicts Starting on Methadone Maintenance," *Lancet*, 1990, 335(8686):424.

Methaminodiazepoxide Hydrochloride *see* Chlordiazepoxide, Blood *on page 542*

Methampex® *see* Methamphetamine, Qualitative, Urine *on this page*

Methamphetamine, Qualitative, Urine

CPT 80101 (screen); 80102 (confirmation)

Related Information

Amphetamine, Qualitative, Urine *on page 534*
Chain-of-Custody Protocol *on page 542*
Drugs of Abuse Testing, Urine *on page 548*

Synonyms "Crank"; Crystal; Desoxyephedrine Hydrochloride; Desoxyn®; Doe; "Ice"; "Meth"; Methampex®; Methedrine®; Speed

Applies to Amphetamines, Urine; Chlorpromazine; d-Methamphetamine; l-Methamphetamine; MDMA; Methylenedioxymethamphetamine; Phentermine; Phenylpropanolamine; Pseudoephedrine; Ranitidine

Test Commonly Includes Amphetamine, methamphetamine

Abstract The d-isomer of this drug is used therapeutically as an anorectic agent and for treatment of hyperactive children. It is also a drug of abuse.

Specimen Random urine

Collection If forensic, observe precautions.

Storage Instructions Refrigerate

Causes for Rejection If forensic, failure to meet temperature check and reasonable urine creatinine concentration

Special Instructions If forensic, use chain-of-custody protocol and form. See test listing Chain-of-Custody Protocol *on page 542* and the Therapeutic Drug Monitoring/Toxicology/Drugs of Abuse Appendix *on page 581*.

Reference Range Negative (less than cutoff); therapeutic, serum: 20-30 ng/mL

Critical Values Cutoff: screen: 1000 ng/mL; confirmation: 500 ng/mL

Use Evaluate for drug abuse, assess toxicity

Limitations Screening test may give false-positives with common cold and antiallergy medications. Qualitative results only (positive or negative); *vide infra*.

Methodology Screening: enzyme immunoassay (EIA), fluorescence polarization immunoassay (FPIA), thin-layer chromatography (TLC); confirmation: gas chromatography/mass spectrometry (GC/MS), gas-liquid chromatography (GLC), high performance liquid chromatography (HPLC)

Additional Information
- Half-life: 10-30 hours
- Volume of distribution: 3-4 L/kg
- Protein binding: 10% to 40%

The most abused drug in this class is d-methamphetamine. The optical isomer, l-methamphetamine, has less pronounced central effects and is used as a nasal decongestant in Vicks Inhaler® (legal, over-the-counter). Amphetamine isomers are present in Dexedrine® and Benzedrine®. These drugs are self-administered orally, I.V., or by smoking. It can be detected in urine within 3 hours of use. The parent drugs are the substances detected by the screening tests. Over-the-counter medication for colds and allergies (Contac®, Dimetapp®, Sine-Off®, Sudafed®) contain phenylpropanolamine or pseudoephedrine which give a positive EIA screening test when the polyclonal antibody is used. This antibody also detects methylenedioxymethamphetamine (MDMA), a controlled substance classed as an hallucinogen and "designer" drug.[1] With the monoclonal EIA test, the above medications are not detected, but phentermine (Adipex®, Fastin®), ranitidine (Zantac®), and chlorpromazine (Thorazine®) give a positive test. Confirmation by GC/MS rules out these false-positives. In order to rule out the false-positive given by l-methamphetamine (legal nasal decongestant), a chiral column or procedure, which separates the "l" and "d" isomers, must be used in the GC/MS confirmation. See Amphetamines, Qualitative, Urine *on page 534* for a discussion of physiological effects.

Methamphetamine is a sympathomimetic amine chemically related to ephedrine and amphetamine. It is used in the management of obesity, to treat certain depressive reactions, and as adjunctive therapy for narcolepsy, epilepsy, attention deficit disorders, and postencephalitic parkinsonism. Methamphetamine is readily absorbed by the GI tract and the effects last from 6-12 hours. Adverse effects include tremor, insomnia, nervousness, anxiety, euphoria or dysphoria, hyper- or hypotension, arrhythmias, circulatory collapse, and nausea and vomiting.

Footnotes

1. Bost RD, "3,4-Methylenedioxymethamphetamine (MDMA) and Other Amphetamine Derivatives," *J Forensic Sci*, 1988, 33(2):576-87.

References

DePace A, Verebey K, and ElSohly M, "Capillary Gas-Liquid Chromatography Separation of Phenethylamines in Amphetamine-Positive Urine Samples," *J Forensic Sci*, 1990, 35(6):1431-5.

Derlet RW and Heischober B, "Methamphetamine. Stimulant of the 1990s?" *West J Med*, 1990, 153(6):625-8.

Ellenhorn MJ and Barceloux DG, "Amphetamines," *Medical Toxicology*, New York, NY: Elsevier, 1988, 625-42.

Gan BK, Baugh D, Liu RH, et al, "Simultaneous Analysis of Amphetamine, Methamphetamine, and 3,4-Methylenedioxymethamphetamine (MDMA) in Urine Samples by Solid-Phase Extraction, Derivatization, and Gas Chromatography/Mass Spectrometry," *J Forensic Sci*, 1991, 36(5):1331-41.

Grinstead GF, "Ranitidine and High Concentrations of Phenylpropanolamine Cross React in the EMIT Monoclonal Amphetamine/Methamphetamine Assay," *Clin Chem*, 1989, 35(9):1998-9.

Methanol *see* Volatile Screen *on page 579*

Methaqualone

CPT 80101 (screen); 80102 (confirmation)

Related Information

Chain-of-Custody Protocol *on page 542*
Drugs of Abuse Testing, Urine *on page 548*

Synonyms Lude®; Ludes

Abstract This drug is a sedative-hypnotic but is currently a DEA schedule II drug. It is a drug of abuse. Taken off U.S. market in 1984.

Specimen Serum, urine

Container Red top tube, plastic urine container

Special Instructions If forensic, use chain-of-custody protocol and form. See test listing Chain-of-Custody Protocol *on page 542* and the Therapeutic Drug Monitoring/Toxicology/Drugs of Abuse Appendix *on page 581*.

Reference Range Urine: negative (less than cutoff); serum: 2-3 µg/mL (SI: 8-12 nmol/L)

Critical Values Cutoff for urine: screen: 300 ng/mL; confirmation: 200 ng/mL

Possible Panic Range Serum values >8 µg/mL (SI: >32 nmol/L) associated with unconsciousness; toxic: >10 µg/mL (SI: >40 nmol/L)

Use Evaluate for toxicity, evaluate for drug abuse

Methodology Immunoassay, gas-liquid chromatography (GLC), UV spectrophotometry, fluorometry; *vida infra*

Additional Information
- Half-life: 10-40 hours
- Volume of distribution: 5-7 L/kg
- Protein binding: 70% to 90%

Methaqualone is a nonbarbiturate sedative-hypnotic. It is rapidly absorbed from the GI tract. Hyperexcitability, coma, and cardiovascular and respiratory depression characterize overdosage. It is a common drug of abuse, and "street" preparations may be adulterated with other pharmacoactive substances. It is extensively metabolized and screening methods must detect metabolites. Enzyme-multiplied immunoassay technique (EMIT) detects four of the most common metabolites.

References
Baselt RC and Cravey RH, *Disposition of Toxic Drugs and Chemicals in Man*, 3rd ed, Chicago, IL: Year Book Medical Publishers Inc, 1989, 524-7.

Beebe DK and Walley E, "Substance Abuse: The Designer Drugs," *Am Fam Physician*, 1991, 43(5):1689-98.

Buckner JC and Mandell W, "Risk Factors for Depressive Symptomatology in a Drug Using Population," *Am J Public Health*, 1990, 80(5):580-5.

Metharbital *see* Barbiturates, Quantitative, Blood *on page 537*

Methedrine® *see* Methamphetamine, Qualitative, Urine *on previous page*

Methoin *see* Mephenytoin *on page 560*

Methotrexate

CPT 80299

Synonyms Amethopterin; Folex®; Mexate®; MTX; Rheumatrex®

Applies to Cerebrospinal Fluid Methotrexate; Citrovorum Factor

Abstract This is a widely used anticancer drug acting as an antimetabolite in DNA synthesis. It is also used for some autoimmune diseases, such as rheumatoid arthritis. It should be monitored in patients receiving high-dose therapy (>100 mg/m²). It is extremely toxic.

Specimen Serum or plasma

Container Red top tube, green top (heparin) tube, or lavender top (EDTA) tube

Sampling Time Will vary according to dosing protocol. Time to peak serum concentration: oral: within 1-2 hours; parenteral: within 30-60 minutes

Storage Instructions Separate and freeze.

Special Instructions Advise laboratory if patient is also on trimethoprim.

Reference Range Therapeutic range is dependent upon therapeutic approach. "High dose" regimens produce drug levels between 10^{-6} M and 10^{-7} M 24-72 hours after drug infusion.

Critical Values Plasma concentrations $>1 \times 10^{-7}$ M, 48 hours postinfusion are associated with increased toxicity. Leucovorin rescue is not complete until plasma concentrations fall below this.

Possible Panic Range Toxic: low-dose therapy: >9.1 ng/mL (SI: >20 nmol/L); high-dose therapy: >454 ng/mL (SI: >1000 nmol/L)

Use Monitor therapeutic drug level of methotrexate, evaluate potential toxicity

Methodology Enzyme immunoassay (EIA), radioimmunoassay (RIA), high performance liquid chromatography (HPLC)

Additional Information
- Half-life: 8-15 hours
- Volume of distribution: 0.4-1.0 L/kg
- Protein binding: 50% to 70%

Methotrexate is an antimetabolite that combines with dihydrofolate reductase and therefore interferes with the synthesis of tetrahydrofolic acid necessary for DNA synthesis. From 40% to 50% of a small dose and up to 90% of a larger dose is excreted unchanged in the urine in 48 hours, a major portion of it during the first 8 hours. Toxicity consists of bone marrow depression with megaloblastosis. Concomitant salicylate administration increases incidence of toxicity, due to diminished renal tubular excretion. The effect of methotrexate on normal cells may be reversed by administration of 5-formyltetrahydrofolate, also called citrovorum factor or leucovorin. This "rescue" makes possible administration of much higher doses of methotrexate than the body would otherwise survive. The initial half-life is 2-4 hours, but the total body clearance (terminal) half-life is 8-15 hours.

Drugs can interfere with the clearance of absorption of methotrexate. Antibiotics may decrease the absorption of methotrexate. Salicylates, sulfonamides, probenecid, and nonsteroidal anti-inflammatory drugs may block the renal clearance of methotrexate, increasing its concentration.

References
Brooks PJ, Spruill WJ, Parish RC, et al, "Pharmacokinetics of Methotrexate Administered by Intramuscular and Subcutaneous Injections in Patients With Rheumatoid Arthritis," *Arthritis Rheum*, 1990, 33(1):91-4.

Fossa SD, Heilo A, and Borner O, "Unexpectedly High Serum Methotrexate Levels in Cystectomized Bladder Cancer Patients With an Ileal Conduit Treated With Intermediate Doses of the Drug," *J Urol*, 1990, 143(3):498-501.

McIvor A, "Charcoal Hemoperfusion and Methotrexate Toxicity," *Nephron*, 1991, 58(3):378.

Minocha A, Dean HA, and Pittsley RA, "Liver Cirrhosis in Rheumatoid Arthritis Patients Treated With Long-Term Methotrexate," *Vet Hum Toxicol*, 1993, 35(1):45-8.

Olsen EA, "The Pharmacology of Methotrexate," *J Am Acad Dermatol*, 1991, 25(2 Pt 1):306-18.

Shiroky JB, Neville C, Esdaile JM, et al, "Low-Dose Methotrexate With Leucovorin (Folinic Acid) in the Management of Rheumatoid Arthritis. Results of a Multicenter Randomized, Double-Blind, Placebo-Controlled Trial," *Arthritis Rheum*, 1993, 36(6):795-803.

Wallace CA, Bleyer WA, Sherry DD, et al, "Toxicity and Serum Levels of Methotrexate in Children With Juvenile Rheumatoid Arthritis," *Arthritis Rheum*, 1989, 32(6):677-81.

Wernick R and Smith DL, "Central Nervous System Toxicity Associated With Weekly Low-Dose Methotrexate Treatment," *Arthritis Rheum*, 1989, 32(6):770-5.

Methylenedioxymethamphetamine *see* Methamphetamine, Qualitative, Urine *on previous page*

Methylmorphine *see* Codeine, Urine *on page 544*

Methylphenobarbital

CPT 80299

Related Information

Phenobarbital, Blood *on page 568*

Synonyms Enphenemalum; Gemonil®; Mebaral®; Mephobarbital; Mephobarbitone

Abstract Mephobarbital is metabolized to phenobarbital, which accounts for most pharmacologic effects. However, mephobarbital has slightly different pharmacokinetics than phenobarbital.

Specimen Serum

Container Red top tube

Sampling Time Consistent sampling time

Reference Range In humans, most of the drug is converted to phenobarbital, and many methods of determination have difficulty distinguishing between the drug and the metabolite. Determination of the total phenobarbital then gives an approximation of antiepileptic drug (AED) level of the parent compound. Very little data exists on reference values for methylphenobarbital. Phenobarbital level should be in the range of 15-40 µg/mL.

Critical Values See Phenobarbital, Blood *on page 568*. Levels >80 µg/mL correlate with decreased mental status.

Use Mephobarbital is used for prophylactic management of tonic-clonic (grand mal) seizures and absence (petit mal) seizures.

Methodology Gas-liquid chromatography (GLC), gas chromatography/mass spectrometry (GC/MS)

Additional Information
- Half-life: 45-55 hours
- Volume of distribution: 2-3 L/kg
- Protein binding: 40% to 60%

Methylphenobarbital has a more linear response between dosage and blood phenobarbital level than does phenobarbital. The limitations and adverse effects of the two drugs are likely to be very similar. Test interactions include an increase in alkaline phosphatase and ammonia, and a decrease in bilirubin and calcium.

References
Pond SM, Olson KR, Osterloh JD, et al, "Randomized Study of the Treatment of Phenobarbital Overdose With Repeated Doses of Activated Charcoal," *JAMA*, 1984, 251(23):3104-8.

Zawada ET, Nappi J, Done G, et al, "Advances in the Hemodialysis Management of Phenobarbital Overdose," *South Med J*, 1983, 76(1):6-8.

Methylphenylethylhydantoin *see* Mephenytoin *on page 560*

Methyl Salicylate *see* Salicylate *on page 573*

Mexate® *see* Methotrexate *on this page*

Mexiletine

CPT 80299

Related Information

Ketoconazole *on page 556*

Phenobarbital, Blood *on page 568*

Phenytoin *on page 569*

pH, Urine *on page 648*

Theophylline *on page 575*

Synonyms Mexitil®

Abstract Mexiletine is an agent used to treat ventricular arrhythmia.
(Continued)

Mexiletine *(Continued)*

Specimen Serum

Container Red top tube

Sampling Time Draw 2-4 hours after last dose for peak level. Draw immediately prior to next dose for trough levels.

Reference Range Therapeutic 0.75-2.00 µg/mL (SI: 4-11 µmol/L)

Possible Panic Range >2.00 µg/mL (SI: >9 µmol/L)

Use Therapeutic monitoring and toxicity assessment. Mexiletine is a class I antiarrhythmic approved for treatment of ventricular arrhythmias. It has no active metabolites. Toxic effects include dizziness, vomiting, confusion, tremor, bradycardia, and hypotension.

Methodology Fluorometry, high performance liquid chromatography (HPLC), gas chromatography (GC)

Additional Information

- Half-life: 7-15 hours
- Volume of distribution: 5-7 L/kg
- Protein binding: 60% to 70%

Metabolism of mexiletine is accelerated by rifampin, phenobarbital, and phenytoin and retarded by cimetidine and ketoconazole. Half-life is urine pH dependent. Acidic urine accelerates elimination.

Mexiletine can increase serum theophylline levels. Phenobarbital, phenytoin, rifampin, and other hepatic enzyme inducers may lower mexiletine plasma levels; cimetidine may increase mexiletine levels. Antacids, narcotics, or anticholinergics may decrease rate of absorption; metoclopramide may increase rate of absorption. Drugs or diets which affect urine pH can increase or decrease excretion of mexiletine. Use with beta-blockers or calcium channel blockers may depress cardiac function. Phenytoin or rifampin can enhance mexiletine metabolism.

References

Frank SE, Snyder JT, "Survival Following Severe Overdose With Mexiletine, Nifedipine, and Nitroglycerin," *Am J Emerg Med*, 1991, 9(1):43-6.

Gottlieb SS and Weinberg M, "Comparative Hemodynamic Effects of Mexiletine and Quinidine in Patients With Severe Left Ventricular Dysfunction," *Am Heart J*, 1991, 122(5):1368-74.

Grech-Belanger O, Barbeau G, Kishka P, et al, "Pharmacokinetics of Mexiletine in the Elderly," *J Clin Pharmacol*, 1989, 29(4):311-5.

Ji SG, Kong QH, Li XL, et al, "Gas Chromatographic Determination of Mexiletine in Human Plasma With Flame Ionization Detection After Reaction With Carbon Disulfide," *Biomed Chromatogr*, 1993, 7(4):196-9.

Manolis AS, Deering TF, Cameron J, et al, "Mexiletine: Pharmacology and Therapeutic Use," *Clin Cardiol*, 1990, 13(5):349-59.

Skluth H, Grauer K, and Gums J, "Ventricular Arrhythmias. An Assessment of Newer Therapeutic Agents," *Postgrad Med*, 1989, 85(6):137-8, 141-8, 153.

Mexitil® *see* Mexiletine *on previous page*

Miltown® *see* Meprobamate *on page 560*

Minute-Gel® *see* Fluoride, Serum *on page 551*

Mist *see* Phencyclidine, Qualitative, Urine *on page 567*

Mitran® *see* Chlordiazepoxide, Blood *on page 542*

Moditen® *see* Fluphenazine *on page 552*

Mole® *see* Caffeine, Blood *on page 539*

Molipaxin® *see* Trazodone *on page 577*

Monoethylglycinexylidide

CPT 80299

Related Information

Lidocaine *on page 558*

Synonyms MEGX

Applies to Lidocaine Metabolite

Test Commonly Includes This is the major active metabolite of lidocaine. It is monitored along with lidocaine as an antiarrhythmic agent.

Abstract Monitored with lidocaine as an antiarrhythmic agent, this drug may also be used to assess donor and recipient organ liver function.

Specimen Serum

Container Red top tube

Sampling Time 15 minutes after subtherapeutic, intravenous dose of 1 mg/kg lidocaine

Reference Range >50 µg/L (SI: >170 nmol/L) when used as liver function test. Lower values are found in women under 45 years of age not on contraceptives.[1]

Critical Values MEGX concentrations depressed by 50% may indicate complications following transplantation.[2] However, the reliability of the test in this role is in question.[3]

Use MEGX is the major metabolite of lidocaine and is used to assess donor and recipient liver function in transplantation of this organ in adults and children. It may be useful in evaluation of liver disease.[4,5] It may have a role as a test in evaluation of shock.[6] Conversion of lidocaine to MEGX after a 1.0 mg/kg dose should result in at least the level indicated in reference range.

Methodology High performance liquid chromatography (HPLC), gas chromatography (GC), fluorescence polarization immunoassay (FPIA)

Additional Information Plasma half-life is 2 hours.

Footnotes

1. Oellerich M, Schutz E, Polzien F, et al, "Influence of Gender on the Monoethylglycinexylidide Test in Normal Subjects and Liver Donors," *Ther Drug Monit*, 1994, 16(3):225-31.

2. Potter JM, Hickman PE, Lynch SV, et al, "Use of Monoethylglycinexylidide as a Liver Function Test in the Liver Transplant Recipient," *Transplantation*, 1993, 56(6):1385-8.

3. Reding R, Wallemacq P, de Ville de Goyet J, et al, "The Unreliability of the Lidocaine/Monoethylglycinexylidide Test for Assessment of Liver Donors," *Transplantation*, 1993, 56(2):323-6.

4. Forte G, Rocco P, Costanzo A, et al, "Monoethylglycinexylidide Production as a Measure in Predicting Hepatic Histology," *Ital J Gastroenterol*, 1994, 26(4):159-62.

5. Huang YS, Lee SD, Deng JF, et al, "Measuring Lidocaine Metabolite - Monoethylglycinexylidide as a Quantitative Index of Hepatic Function in Adults With Chronic Hepatitis and Cirrhosis," *J Hepatol*, 1993, 19(1):140-7.

6. Chandel B, Shapiro MJ, Kurtz M, et al, "MEGX (Monoethylglycinexylidide): A Novel *In Vivo* Test to Measure Early Hepatic Dysfunction After Hypovolemic Shock," *Shock*, 1995, 3(1):51-3.

References

Estes NA 3d, Manolis AS, Greenblatt DJ, et al, "Therapeutic Serum Lidocaine and Metabolite Concentrations in Patients Undergoing Electrophysiologic Study After Discontinuation of Intravenous Lidocaine Infusion," *Am Heart J*, 1989, 117(5):1060-4.

Oellerich M, Raude E, Burdelski M, et al, "Monoethylglycinexylidide Formation Kinetics: A Novel Approach to Assessment of Liver Function," *J Clin Chem Clin Biochem*, 1987, 25(12):845-53.

Schroeder TJ, "A Novel Approach to the Diagnosis of Acute Rejection in Pediatric Liver Allograft Recipients," *J Hepatol*, 1989, 10:616-24.

Morphine, Urine

CPT 83925

Related Information

Chain-of-Custody Protocol *on page 542*

Drugs of Abuse Testing, Urine *on page 548*

Opiates, Qualitative, Urine *on page 566*

Oral Cavity Cytology *on page 298*

Synonyms Astramorph™ PF; Duramorph®; Epimorph Dolcontin®; Heroin Metabolite, Urine; MS Contin®; MSIR®; MST®; OMS®; Oramorph SR®; RMS®; Roxanol™; Roxanol SR™; Sevredol®; Statex®

Test Commonly Includes Codeine, Demerol®, heroin, hydromorphone (Dilaudid®), morphine, and morphine glucuronide

Abstract This drug is widely used therapeutically as an analgesic. Morphine itself is not an extensively used drug of abuse but two derivatives, heroin and codeine, are.

Storage Instructions Refrigerate sample

Special Instructions If forensic, use chain-of-custody protocol and form. See test listing Chain-of-Custody Protocol *on page 542* and the Therapeutic Drug Monitoring/Toxicology/Drugs of Abuse Appendix *on page 581*.

Reference Range Negative (less than cutoff)

Critical Values Cutoff: screen (total opiates): 300 ng/mL; confirmatory: 300 ng/mL

Use Evaluate toxicity or detect drug of abuse. Heroin is metabolized to morphine, but morphine detection may only suggest heroin use. To **prove** heroin use, 6-O-acetyl morphine must be identified in the urine.

Methodology Gas-liquid chromatography (GLC)

Additional Information

- Half-life: 2-4 hours
- Volume of distribution: 2-4 L/kg
- Protein binding: 30% to 40%

Morphine, the major phenanthrene alkaloid of powdered opium, is used for relief of moderate to severe acute and chronic pain after non-narcotic analgesics have failed. It is also used as preanesthetic medication, to relieve the pain of myocardial infarction and to relieve the dyspnea of acute left ventricular failure and pulmonary edema. Peak analgesia is achieved 50-90 minutes after subcutaneous administration and 20 minutes after I.V. injection. Ninety percent of morphine is found in the urine after 24 hours, either free or in the glucuronide conjugated form. Adverse effects include CNS depression, nausea and vomiting, hypotension, bradycardia, histamine release, increased intracranial pressure, miosis, antidiuretic hormone release, and physical and psychological dependence. Naloxone is a specific antidote. Morphine is generally detectable for 1-2 days after use.

Morphine may cause an increase in ALT, AST, and amylase.

References

Baselt RC and Cravey RH, *Disposition of Toxic Drugs and Chemicals in Man*, 3rd ed, Chicago, IL: Year Book Medical Publishers Inc, 1989, 575-9.

Cone EJ, Dickerson S, Paul BD, et al, "Forensic Drug Testing for Opiates: Urine Testing for Heroin, Morphine, and Codeine With Commercial Opiate Immunoassays," *J Anal Toxicol*, 1993, 17(3):156-64.

Lin Z, Lafolie P, and Beck O, "Evaluation of Analytical Procedures for Urinary Codeine and Morphine Measurements," *J Anal Toxicol*, 1994, 18(3):129-33.

McQuay HJ, Carroll D, Faura CC, et al, "Oral Morphine in Cancer Pain: Influences on Morphine and Metabolite Concentration," *Clin Pharmacol Ther*, 1990, 48(3):236-44.

Osborne R, Joel S, Trew D, et al, "Morphine and Metabolite Behavior After Different Routes of Morphine Administration: Demonstration of the Importance of the Active Metabolite Morphine-6-Glucuronide," *Clin Pharmacol Ther*, 1990, 47(1):12-9.

Portenoy RK, Khan E, Layman M, et al, "Chronic Morphine Therapy for Cancer Pain: Plasma and Cerebrospinal Fluid Morphine and Morphine-6-Glucuronide Concentrations," *Neurology*, 1991, 41(9):1457-61.

Portenoy RK, Thaler HT, Inturrisi CE, et al, "The Metabolite Morphine-6-Glucuronide Contributes to the Analgesia Produced by Morphine Infusion in Patients With Pain and Normal Renal Function," *Clin Pharmacol Ther*, 1992, 51(4):422-31.

Sear JW, Hand CW, Moore RA, et al, "Studies on Morphine Disposition: Influence of Renal Failure on the Kinetics of Morphine and its Metabolites," *Br J Anaesth*, 1989, 62(1):28-32.

"Toxicity and Pharmacokinetics of Morphine and Morphine-6-Glucuronide," *Br J Anaesth*, 1991, 67(3):362-3.

Zakowski MI, Ramanathan S, Sharnick S, et al, "Uptake and Distribution of Bupivacaine and Morphine After Intrathecal Administration in Parturients: Effects of Epinephrine," *Anesth Analg*, 1992, 74(5):664-9.

Moxadil® *see* Amoxapine, Blood *on page 533*

MS Contin® *see* Morphine, Urine *on previous page*

MSIR® *see* Morphine, Urine *on previous page*

MST® *see* Morphine, Urine *on previous page*

MTX *see* Methotrexate *on page 563*

Myapap® Drops *see* Acetaminophen, Serum *on page 530*

Mychel-S® *see* Chloramphenicol *on page 542*

Mylepsin® *see* Primidone *on page 570*

Myochrysine® *see* Gold *on page 553*

Mysoline® *see* Primidone *on page 570*

N-Acetyl Procainamide *see* Procainamide *on page 570*

NAPA *see* Procainamide *on page 570*

Napamide® *see* Disopyramide *on page 547*

Narcotics *see* Opiates, Qualitative, Urine *on next page*

Narcotics Drug Screen, Urine *see* Toxicology Drug Screen, Urine *on page 576*

Nativelle® *see* Digitoxin *on page 546*

Nembutal® *see* Barbiturates, Quantitative, Blood *on page 537*

Neopap® *see* Acetaminophen, Serum *on page 530*

Nervocaine® *see* Lidocaine *on page 558*

Neuramate® *see* Meprobamate *on page 560*

Neurontin® *see* Gabapentin *on page 552*

Nipride® *see* Thiocyanate, Blood or Urine *on page 575*

Nitroprusside *see* Thiocyanate, Blood or Urine *on page 575*

Nizoral *see* Ketoconazole *on page 556*

No-Doz® *see* Caffeine, Blood *on page 539*

11-Nor-9-Carboxy-Delta-9-Tetrahydrocannabinol *see* Cannabinoids (Marijuana Metabolites), Qualitative, Urine *on page 539*

Norocaine® *see* Lidocaine *on page 558*

Norpace® *see* Disopyramide *on page 547*

Norpramin® *see* Antidepressants, Cyclic *on page 535*

Norpramin® *see* Imipramine *on page 554*

Norpropoxyphene *see* Propoxyphene, Serum or Urine *on page 571*

Nortrilen® *see* Nortriptyline *on this page*

Nortriptyline

CPT 80182

Related Information

Amitriptyline, Blood *on page 533*
Antidepressants, Cyclic *on page 535*
Disopyramide *on page 547*
Phenytoin *on page 569*
Procainamide *on page 570*
Quinidine, Serum *on page 572*
Warfarin *on page 579*

Synonyms Allegron®; Aventyl® Hydrochloride; Nortrilen®; Norval®; Pamelor®

Abstract This is a cyclic antidepressant.

Specimen Serum

Container Red top tube

Collection Collect specimen immediately prior to next dose unless specified otherwise.

Storage Instructions Separate serum and refrigerate.

Reference Range Therapeutic: 50-150 ng/mL (SI: 190-570 nmol/L)

Critical Values Toxic: >500 ng/mL (SI: >1900 nmol/L)

Possible Panic Range ≥1000 ng/mL

Use Monitor therapeutic drug level; evaluate toxicity, overdoses. Nortriptyline, a tricyclic antidepressant, is a derivative and metabolite of amitriptyline and is used to treat endogenous depression.

Limitations Results not valid if patient receiving imipramine or desipramine

Contraindications Cyclic antidepressants should be avoided in pregnant and lactating women because these drugs have not been established to be safe. Geriatric patients are especially susceptible to orthostasis, urinary retention, constipation, and sedation.

Methodology High performance liquid chromatography (HPLC), liquid chromatography,[1] fluorescence polarization immunoassay[2]

Additional Information

- Half-life: 20-90 hours
- Volume of distribution: 15-23 L/kg
- Protein binding: 90% to 95%

Nortriptyline may be associated with cholestasis and cholestatic jaundice. Hematologic consequences include agranulocytosis, purpura, and thrombocytopenia. Other side effects include a host of GI, endocrinologic, allergic, anticholinergic, cardiovascular, and neurologic disorders. Fulminant hepatic failure may be idiosyncratic.[3]

Nortriptyline is completely absorbed but undergoes some first-pass elimination. The bioavailability of nortriptyline is 45% to 70% with a peak concentration 2-6 hours after an oral dose. It is 90% bound to plasma proteins and is also highly bound to tissues.

Anticholinergic side effects are common with this drug. They are not severe and may diminish with continued therapy or can be treated with other pharmacologic and nonpharmacologic therapies. Anticholinergic side effects are more troublesome in the elderly. Sedation may also decrease with continued use. Nortriptyline can also lower the seizure threshold and cause orthostasis and arrhythmias. Cardiovascular effects are more common in patients with underlying cardiovascular disorders.

Drug interactions are common with the cyclic antidepressants. Since they are cleared by the liver, they are susceptible to decreases in enzyme activity caused by cimetidine, fluoxetine, and antipsychotics resulting in increased concentrations of nortriptyline. Enzyme inducers such as phenytoin, chloral hydrate, smoking, and the barbiturates will decrease nortriptyline concentrations. Additive anticholinergic side effects occur when cyclics are combined with antihistamines, anti-Parkinson drugs, and antipsychotics. The cardiovascular effects of the cyclics are additive with any of the class IA antiarrhythmics (quinidine, procainamide, disopyramide). Direct-acting sympathomimetics (epinephrine, norepinephrine, phenylephrine) are potentiated by cyclics. Monoamine oxidase inhibitors (MAOI) and thyroid hormones potentiate the toxicities of cyclics. Hyperthermia, delirium, convulsions, coma, and fatalities have occurred with the combination of MAOIs and cyclics. These drugs have been used in combination in refractory cases of depression. The cyclics can also affect other drugs. The antihypertensive effects of the central α-agonists (clonidine, methyldopa, guanethidine) are reversed when combined with cyclics. Warfarin anticoagulation effects may be potentiated by the cyclics.

Test interactions include possible increase in glucose and elevation of plasma norepinephrine levels and plasma epinephrine levels threefold to fivefold. EMIT assays for nortriptyline may give false-positive in the presence of diphenhydramine, thioridazine, chlorpromazine, alimenazine, carbamazepine, cyclobenzaprine, or perphenazine.

The cyclic antidepressants are commonly seen in overdose situations. Cardiovascular, anticholinergic and central nervous system toxicities can be lethal. Treatment includes supportive measures and removal of ingested drug by emesis or gastric lavage. This drug is not removed by hemo or peritoneal dialysis.

Footnotes

1. el-Yazigi A and Raines DA, "Concurrent Liquid Chromatographic Measurement of Fluoxetine, Amitriptyline, Imipramine, and Their Active Metabolites Norfluoxetine, Nortriptyline, and Desipramine in Plasma," *Ther Drug Monit*, 1993, 15(4):305-9.

2. Adamczyk M, Fishpaugh JR, Harrington CA, et al, "Immunoassay Reagents for Psychoactive Drugs. Part 4. Quantitative Determination of Amitriptyline and Nortriptyline by Fluorescence Polarization Immunoassay," *Ther Drug Monit*, 1994, 16(3):298-311.

3. Berkelhammer C, Kher N, Berry C, et al, "Nortriptyline-Induced Fulminant Hepatic Failure," *J Clin Gastroenterol*, 1995, 20(1):54-6.

References

Brasfield KH, "Practical Psychopharmacologic Considerations in Depression," *Nurs Clin North Am*, 1991, 26(3):651-63.

Feldman MD, "Therapeutic Blood Monitoring of Tricyclic Antidepressants," *South Med J*, 1994, 87(1):101.

Jerling M and Alvan G, "Nonlinear Kinetics of Nortriptyline in Relation to Nortriptyline Clearance as Observed During Therapeutic Drug Monitoring," *Eur J Clin Pharmacol*, 1994, 46(1):67-70.

Jerling M, Bertilsson L, and Sjoqvist F, "The Use of Therapeutic Drug Monitoring Data to Document Kinetic Drug Interactions: An Example With Amitriptyline and Nortriptyline," *Ther Drug Monit*, 1994, 16(1):1-12.

(Continued)

Nortriptyline *(Continued)*

Kehoe WA, Harralson AF, Jacisin JJ, et al, "Sources of Prediction Error When Using a Bayesian Method to Evaluate Nortriptyline Serum Concentrations," *J Clin Pharmacol*, 1994, 34(8):842-7.

Lipper B and Gaynor BD, "Value of Serum Tricyclic Antidepressant Levels With Massive Nortriptyline Overdose and Persistent Hypotension," *Am J Emerg Med*, 1995, 13(1):107.

Lipper B, Bell A, and Gaynor B, "Recurrent Hypotension Immediately After Seizures in Nortriptyline Overdose," *Am J Emerg Med*, 1994, 12(4):452-3.

Nair NP, Amin M, Holm P, et al, "Moclobemide and Nortriptyline in Elderly Depressed Patients. A Randomized, Multicentre Trial Against Placebo," *J Affect Disord*, 1995, 33(1):1-9.

Shapiro PA, "Nortriptyline Treatment of Depressed Cardiac Transplant Recipients," *Am J Psychiatry*, 1991, 148(3):371-3.

Norval® *see* Nortriptyline *on previous page*

Norverapamil *see* Verapamil *on page 578*

Nose Candy *see* Cocaine (Cocaine Metabolite), Qualitative, Urine *on page 543*

Novocainamidum *see* Procainamide *on page 570*

Novocamid® *see* Procainamide *on page 570*

Novoxapin® *see* Doxepin *on page 548*

6-O-Acetyl Morphine *see* Opiates, Qualitative, Urine *on this page*

Octocaine® *see* Lidocaine *on page 558*

Oil of Wintergreen *see* Salicylate *on page 573*

Omnipres® *see* Amoxapine, Blood *on page 533*

OMS® *see* Morphine, Urine *on page 564*

Opiates, Qualitative, Urine

CPT 80101 (screen); 80102 (confirmation)

Related Information

Chain-of-Custody Protocol *on page 542*
Codeine, Urine *on page 544*
Drugs of Abuse Testing, Urine *on page 548*
Morphine, Urine *on page 564*

Applies to Heroin; Narcotics; 6-O-Acetyl Morphine; Poppy Seeds

Test Commonly Includes Morphine, codeine, hydrocodone (Hycodan®), hydromorphone (Dilaudid®)

Abstract The qualitative detection of urine opiates is used almost exclusively to demonstrate presence of drugs of abuse in this class. Morphine and codeine are used therapeutically for pain.

Specimen Random urine

Collection If forensic, observe precautions (see the Therapeutic Drug Monitoring/Toxicology/Drugs of Abuse Introduction *on page 527*).

Storage Instructions Refrigerate

Special Instructions If forensic, use chain-of-custody protocol and form. See test listing Chain-of-Custody Protocol *on page 542* and the Therapeutic Drug Monitoring/Toxicology/Drugs of Abuse Appendix *on page 581*.

Reference Range Negative (less than cutoff)

Critical Values Cutoff: screen: 300 ng/mL; confirmation: 300 ng/mL of specific opiates

Use Evaluate drug abuse; assess toxicity

Limitations In most immunoassays a number of narcotic drugs can cross react to give a positive screen. Every effort should be made to confirm, by an analytically different and more sensitive method, all presumptive positive opiate screens. See above.

Methodology Screening: immunoassay, thin-layer chromatography (TLC), high performance liquid chromatography (HPLC), gas chromatography (GC); confirmation: gas chromatography/mass spectrometry (GC/MS)

Additional Information For morphine:
- Half-life: 2-4 hours
- Volume of distribution: 2-4 L/kg
- Protein binding: 30% to 40%

A qualitative urine screen for opiates is performed in suspected overdose cases or as part of a drugs-of-abuse program. The test is most sensitive for morphine and codeine, but other drugs will cross react in an immunoassay and give positive results (eg, hydrocodone, hydromorphone). All presumptive positive assays should be confirmed, preferably by GC/MS. Morphine is a prescribed drug for pain relief, a metabolite of heroin, a metabolite of codeine, and a constituent of poppy seeds. Its presence in urine, even after confirmation, must be interpreted very carefully. Ingestion of poppy seeds (bagels, Danish) can cause positive opiate screens at a 300 ng/mL cutoff.[1] The intake of heroin by the user can only be proved by the detection of 6-O-acetyl morphine by the urine confirmatory test.

Opiates in general are a group of drugs (commonly referred to as narcotics) which are used medically to relieve pain, but which also have a high potential for abuse. Some opiates come from a resin taken from the seed pod of the Asian poppy. This group of drugs includes opium, morphine, and codeine. Other opiates are synthesized or manufactured (eg, heroin). Opium appears as dark brown chunks or as a powder, and is usually smoked or eaten. Heroin can be a white or brownish powder which is usually dissolved in water and injected.

Opiates tend to relax the user. When the opiates are injected, the user feels an immediate "rush." Other initial and unpleasant effects include restlessness, nausea, and vomiting. The user may go "on the nod," going back and forth from feeling alert to drowsy. With very large doses, the user cannot be awakened, pupils become smaller, and the skin becomes cold, moist, and bluish in color. Furthermore, breathing slows down and death may occur. Clearance may be slower in geriatric patients.

Footnotes

1. Selavka CM, "Poppy Seed Ingestion as a Contributing Factor to Opiate-Positive Urinalysis Results: The Pacific Perspective," *J Forensic Sci*, 1991, 36(3):685-96.

References

Barsan W, "Narcotic Agents," *Ann Emerg Med*, 1986, 15:1019-20.

Cone EJ, Dickerson S, Paul BD, et al, "Forensic Drug Testing for Opiates. Urine Testing for Heroin, Morphine, and Codeine With Commercial Opiate Immunoassays," *J Anal Toxicol*, 1993, 17(3):156-64.

Gillogley KM, Evans AT, Hansen RL, et al, "The Perinatal Impact of Cocaine, Amphetamine, and Opiate Use Detected by Universal Intrapartum Screening," *Am J Obstet Gynecol*, 1990, 163(5 Pt 1):1535-42.

Montamat SC, Cusack BJ, and Vestal RE, "Management of Drug Therapy in the Elderly," *N Engl J Med*, 1989, 321(5):303-9.

Pettitt BC Jr, Dyszel SM, and Hood LV, "Opiates in Poppy Seed: Effect on Urinalysis Results After Consumption of Poppy Seed Cake-Filling," *Clin Chem*, 1987, 33(7):1251-2.

Storrow AB, Wians FH Jr, Mikkelsen SL, et al, "Does Naloxone Cause a Positive Urine Opiate Screen?," *Ann Emerg Med*, 1994, 24(6):1151-3.

Oramorph SR® *see* Morphine, Urine *on page 564*

Organic Mercury *see* Mercury, Blood *on page 561*

Ormazine® *see* Chlorpromazine, Serum or Urine *on page 543*

Ormazine® *see* Phenothiazines, Serum *on page 568*

Oxazepam, Serum

CPT 80154

Related Information

Benzodiazepines, Qualitative, Urine *on page 538*
Glucose, Fasting *on page 137*

Synonyms Adumbran®; Serax®; Serenid® Forte

Abstract Oxazepam is a benzodiazepine used as an antianxiety agent with alcohol withdrawal and as an anticonvulsant. It is an active metabolite of several other benzodiazepines that are used therapeutically.

Specimen Serum

Container Red top tube

Sampling Time Collect specimen immediately prior to next dose unless specified otherwise.

Storage Instructions Separate serum and refrigerate.

Reference Range 0.2-1.4 µg/mL (SI: 0.7-4.9 µmol/L)

Use Monitor therapeutic drug level; evaluate toxicity

Methodology Gas-liquid chromatography (GLC), high performance liquid chromatography (HPLC)[1] with fluorescence detection[2]

Additional Information
- Half-life: 4-12 hours
- Volume of distribution: 0.5-2.0 L/kg
- Protein binding: 95% to 98%

Oxazepam, a benzodiazepine derivative, is related to chlordiazepoxide and shares many of its qualities. It does, however, have a shorter duration of action and causes fewer adverse effects. It is rapidly eliminated by urinary excretion as a glucuronide conjugate. Oxazepam is used to manage tension and anxiety and to aid in the control of acute withdrawal symptoms in chronic alcoholism. Peak plasma levels are achieved in 2-4 hours. Adverse effects are mild and infrequent. They include drowsiness, vertigo, ataxia, headache, tremor, slurred speech, nausea, hypotension, and leukopenia. Simultaneous alcohol ingestion potentiates some of the effects of benzodiazepines.

Visine®, Drano®, and bleach may cause false-negative urine tests for oxazepam. Oxazepam may interfere in giving falsely elevated glucose results in test serum.

Footnotes

1. Goldnik A, Gajewska M, and Jaworska M, "Determination of Oxazepam and Diazepam in Body Fluids by HPLC," *Acta Pol Pharm*, 1993, 50(6):421-2.
2. Berrueta LA, Gallo B, and Vicente F, "Analysis of Oxazepam in Urine Using Solid-Phase Extraction and High-Performance Liquid Chromatography With Fluorescence Detection by Post-Column Derivatization," *J Chromatogr*, 1993, 616(2):344-8.

References

Baselt RC and Cravey RH, *Disposition of Toxic Drugs and Chemicals in Man*, 3rd ed, Chicago, IL: Year Book Medical Publishers Inc, 1989, 622-3.

Craig CR and Stitzel RE, *Modern Pharmacology*, 3rd ed, Boston, MA: Little, Brown and Co, 1990, 440-6.

Moshkowitz M, Pines A, Finkelstein A, et al, "Skin Blisters as a Manifestation of Oxazepam Toxicity," *J Toxicol Clin Toxicol*, 1990, 28(3):383-6.

Weinberg AD, Pals JK, Marinelli FC, et al, "Oxazepam Overdose Associated With Ethanol Ingestion: Treatment With a Benzodiazepine Antagonist," *Am J Crit Care*, 1994, 3(6):464-6.

Zileli MS, Teletar F, Deniz S, et al, "Oxazepam Intoxication Simulating Nonketo-Acidotic Diabetic Coma," *JAMA*, 1971, 215(12):1986.

Oxazolidinediones

CPT 80299

Synonyms Paradione®; Tridione®; Trimedone

Test Commonly Includes Trimethadione and paramethadione

Abstract Trimethadione and paramethadione can be considered for absence seizures in patients unable to take other medications. However, oxazolidinediones are less effective and have clear teratogenic effects.

Specimen Serum

Container Red top tube

Reference Range Therapeutic monitoring of trimethadione is achieved by measurement of its active metabolite, dimethadione. Reference range: 50-1200 µg/mL. Reference ranges for paramethadione and its metabolites have not been determined. There are no relevant drug interactions reported. Low levels of dimethadione may occur in the first 2 weeks of administration as the metabolite reaches plateau levels.

Possible Panic Range Dose dependent, reversible adverse effects include hemeralopia (night blindness), photophobia, sedation, fatigue, dizziness, and ataxia

Use Monitor for compliance, efficacy, and possible toxicity

Methodology High performance liquid chromatography (HPLC), gas-liquid chromatography (GLC), infrared spectrophotometry

Additional Information Dimethadione has a half-life of 6-13 days. Close monitoring during administration is indicated.

P-450 System see Carbamazepine *on page 540*

Pamelor® see Nortriptyline *on page 565*

Pamelor® see Amitriptyline, Blood *on page 533*

Pamelor® see Antidepressants, Cyclic *on page 535*

Panadol® see Acetaminophen, Serum *on page 530*

Panwarfin® see Warfarin *on page 579*

Paradione® see Oxazolidinediones *on this page*

Paveral see Codeine, Urine *on page 544*

Pb, Blood see Lead, Blood *on page 556*

Pb, Urine see Lead, Urine *on page 557*

PCP see Phencyclidine, Qualitative, Urine *on this page*

Peace Pills see Phencyclidine, Qualitative, Urine *on this page*

Peace Weed see Phencyclidine, Qualitative, Urine *on this page*

Pediaflor® see Fluoride, Serum *on page 551*

Peganone® see Ethotoin *on page 550*

PEMA see Primidone *on page 570*

Pentobarb see Barbiturates, Qualitative, Urine *on page 537*

Pentobarbital see Barbiturates, Quantitative, Blood *on page 537*

Pep Back® see Caffeine, Blood *on page 539*

Percoffedrinol N® see Caffeine, Blood *on page 539*

Percutafeine® see Caffeine, Blood *on page 539*

Permitil® see Fluphenazine *on page 552*

Pertofrane® see Antidepressants, Cyclic *on page 535*

Pertofrane® see Imipramine *on page 554*

Pethidine Hydrochloride see Meperidine, Blood or Urine *on page 560*

PFI-Lith® see Lithium *on page 558*

Pharmaflur® see Fluoride, Serum *on page 551*

Phasal® see Lithium *on page 558*

Phenacemide

CPT 80299

Synonyms Phenurone®

Abstract Phenacemide is used as an antiepileptic drug of last resort for patients with uncontrollable seizures.

Specimen Serum

Container Red top tube

Reference Range 16-75 µg/mL[1]

Possible Panic Range Signs of hepatic, renal, or psychiatric problems regardless of level

Methodology High performance liquid chromatography (HPLC)

Additional Information The half-life is 40 hours with chronic administration. Fatal bone marrow depression, hepatotoxicity, and renal toxicity are reported. Depression and psychotic reactions, including a risk of suicide, are reported with phenacemide. Close medical supervision with administration is required.

Footnotes

1. Coker SB, Holmes EW, and Egel RT, "Phenacemide Therapy of Complex Partial Epilepsy in Children: Determination of Plasma Drug Concentrations," *Neurology*, 1987, 37(12):1861-6.

References

Engel J, *Seizures and Epilepsy*, Contemporary Neurology Series, Philadelphia, PA: FA Davis Co, 1989.

Phenacetin see Acetaminophen, Serum *on page 530*

Phenantoin see Mephenytoin *on page 560*

Phencyclidine, Qualitative, Urine

CPT 80101 (screen); 80102 (confirmation, each procedure); 83992 (quantitative)

Related Information

Chain-of-Custody Protocol *on page 542*
Drugs of Abuse Testing, Urine *on page 548*

Synonyms Angel Dust; Crystal Joint; Elephant Tranquilizers; Goon; Hog; Kay Jay; Killer Weed; Mist; PCP; Peace Pills; Peace Weed; Rocket Fuel; Sheets; Sherm; Snorts; Soma®; Supergrass; Wickistick

Abstract This is a widely used drug of abuse which was formerly sold as a veterinary tranquilizer. All legal manufacture and sale has been stopped. It is classified by DEA as a Schedule II controlled substance. Acute intoxication with phencyclidine may be life threatening. It causes psychosis and other symptoms and signs.[1]

Specimen Random urine

Collection If forensic, observe precautions (see Therapeutic Drug Monitoring/Toxicology/Drugs of Abuse Introduction *on page 527*).

Special Instructions If forensic, use chain-of-custody protocol and form. See test listing Chain-of-Custody Protocol *on page 542* and the Therapeutic Drug Monitoring/Toxicology/Drugs of Abuse Appendix *on page 581*.

Reference Range Negative (less than cutoff)

Critical Values Cutoff: screen: 25 ng/mL; confirmation: 25 ng/mL

Possible Panic Range Excitation: 20-30 ng/mL; coma: 30-100 ng/mL; seizures, fatalities: >500 ng/mL

Use Evaluate presence of phencyclidine, drug abuse, PCP toxicity; determine phencyclidine involvement in unexplained psychoses

Limitations Adulteration with bleach can cause false-negative urine immunoassays for phencyclidine. Doxylamine can cause a false-positive urine gas chromatographic result.

Methodology Immunoassay, thin-layer chromatography (TLC), gas chromatography (GC), gas chromatography/mass spectrometry (GC/MS). Immunoassays are very specific and detect PCP at 25 ng/mL (SI: 100 nmol/L). Polarization fluoroimmunoassay.[2]

Additional Information

• Half-life: 10-50 hours
• Volume of distribution: 5-7 L/kg
• Protein binding: 65% to 80%

Phencyclidine is most often called "angel dust." It was first developed as an anesthetic in the 1950s. It was taken off the market for human use because it sometimes caused hallucinations. PCP is available in a number of forms. It can be a pure white crystal-like powder, a tablet or capsule, and it can be swallowed, smoked (alone or with marijuana), sniffed, or injected. Although PCP is illegal, it is easily manufactured.

Effects depend on how much of the drug is taken, the way it is used, and the individual. Small amounts act as a stimulant, speeding up body functions. For many users, PCP changes how they see their own bodies and things around them. Speech, muscle coordination, and vision are affected; sense of touch and pain are dulled; and body movements are slowed. Time seems to "space out." Effects include increased heart rate and blood pressure, flushing, sweating, dizziness, and numbness. When large doses are taken, effects include drowsiness, convulsions, and coma. Taking large amounts of PCP can also cause death from repeated convulsions, heart and lung failure, or ruptured central nervous system blood vessels. PCP can be detected for 7 days after administration; 2-4 weeks in chronic users.

Footnotes

1. Brust JC, "Other Agents. Phencyclidine, Marijuana, Hallucinogens, Inhalants, and Anticholinergics," *Neurol Clin*, 1993, 11(3):555-61.
2. Gooch JC, Gallacher G, Wright JG, et al, "Detection of Phencyclidine in Urine Using a Polarization Fluoroimmunoassay," *Analyst*, 1994, 119(8):1797-800.

(Continued)

Phencyclidine, Qualitative, Urine (Continued)

References

Chan KM, Matthews WS, Saxena S, et al, "Frequency of Cocaine and Phencyclidine Detection at a Large Urban Public Teaching Hospital," *J Anal Toxicol*, 1993, 17(5):299-303.

Ellenhorn MJ and Barceloux DG, "Phencyclidine," *Medical Toxicology*, New York, NY: Elsevier, 1988, 763-78.

Milhorn HT Jr, "Diagnosis and Management of Phencyclidine Intoxication," *Am Fam Physician*, 1991, 43(4):1293-302.

Wessinger WD and Owens SM, "Phencyclidine Dependence: The Relationship of Dose and Serum Concentrations to Operant Behavioral Effects," *J Pharmacol Exp Ther*, 1991, 258(1):207-15.

Phenemal see Phenobarbital, Blood *on this page*

Phenemalum see Phenobarbital, Blood *on this page*

Phenobarb see Barbiturates, Qualitative, Urine *on page 537*

Phenobarb see Phenobarbital, Blood *on this page*

Phenobarbital see Barbiturates, Quantitative, Blood *on page 537*

Phenobarbital see Valproic Acid *on page 577*

Phenobarbital, Blood

CPT 80184

Related Information

Antidepressants, Cyclic *on page 535*
Barbiturates, Quantitative, Blood *on page 537*
Benzodiazepines, Qualitative, Urine *on page 538*
Chloramphenicol *on page 542*
Cyclosporine *on page 545*
Ethosuximide *on page 549*
Methylphenobarbital *on page 563*
Mexiletine *on page 563*
Phenothiazines, Serum *on this page*
Phenytoin *on next page*
Primidone *on page 570*
Quinidine, Serum *on page 572*
Theophylline *on page 575*
Valproic Acid *on page 577*
Verapamil *on page 578*
Warfarin *on page 579*

Synonyms Barbita®; Comizial®; Fenilcal®; Gardenal®; Luminal®; Phenemal; Phenemalum; Phenobarb; Phenobarbitone; Phenylethylmalonylurea; Solfoton®; Stental Extentabs®

Abstract Phenobarbital is indicated for generalized tonic-clonic and partial seizures.

Specimen Serum or plasma

Container Red top tube, green top (heparin) tube, or lavender top (EDTA) tube

Sampling Time Consistent sampling time is desirable but less important than for other anticonvulsants, due to its long half-life.

Reference Range Infants and children: 15-30 µg/mL (SI: 65-129 µmol/L); **adults:** 20-40 µg/mL (SI: 86-172 µmol/L). See Table A in the Therapeutic Drug Monitoring/Toxicology/Drugs of Abuse Appendix *on page 582*. Low level: Most common cause is noncompliance. Other causes include drug interactions, including antipsychotic medication, chloramphenicol, acetazolamide, and phenytoin. Infants and children may be fast metabolizers. High level: addition of valproic acid to regimen inhibits phenobarbital metabolism (parahydroxylation) and should be accompanied by a cut in phenobarbital dosage. In newborns, unlike older infants, very long half-lives are found which may be associated with high levels.

Critical Values Toxic: >40 µg/mL (SI: >172 µmol/L) but if given intravenously, life-threatening side effects can occur with much lower levels, and patients should be monitored. Toxic effects are mostly neurologic. Adults present with lethargy and coma; children may present with irritability or hyperactivity. Levels >80 µg/mL (SI: >344 µmol/L) are associated with coma. **Fatal:** 50-130 µg/mL (SI: 215-559 µmol/L).

Use Monitor patients for compliance, efficacy, and possible toxicity. Mephobarbital and primidone are metabolized to phenobarbital and, therefore, patients taking these drugs will have detectable levels of phenobarbital on therapeutic monitoring.

Methodology Enzyme immunoassay (EIA), gas-liquid chromatography (GLC), high performance liquid chromatography (HPLC)

Additional Information
- Half-life: 50-140 hours
- Volume of distribution: 0.5-1.0 L/kg
- Protein binding: 40% to 50%

Phenobarbital can affect the metabolism of phenytoin, ethosuximide, and increase the clearance and elimination of chloramphenicol, theophylline, oral anticoagulants (warfarin), cyclosporine, and oral contraceptives; where appropriate, the use of these drugs in patients on phenobarbital should be monitored clinically and through the laboratory.

Phenobarbital may decrease the serum concentration or effect of phenylbutazone, griseofulvin, doxycycline, beta-blockers, theophylline, corticosteroids, tricyclic antidepressants, quinidine, haloperidol, and phenothiazines, valproic acid, methylphenidate, chloramphenicol, propoxyphene. Furosemide may inhibit the metabolism of phenobarbital with resultant increase in phenobarbital serum concentration. Valproic acid and salicylates may also increase phenobarbital concentration. Phenobarbital and benzodiazepines or other CNS depressants may cause an increase of CNS and respiratory depression (especially with I.V. loading doses of phenobarbital). Pyridoxine may reduce serum phenobarbital levels.

Phenobarbital may increase alkaline phosphatase, ammonia, and gamma glutamyl transferase and may decrease bilirubin and calcium in test samples.

References

Ammann H and Vinet B, "Accuracy, Precision, and Interferences of Three Modified EMIT Procedures for Determining Serum Phenobarbital, Urine Morphine, and Urine Cocaine Metabolite With A Cobas-Fara," *Clin Chem*, 1991, 37(12):2139-41.

Bertino J and Reed M, "Barbiturate and Nonbarbiturate Sedative Hypnotic Intoxication in Children," *Pediatr Clin North Am*, 1986, 33(3):703-22.

Kutt H, "Phenobarbital: Interactions With Other Drugs," *Antiepileptic Drugs*, 3rd ed, Levy RH, Dreifuss FE, Mattson RH, et al, eds, New York, NY: Raven Press, 1989, 313-27.

Painter MJ, Minnigh MB, Gaus L, et al, "Neonatal Phenobarbital and Phenytoin Binding Profiles," *J Clin Pharmacol*, 1994, 34(4):312-7.

Winter M, "Phenobarbital," *Basic Clinical Pharmacokinetics*, 3rd ed, Koda-Kimble M and Young L, eds, Vancouver, WA: Applied Therapeutics, Inc, 1994.

Phenobarbitone see Phenobarbital, Blood *on this page*

Phenothiazines see Chlorpromazine, Serum or Urine *on page 543*

Phenothiazines, Serum

CPT 80101 (screen); 80102 (confirmation, each procedure); 84022 (quantitative)

Related Information

Fluphenazine *on page 552*
Phenobarbital, Blood *on this page*

Applies to Chlorpromazine; Compazine®; Etrafon®; Mellaril®; Mesoridazine; Ormazine®; Prochlorperazine; Prolixin®; Serentil®; Stelazine®; Thioridazine; Thorazine®; Trifluoperazine

Abstract The drugs in this class are used as antipsychotic agents and tranquilizers.

Specimen Serum

Container Red top tube

Sampling Time Obtain serum at least 3 hours after last dose.

Reference Range Chlorpromazine: therapeutic: 50-300 ng/mL (SI: 157-942 nmol/L); **thioridazine:** therapeutic: 1.0-1.5 µg/mL (SI: 2.7-4.1 µmol/L); fluphenazine: 2-4 ng/mL; therapeutic response and blood levels have not been established for trifluoperazine

Possible Panic Range Toxic: **chlorpromazine:** >750 ng/mL (SI: >2350 nmol/L); **thioridazine:** >10 µg/mL (SI: >27 nmol/L); **trifluoperazine:** >50 ng/mL (SI: >104 nmol/L); fluphenazine: >20 ng/mL

Use Evaluate phenothiazine toxicity

Limitations Suboptimal assay accuracy and number of drug metabolites make clinical application infrequent. These drugs are not usually monitored because poor correlation exists between serum level and antipsychotic effect.

Methodology Thin-layer chromatography (TLC), gas-liquid chromatography (GLC), radioimmunoassay (RIA), high performance liquid chromatography (HPLC), spectrophotometry

Additional Information
- Half-life: 20-50 hours
- Volume of distribution: 15-25 L/kg
- Protein binding: 70% to 90%

Phenothiazines are tranquilizers frequently used in the treatment of psychoses. They may act by antagonizing postsynaptic dopamine receptors. There are three different classes of phenothiazines: aliphatic (chlorpromazine), piperidine (thioridazine), and piperazine (fluphenazine). All are effective in therapy in appropriate doses, but differ in frequency, type, and severity of side effects. Side effects include drowsiness, ataxia, respiratory depression, hypotension, tachycardia, cardiac arrest, bone marrow depression. There is also a "dysphoric" response by some patients.

The piperazine prochlorperazine (Compazine®) is widely used as an antiemetic.

Phenothiazines can also be measured in urine and gastric contents.

Chlorpromazine and thioridazine cause false-positives for phenylketonuria, urinary amylase, uroporphyrins, and urobilinogen.

References

Adamczyk M, Fishpaugh JR, Harrington CA, et al, "Immunoassay Reagents for Psychoactive Drugs. Part 3. Removal of Phenothiazine Interferences in the Quantification of Tricyclic Antidepressants," *Ther Drug Monit*, 1993, 15:(5)436-9.

Chouinard G, Annable L, and Campbell W, "A Randomized Clinical Trial of Haloperidol Decanoate and Fluphenazine Decanoate in the Outpatient Treatment of Schizophrenia," *J Clin Psychopharmacol*, 1989, 9(4):247-53.

Cooper JK, Hawes EM, Hubbard JW, et al, "An Ultrasensitive Method for the Measurement of Fluphenazine in Plasma by High Performance Liquid Chromatography With Coulometric Detection," *Ther Drug Monit*, 1989, 11(3):354-60.

Knight ME and Roberts RJ, "Phenothiazine and Butyrophenone Intoxication in Children," *Pediatr Clin North Am*, 1986, 33(2):299-309.

Krishel S and Jackimczyk K, "Cyclic Antidepressants, Lithium, and Neuroleptic Agents. Pharmacology and Toxicology," *Emerg Med Clin North Am*, 1991, 9(1):53-86.

Levinson DF, Simpson GM, Singh H, et al, "Fluphenazine Dose, Clinical Response, and Extrapyramidal Symptoms During Acute Treatment," *Arch Gen Psychiatry*, 1990, 47(8):761-8.

Marder SR, Midha KK, Van Putten T, et al, "Plasma Levels of Fluphenazine in Patients Receiving Fluphenazine Decanoate. Relationship to Clinical Response," *Br J Psychiatry*, 1991, 158:658-65.

Midha KK, Hubbard JW, Marder SR, et al, "Impact of Clinical Pharmacokinetics on Neuroleptic Therapy in Patients With Schizophrenia," *J Psychiatry Neurosci*, 1994, 19(4):254-64.

Midha KK, Marder SR, Jaworski TJ, et al, "Clinical Perspectives of Some Neuroleptics Through Development and Application of Their Assays," *Ther Drug Monit*, 1993, 15(3):179-89.

Ryan PM, "Epidemiology, Etiology, Diagnosis, and Treatment of Schizophrenia," *Am J Hosp Pharm*, 1991, 48(6):1271-80.

Phentermine *see* Methamphetamine, Qualitative, Urine *on page 562*

Phenurone® *see* Phenacemide *on page 567*

5-Phenyl-5-Ethylhydantoin (Nirvanol®) *see* Mephenytoin *on page 560*

Phenylethylmalonamide *see* Primidone *on next page*

Phenylethylmalonylurea *see* Phenobarbital, Blood *on previous page*

Phenylpropanolamine *see* Methamphetamine, Qualitative, Urine *on page 562*

Phenytoin

CPT 80185

Related Information

Amiodarone, Serum *on page 532*
Amoxapine, Blood *on page 533*
Antidepressants, Cyclic *on page 535*
Carbamazepine *on page 540*
Chloramphenicol *on page 542*
Cyclosporine *on page 545*
Disopyramide *on page 547*
Ethosuximide *on page 549*
Felbamate *on page 550*
Imipramine *on page 554*
Ketoconazole *on page 556*
Lamotrigine *on page 556*
Mephenytoin *on page 560*
Mexiletine *on page 563*
Nortriptyline *on page 565*
Phenobarbital, Blood *on previous page*
Phenytoin, Free *on next page*
Primidone *on next page*
Quinidine, Serum *on page 572*
Theophylline *on page 575*
Valproic Acid *on page 577*
Vigabatrin *on page 579*

Synonyms Antisacer®; Dilantin®; Dintoina®; Diphenylan Sodium®; Diphenylhydantoin; Ditan®; Epanutin®; Epinat®; Fenitoina; Fenytoin®

Abstract Phenytoin is effective for generalized tonic-clonic and partial seizures. Serum levels should be monitored.

Specimen Serum or plasma

Container Red top tube or lavender top (EDTA) tube

Sampling Time In monitoring patients maintained on chronic therapy, a trough level or consistent sampling time should be used.

Reference Range 10-20 µg/mL (SI: 40-79 µmol/L); toxicity is measured clinically and some patients require levels outside the suggested therapeutic range. Free phenytoin: 1-2 µg/mL (SI: 4-8 µmol/L).

Patients treated for status epilepticus should have levels at or slightly above the upper limit of range. **Low level:** The most common cause of a low level is noncompliance. Absorption problems are most important in young infants (younger than 3 months) or occasionally in patients given phenobarbital, charcoal, or antacids at the same time as the phenytoin.

Pediatric and some adult patients (fast metabolizers), who have breakthrough seizures at the end of the day, require more than once daily dosing. Some formulations other than Kapseals® may require more than once daily dosing, and changing formulations can cause changes in levels. Pregnancy or intercurrent illness such as mononucleosis can cause subtherapeutic levels with seizures. The addition of carbamazepine to a patient taking phenytoin can lower or raise phenytoin level but usually does not cause seizures. Disulfiram administration can increase phenytoin metabolism, lower levels, and may cause seizures. Patients can have lower than expected values if intravenous formulations are given with fluids containing glucose, which precipitates in solution with phenytoin. **High levels**: In patients chronically controlled on phenytoin who become clinically toxic without a change in dose, toxicity can be brought on by a change in formulation, drug interaction, or intercurrent infection. Drugs which can precipitate phenytoin toxicity include chloramphenicol, tricyclic antidepressants, fluconazole, levodopa, and others (see Additional Information). Small dose changes or changes in formulation (including change from one brand to another or to a generic) can cause large changes in antiepileptic drug (AED) levels and toxicity, because phenytoin manifests zero-order kinetics.

Possible Panic Range Toxic: 25-50 µg/mL (SI: 120-200 µmol/L); **lethal**: >100 µg/mL (SI: >400 µmol/L). Toxicity may manifest progressively outside reference range (or occasionally within it) with ataxia, dizziness, nystagmus, and diplopia. Patients can have life-threatening complications with intravenous administration with normal levels; such patients should be placed on a cardiac monitor during intravenous administration of drug.

Use Monitor for compliance, efficacy, and possible toxicity

Limitations See Phenytoin, Free *on page 570*. A systemic allergic reaction characterized by fever, rash, lymphadenopathy, and eosinophilia may include granulomatous features. Necrosis of hepatocytes and cholestasis may occur, a drug-induced hypersensitivity hepatitis. A syndrome including infectious mononucleosis-like features is recognized.[1,2]

Methodology Routine: Enzyme multiplied immunoassay technique (EMIT), enzyme-linked immunosorbent assay (ELISA), and fluorescence polarization immunoassay (FPIA). For physician's office testing, apoenzyme reactive immunoassay (ARIS; Ames Seralyzer®) is rapid, accurate, and may become increasingly important.

Additional Information

- Half-life: adults: 20-40 hours, children: 10 hours
- Volume of distribution: 0.6-0.7 L/kg
- Protein binding: 85% to 95%

Ninety percent of phenytoin is bound to serum proteins. Only the unbound fraction is biologically active. Primary site of action is thought to be the motor cortex, where the promotion of a sodium "efflux" from neurons probably stabilizes the threshold of the neuron against hyperexcitability. Most of a dose of phenytoin is excreted into the bile as inactive metabolites which are then reabsorbed from the intestines and excreted into the urine. Despite normal levels, phenytoin may interfere with the actions of other drugs, including cyclosporine, oral anticoagulants, oral contraceptives, and theophylline; appropriate laboratory monitoring of some of these agents is advised. Teratogenic effects of phenytoin have been proposed but not confirmed; the risks in women of childbearing age should be balanced against the risks of increased seizures.[3]

Phenytoin may decrease the serum concentration or effectiveness of other drugs including valproic acid, carbamazepine, ethosuximide, primidone, corticosteroids, chloramphenicol, rifampin, doxycycline, quinidine, mexiletine, disopyramide, dopamine, or nondepolarizing skeletal muscle relaxants. Protein binding of phenytoin can be affected by VPA or salicylates. Serum phenytoin concentrations may be increased by cimetidine, disulfiram, trazodone, ethanol, halothane, phenylbutazone, azapropazone, ibuprofen, amiodarone, imipramine, miconazole, metronidazole, nifedipine, chloramphenicol, INH, trimethoprim, or sulfonamides and decreased by rifampin, cisplatin, vinblastine, bleomycin, folic acid, or continuous NG feeds, oxacillin, nitrofurantoin. See listing Felbamate *on page 550*.

Footnotes

1. Lee WM, "Drug-Induced Hepatotoxicity," *N Engl J Med*, 1995, 333(17):1118-27.
2. Collins RD, Casey TT, Glick AD, et al, "Lymph Nodes," *Diagnostic Surgical Pathology*, 2nd ed, Chapter 17, Sternberg SS, ed, New York, NY: Raven Press, 1994, 673-734.
3. Dalessio DJ, "Current Concepts: Seizure Disorders and Pregnancy," *N Engl J Med*, 1985, 312(9):559-63.

References

Engel J, "Seizures and Epilepsy," *Contemporary Neurology Series*, Philadelphia, PA: FA Davis Co, 1989.

Lindow J and Wijdicks EF, "Phenytoin Toxicity Associated With Hypoalbuminemia in Critically Ill Patients," *Chest*, 1994, 105(2):602-4.

Phelps SJ, Baldree LA, and Boucher BA, "Neuropsychiatric Toxicity of Phenytoin. Importance of Monitoring Phenytoin Levels," *Clin Pediatr (Phila)*, 1993, 32(2):107-10.

Phenytoin, Free

CPT 80186

Related Information

Phenytoin *on previous page*

Synonyms Free Phenytoin

Abstract Measurement of free phenytoin may be clinically important in situations associated with altered binding of phenytoin.

Specimen Serum or plasma

Container Red top tube or lavender top (EDTA) tube

Reference Range 1-2 µg/mL (SI: 4-8 µmol/L)

Possible Panic Range Toxicity may be progressive >2 µg/mL.

Additional Information

- Half-life (adults): 20-40 hours
- Volume of distribution: 0.6-0.7 L/kg
- Protein binding: 85% to 95%

Phenytoin is 90% bound to serum proteins, but only the free fraction circulates through plasma membranes and is biologically active. Because of rapid equilibration between free and bound portions of drugs, free levels are potentially important only in antiepileptic drugs (AEDs) that are highly bound (ie, phenytoin but not carbamazepine). Measurement of the free fraction is not cost-effective on a routine outpatient basis, but may be clinically relevant in exceptional circumstances associated with alterations in the binding of phenytoin.[1] Binding kinetics may be altered in uremia, hepatic disease, late pregnancy or postpartum, cases of head injury associated with a hypermetabolic state, and certain instances of polypharmacy, described below.[2,3,4] Determination of free levels may also be helpful in overdosages, since only the free portion can be cleared by dialysis.

Most phenytoin is excreted into bile as inactive metabolites which are then reabsorbed by the intestines and excreted into the urine. In renal disease, total phenytoin levels may generate falsely high values, leading to inadequate dosage. Dialysis may increase the amount of free phenytoin available.[5] In hepatic disease, phenytoin competes with endogenous bilirubin for binding sites,[6] and thus the need for a free level may be greatest if the total bilirubin level is high and albumin low. Available liver function tests are not predictive of free phenytoin levels in patients with liver disease.[4]

Drugs which compete for binding sites on albumin and which may displace phenytoin include valproic acid, acetazolamide, high doses of salicylic acid, phenylbutazone, ceftriaxone, nafcillin, and sulfamethoxazole.[7] In a clinical setting in which one of these drugs is used with phenytoin and toxicity is suspected despite normal phenytoin levels, a free level may be useful.

The free phenytoin level can be approximated by the total phenytoin level in cerebrospinal fluid or saliva or other body fluids that are albumin-poor.

Footnotes

1. Theodore WH, Yu L, Price B, et al, "The Clinical Value of Free Phenytoin Levels," *Ann Neurol*, 1985, 18(1):90-3.
2. Levy RH, Dreifuss FE, Mattson RH, et al, *Antiepileptic Drugs*, 3rd ed, New York, NY: Raven Press, 1989.
3. Griebel ML, Kearns GL, Fiser DH, et al, "Phenytoin Protein Binding in Pediatric Patients With Acute Traumatic Injury," *Crit Care Med*, 1990, 18(4):385-91.
4. Dasgupta A, Dennen DA, Dean R, et al, "Prediction of Free Phenytoin Levels Based on Total Phenytoin/Albumin Ratios," *Am J Clin Pathol*, 1991, 95(2):253-6.
5. Dasgupta A and Abu-Alfa A, "Increased Free Phenytoin Concentrations in Predialysis Serum Compared to Postdialysis Serum in Patients With Uremia Treated With Hemodialysis: Role of Uremic Compounds," *Am J Clin Pathol*, 1992, 98(1):19-25.
6. Hooper W, Sutherland J, Bochner F, et al, "Plasma Protein Binding of Diphenylhydantoin. Effects of Sex Hormones, Renal and Hepatic Disease," *Clin Pharmacol Ther*, 1973, 15:276-82.
7. Dasgupta A, Dennen DA, Dean R, et al, "Displacement of Phenytoin From Serum Protein Carriers by Antibiotics: Studies With Ceftriaxone, Nafcillin, and Sulfamethoxazole," *Clin Chem*, 1991, 37(1):98-100.

References

Lenn N and Robertson M, "Clinical Utility of Unbound Antiepileptic Drug Blood Levels in the Management of Epilepsy," *Neurology*, 1992, 42(5):988-90.

Tomson T, Lindbom U, and Ekqvist B, "Epilepsy and Pregnancy: A Prospective Study of Seizure Control in Relation to Free and Total Plasma Concentrations of Carbamazepine and Phenytoin," *Epilepsia*, 1994, 35(1):122-30.

Phos-Flur® *see* Fluoride, Serum *on page 551*

Phyllocontin® *see* Theophylline *on page 575*

Physeptone® *see* Methadone, Urine *on page 561*

Pick-me-up® *see* Caffeine, Blood *on page 539*

Placidyl® *see* Ethchlorvynol *on page 549*

Point-Two® *see* Fluoride, Serum *on page 551*

Poisonous Metals, Blood *see* Heavy Metal Screen, Blood *on page 554*

Poisonous Metals, Urine *see* Heavy Metal Screen, Urine *on page 554*

Poppy Seeds *see* Opiates, Qualitative, Urine *on page 566*

Pot *see* Cannabinoids (Marijuana Metabolites), Qualitative, Urine *on page 539*

Potassium or Sodium Cyanide *see* Cyanide, Blood *on page 544*

Potassium Thiocyanate (KSCN) *see* Thiocyanate, Blood or Urine *on page 575*

Pre-employment Drug Screen *see* Drugs of Abuse Testing, Urine *on page 548*

Presamine® *see* Imipramine *on page 554*

Presamine® *see* Antidepressants, Cyclic *on page 535*

Prevident® *see* Fluoride, Serum *on page 551*

Primaclone *see* Primidone *on this page*

Primidone

CPT 80188

Related Information

Phenobarbital, Blood *on page 568*

Phenytoin *on previous page*

Urinalysis *on page 658*

Valproic Acid *on page 577*

Synonyms Desoxyphenobarbital; Hexamidinum; Majsolin®; Mylepsin®; Mysoline®; Primaclone; Prysolin®

Applies to Metabolites of Primidone; PEMA; Phenylethylmalonamide

Test Commonly Includes Phenobarbital, PEMA

Abstract Primidone is indicated for generalized tonic-clonic and partial seizures. Concurrent monitoring of its active metabolite, phenobarbital, is necessary.

Specimen Serum or plasma

Container Red top tube, green top (heparin) tube, or lavender top (EDTA) tube

Sampling Time Trough or consistent sampling time. Levels of phenobarbital and PEMA can be measured simultaneously.

Reference Range Children younger than 5 years of age: 7-10 µg/mL (SI: 32-46 µmol/L); adults: 5-12 µg/mL (SI: 23-55 µmol/L). Phenobarbital concentration should also be used to guide dosing. Phenobarbital, serum: 15-40 µg/mL.

Critical Values At levels >12 µg/mL (SI: >55 µmol/L) primidone produces CNS depression, vertigo, visual disturbances, areflexia, somnolence, and lethargy. Clinical toxicity correlates with primidone rather than metabolite concentrations. In overdosage, a biphasic peak may be seen with highest toxicity a few hours after ingestion and again 48 hours afterwards. Crystalluria is a feature of overdosage.

Possible Panic Range >15 µg/mL (SI: >69 µmol/L). See Table A in the Therapeutic Drug Monitoring/Toxicology/Drugs of Abuse Appendix *on page 582*.

Use Monitor efficacy, compliance, and possible toxicity

Methodology Enzyme immunoassay (EIA), gas-liquid chromatography (GLC), high performance liquid chromatography (HPLC)

Additional Information

- Half-life: 4-12 hours
- Volume of distribution: 0.5-1.0 L/kg
- Protein binding: 0% to 20%

Since phenobarbital requires a longer interval (48 hours) to achieve therapeutic blood levels, checking both levels can be used to determine chronic compliance. The phenobarbital/primidone ratio normally is 2.5, can be higher (4.3 mean) in patients on other anticonvulsants (phenytoin, carbamazepine) and lower than normal among patients discontinued from those medicines or who are chronically noncompliant. Primidone decreases the effects of oral anticoagulants. Primidone may increase alkaline phosphatase and decrease calcium.

References

Kutt H, "Phenobarbital: Interactions With Other Drugs," *Antiepileptic Drugs*, 3rd ed, Levy RH, Dreifuss FE, Mattson RH, et al, eds, New York, NY: Raven Press, 1989, 313-27.

Schafer H, "Primidone: Chemistry and Methods of Determination," *Antiepileptic Drugs*, 3rd ed, Levy RH, Dreifuss FE, Mattson RH, et al, eds, New York, NY: Raven Press, 1989, 379-90.

Procainamide

CPT 80190

Related Information

Amiodarone, Serum *on page 532*

Amoxapine, Blood *on page 533*

Antinuclear Antibody *on page 368*

Imipramine *on page 554*

Nortriptyline *on page 565*

Quinidine, Serum *on page 572*

Synonyms Biocoryl®; Novocainamidum; Novocamid®; Procaine Amide Hydrochloride; Procan® SR; Pronestyl®; Pronestyl-SR®; Retard®; Rhythmin®

Applies to N-Acetyl Procainamide; NAPA

Test Commonly Includes Procainamide and its metabolite, N-acetyl procainamide (NAPA)

Abstract This drug is an antiarrhythmic with an active metabolite, N-acetyl procainamide. Both should be measured when therapeutic drug monitoring is used.

Specimen Serum

Container Red top tube

Sampling Time Oral treatment: peak: 75 minutes after dose; trough: immediately before next dose. I.V. treatment: immediately after loading dose; 2, 6, 12, and 24 hours after starting I.V. maintenance.

Special Instructions One sample is an inadequate basis for evaluating dosing. Three steady-state levels should be obtained during one dosing interval. For therapeutic drug monitoring, consistently use the same time interval between sampling and dose administration when comparing results from serial samples.

Reference Range Therapeutic: procainamide: 4.0-10.0 µg/mL (SI: 17-42 µmol/L); NAPA: 10-30 µg/mL; sum of procainamide and N-acetyl procainamide: <30 µg/mL (SI: <127 µmol/L). Optimal ranges must be ascertained for individual patients with ECG monitoring.

Possible Panic Range Toxic: procainamide: >14 µg/mL (SI: >59.5 µmol/L); sum of procainamide and N-acetyl procainamide: >30 µg/mL (SI: >127 µmol/L). See Table C in the Therapeutic Drug Monitoring/Toxicology/Drugs of Abuse Appendix *on page 583*.

Use Monitor therapeutic drug level

Limitations Severely hemolyzed, lipemic, or icteric specimens interfere with methods other than HPLC and GC.[1] **Evaluation of toxicity must be made with consideration of patient's clinical status.**

Long-term administration leads to the development of a positive antinuclear antibody test in 50% of patients. A lupus erythematosus-like syndrome may evolve in 20% to 30% of patients.

Methodology Enzyme immunoassay (EIA), fluorescence polarization immunoassay (FPIA), enzyme-multiplied immunoassay (EMIT); high performance liquid chromatography (HPLC), gas chromatography (GC)

Additional Information
- Half-life: procainamide: 2-6 hours, NAPA: 8 hours
- Volume of distribution: 2-4 L/kg
- Protein binding: 10% to 20%

The cardiac actions of this drug are similar to those of quinidine. It is used in a variety of arrhythmias. Procainamide usually is rapidly absorbed from the gastrointestinal tract. Peak blood levels are reached within 1 hour. Optimal plasma sampling time after oral dosage is 1-2 hours. Optimal sampling time after I.V. administration of dose is 30 minutes. The drug is converted by the liver to its active metabolite, N-acetyl procainamide (NAPA). Rate of metabolism is genetically determined (slow and fast acetylator types) contributing to significant inter-individual variability. Impairment of renal function has pronounced effect on drug disposition, especially for NAPA. Patients with severe renal dysfunction generally have prolonged and highly variable half-life characteristics. Elimination half-life may be prolonged in geriatric subjects.[2]

Footnotes
1. Sherwin JE, "Procainamide and N-Acetylprocainamide," *Clinical Chemistry Theory, Analysis, and Correlation*, 2nd ed, Kaplan LA and Pesce AJ, eds, St Louis, MO: Mosby-Year Book Inc, 1989, 1110-3.
2. Montamat SC, Cusack BJ, and Vestal RE, "Management of Drug Therapy in the Elderly," *N Engl J Med*, 1989, 321(5):303-9.

References
Adams LE, Roberts SM, Donovan-Brand R, et al, "Study of Procainamide Hapten-Specific Antibodies in Rabbits and Humans," *Int J Immunopharmacol*, 1993, 15(8):887-97.
Funck-Brentano C, Light RT, Lineberry MD, et al, "Pharmacokinetic and Pharmacodynamic Interaction of N-Acetyl Procainamide and Procainamide in Humans," *J Cardiovasc Pharmacol*, 1989, 14(3):364-73.
Gottlieb SS, Kukin ML, Medina N, et al, "Comparative Hemodynamic Effects of Procainamide, Tocainide, and Encainide in Severe Chronic Heart Failure," *Circulation*, 1990, 81(3):860-4.
Grimm W, Cho JG, and Marchlinski FE, "Effects of Incremental Doses of Procainamide in Patients With Sustained Uniform Ventricular Tachycardia," *J Cardiovasc Electrophysiol*, 1994, 5(4):313-22.
Interian A Jr, Zaman L, Velez-Robinson E, et al, "Paired Comparisons of Efficacy of Intravenous and Oral Procainamide in Patients With Inducible Sustained Ventricular Tachyarrhythmias," *J Am Coll Cardiol*, 1991, 17(7):1581-6.
Yamaji A, Kataoka K, Oishi M, et al, "Simultaneous Determination of Procainamide and N-Acetylprocainamide in Serum by Gas Chromatography With Nitrogen-Selective Detection," *J Chromatogr*, 1987, 415(1):143-7.

Procaine Amide Hydrochloride *see Procainamide on previous page*

Procan® SR *see Procainamide on previous page*

Prochlorperazine *see Phenothiazines, Serum on page 568*

Prolixin® *see Fluphenazine on page 552*

Prolixin® *see Phenothiazines, Serum on page 568*

Pronestyl® *see Procainamide on previous page*

Pronestyl-SR® *see Procainamide on previous page*

Propacet® *see Propoxyphene, Serum or Urine on this page*

Pro-Plus® *see Caffeine, Blood on page 539*

Propoxyphene, Serum or Urine

CPT 80101 (screen); 80102 (confirmation, each procedure)

Related Information

Chain-of-Custody Protocol *on page 542*
Drugs of Abuse Testing, Urine *on page 548*

Synonyms Darvocet-N®; Darvon®; E-Lor®; Genagesic®; Propacet®; Wygesic®

Applies to Norpropoxyphene

Test Commonly Includes Quantitation of propoxyphene and metabolite norpropoxyphene

Abstract Propoxyphene is a narcotic analgesic and is also a drug of abuse.

Specimen Serum (TDM), urine (drugs of abuse)

Container Red top tube, urine container

Sampling Time Urine: random; serum: trough

Special Instructions If forensic, use chain-of-custody protocol and form. See test listing Chain-of-Custody Protocol *on page 542* and the Therapeutic Drug Monitoring/Toxicology/Drugs of Abuse Appendix *on page 581*.

Reference Range Therapeutic: serum: 0.1-0.4 µg/mL (SI: 0.3-1.2 µmol/L) (therapeutic ranges published vary between laboratories and may not correlate with clinical effect); urine (for drugs of abuse): negative (less than cutoff)

Critical Values Cutoff for urine: screen: 0.3 µg/mL; confirmation: 0.2 µg/mL

Possible Panic Range Toxic: serum: >0.5 µg/mL (SI: >1.5 µmol/L); minimal fatal: 1.0 µg/mL (SI: 2.9 µmol/L)

Use Therapeutic monitoring, toxicity assessment, and drug-of-abuse testing

Methodology Immunoassay, gas chromatography (GC), high performance liquid chromatography (HPLC)

Additional Information
- Half-life: 8-24 hours
- Volume of distribution: 10-25 L/kg
- Protein binding: 70% to 80%

Propoxyphene is an analgesic structurally similar to methadone. Its metabolite, norpropoxyphene is also pharmacologically active. Toxic effects include nausea, vomiting, and progressive central nervous system depression. Toxicity is additive with ethanol. Toxicity can be neutralized by narcotic antagonists. Peak serum level occurs 2 hours postoral dose. Propoxyphene can also be measured in urine as part of a drug of abuse screen.

References
Gilman AG, Goodman LS, Rall TW, et al, *The Pharmacological Basis of Therapeutics*, 7th ed, New York, NY: Macmillan Publishing, 1985, 519-20.
Hartman B, Miyada DS, Pirkle H, et al, "Serum Propoxyphene Concentrations in a Cohort of Opiate Addicts on Long-Term Propoxyphene Maintenance Therapy. Evidence for Drug Tolerance in Humans," *J Anal Toxicol*, 1988, 12(1):25-9.
King JW and King LJ, "Propoxyphene and Norpropoxyphene Quantitation in the Same Solid-Phase Extraction Using Toxi Lab Spec VC MP3 System," *J Anal Toxicol*, 1994, 18(4):217-9.
Kurlan R, Majumdar L, Deeley C, et al, "A Controlled Trial of Propoxyphene and Naltrexone in Patients With Tourette's Syndrome," *Ann Neurol*, 1991, 30(1):19-23.
Oles KS, Mirza W, and Penry JK, "Catastrophic Neurologic Signs Due to Drug Interaction: Tegretol® and Darvon®," *Surg Neurol*, 1989, 32(2):144-51.

Propranolol

CPT 84600

Related Information

Flecainide *on page 551*

Synonyms Angilol®; Apsolol®; Beaden®; Bedranol®; Berkolol®; Deralin®; Inderal®

Abstract A relatively short-acting beta-blocker. Propranolol is used as an antianginal agent, an antiarrhythmic, and as an antihypertensive.

Specimen Serum

Container Red top tube

Sampling Time Trough: immediately prior to next dose

Special Instructions The stoppers of some blood collection tubes contain TBEP plasticizers that affect drug distribution in sample. Check with local laboratory.

Reference Range Therapeutic: 50-100 ng/mL (SI: 190-390 nmol/L) at end of dose interval

(Continued)

Propranolol *(Continued)*

Possible Panic Range >1000 ng/mL (SI: >3860 nmol/L); **fatal:** >2000 ng/mL (SI: >7702 nmol/L). See Table C in the Therapeutic Drug Monitoring/Toxicology/Drugs of Abuse Appendix *on page 583*.

Use Monitor therapeutic drug level in patients with cardiac arrhythmias, angina pectoris, and hypertension; evaluate for potential toxicity

Limitations See listing Flecainide *on page 551*.

Methodology Fluorometry, fluorescence polarization immunoassay (FPIA), enzyme immunoassay (EIA), gas-liquid chromatography (GLC), high performance liquid chromatography (HPLC)

Additional Information
- Half-life: 4-6 hours
- Volume of distribution: 3-4 L/kg
- Protein binding: 90% to 95%

Propranolol is well absorbed after oral administration. For therapeutic drug monitoring, consistently use the same time interval between sampling and dose administration when comparing results from serial samples. A number of metabolites have been identified with at least one, 4-hydroxyl propranolol, having pharmacologic activity. Adverse effects of this drug include precipitation of heart failure, bronchospasm, bradycardia, and hypoglycemia. Hyperthyroidism exerts an age-dependent inducing effect on the metabolism of propranolol.[1]

Phenobarbital, rifampin may increase propranolol clearance and may decrease its activity. Cimetidine may reduce propranolol clearance and may increase its effects.

Propranolol may increase thyroxine, cholesterol, and glucose in test samples.

Footnotes
1. Montamat SC, Cusack BJ, and Vestal RE, "Management of Drug Therapy in the Elderly," *N Engl J Med*, 1989, 321(5):303-9.

References

Hall ST, Harding SM, Hassani H, et al, "The Pharmacokinetic and Pharmacodynamic Interaction Between Lacidipine and Propranolol in Health Volunteers," *J Cardiovasc Pharmacol*, 1991, 18(Suppl 11):S13-7.

Nace GS and Wood AJ, "Pharmacokinetics of Long-Acting Propranolol Implications for Therapeutic Use," *Clin Pharmacokinet*, 1987, 13(1):51-64.

Walle T, Walle UK, Cowart TD, et al, "Pathway-Selective Sex Differences in the Metabolic Clearance of Propranolol in Human Subjects," *Clin Pharmacol Ther*, 1989, 46(3):257-63.

2-Propylpentanoic Acid *see* Valproic Acid *on page 577*

2-Propylvaleric Acid *see* Valproic Acid *on page 577*

Protriptyline *see* Antidepressants, Cyclic *on page 535*

Prozac® *see* Fluoxetine *on page 551*

Prozil® *see* Chlorpromazine, Serum or Urine *on page 543*

Prysolin® *see* Primidone *on page 570*

Pseudoephedrine *see* Methamphetamine, Qualitative, Urine *on page 562*

Purgoxin® *see* Digoxin *on page 546*

Purodigin® *see* Digitoxin *on page 546*

Quinaglute® Dura-Tabs® *see* Quinidine, Serum *on this page*

Quinalan® *see* Quinidine, Serum *on this page*

Quinidex® Extentabs® *see* Quinidine, Serum *on this page*

Quinidine, Serum

CPT 80194

Related Information

Amiodarone, Serum *on page 532*
Amoxapine, Blood *on page 533*
Digoxin *on page 546*
Imipramine *on page 554*
Nortriptyline *on page 565*
Phenobarbital, Blood *on page 568*
Phenytoin *on page 569*
Procainamide *on page 570*
Verapamil *on page 578*

Synonyms Biquin®; Cardioquin®; Cin-Quin®; Kiditard®; Kinidin®; Quinaglute® Dura-Tabs®; Quinalan®; Quinidex® Extentabs®; Quini® Durules®; Quinora®; Systodin®

Abstract Quinidine is an antiarrhythmic that is frequently monitored. A great many drug interactions are recognized.

Specimen Serum

Container Red top tube. The stoppers on some tubes contain plasticizers which affect measured drug levels.

Sampling Time Trough: collect just before next dose.

Special Instructions Serum concentration **must be correlated** with patient's clinical status.

Reference Range Therapeutic: 2-5 µg/mL (SI: 6.2-15.4 µmol/L). Patient dependent therapeutic response occurs at levels of 3-6 µg/mL (SI: 9.2-18.5 µmol/L). Optimal therapeutic level is method dependent.[1]

Possible Panic Range Toxic: >8 µg/mL (SI: >24.7 µmol/L). Levels >14 µg/L associated with cardiac toxicity. See Table C in the Therapeutic Drug Monitoring/Toxicology/Drugs of Abuse Appendix *on page 583*.

Use Therapeutic monitoring for quinidine is to provide documentation for adequate dosage[1] as well as toxicity assessment.

Limitations An assay method should be used which also detects active metabolites, in particular dihydroquinidine. Cross reactions occur with EMIT and fluorescence polarization methods.

Methodology Enzyme-multiplied immunoassay technique (EMIT), fluorometry, high performance liquid chromatography (HPLC),[1,2,3,4] gas chromatography (GC)

Additional Information
- Half-life: 6-8 hours
- Volume of distribution: 2-3 L/kg
- Protein binding: 70% to 90%

Optimal resampling time after change in dosage is 1-2 days. **Doses >250 mg/day of quinidine result in increased serum digoxin concentrations about 2.5 times the digoxin concentration before quinidine was added.** The new steady-state of digoxin concentration occurs in 7-14 days, with signs of toxicity beginning to appear in 3-7 days after initiation of quinidine therapy. Therefore, **serum digoxin concentrations should be measured before initiation of quinidine therapy and again in 4-6 days.** Measure trough because of variability of peak interval. Concomitant administration of **phenytoin** increases hepatic metabolism, and therefore decreases half-life and serum quinidine concentrations. Verapamil, amiodarone, alkalinizing agents, and cimetidine may increase quinidine serum concentrations; phenobarbital, and rifampin may decrease quinidine serum concentrations. Beta-blockers and quinidine may cause increased bradycardia; quinidine may enhance coumarin anticoagulants. Cimetidine impairs elimination of quinidine; quinidine and verapamil may result in severe hypotension; nifedipine may reduce serum quinidine levels and quinidine is reported to inhibit nifedipine metabolism.[5] Clearance may be diminished in the elderly.[6] **Renal failure** prolongs apparent half-life, perhaps through accumulation of fluorescent metabolites. Severe heart failure also prolongs half-life, as does liver disease.

Psoriasiform eruption[7] and pneumonitis[8] have been reported.

Footnotes
1. Meineke I, Rohde S, and Gundert-Remy U, "An Inexpensive and Sensitive Method for the Determination of Quinidine in Plasma by High-Performance Liquid Chromatography With Ultraviolet Detection," *Ther Drug Monit*, 1995, 17(1):75-8.
2. Huang JL and Morgan DJ, "Simple Direct Injection High-Performance Liquid Chromatographic Method to Determine Quinidine in Plasma," *J Chromatogr*, 1993, 620(2):278-80.
3. Nielsen F, Nielsen KK, and Brosen K, "Determination of Quinidine, Dihydroquinidine, (3S)-3-Hydroxyquinidine, and Quinidine N-oxide in Plasma and Urine by High-Performance Liquid Chromatography," *J Chromatogr B Biomed Appl*, 1994, 660(1):103-10.
4. Brandsteterova E, Romanova D, Kralikova D, et al, "Automatic Solid-Phase Extraction and High-Performance Liquid Chromatographic Determination of Quinidine in Plasma," *J Chromatogr A*, 1994, 665(1):101-4.
5. Bowles SK, Reeves RA, Cardozo L, et al, "Evaluation of the Pharmacokinetic and Pharmacodynamic Interaction Between Quinidine and Nifedipine," *J Clin Pharmacol*, 1993, 33(8):727-31.
6. Montamat SC, Cusack BJ, and Vestal RE, "Management of Drug Therapy in the Elderly," *N Engl J Med*, 1989, 321(5):303-9.
7. Brenner S, Cabili S, and Wolf R, "Widespread Erythematous Scaly Plaques in an Adult. Psoriasiform Eruption Induced by Quinidine," *Arch Dermatol*, 1993, 129(10):1331-2, 1334-5.
8. Poukkula A and Paakko P, "Quinidine-Induced Reversible Pneumonitis," *Chest*, 1994, 106(1):304-6.

References

Bonavita GJ, Pires LA, Wagshal AB, et al, "Usefulness of Oral Quinidine-Mexiletine Combination Therapy for Sustained Ventricular Tachyarrhythmias as Assessed by Programmed Electrical Stimulation When Quinidine Monotherapy Has Failed," *Am Heart J*, 1994, 127(4 Pt 1):847-51.

Burtis CA and Ashwood ER, *Tietz Textbook of Clinical Chemistry*, Philadelphia, PA: WB Saunders Co, 1994, 1123-5.

Capucci A, Boriani G, Rubino I, et al, "A Controlled Study on Oral Propafenone Versus Digoxin Plus Quinidine in Converting Recent Onset Atrial Fibrillation to Sinus Rhythm," *Int J Cardiol*, 1994, 43(3):305-13.

Eisenman DP and McKegney FP, "Delirium at Therapeutic Serum Concentrations of Digoxin and Quinidine," *Psychosomatics*, 1994, 35(1):91-3.

Giardina EG and Wechsler ME, "Low Dose Quinidine-Mexiletine Combination Therapy Versus Quinidine Monotherapy for Treatment of Ventricular Arrhythmias," *J Am Coll Cardiol*, 1990, 15(5):1138-45.

Gillis AM, Mitchell LB, Wyse DG, et al, "Quinidine Pharmacodynamics in Patients With Arrhythmia: Effects of Left Ventricular Function," *J Am Coll Cardiol*, 1995, 25(5):989-94

Kavanagh KM, Wyse DG, Mitchell LB, et al, "Contribution of Quinidine Metabolites to Electrophysiologic Responses in Human Subjects," *Clin Pharmacol Ther*, 1989, 46(3):352-8.

Kessler KM, Wozniak PM, McAuliffe D, et al, "The Clinical Implication of Changing Unbound Quinidine Levels," *Am Heart J*, 1989, 118(1):63-9.

Oberg KC, O'Toole MF, Gallastegui JL, et al, ""Late" Proarrhythmia Due to Quinidine," *Am J Cardiol*, 1994, 74(2):192-4.

Ujhelyi MR, "Spotlight Article: Quinidine Enhances Digitalis Toxicity at Therapeutic Serum Digoxin Levels," *Heart Lung*, 1993, 22(6):560-2.

Wang L, Sheldon RS, Mitchell LB, et al, "Amiloride-Quinidine Interaction: Adverse Outcomes," *Clin Pharmacol Ther*, 1994, 56(6 Pt 1):659-67.

Quini® Durules® see Quinidine, Serum *on previous page*

Quinora® see Quinidine, Serum *on previous page*

Ranitidine see Methamphetamine, Qualitative, Urine *on page 562*

Red Devils see Barbiturates, Quantitative, Blood *on page 537*

Redutemp® see Acetaminophen, Serum *on page 530*

Repazine® see Chlorpromazine, Serum or Urine *on page 543*

Resposan-10® see Chlordiazepoxide, Blood *on page 542*

Retard® see Procainamide *on page 570*

Retrovir® see Zidovudine *on page 580*

Rheumatrex® see Methotrexate *on page 563*

Rhythmin® see Procainamide *on page 570*

Rhythmodan® see Disopyramide *on page 547*

Ridaura® see Gold *on page 553*

Ritmilen® see Disopyramide *on page 547*

Rivatril® see Clonazepam *on page 543*

RMS® see Morphine, Urine *on page 564*

Rock see Cocaine (Cocaine Metabolite), Qualitative, Urine *on page 543*

Rocket Fuel see Phencyclidine, Qualitative, Urine *on page 567*

Roxanol™ see Morphine, Urine *on page 564*

Roxanol SR™ see Morphine, Urine *on page 564*

Salicylate

CPT 80196

Related Information

Anion Gap *on page 81*
Glucose, Random *on page 138*
Lactic Acid, Blood *on page 156*
pH, Blood *on page 180*
pH, Urine *on page 648*
Potassium, Serum or Plasma *on page 188*

Synonyms Acetylsalicylic Acid, Blood; Anacin®; ASA, Blood; Ascriptin®; Aspergum®; Aspirin, Blood; Bufferin®; Easprin®; Ecotrin®; Empirin®; Measurin®; Salicylic Acid, Blood; Synalgos®; ZORprin®

Applies to Methyl Salicylate; Oil of Wintergreen

Abstract This is the active product produced from aspirin (acetylsalicylic acid) in the body. It is an analgesic, antipyretic and anti-inflammatory drug. Chronic salicylism in pediatric patients causes greater morbidity than acute poisoning, caused by dosing errors and/or dehydration.[1]

Specimen Serum or plasma

Container Red top tube or lavender top (EDTA) tube

Sampling Time Time to peak serum concentration is about 1-2 hours. Optimal sampling time after dosage is 4-6 hours.

Reference Range Therapeutic: <10 mg/dL (SI: <0.72 mmol/L) for analgesic; 15-20 mg/dL (SI: 1.09-1.45 mmol/L) for anti-inflammatory

Possible Panic Range Mild toxicity: 30 mg/dL (SI: 2.17 mmol/L) (tinnitus, dizziness); severe toxicity: >80 mg/dL (SI: >3.62 mmol/L) (CNS effects)

Use Monitor therapeutic drug level, evaluate aspirin toxicity

Limitations Bilirubin (at concentrations of 5-20 mg/dL) has been shown to depress salicylate results by 1-5 mg/dL. Sodium azide will increase results significantly; anticoagulants interfere.

Methodology Photometry, fluorometry, high performance liquid chromatography (HPLC), gas-liquid chromatography (GLC)

Additional Information

- Half-life: 2-3 hours
- Volume of distribution: 0.1-0.3 L/kg
- Protein binding: 90% to 95%

In patients on chronic therapy, small dose changes may produce disproportionate changes in serum level. Serum half-life is 2-3 hours on low-dose therapy, about 10 hours on high-dose treatment but reaches 15-30 hours as higher doses increase elimination half-life. Optimal resampling time after change in dosage is 6 hours. Use of antacids, which increase renal excretion, can lower serum levels. Steady-state concentrations for an individual patient are not adequately predicted from nomograms or standard dose schedules. In salicylate poisoning the following symptoms may occur: initial alkalosis followed by acidosis, ketosis, and possible elevated plasma glucose (see table). Glucose should be measured when levels >25 mg/dL (SI: >1.81 mmol/L) are detected. Salicylate can be done on urine or gastric juice. The Done nomogram is used to estimate

severity of toxicity based on blood level 6 hours or more after a single-dose ingestion, but cannot be used for chronic intoxication.[1] See nomogram. The level measured 4 hours or more following ingestion is plotted. Specimens drawn earlier may not reflect the peak. The nomogram is not useful when accumulation over several ingestions exists. Urine pH and volume hourly is advocated with urine protein quantitation, plasma pH, potassium and other electrolytes, prothrombin time, AST, ALT, serum bilirubin and arterial blood gases for care of serious pediatric salicylate poisoning. The metabolic acidosis includes lactic acid. Ketone bodies, hyperglycemia, and hypoglycemia may be detected. Low CNS glucose can take place in the presence of normal blood glucose. Salicylates are believed to play a role in the hepatonecrosis of Reye's syndrome in children. They are no longer recommended for use in children.

Serum Salicylate: Clinical Correlations

Serum Salicylate Concentration (mg/dL)	Desired Effects	Adverse Effects/ Intoxication
~10	Antiplatelet Antipyresis Analgesia	GI intolerance and bleeding, hypersensitivity, hemostatic defects
15-30	Anti-inflammatory	Mild salicylism
25-40	Treatment of rheumatic fever	Nausea/vomiting, hyperventilation, salicylism, flushing, sweating, thirst, headache, diarrhea, and tachycardia
>40		Respiratory alkalosis, hemorrhage, excitement, confusion, asterixis, pulmonary edema, convulsions, tetany, metabolic acidosis, fever, coma, cardiovascular collapse, renal and respiratory failure

SERUM SALICYLATE LEVEL AND SEVERITY OF INTOXICATION SINGLE DOSE ACUTE INGESTION NOMOGRAM

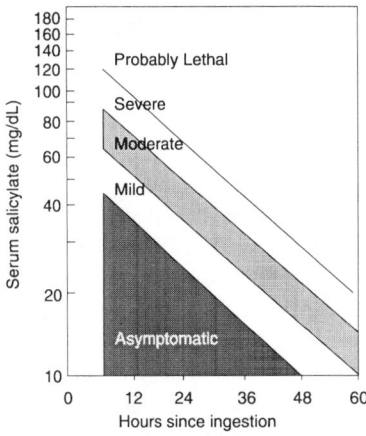

Nomogram relating serum salicylate concentration and expected severity of intoxication at varying intervals following the ingestion of a single dose of salicylate.
From Done AK, "Aspirin Overdosage: Incidence, Diagnosis, and Management," *Pediatrics*, 1978, 62:890-7 with permission.

Signs and symptoms of **acute overdose** may include nausea, vomiting, dehydration, hyperpnea, oliguria, and tinnitus. **Severe poisoning** can include coma, convulsions, severe hyperpnea, and metabolic acidosis.

Symptoms of **chronic salicylism** include fever, vomiting, and tachypnea. It is likely following doses in excess of 100 mg/kg/day for 2 days of more.[1]

Phases of aspirin poisoning:

- Phase I (up to 12 hours after ingestion): Tachypnea and hyperventilation predominate (respiratory alkalosis) with increased renal secretion of sodium, potassium, and bicarbonate resulting in both an alkaline urinary and serum pH.

- Phase II (12-24 hours after ingestion): Urine becomes more acidic as intracellular potassium decreases; while children <4 years of age may develop a pure metabolic acidosis, older patients will have significant respiratory compensation and thus serum pH can be alkalotic; coagulation abnormalities may occur.

- Phase III (over 24 hours after ingestion): Severe potassium and bicarbonate depletion occurs with renal hydrogen ion excretion; acidosis. Infants may reach this phase within 6 hours.

(Continued)

Salicylate *(Continued)*

There is an increased bleeding potential with concomitant warfarin therapy. Salicylate may increase lithium and methotrexate concentrations by decreasing renal clearance and may increase nephrotoxicity of cyclosporine. It may decrease diuretic and hypotensive effects of thiazides, loop diuretics, ACE inhibitors, and beta-blockers.

Salicylate causes false-negative results for glucose oxidase urinary glucose tests (Clinistix®), false-positives using the cupric sulfate method (Clinitest®). May interfere with VMA, 5-HIAA, xylose tolerance test, and some thyroid testing.

Footnotes

1. Mariscalco MM, "Salicylism," *Principles and Practice of Pediatrics*, 2nd ed, Oski FA, DeAngelis CD, Feigin RD, et al, eds, Philadelphia, PA: JB Lippincott Co, 1994.

References

Bailey RB and Jones SR, "Chronic Salicylate Intoxication. A Common Cause of Morbidity in the Elderly," *J Am Geriatr Soc*, 1989, 37(6):556-61.

Chapman BJ and Proudfoot AT, "Adult Salicylate Poisoning: Deaths and Outcome in Patients With High Plasma Salicylate Concentrations," *Q J Med*, 1989, 72(268):699-707.

Done AK, "Aspirin Overdosage: Incidence, Diagnosis, and Management," *Pediatrics*, 1978, 62:890-7.

Dugandric RM, Tierney MG, and Dickinson GE, "Evaluation of the Done Nomogram in the Management of Acute Salicylate Intoxication," *Ann Emerg Med*, 1989, 18(11):1186-90.

Lemesh RA, "Accidental Chronic Salicylate Intoxication in an Elderly Patient: Major Morbiditiy Despite Early Recognition," *Vet Hum Toxicol*, 1993, 35(1):34-6.

Mayer AL, Sitar DS, and Tenenbein M, "Multiple-Dose Charcoal and Whole-Bowel Irrigation Do Not Increase Clearance of Absorbed Salicylate," *Arch Intern Med*, 1992, 152(2):393-6.

Montgomery H, Porter JC, and Bradley RD, "Salicylate Intoxication Causing a Severe Systemic Inflammatory Response and Rhabdomyolysis," *Am J Emerg Med*, 1994, 12(5):531-2.

Pierce RP, Gazewood J, and Blake RL Jr, "Salicylate Poisoning From Enteric-Coated Aspirin. Delayed Absorption May Complicate Management," *Postgrad Med*, 1991, 89(5):61-2, 64.

Sallis RE, "Management of Salicylate Toxicity," *Am Fam Physician*, 1989, 39(3):265-70.

Thallium, Urine or Blood

CPT 82190

Related Information

Abstract Thallium salts have been components of insecticides and rodenticides, but thallium has been excluded as a rodenticide in the U.S. since 1972. It is used also in fireworks, imitation jewelry, lenses, as an alloy and in imaging. It may be found in grain.

Patient Preparation The patient should be instructed to use a plastic bedpan or urinal if necessary, not metal.

Specimen 24-hour urine, serum

Container Plastic urine container, red top tube

Causes for Rejection Specimen allowed to contact metal

Reference Range Urine: <10 µg/24 hours; serum: <10 ng/mL (SI: <49 nmol/L)

Possible Panic Range Blood levels >30 µg/dL are indicative of severe exposure. Toxicity is associated with blood levels of 10 µg/dL or urine levels >20µg/dL. Urine is the major pathway of elimination.

Use Diagnose thallium toxicity: symptoms initially begin with nausea, vomiting, abdominal pain, diarrhea, and gastrointestinal bleeding. A recent case description presented with abdominal colic, paresthesia, and irritability.[1]

Methodology Atomic absorption spectrometry (AA)

Additional Information

- Half-life: 3-15 days

Thallium is radiopaque. Thallium salts have been used in the past as a depilatory. Alopecia may occur several weeks after poisoning. Thallium poisoning following GI symptoms causes polyneuritis, encephalitis, delirium, ophthalmologic symptoms, convulsions, shock, and coma. Mee's lines on nails of hands and feet may appear. Severe poisoning is caused by 1 g or 8 mg/kg body weight. Lethal dose may be 15 mg/kg body weight.

Footnotes

1. Herrero F, Fernandez E, Gomez J, et al, "Thallium Poisoning Presenting With Abdominal Colic, Paresthesia, and Irritability," *J Toxicol Clin Toxicol*, 1995, 33(3):261-4.

References

Graef JW, "Heavy Metal Poisoning," *Harrison's Principles of Internal Medicine*, 13th ed, Isselbacher KJ, Braunwald E, Wilson JD, et al, eds, New York, NY: McGraw-Hill Inc, 1994, 2461-6.

Meggs W, Morasco R, Shih R, et al, "Effects of Prussian Blue and N-Acetylcysteine on Thallium Toxicity," *Vet Hum Toxicol*, 1994, 36:364.

Sabbioni E, Minoia C, Ronchi A, et al, "Trace Element Reference Values in Tissues From Inhabitants of the European Union. VIII. Thallium in the Italian Population," *Sci Total Environ*, 1994, 158(1-3):227-36.

Theophylline

CPT 80198

Related Information

Amiodarone, Serum *on page 532*
Caffeine, Blood *on page 539*
Carbamazepine *on page 540*
Ketoconazole *on page 556*
Lithium *on page 558*
Mexiletine *on page 563*
Phenobarbital, Blood *on page 568*
Phenytoin *on page 569*

Synonyms Aminophylline; Elixophyllin®; Ethylenediamine; Phyllocontin®; Slo-Phyllin®; Sustaire®; Theo-Dur®; Theolair™; Theospan®; Truphylline®

Abstract Theophylline is an antiasthmatic, a bronchodilator useful in asthma and chronic obstructive pulmonary disease (COPD). The drug is tolerated well when serum concentrations are kept within therapeutic range. It is used in neonates for idiopathic apnea/bradycardia. Atrioventricular nodal block induced by adenosine, produced by ischemic myocardium, is reported to respond to theophylline. Theophylline, a methylxanthine derivative, antagonizes cardiac actions of adenosine.

Specimen Serum

Container Red top tube

Sampling Time Measure **trough** and **peak**. Ideally, to measure peak serum theophylline **no** missed doses for previous 48 hours: draw blood at 2 hours after most recent dose for rapid dissolution preparations; 4-6 hours after sustained release preparations. See table. If toxicity is suspected, draw a level any time during a continuous I.V. infusion, or 2 hours after an oral dose.

Guidelines for Drawing Theophylline Serum Levels

Dosage Form	Time to Draw Level
P.O. liquid, fast-release tab	Peak: 1 h post 4th dose
	Trough: just before 4th dose
P.O. slow-release product	Peak: 4 h post 3rd dose
	Trough: just before 3rd dose

Time to peak serum concentration:
Oral: 1 hour
Uncoated tablets: 2 hours
Chewable tablets: 1-1.5 hours
Enteric-coated tablets: 5 hours
Extended-release capsules and tablets: 4-7 hours, in overdoses up to 27 hours
Retention enema: 1-2 hours

Theophylline levels should be initially drawn after 2 days of therapy; repeat levels are indicated 2 days after each increase in dosage or weekly if on a stabilized dosage.

Storage Instructions Refrigerate (do not freeze) a minimum of 0.5 mL serum.

Causes for Rejection Stored specimen not refrigerated

Reference Range Therapeutic: **asthma:** 10-20 µg/mL (SI: 56-111 µmol/L); **neonatal apnea:** 6-13 µg/mL (SI: 33-72 µmol/L)

Possible Panic Range >20 µg/mL (SI: >111 µmol/L); >10 µg/mL (SI: >56 µmol/L) in neonates. High probability of seizures when levels are >40 µg/mL. Chronic overmedication may induce greater risk, even when serum concentrations are in levels considered the range of mild toxicity. In this group, patient age is a sensitive predictor of toxicity. The drug should be used cautiously in elderly subjects.[1]

Use Monitor therapeutic drug level; detect noncompliance and subtherapeutic levels; attempt to predict theophylline toxicity if possible

Limitations Elderly, acutely ill subjects, and patients with severe respiratory problems, pulmonary edema, or liver dysfunction are at greater risk of toxicity because of reduced drug clearance.

Contraindications Uncontrolled arrhythmias, hypersensitivity to ethylenediamine are contraindications to use of this drug.

Methodology Enzyme immunoassay (EIA), high performance liquid chromatography (HPLC), gas chromatography (GC)

Additional Information For adult nonsmoker:
- Half-life: 6-10 hours
- Volume of distribution: 0.4-0.6 L/kg
- Protein binding: 50% to 60%

Theophylline is an alternative, antiarrhythmic drug.

The drug is extensively metabolized with peak serum levels reached 4 hours after oral dose. Troleandomycin and erythromycin may slow theophylline elimination.

Changes in diet may affect the elimination of theophylline. Theophylline may decrease the effects of phenytoin, lithium, and neuromuscular blocking agents. Theophylline increases the excretion of lithium and may

have synergistic toxicity with sympathomimetics. Cimetidine, allopurinol, propranolol, influenza virus vaccine, ciprofloxacin, oral contraceptives, amiodarone, clindamycin, and lincomycin may **increase** theophylline concentrations.

Heart failure, liver disease, prolonged fever, certain infections, and obesity may have similar effects. Prolonged half-life occurs in premature infants. **Dosage should be reduced in these situations.**

By contrast, half-life is shortened in smokers, variable with phenobarbital administration; higher doses tolerated also in acidemia. Smokers on the average are reported to need 1.5 to 2 times as much of the drugs as nonsmokers to achieve the same effects. Marijuana smoking, rifampin, phenobarbital, phenytoin, and aminoglutethimide may **decrease** theophylline concentrations. Optimal resampling time after change in dosage is 48 hours for adults, 1-2 days for children. The half-life varies between individuals. See table.

Theophylline Half-Life

Half-life (h)	Patient Population
6-10	Normal healthy
2-9	Children
15-58	Premature infants
18-24	Severe congestive heart failure
29	Cirrhosis

Studying serum concentrations and toxic effects, Bertino et al found toxicity with peak theophylline concentrations as low as 19.4 mg/L (SI: 108 µmol/L). Recognizing theophylline toxicity over a wide range of theophylline levels, these authors questioned the association between the severity of toxic effects and serum concentrations.[2] Aitken and Martin also found lack of correlation between serum theophylline level and toxic effects.[3]

Blood levels should be interpreted in light of the patient's clinical status and use of other medications.

Toxic effects and signs and symptoms of acute overdose include nausea, vomiting, abdominal pain, tremors, esophageal ulceration, palpitations, anorexia, diuresis, skin rash, insomnia, irritability, atrial fibrillation, tachycardia, paroxysmal supraventricular tachycardia, convulsions, hypotension, visual hallucinations, hypokalemia, hypercalcemia, lactic acidosis, feces discoloration (black), and death.

Footnotes

1. Shannon M, "Predictors of Major Toxicity After Theophylline Overdose," *Ann Intern Med*, 1993, 119(12):1161-7.
2. Bertino JS Jr and Walker JW, "Reassessment of Theophylline Toxicity: Serum Concentrations, Clinical Course, and Treatment," *Arch Intern Med*, 1987, 147(4):757-60.
3. Aitken ML and Martin TR, "Life-Threatening Theophylline Toxicity Is Not Predictable by Serum Levels," *Chest*, 1987, 91(1):10-4.

References

Anderson W, Youl B, and Mackay IR, "Acute Theophylline Intoxication," *Ann Emerg Med*, 1991, 20(10):1143-5.

Bectolet BD, McMurtrie EB, Hill JA, et al, "Theophylline for the Treatment of Atrioventricular Block After Myocardial Infarction," *Ann Intern Med*, 1995, 123(7):509-11.

Butts JD, Secrest B, and Berger R, "Nonlinear Theophylline Pharmacokinetics. A Preventable Cause of Iatrogenic Theophylline Toxic Reactions," *Arch Intern Med*, 1991, 151(10):2073-7.

Emerman CL, Devlin C, and Connors AF, "Risk of Toxicity in Patients With Elevated Theophylline Levels," *Ann Emerg Med*, 1990, 19(6):643-8.

Epstein PE, "Hemlock or Healer? The Mercurial Reputation of Theophylline," *Ann Intern Med*, 1993, 119(12):1216-7.

Greenberger PA, Cranberg JA, Ganz MA, et al, "A Prospective Evaluation of Elevated Serum Theophylline Concentrations to Determine if High Concentrations are Predictable," *Am J Med*, 1991, 91(1):67-73.

Huang D, O'Brien RG, Harman E, et al, "Does Aminophylline Benefit Adults Admitted to the Hospital for an Acute Exacerbation of Asthma?" *Ann Intern Med*, 1993, 119(12):1155-60.

Paloucek FP and Rodvold KA, "Evaluation of Theophylline Overdoses and Toxicities," *Ann Emerg Med*, 1988, 17(2):135-44.

Poe RH and Utell MJ, "Theophylline in Asthma and COPD: Changing Perspectives and Controversies," *Geriatrics*, 1991, 46(4):55-6, 61-5.

Rowe DJF, Watson ID, and Williams J, "The Clinical Use and Measurement of Theophylline," *Ann Clin Biochem*, 1988, 25(Pt 1):4-266.

Ruff F, Santais MC, Callens E, et al, "Effect of Temafloxacin on the Pharmacokinetics of Theophylline," *Am J Med*, 1991, 91(6A):76S-80S.

Schiff G, Regde H, LaCloche L, et al, "Inpatient Theophylline Toxicity: Preventable Factors," *Ann Intern Med*, 1991, 114(9):748-53.

Sessler CN, "Theophylline Toxicity: Clinical Features of 116 Consecutive Cases," *Am J Med*, 1990, 88(6):567-76.

Tsiu SJ, Self TH, and Burns R, "Theophylline Toxicity: Update," *Ann Allergy*, 1990, 64(2 Pt 2):241-57.

Theospan® *see* Theophylline *on this page*

Thiocyanate, Blood or Urine

CPT 84430

Synonyms Ethyl and Methyl Thiocyanate (Thanite® and Lethane®); Potassium Thiocyanate (KSCN)

(Continued)

Thiocyanate, Blood or Urine *(Continued)*

Applies to Cyanide; Nipride®; Nitroprusside

Abstract Thiocyanate is a metabolite of the antihypertensive drug, nitroprusside. It is also a product of cyanide metabolism.

Specimen Serum or plasma, urine

Container Red top tube, lavender top (EDTA) tube, plastic urine container

Reference Range Serum, therapeutic: nonsmoker: 1-4 µg/mL (SI: 0.02-0.07 mmol/L), smoker: 3-12 µg/mL (SI: 0.05-0.21 mmol/L); urine: nonsmoker: 1-4 mg/24 hours, smoker: 7-17 mg/24 hours

Possible Panic Range Serum: >35 µg/mL (SI: >0.60 mmol/L); 200 µg/mL (SI: 3.44 mmol/L) is lethal

Use Evaluate thiocyanate toxicity, nitroprusside poisoning, smoking. Toxic manifestations are psychotic behavior, agitation, and convulsions.

Limitations Because of rapid metabolism of the drug, results are usually meaningless in the clinical setting by the time they are reported.

Methodology Photometry/chromatography

Additional Information Thiocyanate is a major metabolite of cyanide produced in the liver by the enzyme rhodanase. Thiocyanate is present in healthy subjects. It is a component of cigarette smoke, and it can arise from the drug nitroprusside which is sometimes used to control acute hypertension.

References

Balistreri WF, A-Kader HH, Setchell KD, et al, "New Methods for Assessing Liver Function in Infants and Children," *Ann Clin Lab Sci*, 1992, 22(3):162-74.

Hall AH and Rumack BH, "Clinical Toxicology of Cyanide," *Ann Emerg Med*, 1986, 15(9):1067-74.

Thioridazine *see* Phenothiazines, Serum *on page 568*

Thorazine® *see* Chlorpromazine, Serum or Urine *on page 543*

Thorazine® *see* Phenothiazines, Serum *on page 568*

Thrombran® *see* Trazodone *on next page*

Tobramycin, Serum *see* Aminoglycosides *on page 531*

Tocainide

CPT 80299

Related Information

Lidocaine *on page 558*

Synonyms Tonocard®; Xylotocan®

Abstract Tocainide is an antiarrhythmic closely related to lidocaine.

Specimen Serum or plasma

Container Red top tube or green top (heparin) tube; avoid serum separator tube

Sampling Time Peak: 1-1.5 hours after administration; trough: just before next dose

Reference Range Therapeutic: 4-10 µg/mL (SI: 21-52 µmol/L)

Possible Panic Range >12 µg/mL (SI: >52 µmol/L)

Use Therapeutic monitoring and toxicity assessment

Methodology High performance liquid chromatography (HPLC), gas chromatography (GC)

Additional Information

- Half-life: 10-15 hours
- Volume of distribution: 2-4 L/kg
- Protein binding: 10% to 50%

Tocainide is an analog of lidocaine used in the treatment of ventricular antiarrhythmias (class IB). Adverse effects of tocainide are mainly neurological (faintness, tremor) and following overdose coma, seizures, edema and respiratory arrest can occur. Metabolites are inactive.

Decreased effect/levels with cimetidine and rifampin; same possible effect with phenobarbital or phenytoin.

References

Gottlieb SS, Kukin ML, Medina N, et al, "Comparative Hemodynamic Effects of Procainamide, Tocainide, and Encainide in Severe Chronic Heart Failure," *Circulation*, 1990, 81(3):860-4.

Loi CM, Wei X, Parker BM, et al, "The Effect of Tocainide on Theophylline Metabolism," *Br J Clin Pharmacol*, 1993, 35(4):437-40.

Manolis AS, Smith E, Payne D, et al, "Randomized Double-Blind Study of Intravenous Tocainide Versus Lidocaine for Suppression of Ventricular Arrhythmias After Cardiac Surgery," *Clin Cardiol*, 1990, 13(3):177-81.

Roden DM and Woosley RL, "Drug Therapy. Tocainide," *N Engl J Med*, 1986, 315(1):41-4.

Sperry K, Wohlenberg N, and Standefer JC, "Fatal Intoxication by Tocainide," *J Forensic Sci*, 1987, 32(5):1440-6.

Tofranil® *see* Imipramine *on page 554*

Tofranil® *see* Antidepressants, Cyclic *on page 535*

Tonocard® *see* Tocainide *on this page*

Toot *see* Cocaine (Cocaine Metabolite), Qualitative, Urine *on page 543*

Toxic Metals, Blood *see* Heavy Metal Screen, Blood *on page 554*

Toxic Metals, Urine *see* Heavy Metal Screen, Urine *on page 554*

Toxicology Drug Screen, Blood

CPT 80100 (screen); 80102 (confirmation, each procedure)

Related Information

Ketone Bodies, Blood *on page 152*

Toxicology Drug Screen, Urine *on this page*

Synonyms Drug Screen, Comprehensive Panel or Analysis

Applies to Comatose Profile

Test Commonly Includes Amobarbital, butabarbital, butalbital, chlordiazepoxide, diazepam, ethchlorvynol, glutethimide, meprobamate, methaqualone, pentobarbital, phenobarbital, secobarbital, ethanol, methanol, acetone, isopropanol, acetaminophen, phenytoin, salicylates, tricyclics, other drugs could also be analyzed.

Abstract This toxicology screen is carried out by performing individual quantitative tests for each drug or by semiquantitative automated high performance liquid chromatography (Remedi®). Many times urine qualitative screening is faster and more useful in toxicologic emergencies, but both may be needed.

Specimen Serum or plasma

Container Red top tube or lavender top (EDTA) tube

Special Instructions Do **not** collect blood in heparinized tubes.

Reference Range See individual drug listing for therapeutic and toxic ranges.

Use Monitor toxic/overdose situations; most desirable to analyze in conjunction with urine toxicology testing; used to quantitate drug identified qualitatively in urine

Limitations This is not a drugs-of-abuse screen. Evidence for presence of a drug/drug metabolite (screening, qualitative) in the case of most groups of therapeutic agents and drugs of abuse will be found in urine rather than serum. See Toxicology Drug Screen, Urine *on page 576*. **All agents identified in a screening test should be confirmed with a specific test.**

Methodology Immunoassay, thin-layer chromatography (TLC), gas chromatography (GC), high performance liquid chromatography (HPLC), colorimetry, spectrophotometry

Additional Information If only documentation of exposure to toxic drugs or drugs of abuse is desired, a urine drug screen is the most economical approach. See listing Toxicology Drug Screen, Urine *on page 576*. When Toxicology Drug Screen, Blood is ordered, the individual drugs are quantitated in serum. When Toxicology Drug Screen, Urine is ordered, qualitative identification is carried out.

References

Bryson PD, *Comprehensive Review in Toxicology*, 2nd ed, Rockville, MD: Aspen Publishers Inc, 1989, 43-52.

Clark R and Harchelroad F, "Toxicology Screening of the Trauma Patient. A Changing Profile," *Ann Emerg Med*, 1991, 20(2):151-3.

Hepler B, Sutheimer C, and Sunshine I, "Role of the Toxicology Laboratory in Suspected Ingestions," *Pediatr Clin North Am*, 1986, 33(2):245-60.

Puopolo PR, Volpicelli SA, Johnson DM, et al, "Emergency Toxicology Testing (Detection, Confirmation, and Quantification) of Basic Drugs in Serum by Liquid Chromatography With Photodiode Array Detection," *Clin Chem*, 1991, 37(12):2124-30.

Schwartz JG, Zollars R, Okorodudu AO, et al, "Accuracy of Common Drug Screen Tests," *Am J Emerg Med*, 1991, 9(2):166-70.

Wiley JF 2d, "Difficult Diagnoses in Toxicology: Poisons Not Detected By the Comprehensive Drug Screen," *Pediatr Clin North Am*, 1991, 38(3):725-37.

Toxicology Drug Screen, Urine

CPT 80100 (screen); 80102 (confirmation, each procedure)

Related Information

Toxicology Drug Screen, Blood *on this page*

Synonyms Drug Screen, Comprehensive Panel or Analysis, Urine

Applies to Narcotics Drug Screen, Urine

Test Commonly Includes A variety of qualitative screens are in use. Sensitivity and specificity vary and are method dependent. Screens should detect drugs (qualitatively) in the following classes: amphetamines, analgesics, anticonvulsants, antidepressants, antihistamines, cardiacs, narcotics, sedative/hypnotics, tranquilizers, volatiles, and drugs of abuse.

Abstract This is a qualitative screen which with thin-layer chromatography or automated high performance liquid chromatography can detect any of several hundred drugs (Remedi®).

Specimen Random urine. The use of meconium samples from newborns has been shown to be useful.[1]

Storage Instructions Keep refrigerated.

Special Instructions Specify the drug or drugs suspected.

Reference Range None detected or negative (less than cutoff for drugs of abuse)

Use Screen for drug abuse, drug toxicity alone or in conjunction with serum/plasma testing. For typical drugs-of-abuse screening, see Drugs of Abuse Testing, Urine *on page 548.*

Limitations Test provides **only** qualitative detection of drugs, unless laboratory automatically confirms and quantitates drugs detected as a part of the "screening" procedure. Quantitation of urine drug levels is usually not included and is not recommended because urine levels are time and clearance dependent and are not directly related to toxic symptoms seen clinically. Some drugs and/or metabolites are not detected or optimally detected in urine, again relating to method. Serum may be preferable because of clinical and at times technical/kinetic factors (eg, barbiturates, phenytoin). Sensitivity is of the order of 0.5-1.0 µg/mL for TLC of urine. Some substances should be quantitated in blood or serum (eg, iron overdose, methanol, acetaminophen, salicylate, carbon monoxide, ethanol, digoxin, lithium, theophylline, and methemoglobin).

Methodology A variety of methods or combination of methods are in fairly common use and include thin-layer chromatography (TLC), colorimetry/spectrophotometry, enzyme immunoassay technique (EIA), enzyme-multiplied immunoassay technique (EMIT), gas chromatography (GC), gas chromatography/mass spectrometry (GC/MS), high performance liquid chromatography (HPLC).

Additional Information For specific drug blood levels see the listing by specific generic drug name for drug desired. Some toxins (eg, metals, volatiles, gaseous compounds) may require specific methodology (eg, atomic absorption spectrophotometry, gas chromatography). Also see Toxicology, Drug Screen, Blood *on page 576.*

Footnotes
1. Maynard EC, Amoruso LP, and Oh W, "Meconium for Drug Testing," *Am J Dis Child,* 1991, 145(6):650-2.

References
Osterloh JD, "Utility and Reliability of Emergency Toxicologic Testing," *Emerg Med Clin North Am,* 1990, 8(3):693-723.
Osterloh JD and Lee BL, "Urine Drug Screening in Mothers and Newborns," *Am J Dis Child,* 1989, 143(7):791-3.

Toxicology, Volatiles *see* Volatile Screen *on page 579*

Tranquilizers (Valium®, Librium®, etc) *see* Benzodiazepines, Qualitative, Urine *on page 538*

Trazodone
CPT 80299
Related Information
Antidepressants, Cyclic *on page 535*
Synonyms Deprax®; Desyrel®; Molipaxin®; Thrombran®; Trittico®
Abstract This drug is an antidepressant chemically unrelated to the tricyclic or tetracyclic antidepressants.
Specimen Serum or plasma
Container Red top tube or green top (heparin) tube
Sampling Time Trough: just before next dose
Reference Range Therapeutic: 0.5-2.5 µg/mL (SI: 1-6 µmol/L)
Critical Values >2.5 µg/mL (SI: >6 µmol/L)
Possible Panic Range 4 µg/mL (SI: 10 µmol/L)
Use Therapeutic monitoring and toxicity assessment
Methodology High performance liquid chromatography (HPLC), gas chromatography (GC)
Additional Information
- Half-life: 6-15 hours
- Volume of distribution: 0.9-1.5 L/kg
- Protein binding: 85% to 95%

Trazodone is a structurally unique antidepressant that is pharmacologically different from other drugs of this class. The toxicities observed in tricyclic overdose (neuro and cardiotoxicity and respiratory depression) are not seen with trazodone. Chronic toxicity is very low with trazodone although it does have unique side effects including akathisia, allergic reactions, chest pain, delayed urine flow, early and delayed menses, hypersalivation and hypomania, among others. Peak plasma concentrations with average daily dosing is reached in 2-4 hours.

References
Aranow AB, Hudson JI, Pope HG Jr, et al, "Elevated Antidepressant Plasma Levels After Addition of Fluoxetine," *Am J Psychiatry,* 1989, 146(7):911-3.
Carson CC 3d and Mino RD, "Priapism Associated With Trazodone Therapy," *J Urol,* 1988, 139(2):369-70.
Fabre LF, "United States Experience and Perspectives With Trazodone," *Clin Neuropharmacol,* 1989, 12(Suppl 1):S11-7.
Hull M, Jones R, and Bendall M, "Fatal Hepatic Necrosis Associated With Trazodone and Neuroleptic Drugs," *BMJ,* 1994, 309(6951):378.
Ohkubo T, Osanai T, Sugawara K, et al, "High-Performance Liquid Chromatographic Determination of Trazodone and 1-M-Chlorophenylpiperazine With Ultraviolet and Electrochemical Detector," *J Pharm Pharmacol,* 1995, 47(4):340-4.
Spar JE, "Plasma Trazodone Concentrations in Elderly Depressed Inpatients: Cardiac Effects and Short-Term Efficacy," *J Clin Psychopharmacol,* 1987, 7(6):406-9.

Triadapin® *see* Doxepin *on page 548*
Triavil® *see* Amitriptyline, Blood *on page 533*
Tricodein *see* Codeine, Urine *on page 544*
Tricyclic Antidepressants *see* Antidepressants, Cyclic *on page 535*
Tridione® *see* Oxazolidinediones *on page 567*
Trifluoperazine *see* Phenothiazines, Serum *on page 568*
Trimedone *see* Oxazolidinediones *on page 567*
Trittico® *see* Trazodone *on this page*
Tropium® *see* Chlordiazepoxide, Blood *on page 542*
Truphylline® *see* Theophylline *on page 575*
Tylenol® *see* Acetaminophen, Serum *on page 530*
Ty-Pap *see* Acetaminophen, Serum *on page 530*
Uni-Ace® *see* Acetaminophen, Serum *on page 530*
Uppers *see* Amphetamine, Qualitative, Urine *on page 534*
Valium® *see* Diazepam, Blood *on page 546*
Valkote® *see* Valproic Acid *on this page*
Valproate Semisodium *see* Valproic Acid *on this page*
Valproate Sodium *see* Valproic Acid *on this page*

Valproic Acid
CPT 80164
Related Information
Ammonia, Blood *on page 75*
Carbamazepine *on page 540*
Felbamate *on page 550*
Phenobarbital, Blood *on page 568*
Phenytoin *on page 569*
Primidone *on page 570*
Synonyms Depakene®; Depakote®; Depamide®; Dipropylacetic Acid; Divalproex Sodium; Epilim®; Ergenyl®; Leptilan®; 2-Propylpentanoic Acid; 2-Propylvaleric Acid; Valkote®; Valproate Semisodium; Valproate Sodium
Applies to Phenobarbital
Abstract Valproic acid is a first-line anticonvulsant for absence seizures. It is useful for many other seizure types, including primary generalized tonic-clonic, myoclonic, atonic, and mixed seizures.[1,2] It is the drug of choice for mixed absence and generalized seizures and for the epileptic syndromes of juvenile myoclonic epilepsy and generalized tonic-clonic seizures on awakening.
Specimen Serum or plasma
Container Red top tube or green top (heparin) tube
Sampling Time Trough values drawn just before next dose or consistent sampling time in chronic monitoring
Reference Range 50-100 µg/mL (SI: 350-690 µmol/L). Low levels: the most important cause is noncompliance. Phenytoin, phenobarbital, primidone, and carbamazepine decrease the half-life of valproic acid. High levels: carbamazepine and phenytoin can decrease the level of valproic acid by increasing its catabolism.
Critical Values Toxic concentration >200 µg/mL (SI: >1390 µmol/L). Seizure control may improve at levels >100 µg/mL (SI: >690 µmol/L), but toxicity may occur at levels of 100-150 µg/mL (SI: 690-1040 µmol/L). See Table A in the Therapeutic Drug Monitoring/Toxicology/Drugs of Abuse Appendix *on page 582.*
Use Monitor for compliance, efficacy, and possible toxicity
Limitations Since valproic acid is highly bound, drugs that compete for protein binding sites can increase the amount of free valproic acid (biologically active fraction). These include dicumarol, high dose salicylates, and phenylbutazone. If toxicity is suspected, a free valproic acid level should be obtained.
Contraindications Pregnant women in first month are at risk for neural tube defects.
Methodology Enzyme immunoassay (EIA), gas-liquid chromatography (GLC), high performance liquid chromatography (HPLC)
Additional Information
- Half-life (adult): 8-15 hours
- Volume of distribution: 0.1-0.5 L/kg
- Protein binding: 85% to 95%

Valproic acid (VPA) is a broad spectrum antiepileptic that may work by increasing or enhancing the inhibitory neurotransmitter γ-aminobutyric acid (GABA) in the brain. VPA is only commercially available in oral formulations, in the acid form and also as a sodium salt. They are both absorbed rapidly and completely. The bioavailability is 100%. Food will slow absorption. It is highly protein bound to albumin in the serum. VPA (Continued)

Valproic Acid (Continued)

is 90% to 96% bound to albumin, depending upon the concentration of VPA. The free fraction increases as the concentration increases due to nonlinear or capacity-limited binding. This is due to changes in protein binding and the nonlinear binding seen with high concentrations of this drug. The higher the concentration the higher the free fraction and thus the larger the volume of distribution. VPA is almost entirely cleared hepatically and is a low extraction drug, so its clearance is dependent upon enzyme activity and plasma protein binding. The clearance of VPA is also age dependent, children clearing the drug more rapidly than adults. The clearance of valproic acid is also very susceptible to alterations in enzyme activity for its clearance. Valproic acid inhibits the hepatic enzymes that are responsible for the clearance of other drugs. See listing Felbamate on page 550. Hepatic failure has occurred during the first 6 months of therapy. Hepatotoxicity may be preceded by nonspecific symptoms such as malaise, weakness, lethargy, anorexia, and vomiting. Hepatotoxicity may be fatal, but is idiosyncratic and not preventable by routinely monitoring liver enzymes. Hepatotoxicity occurs in very young children, most often those on multiple anticonvulsants.[3] Valproate-induced cytopenias may be dose-related and warrant monitoring of complete blood counts during therapy.[4] Encephalopathy with hyperammonemia without liver function test abnormalities may occur.[5]

Footnotes

1. Penry JK and Dean JC, "Valproate Monotherapy in Partial Seizures," Am J Med, 1988, 84(1A):14-6.
2. Dean JC and Penry JK, "Valproate Monotherapy in 30 Patients With Partial Seizures," Epilepsia, 1988, 29(2):140-4.
3. Dreifuss FE, Santilli N, Langer DH, et al, "Valproic Acid Hepatic Fatalities: A Retrospective Review," Neurology, 1987, 37(3):379-85.
4. Watts RG, Emanuel PD, Zuckerman KS, et al, "Valproic Acid-Induced Cytopenias: Evidence for a Dose-Related Suppression of Hematopoesis," J Pediatr, 1990, 117(3):495-9.
5. Zaret BS, Beckner RR, Marini AM, et al, "Sodium Valproate-Induced Hyperammonemia Without Clinical Hepatic Dysfunction," Neurology, 1982, 32(2):206-8.

References

Addy D, "Serum Valproate Concentrations and Control of Seizures," J Pediatr, 1992, 121(5 Pt 1):835-6.

Engel J, Seizures and Epilepsy, Contemporary Neurology Series, Philadelphia, PA: FA Davis Co, 1989.

Kulick SK and Kramer DA, "Hyperammonemia Secondary to Valproic Acid as a Cause of Lethargy in a Postictal Patient," Ann Emerg Med, 1993, 22(3):610-2.

Levy RH, Wilensky AJ, and Anderson GD, "Carbamazepine, Valproic Acid, Phenobarbital, and Ethosuximide," Applied Pharmacokinetics: Principles of Therapeutic Drug Monitoring, 3rd ed, Evans WE, Schentag JJ, and Jusko WJ, eds, Vancouver, WA: Applied Therapeutics Inc, 1992.

Winter ME, "Valproic Acid," Basic Clinical Pharmacokinetics, 3rd ed, Koda-Kimble MA and Young LY, eds, Vancouver, WA: Applied Therapeutics Inc, 1994.

Valrelease® see Diazepam, Blood on page 546

Vancocin® see Vancomycin on this page

Vancoled® see Vancomycin on this page

Vancomycin

CPT 80202

Related Information

Aminoglycosides on page 531

Antimicrobial Susceptibility Testing, Aerobic and Facultatively Anaerobic Bacteria on page 448

Serum Bactericidal Test on page 496

Synonyms Lyphocin®; Vancocin®; Vancoled®

Abstract Vancomycin is an antimicrobial agent with potent activity against most gram-positive bacteria. Its use has occasionally been associated with nephrotoxicity and/or ototoxicity, though the frequency of these toxicities has decreased as vancomycin preparations have become more purified.

Specimen Serum, body fluid

Container Red top tube, sterile fluid container

Sampling Time Peak: 2 hours following dose; trough: immediately prior to next dose

Storage Instructions Separate serum using aseptic technique and place in freezer

Causes for Rejection Specimen more than 4 hours old

Reference Range Therapeutic concentration: peak: 20-40 µg/mL (SI: 14-27 µmol/L) (depends in part on minimum inhibitory concentration of organism being treated); trough: 5-10 µg/mL (SI: 3.4-6.8 µmol/L)

Possible Panic Range Toxic: >80 µg/mL (SI: >54 µmol/L). See Table B in the Therapeutic Drug Monitoring/Toxicology/Drugs of Abuse Appendix on page 582.

Use Several recent publications have recommended that **routine** monitoring of serum vancomycin levels is unnecessary. Specific situations in which determination of vancomycin levels **might** be helpful include:

- patients receiving vancomycin/aminoglycoside combinations
- anephric patients undergoing hemodialysis who receive infrequent doses of vancomycin

- patients receiving unusually high doses of vancomycin (eg, for treatment of meningitis due to penicillin-resistant pneumococci)
- patients with rapidly changing renal function

Limitations Monitoring serum vancomycin concentration has not been correlated with improved efficacy or decreased toxicity; consequently, the reference and panic ranges listed above must be taken with the proverbial "grain of salt." Vancomycin pharmacokinetics are sufficiently predictable that adequate serum drug concentrations can be obtained with dosing methods that take into account the patient's age, weight, and renal function.

Methodology High performance liquid chromatography (HPLC), gas-liquid chromatography (GLC), immunoassay

Additional Information

- Half-life: 4-8 hours
- Volume of distribution: 0.4-1.3 L/kg
- Protein binding: 50%

Vancomycin is currently being used in its intravenous form to treat a variety of gram-positive bacterial infections, particularly those due to methicillin-resistant staphylococci. Additionally, vancomycin is often used in its oral form to treat pseudomembranous colitis due to Clostridium difficile. The emergence of vancomycin-resistant Enterococcus sp has given substantial motivation to discontinuing this practice; C. difficile colitis should be treated initially with metronidazole. When administered orally, serum vancomycin levels are undetectable due to poor absorption from the gastrointestinal tract. When administered intravenously, vancomycin may be ototoxic and nephrotoxic, though nephrotoxicity is rare with newer preparations. Ototoxicity is seen primarily in patients with extremely high serum concentrations (80-100 µg/mL; SI: 54-68 µmol/L) and rarely occurs when serum concentrations are maintained at ≤30 µg/mL (SI: ≤20 µmol/L). Both oto- and nephrotoxicity are enhanced by concurrent administration of aminoglycosides.

References

Cantu TG, Yamanaka-Yuen NA, and Lietman PS, "Serum Vancomycin Concentrations: Reappraisal of Their Clinical Value," Clin Infect Dis, 1994, 18(4):533-43.

Freeman CD, Quintiliani R, and Nightingale CH, "Vancomycin Therapeutic Drug Monitoring: Is It Necessary?" Ann Pharmacother, 1993, 27(5):594-8.

Moellering RC Jr, "Monitoring Serum Vancomycin Levels: Climbing the Mountain Because It Is There?" Clin Infect Dis, 1994, 18(4):544-6.

Vatran® see Diazepam, Blood on page 546

Veramex® see Verapamil on this page

Verapamil

CPT 80299

Related Information

Carbamazepine on page 540

Cyclosporine on page 545

Digoxin on page 546

Disopyramide on page 547

Lithium on page 558

Phenobarbital, Blood on page 568

Quinidine, Serum on page 572

Synonyms Azupamil®; Calan®; Cordilox®; Ikacor®; Iproveratril Hydrochloride; Isoptin®; Securon®; Veramex®; Verelan®

Applies to Norverapamil

Test Commonly Includes Verapamil and norverapamil (metabolite levels)

Abstract Verapamil is an antihypertensive, antianginal calcium channel antagonist with an active metabolite. It has a role in management of cardiomyopathy. It is used as an antiarrhythmic drug, including therapy of tachyarrhythmias.

Specimen Serum or plasma

Container Red top tube (preferred) or green top (heparin) tube. Do not use serum separator tubes.

Sampling Time Peak: 1-2 hours after last dose

Storage Instructions Centrifuge, separate, and freeze serum (plasma) in a plastic container.

Special Instructions Provide the following information to the laboratory: time specimen drawn, date of last dose, time of last dose, amount of dose, and route administered.

Reference Range Therapeutic: 100-400 ng/mL (SI: 200-815 nmol/L) for parent; under normal conditions norverapamil concentration is the same as parent drug.

Critical Values >400 ng/mL (SI: >815 nmol/L); toxicity proportional to verapamil concentration

Possible Panic Range Toxic: >845 ng/mL; fatal: >2000 ng/mL. A ratio of verapamil/norverapamil >2.3 may be a predictor for fatal outcome.

Use Therapeutic monitoring and toxicity assessment

Limitations Clinical assessment of signs and symptoms is often preferable to use of drug concentrations. Verapamil is commercially available as a racemic mixture. The (S-) enantiomer is the isomer with the greatest pharmacological activity. These enantiomers exhibit stereoselective absorption, binding, and clearance. This makes for a very complex pharmacokinetic picture. It also makes it very difficult to associate measured verapamil concentrations with effect when it cannot differentiate the active (S) enantiomer from the relatively inactive (R) enantiomer.

Methodology Fluorometry, high performance liquid chromatography (HPLC), gas chromatography (GC)

Additional Information
- Half-life: 6-9 hours
- Volume of distribution: 3-5 L/kg
- Protein binding: 85% to 95%

Verapamil is an antiarrhythmic, antihypertensive drug whose main metabolite is norverapamil, which has about 20% of the activity of the parent drug. Verapamil is a calcium channel blocker. Coadministration of verapamil and beta-blockers should be approached with caution. Verapamil increases serum digoxin concentrations 50% to 70%. Toxicity may result when verapamil is used with carbamazepine or lithium.

Increased cardiovascular adverse effects occur with beta-adrenergic blocking agents (especially when administered intravenously), digoxin, quinidine, and disopyramide. Verapamil may increase serum concentrations of digoxin, quinidine, carbamazepine, and cyclosporine necessitating a decrease in dosage. Phenobarbital and rifampin may decrease verapamil serum concentrations by increasing its clearance.

Route of metabolism: hepatic.

References
Carter BL, Noyes MA, and Demmler RW, "Differences in Serum Concentrations of and Responses to Generic Verapamil in the Elderly," *Pharmacotherapy*, 1993, 13(4):359-68.

Hla KK, Latham AN, and Henry JA, "Influence of Time of Administration on Verapamil Pharmacokinetics," *Clin Pharmacol Ther*, 1992, 51(4):366-70.

Hosie J, Hosie G, and Meredith PA, "The Effects of Age on the Pharmacodynamics and Pharmacokinetics of Two Formulations of Verapamil," *J Cardiovasc Pharmacol*, 1989, 13(Suppl 4):S60-2.

MacDonald D and Alguire PC, "Case Report: Fatal Overdose With Sustained Release Verapamil," *Am J Med Sci*, 1992, 303(2):115-7.

Pritza DR, Bierman MH, and Hammeke MD, "Acute Toxic Effects of Sustained-Release Verapamil in Chronic Renal Failure," *Arch Intern Med*, 1991, 151(10):2081-4.

Ramoska EA, Spiller HA, and Myers A, "Calcium Channel Blocker Toxicity," *Ann Emerg Med*, 1993, 19(6):649-53.

Schwartz JB, "Aging Alters Verapamil Elimination and Dynamics: Single Dose and Steady-State Responses," *J Pharmacol Exp Ther*, 1990, 255(1):364-73.

Sporer KA and Manning JJ, "Massive Ingestion of Sustained-Release Verapamil With a Concretion and Bowel Infarction," *Ann Emerg Med*, 1993, 22(3):603-5.

Tom PA, Morrow CT, and Kelen GD, "Delayed Hypotension After Overdose of Sustained Release Verapamil," *J Emerg Med*, 1994, 12(5):621-5.

Verelan® *see Verapamil on previous page*

Vigabatrin

Related Information
Phenytoin *on page 569*

Synonyms Gamma Vinyl GABA

Abstract Vigabatrin is a novel anticonvulsant that increases brain GABA levels by irreversibly inhibiting GABA transaminase and preventing GABA breakdown.

Reference Range There is no direct correlation between plasma concentration and clinical effects. Plasma concentrations of GABA do not reflect CNS concentrations since the blood brain barrier is relatively impermeable to GABA.

Limitations Plasma concentrations of phenytoin are reduced 20% to 30% in patients taking vigabatrin.

Additional Information
- Half-life: 5-8 hours
- Volume of distribution: 1.0-1.5 L/kg

Sedation (drowsiness and fatigue) is common in patients beginning treatment. Oral doses of vigabatrin peak in 1-2 hours, and it is cleared by the kidney by filtration. It increases the enzyme activity used to clear phenytoin. Therefore, phenytoin concentrations will be decreased. Vigabatrin is commercially available as a racemic mixture. The (S+) enantiomer is the isomer with the greatest pharmacological activity.

References
Connelly JF, "Vigabatrin," *Ann Pharmacother*, 1993, 27(2):197-204.

Durham SL, Hoke JF, and Chen TM, "Pharmacokinetics and Metabolism of Vigabatrin Following a Single Oral Dose of 14C Vigabatrin in Healthy Male Volunteers," *Drug Metab Dispos*, 1993, 21(3):480-4.

Grant SM and Heel RC, "Vigabatrin: A Review of Its Pharmacodynamic and Pharmacokinetic Properties, and Therapeutic Potential in Epilepsy and Disorders of Motor Control," *Drugs*, 1991, 41(6):889-926.

Rey E, Pons G, and Olive G, "Vigabatrin Clinical Pharmacokinetics," *Clin Pharmacokinet*, 1992, 23(4):267-78.

Vivactil® *see Antidepressants, Cyclic on page 535*

Vivarin® *see Caffeine, Blood on page 539*

Vivol® *see Diazepam, Blood on page 546*

Volatile Screen

CPT 80101 (screen, single drug class); 80102 (confirmation, each procedure); 84600 (quantitative)

Related Information
Alcohol, Blood or Urine *on page 531*
Anion Gap *on page 81*
Ketone Bodies, Blood *on page 152*
Ketones, Urine *on page 639*
Osmolality, Serum *on page 172*

Synonyms Toxicology, Volatiles

Applies to Acetone; Ethanol; Isopropanol; Methanol

Test Commonly Includes Determination of volatiles by GLC including acetone, ethanol, isopropanol, and methanol

Abstract This screening profile measures ethanol and other possible volatiles.

Specimen Serum or plasma, urine, gastric fluid

Container Red top tube, gray top (sodium fluoride) tube; tightly stoppered container for urine and gastric fluid

Collection All containers should be tightly stoppered and transported on ice. The gray (oxalate/fluoride) tube top is recommended for medicolegal collections and if storage is prolonged. Sodium fluoride (50 mg) can be added as a preservative to urine and gastric samples. Other anticoagulants (eg, heparin EDTA) are acceptable.

Causes for Rejection Specimen leakage

Reference Range None detected

Possible Panic Range Blood: acetone, methanol, isopropanol >500 µg/mL (SI: acetone: >8610 µmol/L, methanol: >15.6 mmol/L, isopropanol: >8.32 mmol/L), ethanol: >2000 µg/mL (SI: >43.4 mmol/L); urine: acetone, methanol, isopropanol >500 µg/mL (SI: acetone: >8610 µmol/L, methanol: >15.6 mmol/L, isopropanol: 8.32 mmol/L), ethanol: >1600 µg/mL (SI: >34.7 mmol/L)

Use Evaluate methanol and isopropanol toxicity, and alcohol drug abuse

Methodology Gas-liquid chromatography (GLC)

Additional Information Both methanol and isopropanol are more intoxicating than ethanol. Methanol is converted to formaldehyde and formic acid, which causes retinal damage leading to blindness and metabolic acidosis. Isopropanol is converted to acetone.

References
Burkhart KK and Kulig KW, "The Other Alcohols. Methanol, Ethylene Glycol, and Isopropanol," *Emerg Med Clin North Am*, 1990, 8(4):913-28.

Jarvie DR and Simpson D, "Simple Screening Tests for the Emergency Identification of Methanol and Ethylene Glycol in Poisoned Patients," *Clin Chem*, 1990, 36(11):1957-61.

Lacouture PG, Heldreth DD, Shannon M, et al, "The Generation of Acetonemia/Acetonuria Following Ingestion of a Subtoxic Dose of Isopropyl Alcohol," *Am J Emerg Med*, 1989, 7(1):38-40.

Litovitz T, "The Alcohols: Ethanol, Methanol, Isopropanol, Ethylene Glycol," *Pediatr Clin North Am*, 1986, 33(2):311-23.

Warfarin

CPT 80299

Related Information
Amiodarone, Serum *on page 532*
Carbamazepine *on page 540*
Imipramine *on page 554*
Ketoconazole *on page 556*
Nortriptyline *on page 565*
Phenobarbital, Blood *on page 568*
Prothrombin Time *on page 262*

Synonyms Athrombin-K®; Coumadin®; Panwarfin®

Applies to Anticoagulants, Oral

Abstract Warfarin is an oral anticoagulant. Serum warfarin concentrations are seldom used to manage therapy. International normalized ratios (INR) and prothrombin times (PT) are more helpful than serum warfarin concentrations in assessing clinical efficacy/toxicity.

Specimen Serum or plasma

Container Red top tube, lavender top (EDTA) tube

Reference Range Therapeutic: 2-5 µg/mL (SI: 6.5-16.2 µmol/L)

Possible Panic Range Toxic: >10 µg/mL (SI: >32.4 µmol/L)

Use Selective therapeutic monitoring and toxicity assessment. Plasma concentrations are only infrequently used in clinical practice. They are typically only used in cases of unusual response.

Limitations This test **does not** measure bishydroxycoumarin and should not be used to monitor this drug.

Methodology High pressure liquid chromatography (HPLC) with fluorescence detection, gas-liquid chromatography (GLC), UV spectrophotometry

Additional Information
- Half-life: 20-60 hours
- Volume of distribution: 0.10-0.15 L/kg

(Continued)

Warfarin *(Continued)*

- Protein binding: 99%

The coumarins, a class of compounds which include warfarin (Coumadin®), are anticoagulants by virtue of their effect on vitamin K metabolism. By inhibition of vitamin K reductases, coagulation proteins II, VII, IX, and X lose their ability to bind calcium and thereby to complex with cofactors on phospholipid surfaces.

Commercial warfarin consists of a racemic mixture of the optically active enantiomers (R) and (S), each of which is metabolized by different isoenzymes of cytochrome P-450. The (S) enantiomer is some five times as active as the (R) form. Chemicals or drugs (eg, ticlopidine, see reference by Gidal et al below) may inhibit the drug metabolizing P-450 enzyme system. In the case of ticlopidine (an antiplatelet agent), R-warfarin is significantly inhibited. S-warfarin, which is more active, is not inhibited with functional coagulation (eg, mean INR values not affected) but with considerable interindividual variation.

Warfarin is used for chronic oral anticoagulation in a variety of clinical settings. Management of warfarin therapy is usually done by following the **prothrombin time** and/or the INR, rather than by measuring serum drug concentrations. Warfarin is subject to a bewildering number and variety of drug interactions, producing increased or decreased clinical effect of itself or other drugs. See listing Prothrombin Time *on page 262* for additional discussion and table. Many of these effects are due to changes in protein binding, hepatic metabolism, and/or availability of vitamin K. Reductions in dosage may be indicated for aging subjects treated for venous thromboembolic or coronary arterial disease, but not in those with peripheral vascular disease, deep vein thrombosis, or valvular heart disease.[1,2]

Warfarin is totally bioavailable. It is very highly protein bound (97% to 99.9%) to albumin. Since it is so highly protein bound, there is a risk for protein binding displacement by drugs or disease. The volume of distribution of warfarin in relatively small 0.13 L/kg. Warfarin is cleared hepatically, which is the main source of drug interactions seen with warfarin. It is particularly sensitive to any hepatic enzyme inducers or inhibitors.

Many drug interactions are associated with warfarin. Changes in protein binding will increase or decrease **free** concentrations only temporarily. For example, if a drug displaces warfarin from its protein binding sites in the plasma, the free concentration will initially increase. By increasing the free fraction, the hepatic clearance of warfarin will also increase. At steady-state, since the increase in free fraction of warfarin will be cleared, there will be no change in free concentration of warfarin but the total concentration will be decreased. **Be careful that you do not increase the dose rate based upon this decreased total concentration**, because it is not representative of the free concentration. Changes in hepatic clearance due to enzyme inhibition or induction will be represented correctly in the total concentration. Consider any inducers or inhibitors to be potential drugs that will cause an interaction with warfarin. Other interactions occur with changes in availability of vitamin K.

Footnotes

1. Montamat SC, Cusack BJ, and Vestal RE, "Management of Drug Therapy in the Elderly," *N Engl J Med*, 1989, 321(5):303-9.

2. James AH, Britt RP, Raskino CL, et al, "Factors Affecting the Maintenance Dose of Warfarin," *J Clin Pathol*, 1992, 45(8):704-6.

References

Bick RL, "Antithrombolytic Therapy," *Disorders of Thrombosis and Hemostasis: Clinical Laboratory Practice*, Chapter 14, Chicago, IL: American Society of Clinical Pathologists, 1992, 291-312.

Cai WM, Hatton J, Pettigrew LC, et al, "A Simplified High-Performance Liquid Chromatographic Method for Direct Determination of Warfarin Enantiomers and Their Protein Binding in Stroke Patients," *Ther Drug Monit*, 1994, 16(5), 509-12.

Gidal BE, Sorkness CA, McGill KA, et al, "Evaluation of a Potential Enantioselective Interaction Between Ticlopidine and Warfarin in Chronically Anticoagulated Patients," *Ther Drug Monit*, 1995, 17(1):33-8.

Middlekauff HR, Stevenson WG, and Gornbein JA, "Antiarrhythmic Prophylaxis vs Warfarin Anticoagulation to Prevent Thromboembolic Events Among Patients With Atrial Fibrillation. A Decision Analysis," *Arch Intern Med*, 1995, 155(9):913-20.

Mortensen M, "Management of Acute Childhood Poisonings Caused By Selected Insecticides and Herbicides," *Pediatr Clin North Am*, 1986, 33(2):421-45.

Poller L and Samama M, "Laboratory Monitoring of Oral Anticoagulant Therapy," *Clin Lab Med*, 1994, 14(4):813-23.

Porter RS and Sawyer WT, "Warfarin," *Applied Pharmacokinetics: Principles of Therapeutic Drug Monitoring*, 3rd ed, Evans WE, Schentag JJ, and Jusko WJ, eds, Vancouver, WA: Applied Therapeutics Inc, 1992.

Redwood M, Taylor C, Bain BJ, et al, "The Association of Age With Dosage Requirement for Warfarin," *Age-Ageing*, 1991, 20(3):217-20.

White Lady *see* Cocaine (Cocaine Metabolite), Qualitative, Urine *on page 543*

Wickistick *see* Phencyclidine, Qualitative, Urine *on page 567*

Wygesic® *see* Propoxyphene, Serum or Urine *on page 571*

Xylocaine® *see* Lidocaine *on page 558*

Xylotocan® *see* Tocainide *on page 576*

Yellow Jackets *see* Barbiturates, Quantitative, Blood *on page 537*

Zarontin® *see* Ethosuximide *on page 549*

Zartalin® *see* Ethosuximide *on page 549*

Zetran® *see* Diazepam, Blood *on page 546*

Zidovudine

CPT 80299

Related Information

Beta$_2$-Microglobulin *on page 371*

CD4/CD8 Enumeration *on page 375*

HIV-1/HIV-2 Serology *on page 403*

Human Immunodeficiency Virus Culture *on page 669*

Synonyms Azidothymidine; AZT; Retrovir®

Abstract Azidothymidine (AZT) is the first FDA-approved drug for the treatment of human immunodeficiency virus (HIV) infection, the cause of AIDS. The drug is a competitive inhibitor of HIV reverse transcriptase; it is incorporated into the viral DNA in place of thymidine and interrupts viral replication because the DNA can no longer elongate.

Specimen Serum or plasma

Container Red top tube preferred, green top (heparin) tube acceptable

Sampling Time Trough level, just before next dose

Collection Volume needed is method dependent (0.1-1 mL)

Causes for Rejection Incorrect specimen sampling time

Reference Range Peak serum level after 200 mg dose: ~0.9 µg/mL

Critical Values Serum level taken 12 hours after a 20 g overdose: 49.4 µg/mL

Use Not established for routine clinical use. Monitoring should probably be limited to studies on pharmacokinetics and efficacy of antiretroviral therapy.

Methodology High performance liquid chromatography (HPLC), radioimmunoassay (RIA), fluorescence polarization immunoassay (FPIA)

Additional Information

- Half-life: 1 hour

Zidovudine is usually administered at a total daily dose of 500 mg (100 mg orally, every 4 hours while the patient is awake); optimal dosing, however, has not been established. Peak serum concentrations are attained within 30-40 minutes after ingestion. The main metabolite is a glucuronide derivative with no antiviral activity that is excreted by the kidneys. The major toxicity associated with zidovudine use is hematologic suppression which may manifest as anemia, leukopenia, and/or granulocytopenia. Monitoring hematologic parameters is the most reasonable approach toward evaluating toxicity; serum levels currently contribute little to evaluating toxic effects of zidovudine. Coadministration of probenecid results in increased serum levels due to competition for glucuronidation pathways. Hepatic and renal failure increases serum levels.

References

Amin NM, "Zidovudine for Treating AIDS. What Physicians Need to Know," *Postgrad Med*, 1989, 86(1):195-6, 201-8.

Collins JM and Unadket JD, "Clinical Pharmacokinetics of Zidovudine. An Overview of Current Data," *Clin Pharmacokinet*, 1989, 17(1):1-9.

Langtry HD and Campoli-Richards DM, "Zidovudine. A Review of its Pharmacodynamic and Pharmacokinetic Properties, and Therapeutic Efficacy," *Drugs*, 1989, 37(4):408-50.

Morris DJ, "Adverse Effects and Drug Interactions of Clinical Importance With Antiviral Drugs," *Drug Saf*, 1994, 10(4):281-91.

Rachlis A and Fanning MM, "Zidovudine Toxicity: Clinical Features and Management," *Drug Saf*, 1993, 8(4):312-20.

ZORprin® *see* Salicylate *on page 573*

The following form is a combination requisition and external chain-of-custody form. The strip at the bottom peels off and is used to seal the urine specimen cup. The number on the strip appears on all 5 copies of the form and serves to positively associate the form with the sample. An internal chain-of-custody form (used in the laboratory and not illustrated here) appears on the back of copy 1.

ACCOUNT NAME AND ADDRESS	ROCKHILL MEDICAL LABORATORY	TOXICOLOGY
		LIS NO.
		ACC NO.

COLLECTOR

IDENTIFICATION	LOCATION	MEDICAL REVIEW OFFICER
	MEDICATIONS WITHIN LAST 30 DAYS	

RESON FOR TESTING:

1 ☐ PRE-EMPLOYMENT
2 ☐ PERIODIC
3 ☐ REASONABLE CAUSE
4 ☐ BLOOD (PROBABLE SUSPICION)

5 ☐ POST-ACCIDENT
6 ☐ RANDOM
7 ☐ OTHER (SPECIFY)_____

PROFILES

DRUGS OF ABUSE SCREEN (THIN LAYER CONFIRMATION)
DRUGS OF ABUSE SCREEN-5 (GC/MS* CONFIRMATION)
DRUGS OF ABUSE SCREEN-10 (GC/MS* CONFIRMATION)
BLOOD ALCOHOL
URINE ALCOHOL
★ GAS CHROMATOGRAPHY/MASS SPECTROMETRY

TEMPERATURE

SPECIMEN TEMPERATURE
Has it been read within 4 minutes? ☐ Yes ☐ No

TEMPERATURE IS WITHIN RANGE OF 32.5°-37.7°C/90.5°-99.8°F
☐ Yes ☐ No - If NOT, record actual temp: _____ °

TO BE COMPLETED BY COLLECTOR

NAME _____ LOCATION _____

I CERTIFY THAT THE SPECIMEN IDENTIFIED ON THIS FORM IS THE SPECIMEN PRESENTED TO ME BY THE APPLICANT/EMPLOYEE SIGNING THIS FORM, AND THAT THE SPECIMEN BEARS AN IDENTIFICATION NUMBER IDENTICAL TO THE NUMBER BELOW, AND THAT IT HAS BEEN COLLECTED, LABELED, AND SEALED WITH THE SECURITY LABEL PROVIDED ON THIS FROM IN THE DONOR'S

SIGNATURE	DATE/TIME	PHONE

TO BE COMPLETED BY DONOR

I HEREBY CONSENT TO HAVE A SPECIMEN OF MY URINE AND/OR BLOOD TAKEN, AND I UNDERSTAND THAT IT WILL BY USED FOR DRUG ANALYSIS BY ROCKHILL MEDICAL LABORATORY. THE RESULTS OF THE TESTS ON MY SPECIMEN WILL THEN BY MADE AVAILABLE TO THE ABOVE NAMED COMPANY/EMPLOYER FOR EMPLOYMENT EVALUATION ONLY. I HEREBY RELEASE ALL PHYSICIANS, MEDICAL FACILITIES, TESTING FACILITIES, THE ABOVE NAMED EMPLOYER/COMPANY, CLINICS, AND THEIR EMPLOYEES, AGENTS AND REPRESENTATIVES FROM ANY AND ALL LIABILITY ARISING FROM THE RELEASE OF THE INFORMATION DISCOVERED FROM MY TEST. IN ADDITION, I HEREBY ACKNOWLEDGE THAT THE SPECIMEN LABELED WITH THE IDENTIFICATION NUMBER BELOW IS MY OWN, AND THE SPECIMEN WAS LABELED AND SEALED IN MY PRESENCE.

SIGNATURE OF APPLICANT _____ TIME/DATE: _____

CHAIN OF CUSTODY

COLLECTOR	RELEASED BY:	RECEIVED BY:	
REASON FOR CUSTODY CHANGE	SIGNATURE/PRINT NAME	SIGNATURE/PRINT NAME	DATE/TIME
PROVIDE SPECIMEN FOR TESTING	DONOR XXXX		
SHIP TO LABORATORY			

LAB USE ONLY

SEAL INTACT YES NO	VOLUME	SPECIMEN IS: ☐ACCEPTED ☐NOT SUITABLE FOR ANALYSIS
COMMENTS		

X _____
COLLECTOR'S SIGNATURE

_____ _____
DONOR'S INITIAL   DATE

PLACE OVER CAP
TOXICOLOGY COPY-1

NAME OR I.D. NUMBER OF DONOR _____

002576

Reprinted with permission from Baptist Medical Center, Kansas City, MO.

Table A. Class of Drug – Anticonvulsants

Name of Drug	Therapeutic Range	Toxic Level	Half-Life	Time to Sample	Protein Binding (%)	Active Metabolites	Route of Excretion	Major Drug Interactions
Carbamazepine	8-12 µg/mL	>12 µg/mL	15-40 h	7-12 d	60-80	10,11-N-epoxide	Hepatic	
Clonazepam	10-50 ng/mL	>100 µg/mL	20-60 h	5-6 d	80-90	7-Amino		
Ethosuximide	40-100 µg/mL	>100 µg/mL	25-70 h	10-13 d	0		Hepatic	
Felbamate	20-100 µg/mL		20-23 h		20-25			
Gabapentin	1-2 µg/mL		5-7 h		<3			
Lamotrigine	2-4 µg/mL		24-30 h		50-60			
Mephenytoin	25-40 µg/mL	>50 µg/mL	8 h		20-50	5-Ethyl, 5-phenyl-hydantoin		
Phenobarbital	20-40µg/mL	>40 µg/mL	50-140 h	20 d	40-50		Hepatic	Hydantoin, valproic acid
Phenytoin	10-20 µg/mL		20-40 h		85-95			
Primidone	5-12 µg/mL	>12 µg/mL	4-12 h	5 d	0-20	Phenobarbital		
Valproic acid	50-100 µg/mL	>100 µg/mL	8-15 h	4 d	85-95		Renal	Phenobarbital, phenytoin
Vigabatrin			5-8 h		0			

Table B. Class of Drug – Antibiotics

Name of Drug	Therapeutic Range*	Toxic Level	Half-Life	Time to Sample (after starting)	Protein Binding %	Route of Excretion
Amikacin	P: 20-30 µg/mL†; T: 4-8 µg/mL	T: >8 µg/mL	2-3 h	15 h	4	Renal
Chloramphenicol	P: 10-25 µg/mL; T: <5 µg/mL	P: >25 µg/mL	1.5-5 h‡	10-15 h‡	50-60	Renal§
Gentamicin	P: 6-10 µg/mL†; T: <2 µg/mL	T: >2 µg/mL	2-3 h	15 h	10	Renal
Tobramycin	P: 6-10 µg/mL†; T: <2 µg/mL	T: >2 µg/mL	2-3 h	15 h	10	Renal
Vancomycin¶	P: 20-40 µg/mL; T: 5-10 µg/mL	P: >80 µg/mL	4 h	24 h	55	Renal

P = peak, T = trough.

*Dependent upon site of infection and individual MIC of drug. See individual drugs.

†Higher peak levels will be attained with once daily dosing.

‡Varies substantially with age.

§Hepatic inactivation very important.

¶Routine monitoring of serum vancomycin levels is necessary.

Table C. Class of Drug — Cardiac Drugs

Name of Drug	Therapeutic Range	Toxic Level	Half-Life	Time to Sample	Protein Binding %	Active Metabolites	Route of Excretion	Major Drug Interactions
Digitoxin	18-35 ng/mL	>35 ng/mL	150-250 h		88	Digoxin	Hepatic	
Digoxin	0.8-2.0 ng/mL	>2.0 ng/mL	20-60 h	5 d	20-30		Renal	Quinidine
Disopyramide	2.8-3.2 µg/mL	>7.0 µg/mL	4-8 h	30 h	30-70	N-desisopropyl	Renal	
Lidocaine	1.5-5.0 µg/mL	>6.0µg/mL	1.5-2 h	5-10 h	60-80	MEGX	Hepatic	Phenobarbital
Procainamide	4-10 µg/mL	>14 µg/mL	2-6 h	20 h	10-20	N-acetylprocainamide	Renal	
Propranolol	50-100 ng/mL	>1000 ng/mL	4-6 h	30 h	90	4-Hydroxy-	Hepatic	
Quinidine	2-5 µg/mL	>8 µg/mL	6-8 h	24 h	90	3-Hydroxy-	Hepatic	Digitalis

TRACE ELEMENTS

Glen R. Willie, MD

Knowledge of trace elements in human toxicity, nutrition, and trace element-related disease states has lagged behind similar knowledge in veterinary medicine, but there have recently been substantial advances.

All trace elements are toxic if given in excessive amounts, and some metals such as thallium, lead, mercury, and arsenic are classically known as "heavy metals" and are covered in the chapter Therapeutic Drug Monitoring/Toxicology/Drugs of Abuse. Other elements have major additional aspects of clinical interest and are included in this chapter, drawn together by the common thread of either their being essential to human health or by the need to monitor them on a regular basis in certain clinical situations (aluminum: patients with chronic renal failure with potential aluminum exposure).

Many essential trace elements have specific binding proteins, and all bind nonspecifically to various serum proteins. Knowledge of these binding characteristics is often essential to properly interpret trace element analyses.

Acknowledgment is given for helpful advice from Phillip H. Stoltenberg, MD, for review of the entries for serum copper and urine copper; and to H. Ray Adams, PhD[1] and Edward D. Harris, PhD,[2] for review of the entire chapter in a prior edition.

Blood Collection Methods for Trace Elements

Since at least 1971, reports have appeared detailing trace metal contamination or alteration of blood and serum samples by blood collection needles, syringes, and vacuum tubes. Problems have included the leaching of chromium or manganese from metal needles; the contamination of the sample by the glass or the rubber parts of syringes or by the rubber stopper; or the adsorption with time of selenium or lead onto ordinary glass blood tubes, leading to falsely low levels for these elements.

Because of these problems, the gold-standard method that evolved was to:
- draw the sample through a plastic catheter preplaced in the vein
- use a syringe (acid-leached, all plastic) that allowed centrifugation in the syringe, or transfer of the blood to a plastic centrifuge tube, and
- transfer or store serum sample or blood in a special acid-leached plastic vial

Although these methods provide reliable results, they are sufficiently cumbersome for clinical practice that alternative methods have been sought.

For several years, Becton Dickinson has marketed a "trace metal" royal blue top tube which has been found satisfactory for most analyses **but not for chromium, manganese, aluminum, and selenium**. Recently, Sherwood Medical Company has marketed a trace metal evacuated blood collection tube that, for clinical purposes, has been found satisfactory for aluminum, arsenic, cadmium, copper, chromium, iron, lead, magnesium, manganese, mercury, selenium, and zinc. Although slight alterations in lead, aluminum, and manganese were noted over a 24-hour period of time of contact, these tubes appear satisfactory for usual clinical practice where brief contact time is anticipated and are recommended for these analyses.

Specifically, if using a vacuum device for drawing blood, we recommend the BD #5175 20-gauge stainless steel needle and a Sherwood Monoject™ trace element blood collection tube, #8881-307006, as a clot tube for serum or #8881-307022 EDTA tube for whole blood. If several tubes of blood are to be drawn together, draw all trace metal tubes first so as not to contaminate the needle by puncture of the ordinary Vacutainer® stoppers. (Vacutainer® rubber stoppers are heavily contaminated by several trace metals.)

If a "butterfly" type needle is needed for a difficult venipuncture, Terumo or Abbot butterfly needles have been found not to contribute trace metals to the sample.

Not reliable are ordinary "red top" clot tubes or the use of needles with metal hubs or syringes with rubber plungers. Directions for obtaining blood samples are briefly summarized for each specific test.

Footnotes
1. H. Ray Adams, PhD, Chief of General Chemistry and Toxicology, Department of Pathology, Texas A&M University Health Science Center College of Medicine, Scott & White Clinic, and Memorial Hospital, Temple, Texas.
2. Edward D. Harris, PhD, Professor of Biochemistry and Biophysics, Texas A&M University, Bryan-College Station, Texas.

References
Moody JR and Lindstrom RM, "Selection and Cleaning of Plastic Containers for Storage of Trace Element Samples," *Anal Chem*, 1977, 49:2264-7.

Moyer TP, Mussmann GV, and Nixon DE, "Blood-Collection Device for Trace and Ultra-Trace Metal Specimens Evaluated," *Clin Chem*, 1991, 37:709-14.

Pragay DA, Howard SF, and Chilcote ME, "Inorganic Ion Contamination in Vacutainer® Tubes and Micropipets Used for Blood Collection," *Clin Chem*, 1971, 17:350-1.

Al, Bone *see* Aluminum, Bone *on this page*

Al, Serum *see* Aluminum, Serum *on this page*

Aluminum, Bone

CPT 82108

Related Information

Aluminum, Serum *on this page*

Calcium, Serum *on page 97*

Deferoxamine Infusion Test *on page 591*

Histopathology *on page 42*

Osteocalcin, Serum *on page 174*

Vitamin D₃, Serum *on page 218*

Synonyms Al, Bone

Applies to Bone Biopsy; Histomorphometry

Test Commonly Includes Aluminum measured on anterior iliac crest bone biopsy specimen

Patient Preparation Tetracycline and Declomycin® fluoresce differently under ultraviolet light and can be separately distinguished under the microscope so as to indicate the amount of bone formed between the two tetracycline labels. **Tetracycline and Declomycin® should be taken between meals, and all antacids, calcium supplements, and phosphate binders should be avoided on the days when these labels are taken.** Days 1, 2 (2 days): tetracycline 500 mg twice daily, midmorning and midafternoon; days 3-12: no tetracycline; days 13, 14, 15, 16 (4 days): Declomycin® 300 mg twice daily, midmorning and midafternoon; days 17, 18 (2 days): no tetracycline; day 19, 20, or 21: do bone biopsy. The dates and times of labels and of biopsy should be recorded and submitted with the specimen to facilitate interpretation.

Specimen The patient's skeleton is prelabeled with tetracycline (see **Patient Preparation**). The timing of the labels and the day of the biopsy is critical to standardize the time between tetracycline labels (which appear fluorescent in the bone) and the day of biopsy. The biopsy specimen is a **0.8 cm diameter core of bone** taken under local or general anesthesia full thickness from the anterior iliac crest in a standardized fashion with a hollow bone biopsy instrument so as to obtain both layers of cancellous bone as well as the internal trabecular bone.

Container Acid-washed plastic vial containing 95% ethanol. **(The surgeon should be requested not to fix the specimen in formalin.)**

Special Instructions Bone aluminum is usually measured in concert with bone histomorphometry and is performed by prearrangement with a reference laboratory specializing in bone histomorphometry. These instructions assume bone histomorphometry will also be performed in parallel with bone aluminum determination.

Reference Range Bone aluminum: <15 µg/g dry weight[1] (see figure). Bone aluminum relates to total body burden of aluminum, whereas **serum aluminum** may be only recently elevated in heavy exposure and may not correlate with aluminum related bone disease (ARBD).

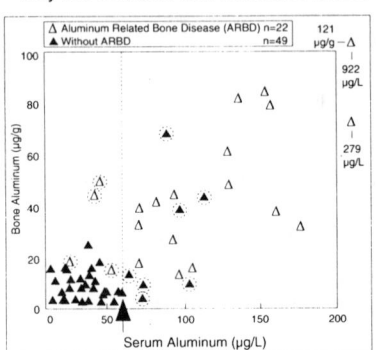 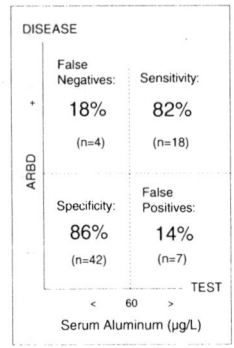

Relationship between serum aluminum, bone aluminum, and aluminum-related bone disease (ARBD). The sensitivity and specificity of a serum aluminum value of 60 µg/L (↑) in the detection of ARBD is illustrated. ▲ without ARBD; △ with ARBD as diagnosed by histochemistry, histology, and bulk analysis; ◬ false-positive; ◿ false negatives.

Histomorphometry normal values:[2]

• Trabecular bone: 3% unmineralized, 97% mineralized

• Osteoid covers 25% bone surface, lined with osteoblasts

• Osteoclasts 4% of trabecular surface

Variations from normal histomorphometry are interpreted by the pathologist as compatible with pure osteitis fibrosa, pure osteomalacia, aplastic bone disease, or mixed bone disease. The measured distance between the two tetracycline labels allows calculation of bone formation rate, which is reduced in aluminum related bone disease. Many feel that an aluminum stain, however, is most specific for aluminum related bone disease if the aluminum is detected on the mineralization front, blocking calcium deposition and resulting in osteomalacia.[3] The rate of bone

formation has been found to be inversely related to the amount of aluminum present.[4]

Use Diagnose or confirm aluminum related bone disease (ARBD) in patients with renal failure (with or without dialysis) or receiving parenteral nutrition. Aluminum bone disease among parenteral nutrition patients is much less of a clinical problem recently as nutritional products for intravenous use are more pure. Intravenous albumin products may still be a significant source of aluminum.[5] Patients with ARBD may have coexisting other types of bone disease from hyperparathyroidism or osteomalacia related to lack of vitamin D.

Limitations Histomorphometry does not always correlate with total bone aluminum content. Secondary hyperparathyroidism relatively protects from clinical aluminum bone disease, despite the presence of substantial aluminum stored in bone. Stainable aluminum at the osteoid mineralization front is taken by some authors as most sensitive for aluminum bone disease, but this is present in many aluminum exposed patients who are without symptoms. Bone aluminum correlates best with aluminum bone disease, but not as well with aluminum related microcytic anemia or encephalopathy, other forms of aluminum toxicity.

Contraindications Bone biopsy should be done with caution in the presence of a coagulopathy; history of allergy to tetracyclines precludes tetracycline labeling.

Methodology Atomic absorption (AA), graphite furnace flameless atomic absorption

Additional Information Aluminum interferes with normal bone formation by several mechanisms, including direct reduction of osteoblast function and population; reduction of parathyroid hormone release, thereby down-regulating bone turnover; and in the presence of citrate, direct inhibition of calcium phosphate crystal growth. Bone serves as a major store of aluminum, and aluminum from bone can be released back to the blood and other tissues during stress, illness, hyperthyroidism, or failed renal transplant, precipitating aluminum encephalopathy.

Footnotes

1. D'Haese PC, Clement JP, Elseviers MM, et al, "Value of Serum Aluminum Monitoring in Dialysis Patients: A Multicentre Study," *Nephrol Dial Transplant*, 1990, 5(11):45-53.
2. Visser WJ and Van de Vyver FL, "Aluminum-Induced Osteomalacia in Severe Chronic Renal Failure (SCRF)," *Clin Nephrol*, 1985, 24(1 Suppl):S30-6.
3. McCarthy JT, Kurtz SB, and McCall JT, "Elevated Bone Aluminum Content in Dialysis Patients Without Osteomalacia," *Mayo Clin Proc*, 1985, 60(5):315-20.
4. Ott SM, Maloney NA, Coburn JW, et al, "The Prevalence of Bone Aluminum Deposition in Renal Osteodystrophy and Its Relation to the Response to Calcitriol Therapy," *N Engl J Med*, 1982, 307:709-13.
5. May JC, Rains TC, Yu LJ, et al, "Aluminum Content of Source Plasma and Sodium Citrate Anticoagulant," *Vox Sang*, 1992, 62(2):65-9.

References

Wills MR and Savory J, "Aluminum and Chronic Renal Failure: Sources, Absorption, Transport, and Toxicity," *Crit Rev Clin Lab Sci*, 1989, 27(1):59-107.

Aluminum, Serum

CPT 82108

Related Information

Aluminum, Bone *on this page*

Calcium, Serum *on page 97*

Deferoxamine Infusion Test *on page 591*

Heavy Metal Screen, Blood *on page 554*

Heavy Metal Screen, Urine *on page 554*

Red Blood Cell Indices *on page 343*

Synonyms Al, Serum

Specimen Serum, dialysis fluid, urine, cerebrospinal fluid

Container Special metal-free Sherwood Monoject™ trace element blood collection tube #8881-307006 for serum separation; acid-washed plastic vials for other samples. See the Trace Elements Introduction *on page 585*.

Collection Use B-D #5175 20-gauge stainless steel needle, or Terumo or Abbot butterfly needle. Draw any trace metal tube prior to any other type of blood sample to prevent contamination of needle by regular rubber stoppers.

Causes for Rejection Contamination by aluminum contact, dust, or ordinary collection tubes or stoppers. Urine must not be contaminated by stool.

Special Instructions The patient should take no aluminum-containing antacids or medicines (such as Amphojel®, Basaljel®, Gelusil®, Maalox®, Mylanta® , Sucralfate) for 24 hours prior to test.

Reference Range Serum (normal patient): 0-6 ng/mL (SI: 0-0.22 µmol/L) (may vary with laboratory); serum (dialysis patients): up to 40 ng/mL (SI: <1.48 µmol/L) without apparent acute effects, >100 ng/mL (SI: >3.7 µmol/L) possible CNS toxicity, >200 ng/mL (SI: >7.4 µmol/L) probable multisystem toxicity; urine: 0-32 ng/day (SI: 0-1.2 µmol/day); dialysate: <0.01 mg/L (AAMI standards)

Use Monitor patients for prior and ongoing exposure to aluminum. Patients at risk include:

• infants on parenteral fluids, particularly parenteral nutrition

- burn patients through administration of intravenous albumin, particularly with coexisting renal failure
- adult and pediatric patients with chronic renal failure, who accumulate aluminum readily from medications and dialysate
- adult parenteral nutrition patients (less so, recently)
- patients with industrial exposure

Monitor dialysate and water to prepare dialysate to prevent aluminum toxicity in dialysis patients. Research use: investigation of amyotrophic lateral sclerosis (in Guam) and Alzheimer's disease.

Limitations Serum levels rise and fall after each dose of aluminum-containing phosphate binder or sucralfate. If renal function is normal, renal clearance of aluminum is prompt with urine levels rising quickly after a course of aluminum-containing antacid is begun and elevated levels persisting for over a week. Urine levels rise after a dose of deferoxamine given for any reason. The degree of rise in serum aluminum after deferoxamine is regarded as reflecting total body aluminum burden (see **Deferoxamine Infusion Test** *on page 591*). Serum aluminum levels <40 ng/mL or even <20 ng/mL do not exclude serious toxicity in dialysis patients. As aluminum exposure of dialysis patients by medications has fallen in recent years, there is a tendency to move the lower limit of normal down toward 10 ng/mL or 12 ng/mL, even for dialysis patients.

Methodology Atomic absorption (AA), inductively coupled plasma atomic emission spectrometry

Additional Information Aluminum toxicity has been recognized in many settings. Risk factors include heavy or prolonged exposure, poor renal function, chronic citrate intake which enhances aluminum absorption, or a previously accumulated bone burden which may be released in stress or illness. Signs and symptoms include:

- encephalopathy (stuttering, gait disturbance, myoclonic jerks, seizures, coma, abnormal EEG)
- osteomalacia or aplastic bone disease (associated with painful spontaneous fractures, hypercalcemia, tumorous calcinosis)
- proximal myopathy
- increased risk of infection
- increased left ventricular mass and decreased myocardial function
- microcytic anemia
- with very high levels, sudden death

Aluminum is ubiquitous in our environment; it is the third most prevalent element in the earth's crust. The gastrointestinal tract is relatively impervious to aluminum, absorption normally being only about 2%. Aluminum is absorbed by a mechanism related to that for calcium. Gastric acidity and oral citrate favors absorption, and H_2-blockers reduce absorption. As is true for several trace elements, transferrin is the primary protein binder and carrier for aluminum in the plasma, where 80% is protein bound and 20% is free or complexed to small molecules such as citrate. Cells appear to take up aluminum from transferrin rather than from citrate. Purified preparations of ferritin from brain and liver have been found to contain aluminum. It is not known if ferritin has a specific binding site for aluminum. Factors regulating the migration of aluminum across the blood-brain barrier are not well understood. Serum aluminum correlates with encephalopathy; red cell aluminum correlates with microcytic anemia;[2] and bone aluminum correlates with aluminum bone disease. Basal PTH when elevated appears to protect bone and thereby favor CNS toxicity. Other factors favoring one form of toxicity over another are not well understood. Aluminum toxicity has been reported to impair the formation and release of parathyroid hormone. The parathyroid glands concentrate aluminum above levels in surrounding tissues. Treatment of aluminum toxicity in renal failure patients often reactivates hyperparathyroidism, which to a certain extent is helpful for bone remodeling and healing.

Footnotes
1. Recommended Maximum Promulgated by the Association for Advancement of Medical Instrumentation, 1990, 33330 Washington Blvd, Suite 400, Arlington, VA 22201.
2. Abreo K, Brown ST, Sella M, et al, "Application of An Erythrocyte Aluminum Assay in the Diagnosis of Aluminum-Associated Microcytic Anemia in Patients Undergoing Dialysis and Response to Deferoxamine Therapy," *J Lab Clin Med*, 1989, 113(1):50-7.

References
Alfrey AC, LeGendre GR, and Kaehny WD, "The Dialysis Encephalopathy Syndrome: Possible Aluminum Intoxication," *N Engl J Med*, 1976, 294:184-8.

Chappuis P, Poupon J, and Rousselet F, "A Sequential and Simple Determination of Zinc, Copper, and Aluminum in Blood Samples by Inductively Coupled Plasma Atomic Emission Spectrometry," *Clin Chim Acta*, 1992, 206(3):155-65.

Ellenberg R, King AL, Sica DA, et al, "Cerebrospinal Fluid Aluminum Levels Following Deferoxamine," *Am J Kidney Dis*, 1990, 16(2):157-9.

Gruskin AB, "Aluminum: A Pediatric Overview," *Adv Pediatr*, 1988, 35:281-330.

Klein GL, "Aluminum in Parenteral Products: Medical Perspective on Large and Small Volume Parenterals," *J Parenter Sci Technol*, 1989, 43(3):120-4.

Monteagudo FS, Cassidy MJ, and Folb PI, "Recent Developments in Aluminum Toxicology," *Med Toxicol Adverse Drug Exp*, 1989, 4(1):1-16.

Russo LS, Beale G, Sandroni S, et al, "Aluminum Intoxication in Undialysed Adults With Chronic Renal Failure," *J Neurol Neurosurg Psychiatry*, 1992, 55(8):697-700.

<rac[Tzamaloukas AH, "Diagnosis and Management of Bone Disorders in Chronic Renal Failure and Dialyzed Patients," *Med Clin North Am*, 1990, 74(4):961-74.

Bone Biopsy *see* Aluminum, Bone *on previous page*

Chromium, Serum
CPT 82495

Related Information
Glucose Tolerance Test *on page 139*
Heavy Metal Screen, Blood *on page 554*
Heavy Metal Screen, Urine *on page 554*
Protein, Quantitative, Urine *on page 649*
Protein, Semiquantitative, Urine *on page 650*
Urinalysis *on page 658*

Synonyms Cr, Serum

Abstract Determination of the amount of chromium in the serum or urine of normal persons is extremely difficult, due to the very low levels present. Levels observed are in the 0.1 ng/mL range, equivalent to one part in 10 billion. Extreme caution must be taken to avoid contamination by dust (from skin, leather, cloth) and contact with steel (which contains chromium). Chromium is felt to be an essential element in the human, with chromium III purported to be an integral part of "glucose tolerance factor," a partially characterized complex that is thought to contain two molecules of nicotinic acid and a small oligopeptide complexed to chromium III. This organic moiety is considered necessary for insulin action on the cell surface. Deficiency of chromium can cause an acquired insulin resistance or diabetes mellitus with associated hyperlipidemia in otherwise well-nourished patients. The classic cases, however, were reported prior to the availability of accurate serum levels of chromium, and reported levels then in "deficiency" were tenfold or more higher than we now know to be "normal". Chromium deficiency with associated glucose intolerance and fasting hypoglycemia has been most often observed during refeeding of malnourished individuals after famine starvation in relief programs. In infants, one or more oral doses of chromium, 250 µg, have been curative. Chromium deficiency with associated glucose intolerance has also been observed in long-term parenteral nutrition when inadequate chromium was included.[1] Neuropathy, encephalopathy, and abnormalities of amino acid profile (serum low in branched-chain amino acids and high in aromatic amino acids) have been noted in conjunction with this condition.[2]

With regard to toxicity, pure metallic chromium is nontoxic. Chromium III is poorly absorbed, and much less toxic than chromium VI. Industrial monitoring for toxicity in the past has relied on air samples largely for total and hexavalent chromium, the major species of concern. Workers are potentially exposed in tanneries, mines, and industries for metal plating, welding, photography, paint, dye, and explosives. Skin exposure may lead to dermatitis, and respiratory exposure to bronchitis, asthma, and lung cancer. Hair contains 1000-fold more chromium than serum or urine, and hair chromium content does correlate with industrial exposure, but more data are needed before hair chromium monitoring can replace industrial air monitoring and samples of blood and urine in cases of suspected toxicity[3] or deficiency. Acute systemic chromate toxicity may cause acute tubular necrosis, acute hepatitis, convulsions, and coma. Acute respiratory or gastrointestinal symptoms relate to the locus of absorption. Intermediate levels of long-term exposure may cause tubular proteinuria in industrial workers.[4]

Chromium supplementation has been shown by some workers to improve glucose tolerance and improve insulin efficiency in glucose intolerant (but not in normal or overtly diabetic) patients on diets equivalent to the lower quartile of ordinary chromium intake in the United States.[5] The implication is that many individuals in the U.S. population have a marginal chromium intake, and that much of glucose intolerance is due to chromium deficiency. Other workers have carefully looked for an effect of "organic chromium" as is found in yeast, and have found **no** effect on glucose tolerance, insulin levels, or glycosylated hemoglobin in stable elderly patients with glucose intolerance.[6] This of course has not deterred a brisk sale of Chromium tablets through the health food stores. We may anticipate even more self-medication and supplementation in the future, and greater medical interest in this trace metal. The literature regarding chromium was for many years confused due to difficulties with analysis and contamination. Much old work needs to be repeated, and this field is still very much in flux.

Patient Preparation Patient should be fasting for basal level.

Specimen Serum

Container Special metal-free, Sherwood Monoject™ trace element blood collection tube #8881-307006. See the Trace Elements Introduction *on page 585*.

Sampling Time A morning fasting sample should be obtained. A glucose load, due to the insulin response it induces, drives chromium levels lower. In the nocturnal total parenteral nutrition patient, the sample should be drawn "fasting" in the afternoon, before the glucose-containing TPN solution is started for the evening.

(Continued)

Chromium, Serum *(Continued)*

Collection Follow specific instructions of laboratory to which sample will be submitted. Contact with steel, dust, ordinary glassware, or plastic is to be avoided. Draw blood through indwelling plastic intracath needle. Some siliconized stainless steel needles have also been found to be acceptable as is the B-D #5175 20-gauge stainless steel needle, or the Terumro or Abbott butterfly needles. Draw trace metal sample prior to any other blood samples. Remove serum with an all-plastic pipette (no internal metal parts) and store serum in plastic vial. Leeching plastic containers in 10% nitric acid for 48 hours removes trace metal contamination if special purpose vials are not available. The containers are then rinsed three times with twice distilled water and air dried in a dust-free environment prior to use.

Storage Instructions Some reference laboratories request specimens to be frozen and sent on dry ice.

Causes for Rejection Improper collection or storage with contact by steel, dust, or ordinary Vacutainer® tubes

Reference Range 0.05-0.15 ng/mL (SI: 1-3 nmol/L).[7] Some laboratories report much higher "normals" because the methods they use or the collection technique is not adequate to prevent substantial contamination. If a laboratory reports "<1 ng/mL" or some similar figure without a lower level for normal, the value can be relied upon to discover toxic states, perhaps, but not deficiency states. Serum levels of 10 ng/mL correspond to short-term atmospheric exposure limit of 0.1 mg/m[3] of chromium trioxide.[8] Serum levels even higher would be expected in acute systemic toxicity. Almost a twofold diurnal variation is noted in serum chromium levels, with the level highest in the morning and falling after each meal as insulin levels rise. Serum chromium levels are about 60% of normal in diabetic patients, which overlaps the normal range.

Use Evaluate suspected chromium toxicity or exposure; follow patients receiving chromium in their parenteral nutrition; evaluate acquired glucose intolerance in refeeding programs, or in parenteral or enteral nutrition; evaluate insulin resistance in the nonseptic patient during parenteral nutrition

Limitations Extreme attention to detail is needed to achieve reliable results; for many laboratories even now a high serum level more often reflects sample contamination rather than excess chromium exposure.

Methodology Any reported levels in biological materials prior to about 1979 are suspect, as the available methods did not have the sensitivity to separate normal values from the "blank." Reported levels were tenfold or more too high. Accurate and independently verified values have been reported with:

- stable isotope dilution, isotope ratio mass spectroscopy
- graphite furnace atomic absorption spectroscopy

All pipettes must have plastic tips and no exposed internal metal parts. Work is done in the laboratory under a laminar flow class 100 work station, free from exposed stainless steel to avoid airborne contamination. This is essential to reduce contamination sufficiently to detect "normal levels" in human serum or urine. Even with these precautions, different laboratories report different normal values.

Additional Information Iron competitively inhibits the binding of chromium III to transferrin. Iron overloaded patients with hemochromatosis poorly retain a radioactive tracer dose of chromium III. It has been suggested that chromium deficiency at a cellular level may play a role in the development of diabetes in hemochromatosis.[9]

Footnotes

1. Jeejecbhoy KN, Chu RC, Marliss EB, et al, "Chromium Deficiency, Glucose Intolerance, and Neuropathy Reversed by Chromium Supplementation, in a Patient Receiving Long-Term Total Parenteral Nutrition," *Am J Clin Nutr*, 1977, 30:531-8.
2. Freund H, Atamian S, and Fischer JE, "Chromium Deficiency During Total Parenteral Nutrition," *JAMA*, 1979, 241:496-8.
3. Randall JA and Gibson RS, "Hair Chromium as an Index of Chromium Exposure of Tannery Workers," *Br J Ind Med*, 1989, 46(3):171-5.
4. Wedeen RP and Qian L, "Chromium-Induced Kidney Disease," *Environ Health Perspect*, 1991, 92:71-4.
5. Anderson RA, Polansky MM, Bryden NA, et al, "Supplemental-Chromium Effects on Glucose, Insulin, Glucagon, and Urinary Chromium Losses in Subjects Consuming Controlled Low-Chromium Diets," *Am J Clin Nutr*, 1991, 54(5):909-16.
6. Uusitupa MI, Mykkanen L, Siitonen O, et al, "Chromium Supplementation in Impaired Glucose Tolerance of Elderly: Effects on Blood Glucose, Plasma Insulin, C-Peptide and Lipid Levels," *Br J Nutr*, 1992, 68(1):209-16.
7. Chappuis P, Poupon J, Deschamps JF, et al, "Physiological Chromium Determination in Serum by Graphite Furnace Atomic Absorption Spectrometry. A Serious Challenge," *Biol Trace Elem Res*, 1992, 32:85-91.
8. Baruthio F, "Toxic Effects of Chromium and Its Compounds," *Biol Trace Elem Res*, 1992, 32:145-53.
9. Sargent T, Lim TH, and Jenson RL, "Reduced Chromium Retention in Patients With Hemochromatosis, A Possible Basis of Hemochromatotic Diabetes," *Metabolism*, 1979, 28:70-9.

References

Brown RO, Forloines-Lynn S, Cross RE, et al, "Chromium Deficiency After Long-Term Total Parenteral Nutrition," *Dig Dis Sci*, 1986, 31(6):661-4.
Hopkins LL Jr, Ransome-Kuti O, and Majaj AS, "Improvement of Impaired Carbohydrate Metabolism by Chromium (III) in Malnourished Infants," *Am J Clin Nutr*, 1968, 21:203-11.

Morris BW, MacNeil S, Stanley K, et al, "The Inter-Relationship Between Insulin and Chromium in Hyperinsulinaemic Euglycaemic Clamps in Healthy Volunteers," *J Endocrinol*, 1993, 139(2):339-45.
Schermaier AJ, O'Connor LH, and Pearson KH, "Semiautomated Determination of Chromium in Whole Blood and Serum by Zeeman Electrothermal Atomic Absorption Spectrophotometry," *Clin Chim Acta*, 1985, 152(1-2):123-34.
Veillon C, "Chromium," *Methods Enzymol*, 1988, 158:334-43.

Chromium, Urine

CPT 82495

Related Information

Glucose Tolerance Test *on page 139*
Heavy Metal Screen, Blood *on page 554*
Heavy Metal Screen, Urine *on page 554*
Urine Collection, 24-Hour *on page 30*

Synonyms Cr, Urine

Abstract Urine chromium levels are extremely low, and until recently, not reliable. Urine chromium assay is used to look for chromium toxicity in cases of potential exposure. As testing becomes more reliable, new applications of the test will arise to determine chromium III nutritional adequacy or deficiency states. See listing Chromium, Serum *on page 587*, for signs and symptoms of toxicity and deficiency states and for additional references.

Specimen 24-hour urine

Container Plastic metal-free container. To prepare, leech 48 hours in 10% nitric acid and wash with distilled water that has had no contact with metal. Dry in quiet air in a metal-free environment.

Collection Care must be taken to avoid contact with metal. Use plastic urinal, prepared as above. Stool contamination must be avoided.

Causes for Rejection Improper collection, contact with metal, ordinary urine container used, stool contamination

Reference Range <1 µg/24 hours[1]. Levels vary with the laboratory and have declined with improved methods of avoiding contamination. Levels two- to threefold above this may reflect supplementation or excess losses. Levels elevated tenfold and higher have been seen in exposed asymptomatic tannery workers. Spot levels of chromium in urine of 30 ng/g creatinine correspond to the short-term atmospheric exposure limit of 0.1 mg/m[3] of chromium trioxide in industrial exposure situations.[2]

Use Evaluate industrial exposure, suspected toxicity; or in conjunction with serum levels, to attempt to detect suspected chromium deficiency, especially in a recent onset of glucose intolerance

Limitations Levels are so low in normal people (on the order of one part in 10 billion in urine) that many laboratories are not able to detect the lower limit of normal, and thus report "less than" some set level as being normal. Thus, for many laboratories, the test can only be used to detect toxicity. Contamination of the specimen may result in a tenfold or more increase in urine concentration being reported, making potential contamination the major limiting factor in the test.

Methodology Atomic absorption (AA) or neutron activation

Additional Information The main excretory pathway for chromium III is renal. Estimated safe and adequate, oral intake recommended by the U.S. National Academy of Sciences range from 50-200 µg/day,[3] but in the U.S. 90% of people eat less, the mean intake being 25-33 µg/day. Such intake recommendations likely derive from the 1980s when average estimated intake was determined to be 50-100 µg/day. With increasingly accurate assays, new recommended ranges may be set lower. Absorption of chromium III is on the order of 0.5%, by radioisotope studies. One hospital pharmacy supplies 12 µg of chromium from MTE5® trace mineral parenteral nutrition supplement per day. We are unaware of a large survey.

As improved methods have progressively reduced the lower level of detection, urine chromium levels have been found to be related to glucose metabolism. Recent studies[4] have demonstrated the metabolic relationships between serum insulin, serum glucose, and serum chromium III in the fasting and postprandial states and the relationship of the postprandial state to urine chromium concentration. Briefly, diabetic patients lose threefold more chromium in the urine than nondiabetics, and despite increased intestinal absorption, diabetic patients on ordinary diets develop and maintain lower serum levels. Chromium loss is not specifically related to micro- or macroalbuminuria and precedes the onset of diabetic nephropathy. Urine chromium rises threefold 40 minutes after a carbohydrate meal and more so with carbohydrates that stimulate higher insulin levels. Serum levels fall after a meal, more so than can be explained by urine loss. Thus, glucose stimulates insulin to take chromium to a cellular location, which favors increased renal excretion.

Footnotes

1. Milni DB, "Trace Elements," *Textbook of Clinical Chemistry*, Tietz NA, ed, Philadelphia, PA: WB Saunders Co, 1994, 1342-4.
2. Baruthio F, "Toxic Effects of Chromium and Its Compounds," *Biol Trace Elem Res*, 1992, 32:145-53.

3. National Research Council, *Recommended Dietary Allowances*, 10th ed, National Academy of Sciences.
4. Morris BW, Blumsohn A, Mac Neil S, et al, "The Trace Element Chromium - A Role in Glucose Homeostasis," *Am J Clin Nutr*, 1992, 55(5):989-91.

Copper, Serum

CPT 82525

Related Information

Ceruloplasmin *on page 107*
Copper, Urine *on next page*
Heavy Metal Screen, Blood *on page 554*
Heavy Metal Screen, Urine *on page 554*
Liver Biopsy *on page 48*
Zinc, Serum *on page 595*

Synonyms Cu, Serum

Applies to Metallothionein; Transcuprein; Zinc Administration

Abstract Our understanding of copper as an essential trace element in human nutrition and a factor in several diseases has advanced substantially over the past few years. Copper is a component of many metalloenzymes including:

- cytochrome C oxidase
- superoxide dismutase
- tyrosinase
- dopamine-β-hydroxylase
- lysyl oxidase
- clotting factor V
- an unknown enzyme that cross-links keratin in hair
- ceruloplasmin, a ferroxidase in serum which also seems to serve as a major transport protein for copper. (See listing Ceruloplasmin *on page 107*.)

Inorganic copper is very reactive and a potent cellular toxin. Its metabolism is complicated. Copper is absorbed in the stomach and duodenum by a process regulated by the metallothionein (MT) concentration in intestinal mucosal cells. MT synthesis is induced by copper. The more MT present, the more copper is trapped in the mucosal cell and is sloughed into the intestinal lumen to be lost in the stool unabsorbed. Thus, copper absorption is partially self-limiting.

Tissue levels of MT are induced by both copper and zinc. Zinc is more poorly bound by MT than copper, but zinc is the better inducer; relatively small excesses of zinc in the food stream markedly inhibit copper absorption by stimulating high levels of MT. Zinc also has an immediate and direct action on copper uptake by the intestinal mucosal cell, blocking transport even before there are changes in the intracellular levels of MT. Cadmium and iron can also inhibit copper absorption, possibly through similar mechanisms. Molybdenum decreases absorption by forming insoluble copper-molybdenum-sulfur compounds. This interaction has been used in the detoxification of certain patients with Wilson's disease by giving oral molybdenum-sulfur compounds.

After absorption, copper appears in the blood, loosely bound to albumin and also as copper-histidine. The liver and other organs take up the copper by membrane-bound ligands and transfer it intracellularly. Linder isolated a binding protein ("transcuprein") which may also serve to transport copper from the intestine to the liver.

In the liver, copper is used to synthesize ceruloplasmin, which appears in a few hours in the blood stream. Copper uptake by various organs depends on the amount of copper in the blood that is incorporated into ceruloplasmin as opposed to that loosely bound to histidine or albumin. About 65% of the copper in peripheral blood is in the form of ceruloplasmin.

Copper, stored in the liver, is secreted in the bile. **Biliary excretion** increases when copper stores are plentiful. Copper has an enterohepatic circulation, but that amount of copper secreted in the bile sequestered in ceruloplasmin fragments resists digestion and is carried out in the stool, poorly reabsorbed by the more distal small bowel. Thus copper excretion is self regulating. Renal tubular reabsorption of filtered copper is efficient, so normally only a small fraction of copper is lost in the urine. Overflow **losses in the urine** are proportional to copper stores except when abnormal urine losses occur as in burns, I.V. administration of amino acids, Menkes' syndrome, and with chelating drugs.

This complicated metabolic pathway explains many features of known human diseases involving copper. Oral zinc administration inhibits absorption of copper and may cause copper deficiency states. Oral zinc can be used to treat copper excess states including Wilson's disease[1] or can inadvertently cause copper deficiency[2] by stimulating excess metallothionein (MT) synthesis. Even after oral zinc therapy is discontinued, high total body zinc stores continue to block oral copper absorption through the MT mechanism.

The genes for Wilson's disease and Menkes' disease have been cloned, and the gene products identified; they provide a model to help us understand all the inherited diseases of copper metabolism. In Wilson's disease there is a defective P-type copper transporting ATPase, which leads to tissue maldistribution of copper. There is a secondary failure of ceruloplasmin synthesis (poor incorporation of copper into ceruloplasmin). This leads to higher free and loosely albumin-bound copper in the blood, which delivers additional copper to brain tissue. The reduced ceruloplasmin synthesis probably additionally decreases biliary excretion of copper[3] and thereby contributes to excess, ultimately toxic hepatic copper. In a later acute hepatitis syndrome, the liver can release so much copper to the blood (unbound to ceruloplasmin) that encephalopathy, acute red blood cell hemolysis and acute renal failure may result.

In both Wilson's disease and Indian childhood cirrhosis (ICC), there are inherited and environmental factors, and toxic accumulation of hepatic copper. ICC had been considered an illness of toxic exposure of the child to milk boiled in brass vessels, especially among poor families where the vessels were not tinned frequently to prevent exposure to the brass. Indeed, the incidence of ICC drops markedly as brass utensils are discarded by a community. There is now, however, good evidence that, like Wilson's disease, this is primarily a genetic disease. In ICC, the basal production and metal-induced synthesis of MT is defective (glucocorticoid-induced MT synthesis is normal). Copper accumulates in the cytoplasm, massively so in the liver. Pathology of the liver in ICC is distinct from Wilson's disease. ICC has been reported in both Europe and the United States, where excess copper intake could not be proven.

Copper deficiency from any cause causes markedly reduced ceruloplasmin synthesis rates and blood levels, and a microcytic or normocytic anemia due to blocks in iron metabolism. This anemia fails to respond to oral or I.V. iron, but brisk reticulocytosis follows copper administration. Copper deficiency can cause a scurvy-like bone disease (probably due to lysyl oxidase deficiency), depigmentation (probably due to tyrosinase deficiency), growth failure, and neutropenia.

Menkes' disease is a severe X-linked copper deficiency syndrome presenting usually by 3 months of age. The gene product is also a P-type copper transporting ATPase. When defective, it results in copper accumulation in intestinal mucosa and kidney with failure to deliver adequate copper to other tissues and resulting functional copper deficiency in terms of symptomatology. There is increased urine copper loss due to failure of renal tubular reabsorption. Effects of cellular copper deficiency are noted in bone, pigmentation, CNS development, growth, and arterial connective tissue. Oral or I.V. inorganic copper is ineffective in treatment, and the condition is usually fatal. Several recent reports[4] of I.V. copper-histidine (plus intermittent penicillamine to prevent copper overload) are encouraging, but difficult to interpret, as some cases are more severe than others, and every family studied has had a different point mutation in the MNK gene.

Occipital horn syndrome (OHS) (Ehlers-Danlos syndrome type IX) has been confirmed as an inherited disorder of copper metabolism. It may be allelic to Menkes' disease. It is usually recognized by its characteristic physical features, but can be confirmed by serum copper, serum ceruloplasmin, and fibroblast lysyl oxidase activity, which are all low. Intestinal absorption of copper is poor. Urine copper has not been reported.

Acute copper toxicity causes gastrointestinal irritation or bleeding (locally) and systemically leads to intravascular hemolysis, hepatic and renal tubular necrosis.

Ceruloplasmin synthesis is stimulated by copper intake, and ordinarily ceruloplasmin carries about 65% of serum copper. Serum copper and serum ceruloplasmin usually parallel each other in the healthy patient and, therefore, do not provide independent information. Red blood cell copper has a similar value to serum, so hemolysis does not interfere with serum copper determination.

There are at least two situations in which ceruloplasmin may not parallel total serum copper. In acute copper toxicity, there may not yet have been time for ceruloplasmin synthesis, so free (or loosely bound) copper is elevated, total serum copper may be elevated, and ceruloplasmin may still be normal. In Wilson's disease, with chronic low levels of ceruloplasmin, more copper in serum may be loosely bound and (total) serum copper may even be normal (10% incidence) rather than low. In this situation, it is especially important to measure both total serum copper and ceruloplasmin. High **urine copper** is also a feature of Wilson's disease. Because no combination of noninvasive tests has proven 100% sensitive and specific for Wilson's disease, molecular genetics will likely be more frequently used in diagnosis within families.

Specimen Serum, cerebrospinal fluid, tissue

Container Royal blue top tube which contains no anticoagulant. Alternate is the Sherwood trace metal tube #8881-307006. See the Trace Elements Introduction *on page 585*.

Collection Use a stainless steel needle (B-D #5175). Draw tube prior to any other blood samples. After centrifugation, pour serum into a metal-free vial for transport to reference laboratory. CSF can be transferred directly to a royal blue top tube.

For liver tissue, follow directions of reference laboratory. Handling instructions have recently been published.[5]

(Continued)

Copper, Serum (Continued)

Reference Range Serum: Approximately 0.7-1.5 µg/mL (SI: 11-24 µmol/L). Mean levels are slightly higher in women and children. There is diurnal variation with peak levels in the morning. Cerebrospinal fluid: 6-35 ng/mL.[6] Levels in CSF are elevated up to threefold in the neurotoxicity of Wilson's disease. Liver tissue: 9-45 ng/g dry weight. Ceruloplasmin levels rise dramatically in the last 2 weeks of pregnancy, and therefore copper levels rise then also.

Use Serum copper is used, along with serum ceruloplasmin and urine copper to screen for Wilson's disease and more often, in monitoring the nutritional adequacy of parenteral or enteral nutrition, especially when copper deficiency may be suspected because of ongoing gastrointestinal losses of the element (see table). The test is done in suspected copper toxicity in premature infants when they are acutely ill and may not be able to assimilate the copper in their prescribed nutrition; in acute copper intoxications; or in Indian childhood cirrhosis (ICC), an inherited illness once considered fatal which is aggravated by high oral intake of copper but not limited to Indian children.[7] The test, along with urine copper, is used to follow such children under therapy with penicillamine. Serum copper is low in Menkes' syndrome and occipital horn syndrome (OHS). Copper in the CSF is reported to mirror the neurotoxicity of copper in Wilson's disease.[6] Serum and urine copper are used to follow copper status in acrodermatitis enteropathica, in which chronic oral zinc therapy puts the patient at risk for symptomatic copper deficiency. The combination of increased hepatic copper and low ceruloplasmin occurs only in Wilson's disease and normal infants, who are born at term with increased copper stores and develop normal ceruloplasmin levels by 3-6 month of age. Copper stores rise during the last trimester of pregnancy, so premature infants may not have elevated liver copper.

Limitations Since ceruloplasmin is an acute-phase reactant protein which binds a large portion of serum copper, both serum copper and ceruloplasmin increase with inflammatory conditions and estrogen. Serum copper is therefore elevated in pregnancy, in patients on estrogens and estrogen-containing contraceptive drugs, in rheumatoid arthritis, and a number of other pathologic entities. It may be low with low serum proteins as in nephrosis, malabsorption, and malnutrition without necessarily reflecting inadequate liver copper stores. It is reduced under the influence of ACTH or glucocorticoids, or valproate[8] therapy. Although serum copper levels are usually ordered to work up possible cases of Wilson's disease, Menkes' syndrome, and ICC, serum copper alone is of only limited value.

Methodology Atomic absorption (AA), inductively coupled plasma atomic emission spectrometry

Additional Information The demand for sensitive noninvasive tests for Wilson's disease, especially for children in families where the disease is known to occur, has stimulated search for newer indices of copper metabolism. Urine copper after penicillamine load has recently been proposed.[9]

Elevations in liver tissue copper are found in Wilson's disease but may occur also in other types of liver disease, especially primary biliary cirrhosis.[4] Liver tissue copper level remains the gold standard for diagnosis of Wilson's disease and Indian childhood cirrhosis (ICC), although even this, though sensitive, is not 100% specific. It remains diagnostic in a sibship because both diseases are inherited disorders, and other etiologies of excess liver copper are rarely in the differential diagnosis within a family. Liver copper is used to confirm Menkes' syndrome and may be measured in liver disease of uncertain etiology. It can confirm ICC in the appropriate setting. Liver copper rises with time in biliary cirrhosis, but does not confirm the diagnosis. The liver biopsy diagnosis of Wilson's disease has been recently reviewed.[5] See listing Liver Biopsy on page 48.

Footnotes

1. Brewer GJ, Dick RD, and Yuzbasiyan-Gurkan V, et al, "Treatment of Wilson's Disease With Zinc. XIII. Therapy With Zinc in Presymptomatic Patients From the Time of Diagnosis," *J Lab Clin Med*, 1994, 123(6):849-58.
2. Hoffman HN II, Phyliky RL, and Fleming CR, "Zinc-Induced Copper Deficiency," *Gastroenterology*, 1988, 94(2):508-12.
3. Lee HH, Hill GM, Sikha VKN, et al, "Pancreaticobiliary Secretion of Zinc and Copper in Normal Persons and Patients With Wilson's Disease," *J Lab Clin Med*, 1990, 116(3):283-8.
4. Nadal D and Baerlocher K, "Menkes' Disease: Long-Term Treatment With Copper and D-Penicillamine," *Eur J Pediatr*, 1988, 147(6):621-5.
5. Ludwig J, Moyer TP, and Rakela J, "The Liver Biopsy Diagnosis of Wilson's Disease: Methods in Pathology," *Am J Clin Pathol*, 1994, 102(4):443-6.
6. Weisner B, Hartard C, and Dieu C, "CSF Copper Concentration: A New Parameter for Diagnosis and Monitoring Therapy of Wilson's Disease With Cerebral Manifestation," *J Neurol Sci*, 1987, 79(1-2):229-37.
7. Weiss M, Müller-Höcker J, Wiebecke B, et al, "First Description of "Indian Childhood Cirrhosis" in A Non-Indian Infant in Europe," *Acta Paediat Scand*, 1989, 78(1):152-6.
8. Kaji M, Ito M, Okuno T, et al, "Serum Copper and Zinc Levels in Epileptic Children With Valproate Treatment," *Epilepsia*, 1992, 33(3):555-7.
9. Martins da Costa C, Baldwin D, Portmann B, et al, "Value of Urinary Copper Excretion After Penicillamine Challenge in the Diagnosis of Wilson's Disease," *Hepatology*, 1992, 15(4):609-15.

References

Cox DW, "Genes of the Copper Pathway," *Am J Hum Genet*, 1995, 56(4):828-34.
Danks DM, "Copper Deficiency in Humans," *Annu Rev Nutr*, 1988, 8:235-57.
Danks DM, "Disorders of Copper Transport," *The Metabolic Basis of Inherited Disease*, 6th ed, Scriver CR, Beaudet AL, Sly WS, et al, eds, New York, NY: McGraw-Hill Inc, 1989, 1411-31.
Kaler SG, Gallo LK, Proud VK, et al, "Occipital Horn Syndrome and a Mild Menkes' Phenotype Associated With Splice Site Mutations at the MNK Locus," *Nat Genet*, 1994, 8(2):195-202.
Pereira GR and Zucker AH, "Nutritional Deficiencies in the Neonate," *Clin Perinatol*, 1986, 13(1):175-89.
Scheinberg IH, "Wilson's Disease and the Physiological Chemistry of Copper," *Inorg Chem Biol Med*, 1980, 21:373-80.
Vulpe CD and Packman S, "Cellular Copper Transport," *Ann Rev Nutr*, 1995, 15:293-322.
Wachnik A, "The Physiological Role of Copper and the Problems of Copper Nutritional Deficiency," *Nahrung*, 1988, 32(8):755-65.
Wakai S, Ishikawa Y, Nagaoka M, et al, "Central Nervous System Involvement and Generalized Muscular Atrophy in Occipital Horn Syndrome: Ehlers-Danlos Type IX. A First Japanese Case," *J Neurol Sci*, 1993, 116(1):1-5.
Waslen TA, Houston CS, and Tchang S, "Menkes' Kinky-Hair Disease: Radiologic Findings in a Patient Treated With Copper Histidinate," *Can Assoc Radiol J*, 1995, 46(2):114-7.
Yuzbasiyan-Gurkan V, Johnson V, and Brewer GJ, "Diagnosis and Characterization of Presymptomatic Patients With Wilson's Disease and the Use of Molecular Genetics to Aid in the Diagnosis," *J Lab Clin Med*, 1991, 118(5):458-65.

Copper, Urine

CPT 82525

Related Information

Ceruloplasmin on page 107
Copper, Serum on previous page
Heavy Metal Screen, Blood on page 554
Heavy Metal Screen, Urine on page 554
Liver Biopsy on page 48
Urine Collection, 24-Hour on page 30

Synonyms Cu, Urine

Abstract Copper is an essential trace element in human nutrition and a component of many metalloenzymes. Urine copper may be used as an aid to detect copper deficiency, Wilson's disease, Menkes' disease, Indian childhood cirrhosis (ICC), and chronic or acute copper toxicity.

Patient Preparation If a bedpan or urinal is necessary for collection, it must be made of plastic. Stool contamination must be avoided.

Specimen 24-hour urine

Container Plastic urine container, no preservative

Collection Collect in acid-washed plastic container, preferably polyethylene. Acidify to pH 2 with hydrochloric or nitric acid.

Causes for Rejection Specimen allowed to contact metal or stool

Reference Range 15-60 µg/24 hours (SI: 0.22-0.9 µmol/day). See figure.

Copper, Serum

	Deficiency, Nutritional	Menkes' Syndrome	Acute Copper Toxicity	ICC and Chronic Copper Toxicity	Wilson's Disease	Smoking, Inflammatory Conditions, Pregnancy, Estrogens
Serum copper	↓	↓	↑, ↑↑	↑	N or ↓	↑, ↑↑
Serum ceruloplasmin	↓	↓	N (early)	↑	Usually ↓; may be N in children	↑, ↑↑
Urine copper	↓	↑	↑	↑	↑, ↑↑	N
CSF copper					N or ↑	N
Liver copper	↓	↓	N (early)	↑, ↑↑	↑↑	N

N = normal, ↑ = increase, ↑↑ = large increase, ↓ = decrease.

URINE COPPER IN WILSON'S DISEASE SIBLINGS

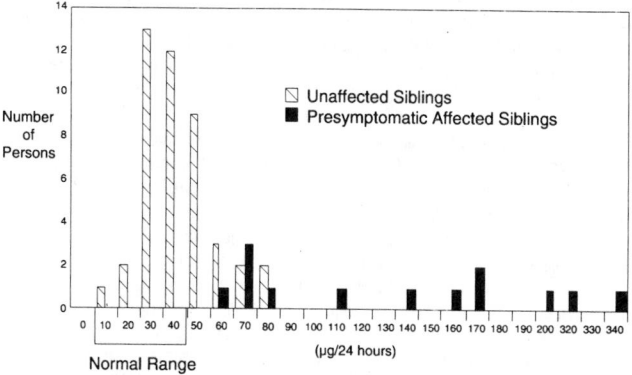

From Yuzbasiyan-Gurkan V, Johnson V, and Brewer GS, "Diagnosis and Characterization of Presymptomatic Patients With Wilson's Disease and the Use of Molecular Genetics to Aid in the Diagnosis," *J Lab Clin Med*, 1991, 118(5):458-65, with permission.

Use Increased urinary copper is found in Wilson's disease, Menkes' syndrome, Indian childhood cirrhosis (ICC), and in chronic and acute copper toxicity states including. The test is also used to follow the effectiveness of chelation therapy for Wilson's disease, or to check copper balance in patients with Wilson's disease on oral zinc therapy, or patients receiving parenteral copper as part of parenteral nutrition.

Copper excretion by the kidneys is abnormally increased with high dose intravenous histidine or mixed amino acids, as in total parenteral nutrition. Captopril and other medications may chelate copper and increase urinary excretion (usually only a tiny fraction of total daily balance). For comparison of urine copper in Wilson's disease sibships, see figure.

Over time, biliary cirrhosis leads to copper accumulation, and since biliary excretion is partly blocked, urinary excretion rises and is usually elevated, leading to diagnostic confusion with Wilson's disease. Serum ceruloplasmin and liver biopsy can distinguish these.

Limitations Increased urinary copper excretion may occur in ICC or with chronic active hepatitis; Wilson's disease and chronic active hepatitis may also resemble one another; thus, parameters in addition to urinary copper excretion, such as ceruloplasmin, serum copper, and sometimes liver biopsy are needed.

Methodology Atomic absorption, inductively coupled plasma atomic emission spectrometry

Additional Information Further information is provided in the listings Copper, Serum *on page 589* and Ceruloplasmin *on page 107*.

References

Petrukhin K and Gilliam TC, "Genetic Disorders of Copper Metabolism," *Curr Opin Pediatr*, 1994, 6(6):698-701.

Yuzbasiyan-Gurkan V, Johnson V, and Brewer GJ, "Diagnosis and Characterization of Presymptomatic Patients With Wilson's Disease and the Use of Molecular Genetics to Aid in the Diagnosis," *J Lab Clin Med*, 1991, 118(5):458-65.

Cr, Serum see Chromium, Serum *on page 587*

Cr, Urine see Chromium, Urine *on page 588*

Cu, Serum see Copper, Serum *on page 589*

Cu, Urine see Copper, Urine *on previous page*

Deferoxamine Infusion Test

CPT 82108 (plus charge for deferoxamine administration)

Related Information

Aluminum, Bone *on page 586*
Aluminum, Serum *on page 586*

Synonyms Desferrioxamine Infusion Test

Test Commonly Includes Determination of serum aluminum prior to and 48 hours postinfusion of deferoxamine

Abstract This test is used in suspected aluminum toxicity, especially among dialysis patients with known aluminum exposure, who lack diagnostically elevated serum aluminum concentrations. It is best used to exclude aluminum bone disease, which a negative test will do. A positive test requires confirmation by bone histomorphometry (See Aluminum, Bone *on page 586*). The test is felt to better reveal the total body burden of aluminum than does serum aluminum, which is more sensitive to recent exposure. Urine aluminum can not be effectively used in patients with renal failure.

Specimen Serum

Container Special metal-free Sherwood Monoject™ trace element blood collection tube #8881-307006. See the Trace Elements Introduction *on page 585*.

Collection Use B-D #5175 20-gauge stainless steel needle, or Terumo or Abbot butterfly needle. Draw any trace metal tubes prior to collecting other blood samples. Serum is separated and stored or submitted to reference laboratory for analysis of serum aluminum *on page 586* in special acid-washed plastic vial.

Special Instructions Most patients for whom this test is indicated are on dialysis, and the test is done in conjunction with their dialysis procedure (hemodialysis or peritoneal dialysis). The patient is instructed to stop any aluminum-containing antacids 3 days prior to the test. The first blood sample is obtained, then 0.5 g deferoxamine is administered in 100 mL 0.9% sodium chloride intravenously during the last 2 hours of dialysis through the venous blood line. Forty-eight hours later, prior to the next hemodialysis, a second blood sample is drawn. The timing is the same for peritoneal dialysis patients, for whom peritoneal dialysis is halted during the 48-hour period.

Reference Range The test is considered positive if the second sample more than triples the first, or exceeds it by 150 ng/mL (SI: 5.6 μmol/L)[1,2]

Critical Values Serum levels >200 ng/mL (SI: >7.4 μmol/L) can be associated with development of aluminum neurotoxicity.

Use Screen patients with known aluminum exposure and abnormal (but not diagnostically elevated) serum aluminum levels for high body burden of aluminum, which is known to be correlated with aluminum bone disease. Patients with serum aluminum levels ≤75 ng/mL are less likely to benefit from the test[3], and patients with persistent serum aluminum levels >150 ng/mL should probably go directly to bone biopsy for confirmation of bone aluminum burden.

Limitations Use of this test is controversial. Originally proposed as a 2 g deferoxamine infusion test[4], complications have been reported, including permanent visual disturbances after a single 2 g dose[5,6] Due to multiple reported complications (ocular, auditory, anaphylaxis, hematopoietic, infectious) of high dose deferoxamine therapy for iron overload in thalassemia and for aluminum overload and toxicity in chronic renal failure, therapeutic doses have generally been reduced. The 0.5 g dose infusion test[2] has so far not been reported to cause complications. Some authors endorse the use of an infusion test[7], others do not. By restricting its use to patients who probably have a moderate but not extreme body burden of aluminum, the test will help select patients needing further study by bone biopsy, a more invasive procedure.[8]

Contraindications When there is a heavy bone burden of aluminum, often reflected by high basal levels, the serum aluminum may acutely rise to toxic levels after deferoxamine dose is given as "challenge" test or as treatment, and encephalopathy may worsen. In cases of actual or anticipated intolerance to deferoxamine, hemoperfusion over specially treated charcoal (an aluminum removal device) would be an alternative treatment modality.

Methodology Atomic absorption (AA), or inductively coupled plasma atomic emission spectrometry

Footnotes

1. Yaqoob M, Ahmad R, Roberts N, et al, "Low-Dose Desferrioxamine Test for the Diagnosis of Aluminum-Related Bone Disease in Patients on Regular Haemodialysis," *Nephrol Dial Transplant*, 1991, 6(1):484-6.
2. De Broe ME, D'Haese PC, Elseviers MM, et al, "Aluminum and End Stage Renal Failure," *Nephrology*, 1988, 2:1086-116.
3. de Vernejoul MC, Marchais S, London G, et al, "Deferoxamine Test and Bone Disease in Dialysis Patients With Mild Aluminum Accumulation," *Am J Kidney Dis*, 1989, 14(2):124-30.
4. Milliner DS, Nebeker HG, Ott SM, et al, "Use of the Deferoxamine Infusion Test in the Diagnosis of Aluminum-Related Osteodystrophy," *Ann Intern Med*, 1984, 101(6):775-9.
5. Bene C, Manzler A, Bene D, et al, "Irreversible Ocular Toxicity From Single "Challenge" Dose of Deferoxamine," *Clin Nephrol*, 1989, 31(1):45-8.
6. Ravelli M, Scaroni P, Mombelloni S, et al, "Acute Visual Disorders in Patients on Regular Dialysis Given Desferrioxamine as a Test," *Nephol Dial Transplant*, 1990, 5(11):945-9.
7. McCarthy JT, Milliner DS, and Johnson WJ, "Clinical Experience With Desferrioxamine in Dialysis Patients With Aluminum Toxicity," *Q J Med*, 1990, 74(275):257-76.
8. DeVita MV, Rasenas LL, Bansal M, et al, "Assessment of Renal Osteodystrophy in Hemodialysis Patients," *Medicine*, 1992, 71(5):284-90.

References

Fournier A, Yverneau PH, Hue P, et al, "Adynamic Bone Disease in Patients With Uremia," *Curr Opin Nephrol Hypertens*, 1994, 3(4):396-410.

Wills MR and Savory J, "Aluminum and Chronic Renal Failure: Sources, Absorption, Transport, and Toxicity," *Crit Rev Clin Lab Sci*, 1989, 27(1):59-107.

Desferrioxamine Infusion Test see Deferoxamine Infusion Test *on this page*

Histomorphometry see Aluminum, Bone *on page 586*

Hypoxanthine, Urine see Molybdenum, Blood *on page 593*

Manganese, Blood

CPT 83785

Related Information

Heavy Metal Screen, Blood *on page 554*
Heavy Metal Screen, Urine *on page 554*
(Continued)

Manganese, Blood (Continued)

Synonyms Mn, Serum

Abstract Manganese is essential to life in many species and is part of many human enzyme systems. For this reason, it is considered essential for human nutrition, even though no well-documented example of a manganese deficiency state has been found in humans.[1] Manganese is routinely included in parenteral and enteral nutrition formulae, in a "multiple trace metals" additive for the former. As in several trace metals that are concentrated in the cellular elements of blood, whole blood manganese or red blood cell manganese may better reflect total body manganese stores than do serum levels in healthy individuals. Recently, monocyte manganese has been reported to vary independently of whole blood or serum manganese, and has been postulated to be a better marker of body stores.[2] In the serum, essentially all manganese is transported bound to transferrin. Transferrin receptors on the cell internalize the manganese as efficiently as iron-transferrin complexes. Once in the cell, manganese is 80% bound to ferritin.[3]

Manganese is implicated as a cofactor in many important cellular enzyme systems, especially mitochondrial superoxide dismutase. In vitro, magnesium or even cobalt, iron, calcium, or zinc may substitute for manganese in some of these enzyme systems. From animal studies, manganese deficiency is involved in osteoporosis and skeletal deformities. In humans, low levels are associated with epilepsy[4] (regardless of type of anticonvulsant) and reported with the skeletal deformities of Perthes' disease.[5] Some have argued that the late hip dislocations in infants may be related to the low manganese content in cow's milk. A single case of suspected inadvertent experimental deficiency was reported to cause hair changes and coagulopathy.

Manganese toxicity causes nausea, vomiting, headache, and psychiatric disturbances with central nervous system damage manifested by disorientation, memory loss, anxiety, and compulsive laughing or crying. In the more chronic form, manganese toxicity resembles Parkinson's disease with akinesia, rigidity, tremors, and mask-like faces. Liver failure in and of itself has been reported to cause classic manganese neurotoxicity in the child.[6] Normalization of serum levels later may reverse the neurological damage. Magnetic resonance imaging shows characteristic manganese deposits in the brains of patients industrially exposed to manganese, and in some patients who have had intravenous manganese as part of their parenteral nutrition. This latter fact suggests standard TPN doses of manganese may be too high.

Several medications are thought to chelate manganese, including valproate and hydralazine. Dialysis lowers manganese levels, and patients on hemodialysis usually have lower basal serum levels. Ninety-nine percent of manganese excretion occurs in the feces, from the bile. When intake is limited, excretion in the urine and feces may fall more than tenfold. Manganese levels rise to two to four times normal (without signs of toxicity) in children given standard amounts in their parenteral nutrition when jaundice occurs. High, potentially toxic levels have been seen after liver transplantation. Recommendations have been made[7] that supplemental manganese be withheld from parenteral nutrition solutions if serum levels cannot be followed in the presence of cholestatic jaundice (some manganese is still present in the ingredients of parenteral nutrition on a contaminant basis). Manganese is present in very small quantities in biological samples. Published normal levels have fallen by more than tenfold with better methods of avoiding contamination and improvements in analytic methods.

Specimen Serum, whole blood

Container Special metal-free Sherwood Monoject™ trace element blood collection tube #8881-307006. For whole blood, use #8881-307022 EDTA tube. See the Trace Elements Introduction on page 585.

Collection Use B-D #5175 20-gauge stainless steel needle; or Terumo or Abbot butterfly needle; draw directly into the trace metal vacuum tube. Draw this and any other trace metal blood sample first before using needle to perforate ordinary rubber stopper of ordinary blood tube. For isolation of serum, allow clotting and centrifuge. Carefully pour serum into special plastic metal-free vial or transfer with acid-washed all-plastic pipet, being careful not to disturb the clot, or any buffy coat. Store sample frozen if it is to be transported to reference laboratory. One author has suggested the use of an aluminum needle, not widely available.

Reference Range Serum: 0.43-0.76 ng/mL (SI: 7.8-13.8 nmol/L)[8]; whole blood: 10-11 ng/mL (SI: 190-200 nmol/L).[2] Levels are about three-fold higher in very low birth weight babies at birth and fall slightly over the first 3 month of life. In a recent report, exposed manganese workers who developed signs of manganese toxicity had whole blood manganese levels of 20-400 ng/mL when measured during on-going exposure.[9] One worker who left the company had a whole blood level of 10 ng/mL 6 months after exposure.

Use Follow manganese therapy in parenteral nutrition, especially in liver disease, or when there are excessive gastrointestinal losses; evaluate suspected manganese toxicity or exposure, especially neurological syndromes and movement disorders

Limitations In evaluating toxicity, the serum level may have returned to normal while neurological damage persists. The human deficiency syndrome is poorly defined, making interpretation difficult. Levels are reportedly reduced mildly in epilepsy, and raised in hepatitis or jaundice. Manganese levels are 60% lower than normal in hemodialysis patients.

Methodology Neutron activation is the most sensitive but does not lend itself to clinical testing. Atomic absorption (AA) spectrophotometry with Zeeman background correction is currently the preferred method.

Additional Information Toxic exposure may occur from dry cells, fungicide (maneb), and in the steel industry or chemical industry. Manganese is present in the coloring agents for glass and soap, in paints, varnish and enamel, and in linoleum. It is used in the manufacture of chlorine gas and now in lead-free gasoline. Industrial manganese poisoning has been recognized since 1837. Some water supplies are sufficiently contaminated by manganese that endemic psychiatric and neurological disease is present. Manganese levels in tears are 50-fold higher than in serum.

Footnotes
1. "Manganese Deficiency in Humans: Fact or Fiction?" *Nutr Rev*, 1988, 46(10):348-52.
2. Matsuda A, Kimura M, Takeda T, et al, "Changes in Manganese Content of Mononuclear Blood Cells in Patients Receiving Total Parenteral Nutrition," *Clin Chem*, 1994, 40(5):829-32.
3. Suarez N and Eriksson H, "Receptor-Mediated Endocytosis of a Manganese Complex of Transferrin Into Neuroblastoma (SHSY5Y) Cells in Culture," *J Neurochem*, 1993, 61(1):127-31.
4. Carl GF, Keen CL, Gallagher BB, et al, "Association of Low Blood Manganese Concentrations With Epilepsy," *Neurology*, 1986, 36(12):1584-7.
5. Hall AJ, Margetts BM, Barker DJ, et al, "Low Blood Manganese Levels in Liverpool Children With Perthes' Disease," *Paediatr Perinat Epidemiol*, 1989, 3(2):131-6.
6. Devenyi AG, Barron TF, and Mamourian AC, "Dystonia, Hyperintense Basal Ganglia, and High Whole Blood Manganese Levels in Alagille's Syndrome," *Gastroenterology*, 1994, 106(4):1068-71.
7. Hambidge KM, Sokol RJ, Fidanza SJ, et al, "Plasma Manganese Concentrations in Infants and Children Receiving Parenteral Nutrition," *J Parenter Enteral Nutr*, 1989, 13(2):168-71.
8. Neve J and Leclercq N, "Factors Affecting Determinations of Manganese in Serum by Atomic Absorption Spectrometry," *Clin Chem*, 1991, 37(5):723-8.
9. Wang JD, Huang CC, Hwang YH, et al, "Manganese Induced Parkinsonism: An Outbreak Due to an Unrepaired Ventilation Control System in a Ferromanganese Smelter," *Br J Ind Med*, 1989, 46(12):856-9.

References
Barlow PJ and Sylvester PE, "Hip Dislocation and Manganese Deficiency," *Lancet*, 1983, 2:685.
Falbe WJ, Brown RO, Luther RW, et al, "Individualized Manganese Supplementation in Patients Receiving Total Parenteral Nutrition," *Clin Pharm*, 1987, 6(3):226-9.
Ferraz HB, Bertolucci PHF, Pereira JS, et al, "Chronic Exposure to the Fungicide Maneb May Produce Symptoms and Signs of CNS Manganese Intoxication," *Neurology*, 1988, 38(4):550-3.
Kondakis XG, Makris N, Leotsinidis M, et al, "Possible Health Effects of High Manganese Concentration in Drinking Water," *Arch Environ Health*, 1989, 44(3):175-8.
Kurkus J, Alcock NW, and Shils ME, "Manganese Content of Large-Volume Parenteral Solutions and of Nutrient Additives," *J Parenter Enteral Nutr*, 1984, 8(3):254-7.
Reynolds AP, Kiely E, and Meadows N, "Manganese in Long Term Paediatric Parenteral Nutrition," *Arch Dis Child*, 1994, 71(6):527-8.

Manganese, Urine

CPT 83785

Related Information

Heavy Metal Screen, Blood on page 554
Heavy Metal Screen, Urine on page 554
Urine Collection, 24-Hour on page 30

Synonyms Mn, Urine

Abstract Urine manganese is used in conjunction with serum manganese to evaluate possible toxicity or deficiency of manganese,[1] an essential mineral which, in high concentration, can cause neurological damage similar to Parkinson's disease. See Manganese, Blood on page 591 for signs and symptoms of deficiency and toxicity, and for additional references.

Specimen 24-hour or random ("spot") urine. Consider simultaneous determination of urine creatinine, especially on "spot" samples.

Container Acid-washed plastic urine container, avoid contamination by stool, dust, and metal.

Causes for Rejection Contamination by metal, stool, or dust

Reference Range <2.0 µg/L (SI: <36 nmol/L) (97.5% confidence).[2] Varies with laboratory. Level may fall to 0.2 µg/L (tenfold) in experimental deficiency.[1] Some of the best data on industrial exposure have been normalized to the creatinine content of urine or to µg/hour excretion due to the impracticality of 24-hour urine samples in the industrial setting.[3] Ten free-living, nonexposed young men in Wisconsin had urinary excretion varying from approximately 0.17-0.66 µg/g creatinine.[2] Levels higher than this but <9.0 µg/g creatinine may reflect increased exposure, not necessarily at a toxic level.[4] Another group of factory workers exposed to manganese, some of whom were symptomatic with parkinsonian signs, had urine levels of manganese varying from 11.2-216.0 µg/L.[5] Bile and feces are the main routes of excretion, accounting for 99% of excretion when intake is low, and excretion rather than absorption appears to be regulated. Urine losses appear to be overflow losses, representing a higher fraction of total loss when intake is high.

Use Confirm manganese exposure, toxicity, or poisoning by documenting excessive urine excretion of the metal. Also used to individualize manganese dosing in long-term parenteral nutrition, especially in liver disease, when biliary excretion is low, or when there is excessive gastrointestinal losses, such as in short bowel syndrome. Has been used to follow the success of chelation therapy with para-aminosalicylate sodium in manganism.

Limitations Levels in urine are so low that considerable error may be introduced by contamination. Manganese toxicity may leave residual neurologic damage after serum and urine levels have returned to normal, masking the original cause.

Methodology Atomic absorption (AA)

Additional Information As much as twofold diurnal variation is present in urine manganese, especially in workers exposed to manganese at work.

Footnotes

1. "Manganese Deficiency in Humans: Fact or Fiction?" *Nutr Rev*, 1988, 46(10):348-52.
2. Greger JL, Davis CD, Suttie JW, et al, "Intake, Serum Concentrations, and Urinary Excretion of Manganese by Adult Males," *Am J Clin Nutr*, 1990, 51(3):457-61.
3. Roels HA, Ghyselen P, Buchet JP, et al, "Assessment of the Permissible Exposure Level to Manganese in Workers Exposed to Manganese Dioxide Dust," *Br J Ind Med*, 1992, 49(1):25-34.
4. Siqueira ME, Hirata MH, and Adballa DS, "Studies on Some Biochemical Parameters in Human Manganese Exposure," *Med Lav*, 1991, 82(6):504-9.
5. Hua MS and Huang CC, "Chronic Occupational Exposure to Manganese and Neurobehavioral Function," *J Clin Exp Neuropsychol*, 1991, 13(4):495-507.

References

Jacob RA, "Trace Elements," *Textbook of Clinical Chemistry*, Tietz NA, ed, Philadelphia, PA: WB Saunders Co, 1986, 965-96.

Metallothionein see Copper, Serum *on page 589*

Metallothionein see Zinc, Serum *on page 595*

Methionine, Serum see Molybdenum, Blood *on this page*

Mn, Serum see Manganese, Blood *on page 591*

Mn, Urine see Manganese, Urine *on previous page*

Mo, Blood see Molybdenum, Blood *on this page*

Molybdenum, Blood

CPT 82190

Related Information

Heavy Metal Screen, Blood *on page 554*
Heavy Metal Screen, Urine *on page 554*

Synonyms Mo, Blood

Applies to Hypoxanthine, Urine; Methionine, Serum; Molybdopterin; S-Sulfocysteine, Urine; Sulfite, Urine; Xanthine, Urine

Abstract Molybdenum is vital to human health through its essential inclusion in at least three human enzymes: xanthine oxidase, aldehyde oxidase, and sulfite oxidase. The active site of each of these binds molybdenum in the form of a cofactor "molybdopterin," a pterin ring similar to folic acid which tightly complexes molybdenum.[1]

Molybdenum interferes with copper metabolism, especially in the presence of dietary sulfides, by the formation of insoluble copper thiomolybdenates in the gut lumen; absorbed thiomolybdenates may also interfere with copper metabolism. Copper deficiency on this basis is common in ruminant animals but so far has not been reported in man. High levels of tungsten in the diet compete with molybdenum in experimental animals so that total body molybdenum deficiency can be created by loading with tungsten. So far this has not been reported to occur in humans, but there is no reason not to anticipate molybdenum deficiency should chronic tungsten exposure occur. The clinical syndromes so far reported for humans involving molybdenum include:

1. **Molybdenum cofactor deficiency**: This is a recessively inherited error of metabolism involving failure to synthesize molybdopterin. It is diagnosed by noting combined xanthine oxidase deficiency (low serum uric acid <1 mg/dL, increased urine hypoxanthine and xanthine) and sulfite oxidase deficiency (marked by increased urinary sulfite, decreased to absent urine inorganic sulfate, increased urinary S-sulfocysteine). These patients have severe neurologic abnormalities from infancy on the basis of the sulfite oxidase deficiency including seizures, anterior lens dislocations, opisthotonos, decreased brain weight, decreased brain myelin, and usually death prior to age 1 year.[2] Molybdenum is virtually absent from the liver of such patients, suggesting that molybdopterin is an important storage form of molybdenum in soft tissues. Molybdenum may not be retained at all in soft tissue without molybdopterin cofactor. Serum molybdenum in this disease is reported to be normal. Screening test to detect this among neonates with intractable seizures is the urine sulfite test.

2. **Parenteral nutrition-associated molybdenum deficiency**: One case of molybdenum deficiency has been reported in this setting in a 24-year-old man with Crohn's disease.[3] Biochemical abnormalities were only corrected by the addition of molybdenum to the total parenteral nutrition (TPN). The biochemical abnormalities were essentially similar to those listed above for molybdenum cofactor deficiency: increased urinary sulfite, thiosulfate, xanthine, and hypoxanthine; decreased urinary sulfate and uric acid. In addition, unlike reported cases of molybdenum cofactors deficiency, this patient showed increased serum levels of methionine. The patient suffered night blindness, tachycardia, tachypnea, central scotomata, and irritability leading to coma over 24-48 hours while on TPN. Symptoms disappeared when amino acid administration was stopped, but recurred with either amino acid infusion or bisulfite infusion until molybdenum was added to the TPN. Unfortunately, serum or whole blood molybdenum was not reported for this case, so we do not know at what reduced level of serum or whole blood molybdenum a patient might become symptomatic. The patient refused liver biopsy to assess hepatic stores of molybdenum.

3. **Molybdenum toxicity**: This has only rarely been reported. Two situations are known to expose human populations chronically to excess molybdenum: industrial exposure and through the food chain in areas of the world with high local soil molybdenum. Two villages in Armenia have a high frequency of patients with hepatosplenomegaly, "kidney disease," and an inflammatory arthritis of the knees and small joints of hands and feet, associated with joint erythema, edema, and deformity. Serum levels of uric acid are modestly elevated and whole blood molybdenum is markedly elevated: 310±20 ng/mL vs 60±10 ng/mL control. Dietary intake for these patients is estimated to be 10-15 mg/day vs 0.15-0.5 mg/day recommended. Asymptomatic subjects in the same villages also with high molybdenum intakes have lower but still markedly elevated blood molybdenum levels of 170±10 ng/mL.[1]

Specimen Whole blood

Container In lieu of authoritative recommendations regarding potential molybdenum contamination from blood-drawing vacuum containers and stoppers, the same methods for containers and blood collection for other trace metals should be employed, that is, use the Sherwood Monoject™ trace metal blood collection tube with EDTA #8881-307022 and draw through a B-D #5175 20-gauge stainless steel needle. If other samples are to be collected at the same blood draw, draw the trace metal tube first so as not to contaminate the needle by puncture through ordinary rubber stoppers. See the Trace Metals Introduction *on page 585*.

Reference Range Whole blood molybdenum: <60 ng/mL; lower limit not established. Blood level parallels molybdenum intake. Apparently normal individuals vary from each other by over a 100-fold from 0.5-60 ng/mL, depending on molybdenum intake. 170 ng/mL appears to border on the toxic level based on the report above. Seventy-five percent of people in the United States have levels ≤5 ng/mL, but some geographical areas show 70% of the population >5 ng/mL.

Limitations Data are new and sketchy for this trace metal, and clinical syndromes poorly defined. Serum or plasma molybdenum norms are still being developed. Levels in apparently healthy people vary enormously based on intake, and blood levels are only significant when extremely high or extremely low levels (yet undefined) are encountered.

Methodology Neutron activation; graphite furnace atomic absorption (AA) spectrophotometry after extraction into 8-hydroxyquinoline[4]

Footnotes

1. Rajagopalan KV, "Molybdenum: An Essential Trace Element in Human Nutrition," *Annu Rev Nutr*, 1988, 8:401-27.
2. Johnson JL, Waud WR, Rajagopalan KV, et al, "Inborn Errors of Molybdenum Metabolism: Combined Deficiencies of Sulfite Oxidase and Xanthine Dehydrogenase in a Patient Lacking the Molybdenum Cofactor," *Proc Natl Acad Sci U S A*, 1980, 77:3715-9.
3. Abumrad NN, Schneider AJ, Steel D, et al, "Amino Acid Intolerance During Prolonged Total Parenteral Nutrition Reversed by Molybdate Therapy," *Am J Clin Nutr*, 1981, 34:2551-9.
4. Morrice PC, Humphries WR, and Bremner I, "Determination of Molybdenum in Plasma Using Graphite Furnace Atomic Absorption Spectrometry," *Analyst*, 1989, 114(12):1667-9.

References

Bougle D, Foucault D, Voirin J, et al, "Molybdenum in the Premature Infant," *Biol Neonate*, 1991, 59(4):201-3.
Bougle D, Voirin J, Bureau F, et al, "Molybdenum: Normal Plasma Values at Delivery in Mothers and Newborns," *Acta Paediatr Scand*, 1989, 78(2):319-20.

Molybdopterin see Molybdenum, Blood *on this page*

Penicillamine see Zinc, Serum *on page 595*

Selenium, Serum

CPT 84255

Related Information

Heavy Metal Screen, Blood *on page 554*
Heavy Metal Screen, Urine *on page 554*

(Continued)

Selenium, Serum *(Continued)*

Synonyms Se, Serum

Abstract The essential nature of selenium in human nutrition is beyond dispute. The element is part of the enzyme that converts T_4 to the active thyroid hormone T_3. It is also part of selenium-dependant glutathione peroxidase, an important antioxidant in blood and tissue. Multiple cases of selenium deficiency have been reported, mostly among patients given parenteral nutrition with no added selenium. Deficiency also occurs endemically in places where soil selenium is low, and low levels are thus present throughout the food chain. Endemic cretinism,[1,2] Balkan nephropathy,[3] Keschan disease[4] (endemic dilated cardiomyopathy), and Kashin-Bek disease[5] (endemic deforming osteoarthritis) are probably all caused by endemic selenium deficiency conditioning the host to poorly tolerate an additional environmental stress (cretinism: iodine deficiency; the others: unknown local toxins). Low selenium blood levels have been shown to be a risk factor for peripartum cardiomyopathy in sub-Sahara Africa.[6] Simple deficiency is marked by whitening of the nailbeds, erythrocyte macrocytosis, cardiomyopathy, painful weak muscles, skin and hair depigmentation, and elevations of transaminase and creatinine kinase.[5,7,8] The cardiomyopathy may be mild and asymptomatic or fulminant and fatal.

Selenium toxicity can occur endemically, again due to high soil levels, or through accidental or industrial exposure. Symptoms include garlic breath, odor, thick brittle fingernails, dry brittle hair, red swollen skin of the hands and feet, and nervous system abnormalities of numbness, convulsions, or paralysis.

Selenium in serum is mostly represented by selenoprotein P, yet when mild deficiency is induced by reducing oral intake of selenium in volunteers by 50%, glutathione peroxidase levels fell, serum selenium levels fell, yet the level of selenoprotein P remained normal.

Specimen Serum, plasma, whole blood

Container Sherwood Monoject™ trace element blood collection tube #8881-307006 or #8881-307022 with EDTA for whole blood. See the Trace Elements Introduction *on page 585.*

Collection Draw blood through B-D #5175 stainless steel needle into special trace metal vacuum tube. Centrifuge and pour serum into special plastic metal-free vial for transport.

Reference Range Serum: 95-165 ng/mL. Approximately 40% higher for whole blood. Serum reflects recent intake; red cells reflect more remote intake. Whole blood therefore reflects an average of recent and remote intake of selenium. (Selenium-dependent glutathione peroxidase activity reflects selenium available for enzyme synthesis - see below.) Levels are depressed in HIV infection,[9] critical illness,[10] kwashiorkor, inflammatory bowel disease,[11] renal failure, hemodialysis status, low protein diet, phenylketonuria, maple syrup urine disease (possibly all in part related to poor protein intake), low birth weight,[12] and premature infants with inadequate selenium intake. Levels are increased mostly with the use of glucocorticoids.[13] Levels >500 ng/mL are associated with toxicity.

Use Monitor selenium nutritional status in long-term parenteral nutrition. Studies have indicated no factor or factors that can accurately predict serum levels to preclude need for measurement. May be used diagnostically in cardiomyopathy of unknown cause, especially where nutritional factors are suspected. Monitor selenium status in children with propionic acidemia who are at risk of deficiency on their special diets. Monitor for acute toxicity states.

Limitations Some controversy exists regarding the "best" marker for selenium status. Since selenium as selenomethionine is incorporated nonspecifically into protein, serum and whole blood selenium concentration increases with increasing selenium intake to different degrees depending on inorganic or organic sources of selenium. Glutathione peroxidase activity is more sensitive to deficiency but the test is not well standardized and therefore not reproducible from laboratory to laboratory. Hair selenium may be contaminated by selenium-containing shampoo. Serum selenium level correlates best with intake and therefore with both deficiency and toxicity states, but a wide range of serum levels is compatible with apparent good health.

Methodology Atomic absorption (AA), fluorometric methods

Additional Information Selenium is excreted in feces from the bile, in sweat and skin losses, and the remaining 50% to 70% in the urine. Significant breath losses occur only in toxic states. Dosages in renal failure need not be modified. Symptoms of the deficiency syndrome may rapidly appear after surgery or other stress following a long asymptomatic but chronic deficiency state.

Footnotes

1. Arthur JR, "The Role of Selenium in Thyroid Hormone Metabolism," *Can J Physiol Pharmacol*, 1991, 69(11):1648-52.
2. Contempré B, Vanderpas J, and Dumont JE, "Cretinism, Thyroid Hormones and Selenium," *Mol Cell Endocrinol*, 1991, 81(1-3):C193-5.
3. Maksimović ZJ, "Selenium Deficiency and Balkan Endemic Nephropathy," *Kidney Int Suppl*, 1991, 34:S12-4.

4. Lockitch G, Taylor GP, Wong LTK, et al, "Cardiomyopathy Associated With Nonendemic Selenium Deficiency in a Caucasian Adolescent," *Am J Clin Nutr*, 1990, 52(3):572-7.
5. Levander OA, "A Global View of Human Selenium Nutrition," *Annu Rev Nutr*, 1987, 7:227-50.
6. Cenac A, Simonoff M, Moretto P, et al, "A Low Plasma Selenium is a Risk Factor for Peripartum Cardiomyopathy. A Comparative Study in Sahelian Africa," *Int J Cardiol*, 1992, 36(1):57-9.
7. Kien CL and Ganther HE, "Manifestations of Chronic Selenium Deficiency in a Child Receiving Total Parenteral Nutrition," *Am J Clin Nutr*, 1983, 37:319-28.
8. Brown MR, Cohen HJ, Lyons JM, et al, "Proximal Muscle Weakness and Selenium Deficiency Associated With Long-Term Parenteral Nutrition," *Am J Clin Nutr*, 1986, 43(4):549-54.
9. Cirelli A, Ciardi M, De Simone C, et al, "Serum Selenium Concentration and Disease Progress in Patients With HIV Infection," *Clin Biochem*, 1991, 24(2):211-4.
10. Hawker FH, Stewart PM, and Snitch PJ, "Effects of Acute Illness on Selenium Homeostasis," *Crit Care Med*, 1990, 18(4):442-6.
11. Fernández-Bañares F, Mingorance MD, Esteve M, et al, "Serum Zinc, Copper, and Selenium Levels in Inflammatory Bowel Disease: Effect of Total Enteral Nutrition on Trace Element Status," *Am J Gastroenterol*, 1990, 85(12):1584-9.
12. Lockitch G, Jacobson B, Quigley G, et al, "Selenium Deficiency in Low Birth Weight Neonates: An Unrecognized Problem," *J Pediatr*, 1989, 114(5):865-70.
13. Marano G, Fischioni P, Graziano C, et al, "Increased Serum Selenium Levels in Patients Under Corticosteroid Treatment," *Pharmacol Toxicol*, 1990, 67(2):120-2.

References

Corvilain B, Contempre B, Longombe AO, et al, "Selenium and the Thyroid: How the Relationship Was Established," *Am J Clin Nutr*, 1993, 57(2 Suppl):244S-8S.

Fleming CR, Lie JT, McCall JT, et al, "Selenium Deficiency and Fatal Cardiomyopathy in A Patient on Home Parenteral Nutrition," *Gastroenterology*, 1982, 83:689-93.

Koller LD and Exon JH, "The Two Faces of Selenium - Deficiency and Toxicity - Are Similar in Animals and Man," *Can J Vet Res*, 1986, 50(3):297-306.

Pentel P, Fletcher D, and Jentzen J, "Fatal Acute Selenium Toxicity," *J Forensic Sci*, 1985, 30(2):556-62.

Persson-Moschos M, Huang W, Srikumar TS, et al, "Selenoprotein P in Serum as a Biochemical Marker of Selenium Status," *Analyst*, 1995, 120(3):833-6.

Robbrecht H and Deelstra H, "Factors Influencing Blood Selenium Concentration Values: A Literature Review," *J Trace Elem Electrolytes Health Dis*, 1994, 8(3-4):129-43.

Vinton NE, Dahlstrom KA, Strobel CT, et al, "Macrocytosis and Pseudoalbinism: Manifestations of Selenium Deficiency," *J Pediatr*, 1987, 111(5):711-7.

Selenium, Urine

CPT 84255

Related Information

Heavy Metal Screen, Blood *on page 554*
Heavy Metal Screen, Urine *on page 554*
Urine Collection, 24-Hour *on page 30*

Synonyms Se, Urine

Abstract Urine selenium is used in conjunction with serum selenium to assess selenium nutrition or potential toxic exposure. Like other 24-hour urine collections of an essential element, this reflects recent intake, assuming the patient is in selenium balance. In the case of selenium, skin and stool losses are significant and amount to 30% to 50% of total losses; nevertheless, urine losses often represent overflow losses and can help indicate whether recent intake has been adequate or possibly toxic. When selenium intake is low to normal, less than approximately 140 µg/day, 24-hour urine may not reflect the 24-hour intake of the previous day. This is especially true when the body stores are low and selenium is retained to fill body stores.[1] At higher levels of intake, the 24-hour urine is well correlated with intake and can be used as evidence of excess intake, adequate intake, or prior toxic exposure. When selenium supplementation normalizes serum selenium and whole blood selenium, and then selenium supplementation is stopped, urine selenium falls back toward baseline much faster than blood or serum levels.[2] Urine selenium has recently been found to be correlated with 24-hour urine urea in critically ill patients. This probably reflects catabolism of protein and release of body stores of selenium, though details of the selenium intake of the patients (proportional to protein intake in tube-fed patients) were not provided.[3]

Specimen 24-hour urine

Container Acid-washed plastic urine container

Collection Avoid contamination by hair since some patients use selenium-containing shampoos.

Reference Range Levels <15 µg/L or >150 µg/L probably represent unusually low or high intake without necessarily representing illness. Values vary widely and in apparently healthy U.S. citizens they have been reported to vary from 7 µg/L (24-hour sample) to 231 µg/L. Intake is partly determined by local soil content of selenium and use of local vegetables as food. Healthy persons in New Guinea have been reported with levels as low as 0.9 µg/L but similar patients have rapidly developed symptomatic selenium deficiency when placed on total parenteral nutrition lacking selenium. Urine levels of 7 µg/L have been reported from China in areas where selenium deficiency is symptomatic. Levels >880 µg/L have been seen in chronic selenosis and >600 µg/L during the first 24 hours after acute selenium intoxication. Levels >500 µg/L probably represent toxicity. See the comprehensive review by Robbrecht and Deelstra.[1] Some authors or laboratories report as µg/day.

Use Monitor nutritional therapy, especially parenteral nutrition; monitor potential toxic exposure

Limitations Selenomethionine is incorporated into body protein nonspecifically as methionine, so it is not as quickly excreted in the urine as inorganic selenium (selenite). Thus, the form of selenium ingested will affect short-term balance estimates. Spot urine selenium is of little value, as urine selenium goes up after each meal related to selenium intake and probably other factors, and dilution in spot urine samples varies.

Methodology Fluorometry, atomic absorption (AA)

Additional Information In addition to serum and urine concentrations of selenium, red cell glutathione peroxidase can be monitored as an example of the activity of a seleno-enzyme. Levels will be depressed in deficiency but will not monitor toxicity.

Footnotes
1. Robberecht HJ and Deelstra HA, "Selenium in Human Urine: Concentration Levels and Medical Implications," *Clin Chim Acta*, 1984, 136(2-3):107-20.
2. Välimäki M, Alfthan G, Vuoristo M, et al, "Effects of Selenium Supplementation on Blood and Urine Selenium Levels and Liver Function in Patients With Primary Biliary Cirrhosis," *Clin Chim Acta*, 1991, 196(1):7-15.
3. Hawker FH, Stewart PM, and Snitch PJ, "Effects of Acute Illness on Selenium Homeostasis," *Crit Care Med*, 1990, 18(4):442-6.

References
Edmonds DK and Letchworth AT, "Selenium Deficiency in Kwashiorkor," *Lancet*, 1982, 1:1312-3.

Levander OA, "A Global View of Human Selenium Nutrition," *Annu Rev Nutr*, 1987, 7:227-50.

Pentel P, Fletcher D, and Jentzen J, "Fatal Acute Selenium Toxicity," *J Forensic Sci*, 1985, 30(2):556-62.

Thomson CD, "Clinical Consequences and Assessment of Low Selenium Status," *N Z Med J*, 1991, 104(919):376-7.

Se, Serum *see* Selenium, Serum *on page 593*

Se, Urine *see* Selenium, Urine *on previous page*

S-Sulfocysteine, Urine *see* Molybdenum, Blood *on page 593*

Sulfite, Urine *see* Molybdenum, Blood *on page 593*

Thymulin Assay *see* Zinc, Serum *on this page*

Transcuprein *see* Copper, Serum *on page 589*

Xanthine, Urine *see* Molybdenum, Blood *on page 593*

Zinc Administration *see* Copper, Serum *on page 589*

Zinc, Serum
CPT 84630

Related Information
Albumin, Serum *on page 66*
Copper, Serum *on page 589*
Heavy Metal Screen, Blood *on page 554*
Heavy Metal Screen, Urine *on page 554*

Synonyms Zn, Serum

Applies to Metallothionein; Penicillamine; Thymulin Assay

Abstract The essential nature of zinc (Zn) in human nutrition was confirmed in 1963 and has been widely studied since then. Many potential markers have been examined in the search for the ideal index of zinc status. The simplest of these is serum zinc, which is reduced in moderate to severe zinc deficiency, but is unfortunately not sensitive to mild deficiency states, and is depressed in other situations, often in parallel with reductions of serum albumin, its major binding protein. Other more sensitive tests each have their own problems in clinical use.[1,2,3] Serum zinc remains useful (although not very sensitive) if knowledge of zinc metabolism is applied in interpretation.

Both primary and conditioned nutritional deficiency is fairly common worldwide, as well as in the United States, and has been described in a large variety of clinical situations: in premature infants born with low hepatic stores; in breast fed premature and full-term infants[4] whose mother's milk is lower than normal in zinc; in growing children, especially boys, whose height velocity has increased while under zinc therapy; in prepubertal boys who display delayed sexual maturity, especially in association with diets low in animal protein and high in phytates from grains[5] (which reduce gastrointestinal zinc absorption); in malabsorption and diarrheal states;[6] in diabetes, nephrotic syndrome, cirrhosis (in each of these hyperzincuria occurs), in AIDS and ARC;[7] in burn patients,[8] and those receiving high doses of oral histidine or I.V. amino acids[9] (as in TPN, especially cysteine or histidine) associated with hyperzincuria; and in geophagia[5] (where zinc absorption is reduced). Pharmacological doses of folate increase stool losses of zinc, and may increase infectious complications of pregnancy (Sandstead reference). The most severe cases of zinc deficiency have occurred in acrodermatitis enteropathica (See below), and in the early days of total parenteral nutrition,[10] when zinc was not specifically included in the formulation.

Zinc is absorbed in the small bowel facilitated by small organic molecules, probably citrate from the diet and/or picolinic acid. Picolinic acid is a molecule synthesized by the pancreas from tryptophan and also present in human milk more so than cow's milk.

Babies with the disease of zinc malabsorption known as **acrodermatitis enteropathica** usually first develop their characteristic facial and diaper rash when weaned.[11] Untreated, symptoms progress and include growth retardation, diarrhea, impaired T-cell immunity, poor wound healing, infections, delayed testicular development in adolescence, and early death. Parenteral or enteral zinc corrects the condition. The classic disease is associated with low serum and urine zinc, but some cases have a normal serum zinc.[12] These cases nevertheless respond to zinc supplementation. A new syndrome that clinically mimics acrodermatis enteropathica, is **not** associated with low zinc levels, and occurs in children with maple syrup urine disease while under treatment, and is due to **isoleucine deficiency** has now been reported.[13]

Zinc absorption appears to be partially regulated, through binding receptors on intestinal mucosal cells shared with copper, and with cross competition by copper. The metallothionein (MT) mechanism also regulates zinc absorption as metallothionein is induced by zinc (more strongly than copper) and by binding excess intracellular zinc it prevents further uptake into the body by increasing the zinc in sloughed mucosal cells. This zinc is less able to be reabsorbed further down the intestinal lumen and adds to zinc fecal excretion. This entire mechanism is shared with copper. (See Copper, Serum *on page 589.*) When oral intake of zinc falls, stool excretion, sweat excretion, and eventually urinary excretion all are reduced.[3] Normally, urine losses are a small proportion of total losses; but under certain situations, high urinary losses are excessive and promote a deficiency state. When there are no excessive losses, healthy adults come into neutral zinc balance with 10-20 mg oral zinc and positive zinc balance with 3 mg I.V. zinc per day.

Assessment of Zinc Status*

Reduced pool size	Low plasma zinc + low plasma metallothionein
Tissue redistribution	Low plasma zinc + high plasma metallothionein

*Differentiation of declines in plasma zinc due to decreases in pool size from tissue redistribution.

From King JC, "Assessment of Zinc Status," *J Nutr*, 1990, 120(Suppl 11):1474-9, with permission.

Recently, it has been proposed to use both serum zinc and serum metallothionein to distinguish reductions in serum zinc due to redistribution (sepsis, stress) from that due to nutritional inadequacy.[3] See table. Alternatively, WBC zinc and an assay of thymulin (a zinc dependent thymic hormone)[14] have been proposed to serve as a marker for zinc status. IL-1 production or lymphocyte ecto 5′-nucleotidase activity can also be used to assess zinc status. None of these have yet proven sensitive in all situations.

Zinc deficiency in adolescents and adults is marked by slow growth or weight loss, altered taste, delayed puberty, dwarfism, impaired dark adaptation, central scotomata, alopecia, emotional instability, tremors, cerebellar ataxia, and a bullous-pustular rash over acral areas. Candidiasis reflects impaired T-cell function. Thymulin apo-hormone is present but inactive due to lack of zinc. In severe cases, lymphopenia may occur; death follows an overwhelming infection.

Specimen Serum or plasma

Container Avoid hemolysis or stasis. Use B-D #5175 stainless steel needle. Avoid contact with rubber. Separate serum and store in metal-free plastic vial. See the Trace Elements Introduction *on page 585.*

Causes for Rejection Improper collection

Reference Range 66-110 µg/dL (SI: 10.0-16.8 µmol/L). Serum zinc, when low in an apparently healthy (nonstressed, nonseptic) patient who has normal serum albumin, can be taken as evidence for low zinc stores, especially if urine zinc is also low, or there is known excessive unregulated zinc loss (diarrhea, nephrotic syndrome, etc). **One should not interpret a normal serum zinc as evidence for adequate zinc stores,** however, as serum zinc is insensitive and may be normal even after symptoms of zinc deficiency are definite.

Use Evaluate suspected nutritional inadequacy, especially in enteral or parental nutrition, critically ill or burn patients; cases of diabetes or delayed would healing; growth retardation; follow therapy in confirmed or potential deficiency states, for example when higher intravenous zinc doses are used to balance ongoing ostomy, biliary, or diarrheal losses as in total parenteral nutrition (TPN); follow oral zinc therapy in Wilson's disease; confirm acrodermatitis enteropathica and follow therapy; evaluate possible zinc toxicity or metal fume fever in possible exposure situations (poisoning, industrial exposure)

Limitations Levels may be low in fever, sepsis, estrogen therapy, stress, or myocardial infarction - reflecting mobilization from serum to the liver by interleukin. Levels are usually low in uremia with normal tissue levels. Levels may be high in familial hyperzincemia without toxicity or high zinc
(Continued)

Zinc, Serum *(Continued)*

stores. Albumin is a binding protein for zinc and levels are usually low in cases of hypoalbuminemia of all causes.

Additional Information Chronic oral zinc supplementation interferes with copper absorption and may precipitate copper deficiency. Copper status should be monitored for patients on long-term zinc therapy.

Footnotes

1. Peretz A, Nève J, Jeghers O, et al, "Interest of Zinc Determination in Leukocyte Fractions for the Assessment of Marginal Zinc Status," *Clin Chim Acta*, 1991, 203(1):35-46.
2. Sandstead HH, "Assessment of Zinc Nutriture," *J Lab Clin Med*, 1991, 118:299-300.
3. King JC, "Assessment of Zinc Status," *J Nutr*, 1990, 120(Suppl 11):1474-9.
4. Khoshoo V, Kjarsgaard J, Krafchick B, et al, "Zinc Deficiency in A Full-Term Breast-Fed Infant: Unusual Presentation," *Pediatrics*, 1992, 89(6 Pt 1):1094-5.
5. Prasad AS, Miale A Jr, Farid Z, et al, "Clinical and Experimental: Zinc Metabolism in Patients With the Syndrome of Iron Deficiency Anemia, Hepatosplenomegaly, Dwarfism, and Hypogonadism," *J Lab Clin Med*, 1963, 61:537-49.
6. MacMahon RA, Parker ML, and McKinnon MC, "Zinc Treatment in Malabsorption," *Med J Aust*, 1968, 210-2.
7. Odeh M, "The Role of Zinc in Acquired Immunodeficiency Syndrome," *J Intern Med*, 1992, 231(5):463-9.
8. Boosalis MG, Solem LD, Cerra FB, et al, "Increased Urinary Zinc Excretion After Thermal Injury," *J Lab Clin Med*, 1991, 118(6):538-45.
9. Zlotkin SH, "Nutrient Interactions With Total Parenteral Nutrition: Effect of Histidine and Cysteine Intake on Urinary Zinc Excretion," *J Pediatr*, 1989, 114(5):859-64.
10. Kay RG, Tasman-Jones C, and Pybus J, "A Syndrome of Acute Zinc Deficiency During Total Parenteral Alimentation in Man," *Ann Surg*, 1976, 183:331-40.
11. Moynahan EJ, "Acrodermatitis Enteropathica: A Lethal Inherited Human Zinc-Deficiency Disorder," *Lancet*, 1974, 2:399-400.
12. Mack D, Koletzko B, Cunnane S, et al, "Acrodermatitis Enteropathica With Normal Serum Zinc Levels: Diagnostic Value of Small Bowel Biopsy and Essential Fatty Acid Determination," *Gut*, 1989, 30(10):1426-9.
13. Giacoia GP and Berry GT, "Acrodermatitis Enteropathica-Like Syndrome Secondary to Isoleucine Deficiency During Treatment of Maple Syrup Urine Disease," *Am J Dis Child*, 1993, 147(9):954-6.
14. Prasad AS, Meftah S, Abdallah J, et al, "Serum Thymulin in Human Zinc Deficiency," *J Clin Invest*, 1988, 82(4):1202-10.

References

Alfrey AC, "Essential Trace Elements," *The Kidney: Physiology and Pathophysiology*, 2nd ed, Seldin DW and Giebisch G, eds, New York, NY: Raven Press, 1992, 2993-3003.

Prasad AS, "Zinc: An Overview," *Nutrition*, 1995, 11(1 Suppl):93-9.

Ruz M, Cavan KR, Bettger WJ, et al, "Development of a Dietary Model for the Study of Mild Zinc Deficiency in Humans and Evaluation of Some Biochemical and Functional Indices of Zinc Status," *Am J Clin Nutr*, 1991, 53(5):1295-303.

Sandstead HH, "Understanding Zinc: Recent Observations and Interpretations," *J Lab Clin Med*, 1994, 124(3):322-7.

Zinc, Urine

CPT 84630

Related Information

Heavy Metal Screen, Blood *on page 554*
Heavy Metal Screen, Urine *on page 554*
Urine Collection, 24-Hour *on page 30*

Synonyms Zn, Urine

Specimen 24-hour urine

Container Plastic urine container, no preservative

Storage Instructions Keep on ice or refrigerated. Laboratory will measure and record volume and remove aliquot for analysis.

Causes for Rejection Specimen allowed to contact rubber.

Special Instructions Avoid contact with rubber during collection such as through rubber catheter. If a urinary catheter is absolutely essential, as in burn patients, consider the use of a silicone catheter, which has been shown to release less zinc than other types. Most catheters contribute zinc to the collection, some to a substantial degree. For critical or research cases, it is advisable to document acceptability of the catheter prior to use.[1]

Reference Range Normal subjects: 0.14-0.80 mg/24 hours. Compliant patients on oral zinc therapy for Wilson's disease: >2.00 mg/24 hours.[2]

Use Evaluate zinc toxicity; evaluate low serum zinc levels; evaluate compliance in oral zinc therapy of Wilson's disease. Low urine zinc levels in the presence of depressed serum zinc tend to confirm zinc deficiency.

Limitations Zinc deficiency is usually accompanied by decreased urine zinc excretion. Zinc deficiency, however, may be in part due to excess urine losses, especially in cirrhosis, hemolytic anemias, sickle cell disease, alcoholism, diabetes, or chronic renal diseases.

Methodology Atomic absorption spectrometry (AA)

Footnotes

1. de Haan KEC and Woroniecka UD, "Bladder Catheters and Zinc Contamination of Urine," *Clin Chem*, 1989, 35(5):888.
2. Brewer GJ, Dick RD, and Yuzbasiyan-Gurkan V, et al, "Treatment of Wilson's Disease With Zinc. XIII. Therapy With Zinc in Presymptomatic Patients From the Time of Diagnosis," *J Lab Clin Med*, 1994, 123(6):849-58.

Zn, Serum *see* Zinc, Serum *on previous page*

Zn, Urine *see* Zinc, Urine *on this page*

TRANSFUSION SERVICE (BLOOD BANK)

Douglas W. Huestis, MD

Contributors:
Lowell L. Tilzer, MD, PhD
Wayne R. DeMott, MD

Dread of AIDS and worry about other transfusion-related infectious diseases have led to public reluctance to permit the use of donor blood and its components. Physicians and surgeons, re-examining their usage of blood, have gradually come to realize that blood transfusions and the maintenance of arbitrary hemoglobin levels are not as important as they were once thought to be. Such trends have also led to some diminution in the use of blood and components, and to increasing demands for the use of autologous blood, and other alternatives to conventional allogeneic transfusion.

As a result, physicians now must explain to their patients why transfusions of blood and components may be necessary, the risks involved (in appropriate perspective), and ways of reducing the risks. Obviously, such information should be available to the patient well ahead of the anticipated event so that there will be time to arrange alternatives to address the patient's concerns. Many blood services now have informative brochures about blood transfusion, its risks, and the alternatives. These materials can be placed in clinics and physicians' offices to provide a basis for informed consent for blood transfusion.

Important: The availability of such brochures does not absolve the physician from responsibility to obtain and document informed consent.

Preparation for Transfusion

1. **Sample Collection.** Ask the patient his or her name and check this against the information on the identification band. If the Transfusion Service uses a special transfusion wristband, label it with the patient's full name, hospital number, and date, and apply it appropriately. At the patient's bedside, label the sample tube with at least the patient's full name, hospital number, and date. Other information may be locally required. The same identification must be on the requisition form, plus the initials of the phlebotomist who certifies that the patient's identity has been properly verified.

   Information on the patient's identification plate must agree fully with that on the wristband or the sample should not be drawn. Adjust procedures for emergencies or disasters with great care to avoid the increased likelihood of mix-ups that is inherent in such situations.

   - The patient's identification band (or bands, if the Transfusion Service uses an additional one) must be attached to an accessible part of the patient's body, not taped to the bed or chart. If the bands have been removed for any reason, the identification procedure must be repeated and another sample obtained.
   - Any identification discrepancies or problems must be corrected promptly.

   Clerical error is the most common cause of blood incompatibility and resultant hemolytic transfusion reactions. Full and correct labeling **at the bedside** is essential for all samples of blood drawn for the Transfusion Service. Wax pencil marking is not acceptable. The Blood Bank must not be permitted to accept unlabeled tubes or those with unattached or loose identification, no matter who presents them. Specimen identification requirements are outlined in a listing bearing that name in the specimen collection chapter.

2. **Issuing Blood.** Unless there is some good reason to do otherwise, the oldest unit crossmatched for a patient is dispensed first. But if a patient has autologous and/or directed as well as allogeneic (homologous) units, issue them in this order: first autologous, then directed, and last allogeneic.

   Remove the selected unit from the refrigerator. Carefully inspect for clots, hemolysis, or discoloration. Quarantine any unit of abnormal appearance.

   Two responsible persons (eg, nurse and technologist) should jointly compare the identifying information on the transfusion request form and on the blood bag. This information includes at least the following:
   - patient's name, hospital number, other identifying data
   - patient's ABO and Rh type
   - donor blood ABO and Rh type
   - donor number, expiration date, component being issued
   - crossmatch result (if applicable)
   - result of antibody screen

   Resolve any discrepancies before releasing blood.

   The nurse and technologist, after verifying all information, should certify in writing that they have done so, and enter the date and time of issue.

   With some exceptions (emergencies, major surgery), issue only one unit of blood at a time for a patient receiving elective transfusions. Otherwise, the second unit may remain at room temperature for an extended period.

   Personnel should never be allowed to pick up two units for two or more different patients at the same time.

Administration of Blood and Blood Components

1. Except in urgent situations, avoid starting transfusions at night for three reasons. First, hospital staffing is thinner at night, making it harder to keep a close watch on patients being transfused. Second, patients need sleep. Third, any untoward reaction will awaken the patient and create turmoil on the ward.

2. If possible, before picking up the blood from the Blood Bank, start an I.V. with a Y-type blood-recipient set having a standard clot filter, using isotonic saline and a needle of 19-gauge or bigger. Smaller needles and special sets may be necessary in pediatrics. Run the saline at a slow drip. With an already existing I.V., check the needle gauge and the I.V. site. Change the I.V. tubing if necessary. If solutions other than isotonic saline have been running, flush with saline.

597

Do not use any other solution which may be incompatible with stored blood. Ringer's, for example, causes formation of small clots that may block the needle, while hypotonic solutions, particularly those containing dextrose, may cause decreased post-transfusion survival of transfused red cells. For the same reasons of pharmacologic compatibility, add no medications to stored blood. The same applies to the tubing containing blood, unless it is flushed with saline before and after the medication.

Check other I.V. medications that may have to be given and try to reschedule them before or after the blood transfusion. If necessary, other I.V.s can be given into another extremity.

3. Correctly identify the intended recipient.

- Compare all information on the transfusion form with that on the patient's identification band or bands, and on the donor blood unit. Make sure that everything conforms.
- The wristband or bands must be attached to the patient's body, not elsewhere. Otherwise, the transfusion should not be given until a new sample has been obtained and crossmatching repeated.

4. Inspect the blood unit looking for hemolysis or other abnormal appearance. In the case of anything out of the ordinary, consult the Blood Bank before starting the transfusion.

5. Record the vital signs, including temperature.

6. Do not attempt to vent plastic blood containers.

7. Once the blood is obtained from the Blood Bank or Transfusion Service, it should be mixed thoroughly by repeatedly inverting the bag, and started at once. Return the blood to the Blood Bank without delay if anything interferes with starting the transfusion.

8. **Do not store blood**, even temporarily, in conventional refrigerators on nursing stations, O.R., E.R., or anywhere other than in blood storage units that are specially and continuously monitored. To do so is contrary to all accreditation standards, including federal regulations.

9. Hang the blood.
- Mix gently.
- Carefully insert the plastic cannula of the infusion set to avoid puncturing the wall of the bag.
- In the case of red blood cells, lower the unit and allow 50-100 mL of saline to run into the bag. This allows easier and faster infusion.

10. Special blood filters may be indicated for some patients. See Filters for Blood *on page 609.*

11. Note the time the blood is started.

12. Remain with and observe the patient for at least the first 5 minutes. Take vital signs again at 15 minutes and at the end of the transfusion. Check the patient frequently.

13. Try not to exceed 2 hours for one unit of RBCs. If there is danger of pulmonary edema or congestive heart failure, or if there is a possible immunologic problem or a history of reactions, the time may be extended to 4 hours. If circumstances require even slower transfusion, it may be better to divide the unit in half and give it as two transfusions.

14. After the transfusion, return the empty blood bags to the Blood Bank. The residual small amounts of blood can be very useful in the event of a reaction.

Release of Blood Set Up for Transfusion, Then Not Used

1. Blood issued for transfusion and then not used can be used for another patient as long as:
- the unit has not been entered or punctured
- the unit has not been warmed
- the unit has been returned to the Blood Bank within 30 minutes of the time it was issued (its temperature must not exceed 10°C)
- the unit has not been stored in an unmonitored refrigerator

2. When blood has been set up for a patient but not used, most hospitals limit the time it can be held for that patient. Otherwise, there is a likelihood the blood would be held indefinitely and would outdate because someone forgot to notify the Blood Bank that the patient no longer needed a transfusion. The time limit may vary according to the needs of the institution, but is usually 24-48 hours, or 24 hours after an indicated surgical procedure.

The foregoing policy should be automatic, but not absolute. Clinicians must have the option of requesting that units be held longer for specific clinical indications, provided that those indications do not violate immunologic principles and thus lead to increased risk of transfusion reactions.

Another exception, at the Blood Bank's option, may be when antigen-negative units have been obtained (often with great difficulty) for a patient with a particular blood group antibody. The likelihood of a continuing need will dictate that such units be reserved for the patient.

3. Patients receiving a series of transfusions are at particular risk of forming blood group antibodies that could cause future transfusion reactions. Because such antibodies can form quickly and unpredictably, standards require that a crossmatch sample be valid only for 3 days, after which a new one must be obtained. This is particularly important in patients who have either been pregnant or had transfusions within the past 3 months. The rule may be waived for those who have not had either such event, but the Blood Bank seldom has such knowledge.

Both the foregoing rules (ie, the 1-day hold of blood and the 3-day hold of crossmatch samples) are best written into the Blood Bank's standard policies so as to form part of the operating routine. Requests for exceptions should be the onus of the clinical physician, referred to the Blood Bank physician if necessary.

Transfusions in Trauma and Other Emergencies

Transfusions may be needed at once in an emergency where delay may result in loss of life. In such a case, somewhat different procedures are essential and some steps, such as the crossmatch, may have to be dispensed with in the interest of time. All abbreviated procedures increase the risk to the patient, but to varying degrees.

In this discussion, understand that "blood" usually means red blood cells (previously also known as "packed cells"). Whole blood may be the preferred transfusion medium in acute blood loss or in hypovolemic shock, but it is seldom available nowadays. Experience in the past 20 or so years has shown that emergencies and massive surgical procedures can be as effectively treated with red blood cells and appropriate plasma expanders as has been the case historically with whole blood.

The following procedures are suggested for different periods of time available.

1. **No sample, blood needed now.** Give type O Rh-negative red cells (packed cells) without delay. Request blood sample. If O Rh-negative blood is in short supply, inform the physician and issue O Rh-positive red cells (packed cells). Better a live, immunized patient than a dead one without antibodies. As soon as the patient's own blood type is known, issue type-specific units.

2. **Blood sample provided, blood needed in 5-10 minutes.** Give blood of the patient's own type without crossmatch. If any blood is needed before the typing is finished, give out two units of O Rh-negative red cells (packed cells) immediately, with type-specific to follow.

   In both the foregoing situations, it is important for all persons involved to understand that **blood issued in this manner may turn out to be incompatible with the recipient.**

3. **Blood sample provided, blood needed in 15-30 minutes.** It may be possible to complete crossmatches within this time, depending on the technique used. It will probably not be possible to complete the antibody screening test on the patient's serum.

4. **Afterwards.** When the emergency is over, finish the antibody screening test and all the crossmatches so that the patient's record will be complete. The Blood Bank physician may add a note to the patient's chart as to the departures from normal transfusion routine and on whose authority they were carried out. Many hospitals require an emergency release form to document the original request. Because of the increased risks, this is a good idea.

5. **Additional thoughts.** Blood Bank and Emergency Room should work out their policies and procedures together, so that surprises do not turn up during emergencies. This should include the importance of sample pickup, identification, and the principles of blood selection. In times of blood shortage, notify the E.R. so they will be prepared.

   A foolproof blood sample identification system is vital in all emergencies, since some of the usual precautions will not be used. The system must also be applicable to the multiple trauma situation (imagine dealing with 4 or 5 people from an accident, all with the same surname) and to the mass casualty disaster.

   Remember that blood samples do not clot immediately, and there may be difficulty with fibrin shreds in incompletely clotted samples.

   Do not use up the community's supply of O Rh-negative blood on a massive trauma case. It is reasonable to switch to Rh-positive early, particularly in the case of a male or older female patient, in whom the effects of immunization are more manageable. Remember that even Rh-negative patients often do not become immunized in that setting. This, too, can be part of an understanding between the Blood Bank and the Emergency Room. The Blood Bank physician should always make sure that such decisions are appropriately documented with the names of the deciding parties.

   See listing, Uncrossmatched Blood, Emergency *on page 627*.

Guidelines for Outpatient Transfusion

With some minor exceptions, mostly concerning the timing of the blood sample and crossmatch, outpatient transfusions are handled the same as for inpatients. The precautions are the same, and if the hospital clinic staff are not accustomed to dealing with transfusions, they must be trained to do so.

1. **Informed consent.** The patient should give informed consent for any transfusion. This is the responsibility of the patient's physician. One consent may be understood to cover a series of transfusions, although it may be well to consult legal counsel on that point.

2. **Pretransfusion testing.** Because all these transfusions are elective, the patient should come in the day before (or within 3 days of) the transfusion. The same strictures apply to sample collection, identification, and banding as for inpatients. Be sure the bands used are waterproof, otherwise washing or bathing may obliterate the identification.

3. **Quantity to be transfused.** Since most of these patients have chronic conditions, and many are elderly, it may not be possible to give their units fast. Also, they must take up a bed in the clinic until the transfusions and an observation period are over. For these reasons, it is seldom practical to give more than two units in 1 day.

4. **Observation.** Observe the patient continuously for the first 15 minutes, frequently thereafter. After the transfusion is over, the patient should remain in the clinic under observation for at least 30 minutes. It is better that a relative or friend be available to accompany the patient home.

   Report any untoward reaction at once to the clinic physician or the patient's physician. In such a case, stop the transfusion and allow a saline drip to continue. Notify the Blood Bank.

5. **Instructions.** It is potentially useful to have a set of printed instructions to give the patient, or an informative brochure.

6. **Follow-up.** The patient's physician should inform the Blood Bank of any delayed untoward reactions to the transfusion, or of any evidence of transfusion-associated infectious disease. It may be helpful to see that the physician gets a copy of the Red Cross-AABB *Circular of Information for the Use of Human Blood and Blood Components*, the latest version, which should be obtainable from the community blood center or hospital transfusion service.

Summary Chart of Blood Components

Component	Major Indications	Action	Not Indicated for –	Special Precautions	Hazards	Rate of Infusion
Whole blood	Symptomatic anemia with large volume deficit	Restoration of oxygen-carrying capacity, restoration of blood volume	Condition responsive to specific component	Must be ABO-identical Labile coagulation factors deteriorate within 24 hours after collection	Infectious diseases; septic/toxic, allergic, febrile reactions; circulatory overload	For massive loss, fast as patient can tolerate
Red blood cells	Symptomatic anemia	Restoration of oxygen-carrying capacity	Pharmacologically treatable anemia Coagulation deficiency	Must be ABO-compatible	Infectious diseases; septic/toxic, allergic, febrile reactions	As patient can tolerate but less than 4 hours
Red blood cells, leukocytes removed	Symptomatic anemia, febrile reactions from leukocyte antibodies	Restoration of oxygen-carrying capacity	Pharmacologically treatable anemia Coagulation deficiency	Must be ABO-compatible	Infectious diseases; septic/toxic, allergic reaction (unless plasma also removed, eg, by washing)	As patient can tolerate but less than 4 hours
Red blood cells, adenine-saline added	Symptomatic anemia with volume deficit	Restoration of oxygen-carrying capacity	Pharmacologically treatable anemia Coagulation deficiency	Must be ABO-compatible	Infectious diseases; septic/toxic, allergic, febrile reactions; circulatory overload	As patient can tolerate but less than 4 hours
Fresh frozen plasma	Deficit of labile and stable plasma coagulation factors and TTP	Source of labile and nonlabile plasma factors	Condition responsive to volume replacement	Should be ABO-compatible	Infectious diseases; allergic reactions; circulatory overload	Less than 4 hours
Liquid plasma and plasma	Deficit of stable coagulation factors	Source of nonlabile factors	Deficit of labile coagulation factors or volume replacement	Should be ABO-compatible	Infectious diseases, allergic reactions	Less than 4 hours
Cryoprecipitated AHF	Hemophilia A, von Willebrand disease, hypofibrinogenemia, factor XIII deficiency	Provides factor VIII, fibrinogen, vWF, factor XIII	Conditions not deficient in contained factors	Frequent repeat doses may be necessary	Infectious diseases, allergic reactions	Less than 4 hours
Platelets	Bleeding from thrombocytopenia or platelet function abnormality	Improves hemostasis	Plasma coagulation deficits and some conditions with rapid platelet destruction (eg, ITP)	Should not use microaggregate filters	Infectious diseases; septic/toxic, allergic, febrile reactions	Less than 4 hours
Granulocytes	Neutropenia with infection	Provides granulocytes	Infection responsive to antibiotics	Preferably ABO-compatible, do not use microaggregate filters	Infectious diseases; allergic, febrile reactions	One apheresis unit over 2- to 4-hour period – closely observe for reactions

Modified from *Circular of Information for the Use of Human Blood and Blood Components*, American Red Cross, Council of Community Blood Centers, and American Association of Blood Banks, 1992, with permission.

ABO Group and Rh Type *see* Pretransfusion Testing *on page 619*

AHF, Lyophilized *see* Factor VIII Concentrate *on page 608*

Albumin and Plasma Protein Fraction for Infusion
CPT 36430
Related Information
Fibrinogen *on page 246*
Prothrombin Time *on page 262*

Applies to Normal Serum Albumin (Human); Plasma Protein Fraction (Human) (PPF)

Abstract Commercially prepared human albumin is 96% pure. Heat inactivation for 10 hours at 60°C destroys viruses. Albumin is available as either 5% or 25% (weight/volume). For volume expansion alone, hydroxyethyl starch or electrolyte solutions are much cheaper and often suitable. **Plasma protein fraction (PPF)** is 83% albumin.

Aftercare Follow blood pressure after rapid administration.

Use Volume expander used mostly for replacement of colloid in emergencies such as burns, pancreatitis, shock due to trauma, hemorrhage, or surgery; adult respiratory distress syndrome; with removal of ascitic fluid and for hypotension related to hemodialysis. Used as standard replacement in therapeutic plasma exchange (q.v.). The 25% albumin is used in patients who are not dehydrated, but it may be used with large volumes of normal saline or lactated Ringer's solution.

Limitations Does not contain clotting factors; brief retention; not effective for nutritional objectives. **Side effects and hazards**: Fast administration can cause fluid overload, especially with the hyperosmotic 25 g/dL albumin. Additional saline must be given to patients who are dehydrated. PPF may contain bradykinins which can cause hypotension on rapid infusion. PPF may also lead to anaphylaxis in IgA-deficient patients.

Contraindications Cardiac failure with congestion; not suitable for nutritional support

Additional Information Albumin is not "salt-poor". Sodium content is 100-160 mmol/L; PPF has 130-160 mmol/L. No hepatitis risk. No antibodies are present. Expensive. In plasma exchange, replacement can usually be part albumin and part isotonic saline.

References
Alexander MR, Alexander B, Mustion AL, et al, "Therapeutic Use of Albumin: 2," *JAMA*, 1982, 247:831-3.
Huestis DW, Bove JR, and Case J, *Practical Blood Transfusion*, 4th ed, Boston, MA: Little, Brown and Co, 1988, 315.
sSwisher SN and Petz LD, "Clinical Use of Blood Substitutes," *Clinical Practice of Blood Transfusion*, 2nd ed, New York, NY: Churchill Livingstone, 1989, 746-56.

Allogeneic Blood Transfusion *replaced by* Autologous Transfusion, Intraoperative Blood Salvage *on page 603*

Alloimmunization, Leukocyte *see* Filters for Blood *on page 609*

Antibody Identification, Red Cell
CPT 86870 (each panel)
Related Information
Antibody Titer *on this page*
Antiglobulin Test, Indirect *on next page*
Cold Agglutinin Screen *on page 605*
Cold Autoabsorption *on page 605*
Hemolytic Disease of the Newborn, Antibody Identification *on page 610*
Pretransfusion Testing *on page 619*

Synonyms Unexpected Antibody Identification

Applies to Elution; Red Cell Antigen Typing

Test Commonly Includes Cold autoabsorption may be necessary to remove cold autoagglutinins, to determine whether or not an unexpected antibody is present. Antibodies identified during prenatal testing and known to cause hemolytic disease of the newborn may be titrated.

Specimen Blood

Container One red top tube and one lavender top (EDTA) tube

Causes for Rejection Gross hemolysis, sample placed in a serum separator tube, specimen tube not properly labeled

Turnaround Time Highly variable

Special Instructions Provide Blood Bank with diagnosis, history of pregnancies and transfusions, and list of medications taken by patient.

Use Antibody identification is necessary before transfusion if antibody screen is positive. Used in obstetric patients for antenatal diagnosis of possible hemolytic disease of the newborn, and in hemolytic anemia when direct or indirect antiglobulin test is positive.

Limitations Antibody may be too weak to be detected or identified. Antibodies to low incidence antigens may not be detected.

Contraindications Remove any autoagglutinins first by cold or warm autoabsorption. Transfusion within the past 3-4 months invalidates warm autoabsorption because of the possibility of removing a significant alloantibody. See also Cold Agglutinin Screen *on page 605* and Cold Autoabsorption *on page 605*.

Methodology Panel of separate, selected red cell samples, each of known antigenic composition, exposed to patient's serum or to eluate. Serum may be absorbed with certain test red cells, followed by a repeat panel with the absorbed serum or with antibody eluted from the absorbing cells. Auto controls are extremely important to rule out autoagglutination.

Additional Information Such immunization to red cell antigens may present crossmatch problems. When a panel seems to identify an antibody in a patient's serum, make sure that the patient's red cells lack the corresponding antigen. If the antibody is clinically significant (see table), donor units must also lack the corresponding antigen. Elution and testing the eluate against a panel may identify the antibody causing a positive direct antiglobulin test. Donor blood compatible with the eluate may be acceptable in the case of an alloantibody. With autoantibody of the warm type, it is often the case that no donor blood is fully compatible.

Clinically Significant Blood Group Antibodies	
General	Antibodies that react by immediate spin
	Antibodies that react at 37°C and by antiglobulin, that show hemolysis *in vitro*, and that have been reported to cause hemolytic reactions
Examples	Anti-A and anti-B; antibodies of the Rh, Kell, Duffy, Kidd systems; also anti-S, -s, -U, and some others reacting as above
Clinically Unimportant Blood Group Antibodies	
General	Antibodies reacting only at room temperature or below, which do not show hemolysis
Examples*	Antibodies of the Lewis, P, MN systems; high-titer low-avidity antibodies; cold agglutinins

*Rare exceptions exist, usually when activity extends to 37°C.

References
Turgeon ML, *Fundamentals of Immunohematology: Theory and Technique*, 2nd ed, Baltimore, MD: Williams & Wilkins, 1995, 365-7.

Antibody Screen *see* Antiglobulin Test, Indirect *on next page*

Antibody Titer
CPT 86886
Related Information
Antibody Identification, Red Cell *on this page*
Prenatal Screen, Immunohematology *on page 618*

Synonyms Titer of Unexpected Antibody

Applies to Hemolytic Disease of the Newborn, Antibody Titer

Test Commonly Includes Antibody detection and identification must be done first; if an antibody is present, then it may be titrated in antenatal work-up.

Specimen Serum

Container Red top tube

Storage Instructions Freeze remaining serum in case subsequent parallel titers are required.

Causes for Rejection Gross hemolysis, sample placed in a serum separator tube, specimen tube not properly labeled

Possible Panic Range An increase of at least two tube dilutions during pregnancy suggests consideration for amniocentesis.

Use Commonly involves Rh antibody titers in Rh_o(D)-negative mothers. Follow the course of Rh or other antibody formation in cases of potential maternal-fetal blood incompatibility to predict hemolytic disease of the newborn. Among other criteria, used to evaluate need for amniocentesis.

Limitations Titers do not reflect the condition of an unborn child. False-negatives and false-positives occur. First-time appearance of antibody or rise of at least two tubes in titer usually means the fetus has the corresponding antigen. Failure of titer to rise is not meaningful. There is an inherent error of plus or minus one tube dilution in test performance within a given laboratory and more between different laboratories. Some laboratories use enhancement techniques such as low ionic strength saline (LISS) or enzymes. **Consistency is extremely important and the same laboratory should be used throughout.**

Contraindications No antibody detected in antibody screening test; biologic father lacking corresponding antigen; antibody identified is not implicated in hemolytic disease of newborn (eg, Lewis)

Methodology Serial dilution with saline, enzyme, or low ionic strength saline followed by antiglobulin. Expressed as reciprocal of highest dilution still giving agglutination visible without a microscope. (Continued)

Antibody Titer *(Continued)*

Additional Information Although an indirect antiglobulin titer of 16-32 or higher has been considered significant for $Rh_o(D)$, such figures are not necessarily applicable to other alloantibodies. A rising titer of an antibody capable of causing hemolytic disease of the newborn is more significant than a single assay. Specific phenotype determinations on the father's red cells may be helpful.

References

Walker RH, *Technical Manual*, 11th ed, Arlington, VA: American Association of Blood Banks, 1993, 442-4, 651-4.

Antiglobulin Test, Direct

CPT 86880

Related Information

Antiglobulin Test, Direct, Complement *on this page*
Cold Agglutinin Screen *on page 605*
Cold Autoabsorption *on page 605*
Cord Blood Screen *on page 605*
Hemosiderin Stain, Urine *on page 637*
Pretransfusion Testing *on page 619*
$Rh_o(D)$ Immune Globulin (Human) *on page 623*
Transfusion Reaction Work-up *on page 625*

Synonyms Coombs' Test, Direct; DAT; Direct Antiglobulin Test

Applies to Antiglobulin Test, Direct, IgG

Test Commonly Includes Direct antiglobulin testing with polyspecific anti-human globulin serum. It may include use of monospecific reagents (anti-IgG, anticomplement) when indicated.

Abstract Patient red cells are tested with reagent antiglobulin.

Specimen Blood

Container One lavender top (EDTA) tube and one red top tube

Causes for Rejection Gross hemolysis, sample placed in a serum separator tube, specimen tube not properly labeled

Special Instructions Provide diagnosis, transfusion history, and pertinent medications to the laboratory.

Reference Range Negative

Use Polyspecific antiglobulin serum detects immunoproteins, IgG or complement on red cells (ie, detection of sensitization of erythrocytes *in vivo*). Used to detect autoimmune hemolytic anemias caused by antibody or complement components bound to patient's red cells (including drug-induced), transfusion reaction, and erythroblastosis fetalis (hemolytic disease of the newborn). In warm autoimmune hemolytic anemias and some drug-induced anemias, the antibody is usually IgG. In cold hemolytic anemias, the cell coating is usually with complement components.

Limitations False-positives may occur with cold autoagglutinins and when the serum contains large amounts of paraprotein. Use of red top tubes or serum separator tubes may cause false-positive reactions, particularly if tubes have been refrigerated. Newborn's cells may have negative direct antiglobulin test in ABO hemolytic disease. Wharton's jelly from cord samples can cause false-positives. Technical factors that can cause false-positive and false-negative reactions include saline stored improperly, cold autoagglutinins, and contaminated glassware.

Methodology Antiglobulin serum. In the **direct antiglobulin procedure**, the test is for antibody attached to the patient's red cells *in vivo*. In the **indirect antiglobulin test**, the antigen-antibody reaction occurs *in vitro* and one tests patient's serum for antibody with reagent red cells (the antigen).

Additional Information Drugs, including the penicillins and cephalosporins, α-methyldopa, levodopa, quinidine, insulin, mefenamic acid, sulfonamides, tetracycline, and others may cause positive direct antiglobulin tests. Many positive direct antiglobulin tests are due to methyldopa. Methyldopa antibodies are predominantly IgG; about 1% of patients on methyldopa develop hemolytic anemia, but as many as 15% develop a positive DAT. Although drugs and alloantibodies may cause a positive direct antiglobulin test, the majority have no such association. It is unusual to find a significant antibody in the eluate from a positive direct antiglobulin test. Broad spectrum or polyspecific antisera contain both anti-IgG and anti-C3d. Anti-IgG may be used to determine if the cells are coated with IgG. If indicated, an indirect test and antibody identification are included in the work-up of a positive direct antiglobulin test. In cases of autoimmune hemolytic anemia, an eluate from the patient's red cells sometimes shows antibody specificity.

References

Bator S, Litty C, Dignam C, et al, "Current Utilization of the Direct Antiglobulin Test Investigation: Results of a Hospital Survey," *Transfusion*, 1994, 34(5):457-8.
Canadian Red Cross Society, *Serological and Immunological Methods of the Canadian Red Cross Blood Transfusion Service*, 8th ed, Toronto, Canada: The Canadian Red Cross Society, 1980.
Freedman J, "False-Positive Antiglobulin Tests in Healthy Subjects and in Hospital Patients," *J Clin Pathol*, 1979, 32:1014-8.

Huh YO, Liu FJ, Rogge K, et al, "Positive Direct Antiglobulin Test and High Serum Immunoglobulin G Values," *Am J Clin Pathol*, 1988, 90(2):197-200.
Judd WJ, Barnes BA, Steiner EA, et al, "The Evaluation of a Positive Direct Antiglobulin Test (Autocontrol) in Pretransfusion Testing Revisited," *Transfusion*, 1986, 26(3):220-4.
Snyder EL and Falast GA, "Significance of the Direct Antiglobulin Test," *Lab Med*, 1985, 16:89-96.
Walker RH, *Technical Manual*, 11th ed, Arlington, VA: American Association of Blood Banks, 1993, 355-87.
Waters AH, "Antiglobulin Test," *Practical Haematology*, 8th ed, New York, NY: Churchill Livingstone, 1995, 457-61.

Antiglobulin Test, Direct, Complement

CPT 86880

Related Information

Antiglobulin Test, Direct *on this page*

Synonyms Complement Direct Coombs' Test; DAT, Complement; Direct Antiglobulin Test, Complement

Test Commonly Includes Antiglobulin test using anticomplement

Specimen Blood

Container One lavender top (EDTA) tube and one red top tube

Storage Instructions Do not refrigerate specimen.

Causes for Rejection Gross hemolysis, sample placed in a serum separator tube, specimen tube not properly labeled

Special Instructions Provide diagnosis and **all** medications received by patient before and after admission to the hospital, to the laboratory.

Reference Range Negative

Use Determine if a positive direct antiglobulin is due to complement coating the patient's red blood cells; for example, in the case of any suspected autoimmune hemolytic anemia. Red cells of 10% to 13% of warm autoimmune hemolytic anemias react only to complement DAT. The complement DAT is used in work-up of the cold agglutinin syndrome and in paroxysmal cold hemoglobinuria. Work-up of drug-induced antibodies, cold autoimmune hemolytic anemia, cold agglutinin disease, paroxysmal cold hemoglobinuria, collagen disease includes complement-active antiglobulin testing.

Limitations Serum separator tubes and red top tubes may cause false-positives due to *in vitro* sensitization with complement. Harmless cold autoagglutinins coating previously refrigerated patient red cells may give weak positive results with such antiglobulin serum. Only a small number of clinically significant antibodies are found by anticomplement. Many transfusion services keep broad spectrum and IgG antiglobulins but not anticomplement.

Methodology Antiglobulin serum, C3

Additional Information Usually done only upon special request or particular indication. A positive polyspecific antiglobulin with a negative IgG implies that the positive direct test is due to complement. IgG DAT alone, without complement DAT, is found in 20% to 40% of instances of warm-reactive autoimmune hemolytic anemia and about 50% or more of such patients have both IgG and complement coating their erythrocytes.

Drug therapy: Some drugs causing antiglobulin positivity (eg, quinidine and phenacetin) are commonly characterized by positivity of complement DAT. Positivity of complement-active direct antiglobulin in a patient receiving methyldopa is evidence that methyldopa is probably not the only problem.

References

Garratty G, "The Clinical Significance (and Insignificance) of Red-Cell-Bound IgG and Complement," *Current Applications and Interpretations of the Direct Antiglobulin Test*, Arlington, VA: American Association of Blood Banks, 1988.
Petz LD and Swisher SN, "Blood Transfusion in Acquired Hemolytic Anemias," *Clinical Practice of Blood Transfusion*, 2nd ed, New York, NY: Churchill Livingstone, 1989, 549-82.
Snyder EL and Falast GA, "Significance of the Direct Antiglobulin Test," *Lab Med*, 1985, 16:89-96.

Antiglobulin Test, Direct, IgG *see* Antiglobulin Test, Direct *on this page*

Antiglobulin Test, Indirect

CPT 86886

Related Information

Antibody Identification, Red Cell *on previous page*
Hemolytic Disease of the Newborn, Antibody Identification *on page 610*
Prenatal Screen, Immunohematology *on page 618*
Pretransfusion Testing *on page 619*

Synonyms Antibody Screen; Coombs', Indirect; IAT; Indirect Antiglobulin Test

Abstract Patient serum is tested for antibodies with known reagent red cells.

Specimen Blood

Container Red top tube

Collection If for use with crossmatch, see Pretransfusion Testing *on page 619.*

Causes for Rejection Gross hemolysis, sample placed in a serum separator tube, specimen tube not properly labeled

Reference Range Negative

Use Screen for unknown antibodies in serum by use of known red cells. Such detection of antibody in patient's serum by normal reagent red blood cells is in very wide use, especially to screen for unexpected antibodies in pretransfusion testing and the first trimester of pregnancy, in Rh-positive as well as in Rh-negative expectant mothers. Evaluate potential cause of hemolysis. The indirect antiglobulin test is used in panels, in titrations, and in full crossmatches. In addition to its use in investigation of unknown antibodies in serum, the indirect antiglobulin test is also the means of antibody identification with elution techniques when antibody is eluted from coated red cells. When the indirect antiglobulin test is used in the crossmatch, neither antigens nor antibodies are known.

Limitations Abnormal proteins and cold autoagglutinins may interfere and cause delays in interpretation. Test will not detect all antibodies (eg, antibodies in low titer, antibodies to low-incidence antigens). In some instances of autoimmune hemolytic anemia, the antibody may be completely adsorbed onto the erythrocytes and not detectable by the indirect antiglobulin test.

Methodology Antiglobulin serum

Additional Information The antibody screen is the "screen" portion of the "type and screen." It is routine in compatibility testing (crossmatch) and on mother's serum during prenatal care and at the time of delivery. A positive indirect antiglobulin test must be followed up with antibody identification. The **indirect antiglobulin** is done on patient serum with red cells of known antigenic type. The **direct antiglobulin** is done on patient red cells. A common **drug cause** of positive indirect antiglobulin tests is methyldopa, which causes as many as 25% of positive DAT reactions in hospital patients. It causes positive indirect reactions in 15% of such patients. Levodopa and mefenamic acid are among other drugs known to cause positive indirect reactions.

References
Snyder EL and Spivack M, "Clinical and Serological Management of Patients With Methyldopa-Induced Positive Antiglobulin Tests," *Transfusion*, 1979, 19:313-6.
Walker RH, *Technical Manual*, 11th ed, Arlington, VA: American Association of Blood Banks, 1993, 175-87.

Antihemophilic Factor (Human) *see* Factor VIII Concentrate *on page 608*

Antiplatelet Antibody *see* Platelet Antibody, Immunohematologic *on page 616*

Anti-Rh Globulin *see* Rh_o(D) Immune Globulin (Human) *on page 623*

Autologous Stem Cells *see* Peripheral Blood Stem Cells, Autologous *on page 613*

Autologous Transfusion, Intraoperative Blood Salvage

CPT 86891

Related Information
Autologous Transfusion, Preoperative Deposit *on this page*

Synonyms Blood Salvage, Intraoperative Autologous Transfusion

Replaces Allogeneic Blood Transfusion

Special Instructions With automated systems, it is usually necessary to reserve or schedule use of the equipment beforehand. In some regions, this service is offered by the community blood center.

Methodology Although **preoperative** autologous blood collection is the best-known way of avoiding a transfusion of homologous blood, a patient's own blood may be saved and returned **during** the operation or immediately **afterwards**.

Three procedures are available:
- Intraoperative hemodilution: Blood is withdrawn from the patient after the induction of anesthesia but before the surgical incision is made. Crystalloids can support the blood volume.
- Intraoperative cell salvage: This procedure is only cost-effective if two or more units of shed blood can be salvaged during surgery. Some red cell savers process the blood in a semicontinuous manner. They wash the blood in normal saline. Most of the plasma and platelets and other debris are removed. A reinfusion bag contains the saline-suspended red cells, which can be transfused back to the patient using a standard filter. The cycle of removal, washing, and resuspension takes about 10 minutes. A specially trained operator is required.

Other systems usually involve collection of shed blood into a container from which it is given back to the patient through a filter. Without a wash step, such systems risk transfusing thromboplastic debris with the collected blood.
- Postoperative cell salvage: The blood from mediastinal drainage and from other sterile operative sites is saved, defibrinogenated, and returned to the patient. Washing and centrifugation gets rid of any microaggregates. The procedure appears to be safe, but the quantities salvaged are often too small to be cost-effective. Infection has not been a problem.

References
Council on Scientific Affairs, "Autologous Blood Transfusions," *JAMA*, 1986, 256(17):2378-80.
Dzik WH and Sherburne B, "Intraoperative Blood Salvage: Medical Controversies," *Transfus Med Rev*, 1990, 4(3):208-35.
"Transfusion Alert: Use of Autologous Blood," National Heart, Lung, and Blood Institute Expert Panel on the Use of Autologous Blood, *Transfusion*, 1995, 35(8):703-11.

Autologous Transfusion, Preoperative Deposit

CPT 86890 (collection processing and storage); 86985 (splitting of blood or blood products, each unit)

Related Information
Autologous Transfusion, Intraoperative Blood Salvage *on this page*
Donation, Blood *on page 607*
Donation, Blood, Directed *on page 608*
Erythropoietin, Serum *on page 124*

Synonyms Autotransfusion; Transfusion, Autologous

Test Commonly Includes Removal of blood or components from a donor for subsequent autologous transfusion. ABO and Rh typing of blood. It is best to use distinctively colored blood bag labels and wristbands. Autologous transfusion alleviates concern about the safety and availability of blood for transfusion. Blood collected from a patient is reserved for that person for elective surgery. There is no risk of transmission of hepatitis, AIDS, or other donor infectious disease, nor of reaction to serum protein or red cell antigens. Alloimmunization cannot occur. But risks do exist, namely those of identification mixup, bacterial contamination, volume overload, plus the possibility of donation reactions and excessive anemia. The patient's bone marrow is usually stimulated to produce red cells faster (increased erythropoietin production).

Categories of autologous programs:
- preoperative phlebotomy (the principal type discussed in this listing)
- immediate preoperative phlebotomy with hemodilution
- intraoperative cell salvage
- postoperative salvage
- combinations of techniques; especially the first and third types are used together successfully.

Patient Preparation Patient should be in generally good health.

Aftercare Replacement of iron is important. Increase fluid intake on the days of donation. Immediately after donating blood, the patient should remain lying down for a few minutes. When moved to a chair **with assistance**, the donor/patient should remain seated for 15-30 minutes. The bandage can be removed 2-4 hours after application.

Container Blood bag, which must be labeled "for autologous use only". A donor classification label or tag is required, "Autologous Donation".[1] Distinctive green color for such labels are helpful.

Collection Collect blood as for regular blood donation (see Donation, Blood *on page 607*), although the patient/donor qualifications will obviously have to allow for some exceptions. In elderly patients or children, who might otherwise suffer hypovolemia on blood withdrawal, an effective preventive measure is to infuse about 500 mL of isotonic saline (less for children) immediately before phlebotomy (isovolemic blood donation).

Storage Instructions Keep blood unit(s) in a monitored Blood Bank refrigerator for up to 42 days, when collected in the AS-1 system. For longer storage, blood may be frozen within 5 days of collection if such facilities are available.

Causes for Rejection Criteria vary. Those for whom elective orthopedic procedures are planned, with intact cardiorespiratory and other systems, are ideal candidates for autologous donation. Some persons who have been disqualified as candidates for homologous donation, for instance those with a history of cancer, may still be candidates for autologous donation.

In all cases, the primary physician and the Blood Bank physician share responsibility for accepting a patient and doing the procedure.

Widely accepted **criteria for disqualification** of a proposed autologous donor include:
- anemia (hematocrit <33%)
- possibility of bacteremia. Patients should be off antibiotics for 48-72 hours or more. Dental work in the prior 72 hours is a contraindication for fear of low-grade bacteremia and contamination of the unit.
- unstable angina
- aortic or subaortic stenosis
- congestive heart failure
- recent infarct of myocardium

(Continued)

Autologous Transfusion, Preoperative Deposit

(Continued)

- significant ventricular arrhythmia
- atrioventricular block
- uncontrolled epilepsy

Other possible criteria for rejection of a proposed autologous donor include:

- pregnancy - autologous or any other transfusion is seldom indicated in uncomplicated pregnancy. Thus, lacking some specific problem, autologous blood donation is usually unnecessary. Nevertheless, it is a reasonably safe procedure, even in pregnancy. Some legal questions exist.
- uncontrolled hypertension

Special Instructions Usually by appointment with Blood Bank. Physician should write out a prescription giving the date of the intended surgery, how many units are to be drawn, and indicating that the patient has been given a prescription for oral iron. An order for Type and Screen is desirable to cover unanticipated blood needs that might exceed the amount of autologous blood.

Use Usually for elective surgery. Eliminates risks of alloimmunization, of transmission of infectious diseases, and of a number of other hazards. Autologous blood may be the only suitable source of blood/components for patients who react adversely to homologous blood, patients of extremely rare blood types, patients who have antibodies to high incidence antigens, or who have multiple antibodies.

Limitations Prephlebotomy hemoglobin concentration should be ≥11.0 g/dL or the hematocrit ≥33%.

Technical problems may prevent return of the donated autologous blood (eg, accidental puncture of the bag, clot formation, or discoloration leading to concern about bacterial growth). Surgery may require use of additional, homologous units. Hypovolemic and vasovagal reactions may occur. Preoperative donations diminish presurgical hemoglobin. Identification procedures are important throughout.

There is usually a charge for each unit of blood collected, even though it may not be transfused.

Blood not used by the autologous donor usually cannot be used for anyone else for the following reasons.

a. The donor, by the nature of his/her illness, may not qualify as a regular donor, and the donor history for an autologous donor may not meet the requirements for conventional (allogeneic) donation. Donor history questions do not cover FDA-mandated AIDS questions.

b. Some of the units collected may not meet the requirements for donor blood (eg, hematocrit).

c. A hospital collecting autologous blood for its own patients need not do all the infectious disease screening tests. In that case, the blood may be used **only** by the patient/donor, may not be released for other patients, and may not be shipped to other facilities. The FDA may require testing for all autologous units in 1996.

d. The cost effectiveness of the procedure has recently been questioned.[4]

Contraindications Donation by high-risk autologous donors has been recognized as safe as donation by those who meet criteria for homologous donation, in a controlled setting.[5] The safety of cardiac patients as predeposit autologous donors is supported.[6]

Methodology Similar to conventional blood donation

Additional Information Some general considerations of an autologous blood program follow.

- Donors/patients should meet the general requirements of a regular blood donor. The patient's age may be younger than 17 at the discretion of the Blood Bank physician.
- The patient should be taking iron for at least 1 week before the first donation. This is especially important if a series of 3 or 4 units is to be drawn.
- Units of blood are normally drawn at weekly intervals.
- Autologous donation stimulates erythropoietin production.
- The use of recombinant human erythropoietin may make autologous donation easier for patients with marginal hemoglobin levels.
- Elderly persons are not necessarily excluded.[7,8]
- Autologous donations in preteen and adolescent patient/donors can be safe and effective.[9] If donor weighs less than 100 pounds, the amount of anticoagulant should be adjusted.
- An old technique called "leapfrog" can be useful if surgery is delayed after some autologous units have already been collected. To prevent the first unit or units from outdating, give the oldest unit back to the patient then collect two fresh ones at the same session. This can be repeated but has obvious limitations.

Except under special circumstances, donations should be no more frequent than every 3 days and not within 72 hours of major surgery.[1]

The following **risks** exist:

- identification mixup
- bacterial contamination
- volume overload
- donation reactions
- anemia

Should autologous blood be transfused on the same strict clinical indications as donor blood? This is a pertinent topic for a hospital blood utilization committee.[10] Most authorities say it should. On the other hand, some surgeons, pathologists, and patients feel that, because autologous blood is the patient's own, it may be transfused postoperatively even if the usual criteria do not hold. Whereas it is axiomatic that a treatment not indicated is contraindicated, whether desired by the patient or not, the risks of autologous blood are clearly less than homologous. So it seems reasonable that the criteria could be eased for autologous. It is important that there be some **clinical** reason for any transfusion and that reason must be documented in the patient's record.

In addition to elective autologous transfusion previously outlined, intraoperative blood salvage procedures are now commonly used.

Footnotes

1. Klein HG, *Standards for Blood Banks and Transfusion Services*, 16th ed, Bethesda, MD: American Association of Blood Banks, 1994, 37-40.
2. Toy PT, Strauss RG, Stehling LC, et al, "Predeposited Autologous Blood for Elective Surgery. A National Multicenter Study," *N Engl J Med*, 1987, 316(9):517-20.
3. Owings DV, Kruskall MS, Thurer RL, et al, "Autologous Blood Donations Prior to Elective Cardiac Surgery. Safety and Effect on Subsequent Blood Use," *JAMA*, 1989, 262(14):1963-8.
4. Etchason J, Petz L, Keeler E, et al, "The Cost Effectiveness of Preoperative Autologous Blood Donations," *N Engl J Med*, 1995, 332(11):719-24.
5. Hillyer CD, Hart KK, Lackey DA 3d, "Comparable Safety of Blood Collection in 'High-Risk' Autologous Donors Versus Non-High-Risk Autologous and Directed Donors in a Hospital Setting," *Am J Clin Pathol*, 1994, 102(3):275-7.
6. Adegboyega PA, "Comparative Safety of Blood Collection in High-Risk Autologous Donors Versus Non-High-Risk Autologous and Directed Donors in a Hospital Setting," *Am J Clin Pathol*, 1995, 103(3):374-5.
7. Haugen RK and Hill GE, "A Large-Scale Autologous Blood Program in a Community Hospital. A Contribution to the Community's Blood Supply," *JAMA*, 1987, 257(9):1211-4.
8. Pindyck J, Avorn J, Kuriyan M, et al, "Blood Donation by the Elderly. Clinical and Policy Considerations," *JAMA*, 1987, 257(9):1186-8.
9. Silvergleid AJ, "Safety and Effectiveness of Predeposit Autologous Transfusions in Preteen and Adolescent Children," *JAMA*, 1987, 257(24):3403-4.
10. Simon TL and Stehling L, "Indications for Autologous Transfusions," *JAMA*, 1992, 267(19):2669.

References

Axelrod FB, Pepkowitz SH, and Goldfinger D, "Establishment of a Schedule of Optimal Preoperative Collection of Autologous Blood," *Transfusion*, 1989, 29(8):677-80.

Cohen JA and Brecher ME, "Preoperative Autologous Blood Donation: Benefit or Detriment? A Mathematical Analysis," *Transfusion*, 1995, 35(8):640-4.

Dzik WH and Sherburne B, "Intraoperative Blood Salvage: Medical Controversies," *Transfus Med Rev*, 1990, 4(3):208-35.

Goodnough LT, Rudnick S, Price TH, et al, "Increased Preoperative Collection of Autologous Blood With Recombinant Human Erythropoietin Therapy," *N Engl J Med*, 1989, 321(17):1163-8.

Kruskall MS, "Autologous Transfusions - Past, Present, and Future," *Mayo Clin Proc*, 1992, 67(4):392-3.

Moore SB, Swenke PK, Foss ML, et al, "Simplified Enrollment for Autologous Transfusion: Automatic Referral of Presurgical Patients for Assessment for Autologous Blood Collections," *Mayo Clin Proc*, 1992, 67(4):323-7.

"Transfusion Alert: Use of Autologous Blood. National Heart, Lung, and Blood Institute Expert Panel on the Use of Autologous Blood," *Transfusion*, 1995, 35(8):703-11.

Popovsky MA, "Autologous Blood Transfusion in the 1990s. Where Is It Heading?" *Am J Clin Pathol*, 1992, 97(3):297-300.

Surgenor DM, "The Patient's Blood Is the Safest Blood," *N Engl J Med*, 1987, 316(9):542-4.

Vamvakas EC and Moore SB, "Total Potential Frequency of Autologous Blood Transfusion in Olmsted County, Minnesota," *Mayo Clin Proc*, 1995, 70(1):37-44.

Autotransfusion *see* Autologous Transfusion, Preoperative Deposit *on previous page*

Blood Components, Irradiated *see* Irradiated Blood Components *on page 611*

Blood Donation *see* Donation, Blood *on page 607*

Blood Donation, Designated *see* Donation, Blood, Directed *on page 608*

Blood Grouping and Rh Typing *see* Pretransfusion Testing *on page 619*

Blood Salvage, Intraoperative Autologous Transfusion *see* Autologous Transfusion, Intraoperative Blood Salvage *on previous page*

Bone Marrow, Autologous

CPT 86915

Related Information

Peripheral Blood Stem Cells, Autologous *on page 613*

Synonyms Bone Marrow Transplant, Autologous

Test Commonly Includes Aspiration of bone marrow from leukemia or cancer patient in remission, frozen storage, and autologous transfusion after tumoricidal therapy that has bone-marrow-ablative side effect

Abstract Patient is in remission from cancer or leukemia, without evidence of residual disease in bone marrow. Marrow aspiration is an operating room procedure. A single session usually produces enough marrow for restoration of normal marrow function. The standard is a minimum of 2×10^8 nucleated cells per kg patient's body weight (in at least 75% of collections); total volume aspirated is less than 1500 mL.

Patient Preparation Because of blood loss in marrow collection, it is customary to collect two units of autologous red cells in preparation.

Storage Instructions Marrow is concentrated, resuspended in dimethyl sulfoxide, and frozen at a controlled rate in liquid nitrogen. Label as comparable autologous blood component. Unless red cells are removed by various techniques, marrow contains a substantial amount of blood. No formal expiration date has been set.

Causes for Rejection Malignant involvement of bone marrow; fibrosis of marrow at usual sites of collection, such as might be caused by prior radiation therapy of the pelvis

Special Instructions Available on scheduled basis only after consultation with Blood Bank physician.

Use Collection and storage of autologous bone marrow make it possible to treat malignant disease with heavy doses of chemotherapy and/or irradiation that would otherwise destroy the patient's marrow function. After such treatment, marrow is repopulated from the stored autologous supply.

Limitations Repopulation of marrow depends on the number of pluripotent stem cells in the stored collection. This can be evaluated only by stem cell culture, which is thus the primary quality control method. Inadequacy of stem cells will mean failure of repopulation.

Methodology The patient/donor is under general or spinal anesthesia. Multiple aspirations of bone marrow from the posterior superior iliac crests are made by means of special needles and syringes until, under cell-count control, enough nucleated cells have been collected. The total volume is usually less than 1500 mL and contains substantial amounts of blood. Blood loss usually requires transfusion of the units of autologous blood that were collected before the procedure. After marrow collection, the harvest is filtered to remove clots and bony spicules.

Additional Information Label the aspirated bone marrow with the same care needed in the preparation of other autologous blood components.

References

Areman EM and Sacher RA, "Bone Marrow Processing for Transplantation," *Transfus Med Rev*, 1991, 5(3):214-27.

Bociek RG, Stewart DA, and Armitage JO, "Bone Marrow Transplantation - Current Concepts," *J Invest Med*, 1995, 43(2):127-35.

Soutar RL and King DJ, "Bone Marrow Transplantation," *BMJ*, 1995, 310(6971):31-6.

Bone Marrow Transplant, Autologous *see* Bone Marrow, Autologous *on previous page*

Cold Agglutinin Screen

CPT 86940 (auto, screen, each); 86941 (incubated)

Related Information

Antibody Identification, Red Cell *on page 601*

Antiglobulin Test, Direct *on page 602*

Cold Agglutinin Titer *on page 384*

Cold Autoabsorption *on this page*

Cold Hemolysin Test *on page 311*

Complete Blood Count *on page 312*

Mycoplasma pneumoniae Diagnostic Procedures *on page 671*

Applies to Cold Autoagglutinins

Specimen Blood

Container Red top tube

Causes for Rejection Gross hemolysis, sample placed in a serum separator tube, specimen tube not properly labeled

Reference Range Negative; titer <32

Use Usually done when the antibody screen or panel indicates that a cold autoagglutinin may be present, interfering with examination for irregular antibodies

Methodology 4°C and room temperature testing

Additional Information A cold agglutinin titer is another serologic test not directly related to transfusion but used as an aid in diagnosis of primary atypical pneumonia and certain hemolytic anemias. When present, cold autoagglutinins may have to be removed to detect a clinically significant unexpected antibody, masked by the cold agglutinins. See listing Cold Autoabsorption *on page 605*. Cold hemagglutinins are in everybody's serum. They react most strongly at 4°C. They are not normally seen in the room temperature crossmatch. When cold agglutinins are present at 20°C or higher they are said to be of "wide thermal amplitude." Such cold agglutinins may cause pain in the extremities,

thrombosis, agglutination, and hemolysis. Cold autoagglutinins are usually of I specificity. Their presence may follow an infection, such as *Mycoplasma pneumoniae*. Cold hemagglutination (autoagglutination) can also occur during cardiac surgery when the temperature of the perfusate may be between 15°C and 32°C.[1,2]

Footnotes

1. Leach AB, Van Hasselt GL, and Edwards JC, "Cold Agglutinins and Deep Hypothermia," *Anaesthesia*, 1983, 38:140-3.

2. Diaz JH, Cooper ES, and Ochsner JL, "Cold Hemagglutination Pathophysiology. Evaluation and Management of Patients Undergoing Cardiac Surgery With Induced Hypothermia," *Arch Intern Med*, 1984, 144(8):1639-41.

References

Heddle NM, "Acute Paroxysmal Cold Hemoglobinuria," *Transfus Med Rev*, 1989, 3(3):219-29.

Mollison PL, Engelfriet CP, and Contreras M, *Blood Transfusion in Clinical Medicine*, 9th ed, Oxford, UK: Blackwell Scientific Publications, 1993, 284-92.

Roelcke D, "Cold Agglutination," *Transfus Med Rev*, 1989, 3(2):140-66.

Cold Autoabsorption

CPT 86975

Related Information

Antibody Identification, Red Cell *on page 601*

Antiglobulin Test, Direct *on page 602*

Cold Agglutinin Screen *on this page*

Cold Agglutinin Titer *on page 384*

Test Commonly Includes Detection of cold autoagglutinin, removal of antibody by absorption at 4°C with autologous RBCs

Specimen Blood

Container One red top tube and one lavender top (EDTA) tube

Causes for Rejection Gross hemolysis, sample placed in a serum separator tube, specimen tube not properly labeled

Turnaround Time Up to 48 hours

Reference Range Negative antibody screen after absorption

Use Removes cold autoagglutinins in order to determine whether or not an unexpected antibody, such as $Rh_o(D)$, is present in the serum of patients needing transfusion, particularly when the cold autoagglutinin is active at 37°C, and to permit identification of such antibody.

Limitations Potent autoagglutinins may not readily absorb out of patient's serum.

Additional Information Often done when there is a positive antibody screen due to cold autoagglutinins, to rule out clinically significant unexpected antibodies, such as Rh antibodies. Such antibodies can be masked by cold autoagglutinins. Cold autoabsorption is a common cause of delay in the availability of compatible blood. In the case of high-titered cold autoagglutinins, prolonged or repeated absorption may be needed. Repeated absorptions are best. Absorb the serum with the patient's washed RBCs for 30 minutes, remove the supernatant, wash the red cells in warm saline, then repeat using the same red cells, until the absorbed serum no longer agglutinates the cells at 4°C. **Warm** autoabsorption is addressed briefly under Antibody Identification, Red Cell. An important alternative is to do crossmatching at 37°C.[1,2]

Footnotes

1. Mallory D, "Controversies in Transfusion Medicine. Prewarmed Tests: Pro - Why, When, and How - Not If," *Transfusion*, 1995, 35(3):268-70.

2. Judd WJ, "Controversies in Transfusion Medicine. Prewarmed Tests: Con," *Transfusion*, 1995, 35(3):271-5.

References

Mollison PL, Engelfriet CP, and Contreras M, *Blood Transfusion in Clinical Medicine*, 9th ed, Oxford, UK: Blackwell Scientific Publications, 1993, 284-92.

Cold Autoagglutinins *see* Cold Agglutinin Screen *on this page*

Complement Direct Coombs' Test *see* Antiglobulin Test, Direct, Complement *on page 602*

Coombs', Indirect *see* Antiglobulin Test, Indirect *on page 602*

Coombs' Test, Direct *see* Antiglobulin Test, Direct *on page 602*

Cord Blood Screen

CPT 86880 (antiglobulin, direct); 86900 (ABO); 86901 (Rh(D))

Related Information

Amniotic Fluid Analysis for Erythroblastosis Fetalis (OD 450) *on page 76*

Antiglobulin Test, Direct *on page 602*

Bilirubin, Neonatal *on page 86*

Hemolytic Disease of the Newborn, Antibody Identification *on page 610*

Newborn Crossmatch and Transfusion *on page 612*

Prenatal Screen, Immunohematology *on page 618*

Rh Genotype *on page 622*

$Rh_o(D)$ Immune Globulin (Human) *on page 623*

Synonyms Type and Coombs', Cord Blood

Test Commonly Includes ABO group, Rh type, direct antiglobulin test on cord blood sample

(Continued)

Cord Blood Screen *(Continued)*

Specimen Cord blood

Container One lavender top (EDTA) tube and one red top tube

Collection Do not overfill lavender top tube with cord blood. Mix well. Patient's identity must be verified and recorded on label and request form.

Causes for Rejection Gross hemolysis, sample placed in a serum separator tube, specimen tube not properly labeled

Use Determine ABO group and Rh type of the newborn. The direct antiglobulin test detects maternal antibody bound to fetal cells in cases of hemolytic disease of the newborn. A negative direct antiglobulin test on Rh-positive baby's cells when the mother has not received antenatal Rh immune globulin and is Rh-negative, is an indication that the mother is a candidate for Rh immune globulin.

Limitations Wharton's jelly may interfere with testing; cells heavily coated with maternal IgG antibodies may give misleading results with many antisera. Accurate results may be impossible if the cord blood specimen is contaminated with maternal red cells. Positive direct antiglobulin results due to anti-D are not a contraindication to postdelivery $Rh_o(D)$ immune globulin, when the mother has been given an antenatal dose of this material.

Additional Information Further investigation may be indicated based on results of this screen. $Rh_o(D)$ immunization is not the only cause of fetal hemolytic disease. In addition to anti-A and anti-B, any blood group antibody of IgG class (especially of subclass 1 and 3) can cross the placenta and cause hemolytic disease. But, other than the ABO situation, these are uncommon.[1]

Footnotes

1. Whittle MJ, "Rhesus Haemolytic Disease," *Arch Dis Child*, 1992, 67(1 Spec No):65-8.

Cryoprecipitate

CPT 36430 (transfusion); 86965 (pooling)

Related Information

Activated Partial Thromboplastin Time *on page 227*
Anticoagulant, Circulating *on page 229*
Factor VIII *on page 240*
Factor VIII Concentrate *on page 608*
Fibrinogen *on page 246*
Fibrin Split Products, Protamine Sulfate *on page 248*
Kidney Stone Analysis *on page 640*
Plasma, Fresh Frozen *on page 615*
Prothrombin Time *on page 262*
Thrombin Time *on page 266*
von Willebrand Factor Antigen *on page 267*

Synonyms Cryoprecipitated Antihemophilic Factor

Applies to Fibrin Glue; Fibrinogen Therapy; Hemophilia A Therapy; von Willebrand Disease Therapy

Abstract Cryoprecipitate is a labile component containing factor VIII, von Willebrand factor, fibrinogen, and factor XIII. Cryoprecipitate is the only available source of fibrinogen for patients with clinical deficiencies of that fraction (eg, disseminated intravascular coagulation (DIC)).

Patient Preparation Prothrombin time, PTT, and fibrinogen assay to document indication (eg, hemophilia). Patient should have transfusion wristband for checking against component container label before administration.

Dosage and administration: Rapid administration of about 10 mL of diluted cryoprecipitate per minute is used as a loading dose for hemophilia, followed by a smaller dose at 12-hour intervals,[1] depending on clinical circumstances. In pooling, single containers are washed with 0.9% saline, so that the volume of six units of cryoprecipitate is 100-150 mL. In the presence of circulating anticoagulants, larger doses or other special measures may be indicated.[1] Factor VIII activity should be greater than 80 units/bag.[2]

A 70 kg patient should have an increase of about 2.5% AHF for each bag of cryoprecipitate given.[3] For minor bleeding, dosage raising the patient's level to 30% to 50% may be used. For major surgical procedures, a preoperative dose sufficient to raise the level to 80% to 100%, followed by postoperative maintenance calculated to keep the level constantly >50% for 10-14 days.

In treatment of **von Willebrand disease**, smaller amounts given less often will usually suffice.[1] When using cryoprecipitates, the factor VIII levels achieved from a calculated dose will vary. Use of factor VIII concentrate is preferred to cryoprecipitate for most von Willebrand patients (those requiring treatment with plasma fractions).[4]

Cryoprecipitate must be given through a filter.

To treat **hypofibrinogenemia**, one bag can be expected to raise plasma fibrinogen level about 7-10 mg/dL. A bag of cryoprecipitate provides at least 250 mg of fibrinogen.[2]

Cryoprecipitate may also be used as a topical **"fibrin glue,"** which can stop local bleeding especially in cardiothoracic surgery.[5,6] Topical thrombin and calcium chloride convert the fibrinogen in the cryoprecipitate to fibrin. The volume of the individual units of cryoprecipitate used for the fibrin glue should not exceed 15 mL.

Aftercare Factor VIII assay and activated partial thromboplastin time can serve as controls in therapy of hemophilia A and von Willebrand disease, and fibrinogen levels and thrombin time when hypofibrinogenemia is being treated.[1] Bleeding time measurements can also be useful in some cases of von Willebrand disease.

Specimen Blood

Storage Instructions (For blood component) Cryoprecipitate requires frozen storage, without thawing, for up to 1 year, preferably at -30°C or below, but not above -18°C. Before infusion, thaw (but do not warm) for up to 15 minutes in a water bath at 37°C in a plastic overwrap, so that the precipitate is dissolved. Pool multiple units before administration. Once thawed, store at room temperature. Transfuse cryoprecipitate ideally within 2 hours or less, but not more than 6 hours after thawing and not more than 4 hours after pooling. Once thawed it cannot be reissued by the Blood Bank.

Causes for Rejection (Of patient sample): Gross hemolysis, sample placed in a serum separator tube, specimen tube not properly labeled

Use Treatment of deficiency of coagulation factor VIII (hemophilia A), von Willebrand disease, and hypofibrinogenemic states. Replacement of fibrinogen should be considered when levels decrease to <100 mg/dL and patient is bleeding. The physician making such decisions should be aware of the coefficient of variation for fibrinogen levels in the laboratory being used. Prolongation of the thrombin time may support indications for infusion of fibrinogen as cryoprecipitate. Cryoprecipitate rather than antihemophilic factor concentrate should serve for treatment of von Willebrand disease. Classical hemophilia usually requires factor VIII concentrate, but cryoprecipitate may be suitable when the need for treatment is only occasional. Cryoprecipitate is useful as a temporary treatment of bleeding tendency in uremia.[7] It also provides factor XIII. Cryoprecipitate may also help remove renal stones ("gravel"). Use 25 mL of cryoprecipitate, 4 mL of topical bovine thrombin, 1 mL of 10% $CaCl_2$. Administer using a #8 Foley catheter with a 22-gauge needle.[7]

Limitations There is considerable variation from bag to bag in factor VIII levels, but a "pool" of six units will help to iron out the variation. Cryoprecipitate is a poor source of factors II, V, IX, X, and XI.[3]

Contraindications Do not use unless laboratory or clinical studies indicate a specific coagulation defect for which cryoprecipitate is appropriate.

Additional Information A crossmatch is not necessary. Many units are sometimes needed. One concentrate per 5 kg body weight may serve as a rough guide to initial dosage. **Hazards**: The risk of hepatitis and other viral infections is less than that of AHF concentrate because each bag comes from a single donor. Febrile and allergic reactions may occur.[1] Large volumes of ABO incompatible cryoprecipitate may result in a positive direct antiglobulin test with mild hemolysis.[1] Presence of acquired inhibitors to factor VIII makes treatment with cryoprecipitate difficult or impossible. Factor VIII concentrates will be needed for such patients.

Footnotes

1. *Circular of Information for the Use of Human Blood and Blood Components*, American Red Cross, Council of Community Blood Centers, American Association of Blood Banks, 1992, 21-3.
2. Ness PM and Perkins HA, "Cryoprecipitate as a Reliable Source of Fibrinogen Replacement," *JAMA*, 1979, 241:1690-1.
3. Huestis DW, Bove JR, and Case J, *Practical Blood Transfusion*, 4th ed, Boston, MA: Little, Brown and Co, 1988, 320-1.
4. Cohen H and Kernoff PB, "ABC of Transfusion. Plasma, Plasma Products, and Indications for Their Use," *BMJ*, 1990, 300(6727):803-6.
5. Lupinetti FM, Stoney WS, Alford WC Jr, et al, "Cryoprecipitate - Topical Thrombin Glue. Initial Experience in Patients Undergoing Cardiac Operations," *J Thorac Cardiovasc Surg*, 1985, 90(4):502-5.
6. Alving BM, Weinstein MJ, Finlayson JS, et al, "Fibrin Sealant: Summary of a Conference on Characteristics and Clinical Uses," *Transfusion*, 1995, 35(9):783-90.
7. Janson PA, Jubelirer SJ, Weinstein MJ, et al, "Treatment of the Bleeding Tendency in Uremia With Cryoprecipitate," *N Engl J Med*, 1980, 303:1318-22.

References

Goodnight SH, "Cryoprecipitate and Fibrinogen," *JAMA*, 1979, 241:1716-7.

Cryoprecipitated Antihemophilic Factor *see Cryoprecipitate on this page*

Cytapheresis, Therapeutic

CPT 36520

Related Information

Plasma Exchange *on page 614*
Platelets, Apheresis, Donation *on page 617*
Sickle Cell Tests *on page 347*

Synonyms Cytoreduction; Therapeutic Cytapheresis

Applies to Erythrocytapheresis; Granulocytapheresis; Leukapheresis, Therapeutic; Red Cell Exchange; Stem Cell Collection; Therapeutic Leukapheresis

Test Commonly Includes Selective removal of platelets or leukocytes by means of a blood cell separator with subsequent return of plasma and red cells to the patient, removal of red cells in the treatment of hemoglobinopathies. Use of a blood cell separator for therapeutic manipulation of blood.

Patient Preparation Excellent vascular access is essential.

Aftercare Monitor patient's vital signs, watch for hypovolemia resulting from removal of large volumes of buffy coat. It is common to process as much as 10 L of patient's blood. Some albumin replacement is sometimes necessary.

Collection Carried out by Blood Bank personnel in apheresis area or patient's room

Causes for Rejection Moribund patient, or one who cannot withstand establishment of an extracorporeal circuit; lack of specific indication for procedure. Decision to do this form of blood manipulation is shared between clinical and Blood Bank physicians.

Special Instructions Usually on scheduled basis, but can be emergent. Consult with Blood Bank physician.

Use Reduce platelets in thrombocythemic patient or leukocytes in hyperleukocytic leukemia; remove abnormal RBC and replace with normal RBCs in sickle cell disease with crisis. See table.

Indications for Therapeutic Cytapheresis

Leukapheresis	
Clinical indication	Evidence of vascular insufficiency (leukostasis), especially pulmonary or cerebral
WBC count (x 10³/mm³)	<100: seldom necessary; 100-200: occasionally*; >200: often urgent* (except in chronic lymphocytic leukemia)
Platelet Apheresis	
Clinical indication	Thrombosis or hemorrhage
Platelet count (/mm³)	>1,500,000 spleen present, not in reactive thrombocytosis
Red Cell Exchange	Sickle cell crisis in pregnancy

*Particularly when there is a high proportion of blasts.

From Huestis DW, Bove JR, and Case J, *Practical Blood Transfusion*, 4th ed, Boston, MA: Little, Brown and Co, 1988, 383, with permission.

Limitations The extent of each procedure will be determined by the Blood Bank physician in consultation with the attending physician. When clinical circumstances so indicate, 10 L or more of patient's blood may be processed. Depends on blood cell separator used.

Additional Information Therapeutic cytapheresis or cytoreduction, the removal of excessive blood cells, is carried out to correct extraordinarily increased leukocytes in various leukemias or platelets in severe thrombocytosis. This procedure is a stopgap method for immediate reduction of these two elements when there is risk of hemorrhage, thrombosis, or pulmonary or cerebral leukostasis. The body's tumor burden can thus be reduced while chemotherapy is initiated. Guidelines are given in the table. Red cell exchange removes defective red cells and replaces these with healthy red cells. This procedure is predominantly to treat sickle cell anemia during pregnancy or before surgery. Peripheral blood stem cell (PBSC) collection is being used to supplement or replace bone marrow transplants in patients with leukemia, lymphoma, and certain solid tumors.

References

Hester J, "Therapeutic Cytapheresis," *Therapeutic Hemapheresis*, Vol II, MacPherson J and Kasprisin DO, eds, Boca Raton, FL: CRC Press, 1985, 143-53.

Nusbacher J, "Therapeutic Hemapheresis: Indications, Efficacy, Complications," *Williams Hematology*, 5th ed, Beutler E, Lichtman MA, Coller BS, et al, eds, New York, NY: McGraw-Hill Inc, 1995, 1663-8.

Wayne AS and Fosburg MT, "Therapeutic Plasma Exchange and Cytapheresis," *Hematology of Infancy and Childhood*, 4th ed, Chapter 53, Nathan DG and Oski FA, eds, Philadelphia, PA: WB Saunders Co, 1993, 1819-31.

Cytoreduction *see* Cytapheresis, Therapeutic *on previous page*

DAT *see* Antiglobulin Test, Direct *on page 602*

DAT, Complement *see* Antiglobulin Test, Direct, Complement *on page 602*

Direct Antiglobulin Test *see* Antiglobulin Test, Direct *on page 602*

Direct Antiglobulin Test, Complement *see* Antiglobulin Test, Direct, Complement *on page 602*

Directed Blood Donation *see* Donation, Blood, Directed *on next page*

Donation, Blood

CPT 86890 (collection processing and storage)

Related Information

Autologous Transfusion, Preoperative Deposit *on page 603*
Donation, Blood, Directed *on next page*
Hepatitis B Core Antibody *on page 396*
Hepatitis C Serology *on page 399*
HIV-1/HIV-2 Serology *on page 403*
HTLV-I/II Antibody *on page 406*
Phlebotomy, Therapeutic *on page 614*
RPR *on page 428*
VDRL, Serum *on page 438*
Whole Blood *on page 627*

Synonyms Blood Donation; Phlebotomy, Blood Donor

Test Commonly Includes Donor phlebotomy, ABO grouping, Rh typing, antibody screen, HB$_s$Ag, hepatitis core antibody, hepatitis C antibody, HIV-1,-2 antibody, and HTLV-I antibody

Patient Preparation Donors should be at least 18 years of age. Depending on state law, donors between 17 and 18 may donate with parental consent. The upper age limit usually is decided by the Blood Bank physician. Donor should weigh at least 110 pounds, should have a light meal before donation, no alcoholic beverages for 12 hours, **be in generally good health**, and afebrile.

Aftercare Activities are restricted for certain hazardous occupations for 24 hours. Donor reactions occur, rarely severe.[1,2]

Specimen Blood

Container Blood bag of appropriate configuration

Collection Drawn by Blood Bank personnel

Causes for Rejection History of hepatitis, history of HB$_s$Ag positivity, drug addiction involving injection, homosexual activity, diabetes requiring insulin, coronary heart disease permanently disqualify. Temporary disqualifications include hypotension, hypertension, anemia, positive syphilis serology (STS), travel to malaria endemic areas, exposure to hepatitis, pregnancy, recent childbirth, recent surgery, recent transfusion, tattoo within 6 months, inmate of penal or mental institution, and certain other medical conditions. Donors who have taken penicillin should be excluded from donation for 7 days. Use of vitamins, thyroid preparations, or oral contraceptives does **not** disqualify donors. Blood Banks now must present would-be donors with educational materials explaining the risk of AIDS in blood transfusion and encouraging self-deferment by those at risk of AIDS. They should also ask donors directly (face to face) about behaviors that might place donors at risk of AIDS (ie, male homosexual activity, I.V. drug use, prostitution, or exchange of sex for drugs or money). The aim is to discourage donors at risk from donating blood as a means of getting an AIDS test.

Use Obtain blood and its components for transfusion to patients.

Limitations Once per 8 weeks. Donations not to exceed six in any 12-month period. Truthful information must be provided by the prospective donor.

Methodology Donor blood must be tested for ABO and Rh type, screen for unexpected antibodies and include HB$_s$Ag, HB core antibody, which may prevent instances of post-transfusion hepatitis and may be a surrogate marker for HIV infection. Other tests include hepatitis C antibody, STS (a serological test for syphilis), anti-HIV-1 and -2, and anti-HTLV-I and -II. The ALT test, formerly a requirement, has been dropped as of 1995.[3,4]

Additional Information Increasing use of blood and components requires more donations to assure adequate supplies for transfusion. Questions often arise as to acceptance or disqualification of would-be blood donors taking various medications.[1,5]

Footnotes

1. Huestis DW, Bove JR, and Case J, *Practical Blood Transfusion*, 4th ed, Boston, MA: Little, Brown and Co, 1988, 1-54.
2. Kasprisin DO, Glynn SH, Taylor F, et al, "Moderate and Severe Reactions in Blood Donors," *Transfusion*, 1992, 32(1):23-6.
3. Desforges JF, "Infectious Disease Testing for Blood Transfusions," *NIH Concensus Statement*, 1995, 13(1):1-27.
4. Busch MP, Korelitz JJ, Kleinman SH, et al, "Declining Value of Alanine Aminotransferase in Screening of Blood Donors in Prevent Post-Transfusion Hepatitis B and C Virus Infection," *Transfusion*, 1995, 35(11):903-10.
5. Ferner RE, Chaplin S, Dunstan JA, et al, "Drugs in Donated Blood," *Lancet*, 1989, 2(8654):93-4.

References

Klein HG, *Standards for Blood Banks and Transfusion Services*, 16th ed, Bethesda, MD: American Association of Blood Banks, 1994, 3-8.

Sayers MH, "Duties to Donors," *Transfusion*, 1992, 32(5):465-6.

Scott EP, "The Safety of Blood Donation - Is It What It Should Be?" *Transfusion*, 1995, 35(9):717-8.

Walker RH, *Technical Manual*, 11th ed, Arlington, VA: American Association of Blood Banks, 1993, 1-28.

Donation, Blood, Directed

CPT 36430 (transfusion); 86999

Related Information

Autologous Transfusion, Preoperative Deposit *on page 603*

Donation, Blood *on previous page*

Irradiated Blood Components *on page 611*

Synonyms Blood Donation, Designated; Directed Blood Donation

Test Commonly Includes Donor phlebotomy, ABO grouping, Rh typing, antibody screen, HB_sAg, HB core antibody, hepatitis C antibody, HIV-1,-2 antibody, and HTLV-I antibody

Abstract Designation of a friend or relative to provide blood donation. Siblings, parents, and children are more likely to provide compatible blood.

Patient Preparation Donors must meet all the requirements of a regular blood donor.

Aftercare Activities are restricted for certain hazardous occupations for 24 hours. Donor reactions occur occasionally.

Specimen Blood

Container Blood bag

Causes for Rejection As for regular blood donation (see Donation, Blood *on page 607*).

Use Obtain blood or components for later use by a designated patient

Limitations Donors recruited by the family and friends of the patient may not be eligible to give blood. They must not have donated blood within the past 8 weeks, they must be in good health, and they must pass all the tests and answer the health questions appropriately .

Other limitations:

• Directed donations cannot supply blood in an emergency.

• Blood from directed donations generally cannot be available in less than 72 hours.

• Directed donors are neither safer nor riskier than regular blood donors.

• Administrative costs increase when directed donors are requested. Telephone calls and unproductive visits to the blood center take up everyone's time.

• Directed donors lose the anonymity of the conventional donor and may become subject to legal complications.

• More units may be needed than the directed donor(s) can provide.

• Rh-negative recipients may have difficulty finding enough Rh-negative directed donors.

• Husband-to-wife transfusions incur increased likelihood of both hemolytic disease of the newborn and transfusion reactions. The reason is that blood group immunization may take place or may already have taken place.

• Graft-versus-host disease (GVHD) occurs occasionally in immunocompetent recipients of directed donations from blood relatives. The FDA mandates that such donated blood should be irradiated with at least 1500 rad (1500 cGy). Many facilities use 2500 rad. Increased potassium occurs in irradiated blood.

• There is little logic in directed donations for general purposes (eg, surgery), but the Blood Bank physician should not take too rigid an attitude to this. First, directed donors continue to provide platelets for cancer and leukemia patients, for somewhat different reasons. Second, many patients have a highly emotional fixation about it and are not moved by logic. Finally, although the procedure is an expensive administrative nuisance, it does make the patient feel better about transfusions. Many physicians request it for themselves.

Methodology Contact the blood center and the hospital Blood Bank to make the arrangements. Send a prescription giving the name of the patient, the number of units of blood requested, the date of surgery, and the name of the hospital.

Additional Information Directed donations are not as safe as the patient's own blood. They are not equivalent to autologous donations.[1]

Footnotes

1. "Transfusion Alert: Use of Autologous Blood. National Heart, Lung, and Blood Institute Expert Panel on the Use of Autologous Blood," *Transfusion*, 1995, 35(8):703-11.

References

Aubuchon JP, "Autologous Transfusion and Directed Donations: Current Controversies and Future Directions," *Transfus Med Rev*, 1989, 3(4):290-306.

Hillyer CD, Tiegerman KO, and Berkman EM, "Evaluation of the Red Cell Storage Lesion After Irradiation in Filtered Packed Red Cell Units," *Transfusion*, 1991, 31(6):497-9.

Kanter M, Selvin S, and Myhre BA, "The Probability of Finding Suitable Directed Donors," *Arch Pathol Lab Med*, 1989, 113(2):174-6.

Starkey JM, MacPherson JL, Bolgiano DC, et al, "Markers for Transfusion-Transmitted Disease in Different Groups of Blood Donors," *JAMA*, 1989, 262(24):3452-4.

Thaler M, Shamiss A, Orgad S, et al, "The Role of Blood From HLA-Homozygous Donors in Fatal Transfusion-Associated Graft-Versus-Host Disease After Open Heart Surgery," *N Engl J Med*, 1989, 321(1):25-8.

Wagner FF and Flegel WA, "Transfusion-Associated Graft-Versus-Host Disease: Risk Due to Homozygous HLA Haplotypes," *Transfusion*, 1995, 35(4):284-91.

Donor Blood Transfusion *see* Red Blood Cells *on page 621*

Donor Plasmapheresis *see* Plasmapheresis, Donor *on page 616*

D^u

CPT 86901

Related Information

Kleihauer-Betke *on page 329*

Prenatal Screen, Immunohematology *on page 618*

Rh Genotype *on page 622*

Rh_o(D) Immune Globulin (Human) *on page 623*

Rosette Test for Fetomaternal Hemorrhage *on page 625*

Synonyms Rh_o Variant; Weak D (D^u)

Applies to Prenatal Testing; Rh; Rosette Test (Erythrocyte)

Test Commonly Includes Rh_o(D) typing; antiglobulin test, direct

Specimen Blood

Container One red top tube and one lavender top (EDTA) tube

Causes for Rejection Gross hemolysis, sample placed in a serum separator tube, specimen tube not properly labeled

Use Determine candidacy for Rh immune globulin and detect massive fetal-maternal bleeds in Rh-negative mothers; distinguish Rh-negative from Rh-positive donor blood

Limitations Does not detect all massive fetal-maternal bleeds (the Kleihauer-Betke and the rosetting tests are superior for this purpose). Contaminating antibodies in anti-Rh_o reagent may cause weak false-positive reactions. D^u typing is not dependable in newborn babies with positive DAT due to ABO incompatibility. D^u cells from newborns are not easily detectable by the rosette test. Do a Kleihauer-Betke test on the maternal specimen when the infant types D^u positive.

Methodology Read microscopically

Additional Information Some people are weakly Rh_o(D)-positive and are called type "D^u".[1] Do test before and after delivery on Rh-negative mothers. If a woman is D^u-negative antepartum but appears D^u-positive immediately postpartum, sufficient fetal Rh-positive RBCs have escaped into her circulation to cause the mother to appear transiently D^u-positive. This is an indication to do a Kleihauer-Betke immediately. Although all antepartum Rh-negative patients should be tested for D^u, the D^u run postpartum misses a significant number of fetal-maternal bleeds for which one dose of Rh_o(D) immune globulin (human) is insufficient. Thus, Rh immunization may still occur, uncommonly, in postpartum women who have had Rh immune globulin in an inadequate dose. In the erythrocyte rosetting test, the endpoint of rosetted red cells detects fetomaternal hemorrhages of 10-15 mL of fetal blood cells.[2,3] See Rosette Test for Fetomaternal Hemorrhage *on page 625*.

Footnotes

1. Szymanski IO and Araszkiewicz P, "Quantitative Studies on the D Antigen of Red Cells With the D^u Phenotype," *Transfusion*, 1989, 29(2):103-5.

2. Stedman CM, Baudin JC, White CA, et al, "Use of the Erythrocyte Rosette Test to Screen for Excessive Fetomaternal Hemorrhage in Rh-Negative Women," *Am J Obstet Gynecol*, 1986, 154(6):1363-9.

3. Taswell HF and Reisner RK, "Prevention of Rh_o Hemolytic Disease of the Newborn: The Rosette Method - a Rapid, Sensitive Test," *Mayo Clin Proc*, 1983, 58:342-3.

Elution *see* Antibody Identification, Red Cell *on page 601*

Emergency Blood *see* Uncrossmatched Blood, Emergency *on page 627*

Emergency Issue of Uncrossmatched Blood *see* Uncrossmatched Blood, Emergency *on page 627*

Emergency Transfusion *see* Uncrossmatched Blood, Emergency *on page 627*

Erythrocytapheresis *see* Cytapheresis, Therapeutic *on page 606*

Exchange Transfusion *see* Newborn Crossmatch and Transfusion *on page 612*

Exchange Transfusion *see* Hemolytic Disease of the Newborn, Antibody Identification *on page 610*

Exclusion of Parentage *see* Paternity Studies *on page 613*

Exsanguinating Emergency *see* Uncrossmatched Blood, Emergency *on page 627*

Factor VIII Concentrate

CPT 36430

Related Information

Activated Partial Thromboplastin Time *on page 227*

Anticoagulant, Circulating *on page 229*

Cryoprecipitate *on page 606*

Factor VIII *on page 240*

Plasma, Fresh Frozen *on page 615*

Synonyms AHF, Lyophilized; Antihemophilic Factor (Human)

Patient Preparation Do factor VIII levels, prothrombin time, and PTT before calculation of dosage if time permits

Reference Range Half-life of factor VIII is 8-12 hours[1] in the absence of inhibitors.

Use Treatment of acute bleeding and sometimes, prophylaxis, in patients with deficiency of clotting factor VIII (hemophilia A) and with acquired factor VIII inhibitors. Heat-treated, solvent-detergent-treated, monoclonal-antibody-purified, and recombinant factor VIII concentrates are purer and cause less immune stimulation than the older concentrates.[1] These newer preparations, though much more expensive, are a great deal safer from the point of view of virus contamination.[1,2]

Limitations The presence of inhibitors to factor VIII make treatment more difficult; refer to physicians experienced in the treatment of such cases.

Contraindications Normal coagulation studies. Factor VIII concentrate is not suitable for treatment of von Willebrand disease.

Additional Information The activated partial thromboplastin time is useful for both hemophilia and von Willebrand disease and may be more readily available than are factor assays. All these tests can guide therapy, as can the clinical response of the patient.

Calculation of dosage: Each bottle is labeled with the number of AHF units it contains. One factor VIII unit per kilogram may raise the level by 2%.[1] The dose required may vary from 10-50 units/kg.[1] In general, deeper hemorrhage and hemarthrosis need higher levels of activity. Still greater levels are necessary for retropharyngeal and retroperitoneal bleeding, even 100% activity for head injuries.[1]

Hazards: Since lyophilized AHF concentrate is a derivative of pooled plasma, the risk of transmitting hepatitis, HIV, and other viral infections is present.[3] Treatment of the product by heat for a prolonged period of time has greatly reduced the risk of transmitting viruses.[1] AHF contains anti-A and anti-B; when large or frequent doses are needed, monitor patients of group A, B, or AB for signs of intravascular hemolysis. Infrequent allergic reactions may occur. See table.

Therapeutic Factor VIII and Factor IX Concentrates

	Demonstrated Viral Disease Transmission?	
	Non-A, Non-B Hepatitis	Human Immunodeficiency Virus
Factor VIII		
Cryoprecipitate	Yes	Yes
"Dry" heat	Yes	Yes
"Wet" heat (pasteurized)	No	No
Monoclonal antibody-purified		
"Dry" heat	No	No
Solvent/detergent-treated	No	No
"Wet" heat in organic solvent	Yes	No
Detergent/solvent-treated	No	No
Factor IX		
"Dry" heat	Yes	?
"Wet" heat in organic solvent	?	No

From Menitove JE, "Preparation and Clinical Use of Plasma and Plasma Fractions," *Hematology*, 4th ed, Williams WJ, Beutler E, Erslev AJ, et al, eds, New York, NY: McGraw-Hill, 1990, 1659-73, with permission.

Footnotes
1. Menitove JE, "Preparation and Clinical Use of Plasma and Plasma Fractions," *Hematology*, 4th ed, Williams WJ, Beutler E, Erslev AJ, et al, eds, New York, NY: McGraw-Hill Inc, 1990, 1659-73.
2. Aronson DL, "The Development of the Technology and Capacity for the Production of Factor VIII for the Treatment of Hemophilia A," *Transfusion*, 1990, 30(8):748-58.
3. Thomas DP, "Reducing the Risk of Virus Transmission by Blood Products," *Br J Haematol*, 1988, 70(4):393-5.

References
Goedert JJ, Kessler CM, Aledort LM, et al, "A Prospective Study of Human Immunodeficiency Virus Type 1 Infection and the Development of AIDS in Subjects With Hemophilia," *N Engl J Med*, 1989, 321(17):1141-8.

Pierce GF, Lusher JM, Brownstein AP, et al, "The Use of Purified Clotting Factor Concentrates in Hemophilia: Influence of Viral Safety, Cost, and Supply on Therapy," *JAMA*, 1989, 261(23):3434-7.

Roberts HR, "The Treatment of Hemophilia: Past Tragedy and Future Promise," *N Engl J Med*, 1989, 321(17):1188-90.

Schimpf K, Brackmann HH, Kreuz W, et al, "Absence of Anti-Human Immunodeficiency Virus Types 1 and 2 Seroconversion After the Treatment of Hemophilia A or von Willebrand's Disease With Pasteurized Factor VIII Concentrate," *N Engl J Med*, 1989, 321(17):1148-52.

Factor IX Complex (Human)
CPT 36430

Related Information
Activated Partial Thromboplastin Time *on page 227*
Anticoagulant, Circulating *on page 229*
Factor VIII *on page 240*
Factor IX *on page 241*
Plasma, Fresh Frozen *on page 615*

Synonyms Prothrombin Complex Concentrates

Test Commonly Includes Factor IX concentrate is a preparation containing high levels of the vitamin K-dependent factors, factor II (prothrombin), VII, IX (PTC, Christmas factor), and X (Stuart-Prower factor).

Abstract A plasma fraction for treatment of hemophilia B (factor IX deficiency) and hemophilia A with inhibitor

Patient Preparation Identification of the deficiency as one of factor II or IX is essential before administration of factor IX complex. Follow manufacturers' instructions on package insert.

Use High risk fraction for patients with severe Christmas disease, hemophilia B (inherited factor IX deficiency) during episodes of traumatic or spontaneous bleeding, or in conjunction with surgery; it may also control deficiency of factor II, VII, X, or factor VIII with inhibitor. **Use fresh frozen or aged plasma**, if possible, unless patient cannot tolerate the larger fluid volumes necessary.[1,2]

Limitations Hazards: Heat and solvent-detergent treatment have reduced the once high risk of hepatitis. Disseminated intravascular coagulation and thrombosis are among the risks. Inhibitors may occur.

Contraindications Do not use in liver disease. Do not use in vitamin K deficiency, for which vitamin K preparations are appropriate, or in patients with overdose of coumarin. See listing Plasma, Fresh Frozen *on page 615*.

Footnotes
1. Menitove JE, Gill JL, and Montgomery RR, "Preparation and Clinical Use of Plasma and Plasma Fractions," *Williams Hematology*, 4th ed, Beutler E, Lictman MA, Coller BS, et al, eds, New York, NY: McGraw-Hill Inc, 1995, 1649-63.
2. Walker RH, *Technical Manual*, 11th ed, Arlington, VA: American Association of Blood Banks, 1993, 412-3.

References
Goedert JJ, Kessler CM, Aledort LM, et al, "A Prospective Study of Human Immunodeficiency Virus Type 1 Infection and the Development of AIDS in Subjects With Hemophilia," *N Engl J Med*, 1989, 321(17):1141-8.

Huestis DW, Bove JR, and Case J, *Practical Blood Transfusion*, 4th ed, Boston, MA: Little, Brown and Co, 1988, 320-6.

Factor V Replacement *see* Plasma, Fresh Frozen *on page 615*

Factor VII Replacement *see* Plasma, Fresh Frozen *on page 615*

Factor IX Replacement *see* Plasma, Fresh Frozen *on page 615*

Factor X Replacement *see* Plasma, Fresh Frozen *on page 615*

Factor XI Replacement *see* Plasma, Fresh Frozen *on page 615*

Factor XIII Replacement *see* Plasma, Fresh Frozen *on page 615*

Febrile Transfusion Reaction *see* Filters for Blood *on this page*

Fetalscreen™ *see* Rosette Test for Fetomaternal Hemorrhage *on page 625*

FFP *see* Plasma, Fresh Frozen *on page 615*

Fibrin Glue *see* Cryoprecipitate *on page 606*

Fibrinogen Replacement *see* Plasma, Fresh Frozen *on page 615*

Fibrinogen Therapy *see* Cryoprecipitate *on page 606*

Filters for Blood
CPT 86999

Related Information
Platelet Concentrate, Donation and Transfusion *on page 616*
Red Blood Cells *on page 621*
Red Blood Cells, Washed *on page 622*
Whole Blood *on page 627*

Synonyms Filters, Microaggregate; Leukocyte Removal

Applies to Alloimmunization, Leukocyte; Febrile Transfusion Reaction; Transfusion Reaction, Febrile

Special Instructions Regular and special blood filters are available, as a rule, at hospital transfusion services or from pharmacy and supplies services.

Use Clots may form in any unit of blood and are readily removed by the clot filters in all regular blood infusion sets. Microaggregate filters remove debris composed of platelets with admixed granulocytes and fibrin in massive transfusions of older stored units of blood. This common usage remains controversial. Leukocyte filters help reduce, but do not eliminate febrile nonhemolytic reactions. Two consecutive febrile reactions may be an indication for leukocyte-poor blood. Leukocyte filters (Continued)

Filters for Blood *(Continued)*

also reduce the likelihood of HLA alloimmunization, and CMV transmission.

Limitations Do **not** use microaggregate filters for platelet or neutrophil transfusions. Filters other than regular clot filters diminish flow when rapid infusion of red cells is necessary. Newer filters remove white cells even though microaggregates have not yet formed. Leukocyte filtration after various periods of storage of RBCs or platelets may not be as effective as at the time of collection. Leukocyte filters are not adequate to prevent graft-versus-host disease in susceptible blood recipients.

Additional Information There are several types of blood filters:

Clot filter (170 micron pore size): All blood and components must be given through this filter, intended to remove clots and fibrin shreds.

Microaggregate filters (20-40 microns pore size).[1] These filters remove the microaggregates of leukocytes and platelets that form in stored blood, particularly in massively transfused patients. The aim is to prevent microembolization and respiratory distress syndrome. This use remains controversial.[1] A volume of literature has developed with regard to best use of microaggregate filters. They did not provide demonstrable benefits in a series of patients with pulmonary dysfunction.[2]

Leukocyte-depletion filters (3-100 micron pore size).[3,4,5] These remove up to 99.9% of WBCs from platelets or RBCs, the intention being to prevent febrile reactions and alloimmunization to leukocyte antigens or to prevent transmission of viruses carried by donor leukocytes (eg, cytomegalovirus). For such purposes, it appears that filtration must be so efficient that platelet or RBC concentrates contain no more than 5×10^6 WBCs per transfusion. Since electronic particle counters are grossly inaccurate in those count ranges, quality control requires special techniques. Furthermore, the efficacy of filtration is in part inversely proportional to the initial WBC count of the concentrate.[5] Leukocyte removal is advantageous for patients receiving many transfusions over time, probably not for those who have only single or occasional transfusion episodes. Cost and other practical matters are still evolving. It seems likely now that filtration before storage is more effective than bedside filtration. For optimal effect, most leukocyte-depleting filters must be carefully used according to the manufacturer's instructions.

Footnotes
1. Snyder EL, Hezzey A, Barash PG, et al, "Microaggregate Blood Filtration in Patients With Compromised Pulmonary Function," *Transfusion*, 1982, 22:21.
2. Steneker I, van Luyn MJ, van Wachem PB, et al, "Electronmicroscopic Examination of White Cell Reduction by Four White Cell-Reduction Filters," *Transfusion*, 1992, 32(5):450-7.
3. Dzik WH, "White Cell-Reduced Blood Components: Should We Go With The Flow?" *Transfusion*, 1991, 31(9):789-91.
4. Wenz B, "Clinical and Laboratory Precautions That Reduce the Adverse Reactions, Alloimmunization, Infectivity, and Possibly Immunomodulation Associated With Homologous Transfusions," *Transfus Med Rev*, 1990, 4(4 Suppl 1):3-7.
5. Freedman J, Blanchette V, Hornstein S, et al, "White Cell Depletion of Red Cell and Pooled Random-Donor Platelet Concentrates by Filtration and Residual Lymphocyte Subset Analysis," *Transfusion*, 1991, 31(5):433-40.

References
Andreu G, Dewailly J, Leberre C, et al, "Prevention of HLA Immunization With Leukocyte-Poor Packed Red Cells and Platelet Concentrates Obtained by Filtration," *Blood*, 1988, 72(3):964-9.
Hill RC, Middaugh RE, Menk EJ, et al, "Clinical Evaluation of Commonly Used Blood Administration Sets," *J Emerg Med*, 1989, 7(2):103-7.
Snyder EL and Bookbinder M, "Role of Microaggregate Blood Filtration in Clinical Medicine," *Transfusion*, 1983, 23:460-70.

Filters, Microaggregate *see* Filters for Blood *on previous page*

"Fresh Blood" *see* Whole Blood *on page 627*

Fresh Frozen Plasma *see* Plasma, Fresh Frozen *on page 615*

Frozen Blood *see* Frozen Red Blood Cells *on this page*

Frozen Red Blood Cells

CPT 36430 (transfusion); 86930 (preparation for freezing); 86931 (with thawing); 86932 (with freezing and thawing)

Synonyms Frozen Blood; Red Blood Cells, Deglycerolized; Red Blood Cells, Frozen

Test Commonly Includes ABO, Rh, antibody screen, and crossmatch

Abstract Glycerol serves as a cryoprotective agent when added to reasonably fresh red blood cells, which can then be frozen at -80°C or lower. After thawing and deglycerolization by washing, some 80% to 90% of the original red cells remain, as a more or less pure suspension in isotonic saline.[1] The hematocrit is usually about 60%. Platelets, leukocytes (except for a few lymphocytes), and plasma constituents are almost completely removed during processing. Frozen storage time can be up to 10 years, although some data support even longer periods.[2,3] Post-thaw storage time is 24 hours at 1°C to 6°C. Volume and hematocrit vary.

Patient Preparation As for transfusion of whole blood or red blood cells

Specimen Blood

Container As in Donation, Blood, for obtaining unit; one red top tube and one lavender top (EDTA) tube for patient testing

Collection A unit of red blood cells is prepared in the usual way from whole blood. The mechanism of transfer to a special freezing container and the addition and concentration of glycerol vary according to the method used. Freezing may be in mechanical freezers or in liquid nitrogen.

Storage Instructions Deglycerolized red blood cells must be transfused within 24 hours after thawing or must be discarded.

Causes for Rejection If a crack is found in the frozen plastic of the container or if there is evidence of leakage, discard the unit.[1]

Turnaround Time Long processing time is a severe disadvantage in emergency settings.

Special Instructions After issue from the transfusion service, blood must be transfused within 2 hours; blood cannot be returned to the Blood Bank for reissue.

Use Restores red cell volume. Frozen red cells are essentially free of plasma proteins; about 0.025% of the original plasma is present. Such properties have more to do with the washing, than with the freezing process itself. Frozen red cells are useful particularly for patients with very rare red cell types and antibodies to high frequency antigens or combinations of antigens.[1]

Long-term storage of autologous red cells.

Rare donor red cell depot.

Limitations About 10% to 15% of the original red cells are lost in processing; expensive - about two to three times the cost of a unit of conventional red blood cells; short dating after thawing - 24-hour shelf-life;[1] not always available even in larger cities; slow and complex. Because of these problems, lack of stat availability for emergencies, and expense, frozen red cells have been somewhat of a disappointment.

Contraindications Sickling hemoglobinopathies and G-6-PD deficiency in donors are contraindications to freezing, since red cell recovery in these conditions has been poor.[1] As for recipients, frozen red cells should generally not be used when anemia and/or hypoxia can be corrected with specific products (eg, iron, B_{12}, folic acid). Not suitable for correction of coagulation deficiencies.

Methodology A number of methods for freezing and thawing red cells are in use.

Additional Information Red blood cells must be ABO and Rh compatible. A crossmatch is necessary. Hepatitis and some other infectious diseases remain a hazard. Infuse within 2 hours of thawing, if possible; more rapidly in urgent situations.

Footnotes
1. Chaplin H Jr, "Clinical Uses of Frozen-Stored Red Blood Cells," *Clinical Practice of Blood Transfusion*, Petz LD and Swisher SN, eds, New York, NY: Churchill-Livingstone, 1989, 315-25.
2. Umlas J, Jacobson M, and Kevy SV, "Suitable Survival and Half-Life of Red Cells After Frozen Storage in Excess of 10 Years," *Transfusion*, 1991, 31(7):648-9.
3. Valeri CR, Pivacek LE, Gray AD, et al, "The Safety and Therapeutic Effectiveness of Human Red Cells Stored at -80°C for as Long as 21 Years," *Transfusion*, 1989, 29(5):429-37.

References
Circular of Information for the Use of Human Blood and Blood Components, American Red Cross, Council of Community Blood Centers, American Association of Blood Banks, 1992.
Walker RH, *Technical Manual*, 10th ed, Arlington, VA: American Association of Blood Banks, 1990, 92-9.

Genetic Studies *see* Paternity Studies *on page 613*

Genotype, Immigration *see* Paternity Studies *on page 613*

Granulocytapheresis *see* Cytapheresis, Therapeutic *on page 606*

Granulocytes, Apheresis, Donation *see* Neutrophils, Apheresis, Donation *on next page*

Granulocytes, Pheresis (FDA) *see* Neutrophils, Apheresis, Donation *on next page*

Granulocytes, Transfusion *see* Neutrophils, Transfusion *on page 612*

Hazards of Transfusion *see* Risks of Transfusion *on page 623*

Hemolytic Disease of the Newborn, Antibody Identification

CPT 86870 (panel); 86885 (screen)

Related Information

Amniotic Fluid Analysis for Erythroblastosis Fetalis (OD 450) *on page 76*

Antibody Identification, Red Cell *on page 601*

Antiglobulin Test, Indirect *on page 602*

Bilirubin, Neonatal *on page 86*

Cord Blood Screen *on page 605*

Newborn Crossmatch and Transfusion *on next page*

Synonyms Newborn/Maternal Antibody Work-up

Applies to Exchange Transfusion

Test Commonly Includes Infant ABO, Rh, and antiglobulin test, direct; mother's ABO, Rh, and antiglobulin test, indirect; antibody identification, red cell

Specimen Blood from mother and newborn

Container Red top tube and lavender top (EDTA) tube

Causes for Rejection Gross hemolysis, sample placed in a serum separator tube, specimen tube not properly labeled

Use Diagnose erythroblastosis fetalis (hemolytic disease of the newborn) and provide the safest possible donor blood for potential exchange transfusion. Test panel for identification of irregular antibodies with mother's serum when her indirect antiglobulin test (antibody screen) is positive.

Limitations If mother is Rh negative, the specimen must be drawn before Rh immune globulin is given if it is indicated.

Additional Information Newborn's antibody is from mother. Hemolytic disease caused by **fetomaternal ABO incompatibility** is common, often subclinical, usually mild and rarely requires exchange transfusion; the direct antiglobulin test in such cases may be positive or negative, spherocytes are often found in the peripheral blood film, and in uncomplicated ABO incompatibility, the maternal serum lacks irregular antibodies. Unlike Rh incompatibility, in which much of the antibody is bound to the red cells, in ABO incompatibility there is often a marked quantitative discrepancy between the maternal and cord anti-A or anti-B antibody. The difference may be explained by the absorption of anti-A or anti-B on to A and B sites other than those on the red cells.[1] The usual situation is an O mother with an A baby. Serologically, diagnosis is not difficult (see table). Whether or not the serologic findings are clinically significant depends on clinical findings.

Blood group antibodies other than ABO and Rh can also cause fetal hemolytic disease and may be even more dangerous because of being unsuspected.[2] The severity of hemolytic disease probably depends more on the biochemical characteristics of the antibody than on its serologic specificity.

Rh hemolytic disease of the newborn is largely preventable[1] but still occurs occasionally. The cause of death *in utero* is anemia. It is now possible to transfuse the baby directly into the umbilical vein under ultrasound monitoring.[3] However, it requires skill and experience to transfuse a baby *in utero*.[4] The more usual treatment for intrauterine disease when the baby cannot survive to maturity is intrauterine transfusion into the fetal abdominal cavity.

Blood Grouping Results in a Typical Case of ABO Erythroblastosis

	Known Serums, Anti-			Known Red Cells			Direct Antiglobulin Test
	A	B	A, B	A	B	O	
Mother	0	0	0	+*	+	0	0
Baby	+	0	+	+	Weak	0	+
Eluate from baby's cells				+	0 or +	0	

*Hemolysis

Note that the mother has hemolytic anti-A and that anti-A was eluted from the baby's red cells. Incompatible maternal anti-A, as well as some anti-B, are present in the baby's serum, an important diagnostic point.

From Huestis DW, Bove JR, and Case J, *Practical Blood Transfusion*, 4th ed, Boston MA: Little, Brown and Co, 1988, 364, with permission.

Footnotes

1. Chavez GF, Mulinare J, and Edmonds LD, "Epidemiology of Rh Hemolytic Disease of the Newborn in the United States," *JAMA*, 1991, 265(24):3270-4.
2. Bowman JM, Pollock JM, Manning FA, et al, "Maternal Kell Blood Group Alloimmunization," *Obstet Gynecol*, 1992, 79(2):239-44.
3. Grannum PA, Copel JA, Plaxe SC, et al, "*In Utero* Exchange Transfusion by Direct Intravascular Injection in Severe Erythroblastosis Fetalis," *N Engl J Med*, 1986, 314(22):1431-4.
4. Queenan JT, "Erythroblastosis Fetalis: Closing the Circle," *N Engl J Med*, 1986, 314(22):1448-9.

Hemolytic Disease of the Newborn, Antibody Titer *see* Antibody Titer *on page 601*

Hemolytic Disease of the Newborn, Crossmatch *see* Newborn Crossmatch and Transfusion *on next page*

Hemophilia A Therapy *see* Cryoprecipitate *on page 606*

IAT *see* Antiglobulin Test, Indirect *on page 602*

Indirect Antiglobulin Test *see* Antiglobulin Test, Indirect *on page 602*

Irradiated Blood Components

CPT 36430 (transfusion); 86945 (irradiation of blood product, each unit)

Related Information

Donation, Blood, Directed *on page 608*

Platelet Concentrate, Donation and Transfusion *on page 616*

Applies to Blood Components, Irradiated; Whole Blood, Irradiated

Test Commonly Includes Irradiation of blood components with a gamma radiation source, usually cesium-137 or cobalt-60

Abstract Graft-versus-host disease (GVHD) may occur when donor T lymphocytes from transfused blood attack recipient tissues.

Patient Preparation Usual pretransfusion testing.

Use Avoid graft-versus-host disease (GVHD) in blood recipients

Limitations Irradiation causes premature release of potassium from red cells. After irradiation, shelf-life is reduced to 28 days.

Methodology Irradiation of blood leads to nonviability of donor lymphocytes. Although 1500 rad has been the dose generally used, at least 2500 may be best.

Additional Information GVHD occurs when viable lymphocytes are transfused into severely immunosuppressed patients. The patient is unable to destroy these incoming lymphocytes, and they attack the host cells, recognizing them as foreign. GVHD also occurs after allogeneic bone marrow transplantation. GVHD may occur in immunocompetent patients if they receive blood from a blood relative who is homozygous for an HLA haplotype for which the patient is heterozygous. Preventive irradiation is a wise resort in the case of directed donations from blood relatives, even if the HLA types are unknown. Irradiation has little effect on RBCs and none on platelets. Available filtration methods of leukocyte removal are not adequate to prevent GVHD. Currently there is no means to prevent GVHD following bone marrow transplantation.

A molecular method has been described to demonstrate donor DNA in subjects with GVHD.[1]

Footnotes

1. Wang L, Juji T, Tokunaga K, et al, "Brief Report: Polymorphic Microsatellite Markers for the Diagnosis of Graft-Versus-Host Disease," *N Engl J Med*, 1994, 330(6):398-401.

References

Linden JV and Pisciotto PT, "Transfusion-Associated Graft-Versus-Host Disease and Blood Irradiation," *Transfus Med Rev*, 1992, 6(2):116-23.

Thorp JA, Plapp FV, Cohen GR, et al, "Hyperkalemia After Irradiation of Packed Red Blood Cells: Possible Effects With Intravascular Fetal Transfusion," *Am J Obstet Gynecol*, 1990, 163(2):607-9.

Leukapheresis, Automated *see* Neutrophils, Apheresis, Donation *on this page*

Leukapheresis, Therapeutic *see* Cytapheresis, Therapeutic *on page 606*

Leukocyte Concentrate *see* Neutrophils, Transfusion *on next page*

Leukocyte Removal *see* Filters for Blood *on page 609*

Leukocytes, Apheresis *see* Neutrophils, Apheresis, Donation *on this page*

Leukocytes, Transfusion *see* Neutrophils, Transfusion *on next page*

Massive Acute Blood Loss *see* Uncrossmatched Blood, Emergency *on page 627*

Massive Transfusions *see* Whole Blood *on page 627*

Neonatal Transfusion *see* Newborn Crossmatch and Transfusion *on next page*

Neutrophils, Apheresis, Donation

CPT 36520 (leukapheresis)

Synonyms Granulocytes, Apheresis, Donation; Granulocytes, Pheresis (FDA); Leukapheresis, Automated; Leukocytes, Apheresis

Test Commonly Includes As for regular blood donation

Patient Preparation The more granulocytes, the more effective the transfusions. To achieve maximal yields, stimulate the donor with corticosteroids (eg, three doses of prednisone, 20 mg each, given respectively at about 18, 12, and 2 hours before donation). Steroid given at the beginning of leukapheresis is useless. The best qualification of a donor for leukapheresis is a history of uneventful regular blood donation.

Specimen Donor granulocytes including therapeutic doses of platelets

Collection Collection of granulocytes is by means of a blood cell separator. Most makes are satisfactory. Methods of collecting granulocytes from fresh whole blood units have been published, but the numbers obtainable this way appear to be too small even for infants. Anticoagulation is by a citrated macromolecular agent, usually hydroxyethyl starch (HES, Hetastarch, Hespan®). Pentastarch, which has a shorter half-life, is now also available. Without such an agent, separation of granulocytes (Continued)

Neutrophils, Apheresis, Donation (Continued)

from RBCs is poor and yields are unacceptably low. The final concentrate must contain at least 10^{10} granulocytes. At least double that number is desirable. To attain the minimum, collections will need to **average** at least twice that, as considerable variation occurs. Each concentrate also contains at least 15 mL RBCs and 3-8 x 10^{11} platelets.

Causes for Rejection As for regular blood donation.

Special Instructions Donors selected for this procedure are often family members (best motivation). ABO and Rh compatibility are desirable but not essential, as RBCs can readily be removed. HLA compatibility is desirable in the case of alloimmunized recipients but is seldom practical. Screening and testing are as for regular blood donations.

Use Granulocytes for transfusion of septic patients with severe neutropenia (ie, granulocyte count <500/mm^3)

Limitations Donation not exceeding twice a week with a 48-hour interval between procedures unless otherwise determined by Blood Bank physician.

Contraindications Donors with intolerance of HES; donors with conditions that might be exacerbated by prednisone (eg, diabetes, history of tuberculosis, peptic ulcer, hypertension). See listing Platelets, Apheresis, Donation *on page 617* for table listing donor reactions specific to leukapheresis.

Methodology Continuous or intermittent flow centrifugation. Exact method depends on separator used.

Additional Information Crossmatch may be desirable if recipient has a positive antibody screen, since most concentrates include considerable RBCs.

References
Hinkley MH and Huestis DW, "Premedication for Optimal Granulocyte Collection," *Plasma Ther Transfus Technol*, 1981, 2:149-52.
Huestis DW and Glasser L, "The Neutrophil in Transfusion Medicine," *Transfusion*, 1994, 34(7):630-46.
Mishler JM IV, *Pharmacology of Hydroxyethyl Starch. Use in Therapy and Blood Banking*, Oxford, UK: Oxford University Press, 1982.

Neutrophils, Transfusion

CPT 86950

Synonyms Granulocytes, Transfusion; Leukocyte Concentrate; Leukocytes, Transfusion; White Cells, Transfusion

Test Commonly Includes Preparations of granulocytes (neutrophils) generally also contain platelets and red blood cells. ABO and Rh type, antibody screen, antibody identification if indicated.

Patient Preparation Unit should preferably be ABO and Rh compatible. Red cell compatibility test is needed, since most units contain sufficient red cells to cause red cell transfusion reaction. However, in case of incompatibility, it is relatively easy to remove almost all the red cells. HLA compatibility is seldom practical. Family members may be the most suitable. Dosage and administration: Give neutrophils for at least 4 days. Mollison's 1993 text recommends functioning granulocytes twice daily for 4-7 days.[1] In the U.S., once daily is the usual dose interval. Use clot filter but not microaggregate filter. During infusion, monitor patient carefully. Administer neutrophils as soon as possible after collection.

Specimen Blood from recipient and donor

Container Red top tube from recipient

Collection (Of sample from intended recipient): As for other red-cell-containing blood components.

Storage Instructions Storage should be at 20°C to 24°C, without agitation, for a maximum of 24 hours.

Causes for Rejection (Of patient sample): Gross hemolysis, sample placed in a serum separator tube, specimen tube not properly labeled

Special Instructions Expiration date is 24 hours.

Use Temporary therapy for severely neutropenic patients, especially newborns, with infection nonresponsive to antibiotic therapy. Criteria for neutrophil transfusion: Absolute neutrophil count ≤500/mm^3 in at least two counts; sepsis or severe local infection; infection caused by gram-negative organism or suspicion of gram-negative infection, in patient with profound neutropenia not responding to at least 3 days of conventional therapy. Use in gram-positive and fungal infections has not been well studied. Neutrophil transfusion is never the sole form of therapy. Do not use prophylactically.

Limitations Expensive. HLA selection may be indicated for alloimmunized recipients. High incidence of febrile and other reactions, which are not necessarily cause for stopping the transfusion. Neutrophil transfusions are seldom used now in adults.[2,3] However, in septic newborns with poor marrow neutrophil production, neutrophils (even a single large infusion) may be lifesaving.

Contraindications Not indicated for infections that can be managed successfully with antibiotics. Stop infusion of neutrophils in the presence of pulmonary distress and give hydrocortisone.[1] Given with amphotericin B, there may be a risk of severe pulmonary reaction.[1] If a minimal dose

comfortably above 10^{10} neutrophils/transfusion cannot be provided, it is probably not worthwhile to give neutrophil transfusions to adults.[3]

Antibiotics and recombinant granulocyte colony stimulation factor (GCSF) may alter utilization of this fraction.

Methodology Cytapheresis, using hydroxyethyl starch with steroid premedication of donor

Additional Information Transfusions are administered at a slower rate than whole blood or red blood cells to prevent reactions. **Hazards**: Chills, fever, allergic reactions, including urticaria; immunization to HLA antigens. Graft-versus-host reactions may occur in immunodeficient or immunosuppressed patients.[1] Units may be irradiated to prevent graft-versus-host disease.[3] **Hazards of transfusion**. Risks of viral hepatitis and other microbiologic hazards exist. Since red cells are present in granulocyte units, immunization and hemolysis can occur.

Footnotes
1. Mollison PL, Engelfriet CP, and Contreras M, "The Transfusion of Platelets, Leukocytes, Hematopoietic Cells, and Plasma Components," *Blood Transfusion in Clinical Medicine*, 9th ed, Oxford, UK: Blackwell Scientific Publications, 1993, 651-2.
2. Lazarus HM, "Granulocyte Transfusions: Have We Learned Anything?" *J Lab Clin Med*, 1990, 115(3):271-2.
3. Huestis DW and Glasser L, "The Neutrophil in Transfusion Medicine," *Transfusion*, 1994, 34(7):630-46.

References
Dahlke MB, Keashen M, Alavi JB, et al, "Granulocyte Transfusions and Outcome of Alloimmunized Patients With Gram-Negative Sepsis," *Transfusion*, 1982, 22:374-8.
Huestis DW, Bove JR, and Case J, *Practical Blood Transfusion*, 4th ed, Boston, MA: Little, Brown and Co, 1988, 337-41.
Schiffer CA, "Granulocyte Transfusions: An Overlooked Therapeutic Modality," *Transfus Med Rev*, 1990, 4(1):2-7.
Sweetman RW and Cairo MS, "Blood Component and Immunotherapy in Neonatal Sepsis," *Transfus Med Rev*, 1995, 9(3):251-9.

Newborn Crossmatch and Transfusion

CPT 36450 (exchange transfusion, blood, newborn); 86921 (incubation technique); 86922 (antiglobulin technique)

Related Information
Cord Blood Screen *on page 605*
Hemolytic Disease of the Newborn, Antibody Identification *on page 610*
Rh$_o$(D) Immune Globulin (Human) *on page 623*
Rosette Test for Fetomaternal Hemorrhage *on page 625*
Warming, Blood *on page 627*

Synonyms Exchange Transfusion; Neonatal Transfusion; Newborn Transfusion; Type and Crossmatch for Exchange Transfusion of Newborn

Applies to Hemolytic Disease of the Newborn, Crossmatch

Test Commonly Includes For exchange transfusion, reasonably fresh donor blood, preferably in storage less than 5 days, compatible with mother's serum. For small transfusions (not exchange), blood less than 2 weeks in storage should be satisfactory. ABO and Rh type of mother and infant, antibody screen on mother's blood, antibody identification if indicated, crossmatch of mother's serum and donor cells. If mother's blood is not available, crossmatch may use newborn's serum and/or eluate from cord red cells.

Patient Preparation For exchange transfusion, blood should be passed through a warming device to raise the temperature of the blood to about 37°C during administration. Do not infuse unfiltered blood. Donor blood must lack the antigen corresponding to the mother's antibody (eg, in Rh erythroblastosis, donor blood must be Rh-negative). When mother and baby are the same ABO type, use group-specific donor blood.[1] Otherwise, use type O Rh-negative donor packed cells or whole blood. If necessary, adjust the hematocrit of donor blood by adding or removing plasma. If adding, use plasma from the same donor if possible. Albumin is also acceptable. For smaller, nonexchange transfusions, select blood as for adults. In the latter case, warming and adjustment of hematocrit are seldom necessary.

Aftercare Citrate toxicity, hypocalcemia, and other metabolic effects may occur. Postexchange serum calcium levels are useful. When exchange transfusion is completed, determinations of hematocrit, electrolytes, calcium, direct antiglobulin test, and bilirubin are often useful.[1]

Specimen Blood from mother and infant

Container 10 mL red top tube from mother; 15-20 blue tip capillaries from baby

Collection (Of sample from mother): As for regular type and crossmatch. Similarly, verify identity of baby and prepare appropriate labels.

Causes for Rejection (Of patient sample): Gross hemolysis, sample placed in a serum separator tube, specimen tube not properly labeled

Special Instructions Advance notice permits collection of appropriate donor blood into a bag with multiple satellites (quad packs). The advantage of such satellite bags is that multiple small transfusions can be given to the infant from the same donor, without exposure of the baby to multiple risks of viral hepatitis. Another way of accomplishing the same end is by subdividing donor blood units by means of a sterile-connecting device. This permits multiple transfusions from a regular blood unit without affecting the dating and at lower cost than quad-pack sets. CMV negative blood should be provided for babies who weigh less than 1200 g, if the mother is also CMV negative or if her status is unknown. There are unresolved questions about transfusions to newborns of blood stored in extended-storage media. It is unlikely that any risk attaches to small-volume supplementary transfusions of such blood. But the situation may be different in premature babies with liver or kidney damage or in massive transfusions, such as exchange transfusion. Even lacking clinical data on harmful effects, the use of unmodified extended-storage blood in such patients might be unwise. Removal of the supernatant and substitution of saline or albumin would be a prudent course.

Reference Range Compatible

Use Hemolytic disease of the newborn is due to transplacental passage of maternal antibodies - ABO, Rh (D, C, c), Kell, Duffy, Kidd, or other blood group system antibodies.

Immediate exchange laboratory criteria for term infants include significant anemia and rapidly increasing hyperbilirubinemia. Consult pediatric literature for more detailed criteria and procedure.[1,2]

A classic indication for exchange transfusion in full-term infants is an indirect bilirubin level ≥20 mg/dL. At this level, brain damage may occur. In premature babies or those with other complications, brain damage may occur at lower levels of bilirubin.[1] An exchange transfusion may then be appropriate at levels <20 mg/dL. Severe bilirubinemia may also occur with hepatic failure, disseminated intravascular coagulopathy,[1] and in the respiratory distress syndrome. In the latter disorder, exchange transfusion aims to shift the oxygen dissociation curve to the right by replacing hemoglobin F with hemoglobin A.

Limitations Clots in the cord blood tube may generate misleading cord hemoglobin and hematocrit. Relatively mild jaundice beginning 1-2 days after delivery with a weakly positive direct antiglobulin test in a baby of type A or B and a mother of type O usually indicates ABO hemolytic disease. Anti-A or anti-B in the baby's serum incompatible with its own RBCs is usually detected. A more definitive test is to elute antibody from the baby's RBCs and test it against A_1, B, and O red cells. Exchange transfusion is seldom necessary in ABO hemolytic disease. Complications of exchange transfusion have been compiled.[1]

Contraindications In hypoxic or acidotic babies receiving exchange transfusion, consider selection of blood known to lack hemoglobin S.[3]

Additional Information Red cell transfusions are not infrequently given to premature infants weighing less than 1300 g for anemia of prematurity and for loss from repeated blood sampling. The use of recombinant human erythropoietin in this group has recently been discussed.[4,5]

Footnotes

1. Sacher RA and Lenes BA, "Exchange Transfusion," *Clin Lab Med*, 1981, 265-83.
2. Klemperer M, "Perinatal and Neonatal Transfusion," *Clinical Practice of Transfusion Medicine*, Petz LD and Swisher SN, eds, New York, NY: Churchill Livingstone, 1989, 615-34.
3. Klein HG, *Standards for Blood Banks and Transfusion Services*, 16th ed, Bethesda, MD: American Association of Blood Banks, 1994, 29.
4. Maier RF, Obladen M, Scigalla P, et al, "The Effect of Epoetin Beta (Recombinant Human Erythropoietin) on the Need for Transfusion in Very-Low-Birth-Weight Infants. European Multicentre Erythropoietin Study Group," *N Engl J Med*, 1994, 330(17):1173-8.
5. Strauss RG, "Erythropoietin and Neonatal Anemia," *N Engl J Med*, 1994, 330(17):1227-8.

References

Hume H and Bard H, "Small Volume Red Blood Cell Transfusions for Neonatal Patients," *Transfus Med Rev*, 1995, 9(3):187-99.
Luban NL, "Massive Transfusion in the Neonate," *Transfus Med Rev*, 1995, 9(3):200-14.
Luban NL, Strauss RG, and Hume HA, "Commentary on the Safety of Red Cells Preserved in Extended Storage Media for Neonatal Transfusions," *Transfusion*, 1991, 31(3):229-35.
Sayers MH, Anderson KC, Goodnough LT, et al, "Reducing the Risk for Transfusion-Transmitted Cytomegalovirus Infection," *Ann Intern Med*, 1992, 116(1):55-62.

Newborn/Maternal Antibody Work-up see Hemolytic Disease of the Newborn, Antibody Identification *on page 610*

Newborn Transfusion see Newborn Crossmatch and Transfusion *on previous page*

Normal Serum Albumin (Human) see Albumin and Plasma Protein Fraction for Infusion *on page 601*

Packed Red Cells, Transfusion see Red Blood Cells *on page 621*

Parentage Studies see Paternity Studies *on this page*

Paternity Studies

CPT 86910

Related Information

Chain-of-Custody Protocol *on page 542*
Haptoglobin, Serum *on page 141*
HLA Typing, Single Human Leukocyte Antigen *on page 405*

Identification DNA Testing *on page 517*
Red Blood Cell Enzyme Deficiency Screen *on page 343*
Tissue Typing *on page 434*

Synonyms Exclusion of Parentage; Genetic Studies; Genotype, Immigration; Parentage Studies; Paternity Testing

Specimen Blood; legal chain-of-custody problems exist. See listing Chain-of-Custody Protocol *on page 542*

Container Red top tube for red cell antigens; containers for other systems as laboratory requests

Collection Obtain witnesses for collection of blood samples from mother, baby, and presumptive father. Use positive identification procedures of persons before drawing samples. Include a photograph of mother, father, and child. Label all samples appropriately.

Causes for Rejection All parties usually must be at the laboratory at the same time, and appointments are required. When a single individual appears for venipuncture for paternity studies, many transfusion centers and blood centers will decline to draw a specimen, for lack of mutual identification.

Special Instructions Exclusion of parentage is a highly specialized area of forensic medicine. It is not a field for amateurs, nor is it part of the procedures involved in the diagnosis or treatment of disease. For these reasons, those without special forensic training are wise to refer paternity studies to experts.

Use Resolve cases of disputed paternity; establish blood relationship of potential immigrant, possible exchange of infants in nursery, and kidnapped child; it can also be used to estimate the chance of monozygosity and dizygosity of twins

Limitations Paternity studies have only ruled out parentage. Although they have not previously proved parentage, the statistical likelihood of paternity can be admitted as evidence in some courts.

Methodology Red cell antigens including ABO, MN, Rh, Duffy, Kell, and Kidd systems, serum protein markers, RBC enzymes, and HLA typing

Additional Information In the future, restriction endonuclease fragment-length polymorphisms and computers may provide near certainty in paternal identity.[1,2] See Identification DNA Testing *on page 517*.

Footnotes

1. Markowicz KR, Tonelli LA, Anderson MB, et al, "Use of Deoxyribonucleic Acid (DNA) Fingerprints for Identity Determination: Comparison With Traditional Paternity Testing Methods," Part II, *J Forensic Sci*, 1990, 35(6):1270-6.
2. Tonelli LA, Markowicz KR, Anderson MB, et al, "Use of Deoxyribonucleic Acid (DNA) Fingerprints for Identity Determination: Comparison With Traditional Paternity Testing Methods," Part I, *J Forensic Sci*, 1990, 35(6):1265-9.

References

Brooks MA, "Paternity Testing," *Modern Blood Banking and Transfusion Practices*, 2nd ed, Harmening D, ed, Philadelphia, PA: FA Davis Co, 1989, 379-89.
Bryant NJ, "Paternity Testing: Current Status and Review," *Transfus Med Rev*, 1988, 2(1):29-39.

Paternity Testing see Paternity Studies *on this page*

Peripheral Blood Stem Cells, Autologous

CPT 86890

Related Information

Bone Marrow, Autologous *on page 604*

Synonyms Autologous Stem Cells; Peripheral Stem Cells; Progenitor Cells

Test Commonly Includes Multiple collections of peripheral stem cells by hemapheresis, frozen storage, and autologous transfusion of stem cells after bone marrow ablative therapy for cancer or leukemia

Abstract Patient first undergoes course of chemotherapy and may also receive hematopoietic growth factor (eg, GM-CSF, G-CSF) stimulation. Using a stem-cell protocol with any suitable blood cell separator, collect 6-8 x 10^8 mononuclears per kg of patient's body weight, by a series of 3- to 4-hour leukaphereses. Three to 12 procedures may be necessary. Procedures are usually done daily. Newer techniques aim at reducing the number of procedures needed. Methods of specifically extracting stem cells by automated immune adsorption are under development.

Patient Preparation Excellent vein access is a daily requirement for which indwelling intravenous catheters (eg, subclavian) are suitable.

Collection As prescribed by the manufacturer of the blood cell separator used.

Storage Instructions Store each collection in liquid nitrogen after concentration and resuspension in dimethyl sulfoxide. Label as for other blood components.

Causes for Rejection Cancer or leukemia cells in peripheral blood

Use Patients with malignant disease not responding to conventional therapy. Concept is to collect enough peripheral stem cells to repopulate patient's bone marrow after heavy chemotherapy and/or irradiation sufficient to obliterate marrow function and, it is hoped, also to destroy remaining malignant cells. The system is also useful for collecting stem cells for gene therapy.

(Continued)

Peripheral Blood Stem Cells, Autologous
(Continued)

Methodology Depends on blood cell separator used

Additional Information This is a relatively new therapy, involving very close coordination between Hematology/Oncology and laboratory physicians. So far, the results have been encouraging. The reconstitution of bone marrow function in this setting depends on many variables involving the patient and the treatment regimen. The mononuclear cell count indicates an endpoint for the collection of stem cells, but the ultimate quality assurance method would be to count stem cells themselves. Actual stem cell culture and quantitation of colony-forming units are the "gold standard," but enumeration of cells positive for CD34 receptor is gaining acceptance. Very interesting work is in progress on the collection of stem cells from the rich source of umbilical cord (placental) blood. This is still experimental, but placental stem cells are already in use for related-sibling and even for unrelated stem cell transplants.

References

Collins RH Jr, "CD34+ Selected Cells in Clinical Transplantation," *Stem Cells*, 1994, 12(6):577-85.

Comenzo RL and Berkman EM, "Hematopoietic Stem and Progenitor Cells From Blood: Emerging Uses for New Components for Transfusion," *Transfusion*, 1995, 35(4):335-45.

Inwards D and Kessinger A, "Peripheral Blood Stem Cell Transplantation: Historical Perspective, Current Status, and Prospects for the Future," *Transfus Med Rev*, 1992, 6(3):183-90.

Roberts GT and Sacher RA, "The Fetus as a Recipient and Donor of Blood Components," *Transfus Med Rev*, 1995, 9(3):260-70.

Wagner JE, "Umbilical Cord Blood Transplantation: Overview of the Clinical Experience," *Blood Cells*, 1994, 20(2-3):227-34.

Peripheral Stem Cells
see Peripheral Blood Stem Cells, Autologous *on previous page*

Phlebotomy, Blood Donor
see Donation, Blood *on page 607*

Phlebotomy, Therapeutic

CPT 99195

Related Information

Blood Gases, Arterial *on page 87*

Blood Volume *on page 306*

Carboxyhemoglobin *on page 541*

Donation, Blood *on page 607*

Erythropoietin, Serum *on page 124*

Iron and Total Iron Binding Capacity/Transferrin *on page 150*

Leukocyte Alkaline Phosphatase *on page 330*

Liver Biopsy *on page 48*

Porphyrins, Quantitative, Urine *on page 186*

Vitamin B$_{12}$ *on page 351*

Synonyms Therapeutic Phlebotomy

Patient Preparation Before the elective removal of blood for polycythemia, the physician should ascertain that an absolute polycythemia actually exists (ie, that a significant absolute increase of red cell mass exists, rather than a decrease of plasma volume). Diagnostic criteria should be fulfilled. The attending physician must make written request and specify amount of blood to be drawn. Approval of the blood bank physician is required as well.[1] Record prephlebotomy and postphlebotomy vital signs. The patient and physician should both understand that therapeutic phlebotomy is an operative procedure, not a blood donation.

Aftercare Advise outpatients to guard against fainting afterwards while driving, working, etc. Avoid strenuous exercise for 24 hours. Tell them also whom to call if they have a reaction at home. Multiple procedures may be needed over a long period.

Causes for Rejection Anemia, patient with blood pressure <90 mm Hg. Phlebotomy is contraindicated in stress polycythemia, in which plasma volume is contracted. Certain conditions may require the presence of the attending physician during phlebotomy (eg, hypertension, cardiac symptoms). The blood bank physician may decline to do the procedure on high-risk patients.

Special Instructions For polycythemia, evaluate the patient's hemoglobin, hematocrit, red cell count, platelet count, WBC count, leukocyte alkaline phosphatase, serum vitamin B$_{12}$, carboxyhemoglobin, and blood volume. In primary polycythemia, erythropoietin levels in blood and urine are decreased. Erythropoietin is increased in secondary polycythemia. Arterial blood gases may be helpful, with significantly decreased pO$_2$ and oxygen saturation pointing to secondary polycythemia.[2,3] Arterial blood oxygen saturation ≥92% is expected in polycythemia vera, and 75% have splenomegaly.

The diagnosis of **hemochromatosis** requires transferrin saturation >55% with serum ferritin >400 μg/L. The "gold standard" is liver biopsy with measured iron concentration.[4]

Use Removal of blood to reduce red cell mass in polycythemia, with the patient's hematocrit >53%, to reduce hematocrit to 42% to 44%; occasionally in acute cardiac failure for emergency reduction of circulatory volume; idiopathic hemochromatosis, for which ferritin levels and/or transferrin saturation are used as monitors; therapy for porphyria cutanea tarda

Limitations In general, take no more than 450 mL of whole blood from a patient at one time. The goal is to reduce the hematocrit to <50% for secondary polycythemia. The procedure may be repeated subsequently. With some exceptions, the blood is not suitable for transfusion (it does not come from a "healthy" donor).

Contraindications Lack of documented increase of red cell mass when polycythemia is considered. Hemoglobinopathies exist in which polycythemia occurs, the abnormal hemoglobin having increased oxygen affinity. Methemoglobinemias may relate to secondary polycythemias. Uncommonly, certain tumors induce erythrocytosis. Renal tumors are the most widely known cause of tumor erythrocytosis. These considerations are the responsibility of the clinical physician.

Additional Information For polycythemia, follow platelet counts as well as hematocrit; platelet counts over 1 million may require special treatment.[1] Blood viscosity increases significantly when hemoglobin increases from 14 g/dL to 16 g/dL.

Phlebotomies for hemochromatosis should lead to decreased serum ferritin, then decreased serum iron. Details are published.[4,5]

Footnotes

1. Klein HG, *Standards for Blood Banks and Transfusion Services*, 16th ed, Bethesda, MD: American Association of Blood Banks, 1994, 10.

2. Landaw SA, "Polycythemia Vera and Other Polycythemic States," *Clin Lab Med*, 1990, 10(4):857-71.

3. Chetty KG, Light RW, Stansbury DW, et al, "Exercise Performance of Polycythemic Chronic Obstructive Pulmonary Disease Patients. Effect of Phlebotomies," *Chest*, 1990, 98(5):1073-7.

4. Edwards CQ and Kushner JP, "Screening for Hemochromatosis," *N Engl J Med*, 1993, 328(22):1616-20.

5. "Case Records of the Massachusetts General Hospital. Weekly Clinicopathological Exercises. Case 31-1994. A 25-Year-Old Man With Recent Onset of Diabetes Mellitus and Congestive Heart Failure," *N Engl J Med*, 1994, 331(7):460-6.

References

Dostik H and Prasad B, "Coulter S Hematocrit and Microhematocrit in Polycythemic Patients," *Am J Hematol*, 1978, 5:51.

England JM, Walford DM, Waters DA, et al, "Reassessment of the Reliability of the Hematocrit," *Br J Haematol*, 1972, 23:247-56.

Plasma Exchange

CPT 36520

Related Information

Cytapheresis, Therapeutic *on page 606*

Plasmapheresis, Donor *on page 616*

Synonyms Plasmapheresis; Plasmapheresis, Therapeutic

Test Commonly Includes Use of blood cell separator to remove pathogenic component from plasma (eg, autoantibody, paraprotein), with simultaneous replacement by protein-containing medium (eg, 5% albumin) and electrolyte solutions

Patient Preparation Excellent vascular access is essential, as most continuous-flow blood cell separators require two venipunctures and a series of procedures is usual.

Aftercare Monitor fluid and electrolyte balance. If infection seems to be a risk, it may be necessary to provide immunoglobulins when the replacement fluid has been albumin. Likewise, observe patient carefully for hemorrhage from loss of clotting factors. Both of these potential complications are rare.

Special Instructions Generally done on scheduled basis, depending on availability of blood cell separator and by consultation with Blood Bank physician. Occasionally emergent; team must be prepared to offer 24-hour, 7-day coverage. Plasma exchange removes the good with the bad in the patient's plasma. This means that blood levels of the patient's medications will be reduced significantly. Adjust medication schedule therefore to allow for effect of plasma exchange. Whenever possible, measure efficacy of exchanges by monitoring levels of some marker that indicates progress or regression of the disease treated (eg, specific antibody, immunoglobulin, abnormal protein). The usual amount of plasma exchanged in a procedure is 40 mL per kg patient's body weight. This figure (about one plasma volume) can be applied to children as well.

Use Treatment of blood diseases, primarily autoimmune. The **clinical indications** for plasma exchange are now fairly well established, but it continues to be applied to some conditions for which its scientific basis is not firm. These two groups are given in the table.

Contraindications Moribund patient or one who cannot withstand the establishment of an extracorporeal circuit; inadequate vascular access; lack of specific indication for the procedure. The decision to do this form

Efficacy of Plasma Exchange

Generally Seems To Be Effective*	Efficacy Debatable or Controlled Studies Lacking
Hyperviscosity syndrome	Systemic lupus erythematosus
Myasthenia gravis	Fulminant crescentic nephritis
Goodpasture's syndrome	Rheumatoid arthritis
Thrombotic thrombocytopenic purpura	Multiple sclerosis
Cryoglobulinemia	Rh hemolytic disease of the newborn
Hemophilia with inhibitor	ABO-incompatible bone marrow transplantation
Guillain-Barré syndrome	Renal transplant rejection
Post-transfusion purpura	Hypercholesterolemia (familial)
Refsum's disease	Cold antibody hemolytic anemia

*Effective = producing significant clinical improvement that is better than transitory.

From Huestis DW, Bove JR, and Case J, *Practical Blood Transfusion*, 4th ed, Boston, MA: Little, Brown and Co, 1988, 377-80, with permission.

of blood manipulation is shared between clinical and Blood Bank physicians.

Methodology Depends on the blood cell separator used. Most available machines can be used successfully, but **continuous-flow** systems are generally quicker, more efficient, and entail a smaller extracorporeal volume of blood. With removal of plasma in quantity approximating one blood volume (40 mL/kg body weight), replace it with a protein-containing medium. This is usually 5% albumin. For first exchanges, albumin need not be used exclusively, but can make up about half the replacement, with the other half isotonic saline. For further exchanges, particularly when doing a large series at short intervals, increase the proportion of albumin to saline, depending on the patient's serum protein values. Electrolyte supplementation is sometimes necessary, as judged by the clinical physician. It might seem logical to use normal plasma for replacement, but plasma causes too many reactions in the volumes used; allergic and citrate reactions are common, and more severe reactions have been reported. Use fresh frozen plasma as a replacement, however, in thrombotic thrombocytopenic purpura, hemolytic uremic syndrome, and other forms of microangiopathic hemolytic anemia where plasma seems to supply normal factors needed in those conditions.

Additional Information Although, when properly carried out for appropriate indications, plasma exchange is a relatively benign procedure; risks of morbidity and even rarely mortality exist.[1,2] Clinical physicians as well as those in transfusion services need to be aware of the risks (see table).

Complications of Plasma Exchange

Vascular Complications		
Hemorrhage, hematoma	Shunts, fistulas:	Catheters:
Sclerosis of veins	surgical procedure needed	perforation
Thrombosis, embolism	Thrombosis	infection
	infection	
	circulatory interference	
Procedural Reactions		
Vasovagal reaction	Citrate effects:	Volume changes:
Chilling	tremors, paresthesias	hypovolemia
Hemolysis, mechanical	Tetany	hypervolemia, overload
Allergy, anaphylaxis	Cardiac arrhythmia, arrest	
Acute pulmonary edema		
Hypoproteinemia		
Delayed Complications		
Clotting factor depletion	Infections:	
Thrombocytopenia	bacterial (sepsis)	
Hemorrhage	viral hepatitis	
Hypoproteinemia		
DIC, thrombosis		

From Huestis DW, "Risks and Safety in Hemapheresis Procedures," *Arch Pathol Lab Med*, 1989, 113:273-8, with permission.

Footnotes

1. Huestis DW, "Risks and Safety Practices in Hemapheresis Procedures," *Arch Pathol Lab Med*, 1989, 113(3):273-8.
2. Pohl MA, Lan SP, and Berl T, "Plasmapheresis Does Not Increase the Risk for Infection in Immunosuppressed Patients With Severe Lupus Nephritis. The Lupus Nephritis Collaborative Study Group," *Ann Intern Med*, 1991, 114(11):924-9.

References

Huestis DW, Bove JR, and Case J, *Practical Blood Transfusion*, 4th ed, Boston, MA: Little, Brown and Co, 1988, 367-89.

Plasma, Fresh Frozen

CPT 36430 (transfusion); 86927 (thawing, each unit)

Related Information

Activated Partial Thromboplastin Time *on page 227*
Cryoprecipitate *on page 606*
Factor V *on page 239*
Factor VII *on page 240*
Factor VIII *on page 240*
Factor VIII Concentrate *on page 608*
Factor IX *on page 241*
Factor IX Complex (Human) *on page 609*
Factor X *on page 242*
Factor XI *on page 243*
Factor XII *on page 243*
Factor XIII *on page 243*
Fibrinogen *on page 246*
Prothrombin Time *on page 262*

Synonyms FFP; Fresh Frozen Plasma

Applies to Factor IX Replacement; Factor VII Replacement; Factor V Replacement; Factor XIII Replacement; Factor XI Replacement; Factor X Replacement; Fibrinogen Replacement

Test Commonly Includes ABO type.[1] Plasma from a unit of whole blood separated from the red blood cells within 6 hours of collection and frozen rapidly. The unit has a volume of 150-275 mL. It contains all coagulation factors except platelets, but it is not a concentrate. A severe deficiency of coagulation factors cannot be corrected by giving FFP. Fluid overload would result.

Abstract FFP is plasma which has been separated and placed at -18°C or lower within 8 hours of collection. Heparin is not acceptable as an anticoagulant for this purpose.[1]

Patient Preparation Use coagulation studies as a guide to transfusion of FFP. **Dosage and administration:** FFP should be ABO compatible,[1] especially when it is to be given to infants.[2] It contains anti-A or anti-B. Rh need not be considered (but see Additional Information). Crossmatch is not necessary. Administer through a filter. The usual unit contains about 200 units of factor VIII,[1] and 250-400 mg of fibrinogen. It contains factor IX as well as other stable and labile coagulation factors. One unit of fresh frozen plasma will raise patient's plasma level of fibrinogen only about 10-13 mg/dL; cryoprecipitate is a better source of fibrinogen. Give FFP at about 10 mL/minute, to a total dose of about 10 mL/kg.[1]

Specimen Blood

Container Red top tube

Storage Instructions Frozen at -18°C or lower, FFP has a shelf-life of 1 year. Examine the frozen plastic bag for cracks, especially the seams. Thaw at 37°C with agitation in a waterbath, using a plastic overwrap.[3] Thawing requires 15-30 minutes depending on the number of units being thawed. Once thawed, store in Blood Bank refrigerator and transfuse within 24 hours.[3] Plasma ideally should be transfused within 2 hours after thawing when the patient requires labile coagulation factors. Once thawed and not transfused, FFP usually cannot be reissued by the Blood Bank. After 24 hours, a thawed unit of FFP becomes a unit of single donor plasma.

Special Instructions Usually available on request. Requires 15-30 minutes to thaw and issue.

Use Treatment of bleeding caused by labile and stable coagulation factor deficiency,[1] in some instances while awaiting specific concentrates or fractions. FFP is a source of factors V, VII, X, XI, XIII, and fibrinogen. Up to a point, FFP may be used to replace factor IX; factor IX concentrates carry a high risk of hepatitis.[3] Used with vitamin K, for bleeding related to vitamin K deficiency; in severe warfarin overdosage, uncommonly; for bleeding patients with severe liver disease.[1] Also used as replacement medium in plasma exchange for thrombotic thrombocytopenic purpura or hemolytic-uremic syndrome.

Limitations Circulatory overload is a hazard of use of FFP in a number of situations. **Fresh frozen plasma is grossly overused.**[4]

Contraindications Do not use FFP prophylactically to prevent dilutional coagulopathy in large transfusions. Do not use it as a plasma expander (unless it is autologous); albumin is better and safer. Do not use FFP if prothrombin time and activated partial thromboplastin time are less than 1.5 times normal and in the absence of abnormal bleeding. Coagulopathies are usually better corrected with specific therapy, such as cryoprecipitate or AHF for hemophilia and for von Willebrand disease.

Additional Information Hazards: Risk of disease transmission (that of any single unit exposure), plasma volume overload, anaphylaxis in IgA deficient recipient is a remote hazard. FFP contains anti-A or anti-B. Although FFP is basically cell-free, it is not without antigens. Recipients
(Continued)

Plasma, Fresh Frozen *(Continued)*

can have mild or severe allergic reactions and sometimes fever. Immunization can take place to soluble constituents as well as to Rh and other red cell antigens,[5] the latter presumably from cell fragments in the plasma. See also the listing Cryoprecipitate *on page 606.*

Footnotes

1. *Circular of Information for the Use of Human Blood and Blood Components*, American Red Cross, Council of Community Blood Centers, American Association of Blood Banks, 1992.
2. Klein HG, *Standards for Blood Banks and Transfusion Services*, 16th ed, Bethesda, MD: American Association of Blood Banks, 1994, 12, 27.
3. Walker RH, *Technical Manual*, 11th ed, Arlington, VA: American Association of Blood Banks, 1993, 402-7.
4. Consensus Conference, "Fresh Frozen Plasma. Indications and Risks," *JAMA*, 1985, 253(4):551-3.
5. Ching EP, Poon M-C, Neurath D, et al, "Red Blood Cell Alloimmunization Complicating Plasma Transfusion," *Am J Clin Pathol*, 1991, 96(2):201-2.

References

Barnette RE, Fish DJ, and Eisenstaedt RS, "Modification of Fresh-Frozen Plasma Transfusion Practices Through Educational Intervention," *Transfusion*, 1990, 30(3):253-7.

Coffin C, Matz K, and Rich E, "Algorithms for Evaluating the Appropriateness of Blood Transfusion," *Transfusion*, 1989, 29(4):298-303.

"Use of Blood Components," *FDA Drug Bulletin*, 1989, 19:15.

Plasmapheresis *see Plasma Exchange on page 614*

Plasmapheresis, Donor

CPT 36520

Related Information

Plasma Exchange *on page 614*

Synonyms Donor Plasmapheresis

Test Commonly Includes Centrifugation of whole blood from a donor, with separation and retention of plasma and return of RBCs to the donor. The procedure may be manual or automated.

Causes for Rejection Of donor: As for regular whole blood donation, except for the donation interval.

Use Obtain plasma for transfusion or laboratory use

Limitations Must meet donor criteria specified by AABB and FDA.

Methodology May be separated manually from whole blood collections with return of RBCs to donors or may be prepared by use of mechanical blood cell separators.

Additional Information Plasma is used as fresh frozen plasma or the starting material for various blood components. It can be obtained either by direct plasmapheresis or harvested from a single donation of whole blood. The products derived from plasmapheresis include fresh frozen plasma, cryoprecipitate, and manufactured derivatives such as plasma protein fraction, albumin, immune globulins, and clotting factor concentrates.

References

Klein HG, *Standards for Blood Banks and Transfusion Services*, 16th ed, Bethesda, MD: American Association of Blood Banks, 1994, 21-2.

Plasmapheresis, Therapeutic *see Plasma Exchange on page 614*

Plasma Protein Fraction (Human) (PPF) *see Albumin and Plasma Protein Fraction for Infusion on page 601*

Platelet Antibody, Immunohematologic

CPT 86022

Related Information

Platelet Antibody *on page 258*

Platelet Count *on page 340*

Synonyms Antiplatelet Antibody; Platelet-Bound IgG, Direct; Platelet-Bound IgG, Indirect

Abstract Increased platelet-associated IgG and/or IgM (surface-bound) generally indicates antibody adsorbed to the platelet membrane and is the platelet equivalent of a direct antiglobulin test on RBCs. The corresponding indirect test, using a patient's serum and a substrate of known reagent platelets, is the equivalent of an indirect antiglobulin test on RBCs. Interpretation of results is similar to that of the RBC tests.

Specimen Blood

Collection Depends on method used

Storage Instructions Depends on method used

Special Instructions Must consult with laboratory in advance.

Use Test for presumably specific auto- or alloantibodies directed against platelet antigens in cases of thrombocytopenia or apparent clinical refractoriness to platelet transfusions. Can also serve as "platelet crossmatch" for refractory patients.

Limitations Unfortunately, these procedures are not well standardized, and the results do not always conform to the clinical situation or correlate with the presence or absence of cytotoxic antibodies. Furthermore, in thrombocytopenic patients, it may be necessary to collect large amounts

of blood to have enough platelets to test. This may make the test impractical.

Contraindications The quantity of blood required for platelet isolation may make the test impractical in children or anemic adults.

Methodology Flow cytometry (FC) is the method of choice for the direct test, and may also be suitable for the indirect test. A problem is to find suitable substrate platelets (analogous to reagent red blood cells in the indirect antiglobulin test). A single sample, even pooled from several donors, is seldom satisfactory. A platelet panel would be ideal but putting one together presents formidable obstacles. Another method for indirect testing is solid-phase, binding platelets to wells in a microplate, exposing them to patient serum, then adding an indicator of IgG-coated RBCs. A commercial testing kit for this is available, although it has a very short shelf-life and is costly. But it does seem to be a good system, has its own small panel of typed platelets, and gives clear positive and negative results.

Additional Information Platelet antigen and antibody testing is still in a developmental stage. Those not prepared to put up with the problems of poorly standardized procedures would be wise to consult with reference or research laboratories working in this field. For additional discussion and from the perspective of immune thrombocytopenia see the listing Platelet Antibody *on page 258*.

References

Finley PR, Williams RJ, and Fletcher C, "Flow Cytometry Analysis of Platelet Antibodies," *J Clin Lab Anal*, 1988, 2:249-55.

George JN, "Platelet Immunoglobulin G: Its Significance for the Evaluation of Thrombocytopenia and for Understanding the Origin of α-Granule Proteins," *Blood*, 1990, 76(5):859-70.

McMillan R, "Clinical Role of Antiplatelet Antibody Assay," *Semin Thromb Hemost*, 1995, 21(1):37-45.

Rachel JM, Sinor LT, Tawfik OW, et al, "A Solid-Phase Red Cell Adherence Test for Platelet Cross-Matching," *Med Lab Sci*, 1985, 42(2):194-5.

von dem Borne AE and Décary F, "Nomenclature of Platelet-Specific Antigens," *Hum Immunol*, 1990, 29(1):1-2.

Platelet-Bound IgG, Direct *see Platelet Antibody, Immunohematologic on this page*

Platelet-Bound IgG, Indirect *see Platelet Antibody, Immunohematologic on this page*

Platelet Concentrate, Donation and Transfusion

CPT 36430 (transfusion); 36520 (donation); 86965 (pooling of platelets)

Related Information

Bleeding Time, Mielke *on page 234*

Filters for Blood *on page 609*

Irradiated Blood Components *on page 611*

Platelet Count *on page 340*

Platelets, Apheresis, Donation *on next page*

Synonyms Platelet Rich Plasma; Platelets; Platelet Transfusion; Pooled Platelets; Random Platelets

Test Commonly Includes ABO and Rh type

Abstract Platelet concentrate consists of platelets, suspended in about 50 mL of plasma, separated from whole blood collected from a single whole blood donation. It contains at least 5.5×10^{10} platelets; the average content should be about 7×10^{10}. Storage life is 5 days. It contains stable coagulation factors and labile factors V and VIII. The presence of these factors may be significant, since a common dose is about 1 concentrate per 10 kg body weight. Platelet apheresis concentrates contain at least 3×10^{11} platelets, with an average of 4×10^{11} or more. The dose is usually one concentrate per adult. The donor plasma should be ABO compatible with erythrocytes of the intended recipient, especially when the recipient is an infant.[1]

Patient Preparation Follow the usual transfusion identification procedures. It is not unusual for a platelet concentrate to have a pink tinge, indicating the presence of some RBCs. Despite this, a red cell crossmatch is not useful. If the patient is likely to receive many platelet transfusions, it is wise to have the patient HLA-typed early, in case platelet refractoriness occurs. **Dosage and administration:** In a bleeding adult with a platelet count <20,000/mm^3, 1 concentrate per 10 kg body weight is a good dose. Use special platelet filters if there is a need for a leukocyte-poor product. Use a 19-gauge needle or larger for administration. Give platelets rapidly, with an average of 10 minutes per platelet concentrate. Isotonic saline may be used to flush the container and filter. Do not warm platelets. Do not add any medications to platelet packs.

Aftercare Close clinical/nursing observation for bleeding, petechiae. **To evaluate efficacy of platelet transfusions, get a platelet count within 1 hour after the transfusions are completed.** This is useful in evaluating the response to platelet transfusions and in calculating the corrected count increment (CCI). The latter expresses the platelet increment per 10^{11} platelets transfused per meter of body surface area (BSA). Where post = post-transfusion platelet count x 10^3/mm^3; pre = pretransfusion platelet count; and PTx = number of platelets transfused (x 10^{11}).

Causes of Refractoriness to Platelet Transfusions

Nonimmune	Immune
Infection, sepsis, fever Hemorrhage, purpura, DIC Splenomegaly Antibiotic therapy Amphotericin B Bone marrow transplant	Alloimmunity; prior transfusions, pregnancy, HLA, platelet-specific ABO (uncommon)

$$CCI \times 10^3 = (post\text{-}pre) \times BSA/PTx$$

A value above 7.5 is usually considered satisfactory. Thus, a patient with a BSA of 1.5 m^2 receives 6 platelet concentrates with a total of 4.2×10^{11} platelets. The pre- and postcounts are 10×10^3 and 40×10^3 respectively.

$$CCI = (40 - 10) \times 1.5/4.2 = 10.7 \times 10^3$$

That would be considered a good response. This formula is not needed if the raw increment is zero or close to it, or if the response is obviously satisfactory. But it is helpful when the patient is small (eg, a child), or when the post counts appear to show small or moderate increments. Poor response to platelet transfusions (refractoriness) is common,[2] usually from nonimmune causes (see table). When refractoriness seems to be due to alloimmunization, then it will be necessary to change from regular platelet concentrates to single-donor platelets (platelets, apheresis) and perhaps to select donors according to HLA type. Alloimmunization to platelets seems to be largely caused by contaminating leukocytes in the concentrates and may be prevented by the removal of leukocytes by special filtration[3] (see Filters for Blood on page 609), or reduced experimentally by ultraviolet-B irradiation of platelet concentrates.

Selection of Platelets for Immune-Refractory Patients

1. Change from random (regular) platelets to single-donor.
2. Recruit blood relatives of patient as donors, if available.
3. HLA type patient, if possible.
4. Test patient for cytotoxic antibodies.
5. Test patient for platelet-specific antibodies.
6. Select platelet donors lacking antigens corresponding to any antibodies detected in steps 4 and 5, if feasible.
7. Check whether ABO compatibility affects outcome. Sometimes it does, especially type A platelets to an O patient.
8. Select donors by HLA type. The HLA does not have to be identical; a reasonable match by cross-reacting groups is usually as effective.
9. Recognize that this is a thorny problem. Any or all of the above may work, not necessarily in the order given; or none of them may be effective.

Specimen Blood

Container Red top tube

Storage Instructions Store at room temperature with continuous agitation for 5 days. Pooled platelets must be transfused within 4 hours after pooling.

Special Instructions May not be kept "on hold." When ordered, transfuse each platelet concentrate at once or it may have to be discarded. Do not refrigerate platelet concentrate.

Use Treatment of bleeding, petechiae, and ecchymoses when platelet count is <20,000/mm^3 or when platelets are functionally abnormal; prophylaxis against bleeding due to thrombocytopenia when platelet count is <20,000/mm^3, especially when platelet count is dropping; in splenectomy for ITP when abnormal bleeding occurs; in acute blood loss with platelet count <50,000/mm^3. Platelet apheresis concentrates can be used for any patient needing platelet transfusions. Single-donor platelets have the advantage of providing an entire platelet transfusion for an adult from one donor, hence with a single antigenic combination and a single donor exposure. Furthermore, the donor can be selected (eg, from a patient's relatives or by HLA type). Single-donor platelets are available from most blood centers and larger hospital blood banks on a more or less regular basis. Some institutions reserve them for patients who regularly receive platelet transfusions or who may be refractory to regular platelet transfusions.[2]

Limitations Hazards: As for transfusion of other blood components. Platelet concentrates always contain both red and white blood cells, so immunization to any of these antigens may occur. If feasible, Rh-negative girls and women younger than age 50 should receive Rh-negative platelets to avoid Rh immunization. Otherwise, consider giving them Rh immune globulin. The dosage can be calculated by knowing that regular platelet concentrates seldom contain more than 0.1 mL RBC each and single-donor platelets rarely more than 2 mL each. Although the ABO antigens are poorly developed on platelets, ABO-incompatible platelets

sometimes have decreased post-transfusion survival.[4] Immunosuppressed patients, and rarely immunocompetent patients, receiving platelets from closely related donors can suffer graft-versus-host disease; this is easily prevented by irradiation of platelet concentrates (see Irradiated Blood Components on page 611). Bacterial contamination and growth during storage are a real risk, as platelets are stored at room temperature.

Contraindications Not usually useful in idiopathic or immune thrombocytopenia, thrombotic thrombocytopenic purpura or certain stages of disseminated intravascular coagulation. Not to be used if bleeding is not caused by thrombocytopenia or abnormal platelet function. Microaggregate filters may remove platelets, but special leukocyte filters effectively remove leukocytes from platelet concentrates.[3]

Additional Information A platelet count of not less than 100,000/mm^3 is desirable for major surgery. One unit of platelet concentrate usually increases the platelet count of an adult with a blood volume of 5000 mL by about 5000/mm^3. Neonatal **alloimmune thrombocytopenia** may be treated with maternal platelet transfusions.

Alloimmune neonatal thrombocytopenia is usually caused by Pl^{A1} antigen inherited from the father by the baby, who then immunizes the mother so that she makes antibody to the baby's platelets (ie, anti-Pl^{A1}). The mother's platelet count is normal, but the baby's platelet count is low. It may not, however, be sufficiently low to cause symptoms, and so the diagnosis may be missed. The first born child may be affected.[5,6] The most serious complication is intracranial hemorrhage, which may occur during pregnancy, but the risk is probably greatest during delivery. If the diagnosis is made after delivery and the baby is unharmed, remember that later babies are also at risk.

For confirmatory diagnosis, send mother's serum and father's platelets (and the baby's if they can be obtained) to a reference laboratory for antibody test and selection of platelets for transfusion.

Treatment: The most convenient and readily available source of compatible platelets is the mother. A large number of platelets, relative to the baby's size, can be obtained by maternal platelet apheresis. Such platelets should last about 7 or 8 days in the baby. Platelet count should be checked daily. A further collection of platelets from the mother can be done if necessary.

Neonatal **autoimmune thrombocytopenia**, in which maternal thrombocytopenia occurs, is treated by steroids or exchange transfusion.

One thing to remember is that with each 10 units of platelets the patient will also receive 500 mL of fresh plasma (in which the platelets are suspended). This volume may need to be reduced for children.

Footnotes

1. Klein HG, Standards for Blood Banks and Transfusion Services, 16th ed, Bethesda, MD: American Association of Blood Banks, 1994, 13, 27.
2. Bishop JF, Matthews JP, McGrath K, et al, "The Definition of Refractoriness to Platelet Transfusions," Transfus Med, 1992, 2(1):35-41.
3. van Marwijk-Kooy M, van Prooijen HC, Borghuis L, et al, "Filtration. A Method to Prepare White Cell-Poor Platelet Concentrates With Optimal Preservation of Platelet Viability," Transfusion, 1990, 30(1):34-8.
4. Lee EJ and Schiffer CA, "ABO Compatibility Can Influence the Results of Platelet Transfusion. Results of a Randomized Trial," Transfusion, 1989, 29(5):384-9.
5. "Management of Alloimmune Neonatal Thrombocytopenia," Lancet, 1989, 1(8630):137-8.
6. Mueller-Eckhardt C, Grubert A, Weisheit M, et al, "348 Cases of Suspected Neonatal Alloimmune Thrombocytopenia," Lancet, 1989, 1(8634):363-7.

References

Buchanan GR, "Hematopoietic Diseases," Principles and Practice of Pediatrics, 2nd ed, Oski FA, DeAngelis CD, Feigin RD, et al, eds, Philadelphia, PA: JB Lippincott Co, 1994, 476-86.
Consensus Conference, "Platelet Transfusion Therapy," JAMA, 1987, 257(13):1777-80.
Gernsheimer T, Stratton J, Ballem PJ, et al, "Mechanisms of Response to Treatment in Autoimmune Thrombocytopenic Purpura," N Engl J Med, 1989, 320(15):974-80.
Kickler TS, Ness PM, and Braine HG, "Platelet Crossmatching: A Direct Approach to the Selection of Platelet Transfusions for the Alloimmunized Thrombocytopenic Patient," Am J Clin Pathol, 1988, 90(1):69-72.
Rachel JM, Summers TC, Sinor LT, et al, "Use of a Solid Phase Red Blood Cell Adherence Method for Pretransfusion Platelet Compatibility Testing," Am J Clin Pathol, 1988, 90(1):63-8.
Welch HG, Larson EB, and Slichter SJ, "Providing Platelets for Refractory Patients. Prudent Strategies," Transfusion, 1989, 29(3):193-5.

Plateletpheresis see Platelets, Apheresis, Donation on this page

Platelet Rich Plasma see Platelet Concentrate, Donation and Transfusion on previous page

Platelets see Platelet Concentrate, Donation and Transfusion on previous page

Platelets, Apheresis, Donation

CPT 36520

Related Information

Cytapheresis, Therapeutic on page 606
Platelet Antibody on page 258
(Continued)

Platelets, Apheresis, Donation *(Continued)*

Platelet Concentrate, Donation and Transfusion *on page 616*
Platelet Count *on page 340*

Synonyms Plateletpheresis; Platelets, Pheresis (FDA); Single-Donor Platelets

Test Commonly Includes Collection of platelets by cytapheresis, using a blood cell separator. Donor screening, blood typing, and testing for infectious diseases as routinely done in regular blood donation.

Storage Instructions Storage of platelets is in their native plasma, at 20°C to 24°C, with continuous gentle agitation. Do not refrigerate.

Causes for Rejection (Of donor): As for regular blood donation. A history of successful regular blood donation is the best qualifying criterion. Platelet concentrates that show any visible aggregation are not suitable for transfusion.

Special Instructions Single-donor platelets are available from most blood centers and larger hospital blood banks on a more or less regular basis. In many institutions they are reserved for patients who regularly receive platelet transfusions, or who may be refractory to regular platelet transfusions. Donors must not (within previous 3 days) have taken any medications that might adversely affect their platelets (eg, aspirin).

Use Single-donor platelets are suitable for any patient needing platelet transfusions. Single-donor platelets have the advantage of providing an entire platelet transfusion for an adult from one donor, hence with a single antigenic combination and a single donor exposure. Furthermore, the donor can be selected (eg, from a patient's relatives or by HLA type).

Limitations FDA guidelines recommend a maximum of 24 donations per year. This is undoubtedly too much for most donors. It is better to limit donations to the same frequency as regular blood donations (ie, every 2 months). In the case of specially selected donors for a particular patient (eg, relatives), donations can be as often as twice a week for limited periods, but this must be authorized on an individual basis by the Blood Bank physician, with careful monitoring of platelet counts and other variables. Reactions to platelet apheresis donation are given in the table.

Reactions Encountered in Hemapheresis Donations

Reaction	Prevention
Procedural reactions	
Vasovagal	Psychology; friendly, professional atmosphere
Hypovolemia	Avoid excessive extracorporeal volume
Hypervolemia	Control inflow to equal outflow
Citrate	Slow blood flow; decrease citrate proportion; use oral calcium or milk
Hemolysis	Avoid kinks in plastic tubing
Chills	Keep donors warm, use blood warmer
Allergy, anaphylaxis	Not avoidable, be prepared for immediate treatment
Reactions specific to leukapheresis*	
Hypervolemia, edema, skin manifestations, HES† accumulation	Avoid too frequent use of HES (eg, several times/week)
Steroid effect	Avoid excessive dosage and frequency
Perineal pain	Avoid filtration leukapheresis
Priapism	Avoid filtration leukapheresis
Complement activation	Avoid filtration leukapheresis
General reaction	
Donor burnout	Do not overuse donors; keep their interest in program; maintain a warm, friendly atmosphere

*Because of the additional risks to the donor in leukapheresis and the dubious value of transfused leukocytes in many situations, granulocyte transfusions should be given only on impeccable clinical indications.

†HES indicates hydroxyethyl starch.

From Huestis DW, "Risks and Safety Practices in Hemapheresis Procedures," *Arch Pathol Lab Med*, American Medical Association, 1989, 113:273-8, with permission.

Methodology Apheresis by continuous- or intermittent-flow centrifugation. Exact procedure depends on the separator used. Platelet apheresis differs from leukapheresis in that a macromolecular agent is not used and there is no need to stimulate the donor with steroids.

Additional Information Single-donor platelets are desirable because of the limitation in donor exposures. But regular platelets are entirely adequate for patients receiving platelets only once or twice (eg, surgical patients). Cancer or leukemia patients, who will receive many transfusions over a long time, may become refractory (ie, fail to show the expected response to regular platelets). Refractoriness has many causes, most of them nonimmune (see Causes for Refractoriness to

Platelet Transfusions in Platelet Concentrate, Donation and Transfusion *on page 617*). Patients with **nonimmune platelet refractoriness** are not likely to have a platelet count increase in response to any platelet transfusions. However, **immune refractoriness** sometimes responds to selection of platelet donors from among a patient's blood relatives, or by HLA type, or lacking an antigen corresponding to the patient's antibody. See table.

Selection of Platelets for Immune-Refractory Patients

1. Change from random (regular) platelets to single-donor.
2. Recruit blood relatives of patient as donors, if available.
3. HLA type patient, if possible.
4. Test patient for cytotoxic antibodies.
5. Test patient for platelet-specific antibodies.
6. Select platelet donors lacking antigens corresponding to any antibodies detected in steps 4 and 5, if feasible.
7. Check whether ABO compatibility affects outcome. Sometimes it does, especially type A platelets to an O patient.
8. Select donors by HLA type. The HLA does not have to be identical; a reasonable match by cross-reacting groups is usually as effective.
9. Recognize that this is a thorny problem. Any or all of the above may work, not necessarily in the order given; or none of them may be effective.

The technology of platelet apheresis is changing rapidly, with increasing emphasis on the reduction or virtual elimination of contaminating leukocytes.[1,2] The aim is to prevent immune refractoriness in patients who must receive repeated platelet transfusions.[2] In the face of existing immune refractoriness, ABO[3] and HLA selection are options. Platelet crossmatching is still a developing field.[4]

Footnotes

1. van Marwijk Kooy M, van Prooijen HC, et al, "Use of Leukocyte-Depleted Platelet Concentrations for the Prevention of Refractoriness and Primary HLA Alloimmunization: A Prospective, Randomized Trial," *Blood*, 1991, 77(1):201-5.
2. Schiffer CA, "Prevention of Alloimmunization Against Platelets," *Blood*, 1991, 77(1):1-4.
3. "ABO Incompatibility and Platelet Transfusion," *Lancet*, 1990, 335(8682):142-3.
4. Kieckbusch ME, Moore SB, Koenig VA, et al, "Platelet Crossmatch Evaluation in Refractory Hematologic Patients," *Mayo Clin Proc*, 1987, 62(7):595-600.

References

"Consensus Conference. Platelet Transfusion Therapy," *JAMA*, 1987, 257(13):1777-85.
McCullough J, Steeper TA, Connelly DP, et al, "Platelet Utilization in a University Hospital," *JAMA*, 1988, 259(16):2414-8.
Slichter SJ, "Controversies in Platelet Transfusion Therapy," *Annu Rev Med*, 1980, 31:509-40.

Platelets, Pheresis (FDA) *see* Platelets, Apheresis, Donation *on previous page*

Platelet Transfusion *see* Platelet Concentrate, Donation and Transfusion *on page 616*

Pooled Platelets *see* Platelet Concentrate, Donation and Transfusion *on page 616*

Prenatal Screen, Immunohematology

CPT 86880 (antiglobulin test, direct); 86885 (antiglobulin test, indirect); 86900 (ABO); 86901 (D^u); 86901 (Rh(D))

Related Information

Amniotic Fluid Analysis for Erythroblastosis Fetalis (OD 450) *on page 76*
Antibody Titer *on page 601*
Antiglobulin Test, Indirect *on page 602*
Cord Blood Screen *on page 605*
D^u *on page 608*
Kleihauer-Betke *on page 329*

Synonyms Prenatal Serologic Testing

Test Commonly Includes Initial screen: ABO, Rh, D^u if D-negative; antibody screen (indirect antiglobulin test), antibody identification (panel) when screen is positive.

Patient Preparation Do prenatal screen at the initial visit in all pregnant women. Multiparity and/or history of prior transfusion are factors that indicate a need to follow antibody screens more closely. In patients with antibody, coordinate titers with possible amniocentesis. It is not usually necessary to do titrations and repeat testing in the case of antibodies that are predominantly IgM or otherwise not clinically significant (eg, Lewis, P, or cold autoagglutinins). American College of Obstetrics and Gynecology recommends ABO and Rh type and antibody screen as early as practical and repeat screens at 28, 32, and 36 weeks if subject is D-negative and not immunized to Rh$_o$(D).[1,2]

Specimen Blood

Container Red top tube

Causes for Rejection Improperly labeled tube, gross hemolysis

Reference Range Indirect antiglobulin test (antibody screen): negative

Use Prenatal screen for possible maternal-fetal blood incompatibility, to identify women at risk of having a baby affected by hemolytic disease of the newborn and to try to predict risk to the fetus. Rh and D^u to work up for possible administration of Rh immune globulin. Do a D^u on all apparently Rh-negative women. Should a prenatal patient be shown to be D^u-negative, but then immediately after delivery appear D^u-positive, an extremely important observation has been made. There may be massive fetal-maternal bleeding from an Rh-positive baby. Do a Kleihauer-Betke stain.

Limitations Will not detect all maternal-fetal incompatibilities or all antibodies present in a patient's serum

Methodology Antibody screening including antiglobulin testing. Titrate IgG-type antibodies known to be associated with hemolytic disease of the newborn.

Additional Information Antibody screen is commonly done for obstetric patients, including those with incomplete abortion or with ectopic pregnancy, and those possibly requiring transfusion. Rh-negative women with miscarriage or ectopic pregnancy are candidates for Rh immune globulin.

Footnotes
1. Huestis DW, Bove JR, and Case J, *Practical Blood Transfusion*, 4th ed, Boston, MA: Little, Brown and Co, 1988, 352-3.
2. "The Selective Use of Rh$_o$(D) Immune Globulin (RhIG)," *ACOG Technical Bulletin Update*, November, 1983.

Prenatal Serologic Testing *see* Prenatal Screen, Immunohematology *on previous page*

Prenatal Testing *see* D^u *on page 608*

Prenatal Testing *see* Rh Genotype *on page 622*

Pretransfusion Testing

CPT 86880 (antiglobulin test, direct); 86886 (antiglobulin test, indirect); 86900 (ABO); 86901 (Rh(D)); 86922 (compatibility test, each unit, antiglobulin)

Related Information
Antibody Identification, Red Cell *on page 601*
Antiglobulin Test, Direct *on page 602*
Antiglobulin Test, Indirect *on page 602*
Rh Genotype *on page 622*
Risks of Transfusion *on page 623*
Uncrossmatched Blood, Emergency *on page 627*

Applies to ABO Group and Rh Type; Blood Grouping and Rh Typing; Rh$_o$(D) Typing; Type and Crossmatch; Type and Screen

Test Commonly Includes ABO group, Rh typing, antibody screen (indirect antiglobulin test), crossmatch, and "type and screen"

Patient Preparation Patient should have a wristband or other positive written identification on the body. This must be physically attached to the body, not on the wall or the bed or clipped to the chart.

Specimen Blood

Container Red top tube, lavender top (EDTA) tube

Collection At the patient's bedside, ask the patient to give his or her name. Compare with the hospital wristband. Label the Blood Bank wristband (if there is one) with the patient's full name, hospital number, date, and initials of the collector. Label sample tube with the same information, including identification number from the wristband. Label requisition form with identification number. The collector signs the requisition, verifying the patient's identity with hospital wristband and Blood Bank wristband. Some hospitals require additional information. It is always best to stamp the requisition with the patient's identification plate to avoid transcription errors. Take extra care with identification of unresponsive patients.

Causes for Rejection Gross hemolysis, sample placed in a serum separator tube, specimen tube not properly labeled

Timetable For Obtaining Emergency Blood From Blood Bank

Time Available (approx minutes)	Blood Bank Can Issue	Extent of Testing Done
<5	Type O RBCs, Rh-neg if possible	None
5-10	RBCs of patient's own ABO and Rh types	Patient's ABO and Rh typing, no crossmatch
15	Crossmatched ABO and Rh-specific RBCs, unexpected IgG antibody not ruled out	ABO and Rh typing, crossmatch,* no antibody screen
45-60†	Serologically compatible RBCs	Full pretransfusion testing, including antibody screen

*Assuming 'immediate-spin' crossmatch
†Assuming no unexpected antibody detected

Turnaround Time In life-threatening emergencies, type O RBCs can be issued immediately to patients whose blood type is unknown. See listing Uncrossmatched Blood, Emergency *on page 627*. But the more complete the pretransfusion testing, the safer the transfusion. In emergencies, blood bank can issue blood at any stage of testing. The time requirements are shown in the table.

Use Determine patient's blood type to enable blood selection before transfusion; detect and, if necessary, identify any unexpected blood group antibodies; detect any incompatibility in donor units before transfusion. ABO, Rh, and antibody screen are also used in prenatal testing of pregnant women to detect maternal-fetal incompatibility that might cause fetal hemolytic disease.

Limitations Abnormal plasma proteins, cold autoagglutinins, positive direct antiglobulin test, and in some cases, bacteremia may interfere. These tests do not assure normal red cell survival, will not detect all antibodies or incompatibilities, do not prevent all transfusion reactions, and do not prevent reactions to blood components other than red cells. Clerical and technical competence is requisite. A great many pitfalls exist, which may cause false-positive or false-negative reactions.

Contraindications See listing Risks of Transfusion *on page 623*.

Methodology Serologic pretransfusion procedures involve separation of serum and RBCs from the patient's blood and subsequent testing of the RBCs with known standardized antiserums, and the serum against suspensions of reagent RBCs of known antigenic composition. These procedures and reagents are common to ABO and Rh typing, to testing of the serum for the presence of unexpected blood group antibodies, and to compatibility testing (crossmatching). All such reagents and procedures are FDA licensed and subject to review and inspection by the FDA and various accrediting agencies. Methods vary according to the reagents and equipment in use; testing may be on glass slides, in test tubes, or by a variety of automated systems. If the laboratory uses a computer for recording test results or for tracking of patients and donor blood components, the program must be appropriately validated to make sure it functions as expected.

ABO typing consists of testing the patient's RBCs with reagent anti-A and anti-B, and usually also anti-AB (type O serum) as a confirmatory procedure. An additional confirmation consists of "reverse grouping," (ie, testing the patient's serum against known A$_1$ and B reagent RBCs).

Rh typing is done by testing RBCs with anti-Rh$_o$(D) as a routine. The term "Rh-positive" (or "Rh-negative") refers only to the presence or absence of Rh$_o$(D). This is the most important antigen of the Rh system. Do not be concerned about the numerous other antigens unless the patient is immunized to one of them (which would usually become apparent from the results of the antibody screen or crossmatch).

As a rule, the Blood Bank issues blood of the patient's own ABO and Rh types. But some leeway is permissible; see table. When difficulties occur in blood selection, consultation will be necessary between the Blood Bank physician and the patient's physician.

Selection of Donor Blood for Transfusion to Recipients of Various ABO and Rh Types

Patient Blood Type	First Choice	Second Choice	Third Choice
O pos	O pos	O neg	None
O neg	O neg	None	O pos
A pos	A pos	A neg	O pos, O neg
A neg	A neg	None	O neg, O pos, A pos
B pos	B pos	B neg	O pos, O neg
B neg	B neg	None	O neg, O pos, B pos
AB pos	AB pos	AB neg, A pos, B pos, A neg, B neg	O pos, O neg
AB neg	AB neg	A neg, B neg	O neg, AB pos, A pos, B pos, O pos

Note: The technologist may always substitute Rh-negative donor RBC for Rh-positive patients, if supplies permit. Physician approval is required for third choice donor blood selection in the event that first and second choice are unavailable. In the case of using A or B for AB, it is either A or B for one patient, not both to the same patient, and before changing the blood type the Blood Bank physician must approve. In this table, "pos" and "neg" refer to Rh-positive and Rh-negative respectively.

Antibody screen: (See listing Antiglobulin Test, Indirect *on page 602*.) This is the procedure used for detecting unexpected IgG antibodies in the serum of a patient before transfusion and for identifying any such antibodies. A negative antibody screen means there is no IgG antibody reacting in the test conditions with the reagent red cells used. The test is (Continued)

Pretransfusion Testing *(Continued)*

not perfect. It can miss weak antibodies and those reacting with antigens not present on the test red cells.

A positive result requires identification of antibody before blood is issued for transfusion. That in turn may require selection of donor units negative for the offending antigen before crossmatching. On the other hand, the test may be positive because of technical interference or irrelevant antibodies that do not cause transfusion reactions. The Blood Bank can resolve such problems.

Basically, the antibody screen is like a crossmatch but uses a selected RBC substrate (type O reagent red blood cells for antibody detection) instead of donor red cells.

Crossmatch: (See listings Antiglobulin Test, Indirect *on page 602* and Uncrossmatched Blood, Emergency *on page 627.*) The crossmatch tests patient serum directly against donor RBCs. Except for the test red cells, it is like an antibody screen. The crossmatch may include various techniques including the indirect antiglobulin test. It must be able to detect clinically significant antibodies.

Alternative method: Since 1984, AABB standards have allowed a crossmatch that is suitable for the detection only of ABO incompatibility (eg, only an immediate spin, without 37°C or antiglobulin phases). Such a crossmatch is acceptable only if:

- the antibody screen includes 37°C and antiglobulin phases
- the reagent red cells are not pooled
- the antibody screen has not detected a clinically significant antibody (see table in Antibody Identification, Red Cell *on page 601*)
- the patient has no record of previous detection of such antibodies.[1]

Because delays in reading such abbreviated crossmatches may permit hemolysis, which is hard to see, it is probably wise to add EDTA to the saline used to suspend the donor RBCs.[2,3]

Increasingly, larger hospitals are using this alternative method because it greatly lessens the amount of laboratory work per unit at little or no increase in risk.[4] For example, crossmatching four units of blood requires four immediate spins for the crossmatch and three or four antiglobulins for the antibody screen by this alternative, as opposed to six or seven indirect antiglobulins the other way. So far, experience supports the safety of the simplified procedure. The real danger in transfusion is ABO incompatibility, not missing an antibody to some low-incidence antigen that is missing from the screening cells.

Some Operations for Which Routine Crossmatching Is Unnecessary and for Which a Type and Screen Can Usually Be Substituted Safely

General Surgery	Face lift*
Anal fissure or fistula repair*	Rhinoplasty*
Appendectomy*	Skin graft (excluding major burns)
Breast biopsy*	
Cholecystectomy	**Gynecology**
Colostomy or closure	Dilation and curettage, with or without conization
Exploratory laparotomy	
Gastroenterostomy	Exploratory laparotomy for infertility
Hemorrhoidectomy*	
Inguinal, femoral or hiatal hernia repair*	Hysterectomy, abdominal or vaginal
Parathyroid excision or exploration	Ovarian cystectomy
	Tuboplasty
Pilonidal cystectomy	Vaginal plastic procedures
Polypectomy	
Pyloroplasty	**Obstetrics**
Sympathectomy	Cesarean section
Thyroidectomy	
Vein stripping	**Neurosurgery**
	Cordotomy
Urology	Hypophysectomy
Ileal conduit	Nerve repair
Marshall-Marchetti procedure	Shunt surgery
Nephrostomy	Sympathectomy
Open biopsy of prostate	
Penile prosthesis	**Orthopedics**
Pyelolithotomy	Knee surgery
Transurethral prostatectomy	Leg amputation
Transurethral resection of bladder tumor	Meniscectomy
	Most open reductions
Ureterolithotomy	Osteotomy or biopsy of bone
Plastic Surgery	Removal of hip pin
Augmentation mammoplasty	Shoulder reconstruction

*In these operations, even the type and screen is usually unnecessary.
From Huestis DW, Bove JR, and Busch S, *Practical Blood Transfusion*, 3rd ed, Boston, MA: Little, Brown and Co, 1981, 236, with permission.

The **electronic or computer crossmatch** is something relatively new. Not a serologic test at all, it is rather a computer match of donor and recipient ABO and Rh types.[5] As such, it is intended to substitute for the immediate-spin crossmatch. With specific precautions, the electronic crossmatch is acceptable to accrediting agencies.

Patients with known or historic unexpected blood group antibodies require a complete serologic crossmatch including the antiglobulin phase. Neither electronic nor immediate-spin crossmatches will suffice for them.

Type and screen: When a patient is undergoing a procedure or treatment in which transfusion is very unlikely, it is wasteful to crossmatch blood and put it aside for that patient. Instead, the type and screen includes ABO and Rh typing and an antibody screen.[6] If this screen is negative and hemorrhage occurs, the Blood Bank may issue blood of the patient's type immediately, without awaiting the crossmatch. Of course, if an unexpected antibody turns up in the type and screen, a crossmatch becomes necessary, and the patient's physician is alerted to the situation beforehand. See table for procedures in which Type and Screen is appropriate.

ADL: Allow additional time for patients known to be immunized to red cell antigens. Unanticipated problems can occur with antibody reidentification and selection of blood of appropriate phenotype. Patients receiving a series of transfusions are at risk of forming red cell antibodies. For this reason, *Standards* require a new blood sample and repeat antibody screening every 3 days.

Footnotes
1. Klein HG, *Standards for Blood Banks and Transfusion Services*, 16th ed, Bethesda, MD: American Association of Blood Banks, 1994, 25-9.
2. Shulman IA and Kent D, "Safety in Transfusion Practice. Is It Safe to Eliminate the Major Crossmatch for Selected Patients?" *Arch Pathol Lab Med*, 1989, 113(3):270-2.
3. Shulman IA and Calderon C, "Effect of Delayed Centrifugation or Reading on the Detection of ABO Incompatibility by the Immediate-Spin Crossmatch," *Transfusion*, 1991, 31(3):197-200.
4. Cordle DG, Strauss RG, Snyder EL, et al, "Safety and Cost-Containment Data That Advocate Abbreviated Pretransfusion Testing," *Am J Clin Pathol*, 1990, 94(4):428-31.
5. Leparc GF, "Electronic Crossmatch. Transfusion Service's New Frontier," *Lab Med*, 1994, 25(12):781-3.
6. Mintz PD, Henry JB, and Boral LI, "The Type and Antibody Screen," *Clin Lab Med*, 1982, 2:169-80.

Progenitor Cells *see* Peripheral Blood Stem Cells, Autologous *on page 613*

Prognosis for Rh Hemolytic Disease of Newborn *see* Rh Genotype *on page 622*

Prothrombin Complex Concentrates *see* Factor IX Complex (Human) *on page 609*

Quality Assurance, Transfusion

Synonyms Quality Control

Applies to Transfusion Review Committee

Test Commonly Includes Peer professional review of clinical transfusion practices

Abstract Physicians practicing in hospitals and using blood services are likely to find their transfusion practices monitored by the institutional Transfusion Review Committee. This is a requirement of the Joint Commission on Accreditation of Healthcare Organizations (JCAHO). The commission requires detailed records of review of transfusion practices, including indications, single-unit transfusions, transfusion reactions, clinical effectiveness, and other aspects. The JCAHO Accreditation Manual for Hospitals covers blood usage and criteria for transfusion in its sections on medical staff, pathology and clinical laboratory services, surgical and anesthesia services, emergency services, special care units, and quality assessment and improvement. Blood Banks and Transfusion Services are also inspected by the Commission on Laboratory Accreditation of the College of American Pathologists and American Association of Blood Banks voluntary peer review programs,[1] the FDA, and by some state agencies.

Use Close peer review of all transfusions of blood and components is a fact of modern hospital practice. Maintenance of perfusion, need for replacement in acute hemorrhage, as well as arterial oxygenation, cardiac output, and blood volume are relevant. Many current publications address indications for transfusion. Hemoglobin level <8 g/dL and hematocrit <24% with clinical signs and symptoms of anemia usually justifies red blood cell transfusion. Use of whole blood, platelets, cryoprecipitate, and fresh frozen plasma is monitored by the transfusion committee.[2] However, the important thing is the patient's clinical status; emphasis upon hemoglobin and other laboratory test results, with insufficient bedside assessment, leads to transfusion overuse.[3]

Additional Information Current concern over the adverse effects of transfusion and the cost of medical care, as well as the current litigious climate in blood transfusion, all justify an important role for quality assurance procedures. A casual attitude to the use of blood is no longer acceptable. The physician must not only follow established guidelines in blood transfusion but must also include in every patient's clinical records the rationale for using blood or its components in the existing circumstances.

Footnotes

1. Klein HG, *Standards for Blood Banks and Transfusion Services*, 16th ed, Bethesda, MD: American Association of Blood Banks, 1994.
2. Silberstein LE, Kruskall MS, Stehling LC, et al, "Strategies for the Review of Transfusion Practices," *JAMA*, 1989, 262(14):1993-7.
3. Carmel R and Shulman IA, "Blood Transfusion in Medically Treatable Chronic Anemia. Pernicious Anemia as a Model for Transfusion Overuse," *Arch Pathol Lab Med*, 1989, 113(9):995-7.

References

Blanchette VS, Hume HA, Levy GJ, et al, "Guidelines for Auditing Pediatric Blood Transfusion Practices," *Am J Dis Child*, 1991, 145(7):787-96.
Carson JL, Poses RM, Spence RK, et al, "Severity of Anemia and Operative Mortality and Morbidity," *Lancet*, 1988, 1(8588):727-9.
"Consensus Conference. Fresh Frozen Plasma Indications and Risks," *JAMA*, 1985, 253(4):551-3.
"Consensus Conference. Perioperative Red Blood Cell Transfusion," *JAMA*, 1988, 260(18):2700-3.
"Consensus Conference. Platelet Transfusion Therapy," *JAMA*, 1987, 257(13):1777-80.
Goldman RL, "The Reliability of Peer Assessments of Quality of Care," *JAMA*, 1992, 267(7):958-60.
Goodnough LT, Johnston MF, Ramsey G, et al, "Guidelines for Transfusion Support in Patients Undergoing Coronary Artery Bypass Grafting," *Ann Thorac Surg*, 1990, 50(4):675-83.
Grindon AJ, Tomasulo PA, Bergin JJ, et al, "The Hospital Transfusion Committee. Guidelines for Improving Practice," *JAMA*, 1985, 253(4):540-3.
Mozes B, Epstein M, Ben-Bassat I, et al, "Evaluation of the Appropriateness of Blood and Blood Product Transfusion Using Preset Criteria," *Transfusion*, 1989, 29(6):473-6.
Salem-Schatz SR, Avorn J, and Soumerai SB, "Influence of Clinical Knowledge, Organizational Context, and Practice Style on Transfusion Decision Making," *JAMA*, 1990, 264(4):471-5.
van Schoonhoven P, Berkman EM, and Lehmann R, *Medical Staff Monitoring Functions-Blood Usage Review*, Fromberg Ed, ed, Chicago, IL: JCAHO, 1987.
Welch HG, Meehan KR, and Goodnough LT, "Prudent Strategies for Elective Red Blood Cell Transfusion," *Ann Intern Med*, 1992, 116(5):393-402.

Quality Control *see* Quality Assurance, Transfusion *on previous page*

Random Platelets *see* Platelet Concentrate, Donation and Transfusion *on page 616*

Red Blood Cells

CPT 36430 (transfusion); 86880 (antiglobulin test, direct); 86885 (antiglobulin test, indirect); 86900 (ABO); 86901 (Rh(D)); 86922 (compatibility test, each unit, antiglobulin)

Related Information

Cold Agglutinin Titer *on page 384*
Filters for Blood *on page 609*
Hematocrit *on page 322*
Hemoglobin *on page 323*
Risks of Transfusion *on page 623*
Whole Blood *on page 627*

Synonyms Packed Red Cells, Transfusion

Applies to Donor Blood Transfusion

Test Commonly Includes A unit of red blood cells has a volume of 230-350 mL. ABO and Rh type, antibody screen, crossmatch, antibody identification when screen is positive (ie, preparation as for other transfusions). Red cells have a hematocrit of approximately 55% to 70% and contain the same mass of red cells as does a unit of whole blood, approximately 200 mL. The expiration date with CPDA-1 anticoagulant is 35 days after the date of collection, when stored continuously between 1°C to 6°C until transfused. With additional adenine supplementation after removal of plasma, AS-1 red blood cells have a hematocrit of 55% to 60% and a storage period of 42 days at 1°C to 6°C. If the hermetic seal is broken during preparation, the red blood cells must be infused within 24 hours or discarded. Storage intervals are those approved by the FDA.

Patient Preparation The patient should have an identification wristband. ER may use special or temporary identification. **Dosage and administration:** Give red cells through a standard 170 micron filter. Most transfusions should not exceed 4 hours duration; 2 hours or less per unit is preferable. Speed up the infusion by adding 50-100 mL of sterile isotonic sodium chloride solution, USP, just before administration.[1] **Do not add or transfuse with lactated Ringer's solution, 5% aqueous dextrose, 5% dextrose in 0.225% saline, or other calcium-containing, hypotonic, or glucose-containing fluids through the same tubing because clumping, hemolysis, or clotting may occur.**[1] Drugs or medications may **not** be added to blood or blood components.

Aftercare One unit should raise the hematocrit of an adult about 4 percentage points. Monitor hemoglobin and hematocrit.

Specimen Blood

Container Red top tube

Collection (Of sample from intended recipient): At the patient's bedside, ask the patient to give his or her name. Compare with the hospital wristband. Label the Blood Bank wristband (if there is one) with the patient's full name, hospital number, date, and initials of the collector. Label sample tube with the same information, including identification number from the wristband. Label requisition form with identification number. The collector signs the requisition, verifying the patient's identity with hospital wristband and Blood Bank wristband. Some hospitals require additional information. It is always best to stamp the requisition with the patient's identification plate to avoid transcription errors. Take extra care with identification of unresponsive patients.

Storage Instructions Store in Blood Bank monitored refrigerator only until issue. When it is not possible to transfuse immediately after issue, return blood to Blood Bank within approximately 30 minutes. Otherwise, blood that has been out of monitored refrigeration must be discarded. Appropriate refrigeration includes specified conditions which include temperature recorders and audible signals.[2] These conditions are regularly intensely inspected by regulatory agencies.

Causes for Rejection (Of patient sample): Gross hemolysis, sample placed in a serum separator tube, specimen tube not properly labeled

Turnaround Time Red blood cells can be ready for transfusion within 30-45 minutes from the time the Blood Bank gets the type and crossmatch sample, if blood of the appropriate type is on hand. Presence of unexpected antibodies may require hours to a day or two for identification.

Special Instructions Blood banks and hospital transfusion services hold crossmatched blood only for 24 hours after which they make it available for other patients. There will be some exceptions. Notify the Blood Bank as soon as possible if the patient will not need transfusion so the blood can be used for some other patient.

Use Replace red cell volume;[3] provide oxygen transport; transfusion of patients with heart, liver, or renal disease in whom restriction of plasma volume or of sodium may be desirable, eg, to decrease the likelihood of volume overload (as compared with effect of whole blood); transfusion of patients with chronic anemias; replace blood lost in surgical operations. Type O RBCs may be given in emergencies to recipients of unknown ABO type (RBCs have less anti-A and anti-B than whole blood). Indications for transfusion include maintenance of perfusion, arterial oxygenation, cardiac output, and blood volume. Hemoglobin <8 g/dL with signs and symptoms of anemia usually justifies transfusion, but in some patients with chronic anemia, hemoglobin of 7 g/dL or even less may provide adequate oxygen carrying capacity.[4,5]

Limitations Red cells prepared in an "open" system expire in 24 hours. Most RBCs, however, are prepared in closed systems with full dating. RBCs often have a slow flow rate, which can be speeded up by adding 50-100 mL of isotonic saline to the bag.

Contraindications Surgeons and many other physicians have been casual in the use of RBCs. With the AIDS epidemic and increasing knowledge of the risks of transfusion, as well as Transfusion Committee surveillance, a casual attitude to transfusion is no longer acceptable. Do not give blood transfusion when anemia and/or hypoxia can be corrected with specific and safer therapy such as iron, B_{12}, or folic acid. For correction of coagulation deficiencies, specific fractions are appropriate. Do not add medications to blood for transfusion; many are incompatible with stored blood.

Additional Information Red blood cells must be ABO and Rh compatible. A crossmatch is necessary unless life-threatening urgency exists. See listing Risks of Transfusion *on page 623*. Advantage of RBCs as compared with whole blood is greater safety in treatment of patients likely to suffer complications of volume excess.

Footnotes

1. *Circular of Information for the Use of Human Blood and Blood Components*, American Red Cross, Council of Community Blood Centers, American Association of Blood Banks, 1992.
2. Klein HG, *Standards for Blood Banks and Transfusion Services*, 16th ed, Bethesda, MD: American Association of Blood Banks, 1994, 18.
3. Consensus Conference, "Perioperative Red Blood Cell Transfusion," *JAMA*, 1988, 260(18):2700-3.
4. "Use of Blood Components," *FDA Drug Bulletin*, 1989, 19:14-5.
5. Viele MK and Weiskopf RB, "What Can We Learn About the Need for Transfusion From Patients Who Refuse Blood? The Experience With Jehovah's Witnesses," *Transfusion*, 1994, 34(5):396-401.

References

Carson JL, Poses RM, Spence RK, et al, "Severity of Anemia and Operative Mortality and Morbidity," *Lancet*, 1988, 1(8588):727-9.
Walker RH, *Technical Manual*, 11th ed, Arlington, VA: American Association of Blood Banks, 1993.

Red Blood Cells, Deglycerolized *see* Frozen Red Blood Cells *on page 610*

Red Blood Cells, Frozen *see* Frozen Red Blood Cells *on page 610*

Red Blood Cells, Washed

CPT 36430 (transfusion); 86985 (splitting of blood products)

Related Information

Filters for Blood *on page 609*

Ham Test *on page 320*

Synonyms Washed Blood Cells

Applies to Transfusion Reaction, Allergic; Transfusion Reaction, Febrile

Test Commonly Includes ABO and Rh type, antibody screen, cross-match, and antibody identification when screen is positive, as for other transfusions. Hematocrit is 65% to 85%.[1] Expiration date is 24 hours from washing.

Patient Preparation Patient should have an identification wristband.

Aftercare Same as for other RBC transfusions.

Specimen Blood

Container One red top tube and one lavender top (EDTA) tube

Collection Of sample from intended recipient: Same as for other RBC transfusions.

Causes for Rejection (Of patient sample): Gross hemolysis, sample placed in a serum separator tube, specimen tube not properly labeled

Turnaround Time Allow about 1 hour after selection of compatible red cells.

Special Instructions Must be used within 24 hours after preparation.

Use Reduction of likelihood of febrile transfusion reaction in patients with history of febrile transfusion reactions. Useful also for patients who have severe allergic reaction to conventional transfusion. Prevention of transfusion reaction to plasma proteins, especially IgA, in patients with IgA immunoglobulin deficiency. Washed red cells are usually used for patients with paroxysmal nocturnal hemoglobinuria (PNH) although some believe this to be a myth.[2] It would seem prudent to use leukocyte-poor red cells for transfusion of patients with PNH[3] and if precautions to avoid reactions resulting in activation of complement cannot be taken, use of saline-washed red cells should be considered.[4]

Limitations High outdating rate (24 hours). Cannot be ordered "on hold." Time consuming and expensive. There is up to 20% loss of red cells.

Methodology Various methods are available. The best is probably a system using a continuous-flow centrifuge and 2-3 L of isotonic saline per unit.

Additional Information This component is comparable to deglycerolized red blood cells, from which 99% of WBCs are removed. The washing process removes most of the plasma proteins, fibrinogen, fibrin, potassium, citrate, ammonia, microaggregates, platelets and leukocytes, including lymphocytes.[3] The effectiveness of washing depends on the method and on the volume of isotonic saline used. Red cells have been shown to have normal survival after washing. See also Filters for Blood *on page 609*. Use of washed RBCs is giving way to leukocyte filters for removal of WBCs, but washed cells are still appropriate for patients who have repeated allergic reactions or who have anti-IgA. Washing RBCs is not satisfactory for the prevention of graft-versus-host disease.

Footnotes

1. *Circular of Information for the Use of Human Blood and Blood Components*, American Red Cross, Council of Community Blood Centers, American Association of Blood Banks, 1992.
2. Brecher ME and Taswell HF, "Paroxysmal Nocturnal Hemoglobinuria and the Transfusion of Washed Red Cells. A Myth Revisited," *Transfusion*, 1989, 29(8):681-5.
3. Mollison PL, Engelfriet CP, and Contreras M, *Blood Transfusion in Clinical Medicine*, 9th ed, Oxford, UK: Blackwell Scientific Publications, 1993, 507.
4. Rosse WF, "Transfusion in Paroxysmal Nocturnal Hemoglobinuria - To Wash or Not to Wash?" *Transfusion*, 1989, 29(8):663-4.

Red Cell Antigen Typing *see* Antibody Identification, Red Cell *on page 601*

Red Cell Exchange *see* Cytapheresis, Therapeutic *on page 606*

Rh *see* D^u *on page 608*

Rh Genotype

CPT 86906

Related Information

Cord Blood Screen *on page 605*

D^u *on page 608*

Pretransfusion Testing *on page 619*

Rh$_o$(D) Immune Globulin (Human) *on next page*

Synonyms Zygosity, Rh

Applies to Prenatal Testing; Prognosis for Rh Hemolytic Disease of Newborn

Test Commonly Includes Rh typing of male partners of pregnant, Rh-immunized women. Testing of RBCs with anti-Rh$_o$(D), -rh'(C), -hr'(c), -rh"(E), and sometimes anti-hr"(e).

Causes for Rejection Hemolyzed blood sample

Special Instructions Some antiserums may be hard to get. Antiserums may contain extraneous antibodies brought out by different techniques,

so use them strictly according to the manufacturer's instructions. For interpretation, get clinical data including ethnic group of subject and whether woman is Rh-immunized.

Reference Range Frequencies of various Rh phenotypes and genotypes vary significantly in different ethnic groups.[1] Most of the published data are for whites of European descent (see table), so make allowance for other ethnic groups.

Frequencies of the More Common Rh-Positive Genotypes

Phenotype		Genotype		Genotype Frequency in the Total Population (%)	Likelihood of Zygosity (%)*	
CDE	Rh	CDE	Rh		Homozygous	Heterozygous
DCce	Rh$_1$ rh	DCe/dce	R^1 r	32.0	6	94
		DCe/Dce	R^1 R^0	2.0		
DCe	Rh$_1$ Rh$_1$	DCe/DCe	R^1 R^1	17.0	96	4
		DCe/dCe	R^1 r'	0.8		
DcEe	Rh$_2$ rh	DcE/dce	R^2 r	11.0	6	94
		DcE/Dce	R^2 R^0	0.7		
DcE	Rh$_2$ Rh$_2$	DcE/DcE	R^2 R^2	2.0	86	14
		DcE/dcE	R^2 r"	0.3		
DCcEe	Rh$_z$	DCe/DcE	R^1 R^2	12.0	89	11
		DCe/dcE	R^1 r"	1.0		
		dCe/DcE	r'R^2	0.3		
		DCE/dce	R^z r	0.2		
Dce	Rh$_0$	Dce/dce	R^0 r	2.0	3	97
		Dce/Dce	R^0 R^0	0.07		

*The figures given are for the random white population. Among blacks, the Dce (R^0) gene is much more common, which will greatly increase the probability of homozygosity, most particularly when the phenotype is DCce (Rh$_1$ rh), DcEe (Rh$_2$ rh), or Dce (Rh$_0$).

From Huestis DW, Bove JR, and Case J, *Practical Blood Transfusion*, 4th ed, Boston, MA: Little, Brown and CO, 1988, 97, with permission.

Limitations Genotype frequencies are given for random populations. Remember that the husbands of Rh-immunized women are a loaded population, with a higher incidence of homozygosity.[2] On the other hand, if any of the children of an Rh-positive/Rh-negative couple is Rh-negative, or if either of the husband's parents is Rh-negative, the husband must be heterozygous.

Methodology Determine the husband's Rh phenotype with the serums mentioned above. Once the phenotype is known, determine the most likely corresponding genotype (and thus the likelihood of homozygosity versus heterozygosity) by consulting a table of known genotype frequencies (such as the table given here).

Additional Information When a woman of childbearing age has Rh antibody, it is important for prognostic purposes to know whether the husband is homozygous or heterozygous for the gene determining D. An infant whose father is homozygous will be Rh-positive, but half the babies of a heterozygous man will be Rh-negative. The D genotype must be estimated indirectly, there being no detectable allele of D. One can usually determine the zygosity for Rh factors other than D directly by testing with appropriate serums. For example, in the case of hemolytic disease due to anti-c, if the husband's red cells are positive for both C and c, then he is heterozygous for c. If his cells are negative for C, then he is probably homozygous. There are occasional exceptions. In reporting, it is always wise to express the conclusion as "probable genotype". Mathematical odds can be given to support the conclusion.

Footnotes

1. Mourant AE, Kopec A, and Domaniewska-Sobczak K, *The Distribution of the Human Blood Groups and Other Biochemical Polymorphisms*, 2nd ed, Oxford, UK: Oxford University Press, 1976.
2. Kanter MH, "Derivation of New Mathematic Formulas for Determining Whether a D-Positive Father Is Heterozygous or Homozygous for the D Antigen," *Am J Obstet Gynecol*, 1992, 166(1 Pt 1):61-3.

RhIG *see* Rh$_o$(D) Immune Globulin (Human) *on next page*

Rh Immune Globulin *see* Rh$_o$(D) Immune Globulin (Human) *on this page*

Rh$_o$(D) Immune Globulin (Human)

CPT 90742

Related Information

Antiglobulin Test, Direct *on page 602*
Cord Blood Screen *on page 605*
D^u *on page 608*
Kleihauer-Betke *on page 329*
Newborn Crossmatch and Transfusion *on page 612*
Rh Genotype *on previous page*
Rosette Test for Fetomaternal Hemorrhage *on page 625*

Synonyms Anti-Rh Globulin; Rh Immune Globulin; RhIG

Test Commonly Includes Rh$_o$(D) type of mother and baby, rosette test, D^u, and antibody screen on mother, direct antiglobulin test on baby. Rh$_o$(D) immune globulin is an immunoglobulin product, an IgG containing anti-Rh$_o$(D). In the U.S., a dose of RhIG contains 300 μg anti-D. Each U.S. vial of injection is sufficient to prevent immunization by 30 mL of whole blood or 15 mL of red cells.

Abstract AABB standards require that all women undergoing delivery, abortion, or invasive obstetric procedures have determination of Rh type, with negative testing for D and D^u leading to designation as Rh negative. Criteria are required to avoid mistyping of Rh-negative mothers as positive when mixed field agglutination in anti-D testing follows large fetomaternal hemorrhage. Rh-negative women should be given. Rh$_o$(D) immune globulin, preferably within 72 hours following delivery, amniocentesis or other procedures that could cause fetomaternal hemorrhage, except when the fetus is Rh negative or immunization to D not caused by antepartum Rh immune globulin is recognized. Testing postpartum of Rh-negative women for sufficiently large fetomaternal hemorrhage to require more than a single dose is required. Subjects who have been given Rh immune globulin must be considered for additional treatment with this material following delivery.

Use of Rh immune globulin following exposure to Rh-positive erythrocytes in Rh-negative recipients, following transfusion including red cells infused with platelets or granulocytes may be appropriate.[1]

Patient Preparation The Kleihauer-Betke test on maternal blood is advisable after delivery to estimate the volume of fetal-maternal hemorrhage. The D^u on maternal blood after delivery, read microscopically, will detect some massive fetal-maternal hemorrhages. It will not detect them all. See listing Rosette Test for Fetomaternal Hemorrhage *on page 625*.

Specimen Blood from both mother and infant

Container Red top tube or capillary tube; lavender top (EDTA) tube

Collection Collected postpartum. Blood required from both mother and newborn. Label each specimen.

Causes for Rejection (Of patient sample): Gross hemolysis, sample placed in a serum separator tube, specimen tube not properly labeled. RhIG is not indicated for newborn Rh-negative, mother Rh-positive or D^u-positive, anti-D present in mother's serum when mother has not had prenatal Rh immune globulin.

Use Given to Rh-negative, D^u-negative women postpartum, or after termination of pregnancy, abortion, or ectopic pregnancy to prevent development of Rh antibody. Such antibody may cause erythroblastosis fetalis (hemolytic disease of the newborn) or years later lead to transfusion reaction if Rh-positive RBCs are transfused. Occasionally, RhIG is given to an Rh-negative person who received Rh-positive red blood cells accidentally or an Rh-positive component (eg, platelets). RhIG has been given to Rh-negative women after amniocentesis. Give RhIG antepartum at 28-32 weeks, as well as within 3 days of delivery. When it is given antepartum, then after delivery there will still be anti-D in the maternal serum. The direct antiglobulin test may be positive on the cord cells; in this setting such findings are not contraindications for a postpartum dose. Give a postpartum dose to the appropriate mother whether or not Rh immune globulin was given antepartum.

Limitations In instances of large fetomaternal hemorrhage, one dose is not sufficient. The D^u test read microscopically will detect some large hemorrhages but miss others that require more than one dose. The rosette test is more sensitive. See preparation discussion in the Kleihauer-Betke *on page 329* test. A smaller Rh immune globulin dose may be used after abortion or miscarriage up to 12 weeks gestation, but not beyond; after 12 weeks of gestation a conventional dose is indicated.

Failures occur. The most common cause of Rh immunization is failure to give RhIG when it is indicated. RhIG is sometimes forgotten in ectopic gestation and in abortion in Rh-negative women. However, 1% to 2% of term mothers develop anti-D in spite of postpartum RhIG properly administered. Postpartum failure may be secondary to fetomaternal hemorrhage in the third trimester (hence, antenatal RhIG)[2] and because of large fetomaternal hemorrhages at delivery (the Kleihauer-Betke test

will detect these). The mother who is a false D^u-positive really needs more than one dose of RhIG. Few fetomaternal hemorrhages are larger than 15 mL of red cells. Some of these patients may become immunized.[3]

Contraindications Do not give RhIG to an Rh-positive or D^u-positive person, or a person already immunized to the Rh$_o$(D) blood factor whose serum contains anti-D. (However, if Rh$_o$(D) immune globulin was given as an antenatal dose to mother, then anti-D detectable in her serum is not a contraindication to postnatal administration of RhIG.) Do not give RhIG to an infant, to the mother of an Rh-negative baby, or when the biological father of the fetus is known with certainty to be Rh negative.

The question of using RhIG for women of type D^u remains debatable. Certainly, the likelihood of a D^u mother making anti-Rh is low, and one might expect that passive anti-Rh would be as likely to attach to the mother's RBCs as to any invading fetal cells. But there is evidence that some administered RhIG does remain unbound,[4] so the question remains open. There are no data as to effectiveness of RhIG in this setting.

Methodology Read package insert.

Additional Information Give RhIG to an Rh-negative mother within 72 hours of delivery, miscarriage, or removal of ectopic pregnancy.

The **Kleihauer-Betke** test done on maternal blood after delivery estimates the volume of fetal-maternal hemorrhage. Calculate the dose of Rh$_o$ immune globulin as follows:

- Percent of fetal red cells x 50 = mL fetal whole blood in maternal circulation.
- Give one dose of RhIG for every 25 mL of fetal maternal hemorrhage.
- This is slightly higher than the usually recommended dose of 300 μg of RhIG per 30 mL of fetal blood. There is a tendency to underestimate because of the poor precision of the Kleihauer-Betke test.

Give RhIG to Rh-negative mothers with negative screens when cord blood is not available (ectopic pregnancies, abortions, etc) unless the father is Rh negative. If the patient refuses, she should sign an appropriate statement to that effect. Although **antenatal doses** may have been given at 28-32 weeks, give a postpartum dose anyway. Transmission of viral infections does not occur with this preparation.

Footnotes

1. Klein HG, *Standards for Blood Banks and Transfusion Services*, 16th ed, Bethesda, MD: American Association of Blood Banks, 1994, 33-4.
2. Bowman JM, "Antenatal Suppression of Rh Alloimmunization," *Clin Obstet Gynecol*, 1991, 34(2):296-303.
3. Sebring ES and Polesky HF, "Fetomaternal Hemorrhage: Incidence, Risk Factors, Time of Occurrence, and Clinical Effects," *Transfusion*, 1990, 30(4):344-57.
4. Lubenko A, Contreras M, and Habash J, "Should Anti-Rh Immunoglobulin Be Given to D Variant Women?" *Br J Haematol*, 1989, 72(3):429-33.

References

Mittendorf R and Williams MA, "Rh$_o$(D) Immunoglobulin (RhoGAM™): How It Came Into Being," *Obstet Gynecol*, 1991, 77(2):301-3.
Zimmerman DR, *Rh. The Intimate History of a Disease and Its Conquest*, New York, NY: Macmillan Publishing Co Inc, 1973.

Rh$_o$(D) Typing *see* Pretransfusion Testing *on page 619*

Rh$_o$ Variant *see* D^u *on page 608*

Risks of Transfusion

Related Information

Alanine Aminotransferase *on page 65*
Automated Reagin Test *on page 370*
Babesiosis Serological Test *on page 370*
Chagas' Disease Serological Test *on page 383*
Cold Agglutinin Titer *on page 384*
Cytomegalovirus Antibody *on page 389*
Hepatitis B Core Antibody *on page 396*
Hepatitis B Surface Antigen *on page 399*
Hepatitis C Serology *on page 399*
HIV-1/HIV-2 Serology *on page 403*
HTLV-I/II Antibody *on page 406*
IgA Antibodies *on page 407*
Immunoglobulin A *on page 408*
Intravascular Coagulation Screen *on page 253*
p24 Antigen *on page 420*
Pretransfusion Testing *on page 619*
Red Blood Cells *on page 621*
RPR *on page 428*
Transfusion Reaction Work-up *on page 625*
VDRL, Serum *on page 438*
Whole Blood *on page 627*
Yersinia enterocolitica Antibody *on page 440*

Synonyms Hazards of Transfusion; Transfusion Complications

Special Instructions Report all adverse effects of transfusion at once to the Blood Bank for follow-up and investigation. The physician in charge
(Continued)

Risks of Transfusion *(Continued)*

of transfusion must in turn investigate **all** reported reactions, with interpretation and recommendations recorded in the patient's chart. The FDA requires a report of all fatal transfusion reactions. Report also any suspected cases of transfusion-associated infectious disease to the Blood Bank so that implicated donors can be traced and investigated. These are obligations written into federal regulations, AABB standards, and those of other accrediting agencies.

Some Risks of Allogeneic Transfusion

Reactions	Disease Transmission	Other
Hemolytic, immediate, delayed	Hepatitis B, C, etc	Alloimmunization RBC, WBC, etc
Febrile	Cytomegalovirus	Marrow suppression
Allergic, anaphylactic	Syphilis	Immunosuppression
Sepsis	Malaria	Storage changes
Overload	Babesiosis	Graft-vs-host disease
Hypothermia, cold	Brucellosis	Dilutional coagulopathy
Air embolism	Chagas disease	Nonimmune hemolysis
Post-transfusion purpura	AIDS	Iron overload

Additional Information

INCOMPATIBLE BLOOD:

Hemolytic transfusion reactions usually result from clerical and other identification errors involving ABO incompatibility.[1,2] This is why unlabeled or improperly labeled sample tubes are unacceptable to the Transfusion Service. Chills, fever, dyspnea, chest or back pain, headache, abnormal bleeding, or shock can all characterize acute hemolytic reactions. Hemoglobinemia heralds **intravascular** hemolysis, followed by hemoglobinuria, then jaundice. This is usually mediated by anti-A or anti-B or both. **Extravascular** hemolysis takes place mostly in the spleen as a result of the action of IgG antibodies, such as those of the Rh system. With these, hemoglobinemia and hemoglobinuria seldom occur. See listing Transfusion Reaction Work-up *on page 625.* Renal shutdown, shock, or hemorrhage may be fatal. When this type of reaction occurs, stop the transfusion at once. Treat shock. Give appropriate fluids and diuretics to maintain urinary output. Treat for incipient renal failure, if indicated.

Delayed hemolytic reactions can occur in some patients with other serologically undetectable antibodies (other than anti-A or anti-B).[3] These are noticed when more blood is ordered a few days after an earlier transfusion of apparently compatible blood. There has usually been a poor clinical response to the prior transfusion. The Blood Bank finds a positive direct antiglobulin test and antibody that is now incompatible with the recently transfused RBCs. The antibody may be either in the patient's serum or in an eluate from the red cells. The diagnosis is easily missed. Delayed hemolytic reactions are not uncommon; they are usually mild, rarely severe.

Remember that **nonimmune hemolysis** can also occur and may be mistaken for an incompatible blood reaction. Some causes include inappropriate I.V. solutions run in the same tubing with blood (eg, hypotonic or dextrose-containing solutions - even water has been used this way); overheating; accidental freezing (eg, packing RBCs in a box with dry ice); irrigation of bleeding surgical surfaces with water (eg, in bladder surgery); accidental infusion of water instead of saline; bacterial contamination of blood; and, rarely, G-6-PD deficiency (either in donor or patient).

Other immune reactions include **febrile nonhemolytic** reactions,[4] usually in patients with antibodies to donor leukocytes, occurring in as many as 1% of transfusions. They are treated symptomatically with antipyretics, and may be prevented by passing RBCs or platelets through leukocyte-removing filters, or by using washed RBCs. **Allergic transfusion reactions** are about as frequent and usually appear in the form of hives (urticaria) without fever. Treatment and prevention is with antihistaminics (given to the patient, not put into the blood container).[1] Anaphylaxis is rare.

TRANSFUSION-ASSOCIATED INFECTIOUS DISEASES:

Viral hepatitis, the incidence of which is changing rapidly.[5,6] Type A is very rare, B now uncommon, and C decreasing significantly.

Cytomegalovirus infection, significant in premature newborns and immunosuppressed adults, including transplant recipients.[7,8] For the latter and for babies weighing less than 1200 g and having CMV-seronegative mothers, use blood from CMV-seronegative donors. Removal of WBCs may reduce and perhaps prevent CMV infections.

Bacterial contamination of blood or components, usually with gram-negatives.[9] This can cause septic shock and death and must be vigorously treated if observed. Currently, there is concern over contamination

with *Yersinia enterocolitica*, particularly in platelets.[10] *Y. enterocolitica* can grow in refrigerated blood.

The following infections are occasionally seen, but should be considered rare: syphilis, malaria (rare in the U.S.), babesiosis (endemic in some areas of the east coast), brucellosis, Chagas' disease (trypanosomiasis, rare in the U.S., common in parts of South America) and, of course, AIDS.

AIDS, as a transfusion hazard, is statistically rare,[5,11] but regarded by the public as a terrifying risk of transfusion. Fear of AIDS gives it a prominence in the public eye that is out of all proportion to the real risk. Most recipients of HIV-infected blood or components will become seropositive and will in time progress to clinical AIDS. Since the onset of testing for anti-HIV-1 in 1985, very few cases of transfusion-associated AIDS have occurred.[12] These depend, for the most part, on donations by persons recently infected with HIV who have not yet formed detectable antibody. Presently more recipients die of HCV than of AIDS following transfusion. The improved sensitivity of present enzyme immunosorbent assays has led to extremely small estimated risk.[13]

Bone marrow suppression of RBC production will occur after the transfusion of RBCs, another reason to avoid giving transfusions to patients whose anemia might respond to conventional medication.

Immunosuppression of varying degree follows allogeneic transfusion.[14] Just as transfusion improves the survival of kidney allografts, so also does it depress the body's natural immunity and resistance. Patients who get transfusions at surgery to remove malignancies seem more likely to have the tumor recur than those who were not transfused.[15] Transfused patients are more likely to have postoperative infections.[16] This phenomenon does not occur with autologous transfusion.

Transfusion-related acute lung injury ("TRALI"). Clinically similar to adult respiratory distress syndrome, seems to be related to leukocyte antibodies in donor plasma, reacting with recipient's antigens, perhaps with release of complement.[17] Unlike ARDS, the condition usually improves quickly with pulmonary support.

Simple **volume overload** of the recipient's circulation may cause pulmonary edema without leukocyte antibodies.

Air embolism can result from any admission of air into intravenous tubing and can have serious consequences.

Anaphylactic reaction: See listings IgA Antibodies *on page 407* and Immunoglobulin A *on page 408.* Nausea, chills, severe abdominal cramps, emesis, diarrhea, dyspnea, flushing with hypotension, and flushing may take place due to donor plasma IgA. IgA-negative blood is available for recipients who lack IgA.

Graft-versus-host disease (GVHD) can result from transfusion of blood components containing living donor lymphocytes. Normally, these would be rapidly eliminated by the host's immune response. But in immuno-compromised patients (transplant recipients, patients receiving immuno-suppressive chemotherapy and, rarely, premature newborns), the donor lymphocytes are able to attack the host tissues, sometimes with fatal results.[18] GVHD occasionally occurs in immunocompetent recipients, which is harder to understand. This is rare in the U.S. but less so in Japan, where homozygous HLA phenotypes are more common. It requires a donor, usually a close relative, who is homozygous for an HLA haplotype for which the recipient is heterozygous. Thus, the recipient does not recognize the donor lymphocytes as foreign, while the donor cells are able to survive and attack the recipient. In general, GVHD is preventable by irradiation of the blood or component to be transfused to a patient at risk[19] (see Irradiated Blood Components *on page 611*). AABB advises irradiation of directed donations from blood relatives of any patient to prevent this rare complication.

Approximate Frequency of Some Transfusion Complications Compared to a Large Study of Hospitalized Patients*

Complication	Approximate Frequency per Unit Transfused
Hepatitis C	1:3300
Hepatitis B	1:200,000
HIV-1 (AIDS)	1:225,000
HTLV-I	1:50,000
Transfusion-associated infections (overall)	3 per 10,000 patients
Febrile or allergic reaction	1:100
Hemolytic transfusion reaction	1:6000
Fatal hemolytic reaction	1:100,000
Accidental and preventable deaths in hospital	6 per 1000 patients

*From Dodd RY, "The Risk of Transfusion-Transmitted Infections," *N Engl J Med,* 1992, 327:419-21, with permission.

Complications of massive transfusion: Hemorrhagic diathesis due to dilution and washout (dilutional coagulopathy) of coagulation factors and platelets.[20] DIC can also occur in the settings in which massive transfusions are given. Rapid laboratory evaluation of hemostasis can be vital. Treatment of abnormal bleeding in this situation is primarily with platelet concentrates, sometimes also with FFP, and less often cryoprecipitate. If fluid balance is not carefully observed, fluid overload or adult respiratory distress syndrome may occur. 2,3-DPG depletion of stored RBCs is a theoretic problem, rarely of any clinical significance. Prevent hypothermia, caused by rapid massive transfusion of cold blood, with blood warmers (see Warming, Blood *on page 627*). With massive transfusions, particularly in trauma, there is often tumult and confusion, which makes an ideal setup for clerical errors and increased likelihood of incompatible blood transfusion. Avoiding errors in such settings is vital.

Footnotes

1. Huestis DW, Bove JR, and Case J, *Practical Blood Transfusion*, 4th ed, Boston, MA: Little, Brown and Co, 1988, 249-68.
2. Mollison PL, Engelfriet CP, and Contreras M, *Blood Transfusion in Clinical Medicine*, 9th ed, Chapters 10, 11, 15, 16, Oxford, UK: Blackwell Scientific Publications, 1993, 499-542, 677-785.
3. Ness PM, Shirey RS, Thoman SK, et al, "The Differentiation of Delayed Serologic and Delayed Hemolytic Transfusion Reactions: Incidence, Long-Term Serologic Findings, and Clinical Significance," *Transfusion*, 1990, 30(8):688-93.
4. Brubaker DB, "Clinical Significance of White Cell Antibodies in Febrile Nonhemolytic Transfusion Reactions," *Transfusion*, 1990, 30(8):733-7.
5. Dodd RY, "The Risk of Transfusion-Transmitted Infection," *N Engl J Med*, 1992, 327(6):419-21.
6. Donahue JG, Muñoz A, Ness PM, et al, "The Declining Risk of Post-transfusion Hepatitis C Virus Infection," *N Engl J Med*, 1992, 327(6):369-73.
7. Eisenfeld L, Silver H, McLaughlin J, et al, "Prevention of Transfusion-Associated Cytomegalovirus Infection in Neonatal Patients by the Removal of White Cells From Blood," *Transfusion*, 1992, 32(3):205-9.
8. Sayers MH, Anderson KC, Goodnough LT, et al, "Reducing the Risk for Transfusion-Transmitted Cytomegalovirus Infection," *Ann Intern Med*, 1992, 116(1):55-62.
9. Goldman M and Blajchman MA, "Blood Product-Associated Bacterial Sepsis," *Transfus Med Rev*, 1991, 5(1):73-83.
10. Morrow JF, Braine HG, Kickler TS, et al, "Septic Reactions to Platelet Transfusions. A Persistent Problem," *JAMA*, 1991, 266(4):555-8.
11. Carson JL, Russell LB, Taragin MI, et al, "The Risks of Blood Transfusion: The Relative Influence of Acquired Immunodeficiency Syndrome and Non-A, Non-B Hepatitis," *Am J Med*, 1992, 92(1):45-52.
12. Conley LJ and Holmberg SD, "Transmission of AIDS From Blood Screened Negative for Antibody to the Human Immunodeficiency Virus," *N Engl J Med*, 1992, 326(22):1499-1500.
13. Lackritz EM, Satten GA, Aberle-Grasse J, et al, "Estimated Risk of Transmission of the Human Immunodeficiency Virus by Screened Blood in the United States," *N Engl J Med*, 1995, 333(26):1721-5.
14. Brunson ME and Alexander JW, "Mechanisms of Transfusion-Induced Immunosuppression," *Transfusion*, 1990, 30(7):651-8.
15. Wobbes T, Joosen KH, Kuypers HH, et al, "The Effect of Packed Cells and Whole Blood Transfusions on Survival After Curative Resection for Colorectal Carcinoma," *Dis Colon Rectum*, 1989, 32(9):743-8.
16. Triulzi DJ, Vanek K, Ryan DH, et al, "A Clinical and Immunologic Study of Blood Transfusion and Postoperative Bacterial Infection in Spinal Surgery," *Transfusion*, 1992, 32(6):517-24.
17. Popovsky MA, Chaplin HC Jr, and Moore SB, "Transfusion-Related Acute Lung Injury: A Neglected, Serious Complication of Hemotherapy," *Transfusion*, 1992, 32(6):589-91.
18. Holland PV, "Prevention of Transfusion-Associated Graft-vs-Host Disease," *Arch Pathol Lab Med*, 1989, 113(3):285-91.
19. Anderson KC, Goodnough LT, Sayers M, et al, "Variation in Blood Component Irradiation Practice: Implications for Prevention of Transfusion-Associated Graft-Versus-Host Disease," *Blood*, 1991, 77(10):2096-102.
20. Sohmer PR, "Transfusion Therapy in Surgery," *Clinical Practice of Transfusion Medicine*, Petz LD and Swisher SN, eds, New York, NY: Churchill-Livingstone, 1989, 363-400.

References

Desforges JF, "Infectious Disease Testing for Blood Transfusions," *NIH Consensus Statement*, 1995, 13(1):1-27.
Gottlieb T, "Hazards of Bacterial Contamination of Blood Products," *Anaesth Intensive Care*, 1993, 21(1):20-3.
Koretz RL, Abbey H, Coleman E, et al, "Non-A, Non-B Post-Transfusion Hepatitis. Looking Back in the Second Decade," *Ann Intern Med*, 1993, 119(2):110-5.
Leslie SD and Toy PT, "Laboratory Hemostatic Abnormalities in Massively Transfused Patients Given Red Blood Cells and Crystalloid," *Am J Clin Pathol*, 1991, 96(6):770-3.
Reichen J, "Long-Term Course of Non-A, Non-B Post-Transfusion Hepatitis," *ACP J Club*, November/December, 1993, 85.
Sazama K, "Bacteria in Blood for Transfusion. A Review," *Arch Pathol Lab Med*, 1994, 118(4):350-65.
Shapiro CN, "Transmission of Hepatitis Viruses," *Ann Intern Med*, 1994, 120(1):82-4.
Tong MJ, El-Farra NS, Reikes AR, et al, "Clinical Outcomes After Transfusion-Associated Hepatitis C," *N Engl J Med*, 1995, 332(22):1463-6.

Rosette Test (Erythrocyte) see D[u] *on page 608*

Rosette Test for Fetomaternal Hemorrhage

CPT 85461

Related Information

D[u] *on page 608*
Kleihauer-Betke *on page 329*
Newborn Crossmatch and Transfusion *on page 612*
Rh[o](D) Immune Globulin (Human) *on page 623*

Synonyms Fetalscreen™

Abstract A postdelivery Rh-negative maternal specimen is screened for the presence of Rh-positive fetal cells.

Specimen Blood

Container One red top tube and one lavender top (EDTA) tube

Sampling Time Specimen used for testing must be a postdelivery specimen.

Causes for Rejection Specimen grossly hemolyzed

Use Determine if fetal maternal hemorrhage of more than 15 mL red cells has occurred

Limitations This is a screening test for the detection of fetal D-positive cells in D-negative maternal blood. An acid-elution test should follow a positive screen to quantify the number of fetal cells present. May be unreliable if the newborn is D[u] type.

Methodology Anti-D is added to the Rh-negative maternal blood and incubated. D-positive cells are then added to the maternal cell-anti-D mixture. Antibody coating is not strong enough to cause direct agglutination, but rosette formation occurs in positive specimens after addition of the D-positive cells.

References

Mollison PL, Engelfriet CP, and Contreras M, *Blood Transfusion in Clinical Medicine*, 9th ed, Oxford, UK: Blackwell Scientific Publications, 1993, 546-53.

Single-Donor Platelets see Platelets, Apheresis, Donation *on page 617*

Stem Cell Collection see Cytapheresis, Therapeutic *on page 606*

Therapeutic Cytapheresis see Cytapheresis, Therapeutic *on page 606*

Therapeutic Leukapheresis see Cytapheresis, Therapeutic *on page 606*

Therapeutic Phlebotomy see Phlebotomy, Therapeutic *on page 614*

Titer of Unexpected Antibody see Antibody Titer *on page 601*

Transfusion, Autologous see Autologous Transfusion, Preoperative Deposit *on page 603*

Transfusion Complications see Risks of Transfusion *on page 623*

Transfusion Complication Work-Up see Transfusion Reaction Work-up *on this page*

Transfusion Reaction, Allergic see Red Blood Cells, Washed *on page 622*

Transfusion Reaction, Febrile see Filters for Blood *on page 609*

Transfusion Reaction, Febrile see Red Blood Cells, Washed *on page 622*

Transfusion Reaction Work-up

CPT 86880 (antiglobulin test, direct); 86900 (ABO); 86901 (Rh(D))

Related Information

Antiglobulin Test, Direct *on page 602*
Antineutrophil Antibody *on page 366*
Risks of Transfusion *on page 623*

Synonyms Transfusion Complication Work-Up

Test Commonly Includes If there is any evidence of significant reaction other than mild urticaria, **stop the transfusion** but keep normal saline dripping in slowly to keep the I.V. open. Report reaction to Blood Bank. Examine label on blood container(s) and all clerical work and records for possible error, and review possible mirror image or other-side-of-the-coin error (is there a roommate also getting blood? If one unit is infused into a wrong patient, what has become of the other unit crossmatched?) Examination of prereaction and postreaction serum or plasma for hemolysis or jaundice. This should be begun by examination of the postreaction blood sample sent very promptly to the Blood Bank.

Direct antiglobulin test on postreaction specimen. (If positive, it must be compared with a pretransfusion specimen.[1])

Repeat ABO and Rh typing on patient and donor blood; compare with previous reports.

If the above are negative and there is no suspicion of incompatibility, additional tests are not essential. Minor reactions (eg, febrile or allergic) need no further work-up. If actual hemolysis is suspected, the following may be done.

Hemoglobin and hematocrit: Look for expected increase from amount of blood infused or lack of increase... was there an appropriate rise? (But in the bleeding patient, for instance, the hemoglobin may not rise anyway.)

Urinalysis for free hemoglobin: A red supernatant in the centrifuged urine specimen, positive for hemoglobin. Watch for brown as well as red (Continued)

Transfusion Reaction Work-up *(Continued)*

urine. Urine dipsticks also provide reactions for bilirubin and urobilinogen. Follow urine output and record it.

Blood container, attached transfusion set, and intravenous solutions must be sent to Transfusion Service.

Serum bilirubin

Culture of remaining donor blood, especially if the patient has fever and shock.

BUN and creatinine

Repeat crossmatch and antibody screen on donor and recipient.

Antibody identification if indicated.

Test for haptoglobin in recipient (but haptoglobin may decrease even following uneventful transfusions).

In case of possible DIC (disseminated intravascular coagulation), baseline studies include platelet count, prothrombin time, PTT, fibrin split products, fibrinogen, and thrombin time. Oozing from venipuncture site or sites or from a surgical wound is an indication for as many of these tests as can be done stat; preferably, all of them. Such microvascular bleeding has often been the only clue to a hemolytic reaction occurring during surgery.

Schedule of Investigation of Reported Transfusion Reactions

A. All reported reactions
  1. Specimens needed
     a. Pretransfusion blood of recipient
     b. Post-transfusion blood of recipient
  2. Investigation (letters refer to specimens listed above)
     - Check donor and patient identification and crossmatch report
     - Repeat ABO and Rh typing (b, and donor bag, if indicated)
     - Direct antiglobulin test (b, if indicated)
     - Examine for visible hemolysis (b); if necessary, compare (b) with (a)

If these procedures reveal no evidence of incompatibility or hemolysis, and there is no additional information to arouse suspicion, no further investigation is needed. Otherwise, proceed as follows:

B. If there is evidence of hemolysis or incompatible transfusion
  1. Specimens needed
     a. Pretransfusion blood of recipient
     b. Post-transfusion blood of recipient
     c. Pilot samples of donor blood
     d. Blood from container implicated in reaction (if available)
     e. Post-transfusion urine
  2. Immunologic investigation
     - Repeat ABO, Rh, and direct antiglobulin test (a, c, d)
     - Repeat crossmatch (a, b, c; d, if indicated) (major; minor only if indicated)
     - Repeat antibody screen (a, b, c) (special, sensitive techniques if necessary)
     - Identification of any unexpected antibody or incompatibility
  3. Other procedures as indicated
     - Serum haptoglobin (a, b)
     - Bacteriologic smear and culture (d)
     - Serum urea and bilirubin (a, b)
     - Urine hemoglobin (e)
     - Urine hemosiderin (e)
  4. Investigation of nonimmune causes of hemolysis

From Huestis DW, Bove JR, and Case J, *Practical Blood Transfusion*, 4th ed, Boston, MA: Little, Brown and Co, 1988, 268, with permission.

Abstract Any adverse reaction which takes place in association with a transfusion must be regarded with suspicion[1] until proven otherwise.

Aftercare As investigation is in progress in the laboratory, those caring for the patient must monitor for evidence of shock, renal shutdown, and/or evidence of DIC (ie, look for oozing, petechiae, or ecchymoses). Vigorous treatment may be needed for any or all of these manifestations, possibly including additional transfusions.

Specimen Blood, urine

Container Red top tube, lavender top (EDTA) tube, and plastic urine container

Causes for Rejection (Of patient sample): Specimen tube not properly labeled

Turnaround Time Examination of pretransfusion and current serum or plasma for hemolysis can be done very rapidly. A repeat ABO and Rh, direct antiglobulin test, and clerical check can be done in minutes.

Special Instructions If patient develops chills, fever exceeding 1.5°C, hypotension, dyspnea, nausea, etc, stop the transfusion, notify physician

and Transfusion Service immediately. **If in doubt about any possible reaction, stop transfusion immediately. Notify physician and Transfusion Service immediately.** Return blood bag to Transfusion Service. If a hemolytic transfusion reaction is suspected, send all I.V. solutions and concurrent medications to Transfusion Service. Report patient's diagnosis, medications, pretransfusion and post-transfusion vital signs to the patient's physician and to the Transfusion Service. Keep I.V. needle open with slowly infusing normal saline, pending physician's instructions. **Blood container**, attached transfusion set, and intravenous solutions must be sent to the Transfusion Service.

Use Investigate cause of possible transfusion reactions. Symptoms and signs of transfusion reaction may include chills, temperature elevation, dyspnea, nausea, pain in lower back, shock, urticaria, and/or hematuria.

Limitations The transfusion reaction work-up will mainly detect those reactions caused by red cell incompatibility and with culture, those caused by bacterial contamination of the infused unit. The conventional investigation may not detect reactions to white cells, platelets, or to plasma proteins such as IgA reactions. Circulatory overload and allergic reactions do not need to be evaluated as possible hemolytic reactions.[1]

Contraindications The two most common complications of transfusion are urticaria and fever. **Urticaria** (hives, rash, itching) occurs in about 1% of transfusions and does not call for a full reaction work-up. An antihistamine by mouth or by vein usually relieves such symptoms. The patient's physician may decide to continue the transfusion after symptomatic medication, bearing in mind the risk of giving more allergen to a demonstrably allergic patient. **Fevers and chills** (a sharp rise of at least 1.5°C, not sustained, without other causes of fever) indicates a **febrile nonhemolytic transfusion reaction**. Most such reactions are caused by a recipient's antibody to donor leukocytes and respond to symptomatic antipyretic medication. Since true hemolytic reactions may start with fever, the investigation must rule out hemolysis. The time needed to do this usually precludes restarting transfusion of the unit implicated. If a patient has repeated febrile reactions, provide washed red cells or filter the blood through special leukocyte filters. Culture of the unit is not indicated. If a patient has sustained high fever, bloody emesis, diarrhea, or signs of **sepsis, toxemia, or "red shock,"** suspect bacteremia or endotoxic shock from contaminated blood. Immediate, intensive treatment is essential for this very dangerous reaction. A Gram's stained smear and culture from the suspected unit and blood culture from the patient will be diagnostic.

Additional Information Most fatal transfusion reactions involve clerical (labeling) error and incompatibility in the ABO system, with intravascular hemolysis.

Hemolytic transfusion reactions are characterized by fever, flushing, a feeling of apprehension, chest or back pain, chills, nausea, vomiting, and in severe cases, shock, oliguria, hemoglobinuria, bleeding, and renal failure. If a hemolytic transfusion reaction is suspected, the transfusion must be discontinued immediately, the Transfusion Service or Blood Bank notified at once, and appropriate clinical measures taken to support circulation, renal failure, and coagulation.

Bacterial pyrogens, circulatory overload, air embolism, faulty blood warming apparatus, inappropriate storage of blood or components before infusion, and medications added to the blood unit or infusion tubing are other causes of transfusion reactions. These are not always detected by the transfusion reaction work-up. Most are prevented by careful transfusion technique.

Delayed transfusion reactions are often missed. They may be detected by unexplained anemia, by a positive direct antiglobulin test, or by the detection of an unexplained antibody, which was absent when the type and screen were done.

Report any case of unexplained **liver dysfunction** occurring 2 weeks to 6 months after transfusion to the Transfusion Service because they may be secondary to post-transfusion hepatitis (hepatitis C, cytomegalovirus, or now rarely, hepatitis B).

See listing Risks of Transfusion *on page 623.*

By federal regulations, all suspected transfusion reactions must be reported to the Transfusion Service and all must be investigated and reported to the patient's physician. Any fatal reaction must be reported to the FDA.

Footnotes

1. Klein HG, *Standards for Blood Banks and Transfusion Services*, 16th ed, Bethesda, MD: American Association of Blood Banks, 1994, 35-6.

References

Huestis DW, Bove JR, and Case J, *Practical Blood Transfusion*, 4th ed, Boston, MA: Little, Brown and Co, 1988, 249-85.

Mollison PL, Engelfriet CP, and Contreras M, *Blood Transfusion in Clinical Medicine*, 9th ed, Chapters 10 and 11, Oxford, UK: Blackwell Scientific Publications, 1993.

Walker RH, *Technical Manual*, 11th ed, Arlington, VA: American Association of Blood Banks, 1993, 471-89.

Transfusion Review Committee *see* Quality Assurance, Transfusion *on page 620*

Type and Coombs', Cord Blood *see* Cord Blood Screen *on page 605*

Type and Crossmatch *see* Pretransfusion Testing *on page 619*

Type and Crossmatch for Exchange Transfusion of Newborn *see* Newborn Crossmatch and Transfusion *on page 612*

Type and Screen *see* Pretransfusion Testing *on page 619*

Uncrossmatched Blood, Emergency

CPT 36430

Related Information

Pretransfusion Testing *on page 619*

Synonyms Emergency Blood; Emergency Transfusion; Universal Donor Blood

Applies to Emergency Issue of Uncrossmatched Blood; Exsanguinating Emergency; Massive Acute Blood Loss

Test Commonly Includes No testing before issue, but as soon as possible do ABO and Rh type, antibody screen, antibody identification if indicated, and crossmatch.

Specimen Venous or arterial blood

Container One or two red top tubes and one lavender top (EDTA) tube

Collection (Of sample from intended recipient): Identify patient by wristband(s) or other system specially set up for identifying unconscious or noncommunicating patients in emergencies. Label tube specimen with the same information, including identification number from the wristband; label requisition form with identification number. Requisition should be signed by collector, indicating that patient's identity has been verified. Positive identification of patient sample is important, even in emergency. If it is impossible to get a blood sample, record this fact.

Causes for Rejection Nonemergent situations

Turnaround Time Although uncrossmatched O Rh-negative red blood cells can be issued immediately if available, ABO and Rh type can be done in only 5-10 minutes. Antibody screen and crossmatch require as much as 1 hour, longer if antibodies are detected. The process is much quicker if patient has already had a type and screen. See listing Pretransfusion Testing *on page 619* for table of times needed for blood issuance in emergencies.

Special Instructions An emergency request for uncrossmatched blood should include name of physician requesting blood and signature of person authorized, name and location of patient, and nature of emergency. There should also be a statement that the situation was sufficiently urgent to require release of blood before completion of testing.

Use Blood replacement in exsanguinating emergency, massive acute blood loss

Limitations Blood issued in life-threatening emergencies is clearly more dangerous than in controlled circumstances. All parties involved need to understand this.

Contraindications Do not use group O whole blood even in emergencies, for patients of other types, because the anti-A and anti-B can cause hemolysis of the recipient's RBCs. In life-threatening trauma or bleeding when the patient is untyped, use O RBCs. Most of the antibodies have been removed from these. The risks of hemolytic transfusion reactions are real and should be carefully weighed against any benefits anticipated.

Methodology When issuing uncrossmatched blood, apply a label indicating uncrossmatched status.

EMERGENCY RELEASE COMPATIBILITY TESTING INCOMPLETE

Additional Information There is no such thing as a "universal donor." Type O blood lacks A and B but has antigens of other blood group systems, any of which may be a problem for a given patient. Blood can be ABO and Rh typed in 5-10 minutes, and the patient then should receive ABO-specific blood. **Volume can be made up temporarily with plasma expanders.** Type O Rh-negative red cells are not always available. Type O Rh-positive red cells (packed cells) are usually available. The risks of the Rh-positive cells include hemolytic transfusion reaction if the patient has anti-D, and immunization to D if the patient is D-negative but not previously immunized. Some trauma centers commonly use O Rh-positive red cells in emergencies[1] or uncrossmatched type-specific blood.[2] Even in emergency ABO and Rh typing, blood sample must clot so that bits of fibrin are not mistaken for specific agglutination, or EDTA (lavender top tube) cells must be washed first. 5-10 minutes are

consumed. Risk is greatly increased when antibody screen and crossmatch are not completed before blood is infused. See also Transfusions in Trauma and Other Emergencies in the Transfusion Service (Blood Bank) Introduction *on page 597*.

Footnotes

1. Schmidt PJ, Leparc GF, and Samia CT, "Use of Rh Positive Blood in Emergency Situations," *Surg Gynecol Obstet*, 1988, 167(3):229-33.
2. Gervin AS and Fischer RP, "Resuscitation of Trauma Patients With Type-Specific Uncrossmatched Blood," *J Trauma*, 1984, 24(4):327-31.

References

Klein HG, *Standards for Blood Banks and Transfusion Services*, 16th ed, Bethesda, MD: American Association of Blood Banks, 1994, 28.

Unkle D, Smejkal R, Snyder R, et al, "Blood Antibodies and Uncrossmatched Type O Blood," *Heart Lung*, 1991, 20(3):284-6.

Unexpected Antibody Identification *see* Antibody Identification, Red Cell *on page 601*

Universal Donor Blood *see* Uncrossmatched Blood, Emergency *on this page*

von Willebrand Disease Therapy *see* Cryoprecipitate *on page 606*

Warming, Blood

Related Information

Cold Agglutinin Titer *on page 384*

Newborn Crossmatch and Transfusion *on page 612*

Abstract Warming should take place, when necessary, during passage through the transfusion set. A visible thermometer is required. An audible warning system is recommended.[1]

Use For very rapid, massive transfusion (above 50 mL/minute). Detection of cold agglutinins may be important in patients in whom cold blood may be used, see listing Cold Agglutinin Titer *on page 384*.

Limitations Uncontrolled warming of donor blood can severely damage RBCs. Although red cells must be heated to 44°C or higher to be damaged, it is probably best not to allow warming above 40°C. Warming may not exceed 42°C.[1]

Contraindications When moderate volumes of blood are given at ordinary rates, warming is unnecessary. It is probably unnecessary also in most patients with cold agglutinin disease or paroxysmal cold hemoglobinuria (warming the patient is more effective).

Methodology A considerable variety of hardware is available for blood warming (listed with commentary in Iserson and Huestis[2]). To be effective, an instrument should be able to warm blood efficiently at a flow rate of at least 150 mL/minute. A simple system, not needing expensive equipment, is to maintain a few 250 mL bags of isotonic saline at 70°C. Add this quantity rapidly to a unit of 4°C RBCs, and it immediately results in a temperature about 37°C, without hemolysis or other damage.[3]

Additional Information Relatively large volumes of blood at refrigerator temperature, infused rapidly, can cause hypothermia and cardiac arrest. During transfusion of blood that is being warmed, the temperature of the blood warmer must be monitored. The temperature of the blood warmer should be recorded at 30 and 60 minutes from the start of the transfusion, if transfusion has not been completed. Blood subjected to excessive heat (ie, above 44°C) may be lethal. A quality assurance protocol is essential for all blood warmers and is required by accrediting agencies.[1]

Footnotes

1. Klein HG, *Standards for Blood Banks and Transfusion Services*, 16th ed, Bethesda, MD: American Association of Blood Banks, 1994.
2. Iserson KV and Huestis DW, "Blood Warming: Current Applications and Techniques," *Transfusion*, 1991, 31(6):558-71.
3. Iserson KV, Knauf MA, and Anhalt D, "Rapid Admixture Blood Warming: Technical Advances," *Crit Care Med*, 1990, 18(2):1138-41.

References

Mollison PL, Engelfriet CP, and Contreras M, *Blood Transfusion in Clinical Medicine*, 9th ed, Oxford, UK: Blackwell Scientific Publications, 1993, 699-700.

Washed Blood Cells *see* Red Blood Cells, Washed *on page 622*

Weak D (Dᵘ) *see* Dᵘ *on page 608*

White Cells, Transfusion *see* Neutrophils, Transfusion *on page 612*

Whole Blood

CPT 36430 (transfusion); 36450 (exchange transfusion, newborn)

Related Information

Donation, Blood *on page 607*

Filters for Blood *on page 609*

Red Blood Cells *on page 621*

Risks of Transfusion *on page 623*

Applies to "Fresh Blood"; Massive Transfusions

Test Commonly Includes A unit of whole blood consists of about 450 mL (±10%) blood including plasma and about 63 mL of anticoagulant

(Continued)

Whole Blood *(Continued)*

preservative such as citrate phosphate dextrose adenine solution (CPDA-1). A typical donor unit has a hematocrit of about 35% to 40%. The expiration date for CPDA-1 blood is 35 days after the date of collection if stored continuously at 1°C to 6°C, unless the seal has been broken. Anticoagulants in use have been recently tabulated.[1] ABO, Rh typing, and antibody screen of donor unit and of patient, and crossmatch are required.

Patient Preparation Identify the patient fully, preferably with a hospital identification band attached to the body, or with an alternative emergency identification. Measure blood loss if possible, as well as fluid intake and output. **Dosage and administration:** Give whole blood through a filter. It can be warmed, if warming is clinically indicated, as with rapid infusion of large volumes of blood at refrigerated temperature. The blood should not be warmed above 38°C. The rate of infusion depends on clinical conditions but should not be slower than 4 hours per unit. **No medications or solutions should be added to blood. Never give Ringer's lactate, hypotonic, or dextrose-containing solutions through the same tubing as blood.** These solutions are incompatible with stored blood, causing clots, aggregates, and shortened cell survival.

Aftercare Many of the important clinical manifestations of transfusion reaction occur during the administration of the first 50-100 mL of blood. Pay close attention to vital signs (ie, temperature, pulse, and blood pressure) before, after, and frequently during the transfusion. Reactions may occur up to several hours after transfusion, and delayed transfusion reactions can occur several days afterwards. Monitor electrolytes, hemoglobin/hematocrit.

Specimen Blood

Container One red top tube and one lavender top (EDTA) tube

Collection (Of sample from intended recipient): At the patient's bedside, ask the patient to give his or her name. Compare with the hospital wristband. Label the Blood Bank wristband (if there is one) with the patient's full name, hospital number, date, and initials of the collector. Label sample tube with the same information, including identification number from the wristband. Label requisition form with identification number. The collector signs the requisition, verifying the patient's identity with hospital wristband and Blood Bank wristband. Some hospitals require additional information. It is always best to stamp the requisition with the patient's identification plate to avoid transcription errors. Take extra care with identification of unresponsive patients.

Storage Instructions Stored in properly monitored Blood Bank refrigerator at 1°C to 6°C until issue. Start blood transfusion immediately after blood is issued, otherwise return blood to Blood Bank within approximately 30 minutes. **Do not store blood in ward/nursing-station refrigerators. They are not monitored and are not safe.**[1]

Causes for Rejection (Of patient sample): Gross hemolysis, sample placed in a serum separator tube, specimen tube not properly labeled

Turnaround Time Because of required testing, the time from blood donation until the blood is available for transfusion varies from about 18-36 hours.

Special Instructions As for other blood components.

Use Nowadays, the principal use of whole blood is to serve as the raw material for blood components. Replace red cell mass and plasma volume in patients in whom there is significant loss or depletion of both, improve oxygen transport (ie, treatment of acute blood loss). Acute bleeding, including massive transfusion in exsanguinating emergencies and some surgical cases. Exchange transfusion. Whole blood can be administered rapidly.

Limitations Usually in short supply because of demand for blood components. Although whole blood provides plasma proteins, other sources of oncotic/coagulation proteins are available. Some components, eg, platelets, factor V, factor VIII (AHF), are labile and not present in sufficient quantity in stored whole blood to provide adequate replacement therapy. Adenine, citrate, sodium, and antibodies are less in red blood cells, which are preferable to whole blood for patients with chronic renal or liver disease.

Contraindications Do not use whole blood for anemia that can be corrected with specific, safer products (eg, iron, B_{12}, folic acid). Whole blood is contraindicated in patients with congestive heart failure, uremia or hepatic failure, or with other chronic decrease of red cell mass. Such patients should receive red cells rather than whole blood if they require transfusion. For exchange transfusion, whole blood should preferably not be more than 5 days old. Replace blood volume deficits more safely and adequately with other volume expanders (saline, Ringer's lactate, albumin, plasma protein fraction). Treat coagulation factor deficiencies with appropriate concentrates (eg, cryoprecipitate or factor VIII or IX). The infusion of large volumes of blood may cause additional bleeding due to dilution of clotting factors or platelets, and may expand blood volume such that therapy with appropriate fractions (eg, FFP) may become hazardous. IgA-deficient patients may have anaphylactic reaction. Donor and recipient should be ABO and Rh compatible, except in unusual, life-threatening emergencies. A crossmatch is necessary unless delay in provision of blood might result in death.

Additional Information Whole blood is often not available. Substitute red blood cells. **Fresh blood** is impossible to define except by reference to whatever labile component is needed. Requests for "fresh" blood necessitate consultation and will usually be filled by issuing the appropriate components or fractions.

Footnotes

1. Klein HG, *Standards for Blood Banks and Transfusion Services*, 16th ed, Bethesda, MD: American Association of Blood Banks, 1994, 18.

References

Circular of Information for the Use of Human Blood and Blood Components, American Red Cross, Council of Community Blood Centers, American Association of Blood Banks, 1992.

Sohmer PR, "Transfusion Therapy in Surgery," *Clinical Practice of Transfusion Medicine*, Petz LD and Swisher SN, eds, 2nd ed, New York, NY: Churchill-Livingstone, 1989, 363-400.

Walker RH, *Technical Manual*, 11th ed, Arlington, VA: American Association of Blood Banks, 1993.

Whole Blood, Irradiated *see* Irradiated Blood Components *on page 611*

Zygosity, Rh *see* Rh Genotype *on page 622*

URINALYSIS AND CLINICAL MICROSCOPY

David S. Jacobs, MD

Wayne R. DeMott, MD

Bernard L. Kasten, Jr, MD

Eugene S. Olsowka, MD, PhD

Analysis of urine dates to ancient times. Clinical microscopy has been practiced for several hundred years. Thus, many of the tests presented are among the most enduring in medicine. Other more recently developed tests, such as dipstick screening procedures for urine glucose, protein, leukocyte esterase, and nitrite, yield significant clinical information rapidly and relatively inexpensively. Some of the other analyses performed on urine are listed in Chemistry introduction *on page 61* and the Therapeutic Drug Monitoring/Toxicology/Drugs of Abuse introduction *on page 527*.

Urine color has been of interest for centuries. Its color is determined by its concentration, the presence of drugs, exogenous and endogenous compounds, and its pH. **Colorless** urine may be normal or secondary to diuretic use, high fluid intake, diabetes insipidus, or diabetes mellitus. **Cloudy or hazy** urine may reflect the presence of phosphates, pyuria, or bacteruria. On oxidation, development of a **black** color is evidence for alkaptonuria.[1] Increased indican may cause the urine to blacken on standing. **Dark** urine is the second most common sign of acute intermittent porphyria. Very rarely, dark urine may indicate the presence of malignant melanoma. **Green** urine may be produced by indigo carmine, methylene blue, phenol, and in some cases of iodochlorhydroxyquin (clioquinol)-induced subacute myelo-opticoneuropathy. Other causes of green urine are reported as *Pseudomonas* bacteremia, urinary bile pigments, amitriptyline hydrochloride or methocarbamol ingestion, and breath freshener abuse.[2] **Red** urine was described elegantly by Berman[3] and is described further in the listing, Blood, Urine. Red plasma and red urine indicate hemoglobin; clear plasma with red urine may indicate myoglobin, but may occur as well in congenital erythropoietic porphyria and cutanea tarda porphyria. **Purple** urine, after standing, may also be due to porphyrins.[4] **Yellow** to **orange** urine may contain bile and should be tested for the presence of bile. Other causes of darker yellow to orange urine include increased concentration of urine or the presence of riboflavin, quinacrine (Atabrine®), rifampin (Rifadin®, Rimactane®), phenazopyridine (Pyridium®), or salicylazosulfapyridine (Azulfidine®). Color and appearance of urine were outlined well by Bradley and Shumann,[5] and by Graff.[6] As in some examples above, **drugs** may cause unusual urine colors.[7] The plastic urine bag may discolor **purple** in the presence of the indican produced by *Providencia* or *Klebsiella* species.[8]

Footnotes

1. Gaines JJ, "The Pathology of Alkaptonuric Ochronosis," *Hum Pathol*, 1989, 20:40-6.
2. Norfleet RG, "Green Urine," *JAMA*, 1982, 247:29.
3. Berman LB, "When the Urine Is Red," *JAMA*, 1977, 237:2753-4.
4. Forland M, "Urinalysis," *Internal Medicine*, 2nd ed, Chapter 85, Stein JH, ed, Boston, MA: Little, Brown and Co, 1987, 724-30.
5. Bradley M and Schumann GB, "Examination of Urine," *Todd-Sanford-Davidsohn Clinical Diagnosis and Management by Laboratory Methods*, 17th ed, Henry JB, ed, Philadelphia, PA: WB Saunders Co, 1984, 380.
6. Graff L, *Examination of Physical Characteristics, A Handbook of Routine Urinalysis*, Philadelphia, PA: JB Lippincott Co, 1982, 10-14.
7. Lubran MM, "Effect of Drugs on Clinical Laboratory Tests," *Clinical Pathology in the Elderly*, Chapter 24, Rochman H, ed, 1988, 193-6.
8. Dealler SF, Belfield PW, Belford M, et al, "Purple Urine Bags," *J Urol*, 1989, 142:769-70.

Acetest® *see* Ketones, Urine *on page 639*

Acetoacetic Acid, Urine *see* Ketones, Urine *on page 639*

Acetone, Semiquantitative, Urine *see* Ketones, Urine *on page 639*

Addis Count, 12-Hour

CPT 81015

Synonyms Urine Sediment, Quantitative

Test Commonly Includes Quantitation of casts, erythrocytes, and leukocytes

Use Primarily of historical interest

Limitations The Addis count is no longer in common clinical use because it is time consuming and is prone to technical inaccuracies. Semiquantitative urinalyses are now more commonly used. Note the dates of the publications listed in the following references. See listing Urinalysis *on page 658*.

References

Addis T, "A Clinical Classification of Bright's Disease," *JAMA*, 1925, 85:163-7.

Addis T, "The Effect of Some Physiologic Variables on the Number of Casts, RBCs, WBCs, and Epithelial Cells in the Urine of Normal Individuals," *J Clin Invest*, 1926, 2:417-21.

Addis T, "The Number of Formal Elements in Urinary Sediment of Normal Individuals," *J Clin Invest*, 1928, 2:409-15.

Albumin: Creatinine Ratio *see* Microalbuminuria *on page 643*

Albumin, Urine *see* Protein, Semiquantitative, Urine *on page 650*

Antispermatozoal Antibody Test *see* Infertility Screen *on page 638*

Bacteria Screen, Urine *see* Leukocyte Esterase, Urine *on page 641*

Bacteria Screen, Urine *see* Nitrite, Urine *on page 645*

Beta-Hydroxybutyric Acid, Urine *see* Ketones, Urine *on page 639*

Bile Fluid Examination

CPT 89050 (cell count, body fluid); 89060 (crystal identification, body fluid); 89100 (intubation, aspiration single specimen plus appropriate test procedure); 89105 (multiple fractional specimens with pancreatic or gallbladder stimulation)

Synonyms Biliary Drainage Examination; Crystal Examination, Biliary Drainage; Duodenal Drainage Examination

Abstract A variety of bile/duodenal content specimens obtained by tube aspiration, endoscopic retrograde cholangiopancreatography, or direct gallbladder puncture are studied for the presence of cholesterol, calcium bilirubinate, calcium carbonate crystals, bilirubin crystals, or parasites (predominantly *Giardia lamblia*). Crystals may support diagnoses of gallbladder and/or pancreatic disease. **Biliary sludge** is usually defined as a suspension of precipitates of cholesterol monohydrate crystals or calcium bilirubinate granules in bile[1] but calcium carbonate microspheroliths may be relevant as well.[2]

Patient Preparation Specimen is obtained by use of a gastroduodenal tube or a fiberoptic endoscopy study, either by direct aspiration or into a trap. Patient must take nothing by mouth after midnight before the test.

Specimen Bile fluid, duodenal drainage specimen

Sampling Time With tube in place and after a few minutes for a basal period Sincalide (Kinevac®-Squibb), a synthetic C-terminal octapeptide of cholecystokinin (CCK) is administered intravenously (I.V.) in a dose of 0.02 µg/kg of body weight and duodenal aspirate collected over the next 20-30 minutes. Alternatively, 100 units of cholecystokinin pancreozymin (the Boots Company, PLC, UK) may be given I.V. over a period of 1 minute.

Collection The collection may be divided into multiple containers, usually three: "A" bile (yellow - common duct origin), "B" bile (viscous and green or green-brown - gallbladder bile), and "C" bile (lighter color - hepatic bile duct origin). Many physicians send only one specimen, either a "pool" or a collection of largely "B" bile. Such "B" bile (gallbladder origin) may have a volume of 30-50 mL.

Reference Range Normal bile should not include any significant number of cholesterin plates (cholesterol crystals), calcium bilirubinate or bilirubin crystals, parasites, or inflammatory cells.

Use Evaluate cholelithiasis and cholecystitis in cases in which a high index of suspicion exists, but in which usual tests such as cholecystogram and ultrasound are negative. To try to improve results of litholytic therapy, cholesterol crystals in bile can identify most cholesterol calculi and calcium bilirubinate granules can be used to identify pigment stones.[3] It may used to detect occult microlithiasis in cases of "idiopathic"

acute pancreatitis.[4] Such fluid may be used to establish the presence of giardiasis. See also Ova and Parasites, Stool *on page 494.*

Limitations Specimen pH <4.5 may produce a false-positive bilirubin precipitate which may be confused with calcium bilirubinate.

This diagnostic approach for identification of crystals and diagnosis of cholelithiasis is not widely used.

Methodology Variation in processing of duodenal bile specimens prior to microscopic examination has contributed to difficulty in comparison of results of published series. The technique used is usually that of Juniper and Burson.[5,6] Each bile fraction is centrifuged at 2000 rpm for 10 minutes and the sediment examined using transmitted and polarized light microscopy, and the number of crystals specified using a grading system of 1-4. Some report crystals per high power field. Neoptolemos et al[7] centrifuged duodenal bile specimens at 3000 G for 10 minutes, examining the sediment at 20°C using direct and polarizing microscopy and examining a second sediment obtained by recentrifuging the supernatant after incubation at 37°C for 24 hours. Ramond et al,[8] studying gallbladder bile obtained by direct puncture at cholecystectomy, found sensitivity was increased by a second microscopic examination at 24 hours. They kept the bile samples at 37°C for at least 1 hour, centrifuged it at 12,000 rpm for 5 minutes, and examined the bile sample and pellet for crystals initially and after a 24-hour incubation at 37°C.

Stones can be classified by quantitative infrared spectroscopy.

Additional Information Microscopy of duodenal drainage bile may be useful in the investigation of cholelithiasis, "idiopathic" pancreatitis, and parasitism.[5,6,7,8,9] Analysis of aspirated stimulated "duodenal bile" can provide presumptive evidence of calculous biliary tract disease in patients with suggestive symptoms but negative gallbladder radiologic and ultrasonic studies.

In studies of gallbladder bile (obtained at cholecystectomy), presence of rhomboidal-shaped, birefringent cholesterol crystals as an indication of cholesterol gallstones has a sensitivity approaching 90% and a specificity of nearly 100%.[8] Reddish brown bilirubinate crystals alone as predictors of pigment stones have a lower level of sensitivity (about 70%) and specificity (slightly >90%).[8] Ramond et al found cholesterol crystals (in the absence of stones) in 4 of 11 patients with biliary stenosis, raising the possibility that bile stasis induces the formation of cholesterol crystals. As duodenal bile is diluted with variable amounts of gastric and small intestinal content, sensitivity of microscopy for crystals is likely somewhat decreased. Van Erpecum et al found the sensitivity (84%) of cholesterol crystals in fresh bile only slightly reduced in dilute gallbladder bile. They note "...examination of fresh bile for cholesterol crystals is a specific and reasonably sensitive test for cholesterol gallstone disease."[9]

Almost 70% of cases of acute pancreatitis are caused by gallstones or alcohol abuse.[1] Duodenal bile crystal analysis has been found useful in the investigation of "idiopathic" pancreatitis.[7] Microscopic examination of centrifuged duodenal bile in patients recovering from an episode of acute pancreatitis found cholesterol, bilirubinate, or calcium carbonate microspheroliths in 67% of cases while bile from postalcoholic pancreatitis patients was negative for crystals.[4] Study of gallbladder bile obtained at cholecystectomy (and/or serial GB ultrasonography) found biliary sludge or microlithiasis in 73% of patients.[4]

Bile cholesterol supersaturation with nearly all patients having cholesterol crystals in their bile has been reported in postcolectomy ulcerative colitis patients.[10]

Nucleation time (time required for the precipitation of cholesterol crystals in gallbladder bile) has been used in studies of the mechanism of gallstone dissolution by chenodeoxycholic acid versus ursodeoxycholic acid[11] and may be of use in predicting the formation of cholesterol gallstones.[12]

A sensitivity of 83% and specificity of 100% for recognition of cholelithiasis has been reported on the basis of microscopic examination of bile samples obtained at endoscopic retrograde cholangiography.[13]

When endoscopic drainage is utilized for initial control of severe acute cholangitis caused by choledocholithiasis, material can be cultured.[14]

While a variety of protozoan, trematode, and nematode parasites have been found in duodenal specimens, *Giardia lamblia* is most frequently encountered.[5] In patients clinically suspected of opisthorchiasis, in whom stool specimens are negative for ova, bile microscopy may be of special importance in establishing the diagnosis.[15]

Footnotes

1. Lee SP, Nicholls JF, and Park HZ, "Biliary Sludge as a Cause of Acute Pancreatitis," *N Engl J Med*, 1992, 326(9):589-93.
2. Steinberg WM, "Acute Pancreatitis - Never Leave a Stone Unturned," *N Engl J Med*, 1992, 326(9):635-7.
3. Agarwal DK, Choudhuri G, Saraswat VA, et al, "Utility of Biliary Microcrystal Analysis in Predicting Composition of Common Bile Duct Stones," *Scand J Gastroenterol*, 1994, 29(4):352-4.
4. Ros E, Navarro S, Bru C, et al, "Occult Microlithiasis in 'Idiopathic' Acute Pancreatitis: Prevention of Relapses by Cholecystectomy or Ursodeoxycholic Acid Therapy," *Gastroenterology*, 1991, 101(6):1701-9.

5. Juniper K and Burson EN Jr, "Biliary Tract Studies: II. The Significance of Biliary Crystals," *Gastroenterology*, 1957, 32:175-211.

6. Burnstein MJ, Vassal KP, and Strasburg SM, "Results of Combined Biliary Drainage and Cholecystokinin Cholecystography in 81 Patients With Normal Oral Cholecystograms," *Ann Surg*, 1982, 196:627-32.

7. Neoptolemos JP, Davidson BR, Winder AF, et al, "Role of Duodenal Bile Crystal Analysis in the Investigation of "Idiopathic" Pancreatitis," *Br J Surg*, 1988, 75(5):450-3.

8. Ramond MJ, Dumont M, Belghiti J, et al, "Sensitivity and Specificity of Microscopic Examination of Gallbladder Bile for Gallstone Recognition and Identification," *Gastroenterology*, 1988, 95(5):1339-43.

9. van Erpecum KJ, van Berge Henegouwen GP, Stoelwinder B, et al, "Cholesterol and Pigment Gallstone Disease: Comparison of the Reliability of Three Bile Tests for Differentiation Between the Two Stone Types," *Scand J Gastroenterol*, 1988, 23(8):948-54.

10. Harvey PR, McLeod RS, Cohen Z, et al, "Effect of Colectomy on Bile Composition, Cholesterol Crystal Formation, and Gallstones in Patients With Ulcerative Colitis," *Ann Surg*, 1991, 214(4):396-401.

11. Sahlin S, Ahlberg J, Angelin B, et al, "Nucleation Time of Gallbladder Bile in Gallstone Patients: Influence of Bile Acid Treatment," *Gut*, 1991, 32(12):1554-7.

12. Marks JW, Broomfield P, Bonorris GG, et al, "Factors Affecting the Measurement of Cholesterol Nucleation in Human Gallbladder and Duodenal Bile," *Gastroenterology*, 1991, 101(1):214-9.

13. Buscail L, Escourrou J, Delvaux M, et al, "Microscopic Examination of Bile Directly Collected During Endoscopic Cannulation of the Papilla - Utility in Patients With Suspected Microlithiasis," *Dig Dis Sci*, 1992, 37(1):116-20.

14. Lai EC, Mok FP, Tan ES, et al, "Endoscopic Biliary Drainage for Severe Acute Cholangitis," *N Engl J Med*, 1992, 326(24):1582-6.

15. Dao AH, Barnwell SF, and Adkins RB Jr, "A Case of Opisthorchiasis Diagnosed by Cholangiography and Bile Examination," *Am J Surg*, 1991, 57(4):206-9.

References

Bockus HL, Shay H, Willard JH, et al, "Comparison of Biliary Drainage and Cholecystography in Gallstone Diagnosis: With Especial Reference to Bile Microscopy," *JAMA*, 1931, 96:311-17.

Janowitz P, Swobodnik W, Wechsler JG, et al, "Comparison of Gallbladder Bile and Endoscopically Obtained Duodenal Bile," *Gut*, 1990, 31(12):1407-10.

Magnuson TH, Lillemoe KD, Scheeres DE, et al, "Altered Bile Composition During Cholesterol Gallstone Formation: Cause or Effect?" *J Surg Res*, 1990, 48(6):584-9.

Paumgartner G and Sauerbruch T, "Secretions, Composition, and Flow of Bile," *J Clin Gastroenterol*, 1983, 12:3-23.

Bile, Urine

CPT 81002 (dipstick, nonautomated); 81003 (dipstick, automated)

Related Information

Bilirubin, Direct *on page 86*
Bilirubin, Total *on page 86*
Urobilinogen, 2-Hour Urine *on page 660*

Synonyms Bilirubin, Urine

Abstract Screen for diseases characterized by increased serum conjugated bilirubin. Only conjugated bilirubin is passed into the urine.

Specimen Random urine

Storage Instructions Refrigeration

Reference Range Negative

Use Detect the presence of bilirubin in urine; screen for some instances of liver disease. In obstructive disease of the biliary tract such as biliary calculi, carcinoma of pancreas or of bile ducts, urine bilirubin is frequently positive. See table.

Differential Diagnosis Using Urine Bilirubin and Urobilinogen Tests

Type of Jaundice	Urine Bilirubin	Urine Urobilinogen
Normal	0	0 - trace
Hepatocellular jaundice (eg, hepatitis, chemical, or drug injury)	↑	↑
Biliary obstruction (extrahepatic and intrahepatic); obstructive jaundice	↑	0
Hemolytic jaundice	0	↑

0 = absent; ↑ = increased

Limitations Occasional false-positives are seen, predominantly in elderly patients. They commonly represent stool contamination of the urine sample. Ponstel® (mefenamic acid) administration and Thorazine®, Ormazine® (chlorpromazine) therapy may result in false-positive reactions. Prolonged standing of the sample, especially at room temperature and in the light, may lead to false-negatives. Pyridium® (phenazopyridine) and Serenium® (ethoxazene hydrochloride) and local anesthetic metabolites give bright reddish orange colors which may mask the reaction of small amounts of bilirubin. Specific urine bile assays, even urine urobilinogen, provide substantial numbers of false-negatives when used as a screen for liver disease as determined by at least one abnormal serum liver function test abnormality. If just used to screen for the presence of raised serum bilirubin, the test is about 79% to 89% specific and has an 89% negative predictive value when used in an emergency room setting.[1] Indoxyl has been reported to interfere with dip-and-read testing for urine bilirubin sufficiently to mask a weak reaction. A more specific test such as the Ictotest® has been recommended when such dip-and-

read results are inconclusive.[2] The manufacturer expresses a need for proper storage of the reagent.

Methodology Diazotization reaction in an acid medium yields a blue to purple color

Additional Information The method detects as little as 0.05-0.1 mg bilirubin/100 mL. The test is exquisitely sensitive for bilirubinuria. However, detection of bilirubinuria is not a sensitive indicator of hepatic disease. In uncomplicated hemolytic anemia serum bilirubin may be normal, or a minimal elevation of indirect bilirubin may be present; **indirect (unconjugated) bilirubin does not readily pass through the glomerulus. Therefore, bile is not usually detectable in the urine in uncomplicated hemolytic anemia.** Similarly, urine bilirubin may not be present with well advanced hepatic disease; serum total bilirubin is not always increased with advanced liver disease. If jaundice is severe, renal excretion becomes significant; and if renal function deteriorates, serum direct bilirubin levels may increase.[3] Urine bile, if positive, carries an implication of elevation of serum conjugated (direct) bilirubin and should be confirmed by measurement of total and direct bilirubin in serum, as well as liver-related enzymes. The liver cell conjugates bilirubin with glucuronic acid.

Footnotes

1. Binder L, Smith D, Kupka T, et al, "Failure of Prediction of Liver Function Test Abnormalities With the Urine Urobilinogen and Urine Bilirubin Assays," *Arch Pathol Lab Med*, 1989, 113(1):73-6.

2. Skjold AC, Freitag JF, and Stover LR, "Indoxyl Sulfate Interferes With Dip-and-Read Urinalysis," *Clin Chem*, 1980, 26(9):1368-9.

3. Fleischner G and Arias IM, "Recent Advances in Bilirubin Formation, Transport, Metabolism, and Excretion," *Am J Med*, 1970, 49:576-89.

Biliary Drainage Examination *see* Bile Fluid Examination *on previous page*

Bilirubin, Urine *see* Bile, Urine *on this page*

Blood, Occult, Stool *see* Occult Blood, Stool *on page 645*

Blood, Occult, Urine *see* Blood, Urine *on this page*

Blood, Urine

CPT 82273

Related Information

Glomerular Basement Membrane Antibody *on page 395*
Hemoglobin, Qualitative, Urine *on page 637*
Hemosiderin Stain, Urine *on page 637*
Kidney Stone Analysis *on page 640*
Myoglobin, Qualitative, Urine *on page 644*
Ova and Parasites, Urine *on page 495*
Platelet Count *on page 340*
Protein, Quantitative, Urine *on page 649*
Prothrombin Time *on page 262*
Urinalysis *on page 658*
Urinalysis, Fractional *on page 659*
Urine Cytology *on page 301*

Synonyms Blood, Occult, Urine; Hemoglobin, Urine; Occult Blood, Urine

Test Commonly Includes Dipstick method for occult blood is usually a part of urinalysis.

Abstract Positive dipstick usually indicates hematuria, hemoglobinuria, or myoglobinuria. When a dipstick is positive for blood, microscopy is desirable to search for RBCs. A definition of pediatric hematuria is 2 cells/hpf in urine sediment. The presence of proteinuria is clinically relevant when hematuria is detected.[1]

In adults, a definition of hematuria has included five or more RBCs/hpf. Hematuria may provide evidence of neoplasm, nephrolithiasis, papillary necrosis, infection (including tuberculosis), renal cysts, and other entities.[2]

Both reagent strips and sediment microscopy are necessary.[3]

Specimen Random urine

Storage Instructions Refrigeration; examination of fresh urine is best.

Causes for Rejection Standing for more than 2 hours at room temperature may be a reason to consider a specimen unacceptable.

Reference Range Negative by dipstick; up to 2-3 red cells/high power field are generally accepted as normal by microscopy.

Use Detect myoglobin, hemoglobin, or red blood cells in urine (detect hematuria, microhematuria, hemoglobinuria, or erythrocyturia). See table.

Limitations Dipstick methods detect myoglobin as hemoglobin. Both intact erythrocytes and free hemoglobin give a positive reaction. Iodine solutions in urine, or applied to patient's skin, are reported to cause false-positives.[4] Certain oxidizing agents such as hypochlorite (bleach) may produce false-positive results if present in the collection vessel. Microbial peroxidase, particularly that produced by gram-negative rods and staphylococci associated with urinary tract infection and leukocyte (Continued)

Blood, Urine (Continued)

Blood, Urine

Causes of Hematuria	Causes of Hemoglobinuria
Renal diseases including:	Hemolysis associated with:
glomerulonephritis	parasites (ie, malaria)
Goodpasture's syndrome	drugs
lupus nephritis	chemicals
arteritis	antibodies
Wegener's granulomatosis	March hemoglobinuria –
stone	secondary to severe exercise
tumor	Transfusion reactions
polycystic kidney	incompatible blood
nfarct	Burns
infection, including	Crush injury
pyelonephritis	Poisoning
necrotizing papillitis	snake or spider bite
trauma	Paroxysmal nocturnal hemoglobinuria
Blood diseases including:	Paroxysmal cold hemoglobinuria
thrombocytopenia	Myoglobin (detected as hemoglobin)
thrombotic thrombocytopenic purpura	
Henoch-Schönlein purpura	
infective endocarditis	
leukemia	
hemophilias	
sickle cell trait	
Bladder diseases including:	
cystitis	
carcinoma	
papilloma	
Prostatic diseases including:	
prostatitis	
BPH (benign nodular and glandular hyperplasia)	
prostatic adenocarcinoma	
Urethral diseases including:	
urethritis	
tumor	
Trauma	
Drugs including:	
Coumadin®	
heparin	
salicylates	
many others	

The number of red cells (grade of microhematuria) does not necessarily correlate with the degree or significance of urologic pathologic findings (ie, a patient with more than 5 unexplained red cells in urine may have an important urologic lesion). Additional studies (such as urine culture, cytology, excretory urography, cystoscopy) may be indicated. Patients on anticoagulants exhibiting gross or microscopic hematuria should be carefully evaluated for carcinoma and calculi.[10] Recognizable genitourinary tract disease is found in most anticoagulated individuals who have microscopic hematuria. Contemporary levels of long-term anticoagulation do not provide explanation for hematuria.[2] The use of nonsteroidal anti-inflammatory drugs including aspirin may be associated with hematuria.[11]

A positive dipstick test for blood without red cells in the urine sediment may indicate hemoglobinuria, myoglobinuria, or the presence of porphyrins. Drugs causing hematuria are listed.[9] Algorithms for diagnosis of hematuria are published for children[12] and adults.[13] Phenytoin does not cause urine to appear red, but uric acid and urate crystals in acid urine may cause a pink to red-brown color.[14] **See Urinalysis Introduction *on page 629* for further information on colored urine.**

In correlation between dipsticks and microscopy in abdominal trauma, some authors feel that microscopy is needed when the dipstick is positive to determine whether or not an IVP is indicated. Others have recommended urine microscopy in all cases of blunt abdominal traumas.[15] Kennedy et al report false-negatives and false-positives but concluded that the safety of dipsticks for hematuria in subjects sustaining blunt or penetrating abdominal trauma is acceptable.[16] Messing and coworkers found that hematuria, even in the presence of significant disease such as urinary tract malignancy, often was intermittent. They have proposed home dipstick screening based upon their study of asymptomatic men older than 50 years of age;[17] others disagree.[18]

Twenty percent of patients older than 40 years with asymptomatic hematuria have significant urologic lesions, of which half are malignant.[19]

An important response to a paper reporting inaccurate results of urine dipstick results[7] emphasizes the need for quality control and perceives the need for laboratory testing to be performed by those well versed in good laboratory practice.[20]

Footnotes

1. Fitzwater DS and Wyatt RJ, "Hematuria," *Pediatr Rev*, 1994, 15(3):102-8.
2. Culclasure TF, Bray VJ, and Hasbargen JA, "The Significance of Hematuria in the Anticoagulated Patient," *Arch Intern Med*, 1994, 154(6):649-52.
3. Bartlett RC, Zern DA, Ratkiewicz I, et al, "Reagent Strip Screening for Sediment Abnormalities Identified by Automated Microscopy in Urine From Patients Suspected to Have Urinary Tract Disease," *Arch Pathol Lab Med*, 1994, 118(11):1096-101.
4. Said R, "Contamination of Urine With Povidone-Iodine. Cause of False-Positive Test for Occult Blood in Urine," *JAMA*, 1979, 242:748-9.
5. Jaffe RM, Lawrence L, Schmid A, et al, "Inhibition by Ascorbic Acid (Vitamin C) of Chemical Detection of Blood in Urine," *Am J Clin Pathol*, 1979, 72:468-70.
6. Brown SH, MacDougall ML, and Wiegmann TB, "Microscopic Hematuria," *Kans Med*, 1986, 87(4):99-101,113.
7. Cohen HT and Spiegel DM, "Air-Exposed Urine Dipsticks Give False-Positive Results for Glucose and False-Negative Results for Blood," *Am J Clin Pathol*, 1991, 96(3):398-400.
8. Yadin O, "Hematuria in Children," *Pediatr Ann*, 1994, 23(9):474-8, 481-5.
9. Abuelo JG, "The Diagnosis of Hematuria," *Arch Intern Med*, 1983, 143:967-70.
10. Schuster GA and Lewis GA, "Clinical Significance of Hematuria in Patients on Anticoagulant Therapy," *J Urol*, 1987, 137(5):923-5.
11. Kraus SE, Siroky MB, Babayan RK, et al, "Hematuria and the Use of Nonsteroidal Anti-inflammatory Drugs," *J Urol*, 1984, 132(2):288-90.
12. Lieu TA, Grasmeder HM 3d, and Kaplan BS, "An Approach to the Evaluation and Treatment of Microscopic Hematuria," *Pediatr Clin North Am*, 1991, 38(3):579-92.
13. Restrepo NC and Carey PO, "Evaluating Hematuria in Adults," *Am Fam Physician*, 1989, 40(2):149-56.
14. Derby BM and Ward JW, "The Myth of Red Urine Due to Phenytoin," *JAMA*, 1983, 249:1723-4.
15. Daum GS, Krolikowski FJ, Reuter KL, et al, "Dipstick Evaluation of Hematuria in Abdominal Trauma," *Am J Clin Pathol*, 1988, 89(4):538-42.
16. Kennedy TJ, McConnell JD, and Thal ER, "Urine Dipstick vs Microscopic Urinalysis in the Evaluation of Abdominal Trauma," *J Trauma*, 1988, 28(5):615-7.
17. Messing EM, Young TB, Hunt VB, et al, "Urinary Tract Cancers Found by Homescreening With Hematuria Dipsticks in Healthy Men Over 50 Years of Age," *Cancer*, 1989, 64(11):2361-7.
18. Woolhandler S, Pels RJ, Bor DH, et al, "Dipstick Urinalysis Screening of Asymptomatic Adults for Urinary Tract Disorders - I. Hematuria and Proteinuria," *JAMA*, 1989, 262(9):1214-9.
19. Chen HH, Shields RC, and Bardsley WT, "68-Year Old Man With Anemia and Renal Failure," *Mayo Clin Proc*, 1996, 71(2):197-200.
20. Cadoff EM, "Inaccurate Results of Urine Dipstick Tests," *Am J Clin Pathol*, 1992, 98(2):269.

peroxidase, may cause a false-positive reaction. Pyridium® (phenazopyridine) and Serenium® (ethoxazene hydrochloride) metabolites may mask the dipstick reaction. Large amounts of nitrite may delay reactions. The sensitivity of the occult blood test is reduced in urines with high specific gravity and/or high ascorbic acid content.[5] High urine protein and formalin are reported to cause false-negatives.[6] Prolonged air exposure of the dipstick (dipstick jar left uncapped) reduces the sensitivity of the dipstick for blood.[7] Transient hematuria can reflect menstruation, catheterization, or strenuous exercise. Urine sediment microscopy should be used to confirm a diagnosis of hematuria suggested by positive dipstick. The dipstick sensitivity for the detection of red cells was reported to be 75.3% and specificity 88.6% in a recent study. Screening asymptomatic adults for microhematuria as a method of detection of subsequent urological cancers was not recommended in a 1994 report.

Methodology Dipstick is based on the pseudoperoxidase activity of hemoglobin. Microscopy is used for recognition of red blood cells and red cell casts.

Additional Information Clues to glomerular origin of hematuria include proteinuria, red cell casts and dysmorphic red cells, hypertension, and evidence of renal dysfunction.[8] The test will detect 0.03 mg/dL free hemoglobin or 10 intact red blood cells/µL. Further tests to work-up hematuria may include CBC, platelet count, urine culture, ESR, ANA, prothrombin time, PTT, serum BUN, creatinine, and other examinations as appropriate. IgA nephropathy is the most common type of glomerular disease related to asymptomatic gross hematuria. More than 3.5 g of protein in a 24-hour urine collection provides indication of glomerular disease;[9] more than 1 g of protein is suggestive.

References

Abarbanel J, Benet AE, Lask D, et al, "Sports Hematuria," *J Urol*, 1990, 143(5):887-90.

Abuelo JG, "Evaluation of Hematuria," *Urology*, 1983, 21:215-25.

Bee DE, James GP, and Paul KL, "Hemoglobinuria and Hematuria: Accuracy and Precision of Laboratory Diagnosis," *Clin Chem*, 1979, 10:1696-9.

Bloom KJ, "An Algorithm for Hematuria," *Clin Lab Med*, 1988, 8(3):577-84.

Bonnardeaux A, Somerville P, and Kaye M, "A Study on the Reliability of Dipstick Urinalysis," *Clin Nephrol*, 1994, 41(3):167-72.

Campbell KL, "Blood, Urine, Saliva, and Dip-Sticks: Experiences in Africa, New Guinea, and Boston," *Ann N Y Acad Sci*, 1994, 709:312-30.

Copley JB, "Isolated Asymptomatic Hematuria in the Adult," *Am J Med Sci*, 1986, 291(2):101-11.

Hiatt RA and Ordonez JD, "Dipstick Urinalysis Screening, Asymptomatic Microhematuria, and Subsequent Urological Cancers in a Population-Based Sample," *Cancer Epidemiol Biomarkers Prev*, 1994, 3(5):439-43.

Lam MH, "False Hematuria Due to Bacteriuria," *Arch Pathol Lab Med*, 1995, 119(8):717-21.

Mohr DN, Offord KP, Owen RA, et al, "Asymptomatic Microhematuria and Urologic Disease. A Population-based Study," *JAMA*, 1986, 256(2):224-9.

Moore GP and Robinson M, "Do Urine Dipsticks Reliably Predict Microhematuria? The Bloody Truth!" *Ann Emerg Med*, 1988, 17(3):257-60.

Smith RF, Mohr DN, Torres VE, et al, "Renal Insufficiency in Community Patients With Mild Asymptomatic Microhematuria," *Mayo Clin Proc*, 1989, 64(4):409-14.

Yoshikawa N, Matsuyama D, Iijima K, et al, "Benign Familial Hematuria," *Arch Pathol Lab Med*, 1988, 112(8):794-7.

Body Fluid, Specific Gravity *see* Specific Gravity, Urine *on page 653*

Breath Hydrogen Analysis *see* Reducing Substances, Stool *on page 651*

Calcium Pyrophosphate Dihydrate Crystal (CPPD) Deposition *see* Synovial Fluid Analysis *on page 656*

Calculus Analysis *see* Kidney Stone Analysis *on page 640*

Casts, Urine *see* Urinalysis *on page 658*

Cervical Mucus Interaction, Cross Hostility Tests *see* Sperm Mucus Penetration Test (Human or Bovine Cervical Mucus) *on page 654*

Clinitest® for Sugar, Urine *see* Reducing Substances, Urine *on page 652*

¹³CO₂ Breath Test *see* Reducing Substances, Stool *on page 651*

Colo-Rect® *see* Occult Blood, Stool *on page 645*

Colo-Screen® *see* Occult Blood, Stool *on page 645*

Concentrating Ability, Urine *see* Concentration Test, Urine *on this page*

Concentration Test, Urine

CPT 81000 (specific gravity, automated); 81002 (specific gravity, nonautomated); 83935 (osmolality)

Related Information
Calcium, Serum *on page 97*
Osmolality, Urine *on page 173*
Potassium, Serum or Plasma *on page 188*
Sodium, Blood *on page 199*
Specific Gravity, Urine *on page 653*

Synonyms Concentrating Ability, Urine; Fishberg Concentration Test; Urine Concentration Test

Applies to Vasopressin Concentration Test

Test Commonly Includes Assessment of concentrating ability of the kidney by determination of specific gravity or osmolality following water deprivation and/or after administration of vasopressin

Abstract Patients with polyuria are sometimes difficult to evaluate, as some have polydipsia with resulting polyuria and normal kidneys; others have polyuria with resultant mild or moderate hypernatremia and therefore polydipsia. To separate these groups, this test evaluates urine output and osmolality (and/or specific gravity) when water is deprived, sufficient to cause mild hypernatremia. Since the kidneys may abnormally excrete water in the face of hypernatremia or even hypovolemia, this test must be closely monitored to prevent patient injury (hyperosmolar state or dehydration).

Patient Preparation The evening meal must be high in protein and contain not more than 200 mL of liquid. Patient is to consume no fluids after the evening meal. On awakening in the morning, the patient voids and saves the specimen in container #1. All further urine passed until 1 hour later is included in specimen #2. All further urine then until 2 hours later is collected as specimen #3. The volume of each voiding and the total volume of each collection is recorded. If urine specific gravity plateaus but a specific gravity of 1.027 or urine osmolality of 850 mOsm/kg is not achieved, vasopressin can be administered.

Protein and radiographic dyes can increase specific gravity despite decreased concentrating ability. The patient must not be taking diuretics.

Aftercare Fluid restriction may decrease plasma volume and have an adverse effect on cardiac output in patients with compromised cardiac function. If diabetes insipidus is present, urine output may remain very high despite fluid deprivation. Body weight and blood pressure should be carefully followed throughout the procedure. If body weight is decreased by 5% or orthostatic hypotension occurs, the procedure should be terminated. Test should be supervised by the physician.

Specimen Urine

Container Three urine containers

Storage Instructions Refrigeration

Reference Range Normal: specific gravity of at least one specimen should be >1.026 or >850 mOsm/kg (SI: >850 mmol/kg); severe renal disease: <400 mOsm/kg (SI: <400 mmol/kg). A random urine collected without water restriction yielding a urine osmolality ≥900 mOsm/kg (SI: ≥900 mmol/kg) or a specific gravity ≥1.027 virtually excludes a defect in concentrating ability, and thus, may be done as a screening procedure before more elaborate deprivation studies are undertaken.[1]

Use Evaluate renal concentrating ability, a test of tubular function; useful in the differential diagnosis of diabetes insipidus,[2] compulsive water drinking, and renal disease

Causes of Symptomatic (Polyuric) Deficiencies in Plasma Vasopressin

Decreased secretion
Destruction of neurohypophysis (neurogenic diabetes insipidus)
  Sporadic
    Idiopathic
    Trauma (surgical, accidental)
    Malignancy
      Primary (craniopharyngioma, dysgerminoma, meningioma, adenoma, glioma, astrocytoma)
      Secondary (metastatic from lung or breast, lymphoma, leukemia, dysplastic pancytopenia)
    Granuloma (sarcoid, histiocytosis, xanthoma disseminatum)
    Infection (viral/bacterial meningitis, encephalitis)
    Vascular (Sheehan's syndrome, carotid aneurysm, hematoma, aortocoronary bypass, ischemic brain death)
    Autoimmune disease
    Dysplasia (septo-optic, microcephaly, porencephaly, etc)
    Metabolic (anorexia nervosa)
  Familial (autosomal dominant)
Excessive water intake (primary polydipsia)
  Psychogenic (schizophrenia, ? neurosis)
  Dipsogenic (abnormal thirst)
    Idiopathic
    Trauma
    Granuloma (neurosarcoid, tuberculous meningitis)
    Autoimmune (multiple sclerosis)
    Chemical (lithium)
Increased metabolism
  Gestational

From Robertson GL and Berl T, "Pathophysiology of Water Metabolism," *The Kidney*, Brenner BM and Rector FC Jr, eds, Philadelphia, PA: WB Saunders Co, 1991, 695, with permission.

Causes of Defects in Antidiuretic Action of Vasopressin

Familial nephrogenic diabetes insipidus
  X-linked recessive
Sporadic nephrogenic diabetes insipidus
  Chemical (lithium, demeclocycline, methoxyflurane)
  Metabolic (hypokalemia, hypercalcemia)
  Mechanical (ureteral obstruction)
  Vascular (sickle cell disease or trait)
  Granulomatous (sarcoid)
  Dysplastic (polycystic disease)
  Infectious (pyelonephritis)
  Infiltrative (amyloid)
  Gestational
  Malignant (fibrosarcoma)
Solute diuresis
  Metabolic (glucosuria)
  Iatrogenic (mannitol, furosemide, radiocontrast dyes, saline loading)
  Mechanical (postureteral obstruction)

From Robertson GL and Berl T, "Pathophysiology of Water Metabolism," *The Kidney*, Brenner BM and Rector FC Jr, eds, Philadelphia, PA: WB Saunders Co, 1991, 699, with permission.

Limitations In polydipsic patients, the urine specific gravity may not rise to 1.026 until after many hours of deprivation. False-positive tests can be avoided by making sure serum sodium is 141-145 mmol/L before termination of the test. The test may have to be extended or adapted to the
(Continued)

Concentration Test, Urine *(Continued)*

patient, and this is best done with a clear understanding of the physiology of vasopressin and of water metabolism. For details see Robertson and Berl reference.[3]

Contraindications Glucosuria invalidates a concentration test by virtue of its diuretic effect; hypernatremia or orthostatic hypotension are contraindications.

Methodology Modified Fishberg procedure

Additional Information Glomerular disorders causing proteinuria result in decreased concentrating ability by producing an osmotic diuresis in the functioning nephrons. Even subtle renal interstitial disorders may impair concentrating ability. Hypokalemia and hypercalcemia decrease renal medullary tonicity and inhibit tubular reabsorption of water. Sickle cell disease decreases medullary blood flow and interferes with loop of Henle sodium transport. Achievement of normal maximal urinary concentration requires a normal or near normal glomerular filtration rate.[1] In central diabetes insipidus, administration of vasopressin will raise urine osmolality. In nephrogenic diabetes insipidus, the urine osmolality will not increase with vasopressin or water deprivation.

Urine color may be used in athletic or industrial settings to determine whether humans are well hydrated, euhydrated, or hypohydrated. Urine osmolality and urine specific gravity can be utilized interchangeably to determine hydration status more accurately and precisely.[4]

Footnotes
1. Haycock GB, "Old and New Test of Renal Function," *J Clin Pathol*, 1981, 34:1276-81.
2. Price JD and Lauener RW, "Serum and Urine Osmolalities in the Differential Diagnosis of Polyuric States," *J Clin Endocrinol Metab*, 1966, 26:143-9.
3. Robertson GL and Berl T, "Pathophysiology of Water Metabolism," *Kidney*, Brenner BM and Rector FC Jr, eds, Philadelphia, PA: WB Saunders Co, 1991, 677-736.
4. Armstrong LE, Maresh CM, Castellani JW, et al, "Urinary Indices of Hydration Status," *Int J Sport Nutr*, 1994, 4(3):265-79.

References
Gupta AK, Kirchner KA, Nicholson R, et al, "Effects of α-Thalassemia and Sickle Polymerization Tendency on the Urine-Concentrating Defect of Individuals With Sickle Cell Trait," *J Clin Invest*, 1991, 88(6):1963-8.

Crystal Examination, Biliary Drainage *see* Bile Fluid Examination on page 630

Crystals, Urine *see* Urinalysis on page 658

Duodenal Drainage Examination *see* Bile Fluid Examination on page 630

Eosinophils, Urine

CPT 85999

Related Information
Ova and Parasites, Urine *on page 495*
Protein, Quantitative, Urine *on page 649*
Urinalysis *on page 658*

Synonyms Eosinophiluria; Hansel's Stain of Urine; Urinary Eosinophils

Abstract A relatively new, nonspecific and poorly standardized marker for interstitial nephritis, eosinophilic cystitis, atheroembolic disease, and probably other entities.

Specimen Clean catch midstream urine specimen[1]

Storage Instructions Test should be done on a fresh specimen.

Causes for Rejection Urine more than 3 hours old from time of collection

Reference Range <100 eosinophils/mL; using Hansel's stain, <1% eosinophils[2]

Use Eosinophils are sought in urine to help confirm suspected cases of interstitial nephritis, eosinophilic cystitis, and renal atheroemboli (cholesterol emboli syndrome).

Limitations Eosinophiluria is not always present or prominent in interstitial nephritis and may be present in other disease entities. In a recent report, 6 of 15 patients with a confirmed diagnosis of acute interstitial nephritis (AIN) had eosinophiluria; however, 10 of 36 patients with other renal diagnosis also had eosinophiluria. Sensitivity was 40%, specificity 72%. Positive predictive value for AIN was only 38%.[2]

Methodology Centrifuged clean catch, midstream urine, stained with Hansel's stain.[3] It is methylene blue and eosin Y in methanol (Lide Labs, Florissant, MO). Wright's stain is no longer recommended, as it is less sensitive, although still specific.
- Spin 10 mL of freshly voided urine at 2000 rpm, 5 minutes.
- Decant supernatant.
- Pipette sediment to a glass slide and air dry.
- Immerse slides in 95% methanol for 5 seconds.
- Apply Hansel's stain, 45 seconds.
- Add 20 drops of distilled water, allow to stand for 30 seconds.
- Remove excess stain with distilled water.
- Decolorize with four drops of methanol for 1-2 seconds.
- Rinse with distilled water.
- After drying, apply a coverslip with a drop of immersion oil.

- Following this protocol, 1% (or more) eosinophils is regarded as positive.[3]

Additional Information There is an uncertain relationship between eosinophiluria and peripheral blood eosinophilia. In only 33% of cases of drug-induced acute interstitial nephritis is the complete syndrome present. The complete syndrome includes fever, rash, eosinophiluria with acute renal failure.[3] Acute interstitial nephritis relates to penicillin derivatives, sulfa drugs, allopurinol, sulfinpyrazone, nitrofurantoin, and erythromycin. Methicillin is also frequently mentioned.[1] Eight of nine patients with biopsy proven atheroembolic renal failure demonstrated eosinophiluria by Hansel's stain. Six of eight of these patients had >5% of leukocytes as eosinophils.[4] Other diseases in which urinary eosinophilia is reported include contrast nephropathy, renal failure, glomerulonephritis, urinary tract infection,[5] and schistosomiasis.[6]

Footnotes
1. Sutton JM, "Urinary Eosinophils," *Arch Intern Med*, 1986, 146(11):2243-4.
2. Ruffing KA, Hoppes P, Blend D, et al, "Eosinophils in Urine Revisited," *Clin Nephrol*, 1994, 41(3):163-6.
3. Nolan CR 3d, Anger MS, and Kelleher SP, "Eosinophiluria - A New Method of Detection and Definition of the Clinical Spectrum," *N Engl J Med*, 1986, 315(24):1516-8.
4. Wilson DM, Salazer TL, and Farkouh ME, "Eosinophiluria in Atheroembolic Renal Disease," *Am J Med*, 1991, 91(2):186-9.
5. Corwin HL, Korbet SM, and Schwartz MM, "Clinical Correlates of Eosinophiluria," *Arch Intern Med*, 1985, 145(6):1097-9.
6. Eltoum IA, Ghalib HW, Sualaiman S, et al, "Significance of Eosinophiluria in Urinary Schistosomiasis - A Study Using Hansel's Stain and Electron Microscopy," *Am J Clin Pathol*, 1989, 92(3):329-38.

References
Brunzel NA, *Fundamentals of Urine and Body Fluid Analysis*, Philadelphia, PA: WB Saunders Co, 1994, 214, 222.
Corwin HL, Bray RA, and Haber MH, "The Detection and Interpretation of Urinary Eosinophils," *Arch Pathol Lab Med*, 1989, 113(11):1256-8.
Nolan CR 3d and Kelleher SP, "Eosinophiluria," *Clin Lab Med*, 1988, 8(3):555-65.

Eosinophiluria *see* Eosinophils, Urine on this page

Esterase, Leukocyte, Urine *see* Leukocyte Esterase, Urine on page 641

Fat, Semiquantitative, Stool

CPT 82705

Related Information
Carotene, Serum *on page 103*
d-Xylose Absorption Test *on page 122*
Fecal Fat, Quantitative, 72-Hour Collection *on page 127*
Meat Fibers, Stool *on page 642*
Methylene Blue Stain, Stool *on page 642*
pH, Stool *on page 648*

Synonyms Fatty Acid, Stool; Fecal Fat Stain; Neutral Fat, Stool; Stool Fat, Semiquantitative; Sudan III Stain, Stool

Applies to Fecal Fat Analysis, 72-Hour; Steatocrit

Abstract In this simple and low cost procedure, fecal fat is stained with Sudan III. The test is used as a screen for the presence of fecal neutral fat and fatty acids and may assist in the determination of the cause of steatorrhea. However, the diagnosis of steatorrhea is defined by a quantitative 72-hour fecal fat.

Patient Preparation Patient should be on diet containing at least 60 g of fat. The patient should not use suppositories or mineral oil before the specimen is collected. Oily material (eg, creams, lubricants, etc) should be avoided prior to collection of the specimen.

Specimen Fresh random stool

Reference Range Neutral fat: <50 fat globules/hpf, reported as normal. Fatty acids: <100 fat globules/hpf is considered normal.

Use Screen for the presence of fecal fatty acids and neutral fat. Increases in neutral fat are commonly associated with pancreatic exocrine insufficiency. Increased stool fatty acids are likely to be associated with small bowel disease.

Limitations Castor oil or mineral oil droplets can mimic neutral fat.

This is not a definitive test; *vide infra*.

Contraindications Administration of barium, bismuth, Metamucil®, castor oil, or mineral oil within 1 week prior to collection of the specimen

Methodology Small amount of stool sample is mixed with two drops of water, two drops of 95% ethanol, and three to four drops of Sudan III stain. Increased yellow-orange refractile fat globules (direct Sudan III stain) identifies neutral fats. Fatty acids and fat soaps are detected after hydrolysis by mixing stool sample with two to three drops each of Sudan III and glacial acetic acid, followed by heating before microscopic examination.

Additional Information The test consists of determination of the presence of neutral fats and of total fats representing fatty acids. The results are reported semiquantitatively. In a comparison of screening tests for enteropathy in children, results of lactose breath hydrogen, 1-hour d-xylose absorption, and 72-hour fecal fat tests were compared with the results of jejunal biopsy. Only the d-xylose and fecal fat tests correlated significantly with biopsy results.[1] See listing Meat Fibers, Stool *on page 642.*

Presence of steatorrhea can be established by the results of a 72-hour fecal fat analysis. Maldigestion or malabsorption may cause steatorrhea. Patients with maldigestion excrete excess triglyceride while patients with malabsorption excrete excess fatty acid. The 72-hour fecal fat determination involves saponification and does not usually provide for selective quantitation of triglyceride and fatty acid. The two-step Sudan III staining procedure (described above) has been considered capable of distinguishing triglyceride from fatty acid (and thereby maldigestion from malabsorption). However, there is evidence that in adults with pancreatic insufficiency, the fecal triglyceride content may be normal. At least, the fecal triglyceride expressed in mg/g of fecal weight is not increased in cases of pancreatic insufficiency.[2] One may not be able to differentiate maldigestion from malabsorption (pancreatic vs intestinal steatorrhea) by comparing fecal triglyceride/fatty acid or fecal fat concentration.[3,4,5,6] The influence of extrapancreatic lipase (eg, gastric lipase) must be considered.[7,8,9] Some experimental work has been performed toward a quantitative Sudan stain based procedure for fecal triglyceride and fatty acid.[10] Cholesterol absorption, in particular the serum level of high-density lipoprotein cholesterol, is decreased with pancreatic insufficiency and is increased as a result of exogenous pancreatic enzyme substitution.[9] The steatocrit, a semiquantitative method for the detection of steatorrhea, has been reported to correlate with chemical methods.[11] A linear relationship exists between the amount of long chain fatty acids consumed and the quantity in the stools.[12]

Footnotes
1. Levine JJ, Seidman E, and Walker WA, "Screening Tests for Enteropathy in Children," *Am J Dis Child*, 1987, 141(4):435-8.
2. Bernstein LH, "Old Insight Into a New Insight Into an Old Test," *Gastroenterology*, 1989, 97(2):552-3.
3. Khouri MR, Ng S-N, Huang G, et al, "Fecal Triglyceride Excretion Is Not Excessive in Pancreatic Insufficiency," *Gastroenterology*, 1989, 96(3):848-52.
4. Lembcke B, Grimm K, and Lankisch PG, "Raised Fecal Fat Concentration Is Not a Valid Indicator of Pancreatic Steatorrhea," *Am J Gastroenterol*, 1987, 82(6):526-31.
5. Bai JC, Andrüsh A, Matelo G, et al, "Fecal Fat Concentration in the Differential Diagnosis of Steatorrhea," *Am J Gastroenterol*, 1989, 84(1):27-30.
6. Kaunitz JD, "Dietary Fat Intake, 72-Hour Excretion, and Sudan Stain for Fecal Fat," *Gastroenterology*, 1989, 97(2):550-1.
7. De Nigris SJ, Hamosh M, Kasbekar DK, et al, "Secretion of Human Gastric Lipase From Dispersed Gastric Glands," *Biochim Biophys Acta*, 1985, 836(1):67-72.
8. Moreau H, Laugier R, Gargouri Y, et al, "Human Preduodenal Lipase Is Entirely of Gastric Fundic Origin," *Gastroenterology*, 1988, 95(5):1221-6.
9. Abrams CK, Hamosh M, Lee TC, et al, "Gastric Lipase: Localization in the Human Stomach," *Gastroenterology*, 1988, 95(6):1460-4.
10. Khouri MR, Huang G, and Shiau YF, "Sudan Stain of Fecal Fat: New Insight Into an Old Test," *Gastroenterology*, 1989, 96(2 Pt 1):421-7.
11. Sugai E, Srur G, Vazquez H, et al, "Steatocrit: A Reliable Semiquantitative Method for Detection of Steatorrhea," *J Clin Gastroenterol*, 1994, 19(3):206-9.
12. Donowitz M, Kokke FT, and Saidi R, "Evaluation of Patients With Chronic Diarrhea," *N Engl J Med*, 1995, 332(11):725-9.

References
Ahnen DJ, "Disorders of Nutrient Assimilation," *Textbook of Internal Medicine*, 2nd ed, Chapter 80, Kelley WN, DeVita VT, Jr, Dupont HL, et al, eds, Philadelphia, PA: JB Lippincott Co, 1992, 479-80.
Roberts IM, Poturich C, and Wald A, "Utility of Fecal Fat Concentrations as Screening Test in Pancreatic Insufficiency," *Dig Dis Sci*, 1986, 31(10):1021-4.
Simko V, "Sudan Stain and Quantitative Fecal Fat," *Gastroenterology*, 1990, 98(6):1722-3 (letter).
Vuoristo M, Väänänen H, and Miettinen TA, "Cholesterol Malabsorption in Pancreatic Insufficiency: Effects of Enzyme Substitution," *Gastroenterology*, 1992, 102(2):647-55.

Fatty Acid, Stool *see* Fat, Semiquantitative, Stool *on previous page*

Fat, Urine
CPT 89125

Related Information
Glucose, Semiquantitative, Urine *on next page*
Kidney Biopsy *on page 47*
Mercury, Blood *on page 561*
Mercury, Urine *on page 561*
Protein, Quantitative, Urine *on page 649*
Urinalysis *on page 658*

Synonyms Free Fat, Urine; Lipiduria

Test Commonly Includes Light and polarized microscopy of urine sediment and staining with Sudan III or IV

Abstract Lipiduria includes oval fat bodies, fatty casts, or free fat. These are found in nephrotic syndromes (proteinuria ≥3.5 g/24 hours).[1] Oval fat bodies are lipid-laden, pathologic, renal tubular epithelial cells which bear a strong association with marked proteinuria.

Patient Preparation Avoid contamination of the specimen with oils and lubricants from catheters and soaps. Avoid contamination with glove powder.

Specimen Random urine

Causes for Rejection Contamination of specimen with oils, soaps, and lubricants

Reference Range Negative

Use Evaluate nephrotic syndrome, renal tubular necrosis, mercury poisoning, ethylene glycol ingestion (which may produce oval fat bodies), and fatty casts in the urine; evaluate bone marrow and fat embolism, which may produce gross fat globules in urine

Limitations Urinary fat globules, like air bubbles and yeasts, can be confused with erythrocytes if Sudan stain is not used.

Methodology Sudan III and IV staining of urine sediment. Microscopically fat globules appear as spherical or ovoid dark glistening bodies. Under polarized light they appear doubly refractile and give a Maltese cross pattern. Maltese cross patterns may also be seen with some crystals, in particular starch granules found in some glove powders. Corn starch contamination may give rise to doubly refractile false urine lipid bodies[2] which are not as regular and round as are free urine lipid bodies. With polarized light the conical configuration of false lipid bodies tends to be off center, "French cross pattern."[3] True urine fat globules are usually seen in urines with increased protein. Lipiduria usually reflects glomerular abnormalities and/or multisystem disease states including diabetic glomerulopathy, amyloidosis, SLE, and cryoglobulinemia.[1]

Additional Information Urinary doubly refractile lipid bodies usually occur with heavy proteinuria. Refractile lipid bodies have been found in nonglomerular renal disease at relatively low levels of proteinuria and, rarely, even in patients without renal disease. The frequency of urine lipid bodies in patients with nonglomerular renal diseases include chronic interstitial nephritis (26%), polycystic kidney disease (38%), prerenal azotemia (20%), acute tubular necrosis (15%), and acute interstitial nephritis (33%). Presence of refractile urine lipid bodies in numbers >5 per 20 high power microscopic fields may be required to differentiate glomerular from nonglomerular renal disease.[4] See **Fatty casts** and **oval fat bodies ("lipiduria")** in the listing Urinalysis *on page 658.*

Footnotes
1. Larson TS, "Evaluation of Proteinuria," *Mayo Clin Proc*, 1994, 69(12):1154-8.
2. Senécal PE and Rochette J, "Misidentification of Urine Lipid Bodies Owing to Use of Starch-Powdered Gloves," *Clin Chem*, 1988, 34(9):1926-7.
3. Hudson JB, Dennis AJ, and Gerhardt RE, "Urinary Lipid and the Maltese Cross," *N Engl J Med*, 1978, 299:586.
4. Braden GL, Sanchez PG, Fitzgibbons JP, et al, "Urinary Doubly Refractile Lipid Bodies in Nonglomerular Renal Diseases," *Am J Kidney Dis*, 1988, 11(4):332-7.

References
Streather CP, Varghese Z, Moorhead JF, et al, "Lipiduria in Renal Disease," *Am J Hypertens*, 1993, 6(11 Pt 2):353S-7S.
Yager HM and Harrington JT, "Urinalysis and Urinary Electrolytes," *The Principles and Practice of Nephrology*, Chapter 28, Jacobson HR, Striker GE, and Klahr S, eds, Philadelphia, PA: BC Decker Inc, 1991, 167-77.

Fecal Fat Analysis, 72-Hour *see* Fat, Semiquantitative, Stool *on previous page*

Fecal Fat Stain *see* Fat, Semiquantitative, Stool *on previous page*

Fecal Leukocyte Stain *see* Methylene Blue Stain, Stool *on page 642*

Fecal Occult Blood Test *see* Occult Blood, Stool *on page 645*

Fecal pH *see* pH, Stool *on page 648*

Fishberg Concentration Test *see* Concentration Test, Urine *on page 633*

Franklin Dukes Test *see* Infertility Screen *on page 638*

Free Fat, Urine *see* Fat, Urine *on this page*

Glomerular Filtration Rate *see* Protein, Quantitative, Urine *on page 649*

Glucose, Dipstick, Urine *see* Glucose, Semiquantitative, Urine *on next page*

Glucose, Qualitative, Urine *replaced by* Glucose, Semiquantitative, Urine *on next page*

Glucose, Quantitative, Urine
CPT 82947

Related Information
Fructosamine *on page 130*
Glucose, 2-Hour Postprandial *on page 136*
Glucose, Fasting *on page 137*
Glucose, Random *on page 138*
Glucose, Semiquantitative, Urine *on next page*
Glucose Tolerance Test *on page 139*
Glycated Hemoglobin *on page 140*
Ketone Bodies, Blood *on page 152*
Ketones, Urine *on page 639*
Osmolality, Urine *on page 646*
Reducing Substances, Urine *on page 652*
Urine Collection, 24-Hour *on page 30*

Synonyms Sugar, Quantitative, Urine; Urinary Sugar Test

(Continued)

Glucose, Quantitative, Urine *(Continued)*

Specimen 24-hour urine or other specific timed collections

Container Plain urine container, sodium fluoride preservative

Storage Instructions If the specimen cannot be processed immediately by the laboratory, it should be refrigerated.

Reference Range ≤100 mg/24 hours (SI: ≤5.6 mmol/day). Excretion <5% of total daily caloric intake has in the past been considered good diabetic control. Excretion >10% of total caloric intake is considered very poor control. Normal ranges are not available on random specimens.

Use Aid in the evaluation of glucosuria, renal tubular defects; manage diabetes mellitus

Limitations With the advent of home glucose monitoring and the usefulness of glycosylated hemoglobin in following the degree of glucose control in a diabetic subject, the measurement of quantitative urine glucose is no longer used for control of diabetic patients.

Methodology Glucose oxidase

Additional Information Tests for ketones in serum and urine are useful adjuncts.

References
Knowles HC, "Evaluation of a Positive Urinary Sugar Test," *JAMA*, 1975, 234:961-3.

Glucose, Semiquantitative, Urine

CPT 81002 (dipstick, nonautomated); 81003 (dipstick, automated)

Related Information
Fat, Urine *on previous page*
Glucose, 2-Hour Postprandial *on page 136*
Glucose, Fasting *on page 137*
Glucose, Quantitative, Urine *on previous page*
Glucose, Random *on page 138*
Glucose Tolerance Test *on page 139*
Glycated Hemoglobin *on page 140*
Ketone Bodies, Blood *on page 152*
Ketones, Urine *on page 639*
Osmolality, Urine *on page 173*
Reducing Substances, Urine *on page 652*
Urinalysis *on page 658*

Synonyms Sugar, Qualitative, Urine; Urinary Sugar Test

Applies to Glucose, Dipstick, Urine; Glucose Tolerance Test Urines; Urines for Glucose Tolerance

Replaces Glucose, Qualitative, Urine

Test Commonly Includes Dipstick glucose is usually a part of urinalysis.

Specimen Random urine, double-void technique preferred

Sampling Time Random or following a glucose load

Storage Instructions If the specimen cannot be processed promptly, it should be refrigerated.

Reference Range None detected

Use Detect glucose (sugar) in the urine. Glycosuria may occur in situations, such as pregnancy, in which the increased filtered load may exceed renal tubular reabsorption capacity. Rarely corticosteroid therapy may cause a combination of mild hyperglycemia and increased renal glomerular filtration, producing glycosuria. Renal glycosuria due to a low renal threshold for glucose occurs. Because these causes of glucosuria are rare and glucosuria usually indicates significant hyperglycemia, a positive screening test for urine glucose is significant and indicates a substantial likelihood of diabetes mellitus in the nonpregnant patient. In the pregnant patient, glucosuria has a 27% sensitivity and only a 7.1% predictive value for gestational diabetes. Its greatest value is to which women should be screened with serum glucose after a 50 g oral glucose load **prior** to 24-28 weeks gestation, the usual recommended time of screening.[1] Urine glucose testing may be used as a monitor in diabetics in concert with plasma glucose and glycosylated hemoglobin. Bedside glucose monitoring has been claimed to replace urine testing for glucose, although these programs themselves may be wanting in performance characteristics.[2]

Limitations Dipstick methods are limited in usefulness as quantitative methods.[3,4] Acquired color vision deficiency caused by diabetic retinopathy may cause erroneous reading of the strip by patients.[5] Each brand of commercial dipsticks lists interfering substances. Such package inserts should be reviewed. Home blood glucose testing has largely replaced qualitative and semiquantitative urine methods for long-term and outpatient monitoring of diabetic therapy.[6] Glucose in urine is detected later in time than the hyperglycemia it indirectly represents by approximately one-half the time between voidings. In renal failure, the time delay may become excessive due to oliguria. Excessive urinary bladder residual volume further limits the test as a reflection of **current** hyperglycemia.

For diagnosis, fasting state urine glucose testing lacks sensitivity (17%) but provides 98% specificity. Postload glucosuria provides only moderate sensitivity and specificity, 70% to 80%.[7]

As a patient-based monitor of control in known diabetics, urine glucose determination does not provide reliable differentiation between current mild elevation, and normality or decrease of blood glucose. Urine glucose testing cannot detect hypoglycemia and lacks sufficient sensitivity for tight control. Urine glucose testing is considered inferior to self-monitoring of capillary glucose for type I diabetics.[7] Levels below the renal threshold of glucose are not subject to evaluation by urine glucose testing. The renal threshold for glucose is variable between different patients.[7]

Large quantities of ketones and ascorbic acid (eg, after ingestion of vitamin C tablets) may depress the color reaction. Contamination of the collection container by hypochlorite, chlorine or peroxide may cause false-positives. Pyridium® metabolites may mask the reaction.

The double enzyme (glucose-specific) method for urine sugar will not detect sugars in the urine other than glucose. For screening for other sugars, see the listing Reducing Substances, Urine *on page 652.*

Urines negative for glucose with properly stored Multistix® (Miles Inc, Elkhart, IN) were trace positive following dipstick air exposure (jars left uncapped).[8]

Methodology Double sequential enzyme analysis, specific for glucose (glucose oxidase/peroxidase). Sensitivity is 50-100 mg glucose/dL (SI: 2.8-5.6 mmol/L) urine.

Additional Information The renal threshold for glucose is 160-180 mg/dL (SI: 8.9-10.0 mmol/L). Thus, reasonable diabetic control can be maintained and the risk of hypoglycemia minimized if urine glucose screening tests are maintained at a trace to 1+ level. High urine specific gravity will decrease sensitivity.

It has been advocated that physicians examining ill-appearing dehydrated infants without any obvious cause for the dehydration should quickly screen the urine for glucose and ketones.[9]

Use of beta-blockers, bisoprolol and atenolol, did not significantly show an increase in glycosuria in untreated noninsulin diabetics.[10]

Footnotes
1. Watson WJ, "Screening for Glycosuria During Pregnancy," *South Med J*, 1990, 83(2):156-8.
2. Jones BA, Bachner P, and Howanitz PJ, "Bedside Glucose Monitoring," *Arch Pathol Lab Med*, 1993, 117(11):1080-7.
3. James GP and Bee DE, "Glycosuria: Accuracy and Precision of Laboratory Diagnosis by Dipstick Analysis," *Clin Chem*, 1979, 25:996-1001.
4. Dyerberg J, Pederson L, and Aagaard O, "Evaluation of a Dipstick Test for Glucose in Urine," *Clin Chem*, 1976, 22:205-10.
5. Bresnick GH, Groo A, Palta M, et al, "Urinary Glucose Testing Inaccuracies Among Diabetic Patients. Effect of Acquired Color Vision Deficiency Caused by Diabetic Retinopathy." *Arch Ophthalmol*, 1984, 102(10):1489-96.
6. Miller PF, Stratton C, and Tripp JH, "Blood Testing Compared With Urine Testing in the Long-Term Control of Diabetes," *Arch Dis Child*, 1983, 58:294-7.
7. Singer DE, Coley CM, Samet JH, et al, "Tests of Glycemia in Diabetes Mellitus: Their Use in Establishing a Diagnosis and in Treatment," *Ann Intern Med*, 1989, 110(2):125-37.
8. Cohen HT and Spiegel DM, "Air-Exposed Urine Dipsticks Give False-Positive Results for Glucose and False-Negative Results for Blood," *Am J Clin Pathol*, 1991, 96(3):398-400.
9. Bland GL and Wood VD, "Diabetes in Infancy: Diagnosis and Current Management," *J Natl Med Assoc*, 1991, 83(4):361-5.
10. Vulpis V, Antonacci A, Prandi P, et al, "The Effects of Bisoprolol and Atenolol on Glucose Metabolism in Hypertensive Patients With Non-Insulin Dependent-Diabetes Mellitus," *Minerva Med*, 1991, 82(4):189-93.

References
Gribble RK, Meier PR, and Berg RL, "The Value of Urine Screening for Glucose at Each Prenatal Visit," *Obstet Gynecol*, 1995, 86(3):405-10.
Knowles HC, "Evaluation of a Positive Urinary Sugar Test," *JAMA*, 1975, 234:961-3.
McCarthy J, "Value of Urine Glucose Tests in the Management of Type II Diabetes Mellitus. Results of a Study of the Double-Void Technique." *Postgrad Med*, 1984, 76(3):204,6,10.

Glucose Tolerance Test Urines *see* Glucose, Semiquantitative, Urine *on this page*

Gram's Stain, Stool *see* Methylene Blue Stain, Stool *on page 642*

Guaiac, Stool *see* Occult Blood, Stool *on page 645*

Hamster (Human + Hamster) Test *see* Sperm Penetration Assay (Human Sperm-Hamster Oocyte) *on page 654*

Hamster Test *see* Sperm Penetration Assay (Human Sperm-Hamster Oocyte) *on page 654*

Hansel's Stain of Urine *see* Eosinophils, Urine *on page 634*

Hema-Chek® *see* Occult Blood, Stool *on page 645*

HemeSelect® *see* Occult Blood, Stool *on page 645*

Hemizona Binding Assay *see* Infertility Screen *on page 638*

Hemoccult® II Sensa *see* Occult Blood, Stool *on page 645*

Hemoccult® II, Stool *see* Occult Blood, Stool *on page 645*

Hemoglobin, Qualitative, Urine

CPT 81002 (dipstick, nonautomated); 81003 (dipstick, automated)

Related Information

Blood, Urine *on page 631*
Glomerular Basement Membrane Antibody *on page 395*
Hemoglobin, Plasma *on page 325*
Hemosiderin Stain, Urine *on this page*
Kidney Biopsy *on page 47*
Myoglobin, Qualitative, Urine *on page 644*
Ova and Parasites, Urine *on page 495*
Urinalysis *on page 658*
Urinalysis, Fractional *on page 659*

Test Commonly Includes Dipstick screening of urine for hemoglobin

Abstract Test for hemoglobin in urine, which also screens for blood in urine. Urine sediment microscopy is needed as well.[1]

Specimen Random urine

Reference Range Negative

Use Hemoglobinuria, the presence of free hemoglobin in the urine, may result from hemolysis. It occurs if the serum haptoglobin binding capacity (100-200 mg/dL Hgb (SI: 1.0-2.0 g/L)) is exceeded and if the renal threshold for tubular reabsorption of hemoglobin (90-140 mg/dL Hgb (SI: 0.9-1.4 g/L)) is exceeded.

Limitations Menstrual or other uterine bleeding may appear as a contaminant in the urine. False-positives may occur with oxidizing contaminants (eg, Betadine® (povidone-iodine)). False-negatives occur with large amounts of ascorbic acid. Formalin in urine can cause false-negative results.[2] Urine dipsticks for blood that are exposed to air lose sensitivity over time. To prevent this, keep dipstick jar tightly capped.

Methodology The peroxidase-like activity of hemoglobin catalyzes the reaction of cumene hydroperoxide and 3,3′,5,5′-tetramethylbenzidine.

Additional Information Hemoglobin is catabolized in the renal tubular cells, and the iron is stored as hemosiderin. See listing Hemosiderin Stain, Urine *on page 637*. The urine in hemoglobinuria may be clear red, clear red-brown, or dark brown. Myoglobinuria also produces a dark or red-orange urine. Both hemoglobin and myoglobin produce positive dipstick tests for blood and must be identified by additional tests.[3] In hematuria, red cells or ghosts (lysed red cells) are observed microscopically.

See listing Blood, Urine *on page 631*.

Footnotes

1. Bartlett RC, Zern DA, Ratkiewicz I, et al, "Reagent Strip Screening for Sediment Abnormalities Identified by Automated Microscopy in Urine From Patients Suspected to Have Urinary Tract Disease," *Arch Pathol Lab Med*, 1994, 118(11):1096-101.
2. Corwin HL and Silverstein MD, "Microscopic Hematuria," *Clin Lab Med*, 1988, 8(3):601-10.
3. Culclasure TF, Bray VJ, and Hasbargen JA, "The Significance of Hematuria in the Anticoagulated Patient," *Arch Intern Med*, 1994, 154(6):649-52.

Hemoglobin, Urine *see* Blood, Urine *on page 631*

HemoQuant® *see* Occult Blood, Stool *on page 645*

Hemosiderin Stain, Urine

CPT 83070 (qualitative); 83071 (quantitative)

Related Information

Antiglobulin Test, Direct *on page 602*
Blood, Urine *on page 631*
Ham Test *on page 320*
Hemoglobin, Qualitative, Urine *on this page*
Iron and Total Iron Binding Capacity/Transferrin *on page 150*
Lactate Dehydrogenase *on page 153*
Sugar Water Test Screen *on page 348*

Synonyms Iron Stain, Urine; Prussian Blue Stain, Urine

Specimen Random urine

Storage Instructions Refrigeration

Use A sign of recent intravascular hemolysis, hemosiderinuria is an important clue in the diagnosis of unexplained anemia. Urine sediment stained for hemosiderin is a screen for increased iron excretion, which can be quantitated and is increased in hemochromatosis, hemolytic anemia, and nephrotic syndrome.

Limitations Hemosiderin is first shed in the urine a few days after hemolysis begins. Hemosiderinuria declines slowly after hemolysis stops. Quantitatively, iron excretion remains slightly elevated for months after replacement of a cardiac valve which has caused hemolytic anemia, although hemosiderinuria is usually absent after a few weeks.

Methodology Microscopic examination of slide stained for hemosiderin (Prussian blue reaction)

Additional Information When haptoglobin is saturated, part of the hemoglobin in the plasma is filtered by the glomerulus and presented to the renal tubular cell. If tubular capacity is not exceeded, all hemoglobin in the urine may be absorbed by the proximal tubular cells, where hemoglobin iron is converted to hemosiderin. When these cells are shed, hemosiderin appears in urine sediment. Hemosiderinuria with or without hemoglobinuria may be seen in chronic hemolytic anemia, paroxysmal nocturnal hemoglobinuria, hemochromatosis, multiple transfusions, and other conditions which result in deposition of iron in the renal parenchyma. Hemosiderinuria may occur when the degree of hemolysis is at such a low level that hemoglobinuria is not detected.[1] Hemosiderin may appear as a brown coarsely granular pigment in tubular epithelial cells, epithelial cell casts, or free in the urine sediment.

Footnotes

1. Pimstone NR, "Renal Degradation of Hemoglobin," *Physiology and Disorders of Hemoglobin Degradation*, Schmid R, Jaffé ER, eds, New York, NY: Grune and Stratton Inc, 1972, 32.

References

Lee GR, "Introduction to the Hemolytic Anemias," *Wintrobe's Clinical Hematology*, Lee GR, Bithell TC, Foerster J, et al, eds, Philadelphia, PA: Lea & Febiger, 1993, 1:944-64.
Tabbara IA, "Hemolytic Anemias. Diagnosis and Management," *Med Clin North Am*, 1992, 76(3):649-68.

Heterologous Ovum Penetration Test *see* Sperm Penetration Assay (Human Sperm-Hamster Oocyte) *on page 654*

Indican, Semiquantitative, Urine

CPT 81005

Synonyms Indoxyl Sulfate, Urine

Applies to Purple Urine Bags

Abstract This simple test can be used to screen for intestinal bacterial overgrowth, malabsorption due to intestinal or biliary obstruction, or Hartnup disease. It can confirm indican as the etiology for a dark or black urine.

Specimen Fresh random urine

Storage Instructions The test must be run on fresh urine specimens. Transport specimen to the laboratory immediately upon collection.

Reference Range Indican is normally present in urine in small amounts; <100 mg/day is normally excreted. It is detected by a semiquantitative color reaction and is reported as "positive" or "negative" (normal).

Use Evaluate intestinal integrity, absorption, and protein catabolism

Limitations Diurnal variation is described in urinary indican excretion.[1] Urine indican is rarely requested.

Methodology Detection of indican depends upon its decomposition and subsequent oxidation of the indoxyl to indigo blue and its absorption by chloroform.

Additional Information Indole is produced by intestinal bacterial action on unabsorbed tryptophan. Although most indole is eliminated in the feces, a small amount is absorbed and detoxified to be excreted as indican (indoxyl potassium sulfate) in the urine. Urinary indican may be increased in biliary obstruction, intestinal obstruction, malabsorption syndromes, and syndromes associated with achlorhydria (eg, gastric carcinoma, pernicious anemia). Hartnup disease patients also have high urine indican. Increased indican may cause the urine to blacken on standing.

Purple urine drainage bags have been reported in a few chronically catheterized, elderly, female patients with urinary tract infection caused by *Providencia* or *Klebsiella*. Urine indican excretion in such subjects was increased.[2]

There is experimental animal evidence that saccharin can induce increase in urinary indican[3] and provide a noninvasive indicator of trypsin inhibitor activity.[4]

Indoxyl sulfate can alter the dip-and-read strip reaction for urinary bilirubin in urines positive for bilirubin, sufficiently to mask a weak reaction. A more specific test such as the Ictotest® has been recommended when dip-and-read bilirubin testing is inconclusive.[5]

Footnotes

1. Kirkland JL, Vargas E, and Lye M, "Indican Excretion in the Elderly," *Postgrad Med J*, 1983, 59:717-9.
2. Dealler SF, Belfield PW, Bedford M, et al, "Purple Urine Bags," *J Urol*, 1989, 142(3):769-70.
3. Sims J and Renwick AG, "Diurnal Variation in the Excretion of Indican in Rats Fed Saccharin-Containing Diet," *Cancer*, 1984, 23(3):259-63.
4. Anderson RL, Maurer JK, Francis WR, et al, "Trypsin Inhibitor Ingestion-Induced Urinary Indican Excretion and Pancreatic Acinar Cell Hypertrophy," *Nutr Cancer*, 1986, 8(2):133-9.
5. Skjold AC, Freitag JF, Stover LR, et al, "Indoxyl Sulfate Interferes With Dip-and-Read Urinary Bilirubin Estimate," *Clin Chem*, 1980, 26(9):1368-9.

Indoxyl Sulfate, Urine *see* Indican, Semiquantitative, Urine *on this page*

Infertility Screen

CPT 89300 (semen analysis presence and/or motility of sperm); 89310 (semen analysis motility and count); 89320 (semen analysis complete; volume, count, motility and differential)

Related Information
Semen Analysis *on page 652*
Sperm Mucus Penetration Test (Human or Bovine Cervical Mucus) *on page 654*
Sperm Penetration Assay (Human Sperm-Hamster Oocyte) *on page 654*

Applies to Antispermatozoal Antibody Test; Franklin Dukes Test; Hemizona Binding Assay; Sperm Agglutination and Inhibition; Sperm Antibodies; Sperm-Oolemma Binding Test

Test Commonly Includes Semen analysis. Specialized infertility/andrology laboratories perform infertility testing, but there is not a standardized test menu.

Abstract Extensive and sophisticated methodology for the evaluation of spermatozoa has been developed during the last decade. Expanding capabilities resulting from continuing growth in artificial insemination/*in vitro* fertilization has provided impetus for the study of sperm function, in particular by specialized andrology laboratories. The following is an overview of infertility evaluation, emphasis largely on the "male factor". It is hoped that the accompanying footnotes and references will provide entry to additional study and to the details of test methodology.

Patient Preparation Follow physician's instructions. Ejaculation should be avoided for 2-3 days prior to collection of the specimen.

Specimen Serum (both partners) and semen

Container Blood: red top tube; semen: clean, dry, wide mouth glass or plastic container known to be free of detergent or other toxic agents

Collection Semen: Postcoital or masturbation using condom-like Silastic seminal fluid collection device (see listing Semen Analysis *on page 652*). There is evidence that some seminal deficiency test parameters are improved by semen collection via intercourse using a seminal collection device as opposed to masturbation.[1]

Storage Instructions Tests should be started as soon as possible after collection of semen at least within 2-3 hours.

Causes for Rejection Semen specimen more than 2 hours old

Special Instructions Semen, as with all blood, urine, and body fluid specimens, because of the risk of AIDS, should be received and handled with care to avoid contamination of laboratory personnel. Gloves must be worn during the handling and manipulation of sperm/semen-containing fluids. Persons with sores/open wounds of the skin must avoid contact with semen. Infertility screen testing is not offered by many routine clinical laboratories. Specialized infertility/andrology laboratories perform infertility testing.

Reference Range Individual test and laboratory dependent

Use Evaluate infertility. The possibility that a couple is infertile can be considered when there is failure to conceive after about 1 year of unimpaired intercourse.

Limitations While the existence of sperm antibodies relating to infertility seems firmly established, methodology of some early testing procedures has not proven to be highly technically reliable. Tests utilizing methanol-fixed spermatozoa may give unpredictable and nonreproducible results.[2]

Methodology Routine semen analysis protocols, semen function tests, computer-assisted sperm morphology/motility studies, Kibrick agglutination assay with or without the use gelatin, method of Franklin and Dukes[3], microagglutination tests, sperm immobilization/cytotoxicity tests (eg, Isojima assay), mixed antiglobulin reaction assay (MAR), enzyme-linked immunosorbent assay (ELISA) using as antigen glutaraldehyde-fixed spermatozoa, Immunobead™ binding assay,[4,5] antisperm antibodies by indirect fluorescence using flow cytometry,[6] fluorescence *in situ* hybridization,[7] human sperm activation assay[8]

Additional Information Approximately 95% of normal couples should conceive within 13-15 months.[9] Many factors may be responsible for infertility. These may be divided into **"female factors"** and **"male factors"**. Common causes of infertility include endometriosis, tubal factors (often pelvic inflammatory disease), ovulation and cervical/uterine factors. A "male factor" is responsible in some 20% of the cases.[9] Basic evaluation (American Fertility Society) includes history and examination of the female, postcoital test, evaluation of tubal patency (hysterosalpingogram), evaluation of hormonal factors, history and examination of the male, and semen analyses.[10] To overcome the effect of transient variables, multiple and/or periodic study of spermatozoa may be necessary. Immunologic factors are a potential important cause of infertility. It has been estimated that 7% to 14% of men attending a fertility clinic have sperm-bound antibodies (as compared to an incidence of 1% to 2% in fertile men without history of vasovasostomy).[11]

This text deals largely with tests that identify "male factor" causes of infertility. The past 15 years has seen increased interest in the evaluation

of spermatozoa, reflecting increased understanding of sperm physiology and increased rate of new test development. Thus, the growing number and capability of fertility/andrology laboratories are usually in support of assisted reproduction programs. The latter include such procedures as *in vitro* fertilization and embryonic transfer (IVF-ET) and gamete-intrafallopian tube transfer (GIFT). The American Fertility Society has published guidelines for human andrology laboratories including recognition of the National Committee for Clinical Laboratory Standards (NCCLS) specified format.[12] An example of a quality control and quality assurance program has been published.[13] An excellent review presents relatively recently developed tests of human sperm function including:[14]

- resistance of sperm to decondensation in sodium dodecyl sulfate
- acidic aniline blue stain for immature sperm nuclei
- acridine orange stain for abnormal nuclear chromatin
- trypan blue or eosin Y membrane dye exclusion test
- follicular fluid induction of acrosome reaction
- calcium ionophore A23187 induction of acrosome reaction
- acrosome assessment by *pisum sativum* agglutinin fluorescein stain
- measurement of acrosomal proteinase activity
- assessment of hyaluronidase activity
- sperm-oolemma binding test
- hypo-osmotic swelling test
- hemizona binding assay
- variety of tests for determination of antisperm antibodies (see below)

Presence of **antisperm antibodies** has not been clearly associated with disease states but bears association with diminished fertility. When clumping of sperm or sperm with poor motility is found, antibodies should be considered.[15] Such antibodies may be found in the circulation, free or as immune complexes, in seminal plasma, and/or attached to the sperm surface. Tests that measure immunoglobulin on the sperm surface have greater sensitivity than assays of serum antisperm antibodies. Some males may have blood negative for sperm antibodies but have demonstrable antibody on the surface of spermatozoa.[2] Sperm-bound antibody measured by ELISA has been found present in a greater percentage of infertile men with varicoceles than infertile men without varicoceles.[16] Results of a modification of the Seminobead™ test (in which the beads are coated with MH61, a monoclonal antibody specific for acrosome-reacted sperm) have been shown to correlate with outcomes of sperm penetration assays (SPA) and IVF.[17]

Antibodies are found in some males with testicular disease. They are also seen in cases of autoimmune aspermatogenesis experimentally induced by immunization with semen, spermatozoa, or testicular homogenates. There may be a cause and effect relationship between spermatozoal antibodies in serum of females and unexplained infertility. Both members of the couple should have their serum tested. The use of a single type of test may not be adequate. Studies indicate that each test has a different incidence of positive results in an infertile population. Repeat of test procedure will at times give different results for a particular serum sample. A number of immunologic based methods for detection of antisperm antibodies have been developed. The Immunobead™ test is currently most commonly employed. Antisperm antibody tests are critiqued in the text by Glover et al including immunofluorescence; gelatin agglutination test (GAT), Kibrick method; tube-slide agglutination test (TSAT), Franklin Dukes method; tray agglutination test (TAT); slide agglutination test (SAT); modified slide agglutination test (MSAT); sperm immobilization test (SIT); mixed antiglobulin reaction (MAR); Immunobead™ test (IBT); enzyme-linked immunosorbent assay (ELISA).[18]

Electro-optical and computer assisted devices and systems are available for the semiautomated/automated study of sperm morphology and motility. These are in use by some andrology laboratories. Some aspects of their application and evaluation are detailed.[19,20,21,22,23,24,25] An editorial comment concerning the risk involved in hypertrophy of technology is especially noteworthy.[21]

A minimum level of extracellular ionized calcium is necessary to the maintenance of normal sperm motility. Spermatozoa appear to be dependent on intracellular translocation of calcium ions rather than on the extracellular concentration of ionized calcium.[26]

Evaluation of spermatozoal function has been approached by measuring surrogate cervical mucus penetration (see also Sperm Mucus Penetration Test (Human or Bovine Cervical Mucus) *on page 654*) and the determination of sperm capacitation index, based on the degree of polyspermy in penetration of zona-free, pellucida-free hamster ova.[27] See also Sperm Penetration Assay (Human Sperm-Hamster Oocyte) *on page 654*.

A study involving 445 men found smoking correlated with decreased semen volume, and coffee drinking correlated with increase in sperm density and number of abnormal forms. Individuals consuming over four cups of coffee per day and who smoked over 20 cigarettes per day had a lower fraction of motile spermatozoa and more dead cells as compared to nonsmoker/coffee drinkers. Alcohol consumption, also studied, did not affect semen quality (by either univariate or multifactorial analysis).[28] A separate study has found use of cocaine associated with low sperm concentration, low sperm motility, and presence of abnormal morphology.[29]

It has been shown that antisperm antibodies will transfer from spermatozoa to immunobeads. It has been proposed that sperm processed using this technique may find application (intrauterine insemination) in the treatment of male immunologic infertility.[30]

Increased frequency of chromosomal as well as numerical abnormalities has been found in sperm from infertile males.[7]

Hypogonadotropic hypogonadism is an uncommon explanation for male infertility, for which therapy is available.[15]

Most cases of male infertility are classified as **idiopathic oligospermia** and **asthenospermia**, defined as <50 million/ejaculate and <50% motility respectively.[15]

Footnotes

1. Zavos PM and Goodpasture JC, "Clinical Improvements of Specific Seminal Deficiencies Via Intercourse With a Seminal Collection Device Versus Masturbation," *Fertil Steril*, 1989, 51(1):190-3.
2. Haas GG Jr, "Antibody-Mediated Causes of Male Infertility," *Urol Clin North Am*, 1987, 14(3):539-50.
3. Franklin RR and Dukes CD, "Further Studies on Sperm-Agglutinating Antibody and Unexplained Infertility," *JAMA*, 1964, 190:682.
4. Bronson R, Cooper G, Hjort T, et al, "Antisperm Antibodies Detected by Agglutination, Immobilization, Microcytotoxicity, and Immunobead™-Binding Assays," *J Reprod Immunol*, 1985, 8(4):279-99.
5. Clarke GN, Elliott PJ, and Smaila C, "Detection of Sperm Antibodies in Semen Using the Immunobead™ Test: A Survey of 813 Consecutive Patients," *Am J Reprod Immunol Microbiol*, 1985, 7(3):118-23.
6. Sinton EB, Riemann DC, and Ashton ME, "Antisperm Antibody Detection Using Concurrent Cytofluorometry and Indirect Immunofluorescence Microscopy," *Am J Clin Pathol*, 1991, 95(2):242-6.
7. Moosani N, Pattinson HA, Carter MD, et al, "Chromosomal Analysis of Sperm From Men With Idiopathic Infertility Using Sperm Karyotyping and Fluorescence In Situ Hybridization," *Fertil Steril*, 1995, 64(4):811-7.
8. Brown DB, Hayes EJ, Uchida T, et al, "Some Cases of Human Male Infertility Are Explained by Abnormal In Vitro Human Sperm Activation," *Fertil Steril*, 1995, 64(3):612-22.
9. Talbert LM, "Overview of the Diagnostic Evaluation," *Infertility - A Practical Guide for the Physician*, 3rd ed, Hammond MG and Talbert LM, eds, Boston, MA: Blackwell Scientific Publications, 1992, 1-10.
10. Taymor ML, *Infertility - A Clinician's Guide to Diagnosis and Treatment*, New York, NY: Plenum Medical Book Company, 1990, 12-3.
11. Glover TD, Barratt CL, Tyler JP, et al, "Seeking Possible Causes of Dysfunction," *Human Male Fertility and Semen Analysis*, San Diego, CA: Academic Press, 1990, 109.
12. Byrd W, Boldt JP, and Wolf DP, *Guidelines for Human Andrology Laboratories*, Birmingham, AL: The American Fertility Society, 1992, 58:11S.
13. Muller CH, "The Andrology Laboratory in an Assisted Reproductive Technologies Program - Quality Assurance and Laboratory Methodology," *J Androl*, 1992, 13(5):349-60.
14. Liu DY and Baker HWG, "Tests of Human Sperm Function and Fertilization In Vitro," *Fertil Steril*, 1992, 58(3):465-83.
15. Howards SS, "Treatment of Male Infertility," *N Engl J Med*, 1995, 332(5):312-7.
16. Gilbert BR, Witkin SS, and Goldstein M, "Correlation of Sperm-Bound Immunoglobulins With Impaired Semen Analysis in Infertile Men With Varicoceles," *Fertil Steril*, 1989, 52(3):469-73.
17. Ohashi K, Saji F, Kato M, et al, "Evaluation of Acrosomal Status Using MH61-Beads Test and Its Clinical Application," *Fertil Steril*, 1992, 58(4):803-8.
18. Glover TD, Barratt CL, Tyler JP, et al, *Human Male Fertility and Semen Analysis*, San Diego, CA: Academic Press, 1990, 137-42.
19. Levine RJ, Mathew RM, Brown MH, et al, "Computer-Assisted Semen Analysis: Results Vary Across Technicians Who Prepare Videotapes," *Fertil Steril*, 1989, 52(4):673-7.
20. Aanesen A and Bendvold E, "Studies on Requirements for Trackpoints in CellSoft* Automated Semen Analysis," *Fertil Steril*, 1990, 54(5):910-6.
21. Williams M, Thompson L, Thomlinson M, et al, "Hypertrophy of Technology," *Fertil Steril*, 1990, 54(6):1188-91.
22. Bartoov B, Ben-Barak J, Mayevsky A, et al, "Sperm Motility Index: A New Parameter for Human Sperm Evaluation," *Fertil Steril*, 1991, 56(1):108-12.
23. Wang C, Leung A, Tsoi W-L, et al, "Computer-Assisted Assessment of Human Sperm Morphology: Comparison With Visual Assessment," *Fertil Steril*, 1991, 55(5):983-8.
24. Kruger TF, DuToit TC, Franken DR, et al, "A New Computerized Method of Reading Sperm Morphology (Strict Criteria) Is as Efficient as Technician Reading," *Fertil Steril*, 1993, 59(1):202-9.
25. Davis RO and Gravance CG, "Standardization of Specimen Preparation, Staining, and Sampling Methods Improves Automated Sperm-Head Morphometry Analysis," *Fertil Steril*, 1993, 59(2):412-7.
26. Aaberg RA, Sauer MV, Sikka S, et al, "Effects of Extracellular Ionized Calcium, Diltiazem and cAMP on Motility of Human Spermatozoa," *J Urol*, 1989, 141(5):1221-4.
27. Smith RG, Johnson A, Lamb D, et al, "Functional Tests of Spermatozoa. Sperm Penetration Assay," *Urol Clin North Am*, 1987, 14(3):451-8.
28. Marshburn PB, Sloan CS, and Hammond MG, "Semen Quality and Association With Coffee Drinking, Cigarette Smoking, and Ethanol Consumption," *Fertil Steril*, 1989, 52(1):162-5.
29. Bracken MB, Eskenazi B, Sachse K, et al, "Association of Cocaine Use With Sperm Concentration, Motility, and Morphology," *Fertil Steril*, 1990, 53(2):315-22.
30. "Abstracts - Scientific Papers to Be Presented at the Forty-Eighth Annual Meeting of the American Fertility Society, November 2-5, 1992, New Orleans, Louisiana," *Fertil Steril*, 1992, 57:S111.

References

Adelman MM and Cahill EM, *Atlas of Sperm Morphology*, Chicago, IL: American Society of Clinical Pathologists, 1989.

Amso NN and Shaw RW, "A Critical Appraisal of Assisted Reproduction Techniques," *Hum Reprod*, 1993, 8(1):168-74.

Auger J, Kunstmann JM, Czyglik F, et al, "Decline in Semen Quality Among Fertile Men in Paris During the Past 20 Years," *N Engl J Med*, 1995, 332(5):281-5.

Bostofte E, Bagger P, Michael A, et al, "Fertility Prognosis for Infertile Couples," *Fertil Steril*, 1993, 59(1):102-7.

Brinsden PR and Rainsbury PA, *A Textbook of In Vitro Fertilization and Assisted Reproduction*, Park Ridge, NJ: The Parthenon Publishing Group, 1992.

College of American Pathologists Conference XX, "New Developments in Reproductive Biology: August 21-23, 1991," *Arch Pathol Lab Med*, 1992, 116(4):323-43.

Comhaire FH, "Sperm Antibodies - ©Gold Standard'?" *Fertil Steril*, 1993, 59(1):242-3.

Damjanov I, "Clinical Evaluation of the Infertile Couple," *Pathology of Infertility*, Chapter 2, St. Louis, MO: Mosby-Year Book Inc, 1993, 7-42.

Green DP, "Mammalian Fertilization as a Biological Machine: A Working Model for Adhesion and Fusion of Sperm and Oocyte," *Hum Reprod*, 1993, 8(1):91-6.

Gwatkin RBL, Collins JA, Jarrell JF, et al, "The Value of Semen Analysis and Sperm Function Assays in Predicting Pregnancy Among Infertile Couples," *Fertil Steril*, 1990, 53(4):693-9.

Haas GG Jr and D'Cruz OJ, "Quantitation of Immunoglobulin G on Human Sperm," *Am J Reprod Immunol*, 1989, 20(2):37-43.

Hamamah S, Seguin F, Barthelemy C, et al, "¹H Nuclear Magnetic Resonance Studies of Seminal Plasma From Fertile and Infertile Men," *J Reprod Fertil*, 1993, 97(1):51-5.

Hellstrom WJ, Overstreet JW, Samuels SJ, et al, "The Relationship of Circulating Antisperm Antibodies to Sperm Surface Antibodies in Infertile Men," *J Urol*, 1988, 140(5):1039-44.

Hurowitz EH, Leung A, and Wang C, "Evaluation of the CellTrak Computer-Assisted Sperm Analysis in Comparison to the Cellsoft System to Measure Human Sperm Hyperactivation," *Fertil Steril*, 1992, 64(2):427-32.

Kjeldsberg CR and Knight JA, *Body Fluids - Laboratory Examination of Amniotic, Cerebrospinal, Seminal, Serous, and Synovial Fluids*, 3rd ed, Chicago, IL: American Society of Clinical Pathologists, 1993, 255-64, 344-66.

Lähteenmäki A, "In-Vitro Fertilization in the Presence of Antisperm Antibodies Detected by the Mixed Antiglobulin Reaction (MAR) and the Tray Agglutination Test (TAT)," *Hum Reprod*, 1993, 8(1):84-8.

Liu DY and Baker HWG, "Morphology of Spermatozoa Bound to the Zona Pellucida of Human Oocytes That Failed to Fertilize In Vitro," *J Reprod Fertil*, 1992, 94(1):71-84.

Mackenna A, Barratt CLR, Kessopoulou E, et al, "The Contribution of a Hidden Male Factor to Unexplained Infertility," *Fertil Steril*, 1993, 59(2):405-11.

McClure RD, Tom RA, Watkins M, et al, "SpermCheck*: A Simplified Screening Assay for Immunological Infertility," *Fertil Steril*, 1989, 52(4):650-4.

McLendon WW, "The American Fertility Society - College of American Pathologists Collaborative Program for Accreditation of In Vitro Fertilization Laboratories: Building Bridges to Enhance Patient Care," *Arch Pathol Lab Med*, 1992, 116(4):317-8.

Menge AC and Beitner O, "Interrelationships Among Semen Characteristics, Antisperm Antibodies, and Cervical Mucus Penetration Assays in Infertile Human Couples," *Fertil Steril*, 1989, 51(3):486-92.

Mortimer D, "The Male Factor in Infertility - Part I: Semen Analysis," *Current Problems in Obstetrics, Gynecology, and Fertility*, Chicago, IL: Year Book Medical Publishers Inc, 1985, 1-87.

Nagler HM and Zippe CD, "Varicocele: Current Concepts and Treatment," *Infertility in the Male*, 2nd ed, Chapter 15, Lipshultz LI and Howards SS, eds, St Louis, MO: Mosby-Year Book, 1991, 313-4.

Pedigo NG, Vernon MW, and Curry TE Jr, "Characterization of a Computerized Semen Analysis System," *Fertil Steril*, 1989, 52(4):659-66.

Rousseaux-Prevost R, De Almeida M, Arrar L, et al, "Antibodies to Sperm Basic Nuclear Proteins Detected in Infertile Patients by Dot-Immunobinding Assay and by Enzyme-Linked Immunosorbent Assay," *Am J Reprod Immunol*, 1989, 20(1):17-20.

Sherins RJ, "Are Semen Quality and Male Fertility Changing?" *N Engl J Med*, 1995, 332(5):327-8.

Visscher RD, "Partners in Pursuit of Excellence: Development of an Embryo Laboratory Accreditation Program," *Arch Pathol Lab Med*, 1992, 116(4):318-9.

Yablonsky T, "Male Fertility Testing. New Tests Yield More Predictive Power: But Are They Useful?" *Lab Med*, 1996, 27(6):378-80.

Intestinal Converted Fraction see Occult Blood, Stool *on page 645*

In Vivo Cervical Mucus Penetration (Postcoital) Test *see* Sperm Mucus Penetration Test (Human or Bovine Cervical Mucus) *on page 654*

Iron Stain, Urine *see* Hemosiderin Stain, Urine *on page 637*

Joint Fluid Analysis *see* Synovial Fluid Analysis *on page 656*

Ketones, Urine

CPT 81002 (dipstick, nonautomated); 81003 (dipstick, automated)

Related Information

Amino Acid Screen, Plasma *on page 74*
Ammonia, Blood *on page 75*
Anion Gap *on page 81*
Glucose, 2-Hour Postprandial *on page 136*
Glucose, Quantitative, Urine *on page 635*
Glucose, Random *on page 138*
Glucose, Semiquantitative, Urine *on page 636*
Ketone Bodies, Blood *on page 152*
Osmolality, Calculated *on page 172*
Osmolality, Serum *on page 172*
Reducing Substances, Urine *on page 652*
Urinalysis *on page 658*
Volatile Screen *on page 579*

Synonyms Acetest®; Nitroprusside Reaction for Ketones, Urine; Urine Ketones

Applies to Acetoacetic Acid, Urine; Acetone, Semiquantitative, Urine; Beta-Hydroxybutyric Acid, Urine

Specimen Random urine

Container Plastic urine container

Storage Instructions If sample cannot be tested immediately, it should be refrigerated.

(Continued)

Ketones, Urine (Continued)

Special Instructions Transport specimen to the laboratory promptly following collection.

Reference Range Negative; in starvation diets or in other instances of abnormal carbohydrate metabolism, ketones appear in the urine in excessively large amounts before serum ketones are elevated.

Use Semiquantitative test to evaluate ketonuria, detect acidosis, ketoacidosis of alcoholism and diabetes mellitus, fasting, starvation, high protein diets, and isopropanol ingestion. Remains useful as a monitor in known diabetics, in type I patients when ill and during marked hyperglycemia and in type II diabetics during acute illness. In pregnancy, the risk of ketosis is increased; all pregnant type I diabetics are advised to monitor urine for ketosis in first morning urine and when blood glucose is >150 mg/dL.[1] A portion of initial assessment for inborn errors of metabolism in infancy and childhood.[2]

Limitations Specimens containing large amounts of ascorbic acid or levodopa metabolites, valproic acid, phenazopyridine (Pyridium®), PSP dye, phenylketones, or phthalein compounds such as are administered for liver and kidney function tests may cause false-positives. Beta-hydroxybutyric acid (the third of the three ketone bodies) is not detected by the nitroprusside method. N-acetylcysteine causes false-positive ketone results.[3,4]

Methodology Nitroprusside reaction, Ketostix® or Acetest®; acetoacetic acid and acetone react with nitroprusside to create a color change, especially the former.

Additional Information In infants and children, ketonuria can occur with febrile illnesses, toxic states with marked vomiting or diarrhea. Genetic disorders resulting in ketonuria include propionyl CoA carboxylase deficiency, glycogen storage disease, branched-chain ketonuria, and methylmalonic aciduria. In adult healthy men, a fast of 18 hours or greater produces ketonemia at a level that would result in detectable ketonuria. Aging is associated with increased susceptibility to fasting-induced hyperketonemia.[5] Ketonuria may be noted in normal pregnancy.[6] Acetoacetic acid, beta-hydroxybutyric acid, and acetone are ketone bodies. In ketosis, usually 80% of total ketones are beta-hydroxybutyric acid. Acetoacetic acid comprises most of the remainder with acetone present in trace amounts. Urine ketones should generally be determined in patients with a positive urine test for urine glucose and followed during the management of diabetes mellitus and ketoacidosis. Ketones detected by Multistix® correlated well with Acetest® results. Specificity 96%, sensitivity 87.5% (63.3% when trace ketonuria was regarded as positive ketonuria). Acetest® confirmation of Multistix® positive ketone results is only necessary for trace ketonuria.[7]

Footnotes

1. Singer DE, Coley CM, Samet JH, et al, "Tests of Glycemia in Diabetes Mellitus - Their Use in Establishing a Diagnosis and in Treatment," *Ann Intern Med*, 1989, 110(2):125-37.
2. Lindor NM and Karnes PS, "Initial Assessment of Infants and Children With Suspected Inborn Errors of Metabolism," *Mayo Clin Proc*, 1995, 70:987-8.
3. Poon R, Hinberg I, and Peterson RG, "N-Acetylcysteine Causes False-Positive Ketone Results With Urinary Dipsticks," *Clin Chem*, 1990, 36(5):818-9.
4. Holcombe BJ, Hopkins AM, and Heizer WD, "False Positive Tests for Urinary Ketones," *N Engl J Med*, 1994, 330(8):578.
5. London ED, Margolin RA, Duara R, et al, "Effects of Fasting on Ketone Body Concentrations in Healthy Men of Different Ages," *J Gerontol*, 1986, 41(5):599-604.
6. Chez RA and Curcio FD, 3d, "Ketonuria in Normal Pregnancy," *Obstet Gynecol*, 1987, 69(2):272-4.
7. Abdelaziz HM and Billett HH, "Follow-up Testing for Ketonuria. Is it Necessary?" *Am J Clin Pathol*, 1994, 101(3):346-8.

References

Foster DW, "Banting Lecture 1984. From Glycogen to Ketones and Back," *Diabetes*, 1984, 33(12):1188-99.
McGarry JD, "New Perspectives in the Regulation of Ketogenesis," *Diabetes*, 1979, 28:517-23.

Kidney Stone Analysis

CPT 82355 (qualitative chemical); 82360 (quantitative chemical); 82365 (infrared spectroscopy); 82370 (x-ray diffraction)

Related Information

Synonyms Calculus Analysis; Nephrolithiasis Analysis

Test Commonly Includes Analysis for calcium, carbonate, cystine, magnesium, oxalate, phosphates, and urates

Abstract Passage of a stone in the urinary tract is often accompanied by hematuria and usually by abrupt, severe, constant pain (acute renal colic). Infection may occur. Up to 80% of renal stones are calcium oxalate, of which about 30% include calcium phosphate (apatite); 3% to 5% are uric acid stones; ≤2% are cystine. Up to 20% are magnesium ammonium phosphate (struvite) (infection stones). Five percent to 20% of Americans will form kidney stones. Recurrence rate is ≤95% at 25 years. Diets rich in protein and salt bear association with nephrolithiasis. Risk factors for stone formation include positive family history, osteoporosis, pathologic fracture, urinary tract infections, gout, magnesium deficiency, and small bowel Crohn's disease with prior resection, as well as age, sex, and climate. Diet and fluid intake are relevant.

Specimen Kidney ureteral stones

Collection Specimen should be washed free of tissue and blood, and submitted in a clean, dry container. If necessary, urine should be filtered to recover gravel or stone.

Storage Instructions Do **not** apply any tape to stones. Adhesives interfere with infrared spectroscopy.

Turnaround Time Usually several days

Special Instructions Urinalysis can provide useful information including detection of crystalluria and presence of red blood cells. Urine culture is often indicated.

Use Evaluate stone composition to decrease morbidity, prevent development of new stones, and support recognition of underlying abnormalities

Limitations Chemical analysis is generally available in most laboratories while x-ray diffraction and infrared spectroscopy are reference laboratory procedures. The relative merits of stone analysis techniques are subject to debate. Chemical analysis is more readily available and has correlated with more sophisticated techniques,[1] but chemical analysis requires 5 mg of stone and is time consuming. X-ray diffraction is able to separately determine the composition of the nidus as well as the major portion of the stone. The composition of the nidus may be unlike that of the cortex.

Methodology Chemical analysis, infrared spectroscopy, x-ray diffraction analysis, crystallographic analysis

Additional Information Urine uric acid excretion reflects purine intake, usually from meats. Phosphate excretion reflects meat and dairy intake primarily. Sulfates reflect meat intake. Urine calcium is correlated with urine sulfate and urine sodium, giving clues to treatment.

A **serum chemistry panel** which includes calcium and phosphorus (for hyperparathyroidism), alkaline phosphatase (for Paget's disease of bone), uric acid, albumin, magnesium, BUN, and creatinine is usually needed. Serum sodium, potassium, chloride, and CO_2, and parathormone (PTH) levels, if indicated, may be useful additional investigations. CBC and vitamin D₃ levels may be helpful.

Urine culture is needed. Urine nitroprusside (for cystinuria), urine volume, and fasting morning urine pH (with electrolytes, for renal tubular acidosis) may be indicated. **Twenty-four hour urine collections** for volume, creatinine clearance, uric acid, oxalate, calcium, sodium, potassium, citrate, ammonium, magnesium, and phosphate are commonly indicated but should be delayed about a month following stone passage or removal.

Cystinuria and xanthinuria are rare causes of renal calculi. See Cystine, Urine *on page 120*. Other uncommon causes of renal stones include sarcoidosis, Cushing's syndrome, excessive calcium or vitamin D ingestion, steroids, immobilization, bone disease, Paget's disease of bone, hyperthyroidism, and glycogen storage disease.[2] An increasing but still low rate of triamterene stones has been noted.[3] Most calcium stones relate to idiopathic hypercalciuria and hyperuricosuria, which may coexist. Hyperoxaluria is a factor requiring evaluation in patients with oxalate nephrolithiasis.[4]

Higher intake of calcium is associated with a reduced risk of nephrolithiasis in selected patients. Such inverse relationship between dietary calcium and kidney stone is probably caused by increased binding of oxalate by ingested calcium.[5] Urinary oxalate excretion falls by 1.1-1.8 mg/day for each increase of 100 mg in calcium ingestion.[6] The risk of calcium nephrolithiasis is related to the free ion concentration product of oxalate and calcium. There are many urinary constituents which can complex calcium, but only calcium complexes and precipitates with oxalate.

Nephrolithiasis is a complication of magnesium deficiency. Decreased magnesium is found in patients with Crohn's disease and in other states; see listings Magnesium, Serum *on page 164* and Magnesium, Urine *on page 165*. Magnesium supplements can diminish risk of calcium oxalate nephrolithiasis in subjects who have fat malabsorption.[7] Potassium and fluid intake are also associated with reduced risk, but intake of animal protein is directly related to risk of kidney stones,[5] probably because sulfated amino acids increase calciuria. Other dietary risk factors include ascorbic acid, oxalate-rich substances (eg, iced tea, chocolate, spinach), and sodium. Males are two to three times more likely to develop stones than females. Whites are three to four times as likely as African-Americans to develop stones.[8]

Careful microscopy of urine sediment may be helpful, especially when done on freshly voided, warm urine.

Footnotes

1. Moriss RH, Bedir MF, and Freeman JA, *Urinary Stone Analysis in Laboratory Medicine/Urinalysis and Medical Microscopy*, 2nd ed, Philadelphia, PA: Lea & Febiger, 1983, 341-4.
2. Talente GM, Coleman RA, Alter C, et al, "Glycogen Storage Disease in Adults," *Ann Intern Med*, 1994, 120(3):218-26.
3. Carr MC, Prien EL Jr, and Babayan RK, "Triamterene Nephrolithiasis: Renewed Attention Is Warranted," *J Urol*, 1990, 144(6):1339-40.
4. Robertson WG and Peacock M, "The Cause of Idiopathic Calcium Stone Disease: Hypercalciuria or Hyperoxaluria?" *Nephron*, 1980, 26:105-10.
5. Curhan GC, Willett WC, Rimm EB, et al, "A Prospective Study of Dietary Calcium and Other Nutrients and the Risk of Symptomatic Kidney Stones," *N Engl J Med*, 1993, 328(12):833-8.
6. Lemann J Jr, "Composition of the Diet and Calcium Kidney Stones," *N Engl J Med*, 1993, 328(12):880-2.
7. Fleming CR, George L, Stoner GL, et al, "The Importance of Urinary Magnesium Values in Patients With Gut Failure," *Mayo Clin Proc*, 1996, 71(1):21-4.
8. Sarmina I, Spirnak JP, and Resnick MI, "Urinary Lithiasis in the Black Population: An Epidemiologic Study and Review of the Literature," *J Urol*, 1987, 138(1):14-7.

References

Coe FL and Favus MJ, "Nephrolithiasis," *Kidney*, Brenner BM and Rector FC, eds, Philadelphia, PA: WB Saunders Co, 1991, 1728-67.

Daudon M, Bader CA, and Jungers P, "Urinary Calculi: Review of Classification Methods and Correlations With Etiology," *Scanning Microsc*, 1993, 7(3):1081-106.

Jones P, "Laboratory Evaluation of Renal Stone Forming Patients: Significant Progress," *Third Annual Progress in Clinical Pathology*, The University of Texas Southwestern Medical Center at Dallas, Sept 30, 1995.

Klugman V and Favus MJ, "Diagnosis and Treatment of Calcium Kidney Stones," *Adv Endocrinol Metab*, 1995, 6:117-42.

Pak CY, "Medical Management of Nephrolithiasis in Dallas: Update 1987," *J Urol*, 1988, 140(3):461-7.

Westbury EJ, "A Chemist's View of the History of Urinary Stone Analysis," *Br J Urol*, 1989, 64(5):445-50.

Ziyadeh FN and Goldfarb S, "XII Nephrolithiasis," *Sci Am*, 1993, 1-10.

Knee Fluid Analysis *see Synovial Fluid Analysis on page 656*

Leukocyte Esterase, Urine

CPT 81002 (dipstick, nonautomated); 81003 (dipstick, automated)

Related Information

Bacterial Culture, Urine, Clean Catch *on page 468*
Gram's Stain *on page 481*
Nitrite, Urine *on page 645*
Urinalysis *on page 658*

Synonyms Bacteria Screen, Urine; Esterase, Leukocyte, Urine

Test Commonly Includes Screening of urine for leukocyte esterase activity by dipstick is usually a part of urinalysis

Abstract A rapid indirect test for detection of bacteriuria. It is a surrogate indicator for the presence of intact or lysed neutrophils. Evaluation of urinary tract infection includes nitrite (also on reagent strips) microscopy, Gram's stain, and other methods.

Specimen Random clean catch urine; preferably midstream, clean catch collection

Storage Instructions If the specimen cannot be processed within 2 hours, it should be refrigerated for other portions of urine evaluation.

Reference Range Negative

Use Detect leukocytes in urine to screen for urinary tract infections. It will detect either intact or lysed white blood cells and therefore can be positive when WBCs are not found on microscopic examination. The lysis of leukocytes that occurs when urine is allowed to stand intensifies the color reaction from release of esterase.

Limitations False-positives may occur in specimens contaminated with vaginal secretions. False-positive results from trichomonads have been controversial. Cephalexin, cephalothin, or large amounts of oxalic acid

(eg, iced tea drinkers) may lead to decreases. High glucose or specific gravity may lead to decreased results. Sensitivity decreases with urinary tract infections characterized by 10^3-10^4 colony forming units/mL. Albumin and ascorbic acid inhibit the method. Tetracycline may cause decreased reactivity or false-negatives. Neutropenia can cause false-negative results. Leukocyte esterase is unacceptable as a screen unless combined at least with nitrite testing. Leukocyte esterase, even combined with nitrite, should not replace microscopy and culture in symptomatic patients. Urine culture is indicated for subjects with symptoms of urinary tract infection. Even with pyuria on microscopy, leukocyte esterase was found to be a poor predictor of positive urine cultures.[1]

Methodology Indoxyl is released by leukocyte esterase if present in the urine specimen. The substrate on the strip is indoxyl carbonic acid ester. Indoxyl is oxidized by atmospheric oxygen to indigo blue. The reaction time is 1 minute, but high sensitivity requires interpretation 5 minutes after immersion in the sample.[2] A package insert provides the following: "Granulocytic leukocytes contain esterases that catalyze the hydrolysis of the derivatized pyrrole amino acid ester to liberate 3-hydroxy-5-phenyl pyrrole. This pyrrole then reacts with a diazonium salt to produce a purple product," copyright Miles Inc.

Additional Information The principal advantage of the method is the ability to identify the presence of leukocyte esterase in dilute urine specimens and in specimens which have been subject to standing with lysis of the white cells. When combined with the nitrite test, in some groups reagent strips provided sensitivity for both tests of up to 85% and specificity of 65%, for infections with 10^5 colony forming units/mL. Of 750 obstetric patients, five had negative screening tests and positive cultures, each a gram-positive organism.[3] Another study for detection of asymptomatic urinary tract infections in an obstetric population found Gram's staining better than reagent strips or urinalysis.[1] Others support use of the Gram's stain.[4,5] See listing Gram's Stain *on page 481*. Urine culture remains the standard for the initial prenatal visit in some practices.[5] Dipstick screening has been compared to Gram's stains of unspun urine[6] and to urine sediment microscopy[7,8,9,10] and culture.[9,11] A 1988 proposal indicates that for screening, a clear yellow specimen negative for blood, leukocyte esterase, nitrite, and with ≤30 mg/dL (SI: ≤0.3 g/L) of protein does not require microscopy, but even such samples should be examined by microscopy when from symptomatic subjects or persons with known renal disease.[10] Goldsmith and Campos found the leukocyte esterase comparable to urine sediment microscopy when negative but not positive with predictive accuracy for urines in the range of 10^4-10^5 bacteria/mL.[12]

The number of leukocytes/hpf used as a criterion of infection in urine sediment microscopy has been controversial in the literature.[13] Others would not do away with urine microscopy based on normal dipstick tests.[14,15,16] Sensitivity and specificity of leukocyte esterase and nitrite screening have been criticized.[1,17] Leukocyte esterase has been used for detection of sexually transmitted disease in males.[18,19,20] Its use for screening urethritis or urethral pathogens in asymptomatic patients is limited by lack of sufficient sensitivity.[21]

The **acute urethral syndrome** includes symptoms of urgency, frequency, and dysuria with low bacterial counts and with positive leukocyte esterase, indicating 8-10 WBC/hpf.[22]

Footnotes

1. Bachman JW, Heise RH, Naessens JM, et al, "A Study of Various Tests to Detect Asymptomatic Urinary Tract Infections in an Obstetric Population," *JAMA*, 1993, 270(16):1971-4.
2. Shaw ST Jr, Poon SY, and Wong ET, "Routine Urinalysis, Is the Dipstick Enough?" *JAMA*, 1985, 253(11):1596-600.
3. Robertson AW and Duff P, "The Nitrite and Leukocyte Esterase Tests for the Evaluation of Asymptomatic Bacteriuria in Obstetric Patients," *Obstet Gynecol*, 1988, 71(6 Pt 1):878-81.
4. Keeler LL Jr, "Tests to Detect Asymptomatic Urinary Tract Infection," *JAMA*, 1994, 271(18):1399.
5. Bachman JW, "A Study of Various Tests to Detect Asymptomatic Urinary Tract Infections in an Obstetric Population," *JAMA*, 1994, 271(18):1399.
6. Sewell DL, Burt SP, Gabbert NJ, et al, "Evaluation of the Chemstrip 9™ as a Screening Test for Urinalysis and Urine Culture in Men," *Am J Clin Pathol*, 1985, 83(6):740-3.
7. Scheer WD, "The Detection of Leukocyte Esterase Activity in Urine With a New Reagent Strip," *Am J Clin Pathol*, 1987, 87(1):86-93.
8. Hamoudi AC, Bubis SC, and Thompson C, "Can the Cost Savings of Eliminating Urine Microscopy in Biochemically Negative Urines Be Extended to the Pediatric Population?" *Am J Clin Pathol*, 1986, 86(5):658-60.
9. Loo SY, Scottolini AG, Luangphinith S, et al, "Performance of a Urine Screening Protocol," *Am J Clin Pathol*, 1986, 85(4):479-84.
10. High SR, Rowe JA, and Maksem JA, "Macroscopic Physiochemical Testing for Screening Urinalysis," *Lab Med*, 1988, 19:174-6.
11. Gutman SI and Solomon RR, "The Clinical Significance of Dipstick-Negative, Culture-Positive Urines in a Veterans Population," *Am J Clin Pathol*, 1987, 88(2):204-9.
12. Goldsmith BM and Campos JM, "Comparison of Urine Dipstick, Microscopy, and Culture for the Detection of Bacteriuria in Children," *Clin Pediatr (Phila)*, 1990, 29(4):214-8.
13. Wilson DM, "Tests to Detect Asymptomatic Urinary Tract Infection," *JAMA*, 1994, 271(18):1399.

(Continued)

Leukocyte Esterase, Urine *(Continued)*

14. Morrison MC and Lum G, "Dipstick Testing of Urine - Can It Replace Urine Microscopy?" *Am J Clin Pathol*, 1986, 85(5):590-4.
15. Nanji AA, Adam W, and Campbell DJ, "Routine Microscopic Examination of the Urine Sediment, Should We Continue?," *Arch Pathol Lab Med*, 1984, 108(5):399-400.
16. Propp DA, Weber D, and Ciesla ML, "Reliability of a Urine Dipstick in Emergency Department Patients," *Ann Emerg Med*, 1989, 18(5):560-3.
17. Wilkins EG, Ratcliffe JG, and Roberts C, "Leukocyte Esterase-Nitrite Screening Method for Pyuria and Bacteriuria," *J Clin Pathol*, 1985, 38(12):1342-5.
18. Sadof MD, Woods ER, and Emans SJ, "Dipstick Leukocyte Esterase Activity in First-Catch Urine Specimens: A Useful Screening Test for Detecting Sexually Transmitted Disease in the Adolescent Male," *JAMA*, 1987, 258(14):1932-4.
19. Shafer MA, Schacter J, Moscicki AB, et al, "Urinary Leukocyte Esterase Screening Test for Asymptomatic Chlamydial and Gonococcal Infections in Males," *JAMA*, 1989, 262(18):2562-6.
20. Tyndall MW, Nasio J, Maitha G, et al, "Leukocyte Esterase Urine Strips for the Screening of Men With Urethritis - Use in Developing Countries," *Genitourin Med*, 1994, 70(1):3-6.
21. Patrick DM, Rekart ML, and Knowles L, "Unsatisfactory Performance of the Leukocyte Esterase Test of First Voided Urine for Rapid Diagnosis of Urethritis," *Genitourin Med*, 1994, 70(3):187-90.
22. Sodeman TM, "A Practical Strategy for Diagnosis of Urinary Tract Infections," *Clin Lab Med*, 1995, 15(2):235-50.

References

Bartlett RC, Zern DA, Ratkiewicz I, et al, "Reagent Strip Screening for Sediment Abnormalities Identified by Automated Microscopy in Urine From Patients Suspected to Have Urinary Tract Disease," *Arch Pathol Lab Med*, 1994, 118(11):1096-101.
Carroll KC, Hale DC, Von Boerum DH, et al, "Laboratory Evaluation of Urinary Tract Infections in an Ambulatory Clinic," *Am J Clin Pathol*, 1994, 101(1):100-3.
Hoffman GC, Green R, and Edinger CA, "Predicting a Positive Microscopic Examination of Urine," *Am J Clin Pathol*, 1990, 93(2):302-3.
Hurlbut TA, 3d and Littenberg B, "The Diagnostic Accuracy of Rapid Dipstick Tests to Predict Urinary Tract Infection," *Am J Clin Pathol*, 1991, 96(5):582-8.
Lachs MS, Nachamkin I, Edelstein PH, et al, "Spectrum Bias in the Evaluation of Diagnostic Tests: Lessons From the Rapid Dipstick Test for Urinary Tract Infection," *Ann Intern Med*, 1992, 117(2):135-40.
Leighton PM and Little JA, "Leukocyte Esterase Determination as a Secondary Procedure for Urine Screening," *J Clin Pathol*, 1985, 38(2):229-32.
Romero R, Emamian M, Wan M, et al, "The Value of the Leukocyte Esterase Test in Diagnosing Intra-Amniotic Infection," *Am J Perinatol*, 1988, 5(1):64-9.
Smalley DL, Kraus AP, and Baddour LM, "Clinical Use of the Leukocyte Esterase Test in Continuous Ambulatory Peritoneal Dialysis," *Lab Med*, 1988, 19:164-6.
Stamm WE and Hooton TM, "Management of Urinary Tract Infections in Adults," *N Engl J Med*, 1993, 329(18):1328-34.
White LV and Kunin CM, "Leukocyte Esterase Tests Detect Pyuria, Not Bacteriuria," *Ann Intern Med*, 1993, 118(3):230.
Yager HM and Harrington JT, "Urinalysis and Urinary Electrolytes," *The Principles and Practice of Nephrology*, Chapter 28, Jacobson HR, Striker GE, and Klahr S, eds, Philadelphia, PA: BC Decker Inc, 1992, 167-77.

Lipiduria *see* Fat, Urine *on page 635*

Meat Fibers, Stool

CPT 89160

Related Information

d-Xylose Absorption Test *on page 122*
Fat, Semiquantitative, Stool *on page 634*
Fecal Fat, Quantitative, 72-Hour Collection *on page 127*
Methylene Blue Stain, Stool *on this page*
pH, Stool *on page 648*
Reducing Substances, Stool *on page 651*

Synonyms Muscle Fiber, Stool; Stool Meat Fibers

Abstract A simple, low cost, nonspecific screen for malabsorption/pancreatic insufficiency

Patient Preparation Patient is required to eat adequate amounts of red meat for 24-72 hours before testing. Specimens obtained with a warm saline enema or Fleet Phospho®-Soda are acceptable. Specimens obtained with mineral oil, bismuth, or magnesium compounds are unsatisfactory. Barium procedures or laxatives should be avoided for 1 week prior to collection of the specimen.

Specimen Stool

Causes for Rejection Purgatives other than saline or Fleet®

Reference Range Negative for muscle fibers

Use Evaluate malabsorption syndromes, pancreatic exocrine dysfunction, or gastrocolic fistula

Methodology Stool is mixed with a 10% solution of eosin in ethanol, stained on a slide for 3 minutes and coverslipped. Only rectangular-shaped fibers with identifiable cross striations are counted.

Additional Information The presence of undigested muscle fibers in patient's stool implies impaired intraluminal digestion. There is good correlation with stool fat determinations. Study of stool for muscle fibers when a high meat intake has been maintained is an inexpensive but necessarily nonspecific test for malabsorption. The presence of fecal muscle fibers cannot differentiate pancreatic insufficiency from other causes of malabsorption.[1] More sophisticated tests of pancreatic exocrine function (secreting ability) include the pancreozymin secretin test, cerulein secretin test, NBT-PABA test, and pancreatic dual-label Schilling test.[2] Muscle fibers reported as present in urine are suggestive of fecal contamination of the specimen.[3]

Footnotes

1. Moore JG, Englert E Jr, Bigler AH, et al, "Simple Fecal Tests of Absorption - A Prospective Study and Critique," *Am J Dig Dis*, 1971, 16:97-105.
2. Chen WL, Morishita R, Eguchi T, et al, "Clinical Usefulness of Dual-Label Schilling Test for Pancreatic Exocrine Function," *Gastroenterology*, 1989, 96(5 Pt 1):1337-45.
3. Graff L Sr, *A Handbook of Routine Urinalysis*, Philadelphia, PA: JB Lippincott Co, 1982, 125.

References

Arvanitakis C and Cooke R, "Diagnostic Tests of Exocrine Pancreatic Function and Disease," *Gastroenterology*, 1978, 74:932-48.
Kao YS and Liu FJ, "Laboratory Diagnosis of Gastrointestinal Tract and Exocrine Pancreatic Disorders," *Todd-Sanford-Davidsohn Clinical Diagnosis and Management by Laboratory Methods*, Chapter 23, Henry JB, ed, Philadelphia, PA: WB Saunders Co, 1991, 541.
Lankisch PG, Brauneis J, Otto J, et al, "Pancreolauryl and NBT-PABA Tests. Are Serum Tests More Practicable Alternatives to Urine Tests in the Diagnosis of Exocrine Pancreatic Insufficiency?" *Gastroenterology*, 1986, 90(2):350-4.

Methylene Blue Stain, Stool

CPT 87205

Related Information

Bacterial Culture, Stool *on page 466*
Clostridium difficile Toxin Assay *on page 473*
Cryptosporidium Diagnostic Procedures *on page 474*
d-Xylose Absorption Test *on page 122*
Entamoeba histolytica Serological Test *on page 391*
Fat, Semiquantitative, Stool *on page 634*
Fecal Fat, Quantitative, 72-Hour Collection *on page 127*
Fungal Culture, Stool *on page 480*
Meat Fibers, Stool *on this page*
Ova and Parasites, Stool *on page 494*
pH, Stool *on page 648*

Synonyms Fecal Leukocyte Stain; Stool, Methylene Blue Stain

Applies to Gram's Stain, Stool; Wright's Stain, Stool

Test Commonly Includes Methylene blue, Gram's, or Wright's stain of stool smear

Abstract Evaluation for fecal leukocytes is a part of the initial evaluation for chronic diarrhea.[1] In general, the presence of fecal leukocytes provides indication for stool culture.

Patient Preparation Collect specimen prior to barium procedures if possible.

Specimen Fresh random stool, rectal swab

Storage Instructions Refrigerate

Reference Range No predominance of yeast, cocci in clusters, or leukocytes

Use Examine fecal specimens for the presence of leukocytes as an indicator of invasive enteric infection. Diarrhea for more than 4 weeks is an indication for evaluation.[1]

Limitations Ten percent to 15% of stools which yield an invasive bacterial pathogen have an absence of fecal leukocytes. Fecal leukocytes are present in idiopathic inflammatory bowel disease.

Methodology Smear of stool (preferably mucus) with one drop methylene blue, coverslip, and observe the presence of leukocytes.

Additional Information Conditions associated with marked fecal leukocytes, blood, and mucus include predominantly bacterial infections including invasive *E. coli*, shigellosis, salmonellosis, *Helicobacter*, *Yersinia* infection, ulcerative colitis, and cases of antibiotic-associated colitis and pseudomembranous colitis. *Salmonella typhi* may evoke a monocyte response. Conditions associated with modest numbers of fecal leukocytes include early shigellosis involving small bowel, and cases of antibiotic-associated colitis. In amebiasis, stool leukocytes are variable. Diarrhea can be watery or bloody.[1] See listing *Entamoeba histolytica* Serological Test *on page 391*. Conditions associated with an absence of fecal leukocytes include toxigenic bacterial infection including *Vibrio cholerae*, giardiasis, and viral infections. The methylene blue stain for polymorpholeukocytes has a high sensitivity (85%) and specificity (88%) for bacterial diarrhea (*Shigella*, *Salmonella*, *Helicobacter*). Positive predictive value is 59%. Negative predicative value is 97%. Combined with a history of abrupt onset, more than four stools per day, and no vomiting before the onset of diarrhea, the stool methylene blue stain for fecal polymorphonuclear leukocytes is a very effective presumptive diagnostic test for bacterial diarrhea.[2] A positive occult blood test may also be suggestive of acute bacterial diarrhea but lacks specificity. Neither method is sufficiently sensitive or specific to pre-empt the use of culture.[3] Similar findings including a sensitivity of 81% and specificity of 74% were observed when both tests were positive.[4]

Footnotes

1. Donowitz M, Kokke FT, and Saidi R, "Evaluation of Patients With Chronic Diarrhea," *N Engl J Med*, 1995, 332(11):725-9.
2. DeWitt TG, Humphrey KF, and McCarthy P, "Clinical Predictors of Acute Bacterial Diarrhea in Young Children," *Pediatrics*, 1985, 76(4):551-6.
3. Huicho L, Sanchez D, Contreras M, et al, "Occult Blood and Fecal Leukocytes as Screening Tests in Childhood Infectious Diarrhea: An Old Problem Revisited," *Pediatr Infect Dis J*, 1993, 12(6):474-7.

4. Siegel D, Cohen PT, Neighbor M, et al, "Predictive Value of Stool Examination in Acute Diarrhea," *Arch Pathol Lab Med*, 1987, 111(8):715-8.

References

Bishop WP and Ulshen MH, "Bacterial Gastroenteritis," *Pediatr Clin North Am*, 1988, 35(1):69-87.

Gilligan PH, Janda JM, Karmali MA, et al, "Laboratory Diagnosis of Bacterial Diarrhea," *Cumitech 12A*, Nolte FS, ed, Washington, DC: American Society for Microbiology, 1992.

Kao YS and Liu FJ, "Laboratory Diagnosis of Gastrointestinal Tract and Exocrine Pancreatic Disorders," *Clinical Diagnosis and Management by Laboratory Methods*, 18th ed, Chapter 23, Henry JB, ed, Philadelphia, PA: WB Saunders Co, 1991, 519-49.

Microalbuminuria

CPT 82043 (quantitative); 82044 (semiquantitative)

Related Information

Glucose, 2-Hour Postprandial *on page 136*

Glucose, Fasting *on page 137*

Glycated Hemoglobin *on page 140*

Protein Electrophoresis, Urine *on page 425*

Protein, Quantitative, Urine *on page 649*

Protein, Semiquantitative, Urine *on page 650*

Urinalysis *on page 658*

Urine Collection, 24-Hour *on page 30*

Applies to Albumin: Creatinine Ratio

Test Commonly Includes Creatinine clearance may be advised from the same urine collection.

Abstract Diabetic nephropathy includes glomerular disease, which is manifested as proteinuria. Small losses initially are detectable as microalbuminuria, developing 10-15 years after hyperglycemia.[1] Microalbuminuria is a test for early increase of proteinuria in diabetes mellitus and in pre-eclampsia, before proteinuria becomes evident by conventional urinalysis. Microalbuminuria may be considered a surrogate marker for renal disease.[2] The leading cause of end stage renal failure in the Western world is diabetic renal disease.[3] About 35% of subjects with insulin-dependent diabetes mellitus develop nephropathy, which is characterized by proteinuria with decreasing glomerular filtration rate.[4]

Specimen 24-hour urine, timed overnight 10-hour collection, or spot AM urine after initial voiding

Turnaround Time Often sent to a reference laboratory

Reference Range <20 mg/L (SI: <0.02 g/L) or ≤30 mg/24 hours (SI: ≤0.03 g/day). For spot AM samples, <.03 mg albumin/mg[5] creatinine

Critical Values "Microalbuminuria" has been defined as albuminuria of 30-300 mg/24 hours, but recently was redefined as ≥40 mg/24 hours.[6]

Use Microalbuminuria is used to detect albuminuria in hypertension and systemic lupus erythematosus. Its major role is to attempt to predict subsequent development of proteinuria, diabetic nephropathy, and early mortality in type I and/or II diabetes.[7] It is proving useful in the management of patients with relatively early diabetes mellitus to try to avoid or delay the onset of diabetic renal disease. Intensive treatment, with tight control of diabetes, has delayed onset and reduced progression of microalbuminuria and albuminuria in subjects with IDDM.[6] The risk of microalbuminuria in such patients increases when hemoglobin A[1] exceeds 10.1% (which is equivalent to hemoglobin A[1c] of 8.1%).[8]

Limitations The relationship between microalbuminuria and glycemia may not be linear.[9]

Methodology Radioimmunoassay (RIA)[7], radial immunodiffusion (RID), enzyme-linked immunosorbent assay (ELISA), immunoturbidimetric methods.[9] Nephelometric and latex particle methods are described. For spot AM sample, determine simultaneous urine creatinine.

Additional Information Of approximately 12 million Americans who have diabetes, 90% have noninsulin-dependent diabetes. Normal albuminuria is <20 mg/L, much less than the sensitivity of current urinalysis with dipstick (150-300 mg/L). Albumin:creatinine ratio ≥3.5 predicts an albumin excretion rate ≥30 μg/minute. A test strip for low concentrations of albumin in urine has been developed ("Micral-Test") and tested.[10] In insulin-dependent diabetes mellitus, detectable diabetic nephropathy begins with onset of microalbuminuria, 40-300 mg albumin in 24 hours. Such microalbuminuria may begin 5 years from onset of diabetes mellitus. In a recent study, the median duration from onset of microalbuminuria to development of diabetic nephropathy was 7 years.[11] In addition to nephropathy, onset of increased hypertension and retinopathy is also preceded by microalbuminuria. The risk of cardiovascular disease is 30-40 times greater in those with nephropathy.[12]

Footnotes

1. Glassock RJ and Brenner BM, "Glomerulopathies Associated With Multisystem Diseases," *Harrison's Principles of Internal Medicine*, 13th ed, Isselbacher KJ, Braunwald E, Wilson JD, et al, eds, New York, NY: McGraw-Hill Inc, 1994, 1306-13.

2. Viberti G, "A Glycemic Threshold for Diabetic Complications?" *N Engl J Med*, 1995, 332(19):1293-4.

3. Viberti G, Mogensen CE, Groop LC, et al, "Effect of Captopril on Progression to Clinical Proteinuria in Patients With Insulin-Dependent Diabetes Mellitus and Microalbuminuria," *JAMA*, 1994, 271(4):275-9.

4. Remuzzi G and Ruggenenti P, "Slowing the Progression of Diabetic Nephropathy," *N Engl J Med*, 1993, 329(20):1496-7.

5. Ellis D, Coonrod BA, Dorman JS, et al, "Choice of Urine Sample Predictive of Microalbuminuria in Patients With Insulin-Dependent Diabetes Mellitus," *Am J Kidney Dis*, 1989, 13(4):321-8.

6. "The Effect of Intensive Treatment of Diabetes on the Development and Progression of Long-Term Complications in Insulin-Dependent Diabetes Mellitus. The Diabetes Control and Complications Trial Research Group," *N Engl J Med*, 1993, 329(14):977-86.

7. Mogensen CE, "Microalbuminuria Predicts Clinical Proteinuria and Early Mortality in Maturity-Onset Diabetes," *N Engl J Med*, 1984, 310(6):356-60.

8. Krolewski AS, Laffel LM, Krolewski M, et al, "Glycosylated Hemoglobin and the Risk of Microalbuminuria in Patients With Insulin-Dependent Diabetes Mellitus," *N Engl J Med*, 1995, 332(19):1251-5.

9. Hindmarsh JT, "Microalbuminuria" *Clin Lab Med*, 1988, 8(3):611-6.

10. Jury DR, Mikkelsen DJ, Glen D, et al, "Assessment of Micral-Test Microalbuminuria Test Strip in the Laboratory and in Diabetic Outpatients," *Ann Clin Biochem*, 1992, 29(Pt 1):96-100.

11. Mathiesen ER, Ronn B, Storm B, et al, "The National Course of Microalbuminuria in Insulin-Dependent Diabetes: A 10-Year Prospective Study," *Diabet Med*, 1995, 12(6):482-7.

12. Nathan, DM, "Long-Term Complications of Diabetes Mellitus," *N Engl J Med*, 1993, 328(23):1676-85.

References

Campbell FM, "Microalbuminuria and Nephropathy in Insulin Dependent Diabetes Mellitus," *Arch Dis Child*, 1995, 73(1):4-7.

Chapman AB, Johnson AM, Gabow PA, et al, "Overt Proteinuria and Microalbuminuria in Autosomal Dominant Polycystic Kidney Disease," *J Am Soc Nephrol*, 1994, 5(6):1349-54.

Chase HP, Jackson WE, Hoops SL, et al, "Glucose Control and the Renal and Retinal Complications of Insulin-Dependent Diabetes," *JAMA*, 1989, 261(8):1155-60.

Chavers BM, Bilous RW, Ellis EN, et al, "Glomerular Lesions and Urinary Albumin Excretion in Type 1 Diabetes Without Overt Proteinuria," *N Engl J Med*, 1989, 320(15):966-70.

Shihabi ZK, Konen JC, and O'Connor ML, "Albuminuria vs Urinary Total Protein for Detecting Chronic Renal Disorders," *Clin Chem*, 1991, 37(5):621-4.

Townsend JC, "Increased Albumin Excretion in Diabetes," *J Clin Pathol*, 1990, 43(1):3-8.

Mucin Clot Test

CPT 83872

Synonyms Synovial Fluid Mucin Clot Test; Synovial Fluid Ropes Test; Synovial Fluid Viscosity

Applies to Synovial Fluid Hyaluronate Concentration

Abstract Qualitative test for the nature of hyaluronic acid in synovial fluid. In rheumatoid arthritis, clot is friable. This test lacks specificity, but bears correlation with the presence of inflammation.[1]

Specimen Synovial fluid

Container Sterile tube or lavender top (EDTA) tube; avoid oxalate anticoagulants.

Storage Instructions Refrigerate if there is delay in analysis.

Reference Range Mucin clot - positive (firm clot)

Use Differential diagnosis of joint disease. Findings are somewhat nonspecific and alone are not diagnostic of a single pathologic entity.

Limitations Results should be assessed with other cellular, chemical, and microscopic joint fluid characteristics as the mucin clot test lacks specificity (ie, not indicative of a single entity). Sibley et al[2] have argued that the mucin clot test should be excluded from the 11 criteria of rheumatoid arthritis by American Rheumatism Association. They feel the low specificity (49%) and positive predictive value (52%) make the test of little value. Others find the mucin clot test to be of questionable value and state that it may be omitted from the "routine" synovial fluid analysis.[3] Similar information may be obtained from measurement of synovial fluid viscosity.

Methodology Evaluate clot formed on reaction of synovial fluid with acetic acid. Equal amounts of fluid and 5% acetic acid are mixed on a glass slide. Quality of the clot may be graded as "good", "fair", or "poor". This test reflects the physical chemical status of hyaluronic acid in a qualitative manner. Inflammation degrades the quality of the mucin clot. Viscosity relates to mucin hyaluronate content and also can be evaluated by the quality of the string produced. Normal (noninflammatory) fluids produce long strings. Inflammatory fluids (low viscosity) produce short strings. Synovial fluid hyaluronate concentration and degree of polymerization as determined by a high performance liquid chromatography (HPLC) procedure has been found to correlate with quality of the mucin clot.[4] It was considered that rheumatology units with HPLC analytic capability could use the more reproducible HPLC determinations to replace older mucin clot test/synovial fluid viscosity studies.

Additional Information In osteoarthritis the clot is firm and the surrounding fluid remains clear even after agitation. In rheumatoid arthritis the clot is friable and the surrounding fluid is turbid. In acute rheumatic fever the clot is firm, and in lupus erythematosus the clot is firm (ie, normal).

Footnotes

1. Bentz JS and Adams B, "Laboratory Examination of Synovial Fluid," *Clin Lab Sci*, 1994, 7(2):90-4.

2. Sibley JT, Harth M, and Burns DE, "The Mucin Clot Test and the Synovial Fluid Rheumatoid Factor as Diagnostic Criteria in Rheumatoid Arthritis," *J Rheumatol*, 1983, 10:889-93.

(Continued)

Mucin Clot Test *(Continued)*

3. Krieg AF and Kjeldsberg CR, "Cerebrospinal Fluid and Other Body Fluids," *Todd-Sanford-Davidsohn Clinical Diagnosis and Management by Laboratory Methods*, Chapter 18, Henry JB, ed, Philadelphia, PA: WB Saunders Co, 1991, 457-63.
4. Saari H and Konttinen YT, "Determination of Synovial Fluid Hyaluronate Concentration and Polymerisation by High Performance Liquid Chromatography," *Ann Rheum Dis*, 1989, 48(7):565-70.

References

Cheek KK and Neely AE, "Synovial Fluid," *Textbook of Urinalysis and Body Fluids*, Ross DL and Neely AE, eds, Norwalk, CT: Appleton-Century-Crofts, 1983, 253-66.

McCarty DJ and Koopman WJ, eds, *Arthritis and Allied Conditions: A Textbook of Rheumatology*, 12th ed, Philadelphia, PA: Lea & Febiger, 1993, 66-7.

Sack U, Kinne RW, Marx T, et al, "Interleukin-6 in Synovial Fluid Is Closely Associated With Chronic Synovitis in Rheumatoid Arthritis," *Rheumatol Int*, 1993, 13(2):45-51.

van Leeuwen MA, Westra J, Limburg PC, et al, "Interleukin-6 in Relation to Other Proinflammatory Cytokines, Chemotactic Activity, and Neutrophil Activation in Rheumatoid Synovial Fluid," *Ann Rheum Dis*, 1995, 54(1):33-8.

Mucin Test for Hyaluronic Acid *see* Synovial Fluid Analysis *on page 656*

Muscle Fiber, Stool *see* Meat Fibers, Stool *on page 642*

Myoglobin, Qualitative, Urine

CPT 83874

Related Information

Blood, Urine *on page 631*
Cocaine (Cocaine Metabolite), Qualitative, Urine *on page 543*
Coccidioidomycosis Antibodies *on page 384*
Creatine Kinase *on page 115*
Hemoglobin, Qualitative, Urine *on page 637*
Lactate Dehydrogenase Isoenzymes *on page 154*
Malaria Smear *on page 332*
Muscle Biopsy *on page 53*
Myoglobin, Blood *on page 167*
Troponin *on page 212*

Synonyms Myoglobin Screen, Urine

Abstract In rhabdomyolysis the urine becomes dark. Urinary myoglobin causes a positive reaction for hemoglobin.

Specimen Random urine

Container Clean, chemical-free, plastic (preferable) urine container

Storage Instructions Stable for 12 days in urine when the pH is adjusted to between 8.0 and 9.5; stable for 1 month in serum.[1]

Reference Range Negative

Use Determine the presence of myoglobinuria; investigate myositis and other entities which damage muscle. Extensive injury to striated muscle

Causes of Myoglobinuria

Metabolic – impaired substrate utilization for energy metabolism	Enzyme deficiencies (LD and others), substrate deficiency, hypokalemia, hypophosphatemia, hypomagnesemia
Excessive muscle use	Severe/unaccustomed exercise, seizures, march hemoglobinuria with myoglobinuria
Hyperpyrexia	Heat stroke, exertional hyperthermia, hyperthermia associated with drug use (eg, cocaine), heat injury
Postinfections	
viral	Influenza A, herpes simplex, Epstein-Barr, coxsackie
bacterial	Fever and sepsis, clostridial with gangrene
Primary muscle disease	Muscular dystrophy, McArdle's disease, polymyositis, dermatomyositis, familial paroxysmal myoglobinuria
Poisoning	
drug	Carbon monoxide, alcohol, barbiturate, cocaine, amphetamine, phencyclidine, neuroleptic malignant syndrome
animal	Hoff's disease (fish poisoning), sea snake bite (*Enhydrina schistosa*), trichinosis
Ischemia	Arterial occlusion, myocardial infarction, thromboembolism, infarction of large muscle, anterior tibial syndrome
Traumatic	Crush injury, wounds, surgical muscle trauma, beatings, electrocution, limb compression with prolonged immobilization due to sleep or coma

is accompanied by high serum **CK** and may be accompanied by myoglobinuria.[2] See table.

Limitations Urine tests for myoglobin may not be reliable. Presence of hypochlorite or microbial peroxidase or other oxidizing contaminants may cause false-positive reactions. Presence of ascorbic acid (high concentrations) may decrease sensitivity. **Serum testing is recommended.**

Methodology Qualitative or screening methods are based on the oxidation of a chromogen (eg, ortho-toluidine) with production of a colored compound. This reaction is catalyzed by hemoglobin or myoglobin. Test sensitivity is about 0.3 mg/dL (SI: 3 mg/L).[3] Specificity for myoglobin can be obtained by the ammonium sulfate test.[3] If initial testing is positive for blood (or myoglobin), preparation of an 80% saturated urine solution of ammonium sulfate will precipitate hemoglobin. On filtering or centrifugation myoglobin stays in solution. Color in the supernatant indicates presence of myoglobin pigment. Electrophoresis can provide definitive differentiation between hemoglobin and myoglobin. Immunoassays (immunodiffusion (ID), isoelectric focusing (IEF), radioimmunoassay (RIA), immunoprecipitation; immunonephelometric; hemagglutination inhibition (HAI)) can also be used in the determination of myoglobin. Four different immunoassays for serum and urine have been compared. Within run coefficients of variability from 5% to 13% with biases seen between assays was reported.[1]

Additional Information Myoglobin (MW approximately 17,000) is released from cardiac/skeletal muscle, filtered by renal glomeruli and excreted in the urine. Resultant urine, depending upon the amount of excreted myoglobin varies in hue and intensity of red/brown/black color and is often referred to as cola colored. Myoglobin causes a false-positive reaction for urine hemoglobin on dipsticks. Serum myoglobin is not bound to haptoglobin and has a renal threshold of 2 mg/dL (SI: 20 mg/L). Muscle injury (metabolic or traumatic, see table) releases myoglobin into the circulation, from which it is rapidly cleared into the urine.

Myoglobinuria has been associated with renal failure. Renal failure itself may cause high serum myoglobin level.[4] Myoglobinuric renal failure commonly complicates rhabdomyolysis of either traumatic and metabolic origin. The mechanism of renal injury is unknown but does not appear to be solely due to nephrotoxicity of myoglobin. The combined effects of toxic products released in rhabdomyolysis with dehydration, hypotension, and electrolyte imbalance may play a role in pathogenesis of the renal failure. Recent studies have suggested that endothelin-1, a potent vasoconstrictor, is responsible, in part, for the massive tubular necrosis that can be observed in myoglobinuric nephropathy.[5]

Cases associated with the use of cocaine may develop as a result of cocaine-induced renal artery vasoconstriction, renal ischemia, and tubular damage.[6] Myoglobinuria may occur with myocardial infarction.[7] Myoglobin deposits in the kidney are demonstrable by immunofluorescent techniques.[8] There are a few reports of rhabdomyolysis-induced renal failure occurring in cases of child abuse.[9] Use of neuroleptic agents in individuals with or without predisposing factors (exhaustion, dehydration, others) may result in the neuroleptic malignant syndrome, a hyperpyrexic syndrome that may be fatal,[10] and associated with myoglobinuria. The dark urine color associated with myoglobinuria develops on standing or in the bladder at acid pH.

The pathophysiology of cocaine- (and other drugs of abuse) induced rhabdomyolysis is not clearly established. In addition to presence of serum and urine myoglobin, there is striking increase in serum **CK** and elevations of **LD (LDH)**, **AST (SGOT)**, and **ALT (SGPT)**. Cocaine blocks presynaptic reuptake of neurotransmitters at postsynaptic receptor sites. In some cases, rhabdomyolysis subsequent to use of cocaine may relate to ischemia of arterial vasoconstriction, to muscle activity associated with dysphoric agitation, and/or to hyperthermia. The most common cause, however, of rhabdomyolysis related to use of abused drugs is limb compression during sleep or coma.[6] Serum CK is usually normal with hemolysis, in which serum LD is generally increased with high LD_1. With circulating myoglobin, serum CK is usually very high, serum LD may be moderately increased, but it is LD_5 that is usually elevated on **LD isoenzyme electrophoresis**. An isomorphic pattern of LD isoenzymes may also be seen. When no specific cause of rhabdomyolysis is apparent, or when precipitating physical exercise was not extreme, or when CPK does not return to baseline, muscle biopsy with measurement of specific muscle enzymes may be indicated. In 77 such muscle biopsies, enzyme deficiencies were noted in 36 patients.[11] A metabolic cause of myoglobinuria is palmitoyl-transferase II deficiency.[12] Psychiatric patients may represent a special risk group for the development of rhabdomyolysis and subsequent myoglobinuria.[13]

Alcoholics may suffer hypokalemic myopathy in which myoglobinuria may be found.

Rhabdomyolysis with myoglobinuria as well as hemoglobinuria may complicate *Plasmodium falciparum* malaria.[14]

Footnotes

1. Wu AH, Laios I, Green S, et al, "Immunoassays for Serum and Urine Myoglobin: Myoglobin Clearance Assessed as a Risk Factor for Acute Renal Failure," *Clin Chem*, 1994, 40(5):796-802.
2. Laios ID, Caruk R, and Wu AH, "Myoglobin Clearance as an Early Indicator for Rhabdomyolysis-Induced Acute Renal Failure," *Ann Clin Lab Sci*, 1995, 25(2):179-84.
3. Race GJ and White MG, "Urinary Pigments," *Basic Urinalysis*, Chapter 12, Hagerstown, MD: Harper & Row Publishers, 1979, 50-1.
4. Feinfeld DA, Briscoe AM, Nurse HM, et al, "Myoglobinuria in Chronic Renal Failure," *Am J Kidney Dis*, 1986, 8(2):111-4.
5. Karam H, Bruneval P, Clozel JP, et al, "Role of Endothelin in Acute Renal Failure Due to Rhabdomyolysis in Rats," *J Pharmacol Exp Ther*, 1995, 274(1):481-6.
6. Pogue VA and Nurse HM, "Cocaine-Associated Acute Myoglobinuric Renal Failure," *Am J Med*, 1989, 86(2):183-6.
7. Levine RS, Alterman H, Gubner RS, et al, "Myoglobinuria in Myocardial Infarction," *Am J Med Sci*, 1971, 262:179-83.
8. Kagan LJ, "Immunofluorescent Demonstration of Myoglobin in the Kidney," *Am J Med*, 1970, 48:649-53.
9. Mukherji SK and Siegel MJ, "Rhabdomyolysis and Renal Failure in Child Abuse," *AJR Am J Roentgenol*, 1987, 148(6):1203-4.
10. Guzé BH and Baxter LR Jr, "Current Concepts. Neuroleptic Malignant Syndrome," *N Engl J Med*, 1985, 313(3):163-6.
11. Tonin P, Lewis P, Servidei S, et al, "Metabolic Causes of Myoglobinuria," *Ann Neurol*, 1990, 27(2):181-5.
12. Venturini E and Pupeschi L, "Myoglobinuria Due to a Deficiency of Carnitine Palmitoyltransferase II. A Clinical Case Report," *Recenti Prog Med*, 1994, 85(5):282-3.
13. Zwettler U, Lippert J, Andrassy K, et al, "Acute Myoglobinuric Kidney Failure as a Consequence of Autoaggressive Behavior in Mental Retardation," *Deutsche Medizinische Wochenschrift*, 1994, 119(28-9):994-8.
14. Knochel JP and Moore GE, "Rhabdomyolysis in Malaria," *N Engl J Med*, 1993, 329(16):1206-7.

References

Schumann GB and Schweitzer SC, "Examination of Urine," *Todd-Sanford-Davidsohn Clinical Diagnosis and Management by Laboratory Methods*, Chapter 17, Henry JB, ed, Philadelphia, PA: WB Saunders Co, 1991, 410-2.

Wu AH, Laios I, Green S, et al, "Immunoassays for Serum and Urine Myoglobin: Myoglobin Clearance Assessed as a Risk Factor for Acute Renal Failure," *Clin Chem*, 1994, 40(5):796-802.

Myoglobin Screen, Urine see Myoglobin, Qualitative, Urine *on previous page*

Nephrolithiasis Analysis see Kidney Stone Analysis *on page 640*

Neutral Fat, Stool see Fat, Semiquantitative, Stool *on page 634*

Nitrite, Urine

CPT 81002 (dipstick, nonautomated); 81003 (dipstick, automated)

Related Information

Bacterial Culture, Urine, Clean Catch *on page 468*
Gram's Stain *on page 481*
Leukocyte Esterase, Urine *on page 641*
Urinalysis *on page 658*

Synonyms Bacteria Screen, Urine

Applies to Urinary Tract Infection Screen; UTI Screen

Test Commonly Includes This test is usually part of a routine urinalysis.

Abstract A rapid screening method for detection of bacteriuria, reacting with those bacteria which reduce urinary nitrate to nitrite. Urine dipstick testing is not consistently more sensitive than Gram's stain and in some studies, does not compare favorably with Gram's staining.[1] Cultures are needed in some clinical circumstances.[2].

Specimen Urine, first morning specimen is preferred; random urine is acceptable; preferably midstream, clean catch collection.

Storage Instructions Refrigeration is important if the specimen cannot be promptly processed.

Reference Range Negative

Use Detect the presence of potentially significant bacteriuria; aid in the diagnosis of cystitis, pyelonephritis, urinary tract infection in concert with leukocyte esterase

Limitations The sensitivity of the nitrite test is decreased with high specific gravity and with high ascorbic acid content. False-negatives can occur when dipsticks are stored at ambient humidity.[3] False-negatives are relatively common and relate to varying retention times of urine in the bladder, varying urinary nitrate concentrations (diet dependent) and the presence and quantity of nitrate reducing organisms present. Storage of sample at room temperature for excessive periods (more than 2 hours) may lead to reduction of nitrite to nitrogen. Some urinary tract infections are caused by organisms which do not contain reductase to convert nitrate to nitrite. Negative results are found when infecting organisms do not convert nitrate to nitrite. These include infections caused by *Streptococcus faecalis* and other gram-positive cocci, *N. gonorrhoeae*, and *M. tuberculosis*. In addition, the urine may not have been retained in the bladder for 4 hours or more to allow adequate reduction of nitrate to occur. In detection of asymptomatic urinary tract infections in obstetric patients, dipstick nitrite testing identified only 50% of the patients with such infections and was less sensitive than Gram's staining. It was reported to be superior to urinalysis.[1]

Methodology This reaction depends upon the conversion of nitrate to nitrite by the action of certain species of urinary bacteria. Nitrite from the urine reacts with *p*-arsanilic acid forming a diazonium compound. The diazonium compound couples with 1,2,3,4-tetrahydrobenzo(h)quinolin-3-ol.

Additional Information A positive nitrite test is strongly suggestive of urinary tract infection (ie, $\geq 10^5$ organisms/mL). Therefore, when positive, a urine culture is recommended, but **urine culture is indicated in any case if the patient is symptomatic**. The use of nitrate and leukocyte esterase together is more extensively discussed in the listing Leukocyte Esterase, Urine *on page 641*. See as well discussion in other tests noted in the related information field above.

Screening Methods for Detection of Urinary Tract Infection

	Sensitivity (%)	Specificity (%)
Leukocyte esterase and nitrite	67	98
Microscopic analysis on spun urine	79	93
Methylene blue stain for pyuria	60	99
Gram's stain for pyuria	45	93
Gram's stain for bacteriuria	65	75

From Carroll KC, Hale DC, Von Boerum DH, et al, "Laboratory Evaluation of Urinary Tract Infections in an Ambulatory Clinic," *Am J Clin Pathol*, 1994, 101(1):100-3, with permission.

Footnotes

1. Bachman JW, Heise RH, Naessens JM, et al, "A Study of Various Tests to Detect Asymptomatic Urinary Tract Infections in an Obstetric Population," *JAMA*, 1993, 270(16):1971-4.
2. Stamm WE and Hooton TM, "Management of Urinary Tract Infections in Adults," *N Engl J Med*, 1993, 329(18):1328-34.
3. Gallagher EJ, Schwartz E, and Weinstein RS, "Performance Characteristics of Urine Dipsticks Stored in Open Containers," *Am J Emerg Med*, 1990, 8(2):121-3.

References

Bartlett RC, Zern DA, Ratkiewicz I, et al, "Reagent Strip Screening for Sediment Abnormalities Identified by Automated Microscopy in Urine From Patients Suspected to Have Urinary Tract Disease," *Arch Pathol Lab Med*, 1994, 118(11):1096-101.

Congdon DD and Fedorko DP, "Evaluation of Two Rapid Urine Screening Tests," *Lab Med*, 1992, 23(9):613-5.

Damato JJ, Garis J, Hawley RJ, et al, "Comparative Leukocyte Esterase-Nitrite and BAC-T-SCREEN Studies Using Single and Multiple Urine Volumes," *Arch Pathol Lab Med*, 1988, 112(5):533-5.

Hallander HO, Kallner A, Lundin A, et al, "Evaluation of Rapid Methods for the Detection of Bacteriuria (Screening) in Primary Healthcare," *Acta Pathol Microbiol Immunol Scand*, 1986, 94(1):39-49.

Hurlbut TA, 3d and Littenberg B, "The Diagnostic Accuracy of Rapid Dipstick Tests to Predict Urinary Tract Infection," *Am J Clin Pathol*, 1991, 96(5):582-8.

Lachs MS, Nachamkin I, Edelstein PH, et al, "Spectrum Bias in the Evaluation of Diagnostic Tests: Lessons From the Rapid Dipstick Test for Urinary Tract Infection," *Ann Intern Med*, 1992, 117(2):135-40.

Rippin KP, Stinson WC, Eisenstadt J, et al, "Clinical Evaluation of the Slide Centrifuge (Cytospin) Gram's Stained Smear for the Detection of Bacteriuria and Comparison With the Filtracheck-UTI and UTIscreen," *Am J Clin Pathol*, 1995, 103(3):316-9.

Nitroprusside Reaction for Ketones, Urine see Ketones, Urine *on page 639*

Occult Blood, Semiquantitative, Urine see Urinalysis *on page 658*

Occult Blood, Stool

CPT 82270

Related Information

Carcinoembryonic Antigen *on page 100*
Colon Cancer, Hereditary Nonpolyposis Type *on page 506*
^{51}Cr Red Cell Survival *on page 314*

Synonyms Blood, Occult, Stool; Colo-Rect®; Colo-Screen®; Fecal Occult Blood Test; Hema-Chek®; HemeSelect®; Hemoccult® II Sensa; Hemoccult® II, Stool; HemoQuant®; Quick-Cult®

Applies to Guaiac, Stool; Intestinal Converted Fraction; Stool Guaiac

Abstract Colorectal carcinoma is the second leading cause of death from cancer in the U.S. Fecal occult blood screening is relatively insensitive as a screen for colorectal neoplasia and is even less sensitive for detection of polyps. Efficacy is poor. Less than 30% of carcinomas and larger polyps bleed sufficiently to be detected by occult blood screening. False-positives, as well as false-negatives occur. In spite of its shortcomings, annual fecal occult blood testing does diminish deaths from colorectal carcinomas. Although screening for stool occult blood is generally not reimbursed by health insurance companies in the U.S.,[1] successful detection and therapy of even a fraction of the approximately 150,000 new U.S. cases annually is meaningful.

(Continued)

Occult Blood, Stool *(Continued)*

Patient Preparation Patient should not receive vitamin C (ascorbic acid) for 5 days prior to occult blood testing by guaiac. Vitamin C does not affect the HemoQuant® test. A high bulk, red meat free diet with restriction of peroxidase-rich vegetables (turnips, horseradish, artichokes, mushrooms, radishes, broccoli, bean sprouts, cauliflower, apples, oranges, bananas, cantaloupes and other melons, grapes) has been recommended for 3-5 days prior to guaiac testing and during testing, to decrease the incidence of false-positives. Ingestion of red meat or use of aspirin or other nonsteroidal anti-inflammatory drugs before or during the collection can affect results for Hemoccult® or HemoQuant®. Alcohol and aspirin, especially together, and other gastric irritants should also be avoided. Social use of ethanol alone is unlikely to cause false-positive HemoQuant® results but therapeutic doses of aspirin may do so.[2] Halogens and cimetidine can cause reactions with guaiac tests. Oral iron is reported to not cause positive guaiac[3,4] or HemoQuant® stool assay results,[5] but it may be well to ask patients to avoid iron supplements for 5 days before and during stool collections for occult blood testing. Positive stool reactions from subjects on therapeutic doses of oral iron should not be dismissed as false-positives.[5]

Collection Stool collection is offensive, unwieldy, and awkward under the best of circumstances. Mostly left to their own inspiration, some patients are unwilling or unable to comply. Up to 75% of blood leaches from the fecal surface into surrounding toilet water in 4-12 minutes. Many toilet sanitizers generate chlorine and are reported to cause false-positive reactions to guaiac tests. False-positives can be traced to toilet bowl water containing blood from menstruation or urine. A collection device has been described.[6]

Storage Instructions Delay in examination can adversely affect Hemoccult® results. Delay does not affect HemoQuant® results.

Special Instructions Tests for stool occult blood are not appropriately applied to detection of blood in gastric juice by virtue of possible ingestion of drugs and the pH of gastric juice.

Reference Range Guaiac: negative. (A positive report has much more significance than does a negative). No consistent fecal hemoglobin level exists above which guaiac tests are reliably positive or below which they are not.[7] HemoQuant®: <2 mg/g is considered normal, 2-4 mg/g is borderline.

Use Detection of gastrointestinal bleeding, especially that from large bowel adenocarcinoma.

Limitations Most methods lack sensitivity to small amounts of blood and might fail to detect slow rates of blood loss. Many adenomas and carcinomas do not bleed. When occult GI bleeding is suspected, at least three samples, preferably of separate bowel movements, should be submitted. Many substances and conditions interfere with guaiac tests. Vitamin C (ascorbic acid) and antacids may cause false-negatives to guaiac tests. False-positive results may be caused by excessive dietary intake of vegetable peroxidases, especially horseradish. Drugs shown to be associated with gastrointestinal blood loss in normal subjects include salicylates (aspirin), steroids, rauwolfia derivatives, all nonsteroidal anti-inflammatory drugs, and colchicine. The sensitivity of the slides is increased by rehydration prior to development. The increment in sensitivity provided by rehydration can be a useful adjunct,[8] but decreases its specificity; *vide infra.*

Ahlquist and Bakken quote Sherlock Holmes' observation that the old guaiacum test is clumsy and uncertain, and they quote his lament of the lack of a reliable test ("A Study in Scarlet"). They describe the still current truth of Arthur Conan Doyle's criticism of guaiac false-positives and negatives,[9] which are outlined in the table. Guaiac tests present a number of additional problems. Acid pH, heat, and dry stools lead to some false-negatives, while watery stools are more apt to test positive. **Intestinal converted fraction** is an expression which describes the fraction of heme converted to porphyrin during fecal transit, a phenomenon which leads to diminished guaiac sensitivity for carcinomas of the more proximal colon.[9,10,11]

Colorectal adenomas and carcinomas cause a minority of positive guaiac tests,[7] 70% of carcinomas and 80% of adenomas larger than 2 cm are missed.[12] The sensitivity of Hemoccult® for detection of intraluminal cancer recurrence, all new primary carcinomas, and Dukes A and B carcinomas was respectively only 21%, 33%, and 29%, and sensitivity for detection of polyps ≥2.0 cm was 20% for Hemoccult® and HemoQuant®.[13] A 1993 *JAMA* editorial concludes that the real limit to occult blood stool testing is likely to be that many asymptomatic carcinomas do not lead to abnormal blood loss.[14] The high incidence of positivity of fecal screening for occult blood, using rehydrated Hemoccult® slides, about 10%, occurs for entities and reasons other than carcinoma or polyp.[15] Ransohoff and Lang express their opinion that sensitivity below about 95% (false-positive rates >5%) are unacceptable, because of the effort and expense of investigation. Hemoccult® II with rehydration has false-positive rates ≥10%.

Methodology Guaiac is a leuko-dye. Commercially generated tests based on it include Colo-Screen® (Helena Laboratories), Colo-Rect® (Roche Diagnostics), Hema-Chek® (Miles Laboratories), Quick-Cult® (Laboratory Diagnostics), Hemoccult® II (SmithKline) and Hemoccult® II Sensa. The peroxidase-like activity of hemoglobin or nonspecific oxidants catalyze the reaction of peroxide and the chromogen ortho-toluidine to form blue oxidized orthotolidine. New methodology, based on heme-derived porphyrin fluorescence, is more expensive (HemoQuant®). It detects peroxidase-negative heme-derived porphyrins, peroxidase-positive hemoglobin, and free heme.[16] HemoQuant® has been described as more expensive and cumbersome. The author expressed his opinion that there is no place for HemoQuant®.[12] Immunologic tests have been developed, but enteric degradation of hemoglobin interferes with immunologic as well as guaiac tests. Immunologic tests do not react with drugs, red meats, or nonhemoglobin peroxidase compounds. HemeSelect® is an immunochemical test for human hemoglobin. See table.

Occult Blood, Stool

	Guaiac	Heme-Derived Porphyrin Fluorescence	Immunoassays
Test	Hemoccult®	HemoQuant®	Antihemoglobin antibodies
Cost	Low	High	Intermediate
Reliability	False-positives, false-negatives	Little better	Intermediate
Specificity	Poor	Specific for heme, little better in practice	Improved over guaiac
Availability	Almost anywhere	Specimens must be sent to a reference laboratory, or application to SmithKline Beecham for a sublicense must be approved.	Limited availability
Recognition of porphyrin derived from heme	No	Yes	N/A
Recognition of bleeding from right colon (intestinal converted fraction)	Like immunologic tests, especially insensitive-enteric heme degradation	Sensitive	Similar to guaiac
Sensitivity deteriorates with time, fecal storage (eg, mailed in specimens)	Yes	No	Similar to guaiac
Such reducing substances as ascorbic acid cause false-negatives	Yes	No	No
Antacids cause false-negatives	Yes	No	No
Dietary (red meats) hemoglobin	Yes	Yes	No
Vegetable peroxidases	False-positives	Not affected	Not affected
Dietary hemoglobin	Yes	Yes	No
Ease of test performance	Not difficult	Complex	Complex - an enzyme immunoassay is available and counter immunoelectrophoresis is described.
Ship to laboratory performing test	Deliver promptly; do not mail.	Ship at 4°C or frozen	Probably best shipped at 4°C

When such paper slides impregnated with guaiac are not promptly processed, drying occurs, which may diminish sensitivity. Such slides may be rehydrated with a drop of deionized water, as was done in a major study.[17] Rehydration increased the number of positives but caused diminution of specificity,[17,18] increasing positivity rates from 2% to 3% to 8% to 16%, with average positivity about 10%. Rehydration is recommended but important criticisms are published.[15,19,20]

Additional Information Methods for guaiac tests of stool for occult blood utilize peroxidation of a chromogen by stool peroxidases. Hemoglobin acts as a peroxidase, but stool may also contain meat, bacterial and plant peroxidases. Normal intestinal blood loss averages 2-2.5 mL. Hemoccult® begins to turn positive at about 5 mg hemoglobin/g feces, which is considered to be the upper limit of normal stool peroxidase activity. This method is capable of detection of 6 mg of added hemoglobin/g feces in 90% of observations, but will fail 80% of the time to detect up to 1.5 mg/g feces. After ingestion of 8 oz of cooked red meat per day, reactions remain negative 95% of the time. Hemoccult® II Sensa is more sensitive in detection of polyps and carcinomas than Hemoccult® II but its specificity is reported to be poor.[21] The heme-derived porphyrin based method (HemoQuant®) has been shown to correlate closely with ^{51}Cr-labeled RBC radioisotope measurements of short-term (12 day) quantitation of fecal blood loss.[22]

Recommendations for screening are published.[23]

Approximately 56,000 deaths occur in the U.S. annually from colorectal cancer.[17,20] 150,000 new cases a year are anticipated. Family history is also relevant when it has been found in first degree relatives.[20]

Alternatives include colonoscopy, which is an expensive gold standard.[20]

See listing Colon Cancer, Hereditary Nonpolyposis Type *on page 506.*

Footnotes

1. Ransohoff DF and Lang CA, "Improving the Fecal Occult-Blood Test," *N Engl J Med*, 1996, 334(3):189-90.
2. Fleming JL, Ahlquist DA, McGill DB, et al, "Influence of Aspirin and Ethanol on Fecal Blood Levels as Determined by Using the HemoQuant® Assay," *Mayo Clin Proc*, 1987, 62(3):159-63.
3. McDonnell WM, Ryan JA, Seeger DM, et al, "Effect of Iron on the Guaiac Reaction," *Gastroenterology*, 1989, 96(1):74-8.
4. Anderson GD, Yuellig TR, and Krone RE Jr, "An Investigation Into the Effects of Oral Iron Supplementation on *In Vivo* Hemoccult® Stool Testing," *Am J Gastroenterol*, 1990, 85(5):558-61.
5. Coles EF and Starnes EC, "Use of HemoQuant® Assays to Assess the Effect of Oral Iron Preparations on Stool Hemoccult® Tests," *Am J Gastroenterol*, 1991, 86(10):1442-4.
6. Ahlquist DA, Schwartz S, Isaacson J, et al, "A Stool Collection Device: The First Step in Occult Blood Testing," *Ann Intern Med*, 1988, 108(4):609-12.
7. Ahlquist DA, "Fecal Blood Testing: Demystifying the Occult," Annual Clinical Conference on Cancer, 30:Gastrointestinal Cancer: Current Approaches to Diagnosis and Treatment, University of Texas System Cancer Center, 1988.
8. Macrae FA, St John DJ, Caligiore P, et al, "Optimal Dietary Conditions for Hemoccult® Testing," *Gastroenterology*, 1982, 82:899-903.
9. Ahlquist DA and Bakken CL, "Fecal Blood Tests," *ASCP Check Sample®*, Chicago, IL: American Society of Clinical Pathologists, 1988.
10. Ahlquist DA, McGill DB, Schwartz S, et al, "HemoQuant®, A New Quantitative Assay for Fecal Hemoglobin," *Ann Intern Med*, 1984, 101(3):297-302.
11. Ahlquist DA, McGill DB, Schwartz S, et al, "Fecal Blood Levels in Health and Disease. A Study Using HemoQuant®" *N Engl J Med*, 1985, 312(22):1422-8.
12. Sandler RS, "Fecal Occult Blood Screening for Colorectal Neoplasia," *ACP J Club*, 1993, 119(Suppl 1):25.
13. Ahlquist DA, Wieand HS, Moertel CG, et al, "Accuracy of Fecal Occult Blood Screening for Colorectal Neoplasia - A Prospective Study Using Hemoccult® and HemoQuant® Tests," *JAMA*, 1993, 269(10):1262-7.
14. Selby JV, "How Should We Screen for Colorectal Cancer?" *JAMA*, 1993, 269(10):1294-6 (editorial).
15. Lang CA and Ransohoff DF, "Fecal Occult Blood Screening for Colorectal Cancer - Is Mortality Reduced by Chance Selection for Screening Colonoscopy?" *JAMA*, 1994, 271(13):1011-3.
16. Selby JV, Friedman GD, Quesenberry CP Jr, et al, "Effect of Fecal Occult Blood Testing on Mortality From Colorectal Cancer," *Ann Intern Med*, 1993, 118(1):1-6.
17. Mandel JS, Bond JH, Church TR, et al, "Reducing Mortality From Colorectal Cancer by Screening for Fecal Occult Blood," *N Engl J Med*, 1993, 328(19):1365-71.
18. Winawer SJ, "Colorectal Cancer Screening Comes of Age," *N Engl J Med*, 1993, 328(9):1416-7.
19. Ahlquist DA, Moertel CG, and McGill DB, "Screening for Colorectal Cancer," *N Engl J Med*, 1993, 329(18):1351.
20. Toribara NW and Sleisenger MH, "Screening for Colorectal Cancer," *N Engl J Med*, 1995, 332(13):861-7.
21. Allison JE, Tekawa IS, Ransom LJ, et al, "A Comparison of Fecal Occult-Blood Tests for Colorectal-Cancer Screening," *N Engl J Med*, 1996, 334(3):155-9.
22. Leahy MB, Pippard MJ, Salzmann MB, et al, "Quantitative Measurement of Faecal Blood Loss: Comparison of Radioisotopic and Chemical Analyses," *J Clin Pathol*, 1991, 44(5):391-4.
23. Levin B, "Colorectal Cancer Screening," *Cancer*, 1993, 72(3 Suppl):1056-60.

References

Bahrt KM, Korman LY, and Nashel DJ, "Significance of a Positive Test for Occult Blood in Stools of Patients Taking Anti-inflammatory Drugs," *Arch Intern Med*, 1984, 144(11):2165-6.
Blebea J and McPherson RA, "False-Positive Guaiac Testing With Iodine," *Arch Pathol Lab Med*, 1985, 109(5):437-40.
Block GE, "Colon Cancer: Diagnosis and Prognosis in the Elderly," *Geriatrics*, 1989, 44(5):45-7, 52-3.
Doyle AC, *A Study in Scarlet*, Philadelphia, PA: JB Lippincott Co, 1902.
Klos SE, Drinka P, and Goodwin JS, "The Utilization of Fecal Occult Blood Testing in the Institutionalized Elderly," *J Am Geriatr Soc*, 1991, 39(12):1169-73.
Losek JD and Fiete RL, "Intussusception and the Diagnostic Value of Testing Stool for Occult Blood," *Am J Emerg Med*, 1991, 9(1):1-3.

Pye G, Jackson J, Thomas WM, et al, "Comparison of ColoScreen Self-Test and Haemoccult Faecal Occult Blood Tests in the Detection of Colorectal Cancer in Symptomatic Patients," *Br J Surg*, 1990, 77(6):630-1.
Solomon MJ and McLeod RS, "Periodic Health Examination, 1994 Update: 2. Screening Strategies for Colorectal Cancer. Canadian Task Force on the Periodic Health Examination," *Can Med Assoc J*, 1994, 150(12):1961-70.
St-John DJB, Young GP, McHutchison JG, et al, "Comparison of the Specificity and Sensitivity of Hemoccult® and HemoQuant® in Screening for Colorectal Neoplasia," *Ann Intern Med*, 1992, 117(5):376-82.
Winawer SJ, Zauber AG, Gerdes H, et al, "Risk of Colorectal Cancer in the Families of Patients With Adenomatous Polyps," *N Engl J Med*, 1996, 334:82-7.

Occult Blood, Urine *see* Blood, Urine *on page 631*

Phenylalanine Test, Urine

CPT 81005

Related Information

Newborn Screen for Phenylketonuria *on page 169*
Phenylalanine, Blood *on page 181*

Synonyms Phenylpyruvic Acid, Urine; PKU, Urine Test

Applies to Tyrosyluria

Specimen Freshly voided random urine

Collection Transport specimen to the laboratory within 1 hour of collection. Container must state date and time of collection.

Reference Range Negative (level of detection with Phenistix® is 5-10 mg/100 mL)

Use Assist in the detection of hyperphenylalaninemia, including phenylalanine hydroxylase deficiency (phenylketonuria, PKU and non-PKU hyperphenylalaninemia), and tetrahydrobiopterin cofactor deficiency.[1] **Urine is not used as an initial screening test for PKU.** See listing Phenylalanine, Blood *on page 181.* **After birth, 2-6 weeks may pass before phenylpyruvic acid is excreted in the urine.**[2] After the diagnosis of PKU has been established, urine screening test may be employed to follow adequacy of dietary control including monitoring of dietary intake of pregnant women who lack phenylalanine hydroxylase.

Limitations Diluted urine may cause false-negatives. The urine screening tests may miss a significant number of cases due to interferences and insensitivity. Tyrosyluria, the result of transitory tyrosinemia in prematures due to immaturity of hepatic metabolism, may result in a positive ferric chloride test.

Contraindications The ferric chloride method should not be used to screen newborns for PKU. Its primary use is to monitor dietary adherence in known cases. The level of phenylalanine in the blood is correlated with urine phenylpyruvic acid in older children.

Methodology Screening tests:
- Ferric chloride method - green color
- Phenistix® urine reagent strips (a ferric chloride method) - a persistent blue-gray to gray-green color is produced with phenylpyruvic acid. (Salicylates or phenothiazine derivatives give pink to purple colors.) Tyrosyluria in the premature or newborn due to liver disease will produce a fading green color with ferric chloride screening tests.[2]

Confirmatory tests may be done by one of several methods:
- high voltage electrophoresis followed by chromatography
- cation exchange column chromatography
- Newer methods are more sensitive and specific, detecting phenylpyruvic acid in the urine by chemiluminescent or fluorometric techniques.[3] High performance liquid chromatography with fluorescent detection is also used, and can detect the low levels of phenylpyruvic acid in normal adults or newborns.

Additional Information The incidence of classic PKU varies considerably in different countries. It occurs in somewhat more than 1 of 11,000 births in the U.S. Mental retardation is the main clinical finding. There are over 170 known mutations at loci of chromosomes that encode components of the phenylalanine hydroxylation reaction.[1] This is the genetic basis for the heterogeneous phenotype of hyperphenylalaninemia. Many mutations result in only transient or variable elevations in blood phenylalanine and presence of urine phenylalanine, tyrosine metabolites, or other amino acids, some are associated with non-PKU hyperphenylalaninemia. Phenylalanine hydroxylase deficient PKU (phenylketonuria) is characterized by impaired postnatal mental and physical development. A blood level of 10-20 mg/dL of phenylpyruvic acid (phenylalanine metabolite) is required to produce a urine level ≥8 mg/dL which is the approximate threshold of the screening tests. **The Guthrie bacterial inhibition test performed on blood is more sensitive and is the preferred and accepted screening procedure.** Positive results of screening tests should be confirmed by a fluorometric method. **The test should be performed after the newborn has had 24 hours of milk feeding.** A metabolite of acetaminophen, has been reported to interfere with chromatographic analyses identifying phenylalanine.[4]

Monitoring of urinary excretion of phenylalanine metabolites (by gas chromatography/mass spectrometry) to avoid neurotoxic effects in children with PKU has been undertaken with the goal of identifying a range (Continued)

Phenylalanine Test, Urine *(Continued)*

of blood phenylalanine that is associated with normal levels of excretion of such products.[5] The importance of controlling blood phenylalanine levels by diet during pregnancy in women with hyperphenylalaninemia (including those with diagnosed and undiagnosed phenylketonuria) has been emphasized in order to decrease the risk of maternal phenylketonuria syndrome.[6]

Footnotes

1. Scriver CR, "Whatever Happened to PKU?" *Clin Biochem*, 1995, 28(2):137-44.
2. Strasinger SK, *Urinalysis and Body Fluids: A Self Instructional Text*, Philadelphia, PA: FA Davis Co, 1985, 116-9.
3. Sano A, Ogawa M, and Takitani S, "Fluorometric Determination of Phenylpyruvic Acid With 1,4-Dimethyl-3-Carbamoylpyridinium Chloride," *Chem Pharm Bull (Tokyo)*, 1987, 35(9):3746-9.
4. Shih VE, Nikiforov V, and Carney MM, "Acetaminophen Metabolite Interferes in Analysis for Amino Acids," *Clin Chem*, 1985, 31(1):148.
5. Michals K, Lopus M, and Matalon R, "Phenylalanine Metabolites as Indicators of Dietary Compliance in Children With Phenylketonuria," *Biochem Med Metab Biol*, 1988, 39(1):18-23.
6. Luder AS and Greene CL, "Maternal Phenylketonuria and Hyperphenylalaninemia: Implications for Medical Practice in the United States," *Am J Obstet Gynecol*, 1989, 161(5):1102-5.

References

American Academy of Pediatrics Committee on Genetics, Newborn Screening Fact Sheets," *Pediatrics*, 1989, 83(3):461-2.
Hilton MA, Sharpe JN, Hicks LG, et al, "A Simple Method for Detection of Heterozygous Carriers of the Gene for Classic Phenylketonuria," *J Pediatr*, 1986, 109(4):601-4.
Scriver CR, Kaufman S, and Eisensmith RC, "The Hyperphenylalaninemias," *The Metabolic and Molecular Basis of Inherited Disease*, 7th ed, Chapter 27, Scriver CK, Beaudet AL, Sly WS, et al, eds, New York, NY: McGraw-Hill Inc, 1995, 1015-75.

Phenylpyruvic Acid, Urine *see Phenylalanine Test, Urine on previous page*

pH, Stool

CPT 83986

Related Information

Clostridium difficile Toxin Assay *on page 473*
Fat, Semiquantitative, Stool *on page 634*
Fecal Fat, Quantitative, 72-Hour Collection *on page 127*
Meat Fibers, Stool *on page 642*
Methylene Blue Stain, Stool *on page 642*
Reducing Substances, Stool *on page 651*

Synonyms Fecal pH; Stool pH

Abstract Evaluation for diarrhea depends first on history and physical examination. Nocturnal diarrhea, weight loss >5 kg, increased ESR, decreased Hgb and Hct as evidence for organic disease. Investigation for chronic diarrhea may include examination for fecal leukocytes, ova and parasites, *C. difficile* toxin assay, stool pH; CBC and differential, ESR, electrolytes, BUN/creatinine, TSH, T_4, gastrin; vasoactive intestinal polypeptide if hypokalemia and diarrhea volume >1 liter/day; assay for *Giardia* antigen and other studies.[1]

Patient Preparation Barium procedures and laxatives should be avoided for 1 week prior to collection of the specimen.

Specimen Fresh random stool

Storage Instructions Refrigerate

Causes for Rejection Specimen contaminated with urine

Reference Range Diet dependent; normal: neutral to slightly alkaline or acid. Stool pH is usually slightly acidic at approximately pH 6. pH is increased with protein breakdown, decreased with carbohydrate or fat malabsorption. Breast-fed infants have slightly acid stools, bottle-fed infants, neutral or slightly alkaline. Acid stool is formed with fat malabsorption. In a South African population of control subjects, the mean stool pH of rural African-Americans was (pH 6.14) significantly lower than that in urban African-American individuals (pH 6.77) and in patients with chronic pancreatitis (pH 6.61).[2]

Critical Values Stool pH <5.3 is diagnostic of carbohydrate intolerance; stool pH >6.8 is evidence of cholerheic enteropathy.[1]

Use Screen for carbohydrate and fat malabsorption; evaluate small intestinal disaccharidase deficiencies

Limitations Limited value due to dependence on stool volume and transit time. The diagnosis of steatorrhea requires 72-hour specimen with diet of 75-100 g fat/24 hours; see listing Fecal Fat, Quantitative, 72-Hour Collection *on page 127*.

Methodology Aqueous stool suspension measured with pH paper

Additional Information Stool pH is dependent in part on fermentation of sugars. Colonic fermentation of normal amounts of carbohydrate sugars and production of fatty acids accounts for the normally slightly acidic pH. If disaccharide intolerance is suspect, simple screening tests may be performed. Slightly alkaline pH may occur in cases of secretory diarrhea without food intake, colitis, villous adenoma, and possibly with antibiotic usage (with resultant impaired colonic fermentation). A stool pH <6 (measured by pH paper) is suggestive evidence of sugar malabsorption. Children and some adults notice that their stools have a sickly sweet

smell as the result of volatile fatty acids and the presence of undigested lactose. Low stool pH also contributes to excoriation of perianal skin which frequently accompanies diarrhea.[3]

Intestinal resections may cause postprandial bile acid diarrhea, cholerheic enteropathy, with stool pH >6.8. It responds to cholestyramine.[4]

Determination of fecal reducing substances is a more reliable screening test for disaccharidase deficiency. See the listings Reducing Substances, Stool *on page 651* and Fat, Semiquantitative, Stool *on page 634*.

High fecal pH may be a risk factor for colorectal cancer.[4,5,6,7,8,] Intake of oat bran (75-100 g/day over a 14-day period) has been shown capable of reducing fecal pH by 0.4 units.[5] There is evidence, however, that high fecal pH may be secondarily rather than primarily related to cancer risk.[6]

Footnotes

1. Donowitz M, Kokke FT, and Saidi R, "Evaluation of Patients With Chronic Diarrhea," *N Engl J Med*, 1995, 332(11):725-9.
2. Riedel L, Walker ARP, Segal I, et al, "Limitations of Faecal Chymotrypsin as a Screening Test for Chronic Pancreatitis," *Gut*, 1991, 32(3):321-4.
3. Cooper BT, "Lactase Deficiency and Lactose Malabsorption," *Dig Dis*, 1986, 4(2):72-82.
4. Kashtan H, Stern HS, Jenkins DJ, et al, "Manipulation of Fecal pH by Dietary Means," *Prev Med*, 1990, 19(6):607-13.
5. Kashtan H, Gregoire RC, Bruce WR, et al, "Effects of Sodium Sulfate on Fecal pH and Proliferation of Colonic Mucosa in Patients at High Risk for Colon Cancer," *J Natl Cancer Inst*, 1990, 82(11):950-2.
6. Thornton JR, "High Colonic pH Promotes Colorectal Cancer," *Lancet*, 1981, 1:1081-3.
7. Malhotra SL, "Faecal Urobilinogen Levels and pH of Stools in Population Groups With Different Incidence of Cancer of the Colon, and Their Possible Role in Its Aetiology," *J R Soc Med*, 1982, 75:709-14.
8. Walker AR, Walker BF, and Walker AJ, "Faecal pH, Dietary Fibre Intake, and Proneness to Colon Cancer in Four South African Populations," *Br J Cancer*, 1986, 53(4):489-95.

References

Lebenthal E, "Small Intestinal Disaccharidase Deficiencies," *Pediatr Clin North Am*, 1975, 20:757-66.
Read NW, "Diarrhea, Chronic," *Difficult Diagnosis*, Taylor RB, ed, Philadelphia, PA: WB Saunders Co, 1985, 109-10.

pH, Urine

CPT 83986

Related Information

Kidney Stone Analysis *on page 640*
Mexiletine *on page 563*
pH, Blood *on page 180*
Salicylate *on page 573*
Urinalysis *on page 658*

Test Commonly Includes pH is part of a routine urinalysis.

Specimen Random urine

Storage Instructions If the specimen cannot be processed promptly, it should be refrigerated.

Reference Range 4.5-7.8; normal kidneys can produce urine with pH from 4.5-8.2, but with ordinary diet, urine pH is about 6.0. Urine becomes more alkaline after meals and is most acidic fasting in the morning.

Use pH is defined as the negative of the log of the hydrogen ion (H^+) concentration. pH is related to the concentrations of undissociated acid and their corresponding anions. pH essentially is a measure of the potential difference which develops between the solution inside a pH electrode and the solution (in this case urine) being measured.

Urine pH is a crude measure of the acid-base balance of the body. It may be helpful in determining subtle presence of distal renal tubular disease or pyelonephritis. Urine pH is useful for identifying crystals in urine and determining predisposition to form a given type of stone. See table. When an accurate pH assessment of acid-base status and renal response is desired, the urine should be collected under circumstances more controlled than is usual. Attention is given to the time of day, the fasting status of the patient, and transfer of sample so as to prevent degasing of sample or growth of bacteria; rapid analysis by pH meter rather than dipstick is indicated. Usually simultaneous serum pH is then also ordered.

Conditions Associated With Acid Urine	Conditions Associated With Alkaline Urine	
Metabolic acidosis	Respiratory alkalosis	Postprandial alkaline tide
Diabetes mellitus	Metabolic alkalosis	(1 hour after meal)
Diarrhea	Urea-splitting bacteria	Fanconi syndrome and
Starvation	(*Proteus* sp)	Milkman's syndrome
Respiratory acidosis	Vegetable diet	(increased urinary loss of
Emphysema	Gastric suction and	bicarbonate)
Sleep	vomiting	Alkali therapy (citrate,
Renal failure with lack of NH_3 buffer	Diuretic therapy	bicarbonate)

Limitations On standing urine becomes alkaline due to the action of urea splitting bacteria (*Proteus* sp).

Methodology Dipstick double indicator principle (methyl red and brom-thymol blue) which gives a broad range of colors covering the urinary pH range 5-9 ±0.5 pH units. A pH meter is the back-up and most accurate method.

Additional Information Dietary factors affect urine pH. Alkaline urine is observed in persons who eat large quantities of citrus fruit and vegetables. Acid urine is observed with high meat intake. Pyridium® metabolites may mask the pH reaction. Urine pH >6.5 indicates presence of bicarbonate while pH <5.5 indicates absence of bicarbonate. Consistently acid urine, pH <5.5, is associated with xanthine, cystine, and uric acid stones. Calcium oxalate and apatite stones are not associated with any particular disturbance of urine pH. Alkaline urine (pH >7) is associated with calcium carbonate, calcium phosphate, and especially magnesium ammonium phosphate stones. In conjunction with serum pH and bicarbonate levels, urine pH may be applied to the study of renal tubular acidification. A recent review detects transport of H^+ ions from cells at a number of sites along the proximal tubule and collecting duct.[1]

The capacity to exchange H^+ for cation is decreased with impaired renal tubular function. In renal tubular acidosis, the distal tubules cannot effectively exchange H^+ for cations. pH of the urine may reflect attempts at correction of metabolic acid-base disturbances. In chronic acidosis such as diabetic ketoacidosis, large amounts of H^+ are excreted. In metabolic alkalosis, high levels of bicarbonate are produced. Compensation of respiratory acidosis and respiratory alkalosis is also associated with increased excretion of H^+ and bicarbonate, respectively.

Footnotes

1. Kleinman JG, "Proton ATPases and Urinary Acidification," *J Am S Nephrol*, 1994, 5(5 Suppl 1):S6-11.

References

Cogan MG and Rector FC Jr, "Acid-Base Disorders," *Kidney*, Chapter 18, Brenner BM and Rector FC Jr, eds, Philadelphia, PA: WB Saunders Co, 1991, 737-804.

Schumann GB and Schweitzer SC, "Examination of Urine," *Todd-Sanford-Davidsohn Clinical Diagnosis and Management by Laboratory Methods*, Chapter 17, Henry JB, ed, Philadelphia, PA: WB Saunders Co, 1991, 398-400.

Ziyadeh FN and Goldfarb S, "XII Nephrolithiasis," *Sci Am*, 1993, 1-10.

PKU, Urine Test *see* Phenylalanine Test, Urine *on page 647*

Protein/Osmolality Ratio *see* Protein, Semiquantitative, Urine *on next page*

Protein, Quantitative, Urine

CPT 84155

Related Information

Blood, Urine *on page 631*
Cadmium, Urine *on page 539*
Chromium, Serum *on page 587*
Creatinine Clearance *on page 117*
Eosinophils, Urine *on page 634*
Fat, Urine *on page 635*
Glycated Hemoglobin *on page 140*
Immunoelectrophoresis, Serum or Urine *on page 408*
Immunofixation Electrophoresis *on page 408*
Kidney Biopsy *on page 47*
Microalbuminuria *on page 643*
Osmolality, Urine *on page 173*
Protein Electrophoresis, Urine *on page 425*
Protein, Semiquantitative, Urine *on next page*
Protein, Total, Serum *on page 194*
Urinalysis *on page 658*
Urine Collection, 24-Hour *on page 30*

Applies to Glomerular Filtration Rate; Tamm-Horsfall Protein

Test Commonly Includes Concomitant creatinine clearance is often indicated. Total urine creatinine should be included to help assure that a complete 24-hour collection was tested.

Abstract Quantitation of urinary protein loss; evaluation of nephrotic syndromes. Favorable explanations for proteinuria include orthostatic proteinuria and benign persistent proteinuria. Persistent proteinuria may indicate serious disease requiring further evaluation.

Specimen 24-hour urine

Container Plain urine container, no preservative

Collection Instruct patient to void at 8 AM and discard the specimen. Then collect all urine including the final specimen voided at the end of the 24-hour collection period (ie, 8 AM the next morning). Label the container with the patient's name and date and time collection started and finished.

Storage Instructions Refrigerate

Reference Range 30-150 mg/24 hours (SI: 0.03-0.15 g/day) (method dependent). Normal urine protein consists of albumin (up to 35 mg/24 hours), other plasma proteins (ie, immunoglobulins, lysozyme, transferrin, haptoglobin, beta$_2$-microglobulin, and light chains), and Tamm-Horsfall glycoprotein secreted by renal tubular cells (may contribute up

to 50 mg/24 hours). Urinary protein normally tends to increase with age, exercise, and standing posture. Proteinuria has been defined as 24-hour urine protein excretion >150 mg/24 hours (SI: >0.15 g/day).[1] In infants and children, different ranges apply and have been published; proteinuria >100 mg/day (SI: >0.10 g/day) in children younger than 10 years of age is regarded as abnormal.[2]

Critical Values Nephrotic syndromes: ≥3.5 g/24 hours[3]

Use Evaluate proteinuria (eg, following urinalysis in which proteinuria is detected); evaluate renal diseases, including proteinuria complicating diabetes mellitus, the nephrotic syndromes (eg, lipoid nephrosis, membranous, proliferative glomerulopathies), metal poisoning (eg, gold, lead, and cadmium), renal vein thrombosis, systemic lupus erythematosus (SLE), constrictive pericarditis, and amyloidosis; work up other renal diseases including hypertension, glomerulonephritis, Goodpasture's syndrome, Henoch-Schönlein purpura, thrombotic thrombocytopenic purpura, collagen diseases, cryoglobulinemia, toxemia of pregnancy, drug nephrotoxicity, hypersensitivity reactions, allergic reactions, and renal tubular lesions; management of myeloma and macroglobulinemia of Waldenström (Bence Jones proteinuria); evaluate hypoproteinemia; tubular proteinurias include Wilson's disease and Fanconi syndrome. In the table shown, some renal lesions are not easily categorized (eg, the glomerular lesions of chrysotherapy) and of toxemia of pregnancy. All important entities are not shown in the table, including for instance absence of one kidney and vasculitis.

Limitations Although evaluation for proteinuria may be the best single test to work up chronic renal disease, proteinuria may wax and wane. In toxemia of pregnancy (pre-eclampsia/eclampsia), magnesium sulfate is used therapeutically. This may result in high urine magnesium levels, depending on methodology. Toxemia is a state in which urine protein excretion is commonly measured. Twenty-four hour urine collections are subject to collection errors. The laboratory method, depending on an aliquot and varying dilutions, is subject to calculation errors. When protein is determined by precipitation methods, x-ray contrast media, tolbutamide, penicillin or cephalosporin analogs and sulfonamides may cause false-positives. Pyridium® interferes with the reaction by causing color interference. Functional and postural proteinuria occur.

Methodology A number of methods are in use including trichloroacetic acid, sulfosalicylic acid precipitation, biuret method with phosphotungstic acid, and Coomassie blue dye binding. The standard for most methodologies is albumin. Different methods are more or less sensitive to globulin than to albumin. Thus, for nonselective proteinurias, in which a variety of proteins are present, different methodologies yield different results.

Additional Information Tests requiring a 24-hour urine collection with no preservative, such as creatinine, may also be performed on the same specimen. Although quantitative protein can be run on a random specimen or timed collections less than 24 hours, 24-hour collections are preferable for evaluation of the nephrotic states and inflammatory renal disorders. Creatinine, creatinine clearance, BUN, serum protein electrophoresis, ANA, anti-DNA antibodies, HIV, hepatitis C antibody, hepatitis B antigen, and complement levels (including total complement, C3, C4) are among useful tests to work up patients with proteinuria. Urine electrophoresis, immunofixation and immunoelectrophoresis are useful in patients older than 35 years of age to investigate possible diagnosis of amyloidosis, myeloma, and Waldenström's macroglobulinemia.

Some patients exhibit orthostatic proteinuria (ie, recumbent urine protein 100-180 mg in a 12-hour overnight urine collection and up to 1 g in the subsequent 12 hours while ambulatory). The presence of urinary protein >200 mg in the overnight specimen or equally increased amounts of urine protein in both specimens indicates need for further work-up.[4]

In a study of blood pressure and the kidney, proteinuria was identified as an independent risk factor for progression of renal disease. Proteinuria was greater in subjects with glomerular disease entities, diabetes, and hereditary nephritis. Proteinuria is a predictor of decline of glomerular filtration rate.[5]

Nephrotic syndromes are the causes of the most severe urinary protein losses. Nephrotic syndrome is defined now usually by degree of proteinuria (ie, proteinuria >50 mg/kg/day or ≥3.5 g/24 hours). After time, additional signs and symptoms occur including hypoproteinemia, hypoalbuminemia, elevation of alpha$_2$-globulin with decreased gamma globulin on electrophoresis, hyperlipidemia, and edema. Urinary albumin is a more sensitive marker of progression and regression of renal disease than urine total protein, especially when urine total protein is <300 mg/g creatinine.[6] In most laboratories, urine albumin is available from protein electrophoresis following concentration procedures. However, this method is not sensitive to low concentrations of albumin.[6]

For low concentrations, see listing Microalbuminuria *on page 643*. The relationship between long-term elevation of glycated hemoglobin, diabetic nephropathy, and protein loss is being addressed.[7,8] About 35% of subjects with insulin-dependent diabetes mellitus develop diabetic nephropathy, which is characterized by proteinuria with decreasing

(Continued)

Protein, Quantitative, Urine *(Continued)*

Outline of Causes of Proteinuria

Normal proteinuria	Albumin ≤35 mg/24 h	
	Tamm-Horsfall ≤50 mg/24 h	
Prerenal proteinuria	Congestive heart failure	
	Orthostatic proteinuria	
	Transient, associated with febrile illness, surgery, anemia, hyperthyroidism, stroke, exercise, seizures	
	Bence Jones proteinuria associated with myeloma, Waldenström's macroglobulinemia, amyloidosis (light chain proteinuria)	
	Lysozyme associated with myelocytic leukemia	
Renal proteinuria	Renovascular hypertension	
	Malignant hypertension of any cause	
	Glomerular Proteinuria >3.5 g/24 h usually reflects a glomerular lesion	Membranous nephropathy and proliferative glomerulonephritis
		Chronic pyelonephritis
		Polycystic disease
		Diabetic nephropathy
		Amyloidosis
		Lupus erythematosus (SLE)
		Goodpasture's syndrome
		Renal vein thrombosis
		Minimal change nephropathy
		High molecular weight proteinuria
	Tubular usually <1 g/24 h	Fanconi syndrome
		Wilson's disease
		Renal tubular acidosis
		Heavy metal poisoning: lead mercury cadmium
		Galactosemia
		Low molecular weight (<60,000) proteinuria
		Beta$_2$-microglobulinemia (molecular weight 11,800)
	Interstitial	Bacterial pyelonephritis
		Uric acid, urate or calcium deposition
		Idiosyncratic drug reaction: methicillin phenindione sulfonamides phenytoin others
		Interstitial diseases generally reflected as tubular defects or mixed tubular interstitial
Postrenal	Tumors of the bladder or renal pelvis	
	<1 g/24 h, IgM excretion significant marker, amount of proteinuria related to size and spread of tumor	
	Cystitis, severe	

glomerular filtration rate. The risk of death is nine times greater than for diabetics who do not suffer this complication. End stage renal failure occurs within 10 years from onset of proteinuria.[9] The leading cause of renal failure in the western world is diabetic kidney disease.[10] Urine electrophoresis may be helpful; see listing Protein Electrophoresis, Urine *on page 425*. See also **fatty casts** and **oval fat bodies** (**"lipiduria"**) in the listing Urinalysis *on page 658*.

Footnotes

1. Epstein M and Oster JR, "Proteinuria," *The Laboratory in Clinical Medicine: Interpretation and Application*, 2nd ed, Halsted JA and Halsted CH, eds, Philadelphia, PA: WB Saunders Co, 1981, 318-23.

2. Kim MS, "Proteinuria," *Clin Lab Med*, 1988, 8(3):527-40.

3. Larson TS, "Evaluation of Proteinuria," *Mayo Clin Proc*, 1994, 69(12):1154-8.

4. Glassock RJ, "Postural (Orthostatic) Proteinuria: No Cause for Concern," *N Engl J Med*, 1981, 305:639-41.

5. Peterson JC, Adler S, Burkart JM, et al, "Blood Pressure Control, Proteinuria, and the Progression of Renal Disease. The Modification of Diet in Renal Disease Study," *Ann Intern Med*, 1995, 123(10):754-62.

6. Shihabi ZK, Konen JC, and O'Connor ML, "Albuminuria vs Urinary Tract Protein for Detecting Chronic Renal Disorders," *Clin Chem*, 1991, 37(5):621-4.

7. Kullberg CE and Arnqvist HJ, "Elevated Long-Term Glycated Haemoglobin Precedes Proliferative Retinopathy and Nephropathy in Type 1 (Insulin-Dependent) Diabetic Patients," *JAMA*, 1993, 36(10):961-5.

8. Viberti G, "A Glycemic Threshold for Diabetic Complications?" *N Engl J Med*, 1995, 332(19):1293-4.

9. Remuzzi G and Ruggenenti P, "Slowing the Progression of Diabetic Nephropathy," *N Engl J Med*, 1993, 329(20):1496-7.

10. Viberti G, Mogensen CE, Groop LC, et al, "Effect of Captopril on Progression to Clinical Proteinuria in Patients With Insulin-Dependent Diabetes Mellitus and Microalbuminuria," *JAMA*, 1994, 271(4):275-9.

References

Ettenger RB, "The Evaluation of the Child With Proteinuria," *Pediatr Ann*, 1994, 23(9):486-94.

Ginsberg JM, Chang BS, Matarese RA, and Garella S, "Use of Single Voided Urine Samples to Estimate Quantitative Proteinuria," *N Engl J Med*, 1983, 309:1543-6.

Levey AS, Madaio MP, and Perrone RD, "Laboratory Assessment of Renal Disease: Clearance, Urinalysis, and Renal Biopsy," *Kidney*, Brenner BM and Rector FC Jr, eds, Philadelphia, PA: WB Saunders Co, 1991, 919-68.

Magil AB, "Tubulointerstitial Lesions in Human Membranous Glomerulonephritis: Relationship to Proteinuria," *Am J Kidney Dis*, 1995, 25(3):375-9.

Maki DD, Ma JZ, Louis TA, et al, "Long-Term Effects of Antihypertensive Agents on Proteinuria and Renal Function," *Arch Intern Med*, 1995, 155(10):1073-80.

Morgensen CE, "Introduction: Nature of Microalbuminuria, Proteinuria, and Progressive Renal Disease," *J Diabetes Complications*, 1995, 9(1):2-6.

Stephenson JM, Kenny S, Stevens LK, et al, "Proteinuria and Mortality in Diabetes: The WHO Multinational Study of Vascular Disease in Diabetes," *Diabet Med*, 1995, 12(2):149-55.

Trachtman H, Bergwerk A, and Gauthier B, "Isolated Proteinuria in Children. Natural History and Indications for Renal Biopsy," *Clin Pediatr (Phila)*, 1994, 33(8):468-72.

Protein, Screen, Urine see Protein, Semiquantitative, Urine *on this page*

Protein, Semiquantitative, Urine

CPT 81002 (dipstick, nonautomated); 81003 (dipstick, automated)

Related Information

Chromium, Serum *on page 587*
Kidney Biopsy *on page 47*
Microalbuminuria *on page 643*
Osmolality, Urine *on page 173*
Protein Electrophoresis, Urine *on page 425*
Protein, Quantitative, Urine *on previous page*
Urinalysis *on page 658*

Synonyms Albumin, Urine; Protein, Screen, Urine; Protein, Urine, Sulfosalicylic Acid; Urine Screen for Albumin; Urine Screen for Protein

Applies to Protein/Osmolality Ratio

Test Commonly Includes Screening for urine protein by dipstick and, in many laboratories, sulfosalicylic acid method for confirmation. This is part of a routine urinalysis.

Abstract Screening test for urinary protein loss. The precipitation methods, including sulfosalicylic acid and trichloroacetic acid, are more sensitive to globulins including light chains, than are dipstick methods. Microscopic examination of urine sediment is essential to evaluate patients with proteinuria: the presence or absence of erythrocytes, red cell casts, leukocytes, white cell casts, eosinophiluria, oval fat bodies, fatty casts, and other abnormalities are relevant.[1]

Specimen Random urine

Collection Early morning specimen is recommended to provide maximally concentrated urine, when Bence Jones urine protein (light chain) detection is important. For other renal disease, daytime urine is satisfactory or even preferred.[2,3] Transport specimen to the laboratory within 2 hours of collection. Container should state date and time of collection.

Storage Instructions If not run promptly, specimen should be refrigerated.

Reference Range Dipstick results include grades negative and trace (10-20 mg/dL) (SI: 0.1-0.2 g/L). The sensitivity of the dipstick is in the range of 150-300 mg/L. It is sensitive mostly for albumin.

Critical Values Dipstick 1+ is about 30 mg/dL, 2+ 100 mg/dL, 3+ (300 mg/dL), or 4+ (1000 mg/dL)

Use Detection of urinary protein; used to screen for nephrotic syndromes, including complications of diabetes mellitus, glomerulonephritis, amyloidosis, and other entities. Proteinuria is probably the single most important indicator of renal disease.

Limitations The dipstick method is sensitive to negatively charged proteins, but much less so to positively charged proteins; thus, dipsticks commonly will not detect Bence Jones (light chain) or myeloma protein, to which sulfosalicylic acid procedures are usually sensitive. False-negatives may be found with highly dilute urines.

False-positive results may be obtained with highly alkaline (pH ≥7) urines on dipsticks, with hematuria, and in highly concentrated urine. Positive protein dipstick results, especially in very alkaline urines, should be confirmed by sulfosalicylic acid testing. Contaminating quaternary ammonium groups or chlorohexidine present in disinfectants may also give false-positive dipstick results. The test area on dipsticks is more sensitive to albumin than to globulin, hemoglobin, Bence Jones protein, or mucoprotein. A negative result, therefore, does not rule out the presence of these other proteins. Pyridium® metabolites may mask the reaction. X-ray contrast media, tolbutamide, nafcillin, massive doses of penicillin, sulfisoxazole (Gantrisin®), para-aminosalicylic acid, and high levels of cephalosporins may cause false-positive reactions with the sulfosalicylic acid method. Dipstick methods may be unreliable in unusually colored urines or when a great deal of sediment is present. The detection limit of Albustix® (Ames Division, Miles Laboratories) is reported as 300 mg/L or 500 mg/day protein. Since normal albuminuria is <20 mg/L, the screening dipstick lacks sensitivity for early detection of protein loss in diabetic nephropathy.[4,5] See listing Microalbuminuria *on page 643.*

Methodology Dipstick, and in some laboratories sulfosalicylic acid, are run on all urinalyses. The dipstick test is based on the color development of indicators, usually bromphenol blue in citric acid buffer. The sulfosalicylic acid test is based on the acid precipitation of protein. Immunofixation or immunoelectrophoresis is indicated when Bence Jones protein is suspected.

Additional Information The protein/osmolality ratio corrects protein concentration for urine osmolality, correcting for dilution effects in a random specimen. It provides a modicum of correlation with 24-hour collections for protein.[1]

If the dipstick for protein is negative and the sulfosalicylic acid test is positive, Bence Jones proteinuria may be present. If clinically indicated, in this situation a urine for electrophoresis and immunoelectrophoresis for light chains or immunofixation should be considered.

Normal newborns may have increased levels of proteinuria during first 3 days of life.

Subclinical increased urinary albumin excretion is thought to be predictive of emergence subsequently of diabetic nephropathy.[2] In many situations beside diabetes, microalbumin determination is much more sensitive to progressing renal disease than is urinary total protein (eg, hypertension, systemic lupus erythematosus). Urine albumin is easier to standardize and should be more sensitive to specific glomerular disease.[6] Following exercise, proteinuria relates more to intensity of exercise than to its duration.[7] In low-risk women with no objective signs of hypertensive disorder, routine dipstick proteinuria screening at each prenatal visit did not provide any clinically important information regarding pregnancy outcome.[8] Discrepancies between protein methods can be recognized in some settings by skilled microscopy of the urinary sediment.

Transient proteinuria may be secondary to fever, congestive heart failure, and following exercise or cold exposure. Repeat collection of first morning urine with sediment microscopy can direct further investigation.[1]

Footnotes
1. Larson TS, "Evaluation of Proteinuria," *Mayo Clin Proc*, 1994, 69(12):1154-8.
2. Risdon P and Shaw AB, "Which Urine Sample for Detection of Proteinuria?" *Br J Urol*, 1989, 63(2):209-10.
3. Harrison NA, Rainford DJ, White GA, et al, "Proteinuria - What Value Is the Dipstick?" *Br J Urol*, 1989, 63(2):202-8.
4. Hindmarsh JT, "Microalbuminuria," *Clin Lab Med*, 1988, 8(3):611-6.
5. Olivarius ND and Mogensen CE, "Danish General Practitioners' Estimation of Urinary Albumin Concentration in the Detection of Proteinuria and Microalbuminuria," *Br J Gen Pract*, 1995, 45(391):71-3.
6. Shihabi ZK, Konen JC, and O'Connor ML, "Albuminuria vs Urinary Total Protein for Detecting Chronic Renal Disorders," *Clin Chem*, 1991, 37(5):621-4.
7. Poortmans JR, "Postexercise Proteinuria in Humans - Facts and Mechanisms," *JAMA*, 1985, 253(2):236-40.
8. Gribble RK, Fee SC, and Berg RL, "The Value of Routine Urine Dipstick Screening for Protein at Each Prenatal Visit," *Am J Obstet Gynecol*, 1995, 173(1):214-7.

References
Schwab SJ, Christensen RL, Dougherty K, et al, "Quantitation of Proteinuria by the Use of Protein-to-Creatinine Ratios in Single Urine Samples," *Arch Intern Med*, 1987, 147(5):943-4.

Protein, Urine, Sulfosalicylic Acid *see* Protein, Semiquantitative, Urine *on previous page*

Prussian Blue Stain, Urine *see* Hemosiderin Stain, Urine *on page 637*

Purple Urine Bags *see* Indican, Semiquantitative, Urine *on page 637*

Quick-Cult® *see* Occult Blood, Stool *on page 645*

RA Cells *see* Synovial Fluid Analysis *on page 656*

Reducing Substances, Stool
CPT 81005
Related Information
d-Xylose Absorption Test *on page 122*
Lactose Tolerance Test *on page 157*
Meat Fibers, Stool *on page 642*
pH, Stool *on page 648*

Synonyms Stool Reducing Substances

Applies to Breath Hydrogen Analysis; $^{13}CO_2$ Breath Test

Test Commonly Includes Stool weight, stool pH, and total reducing substances

Abstract Test for fecal reducing substance (eg, sugars) as an indication of disaccharidase (sucrase, lactase) deficiency

Specimen Fresh random stool

Collection Transport the specimen to the laboratory as soon as possible; delay may cause falsely low results.

Storage Instructions Freeze specimen if testing is delayed.

Causes for Rejection Specimen collected in a diaper or other absorbent surface

Reference Range Normal: <2 mg/g stool; borderline: between 2-5 mg/g stool; abnormal: >5 mg/g stool. Even though premature infants have relative lactase deficiency and pancreatic insufficiency, there is evidence that older (32 weeks gestation) prematures have insignificant fecal loss of intact carbohydrate. Comparison of fecal carbohydrate excretion in infants fed formulas of 50% lactose vs 50% lactose plus 50% glucose polymers found no significant difference. Mean excretion was <0.2 g/day (<1% of carbohydrate intake).[1]

Use Detect deficiency of intestinal border enzymes, primarily sucrase and lactase (disaccharidases) due to congenital deficiency or nonspecific mucosal injury

Limitations Bacterial fermentation may give falsely low results if specimen is not analyzed within 1 hour. In the neonatal period, high Clinitest® results may be observed.

Methodology Clinitest®[2]

Additional Information Sugars should be rapidly absorbed in the upper small intestine. If not, however, they remain in the intestine and cause osmotic diarrhea by the osmotic pressure of the unabsorbed sugar in the intestine, drawing fluid and electrolytes into the gut. Carbohydrate malabsorption is a major cause of the watery diarrhea and electrolyte imbalance seen in patients with the short bowel syndrome. As a result of bacterial fermentation, the stools become acid with a high concentration of lactic acid. The pH measurement reflects this process. The unabsorbed sugars are measured as reducing substances. Although sucrose is not a reducing sugar, it is subjected to acid hydrolysis in the gut, and thus, is also measured as a reducing substance. Idiopathic lactase deficiency is common, occurring in 70% to 75% of Southern European Greeks and Italians, 70% of black adults, >90% of Oriental adults, and 5% to 20% of white American adults. Lactase activity declines with age in humans and is controlled genetically. It is influenced in its phenotypic expression as lactase malabsorption by several nongenetic factors (eg, adaption to nutritional intake of dairy products, biological (circadian) rhythm of enzyme activity, hormones and hormonal changes of the body and the brain, gastrointestinal functions such as motility and the nutritional components of digested food).[3]

The **breath hydrogen analysis** test may provide more definitive information.[4,5] The $^{13}CO_2$ **breath test** is reportedly more sensitive and specific than the H_2 test in the detection of low jejunal lactase activity.[6] There is considerable variation in lactose tolerance between lactase deficient subjects. A 50 g lactose load has been reported to cause symptoms in 75% of lactase deficient adults whereas 10 g causes symptoms in only 50%.[7] A glass of milk has approximately 12 g of lactose. Classically, stools from patients with disaccharidase deficiency are liquid, acid, and frothy in appearance. The use of mucosal disaccharidase enzyme activity as an isolated diagnostic criterion may have limited value.[8]

Footnotes
1. Ameen VZ and Powell GK, "Quantitative Fecal Carbohydrate Excretion in Premature Infants," *Am J Clin Nutr*, 1989, 49(6):1238-42.
2. Kerry KR and Anderson CM, "A Ward Test for Sugars in Feces," *Lancet*, 1964, 1:981.
3. Enck P and Whitehead WE, "Lactase Deficiency and Lactose Malabsorption. A Review," *Z Gastroenterol*, 1986, 24(3):125-34.
4. Rosado JL and Solomons NW, "Sensitivity and Specificity of the Breath Analysis Test for Detecting Malabsorption of Physiological Doses of Lactose," *Clin Chem*, 1983, 29:545-8.
5. Ostrander CR, Cohen RS, Hopper AO, et al, "Breath Hydrogen Analysis: A Review of the Methodologies and Clinical Applications," *J Pediatr Gastroenterol Nutr*, 1983, 2:525-33.
6. Hiele M, Ghoos Y, Rutgeerts P, et al, "$^{13}CO_2$ Breath Test Using Naturally ^{13}C-Enriched Lactose for Detection of Lactase Deficiency in Patients With Gastrointestinal Symptoms," *J Lab Clin Med*, 1988, 112(2):193-200.
7. Cooper BT, "Lactase Deficiency and Lactose Malabsorption," *Dig Dis*, 1986, 4(2):72-82.
8. Calvin RT, Klish WJ, and Nichols BL, "Disaccharidase Activities, Jejunal Morphology, and Carbohydrate Tolerance in Children With Chronic Diarrhea," *J Pediatr Gastroenterol Nutr*, 1985, 4(6):949-53.

References
Ameen VZ, Powell GK, and Jones LA, "Quantitation of Fecal Carbohydrate Excretion in Patients With Short Bowel Syndrome," *Gastroenterology*, 1987, 92(2):493-500.
Gray GM, "Congenital and Adult Intestinal Lactase Deficiency," *N Engl J Med*, 1976, 294:1057-8.
Hammer HF, Fine KD, Santa Ana CA, et al, "Carbohydrate Malabsorption. Its Measurement and Its Contribution to Diarrhea," *J Clin Invest*, 1990, 86(6):1936-44.
Lloyd ML and Olsen WA, "A Study of the Molecular Pathology of Sucrase-Isomaltase Deficiency. A Defect in the Intracellular Processing of the Enzyme," *N Engl J Med*, 1987, 316(8):438-42.

Reducing Substances, Urine

CPT 81005

Related Information

Ammonia, Blood *on page 75*
Glucose, 2-Hour Postprandial *on page 136*
Glucose, Fasting *on page 137*
Glucose, Quantitative, Urine *on page 635*
Glucose, Random *on page 138*
Glucose, Semiquantitative, Urine *on page 636*
Glucose Tolerance Test *on page 139*
Ketone Bodies, Blood *on page 152*
Ketones, Urine *on page 639*

Synonyms Clinitest® for Sugar, Urine

Test Commonly Includes Clinitest® testing of urine

Specimen Random urine

Container Plastic urine container

Storage Instructions If the specimen cannot be processed promptly by the laboratory, it should be refrigerated.

Causes for Rejection Improper labeling, specimen not refrigerated

Reference Range None detected

Use Semiquantitative determination of reducing substances (usually glucose) in urine; detect glycosuria, galactosuria; screen for overt diabetes mellitus; screen for pentosuria; detect renal glycosuria. With the widespread availability and low cost of specific glucose-oxidase test strips for the detection of glucosuria, this test remains useful for the screening of sick newborns and children for various errors of carbohydrate metabolism.[1,2] Positive urine samples that are negative for glucose should be further confirmed by carbohydrate chromatography. In this setting, even trace positive Clinitest® results should be recognized as abnormal.

It has been advocated that physicians examining ill-appearing dehydrated infants without any obvious cause for dehydration should quickly screen the urine for glucose and ketones.[3]

Limitations Clinitest® is not specific for glucose and will react with sufficient quantities of **any** reducing substance in the urine. Glucose, lactose, fructose, galactose, and pentose all cause positive Clinitest®. Large quantities of salicylates, penicillin, ascorbic acid, nalidixic acid, cephalosporins, glucuronic acid, creatinine, uric acid, formaldehyde, and probenecid may cause false-positives.[4] Low specific gravity urines may give slightly elevated results.

Methodology Copper sulfate reacts with reducing substances in urine, converting cupric sulfate to cuprous oxide. The lower limit of glucose detection by Clinitest® is 200 mg glucose/dL (SI: 11.1 mmol/L). Semiquantitation is accomplished by comparison of the color generated with a reference chart. Semiquantitation of urine glucose is also readily accomplished by urine dipstick. This reaction is also utilized in detection of reducing substances in stool.

Footnotes

1. Wannmacher CM, Wajner M, Buchalter MS, et al, "Detection of Inborn Errors of Metabolism in Unselected Patients From Pediatric Intensive Care Units in Porto Alegre, Brazil: Evaluation of Screening Techniques," *Braz J Med Biol Res*, 1987, 20(1):11-23.
2. Lindor NM and Karnes PS, "Initial Assessment of Infants and Children With Suspected Inborn Errors of Metabolism," *Mayo Clin Proc*, 1995, 70:987-8.
3. Bland GL and Wood VD, "Diabetes in Infancy: Diagnosis and Current Management," *J Natl Med Assoc*, 1991, 83(4):361-5.
4. McCue JD, Gal P, and Pearson RC, "Interference of New Penicillins and Cephalosporins With Urine Glucose Monitoring Tests," *Diabetes Care*, 1983, 6:504-5.

Refractive Index, Urine *see* Specific Gravity, Urine *on next page*

Semen Analysis

CPT 89320

Related Information

Arsenic, Blood *on page 536*
Arsenic, Urine *on page 537*
Cannabinoids (Marijuana Metabolites), Qualitative, Urine *on page 539*
Cocaine (Cocaine Metabolite), Qualitative, Urine *on page 543*
Infertility Screen *on page 638*
Lead, Blood *on page 556*
Lead, Urine *on page 557*
Sperm Mucus Penetration Test (Human or Bovine Cervical Mucus) *on page 654*
Sperm Penetration Assay (Human Sperm-Hamster Oocyte) *on page 654*

Synonyms Seminal Cytology; Sperm Count; Sperm Examination; Sperm Morphology Study

Test Commonly Includes A variety of parameters may be included in a "standard" semen analysis, generally an assessment of number, motility, and morphology of the spermatozoa. More specifically, volume of the semen specimen, concentration of sperm, total count, liquefaction status, viscosity, color, odor, assessment of motility, determination of viability, and detection of abnormal morphologic forms. Direct microscopy of wet preparations and/or a modified Papanicolaou method may be utilized.

Abstract Analysis usually consists of a number of measurements including the physical characteristics of the semen and the functional ability of its constituent spermatozoa.

Patient Preparation Ejaculation should be avoided for 2-3 days prior to collection.

Specimen Semen from ejaculate specimen

Container Clean, dry, wide mouth glass or plastic bottle maintained warm and known to be free of detergent or other toxic compounds

Collection Physician will usually provide instruction for collection. Specimen quality is enhanced when collected in physician's office or laboratory obviating delay in testing and exposure to extremes of temperature occasioned by transportation. Alternately, specimen may be obtained at patient's house by coitus interruptus or masturbation and delivered to the laboratory as soon as possible.[1] Collection of semen during intercourse using a seminal collection device may yield a specimen of higher quality as compared to collection by masturbation.[2,3] Use of such a Silastic condom-type seminal pouch (with a small pencil lead-size perforation) to obtain a specimen for analysis in overcoming human infertility is acceptable to and falls within the principles of the Catholic Church.[4]

Storage Instructions Patient should be instructed to bring specimen to the laboratory within 30-60 minutes after collection maintaining warmth (37°C) during transport. Patient should be instructed to transport specimen in a pocket close to the skin. Low temperature during transport may decrease motility of sperm.

Causes for Rejection Specimen more than 2 hours old

Special Instructions Requisition should specify infertility study or postvasectomy study. Semen, as with all blood, urine, and body fluid specimens, because of the risk of AIDS, should be received and handled with attention to universal precautions. Gloves must be worn during the handling and manipulation of sperm/semen containing fluids. Persons with sores/open wounds of the skin must avoid contact with semen.

Reference Range Volume: 2-5 mL; appearance: white, viscid, opaque; clotting and liquefaction: complete in 20-30 minutes; pH: 7.12-8; sperm count: 50-150 million/mL; motility: at least 60% mobile; morphology: at least 70% normal oval-headed forms

Use Infertility studies, postvasectomy studies; diagnose azoospermia, oligospermia

Limitations Lack of standardization of many test parameters

Methodology Macroscopic and microscopic analysis; direct observation, enumeration, and description; systems for computer-assisted study of morphology and motility are available commercially.

Additional Information Sperm counts may be reduced in patients taking cimetidine[5] and possibly other histamine-receptor blockers. The mechanism for sperm count reduction is unknown. LH response to LHRF was reduced and plasma testosterone levels were increased. Other drugs that may be responsible for decrease in sperm count include sulfasalazine, nitrofurantoin, cyclophosphamide, nitrogen mustard, procarbazine, vincristine, methotrexate, and possibly other chemotherapeutics. Estrogens and methyltestosterone may suppress spermatogenesis. Orchitis, testicular atrophy (as after mumps), varicocele, testicular failure, obstruction of vas deferens (as after vasectomy), and hyperpyrexia may be associated with hypospermia or azoospermia and/or morphologically aberrant forms of spermatozoa. The motility of spermatozoa is dependent upon the level of ionized calcium, in particular the intracellular translocation of calcium ions.[6] Cigarette smoking is associated with decrease in volume of semen; coffee drinking with increase in sperm density and percentage of abnormal forms.[7] Alcohol consumption may not affect sperm function at least as measured at semen analysis.[7] Use of cocaine may be associated with low sperm concentration, low sperm motility, and presence of abnormal morphology.[8] Other illicit drugs which may interfere with spermatogenesis include marijuana; anabolic steroids, lead, and arsenic also do so.[9]

In some cases of infertility, cytologically abnormal spermatocytes or spermatogonia may be seen. A number of associations and known etiologies not withstanding the cause of oligospermia in most infertile men remain unknown. Fertility correlates most closely with the parameters of sperm motility and morphology. For high volume testing, automated computer-assisted semen analysis has been introduced.[10] A role for image analysis in selected settings such as oligozoospermia is published.[11]

Testicular biopsy and fine needle biopsy are in use.[12]

Other types of investigation are available as well.

Footnotes

1. Cannon DC and Henry JB, "Seminal Fluid," *Todd-Sanford-Davidsohn Clinical Diagnosis and Management by Laboratory Methods*, 18th ed, Henry JB, ed, Philadelphia, PA: WB Saunders Co, 1991, 497-503.
2. Zavos PM, "Seminal Parameters of Ejaculates Collected From Oligospermic and Normospermic Patients Via Masturbation and at Intercourse With the Use of a Silastic Seminal Fluid Collection Device," *Fertil Steril*, 1985, 44(4):517-20.
3. Zavos PM and Goodpasture JC, "Clinical Improvements of Specific Seminal Deficiencies Via Intercourse With a Seminal Collection Device Versus Masturbation," *Fertil Steril*, 1989, 51(1):190-3.
4. Griese ON, Rev Msgr, *Catholic Identity in Healthcare: Principles and Practice*, The Pope John Center, 1987, 51-3.
5. Fuentes RJ Jr and Dolinsky D, "Endocrine Function After Cimetidine," *N Engl J Med*, 1979, 301:501-2.
6. Aaberg RA, Sauer MV, Sikka S, et al, "Effects of Extracellular Ionized Calcium, Diltiazem, and cAMP on Motility of Human Spermatozoa," *J Urol*, 1989, 141(5):1221-4.
7. Marshburn PB, Sloan CS, and Hammond MG, "Semen Quality and Association With Coffee Drinking, Cigarette Smoking, and Ethanol Consumption," *Fertil Steril*, 1989, 52(1):162-5.
8. Bracken MB, Eskenazi B, Sachse K, et al, "Association of Cocaine Use With Sperm Concentration, Motility, and Morphology," *Fertil Steril*, 1990, 53(2):315-22.
9. Howards SS, "Treatment of Male Infertility," *N Engl J Med*, 1995, 332(5):312-7.
10. Johnson JE, Boone WR, and Shiparo SS, "Determination of the Precision of an Automated Semen Analyzer," *Lab Med*, 1990, 21:33-8.
11. Mazzilli F, Rossi T, Sabatini L, et al, "Superimposed Image Analysis System (SIAS) Software: A New Approach to Sperm Motility Assessment," *Fertil Steril*, 1995, 64(3):653-6.
12. Gottschalk-Sabag S, Weiss DB, Folb-Zacharow N, et al, "Is One Testicular Specimen Sufficient for Quantitative Evaluation of Spermatogenesis?" *Fertil Steril*, 1995, 64(2):399-402.

References

Adelman MM and Cahill EM, *Atlas of Sperm Morphology*, Chicago, IL: American Society of Clinical Pathologists, 1989.
Auger J, Kunstmann JM, Czyglik F, et al, "Decline in Semen Quality Among Fertile Men in Paris During the Past 20 Years," *N Engl J Med*, 1995, 332(5):281-5
Ginsburg KA, Sacco AG, Ager JW, et al, "Variation of Movement Characteristics With Washing and Capacitation of Spermatozoa. II. Multivariate Statistical Analysis and Prediction of Sperm Penetrating Ability," *Fertil Steril*, 1990, 53(4):704-8.
Glover TD, Barratt CLR, Tyler JPP, et al, *Human Male Fertility and Semen Analysis*, San Diego, CA: Academic Press Inc, 1990, 123-45.
Gottschalk-Sabag S, Weiss DB, and Sherman Y, "Assessment of Spermatogenic Process by Deoxyribonucleic Acid Image Analysis," *Fertil Steril*, 1995, 64(2):403-7.
Irvine DS and Aitken RJ, "Seminal Fluid Analysis and Sperm Function Testing," *Endocrinol Metab Clin North Am*, 1994, 23(4):725-48.
Kiessling AA, Lamparelli N, Yin HZ, et al, "Semen Leukocytes: Friends or Foes?" *Fertil Steril*, 1995, 64(1):196-8.
Kjeldsberg CR and Knight JA, *Body Fluids - Laboratory Examination of Amniotic, Cerebrospinal, Seminal, Serous, and Synovial Fluids: A Textbook Atlas*, 3rd ed, Chicago, IL: American Society of Clinical Pathologists, 1993, 255-64, 349-66.
Mansour RT, Aboulghar MA, Serour GI, et al, "The Effect of Sperm Parameters on the Outcome of Intracytoplasmic Sperm Injection," *Fertil Steril*, 1995, 64(5):982-6.
Overstreet JW and Katz DF, "Semen Analysis," *Urol Clin North Am*, 1987, 14:441-9.
Sheriff DS, "Analysis of Semen in a Constantly Changing Social Context of Medicine," *Arch Androl*, 1995, 34(3):125-32.
Sherins RJ, "Are Semen Quality and Male Fertility Changing?" *N Engl J Med*, 1995, 332(5):327-8.
Van Thiel DH, Gavaler JS, Smith WI Jr, et al, "Hypothalamic-Pituitary-Gonadal Dysfunction in Men Using Cimetidine," *N Engl J Med*, 1979, 300:1012-5.
World Health Organization, *WHO Laboratory Manual for the Examination of Human Semen and Semen-Cervical Mucus Interaction*, New York, NY: Cambridge University Press, 1987.
Yablonsky T, "Male Fertility Testing. New Tests Yield More Predictive Power: But Are They Useful?" *Lab Med*, 1996, 27(6):378-80.
Zamboni L, "Clinical Relevance of Evaluation of Sperm and Ova," *Pathology of Reproductive Failure*, Kraus FT, Damjanov I, and Kaufman N, eds, Baltimore, MD: Williams & Wilkins, 1991, 10-31.

Seminal Cytology *see* Semen Analysis *on previous page*

SG, Urine *see* Specific Gravity, Urine *on this page*

SPA, Hamster Zona-Free Ovum Test *see* Sperm Penetration Assay (Human Sperm-Hamster Oocyte) *on next page*

Specific Gravity, Urine

CPT 81002 (dipstick, nonautomated); 81003 (dipstick, automated)

Related Information

Concentration Test, Urine *on page 633*
Osmolality, Urine *on page 173*
Urinalysis *on page 658*

Synonyms Refractive Index, Urine; SG, Urine

Applies to Body Fluid, Specific Gravity

Test Commonly Includes Specific gravity is usually part of Urinalysis.

Specimen Random void urine or body fluid

Collection First morning specimen is recommended, unless part of complete urinalysis.

Storage Instructions Refrigeration

Reference Range Range: 1.003-1.029; adult on normal fluid intake: 1.016-1.022; specific gravity decreases with increasing age

Use Evaluate renal concentrating power, hydration status. Urine specific gravity test strips are effective in home use to help stone formers drink sufficient water to reduce risk of stone formation. The specific gravity of urine indicates the relative proportions of dissolved solid components to the total volume of the specimen. It reflects the relative degree of concentration or dilution of the specimen. Knowledge of the specific gravity is needed in interpretation of results of most tests in urinalysis. Specific gravity must be interpreted in light of presence or absence of glycosuria and/or proteinuria.

Specific Gravity, Urine

Increased >1.020	Decreased <1.009	Fixed 1.010
Water restriction	Excess water ingestion	Severe renal damage, urine concentration fixed at 1.010, the value of glomerular filtrate
Dehydration	Excess I.V. fluids	
Fever	Diuresis	
Sweating	Hypothermia	
Vomiting	Impaired renal concentrating ability	
Diarrhea		
Diabetes mellitus (glycosuria)	pyelonephritis	
	glomerulonephritis	
Proteinuria	diabetes insipidus	
Congestive heart failure		
X-ray dyes		
Adrenal insufficiency		
Inappropriate antidiuretic hormone secretion syndrome		
Tumors-secreting antidiuretic hormone		

Limitations Radiographic dyes in urine increase the specific gravity by hydrometer or refractometer.[1] Glucose or protein also increase specific gravity out of proportion to osmolality, as measured by hydrometer or refractometer. **Strip method urine specific gravity** was reported as having a significant positive bias at urine pH ≤6 and negative bias at pH >7 compared to specific gravity by refractometer.[2] Urine osmolality is considered preferable in some settings. Benitez et al suggest that osmolality is the only accurate measure of urine concentration in newborn infants.[3]

Methodology Refractometer and colorimetric (reagent strip). **Dipstick method** responds to the ionic strength of urine (linear relation to osmolality due to electrolytes). The strip provides a polyionic polymer with binding sites saturated with hydrogen ions that with urine testing are replaced by sodium or potassium cations, consequent release of hydrogen ions (change of pH) affecting an indicator color change; apparent pKa change. Albumin, glucose, and osmotic effects are not measured, and as such a true specific gravity measurement may not be obtained.[4]

When using the **refractometer**, cloudy urines or those with visible particles should be centrifuged, and the supernatant used for refractometer specific gravity determination.

Additional Information Measurement of urine specific gravity is easier and more convenient than direct measurement of osmolality. The two methods correlate well. However, measured osmolality in newborns is generally lower than would be expected by refractometer specific gravity. In newborns, an elevated specific gravity should be confirmed by direct measurement of osmolality when the state of hydration and water balance are being assessed.[3]

Reagent **strip methods** for the determination of urine specific gravity employ a colorimetric method and are sensitive to ions but not undissociated solutes such as urea. The strip method requires a corrected reading for pH ≥6.5 and protein increases the reading.[4] Critical clinical decisions should be based on the more definitive methods. The strip methods are reported to be suitable for urine screening purposes, but not uniformly so. Strip methods are not described as showing a high degree of correlation with refractometer or urinometer methods.[5] Their additional cost as well as bias led Adams to conclude that strip specific gravity methods are neither cost-effective nor clinically useful[2] and Assadi and Fornell to conclude that the magnitude of observed discrepancies places important limitations on strip test SG measurement.[4]

In athletic and industrial settings or field studies urine color indicates hydration status. Urine osmolality as well as urine specific gravity is used to determine hydration status.[6]

Footnotes

1. Smith C and Arbogast PR, "Effects of X-Ray Contrast Media on the Results for Relative Density of Urine," *Clin Chem*, 1983, 29:730-8.
2. Adams LJ, "Evaluation of Ames Multistix® SG for Urine Specific Gravity Versus Refractometer Specific Gravity," *Am J Clin Pathol*, 1983, 80:871-3.
3. Benitez OA, Benitez M, Stijnen T, et al, "Inaccuracy in Neonatal Measurement of Urine Concentration With a Refractometer," *J Pediatr*, 1986, 108(4):613-6.
4. Assadi FK and Fornell L, "Estimation of Urine Specific Gravity in Neonates With a Reagent Strip," *J Pediatr*, 1986, 108(6):995-6.
5. Ciulla AP, Newsome B, and Kaster J, "Reagent Strip Method for Specific Gravity: An Evaluation," *Lab Med*, 1985, 16:38-40.
6. Armstrong LE, Maresh CM, Castellani JW, et al, "Urinary Indices of Hydration Status," *Int J Sport Nutr*, 1994, 4(3):265-79.

(Continued)

Specific Gravity, Urine *(Continued)*

References

Schumann GB and Schweitzer SC, "Examination of Urine," *Todd-Sanford-Davidsohn Clinical Diagnosis and Management by Laboratory Methods*, Chapter 17, Henry JB, ed, Philadelphia, PA: WB Saunders Co, 1991, 396-7.

Sperm Agglutination and Inhibition *see* Infertility Screen *on page 638*

Sperm Antibodies *see* Infertility Screen *on page 638*

Sperm Count *see* Semen Analysis *on page 652*

Sperm Examination *see* Semen Analysis *on page 652*

Sperm Morphology Study *see* Semen Analysis *on page 652*

Sperm Mucus Penetration Test (Human or Bovine Cervical Mucus)

CPT 89330

Related Information

Infertility Screen *on page 638*

Semen Analysis *on page 652*

Sperm Penetration Assay (Human Sperm-Hamster Oocyte) *on this page*

Applies to Cervical Mucus Interaction, Cross Hostility Tests; *In Vivo* Cervical Mucus Penetration (Postcoital) Test

Patient Preparation Follow physician's instructions. Ejaculation should be avoided for 2-3 days prior to collection.

Specimen Liquefied semen. Normal seminal fluid should be liquefied by about 30 minutes after collection (at 37°C). Test should be started within 2-3 hours after collection of the sample.

Container Clean, dry, wide mouth glass or plastic bottle known to be free of detergent or substances toxic to spermatozoa

Collection Postcoital or masturbation using condom-like Silastic seminal fluid collection device (see Semen Analysis *on page 652*) or directly into sterile glass jar.

Storage Instructions Samples should be tested as soon as possible after collection. Time between ejaculation and start of test should not be over 2-3 hours. Human cervical mucus (obtained during time of ovulation) may be stored for some hours at 4°C in the refrigerator.

Causes for Rejection Specimen more than 2 hours old

Special Instructions Semen, as with all blood, urine, and body fluid specimens, because of the risk of AIDS, should be received and handled with close attention to cleanliness. Gloves must be worn during the handling and manipulation of sperm/semen containing fluids. Persons with sores/open wounds of the skin must avoid contact with semen.

Reference Range ≥30 mm penetration by the "vanguard sperm" (Penetrak™ test)

Use Evaluate interaction between spermatozoa and cervical mucus

Limitations Test provides information additional to other semen tests (sperm count, motility, morphology; see Semen Analysis *on page 652*). It is not intended for use without other evaluation.

Methodology Miller and Kurzrok, in 1932, developed and made clinical application of a semen-mucus phase boundary test. A 3 mm-sized fragment of cervical mucus and a similar sized drop of semen were placed 3 mm from each other on a glass slide. A coverslip was applied with minimal motion and the events occurring at the semen-mucus interface were studied by microscopy.[1] In 1965 Kremer described the construction of a "sperm penetration meter" and its use in a cervical mucus sperm penetration test.[2] In the commercially available "Penetrak™" test, bovine cervical mucus is kept frozen in flat sealed capillary tubes. Using a standardized technique, sperm migration through the mucus over a 90-minute period is measured. The distance traveled by the sperm the furthest down the tube (the "vanguard sperm") is measured and reported. The average of duplicate values is reported. If values differ by more than 15 mm, it is recommended that the test be repeated on a different specimen.

Additional Information In a study published in 1981, the bovine CMPT identified a group of individuals with inadequate penetration (<15 mm) who had mean sperm density of $53.8\pm6.8 \times 10^6$/mL (sperm counts within normal limits).[3] Significant numbers of individuals (5%, 10%, and 15% of different groups) had inadequate penetration, but adequate to high sperm counts or levels of motility. Results of *in vitro* tests of sperm penetration have been found to correlate with fertility (pregnancy). Cervical mucus penetration testing has been found of value in assessment of fertility prognosis, in particular when modified to produce a crossmatching penetrability test. The latter study compares results of penetration using cervical mucus of the patient's wife by subject's spermatozoa and additionally with use of semen from fertile donors.[4] The use of hormonally standardized human cervical mucus from female partners has been considered superior to bovine cervical mucus as a penetration

medium and as to ability to provide information about sperm function.[5] There are data to suggest that the ability of cervical mucus to accept spermatozoa is dependent upon the carbohydrate composition of mucus glycoproteins.[6] See listing Sperm Penetration Assay (Human Sperm-Hamster Oocyte) *on page 654*. The SPA uses the zona-free hamster egg, 100% penetration can be achieved by human spermatozoa. Techniques for optimizing and standardizing sperm and ovum preparation have been established. Correlation of SPA test results with human *in vitro* fertilization showed a very low incidence of individuals whose sperm penetrated zona-free hamster ova but did not efficiently penetrate human eggs.[7]

Footnotes

1. Miller EG Jr and Kurzrok R, "Biochemical Studies of Human Semen. III. Factors Affecting Migration of Sperm Through the Cervix," *Am J Obstet Gynecol*, 1932, 24:19-26.
2. Kremer J, "A Simple Sperm Penetration Test," *Int J Fertil*, 1965, 10:209-15.
3. Alexander NJ, "Evaluation of Male Infertility With an *In Vitro* Cervical Mucus Penetration Test," *Fertil Steril*, 1981, 36:201-8.
4. Eggert-Kruse W, Gerhard I, Tilgen W, et al, "Clinical Significance of Crossed *In Vitro* Sperm-Cervical Mucus Penetration Test in Infertility Investigation," *Fertil Steril*, 1989, 52(6):1032-40.
5. Eggert-Kruse W, Leinhos G, Gerhard I, et al, "Prognostic Value of *In Vitro* Sperm Penetration Into Hormonally Standardized Human Cervical Mucus," *Fertil Steril*, 1989, 51(2):317-23.
6. Morales P, Roco M, and Vigil P, "Human Cervical Mucus: Relationship Between Biochemical Characteristics and Ability to Allow Migration of Spermatozoa," *Hum Reprod*, 1993, 8(1):78-83.
7. Smith RG, Johnson A, Lamb D, et al, "Functional Tests of Spermatozoa. Sperm Penetration Assay," *Urol Clin North Am*, 1987, 14(3):451-8.

References

Adelman MM and Cahill EM, *Atlas of Sperm Morphology*, Chicago, IL: American Society of Clinical Pathologists, 1989, 99.

Sperm-Oolemma Binding Test *see* Infertility Screen *on page 638*

Sperm Penetration Assay (Human Sperm-Hamster Oocyte)

CPT 89329

Related Information

Infertility Screen *on page 638*

Semen Analysis *on page 652*

Sperm Mucus Penetration Test (Human or Bovine Cervical Mucus) *on this page*

Synonyms Hamster (Human + Hamster) Test; Hamster Test; Heterologous Ovum Penetration Test; SPA, Hamster Zona-Free Ovum Test

Abstract The SPA is an *in vitro* test that can provide an important measure of the fertilizing capacity of human spermatozoa. The test measures the ability of human sperm to penetrate zona-free hamster oocytes. The test thus reflects the ability of sperm to capacitate, acrosome react, fuse with the oolemma and decondense (within zona-free hamster oocytes).

Patient Preparation Abstinence for a period of at least 48 hours prior to test; less than 48 hours (12 or 24 hours) is associated with reduced penetration potential even though sperm count or motility may not be decreased.[1]

Specimen Semen

Container Clean, wide-mouth glass or plastic container; condom-like device (Silastic seminal fluid collection device - available commercially) placed in a clean jar. Containers should be known free of detergent or other toxic compounds.

Collection Proper collection and handling of the semen specimen is critically necessary to obtain representative results. Semen collection by masturbation in a special room within or adjacent to the laboratory performing the analysis is ideal for some patients. This allows for direct transfer to the laboratory of a fresh specimen without risking degradation of spermatozoa by aging or temperature extremes incurred during transportation.[2] Patient preference, however, may dictate the use of a coital specimen (collected during intercourse) using a Silastic seminal fluid collection device. Commercial sources for such devices include (but may not be limited to) Male-Factor Pak manufactured by Apex Medical Technologies Inc, available from Fertility Technologies Inc, Natick, Massachusetts; HDC Corporation, Mountain View, California. There is evidence that semen quality is improved when collected during intercourse using such a device.[3,4,5] Specimen must be delivered to the laboratory within 30-60 minutes after collection. Avoid exposure to extremes of heat or cold during transport (patient should be instructed to carry specimen in a pocket close to the skin).

Storage Instructions Specimen is maintained in the laboratory at room temperature, allowed to liquefy (usually occurs within 30 minutes, abnormal if not liquefied by 60 minutes), standard semen analysis is commonly initiated, and specimen is buffered (see below) and incubated at 4°C for 18 hours or longer.

Causes for Rejection Question concerning authenticity of specimen identification (label, content), exposure to extreme of temperature, specimen more than 1 hour old (sperm should not stay in contact with seminal fluid for more than 1-2 hours prior to processing)

Turnaround Time Results usually available within 36 hours (dependent upon preincubation time which in current procedures may be as long as 18-22 hours).

Special Instructions Semen, as with all blood, urine, and body fluid specimens, because of the risk of AIDS, should be received and handled with close attention to cleanliness. Gloves must be worn during the handling and manipulation of sperm/semen containing fluids. Persons with sores/open wounds of the skin must avoid contact with semen specimens.

Reference Range Penetration of 21% to 100% - ("good category");[6] penetration index of over 0.2. The terms "penetration index,"[6] "fertilization index,"[7] and "sperm capacitation index,"[8] are a measure of polyspermy (the average number of penetrations per ovum). Earlier procedural protocols found the lower limit of the penetration range for fertile men to vary from 11% to 25%.[7]

Use Evaluate fertilizing capability of human spermatozoa;[8] application to the study of effect that environmental factors have on male fertility; a clinical test of sperm function in conjunction with semen analysis and other studies as a screen for *in vitro* fertilization. The SPA measures components of sperm penetration including capacitation (see below), acrosome reaction, chromatin decondensation, and ability to fuse with oolemma.

Limitations SPA does not assess all functions of human spermatozoa. The test does not measure the ability of sperm to penetrate human ova with granulosa cells and zona pellucida intact. Ability of spermatozoa to bind the zona pellucida is species specific. Thus, semen with a positive SPA result may not necessarily have sperm with normal penetrating ability (false-positive result). Rarely, a patient with a score of zero on SPA will subsequently initiate a pregnancy (false-negative result).[9] The test suffers from lack of standardization and is relatively expensive. Cumulus and zona-free hamster oocytes are not true physiologic models. Extensive experience with the SPA used in conjunction with *in vitro* fertilization, however, indicates that in the great majority of individuals, sperm capable of penetrating zona-free hamster ova can also penetrate intact human eggs.[10]

Methodology The original method of Yanagimachi et al utilized a modified Krebs-Ringer's culture medium developed by Biggers, Whitten, and Whittingham (BWW medium) supplemented with human serum albumin.[11] Ova were obtained from superovulated hamsters and prepared by treatment with bovine testicular hyaluronidase (divests the surrounding cumulus cells). The zona pellucida was removed by treatment with bovine pancreatic trypsin. Human semen, after liquification was diluted with BWW medium, filtered, washed, resuspended, and incubated at 37°C for up to 7.5 hours in air or 5% CO_2. A drop of sperm suspension was placed with ova in BWW medium and examined periodically using phase contrast microscopy for evidence of sperm penetration. Evidence of penetration (fertilization) was presence of swollen sperm heads within the cytoplasm of an oocyte.

The need for maintenance of a hamster colony with production and harvesting of ova on demand and subsequent considerable manipulation and processing places this procedure beyond the capability of most general routine clinical laboratories. The assay has undergone continuing improvement and simplification. Sperm function (capacitation) has been enhanced by use of TES and TRIS (TEST)-yolk-extender buffer (TYB) system, cooling slowly and incubating for 22-42 hours (may be kept up to 96 hours).[6,12,13] The TYB system has increased SPA sensitivity and has allowed specimens to be sent to a reference laboratory. In addition, cryopreserved hamster ova have become commercially available (Cryotech™ hamster ova, Charles River Laboratories, Wilmington, Massachusetts; sales agent Fertility Technologies, Natick, Massachusetts). These are provided in straws, frozen at -150°C (requires liquid nitrogen). Availability of frozen ova simplifies the SPA procedure, logistically allows for ova on demand (can be prepared for use in about 7 minutes) and provides a baseline for use in quality control procedures. The ova (15 per straw) are suspended in propylene glycol (cryoprotectant) in an isotonic salt solution. A sucrose solution, isosmotic to the propylene glycol, is also present in the straw. It acts as an osmotic buffer during dilution of the cryoprotectant out of the ova. The frozen ova were found to be statistically equivalent (% penetration and penetration index) to unfrozen ova in a study of the SPA using 547 frozen hamster ova.[14]

A modification of the SPA uses 10 μL wells of Teraski tissue typing plates allowing the study of very small numbers of spermatozoa as they interact with single hamster ova. This modification may be of value clinically in cases of severe abnormality when few motile spermatozoa can be recovered.[15] Frozen semen is recommended for quality control.[16]

Additional Information There is a lack of consensus and a surprisingly wide variety of opinion concerning the value of the sperm penetration assay in the study of fertility. The 1992 review by Liu and Baker[8] indicates that "the clinical significance of the SPA in predicting male fertility is still disputed" but that "the SPA has been widely used as a clinical test of sperm function." Correlation with the results of *in vitro* fertilization (IVF) has been variable.[6] Over 200 publications dealt with the SPA from 1981-1985.[7] Lack of standardized test parameters, small sample size, and/or variable, often poorly defined parameters of the patient test population characterize many of these reports. Comparisons and conclusions are problematic.

There is unanimity of opinion that the SPA does assess sperm capacitation, acrosome reaction, ability to fuse with oolemma, and chromatin decondensation with head swelling in cytoplasma of the ovum.[6,8] These are major physiologic events necessary to fertilization. The acrosome is a double- layered membrane, an envelope covering the anterior two-thirds of the sperm head. The acrosome contains hydrolytic enzymes including acrosin and hyaluronidase. With the acrosome reaction there is fusion and vesiculation of membranes, formation of pores, and eventual loss of sperm, and outer acrosomal membranous envelope anterior to the equator of the sperm head. The acrosome reaction must occur before the sperm can penetrate the zona pellucida. Round headed spermatozoa (without acrosomes) are thus not capable of fertilization. Before ejaculated spermatozoa are functional, they require a period of time (within the female tract or *in vitro*) before they can fertilize. This process is termed "capacitation" and is followed by an influx of calcium ions leading to the acrosome reaction. Capacitation is not associated with a recognizable morphologic change, thus, the important role of functional based assays such as the SPA.

A large study (241 couples) published in 1992 compared the results of SPA under conditions that enhance sperm capacitation (use of TYB system and cool incubation as detailed in methodology above) with outcome of *in vitro* fertilization.[6] A significant correlation was found between SPA penetration category (poor: 0% to 20%; good: 21% to 100%), and pregnancy rate after IVF. No pregnancy occurred (among eight embryo transfers) in the 31 cases falling into the "poor SPA" category. On the other hand there were 73 pregnancies (34.8%) in the 210 cases falling into the "good SPA" category. Sperm quality (count, motility, and morphology) were all significantly higher in "good SPA" versus the "poor SPA" categories. The authors concluded that the SPA "is a useful screening assay before IVF together with sperm morphology."[6]

Findings from computer-assisted semen analysis have been compared with SPA penetration rates. A study published in 1993 used total motile oval count (TMO), compared to concentration, motility, and technician determined morphology considered independently in predicting the outcome of SPA.[17] TMO was defined as the product of total count, percent motility, and percent normal (oval) forms in the semen specimen. TMO was a greater risk factor than percent sperm with oval morphology in relation to the outcome of SPA. Below 20% penetration in the SPA assay, both TMO and percent oval sperm were comparable predictive factors.

Footnotes

1. Rogers BJ, Perreault SD, Bentwood BJ, et al, "Variability in the Human-Hamster *In Vitro* Assay for Fertility Evaluation," *Fertil Steril*, 1983, 39:204-11.
2. Overstreet JW and Katz DF, "Semen Analysis," *Urol Clin North Am*, 1987, 14(3):441-9.
3. Zavos PM, "Characteristics of Human Ejaculates Collected Via Masturbation and a New Silastic Seminal Fluid Collection Device," *Fertil Steril*, 1985, 43(3):491-2.
4. Zavos PM, "Seminal Parameters of Ejaculates Collected From Oligospermic and Normospermic Patients Via Masturbation and at Intercourse With the Use of a Silastic Seminal Fluid Collection Device," *Fertil Steril*, 1985, 44(4):517-20.
5. Zavos PM and Goodpasture JC, "Clinical Improvements of Specific Seminal Deficiencies Via Intercourse With a Seminal Collection Device Versus Masturbation," *Fertil Steril*, 1989, 51(1):190-3.
6. Soffer Y, Golan A, Herman A, et al, "Prediction of *In Vitro* Fertilization Outcome by Sperm Penetration Assay With TEST-Yolk Buffer Preincubation," *Fertil Steril*, 1992, 58(3):556-62.
7. Rogers BJ, "The Sperm Penetration Assay: Its Usefulness Reevaluated," *Fertil Steril*, 1985, 43(6):821-40.
8. Liu DY and Baker HW, "Tests of Human Sperm Function and Fertilization *In Vitro*," *Fertil Steril*, 1992, 58(3):465-83.
9. Kuzan FB, Muller CH, Zarutskie PW, et al, "Human Sperm Penetration Assay as an Indicator of Sperm Function in Human *In Vitro* Fertilization," *Fertil Steril*, 1987, 48(2):282-6.
10. Smith RG, Johnson A, Lamb D, et al, "Functional Tests of Spermatozoa. Sperm Penetration Assay," *Urol Clin North Am*, 1987, 14(3):451-8.
11. Yanagimachi R, Yanagimachi H, and Rogers BJ, "The Use of Zona-Free Animal Ova as a Test-System for the Assessment of the Fertilizing Capacity of Human Spermatozoa," *Biol Reprod*, 1976, 15:471-6.
12. Johnson AR, Syms AJ, Lipshultz LI, et al, "Conditions Influencing Human Sperm Capacitation and Penetration of Zona-Free Hamster Ova," *Fertil Steril*, 1984, 41(4):603-8.
13. Veeck LL, "TES and TRIS (TEST)-Yolk Buffer Systems, Sperm Function Testing, and *In Vitro* Fertilization," *Fertil Steril*, 1992, 58(3):484-6.
14. Leibo SP, Giambernardi TA, Meyer TK, et al, "The Efficacy of Cryopreserved Hamster Ova in the Sperm Penetration Assay," *Fertil Steril*, 1990, 53(5):906-12.
15. Bronson RA, Oula L, and Bronson SK, "A Microwell Sperm Penetration Assay," *Fertil Steril*, 1992, 58(5):1078-80.

(Continued)

Sperm Penetration Assay (Human Sperm-Hamster Oocyte) *(Continued)*

16. Johnson A, Bassham B, Lipshultz LI, et al, "A Quality Control System for the Optimized Sperm Penetration Assay," *Fertil Steril*, 1995, 64(4):832-7.

17. Brandeis VT, "Importance of Total Motile Oval Count in Interpreting the Hamster Ovum Sperm Penetration Assay," *J Androl*, 1993, 14(1):53-9.

References

Auger J, Kunstmann JM, Czyglik F, et al, "Decline in Semen Quality Among Fertile Men in Paris During the Past 20 Years," *N Engl J Med*, 1995, 332(5):281-5.

Glover TD, Barratt CLR, Tyler JPP, et al, *Human Male Fertility and Semen Analysis*, San Diego, CA: Academic Press Inc, 1990, 123-45.

Howards SS, "Treatment of Male Infertility," *N Engl J Med*, 1995, 332(5):312-7.

Lipshultz LI and Witt MA, "Infertility in the Male," *Infertility: A Practical Guide for the Physician*, 3rd ed, Hammond MG and Talbert LM, eds, Boston, MA: Blackwell Scientific Publications, 1992, 26-55.

Mao C and Grimes DA, "The Sperm Penetration Assay: Can It Discriminate Between Fertile and Infertile Men?" *Am J Obstet Gynecol*, 1988, 159(2):279-86.

Paulson RJ, Sauer MV, Francis MM, et al, "A Prospective Controlled Evaluation of TEST-Yolk Buffer in the Preparation of Sperm for Human *In Vitro* Fertilization in Suspected Cases of Male Infertility," *Fertil Steril*, 1992, 58(3):551-5.

Sherins RJ, "Are Semen Quality and Male Fertility Changing?" *N Engl J Med*, 1995, 332(5):327-8.

Yablonsky T, "Male Fertility Testing. New Tests Yield More Predictive Power: But Are They Useful?" *Lab Med*, 1996, 27(6):378-80.

Zamboni L, "Clinical Relevance of Evaluation of Sperm and Ova," *Pathology of Reproductive Failure*, Kraus FT, Damjanov I, and Kaufman N, eds, Baltimore, MD: Williams & Wilkins, 1991, 10-31.

Steatocrit *see* Fat, Semiquantitative, Stool *on page 634*

Stool Fat, Semiquantitative *see* Fat, Semiquantitative, Stool *on page 634*

Stool Guaiac *see* Occult Blood, Stool *on page 645*

Stool Meat Fibers *see* Meat Fibers, Stool *on page 642*

Stool, Methylene Blue Stain *see* Methylene Blue Stain, Stool *on page 642*

Stool pH *see* pH, Stool *on page 648*

Stool Reducing Substances *see* Reducing Substances, Stool *on page 651*

Sudan III Stain, Stool *see* Fat, Semiquantitative, Stool *on page 634*

Sugar, Qualitative, Urine *see* Glucose, Semiquantitative, Urine *on page 636*

Sugar, Quantitative, Urine *see* Glucose, Quantitative, Urine *on page 635*

Synovial Fluid Analysis

CPT 87070 (culture bacterial); 88104 (cytopathology, smears with interpretation); 89051 (cell count with differential); 89060 (crystal identification)

Related Information

Bacterial Culture, Biopsy or Body Fluid *on page 456*
Body Fluid Analysis, Cell Count *on page 306*
Body Fluid Cytology *on page 286*
Body Fluid Glucose *on page 91*
Body Fluid Lactate Dehydrogenase *on page 92*
Fungal Culture, Biopsy or Body Fluid *on page 476*
Gram's Stain *on page 481*
Lyme Disease Serology *on page 415*
Mycobacterial Culture, Biopsy or Body Fluid *on page 487*
5' Nucleotidase *on page 171*
Rheumatoid Factor *on page 427*
Uric Acid, Serum *on page 213*
Uric Acid, Urine *on page 215*

Synonyms Joint Fluid Analysis; Knee Fluid Analysis

Applies to Calcium Pyrophosphate Dihydrate Crystal (CPPD) Deposition; Mucin Test for Hyaluronic Acid; RA Cells

Test Commonly Includes May vary between laboratories but should include cell count and differential, cultures and Gram's stain for pathogens and microscopic examination for crystals. Other tests, depending on the clinical situation, may be of value including viscosity, clot lysis, uric acid, rheumatoid factor, and cytology.

Abstract Analysis of joint fluid usually includes multiple studies (eg, cell count, microscopic exam, culture) to determine if joint pathology is present and to assess its nature and severity. Analyses are particularly helpful in differentiating traumatic arthritis from the immune-based and crystal-induced arthritides.

Patient Preparation As per physician's usual aseptic aspiration technique

Specimen Joint fluid; simultaneously drawn venous blood in red top tube often helpful, especially with order for serum chemistry profile

Container Capped syringe or three sterile tubes, one with heparin and two red top tubes for joint fluid; one to two red top tubes of venous blood desirable; Thayer-Martin agar is best inoculated with joint fluid at bedside if gonococcal (GC) infection is suspected.

Collection An experienced physician, using sterile technique, obtains the specimen (arthrocentesis). Media appropriate for culture of *N. gonorrhoeae*, *M. tuberculosis*, and other organisms should be available if indicated.

Storage Instructions Testing should be initiated, in most cases, shortly after receipt of the specimen. It may be prudent to save a portion of the specimen for possible additional analyses (eg, bacterial and crystal-induced diseases) if such testing is not performed initially.

Causes for Rejection Some constituent tests of the analysis may not be performed if gross contamination has occurred.

Turnaround Time From hours to days (eg, culture results)

Special Instructions Specimens should be delivered immediately to the laboratory and placed in the hands of a medical technologist. **Physician should indicate clinical impression and indicate tests he/she feels are necessary.** If presence of monosodium urate (MSU) crystals (as are present with gout) is a consideration, alcohol-based fixatives and stains must be used as MSU crystals are water soluble.

Reference Range When synovial fluid can be aspirated, abnormality is probably evident. Normal synovial fluid does not clot spontaneously, because it lacks fibrinogen. Clotting bears an implication of inflammation. There should be <200 WBCs/mm³, 0% to 25% neutrophils, protein should be ≤3.0 g/dL (SI: ≤30 g/L), uric acid should be <8.0 mg/dL (SI: <476 μmol/L) and fluid LD (LDH) should be the same or less than that of the patient's serum drawn at the same time. Glucose is significantly abnormal in the nonfasting subject when it is <40 mg/dL (SI: <2.2 mmol/L). There should be a long string produced normally when synovial fluid is poured from a container and the mucin clot test is normally positive (ie, a firm mucin clot is formed in the presence of acetic acid).

Use Aid the diagnosis of rheumatic disease and diseases which cause joint symptoms, pain, increase in joint fluid or destruction of joint space, including rheumatoid arthritis, joint infection, gout, and pseudogout. In cases with appropriate clinical presentation (see table), synovial fluid analysis using polarized light should be done to confirm presence of a crystal-induced arthropathy.

Limitations Appropriate work-up may not be accomplished unless there is discussion between physician and analyst. Oxalate anticoagulants may lead to problems in crystal identification. If laboratory is unaware of possible gonococcal arthritis, it may not inoculate specimen on Thayer-Martin medium. If GC infection is in the differential consideration, the physician, ideally, should plate out the Thayer-Martin medium at the bedside at time of aspiration. Limited sensitivity and specificity exist overall for synovial fluid analysis.

Methodology Includes polarizing and phase as well as conventional microscopy. Laboratory notes color and presence of clot in centrifuged specimen. Cultures are made from centrifuged sediment and media inoculated for acid-fast bacteria, fungus, routine culture, and Gram's stain smear. Rheumatoid factor titer is desirable in suspected cases of rheumatoid arthritis. Other testing methodologies may be applied as indicated or ordered. The use of Testsimplet™ supravital staining (glass slide precoated with methylene blue and crystal violet) has been found advantageous in microscopy of synovial fluid.[1]

Additional Information Normal fluid is rarely obtained because of its small volume; therefore, any fluid which is aspirated is potentially a diagnostic specimen. When results of analyses are combined with the clinical impression of the physician, a high rate of accurate diagnosis is obtained. Some diagnoses cannot be made without such analysis. Detection of synovial fluid monosodium urate crystals is important in establishing a diagnosis of gout. Heparinized tube is needed for cell count and differential. A red cell count is not necessary, but if grossly bloody, a hematocrit should be ordered. Joint fluid and/or serum uric acid may be helpful in cases of possible gout. Joint fluid uric acid significantly higher than serum uric acid may be diagnostic of gout. Other chemistries are usually of little value with the occasional exception of protein, LD (LDH), and glucose. Decreased fluid glucose indicates inflammation, but the result should be compared to that of serum or plasma. High synovial LD but normal serum LD suggests RA, infectious arthritis, or gout. Synovial LD is normal in degenerative joint disease.

Sediment or fluid may be examined in the cytology laboratory for presence of cartilage. Presence of cartilage cells supports diagnosis of traumatic arthritis or osteoarthritis. While involvement of joints by malignancy is uncommon, both primary and metastatic tumors should be included in the differential consideration.[2] Cytologic examination may support diagnosis of pigmented villonodular synovitis or Reiter's syndrome. While rhomboid cholesterol crystals have been reported in chronic joint effusions of rheumatoid arthritis and osteoarthritis, birefringent lipid bodies (lipid microspherules, liposomes, smectic mesophases, lipid liquid crystals), intra- and extracellular, at least partly formed of cholesterol ester, have been found in fluids from acute and chronic arthritis, traumatic arthritis, and pigmented villonodular synovitis.[3,4] Liposomes (smectic mesophases, lipid liquid crystals), birefringent multilamellated (by EM) lipid microspherules have phospholipid characteristics and have been reported in cases of unexplained acute monoarthritis.[5]

Phase microscopy is used to look for intracellular inclusions in pus cells. These are "RA cells" only if the rheumatoid titer is positive. Synovial fluid in pseudogout, traumatic arthritis and osteoarthritis rarely also may contain intraleukocytic cytoplasmic inclusions. Polarizing microscopy is done to identify crystals of urate and pyrophosphate, the causes of gout and pseudogout. Calcium pyrophosphate dihydrate (CPPD) crystal deposition disease does not equate exclusively with a diagnosis of pseudogout (chondrocalcinosis). It is important to recognize that CPPD disease encompasses an array of disorders occurring largely in the aged.[6] These include asymptomatic chondrocalcinosis, acute pseudogout, and chronic pyrophosphate arthropathy. Cases of CPPD disease may be sporadic, familial, or secondary to degenerative or metabolic disease. Hyperparathyroidism and hemochromatosis may be associated with CPPD deposition. Pyrophosphate salt deposition usually occurs in those of advanced age. As an example, asymptomatic chondrocalcinosis occurs in 10% to 15% in 65-75 years of age and in 30% to 60% of those older than 80 years of age.[6] Cholesterol crystals occur occasionally, indicating RA, and steroid crystals after injection may be found. LE cells may be noted in fluid.

Comparison of Gout and CPPD Crystal Deposition Disease*

Feature	Gout	CPPD Crystal Deposition Disease
Male-female ratio	7:1	1.5:1
Age-group affected	Middle-aged men, postmenopausal women	Elderly
Hereditary forms?	Yes	Yes
Hyperuricemia present?	Yes	No
Clinical picture	Asymptomatic phase, acute and chronic arthritis, tophi, renal disease	Asymptomatic phase, acute and chronic arthritis, tophus-like collections only rarely
Typical joint localization	First MTP joints, midfoot, ankles, knees, wrists	Knees, wrists, MCP joints, elbows, shoulders
Radiologic findings	Erosions with overlying edge of displaced bone	Chondrocalcinosis
Findings on synovial fluid analysis	Evidence of inflammation, MSU crystals	Evidence of inflammation, CPPD crystals
Birefringence of synovial fluid crystals	Strong with negative elongation	Weak with positive elongation
Symptomatic treatment	NSAID, colchicine, corticosteroid (intra-articular or systemic)	NSAID, colchicine (occasionally), corticosteroid (intra-articular)
Definitive treatment	Allopurinol (Zyloprim®) or probenecid (Benemid®) to decrease serum uric acid level	None
Possible underlying disease	Diabetes, obesity, hypertension, hyperlipidemia	Hyperparathyroidism, hemochromatosis, hypomagnesemia, hypophosphatasia, severe hypothyroidism

*Formerly called pseudogout.

CPPD = calcium pyrophosphate dihydrate; MCP = metacarpophalangeal; MSU = monosodium urate; MTP = metatarsophalangeal; NSAID = nonsteroidal anti-inflammatory drugs

From Beutler A and Schumacher HR Jr, "Gout and 'Pseudogout': When Are Arthritic Symptoms Caused by Crystal Deposition?" *Postgrad Med*, 1994, 95(2):103-16, with permission.

Test for viscosity and mucin test for hyaluronic acid measure the physical character of the synovial fluid. Abnormality in either of these tests indicates dilution or inflammation. The viscosity can be evaluated by the quality of stringing; inflammatory fluids of low viscosity produce very short strings, but normal or noninflammatory fluids produce long strings. Viscosity is generally equivalent to mucin hyaluronate content.

The finding of amyloid in synovial fluid (using Congo red stained sections of 10% formol saline fixed, paraffin-embedded, centrifuged sediment) has been considered a sufficient finding to establish a diagnosis of amyloid arthropathy.[7]

More than 2% eosinophils in synovial fluid may be a clue to presence of Lyme disease. Rheumatoid factor negative patients with oligoarthritis of unknown etiology were tested for *Chlamydia trachomatis* utilizing antigen specific synovial T-cell response and detection of bacterial antigen. Antigen specific lymphocyte proliferation was found in the synovial fluid of 34% of such patients. *C. trachomatis* was the most frequent single agent detected. Only chlamydial antigen was found in synovial fluid cells by monoclonal antibody technique.[8]

A variety of cytokines have been found in synovial fluid. Some (IL-6 and IL-8) are increased in cases of inflammatory arthritis (RA) as compared with cases of osteoarthritis.[9]

Individual laboratories may not be proficient in the identification of crystals in synovial fluid. Artifacts and unexplained birefringent materials may be present. Patients with hemarthrosis may develop solid and angular birefringent crystals of two different types. Rectangular hemoglobin-like crystals within red cells are weakly birefringent. Golden brown rhomboid crystals (likely hematoidin) are intensely birefringent with positive or negative elongation. These red cell-derived crystals may be confused with pathogenic crystals.[10]

Advantages have been found in the use of atomic force microscopy (AFM) in the detection of synovial fluid crystals, in particular urate crystals and octacalcium phosphate. Small sample size (only a few microliters are required), minimal sample preparation, and in some cases greater sensitivity (AFM vs polarized light microscopy) have been reported.[11]

Footnotes

1. Reginato AJ, Maldonado I, Reginato AM, et al, "Supravital Staining of Synovial Fluid With Testsimplets," *Diagn Cytopathol*, 1992, 8(2):147-52.
2. Chakravarty KK and Webley M, "Monarthritis: An Unusual Presentation of Renal Cell Carcinoma," *Ann Rheum Dis*, 1992, 51(5):681-2.
3. Ugai K, Kurosaka M, and Hirohata K, "Lipid Microspherules in Synovial Fluid of Patients With Pigmented Villonodular Synovitis," *Arthritis Rheum*, 1988, 31(11):1442-6.
4. Baer AN and Wright EP, "Lipid Laden Macrophages in Synovial Fluid: A Late Finding in Traumatic Arthritis," *J Rheumatol*, 1987, 14(4):848-51.
5. Reginato AJ, Schumacher HR, Allan DA, et al, "Acute Monoarthritis Associated With Lipid Liquid Crystals," *Ann Rheum Dis*, 1985, 44(8):537-43.
6. Bonafede RP, "Evaluating CPPD Crystal Deposition, An Important Disease of Aging," *Geriatrics*, 1988, 43(11):59-68.
7. Muñoz-Gómez J, Gómez-Pérez R, Solé-Arques M, et al, "Synovial Fluid Examination for the Diagnosis of Synovial Amyloidosis in Patients With Chronic Renal Failure Undergoing Haemodialysis," *Ann Rheum Dis*, 1987, 46(4):324-6.
8. Sieper J, Braun J, Brandt J, et al, "Pathogenetic Role of *Chlamydia*, *Yersinia*, and *Borrelia* in Undifferentiated Oligoarthritis," *J Rheumatol*, 1992, 19(8):1236-42.
9. Remick DG, DeForge LE, Sullivan JF, et al, "Profile of Cytokines in Synovial Fluid Specimens From Patients With Arthritis - Interleukin 8 (IL-8) and IL-6 Correlate With Inflammatory Arthritides," *Immunol Invest*, 1992, 21(4):321-7.
10. Tate GA, Schumacher HR Jr, Reginato AJ, et al, "Synovial Fluid Crystals Derived From Erythrocyte Degradation Products," *J Rheumatol*, 1992, 19(7):1111-4.
11. Blair JM, Sorensen LB, Arnsdorf MF, et al, "The Application of Atomic Force Microscopy for the Detection of Microcrystals in Synovial Fluid From Patients With Recurrent Synovitis," *Semin Arthritis Rheum*, 1995, 24(5):359-69.

References

Beutler A and Schumacher HR Jr, "Gout and Pseudogout: When are Arthritic Symptoms Caused by Crystal Deposition?" *Postgrad Med*, 1994, 95(2):103-6, 109, 113-6.

Johnson KD, "Synovial Fluid," *Body Fluids - Laboratory Examination of Amniotic, Cerebrospinal, Seminal, Serous, and Synovial Fluids*, 3rd ed, Chapter 6, Kjeldsberg CR and Knight JA, eds, Chicago, IL: American Society of Clinical Pathologists, 1993, 265-301.

Kerolous G, Clayburne G, and Schumacher HB Jr, "Is It Mandatory to Examine Synovial Fluids Promptly After Arthrocentesis?" *Arthritis Rheum*, 1989, 32(3):271-8.

Lazarevic MB, Skosey JL, Vitic J, et al, "Cholesterol Crystals in Synovial and Bursal Fluid," *Semin Arthritis Rheum*, 1993, 23(2):99-103.

Luukkainen R, Hakala M, Sajanti E, et al, "Predictive Value of Synovial Fluid Analysis in Estimating the Efficacy of Intra-articular Corticosteroid Injections in Patients With Rheumatoid Arthritis," *Ann Rheum Dis*, 1992, 51(7):874-6.

Pascual E, Tovar J, and Ruiz MT, "The Ordinary Light Microscope: An Appropriate Tool for Provisional Detection and Identification of Crystals in Synovial Fluid," *Ann Rheum Dis*, 1989, 48(12):983-5.

Ridderstad A, Abedi-Valugerdi M, Ström H, et al, "Rheumatoid Arthritis Synovial Fluid Enhances T-Cell Effector Functions," *J Autoimmun*, 1992, 5(3):333-50.

Shmerling RH, "Synovial Fluid Analysis. A Critical Reappraisal," *Rheum Dis Clin North Am*, 1994, 20(2):503-12.

Sorsa T, Konttinen YT, Lindy O, et al, "Collagenase in Synovitis of Rheumatoid Arthritis," *Semin Arthritis Rheum*, 1992, 22(1):44-53.

Swan AJ, Heywood BR, and Dieppe PA, "Extraction of Calcium Containing Crystals From Synovial Fluids and Articular Cartilage," *J Rheumatol*, 1992, 19(11):1764-73.

UA *see* Urinalysis *on this page*

Urinalysis

CPT 81000 (nonautomated, with microscopy); 81001 (automated, with microscopy); 81002 (nonautomated, without microscopy); 81003 (automated, without microscopy)

Related Information

Synonyms UA

Applies to Casts, Urine; Crystals, Urine; Occult Blood, Semiquantitative, Urine; Urine Crystals

Test Commonly Includes Opacity, color, appearance, specific gravity, pH, protein, glucose, occult blood, ketones, bilirubin, and in some laboratories, urobilinogen and microscopic examination of urine sediment. Some laboratories include screening for leukocyte esterase and nitrite and do not perform a microscopic examination unless one of the chemical screening (macroscopic) tests is abnormal or unless a specific request for microscopic examination is made.

Abstract The examination of urine is one of the oldest practices in medicine. A carefully performed urinalysis still provides a wealth of information about the patient, both in terms of differential diagnosis, and by exclusion of many conditions when the urinalysis is "normal." Its role in diagnosis and management of renal diseases is pivotal.

Patient Preparation Instructions should be given in method of collection. Both males and females need instruction in cleansing the urethral meatus. "Midstream collections" are performed by initiating urination into the toilet, then bringing the collection device into the urine stream to catch the midportion of the void.

Specimen Urine

Container Plastic urine container

Collection A voided specimen is usually suitable. If the specimen is likely to be contaminated by vaginal discharge or hemorrhage, a clean catch specimen is desirable. If the specimen is collected by catheter, it should be so labeled. The timing of urine collection will vary with the purpose of the test. To check for casts or renal concentration ability, a first voided morning specimen may be preferred. For screening purposes, this is also the best time, as a later and more dilute specimen may make small increases in protein, RBC, or WBC excretion harder to detect. The upright position increases protein excretion by hemodynamic factors. Mid-morning urine is likely to give the highest albumin excretion, but early morning urine is best when attempting to detect Bence Jones protein.

Storage Instructions Transport specimen to the laboratory as soon as possible after collection. If the specimen cannot be processed immediately by the laboratory it should be refrigerated. Refrigeration preserves formed elements in the urine, but may precipitate crystals not originally present. **Examination is best done on freshly voided, warm urine.**

Causes for Rejection Specimen delayed in transport, fecal contamination, decomposition, or bacterial overgrowth

Reference Range See table. **Crystals** are interpreted by the physician. Warm, freshly voided urine sediment from normal subjects almost never

contains crystals, despite maximal concentration. Xanthine, cystine, and uric acid crystal (and stone) formation is favored by a consistently acid urine (pH <5.5-6). Calcium oxalate and apatite stones are associated with no particular disturbance of urine pH. Calcium carbonate, calcium phosphate, and especially magnesium ammonium phosphate stones are associated with pH >7. Urine pH >7.5 may briefly follow meals (alkaline tide) but more commonly indicate systemic alkali intake ($NaHCO_3$, etc) or urine infected by bacteria which split urea to ammonia.

Urinalysis

Test	Reference Range
Specific gravity	1.003-1.029
pH	4.5-7.8
Protein	Negative
Glucose	Negative
Ketones	Negative
Bilirubin	Negative
Occult blood	Negative
Leukocyte esterase	Negative
Nitrite	Negative
Urobilinogen	0.1-1.0 EU/dL
WBCs	0-4/hpf
RBCs	male: 0-3/hpf female: 0-5/hpf
Casts	0-4/lpf hyaline
Bacteria	Negative

hpf = high power field

lpf = low power field

EU = Ehrlich units

Possible Panic Range The presence of massive amounts of oxalate crystals in fresh urine should be reported promptly to the physician, as this finding may represent ethylene glycol intoxication.

Use Screen for abnormalities of urine; diagnose and manage renal diseases, urinary tract infection, urinary tract neoplasms, systemic diseases, and inflammatory or neoplastic diseases adjacent to the urinary tract. Careful microscopy of urine sediment on freshly voided, warm urine is important in evaluation of patients with nephrolithiasis. Urinalysis is pivotal in a wide range of disease states; see Related Information above.

Limitations Insufficient volume, less than 2 mL, may limit the extent of procedures performed. Metabolites of Pyridium® may interfere with the dipstick reactions by producing color interference. High vitamin C intake may cause an underestimate of glucosuria, or a false-negative nitrate test. Survival of WBCs is decreased by low osmolality, alkalinity, and lack of refrigeration. Formed elements in the urine including casts disintegrate rapidly, therefore the specimen should be analyzed as soon as possible after collection. Specific gravity is affected by glucosuria, mannitol infusion, or prior administration of iodinated contrast material for radiologic studies (IVP dye). Some brands of test strips give a "trace positive" protein indication if not stored in dry atmosphere (cap of test strip bottle not on tight). Ambient humidity exposure of the test strips over time also causes some reduction of sensitivity for occult blood and nitrate and increased sensitivity for glucose (false-positive). This can be detected by using tap water as a negative control. False-positive tests for protein can also be due to contamination of the urine by an ammonium-containing cleansing solution. Problems relevant to the sensitivity of protein detection have led to development of methods described in the listing Microalbuminuria *on page 643*.

Methodology The chemical portion of the urinalysis is done by test strip, with confirming chemical method for protein (sulfosalicylic acid precipitation). See individual test entries for further information.

Additional Information

MICROSCOPY:

Crystalluria is frequently observed when urine temperature drops, in urine specimens stored at room temperature or refrigerated, *in vitro* crystal formation. Crystals are most diagnostically useful when observed in warm, fresh urine (*in vivo* crystal formation) in evaluation of microhematuria, nephrolithiasis, or toxin ingestion. Intratubular fluid pH as well as decreased flow are relevant to solute concentration and crystallization. Polarizing microscopy and pH are useful in crystal identification.

Calcium oxalate crystals are classically fairly uniform small double pyramids, base to base, which under the microscope look like little crosses on a square, the octahedral shape of the dihydrate form. Ovoid and dumbbell shapes of oxalate crystals are more easily missed. Polarization helps: oxalate crystals are birefringent, but the red cells and yeasts with which the ovoid forms can be confused are not anisotropic.

Acetic acid (3%) will lyse red cells but not oxalate crystals or yeasts. See listings Oxalate, Urine *on page 174* and Kidney Stone Analysis *on page 640*. In abundance, **calcium oxalate** and/or **hippurate crystals** may suggest ethylene glycol ingestion (especially if known to be accompanied by neurological abnormalities, appearance of drunkenness, hypertension, and a high anion gap acidosis.) Urine is usually supersaturated in calcium oxalate, often in calcium phosphate, and acid urine is often saturated in uric acid. Yet crystalluria is uncommon (in warm, fresh urine) because of the normal presence of crystal inhibitors, the lack of available nidus, and the time factor. When properly observed in fresh urine, crystals may provide a clue to the composition of renal stones even not yet passed, the nidus for such stones, or, as such, have been associated with microhematuria.

Uric acid crystals are reddish brown, rectangular, rhomboidal, or flower-like structures of narrow rectangular petals. **Ammonium urates,** in alkaline urine, are irregular blobs and crescents, sometimes resembling fragmented red cell shapes.

Calcium phosphate crystallizes in urine as flowers of narrow rectangular needles.

Cystine crystals, uniquely in urine, form large irregular hexagonal plates, which may dissolve if alkalinized. They occur only in urine of subjects with cystinuria. (See the listing Cystine, Urine *on page 120*).

Calcium magnesium ammonium phosphate, or "triple phosphate," forms unique "coffin lid" angularly domed rectangles which may be present in massive quantities in alkaline urine. They usually are associated with urine infected by urea splitting bacteria which cause "infection," or "triple phosphate" stones.

Leukocyturia may indicate inflammatory disease in the genitourinary tract, including bacterial infection, glomerulonephritis, chemical injury, autoimmune diseases, or inflammatory disease adjacent to the urinary tract such as appendicitis[1] or diverticulitis.

White cell casts indicate the renal origin of leukocytes, and are most frequently found in acute pyelonephritis. White cell casts are also found in glomerulonephritis such as lupus nephritis, and in acute and chronic interstitial nephritis. When nuclei degenerate, such leukocyte casts resemble renal tubular casts.

Red cell casts indicate renal origin of hematuria and suggest glomerulonephritis, including lupus nephritis. Red cell casts may also be found in subacute bacterial endocarditis, renal infarct, vasculitis, Goodpasture's syndrome, sickle cell disease, and in malignant hypertension. Degenerated red cell casts may be called **"hemoglobin casts"**. Orange to red casts may be found with myoglobinuria as well.

Dysmorphic red cells are observed in glomerulonephritis. "Dysmorphic" red cells refer to heterogeneous sizes, hypochromia, distorted irregular outlines and frequently small blobs extruding from the cell membrane. Phase contrast microscopy best demonstrates RBC and WBC morphology. Nonglomerular urinary red blood cells resemble peripheral circulating red blood cells.[2] Schramek et al have used the presence or absence of dysmorphic red cells to direct the degree of work-up for hematuria and for follow-up.[3] See as well the listing Urinalysis, Fractional *on page 659*.

Crenated RBCs provide no implication regarding RBC source.

Dark brown or smoky urine suggests a renal source of hematuria.

A **pink or red urine** suggests an extrarenal source.

Hyaline casts occur in physiologic states (eg, after exercise) and many types of renal diseases. They are best seen in phase contrast microscopy or with reduced illumination.

Renal tubular (epithelial) casts are most suggestive of tubular injury, as in acute tubular necrosis. They are also found in other disorders, including eclampsia, heavy metal poisoning, ethylene glycol intoxication, and acute allograft rejection.

Granular casts: Very finely granulated casts may be found after exercise and in a variety of glomerular and tubulointerstitial diseases.; coarse granular casts are abnormal and are present in a wide variety of renal diseases.

"Dirty brown" granular casts are typical of acute tubular necrosis.

Waxy casts are found especially in chronic renal diseases, and are associated with chronic renal failure; they occur in diabetic nephropathy, malignant hypertension, and glomerulonephritis, among other conditions. They are named for their waxy or glossy appearance. They often appear brittle and cracked.

Fatty casts and **oval fat bodies ("lipiduria")** are generally found in the nephrotic syndromes, usually glomerular diseases including minimal change disease, focal segmental glomerulosclerosis, membranous glomerulopathy, and membranoproliferative glomerulonephritis. Nephrotic range proteinuria is also found in multisystem diseases including amyloidosis, SLE, cryoglobulinemia, and diabetic nephropathy.[4] Fat droplets originate in renal tubular cells when they exceed their capacity

to reabsorb protein of glomerular origin. See listings Fat, Urine *on page 635* and Protein, Quantitative, Urine *on page 649*.

Broad casts originate from dilated, chronically damaged tubules or the collecting ducts. They can be granular or waxy. **Broad waxy casts** are called "renal failure casts."

Spermatozoa may be seen in male urine related to recent or retrograde ejaculation. In female urine, the presence of spermatozoa may provide evidence of vaginal contamination following recent intercourse.

Automation of the urinalysis is routine in many laboratories.[5,6] Some authors wish to abandon microscopic evaluation of the urine, which is not easily automated, on urine samples testing "normal" by dipstick screening. A urine sample that is normal to inspection and dipstick will be normal to microscopic exam 95% of the time.[7] However, 5% remain. Two recently published volumes may prove helpful.[8,9]

One instrument for automating the entire urinalysis, the Yellow IRIS®, includes a module that automates the microscopic sediment exam. This has been found to be more consistent than the manual method for routine urinalysis and has increased the number of abnormal urines detected.[5,6,10,11]

Tests for **inherited diseases of metabolism** involve blood as well as urine. These subjects are summarized in the listing Inherited Diseases of Metabolism and Cell Structure Tests *on page 327*.

Footnotes

1. Scott JH, "Abnormal Urinalysis in Appendicitis," *J Urol*, 1983, 129:1015.
2. Rizzoni G, Braggion F, and Zacchello G, "Evaluation of Glomerular and Nonglomerular Hematuria by Phase Contrast Microscopy," *J Pediatr*, 1983, 103:370-4.
3. Schramek P, Schuster FX, Georgopoulos M, et al, "Value of Urinary Erythrocyte Morphology in Assessment of Symptomless Microhaematuria," *Lancet*, 1989, 2(8675):1316-9.
4. Larson TS, "Evaluation of Proteinuria," *Mayo Clin Proc*, 1994, 69(12):1154-8.
5. Roe CE, Carlson DA, Daigneault RW, et al, "Evaluation of the Yellow IRIS®. An Automated Method for Urinalysis," *Am J Clin Pathol*, 1986, 86(5):661-5.
6. Wargotz ES, Hyde JE, Karcher DS, et al, "Urine Sediment Analysis by the Yellow IRIS® Automated Urinalysis Workstation," *Am J Clin Pathol*, 1987, 88(6):746-8.
7. Wenz B and Lampasso JA, "Eliminating Unnecessary Urine Microscopy - Results and Performance Characteristics of an Algorithm Based on Chemical Reagent Strip Testing," *Am J Clin Pathol*, 1989, 92(1):78-81.
8. Brunzel NA, *Fundamentals of Urine and Body Fluid Analysis*, Philadelphia, PA: WB Saunders Co, 1994.
9. Ringsrud KM and Linné JJ, *Urinalysis and Body Fluids: A ColorText and Atlas*, St Louis, MO: CV Mosby Co, 1995.
10. Carlson D and Statland BE, "Automated Urinalysis," *Clin Lab Med*, 1988, 8(3):449-61.
11. Bartlett RC, Zern DA, Ratkiewicz I, et al, "Reagent Strip Screening for Sediment Abnormalities Identified by Automated Microscopy in Urine From Patients Suspected to Have Urinary Tract Disease," *Arch Pathol Lab Med*, 1994, 118(11):1096-101.

References

Brock DA and Hundley JM, "Identifying Calcium Oxalate Crystals in Urine," *Lab Med*, 1995, 26(11):733-5.

Cohen HT and Spiegel DM, "Air-Exposed Urine Dipsticks Give False-Positive Results for Glucose and False-Negative Results for Blood," *Am J Clin Pathol*, 1991, 96(3):398-400.

Geyer SJ, "Urinalysis and Urinary Sediment in Patients With Renal Disease," *Clin Lab Med*, 1993, 13(1):13-20.

Haber MH, "Quality Assurance in Urinalysis," *Clin Lab Med*, 1988, 8(3):431-47.

Kiel DP and Moskowitz MA, "The Urinalysis: A Critical Appraisal," *Med Clin North Am*, 1987, 71(4):607-24.

Mariani AJ, Luangphinith S, Loo S, et al, "Dipstick Chemical Urinalysis: An Accurate Cost-Effective Screening Test," *J Urol*, 1984, 132(1):64-6.

Schumann GB, "Cytodiagnostic Urinalysis for the Nephrology Practice," *Semin Nephrol*, 1986, 6(4):308-45.

Schumann GB, *Urine Sediment Examination*, Baltimore, MD: Williams and Wilkins, 1980.

Segasothy M, Lau TM, Birch DF, et al, "Immunocytologic Dissection of the Urine Sediment Using Monoclonal Antibodies," *Am J Clin Pathol*, 1988, 90(6):691-6.

Sheets C and Lyman JL, "Urinalysis," *Emerg Med Clin North Am*, 1986, 4(2):263-80.

Shenoy UA, "Current Assessment of Microhematuria and Leukocyturia," *Clin Lab Med*, 1985, 5(2):317-29.

Wilson DM, "Tests to Detect Asymptomatic Urinary Tract Infections," *JAMA*, 1994, 271(18):1399.

Yager HM and Harrington JT, "Urinalysis and Urinary Electrolytes," *The Principles and Practice of Nephrology*, Chapter 28, Jacobson HR, Striker GE, and Klahr S, eds, Philadelphia, PA: BC Decker Inc, 1991, 167-77.

Urinalysis, Fractional

CPT 81000 (nonautomated, with microscopy); 81001 (automated, with microscopy); 81002 (nonautomated, without microscopy); 81003 (automated, without microscopy)

Related Information

Blood, Urine *on page 631*
Hemoglobin, Qualitative, Urine *on page 637*
Urinalysis *on previous page*

Synonyms Three Glass Test, Urine; Two Glass Test, Urine

Test Commonly Includes Microscopic examination of each fraction

Abstract Sequential urinalysis is performed on the initial urine voided, the midstream urine, and the final passage of urine to gain information regarding the anatomic source of cellular elements in the urine.

Collection Patient voids and the specimen is collected in two or three containers without interrupting the flow of urine. If three containers are (Continued)

Urinalysis, Fractional *(Continued)*

ordered, small amounts of urine are collected in the first and third while the second has the largest volume. Sometimes this method is modified by stopping the flow of urine after the second glass and the third glass is collected after prostatic massage. The exact collection procedure followed should be recorded on the requisition so that the results can be interpreted properly.

Reference Range RBCs: 2-3 cells/high power field; WBCs: 0-5 cells/high power field

Use Define the location of the source of red blood cells and white blood cells present in the urine of male patients. The primary use is in the differential diagnosis of urethritis vs cystitis and pyelonephritis. The test may also contribute to the differentiation of renal vs nonrenal hematuria.

Additional Information Initial hematuria, red blood cells in the first specimen, implies hematuria of urethral origin. Total hematuria, red cells in all three samples, implicates the upper urinary tract. Terminal hematuria, red cells in the last specimen, implies hematuria of prostatic or bladder neck origin. Phase contrast microscopy of urinary red blood cells is used to differentiate hematuria of glomerular vs nonglomerular origin.[1] Glomerular hematuria is characterized by "dysmorphic" urinary RBCs while red cells of nonglomerular origin are "eumorphic." Dysmorphic cells have irregular outlines, granular inhomogeneous cytoplasm (with phase microscopy), uneven cytoplasmic staining and hypochromia (with Wright's stain), and often have small blob-like membrane extrusions (phase microscopy). Eumorphic cells have uniform size and are similar to normal circulating red cells. Nonglomerular hematuria may also be characterized by the presence of red cell "ghosts" (empty membranous sacks which have lost their hemoglobin).[2] Glomerular hematuria is likely when 10% of all urinary RBCs are dysmorphic.[1] If additional evidence of glomerulonephritis is present (edema, proteinuria, renal cellular casts), the glomerular nature of hematuria is essentially established. If all urine red cells are eumorphic, clinical evaluation for extraglomerular sources of hematuria is indicated. Glomerular hematuria does not exclude, in addition, bladder or prostate pathology or malignancy.

Footnotes

1. Stapleton FB, "Morphology of Urinary Red Blood Cells: A Simple Guide in Localizing the Site of Hematuria," *Pediatr Clin North Am*, 1987, 34(3):561-9.
2. Fairley KF and Birch DF, "Hematuria: A Simple Method for Identifying Glomerular Bleeding," *Kidney Int*, 1982, 21:105-8.

References

Schramek P, Schuster FX, Georgopoulos M, et al, "Value of Urinary Erythrocyte Morphology in Assessment of Symptomless Microhaematuria," *Lancet*, 1989, 2(8675):1316-9.

Urinary Eosinophils *see* Eosinophils, Urine *on page 634*

Urinary Sugar Test *see* Glucose, Quantitative, Urine *on page 635*

Urinary Sugar Test *see* Glucose, Semiquantitative, Urine *on page 636*

Urinary Tract Infection Screen *see* Nitrite, Urine *on page 645*

Urine Concentration Test *see* Concentration Test, Urine *on page 633*

Urine Crystals *see* Urinalysis *on page 658*

Urine Ketones *see* Ketones, Urine *on page 639*

Urine Screen for Albumin *see* Protein, Semiquantitative, Urine *on page 650*

Urine Screen for Protein *see* Protein, Semiquantitative, Urine *on page 650*

Urine Sediment, Quantitative *see* Addis Count, 12-Hour *on page 630*

Urines for Glucose Tolerance *see* Glucose, Semiquantitative, Urine *on page 636*

Urobilinogen, 2-Hour Urine

CPT 84580 (quantitative, timed); 84583 (semiquantitative)

Related Information

Bile, Urine *on page 631*
Bilirubin, Direct *on page 86*
Bilirubin, Total *on page 86*

Porphobilinogen, Qualitative, Urine *on page 185*

Synonyms Urobilinogen, Quantitative, Urine

Replaces Urobilinogen, 24-Hour Urine

Abstract This urine screening test detects some but not all instances of hemolytic anemia and liver diseases such as hepatitis and cirrhosis. It is not widely used.

Patient Preparation Alkalinization of the urine by sodium bicarbonate administration increases excretion of urobilinogen. A marked diurnal peak in excretion occurs; therefore an afternoon collection ideally should be scheduled.

Specimen 2-hour urine

Container Dark urine container or foil wrapped container

Collection Have patient void at 2 PM and discard urine. Give patient 500 mL of water to be ingested at once. Collect all urine from 2 PM - 4 PM. Transport promptly to the laboratory. Urobilinogen is sensitive to room temperature and light.

Storage Instructions Refrigerate specimen, protect from light.

Causes for Rejection Specimen exposed to light or not refrigerated

Reference Range Male: 0.3-2.1 mg/2 hours (SI: 0.5-3.6 μmol/2 hours); female: 0.1-1.1 mg/2 hours (SI: 0.2-1.9 μmol/2 hours). Results are sometimes expressed in Ehrlich units, 1 mg urobilinogen = 1 EU.

Use Screen for biliary and liver disease, obstructive jaundice; increased in hemolytic anemia, hepatitis, liver damage with or without jaundice (eg, cirrhosis, congestive heart failure). If a method were in use which could confirm absent urine urobilinogen, then the diagnosis of complete common bile duct obstruction could be supported. See table in the listing Bile, Urine *on page 631.*

Limitations Antibiotics supressing intestinal flora may cause very low levels. Levels may be normal with incomplete obstructive jaundice. Patients with acute porphyria may have an increased value because porphobilinogen also gives a positive result with Ehrlich's aldehyde reagent, as does para-aminosalicylic acid. The absence of or low urobilinogen cannot be determined by dipsticks, a serious drawback, since detection of decreased urine urobilinogen would enhance diagnosis of common duct obstruction. Drugs containing azo dyes may mask the reaction. Like urine bile detection, screen for increased urobilinogen in urine has fairly good specificity. However, the two tests lack great sensitivity when compared with a variety of serum tests related to liver disease.[1]

Methodology Urobilistix®, Watson's method, Ehrlich's aldehyde reagent; para-diethylaminobenzaldehyde reacts with urobilinogen with a color enhancer

Additional Information Urobilinogen is formed in the intestine by the action of bacteria on excreted conjugated (direct) bilirubin. A portion of the urobilinogen is absorbed from the gastrointestinal tract into the bloodstream. It returns to the liver where some is re-excreted in bile (enterohepatic circulation), and the rest (via the general circulation) is excreted into the urine. Urine urobilinogen can be increased as an early indicator of moderate hepatic parenchymal damage. Early toxic injury or hepatitis may also cause increased urine urobilinogen. However, if no bilirubin enters the bile no urobilinogen will be produced; thus, with complete common bile duct obstruction, both urine and fecal urobilinogen will be decreased. Collection time is important because of diurnal variation in urobilinogen excretion. Alkaline pH of urine increases clearance of urobilinogen and increases reliability of results.

Footnotes

1. Binder L, Smith D, Kupka T, et al, "Failure of Prediction of Liver Function Test Abnormalities With the Urine Urobilinogen and Urine Bilirubin Assays," *Arch Pathol Lab Med*, 1989, 113(1):73-6.

Urobilinogen, 24-Hour Urine *replaced by* Urobilinogen, 2-Hour Urine *on this page*

Urobilinogen, Quantitative, Urine *see* Urobilinogen, 2-Hour Urine *on this page*

UTI Screen *see* Nitrite, Urine *on page 645*

Vasopressin Concentration Test *see* Concentration Test, Urine *on page 633*

Wright's Stain, Stool *see* Methylene Blue Stain, Stool *on page 642*

VIROLOGY

Rebecca T. Horvat, PhD

Larry D. Gray, PhD

Contributor: David S. Jacobs, MD

In the last 20 years, demand for laboratory diagnosis of viral infections has increased. Such demands are fueled by increased knowledge of basic biology of viruses, development of monoclonal antibodies and specific antiviral drugs, and the availability of cell culture. In general, viral diagnosis is based on the following principles:

- direct detection of viral antigens in clinical specimens
- isolation of virus from cell culture
- detection of specific antiviral antibodies in serum
- detection of specific viral nucleic acid

A number of biologically different unrelated viruses can be the cause of similar disease syndromes, such as respiratory diseases, diarrhea, or encephalitis. On the other hand, a single type of virus such as herpes zoster can cause a variety of different diseases, including chicken pox, shingles, pneumonitis, and encephalitis. In immunocompromised patients, the extent of disease caused by viral infections can be broader and more diverse than in healthy individuals. Thus, often it is difficult for the clinician to effectively treat patients without information on the infecting virus.

Specimens submitted for viral isolation should be refrigerated, never frozen, and should bear the patient's name, identification number, body site of collection, and date and time of collection with provision of suspected viral infection or symptoms. Material for viral culture should always be submitted in viral-holding media, which prevents the overgrowth of bacteria and fungi and stabilizes viral structure. Specimen collection for virology depends on the specific disease syndrome and the virus suspected. Healthcare providers should contact their laboratory for instructions relevant to collection and transport of virology specimens.

For reference, the Virology Appendix contains:

- a list of antiviral agents and their target viruses
- molecular structures of antiviral agents (Figure 1)
- brief current classification schemes for major viruses (Figures 2 and 3)
- representations of the structures of major viruses (Figure 4)

Other tests relevant to viral diseases can be found in the Immunology and Serology, and Molecular Pathology chapters.

Adenovirus Culture

CPT 87252 (tissue culture, inoculation and observation); 87253 (tissue culture, additional studies, each isolate)

Related Information

Adenovirus Antibody Titer *on page 362*
Bacterial Culture, Conjunctiva *on page 461*
Viral Culture *on page 675*
Viral Culture, Eye or Ocular Symptoms *on page 679*
Viral Culture, Respiratory Symptoms *on page 680*
Viral Culture, Urine *on page 681*
Virus, Direct Detection by Fluorescent Antibody *on page 682*

Synonyms Adenovirus, Rapid Culture; Shell Vial Culture, Adenovirus

Test Commonly Includes Culture for adenovirus only; adenovirus is usually detected in a routine/general virus culture. Rapid culture can be done by staining inoculated shell vials with a specific monoclonal antibody.

Abstract The name "adenovirus" is based on viral isolation from adenoids. The virus is best known for its propensity to infect the upper airway. It is known to persist in lymphoid tissues. Forty-seven or more serotypes exist.

Specimen Midstream urine, stool or rectal swabs, nasopharyngeal secretions, eye exudates, throat swab or tissue, cerebrospinal fluid

Container Sterile container. Swabs should be placed into cold viral transport medium.

Storage Instructions Keep specimens cold and moist. Adenoviruses are more stabile than are most other viruses; however, specimens should not be stored or refrigerated for long periods of time. Specimens should be delivered immediately to the clinical laboratory.

Causes for Rejection Specimen not in proper viral transport medium, specimen not refrigerated during transport

Turnaround Time Variable (1-14 days) and depends on culture method used and amount of virus in the specimen

Reference Range No virus isolated

Use Aid in the diagnosis of disease caused by adenovirus (eg, conjunctivitis, cystitis, gastroenteritis, pneumonia, and pharyngoconjunctivitis)

Limitations Rule out or identify adenovirus **only**

Methodology Conventional culture: Inoculation of specimen into cell cultures, incubation of cell cultures, observation for characteristic cytopathic effect (CPE), and identification by fluorescent monoclonal antibody.

Rapid culture: Specimens are centrifuged onto cell cultures grown on coverslips in the bottoms of 1-dram shell vials. Centrifugation greatly accelerates virus attachment and penetration. After incubation for 2 and/ or 5 days, fluorescein-labeled monoclonal antibodies are applied to the infected cells to detect viral antigens that are expressed in the membranes of the cells. Characteristic fluorescent foci indicate the presence of virus.

Additional Information Adenoviruses are spread directly by oral transmission or infectious aerosols. Infections with adenoviruses occur throughout the year, especially in people who are grouped together such as those in schools, day care centers, nursing home facilities, and hospitals.[1] Adenoviruses can cause severe respiratory infections in children and immunocompromised adults, which sometimes can be fatal.[2] They cause ocular infections in both children and adults. Adenovirus respiratory infections can mimic pertussis.

Adenoviruses type 40 and 41 can cause gastroenteritis in young children and infants but can infect older children and adults. The most common lesion found in intussusception in children is focal lymphoid hyperplasia, found in about half of the cases of intussusception recently reviewed. Intussusception is the most common cause of intestinal obstruction in infants and small children, most commonly found in babies 3-9 months of age. Two types of intranuclear inclusions can be found in hematoxylin and eosin sections, in epithelium overlying adenovirus-infected lymphoid tissue in gastrointestinal tract or elsewhere: Cowdry type B inclusions, poorly demarcated purplish smudges without halos, or Cowdry type A, sharply demarcated red globules surrounded by halos, with peripheral marginated nuclear chromatin. Immunohistochemical reactivity can confirm such infection.[3]

Types 40 and 41 are usually not associated with respiratory illness. Diarrhea can persist for up to 14 days, and during this period virus can be shed.[4] However, culture of type 40 and 41 is more difficult than culture of other adenoviruses and may not be isolated. Stool specimens can be examined for adenovirus type 40 and 41 using an enzyme immunoassay or electron microscopy.[5,6]

Serology to detect adenovirus antibodies is available and is often helpful in establishing a diagnosis. DNA amplification is also currently being investigated.[7]

Footnotes

1. Singh-Naz N, Brown M, and Ganeshananthan M, "Nosocomial Adenovirus Infection: Molecular Epidemiology of an Outbreak," *Pediatr Infect Dis J*, 1993, 12(11):922-5.
2. Hierholzer JC, "Adenoviruses in the Immunocompromised Host," *Clin Microbiol Rev*, 1992, 5(3):262-74.
3. Montgomery EA and Popek EJ, "Intussusception, Adenovirus, and Children: A Brief Reaffirmation," *Hum Pathol*, 1994, 25(2):169-74.
4. Kotloff KL, Losonsky GA, Morris JG Jr, et al, "Enteric Adenovirus Infection and Childhood Diarrhea: An Epidemiologic Study in Three Clinical Settings," *Pediatrics*, 1989, 84(2):219-25.
5. Bhisitkul DM, Todd KM, and Listernick R, "Adenovirus Infection and Childhood Intussception," *Am J Dis Child*, 1992, 146(11):1331-3.
6. Van R, Wun CC, O'Ryan ML, et al, "Outbreaks of Human Enteric Adenovirus Types 40 and 41 in Houston Day Care Centers," *J Pediatr*, 1992, 120(4 Pt 1):516-21.
7. Hierholzer JC, Halonen PE, Dahlen PO, et al, "Detection of Adenovirus in Clinical Specimens by Polymerase Chain Reaction and Liquid-Phase Hybridization Quantitated by Time-Resolved Fluorometry," *J Clin Microbiol*, 1993, 31(7):1886-91.

References

Christensen ML, "Human Viral Gastroenteritis," *Clin Microbiol Rev*, 1989, 2(1):51-89.
Hierholzer JC, "Adenoviruses," *Manual of Clinical Microbiology*, 6th ed, Murray PR, Baron EJ, Pfaller MA, et al, eds, Washington, DC: American Society of Microbiology, 1995, 947-55.
Hierholzer JC, "Adenoviruses - A Spectrum of Human Diseases," *Clin Microbiol Newslet*, 1992, 14(15):113-20.
Hughes JH, "Physical and Chemical Methods for Enhancing Rapid Detection of Viruses and Other Agents," *Clin Microbiol Rev*, 1993, 6(2):150-75.
Khoo SH, Bailey AS, de Jong JC, et al, "Adenovirus Infections in Human Immunodeficiency Virus-Positive Patients: Clinical Features and Molecular Epidemilogy," *J Infect Dis*, 1995, 172(3):629-37.
Martin AL and Kudesia G, "Enzyme-Linked Immunosorbent Assay for Detecting Adenoviruses in Stool Specimens: Comparison With Electron Microscopy and Isolation," *J Clin Pathol*, 1990, 43(6):514-5.
Olsen MA, Shuck KM, Sambol AR, et al, "Isolation of Seven Respiratory Viruses in Shell Vials: A Practical and Highly Sensitive Method," *J Clin Microbiol*, 1993, 31(2):422-5.

Adenovirus Culture, Stool *see* Viral Culture, Stool *on page 680*

Adenovirus, Rapid Culture *see* Adenovirus Culture *on this page*

AIDS Virus Culture *see* Human Immunodeficiency Virus Culture *on page 669*

Amniotic Fluid, Viral Culture *see* Viral Culture, Body Fluid *on page 677*

Body Fluid Viral Culture *see* Viral Culture, Body Fluid *on page 677*

Cerebrospinal Fluid, Viral Culture *see* Viral Culture, Body Fluid *on page 677*

Cerebrospinal Fluid Virus Culture *see* Viral Culture, Central Nervous System Symptoms *on page 677*

Cervical *Chlamydia* Culture *see Chlamydia trachomatis* Culture *on this page*

Cervical Culture for T-Strain *Mycoplasma* *see* Genital Culture for *Ureaplasma urealyticum on page 667*

Cervical Culture for *Ureaplasma urealyticum* *see* Genital Culture for *Ureaplasma urealyticum on page 667*

Cervix, Viral Culture *see* Viral Culture, Urogenital *on page 681*

Chickenpox Culture *see* Varicella-Zoster Virus Culture *on page 675*

Chlamydia trachomatis Culture

CPT 87110

Related Information

Bacterial Culture, Conjunctiva *on page 461*
Bacterial Culture, Endometrium *on page 462*
Bacterial Culture, Genital Specimen *on page 463*
Bacterial Culture, Urine, Clean Catch *on page 468*
Cervical/Vaginal Cytology *on page 290*
Chlamydia Group Titer *on page 383*
Chlamydia trachomatis Direct FA Test *on next page*
Chlamydia trachomatis Genome Detection *on page 505*
Lymphogranuloma Venereum Titer *on page 417*
Synovial Fluid Analysis *on page 656*
Viral Culture, Eye or Ocular Symptoms *on page 679*
Viral Culture, Urogenital *on page 681*

Synonyms Lymphogranuloma Venereum Culture; TRIC Agent Culture

Applies to Cervical *Chlamydia* Culture; Eye Swab *Chlamydia* Culture; Urethral *Chlamydia* Culture

Specimen *Chlamydia* is an intracellular pathogen. Obtain swab specimens containing columnar epithelial cells of urethra, cervix, rectum, conjunctiva, posterior nasopharynx, or throat.

Container Culturette® (dacron) swabs should be used and placed in *Chlamydia* transport medium.

Collection Urethra: Remove mucous/pus. The swab should be inserted 2-4 cm into the urethra. Use firm pressure to scrape cells from the mucosal surface. If possible repeat with second swab. Patient should not urinate within 1 hour prior to specimen collection.

Cervix: Remove mucous/pus with a Culturette® and use firm and rotating pressure to obtain specimen with another swab. May be combined with a urethral swab into same transport medium. This two-swab method is highly recommended.

Rectum: Sample anal crypts with a Culturette®.

Conjunctiva: Remove mucous and exudate. Use a Culturette® and firm pressure to scrape away epithelial cells from upper and lower lids.

Posterior nasopharynx or throat: Collect epithelial cells by using a Culturette®.

Storage Instructions Deliver inoculated transport medium **immediately** to the laboratory. **Specimens must be refrigerated** if stored or transported for 2 days. Specimen must be frozen at -70°C if stored more than 2 days.

Turnaround Time Cultures with no growth usually are reported after 7 days. Rapid culture methods require 48 hours or more.

Special Instructions Availability and specific specimen collection requirements for *Chlamydia* cultures vary between laboratories.

Reference Range No *Chlamydia* isolated

Use Aid in the diagnosis of infections caused by *Chlamydia* (eg, cervicitis, trachoma, conjunctivitis, pelvic inflammatory disease, pneumonia, urethritis, nongonococcal urethritis, pneumonitis, and sexually transmitted diseases)

Limitations Culture may be negative in presence of *Chlamydia* infection. Culture is probably not the gold standard for the detection of *C. trachomatis*. The sensitivity of culture probably is only 70% to 90% because *C. trachomatis* does not always survive transit to the laboratory and because of often inadequate sampling with (multiple) swabs.[1]

Methodology Inoculation of specimen onto McCoy cell, HeLa-229, or Buffalo green monkey cell culture and subsequent detection of *Chlamydia*-infected cells by monoclonal antibody and immunofluorescence

Additional Information

Genital infections due to *C. trachomatis* are the most frequent reportable bacterial sexually transmitted disease in the United States. There are more than 4 million infections reported annually.[2] Many of the cases are asymptomatic or minimally symptomatic. Many will eventually progress to produce serious infections including pelvic inflammatory disease, ectopic pregnancy, and infertility in women.[3,4] Infection with *Chlamydia* during pregnancy places the newborn infant at risk of pneumonia and conjunctivitis.[4]

This organism infects the endocervical columnar epithelial cells and will not be found in the inflammatory cells. In obtaining the specimen, clean the area of inflammatory cells and then attempt to scrape epithelial cells for culturing. Papanicolaou-stained cervical smears are not reliable enough to help establish or exclude the presence of *Chlamydia*. Direct immunofluorescence techniques and enzyme immunoassays are available to detect *Chlamydia* in clinical specimens. These methods usually provide reliable results in high-prevalence populations and detect both viable and nonviable organisms. *Chlamydia* can now be detected by using a DNA probe chemiluminescence test and DNA amplification.[5,6,7,8] These tests appear to be more sensitive than immunoassays and culture.[6] Selection of the most efficient method for recovery of *Chlamydia* depends upon the incidence in the patient population and the local availability of the various methods. Urine culture for *Chlamydia* is not a sensitive procedure and should not be done. Urine samples can be tested for *Chlamydia* using PCR or ligase chain reaction (LCR) rather than culture.[7,8]

Culture should be the test-of-choice in cases of child abuse, ascending pelvic infections, rectal and throat infections, and when a test-for-cure is desired.

Chlamydia is a single genus and consists of the following:
- *C. trachomatis* (serotypes A-K): inclusion conjunctivitis, trachoma, and genital infections
- *C. trachomatis* (serotypes L1-L3): lymphogranuloma venereum
- *C. psittaci*: psittacosis
- *C. pneumoniae* (TWAR): respiratory infections

Serology to detect antibodies to all three species of *Chlamydia* is available.

C. pneumoniae is responsible for approximately 10% of community-acquired pneumonias. However, laboratory diagnosis of *C. pneumoniae* infections is not widely available. The cells (McCoy) usually used to culture *C. trachomatis* will not reliably support the growth of *C. pneumoniae*. Recent studies have shown that other cell lines (H 292 and HEp-2)

are more appropriate.[9] An alternate, widely used method for the laboratory diagnosis of *C. pneumoniae* infection is serology by microimmunofluorescence. Currently, this serological test is the most sensitive and specific laboratory test for *C. pneumoniae* .

Footnotes
1. Harper M and Johnson R, "The Predictive Value of Culture for the Diagnosis of Gonorrhea and *Chlamydia* Infections," *Clin Microbiol Newslet*, 1990, 12:54-6.
2. "False-Positive Results With the Use of *Chlamydia* Tests in the Evaluation of Suspected Sexual Abuse - Ohio, 1990," *MMWR Morb Mortal Wkly Rep*, 1991, 39(51-52):932-5.
3. Stamm WE, "Diagnosis of *Chlamydia trachomatis* Genitourinary Infections," *Ann Intern Med*, 1988, 108(5):710-7.
4. Department of Health and Human Services, Sexually Transmitted Disease Branch, NIH, "Pelvic Inflammatory Disease: Research Directions in the 1990s," *Sex Transm Dis*, 1991, 18(1):46-64.
5. Iwen PC, Blair TMH, and Woods GL, "Comparison of the Gen-Probe PACE2® System, Direct Fluorescent Antibody, and Cell Culture for Detecting *Chlamydia trachomatis* in Cervical Specimens," *Am J Clin Pathol*, 1991, 95(4):578-82.
6. Jaschek G, Gaydos CA, Welsh LE, et al, "Direct Detection of *Chlamydia trachomatis* in Urine Specimens From Symptomatic and Asymptomatic Men By Using a Rapid Polymerase Chain Reaction Assay," *J Clin Microbiol*, 1993, 31(5):1209-12.
7. Lee HH, Chernesky MA, Schachter J, et al, "Diagnosis of *Chlamydia trachomatis* Genitourinary Infection in Women by Lipase Chain Reaction Assay of Urine," *Lancet*, 1995, 345(8944):213-6.
8. Cates W Jr, *ACP J Club*, 1995, 123(1):16.
9. Wong KH, Skelton SK, and Chan YK, "Efficient Culture of *Chlamydia pneumoniae* With Cell Lines Derived From the Human Respiratory Tract," *J Clin Microbiol*, 1992, 30(7):1625-30.

References
Fraiz J and Jones RB, "Chlamydial Infections," *Annu Rev Med*, 1988, 39:357-70.
Grayston JT, "Infections Caused by *Chlamydia pneumoniae* Strain TWAR," *Clin Infect Dis*, 1992, 15(5):757-63.
Le Scolea LJ Jr, "The Value of Nonculture Chlamydial Diagnostic Tests," *Clin Microbiol Newslet*, 1991, 13(3):21-4.
Lombardo JM and Gadol CL, "*Chlamydia trachomatis*: A Perfect Test?" *Clin Microbiol Newslet*, 1990, 12(13):100-2.
Roblin PM, Dumornay W, and Hammerschlag MR, "Use of HEp-2 Cells for Improved Isolation and Passage of *Chlamydia pneumoniae*," *J Clin Microbiol*, 1992, 30(8):1968-71.

Chlamydia trachomatis Direct FA Test

CPT 87206

Related Information

Bacterial Culture, Conjunctiva *on page 461*
Bacterial Culture, Genital Specimen *on page 463*
Cervical/Vaginal Cytology *on page 290*
Chlamydia Group Titer *on page 383*
Chlamydia trachomatis Culture *on previous page*
Chlamydia trachomatis Genome Detection *on page 505*
Lymphogranuloma Venereum Titer *on page 417*
Ocular Cytology *on page 298*
Synovial Fluid Analysis *on page 656*
Viral Culture, Eye or Ocular Symptoms *on page 679*

Synonyms MicroTrak®

Patient Preparation For urogenital specimens, patient should not urinate 1 hour prior to collection.

Specimen Direct smear. Although cumbersome, this is the only *Chlamydia* test applicable to all specimen types, including nasopharyngeal specimens from neonates.

Container Single well (8 mm) glass slide, dacron swabs (one large, one small), one cytobrush, methanol fixative (0.5 mL vial). These items are contained in a commonly used direct detection kit (collection pack) known as MicroTrak®.

Collection Endocervical with cytology brush: Nonpregnant women. Use large swab to remove exudate or mucous from exocervix. Insert cytobrush into cervical os past the squamocolumnar junction. Rest 2-3 seconds, rotate brush 360 degrees to gather columnar cells and withdraw brush. Do not touch vaginal walls with brush, and prepare slides immediately by rotating and twisting brush back and forth across center of slide well.

Endocervical with swab: Pregnant women. Use large swab to remove exudate or mucous from exocervix. Insert another large dacron swab until tip is no longer visible, rotate swab 5-10 seconds, and withdraw swab. Do not touch vaginal walls and prepare slides immediately. Firmly roll one side of swab over top half of well. Turn swab over and roll other side over bottom half of slide well.

Urethral: Males. Patient should not urinate 1 hour before sampling. Remove pus or exudate, insert small swab with wire shaft 2-4 cm into penis. Gently rotate swab to dislodge cells, rest swab 2 seconds, withdraw swab, and prepare slide immediately as above.

Rectal: Symptomatic patients only. Use large swab. Insert approximately 3 cm into anal canal. Move swab from side to side to sample crypts. If fecal contamination occurs, discard swab and obtain another specimen. Prepare slide immediately as above.

Conjunctival: Neonates, symptomatic only. Use large swab to gently remove pus or discharge and discard. If both eyes are sampled, swab (Continued)

Chlamydia trachomatis Direct FA Test *(Continued)*

less affected eye first. Swab inside of lower, then upper lid, and prepare slide immediately as above.

Nasopharyngeal: Neonates, symptomatic only. Use small swab or nasal aspirator. Collect specimen from posterior nasopharynx using standard collection method. If swab was used, prepare slide immediately. If nasal aspirate was collected, deliver to the laboratory technician immediately for slide preparation.

All specimens: Allow specimen to air dry. Lay slide flat and flood with methanol fixative. Let entire quantity evaporate. Refold pack without touching fixed specimen.

Storage Instructions Refrigerate slides at 2°C to 8°C or at room temperature (20°C to 30°C) until taken to the laboratory. Slides must be stained within 7 days of collection.

Causes for Rejection Less than 10 columnar or cuboidal epithelial cells on slide

Turnaround Time The time required to stain and examine the specimen is generally less than 1 hour. Turnaround time depends on staffing within the laboratory.

Special Instructions Specify specimen origin. Include all pertinent information, label slide and collection pack.

Reference Range No *Chlamydia trachomatis* detected

Use Aid in the diagnosis of disease caused by *Chlamydia* (eg, pneumonitis, sexually transmitted disease, inclusion conjunctivitis, trachoma, and pneumonia). In some populations, up to 45% of women who have gonorrheal infection have chlamydial infection as well.[1]

Limitations The direct fluorescent antibody procedure is considerably less sensitive than the cell culture procedure. The number of cells on the slide can be too low for diagnosis. It is cumbersome.

The direct detection of *Chlamydia* in specimens depends largely on the preparation of the cell smear. Smears that are too thick or lumpy can cause false-positive results. Contamination with red blood cells makes the smears difficult to interpret. Smears with too few cells can cause false-negative results. Requires a trained microscopist. This test detects only *Chlamydia trachomatis* major outer membrane protein (MOMP). The test does not distinguish between living and dead organisms. Therefore, the test does not necessarily serve as a test-of-cure.

Methodology The *Chlamydia trachomatis* direct test uses fluorescein-conjugated monoclonal antibodies (reactive with all 15 known serotypes of *C. trachomatis*) to detect elementary bodies in clinical smears.

Additional Information *Chlamydia trachomatis*, primarily a human pathogen, has been implicated in neonatal/infantile conjunctivitis and afebrile pneumonia. Thirty-three percent to 50% of babies born vaginally to mothers with chlamydial infection of the cervix will be infected; the majority of these neonates will develop inclusion conjunctivitis and/or a respiratory tract infection that can lead to the distinctive (afebrile) pneumonia syndrome.

Conjunctivitis: Conjunctivitis in infected neonates usually occurs between the 5th and 12th day after birth. In neonates born to mothers with premature rupture of the membranes, *C. trachomatis* has been detected, in rare cases, as early as the first day following birth.

Afebrile pneumonia: Many neonatal chlamydial infections also involve the respiratory tract. Respiratory infections usually occur secondarily to inclusion conjunctivitis. Rhinitis is often a prodrome for severe lower respiratory tract involvement. Signs of chlamydial pneumonia include cough, tachypnea, inspiratory rales, and, in more severe cases, vomiting and periods of apnea.

Footnotes
1. "Gonorrhea and Chlamydial Infections. ACOG Technical Bulletin Number 190-March 1994," *Int J Gynaecol Obstet*, 1994, 45(2):169-74.

References
Barnes RC, "Laboratory Diagnosis of Human Chlamydial Infections," *Clin Microbiol Rev*, 1989, 2(2):119-36.
Chapin K, "*Chlamydia* Testing," letter, *CAP Today*, Oct 1995, 13-4.
Clarke LM, Sierra MF, Daidone BJ, et al, "Comparison of the Syva MicroTrak® Enzyme Immunoassay and Gen-Probe PACE2® With Cell Culture for Diagnosis of Cervical *Chlamydia trachomatis* Infection in a High-Prevalence Female Population," *J Clin Microbiol*, 1993, 31(4):968-71.
Olsen MA, Sambol AR, and Bohnert VA, "Comparison of the Syva Microtrak® Enzyme Immunoassay and Abbott Chlamydiazyme in the Detection of Chlamydial Infections in Women," *Arch Pathol Lab Med*, 1995, 119(2):153-6.
Schwebke JR, Stamm WE, Handsfield HH, et al, "Use of Sequential Enzyme Immunoassay and Direct Fluorescent-Antibody Tests for the Detection of *Chlamydia trachomatis* Infections in Women," *J Clin Microbiol*, 1990, 28(11):2473-6.
Stamm WE, "Diagnosis of *Chlamydia trachomatis* Genitourinary Infections," *Ann Intern Med*, 1988, 108(5):710-7.

CMV Antigen Detection *see* Cytomegalovirus Antigen Detection *on this page*

CMV, Blood Culture *see* Viral Culture, Blood *on page 677*

CMV, Buffy Coat Culture *see* Viral Culture, Blood *on page 677*

CMV Culture *see* Cytomegalovirus Culture *on this page*

CMV Culture *see* Viral Culture, Blood *on page 677*

CMV Culture, Urine *see* Viral Culture, Urine *on page 681*

Coxsackie A Virus Culture *see* Enterovirus Culture *on page 666*

Coxsackie B Virus Culture *see* Enterovirus Culture *on page 666*

Coxsackie Virus Culture, Stool *see* Viral Culture, Stool *on page 680*

CPE *see* Viral Culture *on page 675*

Cytomegalovirus Antigen Detection

CPT 86313

Related Information
Cytomegalic Inclusion Disease Cytology *on page 293*
Cytomegalovirus Antibody *on page 389*
Cytomegalovirus Culture *on this page*
Cytomegalovirus DNA Detection *on page 508*
Virus, Direct Detection by Fluorescent Antibody *on page 682*

Synonyms CMV Antigen Detection

Test Commonly Includes Detection of CMV antigens in white blood cells

Specimen Blood

Container Green top (heparin) tube or lavender top (EDTA) tube

Collection Transport to laboratory at room temperature within 2 hours of collection.

Storage Instructions Do not freeze.

Use Early diagnosis of CMV infection; monitor patients (ie, transplant or immunodeficient) at risk for severe CMV disease

Limitations Labor-intensive; microscopist must be well-trained to detect positive cells; a minimum of 50,000 cells should be present in order to determine a negative result; CMV may be present for a time following acute infections; some patients with CMV antigenemia are asymptomatic; specimen must be processed quickly to detect viral antigen

Methodology Immunocytochemical detection of CMV antigen (lower-matrix phosphoprotein) in nuclei of peripheral blood mononuclear cells

Additional Information The detection of CMV antigen directly in the peripheral blood leukocytes is a new procedure. It has been compared to conventional and rapid culture methods and shown to be sensitive (91%) and specific (99.4%).

CMV has been found in tissue sections in diffuse interstitial pneumonia by immunohistochemistry and by polymerase chain reaction.[1]

CMV can be detected by PCR from other sources as well (eg, CSF, for neurologic syndromes in AIDS patients and others).

Footnotes
1. Oda Y, Katsuda S, Okada Y, et al, "Detection of Human Cytomegalovirus, Epstein-Barr Virus, and Herpes Simplex Virus in Diffuse Interstitial Pneumonia by Polymerase Chain Reaction and Immunohistochemistry," *Am J Clin Pathol*, 1994, 102(4):495-502.

References
Boeckh M, Woogerd PM, Stevens-Ayers T, et al, "Factors Influencing Detection of Quantitative Cytomegalovirus Antigenemia," *J Clin Microbiol*, 1994, 32(3):832-4.
Erice A, Holm MA, Sanjuan MV, et al, "Evaluation of CMV-vue Antigenemia Assay for Rapid Detection of Cytomegalovirus in Mixed-Leukocyte Blood Fractions," *J Clin Microbiol*, 1995, 33(4):1014-5.
Landry ML and Ferguson D, "Comparison of Quantitative Cytomegalovirus Antigenemia Assay With Culture Methods and Correlation With Clinical Disease," *J Clin Microbiol*, 1993, 31(11):2851-6.
Mazzuli T, Rubin RH, Ferraro MJ, et al, "Cytomegalovirus Antigenemia: Clinical Correlations in Transplant Recipients and in Persons With AIDS," *J Clin Microbiol*, 1993, 31(10):2824-7.

Cytomegalovirus Culture

CPT 87252 (tissue culture, inoculation and observation); 87253 (tissue culture, additional studies, each isolate)

Related Information
Bronchial Washings Cytology *on page 287*
Bronchoalveolar Lavage Cytology *on page 288*
Cervical/Vaginal Cytology *on page 290*
Cytomegalic Inclusion Disease Cytology *on page 293*
Cytomegalovirus Antibody *on page 389*
Cytomegalovirus Antigen Detection *on this page*
Cytomegalovirus DNA Detection *on page 508*
Sputum Cytology *on page 300*
Urine Cytology *on page 301*
Viral Culture *on page 675*
Viral Culture, Blood *on page 677*
Viral Culture, Urine *on page 681*
Virus, Direct Detection by Fluorescent Antibody *on page 682*

Synonyms CMV Culture; Viral Culture, Cytomegalovirus

Test Commonly Includes Culture for CMV only using specific immuno-fluorescence; CMV is usually detected in a routine virus culture

Abstract Cytomegalovirus is a DNA herpes virus which infects up to 90% of the adult population, usually asymptomatically. It is a major problem in immunocompromised patients after renal and other organ transplantation, in allogeneic bone marrow transplantation patients, and in patients with AIDS. Transmission of CMV to neonates may be fatal.

Specimen Urine, throat, bronchoalveolar lavage, bronchial washings, lung biopsy, whole blood, stool

Container Cold viral transport medium for swabs

Collection Urine: A first morning clean catch urine should be submitted in a sterile screw-cap container.

Throat: Rotate swab in both tonsillar crypts and against posterior oropharynx. Place swab in tube of viral transport medium, break off end of swab and tighten cap.

Blood: Collect in a green top Vacutainer® tube containing free heparin.

Storage Instructions Do **not** freeze. Keep specimens cold and moist. Specimens should be delivered to the laboratory and handed to a technologist within 30 minutes of collection. If freezing is absolutely necessary, most specimens can be frozen by adding an equal amount of 0.4M sucrose-phosphate to the specimen before freezing. White blood cells should be isolated from blood specimens before freezing.

Causes for Rejection Dry specimen, specimen not refrigerated during transport, specimen fixed in formalin

Turnaround Time Variable (1-14 days); negative routine viral cultures are usually not reported for 28 days; CMV rapid culture: 1-3 days

Reference Range No virus isolated

Use Aid in the diagnosis of disease caused by CMV (eg, viral pneumonia and gastrointestinal tract involvement in organ transplant-related disease).[1] Clinical manifestations of CMV disease include fever, malaise, arthralgias, hematologic abnormalities, hepatitis, chorioretinitis, skin lesions, Guillain-Barré syndrome, and allograft dysfunction.[1]

Limitations Not available in most routine clinical laboratories; rapid method will only detect specified virus(es); negative culture does not rule out viral infection. CSF cultures are negative in encephalitis and in subjects with AIDS, and are insensitive with CMV myelitis/polyradiculopathy and with ventriculitis in AIDS. CMV culture may be positive in the absence of obvious clinical disease.

Methodology Routine culture detects CMV by cytopathic effect; rapid shell vial specifically detects CMV early viral antigen with immunofluorescence

Additional Information CMV infections are very common in normal individuals and are usually asymptomatic. However, CMV infections are frequently severe and life-threatening in immunocompromised patients, including organ recipients and AIDS patients. CMV is the major viral pathogen following renal transplantation. Blood cultures positive for CMV predict progression.[1] Knowledge of CMV infection is of utmost importance so that ganciclovir can be started as soon as possible.

CMV is the most frequent cause of congenital viral infections in humans and occurs in about 1% of all newborns. Approximately 90% have no clinical symptoms at birth. Ten percent to 20% of these infants will develop complications before school age. Congenital infection may occur as a result of either primary or recurrent maternal infection.

Serology for the detection of cytomegalovirus is available, but the results usually are of limited value. Cytomegalovirus inclusions are recognizable microscopically, and are characterized as owl's eye intranuclear inclusions (Cowdry A inclusions). Cytoplasmic inclusions are found as well.[2] In some settings (eg, gastrointestinal tract), diagnosis can be made from biopsy.[3]

The rapid shell vial method for the detection of CMV has been reported to be more sensitive than and as specific as conventional tube cell culture.[4] The sensitivity of viral culture depends greatly on the type and age of host cells which may vary between laboratories. Several modifications of the shell vial method have been reported to enhance sensitivity.[5] Quantitative results of shell vial procedures sometimes are used to determine the level of viremia in organ and bone marrow transplant recipients.[6,7]

Footnotes

1. Farrugia E and Schwab TR, "Subspecialty Clinics: Nephrology - Management and Prevention of Cytomegalovirus Infection After Renal Transplantation," *Mayo Clin Proc*, 1992, 67(9):879-90.
2. Schwartz DA and Wilcox CM, "Atypical Cytomegalovirus Inclusions in Gastrointestinal Biopsy Specimens From Patients With the Acquired Immunodeficiency Syndrome: Diagnostic Role of *In Situ* Nucleic Acid Hybridization," *Hum Pathol*, 1992, 23(9):1019-26.
3. Goodgame RW, "Gastrointestinal Cytomegalovirus Disease," *Ann Intern Med*, 1993, 119(9):924-35.
4. Gleaves CA, Smith TF, Shuster EA, et al, "Comparison of Standard Tube and Shell Vial Cell Culture Techniques for the Detection of Cytomegalovirus in Clinical Specimens," *J Clin Microbiol*, 1985, 21(2):217-21.
5. Li SB and Fong CK, "Detection of Human Cytomegalovirus Early and Late Antigen and DNA Production in Cell Culture and the Effects of Dimethyl Sulfoxide, Dexamethasone, and DNA Inhibitors on Early Antigen Induction," *J Med Virol*, 1990, 30(2):97-102.
6. Slavin MA, Gleaves CA, Schoch HG, et al, "Quantification of Cytomegalovirus in Bronchoalveolar Lavage Fluid After Allogeneic Marrow Transplantation by Centrifugation Culture," *J Clin Microbiol*, 1992, 30(11):2776-9.
7. Buller RS, Bailey TC, Ettinger NA, et al, "Use of a Modified Shell Vial Technique to Quantitate Cytomegalovirus Viremia in a Population of Solid-Organ Transplant Recipients," *J Clin Microbiol*, 1992, 30(10):2620-4.

References

Ayala E, Martinez EM, Enghardt MH, et al, "An Improved Cytomegalovirus Immunostaining Method," *Lab Med*, 1993, 24:39.

Drew WL, "Nonpulmonary Manifestations of Cytomegalovirus Infection in Immunocompromised Patients," *Clin Microbiol Rev*, 1992, 5(2):104-10.

Mazzulli T, "Improved Diagnosis of Cytomegalovirus Infection by Detection of Antigenemia or Use of PCR Methods," *Clin Microbiol Newslet*, 1993, 15:97-100.

Snydman DR, Rubin RH, and Werner BG, "New Developments in Cytomegalovirus Prevention and Management," *Am J Kidney Dis*, 1993, 21(2):217-28.

Warren WP, Balcarek K, Smith R, et al, "Comparison of Rapid Methods of Detection of Cytomegalovirus in Saliva With Virus Isolation in Tissue Culture," *J Clin Microbiol*, 1992, 30:786-9.

Cytopathic Effect *see* Viral Culture *on page 675*

3-Day Measles Culture *see* Rubella Virus Culture *on page 674*

Direct Detection of Virus *see* Virus, Direct Detection by Fluorescent Antibody *on page 682*

Direct Fluorescent Antibody Test for Virus *see* Virus, Direct Detection by Fluorescent Antibody *on page 682*

EBV Culture *see* Epstein-Barr Virus Culture *on next page*

Echovirus Culture *see* Enterovirus Culture *on next page*

Echovirus Culture, Stool *see* Viral Culture, Stool *on page 680*

Electron Microscopic Examination for Viruses, Stool

CPT 88348

Related Information

Bacterial Culture, Stool *on page 466*
Electron Microscopy *on page 37*
Histopathology *on page 42*
Rotavirus, Direct Detection *on page 674*
Rotavirus Serology *on page 428*
Skin Biopsy *on page 54*
Viral Culture, Stool *on page 680*

Synonyms Enteric Viruses by EM; Gastrointestinal Viruses by EM

Applies to Rotavirus Detection by EM; Skin Viral Disease; Viral Disease in Tissue

Specimen Stool from the acute, diarrheal phase of disease; skin lesions; tissues (biopsy/autopsy)

Turnaround Time Less than 1 day

Reference Range Viruses not observed

Use Demonstrate viral particles (eg, rotavirus, Norwalk virus, calcivirus, astrovirus, and coronavirus) in stool specimens from patients with suspected viral gastroenteritis; examination of tissue from biopsy or autopsy in which immunofluorescent and immunoperoxidase staining is negative.

Limitations Generally, EM visualization of virus particles is not as sensitive as is cell culture, except for detecting nonculturable viruses such as rotavirus. EM can detect viruses if they are present in quantities of 10^6 to 10^7 particles/mL. This sensitivity is appropriate for agents causing diarrhea but is not sufficiently sensitive for the detection of other potential pathogens.[1] It is often difficult to differentiate (by EM) the aforementioned viruses. Very few clinical microbiology/virology laboratories have access to electron microscopes.

Methodology Diluted stool (either with or without being mixed with patient serum) is mixed with an electron-opaque heavy metal solution such as phosphotungstic acid. The stool solution is placed onto an electron-lucent grid support and examined by electron microscopy. Virions or virions agglutinated by specific antibodies (if present in serum) appear as a negative image against a black surrounding background.[1]

Additional Information The electron microscopic observation of viruses is the basis for identification. Electron microscopy is a useful procedure in cases where identification of viruses suspected of causing disease have not been identified by other methods.

Footnotes

1. Drew WL, "Diagnostic Virology," *Clin Lab Med*, 1987, 7(4):721-40.

References

Gray LD, "Novel Viruses Associated With Gastroenteritis," *Clin Microbiol Newslet*, 1991, 13(18):137-44.

Herrmann JE, Taylor DN, Echeverria P, et al, "Astroviruses as a Cause of Gastroenteritis in Children," *N Engl J Med*, 1991, 324(25):1757-60.

Hedberg CW and Osterholm M, "Outbreaks of Food-borne and Waterborne Viral Gastroenteritis," *Clin Microbiol Rev*, 1993, 6:199-210.

(Continued)

Electron Microscopic Examination for Viruses, Stool (Continued)

Lew JF, Moe CL, Monroe SS, et al, "Astrovirus and Adenovirus Associated With Diarrhea in Children in Day Care Settings," *J Infect Dis*, 1991, 164(4):673-8.

Miller SE, "Diagnosis of Viral Infections by Electron Microscopy," *Diagnostic Procedures for Viral, Rickettsial, and Chlamydial Infections*, 7th ed, Lennette EH, Lennette DA, Lennette ET, eds, Washington, DC: American Public Health Association, 1995, 37-78.

Miller SE, "Diagnostic Virology by Electron Microscopy," *Am Soc Microbiol News*, 1988, 54:475-81.

Endocervix, Viral Culture *see* Viral Culture, Urogenital *on page 681*

Enteric Viruses by EM *see* Electron Microscopic Examination for Viruses, Stool *on previous page*

Enterovirus, Blood Culture *see* Viral Culture, Blood *on page 677*

Enterovirus Culture

CPT 87252 (tissue culture, inoculation and observation); 87253 (tissue culture, additional studies, each isolate)

Related Information
Bacterial Culture, Stool *on page 466*
Coxsackie A Virus Titer *on page 387*
Coxsackie B Virus Titer *on page 387*
Enterovirus Genome Detection *on page 510*
Ova and Parasites, Stool *on page 494*
Poliomyelitis I, II, III Titer *on page 423*
Viral Culture *on page 675*
Viral Culture, Blood *on page 677*
Viral Culture, Central Nervous System Symptoms *on page 677*
Viral Culture, Stool *on page 680*
Viral Culture, Urine *on page 681*

Applies to Coxsackie A Virus Culture; Coxsackie B Virus Culture; Echovirus Culture; Poliovirus Culture

Specimen Stool, rectal swab, cerebrospinal fluid, upper and lower respiratory tract specimens, whole blood, throat swab, various organs and tissues (heart, muscle, brain)

Container Sterile container

Sampling Time It is important to obtain specimens very early in the disease; however, virus is shed in the stool for weeks.

Storage Instructions Enteroviruses are rather hardy; however, specimens should be refrigerated or placed into cold virus transport medium and delivered immediately to the clinical laboratory.

Turnaround Time Depends on culture method used and amount of virus in specimen. Negative cultures often are reported after 2 weeks.

Reference Range No virus isolated

Use Aid in the diagnosis of disease caused by enteroviruses (eg, polio, congenital viral infections, viral pericarditis, and meningitis, aseptic)

Limitations Cell culture generally does not support the growth of certain Coxsackie A enteroviruses. Infrequently, aseptic meningitis is caused by Coxsackie A virus types which require animal inoculation for isolation.

Methodology Inoculation of specimens into cell culture, incubation of cultures, and observation for characteristic cytopathic effect (CPE). Enteroviruses are stable at pH 3; rhinoviruses are unstable at this pH. Specimens suspected of containing Coxsackie A virus are inoculated

Clinical Diseases Caused By Enteroviruses

Cardiovascular	Myocarditis
	Pericarditis
Neurologic	Aseptic meningitis
	Encephalitis
	Poliomyelitis
Respiratory	Common cold
	Stomatitis
	Hand-foot-mouth syndrome
	Pharyngitis
	Tonsillitis
	Rhinitis
Miscellaneous	Febrile, exanthematous illness
	Acute hemorrhagic conjunctivitis (Enterovirus 70, Coxsackie A24)

From Rotbart HA, "Nucleic Acid Detection Systems for Enteroviruses," *Clin Micro Rev*, 1991, 4:156-8, with permission.

into suckling mice which are then observed for flaccid paralysis without encephalitis.

Some (usually reference) laboratories can identify specific enteroviruses by using a battery of specific enterovirus-neutralizing antibodies. These antibodies are useful in identifying and typing Coxsackie A, Coxsackie B, echovirus, and poliovirus.

Additional Information Most enteroviral infections are mild and asymptomatic. Clinical diseases in humans can range from a slightly increased temperature to severe CNS disease and paralysis (see table).[1] Humans are the only known reservoir for enteroviruses. Infection occurs by direct contact, the oral-fecal route or the respiratory route. Enteroviral infections most commonly occur from July to September. Children are more likely to become infected than are adults.

The detection of enteroviral nucleic acid directly from specimens seems promising but is not currently used in clinical laboratories.[1,2]

Footnotes
1. Rotbart HA, "Nucleic Acid Detection Systems for Enteroviruses," *Clin Microbiol Rev*, 1991, 4(2):156-8.
2. Thorén A and Widell A, "PCR for the Diagnosis of Enteroviral Meningitis," *Scand J Infect Dis*, 1994, 26(8):249-54.

References
Dowsett EG, "Human Enteroviral Infections," *J Hosp Infect*, 1988, 11(2):103-15.
Modlin JF and Kinney JS, "Perinatal Enterovirus Infections," *Adv Pediatr Infect Dis*, 1987, 2:57-78.
Rotbart HA, "Enteroviruses," *Manual of Clinical Microbiology*, 6th ed, Murray PR, Baron EJ, Pfaller MA, et al, eds, Washington, DC: American Society of Microbiology, 1995, 1004-11.

Enterovirus Culture, Stool *see* Viral Culture, Stool *on page 680*

Epstein-Barr Virus Culture

CPT 87252 (tissue culture, inoculation and observation); 87253 (tissue culture, additional studies, each isolate)

Related Information
Epstein-Barr Virus Serology *on page 392*
Heterophil Agglutinins *on page 401*
Infectious Mononucleosis Screening Test *on page 410*
Lymph Node Biopsy *on page 50*
Viral Culture, Blood *on page 677*

Synonyms EBV Culture

Applies to Lymph Node Culture for EBV; Lymphocyte Culture for EBV

Abstract Epstein-Barr virus (EBV) is a herpesvirus. It was originally isolated from Burkitt's lymphomas. EBV infects a large majority of adults and is transmitted in saliva. Primary infection may be asymptomatic or associated with infectious mononucleosis. Although the most common disease caused by the Epstein-Barr virus (EBV) is infectious mononucleosis, viral culture is rarely indicated in that entity.

Specimen Whole blood, lymph node, spleen, tumor biopsies (eg, portions of nasopharyngeal biopsies), throat garglings (for isolation of excreted virus)

Container Green top (heparin) tube for blood; sterile container for other specimens

Storage Instructions Blood specimen can be maintained at room temperature but should be immediately transported to the laboratory. Biopsy specimen should be sent to the Virology Laboratory immediately after collection.

Turnaround Time Cultures often are observed for 6 weeks before being reported as negative.

Special Instructions The laboratory always should be notified prior to receipt of specimen.

Reference Range No growth of EBV in lymphocyte culture

Use Aid in the diagnosis of EBV which is the cause of a wide spectrum of diseases. These include oral hairy leukoplakia, infectious mononucleosis, undifferentiated nasopharyngeal carcinoma, a portion of cases of Hodgkin's disease, a subset of diffuse large-cell immunoblastic lymphomas in immunocompromised individuals, subsets of peripheral T-cell lymphomas and carcinomas of stomach, rare smooth muscle neoplasms, and Burkitt's lymphomas. It is important in patients following transplantation and in the acquired immune deficiency syndrome. An EBV lymphoproliferative syndrome occurs following transplantation and in other settings.

Limitations Cell culture for EBV is not routinely available and not diagnostically practical because EBV proliferates only in B cells, which often are difficult to obtain and process. In addition, many asymptomatic individuals can shed virus orally. Cell culture requires at least 4 weeks to detect EBV infection. EB virus culture is unnecessary for most cases of infectious mononucleosis (IM). **The diagnosis of IM is based on three pillars: clinical appearance, CBC with differential characterized by lymphocytosis with virocytes, and conventional (Davidsohn) serology.**

Methodology Virus is given opportunity to grow for 4 weeks in a lympho-cyte culture. Virus-infected cells will proliferate; if virus is not present, lymphocytes will die. Positive cultures are confirmed for EBV antigens using monoclonal antibodies.

Additional Information Viral serology (usually immunofluorescence) is the preferred diagnostic method.[1,2] EBV persists regularly in the lymphoreticular system of EBV-infected individuals. EBV-positive lymphoblast lines can be established frequently from peripheral leuko-cytes and lymph node cells from those individuals.

Infectious mononucleosis lymphadenopathy is a recognized entity.[3] EBV is closely associated with Burkitt's lymphoma and with nasopharyngeal carcinomas. The virus is often identified in these samples by gene rear-rangement studies, DNA amplification techniques, in situ hybridization, and immunohistochemical detection.[4,5] It is a problem in organ transplant recipients.[6]

Epstein-Barr virus can be detected by immunochemistry and by poly-merase chain reaction.[7]

See the comparison listings Epstein-Barr Virus Serology on page 392, Heterophil Agglutinins on page 401, and Infectious Mononucleosis Screening Test on page 410.

Footnotes

1. Straus SE, "Epstein-Barr Virus and Human Herpesvirus-6," Practical Diagnosis of Viral Infections, Galasso GJ, Whitley RJ, Merigan TC, eds, New York, NY: Raven Press, 1993, 253-67.
2. Thiele GM and Okano M, "Diagnosis of Epstein-Barr Virus Infections in the Clinical Laboratory," Clin Microbiol Newslet, 1993, 15:41-6.
3. Childs CC, Parham DM, and Berard CW, "Infectious Mononucleosis: The Spectrum of Morphologic Changes Simulating Lymphoma in Lymph Nodes and Tonsils," Am J Surg Pathol, 1987, 11(2):122-32.
4. Tyan YS, Liu ST, Ong WR, et al, "Detection of Epstein-Barr Virus and Human Papillomavirus in Head and Neck Tumors," J Clin Microbiol, 1993, 31(1):53-6.
5. Borisch B, Finke J, Hennig F, et al, "Distribution and Localization of Epstein-Barr Virus Subtypes A and B in AIDS-Related Lymphomas and Lymphatic Tissue of HIV-Positive Patients," J Pathol, 1992, 168(2):229-36.
6. Wu TT, Swerdlow SH, Locker J, et al, "Recurrent Epstein-Barr Virus-Associated Lesions in Organ Transplant Recipients," Hum Pathol, 1996, 27(2):157-64.
7. Oda Y, Katsuda S, Okada Y, et al, "Detection of Human Cytomegalovirus, Epstein-Barr Virus, and Herpes Simplex Virus in Diffuse Interstitial Pneumonia by Polymerase Chain Reaction and Immunohistochemistry," Am J Clin Pathol, 1994, 102(4):495-502.

References

Ambinder RF and Mann RB, "Detection and Characterization of Epstein-Barr Virus in Clinical Specimens," Am J Pathol, 1994, 145(2):239-52.

Chang KL, Chen Y-Y, and Weiss LM, "Lack of Evidence of Epstein-Barr Virus in Hairy Cell Leukemia and Monocytoid B-Cell Lymphoma," Hum Pathol, 1993, 24(1):58-61.

Gratama JW, Oosterveer MA, Lepoutre JM, et al, "Serological and Molecular Studies of Epstein-Barr Virus Infection in Allogeneic Marrow Graft Recipients," Transplantation, 1990, 49(4):725-30.

Lennette ET, "Epstein-Barr Virus," Manual of Clinical Microbiology, 6th ed, Washington, DC: American Society for Microbiology, 1995, 905-10.

Liebowitz D, "Epstein-Barr Virus - An Old Dog With New Tricks," N Engl J Med, 1995, 332(1):55-7.

Eye Swab Chlamydia Culture see Chlamydia trachomatis Culture on page 662

Eye, Viral Culture see Viral Culture, Eye or Ocular Symptoms on page 679

Fluorescent Rabies Antibody Test see Rabies on page 672

FRA Test see Rabies on page 672

Gastrointestinal Viruses by EM see Electron Microscopic Exami-nation for Viruses, Stool on page 665

Genital Culture for Mycoplasma T-Strain see Genital Culture for Ureaplasma urealyticum on this page

Genital Culture for Ureaplasma urealyticum

CPT 87081

Related Information

Bacterial Culture, Endometrium on page 462
Bacterial Culture, Genital Specimen on page 463
Neisseria gonorrhoeae Culture and Smear on page 492
Viral Culture, Central Nervous System Symptoms on page 677

Synonyms Genital Culture for Mycoplasma T-Strain; Mycoplasma T-Strain Culture, Genital; Ureaplasma urealyticum Culture, Genital

Applies to Cervical Culture for T-Strain Mycoplasma; Cervical Culture for Ureaplasma urealyticum; Urethral Culture for T-Strain Mycoplasma

Abstract The class Mollicutes includes the genera Mycoplasma and Ureaplasma.

Specimen Culturette® swab of urethra or cervix

Container Culturette® swab

Collection Contact laboratory to obtain special collection and transport medium. Swab should be agitated in the medium, expressed against the side of the tube, and then removed.

Storage Instructions Keep specimen refrigerated. **Organism is remarkably sensitive to drying**. Swab must be placed promptly into

Culturette® and hand delivered to the Microbiology Laboratory. If stored longer than 24 hours, the specimens should be frozen at -70°C.

Turnaround Time 8 days if negative, up to 2 weeks if positive

Special Instructions Specimen should be collected without contact with lubricants, analgesics, or antiseptics.

Reference Range Less than 10^4 organisms in genital tract

Use Establish the diagnosis of Ureaplasma urealyticum infection in suspected cases of nongonococcal urethritis and cervicitis. It is associ-ated with chorioamnionitis and with perinatal morbidity and mortality. It can be isolated from the central nervous system and the lower respira-tory tract of infected neonates.

Limitations Culture can be negative in the presence of infection, and the presence of Ureaplasma urealyticum or Mycoplasma hominis does not always indicate infection, although there is a significant association with symptomatic disease. Culture is done in only a few specialty laboratories.

Methodology Culture on selective media[1]

Additional Information Frequently isolated from asymptomatic individuals. Ureaplasma and Mycoplasma can be isolated from urethral and genital swabs and from urine of sexually active individuals. Sixty percent or more of all women asymptomatically carry U. urealyticum in their genital tract. Usual prevalence of these organisms in patients with urethral symptoms also is high; thus, conclusions regarding the etiologic role of an isolate in a given patient are difficult to make. U. urealyticum is usually associated with cases of nongonococcal urethritis.

Footnotes

1. Al-Zahawi MF, Kearns AM, Sprott MS, et al, "A Study of Three Blood Culture Media for Isolating Genital Mycoplasmas From Obstetrical and Gynaecological Patients," J Infect, 1990, 21(2):143-50.

References

Carey JC, Blackwelder WC, Nugent RP, et al, "Antepartum Cultures for Ureaplasma urealyticum Are Not Useful in Predicting Pregnancy Outcome," Am J Obstet Gynecol, 1991, 164(3):728-33.

Cassell GH, Waites KB, Watson HL, et al, "Ureaplasma urealyticum Intrauterine Infec-tion: Role in Prematurity and Disease in Newborns," Clin Microbiol Rev, 1993, 6(1):69-87.

Eschenbach DA, "Ureaplasma urealyticum and Premature Birth," Clin Infect Dis, 1993, 17(Suppl 1):S100-6.

Gray DJ, Robinson HB, Malone J, et al, "Adverse Outcome in Pregnancy Following Amniotic Fluid Isolation of Ureaplasma urealyticum," Prenat Diagn, 1992, 12(2):111-7.

Genital Culture, Virus see Viral Culture, Urogenital on page 681

German Measles Culture see Rubella Virus Culture on page 674

Hemadsorbing Virus see Influenza Virus Culture on page 670

Hemadsorbing Virus see Mumps Virus Culture on page 670

Hemadsorbing Virus see Parainfluenza Virus Culture on page 671

Herpes Simplex Virus Antigen Detection

CPT 88346

Related Information

Bacterial Culture, Conjunctiva on page 461
Bacterial Culture, Genital Specimen on page 463
Herpes Cytology on page 296
Herpes Simplex Antibody on page 401
Herpes Simplex Virus Culture on next page
Herpes Simplex Virus DNA Detection on page 514
Oral Cavity Cytology on page 298
Skin Biopsy on page 54
Urine Cytology on page 301
Viral Culture on page 675
Viral Culture, Dermatological Symptoms on page 679
Viral Culture, Urogenital on page 681
Virus, Direct Detection by Fluorescent Antibody on page 682

Synonyms Herpes Simplex Virus by DFA; Herpes Simplex Virus, Direct Immunofluorescence; HSV Antigen Detection, Direct

Applies to Herpes Simplex Virus Antigen Detection by PCR

Test Commonly Includes Direct (nonculture) detection of HSV-infected cells in smears of specimens

Specimen Basal cells of a freshly unroofed lesion rolled onto a clean microscope slide; tissue biopsy of brain; cornea

Sampling Time Preferably within 3 days of lesion eruption. Specimens taken after 5 days are less likely to contain viral particles.

Collection Cells from the bottom of an ulcer or vesicle should be scraped with a swab, scalpel, or curette. Swabs should be **rolled** (**not** smeared) across a small area of the slide several times, and cells scraped with a scalpel should be gently dabbed onto the slide. The best specimen is a collection of the cells at the base of an intact vesicle. Cells from a diseased cornea can also be used. **The smear should be air dried at** (Continued)

Herpes Simplex Virus Antigen Detection
(Continued)

room temperature. The success of direct detection procedures depends on the careful preparation of cell smears. If an EIA method is used, collect specimens as described for HSV viral culture.

Storage Instructions Do not store the specimen. Send it to the laboratory immediately.

Turnaround Time Hours

Special Instructions Operative biopsy specimens and spinal fluid specimens for fluorescent antibody (FA) testing should be **processed immediately.** The laboratory should be **notified in advance** when either of these specimen types will be sent for FA.

Reference Range No herpes simplex virus-infected cells detected

Use Rapid detection of herpes simplex virus

Limitations The efficiency of detection of HSV material depends in great part on the collection of a sufficiently large number of intact infected cells from the lesion. Specimen smears that are too thick can retain or trap the fluorescent reagent and make the test difficult to interpret. If at all possible, it is important to obtain cells from the base of an intact vesicle. The presence of infected cells decreases as the lesion heals, and crusted lesions may have little or no herpes antigenic material remaining. Antigen detection methods have excellent specificity but are less sensitive than culture.

Methodology Direct fluorescent antibody (DFA) or enzyme immunoassay (EIA)

Additional Information In general, this test is only approximately 70% as sensitive as cell culture. In critical situations, clinicians should consider using both methods.[1] Air-dried preparations on slides can also be stained with Giemsa or Diff-Quik™ stains (Tzanck), however, these stains are not specific for HSV. Fixed preparations (usually 95% ethanol) can also be stained with the Papanicolaou or immunoperoxidase methods. Smears fixed with hairspray and subsequently stained with the Papanicolaou stain usually are excellent preparations. The detection of HSV DNA by PCR in CSF and lesion fluid is available in certain laboratories.[2] It is more sensitive than detection of specific antibody for early diagnosis of herpes simplex encephalitis (97% to 99% sensitivity) and provides 95% to 100% specificity.[3]

Polymerase chain reaction was more sensitive than immunocytochemical techniques for detection of herpes simplex virus in formalin-fixed, paraffin-embedded tissue sections from cases of diffuse interstitial pneumonia.[4]

Footnotes
1. Rawls WE, "Herpes Simplex Viruses: Types 1 and 2," *Laboratory Diagnosis of Viral Infections*, Lennette EH, ed, New York, NY: Marcel Dekker Inc, 1992, 443-61.
2. Puchhammer-Stöckl E, Heinz FX, et al, "Evaluation of the Polymerase Chain Reaction for Diagnosis of Herpes Simplex Virus Encephalitis," *J Clin Microbiol*, 1993, 31(1):146-8.
3. ARUP Laboratories, "Herpes Simplex Virus," April 1996.
4. Oda Y, Katsuda S, Okada Y, et al, "Detection of Human Cytomegalovirus, Epstein-Barr Virus, and Herpes Simplex Virus in Diffuse Interstitial Pneumonia by Polymerase Chain Reaction and Immunohistochemistry," *Am J Clin Pathol*, 1994, 102(4):495-502.

References
Arvin AM and Prober CG, "Herpes Simplex Virus," *Manual of Clinical Microbiology*, 6th ed, Murray PR, Baron EJ, Pfaller MA, et al, eds, Washington, DC: American Society of Microbiology, 1995, 876-83.
Smith TF, "Rapid Diagnosis of Viral Infections," *Adv Exp Med Biol*, 1990, 263:115-21.

Herpes Simplex Virus Antigen Detection by PCR see Herpes Simplex Virus Antigen Detection *on previous page*

Herpes Simplex Virus by DFA see Herpes Simplex Virus Antigen Detection *on previous page*

Herpes Simplex Virus Culture

CPT 87140 (culture typing, fluorescent method); 87252 (tissue culture, inoculation and observation); 87253 (tissue culture, additional studies, each isolate)

Related Information

Synonyms HSV 1 and 2 Culture; HSV Culture

Applies to Viral Culture, Eye; Viral Culture, Genital; Viral Culture, Skin

Test Commonly Includes Culture for HSV only; HSV also is detected in a routine viral culture; rapid method includes specific staining with a fluorescent monoclonal antibody

Abstract Herpes simplex viruses cause a wide variety of lesions, including neonatal herpes and encephalitis, entities which are often fatal and which lead to serious sequelae. Herpes infections may be severe in subjects who are immunocompromised. Culture is the method of choice for many clinical presentations, such as vesicles.

Specimen Vesicle fluid, swab of base of lesion, tissue biopsy, nasopharyngeal swab, conjunctival swab

Container Cold viral transport medium for swabs

Collection All specimens should be kept cold and moist. Specimens should be collected in the acute stage of the disease, preferably within 3 days and no longer than 7 days after the onset of illness. Spinal fluid specimens should be submitted in the usual sterile tube; no special transport medium is necessary. All other specimens should be collected on a sterile swab as described and the swab should be placed into cold viral transport medium immediately after collection.

Endocervical: Swab cervix with a rolling/scraping motion to assure obtaining epithelial cells.

Vesicular lesion: Wash vesicles with sterile saline. Carefully open several vesicles and soak up vesicular fluid with swab. If vesicles are absent, vigorously swab base of lesion (specimen should be collected during first 3 days of eruption. Specimens collected later in the course of disease rarely yield virus).

Conjunctival: Using a moistened swab, firmly rub conjunctiva using sufficient force to obtain epithelial cells.

Throat, respiratory, oral: Rotate swab in both tonsillar crypts and against posterior oropharynx.

Storage Instructions Specimens should be delivered to the laboratory and handed to a technologist within 30 minutes of collection. Outpatient specimens: If transport is to be delayed more than 30 minutes after collection, specimen **must** be refrigerated (held at 4°C to 8°C) until it can be transported to the laboratory. If inoculation onto cell cultures is not possible within 48 hours, specimens should be frozen at -70°C. Do not freeze at -20°C.

Turnaround Time Routine culture: 1-14 days; rapid culture: 16 hours to 2 days

Special Instructions Special viral transport medium must be obtained from the laboratory prior to collection of specimen.

Reference Range No virus isolated

Use Aid in the diagnosis of disease caused by HSV. These include gingivostomatitis, herpes labialis, genital herpes, skin lesions, keratoconjunctivitis, neonatal herpes, aseptic meningitis, and encephalitis. Genital transmission of HSV infection to sexual partners and neonates involves subclinical shedding of HSV by women with genital herpes. Such shedding is detectable by viral culture.[1] Culture can provide evidence of acyclovir resistance,[2] and detect potential for transmission of HSV to neonates.[3]

Limitations Standard methods suffer 30% false-negatives for identification of those neonates who subsequently develop neonatal herpes.[3]

Methodology Inoculation of specimen into cell cultures, incubation of cultures, observation for characteristic cytopathic effect (CPE), and identification of HSV by fluorescein-labeled monoclonal antibodies specific for type 1 or 2.[4] In shell vial isolation technique with direct immunofluorescent staining for HSV 1 and HSV 2, characteristic fluorescent foci indicate the presence of virus.

Additional Information HSV can only rarely be cultured from the CSF of patients with HSV 1 encephalitis. The virus is occasionally isolated from spinal fluid of patients with HSV 2 meningitis and of neonates with congenital herpes.

Of other diagnostic approaches for herpes simplex virus encephalitis, PCR is more sensitive for early diagnosis than detection of CSF antibody.[5] Virus can also be isolated from urine in patients with primary genital HSV infections concurrent with cystitis.

Serology for the detection of herpes simplex virus is available, but the results usually are of value only in the diagnosis of primary HSV infections. There is much cross reaction between the antibodies to HSV 1 and HSV 2.

Immunocompromised patients can develop disseminated HSV infections. These infections are characterized by a persistent, severe mucocutaneous infection involving the mouth, face, genital, or perianal areas. Sometimes such infections spread to organs such as the liver, lungs, adrenal glands, and bone marrow. Genital herpes infection has been suggested to be a possible risk factor for HIV-1 infection.[6] At the present time, it is unclear whether this relationship is biological or due to individual sexual habits.

Culture is useful for diagnosis of unusual lesions, such as hepatic glossitis in immunocompromised patients. The buccal mucosa, floor of the mouth, and soft palate may be infected as well.[7]

Footnotes

1. Wald A, Zeh J, Selke S, et al, "Virologic Characteristics of Subclinical and Symptomatic Genital Herpes Infections," *N Engl J Med*, 1995, 333(12):770-5.
2. Kost RG, Hill EL, Tigges M, et al, "Brief Report: Recurrent Acyclovir-Resistant Genital Herpes in an Immunocompetent Patient," *N Engl J Med*, 1993, 329(24):1777-82.
3. Cone RW, Hobson AC, Brown Z, et al, "Frequent Detection of Genital Herpes Simplex Virus DNA by Polymerase Chain Reaction Among Pregnant Women," *JAMA*, 1994, 272(10):792-6.
4. Corey L, "Laboratory Diagnosis of Herpes Simplex Virus Infections: Principles Guiding the Development of Rapid Diagnostic Tests," *Diagn Microbiol Infect Dis*, 1986, 4(3 Suppl):111S-19S.
5. "Herpes Simplex Virus Encephalitis in Pediatrics: Diagnosis by Detection of Antibodies and DNA in Cerebrospinal Fluid," *JAMA*, 1993, 12(12):1001-6.
6. Hook EW 3d, Cannon RO, Nahmias AJ, et al, "Herpes Simplex Virus Infection as a Risk Factor for Human Immunodeficiency Virus Infection in Heterosexuals," *J Infect Dis*, 1992, 165(2):251-5.
7. Grossman ME, Stevens AW, and Cohen PR, "Brief Report: Herpetic Geometric Glossitis," *N Engl J Med*, 1993, 329(25):1859-60.

References

Arvin AM and Prober CG, "Herpes Simplex Virus," *Manual of Clinical Microbiology*, 6th ed, Murray PR, Baron EJ, Pfaller MA, et al, eds, Washington, DC: American Society of Microbiology, 1995, 876-83.

Banks TA and Rouse BT, "Current Approaches and Future Directions in the Treatment of Herpesvirus Infections," *Infect Agents*, 1994, 11(2):148-57.

Brown ZA, Benedetti J, Ashley R, et al, "Neonatal Herpes Simplex Virus Infection in Relation to Asymptomatic Maternal Infection at the Time of Labor," *N Engl J Med*, 1991, 324(18):1247-52.

Forbes BA, "Perinatal Viral Infections," *Clin Microbiol Newslet*, 1992, 14(22):169-72.

Holley HP Jr and Fowler SL, "Update on Herpes Simplex Infections," *Hosp Med*, May 1993, 28-45.

Koelle DM, Benedetti J, Langenberg A, et al, "Asymptomatic Reactivation of Herpes Simplex Virus in Women After the First Episode of Genital Herpes," *Ann Intern Med*, 1992, 116(6):433-7.

Mertz GJ, Benedetti J, Ashley R, et al, "Risk Factors for the Sexual Transmission of Genital Herpes," *Ann Intern Med*, 1992, 116(3):197-202.

Herpes Simplex Virus, Direct Immunofluorescence *see* Herpes Simplex Virus Antigen Detection *on page 667*

Herpesvirus 6 Culture *see* Human Herpesvirus 6 Culture *on this page*

HHV-6 Culture *see* Human Herpesvirus 6 Culture *on this page*

HIV Culture *see* Human Immunodeficiency Virus Culture *on this page*

HSV 1 and 2 Culture *see* Herpes Simplex Virus Culture *on previous page*

HSV Antigen Detection, Direct *see* Herpes Simplex Virus Antigen Detection *on page 667*

HSV Culture *see* Herpes Simplex Virus Culture *on previous page*

HTLV-III Culture *see* Human Immunodeficiency Virus Culture *on this page*

Human Herpesvirus 6 Culture

Related Information

Human Herpesvirus 6 DNA Detection *on page 515*

Human Herpesvirus 6, IgG and IgM Antibodies, Quantitative *on page 406*

Viral Culture, Blood *on page 677*

Synonyms Herpesvirus 6 Culture; HHV-6 Culture

Test Commonly Includes Culture and identification of HHV-6 isolates

Specimen Blood

Container Green top (heparin) tube or lavender top (EDTA) tube

Storage Instructions Transport to laboratory at room temperature. Do not freeze.

Turnaround Time Positive cultures can be detected after 7-10 days; negative cultures are reported after 21 days of culture

Use Confirm the diagnosis of active HHV-6 infection

Limitations Culture for HHV-6 is not routinely done; serology is a better indicator of disease; asymptomatic individuals will shed HHV-6 orally; culture for HHV-6 is tedious and requires at least 3 weeks of culture

Methodology Peripheral blood mononuclear cells are cocultivated with stimulated cord blood lymphocytes or stimulated peripheral blood lymphocytes. In positive cultures, characteristic cytopathic effect can be observed after 7-10 days of culture.

Additional Information HHV-6 causes a common childhood disease called roseola (exanthem subitum). Generally, the disease is mild with fever and rash, but on occasion complications such as seizures and/or encephalitis can occur. HHV-6 can also cause heterophil-negative mononucleosis in adults.

A rapid shell vial method for culture of HHV-6 is under investigation.

References

Cone RW, Hackman RC, Huang ML, et al, "Human Herpesvirus 6 in Lung Tissue From Patients With Pneumonitis After Bone Marrow Transplantation," *N Engl J Med*, 1993, 329(3):156-61.

Pruksananonda P, Hall CB, Insel RA, et al, "Primary Human Herpesvirus 6 Infection in Young Children," *N Engl J Med*, 1992, 326(22):1445-50.

Suga S, Yoshikawa T, Asano Y, et al, "Clinical and Virological Analyses of 21 Infants With Exanthem Subitum (Roseola Infantum) and Central Nervous System Complications," *Ann Neurol*, 1993, 33(6):597-603.

Human Immunodeficiency Virus Culture

CPT 87252 (tissue culture, inoculation and observation); 87253 (tissue culture, additional studies, each isolate)

Related Information

CD4/CD8 Enumeration *on page 375*

HIV-1/HIV-2 Serology *on page 403*

Human Immunodeficiency Virus DNA Amplification *on page 515*

p24 Antigen *on page 420*

Polymerase Chain Reaction *on page 523*

Zidovudine *on page 580*

Synonyms AIDS Virus Culture; HIV Culture; HTLV-III Culture

Specimen Whole blood (20-40 mL), cerebrospinal fluid (10 mL), other body fluids, biopsies.[1] See special precautions in Specimen Collection Introduction *on page 21*.

Container Green top (heparin) tube for blood, sterile container for CSF and other fluids

Collection Routine venipuncture. Invert the tubes several times after drawing the blood to be sure the blood is thoroughly mixed with the heparin.

Storage Instructions Do not freeze or refrigerate blood specimen. Some laboratories require that the specimen be received in the laboratory the same day the specimen is obtained.

Causes for Rejection Specimen leaking from container, blood frozen or refrigerated

Turnaround Time Positive cultures are usually reported after two consecutive positive reverse transcriptase assays. Blood cultures are usually incubated 4 weeks and some laboratories incubate CSF cultures 8 weeks before reporting as negative.

Reference Range No virus isolated

Use Test for active HIV infection

Limitations A negative culture cannot be assumed to rule out the presence of the virus. Fresh human lymphocytes are needed for growth of HIV. These cells are costly and more difficult to maintain than are cell lines. Many laboratories do not have the capability of HIV culture. Culture of HIV poses a risk to laboratory personnel.

Methodology Growth of virus in lymphocyte culture and subsequent (indirect) testing for presence of virus in culture supernatant fluids by enzyme immunoassay (EIA) or reverse transcriptase assay

Additional Information Serology for the detection of HIV antibodies is widely available.[2] Detection of antibodies to HIV is the most common method of HIV testing. It is better suited for routine use in screening patients for exposure to HIV.[3] DNA amplification for detection of HIV (either proviral DNA or viral RNA) is useful in diagnosing HIV in infants of HIV-seropositive mothers[4] and for individuals at high risk for HIV infection.[5] Many laboratories now do a quantitative analysis of amplified viral genome to assess viral load.[6] This is used to follow patients on antiviral therapy.[7]

Footnotes

1. Clarke JR, Williamson JD, Mitchell DM, "Comparative Study of the Isolation of Human Immunodeficiency Virus From the Lung and Peripheral Blood of AIDS Patients," *J Med Virol*, 1993, 39(3):196-9.
2. Abb J, "Diagnostic and Prognostic Significance of Testing for HIV Antigen," *Clin Immunol Newslet*, 1988, 9:185-7.
3. Weniger BG, Quinhões EP, Sereno AB, et al, "A Simplified Surveillance Case Definition of AIDS Derived From Empirical Clinical Data," *J Acquir Immune Defic Syndr*, 1992, 5(12):1212-23.
4. Rogers MF, Ou C-Y, Rayfield M, et al, "Use of the Polymerase Chain Reaction for Early Detection of the Proviral Sequences of Human Immunodeficiency Virus in Infants Born to Seropositive Mothers," *N Engl J Med*, 1989, 320(25):1649-54.
5. Loche M and Mach B, "Identification of HIV-Infected Seronegative Individuals by a Direct Diagnostic Test Based on Hybridization to Amplified Viral DNA," *Lancet*, 1989, 2(8608):418-21.
6. Sei S, Kleiner DE, Kopp JB, et al, "Quantitative Analysis of Viral Burden in Tissues From Adults and Children With Symptomatic Human Immunodeficiency Virus Type 1 Infection Assessed by Polymerase Chain Reaction," *J Infect Dis*, 1994, 170(2):325-33.
7. Kojima E, Shirasaka T, Anderson BD, et al, "Human Immunodeficiency Virus Type 1 (HIV-1) Viremia Changes and Development of Drug-Related Mutations in Patients With Symptomatic HIV-1 Infection Receiving Alternating or Simultaneous Zidovudine and Didanosine Therapy," *J Infect Dis*, 1995, 171(5):1152-8.

References

Erice A, Sannerud KJ, Leske VL, et al, "Sensitive Microculture Method for Isolation of Human Immunodeficiency Virus Type 1 From Blood Leukocytes," *J Clin Microbiol*, 1992, 30(2):444-8.

Jackson JB, "Human Immunodeficiency Virus Type 1 Antigen and Culture Assays," *Arch Pathol Lab Med*, 1990, 114(3):249-53.

Khan NC, Chatterjee S, and Nielson LN, "Pathogenesis of HIV Infection," *Clin Microbiol Newslet*, 1990, 12(23):177-84.

(Continued)

Human Immunodeficiency Virus Culture
(Continued)

Markham PD and Salahuddin SZ, "*In Vitro* Cultivation of Human Leukocytes: Methods for the Expression and Isolation of Human Retroviruses," *BioTechniques*, 1987, 5:432-43.

Influenza Virus Culture

CPT 87140 (culture typing, fluorescent method); 87252 (tissue culture, inoculation and observation); 87253 (tissue culture, additional studies, each isolate)

Related Information
Influenza A and B Titer *on page 411*
Viral Culture *on page 675*
Viral Culture, Respiratory Symptoms *on page 680*
Virus, Direct Detection by Fluorescent Antibody *on page 682*

Applies to Hemadsorbing Virus

Test Commonly Includes Rapid culture for influenza A and B using specific monoclonal antibodies and immunofluorescence. Conventional viral culture will also detect other respiratory viruses (parainfluenza, adenovirus, and respiratory syncytial virus).

Abstract Sputum characterized by acute inflammation without a distinctive bacterial pattern may indicate *Legionella*, RSV, or influenza.[1]

Specimen Throat or nasopharyngeal swab, sputum, bronchial washings, bronchoalveolar lavage

Container Viral transport medium; cold virus transport medium for swabs

Sampling Time Specimens should be collected within 3 days of the onset of illness.

Storage Instructions Specimens should be placed into viral transport medium and kept cold at all times. Specimens should be delivered immediately to the laboratory. Do not freeze specimens.

Causes for Rejection Dry specimen

Reference Range No virus isolated

Use Isolate and identify influenza virus as an etiologic agent in cases of perceived influenza and viral pneumonia. Isolation of influenza viruses permits surveillance of epidemic viral strains and aids in selection of vaccine strains.

Limitations Negative culture does not rule out a viral etiology.

Methodology Routine culture: Inoculation of specimens into cell cultures, incubation of cultures, observation for characteristic cytopathic effect (CPE), and identification/speciation by methods such as hemadsorption and fluorescent monoclonal antibodies specific for influenza virus A or B.

Rapid culture: Inoculation of cells in a shell vial, centrifugation, culture, and staining with an immunofluorescent monoclonal antibody.

Additional Information Influenza is very contagious and is usually transmitted from person to person by inhalation of aerosols, especially in crowded conditions.[2] The peak incidence of influenza infection is between December and March. Both influenza A and influenza B have been implicated in epidemics every 3-6 years.[3]

The shell vial technique to rapidly (within 24 hours) detect viruses has been adopted to detect influenza A and B viruses.[4,5] Serology for the detection of influenza antibodies is available. See listing Influenza A and B Titer *on page 411*. Antibody levels usually peak 4-6 weeks after infection. A single high antibody titer in convalescent serum is suggestive of a recent infection. However, the recommended procedure for a diagnostic antibody titer is comparison of acute and convalescent titers.[6] A commercial and rapid (less than 15 minutes) enzyme immunoassay for the detection of influenza A virus in patient specimen is also available.[7]

Footnotes
1. Yungbluth M, "The Laboratory Diagnosis of Pneumonia. The Role of the Community Hospital Pathologist," *Clin Lab Med*, 1995, 15(2):209-34.
2. Leigh MW, Carson JL, and Denny FW Jr, "Pathogenesis of Respiratory Infections Due to Influenza Virus: Implications for Developing Countries," *Rev Infect Dis*, 1991, 13(Suppl 6):S501-8.
3. Kendal AP, "Epidemiologic Implication of Changes in the Influenza Virus Genome," *Am J Med*, 1987, 82(6A):4-14.
4. Ziegler T, Hall H, Sánchez-Fauquier A, et al, "Type- and Subtype-Specific Detection of Influenza Viruses in Clinical Specimens by Rapid Culture Assay," *J Clin Microbiol*, 1995, 33(2):318-21.
5. Guenthner SH and Linneman CC, "Indirect Immunofluorescence Assay for Rapid Diagnosis of Influenza Virus," *Lab Med*, 1988, 581-3.
6. Harmon MW, Rota PA, Walls HH, et al, "Antibody Response in Humans to Influenza Virus Type B Host-Cell-Derived Variants After Vaccination With Standard (Egg-Derived) Vaccine or Natural Infection," *J Clin Microbiol*, 1988, 26(2):333-7.
7. Waner JL, Todd SJ, Shalaby H, et al, "Comparison of Directigen FLU-A With Viral Isolation and Direct Immunofluorescence for the Rapid Detection and Identification of Influenza A Virus," *J Clin Microbiol*, 1991, 29(3):479-82.

References
Bachman CA, Doyle WJ, and Skoner DP, "Influenza A Virus-Induced Acute Otitis Media," *J Infect Dis*, 1995, 172(5):1348-51.
Couch RB, "Respiratory Diseases," *Practical Diagnosis of Viral Infections*, Galasso GJ, Whitley RJ, Merigan TC, eds, New York, NY: Raven Press, 1993, 143-8.

Kohn MA, Farley TA, Sundin D, et al, "Three Summertime Outbreaks of Influenza Type A," *J Infect Dis*, 1995, 172(1):246-9.
"Prevention and Control of Influenza, Recommendations of the Advisory Committee on Immunization Practices (ACIP). Centers for Disease Control and Prevention," *MMWR Morb Mortal Wkly Rep*, 1995, 44(RR-3):1-22.
Shaw MW, Arden NH, and Maassab HF, "New Aspects of Influenza Viruses," *Clin Microbiol Rev*, 1992, 5(1):74-92.
Ziegler T and Cox NJ, "Influenza Viruses," *Manual of Clinical Microbiology*, 6th ed, Murray PR, Baron EJ, Pfaller MA, et al, eds, Washington, DC: American Society for Microbiology, 1995, 918-25.

Influenza Virus, Direct Detection *see* Virus, Direct Detection by Fluorescent Antibody *on page 682*

Lumbar Puncture Hazards *see* Viral Culture, Central Nervous System Symptoms *on page 677*

Lymph Node Culture for EBV *see* Epstein-Barr Virus Culture *on page 666*

Lymphocyte Culture for EBV *see* Epstein-Barr Virus Culture *on page 666*

Lymphogranuloma Venereum Culture *see* Chlamydia trachomatis Culture *on page 662*

Measles Virus, Direct Detection *see* Virus, Direct Detection by Fluorescent Antibody *on page 682*

MicroTrak® *see* Chlamydia trachomatis Direct FA Test *on page 663*

Mumps Virus Culture

CPT 87252 (tissue culture, inoculation and observation); 87253 (tissue culture, additional studies, each isolate)

Related Information
Mumps Serology *on page 419*
Viral Culture *on page 675*
Viral Culture, Central Nervous System Symptoms *on page 677*
Viral Culture, Urine *on page 681*
Virus, Direct Detection by Fluorescent Antibody *on page 682*

Applies to Hemadsorbing Virus

Test Commonly Includes Mumps virus is isolated from routine viral cultures

Specimen Saliva, urine, cerebrospinal fluid

Container Sterile container for urine and CSF; tube with cold viral transport medium for swabs

Sampling Time At or within 5 days of the onset of illness

Collection It is desirable to collect specimens as early in the disease as possible. Saliva, days one and two after onset; spinal fluid of patients with meningoencephalitis within 6 days after onset. Virus is also excreted in urine for as long as 14 days after the onset of illness. In young patients, saliva is collected by a suitable suction device or by swabbing, especially the area around the orifices of the Stensen duct. The swabs must immediately be placed into cold viral transport medium. Spinal fluid is obtained in the usual manner and put into a sterile tube. For urine specimens, preferably the first voided morning urine is collected in a sterile container. All specimens must immediately be placed on ice and sent to the laboratory.

Storage Instructions Do **not** freeze at -20°C. Storage at -20°C rapidly inactivates the mumps virus. If inoculation is delayed by more than 48 hours, specimens should be frozen at -70°C.

Turnaround Time Variable (5-14 days) and depends on methods used and amount of virus in the specimen. Negative results are reported at 14 days.

Reference Range No virus isolated

Use Aid in the diagnosis of disease caused by mumps virus, especially meningitis

Limitations Negative viral culture does not rule out the involvement of mumps virus in disease process.

Methodology Inoculation of specimen into cell cultures, incubation of cultures, observation for characteristic cytopathic effect (CPE), and identification by methods such as hemadsorption and fluorescent monoclonal antibodies

Additional Information Although virus isolation is the most certain means for establishing the laboratory diagnosis, serologic methods are also useful and technically easier. Demonstration of IgM antibodies in acute serum is diagnostic of primary infection. The incidence of mumps infections has dramatically declined since the introduction of the mumps vaccine in 1967. However, there still remains a significant population of individuals that are unvaccinated or without prior exposure.[1]

Footnotes
1. Hersh BS, Fine PE, Kent WK, et al, "Mumps Outbreak in a Highly Vaccinated Population," *J Pediatr*, 1991, 119(2):187-93.

References

Hierholzer JC, Bingham PG, Castells E, et al, "Time-Resolved Fluoroimmunoassays With Monoclonal Antibodies for Rapid Identification of Parainfluenza Type 4 and Mumps Viruses," *Arch Virol*, 1993, 130(3-4):335-52.

Kleiman MB, "Mumps Virus," *Laboratory Diagnosis of Viral Infections*, Lennette EH, ed, New York, NY: Marcel Dekker Inc, 1992, 549-66.

Swierkosz EM, "Mumps Virus," *Manual of Clinical Microbiology*, 6th ed, Murray PR, Baron ES, Pfaller MA, et al, eds, Washington, DC: American Society for Microbiology, 1995, 963-7.

Mumps Virus Culture, Urine *see* Viral Culture, Urine *on page 681*

Mumps Virus, Direct Detection *see* Virus, Direct Detection by Fluorescent Antibody *on page 682*

Mycoplasma pneumoniae Culture *see Mycoplasma pneumoniae* Diagnostic Procedures *on this page*

Mycoplasma pneumoniae Diagnostic Procedures

CPT 86738 (antibodies); 87109 (culture)

Related Information

Bacterial Culture, Sputum *on page 465*
Cold Agglutinin Screen *on page 605*
Cold Agglutinin Titer *on page 384*
Mycoplasma pneumoniae DNA Probe Test *on page 520*
Mycoplasma Serology *on page 419*

Synonyms *Mycoplasma pneumoniae* Culture

Abstract *Mycoplasma pneumoniae* commonly causes respiratory infections. Most involve the upper respiratory tract, but pneumonia and other manifestations can occur as well.

Specimen Throat or nasopharyngeal swabs

Collection Throat or nasopharyngeal swabs should be placed **immediately** in special transport medium (obtained from the laboratory) and sent immediately to the laboratory. Specimen should be kept at 4°C during transport to the laboratory.

Storage Instructions If storage longer than 24 hours is needed, the specimen should be frozen at -70°C.

Mycoplasma pneumoniae Clinical Manifestations of Infection

Respiratory	Pneumonia
	Pharyngitis
	Otitis media
	Bullous myringitis
	Sinusitis
	Laryngotracheobronchitis
	Bronchiolitis
	Nonspecific upper respiratory symptoms
Neurologic	Meningoencephalitis
	Encephalitis
	Transverse myelitis
	Cranial neuropathy
	Poliomyelitis-like syndrome
	Psychosis
	Cerebral infarction
	Guillain-Barré syndrome
Cardiac	Pericarditis
	Myocarditis
	Complete heart block
	Congestive heart failure
	Myocardial infarction
Gastrointestinal	Pancreatitis
	Hepatic dysfunction
Hematologic	Autoimmune hemolytic anemia
	Bone marrow suppression
	Thrombocytopenia
	Disseminated intravascular coagulation
Musculoskeletal	Myalgias
	Arthralgias
	Arthritis
Genitourinary	Glomerulonephritis
	Tubulointerstitial nephritis
	Tubo-ovarian abscess
Immunologic	Depressed cellular immunity and neutrophil chemotaxis

From Broughton RA, "Infections Due to *Mycoplasma pneumoniae* in Childhood," *Pediatr Infect Dis J*, 1986, 71-85, with permission.

Turnaround Time 2-3 weeks

Reference Range No *Mycoplasma pneumoniae* identified

Use Aid in the diagnosis of pneumonia caused by *Mycoplasma pneumoniae*

Limitations The culture procedure is not often used because it is slow and somewhat insensitive; 2-3 weeks or more are often required for isolation and definitive identification of positive cultures.

Methodology Isolates are cultured in special broth and on special agar media and are identified by biochemical tests and ability to hemolyze erythrocytes. However, the most commonly used and currently recommended method of diagnosis is serology, to measure acute and convalescent antibody levels to *M. pneumoniae*.

Additional Information *Mycoplasma pneumoniae* infection is acquired via the respiratory route from small-particle aerosols or large droplets of secretions. The organism can penetrate the mucociliary barrier of respiratory epithelium and produce cellular injury and ciliostasis which may account for the prolonged cough observed clinically. Most infections are observed in older children and young adults. Early infection in infancy or childhood may increase the severity of subsequent infections. The recently described *M. genitalium* might play a role in the pathogenesis of *M. pneumoniae* disease.[1] Cold agglutinins and *Mycoplasma pneumoniae* serology have been the mainstays of diagnosis because of the limitations and long turnaround time for cultures. However, immunofluorescence techniques and immunoassays to detect antibodies to *M. pneumoniae* are available and are the recommended diagnostic methods. Recently, a DNA amplification method has become available.[2] A number of reference laboratories offer this test as a rapid alternative to culture. See listing *Mycoplasma pneumoniae* DNA Probe Test *on page 520*.

Footnotes

1. Tully JG, "The Current Enigma of *Mycoplasma genitalium*: New Findings That Affect *Mycoplasma* Identification in the Clinical Microbiology Laboratory," *Clin Microbiol Newslet*, 1989, 11:4-6.

2. de Barbeyrac B, Bennet-Poggi C, Febrer F, et al, "Detection of *Mycoplasma pneumoniae* and *Mycoplasma genitalium* in Clinical Samples By Polymerase Chain Reaction," *Clin Infect Dis*, 1993, 17(Suppl 1):S83-9.

References

Cimolai N, Wenstey D, Seear M, et al, "*Mycoplasma pneumoniae* as a Cofactor in Severe Respiratory Infections," *Clin Infect Dis*, 1995, 21:1182-5.

Clyde WA Jr, "Clinical Overview of Typical *Mycoplasma pneumoniae* Infections," *Clin Infect Dis*, 1993, 17(Suppl 1):S32-6.

Mansel JK, Rosenow EC 3d, Smith TF, et al, "*Mycoplasma pneumoniae* Pneumonia," *Chest*, 1989, 95(3):639-46.

"The Changing Role of Mycoplasmas in Respiratory Disease and AIDS," *Clin Infect Dis*, 1993, 17(Suppl 1)S1-315.

Wijnands GJ, "Diagnosis and Interventions in Lower Respiratory Tract Infections," *Am J Med*, 1992, 92(4SA):91S-7S.

Mycoplasma T-Strain Culture, Genital *see* Genital Culture for *Ureaplasma urealyticum* *on page 667*

Negri Bodies *see* Rabies *on next page*

Parainfluenza 1, 2, and 3 Virus Culture *see* Parainfluenza Virus Culture *on this page*

Parainfluenza Virus Culture

CPT 87140 (culture typing, fluorescent method); 87252 (tissue culture, inoculation and observation); 87253 (tissue culture, additional studies, each isolate)

Related Information

Parainfluenza Viral Serology *on page 420*
Viral Culture *on page 675*
Viral Culture, Respiratory Symptoms *on page 680*
Virus, Direct Detection by Fluorescent Antibody *on page 682*

Synonyms Parainfluenza 1, 2, and 3 Virus Culture

Applies to Hemadsorbing Virus

Test Commonly Includes Culture and identification of parainfluenza viruses. Concurrent culture for other respiratory viruses (influenza, adenovirus, and respiratory syncytial viruses)

Abstract Most cases of laryngotracheitis (croup) in infants and children are caused by parainfluenza viruses. They are second only to respiratory syncytial virus as a cause of serious infantile respiratory diseases. These are RNA viruses of the paramyxovirus family.[1]

Specimen Throat or nasopharyngeal swab, nasopharyngeal washes and secretions

Container Viral transport medium; cold viral transport medium for swabs

Collection Place swabs into cold viral transport medium and keep cold. Infants and small children: soft catheters and suction devices (syringes and suction bulbs) can be used to collect nasal secretions from far back in the nose (best specimens). Another excellent method is to introduce 3-7 mL of sterile saline into the child's posterior nasal cavity and immediately aspirate the fluid. **Note**: Do not use **cold** sterile saline when aspirating samples. Warm to room temperature.

(Continued)

Parainfluenza Virus Culture *(Continued)*

Storage Instructions Keep specimens ice cold after collection, but **do not freeze specimens at -20°C**. Specimens that cannot be inoculated into cell culture within 72 hours should be frozen at -70°C.

Turnaround Time Conventional culture: 5-14 days; rapid culture: 2-4 days

Reference Range No virus isolated

Critical Values Positive results

Use Disease caused by parainfluenza virus includes croup (laryngotracheitis), other respiratory illness including laryngitis and pneumonia; bronchopneumonia and bronchiolitis occur in infants. The differential diagnosis includes epiglottitis, bacterial tracheitis, and retropharyngeal abscess.[1]

Limitations Negative viral culture does not rule out viral etiology; rapid methods will only detect specified virus(es)

Methodology Routine culture: Inoculation of specimens into cell cultures, incubation of cultures, observation for hemadsorption or characteristic cytopathic effect (CPE), and identification/speciation by fluorescent monoclonal antibodies specific for types 1, 2, or 3 or by virus neutralization. Rapid culture: Inoculation of cells in shell vial and detection of specific virus with an immunofluorescent monoclonal antibody.

Rapid recognition of viral antigen in nasopharyngeal secretions by immunofluorescent and ELISA methods is available with varying levels of sensitivity.[1]

Additional Information Parainfluenza viruses are rarely isolated from healthy individuals, thus their detection is usually diagnostic. Conventional and rapid cultures will generally detect other respiratory viruses in addition to parainfluenza. Serology for the detection of parainfluenza antibodies is available, but the results are often difficult to interpret.

Most virology laboratories hemadsorb all viral (especially respiratory) cultures at 14 days (prior to discarding the culture) to detect hemadsorbing viruses that have not produced cytopathic effect (CPE) by that time. Positive hemadsorption tests are often reported as "hemadsorbing virus present." This result suggests the presence of influenza, parainfluenza, measles, and/or mumps virus.

Serology for the detection of parainfluenza antibodies is available, but the results are often difficult to interpret. Currently some laboratories do a rapid shell vial assay for detection of several respiratory viruses. This test will detect influenza A and B virus, respiratory syncytial virus, and parainfluenza virus 1, 2, and 3.[2]

Footnotes

1. Long SS, "Parainfluenza Viruses," *Principles and Practice of Pediatrics*, 2nd ed, Oski FA, DeAngelis CD, Feigin RD, et al, eds, Philadelphia, PA: JB Lippincott Co, 1994, 1296-9.
2. Schirm J, Luijt DS, Pastoor GW, et al, "Rapid Detection of Respiratory Viruses Using Mixtures of Monoclonal Antibodies on Shell Vial Cultures," *J Med Virol*, 1992, 38(2):147-51.

References

Costello MJ, Smernoff NT, and Yungblath M, "Laboratory Diagnosis of Viral Respiratory Tract Infections," *Lab Med*, 1993, 24:150-7.

Heilman CA, "From the National Institute of Allergy and Infectious Diseases and the World Health Organization. Respiratory Syncytial and Parainfluenza Viruses," *J Infect Dis*, 1990, 161(3):402-6.

Waner JL, "Parainfluenza Viruses," *Manual of Clinical Microbiology*, 6th ed, Murray PR, Baron EJ, Pfaller MA, et al, eds, Washington, DC: American Society for Microbiology, 1995, 926-31.

Parainfluenza Virus, Direct Detection *see* Virus, Direct Detection by Fluorescent Antibody *on page 682*

Poliovirus Culture *see* Enterovirus Culture *on page 666*

Poliovirus Culture, Stool *see* Viral Culture, Stool *on page 680*

Prostate, Viral Culture *see* Viral Culture, Urogenital *on page 681*

Rabid Animals *see* Rabies *on this page*

Rabies

CPT 88305 (brain/meninges, other than for tumor resection); 88307 (brain biopsy); 88312 (special stains); 88346 (immunofluorescence)

Related Information

Viral Culture, Central Nervous System Symptoms *on page 677*
Virus, Direct Detection by Fluorescent Antibody *on page 682*

Synonyms Rabid Animals

Applies to Fluorescent Rabies Antibody Test; FRA Test; Negri Bodies

Test Commonly Includes Microscopy for Negri bodies, human skin biopsy using direct immunofluorescent antibody

Abstract Rabies, caused by strains of highly neurotropic viruses,[1] has been a recognized disease in humans and animals for more than 25 centuries. Rabies virus is capable of infecting a number of different animal species. Individuals with a high risk of contact with rabid animals (veterinarians, animal control officers, etc) should consider vaccination

against rabies. Human exposure to bats, followed by skunks, foxes, and dogs, has been responsible for all but a single case of rabies acquired in the United States.

Specimen Head of large animal or entire small animal suspected of rabies. Use gloves and mask when handling an animal carcass suspected of rabies.

Human diagnosis is possible through laboratory investigation of cerebrospinal fluid, serum, saliva, or biopsy of brain or nuchal skin.

Container Sealed container

Collection A 6-8 mm full thickness wedge or punch biopsy specimen from the neck containing as many hair follicles as possible should be sampled, snap frozen, and shipped frozen at -70°C to a reference laboratory. Consult with reference laboratory for shipping instructions. False-negative results occur especially after the development of neutralizing antibodies.[1]

Storage Instructions Ideally, animal brain should be examined in the fresh state. Transport using wet ice or place in absorbent material, then in two plastic bags, or, place half the brain in 50% glycerol, half in 10% formalin, depending on instructions from state laboratory. Local state laboratory must be consulted. Rabies virus may also be demonstrated by immunofluorescence in skin biopsies of patients suspected of having rabies (*vide infra*).

Causes for Rejection Unlabeled or improperly packaged specimen

Use Diagnose rabies; evaluate animal bites and exposure to possibly rabid animals for candidacy for rabies immune globulin and/or rabies vaccine.[2,3]

Limitations Negri bodies (viral inclusions in neurons) are found in about 90% of rabid animals.

Contraindications Formalin fixation precludes fluorescent antibody application

Methodology The preferred diagnostic test for rabies is the direct immunofluorescent antibody (DFA) for detection of rabies virus antigen in brain or skin tissue;[4] Negri bodies can be seen in H & E; nucleotide sequence analysis. Inoculation of mice with suspension of brain tissue is not available in routine laboratories.

Additional Information Human exposure to bats, followed by skunks, foxes, and dogs has been responsible for all but a single case of rabies in the U.S. acquired from animals.[2] Animals at risk for rabies include bats, skunks, raccoons, dogs, cats, foxes, and to a lesser extent, jackals, wolves, coyotes, mongooses, weasels, squirrels, cattle, and any escaped wild animal. Twelve of 25 cases of human rabies diagnosed in the U.S. since 1980 are associated with variants of rabies virus related to bats. A clear history of bite was only documented in six.[5] Bites of rabbits, squirrels, hamsters, guinea pigs, gerbils, chipmunks, rats, mice, and other rodents have seldom if ever resulted in human rabies in the United States and are regarded as low risk.

Domestic animals should be kept alive if possible, to be quarantined. Animal bites, when unprovoked, are more likely to transmit rabies.[3] Survival of animal for 10 days makes rabies unlikely. Signs of rabies among wild carnivorous animals cannot be reliably interpreted; any such animal that bites or scratches a person should be killed at once and the head submitted for rabies testing.

The geographic area is important. Although a dog bite along the U.S.-Mexican border is considered a rabies exposure until proven otherwise, such bites in other portions of the U.S. may not require immediate prophylaxis while the animal is confined and observed for 10 days. Dogs in the U.S. are at extremely low risk for rabies with the exception of those along the border with Mexico.[2] Most Americans dying of rabies were exposed in foreign countries. One patient, bitten by a rabid dog in Kenya, had even had pre-exposure prophylaxis with human diploid cell vaccine. This emphasizes the **necessity for postexposure therapy in appropriate cases.**[6] Almost all rabies follows bite exposure. However, rabies virus can enter through nonbite exposure, such as an open wound, or by inhalation of aerosolized bat urine (eg, cave explorers) or by corneal transplantation.[2] The table lists location of exposure to rabid canine bites and extent of exposure as it relates to mortality rates. The proportion of cases for which the source of exposure is not known has been increasing since 1960.[7]

Antemortem rabies virus has been isolated from human saliva, brain tissues, CSF, urine sediment, and tracheal secretions. Rabies virus may also be demonstrated by immunofluorescent rabies antibody staining of skin biopsy tissue. The most reliable and reproducible of the immunofluorescent studies that can aid in patient diagnosis is biopsy of the neck skin.

Footnotes

1. Bernard KW and Fishbein DB, "Rabies Virus," *Principles and Practice of Infectious Diseases*, Chapter 140, Mandell GL, Douglas RG Jr, and Bennett JE, eds, New York, NY: Churchill Livingstone, 1990, 1291-1301.
2. Fishbein DB and Robinson LE, "Rabies," *N Engl J Med*, 1993, 329(22):1632-8.
3. "Mass Treatment of Humans Exposed to Rabies - New Hampshire, 1994," *MMWR Morb Mortal Wkly Rep*, 1995, 44(26):484-6.

Representative Mortality Rates in Nonvaccinated Individuals Following Exposure to Rabid Canines

Location of Exposure	Extent of Exposure	Mortality (%)
Face	Bites (multiple and severe)	60
Other part of head	Bites (multiple and severe)	50
Face	Bite (single)	30
Fingers/hand	Bite (severe)	15
Face	Bites (multiple and superficial)	10
Hand	Bites (multiple and superficial)	5
Trunk/legs	Scratch	3
Hands/exposed skin	Bleeding and superficial wound	2
Skin covered by clothes	Superficial wound	0.5
Recent wound	Saliva	0.1
Wounds >24 h old	Saliva	0.0

From Whitley RJ and Middlebrooks M, "Rabies," *Infections of the Central Nervous System*, Chapter 7, Scheld WM, Whitley RJ, and Durack DT, eds, New York, NY: Raven Press, 1991, 134, with permission.

4. Trimarchi CV and Debbie J, "The Fluorescent Antibody in Rabies," *The Natural History of Rabies*, 2nd ed, Baer GM, ed, Boca Raton, FL: CRC Press, 1991, 219-33.
5. Centers for Disease Control and Prevention, "Human Rabies - Washington 1995," *MMWR Morb Mortal Wkly Rep*, 1995, 44(34):625-7.
6. Centers for Disease Control, "Human Rabies - Kenya," *MMWR Morb Mortal Wkly Rep*, 1983, 32:494-5.
7. Smith JS, Fishbein DB, Rupprecht CE, et al, "Unexplained Rabies in Three Immigrants in the United States. A Virologic Investigation," *N Engl J Med*, 1991, 324(4):205-11.

References
"Human Rabies - Miami, 1994," *MMWR Morb Mortal Wkly Rep*, 1994, 43(42):773-5.
"Human Rabies - New York, 1993," *MMWR Morb Mortal Wkly Rep*, 1993, 42(41):799, 806.
"Raccoon Rabies Epizootic - United States, 1993," *MMWR Morb Mortal Wkly Rep*, 1994, 43(15):269-73.
Mrak RE and Young L, "Rabies Encephalitis in a Patient With No History of Exposure," *Hum Pathol*, 1992, 24(1):109-10.
Mrak RE and Young L, "Rabies Encephalitis in Humans: Pathology, Pathogenesis and Pathophysiology," *J Neuropathol Exp Neurol*, 1994, 53(1):1-10.
Nadin-Davis SA, Casey GA, Wandeler AI, "A Molecular Epidemiological Study of Rabies Virus in Central Ontario and Western Quebec," *J Gen Virol*, 1994, 75(Pt 10):2575-83.
Pearlman ES and Ballas SK, "False-Positive Human Immunodeficiency Virus Screening Test Related to Rabies Vaccination," *Arch Pathol Lab Med*, 1994, 118(8):805-6.
Whitley RJ and Middlebrooks M, "Rabies," *Infections of the Central Nervous System*, Scheld WM, Whitley RJ, and Durack DT, eds, New York, NY: Raven Press, 1991, 134.

Rabies Virus, Direct Detection *see* Virus, Direct Detection by Fluorescent Antibody *on page 682*

Respiratory Syncytial Virus Antigen Detection
CPT 86756

Related Information
Respiratory Syncytial Virus Culture *on this page*
Respiratory Syncytial Virus Serology *on page 426*
Viral Culture, Respiratory Symptoms *on page 680*
Virus, Direct Detection by Fluorescent Antibody *on page 682*

Synonyms RSV Antigen

Test Commonly Includes Detection of RSV antigen in specimens using enzyme immunoassay (EIA)

Abstract Respiratory syncytial virus (RSV), an RNA virus, was first isolated in 1956. It causes most acute lower respiratory disease in infants and young children, and is the cause of most fatal respiratory disease in children younger than 2 years of age. Forty percent of infected children younger than 2 years of age develop lower respiratory tract disease. Hypoxemia is common.

Specimen Nasopharyngeal secretions (nasal washings or aspirates) are preferred; nasopharyngeal swab is acceptable

Collection Swabs must be placed in cold viral transport medium. Soft catheters and suction devices can be used to collect nasal secretions. Nasal washings are done by carefully introducing sterile saline (3-7 mL) into the nasal cavity and aspirating the fluid.

Storage Instructions Can be transported at room temperature without loss of viral antigens.

Turnaround Time 1 day; some laboratories may have a few hours turnaround time

Critical Values Positive results

Use Rapid diagnosis of bronchiolitis, lower respiratory disease caused by RSV, and other disease including otitis media

Methodology Enzyme-linked immunosorbent assay (ELISA), direct fluorescent antibody (DFA) recognize about 85% of cases

Additional Information Respiratory syncytial virus (RSV) is very labile. The detection of RSV antigen allows for detection of virus in specimens in which virus is not culturable. EIA is considered more sensitive than culture. Specimen handling requirements are not as stringent as those required for culture or immunofluorescence. The EIAs used to detect RSV antigen are simple, objective, and quick.

References
Falsey AR, Cunningham CK, Barker WH, et al, "Respiratory Syncytial Virus and Influenza A Infections in the Hospitalized Elderly," *J Infect Dis*, 1995, 172(2):389-94.
Kellogg JA, "Culture Vs Direct Antigen Assays for Detection of Microbi al Pathogens From Lower Respiratory Tract Specimens Suspected of Containing the Respiratory Syncytial Virus," *Arch Pathol Lab Med*, 1991, 115(5):451-8.
Kuzel RJ and Clutter DJ, "Current Perspectives on Respiratory Syncytial Virus Infection," *Postgrad Med*, 1993, 93(1):129-32, 37-8, 41.
Long SS, "Parainfluenza Viruses," *Principles and Practice of Pediatrics*, 2nd ed, Oski FA, DeAngelis CD, Feigin RD, et al, eds, Philadelphia, PA: JB Lippincott Co, 1994, 1296-9.
Olsen MA, Shuck KM, and Sambol AR, "Evaluation of Abbott TestPack RSV for the Diagnosis of Respiratory Syncytial Virus Infections," *Diagn Microbiol Infect Dis*, 1993, 16(2):105-9.
Olsen MA, Shuck KM, Sambol AR, et al, "Performance of the Kallestad Pathfinder Enzyme Immunoassay in the Diagnosis of Respiratory Syncytial Virus Infections," *Diagn Microbiol Infect Dis*, 1993, 16(4):325-9.
Siqueira MM, Nascimento JP, Portes SA, et al, "Enzyme Immunoassay for Respiratory Syncytial Virus: Rapid Detection in Nasopharyngeal Secretions and Evaluation of Isolates Representing Different RSV Subgroups," *J Clin Lab Anal*, 1993, 7(2):130-3.
Smith TF, Wold AD, Espy MJ, et al, "New Developments in the Diagnosis of Viral Diseases," *Infect Dis Clin North Am*, 1993, 7(2):183-201.
van Milaan AJ, Sprenger AJ, Rothbarth PH, et al, "Detection of Respiratory Syncytial Virus by RNA-Polymerase Chain Reaction and Differentiation of Subgroups With Oligonucleotide Probes," *J Med Virol*, 1994, 44(1):80-7.
Walker TA, Khurana S, and Tilden SJ, "Viral Respiratory Infections," *Pediatr Clin North Am*, 1994, 41(6):1365-81.
Waner JL, "Mixed Viral Infections: Detection and Management," *Clin Microbiol Rev*, 1994, 7(2):143-51.

Respiratory Syncytial Virus Culture
CPT 87140 (culture typing, fluorescent method); 87252 (tissue culture, inoculation and observation); 87253 (tissue culture, additional studies, each isolate)

Related Information
Respiratory Syncytial Virus Antigen Detection *on this page*
Respiratory Syncytial Virus Serology *on page 426*
Viral Culture, Respiratory Symptoms *on page 680*
Virus, Direct Detection by Fluorescent Antibody *on page 682*

Synonyms RSV Culture

Test Commonly Includes Conventional culture or rapid culture using specific monoclonal antibodies for respiratory syncytial virus (RSV). May also include concurrent culture for other respiratory viruses (influenza, adenovirus, and parainfluenza viruses).

Abstract Respiratory syncytial virus (RSV) is the most common viral agent causing infant lower respiratory illnesses. By the first year of life, 50% of infants have experienced an RSV infection. Common symptoms are fever, wheezing, lower respiratory tract congestion, cough, and rhinorrhea.

Specimen Throat or nasopharyngeal swab, nasopharyngeal washes and secretions

Container Cold viral transport medium for swabs

Collection Place swabs into cold viral transport medium and keep cold. Infants and small children: soft catheters and suction devices (syringes and suction bulbs) can be used to collect nasal secretions from far back in the nose (best specimens). Another excellent method is to introduce 3-7 mL of sterile saline into the child's posterior nasal cavity and immediately aspirate the fluid. Do not use **cold** sterile saline when aspirating samples. Warm to room temperature.

Storage Instructions Respiratory syncytial virus is extremely labile. **Do not freeze specimens at -20°C.** Send specimens to the laboratory **as soon as possible.** Although less than optimal conditions, specimens can be stored up to 48 hours at 4°C. If necessary specimen can be quickly frozen at -70°C, but freezing will cause loss of infectivity.

Turnaround Time Conventional culture: 1-14 days; rapid culture: 1-2 days

Reference Range No virus isolated

Critical Values Positive results

Use Sputum characterized by acute inflammation, without a distinctive pattern of bacteria, may represent *Legionella*, influenza, or RSV. Culture supports diagnosis of respiratory disease caused by respiratory syncytial virus.

Limitations Culture is not available in many clinical laboratories. Rapid methods will only detect specified virus(es), negative culture does not rule out RSV infection. RSV is a very thermolabile virus and may not survive transport to the laboratory or extreme conditions. Thus, false-negative cultures occur.

Methodology Inoculation of specimen into cell cultures, incubation of cultures, observation for characteristic cytopathic effect (CPE) in 2-7 days, and identification by fluorescent monoclonal antibodies specific for

(Continued)

Respiratory Syncytial Virus Culture *(Continued)*

respiratory syncytial virus. The use of a rapid shell viral culture technique is reported to yield positive culture results overnight.[1]

Additional Information In healthy individuals, the mortality rate due to RSV infection is low; however, in patients with respiratory or cardiac compromise, immune dysfunction, and elderly, the mortality rate is high (~ 37%).[2,3]

Many laboratories offer enzyme immunoassay (EIA) tests for the direct detection of RSV in patient nasopharyngeal swab specimens. In general, these tests are very rapid, sensitive, and specific. Serology is available to detect antibodies to respiratory syncytial virus, but antigen detection from nasopharyngeal washings is better for patient care.[4]

Footnotes
1. Mathey S, Nicholson D, Ruhs S, et al, "Rapid Detection of Respiratory Viruses by Shell Vial Culture and Direct Staining by Using Pooled and Individual Monoclonal Antibodies," *J Clin Microbiol*, 1992, 30(3):540-4.
2. Falsey AR, Cunningham CK, Barker WH, et al, "Respiratory Syncytial Virus and Influenza A Infections in the Hospitalized Elderly," *J Infect Dis*, 1995, 172(2):389-94.
3. Whimbey E, Couch RB, and Englund JA, "Respiratory Syncytial Virus Pneumonia in Hospitalized Adult Patients With Leukemia," *Clin Infect Dis*, 1995, 21(2):376-9.
4. Bruner TA and Fedorko DP, "Opportunities for Rapid Viral Diagnosis," *Clin Microbiol Newslet*, 1993, 15(9):65-9.

References
Hemming VG, Prince GA, Groothuis JR, et al, "Hyperimmune Globulins in Prevention and Treatment of Respiratory Syncytial Virus Infections," *Clin Microbiol Rev*, 1995, 8(1):22-33.

Ottolini MG and Hemming VG, "Respiratory Syncytial Viral Infection: An Old Problem Presents New Challenges," *Infect Med*, 1994, 11(5):342, 347-54, 360.

Takimoto CH, Cram DL, and Root RK, "Respiratory Synctial Virus Infections on an Adult Medical Ward," *Arch Intern Med*, 1991, 151(4):706-8.

Toms GL, "Respiratory Syncytial Virus: Virology, Diagnosis, and Vaccination," *Lung*, 1990, 168 (Suppl):388-95.

Wiedbrauk DL, Freij BJ, and Ruben BE, "Adult Respiratory Syncytial Virus Infections," *Clin Microbiol Newslet*, 1993, 15(8):62-4.

Yungbluth M, "The Laboratory Diagnosis of Pneumonia. The Role of the Community Hospital Pathologist," *Clin Lab Med*, 1995, 15(2):209-34.

Rotavirus Antigen Detection *see* Rotavirus, Direct Detection *on this page*

Rotavirus Detection by EM *see* Electron Microscopic Examination for Viruses, Stool *on page 665*

Rotavirus, Direct Detection

CPT 86313 (immunoassay, multiple step); 86315 (single step)

Related Information
Bacterial Culture, Stool *on page 466*
Electron Microscopic Examination for Viruses, Stool *on page 665*
Ova and Parasites, Stool *on page 494*
Rotavirus Serology *on page 428*
Viral Culture, Stool *on page 680*

Synonyms Rotavirus Antigen Detection

Applies to Viral Antigen Detection, Direct, Stool

Test Commonly Includes Direct (nonculture) detection of rotavirus in stool specimens

Abstract Rotavirus infection is acquired by the fecal-oral route. Generally the incubation period is 1-2 days and the onset is abrupt. Symptoms include vomiting, diarrhea, fever, and abdominal pain. Loss of fluids is the most severe result of rotavirus infection and can lead to severe dehydration. Nosocomial transmission is frequent.[1]

Specimen Stool from the acute, diarrheal phase of disease; rectal swab

Sampling Time 3-5 days after onset

Collection Several specimens during the course of illness should be submitted in an attempt to eliminate false-negative results.

Reference Range No virus detected

Use Evaluation of patients in whom viral gastroenteritis is suspected; differential diagnosis of acute onset winter gastroenteritis, diarrhea, emesis

Limitations A commercially available EIA kit for stool for the detection of rotavirus led to false-positives when used in healthy neonates, but results in symptomatic subjects were reliable.

Methodology Latex agglutination (LA), enzyme immunoassay (EIA), enzyme-linked immunosorbent assay (ELISA), radioimmunoassay (RIA), dot blot technology. RIA and dot blot are definitive procedures but less widely used. Enzyme immunoassays (EIA) is the preferred diagnostic methods. In general, these assays detect the highly conserved internal capsid protein of the rotavirus group.

Additional Information Rotavirus is a common cause of pediatric gastroenteritis. The illness is most likely to occur in winter, is highly contagious, involves 5-8 days of diarrhea, and is rarely fatal.[2] Patients should also be evaluated for possible bacterial gastroenteritis. If available, electron microscopy is a useful technique for detection of rotavirus in stool specimens. Other viral agents causing gastroenteritis are enteric

adenoviruses, caliciviruses, astroviruses, coronaviruses, and Norwalk and Norwalk-like viruses.

Footnotes
1. Christensen ML, "Human Viral Gastroenteritis," *Clin Microbiol Rev*, 1989, 2(1):51-89.
2. Blacklow NR and Greenberg HB, "Viral Gastroenteritis," *N Engl J Med*, 1991, 325(4):252-64.

References
Christensen ML, "Rotaviruses," *Manual of Clinical Microbiology*, 6th ed, Murray PR, Baron EJ, Pfaller MA, et al, eds, Washington, DC: American Society for Microbiology, 1995, 1012-6.

Gray LD, "Novel Viruses Associated With Gastroenteritis," *Clin Microbiol Newslet*, 1991, 13(18):137-44.

Kaplan SL, "Rapid Diagnostic Techniques in Microbiology," *Principles and Practice of Pediatrics*, 2nd ed, Oski FA, DeAngelis CP, Feigin RD, et al, eds, Philadelphia, PA: JB Lippincott, 1994, 1450-3.

RSV Antigen *see* Respiratory Syncytial Virus Antigen Detection *on previous page*

RSV Culture *see* Respiratory Syncytial Virus Culture *on previous page*

Rubella Virus Culture

CPT 87252 (tissue culture, inoculation and observation); 87253 (tissue culture, additional studies, each isolate)

Related Information
Rubella Serology *on page 428*
Viral Culture *on next page*

Synonyms 3-Day Measles Culture; German Measles Culture

Test Commonly Includes Isolation and identification of rubella virus in cell culture

Specimen Two throat swabs, 10 mL urine, cerebrospinal fluid, tissues, amniotic fluid

Container Sterile container or viral transport medium

Sampling Time Virus is more likely to be isolated if specimen is collected within 5 days after onset of illness.

Storage Instructions Specimens should not be stored. Specimens should be delivered immediately to the laboratory. If unavoidable delays occur the specimen can be stored at 4°C for up to 3 days, but there is a loss of infectivity when culture is delayed.

Turnaround Time Positive cultures are usually detected in 3-7 days.

Reference Range No virus isolated

Critical Values Positive culture from amniotic fluid

Use Aid in the diagnosis of disease caused by rubella virus (eg, congenital viral infection)

Limitations Isolation of rubella virus is usually of little help in the diagnosis of rubella except in cases of severe rubella complications, epidemiological purposes, and fatality. Serological diagnosis is much more useful.

Methodology Cell culture, isolation, and confirmation/identification by antibody-specific neutralization

Additional Information The incidence of rubella has been reduced dramatically by the wide use of immunization in children. However, rubella can still occur in older people who were not vaccinated or people who have immigrated to the United States from countries in which vaccination for rubella is not common.[1] Pregnant women, who become infected with rubella, have a very high risk of virus crossing the placenta and infecting the fetus. Congenital rubella infections have disastrous effects, causing fetal death, premature delivery, and severe congenital defects including deafness and congenital heart disease. Neonates with congenital rubella excrete rubella virus in nasopharyngeal secretions and urine for many months after birth. These children pose a risk to susceptible pregnant women.[2] Serology is available for diagnostic purposes. Usually immune status can be determined by examining a single serum sample.

Footnotes
1. Centers for Disease Control, "Rubella and Congenital Rubella Syndrome - United States, January 1, 1994-May 7, 1994," *MMWR Morb Mortal Wkly Rep*, 1994, 43(21):391, 397-401.
2. Herrman KL, "Rubella Virus," *Laboratory Diagnosis of Viral Infections*, Lennette EH, ed, New York, NY: Marcel Dekker Inc, 1992, 731-47.

References
Chernesky MA and Mahony JB, "Rubella Virus," *Manual of Clinical Microbiology*, 6th ed, Murray PR, Baron EJ, Pfaller MA, et al, eds, Washington, DC: American Society for Microbiology, 1995, 968-73.

Shell Vial Culture, Adenovirus *see* Adenovirus Culture *on page 662*

Shingles Culture *see* Varicella-Zoster Virus Culture *on next page*

Skin Viral Disease *see* Electron Microscopic Examination for Viruses, Stool *on page 665*

Synovial Fluid, Viral Culture *see* Viral Culture, Body Fluid *on page 677*

TRIC Agent Culture *see Chlamydia trachomatis* Culture *on page 662*

***Ureaplasma urealyticum* Culture, Genital** *see* Genital Culture for *Ureaplasma urealyticum on page 667*

Urethral *Chlamydia* Culture *see Chlamydia trachomatis* Culture *on page 662*

Urethral Culture for T-Strain *Mycoplasma* *see* Genital Culture for *Ureaplasma urealyticum on page 667*

Urethra, Viral Culture *see* Viral Culture, Urogenital *on page 681*

Varicella-Zoster Virus Culture

CPT 87140 (culture typing, fluorescent method); 87252 (tissue culture, inoculation and observation); 87253 (tissue culture, additional studies, each isolate)

Related Information

Skin Biopsy *on page 54*
Varicella-Zoster Virus Serology *on page 437*
Viral Culture *on this page*
Viral Culture, Central Nervous System Symptoms *on page 677*
Viral Culture, Dermatological Symptoms *on page 679*
Virus, Direct Detection by Fluorescent Antibody *on page 682*

Synonyms Chickenpox Culture; Shingles Culture; VZV Culture

Applies to Viral Culture, Rash; Viral Culture, Skin

Test Commonly Includes Rapid culture by detection of virus using immunofluorescence staining with specific monoclonal antibody. Varicella-zoster virus (VZV) also is usually detected in a routine viral culture.

Abstract Varicella or chickenpox in children and herpes zoster or shingles (reactivated latent infection) in adults are caused by varicella-zoster virus. Persistent pain (postherpetic neuralgia) following zoster can be debilitating.

Specimen Swab specimens of the base of fresh, unroofed lesions, vesicle fluid, vesicle scrapings; blood or bronchial washings (immunocompromised patients); cerebrospinal fluid. In addition, acute and convalescent sera should be collected at appropriate times to document a clinically significant rise in antibody titer.

Container Cold viral transport medium for swab specimens; green top (heparin) tube for blood; sterile CSF tube; syringe or sterile capillary pipet can be used to collect vesicular fluid

Sampling Time Specimens should be collected during the acute phase of the disease (within 3 days of lesion eruption).

Collection Unroofed lesions should be cleaned before specimens are taken. Vesicular fluid from several vesicles can be pooled in a single syringe and sent to the laboratory undiluted. Alternatively, the bases of several freshly unroofed lesions can be vigorously sampled with a sterile swab which subsequently should be placed into cold viral transport medium and sent to the laboratory as soon as possible.

Storage Instructions Keep specimens cold and moist. **Do not freeze specimens at -20°C**. VZV is extremely labile. If immediate inoculation onto cell cultures is not possible, specimens should be frozen quickly at -70°C. Freezing at -70°C will reduce infectivity 10% to 30%.

Turnaround Time Conventional culture: 1-14 days; rapid culture: 2-5 days

Reference Range No virus isolated

Critical Values Positive culture from CSF or blood

Use Aid in the diagnosis of disease caused by varicella-zoster virus (ie, chickenpox and shingles). Varicella-zoster virus is a single virus which causes two diseases: **chickenpox** (varicella) in children and, after reactivation from latency, **shingles** (zoster) in adults.

Limitations Rapid method will only detect specified virus(es), negative culture does not rule out viral infection. VZV is extremely labile and many times cannot be isolated from specimens which have been transported and/or stored in adverse conditions. Cell culture of VZV is less sensitive than direct antigen detection of VZV by immunofluorescence.[1] PCR for VZV DNA is even more sensitive, but it is expensive and turnaround times are likely to be problematic.

Methodology Routine cultures: Inoculation of specimens into cell cultures, incubation of cultures, observation for characteristic cytopathic effect (CPE), and identification by fluorescent monoclonal antibody

Rapid cultures: Specimens are centrifuged onto cell cultures grown on coverslips in the bottoms of 1-dram shell vials. Centrifugation greatly accelerates virus attachment and penetration. After incubation, fluorescein-labeled monoclonal antibodies are applied to the infected cells to detect viral antigens. Characteristic fluorescent foci indicate the presence of virus.

Additional Information Disease caused by VZV is usually self-limited. However, the disease can be life-threatening in pregnant persons, immunocompromised persons, children who receive cancer therapy following organ transplantation, and in fetuses exposed during pregnancy. Complications include dissemination, pneumonitis, myocarditis, cardiomyopathy, hepatitis, and meningoencephalitis. Congenital chickenpox can result in neonatal systemic disease and/or congenital malformations. Congenital varicella syndrome in 2%. People suffering from AIDS can have prolonged reactivated VZV infections.[2,3]

Serology for the detection of VZV antibodies is available. See listing Varicella-Zoster Virus Serology *on page 437*. Rapid turnaround time of serological tests can be especially important in detecting the presence of antibody (prior exposure) in pregnant women who have been exposed to individuals with chickenpox. In these cases VZV-specific immunoglobulin should be given within 3 days (maximum) of exposure.

Footnotes

1. Rawlinson WD, Dwyer DE, Gibbons V, et al, "Rapid Diagnosis of Varicella-Zoster Virus Infection With a Monoclonal Antibody Based Direct Immunofluorescence Technique," *J Virol Methods*, 1989, 23(1):13-8.
2. Glesby MJ, Moore RD, and Chaisson RE, "Clinical Spectrum of Herpes Zoster in Adults Infected With Human Immunodeficiency Virus," *Clin Infect Dis*, 1995, 21(2):370-5.
3. LeBoit PE, Límouá M, Yen TS, et al, "Chronic Verrucous Variella-Zoster Virus Infection in Patients With the Acquired Immunodeficiency Syndrome (AIDS). Histologic and Molecular Biologic Findings," *Am J Dermatopathol*, 1992, 14(1):1-7.

References

Choo PW, Donahue JG, Manson JE, et al, "The Epidemiology of Varicella and its Complications," *J Infect Dis*, 1995, 172(3):706-12.
Houston SH, Sinnott JT 4th, Murphy SJ, et al, "Chickenpox in Pregnancy," *Infect Med*, 1994, 11(8):564-8.
Hughes JH, "Physical and Chemical Methods for Enhancing Rapid Detection of Viruses and Other Agents," *Clin Microbiol Rev*, 1993, 6(2):150-75.
Schirm J, Meulenberg JJ, Pastoor GW, et al, "Rapid Detection of Varicella-Zoster Virus in Clinical Specimens Using Monoclonal Antibodies on Shell Vials and Smears," *J Med Virol*, 1989, 28(1):1-6.
Weller TH, "Varicella and Herpes Zoster: A Perspective and Overview," *J Infect Dis*, 1992, 166(Suppl 1):S1-6.

Varicella-Zoster Virus, Direct Detection *see* Virus, Direct Detection by Fluorescent Antibody *on page 682*

Vesicle Viral Culture *see* Viral Culture, Dermatological Symptoms *on page 679*

Viral Antigen Detection, Direct, Stool *see* Rotavirus, Direct Detection *on previous page*

Viral Culture

CPT 87252 (tissue culture, inoculation and observation); 87253 (tissue culture, additional studies, each isolate)

Related Information

Adenovirus Antibody Titer *on page 362*
Adenovirus Culture *on page 662*
Bacterial Culture, Blood *on page 457*
Bacterial Culture, Conjunctiva *on page 461*
Bacterial Culture, Genital Specimen *on page 463*
Bacterial Culture, Urine, Clean Catch *on page 468*
Body Fluid *on page 89*
Body Fluid Cytology *on page 286*
Bone Marrow *on page 307*
Cervical/Vaginal Cytology *on page 290*
Chlamydia trachomatis Genome Detection *on page 505*
Cytomegalovirus Culture *on page 664*
Enterovirus Culture *on page 666*
Herpes Cytology *on page 296*
Herpes Simplex Antibody *on page 401*
Herpes Simplex Virus Antigen Detection *on page 667*
Herpes Simplex Virus Culture *on page 668*
Herpes Simplex Virus DNA Detection *on page 514*
Histopathology *on page 42*
Influenza Virus Culture *on page 670*
Mumps Virus Culture *on page 670*
Parainfluenza Viral Serology *on page 420*
Parainfluenza Virus Culture *on page 671*
Pemphigus-Like Antibodies *on page 422*
Poliomyelitis I, II, III Titer *on page 423*
Rubella Virus Culture *on previous page*
Skin Biopsy *on page 54*
Skin Biopsy, Immunofluorescence *on page 56*
Urine Cytology *on page 301*
Varicella-Zoster Virus Culture *on this page*
Varicella-Zoster Virus Serology *on page 437*
Viral Culture, Blood *on page 677*
Viral Culture, Body Fluid *on page 677*
Viral Culture, Central Nervous System Symptoms *on page 677*
Viral Culture, Dermatological Symptoms *on page 679*
(Continued)

Viral Culture *(Continued)*

Viral Culture, Eye or Ocular Symptoms *on page 679*
Viral Culture, Stool *on page 680*
Viral Culture, Tissue *on page 680*
Viral Culture, Urine *on page 681*

Applies to CPE; Cytopathic Effect

Test Commonly Includes Inoculation of specimen onto appropriate cell cultures; isolated viruses are identified using specific monoclonal antibodies, neutralization, or hemadsorption

Abstract Some viral diseases can be diagnosed by the isolation of virus in tissue culture cells. However, specimens for viral culture must be collected within the first few days of an illness and specimens should be brought to the laboratory in viral holding media as quickly as possible. This helps to ensure adequate sensitivity of viral culture.

Specimen Whole blood, cerebrospinal fluid, dermal, ocular, genital, mucosal, respiratory, oral, stool, rectal, urine, tissue, biopsy. See table. Whenever a viral etiology is suspected and whenever appropriate, acute and convalescent serum should be collected for viral serology.

Viruses Typically Isolated From Clinical Specimens

Specimen	Virus*
Blood	CMV, enteroviruses†,#, HSV#, VZV#
CSF and CNS tissues	Enteroviruses, mumps virus, HSV, CMV
Dermal lesions	HSV, VZV, adenovirus, enteroviruses
Eye	HSV, VZV, adenovirus, enteroviruses, CMV, *Chlamydia*
Genital	HSV, CMV, *Chlamydia*
Mucosal	HSV, VZV
Oral	HSV, VZV
Rectal	HSV, VZV, enterovirus
Respiratory tract	
upper	Adenovirus, rhinovirus, influenza, parainfluenza, enteroviruses, RSV, reovirus, HSV
lower	Adenovirus, influenza, parainfluenza, RSV, CMV•
Stool	Enteroviruses, adenoviruses
Tissues	CMV, HSV, enteroviruses
Urine	CMV, adenovirus, enteroviruses, mumps

*Abbreviations:

HSV — herpes simplex virus

CMV — cytomegalovirus

VZV — varicella-zoster virus

RSV — respiratory syncytial virus

†Enteroviruses: coxsackie virus, poliovirus, echovirus, and enterovirus.

#Rarely isolated.

•Usually in immunocompromised hosts.

Container Viral transport medium for swabs; sterile screw-cap tube or container for fluids, feces, nasal washings, urine, or biopsy (without preservative); green top (heparin) tube for blood, bone marrow, and buffy coat. **Keep all specimens cold and moist.**

Collection Specimen should be collected during the acute phase of the disease, as follows:

Blood: 5 mL whole blood in heparinized tube

Cerebrospinal fluid: Collect 1 mL CSF aseptically in a sterile dry screw-cap vial. **Keep cold and bring to the laboratory immediately.**

Skin lesions: Open the vesicle and absorb exudate into a dry swab, and/or vigorously scrape base of freshly exposed lesion with a swab to obtain cells which contain viruses. If enough vesicle fluid is available, aspirate the fluid with a fine-gauge needle and tuberculin syringe, and place fluid into cold viral transport medium. Use Virocult® or Culturette® swabs for specimen collection. **Keep cold and bring to the laboratory immediately.**

Eye swab or scraping: Use a Virocult® or Culturette® swab to collect conjunctival material or take conjunctival scrapings with a fine sterile spatula and transfer the scraping to a viral transport medium. **Keep cold and bring to the laboratory immediately.**

Genital swab: See skin. **Keep cold and bring to the laboratory immediately.**

Throat swab: Carefully rub the posterior wall of the nasopharynx with a dry, sterile swab. Avoid touching the tongue or buccal mucosa. Use Virocult® or Culturette® swabs for specimen collection. **Keep cold and bring to the laboratory immediately.**

Feces: Collect 4-8 g of feces (about the size of a thumbnail), and place in a clean, leakproof container. Do **not** dilute the specimen (into virus transport medium) or use preservatives. **Keep cold and bring to the laboratory immediately.**

Rectal swab: Insert a sterile swab 2-4 inches into the rectum and rub the mucosa. Use Virocult® or Culturette® swabs for specimen collection. **Keep cold and bring to the laboratory immediately.** Swab may be placed into cold virus transport medium.

Urine: Collect clean-catch, midstream urine in a leakproof, sterile container. **Keep cold and bring to the laboratory immediately.**

Tissue: Use a fresh set of sterile instruments to collect each tissue. Place each specimen in its own dry, sterile nontoxic leakproof container. Identify each tissue with patient's name, type of tissue, and date collected. **Keep cold and bring tissue to the laboratory immediately.**

Calcium alginate swabs are toxic to *Chlamydia* and many enveloped viruses. **Do not use calcium alginate swabs for viral or chlamydial isolation.**

Storage Instructions Specimen must be kept cold and moist, and must be delivered to the laboratory as soon as possible. If a longer period is required, specimen should be stored or transported according to the laboratory that will receive the specimen. **Do not freeze specimens at -20°C;** if absolutely necessary store specimens at 4°C to 6°C or freeze quickly at -70°C. Specimens to be cultured for influenza virus and cytomegalovirus should be sent on wet ice or with an ice pack.

Causes for Rejection Dry specimen, specimen not refrigerated during transport, specimen fixed in formalin, unlabeled specimen

Turnaround Time The presence of viruses is usually suggested by the characteristic cytopathic effect (CPE) they cause when they infect cell cultures. CPE (and, therefore, positive results) can be observed as soon as 1 day and as late as 28 days postinoculation of the cell culture.[1]

Special Instructions Culture and serological tests for certain specific viruses are available. When possible, the serological tests should be requested at same time as culture. Acute and convalescent blood samples (5 mL) are required for serologic studies. Requisition **must** state specific virus(s) suspected, source of specimen, age of patient, current antibiotic therapy, relevant vaccinations, and pertinent clinical history.

Reference Range No virus isolated

Use Aid in the diagnosis of viral diseases (eg, AIDS, conjunctivitis, congenital viral infections, keratitis, chickenpox, shingles, viral pneumonia, and some diseases characterized by skin vesicles and rashes)

Limitations For all practical purposes, many common viruses are not culturable (see table). Isolation of virus may not be related to the patient's disease. Negative viral culture does not rule out a viral etiology. Some positive cultures are sent to State Health Laboratory for specific virus identification.

Viruses That Are Nonculturable or Require Animal Inoculation or Special Technique

Arenaviruses	Hepatitis D
Astrovirus	Hepatitis E
Calicivirus	Lassa
California encephalitis	Marburg
Coronaviruses	*Molluscum contagiosum*
Coxsackievirus type A	Norwalk agent
Dengue	Papillomaviruses
Eastern equine encephalitis	Parvoviruses
Ebola	Polyomavirus
Filoviruses	Rabies
Hantavirus (Muerto Canyon)	Rotaviruses
Hepatitis A	St Louis encephalitis
Hepatitis B	Western equine encephalitis
Hepatitis C	Yellow fever

Methodology Inoculation of specimen into cell cultures, incubation of cultures, observation for characteristic cytopathic effect (CPE), and identification by methods such as hemadsorption and fluorescent monoclonal antibodies. If specific viruses such as HSV, CMV, VZV, influenza, RSV, or parainfluenza, or adenovirus are suspected, the laboratory might be able to use rapid (1-2 days) culture (shell vial) methods to detect these viruses.

Additional Information Viral cultures: Specimens should be collected in the acute stage of the illness, kept moist, and refrigerated immediately. Whenever possible, specimens should be shipped so they will not arrive in a laboratory over the weekend. Stool specimens should not be placed into viral transport medium or frozen. Spinal fluid and throat washings must be kept cold and must not be frozen. Swabs of lesions or of throat should be rinsed immediately into 1 or 2 mL of viral transport medium; preferably, the swab should be broken off and sent in the medium to the laboratory. Autopsy material should be collected in sterile containers. Urine specimens for CMV culture **must not** be frozen; they should be packed with an ice pack or snow gel, but not with dry ice. **Serological tests:** Give date of onset of illness, date of collection of sera and either a brief clinical description or the provisional diagnosis. The acute serum (5 mL clotted blood or 2 mL serum) should be collected as early as possible, and the second or convalescent serum should be drawn 2-4 weeks later. Paired sera **should** be run in parallel, and a **fourfold rise** in antibody titer is suggestive of a current infection. The ordering physician should see that both specimens are obtained.

Footnotes

1. Yolken RH, "Laboratory Diagnosis of Viral Infections," *Practical Diagnosis of Viral Infections*, Galasso GJ, Whitley RJ, Merigan TC, eds, New York, NY: Raven Press, 1993, 17-67.

References

Forbes BA, "Perinatal Viral Infections," *Clin Microbiol Newslet*, 1992, 14:169-72.

Korones SB, "Uncommon Virus Infections of the Mother, Fetus, and Newborn: Influenza, Mumps, and Measles," *Clin Perinatol*, 1988, 15(2):259-72.

Lennette DA, "Collection and Preparation of Specimens for Virological Examination," *Manual of Clinical Microbiology*, 6th ed, Murray PR, Baron EJ, Pfaller MA, et al, eds, Washington, DC: American Society for Microbiology, 1995, 868-75.

Raj P, "Classification of Medically Important Viruses I: DNA Viruses," *Clin Microbiol Newslet*, 1994, 16(16):121-4.

Raj P, "Classification of Medically Important Viruses II: RNA Viruses," *Clin Microbiol Newslet*, 1994, 16(17):129-34.

Viral Culture, Biopsy see Viral Culture, Tissue on page 680

Viral Culture, Blood

CPT 87252 (tissue culture, inoculation and observation); 87253 (tissue culture, additional studies, each isolate)

Related Information

Bacterial Culture, Blood *on page 457*
Coxsackie A Virus Titer *on page 387*
Coxsackie B Virus Titer *on page 387*
Cytomegalovirus Culture *on page 664*
Enterovirus Culture *on page 666*
Epstein-Barr Virus Culture *on page 666*
Human Herpesvirus 6 Culture *on page 669*
Viral Culture *on page 675*

Synonyms CMV, Blood Culture; CMV, Buffy Coat Culture; CMV Culture; Enterovirus, Blood Culture

Test Commonly Includes Usually includes both rapid shell vial isolation technique (to detect CMV early) and/or conventional cell culture for all major viruses

Patient Preparation Cleanse skin with 70% isopropyl alcohol. Apply povidone-iodine in concentric circles. **Note:** Iodine should remain in contact with skin for at least 1 minute prior to venipuncture to ensure complete antisepsis. Remove iodine with 70% isopropyl alcohol in concentric circles after venipuncture. Obtain 3-6 mL of blood.

Specimen Whole blood

Container Green top (heparin) tube. Some laboratories request that blood be collected in citrate anticoagulant or EDTA. Alternatively, a blood specimen can be obtained in a (previously) heparinized syringe. The heparin should be sterile and free of preservative.

Sampling Time Collect blood during early acute phase of infection.

Storage Instructions Do not store specimen. Send to the laboratory immediately.

Turnaround Time Shell vial rapid isolation: 1-2 days; conventional culture: 2 days to 4 weeks

Use Aid in the diagnosis of systemic viral infections (eg, transplantation-associated viral diseases and congenital viral diseases)

Limitations Blood (serum in particular) is generally not a good specimen from which to recover viruses.

Methodology Inoculation of peripheral blood cells or serum onto cell cultures (either shell vials or tube cultures); identification of virus by cytopathic effect (CPE) and monoclonal antibodies

Additional Information White blood cells can be a source of CMV, and serum has been reported to be a source of enterovirus.[1] A recent study has shown that culture of two separate blood specimens increases the sensitivity of detecting CMV in transplant patients.[2] However, this is a time-consuming and expensive practice. See table in the listing Viral Culture *on page 676*.

Footnotes

1. Hughes JH, "Physical and Chemical Methods for Enhancing Rapid Detection of Viruses and Other Agents," *Clin Microbiol Rev*, 1993, 6(2):150-75.
2. Patel R, Klein DW, Espy MJ, et al, "Optimization of Detection of Cytomegalovirus Viremia in Transplantation Recipients by Shell Vial Assay," *J Clin Microbiol*, 1995, 33(11):2984-6.

References

Jacobson MA and Mills J, "Serious Cytomegalovirus Disease in the Acquired Immunode-ficiency Syndrome (AIDS). Clinical Findings, Diagnosis, and Treatment," *Ann Intern Med*, 1988, 108(4):585-94.

Lennette DA, "Collection and Preparation of Specimens for Virological Examination," *Manual of Clinical Microbiology*, 6th ed, Murray PR, Baron EJ, Pfaller MA, et al, eds, Washington, DC: American Society for Microbiology, 1995, 868-75.

Viral Culture, Body Fluid

CPT 87140 (culture typing, fluorescent method); 87252 (tissue culture, inoculation and observation); 87253 (tissue culture, additional studies, each isolate)

Related Information

Adenovirus Antibody Titer *on page 362*
Body Fluid *on page 89*
Body Fluid Analysis, Cell Count *on page 306*
Body Fluid Cytology *on page 286*
Bone Marrow *on page 307*
Coxsackie A Virus Titer *on page 387*
Coxsackie B Virus Titer *on page 387*
Viral Culture *on page 675*

Synonyms Body Fluid Viral Culture

Applies to Amniotic Fluid, Viral Culture; Cerebrospinal Fluid, Viral Culture; Synovial Fluid, Viral Culture

Specimen Body fluids (eg, cerebrospinal fluid, pleural fluid, pericardial fluid, amniotic fluid)

Collection Specimens obtained aseptically. **Do not place fluids into virus transport medium.** Keep specimens cold (2°C to 8°C) because viruses isolated from body fluids are often labile. Transport to the laboratory as soon as possible.

Turnaround Time Variable (1-28 days)

Reference Range No virus isolated

Use Aid in the diagnosis and differential diagnosis of systemic viral diseases (eg, etiologic agents causing **pericarditis** include adenovirus, enterovirus, coxsackie virus A or B, influenza virus, echovirus type 8, mumps, herpes simplex, and varicella-zoster). Other causes of pericarditis include *H. influenzae, M. tuberculosis*, histoplasmosis, meningococcus, Kawasaki disease, rheumatic fever, myxedema, SLE, scleroderma, rheumatoid arthritis, neoplasm including carcinoma of lung and breast, melanoma, lymphoma including Hodgkin's disease; postirradiation state and myocardial infarct.

Limitations If bacteria are suspected, a separate specimen must be submitted. Often, only a few virus-infected cells are present in fluids. Therefore, larger amounts of fluid are most productive, and specimens should be placed onto cell cultures as soon as possible.

Methodology Inoculation of specimen into cell cultures, incubation of cultures, observation for characteristic cytopathic effect (CPE), and identification/speciation by methods such as hemadsorption and fluorescent monoclonal antibodies. If specific viruses such as HSV, CMV, VZV, or adenovirus are suspected, the laboratory might be able to use rapid (1-2 days) culture (shell vial) methods to detect these viruses.

Additional Information See table in the listing Viral Culture *on page 676*.

References

Braunwald E, "Pericardial Disease," *Harrison's Principles of Internal Medicine*, 13th ed, Isselbacher KJ, Braunwald E, Wilson JD, et al, eds, New York, NY: McGraw-Hill, Inc, 1994, 1094-101.

Lennette DA, "Collection and Preparation of Specimens for Virological Examination," *Manual of Clinical Microbiology*, 6th ed, Murray PR, Baron EJ, Pfaller MA, et al, eds, Washington, DC: American Society for Microbiology, 1995, 868-75.

Smith TF, "Rapid Diagnosis of Viral Infections," *Adv Exp Med Biol*, 1990, 263:115-21.

Viral Culture, Brain see Viral Culture, Central Nervous System Symptoms *on this page*

Viral Culture, Brain see Viral Culture, Tissue *on page 680*

Viral Culture, Bronchial see Viral Culture, Tissue *on page 680*

Viral Culture, Bronchial Wash see Viral Culture, Respiratory Symptoms *on page 680*

Viral Culture, Central Nervous System Symptoms

CPT 87140 (culture typing, fluorescent method); 87252 (tissue culture, inoculation and observation); 87253 (tissue culture, additional studies, each isolate)

Related Information

Bacterial Antigens, Rapid Detection Methods *on page 454*
Bacterial Culture, Cerebrospinal Fluid *on page 460*
California Encephalitis Virus Titer *on page 374*
Cerebrospinal Fluid Analysis *on page 309*
Cerebrospinal Fluid Cytology *on page 290*
Cerebrospinal Fluid Glucose *on page 105*
Cerebrospinal Fluid Lactic Acid *on page 106*
Cerebrospinal Fluid Protein *on page 380*
Coxsackie A Virus Titer *on page 387*
Coxsackie B Virus Titer *on page 387*
Eastern Equine Encephalitis Virus Serology *on page 389*
Enterovirus Culture *on page 666*
Fungal Culture, Cerebrospinal Fluid *on page 477*
(Continued)

Viral Culture, Central Nervous System Symptoms
(Continued)

Synonyms Cerebrospinal Fluid Virus Culture

Applies to Lumbar Puncture Hazards; Viral Culture, Brain; Viral Culture, CSF

Abstract Viral meningitis is the most important cause of aseptic meningitis, a condition which has several clinical presentations and which has both infectious and noninfectious etiologies. Enteroviruses most often cause meningitis in the late summer. Patients are usually children and young adults. Enteroviruses include polioviruses, coxsackie viruses, and echoviruses. Ratzan provides a definition of viral meningitis as part of an aseptic meningitis syndrome characterized by acute disease with signs and symptoms of meningeal inflammation, pleocytosis (usually mononuclear), variable increase in protein content, normal glucose level, and no demonstrable organism by smear and culture of the cerebrospinal fluid.[1] By definition, the cerebrospinal fluid in aseptic meningitis will show a pleocytosis of white blood cells and will be culture-negative.[2]

Specimen Cerebrospinal fluid (do not put into virus transport medium), brain biopsy, lesions, throat or throat washings, stool, urine

Container Sterile CSF tube; sterile screw-cap container for biopsy, tissue, urine, or throat washing; sterile viral transport medium for swab specimens

Sampling Time As soon as possible after the onset of symptoms. Many viruses are more likely to be cultured when samples are obtained early.

Collection Specimen should be collected during the acute phase of the disease, as follows.

Cerebrospinal fluid: Collect 1 mL CSF aseptically in a sterile dry screw-cap vial. **Keep cold and bring to the laboratory immediately.**

The following specimens may be useful for diagnosis of CNS viral infection:

Eye swab or scraping

Skin lesions: Vigorously scrape base of freshly exposed lesion with a swab to obtain cells which contain viruses. Alternatively, open the vesicle and absorb exudate into a dry swab. If enough vesicle fluid is available, aspirate the fluid with a fine gauge needle and tuberculin syringe, and place the fluid into cold viral transport medium. Use Virocult® or Culturette® swabs for specimen collection. **Keep cold and bring to the laboratory immediately.** The clinical appearance of herpes zoster or the vesicles of herpes simplex may suggest the diagnosis. See listings Herpes Cytology *on page 296* and Skin Biopsy *on page 54.*

Throat swab: May be useful for identification of coxsackie, mumps, adenovirus, herpes type 1. Epstein-Barr virus may be recovered from throat washings. Infectious mononucleosis screening test should be done with examination of the peripheral blood smear.

Feces: Enterovirus, adenovirus, cytomegalovirus, herpes simplex, measles, and varicella-zoster virus may be recovered.

Urine: Mumps virus and cytomegalovirus may be recovered.

Genital swab

Storage Instructions Keep all specimens cold and moist. Transport to the laboratory immediately. Enteroviruses are relatively stable from -70°C to 4°C but are labile if allowed to dry or to be at room temperature for several hours. Specimens suspected of having varicella-zoster virus should never be frozen at -20°C or left at room temperature. Freezing at -20°C for 24 hours results in 99% reduction in viral isolation.

Turnaround Time Variable (1-28 days)

Reference Range No virus isolated

Critical Values Growth of virus in CSF

Use Determine etiological agent of viral CNS diseases (eg, aseptic meningitis, meningoencephalitis, polio, and encephalitis)

Limitations The CSF findings in tuberculous meningitis may simulate those of viral meningitis, especially herpes simplex and mumps. Negative viral culture does not rule out viral etiology.

Methodology Inoculation of specimen into cell cultures, incubation of cultures, observation for characteristic cytopathic effect (CPE), and identification/speciation by methods such as hemadsorption and fluorescent monoclonal antibodies. Several specific viruses can be isolated using a rapid (1-2 days) culture (shell vial) method. Bacterial culture, Gram's stain, cell count, glucose, and protein are needed to rule out bacterial meningitis.

Additional Information Arthropodborne (arbo) viruses and reoviruses are not considered culturable and may be detected indirectly by viral serology. See listings Eastern Equine Encephalitis Virus Serology *on page 389*, California Encephalitis Virus Titer *on page 374*, St Louis Encephalitis Virus Serology *on page 432*, and Western Equine Encephalitis Virus Serology *on page 439.*

The seasonal peak of viral meningitis in late summer is widely recognized and clinically significant in differential diagnosis.[1,3] The significance of seasonal curves for viral meningitis (more frequent in summer) versus bacterial meningitis is greater than most physicians recognize.[3] Meningitis caused by HIV, Epstein-Barr virus, CMV, or herpes simplex lacks seasonal variation.

Mumps meningitis is usually self limited and benign.[1] As with lymphocytic choriomeningitis and herpes simplex meningoencephalitis, hypoglycorrhachia may be found.

In the differential diagnosis between viral and bacterial meningitis, much higher CSF WBC count (>1180/mm^3) and protein (>220 mg/dL) are found in many cases of bacterial meningitis. Spanos' reported that in one group of studied patients no patient with acute viral meningitis had glucose <30.6 mg/dL but 43% of the patients with acute bacterial meningitis had glucose levels this low.[3] Although aseptic meningitis is usually characterized by mononuclear cells, PMNs may predominate early in the disease.[4,5,6] Hammer and Connolly summarized the typical CSF laboratory test profile in viral aseptic meningitis as one with WBC count <500/mm^3 with lymphocyte predominance, protein <100 mg/dL, and normal glucose.[6] Blood cultures are desirable because they are usually positive in infants and children with bacterial meningitis.[7] Five patients with mixed viral-bacterial meningitis of 276 patients with viral and/or bacterial culture proven meningitis have been described.[8] Many negative lumbar punctures in babies presenting with fever but without other specific findings have been reported.[9] In a study of 171 children with febrile convulsions, only one child had bacterial meningitis, and four children had aseptic meningitis.[9]

The outcome of chronic idiopathic meningitis is usually benign, but extensive studies are recommended including cultures for viruses, mycobacteria, fungi, and bacteria; cerebrospinal fluid syphilis serology; other cerebrospinal fluid and serum studies; and cerebrospinal fluid cytology.[10]

Complications of lumbar puncture (LP) are between 0.19% and 0.43%, reaching up to 35.5% when minor complications are included. Instances of meningitis and local infection are described following LP in subjects with bacteremia, who may be at risk for meningeal seeding during the puncture.[9,11] Repeat lumbar puncture may fail to identify patients who require further therapy.[11]

Nonviral causes of aseptic meningitis include meningeal carcinomatosis, collagen diseases, sarcoidosis, drugs (including antineoplastic agents and immunosuppressants, and materials used in radiology units), Mollaret's meningitis and many other entities.[5,12]

See table in test listing Viral Culture *on page 676* for the appropriate specimen that should be collected based on the suspected viral infection.

Culture for CMV in central nervous system diseases is relatively insensitive. PCR is becoming available.

Footnotes

1. Ratzan KR, "Viral Meningitis," *Med Clin North Am*, 1985, 69(2):399-413.
2. Polito JM 2d and Stollerman GH, "Aseptic Meningitis: A Case for Clinical Experience," *Hosp Pract (Off Ed)*, 1992, 27(5A):27-39.
3. Spanos A, Harrell FE Jr, and Durack DT, "Differential Diagnosis of Acute Meningitis - An Analysis of the Predictive Value of Initial Observations," *JAMA*, 1989, 262(19):2700-7.
4. Amir J, Harel L, Frydman M, et al, "Shift of Cerebrospinal Polymorphonuclear Cell Percentage in the Early Stage of Aseptic Meningitis," *J Pediatr*, 1991, 119(6):938-41.
5. Rubeiz H and Roos RP, "Viral Meningitis and Encephalitis," *Semin Neurol*, 1992, 12(3):165-77.
6. Hammer SM and Connolly KJ, "Viral Aseptic Meningitis in the United States: Clinical Features, Viral Etiologies, and Differential Diagnosis," *Curr Clin Top Infect Dis*, 1992, 12:1-25.
7. Sáez-Llorens X and McCracken GH Jr, "Bacterial Meningitis in Neonates and Children," *Infect Dis Clin North Am*, 1990, 4(4):623-44.
8. Sferra TJ and Pacini DL, "Simultaneous Recovery of Bacterial and Viral Pathogens From Cerebrospinal Fluid," *Pediatr Infect Dis J*, 1988, 7(8):552-6.
9. Levy M, Wong E, and Fried D, "Diseases That Mimic Meningitis. Analysis of 650 Lumbar Punctures," *Clin Pediatr (Phila)*, 1990, 29(5):254-5, 258-61.
10. Smith JE and Aksamit AJ Jr, "Outcome of Chronic Idiopathic Meningitis," *Mayo Clin Proc*, 1994, 69(6):548-56.
11. Fishman RA, *Cerebrospinal Fluid in Diseases of the Nervous System*, 2nd ed, Philadelphia, PA: WB Saunders Co, 1992, 266, 277-343.
12. Connolly KJ and Hammer SM, "The Acute Aseptic Meningitis Syndrome," *Infect Dis Clin North Am*, 1990, 4(4):599-622.

References

Behrman RE, Kliegman RM, Nelson WE, et al, *Nelson Textbook of Pediatrics*, 14th ed, Philadelphia, PA: WB Saunders Co, 1992, 664-6.

Chonmaitree T, Baldwin CD, Lucia HL, et al, "Role of the Virology Laboratory in Diagnosis and Management of Patients With Central Nervous System Disease," *Clin Microbiol Rev*, 1989, 2(1):1-14.

Greenlee JE, "Approach to Diagnosis of Meningitis - Cerebrospinal Fluid Evaluation," *Infect Dis Clin North Am*, 1990, 4(4):583-98.

Lennette DA, "Preparation of Specimens for Virological Examination," *Manual of Clinical Microbiology*, 5th ed, Balows A, Hausler WJ Jr, Herrmann KL, et al, eds, Washington, DC: American Society for Microbiology, 1991, 818-21.

Walsh-Kelly C, Nelson DB, Smith DS, et al, "Clinical Predictors of Bacterial Versus Aseptic Meningitis in Childhood," *Ann Emerg Med*, 1992, 21(8):910-4.

Viral Culture, CSF *see* Viral Culture, Central Nervous System Symptoms *on page 677*

Viral Culture, Cytomegalovirus *see* Cytomegalovirus Culture *on page 664*

Viral Culture, Dermatological Symptoms

CPT 87140 (culture typing, fluorescent method); 87252 (tissue culture, inoculation and observation); 87253 (tissue culture, additional studies, each isolate)

Related Information
Herpes Cytology *on page 296*
Herpes Simplex Virus Antigen Detection *on page 667*
Herpes Simplex Virus Culture *on page 668*
Skin Biopsy *on page 54*
Skin Biopsy, Immunofluorescence *on page 56*
Varicella-Zoster Virus Culture *on page 675*
Viral Culture *on page 675*
Viral Culture, Urogenital *on page 681*

Synonyms Vesicle Viral Culture; Viral Culture, Lesion; Viral Culture, Pustule; Viral Culture, Rash; Viral Culture, Skin/Dermatological Specimen; Viral Culture, Skin Scrapings; Viral Culture, Ulcer

Patient Preparation Do not prep skin with alcohol, iodine, or Betadine® prior to collection.

Specimen Scraping, swab, fluid of lesion

Container Viral transport medium for swabs

Sampling Time Preferably within 3 days of dermatological symptoms

Collection Specimen should be collected during the acute phase of the disease, as follows. **Skin lesions:** Open the vesicle and absorb exudate into a dry swab, and/or vigorously scrape base of freshly exposed lesion with a swab to obtain cells which contain viruses. If enough vesicle fluid is available, aspirate the fluid with a fine-gauge needle and tuberculin syringe, and place the fluid into cold viral transport medium. Use Virocult® or Culturette® swabs for specimen collection. **Keep cold and bring to the laboratory immediately,** especially if varicella-zoster virus is suspected.

Reference Range No virus isolated

Critical Values Isolation of varicella-zoster virus (VZV) or genital herpes simplex virus (HSV) from pregnant woman

Use Determine etiological agent of viral dermatological infections (eg, chickenpox, shingles, herpes, and vesiculobullous diseases of skin in which viral etiology is within the differential diagnosis)

Limitations Virus cannot always be cultured from skin lesions. Crusted lesions do not contain viral particles. For all practical purposes, measles virus is not culturable from patients.

Methodology Inoculation of specimen into cell cultures, incubation of cultures, observation for characteristic cytopathic effect (CPE), and identification/speciation by fluorescent monoclonal antibodies. If specific viruses such as HSV, VZV, or adenovirus are suspected, the laboratory might be able to use rapid (1-2 days) culture (shell vial) methods to detect these viruses.

Additional Information Virus shedding often diminishes rapidly after the onset of illness; therefore, it is important to collect specimens as early as possible after onset of symptoms.

Usually, only dermatological specimens are collected if rash is not associated with systemic disease (eg, HSV, VZV, and some enteroviruses). If systemic disease is associated with the rash, throat swab, rectal swab, stool, or serum can be taken for the isolation of other viruses (eg, enteroviruses, mumps virus, measles virus, and rubella virus). See table in the listing Viral Culture *on page 676*.

References
Nahass GT, Goldstein BA, Zhu W, et al, "Comparison of Tzanck Smear, Viral Culture, and DNA Diagnostic Methods in Detection of Herpes Simplex and Varicella-Zoster Infection (PCR)," *JAMA*, 1992, 268(18):2541-4.

Siegel CS, "Measles - A Review of the Virological and Serological Methods for Early Detection," *Clin Microbiol Newslet*, 1991, 13(23):177-84.

Straus S, "Clinical and Biological Differences Between Recurrent Herpes Simplex Virus and Varicella-Zoster Virus Infections," *JAMA*, 1989, 262(24):3455-8.

Viral Culture, Eye *see* Herpes Simplex Virus Culture *on page 668*

Viral Culture, Eye or Ocular Symptoms

CPT 87140 (culture typing, fluorescent method); 87252 (tissue culture, inoculation and observation); 87253 (tissue culture, additional studies, each isolate)

Related Information
Adenovirus Culture *on page 662*
Bacterial Culture, Conjunctiva *on page 461*
Chlamydia trachomatis Culture *on page 662*
Chlamydia trachomatis Direct FA Test *on page 663*
Chlamydia trachomatis Genome Detection *on page 505*
Herpes Simplex Virus Culture *on page 668*
Ocular Cytology *on page 298*
Viral Culture *on page 675*

Synonyms Eye, Viral Culture

Patient Preparation Local anesthesia might be necessary. Corneal and sclera specimens should be taken only by an ophthalmologist or other properly trained physician.

Specimen Conjunctival scrapings or swabs, eye exudate, vitreous washings, corneal biopsy

Container Cold and sterile viral transport medium for swabs; sterile container for washings or biopsy

Collection Pus should be removed with a sterile swab. Obtain conjunctival scrapings with a sterile spatula. Collect eye exudate by rubbing palpebral conjunctiva with sterile moist swab. Place swab into cold viral transport medium. Conjunctivitis due to *Chlamydia trachomatis* should be collected with a swab and media specific for chlamydial infections; see *Chlamydia* listings.

Storage Instructions Specimen should be kept cold and transported to the laboratory immediately.

Reference Range No virus isolated

Use Ascertain etiological agent of viral ocular infections (eg, conjunctivitis and keratitis)

Methodology Inoculation of specimen into cell cultures, incubation of cultures, observation for characteristic cytopathic effect (CPE), and identification/speciation by fluorescent monoclonal antibodies. If specific viruses such as HSV, CMV, VZV, or adenovirus are suspected, the laboratory might be able to use rapid (1-2 days) culture (shell vial) methods to detect these viruses; see appropriate listings.

Additional Information Adenovirus, VZV, and HSV are the most common viral etiological agents that cause eye infection. Viral serology can be helpful to establish a diagnosis. See table in the listing Viral Culture *on page 676*.

References
Kowalski RP and Gordon YJ, "Comparison of Direct Rapid Tests for the Detection of Adenovirus Antigen in Routine Conjunctival Specimens," *Ophthalmology*, 1989, 96(7):1106-9.

Liesegang TJ, "Diagnosis and Therapy of Herpes Zoster Ophthalmicus," *Ophthalmology*, 1991, 98(8):1216-29.

Martin AL and Kudesia G, "Enzyme-Linked Immunosorbent Assay for Detecting Adenoviruses in Stool Specimens: Comparison With Electron Microscopy and Isolation," *J Clin Pathol*, 1990, 43(6):514-5.

Pavan-Langston D, "Major Ocular Viral Infections," *Practical Diagnosis of Viral Infections*, Galasso GJ, Whitley RJ, Merigan TC, eds, New York, NY: Raven Press, 1993, 69-108.

Viral Culture, Genital *see* Viral Culture, Urogenital *on page 681*

Viral Culture, Genital *see* Herpes Simplex Virus Culture *on page 668*

Viral Culture, Heart *see* Viral Culture, Tissue *on next page*

Viral Culture, Kidney *see* Viral Culture, Tissue *on next page*

Viral Culture, Lesion *see* Viral Culture, Dermatological Symptoms *on this page*

Viral Culture, Lung *see* Viral Culture, Tissue *on next page*

Viral Culture, Muscle *see* Viral Culture, Tissue *on next page*

Viral Culture, Nasopharyngeal *see* Viral Culture, Respiratory Symptoms *on next page*

Viral Culture, Pulmonary Biopsy *see* Viral Culture, Respiratory Symptoms *on next page*

Viral Culture, Pustule *see* Viral Culture, Dermatological Symptoms *on this page*

Viral Culture, Rash *see* Viral Culture, Dermatological Symptoms *on this page*

Viral Culture, Rash *see* Varicella-Zoster Virus Culture *on page 675*

Viral Culture, Respiratory Symptoms

CPT 87140 (culture typing, fluorescent method); 87252 (tissue culture, inoculation and observation); 87253 (tissue culture, additional studies, each isolate)

Related Information
Adenovirus Antibody Titer *on page 362*
Adenovirus Culture *on page 662*
Bacterial Culture, Bronchoscopy Specimen *on page 459*
Bacterial Culture, Sputum *on page 465*
Bronchial Washings Cytology *on page 287*
Bronchoalveolar Lavage Cytology *on page 288*
Coxsackie A Virus Titer *on page 387*
Coxsackie B Virus Titer *on page 387*
Fungal Culture, Sputum *on page 479*
Influenza Virus Culture *on page 670*
Mycobacterial Culture, Sputum *on page 490*
Parainfluenza Viral Serology *on page 420*
Parainfluenza Virus Culture *on page 671*
Pneumocystis carinii Preparation *on page 299*
Respiratory Syncytial Virus Antigen Detection *on page 673*
Respiratory Syncytial Virus Culture *on page 673*
Respiratory Syncytial Virus Serology *on page 426*
Sputum Cytology *on page 300*
Virus, Direct Detection by Fluorescent Antibody *on page 682*
Viscosity, Serum/Plasma *on page 350*

Synonyms Viral Culture, Bronchial Wash; Viral Culture, Nasopharyngeal; Viral Culture, Pulmonary Biopsy; Viral Culture, Throat Swab

Abstract Viral agents cause 2% to 15% of cases of pneumonia; most common is influenza virus; parainfluenza virus and adenovirus are less common.[1]

Patient Preparation Local anesthesia might be necessary

Specimen Throat swab; throat washing; nasopharyngeal washing, aspirates, or secretions; sputum; bronchial washings or lavage; lung biopsy

Container Cold and sterile viral transport medium for swabs; sterile container for washings, aspirates, and sputum

Sampling Time As soon as possible after onset of illness

Collection Methods are the same as those used for collecting most respiratory specimens (see Specimen). If respiratory syncytial virus or parainfluenza virus is suspected, see collection techniques for these viruses.

Storage Instructions Keep specimen cold and moist. Transport to the laboratory immediately. Can be stored at 4°C up to 48 hours. If longer storage is required freeze quickly at -70°C. **Do not freeze at -20°C.**

Turnaround Time Variable (1-14 days)

Reference Range No virus isolated

Use Determine etiological agent of pneumonia, pneumonitis, croup, and influenza. Viruses to be considered as causes of viral respiratory illness include influenza virus, parainfluenza virus, rhinovirus, RSV, adenovirus, CMV, and reovirus. Immunocompromised patients can also have respiratory illness due to HSV or VZV.

Limitations Presence of nonculturable, disease-causing virus (eg, encephalitis, hepatitis, and gastroenteritis viruses); invasive procedures. Many asymptomatic persons carry and shed viruses which might not be related to illness.

Methodology Inoculation of specimen into cell cultures, incubation of cultures, observation for characteristic cytopathic effect (CPE), and identification/speciation by methods such as hemadsorption and the use of fluorescent monoclonal antibodies. Many laboratories use rapid (1-2 days) culture (shell vial) methods to detect respiratory viruses. Identification is based on reaction with a specific fluorescent-monoclonal antibody.[2,3]

Additional Information See table in the listing Viral Culture *on page 676*. Contact the Virology Laboratory and inform the staff if influenza or parainfluenza is suspected. Rapid detection of several respiratory viruses by using mixtures of monoclonal antibodies and shell vial cultures are often used.[2,3]

Footnotes
1. Bartlett JG and Mundy LM, "Community-Acquired Pneumonia," *N Engl J Med*, 1995, 333(24):1618-24.
2. Schrim J, Luijt DS, Pastoor GW, et al, "Rapid Detection of Respiratory Viruses Using Mixtures of Monoclonal Antibodies on Shell Vial Cultures," *J Med Virol*, 1992, 38(2):147-51.
3. Olsen MA, Shuck KM, Sambol AR, et al, "Isolation of Seven Respiratory Viruses in Shell Vials: A Practical and Highly Sensitive Method," *J Clin Microbiol*, 1993, 31(2):422-5.

References
Costello MJ, Smernoff NT, and Yungbluth M, "Laboratory Diagnosis of Viral Respiratory Tract Infections," *Lab Med*, 1993, 24:150-7.
Lennette DA, "Collection and Preparation of Specimens for Virological Examination," *Manual of Clinical Microbiology*, 6th ed, Murray PR, Baron EJ, Pfaller MA, et al, eds, Washington, DC: American Society for Microbiology, 1995, 868-75.

Takimoto S, Grandien M, Ishida MA, et al, "Comparison of Enzyme-Linked Immunosorbent Assay, Indirect Immunofluorescence Assay, and Virus Isolation for Detection of Respiratory Viruses in Nasopharyngeal Secretions," *J Clin Microbiol*, 1991, 29(3):470-4.

Viral Culture, Skin *see* Herpes Simplex Virus Culture *on page 668*

Viral Culture, Skin *see* Varicella-Zoster Virus Culture *on page 675*

Viral Culture, Skin/Dermatological Specimen *see* Viral Culture, Dermatological Symptoms *on previous page*

Viral Culture, Skin Scrapings *see* Viral Culture, Dermatological Symptoms *on previous page*

Viral Culture, Stool

CPT 87140 (culture typing, fluorescent method); 87252 (tissue culture, inoculation and observation); 87253 (tissue culture, additional studies, each isolate)

Related Information
Bacterial Culture, Stool *on page 466*
Electron Microscopic Examination for Viruses, Stool *on page 665*
Entamoeba histolytica Serological Test *on page 391*
Enterovirus Culture *on page 666*
Poliomyelitis I, II, III Titer *on page 423*
Rotavirus, Direct Detection *on page 674*
Viral Culture *on page 675*
Yersinia enterocolitica Antibody *on page 440*
Yersinia pestis Antibody *on page 440*

Applies to Adenovirus Culture, Stool; Coxsackie Virus Culture, Stool; Echovirus Culture, Stool; Enterovirus Culture, Stool; Poliovirus Culture, Stool

Specimen Stool or rectal swab. Freshly passed stool is preferable to a rectal swab.

Collection Collect stools into plastic screw-cap container; do not use cardboard or waxed containers.

Insert swab gently into rectum and hold there for 10-15 seconds, moisten with contents of Culturette® bulb, and send to the laboratory in cold viral transport medium.

Storage Instructions Keep specimens cold.

Turnaround Time Variable (usually 1-14 days)

Reference Range No virus isolated

Use Identify carriage or excretion of a virus in stool; isolate and identify an enterovirus which could be the cause of meningitis. The viruses most likely to be isolated from stool specimen are those which are extremely hardy and which do not have a lipid membrane envelope (ie, enterovirus, polio, coxsackie, and echoviruses).

Limitations Cannot detect the presence of nonculturable, disease-causing virus (eg, Norwalk group, calicivirus, and gastroenteritis viruses). Some bacterial toxins in fecal specimens, such as *Clostridium difficile* toxin A, can mimic viral cytopathic effect (CPE) in many cell lines, leading to false-positives.

Methodology Inoculation of specimen into cell cultures, incubation of cultures, observation for characteristic cytopathic effect (CPE), and identification/speciation by methods such as hemadsorption and fluorescent monoclonal antibodies

Additional Information Isolation of virus from stool specimens may be of diagnostic help. It is important to be aware of viral shedding to avoid transmission to other people. Children recently vaccinated against polio can shed poliovirus in the stool for months after vaccination. Children convalescing from upper respiratory illness or aseptic meningitis can shed virus in the stool for weeks. See table in the listing Viral Culture *on page 676* for viruses most likely to be isolated from stool specimens. Many viruses responsible for diarrhea can be detected with immunoassays or electron microscopy.

References
Bhan MK, Raj P, Bhandari N, et al, "Role of Enteric Adenoviruses and Rotaviruses in Mild and Severe Acute Enteritis," *Pediatr Infect Dis J*, 1988, 7(5):320-3.
Blacklow NR and Greenberg HB, "Viral Gastroenteritis," *N Engl J Med*, 1991, 325(4):252-64.
Lennette DA, "Collection and Preparation of Specimens for Virological Examination," *Manual of Clinical Microbiology*, 6th ed, Murray PR, Baron EJ, Pfaller MA, et al, eds, Washington, DC: American Society for Microbiology, 1995, 868-75.

Viral Culture, Throat Swab *see* Viral Culture, Respiratory Symptoms *on this page*

Viral Culture, Tissue

CPT 87140 (culture typing, fluorescent method); 87252 (tissue culture, inoculation and observation); 87253 (tissue culture, additional studies, each isolate)

Related Information

Histopathology *on page 42*

Human Immunodeficiency Virus DNA Amplification *on page 515*

Human Papillomavirus DNA Probe Test *on page 516*

Immunoperoxidase Procedures *on page 43*

Viral Culture *on page 675*

Applies to Viral Culture, Biopsy; Viral Culture, Brain; Viral Culture, Bronchial; Viral Culture, Heart; Viral Culture, Kidney; Viral Culture, Lung; Viral Culture, Muscle; Viral Culture, Trachea

Specimen Biopsy, swab, brush, or scrape specimen from any suspect organ, site, lesion, or tissue

Container Sterile, screw-cap container

Sampling Time As soon as possible after onset of illness

Collection Specimen should be collected during the acute phase of the disease, as follows.

Tissue: Use a fresh set of sterile instruments to collect each tissue. Place each specimen in its own dry, sterile nontoxic leakproof container. Identify each tissue with patient's name, type of tissue, and date collected. **Keep cold and bring tissue to the laboratory immediately.**

Biopsy, lung, kidney, heart muscle, brain: Specimens should be placed into a sterile container and kept cold or placed directly in cold viral transport medium.

Tracheal or bronchial tissue or brushings: If possible, brushes should be placed into cold viral transport medium.

Storage Instructions Specimens should be kept cold and moist. If specimen is to be stored longer than 48 hours it should be frozen at -70°C. **Do not freeze at -20°C.** Tissues can be put into viral transport medium.

Turnaround Time Variable (usually 1-14 days)

Reference Range No virus isolated

Use Aid in the diagnosis of disseminated viral diseases (eg, encephalitis and meningitis)

Limitations Presence of nonculturable, disease-causing virus (eg, encephalitis, hepatitis, and gastroenteritis viruses); invasive procedures

Methodology Inoculation of specimen into cell cultures, incubation of cultures, observation for characteristic cytopathic effect (CPE), and identification/speciation by methods such as hemadsorption and fluorescent monoclonal antibodies. If specific viruses such as HSV, CMV, VZV, or adenovirus are suspected, the laboratory might be able to use rapid (1-2 days) culture (shell vial) methods to detect these viruses.

Additional Information See table in the listing Viral Culture *on page 676* for the viruses most likely to be isolated from clinical specimens and for the list of viruses not routinely cultured. Viral DNA can now be detected using nucleic acid amplification procedures or *in situ* hybridization. These techniques are very sensitive and specific. In some viral diseases, such tests can be diagnostically useful (eg, hepatitis). However, other viruses can reside in the host in a latent form without causing disease (CMV, HSV, VZV). Such latent viruses can produce false-positive results if amplification of DNA in these viruses is used in a diagnostic test.

References

Hughes JM, "Physical and Chemical Methods for Enhancing Rapid Detection of Viruses and Other Agents," *Clin Microbiol Rev*, 1993, 6(2):150-75.

Lennette DA, "Collection and Preparation of Specimens for Virological Examination," *Manual of Clinical Microbiology*, 6th ed, Murray PR, Baron EJ, Pfaller MA, et al, eds, Washington, DC: American Society for Microbiology, 1995, 868-75.

Wiedbrauk DL and Johnston SLG, "Specimen Collection and Processing," *Manual of Clinical Virology*, New York, NY: Raven Press, 1993, 22-32.

Viral Culture, Trachea *see* Viral Culture, Tissue *on previous page*

Viral Culture, Ulcer *see* Viral Culture, Dermatological Symptoms *on page 679*

Viral Culture, Urine

CPT 87140 (culture typing, fluorescent method); 87252 (tissue culture, inoculation and observation); 87253 (tissue culture, additional studies, each isolate)

Related Information

Adenovirus Culture *on page 662*

Bacterial Culture, Urine, Clean Catch *on page 468*

Cytomegalic Inclusion Disease Cytology *on page 293*

Cytomegalovirus Culture *on page 664*

Enterovirus Culture *on page 666*

Mumps Virus Culture *on page 670*

Urine Cytology *on page 301*

Viral Culture *on page 675*

Applies to CMV Culture, Urine; Mumps Virus Culture, Urine

Specimen Urine

Sampling Time Shedding of CMV can be intermittent. Therefore, several specimens should be collected, if possible.

Collection Clean catch, midstream urine in sterile, screw-cap container

Storage Instructions Refrigerate if delay of more than 1 hour in transit to the laboratory. Specimen may be stored up to 72 hours at 4°C before inoculation onto cell culture. **Do not freeze specimens at -20°C.** Some viruses are inactivated by freezing at -20°C. Specimens that need to be stored longer than 72 hours can be frozen at -70°C or below in the presence of 30% sorbitol.[1]

Turnaround Time Variable (1-28 days)

Reference Range No virus isolated

Use The viruses most frequently isolated from urine are CMV, mumps, and adenoviruses.

Limitations Urine can be toxic for cell cultures and can result in inconclusive results

Methodology Inoculation of specimen into cell cultures, incubation of cultures, observation for characteristic cytopathic effect (CPE), and identification/speciation by hemadsorption and/or fluorescent monoclonal antibodies. If specific viruses such as CMV or adenovirus are suspected, the laboratory might be able to use rapid (1-2 days) culture (shell vial) methods to detect these viruses.

Additional Information See table in the listing Viral Culture *on page 676*.

Footnotes

1. Fedorko DP, Ilstrup DM, and Smith TF, "Effect of Age of Shell Vial Monolayers on Detection of Cytomegalovirus From Urine Specimens," *J Clin Microbiol*, 1989, 27(9):2107-9.

References

Lennette DA, "Collection and Preparation of Specimens for Virological Examination," *Manual of Clinical Microbiology*, 6th ed, Murray PR, Baron EJ, Pfaller MA, et al, eds, Washington, DC: American Society for Microbiology, 1995, 868-75.

Wiedbrauk DL and Johnston SLG, "Specimen Collection and Processing," *Manual of Clinical Virology*, New York, NY: Raven Press, 1993, 22-32.

Viral Culture, Urogenital

CPT 87140 (culture typing, fluorescent method); 87252 (tissue culture, inoculation and observation); 87253 (tissue culture, additional studies, each isolate)

Related Information

Bacterial Culture, Genital Specimen *on page 463*

Cervical/Vaginal Cytology *on page 290*

Chlamydia trachomatis Culture *on page 662*

Chlamydia trachomatis Genome Detection *on page 505*

Herpes Simplex Virus Antigen Detection *on page 667*

Herpes Simplex Virus Culture *on page 668*

Human Papillomavirus DNA Probe Test *on page 516*

Viral Culture, Dermatological Symptoms *on page 679*

Synonyms Genital Culture, Virus; Viral Culture, Genital

Applies to Cervix, Viral Culture; Endocervix, Viral Culture; Prostate, Viral Culture; Urethra, Viral Culture

Specimen Cervical, urethral, and genital lesions, surgical and biopsy tissue

Container Sterile and cold viral transport medium

Sampling Time As soon as possible after the eruption of vesicles or lesions, preferably within 3 days of lesion eruption. Only occasionally can HSV be isolated as late as 7-10 days after onset.

Collection Disinfection of site prior to collection is generally not recommended. Use a Culturette® swab, spatula, or scalpel blade to scrape away cells from the base of freshly unroofed lesions, and place the swab or collected cells immediately into cold viral transport medium. Vesicular fluid is an excellent specimen, and can be collected by using a tuberculin syringe and a 26-gauge needle. Rinse contents of syringe into cold viral transport medium.

Storage Instructions Keep all specimens cold and moist. Specimens which cannot be inoculated onto cell cultures within 48 hours should be frozen at -70°C.

Turnaround Time Variable (1-14 days)

Reference Range No virus isolated

Critical Values Positive viral culture for HSV during pregnancy.[1]

Use Aid in the diagnosis of viral entities including sexually transmitted diseases. The detection of virus such as HSV or CMV in pregnant women is important to prevent the complications of neonatal infections.[1,2] Infants are at risk of infection during delivery even if the mother is asymptomatic. Human papillomavirus (HPV) causes genital warts and some strains of HPV are associated with cervical cancer. This virus can be detected using *in situ* hybridization, Southern blot analysis, or DNA amplification.[3]

Limitations Some laboratories use methods which detect only HSV in genital specimens; some disease-causing virus (eg, papillomavirus) are nonculturable (see table in Viral Culture *on page 676*); invasive procedures
(Continued)

Viral Culture, Urogenital *(Continued)*

Methodology Inoculation of specimen into cell cultures, incubation of cultures, observation for characteristic cytopathic effect (CPE), and identification/speciation by fluorescent monoclonal antibodies. If specific viruses such as HSV, CMV, or adenovirus are suspected, the laboratory might be able to use rapid (1-2 days) culture (shell vial) methods to detect these viruses.

Additional Information Urogenital, dermal, oral, and mucosal specimens often yield the same viruses. See table in the listing Viral Culture *on page 676.*

Footnotes

1. Prober CG, Corey L, Brown ZA, et al, "The Management of Pregnancies Complicated by Genital Infections With Herpes Simplex Virus," *Clin Infect Dis*, 1992, 15(6):1031-8.
2. Pass RF, Little EA, Stagno S, et al, "Young Children as a Probable Source of Maternal and Congenital Cytomegalovirus Infection," *N Engl J Med*, 1987, 316(22):1366-70.
3. Schiffman MH, Bauer HM, Lorincz AT, et al, "Comparison of Southern Blot Hybridization and Polymerase Chain Reaction Methods for the Detection of Human Papillomavirus DNA," *J Clin Microbiol*, 1991, 29(3):573-7.

References

Arvin AM and Alford CA, "Chronic Intrauterine and Perinatal Infections," *Practical Diagnosis of Viral Infections*, Galasso GJ, Whitley RJ, Merigan TC, eds, New York, NY: Raven Press, 1993, 211-42.

Moscicki AB, "Human Papillomavirus Infections," *Adv Pediatr*, 1992, 39:257-79.

Viral Disease in Tissue *see* Electron Microscopic Examination for Viruses, Stool *on page 665*

Virus, Direct Detection by Fluorescent Antibody

CPT 88346

Related Information

Adenovirus Antibody Titer *on page 362*

Adenovirus Culture *on page 662*

Bronchial Washings Cytology *on page 287*

Bronchoalveolar Lavage Cytology *on page 288*

Cytomegalovirus Antigen Detection *on page 664*

Cytomegalovirus Culture *on page 664*

Frozen Section *on page 41*

Herpes Simplex Virus Antigen Detection *on page 667*

Herpes Simplex Virus Culture *on page 668*

Histopathology *on page 42*

Influenza A and B Titer *on page 411*

Influenza Virus Culture *on page 670*

Measles Antibody *on page 417*

Mumps Serology *on page 419*

Mumps Virus Culture *on page 670*

Parainfluenza Viral Serology *on page 420*

Parainfluenza Virus Culture *on page 671*

Rabies *on page 672*

Respiratory Syncytial Virus Antigen Detection *on page 673*

Respiratory Syncytial Virus Culture *on page 673*

Respiratory Syncytial Virus Serology *on page 426*

Sputum Cytology *on page 300*

Varicella-Zoster Virus Culture *on page 675*

Varicella-Zoster Virus Serology *on page 437*

Viral Culture, Respiratory Symptoms *on page 680*

Synonyms Direct Detection of Virus; Direct Fluorescent Antibody Test for Virus; Virus Fluorescent Antibody Test

Applies to Influenza Virus, Direct Detection; Measles Virus, Direct Detection; Mumps Virus, Direct Detection; Parainfluenza Virus, Direct Detection; Rabies Virus, Direct Detection; Varicella-Zoster Virus, Direct Detection

Test Commonly Includes Direct (nonculture) detection of virus-infected cells using immunofluorescence

Specimen Impression smears of tissues, lesion scrapings and swabs, frozen sections, cell suspensions, upper respiratory tract swabs

Turnaround Time Less than 1 day

Special Instructions Make at least four impression smears or place four frozen sections on four separate slides. Cell suspensions should be centrifuged, resuspended to slight turbidity, and applied to prewelled slides.

Reference Range No virus detected

Possible Panic Range Positive detection of rabies

Use Useful in the rapid diagnosis of HSV, VZV, RSV, parainfluenza, influenza, adenovirus, CMV, measles, mumps, and rabies infections

Limitations It is possible for the test to be negative in the presence of viral infection. Expertly trained and experienced personnel, excellent quality reagents, and adequate numbers of cells are required. **Contact laboratory prior to requesting test to determine if laboratory offers this/these tests.** Generally this test is not as sensitive as cell culture.

Methodology Monoclonal antibody reagents and immunofluorescence microscopy are used to detect viruses/viral antigens in specimen cells.

Additional Information Direct detection of viruses in respiratory secretions can be diagnostically helpful because cell culture results often take several days to weeks.[1]

PCR is becoming available. Its sensitivity for CMV and other entities deserves consideration.

Footnotes

1. McIntosh K, Halonen P, and Ruuskanen O, "Report of a Workshop on Respiratory Viral Infections: Epidemiology, Diagnosis, Treatment, and Prevention," *Clin Infect Dis*, 1993, 16(1):151-64.

References

Costello MJ, Smernoff NT, and Yungbluth M, "Laboratory Diagnosis of Viral Respiratory Tract Infections," *Lab Med*, 1993, 24:150-7.

Smith TF, "Rapid Diagnosis of Viral Infections," *Adv Exp Med Biol*, 1990, 263:115-21.

Virus Fluorescent Antibody Test *see* Virus, Direct Detection by Fluorescent Antibody *on this page*

VZV Culture *see* Varicella-Zoster Virus Culture *on page 675*

Antiviral Agents and Their Target Virus(es)

Antiviral Agent	Target Virus(es)
Nucleoside Analogs	
Acyclovir*	HSV, VZV, EBV, CMV
Bromovinyldeoxyuridine (BVDU)	Some herpesviruses
Buciclovir	HSV
Didanosine (ddI)	HIV
Dideoxoycytidine (Ddc)*	HIV
Dideoxyinosine (Ddi)*	HIV
Famciclovir	VZV
Fluoroiodoaracytosine (FIAC)	Some herpesviruses
Ganciclovir (DHPG)*	CMV
Idoxuridine (IDU)*	HSV
Trifluridine (TFT)*	HSV
Vidarabine (ara-A)*	HSV, VZV
Zalcitabine (ddc)	HIV
Zidovudine (AZT)*	HIV
Nucleoside-like Analogs	
Ribavirin*	Influenza virus, parainfluenza virus, HSV, Lassa fever virus, hepatitis A virus, respiratory syncytial virus
Other Antiviral Agents	
Amantadine*/rimantadine	Influenza virus
Antimoniotungstate (HPA-23)	Retroviruses
Castanospermine	Retroviruses
Disoxaril (Win 51711)	Rhinoviruses, enteroviruses
Phosphonoformate (foscarnet)*	Retroviruses, influenza virus, HSV, CMV
Suramin	Retroviruses
Immunomodulators	
Ampligen	Retroviruses
Interferons	Several viruses

*Agent is FDA-approved for clinical use but not necessarily for use in disease(s) caused by all of the viruses given for that agent. Consult pharmacist and package inserts for indications.

Figure 1
Molecular Structures of Representative Antiviral Agents

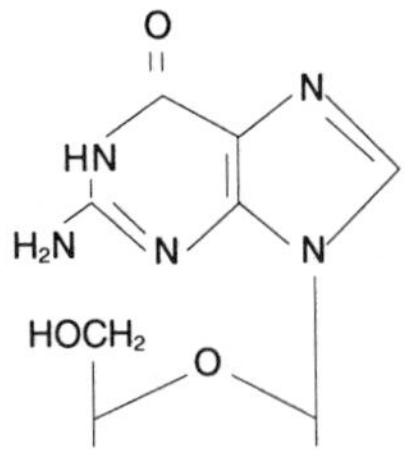

acyclovir

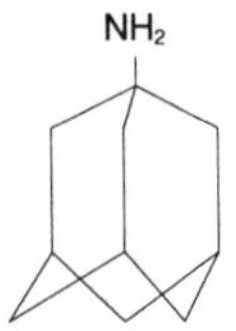

amantadine

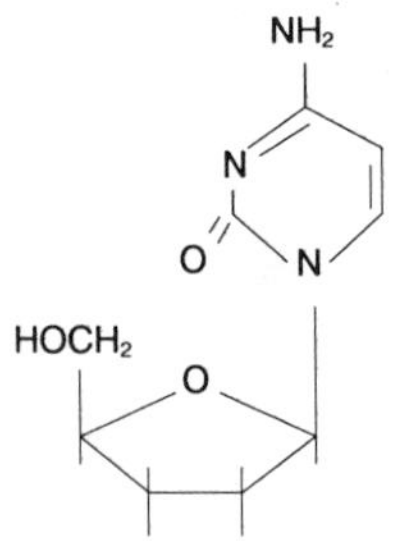

dideoxycytidine

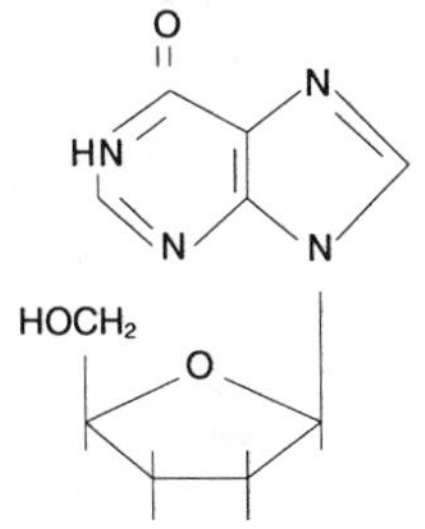

dideoxyinosine

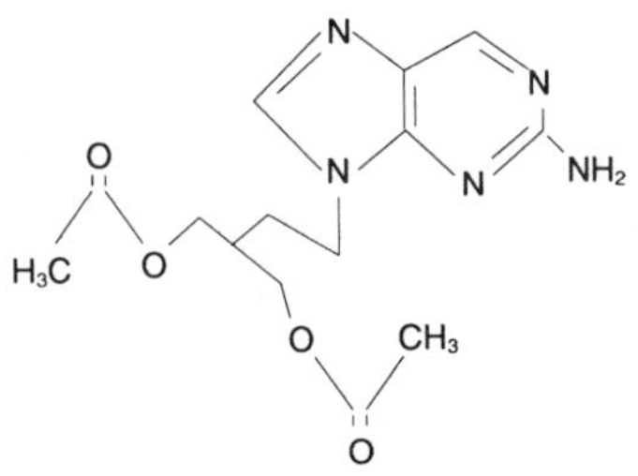

famciclovir

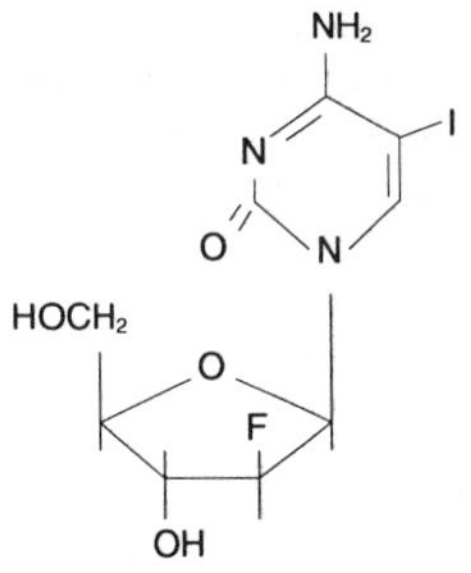

fluoroiodo-
aracytosine

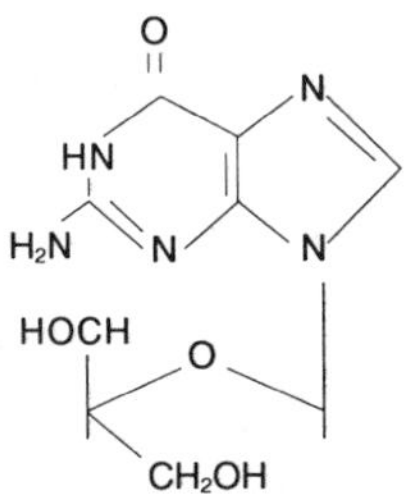

ganciclovir

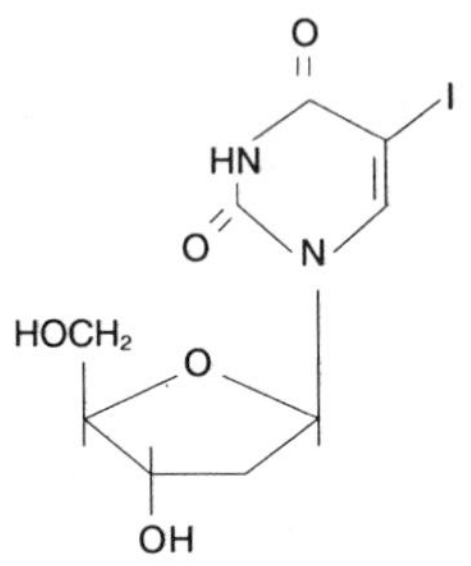

idoxuridine

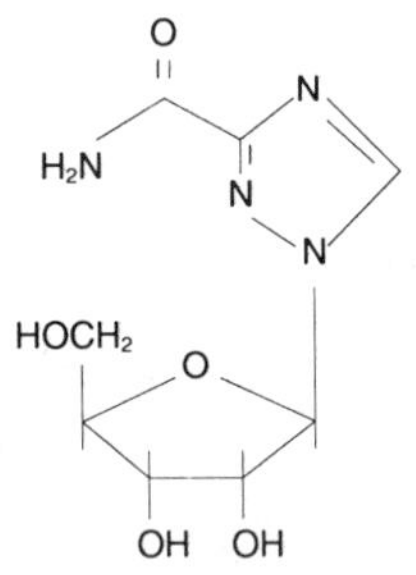

ribavirin

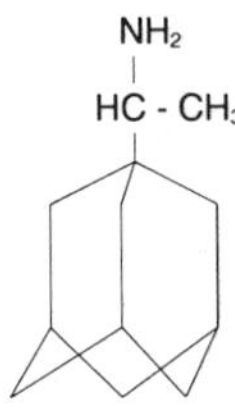

rimantadine

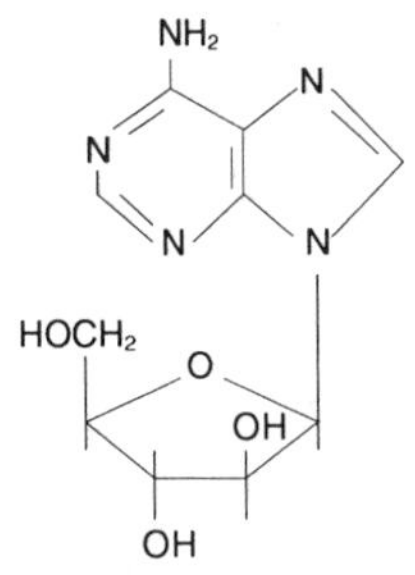

vidarabine

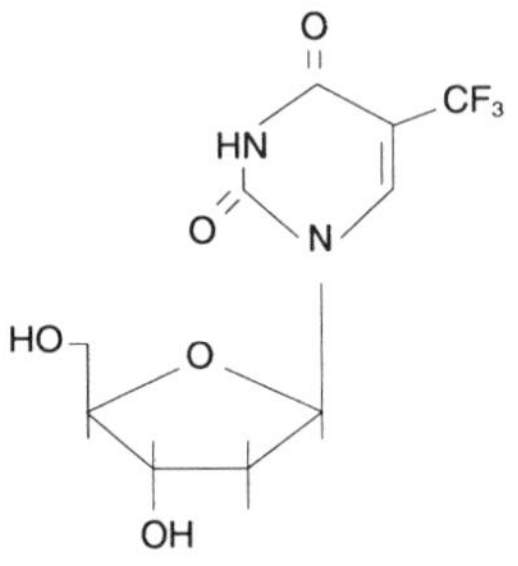

trifluridine

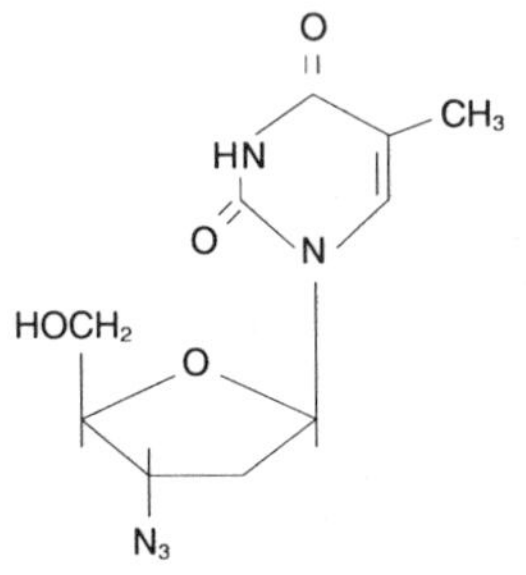

zidovudine

Figure 2

Classification of DNA-Containing Viruses

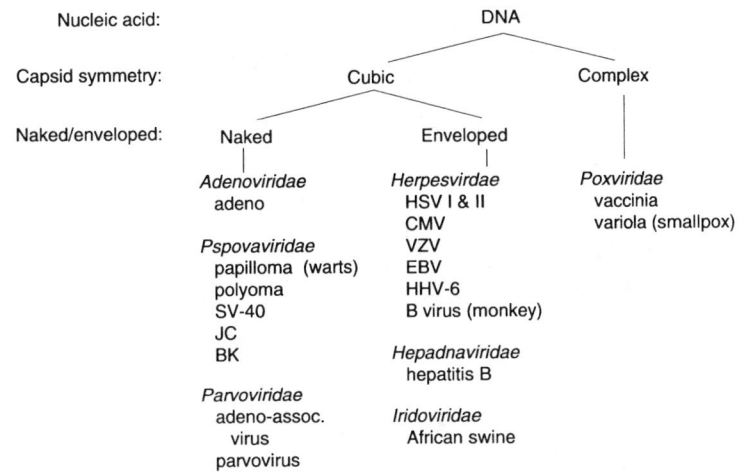

	DNA	
Nucleic acid:		
Capsid symmetry:	Cubic	Complex
Naked/enveloped:	Naked Enveloped	

Adenoviridae
adeno

Pspovaviridae
papilloma (warts)
polyoma
SV-40
JC
BK

Parvoviridae
adeno-assoc.
virus
parvovirus

Herpesvirdae
HSV I & II
CMV
VZV
EBV
HHV-6
B virus (monkey)

Hepadnaviridae
hepatitis B

Iridoviridae
African swine

Poxviridae
vaccinia
variola (smallpox)

Figure 3

Classification of RNA-Containing Viruses

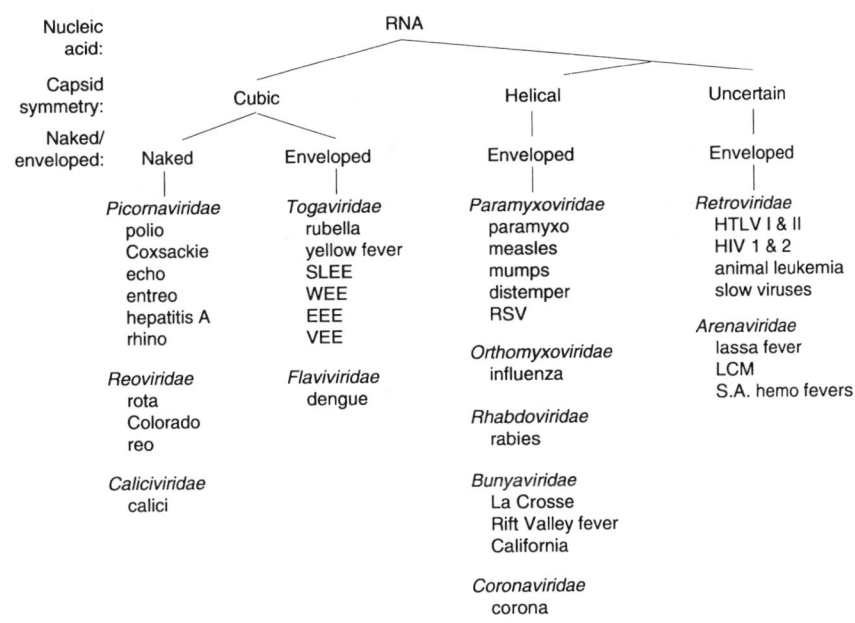

Nucleic acid: RNA

Capsid symmetry: Cubic   Helical   Uncertain

Naked/enveloped: Naked   Enveloped   Enveloped   Enveloped

Picornaviridae
polio
Coxsackie
echo
entreo
hepatitis A
rhino

Reoviridae
rota
Colorado
reo

Caliciviridae
calici

Togaviridae
rubella
yellow fever
SLEE
WEE
EEE
VEE

Flaviviridae
dengue

Paramyxoviridae
paramyxo
measles
mumps
distemper
RSV

Orthomyxoviridae
influenza

Rhabdoviridae
rabies

Bunyaviridae
La Crosse
Rift Valley fever
California

Coronaviridae
corona

Retroviridae
HTLV I & II
HIV 1 & 2
animal leukemia
slow viruses

Arenaviridae
lassa fever
LCM
S.A. hemo fevers

Figure 4

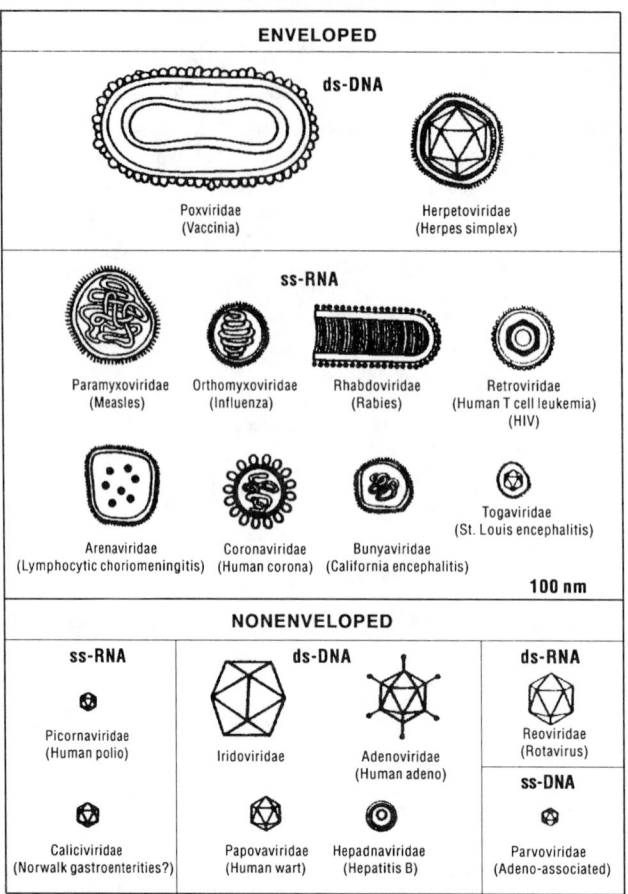

Diagram illustrating the shapes and relative sizes of animal viruses of the major families (bar = 100 nm). Representative members that infect humans are listed in parentheses. Iridoviridae are not known to infect humans. From Melnick JL, "Structure and Classification of Viruses," *Textbook of Human Virology*, Belshe RB, ed, Chicago, IL: Yearbook Medical Publishers, 1984, 1-28, with permission.

ACRONYMS AND ABBREVIATIONS GLOSSARY

This glossary provides a useful listing of many acronyms and abbreviations commonly associated with laboratory medicine. We offer this glossary not as an exhaustive authoritative list, but more as a guide to assist in interpreting frequently used terminology.

a ... atto (10^{-18})
A ... apical; artery
A_1 ... blood group antigen
A_1AT ... alpha$_1$ antitrypsin
A_2 ... aortic second sound; blood group antigen
aa ... of each (ana)
AABB ... American Association of Blood Banks
AAC ... antibiotic associated colitis
AACC ... American Association of Clinical Chemistry
AaG ... alveolar arterial gradient
AAL ... anterior axillary line
AAP ... American Academy of Pediatrics
AAPC ... antibiotic associated pseudomembranous colitis
AAPCC ... American Association of Poison Control Centers
AAS ... acute abdominal series; atomic absorption spectrometry
AAT ... alpha antitrypsin
Ab ... antibody
AB ... abort; antibiotic
ABC ... avidin-biotin complex
ABE ... acute bacterial endocarditis
ABG ... arterial blood gas
ABL ... abetalipoprotein
ABLB ... alternate binaural loudness balance
ABMT ... autologous bone marrow transplantation
ABO ... ABO blood group
ABPA ... allergic bronchopulmonary aspergillosis
ABR ... auditory brainstem response
ABS ... alkylbenzene sulfonate
ac ... before meals (ante cibum)
Ac ... actinium
AC ... air conduction; alternating current
ACA ... anticardiolipin antibody; Du Pont chemistry analyzer
ACC ... amylase creatinine clearance
ACD ... acid-citrate-dextrose
ACE ... angiotensin converting enzyme
AChR ... acetylcholine receptor antibody
ACLS ... advanced cardiac life support
ACOG ... American College of Obstetrics and Gynecology
AcP ... acid phosphatase
ACT ... activated clotting time
ACTH ... adrenocorticotropic hormone
ad ... right ear; up to (ad)
ADA ... adenosine deaminase
ADCC ... antibody-dependent cell-mediated cytotoxicity
ADDH ... attention deficit disorder with hyperactivity
ADH ... alcohol dehydrogenase; antidiuretic hormone
ADHD ... attention deficit hyperactive disorder
ADL ... active daily living
ad lib ... as desired (ad libitum)
ADM ... admission
ADNase ... anti-DNAse
ADP ... adenosine 5-diphosphate
ADR ... acceptable dental remedies; acute dystonic reaction; Adriamycin
ADT ... adenosine triphosphate; alternate-day treatment
AED ... anticonvulsant drugs
AEP ... average evoked potential
AF ... acid-fast; amniotic fluid; artrial fibrillation
AFB ... acid-fast bacillus
AFP ... alpha-fetoprotein
Ag ... antigen; silver
A/G ... albumin/globulin ratio
AGA ... accelerated growth area
AGN ... acute glomerular nephritis
$AgNO_3$ ... silver nitrate
AGS ... adrenogenital syndrome
AH ... antihyaluronidase
A-H ... atrial-HIS
AHA ... acquired hemolytic anemia; autoimmune hemolytic anemia
AHBC ... hepatitis B core antibody
AHF ... antihemophilic factor
AHFS ... American Hospital Formulary Service
AHG ... antihemophilic globulin
AHT ... antihyaluronidase titer
AI ... allergy index; aortic insufficiency
AICC ... anti-inhibitor coagulant complex
AIDS ... acquired immune deficiency syndrome
AIHA ... autoimmune hemolytic anemia
AIP ... acute intermittent porphyria; average intravascular pressure
AJ ... ankle jerk
AK ... adenylate kinase; above the knee
Al ... aluminum
ALA ... aminolevulinic acid
alb ... albumin
alk ... alkaline
AlkP ... alkaline phosphatase
ALL ... acute lymphoblastic leukemia; acute lymphocytic leukemia
$Al(OH)_3$ ... aluminum hydroxide
AlP ... alkaline phosphatase
AlPI ... alkaline phosphatase isoenzymes
ALS ... advanced life support; amyotrophic lateral sclerosis; antilymphocyte serum
ALT ... alanine aminotransferase
Am ... americium
AM ... morning
AMA ... against medical advice; American Medical Association; antimitrochondrial antibody
AMI ... acute myocardial infarction
AML ... acute myeloblastic leukemia; acute myelogenous leukemia
AMP ... adenosine monophosphate
AMPS ... acid mucopolysaccharide
AMPT ... alpha-methyl-p-tyrosine
ANA ... antinuclear antibody
ANC ... absolute neutrophil count
ANCA ... antineutrophil cytoplasmic antibodies
ANF ... antinuclear factor
ANLL ... acute nonlymphocytic leukemia
ANP ... atrial natriuretic peptide
anti-TB ... antituberculosis
A & O ... alert and oriented
AODM ... adult onset diabetes mellitus
AOS ... acridine orange staining
AP ... antepartum; anteroposterior
A & P ... anterior and posterior; assessment and plans
APCA ... antiparetial cell antibody
APhA ... American Pharmaceutical Association
APP ... alum-precipitating pyridine
APSAC ... anisoylated plasminogen streptokinase activator complex
APTT ... activated partial thromboplastin time
APUD ... amine precursor uptake and decarboxylation
aq ... water (aqua)
Ar ... argon
ARA ... antireticulin antibody
ARD ... antimicrobial removal device; acute respiratory distress
ARDS ... adult respiratory distress syndrome
ARF ... acute renal failure
Ars ... arylsulfatase
ART ... arterial line
as ... left ear
As ... arsenic
AS ... anal sphincter; ankylosing spondylitis; aortic stenosis
AsA ... arylsulfatase A
ASA ... acetylsalicylic acid
ASAP ... as soon as possible
AsB ... arylsulfatase B
ASCP ... American Society of Clinical Pathologists
ASCVD ... arteriosclerotic cardiovascular disease
ASD ... atrial septal defect
ASHD ... arteriosclerotic heart disease
ASHP ... American Society of Health-System Pharmacists
ASK ... antistreptokinase
ASKA ... antiskeletal antibody
ASLO ... antistreptolysin O
ASMA ... antismooth muscle antibody
ASO ... antistreptolysin O; arterioselerosis obliterans
AST ... aspartate aminotransferase
ASVD ... arteriosclerotic vascular disease
At ... astatine
ATG ... antithymocyte globulin
AT-III ... antithrombin III
ATN ... acute tubular necrosis
ATP ... adenosine triphosphate
ATPase ... adenosine triphosphatase
ATS ... American Thoracic Society
au ... each ear (auris utro)
Au ... gold
^{198}Au ... radioisotope of gold
A-V ... arteriovenous; atrioventricular; audiovisual
AVA ... availability
AVM ... arteriovenous malformation
AVP ... arginine vasopressin
A & W ... alive and well
Ax ... axillary
AZT ... zidovudine

B ... boron
Ba ... barium
BA ... Bachelor of Arts
BAC ... blood alcohol concentration
BAE ... barium enema

BAEP . . . brainstem auditory evoked potential
BAER . . . brainstem auditory evoked response
BAL . . . bronchial alveolar lavage
BAO . . . basal acid output
BB . . . Blood Bank
BBB . . . blood-brain barrier; bundle branch block
BBPRL . . . big big prolactin
BBT . . . basal body temperature
BC . . . bone conduction
BCG . . . bacillus Calmette-Guérin
BCM . . . bovine cervical mucus
BCP . . . birth control pills; blood cell profile
BCPs . . . birth control pills
bcr . . . breakpoint cluster region
BD . . . bronchodilators
Be . . . beryllium
BE . . . bacterial endocarditis; barium enema
benzodiazepine-GABA . . . gamma-aminobutyric acid
BEP . . . brainstem evoked potential
BERA . . . brainstem evoked response auditory
BF . . . black female
BFS . . . blood fasting sugar
BFT . . . bentonite flocculation test
BGP . . . bone GLA protein
BHB . . . beta-hydroxybutyrate
BHI . . . brain heart infusion
BHT . . . butylated hydroxytoluene
Bi . . . bismuth
bid . . . twice a day (bis in die)
BJ . . . Bence Jones; biceps jerk; bone and joint
Bk . . . berkelium
BK . . . below knee
Bl Obs . . . bladder observation
BLS . . . basic life support
BM . . . black male; bone marrow; bowel movement; breast milk
BMA . . . bone marrow aspirate
BMR . . . basal metabolic rate
BMT . . . bone marrow transplantation
BNO . . . bladder neck obstruction
BP . . . blood pressure
BPD . . . biparietal diameter
BPH . . . benign prostatic hyperplasia
Br . . . bromine; bromide
BR . . . bathroom; bedrest
BrdU . . . 5-bromodeoxyuridine
BRP . . . bathroom privileges
BRU . . . bromide urine
BS . . Bachelor of Science; blood sugar; bowel sounds; breath sounds
bsa . . . body surface area
BSEP . . . brainstem evoked potential
BSO . . . bilateral salpingo-oophorectomy
BSP . . . bromsulfophthalein
BTG . . . beta thromboglobulin
BTL . . . bilateral tubal ligation
BTPS . . body temperature, ambient pressure, and saturated with water vapor (gas)
BU . . . bethesda units
BUN . . . blood urea nitrogen
BVL . . . bilateral vas ligation
BW . . . birth weight; body weight
Bx . . . biopsy

c . . . with (cum)
C . . . carbon
C_2 . . . second cervical vertebra
Ca . . . calcium
CA . . . cancer antigen; cardiac arrest; chronological age
CA 15-3 . . . tumor marker antigen
CA 19-9 . . . tumor marker antigen
CA 50 . . . tumor marker antigen
CA 125 . . . tumor marker antigen
CAB . . . coronary artery bypass
CABG . . . coronary artery bypass graft
CAC . . . circulating anticoagulant
CaCl . . . calcium chloride
$CaCO_3$ . . . calcium carbonate
CAD . . . coronary artery disease
CaEDTA . . . calcium disodium edetate
CAH . . . chronic active hepatitis
CALLA . . . common acute lymphoblastic leukemia antigen
cAMP . . . cyclic AMP
CAPD . . . chronic ambulatory peritoneal dialysis
CASA . . . computer-assisted semen analysis
CAT . . . computed axial tomography
CBAT . . . Coag battery; Coulter battery
CBC . . . complete blood count
CBD . . . common bile duct
CBF . . . cerebral blood flow
CBG . . . capillary blood gases
CBIL . . . conjugated bilirubin
CBS . . . chronic brain syndrome
CBT . . . computerized body tomography
CC . . . chief complaint; closing capacity; colony count
CCI . . . corrected count increment
CCK . . . cholecystokinin
CCK-OP . . . cholecystokinin-octapeptide
CCU . . . cardiac care unit; coronary care unit
Cd . . . cadmium
CDA . . . congenital dyserythropoietic anemia
CDC . . . Centers for Disease Control
CDDP . . . cis-diamminedichloroplatinum
CDP . . . continuous distending pressure; cytidine diphosphate
CDU . . . cumulative dose unit
Ce . . . cerium
CEA . . . carcinoembryonic antigen
CES . . . conjugated estrogenic substances
Cf . . . californium
CF . . . cardiac failure; caucasian female; complement fixation; cystic fibrosis
CFU . . . colony forming units
CG . . . chorionic gonadotropin
CGL . . . chronic granulocytic leukemia
CH . . . congenital hypothyroidism
CHBHA . . . congenital Heinz body hemolytic anemia
CHD . . . congenital heart disease
CHF . . . congestive heart failure
CHS . . . central hypoventilation syndrome
CI . . . cardiac index; color index; confidence intervals
CIC . . . circulating immune complexes
CIE . . . counterimmunoelectrophoresis
CIF . . . clone-inhibiting factor
CIN . . . cervical intraepithelial neoplasia
CIP . . . cellular immunocompetence profile
CIPD . . . chronic inflammatory demyelinating polyradiculoneuropathy
CJD . . . Creutzfeldt-Jakob disease
CK . . . creatine kinase
Cl . . . chlorine
Cla . . . clarithromycin
CLA . . . certified laboratory assistant
CLL . . . chronic lymphocytic leukemia
CLS . . . clinical laboratory scientist
cm . . . centimeter
cm^2 . . . square centimeter
Cm . . . curium
CM . . . caucasian male; contrast media; culture media
CMG . . . cystometrogram
CMI . . . carbohydrate metabolism index; cell-mediated immunity
CML . . . cell mediated lysis; chronic myelogenous leukemia
cmm . . . square centimeter cm^2
CMP . . . cardiomyopathy; cervical mucus penetration
CMPT . . . cervical mucous penetration test
CMV . . . cytomegalovirus
CMV-IGIV . . . cytomegalovirus immune globulin intravenous
CMVS . . . culture midvoid specimen
CN . . . cyanogen
CNS . . . central nervous system; coagulase negative staph
CNSHA . . . congenital nonspherocytic hemolytic anemia
Co . . . cobalt
^{57}Co . . . radioisotope of cobalt
^{58}Co . . . radioisotope of cobalt
^{60}Co . . . radioisotope of cobalt
CO . . . carbon monoxide; cardiac output
C/O . . . complaint of
CO_3 . . . carbonate
coag . . . coagulation
COHb . . . carboxyhemoglobin
COLD . . . chronic obstructive lung disease
COMT . . . catechol-o-methyltransferase
COP . . . chronic obstructive pulmonary
COPD . . . chronic obstructive pulmonary disease
C & P . . . cystoscopy and pyelogram
CPA . . . carotid phonoangiography
CPAP . . . continuous positive airway pressure
CPB . . . cardiopulmonary bypass
CPD . . . cyst disease protein; citrate phosphate dextrose
CPDA . . . citrate phosphate dextrose adenine
CPE . . . cytopathogenic effects
CPI . . . coronary prognostic index
CPK . . . creatine phosphokinase
cpm . . . counts per minute

CPP . . . cerebral perfusion pressure
CPPB . . . continuous positive pressure breathing
CPPD . . . calcium pyrophosphate dihydrate
CPR . . . cardiopulmonary resuscitation
cps . . . cycles per second
CPS . . . Compendium of Pharmaceuticals and Specialties
CPT . . . chest physiotherapy
Cr . . . chromium
^{51}Cr . . . radioisotope of chromium
CRA . . . central retinal artery
Cre . . . creatinine
creat . . . creatinine
CRF . . . chronic renal failure; corticotropin releasing factor
CRM . . . cross reacting material
CRP . . . C-reactive protein
CRS . . . catheter related sepsis
CRST . . . calcinosis, Raynaud's phenomenon, sclerodactylia, telangiectasis
CRT . . . cathode ray tube
Cs . . . cesium
CS . . . cesarean section; coronary sclerosis
C & S . . . culture and sensitivity
CSA . . . cyclosporin A
CS & CC . . . culture, sensitivity and colony count
CSF . . . cerebrospinal fluid
CSP . . . chemistry screening profile
CSR . . . corrected sedimentation rate
CT . . . circulation time; clotting time; computerized tomography
CTA . . . Committee on Thrombolytic Agents
CTAB . . . cetyltrimethylammonium bromide
CTD . . . carpal tunnel decompression; congenital thymic dysplasia
CTM . . . *Chlamydia* transport media
CTT . . . computerized transaxial tomography
CTX . . . cytoxan
Cu . . . copper
CUC . . . chronic ulcerative colitis
CV . . . cardiovascular; coefficient of variation; conjugata vera
CVA . . . cerebrovascular accident
CVD . . . cardiovascular disease
CVE . . . cerebrovascular evaluation
CVI . . . cerebral vascular insufficiency; continuous venous infusion
CVP . . . central venous pressure
CVS . . . cardiovascular system; clean voided specimen
Cx . . . cervical; cervix
CXR . . . chest x-ray
CYT . . . cyclophosphamide

D_5W . . . 5% dextrose in water solution
DALA . . . delta aminolevulinic acid
DAT . . . direct antiglobulin test
db . . . decibel
DB . . . deep breath
DBI . . . development at birth index
DBP . . . diastolic blood pressure
DC . . . direct current
D & C . . . dilatation and curettage
DCG . . . dynamic electrocardiogram
DCH . . . delayed and cutaneous hypersensitivity
DD . . . differential diagnosis
DDD . . . degenerative disc disease
DDI . . . dideoxyinosine; dressing dry and infact
DDP . . . diamminedichloroplatinum
DDS . . . diaminodiphenylsulfone
DDT . . . dichloro-diphenyltrichloroethane
DDX . . . differential diagnosis
DEA . . . Drug Enforcement Agency
DEAE . . . diethylaminoethyl
DER . . . dermatome evoked response
DFA . . . direct fluorescent antibody
DFMO . . . difluoromethylornithine
DFP . . . diisopropylfluorophosphonate
dg . . . decigram
DH . . . dermatitis herpetiformis
DHA . . . dehydroepiandrosterone
DHAD . . . dihydroxybisaminoanthraquinone dihydrochloride
DHEA . . . dehydroepiandrosterone
DHEA-S . . . dehydroepiandrosterone sulfate
DHL . . . diffuse histiocytic lymphoma
DHS . . . duration of hospital stay
DHT . . . dihydrotestosterone
DI . . . diabetes insipidus
DIC . . . disseminated intravascular coagulation
diff . . . differential
DIP . . . dichlorophenolindophenol
DISIDA . . . diisopropyl-iminodiacetic acid
DJD . . . degenerative joint disease
DKA . . . diabetic ketoacidosis
dL . . . deciliter
D-L . . . Donath-Landsteiner
DLCO . . . diffusing capacity of the lung for carbon monoxide
DLE . . . discoid lupus erythematosus
DLF . . . digoxin-like factors
dm . . . decimeter
DM . . . diabetes mellitus; diastolic murmur
DMO . . . dimethyloxazolidinedione
DMSO . . . dimethylsulfoxide
DNA . . . deoxyribonucleic acid
DNase . . . deoxyribonuclease
DNBT . . . dinitroblue
DNP . . . deoxyribonucleoprotein
DNPH . . . dinitrophenylhydrazine
DOA . . . date of admission; dead on arrival
DOB . . . date of birth
DOC . . . deoxycorticosterone
DOE . . . dyspnea on exertion
DOI . . . date of injury
dos . . . dose (dosis)
DOSS . . . diocytl sodium sulfosuccinate
DP . . . diastolic pressure
DPE . . . dipivalyl epinephrine
DPG . . . diphosphoglycerate
DPH . . . diphenylhydantoin
DPPC . . . dipalmitoylphosphatidylcholine
DPT . . . diphtheria toxoid, pertussis vaccine, tetanus toxoid
DQ . . . developmental quotient
Dr . . . doctor
DR . . . donor related
DRG . . . diagnostic related group(s)
DSA . . . digital subtraction angiography
DSC . . . decussation superior cerebellar; differential scanning colorimeter
DSCG . . . disodium cromoglycate
DSD . . . discharge summary dictated; dry sterile dressing
ds-DNA . . . double-stranded DNA
DSF . . . disulfiram
DST . . . dexamethasone suppression test
DT . . . delirium tremons; duration tetany; dye test
dtd . . . let such doses be given (dentur tales doses)
DTM . . . dermatophyte test medium
DTO . . . deodorized opium tincture
DTP . . . diphtheria-tetanus pertussis
DTR . . . deep tendon reflex
dU . . . deoxyuridine
DV . . . deep vein
DVT . . . deep vein thrombosis
dw . . . dry weight
Dx . . . diagnosis
Dy . . . dysprosium

E . . . exa (10^{18})
EA . . . early antigen
EAC . . . external auditory canal
EACA . . . epsilon-aminocaproic acid
EB . . . Epstein-Barr
EBEA . . . Epstein-Barr early antigen
EBNA . . . Epstein-Barr nuclear antigen
EBV . . . Epstein-Barr virus
EBVCA . . . Epstein-Barr virus, capsid antigen
EBVEA . . . Epstein-Barr virus, early antigen
EBVNA . . . Epstein-Barr virus, nuclear antigen
EC . . . *Escherichia coli*; extracellular
ECA . . . external carotid artery
ECG . . . electrocardiogram
ECT . . . emission computed tomography
EDTA . . . ethylenediaminetetraacetic acid
EDX . . . electrodiagnosis
EEG . . . electroencephalogram
EENT . . . eyes, ears, nose, throat
EF . . . ejection fraction; extended-field
EFA . . . essential fatty acids
EFM . . . external fetal monitoring
eg . . . example
EGA . . . estimated gestational age
EGD . . . esophagogastroduodenoscopy
EGFR . . . epidermal growth factor receptor
EH . . . enlarged heart; essential hypertension
EHDP . . . ethanehydroxydiphosphonic acid
EHEC . . . enterohemorrhagic *E. coli*
EIA . . . enzyme immunoassay
EID . . . electroimmunodiffusion

EIEC . . . . enteroinvasive *E. coli*
EKG . . . . electrocardiogram
ELISA . . . . enzyme-linked immunosorbent assay
ELT . . . . euoglobulin lysis time
EM . . . . electron microscopy
EMA . . . . endomysial antibody
EMG . . . . electromyogram
EMIT . . . . enzyme-multiplied immunoassay technique
EMS . . . . eosinophil myalgia syndrome
ENA . . . . extractable nuclear antigen
ENG . . . . electronystagmography
ENT . . . . ear, nose, and throat
EOG . . . . electro-oculogram
eos . . . . eosinophil
EPA . . . . Environmental Protection Agency
EPBI . . . . exercise penile-brachial index
EPEC . . . . enteropathogenic *E. coli*
EPEG . . . . etoposide
EPIS . . . . episiotomy
EPP . . . . erythropoietic protoporphyria
EPS . . . . electrophysiologic studies
EPSEs . . . . extrapyramidal side effects
EPT . . . . early pregnancy test; Eidetic Parents Test; endoscopic
papillotomy
Eq . . . . equivalent
Er . . . . erbium
ER . . . . emergency room; estrogen receptors
ERA . . . . estrogen receptor assay; evoked response audiometry
ERCP . . . . endoscopic retrograde cholangiopancreatography
ERG . . . . electroretinogram
ERPF . . . . effective renal plasma flow
ERV . . . . expiratory reserve volume
Es . . . . Einsteinium
ES . . . . electrical stimulation
ESP . . . . extrasensory perception
ESR . . . . erythrocyte sedimentation rate
ESRD . . . . end-stage renal disease
EST . . . . electroshock therapy
et . . . . and (et)
ETEC . . . . enterotoxigenic *E. coli*
EtOH . . . . ethyl alcohol
ETS-2
. . . . Educational Testing Service; electrical transcranial stimulation;
ETT . . . . extrathyroidal thyroxine
EU . . . . Ehrlich unit
EVI . . . . endocardial, vascular, and interstitial

f . . . . femto (10^{-15})
F . . . . fluorine
FA . . . . fatty acid; filterable agent; fluorescent antibody
FAB . . . . French-American-British
FACP . . . . Fellow of the American College of Physicians
FAD . . . . flavin adenine dinucleotide
FAMA . . . . fluorescent antibody to membrane antigen
FANA . . . . fluorescent antinuclear antibody
FAS . . . . fetal alcohol syndrome
FB . . . . finger breadths; foreign bodies
FBC . . . . functional bactericidal concentration
FBP . . . . fibrin breakdown product
FBS . . . . fasting blood sugar
Fc . . . . portion of antibody molecule bound by membrane receptors
FD . . . . food and drug
FDA . . . . Federal Drug Administration
FDP . . . . fibrin degradation product; fructose diphosphate
Fe . . . . iron
FeCl₃ . . . . ferric chloride
FEF . . . . forced expiratory flow
FENa . . . . fractional excretion of sodium (Na)
FEP . . . . free erythrocyte protoporphyrin
FES . . . . functional electrical stimulation
FETI . . . . fluorescent energy transfer immunoassay
FEV . . . . forced expiratory volume
FF . . . . filtration fraction; force fluids
FFA . . . . free fatty acids
FFP . . . . fresh frozen plasma
fg . . . . femtogram
FH . . . . family history
FHH . . . . familial hypocalciuric hypercalcemia
FHR . . . . fetal heart rate
FHS . . . . fetal heart sounds
FIC . . . . functional inhibitory concentration
FIF . . . . forced inspiratory flow
FITC . . . . fluorescein isothiocyanate
FIVC . . . . forced inspiratory vital capacity
fL . . . . femtoliter; fluid

Fm . . . . fermium
fmol . . . . femtomole
FMULC . . . . free monoclonal urinary light chains
FNA . . . . fine needle aspiration
FOB . . . . fiberoptic bronchoscopy
FOS . . . . fiberoptic sigmoidoscopy
FP . . . . false-positive
FPIA . . . . fluorescence polarization immunoassay
Fr . . . . francium
FRA . . . . fluorescent rabies antibody
FRC . . . . functional residual capacity
FS . . . . frozen section
FSH . . . . follicle stimulating hormone
FSI . . . . foam stability index
FSP . . . . fibrin split products
ft . . . . make (fiat, fiant)
FTA . . . . fluorescent treponemal antibody
FTA-ABS . . . . fluorescent treponemal antibody absorption
FTI . . . . free thyroxine index
FTND . . . . full-term normal delivery
FU . . . . fluorouracil
FUDR-MP . . . . floxuridine monophosphate
FUO . . . . fever of undetermined origin
FVC . . . . forced vital capacity
Fx . . . . fracture
FX . . . . factor X

g . . . . gram
G . . . . giga (10^9)
G-6-PD . . . . glucose 6-phosphate dehydrogenase
Ga . . . . gallium
GABA . . . . gamma-aminobutyric acid
GAL . . . . galactosemia
GAW . . . . airway conductance
GAZT . . . . glucuronide derivative of azidothymidine
GB . . . . gallbladder
GBM . . . . glomerular basement membrane
GC . . . . . . geriatric chair; gonorrhea culture; gas chromatography
GC/MS . . . . gas chromatography/mass spectrometry
G-CSF . . . . granulocyte colony stimulating factors
GCV . . . . ganciclovir
Gd . . . . gadolinium
g/dL . . . . gram percent
gdw . . . . gram dry weight
Ge . . . . germanium
GE . . . . gastroesophageal
GFR . . . . glomerular filtration rate
GGCT . . . . ground glass clotting time
GGT . . . . gamma-glutamyltransferase
GH . . . . growth hormone
GHB . . . . glycohemoglobin
GI . . . . gastrointestinal
GIH . . . . gastric inhibitory hormone
GIP . . . . gastric inhibitory polypeptide
GIS . . . . gastrointestinal series
GK . . . . galactokinase
GLC . . . . gas-liquid chromatography
GM . . . . geometric mean
GMS . . . . Grocott-Gomori methenamine-silver
Gn . . . . gonadotropin
GnRH . . . . gonadotropin releasing hormone
GOT . . . . glutamic-oxaloacetic transaminase
GP . . . . glycoprotein
GPK . . . . guinea pig kidney
GPT . . . . glutamic-pyruvic transaminase
GPUT . . . . glactose phosphate uridyl transferase
GR . . . . glutathione reductase
GSA65 . . . . gross virus antigen
GSD . . . . glycogen storage disease
GSH . . . . glutathione; growth stimulating hormone
GSR . . . . . . galvanic skin response; generalized Schwartzman reaction
GSSR . . . . . . generalized Sandarelli-Shwartzman reaction
GT . . . . gait training; gamma-glutamyltransferase
GTP . . . . glutamyl transpeptidase
gtt(s) . . . . drop(s) (gutta)
GTT . . . . glucose tolerance test
GU . . . . genitourinary; gastric ulcer; gonococcal urethritis
GVHD . . . . graft versus host disease
GXT . . . . graded exercise test
gyn . . . . gynecological

h . . . . hour (hora)
H . . . . hydrogen
Ha . . . . hahnium

691

HA	headache; hemagglutination
HAA	hepatitis-associated antigen
HABA	hydroxybenzeneazobenzoic acid
HAI	hemagglutination inhibition
HANE	hereditary angioneurotic edema
HAV	hepatitis A virus
HAVAB	hepatitis A virus antibody
Hb	hemoglobin
HBAb	hepatitis B antibody
HBAg	hepatitis B antigen
HB$_c$	hepatitis B core
HBD	hydroxybutric dehydrogenase
HBDH	hydroxybutyrate dehydrogenase
HB$_e$Ag	hepatitis B e antigen
HBP	high blood pressure
HB$_s$Ag	hepatitis B surface antigen
HBV	hepatitis B virus
HC	homocystinuria
HCFA	Health Care Financing Administration
hCG	human chorionic gonadotropin
HCl	hydrochloric acid
HCO$_3$	bicarbonate
HCS	human chorionic somatomammotropin
Hct	hematocrit
HD	Hodgkin's disease
HDL	high density lipoprotein
HDLC	high density lipoprotein cholesterol
HDLs	high density lipoproteins
HDN	hemolytic disease of the newborn
HDP	hydroxydimethylpyrimidine
He	helium
HEMPAS	here. erythroblastic multinuclearity with positive acidified serum
HEp	human epithelial cells
HES	acute hypereosinophilic syndrome
Hf	hafnium
HFI	hereditary fructose intolerance
Hg	mercury
^{197}Hg	radioisotope of mercury
^{203}Hg	radioisotope of mercury
HG	herpes gestationis
HGA	homogentisic acid
Hgb	hemoglobin
HGG	human gamma globulin
HGH	human growth hormone
HGPRT	hypoxanthine guanine phosphoribosyl transferase
HHC	home health care
HHD	hypertensive heart disease
HHH	hyperornithinemia, hyperammonemia-homocitrullinuria
HHM	humoral hypercalcemia of malignancy
HHT	head holter traction
HI	hydriodic acid
HIAA	hydroxyindoleacetic acid
HIB	*Haemophilus influenzae* B
HIDA	acetanilidoiminodiacetic acid
HIP	humoral immunocompetence profile
HIV	human immunodeficiency virus
HK	hexokinase
HL	hearing level
HLA	human leukocyte antigen
HMB	homatropine methylbromide
HMM	hexamethylmelamine
HMO	Health Maintenance Organization
HMS	hexose monophosphate shunt
HMW	high molecular weight
HMWK	high molecular weight kininogen
HN	head nurse
Ho	holmium
HO	house officer
H/O	history of
HOB	head of bed
HP	hot packs
H & P	history and physical
hpf	high power field
HPFH	hereditary persistence of fetal hemoglobin
HPI	history of present illness
HPL	human placental lactogen
HPLC	high-performance liquid chromatography
HPN	home parenteral nutrition
HPP	human pancreatic polypeptide
HPPA	hydroxyphenylpyruvic acid
HPPH	hydroxyphenyl-phenylhydantoin
HPT	hyperparathyroidism
hPTH	human parathyroid hormone
HPV	human papillomavirus

HR	heart rate; hospital record
HRANA	histone reactive ANA
HRLM	high resolution light microscopy
hs	at bedtime (hora somni)
HS	herpes simplex; hereditary spherocytosis
HSA	human serum albumin
HSV	herpes simplex virus
HT	hypertension; hypodermic tablet
HTLV	human T-lymphotropic virus
HTN	hypertension
HTP	hydroxytrytophan
HTVD	hypertensive vascular disease
HUS	hemolytic-uremic syndrome; hyaluronidase unit for semen
H-V	HIS-ventricular
HVA	homovanillic acid
Hx	history
HXM	hexamethylmelamine
Hz	hertz

I	indeterminate; intermediate; iodine
^{125}I	radioisotope of iodide
^{131}I	radioisotope of iodide
I-3-AA	indole-3-acetic acid
Ia	antigen
IAA	indole acetic acid
IABP	intra-aortic balloon pump
IADH	inappropriate antidiuretic hormone
IAT	indirect antiglobulin test
Ib	a glycoprotein
IBC	iron binding capacity
IBW	ideal body weight
IC	immune complexes; inspiratory capacity
ICA	internal carotid artery
ICD	isocitrate dehydrogenase
ICDH	isocitrate dehydrogenase
ICF	intracellular fluid
ICG	indocyanine green
ICN	intensive care neonatal
ICS	intercostal space
ICSH	interstitial cell stimulating hormone
ICT	indirect Coombs' test
ICU	intensive care unit
ID	identification; immunodiffusion; infectious disease; intradermal(ly)
IDA	iron deficiency anemia; image display and analysis
IDAT	indirect antiglobulin test
IDDM	insulin dependent diabetes mellitus
IDL	intermediate-density lipoprotein
IEF	isoelectric focusing
IEM	inborn errors of metabolism
IEP	immunoelectrophoresis
IF	immunofluorescence; inspiratory force; interstitial fluid; intrinsic factor
IFA	indirect fluorescent antibody
IFIX	immunofixation
IFLrA	recombinant human leukocyte interferon A
Ig	immunoglobulin
IGIM	immune globulin intramuscular
IGT	impaired glucose tolerance
IHA	indirect hemagglutination
IHSS	idiopathic hypertrophic subaortic stenosis
IIb-IIIa	glycoproteins found on platelet membranes
IIF	indirect immunofluorescence
I.M.	intramuscular
IMD	inherited metabolic disorders
IMIG	intramuscular immunoglobulin
IMP	impression
IMV	intermittent mandatory ventilation
In	indium
IND	investigational new drug
INH	isonicotinic acid hydrazide; isoniazid
INR	international normalized ratio
IOFNA	intraoperative fine needle aspiration
IOL	intraocular lens
IOP	intraocular pressure
IOT	intraocular tension
IP	intraperitoneal(ly)
I-PAO	insulin induced peak acid output
IPF	idiopathic pulmonary fibrosis
IPG	impedence phlebograph
IPPB	intermittent positive pressure breathing
Ir	iridium
IR	infrared
IRDS	infant respiratory distress syndrome
IRG	immunoreactive glucose
IRGH	immunoreactive growth hormone

IRI . . . . immunoreactive insulin
IRMA . . . . immunoradiometric assay
IRT . . . . immunoreactive trypsinogen
ISD . . . . isosorbide dinitrate
ISDN . . . . isosorbibe dinitrate
ISE . . . . ion-selective electrode
IT . . . . inhalation therapy; intrathecal(ly)
ITP . . . . idiopathic thrombocytopenic purpura
ITT . . . . insulin tolerance test
IU . . . . International unit
IUD . . . . intrauterine device
IUGR . . . . intrauterine growth retardation
IUP . . . . intrauterine pregnancy
I.V. . . . . intravenous
IVAC . . . . I.V. infusion control device
IVAD . . . . implanted vascular access device
IVC . . . . inferior vena cava; intravenous cholangiography
IVH . . . . intraventricular hemorrhage
IVIG . . . . intravenous immune globulin
IVP . . . . intravenous push; intravenous pyelogram
IVPB . . . . intravenous piggyback
IVSD . . . . intraventricular septal defect

JODM . . . . juvenile-onset diabetes mellitus
JRA . . . . juvenile rheumatoid arthritis
JVD . . . . jugular-venous distenion
JVP . . . . jugular venous pressure; jugular venous pulse

k . . . . kilo (10^3)
K . . . . potassium
K-B . . . . Kleihauer-Betke
kcal . . . . kilocalorie
KCl . . . . potassium chloride
KCN . . . . potassium cyanide
kg . . . . kilogram
KGS . . . . ketogenic steroids
kL . . . . kiloliter
km . . . . kilometer
KO . . . . keep open
KOH . . . . potassium hydroxide
Kr . . . . krypton
KS . . . . ketosteroids; Kaposi's sarcoma
KU . . . . Karmen units
KUB . . . . kidney and urinary bladder
KVO . . . . keep vein open
KW . . . . Keith-Wagener

L . . . . left; liter; lumbar
L₂ . . . . second lumbar vertebra
La . . . . lanthanum
LA . . . . . latex agglutination; left artrium; local anesthetic
LAD . . . . left anterior descending (artery)
LAI . . . . labioincisal
LAO . . . . left anterior oblique
LAP . . . . leucine aminopeptidase; leukocyte alkaline phosphatase
Lap . . . . laparotomy
LASA . . . . lipid-associated sialic acid
LATS . . . . long-acting thyroid stimulating hormone
LBBB . . . . left bundle branch block
LBM . . . . lean body mass
LBW . . . . low birth weight
LC . . . . lethal concentration
LCI . . . . lung clearance index
LCIS . . . . lobular carcinoma *in situ*
LCM . . . . lymphocytic choriomeningitis
LCS . . . . Leydig cell stimulation
LD . . . . . . lactate dehydrogenase; lethal dose; light difference
LD₁ . . . . lactate dehydrogenase fraction 1
LDH . . . . lactate dehydrogenase
LDHI . . . . LDH isoenzymes
LDL . . . . low density lipoprotein
LDLC . . . . low density lipoprotein cholesterol
LDLs . . . . low density lipoproteins
LDT . . . . lactate dehydrogenase total
LDV . . . . lactate dehydrogenase virus
Le . . . . Lewis antigen
LE . . . . lower extremity; lupus erythematosus
LEA . . . . lower extremity arterial
LES . . . . lower esophageal sphincter
LEV . . . . lower extremity venous
LFT . . . . liver function test
LGV . . . . lymphogranuloma venereum
LH . . . . luteinizing hormone
LHRF . . . . luteinizing hormone releasing factor

LHRH . . . . luteinizing hormone releasing hormone
LHV . . . . left ventricular hypertrophy
Li . . . . lithium
LISS . . . . low ionic strength saline
L-J . . . . Löwenstein-Jensen
LKM . . . . liver/kidney microsomes
LKS . . . . liver, kidneys, spleen
LLA . . . . lupus like anticoagulant
LLDH . . . . liver lactate dehydrogenase
LLL . . . . left lower lobe
LLQ . . . . left lower quadrant
LM . . . . light microscopy
LMN . . . . lower motor neuron
LMP . . . . last menstrual period
LMWH . . . . low molecular weight heparin
LOA . . . . left occipital anterior
LOM . . . . limitation of motion
LOS . . . . length of stay
LP . . . . light perception; lumbar puncture
LPC . . . . leukocyte-poor cells (leukocyte depleted)
lpf . . . . low power field
LPO . . . . left posterior oblique
LPRBC . . . . leukocyte-poor red blood cells
LRC . . . . Lipid Research Clinic
LRH . . . . lutenizing releasing hormone
L/S . . . . lecithin/sphingomyelin ratio
LSD . . . . lysergic acid diethylamide
LSG . . . . labial salivary gland
LTC . . . . long-term care
LTCPs . . . . L-tryptophan-containing products
LTT . . . . lymphocyte transformation test
Lu . . . . lutetium
LUL . . . . left upper lobe
LUQ . . . . left upper quadrant
LV . . . . lung volume
LVET . . . . left ventricular ejection time
LVH . . . . left ventricular hypertrophy
LVOT . . . . left ventricular outflow tract
LVW . . . . lateral vaginal wall
Lw . . . . lawrencium
L & W . . . . living and well
Lytes . . . . electrolytes

m . . . . meter; milli (10^{-3})
m² . . . . square meter
m³ . . . . cubic meter
M . . . . mega (10^6); mix (misce)
mA . . . . milliampere
MA . . . . Master of Arts
M/A . . . . mood and/or affect
MA-1 . . . . a type of respirator
MAA . . . . microaggregatedalbumin
MAI . . . . *Mycobacterium avium-intracellulare*
MAO . . . . maximal acid output; monoamine oxidase
MAR . . . medication administration record; mixed antiglobulin reaction
MB . . . . a fraction of creatine kinase
MBA . . . . Master of Business Administration
MBC . . . . minimum bactericidal concentration; maximum breathing capacity
MBD . . . . maximum bactericidal dilution
MBP . . . . myelin basic protein
mc . . . . millicurie
MC-Ab . . . . monoclonal antibody
MCAD . . . . medium chain ACYL CO-A dehydrogenase
mcg . . . . microgram
MCH . . . . mean corpuscular hemoglobin
MCHC . . . . mean cell hemoglobin concentration
mCi . . . . millicurie
MCL . . . . midclavicular line; midcostal line
MCT . . . . medium chain triglycerides
MCTD . . . . mixed connective tissue disease
MCV . . . . mean corpuscular volume
Md . . . . mendelevium
MD . . . . medical doctor
MDIs . . . . metered dose inhalers
MDM . . . . minor determinant mixture
MDP . . . . mentodextra posterior
MDR . . . . minimum daily requirement
MDS . . . . materials distribution system
MDV . . . . multiple dose vial
MEA . . . . mercaptoethylamine; multiple endocrine adenomatosis
MED . . . . minimal erythemal dose
MEET . . . . multistage exercise electrocardiographics test
MEIA . . . . microparticle enzyme immunoassay
MEN . . . . multiple endocrine neoplasia

mEq	milliequivalent
METS	metastases
MF	mycosis fungoides
MFC	minimum fungicidal concentration
mg	milligram
Mg	magnesium
MgCl$_2$	magnesium chloride
MgCO$_3$	magnesium carbonate
MGP	methyl green pyronine
MgSO$_4$	magnesium sulfate
MH	malignant hyperthermia; marital history; menstrual history; mental health
MHA	microhemagglutination
MHA-TP	microhemagglutination *Treponema pallidum*
MHC	major histocompatibility complex
MHPG	methoxyhydroxyphenylglycol
MHz	megahertz
MI	myocardial infarction; maturation index
MIC	minimum inhibitory concentration
μg	microgram
μL	microliter
μm^3	cubic micrometer
μ	micro (10^{-6})
μm	micrometer
μmol	micromole
μmol/L	micromolar
μOsm	micro-osmolar
μU	microunit
MID	maximum bactericidal dilution
MIF	merthiolate-iodine-formalin; migration inhibitory factor
MIT	migration inhibition test
mIU	milli International unit
mL	milliliter
MLC	mixed leukocyte culture; mixed lymphocyte culture
MLD	metachromatic leukodystrophy; minimum lethal dose
MLR	mixed lymphocyte reaction
MLT	medical laboratory technician
MLV	monitored live voice
mm	millimeter
mm^2	square millimeter
mm^3	cubic millimeter
MMA	methylmalonic acid
MMC	minimal medullary concentration
MMEF	mean midexpiratory flow
MMF	maximal midexpiratory flow rate
mm Hg	millimeters of mercury
mmol	millimole
mmol/L	millimolar
MMPI	Minnesota multiple personality inventory
MMR	measles, mumps, rubella
MMT	manual muscle test
Mn	manganese
MNS	MNS blood group
Mo	molybdenum
MO	mesio-occlusal
MOA-B	monoamine oxidasetype-B inhibitor
mol	mole
mol/L	molar
MOPP	mustargen oncovin procarbazine and prednisone
mOsm	milliosmole
mph	miles per hour
MPH	Master of Public Health
MPHD	methoxyhydroxphenolglycerol
MPS	mucopolysaccharidosis
MPV	mean plasma volume; mean platelet volume
MR	moderately resistant
mrad	millirad
MRI	magnetic resonance imaging
MRSA	methicillin-resistant *S. aureus*
MS	mental status; mitral stenosis; multiple sclerosis
MSAFP	maternal serum alpha fetoprotein
MSD	metabolic screening disorders
msec	millisecond
MSH	melanocyte stimulating hormone
MSL	midsternal line
MSLT	multiple sleep latency test
MSTA	mumps skin test antigen
MSUD	maple syrup urine disease
mt	send of such (mitte talis)
MT	medical technologist
MTB	mycobacterium tuberculosis
MTC	mitomycin-C
^{99m}Tc	radioisotope of technetium Tc 99m
MTHF	5-methyl-tetrahydrofolate
MTRX	methotrexate

MTX	methotrexate
MTX's	methotrexate
mU	milliunit
MUGA	multiple gated scan
MUP	monitor unit potential
MV	minute volume
MVP	mitral valve prolapse
MVV	maximum voluntary ventilation
MW	molecular weight
MZ	monozygotic
n	nano (10^{-9})
N	nitrogen; normal
Na	sodium
NA	not applicable; nursing assistant
Na$_2$CO$_3$	sodium carbonate
NACI	National Advisory Committee on Immunization
NaCl	sodium chloride
NAD	nicotinamide adenine dinucleotide; no acute distress; no apparent distress
NADH	reduced form of NAD
NADP	nicotinamide adenine dinucleotide phosphate
NADPH	reduced form of NADP
NaF	sodium fluoride
NaOH	sodium hydroxide
NAPA	n-acetylprocainamide
NAS	no added salt
NATP	neonatal autoimmune thrombocytopenic purpura
Nb	niobium
NBIL	neonatal bilirubin
NBT	nitro blue tetrazolium
NC	nerve conduction
NCA	National Certification Agency; nonspecific cross reacting antigen
NCCLS	National Committee for Clinical Laboratory Standards
NCEP	National Cholesterol Education Program
NCI	National Cancer Institute
NCS	nerve conduction study
NCV	nerve conduction velocity
Nd	neodymium
Ne	neon
ng	nanogram
NGU	nongonococcal urethritis
NH$_4$Cl	ammonium chloride
NH$_4$OH	ammonium hydroxide
Ni	nickel
NICU	neonatal intensive care unit
NIH	National Institutes of Health
NK	natural killer
NKA	no known allergies
nL	nanoliter
NL	normal
nm	nanometer
NMJ	neuromuscular junction disease
nmol	nanomole
nmol/L	millimicromolar
NMR	nuclear magnetic resonance
NMS	neuroleptic malignant syndrome
No	nobelium
noc	in the night (nocturnal)
non rep	do not repeat; no refills
NOS	no organisms seen
Np	neptunium
NP	nasopharynx
NPO	nothing by mouth
NPT	nocturnal penile tumescence
NPTM	nocturnal penile tumescence monitoring
nr	do not repeat (non repetatur)
NRBCs	nucleated red blood cells
NRC	National Research Council; Nuclear Regulatory Commission
NS	normal saline; not seen; not significant
NSA	no salt albumin
NSAID-induced	nonsteroidal anti-inflammatory drug
NSE	neuron specific enolase
NSR	normal sinus rhythm
NST	nonstress test
NSU	nonspecific urethritis
NSVD	normal spontaneous vaginal delivery
NT	nasotracheal
N & T	nose and throat
NTG	nitroglycerine
NTI	nonthyroidal illness; nonthyroidal index
N & V	nausea and vomiting
NVD	nausea, vomiting, diarrhea
NYD	not yet diagnosed

O ... oxygen
OB ... obstetrics; occult blood
OBS ... organic brain syndrome
OC ... on call; oral contraceptive
OCD ... obsessive-compulsive disorder
OCG ... oral cholecystogram
OCs ... oral contraceptives
OCT ... ornithine carbamyl transferase
od ... right eye (oculus dexter)
OD ... overdose
ODC ... oxygen dissociation curve
ODE ... O-desmethylencainide
ODm ... ophthalmodynamometry
O/E ... on examination
OGTT ... oral glucose tolerance test
OH ... hydroxide; hydroxyl
OHCS ... hydroxycorticosteroid
17-OHCS ... 17-hydroxycorticosteroids
OHP ... oxygen under high pressure
OIF ... oil immersion field
OKT ... a group of monoclonal antibodies for typing lymphocytes
OM ... otitis media
OOB ... out of bed
OPG ... ocular plethysmography
OPV ... out patient visit; oral polio vaccine
O.R. ... operating room
os ... left eye (oculus sinister)
Os ... osmium
OT ... old tuberculin
OTC ... ornithine transcarbamylase
ou ... each eye (oculus uterque)
ov ... ovarian

p ... pico (10^{-12})
P ... peta (10^{15}); phosphorus; pulse
p24 ... antigen in HIV infection
^{32}P ... radioisotope of phosphorus
p50 ... half saturation (oxygen)
Pa ... protactinium
PA .. phenylalinine; platelet associated; pernicious anemia; physician's assistant
P & A ... percussion and auscultation
PABA ... para-aminobenzoic acid
PAC ... premature atrial contraction
PAH ... phenylalanine hydroxylase
PAI ... plasminogen activator inhibitor
PAO ... peak acid output
Pap ... Papanicolaou's stain
PAP ... peroxidase antiperoxidase; pri. atypical pneum.; prostate acid phosphatase
PAR ... pulmonary arteriolar resistance
PAS ... para-aminosalicylic acid; periodic acid Schiff stain
PAT ... paroxysmal atrial tachycardia; preadmission testing
Pb ... lead
PBC ... primary biliary cirrhosis
PBG ... porphobilinogen
PBI ... protein-bound iodine
PBL ... peripheral blood lymphocytes
PBS ... peripheral blood smear
pc ... after meals (post cibum)
PC ... porto-caval; present complaint
pc1 ... platelet count pretransfusion
pc2 ... platelet count post-transfusion
PCA ... parietal cell antibody; percutaneous coronary angioplasty
PCB ... polychlorinated biphenyls
PCD ... polycystic disease; posterior corneal deposits
PCE ... pseudocholinesterase
PCG ... pneumocardiogram
PCH ... paroxysmal cold hemoglobinuria
PCHE ... pseudocholinesterase
PCI ... prothrombin consumption index
PCMX ... parachlorometaxylenol
PCNS ... penicillins
pCO_2 ... carbon dioxide partial pressure (tension)
PCP ... phencyclidine
PCR ... polymerase chain reaction
PCT ... prothrombin consumption test
PCU ... patient care unit
PCV ... packed cell volume
PCWP ... pulmonary capillary wedge pressure
Pd ... palladium
PD ... postural drainage
PDR ... *Physician's Desk Reference*
PDW ... platelet distribution width
PE ... physical examination; pleural effusion; pulmonary embolism
PEEP ... positive end-expiratory pressure
PEF ... peak expiratory flow
PEFR ... peak expiratory flow rate
PEFT ... peak expiratory flow time
PEG ... polyethylene glycol
PEP ... phosphoenolpyruvate
PERLA ... pupils equal, reactive to light and accommodation
PET ... positron emission tomography; pre-eclamptic toxemia
PF ... platelet factor; preservative free
PFA ... phosphonoformatic acid; profunda femoris artery
PFK ... phosphofructoaldolase
PFS ... penile flow study; prefilled syringe
PFT ... pulmonary function test
PFU ... plaque forming units
pg ... picogram
PG ... phosphatidyl glycine
PGD ... phosphogluconate dehydrogenase
PGI ... phosphoglucose isomerase
PGK ... phosphoglycerokinase
PgR ... progesterone receptor
PGs ... prostaglandin; pyoderma gangrenosum
pH ... measurement of acidity or alkalinity
pHa ... arterial blood pH
PHA ... phytohemagglutinin activation
PhD ... Doctor of Philosophy
PHI ... phosphohexoseisomerase
PHP ... persistent hyperphenylalaninemia
PHT ... peroxide hemolysis test
pi ... platelet count increment
PI ... phosphatidylinositol; protamine insulin; pulmonary infarction
PID ... pelvic inflammatory disease
PIO ... progesterone in oil
PIV ... parainfluenza virus
PK ... pyruvate kinase
PKU ... phenylketonuria
Plt ... platelet
PLT ... psittacosis-lymphogranuloma venereum-trachoma
Pm ... promethium
PM ... afternoon
PM-1 ... polymorph; postmortem
PMD ... primary myocardial disease; progressive muscular dystrophy
PMH ... past medical history
PM-I ... platelet membrane antigen
PMN ... polymorphonuclear neutrophil
pmol ... picomole
PMP ... previous menstrual period
PM & R ... physical medicine and rehabilition
PMS ... premenstrual syndrome
PNH ... paroxysmal nocturnal hemoglobinuria
PNP ... nonprotein nitrogen
pNPP ... paranitrophenylphosphate
Pnx ... pneumothorax
po ... by mouth (per os)
Po ... polonium
pO_2 ... oxygen partial pressure (tension)
POA ... pancreatic oncofetal antigen
POMR ... problem oriented medical record
POR ... problem oriented record
PP ... postprandial
PPA ... phenylpropanolamine
PPBS ... postprandial blood sugar
PPD ... purified protein derivative
PPF ... plasma protein fraction
PPG ... photoplethysmography
PPL ... penicilloye-polylysine
PPLO ... pleuropneumonia-like organisms
ppm ... parts per million
ppt ... precipitate
Pr ... praseodymium; presbyopia
PR ... per rectum
PRA ... plasma renin activity; progesterone receptor assay
PRBCs ... packed red blood cells
PRG ... phleborheography
PRL ... prolactin
prn ... as needed (pro re nata)
PROM ... premature rupture of membranes; prolonged rupture of membranes
PRP ... polyribophosphate
PRSM ... peripheral smear
PS ... periodic syndrome; phosphatidylserine; population sample; Porter-Silber; pulmonary stenosis; pyloric stenosis
PSA ... prostate specific antigen
PSG ... polysomnography
PSIS ... posterior/superior iliac spine
PSP ... phenolsulfonphthalein

PSRO	Professional Standards Review Organization
PSS	progressive systemic sclerosis
PS-VER	pattern shift - visual evoked response
PSVT	paroxysmal supraventricular tachycardia
Pt	platinum
PT	physical therapy; prothrombin time
P & T	Pharmacy & Therapeutics
PTA	platelet thromboplastin antecedent; prothrombin activity
PTAH	phosphotungstic acid hematoxylin
PTC	phenylthiocarbamide; plasma thromboplastin component
PTCA	percutaneous transluminal angioplasty
PTH	parathyroid hormone
PTP	prothrombin-proconvertin
PTS	pneumatic tube system
PTT	partial thromboplastin time
Pu	plutonium
PU	peptic ulcer
PUD	peptic ulcer disease
pulv	a powder (pulvis)
PUVA	pulsed ultraviolet actinotherapy
PV	plasma volume
PVA	polyvinyl alcohol
PVC	premature ventricular contraction
PVD	peripheral vascular disease
PVR	pulse volume recording
PVT	paroxysmal ventricular tachycardia
PWM	pokeweed mitogen
Px	physical
PYP	pyrophosphate

q	every (quaque)
QBCA	quantitative buffy coat analysis
qd	every day (quaque die)
qh	every hour (quaque hora)
qhr	every hour (quaque hora)
qid	four times a day (quarter in die)
QNS	quantity not sufficient
qod	every other day
qs	sufficient quantity (quantum sufficiat)
qs ad	sufficient quantity to make (quantum sufficiat ad)
QTC	quantitative tip culture
qv	as much as you will (quam volveris)

R	respiration; right
Ra	radium
RA	rheumatoid arthritis; right atrium
RAC	right atrial catheter
RAD	radiation absorbed dose
RAF	rheumatoid arthritis factor
RAI	radioactive iodine
RAO	right anterior oblique
RAP	rheumatoid arthritis precipitins
RAW	airway resistance
Rb	rubidium
RBC	red blood cell
RBP	retinol binding protein
RC	red cell; retrograde cystogram
RC100	red cell; red cell casts
RCM	radiographic contrast media; right costal margin
RCMI	red cell morphology index
rd	rutherford
RDS	respiratory distress syndrome
RDW	red cell distribution width
Re	rhenium
REM	rapid eye movement
repet	to be repeated (repetatur)
Rf	rutherfordium
RF	renal failure; rheumatoid factor
rGM-CSF	granulocyte-macrophage colony stimulating factor
Rh	antigen; blood group; rhodium; rhesus
RhIG	$Rh_o(D)$ immune globulin
$Rh_o(D)$	red cell antigen
RI	reticulocyte index
RIA	radioimmunoassay
RID	radial immunodiffusion
RIPA	radioimmunoprecipitation
RISA	radioiodinated serum albumin
RK	radial keratotomy
RLL	right lower lobe
RLQ	right lower quadrant
RMSF	Rocky Mountain spotted fever
Rn	radon
RN	registered nurse
RNA	ribonucleic acid

RNP	ribonucleoprotein
RO	routine order
R/O	rule out
RODAC	replicate organism detection and counting
ROM	range of motion
ROS	review of symptoms; review of systems
RPBI	resting penile-brachial index
RPF	renal plasma flow
RPGN	rapidly progressive glomerulonephritis
RPI	reticulocyte production index
rpm	revolutions per minute
RPO	right posterior oblique
RPR	rapid plasma reagin
RPT	right occipital transverse
RQ	respiratory quotient
RR	recovery room; respiratory rate
RRA	right renal artery
RSV	respiratory syncytial virus
RTA	renal tubular acidosis
Ru	ruthenium
RUG	right upper quadrant
RUL	right upper lobe
RUQ	right upper quadrant
RV	reserve volume
RVH	right ventricular hypertrophy
RVVT	Russell viper venom test
Rx	a recipe

s	without (sine)
S	sulfur
S_1	first heart sound
S_2	second heart sound
SA	surface area; sinoatrial
S-A	sinoatrial
SACE	serum angiotensin converting enzyme
SAH	subarachnoid hemorrhage
SAL	suction assisted lipectomy
SASA	sulfapyridine and 5-aminosalicylic acid
Sb	antimony
SBB	small bowel biopsy; specialist in Blood Bank technology
SBE	subacute bacterial endocarditis
SBL	serum bactericidal level
SBP	systemic blood pressure; systolic blood pressure
Sc	scandium
SC	sickle cell; subclavian; subcutaneous
SCAT	sheep cell agglutination test
SCC	squamous cell carcinoma
SCE	sister chromatid exchange
SCID	severe combined immunodeficiency
Scl	scleroderma; scleroderma antibody
SD	senile dementia; spontaneous delivery; standard deviation
S-D	strength duration
SDA	same day admission
SDAS	same day admission for surgery
SDFP	single donor frozen plasma
SDS	same day surgery
Se	selenium
SEM	scanning electron microscopy; standard error of the mean
SEP	serum electrophoresis; somatosensory evoked potential
SER	somatosensory evoked response
SF-EMG	single fiber electromyography
SG	specific gravity
SGOT	serum glutamic oxaloacetic transaminase
SGPT	serum glutamic pyruvic transaminase
SH	serum hepatitis
SHBG	sex hormone binding globulin
Si	silicon
SI	Système International (SI) units
SIADH	syndrome of inappropriate antidiuretic hormone
SIDS	sudden infant death syndrome
Sig	mark, write (signa)
SISI	short increment sensitivity index
SK	streptokinase
SKAB	skeletal antibody
SKSD	streptokinase-streptodornase
SL	sublingual(ly)
SLCG	sulfolithocholylglycine
SLE	systemic lupus erythyematosus
Sm	samarium; Smith antigen
SMA	sequential/serial multiple analysis; smooth muscle antibody
SMX	sulfamethoxazole
Sn	tin
SNF	skilled nursing facility
SOAP	subjective, objective, assessment and plans
SOB	short of breath

SOD	superoxide dismutase
sos	if there is need (si opus sit)
SPC	standard plate count
SPCA	serum prothrombin conversion accelerator
SPECT	single-photon emission tomography
SPEP	serum protein electrophoresis
SPI	selective protein index
SPL	sound pressure level
SPS	sodium polyanetholsulfonate; sulfite polymyxin sulfadiazine
SQ	subcutaneous(ly)
Sr	strontium
SR	sedimentation rate; sustained release; systems review
SRAW	specific airway resistance
SRIF	somatotropin releasing inhibiting factor
SRT	speech reception threshold
ss	one-half (semis)
SS	*Salmonella-Shigella*; saturated solution; subaortic stenosis
SS-A	Sjögren's syndrome A antibody
SS-B	Sjögren's syndrome B antibody
SS-DNA	single-stranded DNA
SSEP	somatosensory evoked potential
SSKI	saturated solution of potassium iodide
SSN	severely subnormal
SSPE	subacute sclerosing panencephalitis
stat	at once (statim); immediately
STD	skin test dose; sexually transmitted disease
STH	somatotropic hormone
STI	systolic time intervals
STIC	serum trypsin inhibitory capacity
STP	standard temperature and pressure
STS	serologic test for syphillis
supp	suppository (suppositorium)
SVC	slow vital capacity
SVR	systemic vascular resistance
SW	short wave
SWI	sterile water injection
Sx	signs; symptom(s)
syr	syrup (syrupus)

T	temperature; tera (10^{12})
T$_3$	tri-iodothyronine
T$_4$	thyroxine
Ta	tantalum
TA	thyroglobulin autoprecipitins
T & A	tonsillectomy and adenoidectomy
tab	tablet (tabella)
TAb	therapeutic abortion
TAD	tricyclic antidepressant drug
TAH	total abdominal hysterectomy
tal	such
tal dos	such doses
TAT	thematic apperception test; toxin-antitoxin; turnaround time
Tb	terbium
TB	tuberculosis
TBA	to be administered; to be admitted
TBG	thyroxine binding globulin
TBGI	thyroid binding globulin index
TBI	thyroid binding index; thyroxine binding index
TBL	total body load
TBM	tuberculous meningitis
TBPA	thyroxine binding prealbumin
TBW	total body water
Tc	technetium
TC	throat culture; total cholesterol
T & C	type and crossmatch
TCA	trichloracetic acid
TCBS	thiosulfate citrate bile salts sucrose
TCE	trichloroethanol
TCM	tissue culture medium
TCT	thrombin clotting time
TDM	therapeutic drug monitoring
TdT	terminal deoxynucleotidyl transferase
Te	tellurium
TEAC	tetraethylammonium chloride
TeBG	testosterone-estradiol-binding globulin
TEE	transesophageal echocardiography
TEG	thromboelastogram
TENS	transcutaneous electrical nerve stimulation
TET	treadmill exercise test
TG	triglyceride
TGT	thromboplastin generation test
TGV	thoracic gas volume
th	thoracic
Th	thorium
THA	transient hemispheric attack

THb	total hemoglobin
THC	tetrahydrocannabinol
TI	total iron
Ti	titanium
TIA	transient ischemic attack
TIBC	total iron binding capacity
tid	three times a day (ter in die)
TIUV	total intrauterine volume
TK	transketolase
TKO	to keep open
TL	tubal ligation
Tl	thallium
TLA	translumbar aortogram
TLC	thin-layer chromatography; total lung capacity
Tm	thulium
TMB	transient monocular blindness
TMJ	temporomandibular joint
TMP	trimethoprim
TMP-SMX	trimethoprim-sulfomethoxazole
TNS	transcutaneous nerve stimulation
TOS	thoracic outlet syndrome
TP	total protein
TPA	tissue plasminogen activator; *Treponema pallidum* agglutination
TPC	telescoping plugged catheter
TPI	*Treponema* immobilization test; triose phosphate isomerase
TPN	total parenteral nutrition
TPP	thiamine pyrophosphate
TPR	temperature, pulse, respiration
TR	turbidity-reducing
TRAP	tartrate resistance leukocyte acid phosphatase
TRH	thyroid releasing hormone
TRIC	trachoma inclusion conjunctivitis
trig	triglycerides
TRIS	tris(hydroxymethyl)aminomethane
trit	triturate (tritura)
TRP	tubular reabsorption of phosphorus
TS	total solids
TSB	trypticase soy broth
TSH	thyroid stimulating hormone
TSI	thyroid stimulating immunoglobulin; total serum iron
tsp	teaspoon
TT	thrombin time
TTP	thrombotic thrombocytopenic purpura
TU	thiouracil; Todd unit; toxic unit; tuberculin unit
TUR	transurethral resection
TURP	transurethral resection of prostate
TV	tidal volume; total volume
TVC	triple voiding cystogram
Tx	therapy; treatment

U	uranium
UA	uric acid; urinalysis
UAO	upper airway obstructions
UB12BC	unsaturated B$_{12}$ binding capacity
UBBC	unsaturated vitamin B$_{12}$ binding capacity
UBBST	universal blood and body substance technique
UBC	unsaturated binding capacity
UCG	urinary chorionic gonadotropin
ud	as directed (ut dictum)
UDP	uridine diphosphate
UDPG	uridinediphosphoglucose
UEA	upper extremity arterial
UES	upper esophageal sphincter
UFC	urinary free cortisol
UGI	upper GI
UIBC	unbound iron binding capacity
U-I-S	uroporphyrinogen-I-synthetase
UK	urokinase
UMN	upper motor neuron
ung	ointment (unguentum)
UP	universal precautions
URI	upper respiratory infection
US	ultrasound
U.S.	United States
USAN	United States Adopted Names
USP	United States Pharmacopeia
ut dict	as directed (ut dictum)
UTI	urinary tract infection
UUN	urine urea nitrogen
UV	ultraviolet
UVA	ultraviolet

V	vanadium
VA	visual activity

VAD . . . . vascular access device; venous admixture
VBG . . . . venous blood gases
VC . . . . vena cava; vital capacity
VCA . . . . viral capsid antigen
VCA-EB . . . . viral capsid antigen, Epstein-Barr
VCG . . . . vectorcardiogram
VCR . . . . vincristine
VCT . . . . venous clotting time
VCU . . . . voiding cystourethrogram
VCUG . . . . voiding cystourethrogram
VD . . . . venereal disease
VDRL . . . . Venereal Disease Research Laboratory; test for syphilis
VE . . . . visual efficiency
VEP . . . . visual evoked potential
VER . . . . visual evoked response
VF . . . . ventricular fibrillation; vision field
VIP . . . . vasoactive intestinal polypeptide
VLDL . . . . very low density lipoprotein
VLM . . . . visceral larva migrans
VMA . . . . vanillylmandelic acid
vo . . . . verbal order
VP . . . . venous pressure
VPA . . . . valproic acid
VPCs . . . . ventricular premature complexes
VS . . . . vital signs
VSD . . . . ventricular septal defect
VSS . . . . vital signs stable
VSV . . . . vesicular stimatitis virus
VT . . . . ventricular tachycardia
VTM . . . . virus transport media
VU . . . . voltage unit
vW . . . . von Willebrand
vWD . . . . von Willebrand's disease
vWF . . . . von Willebrand factor
V-Z . . . . varicella-zoster
VZIG . . . . varicella-zoster immune globulin

VZV . . . . varicella-zoster virus

W . . . . tungsten
wa . . . . while awake
WB . . . . weight bearing; whole blood
WBC . . . . white blood cell
WD . . . . well developed
WDHA . . . . watery diarrhea-hypokalemia-achlorhydria
WDHH . . . . watery diarrhea-hypokalemia-hypochlorhydria
WF . . . . white female
W-F . . . . Weil-Felix
WM . . . . white male
WN . . . . well nourished
WNL . . . . within normal limits
WP . . . . whirlpool
WPW . . . . Wolff-Parkinson-White syndrome
WSR . . . . Westergren sedimentation rate

Xe . . . . xenon
XO . . . . gonadal dysgenesis of Turner type

Y . . . . yttrium
y . . . . year
YAG . . . . yttrium-argon-garnet - a type of laser
Yb . . . . ytterbium

Z-E . . . . Zollinger-Ellison
ZIG . . . . zoster immune globulin
ZIP . . . . zoster immune plasma
Zn . . . . zinc
ZPP . . . . zinc protophorhyrin
Zr . . . . zirconium
ZSR . . . . zeta sedimentation rate

KEY WORD INDEX

The Key Word Index is not intended in any way to suggest patterns of physicians' orders, nor is it complete. Rather, it is the intent of the authors and editors to make information easier to find and utilize in order to support better patient care.

The Key Word Index provides a reference to test names based on a diagnostic property, disease entity, organ system, or syndrome for which the test may be useful. It provides lists of specific tests. Some may support possible clinical diagnoses or help to rule out other diagnostic possibilities.

Each laboratory test which may be relevant to the indexed diagnosis is listed and weighted. Two symbols (••) indicate that the test strongly supports a diagnosis or entity, that is, it significantly contributes to documentation of the diagnosis if the expected result is found. A single symbol (•) indicates a test frequently used in the diagnosis or management of the particular disease. The other listed tests may be useful on a selective basis with consideration of clinical factors and specific aspects of the case. A negative laboratory test result can be, and frequently is, highly relevant in the practice of medicine.

Clinical diagnosis is determined following history, physical examination, and usual laboratory investigation with selected additional tests. Complete blood count (CBC) with differential, urinalysis, and a basic chemistry profile are not only good medicine, they are in fact cost effective. Thus, these basic tests are excluded from much of the Key Word Index.

Diagnoses with *International Classification of Disease—Ninth Revision—Clinical Modification* (ICD-9-CM) codes are indicated within the [ ] symbol.

MACROCYTOSIS see ANEMIA (MACROCYTIC/ MEGALOBLASTIC)

MACROGLOBULINEMIA (ESSENTIAL) [273.3]

MACROGLOBULINEMIA OF WALDENSTRÖM [273.3] see also HYPERGAMMAGLOBULINEMIA, HYPERVISCOSITY, LYMPHOMA, MYELOMA

MALABSORPTION [579.9] see also CELIAC DISEASE, CROHN'S DISEASE, DIARRHEA, SMALL INTESTINE, VITAMINS, VOMITING

MALARIA [084.6] see also ANEMIA (HEMOLYTIC), FEVER UNDETERMINED ORIGIN (FUO), PARASITIC INFESTATIONS

MALIGNANT HYPERTHERMIA see HYPERTHERMIA (MALIGNANT)

MALNUTRITION [263.9] see also CYSTIC FIBROSIS, DIARRHEA, MALABSORPTION, VITAMINS, WEIGHT LOSS

MALTASE DEFICIENCY see POMPE'S DISEASE

MAPLE SYRUP URINE DISEASE [270.3] see also ACIDOSIS/ ALKALOSIS (ACID-BASE BALANCE), KETOSIS/ KETONURIA/KETOACIDOSIS

MARIE-STRÜMPELL DISEASE see SPONDYLITIS (ANKYLOSING)

MASTOCYTOSIS [757.33] see also ANAPHYLACTIC SHOCK, ANGIOEDEMA, PEPTIC ULCER

CPT INDEX

CPT codes are provided with each test for reference, as a basis for documentation of diagnostic procedures performed and to facilitate financial and patient record keeping. The codes are current. Applications of codes may vary by region of the country and in some instances the application of a specific code to a given procedure is a matter of individual interpretation.

Any five-digit numeric Physicians' **Current Procedural Terminology**, (CPT) codes service descriptions, instructions and/or guidelines are Copyright 1995 American Medical Association. All rights reserved.

CPT is a listing of descriptive terms and five-digit numeric identifying codes and modifiers for reporting medical services performed by physicians. This presentation includes only CPT descriptive terms, numeric identifying codes and modifiers for reporting medical services, and procedures that were selected by Lexi-Comp Inc for inclusion in this publication.

The most current CPT is available from the American Medical Association.

No fee schedules, basic unit values, relative value guides, conversion factors or scales or components thereof are included in CPT.

Lexi-Comp has selected certain CPT codes and service/procedure descriptions and assigned them to various specialty groups. The listing of a CPT service or procedure description and its code number in this publication does not restrict its use to a particular specialty group. Any procedure or service in this publication may be used to designate the services rendered by any qualified physician.

The AMA assumes no responsibility for the consequences attributable to or related to any use or interpretation of any information or views contained in or not contained in this publication.

ALPHABETICAL INDEX

The most expedient method for locating a given test is the Alphabetical Index in the last section of this handbook. Test names and synonyms are listed and the page number on which the test description may be found is indicated.

NOTES

NOTES

NOTES

NOTES